THE
OXFORD MEDICAL
COMPANION

THE
OXFORD MEDICAL
COMPANION

EDITED BY

JOHN WALTON
(*Lord Walton of Detchant*)
JEREMIAH A. BARONDESS
and
STEPHEN LOCK

Oxford   New York   Tokyo
OXFORD UNIVERSITY PRESS
1994

Oxford University Press, Walton Street, Oxford OX2 6DR
Oxford   New York
Athens   Auckland   Bangkok   Bombay
Calcutta   Cape Town   Dar es Salaam   Delhi
Florence   Hong Kong   Istanbul   Karachi
Kuala Lumpur   Madras   Madrid   Melbourne
Mexico City   Nairobi   Paris   Singapore
Taipei   Tokyo   Toronto
and associated companies in
Berlin   Ibadan

Oxford is a trade mark of Oxford University Press

Published in the United States by
Oxford University Press Inc., New York

© Oxford University Press, 1994

A catalogue record for this book is available from the British Library

Library of Congress Cataloging in Publication Data
(Data available)
ISBN 0 19 2623559

Typeset by Electronic Book Factory Ltd, Fife
Printed in Great Britain by
Butler & Tanner Ltd, Frome

PREFACE

THE idea of the original *Oxford Companion to Medicine* was conceived in conversations between the late Sir Ronald Bodley Scott and Professor Paul Beeson in the late 1970s. They recognized that medicine affects everybody and that the interest of the general public was continuing to grow. The proposal was, therefore, that an Oxford *Companion* should be prepared in encyclopaedic format: a comprehensive reference book covering the knowledge base and the practice of medicine for both health professionals and laymen.

Initially, a substantial headword list was drawn up of proposed entries and the editors agreed that the book would contain essays, each written by an authority, on the origin, development, and present state of the medical sciences and medical practice. They also proposed to include articles on medical and nursing practice; on the academic, educational, and administrative structure of the profession and its relation to government and the law in Britain, Canada, and the USA; and on many points of contact between the health professions and the public, including medical ethics and experimental method. Another plan was also to include short biographies of those who had contributed significantly to medicine and medical science as well as of doctors distinguished or notorious in other fields.

For a time the project lay fallow because of the untimely death of Sir Ronald Bodley Scott, but eventually one of us (JW) took on the task of senior editor and with Paul Beeson (formerly Nuffield Professor of Medicine in Oxford), who by this time had returned to the USA, continued to recruit contributors. Dr S. G. Owen, former Second Secretary of the Medical Research Council, and Professor Philip Rhodes, former Postgraduate Dean and Professor of Postgraduate Medical Education at the University of Southampton and in the Wessex Region of the NHS, kindly agreed to become associate editors and between them wrote very many of the shorter contributions. In addition, important contributions were made by Sir Douglas Black and Dr William Gibson of Vancouver. The two-volume *Oxford Companion to Medicine* was published in 1986.

In the early 1990s Oxford University Press thought that it was time to consider the production of a second edition. The original *Companion* had received an almost uniformly favourable reception in the medical and in some of the lay press. Nevertheless Dr Paul Beeson, Dr Owen, and Professor Rhodes no longer wished to be involved, and hence John Walton was delighted when Stephen Lock (former editor of the *British Medical Journal*) and Jeremiah A. Barondess (President of the New York Academy of Medicine) agreed to become co-editors of a completely new and revised *Companion*. Both we and the publishers thought that the relatively expensive, long, and encyclopaedic *Companion* in two volumes had not perhaps been absolutely appropriate for the intelligent reading public as well as a general medical audience. Partly perhaps this was because of its length (1 250 000 words), partly because of its cost, and partly because it was thought too specialized to be reviewed in the quality daily and Sunday newspapers.

Hence, all agreed that the new *Companion* should be slimmed down to occupy a single volume, while retaining the alphabetical format of the original. We also agreed that the content of the articles would be substantially revised by the original contributors who wished to be associated with the new book, but that other articles would be added. Some of these would relate to medicine in many parts of the world other than the United Kingdom, the former British Commonwealth, and the United States of America.

We also agreed on some other major principles. First, some superfluous, outdated, and redundant entries from the first *Companion* should be deleted. Secondly, new biographies of prominent people in medicine and medical science who had died since 1986 should be included. Thirdly, articles on new topics should be commissioned from new authors. Of the shorter entries, some have been written by one or other of us, but many of those written by Dr Owen or Professor Rhodes for the original *Companion*, some shortened, others updated where necessary, are included.

We are happy to present the outcome, based on extensive consultation and correspondence not only with our willing and able contributors but also with many others. We trust that many will read and enjoy the book and find it helpful. In particular, we hope that non-medical members of the public will find it useful, while health professionals will not feel that its value has been diminished by a substantial reduction in length.

We owe a particular debt of gratitude to Rosemary Allan, John Walton's secretary in Oxford, who has carried out an invaluable task in keeping track of the individual contributions, in making innumerable adjustments to the headword list, and in keeping a watchful eye on the peccadilloes of the editors.

We also thank the staff of Oxford University Press, who have so skilfully steered the work through the press.

Oxford
London
New York

JOHN WALTON
STEPHEN LOCK
JEREMIAH A. BARONDESS

CONTRIBUTORS

Johan A. Aarli, MD; Professor of Neurology, University of Bergen, Norway; Chairman, Department of Neurology, Haukeland Hospital, Bergen, Norway

H. L. Abrams, AB, MD, DABR, FACR, FACC, FRCR, FRCS; Philip H. Cook Professor and Chairman of Radiology Emeritus, Harvard Medical School, Boston, MA, USA; Professor of Radiology, Stanford University School of Medicine, Stanford, CA, USA

Michael Abrams, CB, FRCP, FFPHM; Formerly Deputy Chief Medical Officer, Department of Health, London, UK

K. G. M. M. Alberti, MA, DPhil, FRCP, FRCP (Edin), FRCPath; Professor of Medicine, University of Newcastle upon Tyne, Newcastle upon Tyne, UK; Director of Research and Development, Northern Regional Health Authority, UK

Anthony Allibone, MBE, MB, BS, FRCGP; Retired General Practitioner; Chairman Health Committee, General Medical Council 1988, London, UK

D. G. Altman, BSc, CStat; Head, Medical Statistics Laboratory, Imperial Cancer Research Fund, PO Box 123, Lincoln's Inn Fields, London, UK

John Anderson, MB, BS, FRCP, FRCOG, FRCP, FRCPS (Glas); Postgraduate Dean and Director, Regional Postgraduate Institute for Medicine and Dentistry, University of Newcastle upon Tyne, and Northern Regional Health Authority, UK; Professor of Medical Education, University of Newcastle upon Tyne, UK

Roger N. Arber; Secretary, Cremation Society of Great Britain, UK; Secretary-General, International Cremation Federation; Editor, *Pharos International*; Managing Director, London Cremation Company plc, London, UK

J. K. Aronson, MA, MB, ChB, DPhil, FRCP; Clinical Reader in Clinical Pharmacology, University of Oxford, Oxford, UK; Honorary Consultant Physician, Oxfordshire Health Authority, Oxford, UK

E. E. P. Barnard, MB, BS, DPhil, FFCM; Retired; formerly Surgeon Rear-Admiral (Operational Medical Services), Royal Navy, UK

J. H. Baron, DM, FRCP, FRCS; Senior Lecturer, Royal Postgraduate Medical School, Hammersmith Hospital, London, UK; Consultant Physician, St Mary's Hospital and Medical School, London, UK

Jeremiah A. Barondess, MD; President, New York Academy of Medicine, New York, NY, USA; Professor Emeritus of Clinical Medicine, Cornell University Medical College, New York, USA

D. Nicholas Bateman, BSc, MD, FRCP; Consultant Physician, Freeman Hospital, Newcastle upon Tyne, UK; Reader in Therapeutics, University of Newcastle upon Tyne, UK

Mongi Ben Hamida, MD; Professor of Neurology, Institut National de Neurologie, Tunis, Tunisia

George Bentley, MB, ChB, ChM, FRCS; Professor of Orthopaedics and Director, Institute of Orthopaedics, University College, London, UK; Honorary Consultant Orthopaedic Surgeon, Royal National Orthopaedic and Middlesex Hospitals, London, UK

Beulah R. Bewley, MA, MD, FRCP, FFPHM, MSc (Soc Med); Reader in Public Health

Medicine, Department of Public Health Sciences, St George's Hospital Medical School, London, UK

Sir Douglas Black, MD, FRCP; Emeritus Professor of Medicine, University of Manchester, Manchester, UK; formerly President, Royal College of Physicians of London, UK

Robert J. Blendon, ScD; Roger I. Lee Professor and Chairman, Department of Health Policy and Management, Harvard School of Public Health, Boston, MA, USA

Robert Blyth, MBE, FRPharmS; Formerly Editor, *The Pharmaceutical Journal*, UK

K. Boddy, OBE, PhD, DSc, FIPSM, CPhys, FInstP, FRSE; Head, Regional Medical Physics Department, Northern Regional Health Authority, UK; Head of Department of Medical Physics, University of Newcastle upon Tyne, UK

Sir Walter Bodmer, PhD, FRCPath, FRS; Director-General, Imperial Cancer Research Fund, PO Box 123, Lincoln's Inn Fields, London, UK

L. E. Böttiger, MD, FRCP; Formerly Professor and Chairman, Department of Internal Medicine, Karolinska Institute and Hospital, Stockholm, Sweden

Robert D. H. Boyd, MA, MB, FRCP; Professor of Paediatrics, University of Manchester, UK

B. Bracegirdle, BSc, PhD, FSA, FRPS; Formerly Keeper, Wellcome Museum of the History of Medicine, London, UK; President, Association Européenne de Musées de I'Histoire des Sciences Médicales

R. D. C. Brackenridge, MD, FRCP (Glas); Chief Medical Officer, Mercantile and General Reinsurance, London, UK

David J. Bradley, MA, DM, FRCP, FRCPath, FFPHM, FIBiol, Hon. FIWEM; Professor of Tropical Hygiene, London School of Hygiene and Tropical Medicine, University of London, UK

Diana J. Brahams, Barrister-at-law; Practising at 15 Old Square, Lincoln's Inn, London WC2, UK specializing in medico-legal work; Legal Correspondent to *The Lancet* from 1981; Editor, *Medico-Legal Journal* from 1983; Honorary Senior Lecturer, Department of Adult Psychiatry, St George's Hospital Medical School, London, UK; Member of Ethics Committee RCGP, London, UK

Thurstan B. Brewin, FRCP, FRCR; Member, Executive Committee of Health Watch; formerly Consultant in Radiotherapy and Oncology, Glasgow, UK

Pamela J. Brink, RN, PhD, FAAN; Professor and Associate Dean, Research Faculty of Nursing, University of Alberta, Edmonton, Alberta, Canada; Adjunct Professor, College of Nursing, University of Iowa, Iowa City, IA, USA; Joint appointment, Department of Anthropology, University of Alberta; Executive Editor, *Western Journal of Nursing Research*

William H. Brock. BSc, MSc, PhD; Reader in History of Science, University of Leicester, Leicester, UK

A Bartley Bryt, MD, FAAP; Fellow in Pediatrics and Public Health, Cornell University Medical College/New York Hospital, New York, USA

Julia W. Buchanan, BS; Division of Nuclear Medicine, The Johns Hopkins Medical Institutions, Baltimore, MD, USA

A. J. Buller, ERD, BSc, PhD, MB, FRCP; Emeritus Professor of Physiology, University of Bristol, UK

G. M. Bydder, MB, ChB, FRCP; Professor of Diagnostic Radiology, Department of Radiology, Nuclear Magnetic Resonance Unit, Royal Postgraduate Medical School, University of London, London, UK

W. F. Bynum, MD, PhD, MRCP; Professor, History of Medicine, University College London, UK; Director, Academic Unit, Wellcome Institute for the History of Medicine, London, UK

Sir Roy Calne, MA, MS, FRCS, FRS; Professor of Surgery, University of Cambridge, Cambridge, UK; Honorary Consultant Surgeon, Addenbrooke's Hospital, Cambridge, UK

W. G. Cannon, MA, FHA; Formerly House Governor and Secretary, Addenbrooke's Hospital, Cambridge, UK; Director, King's Fund Centre, London, UK

Antonlo Carreras Panchon; Department of History of Medicine, University of Salamanca, Spain

T. C. Chalmers, MD; Distinguished Service Professor and Head of Clinical Trials Unit, Mount Sinai School of Medicine, New York, USA; Visiting Professor, Department of Health Policy and Management, Harvard School of Public Health, Boston, Massachusetts, USA.

Jocelyn Chamberlain, MB, BS, FRCP, FFPHM; Professor of Community Medicine, Institute of Cancer Research, University of London, London, UK

W. H. Chapman, BS, MD; Emeritus Professor of Urology, University of Washington, Seattle, WA, USA

Jagjit S. Chopra, DCH, FRCP, PhD, FAMS; Director Principal, Government Medical College, Chandigarh, India; Honorary Professor of Neurology, Postgraduate Institute of Medical Education and Research, Chandigarh, India

Dame Barbara Clayton, DBE, MD, PhD, HonDSc (Edin), Hon DSc (Southampton), FRCP, FRCP(Edin), FRCPath; Honorary Research Professor in Metabolism, University of Southampton, UK

A. L. Cromble, MB, ChB, FRCS (Edin), FRCOphth; Dean of Medicine and Professor of Ophthalmology, University of Newcastle upon Tyne, UK

W. J. Darby, MD, PhD; Emeritus Professor of Biochemistry (Nutrition), School of Medicine, Vanderbilt University, Nashville, TN, USA

R. L. DeHart, MD, MPH, MS, FACPM, FAAFP, FACOEM; Professor, University of Oklahoma Health Sciences Center, College of Medicine, Department of Family Medicine, USA; Director, Division of Occupational and Environmental Medicine, Oklahoma City, OK, USA

Michael Donaghy, BSc, PhD, MA, DPhil, MB, BS, FRCP; Clinical Reader in Neurology, University of Oxford, Oxford, UK; Consultant Neurologist, Radcliffe Infirmary, Oxford, UK; Senior Tutor, Green College, Oxford, UK

Liam Donaldson, MSc, MD, FRCS (Edin), FFPHM; Regional General Manager and Director of Public Health, Northern Regional Health Authority; Professor of Applied Epidemiology, University of Newcastle upon Tyne, UK

Simon Donell, MB, BS, FRCS, FRCS (Orth); Senior Lecturer in Orthopaedics, University College, London, UK; Honorary Consultant Orthopaedic Surgeon, Royal National Orthopaedic Hospital and Well House Trust, London, UK

T. L. Dorpat, BS, MD; Training Analyst, Seattle Psychoanalytic Institute, USA; Clinical Professor, Department of Psychiatry, School of Medicine. University of Washington, Seattle, WA, USA

James O. Drife, MD, FRCS(Edin), FRCOG; Professor of Obstetrics and Gynaecology, University of Leeds, Leeds, UK; Consultant Obstetrician and Gynaecologist, The General Infirmary at Leeds, UK

James M. Dunlop, MA, FRCP, FFPHM; Formerly Director of Public Health, Hull Health Authority, Hull, UK

M. T. Edgerton, BA, MD; Professor of Plastic and Maxillofacial Surgery, University of Virginia Medical Center, VA, USA; former Chairman, Department of Plastic and Maxillofacial Surgery, University of Virginia Medical School, Charlottesville, VA, USA; former Chairman, Division of Plastic Surgery, Johns Hopkins University School of Medicine, Baltimore, MD, USA

Alan E. H. Emery, MD, PhD, DSc, FRCP, FLS, FRS (Edin); The Medical School, University of Edinburgh, Edinburgh, UK; Research Director, European Neuromuscular Center, Baarn, The Netherlands

Marcia H. Emery, BA, MSc; The Medical School, University of Edinburgh, UK; Research Assistant.

Liz Evans, PhD; Secretary, Human Genome Organisation (HUGO) Europe, London, UK

Holly Michaels Fisher, MPH, MSUP; New York Academy of Medicine, New York, NY, USA

Mark J. Flannagan, MA (Hons); MIPR (Member of the Institute of Public Relations); Assistant Director, Action on Smoking and Health, London, UK

A. M. Geddes, MB, ChB, FRCP, FRCP (Edin); Professor of Infection, School of Medicine, University of Birmingham, Birmingham, UK; Honorary Consultant Physician, South West and East Birmingham Health Authorities, Birmingham, UK; Consultant Advisor in Infectious Diseases, Department of Health, London, UK

M. G. Gelder, MA, DM, FRCP, FRCPsych; Professor of Psychiatry, University of Oxford, Oxford, UK; Fellow, Merton College, Oxford, UK

Douglas Gentleman, BSc, MB, ChB, FRCS (Eng). FRCS (Glas); Consultant Neurosurgeon, Dundee Royal Infirmary, Dundee, UK; Honorary Senior Lecturer in Neurosurgery, University of Dundee, UK

Marie Victoria Gianelli; Associate Professor, Department of Neurology, University of Genova, Italy

W. C. Gibson, MD, DPhil, FRCP; Chancellor Emeritus, University of Victoria, Victoria, British Columbia, Canada; Professor Emeritus of the History of Medicine and Science, University of British Columbia, Vancouver, Canada

F. B. Glaser, MD, FRCP (C), FAPA; Director, University of Michigan Substance Abuse Center, MI, USA; Coordinator, University of Michigan Initiative on Alcohol and Other Drugs, MI, USA; Professor of Psychiatry, University of Michigan Medical Center, MI, USA

R. J. Glaser, SB, MD, ScD, LHD; Trustee and Director for Medical Science, Lucille P. Markey Charitable Trust, Menlo Park, CA, USA; Consulting Professor of Medicine, Stanford University, Stanford, CA, USA

Chris Glynn, MA, MB, BS, DCH, FFARCS, MSc; Consultant in Pain Relief, Oxford Regional Pain Relief Unit, Churchill Hospital, Headington, Oxford, UK

Shane Godbolt, BA, FLA; Regional Librarian, Northwest Thames Regional Library and Information Service (in association with the British Postgraduate Medical Federation, University of London), UK; formerly Librarian, Charing Cross and Westminster Medical School, London, UK; Editor, *Health Libraries Review*, UK

K. A. M. Grant, MB, CLB, FFPHM, DTPH, DCH; Health Care Consultant and Partner, Health and Life Sciences partnership, London, UK

Susan A. Greenfield, MA, DPhil; University Lecturer in Synaptic Pharmacology, University of Oxford, Oxford, UK; E. P. Abraham Fellow and Tutor in Medicine, Lincoln College, Oxford, UK

J. Grimley Evans, MA, MD, FRCP, FFPHM; Professor of Clinical Geratology, University of Oxford, UK

Jennifer M. Gurd BEd, Cert Special Ed, MA, DPhil; Research Fellow, Neuropsychology Unit, University Department of Clinical Neurology, Radcliffe Infirmary, Oxford, UK

A. P. Haines, MD, FRCGP, FRCP, FFPHM; Professor of Primary Health Care, University College London Medical School, London, UK; Director of Research and Development, North East Thames Regional Health Authority, UK; General Practitioner, Islington, London, UK

Sir Donald Harrison, MD, MS, PhD, FRCS, FRCOpth; Emeritus Professor of Laryngology, University of London, London, UK; Emeritus ENT Consultant, Moorfields Eye Hospital, London, UK

P. Hassett, FRCOphth, MSc; Senior Registrar in Ophthalmology, Oxford Eye Hospital, Radcliffe Infirmary, Oxford, UK

Keith Hawton, DM, FRCPsych, DPM; Consultant Psychiatrist, Warneford Hospital,

Oxford, UK; Clinical Lecturer, University Department of Psychiatry, Warneford Hospital, Oxford, UK; Fellow, Green College, Oxford, UK

†Winifred E. Hector, Hon DSc, MPhil, RNT, FRCN; Late Principal Tutor, School of Nursing, St Bartholomew's Hospital, London, UK; formerly Senior Lecturer, University of London, UK

N. Hershey, LLB; Professor of Health Law, University of Pittsburgh, Pittsburgh, PA, USA; Counsel, Markel, Schafer & Means, Attorneys, Pittsburgh, PA, USA; Post & Schell, Attorneys, Philadelphia, PA, USA

Robin Higgins, MB, BCh, DPM, BMus; Laban Centre for Movement and Dance, New Cross, London, UK

S. J. J. Hildrey, MA; Editorial/Research Assistant, Department of Public Health Medicine, United Medical and Dental Schools of Guy's and St Thomas's Hospitals, London, UK

R. L. Himsworth, MD, FRCP (Lond, Edin, and Glas); Professor of Research and Development, University of Cambridge, UK; formerly Regius Professor of Medicine, University of Aberdeen, UK

Shigeaki Hinohara, MD, Hon FACP, FACC; President of St Luke's International Hospital; Chairman of the Board, The Life Planning Center, Tokyo, Japan

J. D. H. Holland, MA; Research Assistant, Department of Endocrinology and Chemical Pathology, United Medical and Dental Schools of Guy's and St Thomas' Hospitals, Lambeth Palace Road, London, UK

Walter W. Holland, CBE, MD, BSc, FRCP (Edin), FRCP, FRCGP, FRCPath, FFPHM; Professor of Public Health Medicine, United Medical and Dental Schools of Guy's and St Thomas's Hospitals, University of London; Past President of the Faculty of Public Health Medicine of the Royal College of Physicians of the United Kingdom

Anthony Hopkins, MD, FRCP, FFPHM, FACP; Director, Research Unit, Royal College of Physicians, London, UK; Consultant Neurologist, St Bartholomew's Hospital, London, UK

John Horder, CBE, MA, MD (Hon), FRCP, FRCP (Edin), FRCGP, FRCPsych; Formerly President, Royal College of General Practitioners, UK

Tracey Stelzer Hyams, JD, MPH; Deputy Director, Harvard Program on the Future of Health Care, Harvard School of Public Health, Boston, MA, USA

Sir Donald Irvine, CBE, MD, FRCGP; General Practitioner, Lintonville Medical Group, Ashington, Northumberland, UK; Chairman, Committee on Standards and Medical Ethics, General Medical Council, London, UK

O. Wayne Isom, MD; Professor of Cardiothoracic Surgery, Cornell Medical College, USA; Chairman, Department of Cardiothoracic Surgery, New York Hospital/Cornell Medical Center, New York, NY, USA

A. Jones, MD, FRCP, FRCS, FRCR, FACR; Emeritus Professor of Radiotherapy, University of London, London, UK; Honorary Consulting Physician, Department of Radiotherapy, St Bartholomew's Hospital, London, UK

Reg Jordan, BSc, PhD; Reader in Anatomy and Immunology and Academic Sub-Dean of the Medical School, University of Newcastle upon Tyne, UK

R. J. T. Joy, BS, MA, MD, FACP; Professor and Chairman, Section of Medical History, Uniformed Services University of Health Sciences, Bethesda, MD, USA

D. G. Julian, MD, FRCP, FRACP, FRCP (Edin); Former Consultant Medical Director, British Heart Foundation; Emeritus Professor of Cardiology, Newcastle upon Tyne, UK

G. Kazantzis, PhD, MB, BS, FRCS, FRCP, FFOM, FFCM; Emeritus Professor of Occupational Medicine, University of London, London, UK; Visiting Professor, Imperial College of Science, Technology and Medicine, London, UK; Emeritus Consultant Physician, Middlesex Hospital, London, UK

D. N. S. Kerr, CBE, MSc, FRCP, FRCP (Edin); Former Professor of Medicine, University of Newcastle upon Tyne; former Dean, Royal Postgraduate Medical School, University of London, UK

N. Kessel, MA, MD, FRCP(Lond and Edin), FRCPsych; Emeritus Professor of Psychiatry, University of Manchester, Manchester, UK; Consultant, Manchester Royal Infirmary, Manchester, UK; formerly Dean and Postgraduate Dean, Manchester Medical School, Manchester, UK; Member, General Medical Council, London, UK

Sir Robert Kilpatrick, MD, FRCP (Edin), FRCP; President, General Medical Council, London, UK

B. Knight, MD, MRCP, FRCPath, DMJ (Path); Barrister; Professor of Forensic Pathology, University of Wales College of Medicine, Cardiff, UK; Home Office Pathologist, UK

J. Komender, MD, PhD; Professor of Histology and Transplantology, Deputy Secretary of the Medical Division of the Polish Academy of Sciences, Warsaw, Poland

Peter Lachmann, ScD, FRCP, PRCPath, FRS; Professor of Immunology, University of Cambridge, UK; Honorary Director, MRC Molecular Immunopathology Unit, Cambridge, UK

John Gerard Garvin Ledingham, MA, DM (Oxon), FRCP; May Reader in Medicine, University of Oxford, UK; Director of Clinical Studies, University of Oxford, UK

S. Leibowitz, BSc, MD, FRCPath; Emeritus Professor of Neuroimmunology, UMDS, Guy's Hospital, London, UK

M. H. Lessof, MA, MD, FRCP; Emeritus Professor of Medicine, United Schools of Guy's and St Thomas' Hospitals, London, UK

Donald W. Light, BA, MA, PhD; Professor of Comparative Health Care Systems, University of Medicine and Dentistry of New Jersey, NJ, USA; Adjunct Senior Fellow, Leonard Davis Institute of Health Economics, USA

Stephen Lock, CBE, MA, MSc, MD, FRCP, FRCP (Edin), FRCP (Irel), FACP; Former Editor, *BMJ* 1975–1991; Research Associate, Wellcome Institute for the History of Medicine, London, UK

Don M. Long. MD, PhD; Professor and Director, Department of Neurosurgery, Johns Hopkins University Medical School; Neurosurgeon-in-Chief, Johns Hopkins Hospital, Baltimore, MD, USA; American Association of Neurological Surgeons, USA; Congress of Neurological Surgeons; Society of Neurological Surgeons, USA

I. S. L. Loudon, DM, FRCGP, D (Obst) RCOG; Medical Historian; formerly Wellcome Research Fellow in the Wellcome Unit for the History of Medicine in the University of Oxford, UK

K. G. MacLean, BA, AIMI; Head of Medical Photography and Illustration, Leicester Royal Infirmary NHS Trust, Leicester, UK

D. L. McLellan, MA, MB, BChir, PhD, FRCP; Professor of Rehabilitation, University of Southampton and Consultant in Neurology and Rehabilitation Medicine, Southampton and Portsmouth Health Districts, UK

R. Mahoney, BA, LLB, BCL (Oxon); Member of the Bars of British Columbia and New Zealand; Senior Lecturer, Faculty of Law, University of Otago, New Zealand

Janice Main, MB, ChB, MRCP (UK); Senior Lecturer in Infectious Diseases and General Medicine, St Mary's Hospital, London, UK

James S. Malpas, DPhil, FRCP, FRCR, FFPM; Professor of Medical Oncology, ICRF Department of Medical Oncology, St Bartholomew's Hospital, West Smithfield, London, UK; Honorary Consultant Physician, St Bartholomew's Hospital, London, UK

Marshall Marinker, OBE, MD, FRCGP; Visiting Professor of General Practice, UMDS, London, UK; Director of Medical Education, Merck Sharp and Dohme Ltd, UK

S. G. Marketos, MD, MP; Professor and Chairman, Department of the History of Medicine, National University of Athens School of Medicine, Athens, Greece; President of the International Hippocratic Foundation, Kos, Greece

John C. Marshall, BA, MA, PhD; External Scientific Staff of the Medical Research Council; Director, Neuropsychology Unit, University Department of Clinical Neurology, Radcliffe Infirmary, Oxford, UK

Adrian Marston, MA, DM, MD, MCh, FRCS; Emeritus Consultant Surgeon, Middlesex and University College Hospitals, London, UK; Senior Lecturer in Surgery, University of London, UK

Robert J. Maxwell, CBE, PhD, FCMA; Secretary and Chief Executive, King's Fund, London, UK

A. Maynard, BA, BPhil; Professor of Economics and Director of the Centre for Health Economics, University of York, UK

Peter Maynard, ACII; Research Officer, Mercantile and General Reinsurance, Cheltenham, UK

H. B. Meire, MB, BS, LRCP, MRCS, DMRD, DObstRCOG, FRCR; Consultant Radiologist, King's College Hospital, London, UK; Director of Ultrasound, Portland Hospital, London, UK.

D. W. Millard, MA, MB, ChB, FRCPsych; Consultant Psychiatrist, Oxford Health Authority, UK; Emeritus Fellow, Green College, Oxford, UK; formerly Lecturer in Applied Social Studies, University of Oxford, UK

Sir Godfrey Milton-Thompson, KBE, FRCP; Formerly Surgeon General, Defence Medical Services, UK

†R. S. Mitchell, AB, MD, FACP; Late Professor of Medicine Emeritus, University of Colorado School of Medicine, USA; formerly Director, Webb-Waring Lung Institute, USA

Thomas Q. Morris, MD; Vice President for Program, New York Academy of Medicine, New York, NY, USA; Professor of Clinical Medicine, College of Physicians and Surgeons of Columbia University, New York, NY, USA

M. J. Mossakowski, MD, PhD, Dr hc; Professor of Neuropathology, Scientific Secretary of Medical Section of the Polish Academy of Sciences, Poland; Director of Medical Research Centre and Head, Department of Neuropathology, Medical Research Centre of Polish Academy of Sciences, Warsaw, Poland

J. M. Murray, BA (Hons); British Red Cross Society, London, UK

M. N. Naylor, RD, DL, BSc, BDS, PhD, FDSRCS, Hon. FDSRCPS (Glas); Emeritus Professor of Preventive Dentistry, University of London, London, UK; Honorary Senior Research Fellow, Institute of Dental Surgery, London, UK

I. Oswald, MA, MD, DSc, FRCPsych; Emeritus Professor of Psychiatry, University of Edinburgh, UK

Stephen A. Paget, MD, FACP, FACR; Associate Professor of Clinical Medicine and Associate Attending Physician, New York Hospital/Cornell Medical Center, The Hospital for Special Surgery, New York, USA

Christopher Pallis, DM, FRCP; Reader Emeritus in Neurology, Royal Postgraduate Medical School, London, UK; Senior (Honorary) Consultant Neurologist, Hammersmith Hospital, London, UK

C. P. Panayiotopoulos, MD, PhD; Consultant in Clinical Neurophysiology and Epilepsy, St Thomas' Hospital, London SEI, UK; formerly Clinical Professor of Neurology, University of Colorado, USA

Alex Paton, MD, FRCP; Former Consultant Physician and Postgraduate Dean, UK

†Sir William Paton, CBE, MA, DM, FFARCS, FRCP, FRS; Late Emeritus Professor of Pharmacology, University of Oxford, UK; formerly Honorary Director, Wellcome Institute for the History of Medicine, London, UK

John Hemsley Pearn, AM, RFD, MD, BSc, PhD (Lond), FRACP, FRCP (UK), DCH, FACTM; Professor of Child Health, Royal Children's Hospital, Brisbane, Australia; formerly Florey Fellow, The Royal Society (London); National Director of Training,

St John Ambulance, Australia; Colonel Consultant (Medical Research), Office of the Surgeon General, Australian Defence Force, Australia

Alessandro Polleri, MD; Head, Department of Endocrinological and Metabolic Sciences, University of Genoa, Italy

R. S. Porter, MA, PhD; Professor of the History of Medicine, Wellcome Institute for the History of Medicine, London, UK

Alberto Portera-Sanchez, MD, Professor of Neurology, Complutense University of Madrid, Member of the Spanish Royal Academy of Medicine, Madrid, Spain

Sudesh Prabhakar, MD (Medicine), DM (Neuro), MAMS; Additional Professor and Head, Department of Neurology, Postgraduate Institute of Medical Education and Research, Chandigarh 160012, India

S. J. Proctor, FRCP, FRCPath; Professor of Haematological Medicine, University of Newcastle upon Tyne, Newcastle upon Tyne, UK

David Pyke, CBE, MD, FRCP; Formerly Physician to the Diabetic Department, King's College Hospital, London, UK; Registrar, Royal College of Physicians, London, UK

Sir Philip Randle, Kt, MA, PhD, MD, FRCP, FRS; Professor of Clinical Biochemistry, University of Oxford, John Radcliffe Hospital, Oxford, UK

M. D. Rawlins, BSc, MD, FRCP (Lond), FRCP (Edin), FFPM; Chairman, Committee on Safety of Medicines; Ruth and Lionel Jacobson Professor of Clinical Pharmacology, University of Newcastle upon Tyne, UK; Honorary Consultant Clinical Pharmacologist, Freeman Hospital and Royal Victoria Infirmary, Newcastle upon Tyne, UK

Peter Richards, MA, MD, PhD, FRCP; Pro Rector (Medicine), Imperial College of Science, Technology, and Medicine, London, UK; Dean, St Mary's Hospital Medical School, London, UK

Colin H. Roberts, BSc, CQSW, MA (Oxon); Director of Social Work Studies in the Department of Applied Social Studies and Social Research, University of Oxford, UK; Dean and Fellow of Green College, Oxford, UK

David E. Rogers, MD, MACP; The Walsh McDermott University Professor of Medicine, Cornell University Medical College, New York, NY, USA; Vice Chairman (United States) National Commission on AIDS, USA

†G. Rose, CBE, MA, DM, DSc, FRCP, FFPHM, FRCGP; Late Emeritus Professor of Epidemiology, London School of Hygiene and Tropical Medicine, London, UK; former Honorary Consultant Physician, St Mary's Hospital, London, UK

Todd K. Rosengart, MD; Assistant Professor of Cardiothoracic Surgery, Assistant Attending Cardiothoracic Surgeon, New York Hospital/Cornell Medical Center, New York, USA

M. N. Rossor, MA, MD, FRCP; Consultant Neurologist, St Mary's Hospital and National Hospital for Neurology and Neurosurgery, London, UK; Senior Lecturer, Institute of Neurology, London, UK

Dame Rosemary Rue, OBE, MB, BS, DCH, FFPHM; Formerly Regional General Manager and Regional Medical Officer, Oxford Regional Health Authority, UK

T. Michael Ryan, MA, PhD; Senior Lecturer, Department of Politics, University of Wales, Swansea, UK

Dame Cicely Saunders, OM, DBE, MA, FRCP; Chairman, St Christopher's Hospice, Sydenham, London, UK

Uido Schagen, Dr Med, Sozialmedizin; Leiter der Forschungsstelle Zeitgeschichte im Institut für Geschichte der Medizin (Head of Department of Contemporary History, Institute of History of Medicine), Lehrbeauftragter für Sozialmedizin (Lecturer Social Medicine), Freie Universität Berlin (Free University of Berlin), Germany

†Sir Ronald Bodley Scott, MA, DM, FRCP; Late Consulting Physician, St Bartholomew's Hospital and King Edward VII Hospital for Officers, London, UK

Georges Serratrice, MD; Professor of Neurology; Member of the French Academy of

Medicine; Chairman of Clinique des Maladies du Systeme Nerveux et de I'Appareil Locomoteur, Centre Hospitalier Universitaire de la Timone, Marseille, France

Ra'ad A. Shakir, MB, ChB, MSc, FRCP, FRCP (G), FRCP (E); Consultant Neurologist, Middlesborough General Hospital, Middlesbrough, UK; Lecturer in Neurology, University of Newcastle upon Tyne, UK

W. B. Shelley, MD, PhD, MACP; Professor of Dermatology, University of Ohio, Toledo, OH, USA

J. C. Sherris, MD. FRCPath; Professor Emeritus, Department of Microbiology and Immunology, University of Washington, Seattle, WA, USA

Sir Stanley Cllfford Simmons, FRCS, FRCOG, FRAOG (Honorary); Past-President, Royal College of Obstetricians and Gynaecologists; formerly Consultant Obstetrician, Windsor, Oxford Regional Health Authority, UK

A. David Smith, MA, DPhil; Professor of Pharmacology, University of Oxford, Oxford, UK; Honorary Director, MRC Anatomical Neuropharmacology Unit, University of Oxford, Oxford, UK

Dale C. Smith, PhD; Section of Medical History, Uniformed Services University of the Health Sciences, Bethesda, MD, USA

James M. Smith, PhD, MRPharmS, MCCP, MIInfSci; Regional Pharmaceutical Adviser, Northern Regional Health Authority, UK; Director of Pharmacy, Northern Regional Drug and Therapeutics Centre, UK; Lecturer in Clinical Pharmacy, University of Newcastle upon Tyne, UK

Richard Smith, FRCPE, MFPHM, MSc; Editor, *British Medical Journal*, London, UK

Roger Smith, MD, PhD, FRCP; Consultant Physician (Metabolic Medicine), John Radcliffe Hospital and Nuffield Orthopaedic Centre, Oxford, UK

J. C. Snyder, AB, MD, LLD; Professor of Population and Public Health, Emeritus; former Dean of the Faculty of Public Health, Harvard University School of Public Health, Boston, MA, USA

Peter Sönksen, MD, FRCP; Professor of Endocrinology, United Medical and Dental School of Guy's and St Thomas' Hospitals, London, UK

Lord Soulsby of Swaffham Prior, MA, PhD, AM (hc), DSc (hc), DVM (hc), DVMS (hc), DVSM, MRCVS; Emeritus Professor of Animal Pathology, University of Cambridge, Cambridge, UK; Emeritus Fellow, Wolfson College, Cambridge, UK; formerly Head, Department of Clinical Veterinary Medicine, University of Cambridge, UK

R. E. Steiner, CBE, MD, FRCP, FRCR; Emeritus Professor of Radiology, University of London, London, UK; Nuclear Magnetic Resonance Unit, Royal Postgraduate Medical School, University of London, UK

Edward J. Stemmler, MD; Master, American College of Physicians, Philadelphia, PA, USA; Emeritus Robert G. Dunlop Professor of Medicine and Dean Emeritus, University of Pennsylvania School of Medicine, Philadelphia, PA, USA; Executive Vice President, Association of American Medical Colleges, Washington, DC, USA

Rosemary A. Stevens, PhD; Dean and Thomas S. Gates Professor, School of Arts and Sciences; Professor, Department of History and Sociology of Science, University of Pennsylvania, Philadelphia, PA, USA

J. C. Stoddart, MD, FRCA; Consultant Anaesthetist in Charge, Intensive Therapy Unit, Royal Victoria Infirmary, Newcastle upon Tyne, UK; Consultant in Intensive Therapy, Northern Region of the National Health Service, UK

J. D. Swales, MA, MD, FRCP; Professor of Medicine, University of Leicester, UK

G. Teeling Smith, BA, FRPharmS; Former Director, Office of Health Economics, London, UK; Professor Associate, Brunel University, Uxbridge, Middlesex, UK

H. C. Thomas, BSc, PhD, FRCP, FRCPS, FRCPath; Professor and Chairman of Medicine, Department of Medicine, St Mary's Hospital, Imperial College of Science, Technology, and Medicine, London, UK

A. C. Upton, BA, MD; Professor Emeritus, Department of Environmental Medicine, New York University School of Medicine, New York, NY, USA; Clinical Professor of Pathology and Radiology, University of New Mexico School of Medicine, Albuquerque, NM, USA

L. D. Vandam, PhB, MD, MA; Professor of Anaesthesia Emeritus, Harvard University, Cambridge, MA, USA; Anesthesiologist, Brigham and Women's Hospital, Boston, MA, USA

A. Viriyavejakul, MD, LLB, FRCP; Head, Division of Neurology, Faculty of Medicine, Siriraj Hospital; Vice President for Research and International Relations, Mahidol University, Bangkok, Thailand

Henry N. Wagner, Jr, MD; Professor of Medicine, Radiology and Environmental Health Sciences; Director, Divisions of Nuclear Medicine and Radiation Health Sciences, The Johns Hopkins Medical Institutions, Baltimore, MD, USA

H. A. Waldron, PhD, MD, FRCP, FFOM; Consultant Physician, Department of Occupational Health, St Mary's Hospital, London, UK; Honorary Research Fellow in Palaeopathology, Institute of Archaeology, University College, London, UK

Paul Francis Walker; Executive Director, Muscular Dystrophy Group of Great Britain and Northern Ireland 1973–1991; President of the Neuromuscular Centre; Trustee of Child Rescue International, the Stackpole Trust; Advisor to the Royal College of Pathologists, Friends for the Young Deaf, MacIntyre, the Elizabeth Harwood Memorial Trust, and the Richard Lewis Award Trust, UK

Lord Walton of Detchant, TD, MA, MD, DSc, FRCP, FRCP (Edin), FACP, FRCP (C), FRCPath, FRCPsych; President, World Federation of Neurology; formerly Professor of Neurology, University of Newcastle upon Tyne, UK; formerly Warden, Green College, Oxford, UK

D. A. Warrell, MA, DM, DSc, FRCP; Professor of Tropical Medicine and Infectious Diseases, University of Oxford, UK

M. A. Waugh, MB, BS, MRCPI, DHMSA, Dip Ven, AAC Ven; Consultant Genito-urinary Physician, General Infirmary, Leeds, UK; formerly President, Medical Society for the Study of Venereal Diseases; Secretary General, International Union Against the Venereal Diseases and Treponematoses; Board Member, European Academy of Dermatology and Venereology

Sir David Weatherall, FRS; Regius Professor of Medicine and Honorary Director, Institute of Molecular Medicine, University of Oxford, UK

W. F. Whimster, MA, MD, FRCP, FRCPath; Professor of Histopathology, King's College School of Medicine and Dentistry, King's College, University of London, London, UK

H. White, MA, DM, MCh, FRCS; Consulting Surgeon, Royal Marsden Hospital and King Edward VII Hospital for Officers, London, UK

T. P. Whitehead, CBE, PhD, MRCP, FRCPath, FRSC; Emeritus Professor of Clinical Chemistry and formerly Dean of the Faculty of Medicine and Dentistry, University of Birmingham, Birmingham, UK

J. E. A. Wickham, MS, BSc, FRCS, FRCP, FRCR; Director, Institute of Urology, University of London, London, UK; Senior Research Fellow and Surgeon, Minimally Invasive Surgery Unit, Guy's Hospital, London, UK; formerly Senior Urological Surgeon, St Bartholomew's, St Peter's and King Edward VII Hospitals, London, UK

J. L. Wilkinson, OBE, MD, FRCS, DTM&H; Formerly Medical Superintendent and Surgeon Specialist, Nixon Memorial Hospital, Sierra Leone; Senior Lecturer, Anatomy Department, University of Wales, Cardiff, UK.

J. G. P. Williams, MD, MSc, FRCP, FRCS; Consultant in Rehabilitation Medicine, East Berkshire Health Authority; former Medical Director, Farnham Park Rehabilitation Centre, Farnham Road, Slough, Berkshire, UK; Civil Consultant in Rehabilitation Medicine, Royal Navy, UK

P. O. Williams, CBE, DM, DSc, FRCP; Formerly Director, The Wellcome Trust, London, UK

P. J. Willis, MA; Curator, Museum of the Order of St John, London, UK

Michael Worboys, BSc, MSc, DPhil; Reader in the History of Medicine, Sheffield Hallam University, Sheffield, UK

Peter H. Worlock, DM, FRCS; Consultant Trauma and Orthopaedic Surgeon, John Radcliffe Hospital, Oxford, UK; Chairman, Oxford Critical Care Centre, John Radcliffe Hospital, Oxford, UK

MAIN ENTRIES

The list below gives the titles of the main entries that can be found within the Companion.

Aerospace medicine
AIDS and HIV
Alchemy
Allergy
Anaesthesia (anesthesia)
Anatomy
Anti-infective drugs
Armed forces of the USA: medical services
Art and medicine
Arteries, veins, their diseases and vascular
  surgery

Biochemistry
Bovine spongiform encephalopathy
Boxing
Brain (stem) death

Cardiology
Cardiothoracic surgery
Cell and cell biology
Chemistry, clinical
Chernobyl
Chest medicine
Classification
Clinical investigation
Clinical trials of treatment
Colposcopy
Communication between doctors and
  patients
Complementary (alternative) medicine
Computers in medicine
Cremation

Death, dying, and the hospice movement
Defence medical services (UK)
Dentistry in the UK and USA
Dermatology
Diabetes mellitus
Diagnosis
Doctors as patients
Doctors as truants to literature
Doctors in literature

Doctors in other walks of life (medical
  truants)

Endocrinology
Environment and medicine: I. Physical
  effects
Environment and medicine: II. Poverty and
  health—a global perspective
Epidemiology
Ethical issues in modern health care
Experimental method

Forensic medicine
Foundations and charities in Canada
Foundations and charities supporting
  medical care in the UK
Foundations, charities and grant-making
  bodies supporting medical research in the
  UK (with a brief note on Europe)
Foundations in the USA: their role in
  medicine and health
Fraud and misconduct in medical research

Gastroenterology
General Medical Council
General ophthalmic services
Genetic engineering
Genetics and medical practice
Geriatric medicine (geriatrics)
Government and medicine in the UK
Government and medicine in the USA

Haematology (hematology) and blood
  transfusion
Health care economics
Health care systems and their financing
Historiography of medicine
History of medicine
Hospitals in the UK
Hospitals in the USA: their development
  and organization: historical perspective
Hypertension

A NOTE TO THE READER

Entries are listed in a simple letter-by-letter alphabetical order, with spaces, hyphens, and the definite and indefinite articles being ignored. Names beginning with Mc are ordered as if spelt Mac and St as if spelt Saint. In addition, biographies of individuals whose surnames have a prefix (de, van, von, etc.) occur under the capital letter of the main surname. The Companion contains a system of cross-references that is designed to inform the reader of related entries; this should be particularly useful for anyone less familiar with the more specialized medical vocabulary encountered in some of the entries. A cross-reference is shown in three ways: (i) by the use of an asterisk before a word (e.g. *biochemistry), indicating that there is an entry for that word; (ii) by the use of 'See' followed by the entry title in SMALL CAPITALS, indicating that further discussion will be found under that entry; and (iii) by the use of 'See also' followed by the entry title in SMALL CAPITALS, indicating that there is a related entry that might interest the reader. The cross-referencing does not attempt to be comprehensive but aims to guide the reader towards entries that might enhance the understanding of the entry being consulted. Thus the absence of a cross-reference does not necessarily imply that there is no related entry, and the reader may benefit from checking. A cross-reference is given the first time a particular word appears in an entry but not thereafter, regardless of the length of the entry (save in a few exceptional circumstances). In order to save space the titles of various entries have been abbreviated when they appear in cross-references. As a general rule SI units have been used throughout the text, and these units are described in the entry SI UNITS. Occasionally non-SI units have been used where this reflects common medical practice, for example, millimetres of mercury (mmHg) to record blood pressure. Appendix I contains a list of medical qualifications and Appendix II a list of common medical abbreviations.

ABBOTT, MAUDE ELIZABETH SEYMOUR (1869–1940). Canadian physician, fellow in pathology at McGill and later research professor (1912–23). An authority on *congenital heart disease and a medical historian. She published a valuable *Atlas of congenital cardiac disease* (1936).

ABDERHALDEN, EMIL (1877–1950). Swiss biochemist, professor of general physiology in Berlin in 1904 and of physiology in Halle in 1911. In 1947 he received the emeritus chair of physiological chemistry in Zurich. He contributed notably to the technique and methodology of *biochemistry.

ABDOMEN. That part of the mammalian body, also known as the belly, which lies between the *thorax and the *pelvis. Its cavity is lined by a serous membrane (the *peritoneum) and contains the viscera. It is bounded by the abdominal wall formed by the abdominal muscles, the iliac bones, and the vertebral column; and is separated from the thoracic cavity by the muscular *diaphragm.

ABDUL KASIM (Abu-al-Qasim Khalaf ibn-Abbas al Zahrawi; Albacusis) (*c.* 936–*c.* 1013). Spanish-Arabian physician. Born near Cordoba, he rose to become court physician to the Caliph Abd-ar-Rahman III. His encyclopaedic work *al-Tasrif*, in 30 volumes, exerted great influence in Latin Europe and was the leading text for 500 years.

ABEL, JOHN JACOB (1857–1938). American biochemist. He was professor of *pharmacology at the University of Michigan, 1891–3, and then at *Johns Hopkins Hospital, Baltimore, 1893–1932. Among his accomplishments were the isolation of epinephrine (*adrenaline) and the first preparation of *insulin in crystalline form.

ABERNETHY, JOHN (1764–1831). British surgeon at *St Bartholomew's Hospital, London. His lectures drew such large audiences that the hospital governors built a lecture theatre for him in 1791, thus founding the medical school. His charismatic personality dominated British surgery at the turn of the 19th century.

ABIOTROPHY is tissue *degeneration with loss or disturbance of function, particularly in diseases of genetic origin.

ABLATION. Removal or destruction by physical means such as irradiation or surgical excision, particularly of a whole part, organ, or tissue.

ABORTION is termination of *pregnancy, with expulsion of the products of conception, before the *fetus has reached viability (in the UK, legally taken to be at 24 weeks' *gestation). Abortion may be accidental (spontaneous) or induced (artificial). Induced abortion is either criminal (in a legal sense) or therapeutic (justifiable).

The law relating to abortion in the UK was liberalized by the Abortion Act of 1967, implemented in 1968. Abortion, long an offence against Canon Law, became a statutory crime in England and Wales in 1803; and under the Offences against the Person Act of 1861 it was a felony punishable by life imprisonment.

The new Act provided that abortion would not be an offence when two registered medical practitioners certified in good faith that continuation of *pregnancy would constitute a risk to the life or health of the pregnant woman or her existing children greater than that of termination; nor when there was a risk that the child, if born, would suffer serious mental or physical handicap. Doctors or nurses objecting on grounds of conscience would not have to take part in such operations. In 1992 the law was amended to reduce the legal limit from 28 to 24 weeks, save in cases in which continuation of pregnancy would endanger the pregnant woman's life or seriously damage her health, or in which serious fetal abnormality is involved; in such circumstances there is no legal limit but termination beyond 24 weeks can be carried out only in hospitals of the National Health Service and all such must be reported to the Department of Health. Mifepristone has been licensed as an abortion-inducing drug for use in such hospitals in the UK and can be used in France but not in the USA.

Most Western European countries (e.g. France) have introduced similarly liberal laws; only in Portugal, Spain, and Ireland is abortion still illegal under most circumstances. Abortion has long been legal in most of Eastern Europe.

In the USA, abortion is, in general, legally allowable but the position varies from state to state. In some, specific laws permit abortion to be carried out in cases where there is a threat to health; in others, judicial construction of legislation is required for the purpose. Practice also varies, but the principle of preserving health is sometimes extended to instances of rape, and where a defective child is the likely outcome of a pregnancy.

ABORTUS FEVER. See BRUCELLOSIS.

ABREACTION is the liberation of emotional tension or *anxiety by recalling or re-experiencing the repressed stressful situation or event thought to be responsible for it. An early technique of *psychotherapy, it is associated with C. G. *Jung.

ABSCESS. A collection of *pus, usually confined within a capsule, forming a cavity within inflamed tissue. See also INFLAMMATION.

ABSENCE. Temporary loss of awareness, characteristic of the form of minor epilepsy also known as *petit mal.

ABSINTHE is a strongly alcoholic drink produced by distillation and flavoured by wormwood (*Artemisia absinthium*), prolonged addiction to which notoriously results in mental and neurological changes. These may have been related in part to its containing significant amounts of *methanol. The recipe was associated with the name of Pernod, who in 1797 acquired it from a Frenchman living in Switzerland called Dr Ordinaire. After absinthe became illegal in France and Switzerland (and in the USA), the Pernod firm continued to produce and market an eponymous aperitif flavoured with aniseed rather than absinthium.

ABSTEM® is a proprietary name for citrated calcium carbimide, used as an adjunct in *alcoholism. As with *disulfiram, the ingestion of even small amounts of alcohol after Abstem® leads to production in the body of *acetaldehyde and an extremely unpleasant reaction.

ACADEMIC MEDICINE is that branch of medicine concerned with teaching and research as well as medical practice, residing largely in universities, academies, and other institutions of higher learning. Those engaged in academic medicine usually have university titles (professor, reader, lecturer, etc.) and are often full-time university employees.

ACADEMIE DE MEDECINE, PARIS. It was created by royal ordinance on 20 December 1820. It was charged 'de répondre aux demandes du Gouvernement sur tout ce qui intéresse la santé publique et principalement sur les épidémies, les maladies particulières à certains pays, les épizooties, les différents cas de médicine légale, la propagation de la vaccine, l'examen des remèdes nouveaux et des remèdes tant internes qu'externes, les eaux minérales naturelles ou factices . . .'.

It was intended that the Academy should continue the work of both the Société Royale de Médecine and the Academy of Surgery, which had been suppressed by the Convention in 1793. Its formation ended the feuding between physicians and surgeons which had characterized French medicine in the 18th century. Its authority was further strengthened by the inclusion of pharmacists and veterinarians among its membership.

ACADEMIES are societies or institutions for the cultivation and promotion of literature, the arts or science, or of some particular branch of science such as medicine, e.g. *Académie de Médecine, Paris; *National Academy of Sciences, Washington.

The UK has no overall academy of medicine or medical sciences, though it has sometimes been suggested that one be formed by uniting the several Royal Colleges (see MEDICAL COLLEGES, ETC. OF THE UK), with other individual societies and associations.

ACANTHOCYTOSIS is a condition in which the red blood cells show a characteristic 'thorny' or 'spiny' deformity (*akantha* is Greek for thorn). The usual cause is a defect of fat absorption in which chylomicron formation (see CHYLE) is disordered, and beta-*lipoproteins are absent from the serum (abetalipoproteinaemia).

ACANTHOMA. A tumour of *epidermal cells.

ACARUS. A mite. The genus *Acarus* contains several species which may infest man, burrowing under the skin and causing *dermatitis. They include *Acarus scabiei*, also known as *Sarcoptes scabiei*, the itch mite which causes *scabies.

ACCOMMODATION. See OPHTHALMOLOGY.

ACCOUCHEMENT. Labour, childbirth, lying-in, or confinement.

ACCOUCHEUR. *Obstetrician. The female form, *accoucheuse*, traditionally means midwife although there are many female obstetricians.

ACCREDITATION. Certification of achievements of official requirements for the completion of higher specialist training (in the UK, and only in certain specialties). The term is also used in North America (less often in the UK) to certify official recognition of hospitals and other health-care institutions.

ACETALDEHYDE (CH₃CHO) is a colourless liquid with a characteristic pungent smell, also known as ethanal. It is produced by oxidation of *ethanol and is thus an intermediate product in alcohol metabolism; its stale smell on the breath is a delayed sign of alcohol indulgence. Like alcohol, acetaldehyde is a general tissue poison.

ACETAZOLAMIDE is a drug (a proprietary name is Diamox®) which inhibits the enzyme *carbonic anhydrase and acts as a weak *diuretic. As it inhibits the formation of aqueous humour in the eye, it is of value in treating *glaucoma.

ACETONE. Also known as dimethyl ketone or propranone, acetone is a colourless inflammable liquid with the chemical formula CH₃COCH₃; it has a characteristic sweet smell. It is used as a solvent for fat and other substances, and sometimes as a skin-cleansing agent. It appears in excess in the blood and urine of certain patients, particularly in *diabetes mellitus and *starvation.

ACETYLCHOLINE (ACh) is the body's most important neurotransmitter, i.e. a chemical substance liberated at nerve endings which transmits nervous impulses to muscle or other nerve cells. Nerve fibres transmitting in this way are termed cholinergic; they include many within the central nervous system and all those outside it except the sympathetic (post-ganglionic) nerves, which release *adrenaline and *noradrenaline and are termed adrenergic. Acetylcholine is normally rapidly destroyed in the body by the enzyme *cholinesterase; its action is thus enhanced and prolonged by drugs having an anticholinesterase action (e.g. *neostigmine). Other drugs (e.g. *curare) block cholinergic conduction by competitive inhibition, i.e. by competing for receptor sites.

Several scientists elucidated the role of acetylcholine, discovered in 1906. Notable were Sir Henry *Dale (1914) and Otto *Loewi (1921), who shared the 1936 *Nobel prize for medicine.

ACETYLSALICYLIC ACID, more widely known as aspirin, is a drug with the chemical formula CH₃COOC₆H₄COOH. Since its discovery in Germany in 1853, it has been widely used for its *analgesic, *antipyretic, anticoagulant, and antirheumatic properties. Except for a few people who are unduly sensitive to its irritant action on the stomach mucous membrane, aspirin remains one of the safest and most effective drugs in medicine.

ACh. See ACETYLCHOLINE.

ACHALASIA is, literally, failure of relaxation. The term is usually applied to a condition in which the ring of muscle around the junction of the *oesophagus and *stomach (the cardiac *sphincter) fails to relax normally on swallowing. There is difficulty in swallowing, with

food retained in the lower part of the oesophagus. The condition is called 'achalasia of the cardia' or 'cardiospasm'.

ACHILLES TENDON. The large tendon behind the ankle, also called the tendo calcaneus, anchors the powerful muscles of the calf to the heel-bone or calcaneus. Accidental rupture, which occasionally occurs during sport, usually requires surgical repair. In Achilles himself, the tendon was pierced by an arrow from the bow of Paris.

ACHLORHYDRIA is absence of *hydrochloric acid from the *gastric juice despite maximal stimulation of gastric secretion.

ACHONDROPLASIA is one of the commonest forms of *dwarfism, giving the characteristic appearance of short arms and legs with a relatively normal trunk; the facial appearance is also typical as the bridge of the nose is flattened and the forehead prominent. The condition, inherited as an autosomal dominant trait (see GENETICS), is due to defective growth of bones which normally develop from *cartilage. Achondroplastic dwarfs are normal in all respects other than the bony deformity.

ACHYLIA. Literally, absence of juice. Sometimes applied to the condition in which the *gastric juice contains neither *hydrochloric acid nor *pepsin. See also ACHLORHYDRIA.

ACID–BASE EQUILIBRIUM is the physiological state of *homeostasis, or acid–base balance, which exists within the body's internal environment with respect to *hydrogen ion concentration (pH). Any tendency to change this is counteracted and limited by the intrinsic buffering capacity of tissues and body fluids and by respiratory and renal compensatory mechanisms (see ACIDOSIS; ALKALOSIS).

ACID-FAST describes certain bacteria, notably *mycobacteria, which resist decolorization by acid after staining.

ACIDOSIS is any condition in which the *hydrogen ion concentration of blood and body tissues is increased, i.e. the *pH is lowered, the normal range for blood being 36 nmol/l (pH 7.45) to 43 nmol/l (pH 7.36). The term respiratory acidosis refers to that resulting from carbon dioxide retention by the lungs. Metabolic acidosis implies either retention of non-volatile acids (as in *renal failure or diabetic *ketosis) or loss of base (as in severe *diarrhoea). 'Compensated' acidosis is a state in which either respiratory (in metabolic acidosis) or renal (in respiratory acidosis) compensatory mechanisms have returned the hydrogen ion concentration towards normal.

ACKEE POISONING is Jamaican vomiting sickness, due to eating unripe fruit of the tree *Blighia sapida*. The toxin responsible is hypoglycine, which inhibits gluconeogenesis (see BIOCHEMISTRY) in the liver.

ACNE is a common skin disorder occurring mainly at *puberty and in early adolescence; characterized by greasiness, pimples, blackheads, and pustules it may lead to disfiguring scarring. The areas most affected are those where *sebaceous glands are most numerous, notably the face and the upper back. Hormonal factors are certainly important and diet, drugs, stress, micro-organisms, and heredity may also be involved. The full name, acne vulgaris, distinguishes it from other skin diseases.

ACONITE is the common name for a genus of poisonous plants belonging to the Ranunculaceae. Monkshood is the dried tuberous root of *Aconitum napellus* L. Wolfsbane is derived from *Aconitum eycoctonum*. Both contain the poisonous alkaloid *aconitine.

ACOUSTICS is the science of sound and hearing.

ACQUIRED IMMUNE DEFICIENCY SYNDROME. See AIDS.

ACRIMONY OF HUMOURS. See HUMOURS.

ACROCYANOSIS is persistent symmetrical *cyanosis of the extremities, most often the hands. The blueness may be unaccompanied by other manifestations, or the patient may complain of coldness and sweating. It is associated with slow blood circulation through the skin *capillaries and the subpapillary venous *plexuses; it disappears on warming the parts to speed up blood flow.

ACRODERMATITIS is inflammation of the skin of the extremities. Acrodermatitis enteropathica is an inherited *recessive disease associated with *zinc deficiency in young children; the skin around the mouth and that of the hands and feet is affected, and there are associated disturbances of growth, intestinal function, and immunity.

ACRODYNIA is a condition of infancy and early childhood characterized by pain and pinkness of the extremities together with features such as *apathy, *insomnia, irritability, and failure to thrive. Also known as 'pink disease', it was for long of unknown cause but since it was found to be due to repeated use of, or sensitivity to, *mercury in teething powders it has disappeared.

ACRODYSTROPHY is deformation of the extremities, particularly the feet, occurring in some forms of peripheral sensory *neuropathy.

ACROMEGALY is a condition caused by prolonged and excessive secretion of pituitary *growth hormone occurring after maturity, i.e. after the *epiphyses of the long bones have fused so that they cannot grow further in length (cf. *gigantism). The term refers to enlargement of the nose, jaws, hands, and feet, which gives a characteristic and immediately recognizable appearance. There is, however, overgrowth of virtually all organs and tissues. Most patients have a tumour (adenoma) involving the acidophilic cells of the *pituitary gland which produce growth hormone.

ACROPARAESTHESIAE (ACROPARESTHESIAE). Tingling, pins and needles, numbness, or burning in the extremities, especially the fingers. It is rarely vascular, more often of neurological origin. The commonest cause in the hands is compression of the *median nerve in the carpal tunnel.

ACTH (adrenocorticotrophic hormone). See CORTICOTROPHIN.

ACTIN is one of the principal protein constituents of the muscle fibre. See MYOSIN.

ACTINODERMATITIS is any inflammation of the skin caused by *radiation. This term is usually applied to the effects of overexposure to ultraviolet light (see SUNBURN).

ACTINOMYCIN is one of a group of *antibiotic substances originally isolated by S. A. *Waksman and H. B. Woodruff from soil micro-organisms. The actinomycins also have *cytotoxic properties and are used as anticancer agents.

ACTINOMYCOSIS is a chronic suppurative infection, most often of the head and neck but sometimes affecting the lung, abdomen (especially the liver), and uterus, caused by various species of filamentous *bacteria normally present in the mouth and belonging to the genus *Actinomyces*.

ACTINOTHERAPY is treatment with *ultraviolet radiation.

ACTOMYOSIN is a reversible complex of two muscle proteins, *actin and *myosin, involved in muscular contraction and relaxation.

ACUITY. Sharpness, particularly of vision (see OPHTHALMOLOGY).

ACUPUNCTURE involves puncturing the skin with needles to induce *anaesthesia for surgery, *analgesia in painful disorders, or sometimes for more general treatment. The technique, which originated in China and is widely practised there, has adherents among the medical profession in other countries, including the UK. Traditionally specific insertion points are used, along with vibration, rotation, or electrical stimulation of the needles.

A firm scientific basis for the method is not yet established. The peripheral nerves may be stimulated or the treatment may merely induce hypnosis. There is, however, some objective evidence that the analgesic effect is greater than can be accounted for by suggestion alone and that acupuncture may stimulate production of the body's own intrinsic analgesic substances, called *endorphins.

ACUTE YELLOW ATROPHY, also known as massive hepatic *necrosis, describes the post-mortem appearance of the liver in patients dying from fulminant *hepatitis. It is a rare complication of viral hepatitis, but may also be due to drug overdosage (e.g. *paracetamol) or to other hepatotoxic substances (e.g. *carbon tetrachloride, *poisonous fungi).

ACYCLOVIR. An antiviral agent effective in controlling the orofacial, ocular, and genital manifestations of recurrent *herpes simplex virus (HSV) infection, though not in permanently eradicating it. Acyclovir can be given by mouth as tablets or by intravenous injection, and is also active when applied as an ophthalmic ointment (3 per cent) or as a cream (5 per cent) in the case of facial and genital lesions. When given systemically it is also effective in herpes simplex encephalitis.

ADAMS, ROBERT (1791–1875). Irish surgeon. He was surgeon to the Jervis Street and Richmond Hospitals and was one of the founders of the medical school at the latter. With *Stokes he described syncopal attacks due to *heart block with very slow heart rates (Stokes–Adams syndrome) in 1827.

ADAMS–STOKES ATTACKS. See STOKES–ADAMS ATTACKS.

ADAPTATION is the process of becoming more suited to prevailing conditions, as, for example: dark adaptation; genetic adaptation; immunological adaptation; enzymatic adaptation, etc.

ADDENBROOKE'S HOSPITAL. The district general hospital that serves the town of Cambridge, England, and the surrounding area and which through its associated medical school provides teaching hospital facilities for the University of Cambridge. See also MEDICAL COLLEGES, ETC. OF THE UK.

ADDICT. One who is physically dependent on a drug, i.e. who experiences symptoms and exhibits signs if its regular administration is discontinued. See also SUBSTANCE ABUSE.

ADDISON, CHRISTOPHER, 1st Viscount Addison of Stallingborough (1869–1951). British anatomist and statesman. He taught anatomy at Sheffield, *Charing Cross Hospital and later *St Bartholomew's. He was elected Liberal Member of Parliament for Hoxton in 1910 and worked with Lloyd George on the *National Health Insurance Act of 1911. As president of the Local Government Board he introduced the bill establishing the *Ministry of Health, becoming the first minister in 1919. In 1948 he was appointed chairman of the *Medical Research Council, a body which he had helped evolve in 1920 and on the independence of which he had insisted. Addison is the only medical recipient of the Order of the Garter.

ADDISON, THOMAS (1793–1860). British physician. He was elected assistant physician to *Guy's Hospital, London, in 1824 and physician in 1837. In 1849 he described suprarenal (adrenal) insufficiency (*Addison's disease) and in 1855, in a monograph on the subject, remarked on the need to distinguish it from 'idiopathic anaemia' now known as *pernicious or Addisonian anaemia.

ADDISON'S DISEASE is due to chronic insufficiency of the *adrenocortical gland, first described by Thomas *Addison in 1849. *Atrophy of the gland is usually due to *autoimmunity (when other *endocrine deficiencies may be present) and occasionally to destructive processes such as *tuberculosis. The cardinal manifestations are extreme weakness, weight loss, brown pigmentation of the skin and mucous membranes, low *blood pressure, and gastrointestinal disturbances. Though the condition may progress for years, the outcome without treatment (with *corticosteroids) is ultimately fatal. (The condition must not be confused with Addisonian anaemia, a synonym for *pernicious anaemia.)

ADENITIS. Inflammation of a *gland or *lymph node.

ADENOCARCINOMA. A *carcinoma deriving from glandular tissue.

ADENOIDS. Gland-like lymphoid tissue present in the *nasopharynx of children, disappearing in adult life. Also called the nasopharyngeal tonsil, this tissue, like the *tonsils themselves, may enlarge as a result of repeated upper respiratory tract infections, when obstructive effects such as *sinusitis and *middle ear infection may ensue. Adenoid *curettage when indicated is usually combined with *tonsillectomy ('tonsils and adenoids').

ADENOMA. A benign new growth deriving from glandular tissue.

ADENOPATHY is any disorder of a *gland or *lymph node; normally used to describe lymph node enlargement.

ADENOSINE DIPHOSPHATE/ADENOSINE TRI-PHOSPHATE (ADP/ATP). The relationship between these two substances plays a central role in energy metabolism (see BIOCHEMISTRY).

ADENOSINE TRIPHOSPHATE (ATP), is an energy-storing nucleotide present in all cells. The removal of one phosphate molecule from ATP under physiological conditions to form adenosine diphosphate (ADP) releases 7.3 kcal (0.03 MJ) per mole (see BIOCHEMISTRY).

ADENOVIRUS. One of a large group of *viruses responsible for upper respiratory and conjunctival infections in man and animals, so named because the first reported isolation was from human *adenoid tissue.

ADENYL CYCLASE is a membrane-bound *enzyme, which catalyses the conversion of *adenosine triphosphate (ATP) to the intracellular messenger compound *cyclic AMP (cAMP). It functions only in cell membranes, where it mediates the action of hormones, e.g. *adrenaline.

ADH. See ANTIDIURETIC HORMONE.

ADHESIONS are unions between membranes or organs which have become bound together by fibrous tissue as a late result of inflammation, *trauma, or surgical operations.

ADIPOSE TISSUE is *connective tissue in which fat-containing cells predominate.

ADIPOSITY is accumulation of excessive *fat, either localized to a particular organ or tissue, or generalized; generalized adiposity is *obesity.

ADJUVANT. A term now used in immunology to mean any material which enhances the response of the *immune system to a simultaneously administered *antigen. The diverse substances which can act in this way include bacterial products, particularly *mycobacteria and bacterial *endotoxins, metal salts such as aluminium hydroxide, polyanions such as *dextran, oil emulsions, and some others. Some adjuvants act by stimulating and activating macrophages and T and B *lymphocytes, whereas others exert their primary effect on the administered antigen, enhancing and prolonging its antigenicity. When a maximal adjuvant effect is desired, a mixture of substances is employed.

ADLER, ALFRED (1870–1937). Austrian psychiatrist. A close associate of *Freud and president of the Vienna Psychoanalytical Society. In 1911 he seceded to form his own movement of 'individual psychology'. He developed the notion of the 'inferiority complex' and held that the driving force was not sex, as Freud believed, but a need for superiority and power.

ADP/ATP. See ADENOSINE DIPHOSPHATE/ADENOSINE TRIPHOSPHATE.

ADRENAL GLAND. One of a pair of small, flattened, triangular organs situated in close proximity to the upper pole of each kidney. Each gland has two developmentally and functionally distinct parts, an outer cortex and an inner medulla. The cortex, under the hormonal control of the anterior *pituitary gland, secretes the important substances known as *corticosteroids. The medulla responds to stimulation by the *sympathetic nervous system and is functionally part of that system; it secretes the catecholamines *adrenaline (epinephrine in the USA) and *noradrenaline (norepinephrine) which mimic the effects of sympathetic stimulation throughout the body, i.e. they are 'sympathomimetic'.

ADRENALINE is one of the two main *hormones secreted by the adrenal medulla (the other being *noradrenaline), which are jointly responsible for 'sympathomimetic' physiological effects (see ADRENAL GLAND; SYMPATHETIC NERVOUS SYSTEM). They are also released at the terminals of sympathetic (post-ganglionic) nerves, which are thus termed 'adrenergic' (see ACETYLCHOLINE). In the USA, the substances are called 'epinephrine' and 'norepinephrine' respectively.

ADRENERGIC BLOCKADE. Inhibition by drugs of the effects of stimulation of the *sympathetic nervous system or of those of the circulating *catecholamines *adrenaline and *noradrenaline. Some agents, known as alpha-blockers and exemplified by *phentolamine and the *ergot alkaloids, selectively block effects at a class of adrenergic *receptor known as alpharecptors, which mediate contraction of vascular smooth muscle and hence *vasoconstriction. Others, the beta-blockers, selectively inhibit sympathetic beta-effects, which include cardiac stimulation and bronchodilatation; *propranolol is the prototype of this widely used group of drugs. Beta-blockers relieve anxiety and reduce blood pressure; they are often prescribed in heart disease.

ADRENOCORTICAL. Pertaining to the cortex of the *adrenal gland.

ADRENOCORTICOTROPHIC HORMONE (ACTH). See CORTICOTROPHIN.

ADRIAN, EDGAR DOUGLAS, 1st Baron Adrian of Cambridge (1889–1977). British neurophysiologist. His work was concerned with the conduction of the nervous impulse. In 1932 he shared the *Nobel prize for medicine with *Sherrington.

ADVERSE REACTIONS. Unwanted, often unexpected, and sometimes dangerous reactions may occur to almost any of the wide variety of potent drugs and vaccines available to modern medicine (see PHARMACOLOGY). The Cutter *poliomyelitis catastrophe of 1955 and the *thalidomide tragedy of the 1960s are but two of the more notorious examples.

AEDES. A genus of biting *mosquitoes, important medically as some species are vectors of viral and parasitic diseases (see MICROBIOLOGY). Notable among these are *yellow fever, *dengue, equine *encephalomyelitis, and *filariasis.

AEROBIC. Requiring free (i.e. gaseous or dissolved) *oxygen for *respiration.

AEROSOL. A gas containing finely dispersed particles (of a liquid or solid).

AEROSPACE MEDICINE is the practice of the art and science of medicine as it relates to man's functioning in the flight environment. The activity of flight, whether in air or space, produces stresses and hazards not otherwise experienced.

Classically, medicine has been concerned with the care and cure of the patient experiencing disease in terrestrial surroundings. Disease in this context can be considered to be the demonstration of a disruptive or abnormal *physiology. Thus the patient is usually viewed as experiencing abnormal physiology in a normal environment.

In contrast, aerospace medicine often deals with a healthy individual; the medical selection process for aviators presupposes health. While the patient in classic medicine is comfortable in a terrestrial environment, the aviator must contend with an entirely different, demanding, dynamic, and at times totally hostile, environment. Thus, in aerospace medicine, we deal with normal physiology in an abnormal environment. Health maintenance with minimal therapeutic intervention is the *sine qua non* for the practitioner. In aerospace medicine concern is not limited to the care of aircrew members: ramifications extend to the millions of airline passengers who are flying every day and the ground crews and support personnel who keep them flying.

The past

The discipline of aerospace medicine has been recognized only recently as an area of special competence. Although the number of practitioners in the field remains relatively small, interest and participation by physicians in aeronautics and astronautics have dated from the earliest manned flights.

Man-carrying balloons, kites, and gliders interested many. Slowly an engineering technology began to evolve where lift and drag became a concern, and the aerofoil a solution. The concept slowly evolved of putting an engine on such a craft to try to establish sustained flight. This effort proved feasible at Kill Devil Hill near Kitty Hawk, North Carolina, when on 17 December 1903 the Wright brothers attained sustained controlled powered flight. By the time that man had experienced powered flight, he had already been exposed to low temperature, *hypoxia, alterations in pressure, *motion sickness, crash injury, and death.

The rapid development of aviation as an arm of combat in the First World War led to a parallel development of aviation medicine. One year after the onset of hostilities, the UK reviewed its casualty list. Out of every 100 aviators killed, only 2 had met their deaths at the hands of the enemy, 8 from defects in their aircraft, and an astounding 90 were ascribed to individual deficiencies, including physical defects, recklessness, and carelessness. Further study showed that 60 per cent of the aviation casualties were due to physical defects in the aviators that could have been detected by a careful physical examination. Hence, the British developed a special service for 'the care of the flyer'. The results of this innovative aviation medicine programme were spectacular, with deaths in the second year due to physical defects reduced from 60 to 20 per cent, and by the third year to 12 per cent.

Current aerospace medical activities

The world-wide air transportation system is an important element of international commerce. Within the USA, nearly 90 per cent of long-distance travel in public carriers occurs on airliners. World airline traffic will carry 1400 million passengers in 1995. Internationally, 95 per cent of travel is now aboard aircraft. Approximately 300 million passengers will board international flights flying a combined total of 455 thousand million miles (International Civil Aviation Organization 1992).

The flying environment

Stressors, either single or multiple, can affect the aircrewman and exceed the physiological capability to compensate. The result can be decreased performance, unconsciousness, and death. The stressors are generated by both the medium of flight and the physics of aeronautics. The medium of the atmosphere generates potential stressors resulting from oxygen deprivation, atmospheric pressure alteration, temperature extremes, ozone exposure, and cosmic ray bombardment. The laws of physics produce stress when interacting with physiology because of acceleration, impact, noise, and misinformation to the sensory system.

The atmosphere

The atmosphere is simply an ocean of air enveloping the Earth. Several characteristics of the atmosphere are important as one ascends in flight. Generally, the proportion of gases in the atmosphere remains constant during ascent (Table 1). As altitude increases,

Table 1 Partial pressure (P_x) (mmHg) and percentage of constituents of the atmosphere at selected altitudes

	Altitude in metres								
	Sea-level		1524		3048	4572	10058	14021	
Constituent	%	P_x	%	P_x	P_x	P_x	P_x	%	P_x
Nitrogen (N_2)	78.09	600	79	498	413	339	155	79	84
Oxygen (O_2)	20.95	159	21	134	110	90	41	21	22
Argon (Ar)	0.92	0.7							
Carbon dioxide (CO_2)	0.03	0.2	negligible						
Other	0.01	0.1							
Total	100	760	100	632	523	429	196	100	106

less atmospheric mass pushes on the body; pressure changes occur more rapidly at lower than at higher altitude because of increased air density near the Earth's surface. Problems are caused by (a) lack of oxygen and (b) decrease in pressure.

(a) Oxygen. The percentage composition of oxygen in the Earth's atmosphere is essentially constant up to an altitude of 90 km. As the atmospheric pressure decreases with altitude, so does the availability of oxygen. The normal ambient oxygen partial pressure (pO_2) of about 160 mmHg at sea-level is reduced to 80 mmHg at 5.5 km, 40 mmHg at 11 km, etc.

Even when breathing 100 per cent oxygen, one reaches an altitude where it is impossible to prevent hypoxia. For example, at an altitude of 15 000 m, the combined pressure of water vapour and carbon dioxide in the lung essentially equals the total barometric pressure; thus it becomes impossible to effect any respiratory exchange even with 100 per cent oxygen available. The first subtle effects of hypoxia become noticeable in the unacclimatized individual at altitudes as low as 2000 m where subtle decrements in night vision have been measured. Depression of simple neuromuscular reflexes becomes evident at about 3000 m.

To compensate for inadequate oxygen at altitude, passengers and aircrew are provided with auxiliary oxygen when flying in unpressurized aircraft, and emergency oxygen for pressurized aircraft. Breathing 100 per cent oxygen will provide protection up to 12 000 m (40 000 ft) which is physiologically the same as ascending to 3000 m (10 000 ft) without oxygen.

In commercial flying, passengers do not routinely require supplemental oxygen, although the jet liner may be above 10 000 m, as the pressure inside the cabin of the aircraft is maintained at a safe and comfortable 2000 m equivalent altitude. In the event of an emergency loss of pressure, oxygen would be immediately required for all in the aircraft. Thus, emergency oxygen units are available to all airline passengers in the event of a rapid

pressure change, and the oxygen supply is sufficient to maintain the passenger until a lower, safe altitude is reached.

(b) Pressure. At sea-level the atmospheric pressure is, on average, 101.325 kPa (760 torr, or 1013.25 millibars). With increasing altitude, density decreases in a near-exponential fashion when temperature is held constant. This change in density and, thus, in pressure is illustrated in Fig. 1. Within the cavities of the body such as the *middle ear, the *sinuses, and the gastrointestinal tract, there is a volume of undissolved gas. The gas within these cavities responds to changes in atmospheric pressure in accordance with Boyle's law: at constant temperature, the volume of the gas varies inversely with pressure. Thus, when one ascends in an unpressurized aircraft, air in these cavities will expand. This explains fullness in the ears during ascent due to expansion of the gas trapped in the middle ear. If there is a marked change in altitude, this expansion can be significant. For example, at 5800 m, the volume of trapped

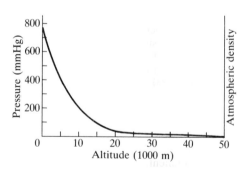

Fig. 1 Atmospheric density as a function of altitude. The rapid decrease in density is correlated with a decrease in both atmospheric pressure and partial pressure of oxygen.

gas will double. It will double again at 10 000 m, and yet again at 16 000 m. This phenomenon is reversed as one descends. It is this expansion, or contraction, of trapped gas with changing pressures which produces signs and symptoms of ear block, *sinusitis, and gastrointestinal discomfort. Entrapment of air within the body in disease states, such as *emphysema, *pneumothorax, *gas gangrene, or intestinal obstruction can be catastrophic.

With altitude change, gas movement is not limited to ventilation of body cavities, but gas moves in and out of body fluids as well. Flying personnel who are decompressed from a lower altitude to a higher altitude, as from sea-level to 8000 m, when that altitude transition is rapid, may exhibit altitude *decompression sickness or 'aviator bends'. The sudden release of gas from solution can produce various symptoms depending on the location of the evolved gas. Most often, discomfort occurs deep in the joints, bones, or muscles of a limb. Whatever the site, the pain is generally diffuse and poorly localized. *Paraesthesiae and sensations of hot or cold have been described. When evolving gas reaches the pulmonary circulation, a condition called 'the chokes' may occur. This condition gives substernal distress (pain beneath the breast bone), accompanied by a burning, gnawing, or piercing pain, generating a dry, non-productive cough. These symptoms are ominous, as they often presage circulatory collapse. Neurological symptoms may develop due to release of gas in the central nervous system. Many symptoms have been observed but visual disturbances are most common, although *hemiplegia and *monoplegia have been described. Such a symptom-complex must be taken seriously as permanent neurological damage may result, as well as shock, collapse, and death.

Until recently, decompression illness was not seen unless the individual had ascended above 6000 m. With the growing popularity of recreational compressed-air diving (scuba), a situation is created where manifestations of the 'bends' may occur at far lower altitudes. An individual who spends an enjoyable afternoon diving to a depth of 20 m, using scuba equipment, has supersaturated body tissues and fluids with nitrogen. Should that person, a few hours later, depart on a commercial airliner, albeit properly pressurized, he or she will experience a sufficient pressure change for nitrogen to be released into the circulation. 'Bends' requiring recompression therapy has been reported at altitudes as low as 1200 m. (See also ENVIRONMENT AND MEDICINE I.)

Physics and physiology
(a) *G force.* An understanding of the biomedical effects of acceleration on the human body is important. In the military environment, high sustained acceleration results in a force acting on the body which is related to gravitational force and is called 'G force'. In space flight, the astronaut experiences the reverse phenomenon as the orbital acceleration neutralizes the Earth's gravitational force and, thus, the space-craft occupants experience zero G. This accelerative environment also generates vector cues to the sensory system, resulting in spatial *disorientation in the aircrew member, particularly when visual cues are not available.

Under terrestrial conditions, the 30 cm blood column from the heart to the brain exerts a hydrostatic pressure of 22 mmHg. With a systolic arterial blood pressure at the heart of 120 mmHg, the arterial pressure at the base of the brain will have been reduced to 98 mmHg. For each additional G, the blood pressure at brain level will be reduced by 22 mmHg, eventually reaching a theoretical pressure of zero at approximately 5.5 G (Ernsting and King 1988). Thus a major physiological result of acceleration can be loss of consciousness.

To increase tolerance, pilots are equipped with a G suit, a garment that covers the abdomen and lower extremities and contains five bladders pressing on the calves, thighs, and abdomen when air pressure inflates the suit. This device can increase tolerance by 2 G through increasing the available circulating blood by preventing abdominal and lower extremity pooling. Physical straining and the use of a tight vest and increased mask pressure are additional techniques for increasing G tolerance.

(b) **Impact and vibration.** Whether called a jolt or a jerk, sudden short-duration impact and vibration forces are experienced by all in the aviation environment, both crew and passengers. Whether in the turbulence of a storm, or the unexpected turbulence that occurs periodically in clear air, the individual is thrown about his seat. Restraint systems have been designed for the protection of both crew and passengers. Far fewer individuals experience the high-magnitude force generated in an accident or crash. Phenomenal improvement has occurred recently in both cabin design and restraint systems used for passengers and aircrew. These improvements have greatly improved the survival rate from accidents which are not catastrophic.

(c) **Noise.** The jet engine has been defined (partly in jest) as a converter of petroleum to noise. Noise generates potential for hearing loss, interference with voice communication, and an intrusion in most communities near military and civil airfields. Concern for the effects of the acoustic energy generated in aerospace systems is appropriate as they probably generate the most severe noise environments to which individuals are repeatedly exposed.

In the 1970s, the airline industry went to considerable expense to develop and acquire propulsion systems designed to reduce acoustic energy. Communities around airports have created compatible-use zones which take into consideration disruptive effects of aircraft noise and control the build-up of residential, school, and hospital facilities in these zones. Acoustic barriers are common considerations in the design of all commercial aircraft. As a result seat-mates in commercial airlines can carry on conversation at a comfortable loudness level. Even with these precautions, noise remains an industrial hazard which costs governments and the aerospace industry large sums in compensation per year.

(d) Acceleration-induced illusions. The three *semicircular canals which maintain spatial orientation of the body are remarkable organs but are designed for terrestrial function. Because of accelerative stimuli in flight, perceptual errors may arise in the vestibular system, resulting in perceptions of spatial orientation which differ from reality. In addition, the otolith organs, which are subjected to linear or gravitational acceleration, are particularly susceptible to miscues in flying. Rarely is the direction of force acting on the otolith membrane in a true vertical direction when flying other than straight and level. The proprioceptive sensors responding to pressure and stretch can be readily misled with misinterpretation of sensory cues. Without visual reference, either to the Earth's horizon or to cockpit instrumentation, no pilot can maintain proper flight attitude and direction for very long.

Aircrew selection
Recognizing the demands that flying makes on a physiological system, national authorities require medical assessment of potential aircrew members.

Flying taxes all the senses and places a premium on neuromuscular co-ordination and dexterity. The intellectual function and time relationships require an individual possessing full cerebral functioning. A prospective pilot cannot suffer from an organic disease which could cause sudden unconsciousness. Bilateral visual acuity should be optimized and, if corrective lenses are required, their use should be a required condition of flight. Unless he or she intends to be restricted in flying activities, a candidate must have adequate night and normal colour vision (see COLOUR BLINDNESS). Hearing must be adequate to understand instructions from ground control or from other aircraft. The cardiovascular system must be free of disorders which could result in sudden incapacitation or could compromise the aviator in an acceleration environment. Thus, *coronary heart disease, *arrhythmia, and *valvular heart disease must be approached not just from the standpoint of the patient flying without endangering a medical condition, but rather, flying without compromising safety of flight. An individual with reduced pulmonary reserve from whatever cause, represents a hazard to flight safety when flying at altitude where he or she may experience a significantly reduced oxygen partial pressure. The gastrointestinal system should be free of disease that is aggravated by stress; it requires little imagination to picture the consequences of a bleeding *peptic ulcer at altitude. Most flying requires full function, both in strength and motion, of the limbs, although some experienced pilots have returned to the cockpit with *prostheses. Oral–nasal disease can have ramifications in flight. Disease that compromises the ventilation of dental cavities, the nasal sinuses, and the middle ear can cause excruciating pain when undergoing rapid altitude changes. The sensorium must be clear and not compromised by the side-effects of drugs, the after-effects of alcohol, or manifestations of another disease process within the body.

Because of the medical selection process, aircraft crews and astronauts are much healthier than the average population. The rigorousness of the physical assessment is usually determined by the stressors involved in the specific flight regimen and the responsibility involved. For example, an astronaut or a military test pilot will receive a far more thorough medical examination than would normally be expected for a general aviator who flies purely for recreation. This 'healthy worker effect' has been documented in several longitudinal studies which reviewed the medical and health circumstances of aircrew (Rayman 1982). Both age-specific *mortality and *morbidity are considerably below those found in the general population.

Health maintenance
The physician's most important role in aerospace medicine is in maintaining the health of aircrew. The goal is to prevent, when possible, or treat medical conditions of aircrew in order to maintain both flight safety and aviation careers.

The periodic examination
All aircrew are required to undergo periodic physical examination to ensure their continued fitness for flight. Unlike the ordinary patient, an aircrew member may not be able to take long-term medication for control of a pathological process, and yet retain his or her flying status. Minor illnesses such as sinusitis and the common cold, readily managed in a terrestrial environment, can result in an acute medical emergency in the flight environment. A military pilot with progressive but asymptomatic aortic valvular disease may have his *G* tolerance compromised and become an unexplained aircraft accident statistic. The physician should therefore advise the aircrew member on measures to reduce risk of illness.

Self-imposed stress
As should be evident in reviewing the flight environment, aviation imposes some degree of stress upon aircrew, even under the most benign conditions. Although the selection process may ensure the fitness of an individual for aircrew duty, the pilot may degrade this fitness through a self-imposed unhealthy life-style.

(a) Self-medication. The side-effects of common medications are well known to practitioners. Physicians dealing with aircrew must be especially aware of the actions of any drugs they may be prescribing. The primary pharmacological effect or side-effect of a particular drug may cause impaired visual acuity, impaired co-ordination, increased reaction time, drowsiness, or *hypotension. Of particular concern are drug classes which include *antihistamines, *anticholinergics, *tranquillizers, *sedatives, antihypertensives, and *analgesics. The physician must be alert, as well, to the over-the-counter medication which the pilot may acquire and self-administer without seeking professional medical advice.

(b) Alcohol and illicit drug abuse. In recent decades the use of illicit drugs has become a global social phenomenon. This use and the abuse of alcohol create a real and present danger to flying safety and to the lives of the aircrew and their passengers. Illicit drugs may cause drowsiness, euphoria, impairment, hallucinations, and flashbacks—a situation totally incompatible with life in the cockpit. Periodically, aircrew may attempt to fly their aircraft while still under the influence of alcohol or while suffering the physiological after-effects of overindulgence. It is incumbent upon the physician who becomes aware of such intolerable situations to intercede medically or administratively. It has been well established that even small amounts of blood alcohol, in the 20–70 mg/dl range, can produce significant performance decrement when compounded by the stress of flight.

(c) Smoking. The compromise to health created by cigarette-smoking centres on coronary artery disease, cancer, or chronic lung disease. These reasons alone should act as a stimulus for the physician, as a practitioner of *preventive medicine, to discourage patients from smoking. In the flight environment, yet another consideration emerges. A by-product of cigarette smoke, *carbon monoxide, has an affinity for *haemoglobin 200 times that of oxygen. This competition for haemoglobin compromises the airman's acclimatization to altitude and significantly increases susceptibility to hypoxia.

Operational stress

In addressing the environment of flight, we have reviewed several stressors which can act upon pilot, crew, and passenger. Additional factors require elaboration.

(a) Temperature and humidity. Modern systems have been designed to provide a comfortable environment for the occupant. However, there are situations when poor environmental control occurs and the aircrew are forced to adapt to rapidly changing hot and cold temperatures. Adequate temperature control is a far greater problem in military aircraft than is usually experienced in the commercial sphere.

More subtle than temperature variation, but certainly of importance in the commercial airliner, is the lack of humidity. By the time that the cabin pressurization system has taken the rarefied air of altitude, compressed it (generating heat), and cooled it, the air is essentially devoid of moisture. Passengers on flights of more than a few hours often complain of thirst and dry mucous membranes. Not infrequently, passengers who have flown for many hours are seen days later with symptoms suggesting an upper respiratory tract infection. This increased susceptibility of mucous membranes to irritation and perhaps infection is appropriately attributed to a low humidity. The establishment of 'No Smoking' zones within aircraft has significantly reduced such irritation and passenger complaints. It is anticipated that soon a non-smoking policy will apply to all commercial flights.

(b) Circadian rhythm. Within the last few decades, individuals involved in international travel have added the term *circadian rhythm to their vocabulary (Randel 1972). The desynchrony in the work–rest cycle occurring when crossing time zones is a significant contributor to post-flight fatigue. This well-known 'jet lag' is a phenomenon with a well-established physiological basis. For politicians, statesmen, athletes, and executives, this alteration in the body synchronization must be considered when travelling to engage in significant negotiations, discussions, or sporting events. An individual experiences less disruption when moving across time zones from east to west. It is recommended that a 36- to 48-hour period of adjustment be planned when important activities are scheduled at the destination after crossing more than four zones.

Aeromedical concerns of air travel

As air travel continues to increase, individuals who, for a variety of reasons, including medical, have been hesitant will venture aboard an airliner. The environment of flight can complicate pre-existing medical conditions: thus, the physician should counsel the individual with medical or surgical problems.

The passenger

The passenger with dental disease, upper respiratory tract infection, or sinusitis, may find that he or she cannot achieve pressure equalization and suffers acute localized pain.

With the advent of the high-flying Boeing 747 and the Concorde, there have been incidents of significant upper respiratory irritation. This phenomenon has been related to increased ozone concentration which can be found in altitudes in excess of 16 000 m. To prevent this clinical syndrome, catalytic converters have been

Table 2 Medical and surgical conditions requiring special considerations for aeromedical transfer

---

Cardiac failure
Severe asthma
Respiratory embarrassment
Trapped gas in body cavities
CNS surgery or diagnostic procedures
Severe anaemia
Psychotic orientation
Facial injury with wired jaw
Facial or respiratory burns
Premature infant

---

installed in environmental control systems to neutralize the ozone.

A passenger with compromised coronary artery flow (coronary insufficiency) may develop symptoms if there is a significant fall in the partial pressure of oxygen. This fall in pressure would not be expected to occur in a commercial airliner unless there is an emergency decompression, at which time oxygen would be available.

Individuals suffering chronic obstructive pulmonary disease, if reasonably mobile, can be expected to travel satisfactorily by air. If the flight is long, it may prove advisable to have a small atomizer available to increase periodically the moisture of the mucous membranes. Oxygen would need to be available in the event of exposure to high ambient altitudes.

Those with mild *anaemia, a haemoglobin above 8 g/dl, should experience no problems on a routine flight. Should an individual suffer from *sickle-cell anaemia, it would be advisable to travel as a patient rather than as a routine passenger; low partial pressures of oxygen could initiate a crisis.

Motion sickness is no longer a common event on large commercial aircraft. Both airlines and flight captains take every precaution to ensure a smooth flight and avoid turbulence. Should an individual be highly susceptible to motion sickness, then pre-flight treatment with an appropriate anti-motion sickness drug, seat selection over the wing, and flying in a reclined position when possible, are all appropriate.

Provided that the expectant mother remains a passenger and does not become a patient with the onset of labour, there is no contraindication to commercial air travel. However, it must be remembered that the seat belt crosses the abdomen and should there be violent turbulence, incidental trauma is a distinct possibility.

Infants more than seven days old have fully developed respiratory systems and therefore make satisfactory passengers. On a long flight it is advisable to ensure adequate hydration by increased feeding of juice, water, or dilute feeds as appropriate. During descent, it is advisable to have the infant awake to assist in pressure equalization.

Passengers who are obviously inebriated, under the influence of drugs, or whose behaviour is in question should be denied passage by the aircraft captain.

The patient

The movement of patients under medical supervision to and between medical treatment facilities by air transportation is becoming more common. Both private and government air ambulance services are joining the military in air evacuation of patients. With appropriate arrangements, many commercial air carriers will make special provision for the transport of patients on commercial flights, provided that there is no undue disturbance to other passengers. Those who are selected for transportation by air require a physician who is aware of the environmental hazards of flight. Although there are no absolute contraindications to aeromedical evacuation, as long as special considerations are given, the attending aeromedical team needs to be fully aware of a number of conditions (Table 2) (Johnson 1977).

Special management of medical and surgical conditions may be required to prepare the patient for evacuation. Plaster casts should be bivalved (divided down one side) to allow for soft-tissue expansion at altitude, particularly if newly applied. Chest tubes may be left in place but require the application of a Hemlich valve. Traction provided by swinging weights is both unreliable and unsafe. Patients travelling with wired jaws should carry surgical scissors around their neck to facilitate release in case of motion sickness. Psychologically disturbed patients should be sedated and restrained. *Colostomy patients should be supplied with an extra supply of bags and wraps due to increased flow often associated with intestinal gas expansion. Eye-injury patients should be transported on a stretcher and not allowed to sit up. Patients can be moved safely and expeditiously by air provided that thought and precautions go into preparation for transport.

The future

Science and technology have opened the way to unconstrained use of both air and space. The medical practitioner, like his or her scientific and engineering colleagues, will be challenged to contribute collectively to each new and exciting advance in aerospace technology. The physician practising the art and science of medicine and, more especially, of aerospace medicine, should recall the oft-quoted phrase, 'It is unwise to treat of any medical subject as if it were complete'.

R. L. DeHART

References

DeHart, R. L. (ed.) *Fundamentals of aerospace medicine*, 2nd edn. Philadelphia. (In press.)
Ernsting, J. and King, P. (ed.) (1988). *Aviation medicine*. London.
International Civil Aviation Organization (ICAO) (1992). Forecast. Montreal.

Johnson, A. (1977). Treatise on aeromedical evacuation. *Aviation, Space and Environmental Medicine*, **48**, 546-54,
Randel, H. W. (ed.) (1972). *Aerospace medicine*. Baltimore.
Rayman, R. B. (1982). *Clinical aviation medicine*. New York.

AESCULAPIUS (or Asclepius). Greek god. Appeared in Homer as the son of Apollo, the pupil of Chiron the Centaur, and the father of Machaon and Podalirius, physicians to the force which invaded the Troad. Later legend made him a native of Epidaurus, and the victim of a thunderbolt launched by Zeus. Certainly Epidaurus became a notable centre of his cult, as were Cos and Cnidus. The priestly order of Asclepiadae practised throughout antiquity, using herbs and sacred serpents. Socrates, before taking the hemlock, observed the custom of sacrificing a cock to Aesculapius. Aesculapius became the Greek god of medicine because of the activities of his priestly order in healing the sick.

AETIOLOGY (ETIOLOGY) is the science and study of disease causation.

AFFECT. In psychiatric usage, the mood, feeling, or emotion attached to ideas.

AFFECTIVE DISORDERS. Disorders of mood, feeling, or emotion, such as *manic-depressive psychosis.

AFLATOXINS are a group of powerfully carcinogenic (in experimental animals) substances caused by the contamination of foodstuffs with certain moulds (species of *Aspergillus*). They are suspected of being implicated in the high prevalence of primary liver cancer in some parts of Africa.

AFTERBIRTH. The *placenta and membranes expelled from the uterus during the third stage of *labour.

AGAR. A preparation of complex *polysaccharides derived from red marine algae, particularly species of *Gelidium*. Soluble in boiling water, it swells and sets into a gelatinous mass on cooling. Being resistant to the digestive action of most bacteria, it is valuable as the basis of solid bacterial *culture media, and in biochemical and immunological techniques requiring gel diffusion. It may also be used as a bulk-forming *laxative.

AGE CONCERN, a UK charity, arose from the recognition of hardship and poverty in the elderly during evacuation from large cities, under threat of bombing in the Second World War. A committee was set up, which by 1955 had become the National Old People's Welfare Council. Smaller similar committees began all over the UK by local initiative. In 1971 the NOPWC became independent of the National Council of Social Service and took the name of Age Concern. In 1974 this became Age Concern England, and similar bodies were started for Northern Ireland, Scotland, and Wales.

The work of this charity concerns welfare of retired and elderly people. It relies greatly on donations. It helps local organizations with financial advice which is available to individuals too. Information is disseminated widely and booklets are published on such matters as 'Your Rights', 'Your Taxes and Savings', and 'Your Holidays in Retirement'. It is also involved in parliamentary lobbying in relation to the affairs of the elderly. A Research Unit, founded in 1976, investigates problems such as those of ethnic minorities, of bereavement, and of voluntary service. Counsellors are trained.

AGEING is the process of growing older; towards the end of life there may be progressive and generally unfavourable physical and mental changes, terminating in death. The desire for youthfulness and immortality have led to countless theories of ageing (gerontology) but little is known about how deterioration in function is related to cellular and molecular changes. *Geriatrics (medical gerontology) is the medical discipline concerned with care of ageing patients.

AGENESIS. Failure of an organ to develop or appear.

AGGLUTINATION. The aggregation or coalescence of bacteria, cells, or other particulate matter in suspension. See also AGGLUTININS.

AGGLUTININS are *antibodies which by combining with particulate *antigens (e.g. on *bacteria, *erythrocytes, etc.) lead to their aggregation. Substances other than antibodies may also act as agglutinins. 'Cold agglutinins' are haemagglutinating antibodies which cause red cells to agglutinate inside the blood vessels of some patients exposed to cold.

AGGRESSION is self-assertive or frankly hostile behaviour towards others, sometimes held to represent compensation for concealed feelings of inadequacy or inferiority.

AGNOSIA was *Freud's term for loss of perception, now used to mean specific inability to attach meaning to or to recognize sensory information.

AGONIST. In pharmacology, an agonist is a *ligand (that is, a specific chemical substance with an affinity for a specific cell *receptor) which produces an effect resembling that caused by a naturally occurring endogenous substance, such as a *hormone or *neurotransmitter. An antagonist, by contrast, is a ligand which binds to its receptor without producing a biological response. (For examples, see PHARMACOLOGY.) The terms are used in a different sense in physiology to describe the actions of muscles, an agonist being a prime mover, an antagonist one which opposes an action.

AGORAPHOBIA is a morbid and incapacitating aversion to open spaces. It may result in inability to leave one's own home, as in the familiar syndrome of the 'house-bound housewife'.

AGRANULOCYTOSIS. Deficiency of granular *leucocytes (i.e. the non-lymphoid white blood cells) in the circulation.

AGRAPHIA is loss of the ability to write, which may be due to a focal lesion of the *cerebral cortex or to more widespread cerebral dysfunction. Agraphia may or may not be accompanied by *alexia.

AGRIPPA, HEINRICH CORNELIUS (otherwise Heinrich von Nettesheim) (1486–?1535). German philosopher, occultist, alchemist, and physician. He practised in Fribourg, where he interested himself in alchemy and hypnosis.

AGUE. Originally (e.g. in the Authorized Version of the Bible) meaning any acute fever, 'ague' came to be applied to a fever with hot and shivering phases, often used synonymously with *malaria.

AIDS AND HIV. The term acquired immune deficiency syndrome (AIDS) is a spectrum of diseases associated with human immunodeficiency virus (HIV), a viral infection which produces a slowly progressive weakening in the cellular immune system. To date it has been uniformly fatal. AIDS was first recognized in 1981 in homosexual men in New York and Los Angeles. In 1984, it was demonstrated that the HIV virus (formerly lymphadenopathy-associated virus (LAV), or human T-cell lymphotropic virus type III (HTLV III)) was the probable cause of AIDS. Since then, the definition of the syndrome has undergone many changes and will probably continue to do so.

There is a global *epidemic of AIDS and HIV infection. World-wide, the *World Health Organization (WHO) estimates that there are between 5 and 10 million people infected with the HIV virus, and the numbers are rising rapidly. The greatest number of cases have been reported in selected areas of North and South America, Central Africa, and Western Europe. Recently, large numbers of cases have been appearing in Asia. In the USA, there are thought to be more than 1 million persons infected with the HIV virus, and almost 250 000 cases of AIDS have been reported. The disease has become a leading cause of death in men and women under the age of 45 and in children under 5 years old.

The ways in which HIV infection is transmitted have been well characterized: by sexual intercourse, by blood, and by the birth process through extensive exposure to infected blood and bodily fluids. The transmission of HIV infection through school, household, workplace, insect bites, or the closest of 'casual' social contacts has not been documented. Therefore school, work, and social contact with HIV-infected individuals poses no known risk for HIV infection.

The great majority of HIV/AIDS cases are sexually transmitted. Anal intercourse seems to carry the highest risk. Man-to-woman transmission is more common than woman-to-man transmission, but any person who is sexually active with partners who are infected or who are of unknown infectivity are at risk for HIV infection.

The *virus is also transmitted by blood or blood products. Intravenous drug users who share needles or use unsterile needles are at high risk of becoming infected with the HIV virus (see also SUBSTANCE ABUSE). Before 1985 more than 95 per cent of patients receiving a *blood transfusion contaminated with the HIV virus became infected. Since mid-1985 screening of all donated blood and blood products has all but eliminated the risk of transfusion-related HIV/AIDS. The chance of a unit of blood containing HIV is now estimated to be between 1 in 40 000 and 1 in 250 000. Antihaemophiliac preparations now appear free of the virus and are non-infectious.

The most common means of infection to children is through the *placenta *in utero* or from vaginal secretions and exposure to blood during childbirth. An infant born to an infected mother has a 25–35 per cent chance of becoming infected. There is no evidence that Caesarean deliveries are protective. There is evidence that infants can rarely become infected while breast-feeding. At this time in the developed world where there are adequate supplies of supplemental infant nutrition, breast-feeding by HIV-infected mothers should be discouraged.

Health-care workers are at low, but not non-existent, risk of HIV infection. A person suffering a hollow bore needle-stick injury with an HIV-contaminated needle has less than a 0.3 per cent risk of becoming infected. Five health-care workers in the USA (i.e. 0.001 per cent of all US cases) are reported to have become infected without a needle-stick injury following exposure of mucous membranes or non-intact skin to infectious blood and bodily fluids.

In the USA approximately 60 per cent of AIDS cases are seen in homosexual or bisexual men, 28 per cent of people infected have a history of illicit intravenous drug use, 5 per cent of cases have heterosexual contact as their only risk factor, 3 per cent have received a contaminated blood transfusion or organ *transplant, 1 per cent have *haemophilia or other coagulation disorders and have received contaminated blood product transfusions, and 3 per cent of AIDS cases are children or have an undetermined exposure. This pattern of infection is similar to the patterns in Canada, Western Europe, Australia, and New Zealand. In Central Africa and the Caribbean, the pattern of spread of the disease is thought to be overwhelmingly via heterosexual intercourse.

In the general population in the USA who do not knowingly practise high-risk behaviour, less than 0.04 per cent of people screened randomly are infected with the HIV virus. This is in stark contrast to general population rates of HIV infection in Central Africa, which may be as high as 3–5 per cent.

Among the groups at high risk for HIV infection and AIDS in the USA, homosexuals may have infection rates as high as 50–70 per cent in high-incidence areas such as New York and San Francisco. Intravenous drug users may also have rates as high as 70 per cent and higher in some high-risk areas. Although haemophiliacs are no longer at increased risk of contracting HIV infection, their infection rate as a group is very high (greater than 70 per cent), because of contaminated clotting factors and transfusions received in the pre-blood screening era.

AIDS develops in HIV-infected persons because of direct HIV viral effects and secondary effects, such as opportunistic infections and tumours, which result from the infected person's depleted immune system. HIV-1 and HIV-2, the only two types of HIV virus identified, are retroviruses. The virus preferentially infects cells of the immune system and the predominant result is a quantitative and qualitative defect in a population of immune cells called T-4 *lymphocytes. These T-4 lymphocytes are largely responsible for the activation of the immune system (see also IMMUNOLOGY). Normally, when the body is infected with a virus, antibodies against the virus are produced, and the infection is effectively resolved. For unknown reasons, the antibodies produced in response to infection with HIV are ineffective. The immune system is not only responsible for defending the body against invading infections, but it is also responsible for keeping *neoplasms in check. As a result, HIV-infected people get infections and tumours more easily than people with an intact immune system. The HIV virus also has direct effects on many of the body's other systems.

The expression of HIV infection varies greatly. Most people infected have initially no symptoms or signs of their illness. Three to six weeks after infection, some develop an acute illness that resembles *mononucleosis or *influenza (the flu) with fever, chills, sore throat, fatigue, muscle and joint aches, headache, rashes, and gastrointestinal complaints. This episode lasts 2–3 weeks and resolves spontaneously in almost all cases. In the following month or two (three months after presumed exposure and infection), the patient produces antibodies, and blood tests are able to detect the antibodies, a sign of HIV infection. The person is now said to have seroconverted. In groups who develop the flu-like illness, the time from resolution of the flu-like state to the development of overt disease varies greatly from individual to individual and from young to old. The period can be shorter than a year or as long as 15 years.

When the immune system is seriously suppressed the disease becomes full-blown. HIV/AIDS patients commonly develop what are called opportunistic infections, because in people with normal immune systems the

organisms that cause these infections are present but kept at bay. Opportunistic infections such as *candidiasis, *Pneumocystis carinii* *pneumonia (PCP), viral infections due to *herpes or *cytomegalovirus (CMV), *toxoplasmosis, *tuberculosis, and opportunistic malignancies such as *lymphoma and *Kaposi's sarcoma are common and life-threatening to the patient.

HIV-infected patients are also prone to haematological or blood problems. Patients commonly have thrombocytopenia (too few *platelets), neutropenia (too few white blood cells (*leucocytes) other than the ones directly affected by the HIV virus) and anaemia (too few red blood cells). (See also HAEMATOLOGY.) These deficiencies result from direct action of the virus, as well as from complications and side-effects of medications prescribed to treat the aforementioned opportunistic infections.

The nervous system is subject to direct attack by the HIV virus and there are many presentations of HIV-related neurological disease. Subacute *encephalitis, AIDS *encephalopathy, or the AIDS–*dementia complex are the most common. These may be the first signs of AIDS or among the later manifestations, and are characterized by changes in mentation, motor skills, and behaviour. Sooner or later, these disorders are found in more than two-thirds of AIDS patients.

Most organ systems in the body are adversely affected by HIV infection. The pulmonary system in most patients is subject to repeated opportunistic infections, such as PCP, CMV, *fungi, *bacteria, and, importantly, *Mycobacterium tuberculosis*. The gastrointestinal system is also affected by tumours or infections in most HIV/AIDS patients. The oesophagus is involved in many patients and infection of this organ is a cause of *dysphagia. Diarrhoea occurs in more than 50 per cent of patients. Both dysphagia and diarrhoea contribute to the problem of weight loss and wasting that is seen in people with HIV/AIDS. The eyes are affected in 75 per cent of AIDS patients and blindness may result from opportunistic infections. Rheumatological problems as well as problems with the cardiovascular, renal, and endocrine systems may also be a part of HIV/AIDS.

The diagnosis of HIV infection is straightforward. Testing for antibodies to the HIV virus, if done properly, makes the diagnosis. The test was developed in 1984. Since then other methods to diagnose infection have been developed. The most frequently used screening test is the enzyme-linked immunosorbent assay (ELISA), which measures antibody against the HIV virus. The test is very sensitive and specific for HIV, but if the result is positive, the Western blot assay, a different and even more specific test, must be run for confirmation. Most patients have a positive ELISA 1–3 months after they are infected, and 95 per cent of tests of infected people are positive 5 months after infection. Newer techniques such as the polymerase chain reaction (PCR) and the growth of the HIV virus in culture are now also employed in diagnosis.

There is as yet no effective *vaccine against the HIV virus and there is no curative treatment for AIDS. Treatment and management of HIV/AIDS patients require a combination of medical, educational, and psychosocial approaches. There are various antiretroviral therapies, such as *zidovudine, ddI, and ddC, numerous antiparasitic and antibacterial prophylactic supportive therapies, and several antineoplastic therapies used in the treatment of already infected persons. Work on other therapies, medications, and a vaccine progresses.

For persons not infected with the virus, education and behaviour modification are the most important aims of the anti-HIV/AIDS effort. Everyone must use safe sexual practices (condoms offer substantial protection) or abstain altogether. Intravenous drug users need education, rehabilitation, and/or clean needles. Health-care workers must practise universal precautions. We must strive to take compassionate care of those who are infected while we are working to develop better therapeutic agents and a vaccine. We should be clear about the fact that even the most close and prolonged casual social contact by adults or children does not spread HIV/AIDS.

A. BARTLEY BRYT
DAVID E. ROGERS

Further reading
Edelson, P. J. (ed.) (1991). Childhood AIDS. *The Pediatric Clinics of North America*, **38**, 1.
Fauci, A. S. and Lane, C. H. (1991). The acquired immunodeficiency syndrome (AIDS). In *Harrison's principles of internal medicine*, (ed. J. D. Wilson *et al.*) pp. 1402–10, McGraw Hill, New York.
Holmes, K. K. *et al.* (ed.) (1990). *AIDS Dx/Rx*. McGraw Hill, New York.
Rubin, R. H. (1992). Acquired immunodeficiency syndrome. In *Medicine*, (ed. F. Rubenstein and D. D. Federman), pp. 1–21. Scientific American, New York.
White, D. A. and Gold, J. W. M. (ed.) (1992). Medical management of AIDS patients. *The Medical Clinics of North America*, **76**, 1.

AIDS FOR THE DISABLED AND HANDICAPPED. Physical aids for the disabled range from simple mechanical devices to assist painful or limited joint movement to the sophisticated and complex products of biomedical engineering (bio-engineering) represented by complete powered artificial limbs. Their provision in the UK is the responsibility of the Department of Health and many other governments make similar arrangements. Topics of recent research and development include urinary incontinence, orthotics, artificial limbs, hearing impairment (including *tinnitus maskers and communication aids), personal transport, and many more. See also REHABILITATION.

AIR. The gaseous envelope surrounding the Earth varies slightly in composition according to locality and altitude. Average percentage values by volume for dry air at sea-level are: *nitrogen 78.08, *oxygen 20.95, argon 0.93, *carbon dioxide 0.03, neon 0.0018, helium 0.0005, krypton 0.0001, and xenon 0.00001. In addition, air normally contains small but variable amounts of water vapour, *hydrocarbons, hydrogen peroxide, *sulphur compounds, *ammonia, and dust particles.

AIR AMBULANCE. An aircraft used for conveying patients, adapted to take stretchers and emergency equipment.

AIR BED. An inflatable mattress.

AIR FORCE, ROYAL: MEDICAL SERVICES. See DEFENCE MEDICAL SERVICES IN THE UK.

AIR HUNGER is a striking form of *hyperventilation, also known as *Kussmaul breathing, characteristic of severe acute metabolic *acidosis.

AIRWAY. The passage by which atmospheric air reaches the lungs, formed by the oral and nasal cavities, the *pharynx, *larynx, *trachea, and *bronchi. Also, a tube which keeps the passage open in situations (e.g. unconsciousness) where it might otherwise become obstructed.

AKINESIA is absence or paucity of spontaneous movement, seen for example, in *parkinsonism.

ALASTRIM was a mild form of smallpox, also known as *variola minor*. The word is thought to be of Brazilian origin. Alastrim was common during the Middle Ages, and became prevalent again during the early years of the 20th century.

ALBEE, FRED HOUTLETT (1876–1945). American orthopaedic surgeon. He was among the first to use living bone grafts as internal splints.

ALBERS-SCHÖNBERG, HEINRICH ERNST (1865–1921). A pioneer German radiologist. He became the first 'Ordinarius' in this specialty in Germany in 1919. He died from radiation injury. His *Röntgenstechnik* (1903) was the first authoritative textbook; he founded the first German radiological journal as well as the German association of radiologists. He invented the compression diaphragm, showed the harmful effects of X-rays on spermatogenesis, and devised a lead protective screen. He described *osteopetrosis or 'marble-bones'.

ALBERTUS MAGNUS, SAINT (otherwise Albert von Bollstädt) (1206–80). German theologian and natural scientist, canonized 1931. He came from a wealthy Swabian family. After studying at Padua he joined the Dominican order and gained his master's degree in theology at Paris in 1244. From 1248 he was director of studies at Cologne, where St Thomas Aquinas was one of his pupils. St Albertus rediscovered *Aristotle and was largely responsible for introducing Greek and Arabian sciences to Europe. He studied embryology and reproduction, classified plants, and published two influential books *De vegetabilibus et plantis* and *De animalibus*.

ALBINISM is the absence of the normal pigment (*melanin) responsible for coloration of the skin, hair, and eyes. The condition is genetically determined, being inherited as an autosomal recessive trait (see GENET-ICS). It is due to absence of an enzyme (tyrosinase) essential for melanin production. Albinos (i.e. those with albinism) are readily recognized by their snowy-white hair, pink skin, and red eyes. They are abnormally sensitive to light, have various visual difficulties, and an increased incidence of malignant skin tumours.

ALBINUS, BERNHARD SIEGFRIED (1697–1770). Dutch anatomist. A pupil of *Boerhaave in Leiden, he became extraordinary professor of anatomy and surgery in 1718. The leading descriptive anatomist of his time, he published *Tabulae anatomicae sceletti et musculorum corporis humani* (1747) with superb illustrations drawn under his supervision.

ALBRIGHT, FULLER (1900–69). American physi-cian who worked at the *Massachusetts General Hos-pital. He was one of the first to recognize the clinical manifestations of *hyperparathyroidism, and demon-strated that *parathyroid hormone influences excretion of phosphate by the kidney. He described a syndrome of bone disease, skin pigmentation, and precocious puberty in young women.

ALBUMIN (ALBUMEN) is a soluble *protein of high molecular weight and the most abundant protein con-stituent of blood serum in vertebrates. It is the principal factor in maintaining the osmotic pressure of the circu-lating blood (see OSMOSIS) and acts as a carrier for many other substances, such as *hormones, *lipids, *drugs, and *haptens. The first spelling is now preferred. The alternative, 'albumen' is reserved for the related protein comprising egg-white in birds and some reptiles.

ALBUMINURIA is the presence of albumin in the *urine, most easily demonstrated by the production of a white coagulate on heating. The term proteinuria is used synonymously.

ALCHEMY. The possibility of manipulating matter into substances of commercial value, such as silver and gold, on the one hand, or of spiritually uplifting value, such as an elixir of life, on the other led to alchemy. It was, in turn, one of the roots of chemistry and *bio-chemistry as well as *chemotherapy. Alchemists derived much of their apparatus and manipulative techniques from the equipment used and developed by artisans,

technologists, and *pharmacists, whose heating, cook-ing, subliming, and distillation techniques were grist to the mill of chemists in the 16th century. Alchemy also provided chemistry with the idea of a symbolic language for practitioners of the art. Here, however, the use of a multiplicity of synonyms for the same thing served not merely to obscure matters for the uninitiated but (according to some historians) to increase greatly the degree of symbolic allusion—to the mystification of later readers and interpreters. For example, according to one Greek alchemical lexicon, mercury was 'seed of the dragon', 'talc of the dragon', 'dew', 'milk of the black cow', 'Scythian water', 'water of silver', 'water of the moon', 'river water', and 'divine water'. A Persian source lists over 80 synonyms for the philosopher's stone, a mysterious seed which supposedly precipi-tated an instant transmutation. Given that the same synonyms were also used for different substances, the resulting poetic mysticism must have been as confusing for alchemical practitioners as it is for the historian. *Newton, for example, spent years compiling an 'Index Chemicus' in an attempt to make sense of alchemical allegory.

Historians have delineated three principal traditions underlying alchemical thought and practice: technical, theoretical, and religious (or psychological). Egyptian and Greek dyers, metallurgists, jewellers, and phar-macists are known to have engaged in tincturing and colouring metallic surfaces from at least the 4th century BC onwards. Such procedures, some of whose recipes have come down to us, were not necessarily fraudulent, but were probably equivalent to the modern production of cheaper synthetic products. Needham, the historian of Chinese alchemy, has usefully called this technology aurifiction. Fraud, fakery, and deliberate deceit were only too possible, and much of the rich and entertaining literature of alchemy, such as Ben Jonson's play *The Alchemist* (1610), hinges on trickery, human frailty, and greed.

Faced by such apparently realistic and successful examples of transmutation by artisans, Greek philoso-phers saw these as aurifactions, that is, as real transfor-mations similar to the change of water into air or an acorn into an oak tree. In the hands of Aristotelian philosophers, transmutation of one metal into another was explained as the transfer of forms and qualities on to a basic, formless, underlying matter. To this esoteric workshop-based aurifiction and aurifaction was added, in the melting-pot of religious and philosophical move-ments of the 2nd and 1st centuries BC, a religious and symbolic interpretation of alchemical transmutation. In this esoteric alchemy, the art became a language and ritual concerned more with an individual's quest for spir-itual enlightenment and transmutation than with real metallurgy. Indeed, it is by no means clear from the sur-viving Greek writings whether the chemical experiments described were imaginary or, if carried out, merely a means to a spiritual end.

In most cultures (for alchemy seems to have been a universal technical and spiritual experience) transformations of matter, or of the human condition, were believed to be achieved through the use of a material substance such as 'the philosopher's stone', or elixir, or by combining spiritual practices with revealed knowledge. Whereas Greek alchemy laid stress upon silver and gold as the most perfect metals, or on significant colour changes in the search for the stone, Chinese alchemy stressed the role of cinnabar (mercuric sulphide) and potable gold. Needham has also suggested that Chinese alchemists, in developing spiritual and physical exercises for their inner perfection, hit upon ways of preparing sex *hormones from human urine (macrobiotics). Modern experimentation has, however, failed to confirm that the Chinese would have been able to prepare sufficient concentrations of *steroids to have been of physiological benefit.

On the other hand, Greek, Indian, and Chinese alchemists undoubtedly perfected the art of distillation; so much so, that when the practices were passed to the Arabic civilization from the 9th century onwards, they were able to isolate mineral acids such as nitric and hydrochloric acids, as well as *alcohol. When knowledge of Greek and Arabic alchemy passed to the Latin West, these new substances were gradually put to use in the preparation of medicinal materials by, among others, John of Rupescissa (*fl.* 1340), whose preparations of 'quintessences' proved useful to *Paracelsus (1493–1541) and his followers. Paracelsus not only expanded the Arabic doctrine that two principles, sulphur and mercury, were the roots of all things by adding a third principle, salt, but he taught that the universe itself functioned like a chemical laboratory. Indeed, God, the Creator, was a divine alchemist whose macrocosmic drama was mirrored in the microcosmic world of man and earthly creatures. It followed that physiological and pathological processes were chemical in nature and that treatments of diseases were best effected by chemical medicines rather than by the herbal ones of the ancients.

The ramifications of this iatrochemical movement were far-reaching. For the Paracelsians, alchemy—or rather chemistry, as it was being called by the 16th century—was to be the handmaiden of medicine. Most notably it meant that chemistry, or at least pharmaceutical chemistry, became part of the European medical curriculum. This was to prove of mutual benefit both for the advancement of medicine and for the emergence of chemistry from the spiritual blanket of esoteric alchemy. Less popular than astrology, the latter continues to inform the doctrines and practices of occultists.

W. H. BROCK

Further reading
Multhauf, R. P. (1966). *The origins of chemistry*. Oldbourne, London.

Needham, J. (1974) *Science and civilisation in China*, Vol. 5 (in 10 parts). Cambridge University Press, Cambridge.
von Martels, Z. R. W. H. (ed.) (1990). *Alchemy revisited*. E. J. Brill, Leiden.

ALCMAEON, of Crotona (*fl.* 535 BC). Greek natural philosopher. He was a pupil of Pythagoras and probably not a physician although he had much influence on medical thought. He probably undertook dissection for he was the first to describe the *optic nerves and the *Eustachian tubes.

ALCOHOL. Any of a group of organic compounds derived from *hydrocarbons by replacing one or more of the hydrogen atoms with hydroxyl (–OH) groups. When otherwise unqualified, alcohol means *ethanol (C_2H_5OH, theoretically derived from ethane, C_2H_6). See also METHANOL.

ALCOHOLICS ANONYMOUS, AA is a fellowship of former alcoholics. It originated in the USA (in Akron, Ohio in 1935), and is now world-wide. The encouragement, comradeship, and mutual social support offered to new members of this fraternity have proved of enormous value in the rehabilitation of patients recovering from *alcoholism and in maintaining their abstinence. The success of AA has led to adoption of the self-help group concept in other spheres (e.g. Gamblers Anonymous).

ALCOHOLISM is pathological dependence on alcohol, together with physical and/or mental changes attributable to chronic *alcohol poisoning. See SUBSTANCE ABUSE.

ALDEHYDE. Any of a large class of organic compounds having the general formula RCHO, where R is an alkyl or aryl *radical. An example is *acetaldehyde (ethanal, CH_3CHO), produced by the oxidation of *ethanol.

ALDEROTTI, TADDEO (otherwise Thaddeus Florentinus) (1223–1303). Italian physician and the founder of the Bolognese school. He wrote voluminous commentaries on *Galen and the Greek and Arabian texts, and a series of *Consilia*—case reports with recommendations for treatment. He is mentioned by Dante (*Paradisio* XII. 83).

ALDOSTERONE is one of the two major hormones of the adrenal cortex, the other being *hydrocortisone or cortisol. The essential function of aldosterone is to enable the body to withstand *salt deprivation. Acting principally on the convoluted tubule of the *nephron, it promotes the retention of *sodium and water, and the excretion of *potassium. Thus hyperaldosteronism (often called *Conn's syndrome) leads to sodium retention, expansion of extracellular fluid volume, *hypertension, and *hypokalaemia; conversely, deficiency of aldosterone causes sodium depletion, loss of extracellular fluid, hypovolaemia, *hypotension, and *hyperkalaemia. Aldosterone secretion is stimulated by *angiotensin II, by potassium, and by *corticotrophin or ACTH.

ALEXANDER of Tralles (525–605). Byzantine physician. He described *migraine, *epilepsy, and intestinal *worms and was the first to recommend *colchicum for *gout and rhubarb as a laxative.

ALEXIA is word-blindness, inability to see or to understand written or printed language in one whose vision is otherwise normal. Like *aphasia, alexia is usually due to damage to the left (dominant) hemisphere of the brain.

ALIBERT, JEAN LOUIS MARC (1768–1837). French dermatologist. In 1807 he became the chief physician at the Hôpital St. Louis, where he started the first dermatological clinic. In 1823 he was made the first professor of therapeutics and *materia medica in the Paris Faculty. He described *mycosis fungoides (1806), *keloid (1810), and cutaneous *leishmaniasis (Aleppo boil, 1829).

ALIENISM. The study and treatment of mental disorders; *psychiatry.

ALIMENTARY TRACT is the collective term for the mouth, *pharynx, *oesophagus, *stomach, and *intestine.

ALKALINE PHOSPHATASE. Any of a number of *phosphatases active at alkaline pH which are normally measured collectively in blood serum; they derive principally from bone, liver, intestine, and, when present, *placenta. Serum activities are raised in various conditions, most markedly in some bone diseases (particularly *Paget's disease of bone and *osteomalacia) and in hepatobiliary disorders (particularly biliary tract obstruction and destructive lesions of the liver).

ALKALOIDS. A group of basic nitrogen-containing organic compounds found in some dicotyledonous plants. Many are bitter-tasting and have powerful pharmacological actions. The first to be discovered was *morphine, in 1817. The names (which all end in -ine) of the many others include *atropine, *caffeine, *cocaine, *codeine, conitine, *nicotine, *quinine and *strychnine. See also POISONOUS PLANTS.

ALKALOSIS. Any condition in which the *hydrogen ion concentration of blood and body tissues is lowered (i.e. in which *pH is increased), the normal range for blood being 36 nmol/l (pH 7.45) to 43 nmol/l (pH 7.36). Respiratory alkalosis results from excessive *carbon dioxide loss by the lungs, as occurs in *hyperventilation, whereas metabolic alkalosis implies either accumulation of *base or loss of non-volatile acids by the body. 'Compensated' alkalosis describes a state in which the pH is returned towards normal by either respiratory (in the case of metabolic alkalosis) or renal (in the case of respiratory alkalosis) compensatory mechanisms.

ALKAPTONURIA is the excretion in the urine of homogentisic acid, which causes the urine to blacken on standing. It is due to a recessively inherited disorder of *tyrosine metabolism which usually causes no other symptoms.

ALKYLATING AGENTS are chemical substances which, because they form covalent bonds with *nucleic acids, damage *deoxyribonucleic acid (DNA) and interfere with cell replication. They are therefore *cytotoxic, *mutagenic, and *carcinogenic. Despite their unwanted potent side-effects, which include infertility due to impaired *gametogenesis and induction of acute myeloid *leukaemia, these agents have an important role in the treatment of malignant disease (see ONCOLOGY), the first so used having been *nitrogen mustard. Others include *cyclophosphamide, chlorambucil, melphalan, and busulphan.

ALLBUTT, SIR (THOMAS) CLIFFORD (1836–1925). British physician, who became regius professor of physic at Cambridge. Allbutt was a physician of deep erudition and culture—he was probably the prototype of Dr *Lydgate in George Eliot's *Middlemarch*. He devised the short clinical thermometer (1866), first separated 'hyperpiesia' (essential *hypertension) from renal hypertension (1921), and edited with Sir Humphry *Rolleston *A system of medicine* (8 vols, 1896–9).

ALLELE, ALLELOMORPH. See GENETICS.

ALLERGEN. Any substance capable of inducing *allergy.

ALLERGIST. A doctor specializing in allergic disorders. See also ALLERGY.

ALLERGY
Allergy through the ages
The notion of allergy was introduced in 1906 by the Austrian paediatrician Clemens von Pirquet as a means of describing the altered reactions that can develop when the body is exposed to specific foreign substances on more than one occasion. What we now recognize as abnormal allergic reactions to harmless inhaled grass pollen ('*hay fever') or to common foods such as cow's milk were certainly regarded in a different light in earlier centuries.

When Maimonides wrote his *Treatise on asthma* in

the 12th century, *asthma was regarded as a difficulty in breathing or a pain in the chest, and the question of an external cause was hardly considered. By the middle of the 16th century, however, reactions to external agents had begun to attract attention and there were several reports of 'rose fever'. A patient of Leonardo Botallo's found that roses made him sneeze, made his nose itch, and gave him headaches. Pietro Mattioli had a patient who was so sensitive to cats that he became ill on entering a room in which a cat was concealed without his knowledge. Soon afterwards there was a report of food intolerance in a young count, whose lips swelled when he ate eggs. Indeed, Pierre Borel, in 1656, confirmed a patient's sensitivity to egg by applying some to his skin and showing that it raised a blister. *Skin tests for allergy therefore have a long tradition.

Bronchial asthma

Most asthmatics wheeze, and Sir John Floyer observed in 1697 that 'Any kind of smoak offends the spirits of the asthmatic'. It was left to Bernardino Ramazzini, however, to emphasize the relevance of specific contact with outside agents, when he described the first example of industrial asthma, occurring in bakers who were in contact with flour. The hazards of industrial asthma have increased throughout the 20th century, and the small number of asthma sufferers in agriculture and in the food industry have been joined by a number of workers in the chemical, plastics, and pharmaceutical industries. In modern Japan, up to 15 per cent of cases of asthma in males are suspected of having an industrial origin.

*Spasm of smooth muscle and reversible airways obstruction are both hallmarks of the acute asthma attack. This kind of 'twitchy lung' reaction can be triggered by allergic sensitivity (extrinsic asthma) or can occur without evidence of allergy in those whose bronchial smooth muscle overreacts for other reasons (intrinsic asthma). Apart from allergy, the factors that can precipitate asthma range from viruses and the inhalation of sulphur dioxide to exercise and emotion. The effect of emotion, in particular, has long been recognized. The 19th century French physician Trousseau knew that he was sensitive to horses. He could enter the stables with impunity, but if he lost his temper with his coachman while he was there, the combination of allergy and emotion would bring on an asthmatic attack.

Wheezing does not always signify asthma but can also be caused by narrowed airways due to retained secretions or *inflammation and thickening of the bronchial lining, for example in chronic *bronchitis. For the diagnosis of asthma, tests are therefore carried out to see if there is a reversible spasm of smooth muscle.

Hay fever

The 'summer *catarrh' which had at first been attributed to roses came to be better understood by the 19th century. In 1831 John Elliotson's lectures in the *London Medical Gazette* laid the blame 'upon the flower of grass, and probably upon the pollen'.

In 1835 W. P. Kirkman, an asthmatic physician, sniffed at some pollinating grass in his hothouse in December and suffered a severe asthmatic attack. Charles Blackley came close to repeating Kirkman's experiment when he disturbed a vase of dried grasses during the winter of 1871 and gave himself an unseasonal attack of hay fever. He then scratched pollen into his skin, causing considerable swelling and a very vigorous local reaction. The evidence of his sensitivity to pollen was thus confirmed.

Blackley suspected that the pollen wafted through the atmosphere at a considerable height. He therefore invented a trap with a timed shuttering device, containing sticky slides, which was borne aloft on a tandem series of kites. The sticky slides collected pollen even at a height of 500 m, thus proving Blackley's point and providing the basis for the present-day atmospheric pollen counts.

At this stage, Blackley went on to draw some remarkable conclusions. He advised his patients to spend the summer season either on a peninsula or on a yacht. Having shown that tiny amounts of pollen could cause a reaction, he also reviewed his entire approach to the practice of medicine and spent the rest of his career as a *homoeopathist.

Skin reactions

The familiar nettle *rash occurs when *histamine is pricked into the skin by hairs of the nettle. It is similar in appearance to the rash of *urticaria, which can have several causes and is one of the most rapidly developing allergic reactions—so rapid that the cause, whether it is a food, a drug, a hot bath, or an insect sting, is often recognized by the person who is affected. In contrast, the raw, weeping rash of *eczema develops much more slowly and presents a far greater diagnostic challenge. In 1895, a German *dermatologist called Joseph Jadassohn suspected that eczema might be caused by a specific sensitivity of the skin and tested this by strapping patches of lint to the skin after they had been soaked in various test solutions. Where a patch of inflammation developed, this showed a specific sensitivity. The method is still in use.

The tendency to develop eczematous skin reactions appears most often in early childhood, when the child can become sensitized to the foreign *protein in a food such as cow's milk or to the dust mites that are present in mattress dust and in bedclothes. Even in childhood, however, more than one provoking agent can contribute, and the omission of a single food is unlikely to be followed by a complete cure.

Allergy and anaphylaxis

Von Pirquet based his observations on allergy upon the unpleasant reactions that followed when horse *serum was administered during the treatment of *diphtheria. Charles Richet then discovered an even more extreme form of the same reaction when he injected a dog with the *venom of a poisonous jellyfish, the Portuguese man-of-war. Instead of finding, as he had hoped, that increasing doses of venom could be tolerated when the venom was given a second or third time, the dog died. What was intended to be protective *prophylaxis proved to be the opposite, and in 1903 he called this *anaphylaxis.

Anaphylaxis is by no means confined to horse serum reactions and can be provoked by insect stings or by food and drug reactions. Harper (1980) has quoted an account written in 1765 of a fatal reaction to a bee sting in a villager who had lost consciousness after two previous stings. On the third occasion he fell to the ground at once and was dead within a few minutes.

There are varying grades of severity of anaphylaxis, ranging from flushing of the skin to more severe reactions including asthma, *shock, and *coma. Every year there are about four fatal reactions to the stings of bees, wasps, or similar insects in the UK and 10 times that number in the USA.

Current views

In the early part of the 20th century it was assumed that a special type of chemical *antidote or '*antibody' was responsible for the effects of immediate allergic reactions, but as yet there was no proof. In a classic experiment, the serum of H. Küstner, who was allergic to fish, was injected into the arm of C. Prausnitz. The next day fish extract was injected into the same place and this led to a hypersensitive skin reaction. Küstner's serum thus contained a 'reagin', which was capable of transferring specific sensitivity. There was thought to be an inherited tendency to produce reagins, which A. F. Coca called *atopy. Forty years later, these reagins were identified as heat-labile *immunoglobulin-E (IgE) antibodies. These antibodies were shown by the Ishizakas in the USA and by Johansson and Bennich in Sweden to be present in serum in tiny amounts which were sufficient to sensitize the skin and other body surfaces.

Mast cell and basophils

The catalysts for the skin-sensitizing process turned out to be the *mast cell and the basophilic *leucocyte, a type of white blood cell. Their functions had remained a mystery after their description by *Ehrlich in 1877, although by 1953 they were known to contain both *heparin and histamine. What is now clear is that IgE antibodies stick to the surface of these cells, from where they can activate the release of a whole range of highly active biological mediators. Since mast cells are located mainly below the skin and lining membranes of the body, any substance penetrating the body surface will come in contact with them. If that substance is one to which the body has produced IgE antibodies, it will combine with

IgE on the surface of the mast cell and cause a discharge of histamine and the synthesis of powerful stimulating substances derived from arachidonic acid. Even in minute amounts, the *leukotrienes, *prostaglandins, and *thromboxanes, which are the substances concerned, can cause smooth muscle contraction or relaxation, can start or stop the clot-promoting activity of platelets, and can attract highly active white blood cells to the scene. The crescendo effects of all these changes could be highly damaging, were it not for the powerful switch-off enzymes that normally limit this activity to a useful level.

Approaches to treatment

In 1901, *adrenaline (epinephrine) was discovered, and within 2 years it had been synthesized. Not only is it the body's main defensive product when anaphylaxis threatens, but it has provided a blueprint from which anti-allergic drugs can be designed. The discovery of histamine before the First World War drew attention to another of the body's chemical products, a specific mediator that could trigger the onset of anaphylaxis. In due course, and with some difficulty, chemical engineers designed a large series of *antihistamine drugs which proved to be useful in hay fever and in allergic skin eruptions of the nettle rash (urticaria) type. They were, however, strangely ineffective in the treatment of bronchial asthma. Eventually, with the identification of other mediators, including those derived from arachidonic acid, a whole series of new, biologically active agents came to be identified, with molecular patterns that have since been modified and tested in the hope of providing additional 'designer' drugs for the treatment of allergy.

Drugs that are absorbed into the body tend to have side-effects that are not intended. There is therefore some logic in the use of locally applied agents for skin disease and inhaled drugs for asthma, including adrenaline-like drugs and sodium cromoglycate. Similarly, although their action is weakened, *cortisone-like drugs have fewer side-effects when they are inhaled than when given by mouth or injection, and these have become increasingly popular in the treatment of asthma. *Hydrocortisone, the natural hormone produced by the *adrenal gland, can interfere with the release of arachidonic acid from the cell membrane and its subsequent metabolism. This is probably the main reason for its beneficial effect in allergic disease.

The *vaccine treatment of allergy

In 1911, L. Noon developed a new treatment for hay fever which was based on the belief that pollen contained a *toxin that was responsible for the patient's symptoms. He reasoned, as Richet had done before him, that repeated injection of a toxin might accustom the body to its presence and reduce its adverse effects. He used very dilute extracts, and, though the theory was wrong, he showed that the reaction to measured amounts of pollen was reduced or abolished after the vaccine treatment.

Subsequently, the method was applied to other types of allergy. For example, insect sting allergy came to be treated by injecting extracts of the bodies of bees or wasps. The patient's sensitivity was, however, to the venom and not the insect, as Lichtenstein and his colleagues showed in the 1970s, when they demonstrated that treatment with venom was effective but that body extracts were no better than a placebo and can be harmful. Vaccine treatment has come under particular scrutiny in the UK, where the *Committee on Safety of Medicines has warned of the dangers and advised that strict safety guidelines should be followed.

Unconventional concepts and doubtful tests

The notion that all adverse reactions are allergic is clearly wrong. Nevertheless, ecologists and environmentalists who are concerned about food contamination and environmental *pollution have often used the word 'allergy' in an undefined sense, to be applied whenever people are adversely affected by food or by a smoky atmosphere. In 1982 there emerged a concept of '*total allergy', which proved to be neither allergic nor total but nevertheless became the subject of much public interest and debate. This centred on the question of whether food allergy or other immune reactions could be so troublesome that it became necessary to provide a specially ventilated atmosphere and specially prepared uncontaminated food to protect the affected person. Although very severe allergies can exist, there was no evidence that allergy was responsible for these problems, which were nevertheless much publicized through the press and television.

The separation of fact and fiction deserves some attention. The main thrust of the 'total allergy' claims concerned food allergy, an important allergic disorder with effects that are not necessarily confined to the bowel itself. Food allergy can, however, be diagnosed only when the condition is caused by the specific mechanisms of hypersensitivity, and in such cases it is often accompanied by asthma, eczema, or other clear manifestations of an allergic response. Most cases of food intolerance are due to other mechanisms, such as a lack of enzymes, the effects of irritant or toxic substances, or associated disorders such as gall-bladder disease. The mechanism for these reactions is not always clear, and the relationship between food and the onset of migraine or joint pains is not fully explained. This is not the same, however, as the cases in which a variety of symptoms are blamed on food but are part of a psychological illness or food fad, sometimes made worse by overbreathing, an unconscious habit which can cause symptoms of giddiness, tingling, or malaise.

By the 1990s, many members of the public were not concerned with these precise definitions. Patients whose problems had not been solved by the medical profession were encouraged to consult unorthodox practitioners who offered to identify 'allergies' from a sample of hair by using radionic equipment, by a 'cytotoxic test' of the blood, or by the pulse changes after a particular food was eaten. Treatments were prescribed which ranged from severe dietary restriction to the administration of food drops under the tongue and, in some cases, to the injection of the patient's own urine. In none of these cases were the test methods validated or the treatment shown to be efficacious. In some, false hopes were raised, nutritionally inadequate diets given, and potentially treatable diseases left undiagnosed.

It does not follow that claims that are made for new methods of treatment should be ignored. They should, however, be evaluated carefully before they are generally adopted. When John Elliotson, in 1831, identified 'the flower of grass' as the cause of hay fever, he proved to be right, but when he espoused mesmerism as a method of treatment he was not. Charles Blackley, whose original technique for the diagnosis of allergy is still in use 100 years later, turned to *homoeopathy in his later years on a totally false premise. A continuous assessment of the methods of diagnosis and treatment is as necessary now as it was then.

MAURICE LESSOF

Further reading
Harper, D. S. (1980). *Footnotes on allergy.* Uppsala.
Lessof, M. H. (1992). *Food intolerance.* James & James, London.
Royal College of Physicians (1992). *Allergy, conventional and alternative concepts.* RCP, London.

ALLGEMEINES KRANKENHAUS, VIENNA was founded in 1794 as a result of the 18th century development of the '*Old Vienna School' of medicine. The energy of the pathologist Carl *Rokitansky, appointed prosector in 1832, complemented on the clinical side by Josef *Skoda, made this the world centre for studies in pathological anatomy and clinicopathological correlations during the 19th century.

ALLOGRAFT. A transplant of an organ or tissue between non-identical individuals of the same species, formerly termed 'homograft' (cf. 'autograft': within the same individual; 'syngraft': between genetically identical individuals, which in man means between uniovular twins; 'xenograft': between individuals of different species).

ALLOPATHY is a term for orthodox medical practice introduced by *Hahnemann to distinguish such practice from *homoeopathy. It implies treatment of disease by methods and drugs antagonistic to the effects of the disease being treated.

ALLOPURINOL is a drug used in the treatment and prevention of *gout; it limits the production of *uric acid. It does so by inhibiting the enzyme xanthine oxidase, which converts xanthine and hypoxanthine into uric acid. It is taken by mouth and must be continued indefinitely.

ALMEIDA LIMA, PEDRO MANUEL DE (1903–83). Portuguese neurosurgeon, formerly professor of neurosurgery and neurology at the Centro de Estudos, Lisbon. Lima's well-known collaboration with Egas *Moniz began in 1926. Moniz was experimenting with cerebral angiography and Lima's interest in neurosurgery was thus stimulated. He developed his experience and skill at the *London Hospital under Sir Hugh *Cairns. Returning to Portugal in 1934, Lima proceeded to found the first such unit in that country. Among his contributions, the development of cerebral *angiography must be reckoned of major importance. In 1935 Almeida Lima gave the first account of the vascular architecture of *meningiomas. He was responsible, with Egas Moniz, for the introduction of *psychosurgery in 1935 by performing the first frontal *leucotomy for treatment of psychosis (see NEUROSURGERY).

ALMONER. Until recently, a hospital official with duties relating to patients' welfare (and formerly with payments to them). The term is now obsolete, having been replaced by 'medical social worker' (see SOCIAL WORK).

ALOPECIA is loss of hair from the head or other hair-bearing areas. The word is Greek for 'fox-mange'.

ALPHA-FETOPROTEIN is a high molecular weight *protein synthesized by the human fetus but normally detectable only in minute quantities in the blood beyond the first year of life. Its importance is twofold. First, its presence in the *amniotic fluid indicates a fetal neural tube defect such as *spina bifida or *anencephaly, allowing antenatal diagnosis of such defects through *amniocentesis and examination of the fluid. Secondly, an elevated serum level occurs in most adult patients with hepatocellular *carcinomas, teratocarcinomas, and embryonal cell carcinomas.

ALPHA-RAYS (α-RAYS) are streams of fast-moving α-particles, each composed of two *protons and two *neutrons (a helium nucleus) and possessing a double positive charge. α-particles are emitted by certain radioactive isotopes of the heavier elements. α-rays produce intense *ionization in gases through which they pass and are easily absorbed by matter, penetration being less than 0.1 mm in water or living tissue. α-rays produce fluorescence on a fluorescent screen.

ALS. See ANTILYMPHOCYTE SERUM. Also an acronym (in the USA) for amyotrophic lateral sclerosis (*motor neurone disease).

ALTERNATIVE MEDICINE. See COMPLEMENTARY (ALTERNATIVE) MEDICINE.

ALTITUDE is height above sea-level, normally expressed in metres or feet. With greater altitude, the atmospheric pressure, and hence the partial pressure of *oxygen, fall. Acute exposure to altitudes above 3000 m causes arterial *hypoxia giving *altitude sickness. In the longer term, physiological adaptation, notably an increase in circulating *haemoglobin concentration and hence in blood oxygen-carrying capacity, normally leads to acclimatization. See also AEROSPACE MEDICINE.

ALTITUDE SICKNESS. Altitude (or mountain) sickness occurs in normal human subjects who ascend to 3000 m or more, unless they do so in commercial aircraft, which are pressurized to the equivalent of 2500 m or less. Features vary according to speed of ascent, age, fitness, exertion, acclimatization, and individual susceptibility, and are due to *hypoxia leading to *hyperventilation, hypocapnia, and respiratory *alkalosis. They include mental impairment (which may be unnoticed by the subject), headache, breathlessness, nausea, vomiting, diarrhoea, abdominal pain, and insomnia. Loss of consciousness is usual in unacclimatized persons after several hours at 5500 m. Altitude sickness may be complicated by cerebral or pulmonary *oedema. See also ENVIRONMENT AND MEDICINE I; AEROSPACE MEDICINE.

ALUMINIUM (ALUMINUM) is a metallic element (symbol Al, atomic number 13, relative atomic mass 26.982) of no known physiological role. Various compounds containing aluminium are widely used in *antacid mixtures and in *astringent and antiperspirant preparations. Aluminium poisoning may cause a severe and sometimes fatal encephalopathic syndrome reported in association with repeated *renal dialysis. It has been suggested that the element may play a minor causative role in *Alzheimer's disease but this is unproven.

ALVEOLUS. The air sac, the functional unit of the lung, across the epithelial wall of which gas exchange occurs between the air in the alveolar space and the blood in the lung capillaries.

Alveolus is also used to denote any small sac-like dilatation. Dental alveoli are the sockets in the jaw bones in which the roots of the teeth are attached.

ALZHEIMER, ALOIS (1864–1915). German neurologist. He described the disease that was named after him and its pathology.

ALZHEIMER'S DISEASE is a common form of *dementia, beginning in middle age or later and formerly known as presenile dementia. It is now clear that it is also the commonest cause of dementia in old age (senile dementia). Intellectual impairment is the major manifestation, the first indication being defective memory for recent events; loss of other intellectual functions follows insidiously but remorselessly. Evidence of localized brain dysfunction (e.g. *aphasia, *apraxia, *epilepsy) occurs in some cases. Pathologically, there is loss of nerve cells, causing cerebral *atrophy, and senile plaques are found in profusion in the cerebral cortex. An uncommon inherited variety is now known to be due to a gene lying on chromosome 21, and abnormalities of β-amyloid have been implicated in causation. Certain classes of *cholinergic drugs are being tested for their usefulness in treatment of this disease.

AMALGAM. Any alloy of *mercury. Amalgams are widely used in dental conservation.

AMANITA is a genus of large fungi with white gills, some species of which are deadly poisonous and some edible. Among the former are the notorious *Amanita phalloides* (death cap), *A. virosa* (destroying angel), and *A. pantherina*; the attractive *A. muscaria* (fly agaric) is poisonous but rarely fatal. The edible species include *A. vaginata* (grisette), *A. fulva* (tawny grisette), and, when cooked, *A. rubescens* (the blusher). Other species, though harmless, are unpleasant to eat. See also POISONOUS FUNGI.

AMANTADINE is an antiviral drug of limited use in the prophylaxis and treatment of *influenza A infections. It also has dopaminergic properties, and benefits some patients with *parkinsonism.

AMAUROSIS is blindness from other than local ocular causes.

AMAUROTIC FAMILY IDIOCY. See TAY–SACHS DISEASE.

AMBLYOPIA. Impairment of vision.

AMBULANCE. Any vehicle adapted for the transport of sick or wounded persons.

AMENORRHOEA (AMENORRHEA). Failure of *menstruation.

AMENTIA is severe mental handicap dating from birth or very early childhood (cf. *dementia). The word has also been used to describe a psychotic state of extreme hallucinatory confusion.

AMERICAN MEDICAL ASSOCIATION was founded in 1847 under the impetus of Dr Nathan Smith *Davis in Philadelphia. The aim was and is 'To promote the science and art of medicine and the betterment of the public health'. See also MEDICAL COLLEGES ETC. IN NORTH AMERICA.

AMES TEST. An *in vitro* screening test for *mutagenicity. A strain of *Salmonella* bacteria lacking the enzyme necessary to synthesize the *amino acid histidine is inoculated into a culture medium in which it cannot grow without that capacity. The suspected mutagen is then added. The appearance and number of bacterial colonies indicate the extent to which mutations have occurred enabling some bacteria to regain the ability to synthesize histidine. The test is important as many mutagens are *carcinogenic.

AMETROPIA is any refractive error of the eye. See OPHTHALMOLOGY.

AMIDOPYRINE is an *analgesic and *antipyretic drug (also known as 'aminopyrine') introduced in 1889 and once widely available to the general public. In 1934, however, it was found to cause *agranulocytosis and over-the-counter sales were prohibited in the UK in 1936 and the USA in 1938.

AMINO ACID. Amino acids are organic compounds containing both basic amino (NH_2) and acid carboxyl (COOH) groups. The general formula is $RCH(NH_2)$ COOH, where R is a variable grouping of atoms (fundamentally a carbon atom, chain, or ring). More than 20 different amino acids occur in nature; the simplest is glycine, with the formula $CH_2(NH_2)COOH$. These molecules are of fundamental importance to life, as hundreds or thousands combine in *polypeptide chains to make each *protein molecule. Of those known, eight are 'essential', i.e. they cannot be synthesized by the human organism and must therefore, like vitamins, be obtained from the environment. These are valine, leucine, phenylalanine, tryptophan, lysine, isoleucine, methionine, and threonine (see BIOCHEMISTRY).

AMINOGLYCOSIDES. A collective term, based on chemical structure, for the important group of *antibiotics that includes *gentamicin, *streptomycin, and *neomycin (other members being kanamycin, tobramycin, netilmicin, and amikacin). They have a wide spectrum of bactericidal action against both Gram-positive and Gram-negative infections. They are not absorbed from the alimentary tract and are therefore, except in intestinal infections, ineffective by mouth. Because of their ototoxic and nephrotoxic side-effects, they must be administered with caution and with reference to drug plasma levels. Particular care is needed in the elderly and in those with impaired renal function; the risk of damage to the fetal *auditory nerve makes their use in pregnancy undesirable. See also ANTIBIOTICS.

AMIODARONE is a drug used to treat rapid cardiac *arrhythmias.

AMITOSIS is cell division occurring without *mitosis; the nucleus divides by simple constriction into two halves without spindle formation, dissolution of nuclear membrane, or the appearance of chromosomes (see CELL AND CELL BIOLOGY).

AMITRYPTYLINE is an effective and widely used *antidepressant drug.

AMMONIA (NH_3) is a pungent and very soluble gas giving an alkaline solution containing ammonium hydroxide, NH_4OH.

AMMON'S HORN. See HIPPOCAMPUS.

AMNESIA is loss of memory.

AMNIOCENTESIS is the sampling of *amniotic fluid, usually by percutaneous puncture with the help of *ultrasonic equipment and, for diagnosis, it is undertaken early in the second trimester of pregnancy. As the procedure carries a small but finite risk to the pregnancy, its performance must be justified. It cannot be regarded as a screening procedure except in mothers at high risk of producing an offspring with, e.g. *Down's syndrome or *spina bifida. Examination of the fluid and of the fetal cells it contains allows: (i) measurement of *alphafetoprotein levels to detect *neural tube defects; (ii) sex determination; (iii) antenatal diagnosis of certain inherited disorders and (iv) chromosomal analysis and detection of chromosomal aberrations.

AMNION. The innermost epithelial membrane enveloping the embryo of amniote vertebrates, i.e. reptiles, birds, and mammals.

AMNIOTIC FLUID. The fluid contained within the *amnion, in which the fetus floats. Sampling of the fluid helps in prenatal diagnosis (see AMNIOCENTESIS). It is also called liquor amnii.

AMOEBA (AMEBA). A group of Protozoa, i.e. animals consisting of a single nucleated cell. Amoebae are of irregular and constantly changing shape, moving and feeding through protoplasmic projections known as pseudopodia. Some species are parasitic in man, especially *Entamoeba histolytica*. See AMOEBIASIS.

AMOEBIASIS (AMEBIASIS) is infection with the protozoan parasite *Entamoeba histolytica*. It exists world-wide, but infection is greater in developing countries because of poorer sanitation and hygiene. The parasite exists in two forms, cyst (infective) and trophozoite (active). Infection is by mouth and, as the cysts are destroyed by cooking, transmission is usually by eating uncooked vegetables and unpeeled fruits; these are best avoided in *endemic areas.

　Often infection produces no symptoms at all. When it does, they may range from mild watery *diarrhoea to explosive bloody *dysentery. Untreated, the condition can persist for many years characteristically causing bouts of diarrhoea separated by complete remissions. Sometimes the infection spreads beyond its primary site in the large intestine to involve other organs, particularly the liver (amoebic liver abscess). Metronidazole, emetine, and various *antibiotics are effective in treatment.

AMOK is a word of Malayan orgin, used as an adjective or adverb to signify a state of frenzied and murderous rage.

AMPHETAMINE is a drug, also called Benzedrine®, with central nervous system stimulant, euphoriant, and appetite-suppressing effects. It, and related compounds such as dexamphetamine (Dexedrine®) and methylamphetamine (Methedrine®), are powerfully addictive (see SUBSTANCE ABUSE). Their medical use is now restricted to a small, well-defined group of patients such as those with *narcolepsy. They should not be used to treat obesity or depressive illness.

AMPHOTERICIN is an antifungal, *antibiotic drug. It is not absorbed from the gastrointestinal tract, and is used either intravenously in systemic fungal infections or topically in local conditions. It penetrates body tissues and fluids poorly. Because of its toxic effect on the kidney it must be used with caution with careful monitoring of renal function.

AMPICILLIN is a broad-spectrum *antibiotic of the *penicillin group, also known as Penbritin, which can be given either by mouth or by injection. It is inactivated by many bacterial penicillinases so that many common bacteria, including most *staphylococci, are now resistant to it.

AMPULLA. An ancient Roman vessel; it is a globular flask with two handles. Anatomically, the dilated end of a tubular structure such as a canal or duct.

AMPUTATION is the removal, in whole or in part, of a limb, breast, or other body appendage.

AMULET. A charm worn to prevent disease, mischief, or witchcraft. An 'amuletic' medicine was one believed to work by occult means.

AMUSIA is the inability to appreciate musical notes or tones, and/or to produce them.

AMYGDALA. An almond-shaped group of nuclei in the temporal lobe of the brain, forming part of the *limbic system.

AMYLASE. One of many *enzymes found in plants and animals which catalyse the splitting of *starch and *glycogen into *sugars. In man, amylases occur in *saliva and in *pancreatic juice.

AMYL NITRITE is an organic nitrite, a clear yellow volatile inflammable fluid dispensed in crushable glass capsules and administered by inhalation. It is a powerful smooth muscle relaxant and vasodilator, employed chiefly in the prophylaxis and treatment of *angina pectoris as a rapidly acting (10 seconds) alternative to sublingual *glyceryl trinitrate or other nitrite preparations. It has also been used in renal and biliary *colic, and also to treat *cyanide poisoning; it has also been abused as a sexual stimulant. Its action is short-lived (about 5 minutes). It is inactive by mouth.

AMYLOIDOSIS is a condition in which an abnormal proteinaceous substance (originally termed 'amyloid' because its staining reaction with *iodine resembles that of *starch) is deposited in organs and tissues, interfering with their function. It is often a complication of other chronic diseases such as *rheumatoid arthritis, *tuberculosis, *leprosy, chronic suppurative infections, *ulcerative colitis, malignant *lymphoma, or *carcinomatosis. There is also an association with *myelomatosis, or the condition may apparently be 'primary'. Familial and age-related varieties occur. The clinical manifestations vary; renal involvement is very common, and cardiac, hepatic, alimentary, neurological, endocrine, and joint disturbances may all occur. Its cause remains obscure. Unless an underlying cause can be identified and successfully treated, it is likely to be progressive.

AMYOTONIA is lack or loss of muscle tone. A disorder known as 'amyotonia congenita' causing muscular weakness and *hypotonia from birth was described by *Oppenheim in 1900. The term is now obsolete. See also NEUROMUSCULAR DISEASE.

AMYOTROPHIC LATERAL SCLEROSIS. See MOTOR NEURONE DISEASE; NEUROMUSCULAR DISEASE.

AMYOTROPHY. *Atrophy of muscle.

ANABOLIC STEROIDS are a group of synthetic *steroids, related to *testosterone, which promote *protein synthesis (anabolism) and increased muscle bulk and power, but which have a relatively weak *androgenic (masculinizing) effect. Prolonged use may cause cysts or cancer of the liver.

ANABOLISM is the synthesis by living organisms of complex organic molecules from simpler ones, involving utilization of energy. The reverse process is termed '*catabolism'.

ANAEMIA (ANEMIA) is 'a reduction below normal in the concentration of circulating *haemoglobin and hence in the oxygen-carrying capacity of blood'. This must be due to a reduction in the concentration of circulating *erythrocytes (red blood cells), or in their haemoglobin content, or in both. As with any continuously distributed variable, arbitrary limits must be set to the normal range of values. The *World Health Organization suggests lower normal limits of 12 g/dl haemoglobin for women and 13 g/dl for men. When the plasma volume is not normal, this does not apply. For example, in acute haemorrhage, blood volume and haemoglobin go down, so that the haemoglobin concentration remains temporarily normal. See also HAEMATOLOGY.

ANAEROBIC (ANEROBIC). Living in the absence of free *oxygen, gaseous or dissolved. Anaerobic respiration is the liberation of energy by breakdown of substances not requiring oxygen consumption.

ANAESTHESIA (ANESTHESIA). As strictly defined, anaesthesia means loss of feeling, and analgesia, loss of painful sensation; this article will deal with the specialty of surgical anaesthesia. Humans and all warm-blooded creatures perceive the sensation of *pain, whether caused by disease, injury, or surgical treatment. Before describing the development of methods to ease surgical pain, it is necessary to explain the phenomenon of pain.

Pain
Everyone has experienced pain, which is a purely subjective matter, for no one can comprehend the pain experienced by another. As there is no universally identifiable stimulus for pain, in contrast to the other senses—seeing, hearing, touch, taste, and smell—pain is usually described according to prior experiences: burning, stabbing, cutting, aching, throbbing, pricking, and the like. Surely the perception and reaction to pain are coloured by one's emotional state and ethnic origins. A confusing factor is that intensification of the classic sensations results in pain: bright light, loud sound, hot and cold, strong tastes, and heavy pressure. Pain is disagreeable and often intolerable: although it is meant to protect against injury, when chronic it can ultimately destroy the sufferer.

Specific receptors for pain exist in the form of naked nerve endings throughout the body, which are dense on the surface and sparse internally; this is why superficial pain is described and located so much more accurately than internal pain. A potentially destructive stimulus is transduced into electrical energy, travelling over a spectrum of specific nerve fibres to the central nervous system, there being decoded and eliciting an appropriate response. According to this schema, pain can be prevented or alleviated peripherally with medications, as in the use of aspirin for treatment of arthritis, or a locally injected anaesthetic to dull the effects of the surgeon's scalpel. Centrally acting drugs can alter the perception and significance of pain, as occurs when morphine or other opioids are given. It is just one step further to induce insensibility with a general anaesthetic.

Surgery before anaesthesia

Surgical operations were performed far back in antiquity by sorcerers, religious adherents, and itinerant technicians, but always for superficial illness; a fractured bone; limb amputation; *trephining the skull to relieve intracranial pressure; to dislodge an ocular lens *cataract; or to crush or extract a urinary bladder stone. Other ailments not visible to the eye were assumed, according to galenical concepts (see GALEN), to result from an internal imbalance among four humours: blood, phlegm, yellow bile, and black bile. Accordingly, treatments to restore the balance comprised blood-letting or *leeching, *purging, use of *enemas, induction of *emesis, and application of heat or cold. Although those practitioners were largely inattentive to the suffering wreaked by surgery, efforts were made to relieve pain through incantation, *hypnosis, *acupuncture, heavy intoxication with alcohol, or inhaling from or sucking upon sponges saturated with extracts of the *poppy, *henbane, and *mandragora root.

Antecedents of anaesthesia

The established route for medication was the gastrointestinal tract, even *c.* 1540 when *Paracelsus of Switzerland sweetened the feed of fowl with sweet oil of vitriol, a compound later called ether by Frobenius. The vapour of this liquid was to be inhaled by many a patient over the 130 years following the eventual introduction of surgical anaesthesia.

Two centuries later the introduction of anaesthesia was prepared for by an emerging comprehension of the physiology of *respiration and the circulation to the lungs. *Harvey, during his observations on the circulation, noticed the change in colour—from dark to florid—when blood traversed the lungs. In 1672 Robert *Boyle, in exhausting air from a vessel containing both a lighted taper and a living bird, succeeded in extinguishing the life of both, thus corroborating the vital nature of a substance in air. Joseph *Priestley, in 1774, while heating mercuric oxide, liberated oxygen, which sustained life to a remarkable degree. Incidentally, Priestley also obtained nitrous oxide from nitric oxide. Antoine *Lavoisier observed that exhaled air caused a precipitate in lime water, and so must consist in part of chalky-air, or carbon dioxide. Thence it was but a step to conclude that the main purpose of respiration was not only to sustain life with oxygen, but also, to change that element into carbon dioxide.

Eventually, the recognition of these gases and vapours led to the practice of pneumatic medicine and, for the first time, utilization of the lungs as an avenue of therapy, a forerunner of *inhalation anaesthesia. Around 1794 a group of physicians and scientists established the Pneumatic Institution at Clifton, Bristol, and chose as superintendent of the Institution a youthful chemist and physicist, Humphry *Davy. While breathing nitrous oxide, Davy found that a headache associated with indigestion and the pain of an erupting wisdom tooth were considerably diminished. Simultaneously, he experienced a 'thrilling' and an uneasiness swallowed up in pleasure. He was led to write, 'As nitrous oxide in its extensive operation appears capable of destroying pain, it may probably be used with advantage during surgical operations.' Davy's remarks went unheeded, with perhaps one exception. Henry Hill *Hickman, general practitioner and surgeon of Shifnal in Shropshire, performed a number of experiments on animals, using carbon dioxide in an asphyxial manner but not for so long that they failed to survive. No matter to whom the glory is accorded, Hickman must be credited with the concept of surgical anaesthesia, unfortunately employing the wrong agent.

The introduction of anaesthesia

A fortuitous outcome of Davy's suggestion, plus his repeated demonstration to friends of the exhilarating effects of nitrous oxide, was the public indulgence in frolics, inhaling ether as well. Crawford W. *Long participated in such revels and while in practice in Jefferson, Georgia, introduced that wild party to friends, so that one of them, James Venable, underwent excision of a tumour from the nape of the neck in 1842, while under the influence of ether.

Another sequence of events took place on 10 December 1844 in Hartford, Connecticut, where Gardner Quincy Colton took a travelling medicine show to allow one and all to experience the effects of inhaling nitrous oxide. The fact that one of the volunteers, Samuel A. Cooley, hurt his leg without noticing it while in the excitement phase of nitrous oxide intoxication intrigued a dentist, Horace *Wells, in the audience. On the very next day, while inhaling Colton's nitrous oxide, Wells had one of his own carious teeth painlessly removed by a fellow dentist. Through the mediation of his former dental pupil, William Thomas Green *Morton (Fig. 1), then practising in Boston, Wells was accorded the opportunity of demonstrating the benefits of nitrous oxide before a group of Harvard University medical students. But the event, in January 1845, proved to be a shattering defeat for Wells, for the volunteer student cried out in pain as a tooth was extracted, though later claiming no awareness or experience of pain. Undoubtedly, in this case anaesthesia failed to progress beyond the excitement phase. This stage of *delirium explains why, under less threatening circumstances, nitrous oxide is called laughing gas.

W. T. G. Morton, a keen witness to Wells's demonstration, was enrolled at that time in a course of Harvard medical school lectures and had become an expert on dental *prosthetics, devising a plate that could be applied to the gums only after the rotted tooth roots had been removed, which was far too painful a venture for all but the most hardy. He accepted the suggestion of Charles T. Jackson, eccentric geologist and chemist, that ether, applied to the gums, would supply, through evaporation, a degree of cold analgesia.

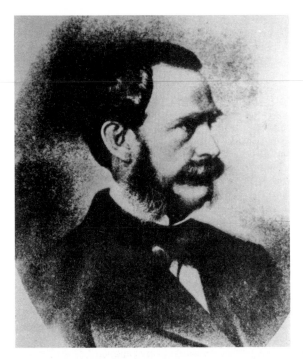

Fig. 1 William Thomas Green Morton, anaesthetist at the first public demonstration of ether anaesthesia. (Reproduced with permission from the collection of the Boston Medical Library in the Francis A. Countway Library of Medicine.)

Following experiments on ether inhalation in several animals, in September 1847 Morton, in his Boston office, painlessly extracted an *abscessed tooth from the jaw of Eben H. Frost, a merchant of that city. The event, reported in a newspaper on the next day, caught the eye of Henry Jacob *Bigelow, an attending surgeon at the Massachusetts General Hospital, who then arranged for a trial at the hospital. The surgeon would be the renowned John Collins *Warren, then aged 68, the patient Edward Gilbert Abbott, a young printer with a congenital tumour below the angle of the jaw. On Friday 16 October 1846 the blood vessels leading to the tumour were ligated, with Morton employing a hastily devised glass inhaler containing a sea sponge saturated with ether (Fig. 2). On termination of the usual rapid operation, Warren was led to exclaim to the gallery, 'Gentlemen, this is no humbug'.

Although surgical anaesthesia was now publicly launched, an interminable period of rancorous controversy ensued over who should be given credit for the discovery. When requested to name the phenomenon, Oliver Wendell *Holmes suggested *anaesthesia*, from the Greek connoting lack of feeling.

News of the discovery soon reached England so that within 64 days the first operations were being performed with the aid of ether anaesthesia. John *Snow (Fig. 3), general practitioner, clinical investigator, and epidemiologist, became the first of a long line of English physician anaesthetists, indeed the first anywhere. Using ether primarily, with a refined apparatus, he was able within several months to report on his experience in a text concerning *The inhalation of the vapour of ether*. Toward the end of 1847, James Young *Simpson abandoned ether as a means of relieving the pain of childbirth, in favour of *chloroform. As chloroform was more pleasant to inhale than ether, and more potent with a consequent rapid induction and emergence, it became the more popular anaesthetic in England.

Subsequent developments
After the introduction of anaesthesia, surgery made little progress in either the USA or the UK, because the prevailing humoral theory of disease had to be modified to embrace the possibility that medical ailments might be cured by surgical treatment. This attitude changed with the development of pathological anatomy and performance of *post-mortem examinations. Next, as the concept of the *bacterical origin of infection was unknown, postsurgical *sepsis was rife after operation. This situation was altered toward the end of the century with acceptance of *Lister's technique of *antisepsis followed by *asepsis, as practised today. Many deaths due to chloroform were reported early on, as was extensive destruction of the liver. The question was whether sudden, intraoperative death might be related to respiratory standstill or heart failure. Fibrillation of the heart, resulting in circulatory arrest, was later recognized as the cause of death, rather than respiratory failure.

Local anaesthesia
Another approach to anaesthesia arose in Vienna in 1884, where Karl Koller and Sigmund *Freud were experimenting with agents for the treatment of morphine *addiction. Koller applied *cocaine, one of the drugs under investigation, to a frog's eye, and noticed that insensitivity to pain resulted. Cocaine, an alkaloid of the coca plant, had been chewed by Peruvian natives for centuries in the course of their labours, numbing the tongue and causing stimulation and exhilaration. Thus the stage was set for the development of local anaesthesia, in contrast to the general method. Within the year, Leonard J. Corning, neurologist of New York City, injected a solution of cocaine into the vicinity of the spinal cord of a man suffering from seminal incontinence and anaesthesia of the lower half of the body developed. Harvey *Cushing later extended the technique to other areas of the body, and coined the term 'regional anaesthesia', in contrast to general anaesthesia. In 1898, August *Bier had spinal anaesthesia with cocaine administered to himself by an assistant: a severe lumbar puncture headache developed as a result of extensive cerebrospinal fluid leakage. All manner of regional anaesthetic techniques were then devised

in the first decade of the 20th century, ranging from mere subcutaneous infiltration of solutions of cocaine, to injection into the major nerves supplying the head, torso, and extremities, and into the large nerve plexuses of the arm and leg. Adrenaline, newly synthesized, was added to the anaesthetic mixture to produce *vasoconstriction, to afford a bloodless surgical field, and to prolong nerve block.

However, the cocaine molecule was unstable, the solution was not easily sterilized, and it soon became well known for its central exhilarating and stimulating properties that led to addiction. William S. *Halsted, America's leading surgeon, who became an addict during self-experimentation with the drug, spent a major part of his career trying to break the habit. Apparently a substitute for cocaine was needed and this came with Alfred Einhorn's synthesis of *novocaine, a short-acting anaesthetic lacking topical activity. A series of amides: lidocaine, mepivacaine, lignocaine, bupivacaine, and etidocaine followed. The advantages of regional anaesthesia lie in its local effect on specific body areas, in contrast to the possible untoward effects on brain, heart, lungs, liver, and kidneys of general anaesthesia. Thus, with local anaesthesia, fewer systemic sequelae are apt to develop.

Theories of narcosis

From the beginning, scientists had pondered on how anaesthetics might act on the brain to produce *narcosis. Claude *Bernard, in about 1870, reasoned that narcosis represented a reversible semicoagulation of the substance of the cell, which returned to its original normal state upon elimination of the anaesthetic. The potent anaesthetics are highly lipid-soluble, and Meyer and Overton, around the turn of the century, independently proposed the *lipid solubility theory of narcosis, which postulated physical effects of anaesthetics on lipid-containing cell membranes. A strong correspondence exists between lipid solubility and anaesthetic potency. Perhaps this physical alteration affects *synaptic transmission between nerve cells in the brain, so that clinical anaesthesia results. Local anaesthetics

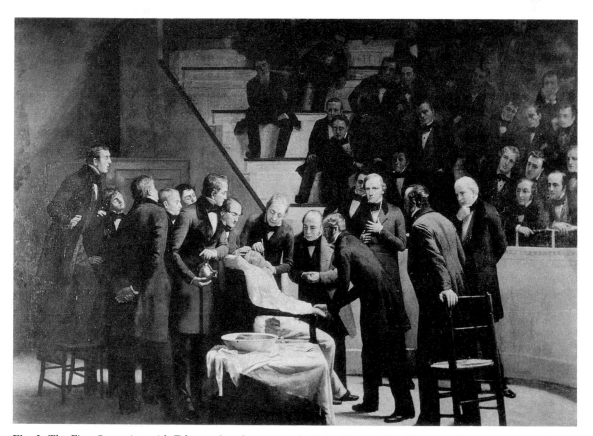

Fig. 2 *The First Operation with Ether*, painted retrospectively by Robert Hinckley over the years 1882–93, begun in Paris and finished in Washington, DC, USA. (Reproduced with permission from the collection of the Boston Medical Library in the Francis A. Countway Library of Medicine.)

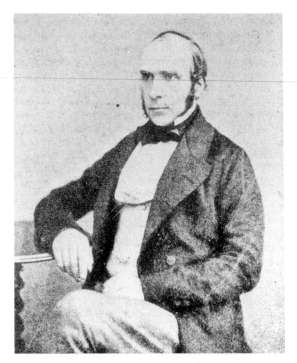

Fig. 3 John Snow. (Reproduced with permission from
B. M. Duncan (1947). *Development of inhalation
anaesthesia*, London.)

are also highly soluble in the lipid-containing membranes of nerves.

Newer anaesthetics and techniques
During the first half of the 20th century, as chloroform
waned in popularity, a number of new anaesthetics were
introduced into practice. Ether then shared the same
fate as chloroform, so that of the original agents, only
nitrous oxide remained. New halogenated hydrocarbons
appeared on the scene; these were distantly related to
chloroform but with the incorporation of the fluorine
molecule rendering the agent more potent, more stable,
and practically non-flammable.

Nowadays, anaesthetic practice does not consist in
the mere giving of a single inhalation agent, as was
originally the case, but in the utilization of several
agents, each ingredient offering one of the desiderata of
anaesthesia (a unitary term which is no longer an accurate description of the phenomenon): analgesia; lack
of awareness and unconsciousness; muscle relaxation;
and obtundation of *reflex responses to surgical stimuli.
The practice of employing multiple agents began, perhaps, with Claude Bernard's experiments, showing that
morphine injected into the dog lessened the amount of
chloroform subsequently needed for anaesthesia. This
experiment antedated the use of preanaesthetic medications, which utilized not only opioids but sometimes

atropine or scopolamine, both of which reduce respiratory tract secretions.

When regional anaesthesia was combined with general anaesthesia and with preanaesthetic medication,
a balanced technique resulted. Synthesis of the short-acting thiobarbiturates resulted in the use of sodium
thiopental for intravenous induction of anaesthesia,
leading to rapid loss of consciousness. In 1942, the
use by Griffith and Johnson of intravenous *curare
(the South American paralysing arrow-poison) for the
first time provided still another essential ingredient. In
purified form this came to be used frequently during
general anaesthesia, to avoid excessive depth of narcosis, while giving the patient the muscle relaxation
necessary for operation. As the abdominal muscles
were paralysed, so were those of respiration—the *diaphragm and intercostals. The *apnoeic patient therefore required assistance or control of respiration via a
mechanical *respirator. Better and safer control was
afforded by insertion of a tracheal tube attached to the
breathing circuit.

Other intravenous agents increased the dimensions
of balanced anaesthesia. Some were used as preanaesthetic medicaments, to supplement regional anaesthesia
or to prevent awareness during operation in the paralysed patient. Newer opioids, such as fentanyl, were
much more potent and offered fewer adverse effects
than the traditional morphine derivatives.

Anaesthetists have been responsible for the development of multidisciplinary pain therapy clinics. However, this class of medical specialist is still largely concerned with the overall care of surgical patients even
though, of necessity, special expertise is needed in cardiac surgery, pulmonary operations, neuroanaesthesia,
obstetrics, paediatrics, orthopaedics, and ambulatory
(out-patient) surgical clinics. Finally, the benefits of
training in anaesthesia are evident in critical (*intensive)
care medicine, resuscitation, and neonatology.

                                            L. D. VANDAM

Further reading
Cartwright, F. F. (1952). *The English pioneers of anaesthesia*.
   Wright, Bristol and Simpkin Marshall, London.
Duncum, B. M. (1947). *The development of inhalation anaesthesia*. Oxford University Press, London.
Keys, T. E. (1963). *The history of surgical anesthesia*. Dover,
   New York.

ANAESTHETIC (ANESTHETIC). Any agent employed to produce *anaesthesia, local or general, i.e.
to abolish sensation.

ANAESTHETIST (ANESTHETIST). In the UK, a
doctor specializing in *anaesthesia; in the USA, a nurse
or technician trained to administer anaesthetic agents,
one who is medically qualified being termed an 'anesthesiologist'.

ANALGESIA. Insensibility to pain.

ANALGESIC. Relieving pain; an agent that removes or diminishes sensibility to pain.

ANALYSIS. Separation or resolution into component parts. See also PSYCHOANALYSIS.

ANAMNESIS is the recall of things past, and is used in two specific medical senses: first, to mean a patient's recollection of symptoms and past illnesses as recounted in the history; secondly, to mean immunological memory, as in the rapid reappearance of an *antibody in response to an *antigen to which an immune response has occurred previously (see IMMUNOLOGY).

ANAPHYLAXIS is an alarming and occasionally fatal reaction following an injection or exposure to a foreign substance (e.g. insect sting, venom, or drug such as penicillin) to which the individual has become abnormally sensitive because of previous exposure. This is due to production of *antibody (of the IgE class) bound to *basophils and *mast cells; subsequent contact with the antigenic substance causes the cells to release substances called mediators (*histamine, *serotonin, *kinins, *prostaglandins) which produce the reaction. Manifestations include shock, hypotension, urticaria, oedema of the face and throat, bronchospasm, and vomiting. The mechanism is like that operating in *allergy except that the latter is due to *local* contact of the allergen with, e.g. the eye, nose, and bronchi, and the reaction is accordingly local (conjunctivitis, hay fever, and asthma). The mechanism was recognized in the early 1900s, when the term anaphylaxis was introduced, although the first recorded case is that of King Menes of Egypt, who died following a wasp sting in the 26th century BC.

ANAPLASIA is loss of differentiation of cells and of their orientation within a tissue. It is a characteristic of malignant *neoplasms.

ANARTHRIA is loss of speech due to inability to articulate.

ANASTOMOSIS. An opening between, or a joining of, two (or more) channels, vessels, organs, or spaces, either occurring naturally or created by surgery, trauma, or pathological processes.

ANATOMICAL NOMENCLATURE. Official anatomical names are laid down in the *Nomina Anatomica (NA)*, revised by the International Anatomical Nomenclature Committee appointed by the Fifth International Congress of Anatomists held at Oxford in 1955, and reaffirmed by the same body on several subsequent occasions.

ANATOMIST. One studying or skilled in *anatomy.

ANATOMY is the scientific study of the structural organization of the body. Aristotle, one of the earliest students of the subject, gave the science its name, *anatome*, some 2400 years ago. Literally this term means cutting up, and while Aristotle probably studied animals rather than man, dissection has remained the essential method for the study of human anatomy through the ages.

For centuries, anatomy meant *gross anatomy*, the structure of the body as seen by the naked eye, but in the last 300 years the boundaries of the subject have widened. Some aspects of studies in physical anthropology are still closely associated with gross anatomy; but through the use of the *microscope the field of anatomy has come to include *microanatomy*, or **histology*, and the study of development before birth, or *embryology*. With the use of radiant energy for *diagnosis and treatment, *radiological anatomy* was included, and some new subspecialties, such as *neuroanatomy*, have emerged. Just as gross anatomy is recognized as the basic science of *surgery, so histology grew up closely related to histopathology, the study of the microscopic changes in cells and tissues in disease. Studies of the microanatomy of tissues extended the understanding not only of structure but also function. Now the subject of histology is an integral part of physiological study and teaching, as well as a logical extension of gross anatomy to the study of cells and tissues forming the structural basis of the body.

Advances in histological studies depended not only on improved microscopes, but on mechanical means for obtaining thin sections, techniques for the fixation of tissues so that they retained orderly structure, albeit changed from that when living, and of stains to enable components of tissues to be differentiated. Later developments included the development of *histo-* and *cytochemistry*, the demonstration of chemical compounds, including *enzymes, within tissues and cells, and the growing of cells and tissues outside the animal body, in culture. The development of the electron microscope, in which use of a beam of electrons instead of light tremendously increased the resolving power, and hence the useful magnifications possible, gave rise to the subject of *cytology*. These and other techniques have enabled anatomical research, now largely based on experiment, to extend its boundaries so that the demarcation between it and other biological sciences has largely disappeared.

Present understanding of the normal structure (and function) of the human body derives from the work of many, but the contribution of the Flemish anatomist Andreas *Vesalius (1514–64) must be considered seminal so that, in retrospect, it is possible to see the history of anatomy as divided into a pre- and post-Vesalian period.

History: before Vesalius
Religious feelings, customary disposal of the dead by burial, *cremation, or other ritual means, the belief that corpses were unclean and contact with them defiled, have all inhibited anatomical study, and the systematic practice of human dissection remained condemned until the 20th century.

The ancient civilizations of Greece and Rome were opposed to dissection and, although medicine was taught in China as early as about the 4th century BC, the effective study of systematic human anatomy dates from about the year 300 BC. For at least 2000 years the Egyptians practised the techniques of embalming the dead. Such preservation was religious in its motivations, but the embalmer needed some familiarity with the anatomical basis of his work. It was against this Egyptian background of centuries of familiarity with human cadavers that, with the approval and support of Ptolemy I, the study of human gross anatomy by dissection began at Alexandria. The corpses of criminals were made available to the Alexandrian anatomists, the best known of whom are *Herophilus (c. 350–280 BC) and *Erasistratus (c. 310–250 BC). The original writings of these and others of the period have long since been lost, and their work has endured only through later writers such as *Galen.

Paradoxically the role of anatomy in medicine apparently diminished over this period. Dissection of cadavers came to be regarded as unnecessary and degrading in Alexandria, as it was elsewhere. Moreover, dissection was held to give false information, a view ascribed to the 'Empiricists', a group of *physicians who allowed that only chance anatomical observations, such as those made on wounded men, were permissible. The study of anatomy was also opposed by another sect, the 'Methodists', whose members were fiercely anti-scientific. This opposition contributed to the decline in anatomical studies and, following the withdrawal of royal patronage, the scholars were finally driven out of Alexandria. Despite this decline, something of the tradition established in the early years persisted until the time of Marinus of Tyre (c. AD 130), and from him a line of teachers can be traced directly to Galen (AD 130–c. 200), a notable figure in any history of medicine.

Galen studied anatomy for more than 10 years, first at Pergamon under Satyros (an anatomist from Smyrna), then in Smyrna itself, and in Corinth and Alexandria. He studied medicine also, and for about 3 years from AD 159 served as physician to the gladiators at Pergamon. This appointment no doubt provided many opportunities to him for the learning of 'anatomy by chance' from the often severely wounded men.

Although skeletons were available for study in Galen's time, human dissection was still not possible in Greek cities, although corpses of enemy soldiers killed in battle, of executed criminals, and of stillborn or exposed children might have been subject to some kind of examination. Anatomical writings from the Alexandrian school were available, however, and Galen himself 'condensed' a treatise by Marinus from 20 books to four. He also practised extensively the dissection of animals. He was a prolific writer, not only on anatomy, but also on *physiology, surgery, and other aspects of medicine. His anatomical texts formed the basis of teaching in this subject for many centuries, surviving

the 'Dark Ages' and still being expounded in the 16th century.

Since studies of practical anatomy based on human dissections were not possible during most of this time, Galen's errors were not recognized, in part from ignorance, but also from adherence to Galen's view that the parts of the body could not be improved upon, and thus further study was not necessary. Thus both his knowledge and his faults were perpetuated. Later teachers encountered, in addition, the problems and complications associated with the handing down of Galen's texts over the centuries. Nevertheless Galenic works, errors and all, exerted a great influence on the development of medicine in Western Europe well into the 17th century.

During the Dark Ages, there was a regression rather than any advance in anatomical and medical knowledge generally. The library and school at Alexandria had been destroyed, and in both Arab and European countries the teaching of medicine, anatomy, and whatever physiology there was continued for centuries to be based on texts such as those of *Hippocrates and Galen. The religious creed of the Muhammadans forbade dissection of human subjects, and little, if any, dissection was carried out in Europe.

Outside the Arab world, the earliest medical school was that founded at *Salerno, probably as early as the 9th century. From the 13th century universities began to be established throughout Western Europe, and in many of these, faculties of medicine were developed. In 1240 the importance of anatomy was recognized when Emperor Frederick II pronounced that surgeons, before being allowed to practise, had to show knowledge of the anatomy of the human body; but the teaching of anatomy continued to be based on established texts and any anatomical dissection carried out was generally in private.

*Bologna occupies a notable place as far as the history of anatomy is concerned. The university was already established by the time of the 13th century, but the medical faculty was not well known until after 1280. A limited amount of human dissection was by that time being carried out, although the purpose of this was to determine the cause of death, as a *post-mortem examination is performed today, rather than to further anatomical knowledge. In 1306 Mondino de Luzzi (*Mundinus) was appointed to the teaching staff of the university, and, despite opposition from the Church, carried out some human dissection in public during the next few years. He dissected in person, not teaching *ex cathedra* with a demonstrator pointing out the structures revealed in the cadaver by the menial dissector. Mondino wrote a practical text, the *Anathomia*, which appeared in 1316. This contained basic, but often inaccurate, descriptions of organs, but has been regarded as inaugurating a new phase in the study of human anatomy. Another work of equal importance, originating at about the same time, was that of Henri *de Mondeville, who lived c. 1270–1320. He was a Norman, a contemporary of

Mondino, and also studied at Bologna before lecturing at *Montpellier in the early years of the 14th century. In his lectures he used full-length anatomical pictures and illustrations showing separate organs.

This period, the beginning of the 14th century, marked a renaissance of learning in Europe, which was associated with considerable changes in the scope of medical education, notably the spread of practical anatomical studies. Mondino's *Anathomia* was followed in 1345 by the publication of a text by Guido de Vigevano which, although illustrated by figures showing dissection, noted that the practice was prohibited by the Church. Gradually, albeit with some reluctance on the part of Church and State, however, the proscription was relaxed. In 1377, public dissections were authorized by decree at Montpellier, and similar recognition followed at Padua in 1429 and at Paris in 1478. Pope Sixtus IV, who held office from 1471 to 1484, permitted dissection provided that permission of the Church authorities was obtained.

The corpses made available for public dissection were those of executed criminals, a practice which continued into the 19th century in Western Europe. Even when opposition of the Church to the practice had weakened, general distaste and even revulsion hindered anatomical progress. There were also other major problems: first, the number of cadavers officially made available to anatomists was limited, sometimes to one per year or less. Secondly, since there was no means of preserving the cadavers, decomposition was rapid, particularly in the warmer countries of the Mediterranean. Dissections had to be carried out rapidly, perhaps without ceasing over several days, and the most perishable organs, such as the abdominal viscera, were demonstrated first. Mid-winter was commonly the season for dissections since at that time decomposition would proceed more slowly than at other times. The public 'anatomies' were generally directed towards the demonstration of the truth of Galenic texts, and little was done to discover and correct their errors.

There seems to have been a considerable stirring of interest in human anatomy at the very end of the 15th century. An increase and wider dissemination of anatomical knowledge resulted from the development of printing and of techniques for the reproduction of illustrations. 'Anatomies' with illustrations began to be available to students. Among texts appearing before the end of the 15th century was a commentary, with some additions, on the work of Mondino by Allessandro Achillini (1463–1512). Another text was that published by Alessandro Benedetti (*c.* 1455–1525) whose *Five books on anatomy, on the history of the human body* appeared in 1493. These and other texts, in the same way as the public dissections, generally perpetuated the still prevalent ideas of Galen, and in 1531 a Latin version of his *On anatomical procedures*, translated from Greek, was published by Johannes Gunther of Andernach (1487–1574).

Although interest in practical anatomy was growing throughout the late 15th and early 16th centuries, the topic was not a major concern of all medical scholars. A 'Humanist' school flourished about this period, whose members held texts to be more valuable than dissections. Books of anatomy based on early writings contained virtually nothing new gained by observation, nor were the texts amended. The early 16th century was thus a time of historically based anatomical scholarship; but contemporaneously, in some centres of learning, awareness of the importance of practical studies was developing.

In 1514 one of the outstanding figures in the history of anatomy, Andreas Vesalius, was born at Brussels. As a young man, he was taught Galenic-based anatomy by Gunther and *Sylvius in Paris, where some (probably surreptitious) dissections were being carried out. In 1537 he was appointed to the chair of anatomy at Padua and, like Mondino, broke established tradition by performing the winter dissection of that year himself. Vesalius published a number of anatomical works. An early one was the *Tabulae anatomicae sex* (1538) which consisted of three drawings of the vascular system and three views of the skeleton. His most famous work appeared in 1543: this was the *De humani corporis fabrica*, which proved to be one of the most important and significant anatomical texts ever published (Figs 1 and 2). The seven books of the *Fabrica* contain large and splendid plates, one series showing progressive

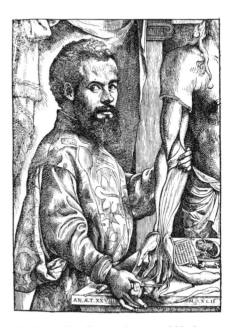

Fig. 1 Andreas Vesalius at the age of 28, from *De humani corporis fabrica*, 1543 (reproduced by permission of the Francis D. Countway Library of Medicine, Boston).

Anatomy

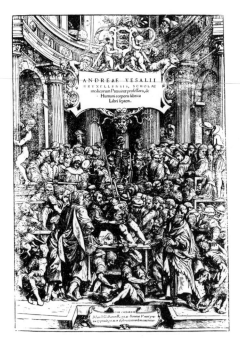

Fig. 2 The title page of *De humani corporis fabrica*, 1543 (reproduced by permission of the Francis D. Countway Library of Medicine, Boston).

stages of dissection from the exposure of superficial structures by removal of skin and underlying connective tissue, through the layers of muscles down to the ligaments and bones. Vessels are shown displayed systematically, suggesting that injected preparations had been made. The drawings were published with terminology in Greek, Latin, Hebrew, and Arabic, in an attempt to reduce the confusion which had resulted from centuries of translation and re-translation of early texts. The *Fabrica* was intended to be an integral work of text and illustrations, both to be appreciated together. He also published, again in 1543, the *Epitome*, intended to form a guide for students, with little actual description of the plates; this, probably because it was cheaper and simpler, became more popular than the *Fabrica*. The changes in anatomical ideas which followed the publication of the *Tabulae sex*, the *Fabrica*, and the *Epitome* were to transform the subject.

History: after Vesalius

The great changes in outlook which eventually followed publication of the Vesalian texts were neither immediate nor universal. The *Fabrica* was ill-received in Louvain, and in Paris his former teacher Sylvius took it as an affront. In the schools of Padua, Bologna, and Pisa, however, the work was greeted with approval and Vesalius was invited to conduct anatomies in these places.

The outstanding contribution made by Vesalius to human anatomy lay not only in his texts, but in the size, extensive annotation, and outstanding quality of his illustrations, which were far ahead of anything that had previously appeared, and in the integration of the text and the figures. Subsequently, as anatomical knowledge increased and texts multiplied, so the quality of the illustrations improved. Practising artists were commonly involved. Indeed, it is generally held that the bulk of the illustrations for the *Fabrica* were executed in Titian's studio. This work marked the beginning of a long and close association between *art and anatomy. Besides the illustration of anatomical texts, a number of renaissance artists studied human anatomy and are known to have dissected, among them Raphael, Michelangelo, and Albrecht Dürer. Leonardo da Vinci left ample evidence of his knowledge of comparative and human anatomy in his notebooks and drawings, often emphasizing the mechanical principles of anatomical features rather that their pure morphology.

The authors of many anatomical works remained familiar to teachers and students, long after their texts had passed out of use, but the extensive eponymous nomenclature that characterized human anatomy was used well into the 20th century. Indeed, it is only in relatively recent years that the International Committee on Anatomical Nomenclature, through its publications, the *Nomina Anatomica*, has introduced a more scientific terminology. In 1955 it was decided that no eponyms should be printed. Yet they persist; although up-to-date anatomical texts may be free of them, their usage has been handed on to students by generations of anatomists and clinicians.

During the 14th century, legal permission to dissect cadavers had been granted to a number of schools in Italy and, as already noted, dissections had been carried out in Bologna as early as the 13th century. However, the practical teaching of anatomy developed more slowly in other countries. Public dissections took place in Paris from 1478, and by the end of the 16th century in Basel and The Netherlands. In England, the universities of Oxford and Cambridge were established early and for a long time were the main centres of medical education. It is not certain when the teaching of anatomy first began, but lectures without dissection were probably given in the 14th century, and a number of manuscripts of anatomical importance have survived from that period. David Edwards, who is said to have made the first dissection in England in 1531, was also the first English author of an anatomical text.

Among the notable teachers concerned in early medical teaching in England was John *Caius, master of Gonville College, Cambridge. Caius, who studied with Vesalius in Padua, obtained a grant from the Crown for the dissection of one subject each year at Gonville. Meanwhile a Royal Commission examined the system of education at Oxford and formulated revised regulations under which a student of medicine during his 6 years was to attend two dissections, two disputations, and an examination before being awarded a Bachelor's degree. Further attendance at dissections was required before proceeding to a Doctorate.

During the first half of the 17th century the teaching of anatomy in the two universities fell into neglect, and in 1646 the Senate of the University of Cambridge passed a Grace (a formal decree) to remedy this situation. At the time of the Commonwealth in the mid-17th century, great interest developed in science at Oxford, and in anatomy in particular. Christopher *Wren was one who studied the subject, and in 1664 there appeared Thomas *Willis's *Cerebri anatome*, with Wren's plates. Even in the early days the privilege of anatomical teaching had not been held exclusively by the universities of Oxford and Cambridge.

In the early 14th century the practice of, and training in, surgery in the City of London were in the hands of two groups, the Company of Barbers and the Fellowship of Surgeons. Members of the former were concerned with shaving, bleeding, and surgery; the Guild of Surgeons was a smaller select body whose members practised surgery only. The Barbers in due course acquired the title of the Barber-Surgeons Company, and in 1540 the two groups united. The united company undertook the provision of lectures and demonstrations in anatomy, and was entitled to the corpses of four malefactors each year for dissection. The 'anatomies' and anatomical lectures were held in Barber-Surgeons Hall. Dissections were public and attendance by surgical freemen and by apprentices was compulsory. As the practice of surgery increased over the years and the demand for instruction grew, private schools flourished, and with them came increased competition for the limited number of subjects available for dissection. The Company of Barber-Surgeons encountered difficulties in obtaining the bodies to which it was legally entitled, as legal officers often found it more profitable to sell the bodies for private study.

In Edinburgh, instruction in anatomy before the foundation of the medical faculty in 1726 was the responsibility of the surgeons and the Town Council. In Aberdeen two foundations, Marischal College and St Mary's, later King's College, taught medicine, including anatomy, from an early date, but there is no record of human dissection until 1636. In Glasgow a chair of anatomy was established in 1720, and, in Ireland, the teaching of anatomy was taking place in Dublin at about the same time.

Since the centuries-old tradition was that students themselves did not dissect, and their instruction depended on a clear view of the proceedings, many schools built custom-designed anatomical theatres. A permanent anatomical theatre was built at Padua in 1594, and a successor, opened in 1783, still exists. Edinburgh had an anatomical theatre founded by the Guild of Surgeons in 1697 and in London the Surgeons Hall was built for the teaching of anatomy. Hogarth's print, the fourth and final stage in the series *The reward of cruelty*, shows a scene of dissection which is probably based on the Cutlerian Theatre of the *Royal College of Physicians, London. This theatre, designed by Robert Hooke, was opened in 1674.

Meanwhile, new technical methods had come to be applied to the study of anatomy, among them the use of injection to prevent putrefaction and to solidify specimens. Injected specimens were among the many preparations collected and displayed in anatomical museums from the 18th century onwards. Of note is the remarkable collection of some 14 000 exhibits assembled by John *Hunter and presented to the *Royal College of Surgeons of London after his death in 1832.

Gradually it was accepted that there was a need for practical anatomical study, at any rate for those training to practice surgical procedures, and the proscription or severe restriction of human dissection was eased. However, the number of corpses granted was small: often only one per year was available. Officially approved occasions for anatomical dissection were thus few, and this constituted a great hindrance to detailed study and teaching. The shortage of legally provided subjects for dissection led to anatomists taking into their own hands the acquisition of additional material for their needs, either by bribing the Sheriff and hangman to provide corpses which should legally have gone to the surgeons and official schools, or ultimately by grave-robbing.

In the UK the growth of *medical education continued throughout the 18th and 19th centuries. More surgeons were needed as the population grew. Inevitably, more surgeons meant a greater demand for anatomical teaching, and students unable to find a place to study at home travelled abroad. After the peace of 1815 there were many English students in Paris, a major attraction being that the 'Paris' method allowed students to dissect for themselves. The shortage of cadavers led anatomists and surgeons to set about procuring corpses for themselves; grave-robbing increased. The demand for subjects for dissection was further increased when, in due course, medical students were allowed, and later required, to dissect for themselves. Since teachers of anatomy had either to provide bodies for dissection or lose their students and their fees, professional grave-robbers appeared to supply the material required. The attention paid to the grave-robbers ('resurrectionists') stems in part from the unsavoury nature of their work; but they played an important, if unpleasant, part in the development of the teaching of practical human anatomy. Legal dissection of hanged felons had long given rise to much ill feeling in their relatives; but the robbing of graves led to much wider revulsion and anger, not directed solely at the robbers, but also at the anatomists to whom they sold their bodies.

Grave-robbing occurred widely in the British Isles, from Aberdeen to London, and also in Ireland. The practice was prevalent in the US where it was first reported in the first decade of American independence.

With the exception of Massachusetts, America was slow to legislate for the provision of the considerable number of cadavers needed for teaching, and grave-robbing continued much later than in Britain, where introduction of the Anatomy Act of 1832 curbed the practice.

The fresher the corpse, the more saleable, and the higher the price; and this led a few body-snatchers to murder. The most widely known series of incidents, set in Edinburgh, is that associated with Burke and Hare in 1827. Sixteen victims were killed in 10 months, and supplied to the Edinburgh anatomist Dr Robert Knox. After the Edinburgh murders, the already strong feeling against both grave-robbers and their clients increased, and led to Parliament passing the Anatomy Act. It empowered the Secretary of State to grant licences to teachers of anatomy and allowed such persons to receive any dead body for anatomical examination in suitable licensed premises.

Gradually over the early decades of the 20th century individuals began to bequeath their bodies for anatomical purposes after death. This, coupled with modern techniques of preservation, essentially relieved the shortage of subjects for dissection. If dissection is now disappearing from medical curricula, it is not for want of cadavers, but because of fundamental revisions in medical education.

Current practice

Although anatomy is still occasionally studied as a discipline in its own right, it remains essentially a vocational subject for students of medicine and dentistry. World-wide, medical education is undergoing a major reorientation. With the exponential growth of medical scientific knowledge, older subject disciplines, such as anatomy and physiology, have become increasingly complex and new ones have been recognized in their own right. Consequently the undergraduate curriculum has become overburdened, and it is recognized that there is a pressing need to re-define the core knowledge, skills, and attitudes required of tomorrow's doctors.

There is a move away from separate discipline-based courses of study in favour of some form of integrated multidisciplinary teaching in which groups of teachers deal with various aspects of the structure, function, *pathology, dysfunction, and therapy relating to a particular system or topic. Such an approach was introduced first at Western Reserve Medical School, USA, in the 1960s, and similar approaches have been introduced subsequently in other centres. The impact of this new approach on the study of teaching of anatomy has been considerable. Indeed, in those schools that have introduced fully integrated curricula, anatomy as a distinct, separately taught subject has virtually disappeared. In most others, the disproportionate time previously allotted in total to the subject, including not only gross anatomy, but the associated topics of neuroanatomy, histology, cytology, and embryology, has been reduced significantly.

One consequence of this reduction in allotted time is that in most schools students are no longer expected to dissect. Instead they study *prosections* prepared by demonstrators, often trainee surgeons. Some authorities claim that losing the chance to dissect, and thereby the opportunity for unhurried exploration of the complexity of the human body, diminishes the educational experience. Others hold that the lost opportunity has no effect, as dissection itself does little to enhance students' core knowledge and understanding of *clinical anatomy*. Indeed, there can be little doubt that in today's medical curriculum there is a need to concentrate anatomical learning upon the principles and concepts essential to the practice of modern medicine and to reduce the teaching of irrelevant and unnecessary detail.

Because of its long and distinguished history, anatomy and its practitioners have recently attracted a reputation for conservatism and resistance to change that is not entirely justified. While the gross structure of the human body and its variations have been well understood since the 19th century (the standard reference Gray's *Anatomy* was first published in 1858), anatomists have been quick to embrace new educational technologies (e.g. multi-media applications of information technology) and exploit new approaches to learning (e.g. problem-based learning). Anatomy has always been taught in relation to clinical medicine and surgery, and its practitioners have responded rapidly to the changing requirements of clinical practice. One recent example of this is the development in a number of schools of clinical and surgical skills laboratories, based upon the use of anatomical models and simulators. Another is the re-introduction of *cross-sectional anatomy* to meet the needs of modern medical imaging techniques such as *computerised axial tomography and *nuclear magnetic resonance.

As for anatomical research, there are few boundaries between this and other biological investigations. Like medical education, much of current medical research is multi-disciplinary in nature. Anatomical science still has its place, and while the scalpel is seldom used now, dissection, in the literal sense of 'cutting up', remains the essential reductionist approach to the elucidation of structure. With the advent of new technologies, morphological research has embraced successive levels of structure from the macroscopic to the molecular, and the study of structure has become inextricably associated with the exploration of function. Moreover, anatomical science, now experimentally based, has spawned more new disciplines than any other. *Embryology*, that branch of anatomy dealing with the study of development before birth, is a good example of this.

Modern embryology has advanced beyond descriptions of the development of tissues, organs, and the individual as a whole, to a realization of the importance of *genetics, *molecular biology, and *biochemisty. Embryological research is now concerned with the complex processes that result in normal and abnormal complex processes that result in normal and abnormal development, and investigation has perforce been directed into a series of related subdisciplines, e.g. teratology. *Teratology* is that branch of embryology which deals with abnormal development. Although Aristotle probably should be considered the father of teratology, only in the 20th century, largely as a result of the *thalidomide episode, has this field of research been recognized properly in its own right. In turn, the prevalence of genetically related congenital defects, the ability to detect certain genetic and chromosomally caused defects, and the developments in *amniocentesis have spawned yet another new discipline: genetic counselling, combining the fields of teratology and genetics.

Other disciplines have at least some of their roots in anatomical science. *Immunology*, for example, employs anatomical techniques, although they may be barely recognized as such; the highly sophisticated flow cytometer bears little resemblance to a fluorescence microscope but its use in examining cells is based on the same principles. If study of anatomy has led to the development of new disciplines, then anatomical science and its approaches have been enriched and developed in consequence. A better understanding of immunological recognition has led directly to the development of sophisticated *immunocytochemical techniques now widely employed in other anatomical fields, e.g. neuroanatomy.

Neuroanatomy is one field where pure structural studies still have a contribution to make. Although the gross topography of the brain and spinal cord were accurately described many years ago, elucidating the fine structure and function of the brain remains one of biology's greatest challenges.

Today, human anatomy still forms an essential part of the scientific basis of medicine and allied skills. Those whose concern is the promotion of health and the prevention and treatment of disease must surely continue to work from knowledge of the normal structure and, inseparable from this, the normal function of the human body.

REG JORDAN

Further reading
Association of American Medical Colleges (1992). *Education of medical students*. Washington.
Ball, J. M. (1928). *The sack 'em up men*. Oliver and Boyd, Edinburgh.
Belvin, C. E. and Cahill, D. R. (1973). Gross anatomy: current courses, training programs and prospective needs. *Journal of Medical Education*, **48**, 264–70.
Cave, A. J. E. (1950). Ancient Egypt and the origin of anatomical science. *Proceedings of the Royal Society of Medicine*, **43**, 508–71.
Choulant, L. (transl. Frank, M.) (1945). *History and bibliography of anatomic illustration*. Schuman's, New York.
Dobson, J. (1953). Some eighteenth century experiments in embalming. *Journal of the History of Medicine*, **8**, 431–41.
Dooley, J. (1974). The rediscovery of anatomy. *Proceedings of the Royal Institution*, **47**, 191–231.
General Medical Council (1993). *Tomorrow's doctors: recommendations of undergraduate medical education*. London.
Kaufman, M. (1976). *American medical education*. Greenwood Press, Westport, Connecticut.
Morton, L. T. (1970). *A medical bibliography*. London.
Saunders, J. B. de C. M. and O'Malley, C. D. (1950). *The illustrations from the works of Andreas Vesalius of Brussels*. World Publishing, Cleveland.
Singer, C. (1957). *A short history of anatomy from the Greeks to Harvey*, (2nd edn). Dover, New York.

ANATOMY ACT 1832. Under the Anatomy Act of 1832, as amended in 1871, institutions in the UK with the lawful custody of inmates who have no known relatives may provide bodies for schools of anatomy. Where a body is bequeathed, the undertaker, having obtained a disposal certificate from the Registrar, removes the body to the donee, a medical school. The school must, within 2 years, arrange final burial according to the religion of the deceased (or cremation since the Anatomy Regulations 1940).

ANDERSON, ELIZABETH GARRETT (1836–1917). British physician. Née Elizabeth Garrett, she was the first woman to qualify in medicine in the UK (see WOMEN IN MEDICINE). Refused entry to medical school, she trained privately, and in 1865 was granted the diploma of Licentiate of the Society of Apothecaries (LSA). The following year she was appointed physician to the Marylebone Dispensary for Women and Children, which later became the New Hospital for Women and finally the Elizabeth Garrett Anderson Hospital, staffed by women; she served as senior physician from 1866 to 1892. She was part founder of the London School of Medicine in 1874. The school was attached to the London (later Royal) Free Hospital, which she served as lecturer in medicine (1875–97) and dean (1883–1905). In 1876 she became the first woman member of the British Medical Association, and was president of the East Anglian branch for 1896–7.

ANDROGENS. Masculinizing substances, i.e. the male sex-hormones and synthetic analogues of these. *Testosterone is the main such hormone, produced by the interstitial (Leydig) cells of the *testis when stimulated by the *luteinizing hormone (LH) of the anterior *pituitary gland.

ANDROGYNE. A female pseudohermaphrodite, i.e. a true female who exhibits some *secondary sexual characteristics of the male.

ANENCEPHALY is a *congenital abnormality in which the roof of the skull is defective and the underlying *cerebral hemispheres are underdeveloped or absent. It is incompatible with life for more than a few days after birth. It is commoner in female fetuses, and tends to recur in subsequent pregnancies. Prenatal diagnosis is possible (see ALPHA-FETOPROTEIN; AMNIOCENTESIS).

ANESTHESIOLOGIST. See ANAESTHETIST.

ANEURIN. See THIAMINE.

ANEURYSM. An abnormal sac-like dilatation of an *artery or part of the wall of the heart.

ANGIITIS. Inflammation of blood or lymph vessels.

ANGINA PECTORIS. Chest pain, characteristically induced by exertion or excitement and relieved by rest, caused by an inadequate supply of oxygen to the heart muscle. It is usually, although not invariably, due to obstructive disease of the coronary arteries. See CORONARY HEART DISEASE.

ANGINA. When otherwise unqualified, angina means *angina pectoris. It can be applied to similar types of pain in other parts of the body, as in angina cruris (see INTERMITTENT CLAUDICATION), produced by a similar mechanism. The word derives from the Greek for 'strangling', and is also used, although now less often, for severe infections of the mouth, throat, and larynx (e.g. diphtheritic angina).

ANGIOCARDIOGRAPHY is radiographic visualization of the heart and great vessels by serial exposures after injecting a contrast agent into the circulation.

ANGIOGRAPHY is the radiographic visualization of blood vessels using a contrast agent.

ANGIOLOGY is the study of *blood and lymph vessels.

ANGIOMA. Any *tumour deriving from, or made up of, blood or lymph vessels.

ANGIONEUROTIC OEDEMA (EDEMA) is an immunological tissue reaction, also known as angioedema and giant urticaria. It resembles *urticaria in producing patches of erythematous oedema of skin and mucous membranes, but it simultaneously involves deeper tissues. The skin of the eyes and lips and the mucous membranes of the mouth and respiratory tract are often affected. The condition is dangerous because of the possibility of death by asphyxia. An inherited (autosomal dominant) form occurs, due to congenital absence of an inhibitor of the *complement system.

ANGIOPLASTY. See ARTERIES AND VEINS: THEIR DISEASES AND VASCULAR SURGERY.

ANGIOTENSIN is a physiological vasoconstrictor substance formed by the action of an enzyme, *renin, released from the kidney, on a fraction of the plasma *globulin. The immediate product, angiotensin I, is a *polypeptide with 10 amino acids having little activity; this is reduced by a converting enzyme in the lungs to angiotensin II, an octapeptide. Angiotensin II has a powerful direct constricting effect on blood vessels, raising *blood pressure; it also stimulates secretion of *aldosterone by the *adrenal gland.

ANGOR ANIMI is a feeling of impending doom, typically experienced by patients suffering a serious vascular catastrophe, such as massive pulmonary embolism, myocardial infarction, etc.

ANGSTROM. A unit of length (symbol Å) equal to 10^{-10} m, formerly used to measure wavelengths of electromagnetic radiation such as light and intramolecular distances. In the SI system it has been replaced by the nanometre (10^{-9} m; 10 Å = 1 nm).

ANHIDROSIS. Absence of, or deficiency of, sweat.

ANIMAL MAGNETISM. See HYPNOTISTS.

ANIMALS AS CARRIERS OF DISEASE. See BIRDS AS CARRIERS OF DISEASE; CATS AS CARRIERS OF DISEASE; DOGS AS CARRIERS OF DISEASE; GOATS AS CARRIERS OF DISEASE; INSECTS AS VECTORS OF DISEASE; ZOONOSIS.

ANIMALS SCIENTIFIC PROCEDURES ACT 1986. See CRUELTY TO ANIMALS ACT 1876.

ANIMISM is the attribution of a living soul to inanimate objects and natural phenomena.

ANION. An *ion carrying a negative electric charge.

ANISOCYTOSIS. Abnormal variation in size of *erythrocytes.

ANISOPHORIA is latent inequality of the ocular visual axes in a horizontal plane, i.e. one axis deviates upwards or downwards relative to the other when visual stimuli are eliminated.

ANISOCORIA. Inequality of the *pupils.

ANKH. A cross with a ring or handle replacing the upper arm, also known as a *crux ansata*: used in ancient Egyptian art as a symbol of life.

ANKYLOSING SPONDYLITIS is an inflammatory condition of the spine formerly thought to be closely related to *rheumatoid arthritis (it is also called rheumatoid spondylitis or Marie–Strümpell disease). It occurs predominantly in young males; there is a genetic component and a strong association with the antigen *HLA-B27. Beginning usually with inflammation of the sacroiliac joints, in progressive cases the spine eventually becomes completely rigid ('poker back') with X-ray appearances aptly described as 'bamboo spine'. Peripheral joints may also be involved, and associated features may include iridocyclitis (up to 40 per cent of patients), cardiac conduction defects, aortic valve incompetence, pulmonary fibrosis, ulcerative colitis, and amyloidosis.

ANKYLOSIS. Fixation and immobility of a joint.

ANKYLOSTOMIASIS (ANCYLOSTOMIASIS) is infestation with hook worms—small (about 1 cm length) *nematode worms of the genus *Ancylostoma*. Two species affect man: *A. duodenale*, endemic in the Far East, the Mediterranean littoral, and other parts of Africa; and *A. americanum* (or *Necator americanus*), also found in Africa but occurring mainly in the Americas; it was a major problem in the Southern states of the USA until about 1920. Adult worms inhabit the small intestine and cause iron-deficiency *anaemia in those with malnutrition. There is no animal reservoir or intermediate host. Ova are excreted in the faeces, become larvae in warm soil, and penetrate intact human skin (causing hookworm dermatitis, or 'ground itch'). They arrive in the intestine via the lungs, bronchi, and upper alimentary tract.

ANODYNE. Anything that relieves pain.

ANOPHELES is a genus of biting *mosquitoes, containing many species. Some are important vectors of *malaria. Anopheline mosquitoes, which can also transmit *filariasis and *arbovirus infection, are thus pests of world-wide medical, social, and economic significance.

ANORECTICS are substances that depress appetite. They fall into two main categories: bulk-forming agents, like methylcellulose and sterculia, which are claimed to promote feelings of satiety; and centrally acting appetite suppressants, which, although effective in the short term, cause central nervous system stimulation and hence carry a risk of drug dependence (see SUBSTANCE ABUSE), e.g. diethylpropion, phentermine, and mazindol. *Amphetamine and related drugs also suppress appetite, but are too addictive to be safely used in treating *obesity.

ANOREXIA. Lack of appetite. See also ANOREXIA NERVOSA.

ANOREXIA NERVOSA, often called the 'slimmer's disease', is nine times commoner in women, usually young, than men. Between 5 and 10 per cent of sufferers die as a direct or indirect result of *starvation. The essential feature is an overwhelming desire to achieve and maintain a low body weight. In about one-third of cases, fasting is periodically interrupted by eating 'binges' (*bulimia) followed by induced vomiting; some bulimic individuals are sexually overactive, although in all wasted patients anovulatory *amenorrhoea is the rule. Less constant features are sleeplessness and obsession with exercise. The condition was described by *Gull in 1868.

ANOSMIA is inability to smell; it may be congenital or due to several acquired causes, including local conditions of the *nasopharynx. Lesions of the olfactory tract (which carries smell sensation to the brain) can occur in brain disease and may follow head injury. It can also be due to *cadmium poisoning.

ANOXIA. Lack of *oxygen.

ANTABUSE®. See DISULFIRAM.

ANTACID. Any substance given to counteract gastric acidity and to relieve symptoms of gastro-oesophageal reflux, gastritis, and peptic ulcer (see GASTROENTEROLOGY), and to promote healing of a *peptic ulcer. Numerous official and proprietary preparations are available, almost all being weak basic compounds of sodium, calcium, aluminium, or magnesium, or mixtures of these. They neutralize hydrochloric acid in the stomach and inactivate *pepsin. Their action is normally brief. In the longer term they raise the volume and acidity of gastric secretion by stimulating the release of *gastrin.

ANTENATAL CLINICS. See MATERNITY SERVICES; OBSTETRICS.

ANTENATAL DIAGNOSIS (or prenatal diagnosis) of fetal diseases and abnormalities by means of various techniques is an ever-widening subject. Many (e.g. *rhesus factor incompatibility, abnormal fetal positions) are revealed during normal antenatal care. Others (e.g. *spina bifida, *Down's syndrome, and a growing number of genetically determined disorders) require special investigations (such as *amniocentesis, *fetoscopy, or chorionic biopsy); these are not entirely without risk to continuation of the pregnancy and are thus reserved for cases where the likelihood of fetal abnormality is above average. See also OBSTETRICS.

ANTERIOR TIBIAL SYNDROME. Pain and swelling in the front of one or both lower legs, usually following unaccustomed exercise. It is due to swelling of the tibialis anterior muscle, causing *ischaemia as blood vessels are compressed; rarely ischaemic *necrosis occurs. The condition is also called the anterior tibial compartment syndrome, 'shin splints', or the tibialis anterior (anticus) syndrome.

ANTHELMINTHICS are drugs used to destroy or eliminate parasitic worms (*helminths). Compounds used for treating the commoner varieties of *helminthiasis include mebendazole (*threadworm, *roundworm, and *hookworm infestations), piperazine (threadworm, roundworm), thiabendazole (threadworm, roundworm, hookworm, and *strongyloides), bephenium (roundworm and hookworm), niclosamide (*tapeworm), tetrachloroethylene (hookworm), pyrantel (hookworm), niridazole (*bilharzia, *guinea worm), oxamniquine (bilharzia), metrifonate (bilharzia), stibocaptate (bilharzia), and diethylcarbamazine (all forms of *filariasis including *onchocerciasis).

ANTHRACOSIS is deposition of *carbon particles or coal dust in the lungs, also called coalminer's lung. This form of *pneumoconiosis, unlike that associated with silicon deposition, leads to little or no impairment of function and is usually asymptomatic.

ANTHRAX is a zoonotic (see ZOONOSIS) bacillary infection primarily of herbivorous animals; it may be acquired by man from infected carcasses or hides. Most cases are cutaneous ('malignant pustule') but dangerous and even fatal infections can involve the lungs ('wool-sorters' disease'), intestine, and central nervous system. The causative organism, *Bacillus anthracis*, is *spore-forming and toxigenic. It is sensitive to *penicillin and other antibiotics. Although cutaneous anthrax has a significant mortality, intestinal anthrax is more often fatal than not, and pulmonary infection almost always so.

ANTHROPOLOGY is the study of man in the widest sense, including his origins, historical and cultural development, and racial characteristics.

ANTHROPOMETRY is the measurement and study of the physical characteristics of the human body; a branch of anthropology.

ANTIBACTERIAL CHEMOTHERAPY is the treatment of bacterial infections with chemical compounds which destroy or inhibit the growth of the micro-organisms concerned without disturbing the metabolism of normal tissue. See also SULPHONAMIDES; PHARMACOLOGY.

ANTIBIOTIC. Any of a class of substances produced by living organisms and having the capacity to destroy or to inhibit the growth of micro-organisms. The term is also applied to synthetic analogues of such substances used in the treatment of infections. See also ANTI-INFECTIVE DRUGS; INFECTIOUS DISEASE; PHARMACOLOGY.

ANTIBODY. Any of a class of *proteins able to react with and neutralize specific *antigens. Antibodies are *serum *globulins with a wide range of specificity for different antigens. See also IMMUNOLOGY.

ANTICHOLINERGIC. Having an action that interferes with impulse transmission in the *parasympathetic nervous system, thus opposing the action of *acetylcholine.

ANTICHOLINESTERASE. Any drug that inhibits the *enzyme (acetylcholinesterase) responsible for destroying the neurotransmitter *acetylcholine, thereby potentiating the latter's action.

ANTICOAGULANTS inhibit blood *coagulation. They are used to treat conditions where there is undesirable or excessive clotting, such as *thrombophlebitis and pulmonary *embolism, or when there is an increased risk of such clotting (e.g. certain surgical operations, including the insertion of prosthetic heart valves). The usual agent employed is either *heparin, which is short acting and must be given by injection, or an oral anticoagulant, which inhibits the hepatic synthesis of the vitamin-K-dependent coagulation factors (prothrombin, factors VII, IX, and X), such as *warfarin sodium. Their principal benefit is in the prevention and treatment of venous thrombosis. In *arteries, where flow is faster, thrombi consist mainly of *platelets with little *fibrin. Any success anticoagulants have had in lessening mortality after *myocardial infarction is probably due to a decreased incidence of deep-vein thrombosis rather than to limiting thrombosis in the coronary arteries themselves.

ANTICONVULSANT. Any drug or method that prevents or reduces the frequency of *epileptic fits.

ANTIDEPRESSANTS are drugs used to combat psychiatric *depression. There are two main groups: the tricyclic and related antidepressant drugs (such as amitriptyline, imipramine, chlomipramine, etc.) and the *monoamine-oxidase inhibitors (MAOI), such as phenelzine, iproniazid, tranylcypromine, etc.). The former are preferred because of their greater effectiveness, and because the MAOIs may have troublesome interactions with other drugs and certain foodstuffs.

There is now general agreement that cerebral *stimulants should not be used to treat depression; although they may elevate mood, they are dangerous, and dangerously addictive (e.g. *amphetamines, *cocaine). See also PSYCHIATRY.

ANTIDIURETIC HORMONE, ADH, is one of the hormones stored and released by the neurohypophysis or posterior *pituitary gland. ADH, also known as vasopressin, stimulates renal retention of water and raises the arterial *blood pressure.

ANTIDOTE. A substance that counteracts a poison.

ANTIGEN. Any substance recognized by the immune system as 'non-self' and thus able to elicit a specific immune response, i.e. the production of specific *antibody and/or sensitized *lymphocytes. Antigens may be soluble or particulate, and are either *proteins or *polysaccharides. See also IMMUNOLOGY.

ANTIHISTAMINES are drugs that oppose the action of *histamine and are therefore used in conditions associated with *allergy or *anaphylaxis. There are many examples and numerous trade names; many are equally effective. They are of value in urticaria, allergic rashes, hay fever, vasomotor rhinitis, insect bites, and drug allergy, and also have antiemetic qualities. Some have the disadvantages of causing drowsiness, impairing driving performance, and enhancing the effects of alcohol. See also H₂ RECEPTOR ANTAGONISTS.

ANTI-INFECTIVE DRUGS. Drugs used in the treatment of infections can be divided into eight categories: (1) antibacterial drugs; (2) antiviral drugs; (3) antiprotozoal drugs; (4) anthelminthic drugs; (5) antitrematodal drugs; (6) antifungal drugs; (7) monoclonal antibodies; (8) adjuvant drugs.

Antibacterial drugs

Antibacterial drugs include antibiotics and chemotherapeutic agents. The strict definition of an *antibiotic is a substance produced by living organisms, which is capable of destroying or inhibiting the growth of *micro-organisms. However, the term is loosely applied to any drug used in the treatment of bacterial infections, including various chemically synthesized drugs, such as the sulphonamides, trimethoprim, and some antituberculous drugs. The main classes of antibacterial drugs are listed in Table 1, along with some examples of drugs belonging to those classes, and the infections treated by these drugs. The modes of action of some anti-infective drugs are shown in Fig. 1.

*Penicillins

Although the anti-infective actions of certain moulds had been known for several centuries, it was not until *Fleming's observations in 1929 that it was appreciated that anti-infective agents might be isolated from moulds. The original penicillin, benzylpenicillin or penicillin G, was isolated from *Penicillium notatum* in Oxford in 1940 by *Florey, *Chain, and Heatley, and was first used in the treatment of infections in 1941, again in Oxford.

Since then many forms of penicillin have been synthesized, and many are in current use. Penicillin G and its oral equivalent, penicillin V, are effective against many *staphylococci, *streptococci, *meningococci, and *gonococci. They are also effective in *spirochaete infections (for example, *syphilis) and in infections caused by actinomycetes (*actinomycosis). Ampicillin and amoxycillin are not as effective against cocci, but have additional effects against certain Gram-negative organisms, including *Escherichia coli*. However, resistance to the penicillins has developed among certain organisms, for which new varieties of penicillins have been developed. In particular, the emergence of resistant staphylococci has led to the development of flucloxacillin, which is very specific in its action, and difficulties in treating infections with *Pseudomonas aeruginosa* have led to the development of piperacillin, ticarcillin, and other similar compounds. (See also adjuvant drugs below.)

The penicillins are very safe and can be given in large doses without risk of major toxicity. However, in about 10 per cent of people they may cause *allergic reactions, and this precludes their use in those people.

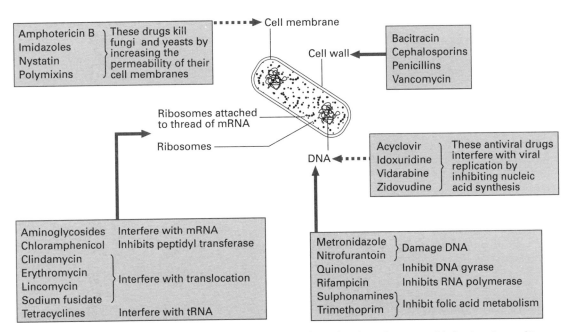

Fig. 1 A stylized representation of a bacterium, showing the sites of action of some anti-infective drugs. (From Grahame-Smith, D. G. and Aronson, J. K. (1992). *The Oxford textbook of clinical pharmacology and drug therapy*, 2nd edn. Oxford University Press.)

Table 1 Some antibacterial drugs, the organisms that are usually sensitive to them, and the infections for which they are usually first choice

Penicillins
 Benzylpenicillin
  Streptococcus pyogenes   Acute follicular tonsillitis
                                    Cellulitis/erysipelas
                                    Acute otitis media (over 5 yr; see also co-amoxiclav)
  'Viridans' streptococci   Endocarditis (+ gentamicin)
  Streptococcus pneumoniae   Pneumococcal pneumonia
  Enterococcus faecalis   Endocarditis (+ gentamicin)
  Neisseria gonorrhoeae   Gonorrhoea
  Neisseria meningitidis   Meningococcal meningitis
  Treponema pallidum   Syphilis

 Amoxycillin
  Streptococcus pneumoniae   Exacerbations of chronic bronchitis, acute bronchitis/pneumonia
  Streptococcus pyogenes   Acute otitis media (under 5 yr)
  Streptococcus pneumoniae   Sinusitis
  Streptococcus pyogenes   Sinusitis
  Escherichia coli   Urinary tract infection (+ clavulanic acid if resistant)
  Enterococcus faecalis   Urinary tract infection (+ clavulanic acid if resistant)
  Listeria monocytogenes   Listerial septicaemia and meningitis

 Co-amoxiclav (amoxycillin + clavulanic acid)
  Haemophilus influenzae   Exacerbations of chronic bronchitis, acute bronchitis, acute
                                       pneumonia, sinusitis, acute otitis media (under 5 yr)

 Flucloxacillin
  Staphylococcus aureus   Wounds, boils (if necessary), and abscesses (penicillin-resistant)
                                    Septic arthritis
                                    Osteomyelitis
                                    Pneumonia
                                    Endocarditis
                                    Impetigo

 Piperacillin
  Pseudomonas aeruginosa   Septicaemia (+ gentamicin)
                                    Urinary tract infection
                                    Pneumonia (+ gentamicin)

Tetracyclines (for example, tetracycline, oxytetracycline, doxycycline)
  Coxiella burnetti   Q fever
  Rickettsiae   Typhus
  Chlamydiae   Trachoma
                                    Psittacosis
                                    Lymphogranuloma venereum
                                    Non-specific urethritis

Aminoglycosides (for example, gentamicin, amikacin, tobramycin)
  'Viridans' streptococci   Endocarditis (+ benzylpenicillin)
  Enterococcus faecalis   Endocarditis (+ benzylpenicillin)
  Escherichia coli
  Klebsiella
  Enterobacter   ⎫   In severe infections, for example septicaemia, acute
  Proteus   ⎬   pyelonephritis, pneumonia, biliary tract infection
  Pseudomonas aeruginosa   ⎭   Urinary tract infection
  (+ azlocillin)   Pneumonia

Table 1 (*cont.*)

Macrolides (for example, erythromycin)	
Legionella pneumophila	Legionnaires' pneumonia
Mycoplasma pneumoniae	Mycoplasmal pneumonia

Trimethoprim
Escherichia coli	Pyelonephritis
	Urinary tract infection
Haemophilus influenzae	Exacerbations of chronic bronchitis
Streptococcus pneumoniae	Exacerbations of chronic bronchitis

Chloramphenicol
Salmonella typhi	Typhoid fever
Haemophilus influenzae	Meningitis

Metronidazole
Anaerobic organisms	Intra-abdominal infections, for example:
(for example *Bacteroides* spp.)	liver abscess
	pelvic inflammatory disease
	cholangitis
	peritonitis
	female genital tract infections
	Lung abscess
	Brain abscess
	Endocarditis
Clostridium difficile	Antibiotic-associated diarrhoea

Vancomycin
Staphylococcus aureus	Infections resistant to methicillin
Coagulase-negative staphylococci	All infections
Clostridium difficile	Antibiotic-associated diarrhoea resistant to metronidazole

Cephalosporins

Searching for organisms that might produce antibiotics, Giuseppe Brotzu discovered a mould, *Cephalosporium acremonium*, in the sea water near a Sardinian sewer. Following his preliminary experiments, cephalosporins were extracted from the mould juice in Oxford in 1949, and numerous derivatives have since been developed. They are effective against a wide range of bacteria, and are particularly useful in the treatment of infections caused by *Haemophilus influenzae* and *Pseudomonas aeruginosa*, in addition to infections by organisms that are sensitive to the penicillins. They are generally used as second-line or third-line agents, but are sometimes used as first-line treatment in severe infections in hospitals. The cephalosporins rarely cause adverse effects, except for allergic reactions, which may occur in 5 per cent of individuals.

Tetracyclines

Tetracyclines were first isolated from *Streptomyces aureofaciens* in 1945. They are effective against a wide range of organisms, and are used in first-line treatment in infections caused by *Coxiella burnetti* (*Q fever), other rickettsiae (*typhus diseases), *Chlamydia psittaci*

(*psittacosis), and other chlamydiae (e.g. in *lymphogranuloma venereum and *trachoma). They are also commonly used in infections of the skin. Their main adverse effects are nausea, vomiting, and diarrhoea, and if they cause dehydration in patients with impaired renal function they may cause acute renal failure. They should not be used in children or pregnant women, because they are deposited in growing bones and teeth, and cause damage there.

Aminoglycosides

The first clinically useful aminoglycoside, streptomycin, was isolated from *Streptomyces griseus* by Selman *Waksman in 1943. It was found to be effective in guinea-pigs infected with *tuberculosis, and this led to its successful introduction into clinical practice. Since then several other antibiotics of this group have been discovered, including gentamicin, amikacin, and netilmicin. Streptomycin apart, they are used in the treatment of severe systemic infections, especially those caused by *Escherichia coli*, *Proteus mirabilis*, *Pseudomonas aeruginosa*, and *Klebsiella pneumoniae*. They are also used in combination with penicillin in the treatment of streptococcal endocarditis. Neomycin is used in a variety of local infections of the skin, ears, and eyes. These drugs are very toxic after systemic administration, and must be used carefully. Their main adverse effects are renal damage and damage to the eighth cranial nerve, which controls hearing and some aspects of balance.

Macrolides

The most commonly used macrolide, erythromycin, was isolated from *Streptomyces erythreus* in 1952. For many years it was reserved for the treatment of infections in patients who would have been treated with a penicillin, were it not for allergy. However, in recent years it has come to be used as the treatment of choice for infections caused by *Legionella pneumophila* (*Legionnaires' disease) and *Mycoplasma pneumoniae*. Although erythromycin was for some time the only example of a macrolide antibiotic in general clinical use, its new uses have stimulated research into new varieties of macrolides, including azithromycin and clarithromycin. The major adverse effects of these drugs are liver damage and, more commonly, nausea, vomiting, and anorexia.

Quinolones

The quinolones are examples of synthetic antibacterial drugs. The first example, *nalidixic acid, was synthesized as an analogue of a by-product of *chloroquine synthesis, and was introduced in the treatment of urinary tract infections in 1962. In recent years, analogues, of which ciprofloxacin is the most commonly used, have emerged and are effective in the treatment of infections due to a wide range of organisms, including *Staphylococcus aureus*, *Neisseria gonorrhoeae*, *Escherichia coli*, *Haemophilus influenzae*, *Pseudomonas aeruginosa*, *Campylobacter*, *Shigella*, and *Salmonella*. Although they are widely used, they are not generally indicated as first choice in those infections. The quinolones commonly cause nausea, vomiting and diarrhoea, headache, dizziness and tiredness, and occasionally skin eruptions. They may worsen *epilepsy and they are not given to infants or pregnant women because of evidence from animal studies that they may damage the joints. In patients whose red blood cells are deficient in the enzyme *glucose 6-phosphate dehydrogenase they may cause haemolysis.

Sulphonamides

The sulphonamides, the first clinically effective anti-infective drugs, were introduced by Gerhard *Domagk in 1935, following his experiments with azo dyes and their effects on bacterial growth. The first sulphonamide, Prontosil Rubrum, was in fact an inactive compound that was metabolized to the active drug after administration. However, active sulphonamides were subsequently synthesized and were widely used in the treatment of a large number of infections. They were gradually superseded by the penicillins and other antibiotics in the 1940s and after, and they are now little used, apart from sulphamethoxazole, which in combination with trimethoprim is known as co-trimoxazole. This is used in treating infections due to *Haemophilus influenzae* and in the treatment of pneumonia due to *Pneumocystis carinii*, an infection which is a serious complication of *AIDS. The sulphonamides have many adverse reactions, including allergy, renal damage, and *bone-marrow toxicity. This has been a contributory factor to the decline in their use.

Trimethoprim

The discovery in 1952 that dihydrofolate reductase was a key enzyme in the utilization of *folic acid by bacteria led to the development of a series of reductase inhibitors, of which trimethoprim was found to be antibacterial. For some years it was used in combination with sulphonamides in the treatment of infections of the urinary tract by organisms such as *Escherichia coli* and *Proteus mirabilis*, but it is now used on its own for that purpose. It has few adverse effects.

Metronidazole

Metronidazole is a chemically synthesized drug, one of a group of imidazoles. It was first synthesized in 1957 and was used initially for the treatment of infections caused by the protozoan *Trichomonas vaginalis*. However, it has since been found to be effective against anaerobic organisms, such as species of *Bacteroides*, for which it is the treatment of first choice. It is also used in the treatment of other protozoan infections, including *amoebiasis and *giardiasis. Other imidazoles (see below) are used in the treatment of fungal infections. Metronidazole rarely causes adverse effects during short-term therapy but produces a severe reaction if the individual taking it drinks *alcohol.

Chloramphenicol

Chloramphenicol was isolated in 1947 from *Streptomyces venezuelae*. It was the first so-called broad-spectrum antibiotic, having activity against a very wide range of organisms, including cocci, bacilli, rickettsiae, and chlamydiae. However, its use was limited because of its severe adverse effects, particularly bone-marrow damage, an idiosyncratic reaction that occurs in about 1 in 250 000 individuals. Nevertheless, it is still the drug of first choice in meningitis due to *Haemophilus influenzae* and in acute *typhoid fever. It is also very commonly used for local treatment of infections of the eyes.

Antituberculous drugs

The rifamycins were isolated from *Streptomyces mediterranei* in 1959. One of these, rifampicin, was found to be effective in the treatment of tuberculosis and has since become one of the mainstays of treatment. Other compounds have been developed as a result of studies of chemical compounds with known tuberculostatic activity. Thiacetazone was developed in the 1940s from a group of compounds called thiosemicarbazides.

Although it was subsequently replaced by safer drugs, it has again recently emerged as a valuable addition to treatment. In 1951 a hydrazide derivative, isoniazid, was synthesized and it is still used in the treatment of tuberculosis. Further investigation of these types of compounds led to the development of pyrazinamide, now a first-line drug in developing countries, and ethionamide, a third-line drug (because of its toxicity). The discovery in 1940 that salicylic acid affected oxygen utilization in the tuberculosis bacterium led to the development of *para*-aminosalicylic acid (PAS), which was used for many years in the treatment of tuberculosis, but which has now been superseded by modern drugs. Ethambutol was developed following the discovery that the ethylenediamines had antitubercular activity. It is still used in combination with rifampicin, isoniazid, and pyrazinamide as standard first-line treatment. The antitubercular drugs have varying adverse effects, but most of them can cause liver damage and have to be used with care in people who have *cirrhosis, in whom tuberculosis is not uncommon. Other effects include damage to the eyes (ethambutol), peripheral nerves (isoniazid), and hearing (streptomycin).

Antiviral drugs

One of the disappointments of the antibiotics was their total ineffectiveness against infections with viruses. However, during the search for antitumour drugs in the 1950s, investigations on halogenated nucleosides showed that idoxuridine had therapeutic efficacy against *Herpesvirus* infections. Nucleosides are important structural components of the nucleic acids, *DNA and *RNA. Modern antiviral drugs are almost all based on the structures of these nucleosides (notably thymidine), but these analogues require activation by intracellular metabolism, and this is generally done with greater specificity by viruses than by human cells. This confers therapeutic activity on such agents with minimal toxicity. Drugs of this kind include acyclovir, used for treating *Herpesvirus* infections, ganciclovir (*cytomegalovirus infection), idoxuridine (*Herpesvirus* infections), tribavirin (infection caused by the respiratory syncytial virus), vidarabine (*Herpesvirus* infections), and zidovudine and didanosine (*HIV infection).

Antiprotozoal drugs

It has been known since the 17th century that Jesuits' bark, the active ingredient of which is *quinine, is effective in the treatment of 'ague', i.e. *malaria. However, it was not until the synthesis of pamaquin in 1925 that the modern series of antimalarial drugs was developed. This group of drugs includes mepacrine, chloroquine, and primaquine, all structurally related to quinine. Their mode of action is unknown, but they seem to bind to components of the DNA of the parasite. Investigations of other structures in the 1940s yielded the unrelated compounds proguanil and pyrimethamine. The antimalarial drugs have relatively few

adverse effects, but they can cause haemolysis in people whose red cells are deficient in the enzyme *glucose 6-phosphate dehydrogenase. Occasionally there may be allergic reactions. During long-term therapy, chloroquine can damage the retina.

A major problem in the treatment of malaria is the rapid development of resistance of the malarial parasite to currently used drugs. Indeed, the rate of emergence of resistance is currently outstripping the emergence of new effective drugs. One promising group of agents are those that are based on compounds found in *Artemisia* species (for example artemether), but it is not clear how long these drugs will prove effective against the parasite.

Other important protozoan diseases include amoebiasis and giardiasis, for which the imidazoles metronidazole (see above) and tinidazole are effective.

With the discovery in 1906 of the effectiveness of salts of antimony in the treatment of *leishmaniasis, various antimonials were developed for the treatment of this protozoan disease. Currently in use are the pentavalent antimony salts (sodium stibogluconate and meglumine antimoniate). An unrelated drug, pentamidine, is also used.

Anthelminthic drugs

The imidazoles were first identified as having antiinfective properties when a substance called azomycin was isolated from a species of *Streptomyces* in 1953. The nitroimidazole metronidazole was subsequently synthesized in 1957, and since then many related compounds have been synthesized. These include mebendazole, albendazole, and niridazole. Cousins of these compounds, the aminothiazoles, have also been developed, and of these levamisole is in current use. These drugs are used variously in the treatment of infestations with *worms, including roundworm, whipworm, hookworm, threadworm, pinworm, and tapeworm.

Antitrematodal drugs

Older drugs, such as oxamniquine and lucanthone, have been superseded by praziquantel. It is used in the treatment of infections with trematodes, including *schistosomiasis, liver- *fluke infections (for example, opisthorchiasis, clonorchiasis, and fascioliasis), intestinal infections (for example, fasciolopsiasis and echinostomiasis), and lung-fluke infections (paragonimiasis).

Antifungal drugs

In 1950 a substance called nystatin was isolated from *Streptomyces noursci* at the New York State Department of Health (hence the name of the compound). It was followed 3 years later by the isolation of a similar compound, amphotericin, from *Streptomyces nodosus*. Both of these drugs were found to be effective against fungi, intravenous infusions of amphotericin being used for the treatment of severe systemic infections.

Several imidazoles, developed since the initial discovery of metronidazole, are now also used for the treatment of fungal infections. These include clotrimazole, econazole, fluconazole, itraconazole, ketoconazole, miconazole, and tioconazole. They are used to treat infections with *Candida albicans* and a variety of dermatophytes, including *Tinea cruris, pedis, corporis, capitis,* and *versicolor.* These drugs are also used in the treatment of systemic fungal infections, including candidiasis, histoplasmosis, coccidioidomycosis, blastomycosis, cryptococcosis, and aspergillosis. Of the antifungal drugs, amphotericin is the most toxic and, in particular, can cause renal damage. The imidazoles can cause liver damage.

Monoclonal antibodies
The discovery, in recent years, of monoclonal antibodies has led to the development of antibodies that are effective against the shock-causing toxins that are produced by some organisms, notably Gram-negative bacteria. These antibodies are under investigation.

Adjuvant drugs
One mechanism whereby bacteria become resistant to the actions of penicillins is by breaking them down with an enzyme, penicillinase. Clavulanic acid, although not itself antibacterial, inhibits the penicillinase and thus reverses this form of resistance. Other drugs are used to prolong the actions of antibacterial drugs in the body by inhibiting their elimination. For example, probenecid inhibits the renal excretion of the penicillins, and cilastatin inhibits the inactivation in the kidney of imipenem, a drug related to the penicillins.

J. K. ARONSON

ANTILYMPHOCYTE SERUM, or ALS, is an *immunosuppressive agent prepared by immunizing animals against human *lymphocytes. ALS, formerly but no longer used to combat rejection in organ transplantation, exerts its effect mainly by depleting the T-lymphocyte pool.

ANTIMETABOLITES are drugs that interfere with cell metabolism and are therefore used to treat various *cancers and *leukaemias. Antimetabolites act either by becoming incorporated into new nuclear material or by combining irreversibly with vital cellular *enzymes. An example is methotrexate, which inhibits the enzyme dihydrofolate reductase. Others include cytarabine, fluorouracil, mercaptopurine, thioguanine, and azathioprine (the last is commonly used as an *immunosuppressant). See also PHARMACOLOGY; ONCOLOGY.

ANTIMONY is a metallic element (symbol Sb, atomic number 51, relative atomic mass 121.75). It has no physiological role, but some compounds are used to treat protozoal and parasitic diseases, notably *trypanosomiasis, *leishmaniasis, and *schistosomiasis. Industrial antimony dust may be a carcinogen.

ANTINEOPLASTIC drugs are given to inhibit the growth of *cancers.

ANTINEOPLASTIC CHEMOTHERAPY is the treatment of *cancer with chemical agents; most are *cytotoxic drugs which destroy or inhibit the growth of rapidly dividing cells, whether normal or neoplastic. They are often more effective when used in combination rather than singly. Strictly speaking, the use of *corticosteroids and sex *hormones in treating certain malignant disorders also falls under this term. See also ONCOLOGY.

ANTIPHLOGISTIC. A medicinal agent intended to alleviate inflammation.

ANTIPYRETIC. Any medicine or procedure designed to reduce fever.

ANTISEPSIS is the prevention of infection by destroying or inhibiting the growth of pathogenic microorganisms.

ANTISEPTICS are agents that inhibit the growth of (although they may not destroy) micro-organisms such as bacteria and viruses. Many chemicals possess this action, including familiar substances such as *ethanol (surgical spirit), *zinc sulphate lotion, *potassium permanganate solution. There are very many trade names, e.g. Dettol® (chloroxylenol), Hibitane® (chlorhexidine gluconate), Cetavlon® (cetrimide), etc. Antiseptics are used to prepare the skin before operations, and whenever it is desired to achieve 'surgical cleanliness'.

ANTISERUM is *serum containing known *antibody, which may be of human or animal origin.

ANTISPASMODIC. Any drug used to counteract *spasm of smooth muscle, usually in the gastrointestinal tract. Antispasmodic drugs are either *anticholinergic agents such as atropine or propantheline; or spasmolytics like papaverine, alverine, and mebeverine, which act directly on smooth muscle but are not anticholinergic.

ANTITHROMBIN. Any of a number of substances, some being physiological, the action of which is opposed to that of thrombin and which therefore tends to inhibit blood *coagulation.

ANTITOXIN. Antibody to a *toxin, which may be bacterial (diphtheria, tetanus, botulism), animal (snake, scorpion, spider, bee), or plant (fungi).

ANTIVIVISECTIONISTS. Those opposed to experiments on living animals.

ANURIA is total failure of *urine production.

ANUS. The posterior opening of the *alimentary canal.

ANXIETY is an unpleasant mental state of foreboding, uneasiness, and apprehension approaching fear; it may be accompanied by signs of sympathetic overactivity such as *tremor, *sweating, and *tachycardia. In appropriate circumstances, such a state may be simply a physiological preparation for whatever ordeal or difficult task lies ahead. When inappropriate, excessive, or prolonged, it is a symptom of mental disorder.

AORTA. The main trunk of the arterial system. The term was first applied to this vessel by *Aristotle. The aorta arises from the left ventricle of the heart, passes upwards (ascending aorta), bends (aortic arch), and then proceeds downwards through the thorax and abdomen (descending aorta), ending at the level of the fourth lumbar vertebra by dividing into the right and left common iliac arteries.

AORTIC ARCH. See AORTA.

AORTIC INCOMPETENCE is present when a structural defect of the aortic *valve allows retrograde flow or regurgitation from the *aorta back into the left *ventricle during the *diastolic phase of the cardiac cycle, when the valve is normally tightly shut. Diastolic filling of the ventricle is thus increased and the chamber needs to pump a correspondingly increased *stroke volume; this overload may eventually cause left ventricular failure. Aortic incompetence can occur acutely during bacterial *endocarditis, but in most instances has been present for some time before symptoms develop. The lesion is most often a late result of cardiac damage by *rheumatic fever (about 50 per cent of cases); other causes are congenital defect (about 10 per cent), *syphilis (decreasing but still about 10 per cent), and some less common conditions including *ankylosing spondylitis and *Reiter's syndrome.

AORTOGRAPHY is radiographic visualization of the *aorta and its branches by serial exposures after injecting into the circulation a radiopaque medium.

APATHY. Absence of feeling, emotion, or interest; indifference.

APES. Monkeys; primates (excluding man). More particularly, they are the larger tailless monkeys, including the gorilla, chimpanzee, orang-utan, and gibbon, comprising the family Pongidae. In the evolutionary system they are the closest surviving relatives of man.

APGAR SCORE. A method of quantifying the condition of a newborn infant by assessing several physiological values, such as heart rate, muscle tone, etc., on an agreed scale and deriving an overall numerical value (named after Dr Virginia Apgar who introduced the method).

APHAKIA. Absence of the lens of the eye.

APHASIA is loss or impairment of language function due to brain damage, causing defective speech, reading, comprehension of speech, and writing. Since in most right-handed subjects language function resides in the left half of the brain, aphasia is most often produced by damage to the left *cerebral hemisphere. See LANGUAGE, COGNITION, AND HIGHER CEREBRAL FUNCTION.

APHONIA. Loss of voice; inability to phonate.

APHRODISIAC. A substance that induces sexual arousal.

APLASIA is partial or complete failure of development of a tissue or organ.

APLASTIC ANAEMIA (ANEMIA) is a serious form of *anaemia due to depression of blood formation in the *bone marrow. It can result from many genetic and environmental causes.

APNOEA (APNEA) Cessation of breathing; respiratory arrest. See also SLEEP APNOEA.

APOCHROMATIC. Free, or relatively so, from *chromatic aberration.

APOLLO was the Greek sun-god, the father of *Aesculapius and a patron *inter alia* of medicine, although he was also the god who sent plagues.

APOMORPHINE is an *opium alkaloid. It has a specific stimulant effect on the vomiting centre, and is a powerful *emetic.

APOPLEXY. A stroke; a sudden impairment of brain function due to haemorrhage from, or obstruction of, cerebral blood vessels. The term is also applied to vascular catastrophes in other organs (e.g. pituitary apoplexy, ovarian apoplexy).

APOTHECARIES. 'Apothecary' was an early term for one who prepared and sold medicinal substances. Since about 1800, this has been done by druggists and *pharmacists. In the 18th century apothecaries were also general medical practitioners, and the term may still be legally applied to those who belong to the Society of Apothecaries or who hold a medical qualification from that Society (see MEDICAL COLLEGES, ETC. OF THE UK).

APOTHECARIES ACT 1815. This enactment required all apothecaries in England and Wales, except those already in practice, to be examined and licensed by the *Society of Apothecaries after serving 5 years' apprenticeship. The Society was empowered to prosecute offenders. The Act was a major landmark in the control of medical practice, imposing for the first time some uniformity of standard. The Society later required for licensing not only the 5 years' apprenticeship, but also certificates of attendance at courses of lectures in anatomy, physiology, and the theory and practice of medicine. In addition, it introduced a rule that candidates for examination must have 'walked the wards' of a recognized hospital for at least 6 months.

APPENDICITIS is inflammation of the *appendix, a common cause of acute abdominal illness.

APPENDIX. Unless otherwise qualified, this term refers to the vermiform appendix, a worm-like, and apparently functionless appendage attached to and continuous with the *caecum of the large intestine; it is a common site of inflammation.

APPERCEPTION is perception accompanied by recognition, identification, and assimilation of pre-existing knowledge; some educational psychologists regard it as the fundamental process in acquiring new knowledge.

APPRENTICESHIP. The principle of apprenticeship has been central to medical training from the earliest days of the profession, as exemplified in the opening phrases of the *Hippocratic Oath. In the UK, it was formalized by the *Apothecaries Act of 1815, and only towards the end of the 19th century did apprenticeship begin to assume a place secondary to academic medical school training in medical education. The tradition persists in the grouping of present-day clinical students into 'firms' attached to individual physicians and surgeons in teaching hospitals.

APPROVED NAMES are the official names of medicinal substances, also known as generic or non-proprietary names. In the UK these are agreed by the *British Pharmacopoeia Commission. They may be followed by an indication of the status of the name e.g. BP, BPC, BNF, etc. See also PHARMACY AND PHARMACISTS.

APRAXIA is a specific inability to perform particular voluntary learned acts in the absence of primary motor or sensory impairment. It indicates organic brain damage to the dominant *cerebral hemisphere.

APUD CELLS. Cells of neuroectodermal origin found in various endocrine tissues and acronymically named for their property of amine precursor uptake and decarboxylation. They occur in association with certain tumours in which ectopic *hormone production is a feature (e.g. oat cell carcinoma of the lung, *argentaffinoma, thymoma), and are also thought to be involved in the pathogenesis of certain genetically determined syndromes of multiple endocrine gland hyperfunction.

AQUEDUCT OF SYLVIUS. The cerebral aqueduct, a short narrow passage in the *midbrain connecting the cavities of the third and fourth *cerebral ventricles.

ARACHNID. Any member of the class Arachnida (phylum Arthropoda). Of the 12 classes of arthropods, the Arachnida and the Insecta (*insects) are the two of most medical significance. Arachnids include *scorpions, *spiders, *mites, *ticks, harvestmen, and king-crabs.

ARACHNODACTYLY is literally 'spider fingers', a condition in which the fingers and toes are abnormally long and hyperextensible. It may be associated with other skeletal abnormalities, and with ocular, cardiac, and aortic defects (Marfan's syndrome). It is inherited as an autosomal dominant trait, although many cases occur sporadically.

ARACHNOID means literally resembling a spider's web; when otherwise unqualified, the word is taken to mean arachnoid mater, the fine serous membrane which is the middle of the three covering the brain and spinal cord. See MENINGES.

ARACHNOIDITIS. Inflammation of the *arachnoid.

ARBOVIRUS. A member of a group of *viruses transmitted by arthropods (see ARACHNID); the name is a contraction of the words *arthropod-borne virus*. An arbovirus is one that multiplies in an arthropod and is thereafter transmitted to a vertebrate. About 100 arboviruses are known to infect man. They include the agents of *yellow fever, *dengue, *sandfly fever, virus *encephalitides, and viral haemorrhagic fevers.

ARBUTHNOT, JOHN (1667–1735). British physician and writer. A wit and a friend of Pope, Gay, and Swift, he contributed to *The Memoirs of Martinus Scriblerus* (1714) and wrote *The History of John Bull* (1712), being the first to use this name for the archetypal Englishman.

ARCHAEUS. The immaterial principle proposed by *Paracelsus as the force that energizes all living matter.

ARCHETYPE. An original model or pattern; a prototype. In jungian *psychology, archetype is a pervasive symbol, idea, or image that forms part of the collective unconscious.

ARCHIATRUS. A chief physician, especially one appointed to attend a monarch.

ARDERNE, JOHN OF (*fl.* 1370). British surgeon. John of Arderne was a layman untrained in medicine, but a passable scholar. He was probably the first British surgeon. He was patronized by the Black Prince and is said to have been at Crécy. He wrote *De arte medica* (1370) and *Liber de fistula* (1370).

ARENAVIRUS. Any member of a genus of pleomorphic *ribonucleic acid (RNA) viruses so designated because of their sandy appearance on *electron microscopy. Their natural hosts are various wild rodents, from which man becomes infected. Examples are the agents of benign lymphocytic *meningitis (associated with the house mouse *Mus musculus*) and *Lassa fever (associated with the multimammate rat *Mastomys natalensis*).

ARETAEUS, OF CAPPADOCIA (*fl.* 2nd century AD). Greek physician. He noted the decussation of the pyramidal (corticospinal) tracts, first suggested the term '*diabetes', and insisted that the physician must show compassion for his patient.

ARGELLATA, PIETRO D' (?–1423). Italian surgeon. The most distinguished of Guy de *Chauliac's pupils, he taught surgery at Bologna. A skilled surgeon who used *sutures and drainage tubes, he was also a competent dentist. He wrote *Cirurgia* in six volumes (Venice, 1480).

ARGENTAFFINOMA. A *tumour arising from argentaffin cells (cells whose granules stain readily with silver and chromium salts and which synthesize and store *serotonin). Such neoplasms arise most often in the lower ileum, but also occur elsewhere in the gastrointestinal tract, bronchi, pancreas, bile duct, and ovaries. When malignant, they may cause extensive hepatic metastases and produce the 'carcinoid syndrome', a characteristic constellation of features (cyanotic flushing attacks, diarrhoea, bronchoconstriction, hypotension, oedema, etc.) due to excessive secretion of serotonin and related substances.

ARGYLL ROBERTSON, DOUGLAS MORAY COOPER LAMB (1837–1909). Scottish ophthalmologist. He described the classical sign, found in *neurosyphilis, especially *tabes dorsalis, that now bears his name. Argyll Robertson pupils are small, irregular, and unequal. They constrict as normal when the patient accommodates to near vision but do so poorly or not at all in response to light.

ARGYRIA is a grey discoloration of the skin due to the prolonged ingestion of silver salts.

ARISTOTLE (384–322 BC). Greek philosopher, biologist, psychologist, and logician. Born at Stagira on the north-west Aegean coast, the son of an Aesclepiad physician, he was a pupil of *Plato in Athens from the age of 17. When Plato died in 347 BC, Aristotle left Athens. He spent 2 years in Lesbos (Mytilene) undertaking biological research. Later he was summoned by Philip of Macedon to teach his son Alexander. When Alexander succeeded on his father's death, Aristotle returned to Athens and taught in the Lyceum, founding what became known as the Peripatetic School.

Aristotle has had a profound and lasting influence on scientific thought. He was the first to study the observable facts of nature, analysing and recording them precisely and in meticulous detail. Once data were assembled and classified he tried to find an explanation that would fit them all and, in thus deriving the universal from the particular, to construct an intelligible universe. His invention of the science of logic established scientific method. He divided reality into spheres of physics, biology, ethics, politics, and psychology, subjecting each to searching analysis. Aristotle is justifiably regarded as the founder of biology, zoology, comparative anatomy, embryology, and psychology.

ARLT, FERDINAND CARL, RITTER VON (1812–87). Austrian ophthalmologist. He made fundamental studies of ocular physiology and pathology. He devised many operations and designed numerous instruments used in ophthalmic surgery.

ARMED FORCES OF THE USA: MEDICAL SERVICE. Military medicine includes those aspects of *medical practice and *public health directed to diseases and injuries restricted to, or more common among, personnel in the armed forces, particularly during wartime. More so than in civilian life, the organization and management of medical systems play a very significant role in prevention and treatment. The medical programmes and people must be integrated into the operations of the armed forces they are supporting; they must be an accepted part of the army, navy, and air force to which they belong.

Origins
In the United States, military medicine began in the army under George Washington in 1775. On 27 July the Continental Congress established a 'hospital' and specified the pay and duties of a director-general and of *surgeons, nurses, etc. The director-general was to organize and control medical affairs after the British model, but he had authority only over the general hospitals; the regimental surgeons reported directly to their colonels. In contrast to Britain, there was no central organization for American navy medicine; each ship's surgeon was independently assigned to his ship in the Continental Navy.

Dr Benjamin Church, the first director-general, introduced examinations for appointment as surgeons and surgeon's mates in the army, and tried to centralize the purchase and distribution of drugs and supplies. His attempts to control the regimental medical system began a running feud that lasted beyond his brief tenure; discovered in treasonous correspondence with the British forces in Boston, he was court-martialled, jailed, released, and drowned when the ship taking him to the West Indies was lost.

Church's successors, John Morgan and William Shippen (who founded the first American medical school in Philadelphia in 1765), typified the approximately 400 American physicians holding the MD degree; the remaining 3000 practitioners were apprentice-trained. Most of the educated medical men in America served in the army. Both Morgan and Shippen were discharged as director-general, in part for active political roles and in part for persistent logistic failures and quarrels with line commanders. Not until 1781, under John Cochran, did the Medical Department acquire an organized, non-political direction, which paralleled the growth of similar organization and professionalism in the combat arms of the army.

The war inspired the publication of the first American medical texts, largely abstracts and compendia of European books, and an original text by Benjamin Rush, educating line officers about camp sanitation and their responsibility for the health of their commands. In 1777, Washington ordered that the army be inoculated against *smallpox. This was the first non-voluntary *immunization of an army, and resulted in a significant reduction of the death rate from smallpox over the next 6 years.

With peace and independence in 1783, the new nation reduced the entire army to a few hundred men and terminated the navy. The navy was re-established in 1794 for the quasi-war with France; naval officers continued to seek a permanent department, which materialized in 1798. Jennerian vaccination for smallpox and lemon juice for *scurvy were used on some ships by 1800. Each naval surgeon remained independently responsible to the captain of his ship, and there was no central medical organization.

Subsequent organization

Congress re-established a medical department during the war with Britain in 1812, and made it permanent in 1818. The *miasma theory of disease transmission led in 1818 to a requirement for medical officers to collect weather and disease data for each unit and post. Published by the surgeon-general, these were the first national health and meteorological *statistics. The medical department collected weather data until 1870, when the task was transferred to other agencies. 'Health of the army' reports began to be issued by the surgeon-general in 1818, the year in which medical officers were given relative military rank.

After the war of 1812, the expansion to the West began. In 1823, William *Beaumont, in a frontier post, began the 10 years of study of Alexis St Martin's gastric

fistula that brought him international fame when he published *Observations on the gastric juice* in 1833. Competitive entry examinations were reintroduced for the army medical corps in 1834; they had existed in the navy since 1828. For over 30 years these examinations were the only persisting licensing examinations in the United States; medical officers were examined for appointment until the Second World War.

The Barbary Coast Wars (1801–16) in the Mediterranean saw the establishment of the first naval hospitals and hospital ships; in the 1820s naval hospitals were established in Washington and Boston; by 1830, permanent naval hospitals were established at Portsmouth and Philadelphia. In 1842 the navy finally achieved centralized medical direction, with the establishment of a Bureau of Medicine and Surgery and the appointment of William P. C. Barton as chief of the bureau (the title of Surgeon-General was added in 1871). Relative rank for navy medical officers was granted in 1846, although regular commissions would not be awarded until 1899.

The Mexican–American War, the first major use of armed force for national expansion, was marked by the first military use of *ether in 1847, 6 months after Morton had demonstrated its use in Boston. That year, army medical officers were granted regular commissions as officers.

Consolidation

The Civil War (1861–65) found the army and navy and their medical departments woefully unprepared. The navy made a smoother transition to war, largely because there was essentially no Confederate navy to fight. Naval support of the army on the Mississippi River, which included the navy's first steam-propelled modern *hospital ship, provided the greatest naval medical challenge.

In the army, the Civil War saw great organizational reform and advances in the management of mass casualties. The first 'modern' war in terms of mass armies and technology was the last major combat before the 'germ theory' and the scientific method entered medicine. Basic field *hygiene and *sanitation, the importance of adequate rations, and the pivotal place of *nursing were lessons available from the medical disasters of the Crimean War. Surgeon-General William A. Hammond, appointed in 1862, reformed the supply system, supported the United States Sanitary Commission (similar to the modern *Red Cross), and insisted on the construction of large general hospitals. He produced a medical department that, by 1863, was efficient and effective.

Among his appointments in 1862 was that of Jonathan Letterman as the medical director of the Army of the Potomac, the most important of the Union Armies. Letterman, an experienced regular army physician, further developed the concepts of Dominique Larrey from the Napoleonic campaigns, but added new and innovative procedures and policies. In a 2 year period,

Letterman installed medically controlled *ambulance evacuation, required echeloned surgical *triage and treatment, established centralized field medical logistics, directed structured *preventive medicine inspections, developed simplified and rapid methods for collecting and reporting medical data, and organized large mobile field hospitals in tents. In short, Letterman, with Hammond's support, built a *system* for the management of casualties. The 'Letterman system' is today the basis for the organization and operation of military medical systems in all armies.

Hammond was responsible for two further medical contributions in 1862. He established the Army Medical Museum in Washington to collect and study pathological specimens from the military hospitals. It was the only federally supported medical research institution until 1902. The Museum evolved into the internationally recognized Armed Forces Institute of *Pathology, now the national pathology reference laboratory for the United States. Hammond also ordered the writing of a medical and surgical history of the war. Six mammoth volumes, published over 18 years, were the first complete accounts of the medical data of a war that saw the army establish the largest military medical system that had as yet existed.

The scientific base

Following the Civil War, during the 30 year final settlement of the American West, army medical officers accompanied the troops sent to ensure the success of the migration. Some of them became naturalists of a high order, as ornithologists, anthropologists, mammologists, and so on, often in collaboration with the Smithsonian Museum.

Following his service in the Civil War, John Shaw *Billings took control of the Army Medical Library and built its collections into the largest in the world; in 1956 it became the National Library of Medicine in the Department of Health, Education and Welfare. In 1879, he began *The index catalogue* and *The index-medicus*—indispensable and innovative author–subject guides to the world medical literature. Billings was instrumental in the construction of *Johns Hopkins Hospital, and the selection of the faculty of what was to become the model for American medical schools. His contributions to library science, public health, hospital planning, vital statistics, medical history, and the concepts underlying modern computers are too numerous to detail. He was probably the most influential physician in America for 25 years.

An Army Hospital Corps of formally trained enlisted men was established in 1887. This began the recognition, sporadic at best in the past, of the critical importance of educated, permanently assigned enlisted personnel in the medical department. In 1893, George M. Sternberg became surgeon-general of the army. Already recognized as one of the leading *bacteriologists in the country (he had written the first American textbook), he

founded the Army Medical School in 1893 as a postgraduate institution to teach the 'new ideas' in hygiene, science, and public health. Taught by the staff of the Army Medical Museum and the Library, with attendance required of all new medical officers, the school was in fact the first school of public health in America. Today, as the Walter Reed Army Institute of Research, it is the oldest and largest *tropical medicine research laboratory in America.

In 1902, the Navy Medical Corps began a similar programme of instruction for new medical officers at the Naval Medical School. Following the Civil War the navy was permitted to wither, even though it had pioneered the new ironclad warships. In the 1880s the nation began to build the new 'steel navy'. Navy medical officers faced new problems in *trauma and disease as steam propulsion and coal replaced wind and sail. In 1898 an enlisted Hospital Corps was established and the *Solace* was commissioned as a hospital ship to steam with the new fleet.

During and after the short Spanish–American War of 1898, Walter Reed directed his two great studies. The study of *typhoid fever in recruit camps led to the discovery of the *carrier state, and forced line officers to accept responsibility for the health of their commands and to begin teaching troop hygiene at the Military Academy at West Point. The work of the *Yellow Fever Board in proving mosquito transmission is too well known to be repeated in detail. In only a few months it documented Finlay's theory of *mosquito transmission of the disease. The first human experimental transmission of a filterable *virus was a part of those studies. Bailey Ashford in 1898, in Puerto Rico, discovered the American hookworm (*ankylostomiasis) and began a successful eradication campaign, later copied for the American South in a programme supported by Rockefeller philanthropy.

The modern era

The yellow fever data were applied by William Gorgas in Panama as early 20th century America followed its 'manifest destiny' to build the Canal, colonize in the Caribbean and the Philippines, and reach out to become a world power. As was true for European nations, the drive for tropical colonies meant the employment of the army and navy and the involvement of army and navy medical officers in studies of tropical diseases. Edward Stitt of the navy wrote a textbook of tropical medicine that was in print from 1914 to 1946. Army physicians in the Philippines proved the viral origin of *dengue, while Frederick Russell in 1909 at the Army Medical School developed a typhoid vaccine so useful that in 1911 the American armed forces became the first in the world to be universally immunized against the disease—which disappeared from the American military community. Carl Darnell, also at the Army Medical School, introduced the anhydrous chlorine method for water purification in 1910; a technology now used world-wide.

An Army Nurse Corps (1901) and a Navy Nurse Corps (1908) were established, although actual commissions would not be permitted until after the First World War, nor regular commissions until after the Second World War. However, the first female general officer in American history was Brigadier General Anna May Hays as Chief of the Army Nurse Corps in 1970.

Military physicians may have reached the apogee of command influence in the years just before the First World War. Presley Rixey, surgeon-general of the Navy, won medical officers the right to command hospital ships at sea in 1907—an authority exercised until 1921. Fred Ainsworth of the Medical Corps was the adjutant general of the army (1904–12) when Leonard Wood, an army medical officer early in his career, became chief of staff of the Army (1910–1914). Although these specific examples were unique in time and person, they signify the final arrival of the military physician as an accepted part of the military command structure and officer corps. While there would be episodes of line–medical tensions in the future, there would never again be a challenge to the basic right of the physician to be an officer.

Just before the First World War, the army (1911) and the navy (1912) established a Dental Corps; the army gave corps status to its veterinarians in 1916. Foreseeing the need for a pool of medical manpower in war, the army established a Medical Reserve Corps of civilian physicians in 1908. In 1916, this law was copied to provide a similar pool of combat arms officers for mobilization.

The First World War saw the massive application of the new modern medicine—widespread immunization, advanced surgery, motor ambulances, management of *shock, definition of '*shell shock' as a psychiatric disorder, prevention and treatment of chemical warfare casualties, and so on. This was the first American war in which the deaths from enemy action equalled those from disease; a clear reflection of the application of the international advances in microbiology and public health during the preceding 50 years.

Two new weapons of war, the submarine and the aeroplane, introduced new medical problems. For the submarine, the physiological and clinical problems inherent in closed, often toxic, atmospheres, the behavioural issues related to confinement, and the high level of technical expertise required in the crew, imposed a selection and prevention programme on navy medicine, but one that did not come to fruition until after the war.

Theodore Lyster, drawing heavily upon British Flying Corps experience early in the First World War, established a physical examination system for pilots and a medical research laboratory for aviation medicine in 1917, to study altitude *physiology, visual and vestibular function, and cardiovascular stress testing, and introduced to American medicine the concepts of the dynamic physical examination and the combination of physiological and performance testing. Flight surgeons

were trained at the research laboratory to support both mobilization and the force in France in 1917.

Between the First and Second World Wars, the medical departments somewhat avoided the stagnation and national indifference suffered by the line. Patient care followed the civilian models, with a very gradual increasing interest in specialization. Limited but significant attention was paid to the lessons of the First World War. An Army Medical Field Service School was established in 1922 to provide practical field instruction in administration, public health, and staff and command operations. The navy and army medical schools taught tropical and military medicine to all entering physicians, and postgraduate, 1 year internships began in service hospitals. Tropical medicine research continued. The School of Aviation Medicine expanded and the discipline, with new textbooks and journals, became a specialty. As the high-speed, high-altitude aircraft of the 1930s were developed, research was done on decompression, pressurized cabins, and gravitational forces in flight. Malcolm Grow and Harry Armstrong pioneered studies in man–machine interactions and human factors research at a new (1937) Air Corps laboratory in Ohio. A Navy School of Aviation Medicine and research laboratory began in Florida in 1939; that same year Armstrong published his seminal textbook, and his determination of the 'Armstrong line'—the 63 000 foot (19 200 m) altitude at which life cannot exist outside a pressurized environment.

The Second World War was fought on so vast a scale that describing military, naval, and aviation medicine in any detail is nearly impossible. The American military medical communities may take just credit for introducing *DDT, especially for prevention of epidemic *typhus; for developing and employing new antimalarial prophylactic drugs; for the multicentre *clinical trials and then use of *penicillin; and for developing systems for the large-scale collection, distribution, and use of whole blood. The army developed the *burn centre concept; after the war it was the leader in the management of burned patients for a number of years. The pre-war planning of William Mann of the navy developed the new operational doctrine for medical support of large amphibious assaults, culminating in the major island battles in the Pacific and the 1944 landings in France. Aeromedical evacuation, within the combat zone, and from overseas to the United States, was employed in an increasingly larger and more sophisticated manner. Physiological studies in the air force led to marked improvements in pressure suits, pilot protection, oxygen systems, etc. The inservice programmes were tightly interwoven with civilian industry and academia through the co-ordination of the National Academy of Sciences and the National Research Council. The development of the atomic weapon posed entirely new problems for military physicians, such as *radiation effects on individuals and the conceptual approaches to the management of mass casualties on a scale never before envisaged.

Consideration of these issues led to the establishment of the Tri-Service Armed Forces Radiobiology Research Laboratory in 1961 to pursue these subjects.

The experience with joint and unified commands during the Second World War led to a major reorganization of the American armed forces after the war. In 1947, the air force became an independent service, and the Department of Defense was established. An attempt to have the Army Medical Department continue to be responsible for the medical care of the air force was not a success, and a separate Air Force Medical Service was established in 1949.

Only a year later the Korean War erupted. The medical and surgical experiences of the Second World War were still reasonably fresh, although the medical services participated in the general unreadiness for the war. The artificial kidney was first used in a battle zone, and *vascular surgery was introduced in the new MASH (mobile army surgical hospital) units. The use of the helicopter as a front-line ambulance was instituted, initially for the severely wounded, and later for more routine evacuation.

The present position

After the Korean War, the United States, for the first time in peacetime, maintained large, active-duty military forces with conscription, and spent great sums of money to build and maintain a world-wide military presence. The medical departments of the army, navy, and air force participated in this expansion and relied on a doctor draft that saw over 90 per cent of all graduating physicians and dentists serve on active duty for 2 years. New hospitals were built, expanded graduate education programmes for residents and fellows were established after civilian models, nursing programmes were enlarged, and routine administration of the system (but not command and control) was largely transferred to the newly established Medical Service Corps in all three medical departments.

Medical research programmes shared in this expansion. The continuing army and navy programmes in tropical medicine and *infectious diseases were enhanced by newly established overseas laboratories in Taiwan, Thailand, Malaysia, Egypt, and elsewhere. From studies in the United States and abroad came *antibiotic cures for typhoid and scrub typhus, new antimalarial drugs, and *vaccines for *adenovirus, meningococcal *meningitis, and Venezuelan equine *encephalitis, among others. The air force began its research programme in space medicine; the basic work for medical support of the astronauts was largely done at the Air Force School of Aerospace Medicine. The crash research of John Paul Stapp, studying the effects of high-speed ejection from the new jet aircraft, was the foundation for civilian automobile crash safety. In the navy, the nuclear submarine brought research on long-term confinement and the study of the *toxicology of trace elements and isotopes in closed environments.

Pioneering work in blood preservation by freezing and in saturation diving expanded the type of navy studies. Robert Phillips of the navy brought the new understanding of body fluid and *electrolyte metabolism to the study of *cholera in work that revolutionized the treatment of the disease.

Although Congressional hearings and various studies had suggested the need for central co-ordination, if not direction, of all armed forces medical programmes, it was not until 1953 that the position of Assistant Secretary of Defense (Health and Medical) was established. Now called Health Affairs, the appointment has always been held by politically appointed civilian physicians. The Assistant Secretaries have continued to move toward an expanded role in operational control and direction of armed forces medicine, albeit in fits and starts, largely determined by the philosophies of the incumbent and the Secretary of Defense. As systems analysis techniques and cost–benefit studies became a way of life in the Department of Defense, the medical systems have been scrutinized and analysed at regular intervals. Two fundamentally opposed philosophies keep emerging; the status quo (however modified) with a surgeon-general and considerable professional and managerial autonomy for each military department, versus a totally unified and centralized medical system, with one surgeon-general, as in the Canadian and some European models. Central policy direction and control to include construction, financing, and training is increasing. Perhaps only the size and complexity of the system have so far deterred unification.

In the long conflict in Vietnam, from 1964 to 1972, medical support of an incredibly sophisticated nature was deployed in fixed facility hospitals with staff and equipment equal to those of academic medical centres in America. The helicopter essentially replaced the motor ambulance for evacuation, and air evacuation to the United States became routine. Preventive medicine kept the infectious disease and non-effectiveness rates at the lowest levels of any war, while rapid evacuation and advanced surgery reduced the died-of-wounds rate to a new low of 2.5 per cent.

The automatic conscription of physicians, which began in 1950, ended in 1973 when the draft law was repealed. In anticipation of this, a military medical school and a scholarship programme in civilian medical schools were established by Congress in 1972 to provide physicians for the armed forces. The medical school, the Uniformed Services University of the Health Sciences, was the first federal medical school to award the MD degree. Graduating its first class in 1980, it now admits 165 students a year to a 4 year course at no cost. Graduates are obligated to serve 7 years active duty and 3 reserve years beyond residency training. The school year is 11 months long; 2 months of this are devoted to special education in military medicine. It is anticipated that graduates of the school will provide about 25 per cent of the peacetime requirements for physicians in the

Department of Defense, with the rest coming from the scholarship students in civilian schools.

The present organization of each of the three medical departments is slightly different. All the surgeons-general are the senior medical staff officers and policy advisers to their service. The surgeon-general of the army commands the research programme as well as being the executive manager of several triservice medical agencies. Army hospital operations in the United States are centralized in a Health Services Command, commanded by the surgeon-general. The surgeon-general of the navy commands medical research and all navy hospitals through the Bureau of Medicine and Surgery. The surgeon-general of the air force is primarily a staff officer; the hospitals and research laboratories are assigned within and under the control of the major commands in the air force. All surgeons-general have technical direction of professional matters, and manage the careers, education, and assignments of officer personnel. In all services, medical people and resources assigned to combat operating units (division, fleet, wing) are under the command of those units. The hospitals and medical people outside the United States fall under the command of the major overseas line commander in the area.

At the time of writing (1992) the Department of Defense is being reduced in size, with bases closed, budgets reduced, and personnel released. By 1995, the services will be trimmed to 80 per cent of their present size; the army will be reduced the most, by 25 per cent. Further reductions are possible. Inevitably, this will have an impact on the medical departments. These now support 9.1 million active duty, retiree, and dependent people; by 1995 this is projected to be 8.4 million, but with an increase in the percentage of retired members theoretically entitled to care.

The military actions in Grenada, Panama, and the Persian Gulf have increased interest in medical preparation for war. Levels of medical support in combat can be described in a similar way to present military descriptions of war, with tactical, operational, and strategic components. Direct patient care of the sick and wounded and operation of the patient evacuation system are the essential tactical tasks and are under the command and control of medical department officers. This level of care is largely left to reserve units, after initial deployment of active forces. Medical and line interactions at the operational level have the most impact on preventing disease and injury. The battle plans, casualty estimates, and logistic capabilities come from the combat arms staff and command elements. The medical staff then recommends medical unit requirements, medical supplies, evacuation systems, and preventive medicine specifics. In overall planning and operation, command and medical elements must have pre-war and wartime knowledge of requirements so they can communicate and collaborate. It is at this level of war that the line commander is primarily responsible for medical support. Medical strategic planning includes medical intelligence about disease threats, research on drugs and vaccines for disease prevention, assembly of deployment supply packages, and structured information on the national medical assets available for mobilization and deployment.

All three medical departments are responding to these requirements, with specialized hospital and logistic units, with targeted research, with increased automation, with heightened interest in training, especially of the reserves, and so on. There is increasing study of joint military medical operations, to parallel the combat arms war planning.

As is true nationally, medical policy in defence is fiscally driven. Medical costs are about 3–5 per cent of the defence budget, increase above the inflation rate, and arouse persistent Congressional interest. Officer- and labour-intensive medical care is troublesome as personnel strength dwindles; the army now has 20 per cent of *all* of its officers in the medical department. Military medicine in the United States is in flux but will survive.

In summary, for 217 years the medical departments of the American armed forces have shared the triumphs and vicissitudes of their parent military services, have gained acceptance as members of both professions, medical and military, and are now at their greatest peacetime size in American history. The men and women of the medical departments have made contributions to the advancement of medicine and science far in excess of their numbers; only some of these are described here. The soldier, sailor, airman, and marine have always had medical care equal to that in civilian medicine and certainly, earlier in our history, superior to that available in the general community. As the medical departments enter their third century, they may justifiably look on their past with pride and to their future with hope and confidence.

R. J. T. JOY

Further reading
OFFICIAL HISTORIES

Cosmas, G. and Cowdrey, A. E. (1992). *Medical service in the European theater of operations*, Washington, Center of Military History. US Government Printing Office.

Cowdrey, A. E. (1987). *The medic's war: Korea*, Washington, Center of Military History. US Government Printing Office.

Link, M. M. and Coleman, H. A. (1955). *Medical support of the army air forces in World War II*. Office of the Surgeon General of the United States Air Force, Washington.

Medical and surgical history of the Rebellion (1870–88), 6 vols. Prepared under the direction of Surgeon General Joseph K. Barnes, United States Army, published in parts. Government Printing Office, Washington.

Smith, C. M. (1956). *The Medical Department: hospitalization and evacuation, zone of interior*, Washington, Center of Military History. US Government Printing Office.

Strott, G. G. (1947). *The Medical Department of the United States Navy in World War I*. US Navy Department, Washington.

The history of the Medical Department of the United States Navy in World War II. Prepared under the direction of the Surgeon General of the Navy. (1950–53), 3 vols. Government Printing Office, Washington.
The history of the Medical Department of the United States Navy, 1945–1955, 1957, (BuMed P-5057). Bureau of Medicine and Surgery, Washington.
The Medical Department of the United States Army in the World War (1921–29), 15 vols in 17. Prepared and published under the direction of Major General Merritte W. Ireland, Surgeon General of the Army. Government Printing Office, Washington.
The Medical Department of the United States Army in World War II (1954–76), 41 vols. Prepared and published under the direction of the Surgeon General of the Army. Government Printing Office, Washington.
The Medical Department of the United States Army in Vietnam (1977–82), 2 vols (to date). Office of the Surgeon General and Center of Military History.
Wiltse, C. M. (1965). *The Medical Department: medical service in the Mediterranean and minor theaters*, Washington, Center of Military History. US Government Printing Office.

SECONDARY SOURCES

Ashburn, P. M. (1929). *A history of the Medical Department of the United States Army*. Houghton Miffin, Cambridge.
Bayne-Jones, S. (1968). *The evolution of preventive medicine in the United States Army, 1607–1939*. US Government Printing Office, Washington.
Gillett, M. C. (1981). *The Army Medical Department, 1775–1818*, Center of Military History. US Government Printing Office, Washington.
Gillett, M. C. (1987). *The Army Medical Department, 1818–1865*, Center of Military History. US Government Printing Office, Washington.
Holcomb, R. C. (1930). *A century with Norfolk Naval Hospital*. Printcraft, Portsmouth, Virginia.
Peyton, G. (1968). *Fifty years of aerospace medicine*. Air Force Systems Command, San Antonio, Texas.
Engle, E. and Lott, A. (1979). *Man in flight*. Leeward, Annapolis, Maryland.

ARMSTRONG, GEORGE (1720–89). British physician. In 1769 he founded a charitable dispensary for children which failed after 12 years through lack of funds. He may be regarded as the first British *paediatrician. He wrote *An essay on diseases most fatal to infants* (1767).

ARMY, BRITISH: MEDICAL SERVICES. See DEFENCE MEDICAL SERVICES (UK).

ARNOLD, OF VILLANOVA (?1235–1311). Catalan physician. He introduced brandy into therapeutics and devised the preparation known as a *tincture.

ARNOLD–CHIARI MALFORMATION is a developmental anomaly causing downwards displacement of the *cerebellum and *medulla oblongata through the *foramen magnum. There is usually obstruction to the circulation of *cerebrospinal fluid producing *hydrocephalus, and other congenital defects may also be present.

ARNOTT, NEIL (1788–1874). British physician and natural philosopher. He was one of the founders of the University of London in 1836 and became a member of the Senate the following year. A pioneer in public health and hygiene, he was also interested in physics on which he lectured and published a textbook. He invented the *waterbed and the smokeless 'Arnott stove'.

ARRHYTHMIA is any disturbance of cardiac *rhythm, varying from the physiological and innocent (e.g. sinus arrhythmia, a cyclical variation in heart rate with breathing; or isolated *extrasystoles) to dangerous and sometimes fatal disorders (e.g. *ventricular fibrillation; *heart block).

ARSENIC is a metallic element of atomic number 33 and relative atomic mass 74.922. It has no physiological role; its compounds, which block the action of *enzymes, are highly toxic to all body tissues. Now that they are no longer used in treatment (before *penicillin they were used to treat *syphilis; and arsenic salts were an ingredient of 'tonic' mixtures for many years), arsenic poisoning is likely to be encountered only in an occupational or possibly a criminal context. Acute arsenic poisoning is treated with *dimercaprol.

ARSPHENAMINE. An arsenical preparation, once widely used in treating *syphilis.

ART AND MEDICINE
Introduction
From earliest times human disease and its treatment has attracted the attention of artists. This may have been because of the supposed mystical significance of certain diseases, but in most cases because the subject itself was intrinsically fascinating. Attitudes to *malformations and diseases, however, have not always been the same. For example, dwarfs in Pharaonic Egypt were characterized by normal faces and very short limbs, in Ancient Greece by snub-noses and prominent foreheads, and in Rome they were often depicted with an over-large phallus. More recently, as in many of Velazquez's (1599–1660) paintings, dwarfs are shown much more sympathetically, as well as more realistically. Furthermore, the artist's intention has sometimes been to use allegorical allusions for a very specific purpose in portraying medical matters. This is particularly true in Dutch genre paintings of the 17th century. In more modern times, as art has become less representational, so paintings have increasingly come to reflect the artist's *subjective impression* of disease and its treatment.

Disorders in the artist
Artists have, not infrequently, suffered from medical conditions themselves, which in some instances have significantly affected their work. This is most obvious in the case of eye disease.

El Greco's (1541–1614) purported *astigmatism is now very much in doubt, but red–green *colour blindness certainly afflicted Fernand Léger (1881–1955) and Piet Mondrian (1872–1944). It could well be that their particular styles were directly influenced by this. Failing sight leading ultimately to blindness is well documented in Malcolm Drummond (1880–1945) and the Russian painter Mikhail Vrubel (1856–1910), and in the case of Percy Wyndham Lewis (1882–1957) this was due to a *pituitary tumour, for which he refused surgery and from which he eventually died. Figure and colour distortion in the later stages of increasing blindness would be expected. Pierre Auguste Renoir's (1841–1919) sight also began to fail in later life, but he was by then severely crippled with *arthritis, which could have influenced his style of painting.

Paul Klee (1879–1940) was very severely disabled in later years by progressive scleroderma (*systemic sclerosis). His anguish is expressed vividly in the painting (?self-portrait) in the year of his death, entitled *Death and Fire*, which shows a pale face leering at the observer—the mouth represented by the letter 'T', one eye as 'o' and the other as 'd', thus signifying death.

Just as traumatic as blindness must also be the loss of an artist's painting hand. This is starkly and dramatically portrayed by the German expressionist painter, Ernst Ludwig Kirchner (1880–1938) in his self-portrait as a soldier in 1915.

The influence of *mental disease on creativity has been much researched. It is tempting to imagine that madness could, in certain circumstances, lead to heightened artistic creativity. Certainly Richard Dadd's (1819–1887) early paintings were attractive but conventional, and it was only after the onset of insanity (which led to his murdering his father and his resultant incarceration in 1844 in Bethlem and later Broadmoor Hospitals for the rest of his life) that his paintings took on an idiosyncratic strangeness, which has attracted considerable attention ever since. But whether or not his later paintings were actually an improvement and more artistic is debatable. Anthony Storr has argued cogently that in severe bipolar *psychosis and *schizophrenia, creativity, rather than being enhanced in some way, is in fact often significantly impaired.

Self-portraits

Self-portraits can sometimes reveal medical disorders in the artist himself. For example, Albrecht Dürer (1471–1528) had a divergent *squint, clearly evident in his self-portraits of 1491 and 1498, as well as in several of his other portraits, including his *Mother (1514), Caspar Sturm* (1520), and *Laughing Peasant Woman* (1505).

Henri de Toulouse-Lautrec (1864–1901) frequently portrayed his own deformities in various caricatures as well as in the painting *Au Moulin Rouge* (1892). His deformities have been convincingly attributed to autosomal recessive pyknodysostosis, on the basis of his short stature, bony fractures, and possibly a large

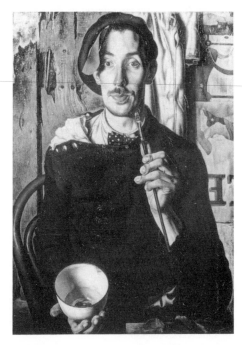

Fig. 1 *Self-portrait* (1939), Dick Ket (reproduced by kind permission of Dr J. R. de Groot, Keeper, Department of Paintings, Gemeentemuseum, Arnhem).

fontanelle, prompting him to wear a hat much of the time, and his parents were first cousins.

The Dutch painter, Dick Ket (1902–40), probably suffered from *Fallot's tetralogy with *dextrocardia, and his many self-portraits clearly show finger clubbing, *cyanosis, plethora and possibly some precordial fullness (Fig. 1).

However, not all artists have been so openly honest. The French painter Jacques-Louis David (1748–1825), had a disfiguring deformity of the left side of his face, which he was very careful to hide in self-portraits, and his pupil, Pierre Langlois, also took care to mask this side of David's face in his portrait of his teacher.

Portraits of the famous

Detailed and careful portraits of the famous have often revealed evidence of medical disorders, which may not have been fully appreciated or even recognized at the time. For example the plethoric appearance of King George III in the portrait by Johann Zoffany (1733–1810) may reflect the possibility of the King having *porphyria. More convincing is the portrayal of Prince Alexandre Ypsilante on a Greek stamp commemorating the liberation of Greece. This clearly illustrates his frontal baldness and a somewhat lugubrious expression, associated with his having myotonic dystrophy (see NEUROMUSCULAR DISEASE). But, as in self-portraits, sometimes an artist has consciously hidden a disfigurement, in this case in order to avoid offending a benefactor. The classic example is the portrait (*c.* 1465) of Federigo da Montefeltro, the Duke of Urbino, by Piero della Francesca (*c.* 1416–92). Here the artist has portrayed his subject in left profile in order to hide the serious and disfiguring injuries to the right side of his face, including the loss of his right eye, sustained in a jousting match. The Emperor Charles V inherited the so-called 'Hapsburg jaw' with 'gross mandibular *prognathism and malocclusion, flat malar areas, and a sloping forehead', but these abnormalities are not at all obvious in the famous portrait by Titian (*c.* 1487–1576). Thus in portraits, whether of the artist himself or of another, disfigurements, deformities, or disease may, in some cases, have been deliberately obscured.

Disorders in art

When the manifestations of a disease are clearcut and unmistakable, as in the case of *smallpox or crippling arthritis, they can often be identified in paintings from the past. This is also true of certain well-defined congenital malformations and genetic disorders. The most noted examples are those of various dwarfs in the court of King Philip IV of Spain, depicted by Velazquez (1599–1660). They include *achondroplasia in a woman in *Las Meninas* (1656) and in a boy in *El Niño de Vallecas* (1637), and possibly pseudoachondroplasia in *Sebastian de Morra* (*c.* 1644) and *El Primo* (1644). Some other fairly well-documented examples are listed in Table 1.

However, what may seem obvious on superficial examination may, in fact, prove to be quite different on more careful study. For example, the simplest interpretation of Jusepe de Ribera's (1591–1652) *The Clubfooted Boy* is that this merely represents *talipes equinovarus. But the boy shown also appears to have a right *hemiplegia, a suspicion of left facial weakness and the note he holds in his hand explains that he cannot speak. Thus, he may well have had some form of *cerebral palsy.

It is equally possible to dismiss a depicted peculiarity as merely a figment of the artist's imagination, when in fact it represents a true likeness of an unusual condition. An excellent example is L. S. Lowry's (1887–1976) *Woman with a Beard*, which the artist actually drew from life (Fig. 2). It seems that Lowry was often fascinated by such tragic characters seen in Northern industrial towns.

Medical diagnosis in art

As cultural, economic, and intellectual life in Europe began to flourish in the late Middle Ages, examples are increasingly found of paintings depicting various diagnostic procedures. Pulse-taking and uroscopy were frequent themes, especially in the 17th and 18th centuries. In more recent times, however, other techniques

have been portrayed. For example there is Théobald Chartran's (1849–1907) painting of René *Laënnec (1781–1826), a French physician credited with having developed the first *stethoscope by rolling sheets of paper into a cylinder and later by using a wooden tube. In this painting, Laënnec is seen listening to a patient's heart using the traditional method of putting his ear to the chest. But in his left hand, ready for use, he is holding his cylindrical stethoscope.

Medical treatment in art

Miracle treatments have also frequently featured in paintings, for example in Hogarth's *The Pool of Bethesda* (*c.* 1735) and *The Good Samaritan* (1737), on the staircase of St Bartholomew's Hospital, London. Here we are concerned only with the depiction of treatment as actually practised at the time, a tradition that can be traced back to the art of Pharaonic Egypt and Ancient Greece, and early Arabic texts. The latter are often in the form of text ornamentation, but these, and illuminated manuscripts and engravings, have been excluded from the present discussion, where the emphasis is on painting.

Bloodletting and cupping formed an important part of the physician's armamentarium from Pharaonic times. In Quirijn van Brekelenkam's (*c.* 1620–68) painting *The Bloodletting*, an older woman applies a *leech to the forearm of a young woman in a quiet domestic interior. This sensitive and sympathetic rendering is in stark contrast to many of the satirical carnival-like scenes of treatments by medical quacks painted by

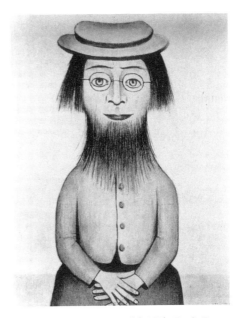

Fig. 2 *Woman With a Beard* (1957), L. S. Lowry (reproduced by kind permission of Mr Martin Bloom).

Table 1 Congenital malformations and genetic disorders depicted in paintings

Disorder	Painting		Artist
	Title (date)	Location	
Albinism	*Nude Girl on a Fur* (1932)	National Gallery of Modern Art, Edinburgh	Otto Dix (1891–1969)
Blindness	*Parable of the Blind* (1568)	Museo Nazionali, Naples	Pieter Brueghel (*c.* 1525–69)
	The Blind Man of Gambazo or *The Sense of Touch* (1632)	Prado, Madrid	Jusepe de Ribera (1591–1652)
Clubfoot	*Feeding the Hungry* (1504) (from the *Altarpiece of the Seven Works of Mercy*)	Rijksmuseum, Amsterdam	Master of Alkmaar (active 1490–1520)
Congenital heart disease	Various self-portraits (see text)	Gemeentemuseum, Arnhem	Dick Ket (1902–40)
Craniosynostosis (?Crouzon's disease)	*Count N. D. Guriev* (1821)	Hermitage, St Petersburg	Jean-Auguste-Dominique Ingres (1780–1867)
Digital abnormalities			
Absent digit	*Ernest Reinhold* (1908)	Musée des Beaux-Arts, Brussels	Oskar Kokoshka (1886–1980)
Polydactyly	*Self Portrait* (1912)	Stedelijk Museum, Amsterdam	Marc Chagall (1887–1985)
Syndactyly	*Portrait of a Canon* [identified as Nicolai Aegidius] (1517)	Royal Museum of Arts, Antwerp	Quentin Massys (*c.* 1465–1530)
Thumb deformity	*Erasmus* (1517)	Galleria Nazionale d'Arte Antica, Rome	
Down's syndrome (?)	*Adoration of the Shepherds* (*c.* 1617)	Grenoble Museum	Jacob Jordaens (1593–1678)
	The Peasant and the Satyr (*c.* 1638)	Staatliche Kunstsammlungen, Kassel	
	A Child with Nondisjunction (nd)	Private collection	Josef Warkany (1902–92)
Duchenne muscular dystrophy (?)	*The Transfiguration* (1520)	Vatican Museum, Rome	Raphael (1483–1520)
	Sick Boy (1915)	Formerly Städtische Kunstsammlung Chemnitz, Karl-Marx-Stadt, Germany	Karl Schmidt-Rottluff (1884–1976)

Table 1 (*cont.*)

Disorder	Painting		Artist
	Title (date)	Location	
Dwarfism			
Achondroplasia	Fresco *Camera degli Sposi* (1474)	Palazzo Ducale, Mantua	Andrea Mantegna (*c.* 1431–1506)
	The Dwarf Morgante (*c.* 1552)	Deposita della Soprintendenza, Florence	Angelo di Cosimo Bronzino (1503–72)
	The Finding of Moses (1570–80)	Prado, Madrid	Paolo Veronese (*c.* 1528–88)
	Apollo Killing the Cyclops (1616–18)	National Gallery, London	Domenichino (Domenico Zampieri) (1581–1641)
	Artist's Studio (not dated)	Bode Museum, Berlin	Jan Miense Molenaer (*c.* 1610–68)
	Peter's Denial of Christ (1636)	Szépmüvészeti Múzeum, Budapest	
	Various (see text)	Prado, Madrid	Velazquez (1599–1660)
	Il Cavadenti (*c.* 1730)	Brera Gallery, Milan	Pietro Longhi (1702–85)
	Francesco Ravai called Bajocco (1773)	Kunstmuseum, Copenhagen	Jens Juel (1745–1802)
	The Dwarf Dona Mercedes (1899)	Musée d'Orsay, Paris	Ignacio Zuloaga (1870–1945)
Pituitary disorders	*Adoration of the Magi* (*c.* 1472)	National Gallery, London	Sandro Boticelli (1445–1510)
	Cardinal Granvella's Dwarf and Dog (1560)	Louvre, Paris	Anthonis van Dashorst (called Antonio Moro) (1519–75)
	The Family of Darius before Alexander (*c.* 1570)	National Gallery, London	Paolo Veronese (*c.* 1528–88)
	Isabella Clara Eugenia with her Dwarf (*c.* 1580)	Prado, Madrid	Follower of Alonso Sanchez Coello (*c.* 1531–88)
	Aletheia Talbot and her Train (*c.* 1630)	Alte Pinakothek, Munich	Peter Paul Rubens (1577–1640)

Table 1 (*cont.*)

Disorder	Painting		Artist
	Title (date)	Location	
Dwarfism (*cont.*)	*Queen Henrietta and her Dwarf Sir Jeffrey Hudson* (*c.* 1633)	National Gallery, Washington	Anthony Van Dyck (1599–1641) (Hudson was also painted by Daniel Mytens in 1630)
Spondylo-epiphyseal dysplasia (?) ?type	*Aragonese Dwarf* (1825)	Fogg Art Museum, Cambridge, Mass.	Vicente Lopez-y-Portana (1772–1850)
	Dwarf with a Dog (1643)	Formerly in Lederer Collection, Vienna	Jusepe de Ribera (1591–1652)
	Jacoba Maria van Wassenaer or *Bernardina Margriet van Raesfeld* (1660)	Mauritshuis, The Hague	Jan Steen (*c.* 1625–79)
Various	*Boys with Dwarfs* (1646)	Stedelijk van Abbe-museum, Eindhoven	Jan Miense Molenaer (*c.* 1610–68)
Epidermolysis bullosa (?)	*Heritage* (1899)	Munch Museum, Oslo	Edvard Munch (1863–1944)
Epilepsy (Madness)	*The Cure for Folly* (*c.* 1480)	Prado, Madrid	Hieronymus Bosch (*c.* 1450–1516)
	Healing of the Madman (*c.* 1496)	Accademia, Venice	Vittore Carpaccio (*c.* 1465–1525)
	The Cure of Folly (*c.* 1556)	Prado, Madrid	Jan Sanders van Hemessen (*c.* 1500–75)
Female hirsutism	*The Bearded Woman of Peñaranda* (*c.* 1590s)	Prado, Madrid	Juan Sánchez Cotán (1561–1627)
	Magdalena Ventura (1631)	Lerma Foundation, Toledo	Jusepe de Ribera (1591–1652)
	Woman with a Beard (1957)	Private collection (UK)	L. S. Lowry (1887–1976)
Hapsburg jaw	*Emperor Charles V at Mühlberg* (1547)	Prado, Madrid	Titian (*c.* 1487–1576)
Hare-lip	*Boy with Cleft Lip* (1902)	Tretiakov Gallery, Moscow	Mikhail Vrubel (1856–1910)
Hemiplegia	*The Clubfooted Boy* (1642)	Louvre, Paris	Jusepe de Ribera (1591–1652)

Table 1 (*cont.*)

Disorder	Painting		Artist
	Title (date)	Location	
Hypertrichosis universalis	*Portrait of Peter Gonzales and his Children* (*c.* 1582)	Kunsthistorisches Museum, Vienna	Bavarian (Artist unknown)
Klippel–Feil anomaly	*Illustrations of the Book of Job* (1825)	–	William Blake (1757–1827)
Lesch–Nyhan syndrome (?)	*Three Miracles of Saint Zenobius* (*c.* 1490–1510) (Zenobius exorcizes two young men gnawing their own flesh)	National Gallery, London	Sandro Botticelli (1445–1510)
Noonan's syndrome (?)	*Among those Left* (1929)	Museum of Art, Carnegie Institute, Pittsburgh	Ivan Le Lorraine Albright (1897–1983)
Pectus carinatum	*Agosta the Pigeon–Chested Man and Rasha the Black Dove* (1929)	Private Collection	Christian Schad (1894–1982)
Phocomelia	*Girl with Wooden Leg and No Arms* (1514) (?gross trauma)	Public Art Museum, Basle	Urs Graf (*c.* 1485–1527/28)
	Charles Emmanuel I of Savoy as a Child Accompanied by a Dwarf (1573)	National Gallery, Turin	Giacomo Vighi, called Argenta(?–1573)
	Mother with Deformed Infant (*c.* 1805)	Louvre, Paris	Francisco de Goya (1746–1828)
Prader–Willi syndrome (?)	*Eugenia Martinez Vallejo, La Monstrua* (*c.* 1680)	Prado, Madrid	Juan Carreño de Miranda (1614–85)
Pyknodysostosis	Various self-portraits	–	Henri de Toulouse-Lautrec (1864–1901)
Spastic paraplegia	*Child on all Fours (after Muybridge)* (1961)	Gemeentemuseum, The Hague	Francis Bacon (1909–92)
Strabismus	Various portraits (see text)	–	Albrecht Dürer (1471–1528)
	Fedra Inghirami (1516)	Pitti, Florence	Raphael (1483–1520)
	Margrave Albrecht von Brandenburg, Duke of Prussia (1528)	Herzog Anton Ulrich Museum, Brunswick	Lucas Cranach (1472–1553)
	Little Girl with a Squint (*c.* 1961)	Gracefield Art Centre, Dumfries	Joan Eardley (1921–63)

Table 1 (*cont.*)

Disorder	Painting		Artist
	Title (date)	Location	
Synophrys	Various self-portraits	–	Frida Kahlo (1907–54)
Thoracopagus	*Joined Twins* (not dated)	Gemeentemuseum, The Hague	E. C. van der Mass (1577–1656)
White forelock (?acquired)	*James McNeill Whistler* (1885)	Metropolitan Museum, New York	William Merritt Chase (1849–1916)

van Brekelenkam's Dutch contemporaries. The latter were often at pains to ridicule the medical profession, whom they viewed as quacks and charlatans, or to make a particular moral point. Thus Dutch genre painters often took the theme of delousing, for example, as having meanings on two levels: outward cleanliness on the one hand and spiritual order and virtue on the other. Furthermore, Dutch genre paintings frequently remind the viewer of patients' gullibility. This is illustrated, for example, in paintings of quacks purporting to treat mental illness.

Some modern artists also appear to view current treatment for mental illness with scepticism, as, for example, in Edvard Munch's (1863–1944) *Electric Shock Treatment.*

Physician and patient in art

This was again an important subject of Dutch genre paintings. A particular exponent was Jan Steen (*c.* 1626–79) who painted almost 40 different versions on the theme of 'The doctor's visit', and whose work was much appreciated at the time. His approach was often humorous, but almost always barbed with a warning or moral admonition. The doctor is usually attired in a way that at the time would clearly have been recognized as antiquated and theatrical. He is often seen assuming a pompous pose. The patient is usually a lovesick maiden, at a time when repressed or unrequited love was believed to cause melancholy. Other elements within the painting often emphasize the theme of love-sickness: a background painting or statue of Cupid or of Venus and Adonis. A ribbon burning in a dish is often included, as nausea induced in the patient in this way was believed to be a test for pregnancy. The doctor is often taking the patient's pulse or inspecting her urine, as these were also believed to be important measures for diagnosing the patient's condition. For example, a sudden increase in pulse rate on an unexpected visit from a lover would be considered diagnostic. In one painting, an additional character holds a herring along with two onions (Fig. 3), which clearly also has sexual connotations. In regard to uroscopy and pregnancy, in

Godfried Schalcken's (1643–1706) *The Medical Examination* the painter makes the meaning quite explicit by including a tiny *embryo in the flask of urine being examined by the physician.

In some genre paintings there are clear warnings against licentiousness and unbridled passion. In Steen's *The Lovesick Girl* (*c.* 1665), currently in the Metropolitan Museum of Art in New York, the artist included a pair of copulating dogs to emphasize his point, and this

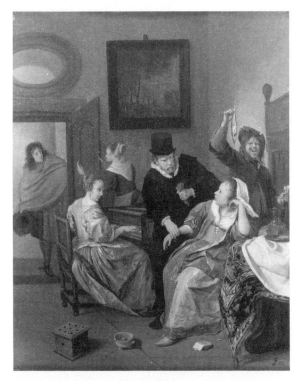

Fig. 3 *The Doctor's Visit* (1663–65), Jan Steen (reproduced by kind permission of the Philadelphia Museum of Art: The John G. Johnson Collection).

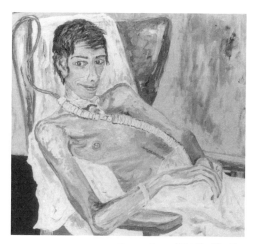

Fig. 4 *Boy After a Liver Transplant* (1989), Sir Roy Calne. (Reproduced by kind permission of the artist).

offending motif was once painted out by a censorious restorer.

In Victorian times, paintings of physicians attending their patients became very popular and were often dramatic, even bordering on the sentimental, as in *The Doctor* by Sir Luke Fildes (1844–1927). Many paintings show the physician in a sympathetic light, bringing comfort and reassurance to his patient.

The artist's interest in portraying medical matters continues to the present day. An excellent example is Sir Roy Calne, Professor of Surgery at the University of Cambridge who helped pioneer liver *transplantation and who is himself also a noted artist. One of his early patients was the Scottish painter John Bellany, who subsequently influenced Calne's technique. The latter's painting of a boy with *Wilson's disease who had undergone liver transplantation, clearly demonstrates the compassion and understanding the artist felt for his subject (Fig. 4).

Other aspects of medicine and art

Many other aspects of medicine and art could be considered, including the association of art with anatomy, dentistry, surgery, and military medicine. Furthermore, the therapeutic value of art for patients themselves is an important topic in its own right, as is the role of medical *illustration and medical photography in current medical practice.

Conclusions

In this brief review of medicine and art, the emphasis has been on paintings and the effects disease may have on the artist's work, as well as the depiction of disease and its diagnosis and treatment in art. Until comparatively recently, paintings have been essentially representational. But in more recent times, they have increasingly

come to reflect the artist's *subjective impression* of disease and its treatment. This is particularly well seen in the work of Frida Kahlo (1907–54), the highly original Mexican painter who was severely injured in her youth and whose subsequent pain, anguish, and frustration are clearly expressed in her paintings, especially her self-portraits. This recent development will provide an interesting and challenging topic for future studies of the relationship between medicine and art.

ALAN E. H. EMERY
MARCIA L. H. EMERY

Further reading
Emery, A. E. H. (1991). Medicine, genetics and art. *Proceedings of the Royal College of Physicians Edinburgh*, **21**, 33–42.
Emery, A. E. H. and Emery, M. (1992). Medicine and art: diagnosis and medical treatment. *Proceedings of the Royal College of Physicians Edinburgh*, **22**, 519–42.
Kunze, J. and Nippert, I. (1986). *Genetics and malformations in art.* Grosse Verlag, Berlin.
MacGregor, J. M. (1989). *The discovery of the art of the insane.* Princeton University Press, Princeton.
Trevor-Roper, P. D. (1988). *The world through blunted sight.* Allen Lane, Penguin Press, London.
Watkins, J. I. (ed.) (1984). *Masters of seventeenth century Dutch genre painting.* Weidenfeld and Nicolson, London.

ARTERIES are the vessels that carry blood away from the heart. With the exception of the pulmonary arteries, which carry deoxygenated blood from the right ventricle of the heart to the lungs, they distribute oxygenated blood from the left side of the heart to all organs and tissues. Left ventricular contraction causes flow within them to be pulsatile and under high pressure (arterial *blood pressure); arterial walls are therefore relatively thick, containing elastic tissue and muscle. The branching arterial tree begins with a single large vessel (the *aorta) arising from the left ventricle, and terminates in innumerable tiny vessels (the *arterioles), leading to the *capillary networks.

ARTERIES AND VEINS: THEIR DISEASES AND VASCULAR SURGERY
Introduction

If the central and peripheral nervous systems can be considered as the electrical messengers of the body, then the blood vessels represent the plumbing. Like a house, the human body is full of pipes, on which it depends for its function. These pipes fulfil four purposes:

1. They carry *oxygen, nutrient materials, and *hormones from the heart to the body tissues.
2. They clear away the waste products of *metabolism, in particular *carbon dioxide and acids, into the lungs and *kidneys.
3. They operate as a reservoir, from which blood can be directed to various parts of the body, according to need. A number of complicated switching mechanisms exist to bring this about.

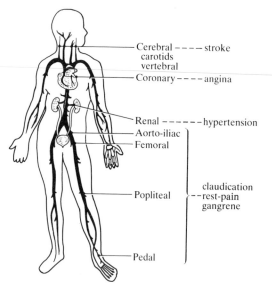

Fig. 1 The main arterial pathways.

4. They are concerned with the regulation of temperature. Our bodies can operate only within a narrow temperature range, but we are, none the less, capable of surviving anywhere from the North Pole to the Sahara. For this to be possible, it is necessary to control and alter blood flow through the skin (see HOMEOSTASIS).

There are two systems of conducting pipes in the body, the arteries and the veins, which have different functions. (The third system, the *lymphatics, lies outside the scope of this article).

The arteries
Arteries (see Fig. 1) are thick-walled muscular tubes that convey oxygenated blood from the left side of the heart to every part of the body, from the brain to the toes. The total amount of arterial tissue is less than 0.5 per cent of the body weight, so that the average man weighing 70 kg contains about 350 g of artery. None the less, damage to this system of tubes represents the commonest cause of death in Western society; it is possible that if everyone was adequately fed, and cancer and infection were eliminated throughout the world, arterial disease would stand between us and immortality. The arteries work at high pressure, with high resistance and fast flow. It is an observed fact that as a man (and to a lesser extent a woman) grows older, the arteries become rougher, thicker, and prone to block, but why this should be is uncertain. Two basic approaches to the problem have emerged. Some scientists relate this change to dietary handling of *cholesterol and related substances. Certainly, families who have an abnormal

cholesterol metabolism show a high incidence of arterial disease, but how far this applies to the population at large is debatable. Others concentrate on chemical factors related to the smooth muscle and lining cells of the artery, which include platelet-activating factor (PAF), *prostaglandins, and an endothelium-derived relaxing factor (EDRF), which is nitric oxide. The mechanisms are complicated, and it is often difficult to separate cause and effect. However, one risk factor has been proved beyond all doubt, and moreover it is controllable: tobacco smoking in any form worsens and accelerates arterial disease.

When an artery is blocked, harm results. A tissue, especially muscle, receiving less than its ideal requirement of blood and oxygen often generates pain. This situation is termed *ischaemia. Examples include pain in the heart due to narrowed coronary arteries, and pain in the legs on walking, due to impairment of flow through the femoral artery or its branches (see Fig. 1). Total blockage of an 'end-artery' (the final route of supply to an organ) results in local death or *gangrene, unless there is a way around the block (the collateral circulation) or the surgeon can restore flow. This is called *infarction. If the infarct affects an arm or a leg, that limb may be lost, which is bad enough, but if the artery supplies the heart muscle or the brain, the results can be devastating or even fatal.

In order to tell whether an artery is narrowed or blocked, and whether it is possible to open it up, it is necessary to 'image' the vessel by some form of X-ray or scan. Formerly, the only way this could be done was to inject radiopaque material directly into the artery, but the development of *ultrasound and

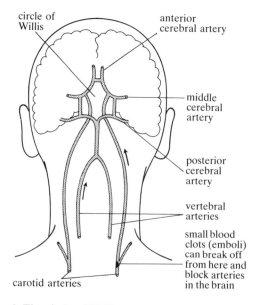

Fig. 2 The circle of Willis.

*magnetic resonance techniques has made this necessary less often, and it is now possible to produce very accurate images with greater safety and much less discomfort.

The brain

The heart gives off four arteries to the brain, two in front and two at the back: the carotid and vertebral arteries, respectively. These form a circle at the base of the skull, called the *circle of Willis, after Queen Elizabeth I's physician, Thomas *Willis, who discovered it (Fig. 2). The circle acts as a safety device, in that if one or more of the four routes into it is closed, the others can maintain flow. From the circle, smaller vessels run up into the brain substance. Interruption of these end-arteries can be very serious, because a part of the brain then ceases to function, resulting in paralysis or death. This is one cause of *stroke, *haemorrhage into the brain being another.

Rather than the small arteries within the brain, the arteries in the neck, accessible to the surgeon, often determine events higher up, sometimes because loose clots, called emboli, become dislodged. Operations on the carotid arteries can stop this happening, but it is not easy to predict who is at risk, and the operations themselves can cause problems. However, multicentre studies carried out in Europe and the USA have now shown beyond doubt that for certain groups of patients such surgery confers a real benefit.

The heart

Perhaps the most crucial arteries in the body, in terms of sustaining life, are the very first branches of the *aorta, the coronary arteries which supply the heart muscle itself. Obstruction (coronary thrombosis) or narrowing of these vessels results in two types of illness. First is the condition known as *angina pectoris, which means pain in the chest on exertion. Angina may be consistent with a relatively normal life, but it always means trouble, and some affected patients progress to the next stage of ischaemic heart disease, the acute 'myocardial infarct' (see CARDIOLOGY). This type of heart attack means that the ischaemia has become critical, in that the blood flow has fallen to a level where part of the cardiac muscle has actually died. If this involves a large area, the heart may fail totally, but more often only a small portion is affected, and the muscle is eventually replaced by a fibrous scar.

If treated early, it is often possible to open up the coronary artery by giving drugs, such as *streptokinase (an enzyme produced by certain bacteria), which dissolve blood clots. Further clotting in the vessel can be discouraged by the use of aspirin, which has a specific effect on the blood *platelets. People with long-standing occlusions in their heart vessels require more radical treatment, which may involve inflating a small, tough balloon inserted into the artery (this can be done through the femoral artery, under a local anaesthetic) or by carrying out a surgical bypass, which involves taking a small vein from the leg and inserting it between the aorta and the coronary artery beyond the block. Coronary artery bypass graft (CABG) (see CARDIOVASCULAR SURGERY), which until quite recently was viewed as a 'high-tech' procedure available only in special centres, is now a routine operation, with a very low mortality. We know that it both relieves symptoms and may prolong life, but whether such surgery will stand the test of time remains to be seen. Clearly, the effective long-term answer must be some means of preventing the accumulation of deposits in the arterial wall, or of dissolving them once they have formed. Alterations in life-style are important, and have brought about a significant reduction in the frequency of ischaemic heart disease. The important risk factors are once again tobacco smoking, *obesity, and high blood pressure.

The kidney

Arteries bring blood to the kidney for purification, as already explained, but the kidney also has a function in regulating blood pressure. If the flow through its main artery falls below a certain level, then its cells produce 'pressor' substances, such as the hormone *angiotensin, which constrict vessels all over the body, thus raising the blood pressure and restoring the kidney's supply of oxygen. However, hypertension is a potentially killing disease, as is discussed elsewhere, and it would seem sensible to attack the problem at source by identifying narrowed or blocked areas in the renal arteries, and correcting them if at all possible. Operations designed to do exactly this were once widely practised, but were superseded by the arrival of a range of very effective drugs which can control blood pressure without recourse to surgery. However, the long-term effects of such drugs are not known, and there has been a recent reawakening of interest in a direct attack on the artery, using the balloon angioplasty techniques already described in relation to the heart. It is too early to tell whether the initially promising results will last, or whether we will develop even more effective ways of controlling blood pressure. The use of '*biofeedback' methods, whereby one can influence ones' body processes by deliberate introspection, has great possibilities here.

The limbs

Arms are almost never ischaemic (unless injured) but the legs are different, and in fact provide the vascular surgeon with most of his work. Why this should be so is not immediately obvious, but certainly the legs work much harder, in the sense of carrying weight around, than do the arms, and also their collateral blood supply is not so well developed.

When the arteries to the lower half of the body start to fail, typical symptoms develop. The first problem the patient notices is that of '*intermittent claudication', which means pain in the calf muscles coming on after a certain walking distance, and relieved by rest. This happens because the blood flow to the muscles, although adequate for resting conditions, cannot be raised (due to the blockage in the artery) to meet the requirements of exercise. Many people with this problem get better without treatment. Before any complicated tests, let alone operations, are carried out, nature must be given every chance to put matters right by spontaneous opening up of the collateral circulation. However, in an unlucky minority of people (particularly if they continue to smoke) this does not happen, and the condition deteriorates to the point that they start to have pain at rest, especially at night, when the blood pressure falls off. This renders life intolerable, and demands relief, either by surgery or by one of the newer interventional radiological procedures (see RADIOLOGY). Quite apart from the pain, if nothing is done there is a very real risk that the leg will be lost.

Eventually, the circulation may fail completely, so that the foot or leg is irrecoverable. Given this, the only possible course is an *amputation which, not only to the victim but also to the surgeon (whose job it is to restore flow to arteries and to save limbs), seems an act of despair. Nevertheless, amputation can be

a life-enhancing operation as it immediately relieves the intense pain of severe ischaemia, and halts the absorption of toxic materials from the dead tissue, which greatly affect both physical and mental well-being. Helped by the provision of a modern lightweight artificial limb, amputation can often be a passport to a new life (see REHABILITATION).

Aneurysms

Curiously, the same disease process (*atheroma) that leads to narrowed and blocked arteries, can also produce vessels that expand under the pressure of the blood within them. A dilated artery is called an *aneurysm (in contrast to a *varix, which is a dilated vein). Aneurysms are dangerous, because as the wall enlarges it becomes steadily weaker and eventually ruptures. This catastrophe can be prevented by early surgery. The abdominal aorta is the vessel most frequently affected, and replacement of aneurysms at that site is nowadays a standard operation. Once the aneurysm has ruptured the mortality is very high, and many such patients die even before they reach hospital, but a planned repair is extremely safe. Moreover, the life expectancy of someone who has had the aneurysm put right is the same as that of a normal person of the same age—this is in contrast to the patient with blocked arteries, who in actuarial terms is 10 years older than his recorded birth date.

The techniques of arterial reconstruction

There are two basic ways of restoring flow to a blocked artery. The first is termed '*endarterectomy' and depends on the fact that as arteries become older they develop a split or plane in the wall. The operation consists in dissecting up this plane and removing the central core that is causing the obstruction (see Fig. 3). When the obstruction is removed, it leaves a relatively smooth surface behind. A remarkable feature of the operation is that the remaining thin outer tube is strong enough to resist the blood pressure and does not bulge out to form an aneurysm. Endarterectomy can now be done in the X-ray department with flexible rotating devices, much as are used to clear blocked drains. These techniques are still being developed.

The other way to deal with a closed artery is to introduce a bypass channel above and below the obstruction. The best material to use for a bypass is a person's own vein, and there is a particular vein in the leg, the long saphenous vein, which is ideal for this purpose, as it is both long and strong, and can be safely removed without any ill-effects. The saphenous, which is easily seen lying under the skin of the leg (the Arabic word *saphena* means easily seen), is used in the heart to bypass the coronary artery, and in the leg to replace the blocked femoral. However, some patients who require a bypass do not have a suitable vein available, either because it has been used already, or because it is anatomically unsuitable. It then becomes necessary to introduce some kind of synthetic conduit. For many

For short blocks of large vessels
aorto-iliac
carotid　　　　　endarterectomy

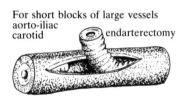

For long blocks of large vessels
aorto-femoral

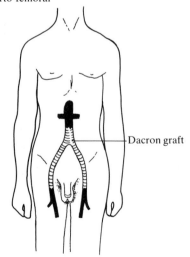

Dacron graft

Fig. 3 Some techniques of arterial reconstruction.

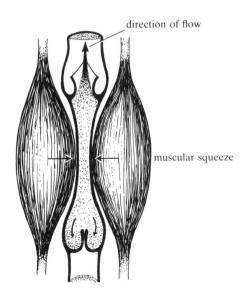

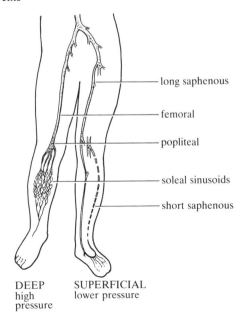

Fig. 4 The venous valves.

Fig. 5 The leg veins, seen from the front.

years scientists have tried to devise an artificial artery that would perform as well as a natural vein, but no one has yet succeeded. Arteries are pulsating, elastic structures with a smooth, glistening lining, which the blood slips over, without any tendency to stagnate or to clot. The engineer attempting to compete with nature has to provide a tube which remains elastic and supple, and at the same time discourages clotting. Of the two requirements, the quality of the lining seems to be the more important, and work is under way to induce living human cells from the inside of blood vessels to grow on these plastic grafts and provide a lining with the right qualities. Such cells produce substances called *prosta-cyclins, which are potent inhibitors of clotting and dilate the vessels, so they would form an ideal covering for the graft. This type of research is exciting, but is still at an early stage.

The veins

In contrast to the high-speed, high-pressure delivery system constituted by the arteries, the veins are thin-walled, low-pressure tubes, whose main function is to return blood from the tissues, via the heart, to the lungs, for discharge of *CO_2 and replenishment of oxygen. They contain one-way valves to direct their flow. The veins contain 80 per cent of the total blood volume, and function as a reservoir in the pumping system, capable of expansion or contraction in response to the body's needs.

If a person stands immobile for more than a few minutes, the circulation to the brain may fail and he will faint and fall over. The reason for this is that the force generated by the heart is not enough to overcome gravity and drive blood up to the top of the body. A

mechanism in the veins of the legs ensures that, as their muscles contract, blood is propelled upwards in the right direction, to re-enter the arterial circulation via the heart (see Fig. 4). But these one-way return valves are subjected to great pressure and, if they are not perfectly co-ordinated, may fail.

There are two systems of veins in the legs (see Figs 5 and 6). The deep veins lie inside the muscles and, because they are squeezed by them, they operate at higher pressure, whereas the superficial veins run in the fatty tissue under the skin, and are not squeezed, so have a much lower pressure. At certain points the two systems connect. These connections are guarded by valves, which prevent high-pressure deep-venous blood from being forced into the superficial veins. Should

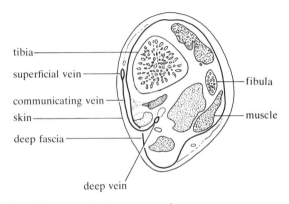

Fig. 6 The leg veins in cross-section.

these valves fail, then the veins under the skin become congested and enlarged, resulting in the appearance of varices. *Varicose veins are extremely common—indeed most people over the age of 40 have some dilated veins on their legs. Whether such an anatomical fault can properly be called a 'disease' is a matter of definition. Certainly, there is little relation between the size of the veins and the symptoms attributed to them, in that some individuals report severe discomfort from quite small veins, whereas more stoical people tolerate enormous bunches of veins apparently without complaint. The cosmetic aspect is perhaps the most important, although it is true that varicosities can at times lead to *ulceration.

Treatment of varicose veins consists either in injecting an irritant solution into the compressed vein, so as to cause its walls to adhere and eliminate the unsightly bulge, or to remove the vein surgically. Care must be taken to preserve the saphenous vein if at all possible, because it may be needed later for artery replacement in the heart or the leg.

In contrast to the common, but relatively innocent, problem of varicose superficial veins, disease in the deep venous system is a threat to health or even sometimes to life.

The deep veins in the legs are arranged in a sort of honeycomb, in which the blood can easily stagnate and clot (a deep vein *thrombosis, or DVT). A patient immobilized in hospital, perhaps because of an operation, is at risk of a silent accumulation of DVT starting in the calf but later extending up into the thigh. This can be very serious, as it may result in a clot becoming dislodged from the leg vein into the lung, causing anything from a slight transient pain in the chest to sudden death. This is known as a pulmonary *embolus. Prevention of this disaster concentrates on mobility, protection of the veins, and anticoagulant therapy designed to keep the blood from clotting, without at the same time causing a risk of haemorrhage. Apart from the acute problem of a pulmonary embolus, DVT can, by destruction of the valves, lead to later tissue changes in the legs, such as swelling, *eczema, and ulceration.

The small vessels

As mentioned at the outset, one of the functions of the circulation is to regulate body temperature by altering flow through the skin. This is done by nervous impulses contracting the muscular walls of the vessels, and by various chemical substances in the blood which directly affect the muscle tone. There is a striking difference in the behaviour of the skin vessels in the two sexes. In men the vessels tend to remain open, and men lose some 10 per cent more of their body heat through the skin than do women, whose arterioles are more reactive and sensitive. The various reflexes influencing the state of the skin vessels were elucidated by Sir Thomas *Lewis in the 1920s, using no more sophisticated equipment than pins, rubber bands, and warm water. Given

how commonly these reflexes are disturbed, leading to *chilblains, vasospasm, and excessive sweating, it is surprising how little our knowledge has advanced since then.

Most problems in the skin circulation arise from spasm in the small vessels, leading to coldness, blueness, and even ulceration. They were originally described in the 19th century by the French physician Maurice *Raynaud, and are sometimes referred to as Raynaud's disease. Other names are *erythromelalgia, *erythrocyanosis, and *acrocyanosis. These long Greek words add nothing to our real understanding of the basic mechanisms of the conditions or of ways of treating them, and on the whole the best we can do is to control the symptoms.

Specific treatment, so far as it goes, may be by drugs or surgery. 'Vasodilators' are agents designed to relax the spasm in the small vessels to the skin and hence to improve flow, but there is little evidence, either from laboratory or field trials, that they actually help. There is much commercial pressure, and it is unfortunately the case that, when doctors have no effective remedy for a disease, they tend to use an ineffective one rather than nothing at all. However, further drugs designed to improve flow are being developed.

The other line of treatment is a *sympathectomy, which consists of cutting or destroying the nerves responsible for constricting the vessel wall. Although sometimes dramatically successful, the improvement is often transient and after a few months the vessels regain their tone and the symptoms come back.

Summary
Although the arteries and veins comprise a small portion of the body mass, they are critical to health, and this applies particularly to the arteries, whose role is to sustain and nourish the vital tissues and organs. Impairment of arterial flow can result in a whole spectrum of disorders, ranging from chilblains to stroke. Problems in the veins can result in cosmetic difficulties such as leg varicosities, but may also extend to a life-threatening pulmonary embolus.

Vascular diseases can, to an extent, be foreseen and prevented by attention to life-style and by avoidance of the main risk factors, including smoking and obesity, but once damage has occurred, modern techniques can often overcome or compensate for some of the worst effects.

A. MARSTON

ARTERIOGRAPHY is the radiographic visualization of arteries after the injection of an appropriate radio-paque medium into the circulation.

ARTERIOLE. The smallest subdivision of the arterial system, these are the branches that connect the *arteries proper to the *capillary bed. The state of the arterioles is the chief determinant of *peripheral vascular resistance and the means whereby selective distribution of the circulation to regions, organs, and tissues is achieved.

ARTERIOSCLEROSIS is literally 'hardening of the *arteries'; it is an inexact term which embraces all pathological processes associated with thickening and loss of elasticity of arterial walls, the commonest being *atherosclerosis.

ARTERITIS. Inflammation of an *artery.

ARTHRITIS. Inflammation of a joint or joints. In common usage, the term covers joint conditions other than those due solely to inflammation, the commonest being '*osteoarthritis' (strictly 'osteoarthropathy'), a degenerative condition.

ARTHRODESIS. Surgical fixation of a joint.

ARTHROGRAPHY is the radiographic visualization of a joint cavity and its internal surfaces after injection of air or a radiopaque contrast material.

ARTHROPATHY is any pathological condition affecting one or more joints.

ARTHROPLASTY. Plastic surgery of a joint; the construction of an artificial joint.

ARTHROPODS are members of the Arthropoda, the most numerous phylum of the animal kingdom; it contains 85 per cent of all known animal species. Of the 12 component classes, the two most important medically are the Insecta (insects) and the Arachnida (scorpions, spiders, ticks, mites, harvestmen, and king-crabs); the Crustacea should also be mentioned. Many arthropods are either vectors of infectious disease, or are parasitic on man. See also ACARUS; ANOPHELES; ARACHNID; ARBOVIRUS; INSECTS AS VECTORS OF DISEASE; SCORPIONS; etc.

ARTHROSCOPY is the inspection of the internal surfaces of a joint with an endoscopic instrument (see ENDOSCOPY). It is also now possible to carry out surgical operations on the interior of the knee joint through an arthroscope.

ARTHUS, NICOLAS MAURICE (1862–1945). French physiologist. Between 1903 and 1906 he showed that if an *antigen is injected into the skin when *antibody to that antigen is already present, an inflammatory lesion develops leading on to haemorrhage, necrosis, and ulceration. This example of immediate *hypersensitivity is called the Arthus reaction (see ALLERGY). Other forms of hypersensitivity due to antigen–antibody unions, such as *serum sickness, *glomerulonephritis, and *farmer's lung, may be called Arthus-type reactions.

ARTICULATION has two meanings: the enunciation of speech; and a joint, or the process of jointing.

ARTIFICIAL INSEMINATION is the artificial introduction of *semen into the vagina or cervix; the semen (either fresh or previously frozen with glycerol) is obtained by *masturbation from the patient's husband (AIH) or from another donor (AID). The procedure is undertaken during the menstrual cycle at about the time of ovulation, as indicated by body temperature and/or biochemistry.

ARTIFICIAL PNEUMOTHORAX is a procedure formerly employed in the treatment of pulmonary *tuberculosis and sometimes now of value in diagnostic *radiology. See PNEUMOTHORAX.

ARTIFICIAL RESPIRATION. A term commonly used to mean *ventilation of the lungs (i.e. inspiration and expiration) by artificial means. Of the many techniques devised the mouth-to-mouth method is now preferred as being both effective and easy to perform. In hospital, mechanical devices are available, most of which depend on pumping air or oxygen into the lungs via a tube inserted into the trachea (wind-pipe). See also FIRST AID; INTENSIVE CARE; RESUSCITATION

ASBESTOSIS is a dangerous form of *pneumoconiosis caused by inhalation of asbestos fibres. It is characterized by interstitial pulmonary fibrosis and pneumonitis, and is associated with malignant growths of the pleura and peritoneum (*mesothelioma), of the bronchi (bronchial carcinoma), and occasionally of other sites.

ASCARIASIS is infestation with the *nematode parasite *Ascaris lumbricoides*, common in many parts of the world, particularly in children. It is spread between humans by faecal contamination of the environment; no intermediate host is involved, but to become infective, the fertilized ova excreted by one individual require maturation in soil (about 10 days) before ingestion by another. After being swallowed, they hatch in the *duodenum and penetrate into the veins, then undertaking a remarkable odyssey (venous circulation–lungs–alveoli–bronchi–trachea–pharynx) before being re-swallowed into the small *intestine. Here they develop into male and female adults, and live for about 18 months if undisturbed. The intestinal upset they produce is variable and may be mild; it includes attacks of diarrhoea and vomiting, with malabsorption and consequent malnutrition. Complications may arise because of their continued tendency to wander (e.g. biliary or pancreatic tract obstruction, intestinal perforation, liver abscess, appendicitis); a tangled mass of worms may also cause intestinal obstruction. During the original infection, the larval forms may produce clinically apparent *pneumonitis (inflammation of the lung) with *eosinophilia (Loeffler's syndrome).

ASCARIS. A genus of *nematodes (roundworms), species of which are parasitic in man and animals. The important human parasite is *Ascaris lumbricoides* (see ASCARIASIS); this is the largest nematode to infest man, adults being from 25 to 50 cm long.

ASCHHEIM, SELMAR (1878–1965). German physician. With *Zondek he devised the first reliable *pregnancy test (1928).

ASCHOFF, KARL ALBERT LUDWIG (1866–1942). German pathologist in the *Virchow tradition. He described the Aschoff bodies in the rheumatic myocardium (1904) and put forward the notion of the *reticuloendothelial system (1913).

ASCITES is the accumulation of fluid within the *peritoneal cavity, with resultant distension of the abdomen. Ascites has many causes; among the commonest are chronic liver disease, malignant invasion (cancer) of the peritoneum, tuberculosis, and generalized fluid retention.

ASCORBIC ACID ($C_6H_8O_6$) is a water-soluble *vitamin also known as vitamin C. It is an essential component of the diet of man (although of few other animals), the recommended daily allowance for adults being 60 mg. Adequate intake is necessary for normal wound healing and resistance to infection; deficiency causes *scurvy. There is little or no evidence to substantiate the claim that in 'megadosage' it is effective in the prophylaxis and treatment of the common cold.

ASELLI, GASPARE (1581–1625). Italian anatomist. In 1622 he rediscovered the *chylous (lymphatic) vessels or lacteals, which had been known to *Herophilus and *Erasistratus in the 4th century BC.

ASEPSIS. Freedom from, or prevention of *infection with micro-organisms.

ASHER, RICHARD ALAN JOHN (1912–69). Influential writer and stylist, as well as physician at the Central Middlesex Hospital, he was the first to describe *Münchausen's syndrome, as well as to emphasize the frequency of mental changes in *thyroid disease ('myxoedematous madness') and the dangers of the, then, panacea of bed rest.

ASKLEPIOS (AESCULAPIUS), OF BYTHNIA (?130–?40 BC). Greek physician. He practised in Rome, rejected the Hippocratic humoralism, and imported the atomic views of Democritus into medicine, to become the founder of *solidism. He believed all disease resulted from an abnormal arrangement of the 'atoms' relative to the 'pores', which were the physical basis of the body.

He advocated the humane treatment of the insane, was a fervent believer in *hydrotherapy, and the first to mention *tracheostomy.

ASPERGILLOSIS is one of the *opportunistic *mycoses (i.e. fungal infections), occurring mostly in patients whose immune defence mechanisms are impaired. *Aspergillus* species, of which there are many, are common moulds, widely distributed in the environment, but are not normally pathogenic to man (except occasionally in allergic conditions).

ASPHYXIA. Originally and literally meaning 'stoppage of the pulse', asphyxia is now synonymous with *suffocation from lack of inspired oxygen.

ASPIRATION is the action or process of drawing fluids, gases, etc. in, out, or through by suction. An aspirator is an apparatus for removing material by suction from the respiratory tract or other body cavity.

ASPIRIN. See ACETYLSALICYLIC ACID.

ASSAY. Measurement of amount, particularly with reference to the biological or pharmacological activity of a substance.

ASSOCIATION OF AMERICAN MEDICAL COLLEGES (AAMC), after a faltering start in 1876, was re-formed in 1890 and its work continues. It was, and is, a coming-together of all the medical schools and colleges. Its functions have become increasingly formal in maintaining standards in all stages of medical education, both of undergraduates and graduates. The AAMC now has four constituent bodies—a Council of Deans, a Council of Academic Societies, a Council of Teaching Hospitals, and the Organization of Student Representatives—which meet as an Assembly, the Association's legislative and policy-making body. A major fillip to its power was given especially by the *Flexner Report* of 1910, which criticized the standards of medical education in the USA (and elsewhere), often in the inadequate money-making schools which had sprung up outside reputable institutions. The result was that these were closed down, largely because their inadequacy was exposed by both the AAMC and the *American Medical Association (AMA), who inspected premises, facilities, and faculty. Now the AAMC and the AMA join in a Liaison Committee on Medical Education which inspects and accredits medical schools. Apart from its prime function in medical education, the AAMC has Groups concerned with Business Affairs, Institutional Planning, Public Affairs, and Student Affairs.

The AAMC is also responsible for the Medical College Admission Test, a national test taken by virtually all applicants for admission to medical schools in the USA and some in Canada. They also run the American Medical College Application Service, which allows applicants to use only a single form for admission to several schools. Obviously, the AAMC is a clearing house for information on medical education to all its constituent bodies and other corporations. With others it helps organize the examinations of the Educational Commission for Foreign Medical Graduates and the Visa Qualifying Examination, designed to test the capabilities of overseas doctors who wish to practise in the USA. These are usually accepted by the licensing bodies of the various states.

Working with others, the AAMC accredits hospitals, and programmes of education for younger graduates and for continuing education for the more senior. There is an Accreditation Council for Graduate Medical Education and one for Continuing Medical Education. All advanced countries have felt it imperative to preserve standards of medical practice by controlling medical education by methods such as those outlined. The principles are ubiquitous, although the methods of achieving the objectives vary from country to country in accordance with differing historical developments. (See also MEDICAL EDUCATION IN THE USA AND CANADA.)

ASTHENIA. Lack (or impairment) of strength; debility.

ASTHMA is a paroxysmal breathlessness, usually associated with widespread narrowing of the airways (bronchoconstriction) and obstruction to breathing ('bronchial asthma'). 'Cardiac asthma' is a term sometimes given to paroxysmal breathing difficulty of a quite different cause, namely episodic failure of the left ventricle of the heart.

ASTIGMATISM is a common refractive error of the eye, due to unequal radii of curvature of the refracting surfaces of the lens. It can be readily corrected by spectacles with appropriate lenses (see OPHTHALMOLOGY).

ASTRINGENT describes pharmaceutical preparations which when applied locally, exert a shrinking action on the skin and superficial tissues; by precipitating proteins, they also form a hard protective layer. The main astringents are tannins and aluminium and zinc salts.

ASTROCYTOMA. A brain tumour arising from astrocytes, cells forming part of the ectodermal component of *neuroglia. Although astrocytomas can be classified pathologically into varying degrees of malignancy on the basis of cell differentiation (the most malignant type usually being termed glioblastoma multiforme), they almost invariably, sooner or later, cause the death of the patient. See CEREBRAL TUMOUR; NEUROSURGERY.

ASTROLOGY is a pseudo-science based upon the supposed influence of the stars and planets on human affairs. Physician–astrologers flourished in the 14th and 15th centuries. One system related the seven planets to the major organs, the days of the week, and the seven metals, and so to diagnosis, treatment, and prognosis. Chaucer's portrait of a 'Doctor of Phisyck' in *The Canterbury Tales* (*c*. 1397) is not untypical of the period.

ASYLUMS. An asylum is a secure place of refuge, shelter, or retreat, originally for criminals and debtors, now more often used in respect of political dissidents and refugees. It was literally and originally a place where pillage was forbidden (Greek *sulon*, right of pillage); the ancients set aside certain places of refuge where the vilest criminals were protected from both private and public assaults. The term also came to mean a benevolent institution for the shelter of some classes of the afflicted, the unfortunate, or the destitute; in popular usage it was often restricted to 'lunatic asylum'. The use of 'asylum' to mean mental institution or hospital is now obsolete.

ASYMBOLIA is the inability, due to cerebral damage, to use or comprehend symbols, including words and signs; it is a form of *aphasia.

ASYNERGY is a lack of co-ordination of parts or organs which normally act in concert, exemplified by cerebellar *ataxia.

ASYSTOLE is *cardiac arrest, i.e. the absence of heartbeat.

ATAXIA is lack of co-ordination, resulting in unsteadiness of posture, gait, and movements, including eye movements and speech. Ataxia can be broadly classified into *sensory* (or proprioceptive) forms, in which joint position sense (proprioception) is impaired; and *motor* ataxia, due to disturbance of cerebellar or vestibular function. The former is aggravated when the eyes are shut because visual input normally counteracts the proprioceptive defect.

ATELECTASIS is failure of expansion of part or all of a lung in newborn infants. It is often, although less correctly, used to mean collapse of lung tissue at any age.

ATHEROMA is a common degenerative arterial condition in which *lipid-rich yellowish plaques (the term 'atheroma' derives from a fancied resemblance to porridge) are deposited in the lining (*intima) of large and medium-sized *arteries, leading to changes collectively known as *atherosclerosis.

ATHEROSCLEROSIS is thickening, loss of elasticity, and narrowing of *arteries as a result of pathological changes in the vessel walls due to the deposition of *atheroma. Atherosclerosis is much the commonest arterial disease, and is present in some degree in virtually the entire adult male population of Western societies. It is less common in females. Its effect, which varies with its extent and distribution, is to impair the blood supply to organs and tissues, i.e. to cause *ischaemia. It predisposes to the formation of intra-arterial *thrombus and so may cut off circulation altogether. Atherosclerosis is the usual cause of *coronary heart disease (*angina and *coronary thrombosis causing *myocardial infarction) and *stroke, and plays a major role in many other diseases of middle and old age. Its aetiology is complex, but several 'risk factors' have been identified: these include increasing age; being male; high level of circulating blood *lipids; cigarette smoking; high blood pressure (*hypertension); obesity; lack of physical exercise; genetic predisposition; and stress. Diet may also be important.

ATHETOSIS. Slow involuntary movements, often described as writhing, affecting particularly the hands and feet. It occurs in brain-damaged children, and is most often seen in *cerebral palsy.

ATHLETE'S FOOT, or tinea pedis, is a common *fungal infection of the skin of the foot. The name derives from the fact that it may be acquired in showers, changing-rooms, etc.

ATHLETICS. See DOCTORS AS ATHLETES; SPORT AND MEDICINE.

ATKINS, JOHN (1685–1757). British naval surgeon. His book *The Navy surgeon* (1732) went through several editions and contained the first description of *trypanosomiasis (sleeping sickness).

ATMOSPHERIC POLLUTION. Chemical pollution of the urban atmosphere arises chiefly from combustion of fossil fuels, i.e. coal, oil, and petroleum products. The products include particulate carbon, *carbon monoxide, *carbon dioxide, *hydrocarbons, *sulphur, and lead compounds. Although the medical consequences of these pollutants are often not fully established (note the controversies surrounding the possible influence of lead on intellectual development, or of carbon and sulphur products on common cardiopulmonary diseases), few would deny that the quality of life has improved in many great cities because of various clean-air enactments of recent years or that pollution control is socially desirable. See also ENVIRONMENT AND DISEASE; POLLUTION

ATMOSPHERIC PRESSURE. At sea-level and 0 °C the pressure of the atmosphere fluctuates about an average value of 101 325 pascals (Pa) (newtons per square metre, N/m^2) or approximately 14.72 lb/in^2. This value, a unit of 1 atmosphere, can support a column of mercury 760 mm high (29.92 in).

ATOPY is an inherited predisposition to *allergy and allergic disorders sometimes termed an 'allergic diathesis' or 'hereditary allergy'.

ATP/ADP. See ADENOSINE TRIPHOSPHATE.

ATRESIA is the congenital obliteration or developmental absence of an orifice, duct, or other passage.

ATRIAL FIBRILLATION is one of the commonest disorders of cardiac rhythm. Contractions of the atrial *myocardium are rapid (350–600 per minute) and uncoordinated, and thus irregular and ineffective. Ventricular response, and hence the arterial pulse, is also rapid and irregular; without treatment, the pulse rate is usually between 120 and 180 per minute. See also CARDIOLOGY.

ATRIAL FLUTTER is a cardiac *arrhythmia in which atrial contractions occur at the abnormally rapid rate of about 300 per minute but are regular and co-ordinated (cf. *atrial fibrillation). This is usually too rapid for the atrioventricular conducting system, so that a ventricular response occurs to only every second, third, or even fourth atrial impulse, producing arterial *pulse rates of about 150, 100, or 75 per minute, respectively. Atrial flutter is sometimes an established and sometimes a paroxysmal rhythm. Diagnosis by *electrocardiography is easy, but may also be made by comparing the frequency of 'f' or flutter waves in the cervical venous pulse with that of the arterial pulse.

ATRIOVENTRICULAR NODE. Part of the specialized conducting system of the *myocardium, lying beneath the endocardium in the right posterior interatrial septum, close to the *tricuspid valve. The atrioventricular (AV) node receives the cardiac excitation wave from the atrial myocardium and rapidly transmits it to the *bundle of His, with which it is continuous, thence to the two bundle branches, the subendocardial *Purkinje network of fibres, and so to the ventricular myocardium.

ATRIUM. Any anatomical structure that acts as an antechamber. When otherwise unqualified, an atrium is one of the two upper chambers (right and left) of the heart (formerly termed auricles).

ATROPHY. Wasting, diminution in size.

ATROPINE ($C_{17}H_{23}NO_3$) is an *alkaloid that blocks the effects of the *parasympathetic nervous system on smooth muscle, cardiac muscle, and glandular cells. Because it opposes the action of *acetylcholine, it is termed an anticholinergic agent. It thus paralyses visual accommodation, decreases salivary secretion, increases heart rate and pulmonary ventilation, and decreases digestive activity (i.e. is an *antispasmodic). It is widely used in treatment.

ATTACK. Any accession of illness.

AUDIOLOGY is the science of *hearing, particularly the study of hearing loss. See OTORHINOLARYNG-OLOGY.

AUDIOMETRY is measurement of the sensitivity of the ear to sounds of different frequencies and intensities. See OTORHINOLARYNGOLOGY.

AUDIT in medicine has been defined as 'The systematic critical analysis of medical care, including the procedures used for diagnosis and treatment, the use of resources and the resulting outcome and quality of life for the patient.' (UK NHS Review; working paper 6, 1991.)

AUDITORY NERVE. The eighth *cranial nerve, also known as the vestibulocochlear nerve. It has two functionally separate divisions: the vestibular nerve carries afferent fibres from that part of the inner ear concerned with balance (the vestibule of the *labyrinth and the *semicircular canals); the cochlear nerve carries fibres from the essential organ of hearing (the organ of Corti) in the *cochlea. The two divisions run together from the internal auditory meatus in the *temporal bone to enter the *brainstem in the angle between the *cerebellum and the *pons (the cerebellopontine angle).

AUENBRUGGER, JOSEPH LEOPOLD (1722–1809). Austrian physician, the son of an inn-keeper, his most noteworthy contribution was to discover the diagnostic value of *percussion. Traditionally it was attributed to seeing his father tapping on barrels to determine the levels of wine they contained. He was also a keen musician and even wrote the libretto for his friend Antonio Salieri's comic opera *Der Rauchfangkehrer (The Chimney Sweep)*.

AUERBACH, LEOPOLD (1828–97). German anatomist and neurologist. He described the myenteric plexus (Auerbach's plexus) in 1862. This is a network of *autonomic nerve fibres and *parasympathetic ganglia distributed through the muscular coat of the intestinal wall.

AUGUSTINIAN SISTERS OF HOTEL DIEU, the oldest purely nursing order of nuns, staffed the *Hôtel Dieu (founded by Landry, Bishop of Paris, in AD 651) from its earliest history and continued to work there until 1908. Their record of over 12 centuries of service to the hospital constitutes the longest history of *nursing by any Order. The sisters were united into a strict Order under Augustinian rule by Pope Innocent IV in the 15th century. As records of the Hôtel Dieu are available from the 12th century, much is known about the dedication of the sisters and the rigours they were required to endure.

AURA is a term used in medicine to describe a premonitory sensation that warns of the impending onset of a periodic disorder, particularly of *epilepsy but also of *migraine.

AURICLE is the external ear; it was also formerly used for the two upper chambers of the heart but has been superseded by (right and left) '*atrium'.

AURISCOPE. An instrument for examining the ear.

AUSCULTATION is the act of listening, either directly with the ear (direct auscultation) or indirectly with a *stethoscope (mediate ausculation) to sounds generated within the body arising in the heart, lungs, pleura, blood vessels, intestine, fetus, etc. See also LAENNEC.

AUTISM is a disorder of mental and emotional development of uncertain nature, characterized by withdrawal and failure of social communication. The name derives from the patient's apparent preoccupation with self-centred and subjective patterns of thought. Repetitive and seemingly meaningless actions may also be a feature. The condition usually begins in early childhood and is thought by some to be a childhood variant of *schizophrenia; others regard it as an expression of mental handicap. Yet another view holds that the impenetrable aloofness conceals a significant capacity for intellectual development.

AUTOANALYSIS is self-analysis, especially exploration by a person of his own conscious or unconscious mind; it is advocated in the treatment of *psychoneurosis as a form of *psychoanalysis.

AUTOANTIBODY. *Antibody directed against an *antigen which is a normal constituent of the body. See also IMMUNOLOGY.

AUTOCLAVE. An apparatus that sterilizes objects by subjecting them to steam under high pressure.

AUTOGRAFT. A transplant of tissue to another part of the same individual (cf. *allograft).

AUTOIMMUNE DISEASE is any disease in which *autoimmunity is known or suspected to be involved in causation or pathogenesis, e.g. *pernicious anaemia, *myasthenia gravis, some forms of *haemolytic anaemia, *Hashimoto's disease and some other *thyroid disorders, *glomerulonephritis, *rheumatoid arthritis, *ulcerative colitis, and many others. See IMMUNOLOGY.

AUTOIMMUNITY is any condition in which an 'immune' response, cellular and/or humoral, is directed against one or more of the body's own constituents. See IMMUNOLOGY.

AUTOINTOXICATION is poisoning by, or resulting from, *toxin produced in the body.

AUTOLYSIS is enzymatic self-digestion of cells or tissues following death or injury.

AUTOMATISM is the performance of complex (i.e. non-reflex) acts without consciousness or volition.

AUTONOMIC NERVOUS SYSTEM. That part of the nervous system regulating the involuntary or 'self-governing' activity of glands, smooth muscle, and cardiac muscle. It comprises *sympathetic and *parasympathetic systems, which have generally opposing actions, and which derive respectively from the thoracolumbar and the craniosacral parts of the nervous system (neuraxis).

AUTOPSY (literally 'seeing for oneself') is the postmortem dissection of a dead body and its structures in order to determine the cause of death and the nature of the pathological changes that brought it about. Synonymous with necropsy.

AUTORADIOGRAPHY is a technique for localizing *radioactive material (particularly that labelled with tritium (^{3}H) or carbon-14) within tissues and individual cells. These nuclides decay by emitting beta particles, producing a latent image on a photographic film or plate brought into contact with a smear or thin tissue section after it has been treated with, e.g., triturated thymidine. The histological and radiographic appearances are then compared.

AUTOREGULATION is the automatic adjustment of local physiological variables, such as vascular resistance, in order to maintain constancy of local tissue or organ *perfusion, or constancy of the relationship between perfusion and metabolic activity; it is a particular example of *homeostasis.

AVELING, JAMES HOBSON (1829–92). British obstetrician, one of the founders of the Chelsea Hospital for Women. He was an early exponent of direct *blood transfusion, for which he devised an ingenious apparatus.

AVENZOAR (Abu Merwan Abdul-Malik ibn Zuhr) (fl. 1162). Moorish physician. He first described the itch-mite (*Acarus scabiei*) of *scabies.

AVERY, OSWALD THEODORE (1877–1955). American microbiologist and immunologist. Nearly all his professional life was spent as a member of the *Rockefeller Institute, where he focused attention on one bacterium: the *pneumococcus. With McLeod and McCarty he demonstrated that DNA is the genetic substance.

AVICENNA (Abu Ali al-Hussein ibn Abdullah ibn Sina) (980–1037). Persian physician and philosopher. He wrote many philosophical books but his great legacy to medicine was his *Canon of Medicine*, a vast encyclopaedia in which he attempted to correlate the views of *Hippocrates, *Galen, and *Aristotle. It was first translated into Latin in the 12th century and was a much consulted textbook of medicine up to the 17th century. Avicenna was the first to describe the *guinea worm (*Dracunculus medinensis*) and *anthrax ('Persian fire'). He is also said to have noted the sweet taste of diabetic urine.

AXENFELD, THEODOR (1867–1930). German ophthalmologist. He advanced the surgical techniques of ophthalmology and described the Morax–Axenfeld bacillus of chronic *conjunctivitis (1896–97).

AXON. The delicate thread-like extension of a *neurone (nerve cell) which conducts impulses away from the cell body and which constitutes a nerve fibre. The larger axons are surrounded by sheaths of a fatty substance called *myelin which provide high-resistance insulation. At the termination of the axon the impulses are transmitted to other neurones or to effector organs.

AYERZA, ABEL (1861–1918). Argentinian physician. He described a disease in which there is *arteriosclerosis of the pulmonary artery, leading to *cyanosis, difficult breathing (dyspnoea), breathlessness on lying down (orthopnoea), and an enlarged liver and spleen with a compensatory increase in the number of circulating red blood cells.

AYURVEDIC MEDICINE is the traditional Hindu medical science (see MEDICINE IN INDIA). Although this declined with the Moslem conquest of India, much medical knowledge had spread to Mediterranean countries from about the beginning of the first millennium BC.

AZATHIOPRINE is a *cytotoxic *immunosupressive drug used to prevent *transplant rejection and also to treat many *autoimmune and *collagen disorders.

AZOOSPERMIA is the absence of *spermatozoa from the *semen.

AZOTAEMIA (AZOTEMIA) is an excess of urea and other nitrogenous compounds in the blood, synonymous with uraemia. The normal range for blood urea is 2.6–6.5 nmol/l (15–40 mg/dl).

BABINSKI, JOSEPH FRANCOIS FELIX (1857–1932). Franco-Polish neurologist. In 1896 he described the extensor plantar reflex (Babinski's sign) characteristic of an upper motor neurone lesion.

BABKIN, BORIS PETROVITCH (1877–1950). Russian gastroenterologist and neurophysiologist. Despite his close association with *Pavlov, Babkin was *imprisoned in 1922 by the Soviet authorities with whose policies he disagreed. On release he joined Professor Ernest *Starling in London for two years. He was appointed to the chair of physiology at Dalhousie University in Halifax, Nova Scotia in 1924 and four years later to a research chair at McGill. Babkin was a talented musician and composer; his earliest composition at the age of 15 was entitled 'The Pussy Cat Gavotte'.

BACILLE CALMETTE–GUERIN (BCG) is a permanently attenuated strain of the bovine *tuberculosis bacillus (*Mycobacterium bovis*) widely employed as a vaccine for active *immunization against tuberculosis. It was developed at the *Pasteur Institute by L. C. A. *Calmette and C. *Guérin beginning in 1906 and was introduced into human and veterinary medicine during 1921–4. It reduces the incidence of tuberculosis by up to 80 per cent, protection lasting from 7 to 10 years.

BACILLUS is generally applied to any rod-shaped bacterium, though modern classification restricts the name to 33 large aerobic *spore-forming Gram-positive species of the genus *Bacillus*.

BACKACHE and back pain are very common complaints and have a multiplicity of causes. Backache commonly occurs, for example, whenever the body temperature is raised, or after a spell of unaccustomed digging or other exertion. Nevertheless, it may also be a manifestation of important disease and for that reason should always receive serious attention.

Four out of five adults suffer at some time from back pain. A recent estimate (1980) for working days lost in a year in England and Wales as a result of this complaint was 39.5 million.

BACON, ROGER (1214–94). English philosopher. Educated at Oxford and Paris, he wrote on philosophy,

physics, and alchemy. He helped to release doctors from the dogmas forged in antiquity that persisted through the Dark and Middle Ages, and indeed remained of some influence even in the days of Thomas *Linacre and William *Harvey.

BACTERAEMIA (BACTEREMIA) means bacteria in the blood.

BACTERIAL ENDOCARDITIS. See INFECTIVE BACTERIAL ENDOCARDITIS.

BACTERIOLOGY is the study of bacteria, part of the more general science of micro-organisms known as *microbiology.

BACTERIOLYSIS is the process of dissolution of bacterial cells, also known as bacterioclasis.

BACTERIOPHAGE, also known simply as 'phage', is a *virus that requires a *bacterium in which to replicate. It has a polyhedral head containing *deoxyribonucleic acid (DNA) (sometimes *ribonucleic acid (RNA)) enclosed by a wall of *protein prolonged into a hollow tail. Having penetrated the bacterium, the phage DNA uses the bacterial genetic machinery to reproduce itself.

BACTERIUM. Any one of a class (Schizomycophyta) of microscopic, cellular (usually unicellular), *prokaryotic (no nuclear membrane, unpaired *chromosomes) organisms which lack *chlorophyll and are thus incapable of *photosynthesis. Reproduction is usually by *mitosis. Bacteria are usually classified with plants rather than animals, but are distinct from both. See also MICROBIOLOGY.

BAER, KARL ERNST RITTER VON (1792–1876). Russian embryologist and anthropologist, the father of comparative *embryology, who described the germ-layers, the notochord, and the neural tube in the embryo. In 1827 he discovered the mammalian ovum. He first used the word '*spermatozoa' and in 1827 published *De ovi mammalium et hominis genesi*.

BAGASSOSIS is a form of occupational *hypersensitivity *pneumonitis similar to *farmer's lung' but due to the inhalation of the dust of dried sugarcane containing the antigenic mould *Thermoactinomyces saccharii*.

BAILLIE, MATTHEW (1761–1823). British physician and morbid anatomist. Baillie married the sister of John and William *Hunter and worked at the *Great Windmill Street School, which he inherited on William's death. He was the greatest early British morbid anatomist and published the first work on the subject: *The morbid anatomy of some of the most important parts of the human body* (1793).

BAILLOU (OR BAILLON), GUILLAUME DE (1583–1616). French physician. Baillou was a skilled clinician, the first to describe *whooping cough (1578), to distinguish *measles from *smallpox, and to use the word '*rheumatism'.

BAKER, SIR GEORGE (1722–1809). British physician. Between 1785 and 1795 he was elected president of the Royal College of Physicians of London nine times. Baker was an elegant classical scholar whose *Essays on the cause of the colic of Devonshire and Poitou* (1767) showed that *lead poisoning was responsible and led to him being reviled as a disloyal son of Devon.

BAL. See BRITISH ANTI-LEWISITE.

BALANCE has various senses, but means particularly: the relationship between the body's intake of a substance and its output (as in *calcium, fluid, *acid–base balance, etc). It is also the faculty involved in maintaining postural equilibrium.

BALFOUR, SIR ANDREW (1873–1931). British physician, hygienist, and novelist. In 1902 he became director of the Wellcome Tropical Research Laboratories, Khartoum, and in 1913 founded the Wellcome Bureau of Scientific Research in London. In 1923 he became the first director of the *London School of Hygiene and Tropical Medicine. In his younger days he published several novels, of which *The golden kingdom* (1903) was the most successful.

BALLANCE, SIR CHARLES (1856–1936). English surgeon. He was a pioneer in the management of intracranial complications of middle ear disease and in mastoid surgery.

BALLISTOCARDIOGRAPHY records the movements of the body caused by the ejection of blood from the *ventricles at each cardiac contraction.

BALLOTTEMENT is the sensation felt on palpating a floating object, such as a fetus *in utero*.

BALNEOTHERAPY is treatment of disease by baths or medicinal springs. See also MINERAL SPRINGS.

BANCROFT, JOSEPH (1836–94). English-Australian physician. He recognized *leprosy in Queensland, and discovered the worm that causes *filariasis, later named *Wuchereria bancrofti*. He also studied the culture and diseases of plants, and invented a process for drying meat which yielded pemmican.

BANDAGE. Any strip of cloth or other material used for wrapping around part of the body for purposes of protection, immobilization, etc.

BANG, BERNHARD LAURITS FREDERIK (1848–1932). Danish veterinary surgeon. In 1897 he discovered the bacterial cause of infectious abortion in cattle, *abortus fever, now known as *Brucella abortus*.

BANISTER, RICHARD (d. 1626). British '*oculist'. He published in 1622 a second translation of Guillemeau's *Traité des maladies de l'oeil*, which was the earliest textbook of *ophthalmology in English and became known as Banister's *Breviary of the eyes*.

BANK. A store of human tissues, organs, or other material for future use (e.g. *blood, *milk, *sperm, *cornea, *skin, fetal tissue for tissue culture, etc.).

BANTING, SIR FREDERICK GRANT (1891–1941). Canadian orthopaedic surgeon and physiologist. After qualification he served with the Canadian Army Medical Corps in France from 1916 to 1918 and was awarded the Military Cross. He then trained as an orthopaedic surgeon, but in his spare time did research in J. J. R. Macleod's department of physiology. Here in November 1921, working with Charles H. *Best, he isolated *insulin. Two months later the first diabetic patient was treated with this hormone. For this work Banting and Macleod were awarded the *Nobel prize for 1923. In 1939 he became head of the medical research committee of the National Research Council of Canada. He was killed in an aircraft crash when flying to Europe in 1941.

BANTING, WILLIAM (1797–1878). British undertaker, so incommoded by obesity that he went on a diet of 'meat, fish, and dry toast', and rapidly lost 21 kg (46 lb). His improved health led him to publish *A letter on corpulence addressed to the public* (1863). It was a best seller and to 'bant' became a household word.

BARANY, ROBERT (1876–1936). Austrian otologist. His researches into the function of the *labyrinth won him the Nobel prize in 1914. An army medical officer in the First World War, he was captured by the Russians in 1915 and moved to Sweden to take charge of the department of otology at Uppsala. He devised several methods for testing labyrinthine function, which are still widely used. See also OTORHINOLARYNGOLOGY.

BARBER-SURGEON is a term reflecting the association of these two trades before the Royal Charter of Henry VIII of 1540 (see BARBER-SURGEONS, COMPANY OF), when minor surgery was traditionally done by barbers. Guilds or similar associations of barber-surgeons, denied the university education available to physicians, came into being throughout Europe. See also SURGERY, GENERAL.

BARBER-SURGEONS, COMPANY OF. Granted a Royal Charter by Henry VIII in 1540 at the behest of his personal barber-surgeon Thomas *Vicary, the United Company of Barber-Surgeons took the first step in separating the two trades (not complete for another 200 years) and brought together various guilds (such as 'The Mystery and Commonalty of the Barbers and Surgeons of London') which had been scattered and separate. Surgeons were no longer required to be barbers, and barbers were limited to dental surgery. Rules of apprenticeship were laid down, and fines for unlicensed practitioners specified. The Company was empowered to receive the bodies of four executed criminals each year for dissection and anatomical study (see ANATOMY). The new Company, however, was unable to narrow the gulf between surgeon and physician.

BARBITURATES are salts of barbituric acid (2,4,6-trioxohexahydropyrimidine), a group of central-nervous-system-depressant drugs long used as *hypnotics, *sedatives, and anxiolytics, of which barbitone (or barbital) was the first. Because of their dangers (addiction, suicide), they have been largely replaced by the safer *benzodiazepines. Their chief remaining uses are in *epilepsy (long-acting preparations like *phenobarbitone) and intravenous *anaesthesia (short-acting).

BARCROFT, SIR JOSEPH (1872–1947). Anglo-Irish physiologist. His researches were chiefly into *respiration, *haemoglobin, and fetal *metabolism. He devised the blood gas *manometer. From 1917 to 1919 he was chief physiologist to the gas warfare centre at Porton. He wrote *The respiratory function of the blood* (1914). A man of immense charm, and a brilliant lecturer, his book *Features in the architecture of physiological function* (1934) is an ageless classic. In 1952, a 3970 m (13 020 ft) peak in the White Mountains of California was named Mount Barcroft, the location of a high-altitude laboratory.

BAREFOOT DOCTORS. According to the official Chinese definition, barefoot doctors were 'peasants trained to give medical treatment locally, without leaving their farmwork'. During the 'cultural revolution', they received official recognition and were given some instruction in Western as well as traditional medicine. They treated minor complaints, and were responsible for a variety of preventative health and hygiene programmes (e.g. sanitation, birth control). In 1985, the Chinese government announced that they were to be disbanded.

BARGER, GEORGE (1878–1939). Anglo-Dutch chemist. He was associated with Sir Charles *Harrington in the synthesis of *thyroxine; he isolated *ergotoxin and *histamine, and invented the word *sympathomimetic'.

BARIUM is a metallic element (symbol Ba, atomic number 56, relative atomic mass 137.34). Its compounds resemble those of *calcium but are poisonous and have no place in modern therapeutics. Barium sulphate ($BaSO_4$), however, is a tasteless white insoluble powder, which in suspension provides a useful medium for contrast *radiography of the intestinal tract (see BARIUM ENEMA; BARIUM MEAL).

BARIUM ENEMA. A *radiopaque suspension of barium sulphate introduced into the large intestine through the rectum and retained during radiological examination. This is a standard technique for demonstrating abnormalities of the large intestine, such as *diverticula, *neoplasms, etc.

BARIUM MEAL. A *radiopaque suspension swallowed by the patient and retained in the proximal part of the alimentary tract long enough to allow radiological examination of the oesophagus, stomach, and proximal intestine. This is a standard radiological method for the diagnosis of *gastric and *duodenal ulcer, gastric carcinoma, etc.

BARLOW, SIR THOMAS (1845–1945). British physician. He first distinguished infantile *scurvy ('Barlow's disease') from 'acute' *rickets (1883) and described with Samuel *Gee 'post-basic' *meningitis ('cervical opisthotonos of infants', 1878).

BARNARDO, THOMAS JOHN (1845–1905). British physician and philanthropist. He began evangelical work in Dublin where he was born, but in 1866 entered the *London Hospital to train as a medical missionary to China. However, experience in a *cholera epidemic led him to work for homeless children in England. In 1867, with the patronage of Lord Shaftesbury, he founded the East End Juvenile Mission.

BARNARDO'S HOMES were homes for waifs, founded by Thomas John *Barnardo. He established the first of these, the Boys' Home, in Stepney in 1870, followed in 1876 by the Girls' Village Home in Barkingside, Essex. Many homes were established, and by his death in 1905 59 384 destitute children had been rescued. After his death, a fund was organized in his memory which freed his homes from debt.

The Barnardo organization is now responsible for caring for 'destitute, orphan, and forsaken children.'

There are over 150 projects in the UK involving 22 000 children.

BAROCEPTOR. A receptor sensitive to changes in hydrostatic pressure, e.g. stretch receptors found in arterial walls (as in the *carotid sinus).

BAROTRAUMA is injury due to abrupt change in ambient (barometric) pressure, such as that occurring on sudden decompression of the passenger compartment of an aircraft (e.g. rupture of the eardrum). See AEROSPACE MEDICINE.

BARR BODY. See NUCLEAR SEXING.

BARRIER NURSING separates the immediate microbiological environment of the patient from that of the hospital so as to prevent contamination of the latter with potentially dangerous micro-organisms; such techniques are necessary when patients are suffering, or suspected to be suffering, from serious communicable diseases. 'Reverse barrier nursing' refers to the similar methods adopted to protect patients (whose normal immune defences may be compromised) from infection by one or more of the micro-organisms present in any hospital.

BARTHOLIN, CASPAR (1655–1738). Danish anatomist. Born in Copenhagen, he was the son of Thomas *Bartholin. He discovered glands, now named after him, at the rear end of the vulva, with a duct opening separately there. He showed that the glands secreted a milky fluid only during coitus or masturbation.

BARTHOLIN, THOMAS (1616–80). Danish anatomist. He made many original pathological observations, showing, for example, that the *lymphatic system was separate from the vascular system of the blood. He claimed to have discovered the *thoracic duct, although Olof Rudbeck (1651) is generally credited with the priority. He was responsible for the royal decrees of 1672 which determined the organization of Danish medicine for a century, and was also responsible for the publication of the first Danish medical journal.

BARTONELLA is the causal organism of South American *Oroya fever. The genus *Bartonella* contains only one species, *Bartonella bacilliformis*, a small *bacillus-like Gram-negative *bacterium which can parasitize red blood cells.

BASAL GANGLIA. The large masses of grey matter embedded deep in the *cerebral hemispheres and the *midbrain (the caudate and lenticular nuclei, which together constitute the corpus striatum; the subthalamic nucleus; and the substantia nigra of the midbrain). The basal ganglia have complex connections with the cerebral cortex, thalamus, and other parts of the central nervous system; they are concerned with the regulation of movement and form part of the 'extrapyramidal' motor system. Disease or degeneration of the basal ganglia and their connections gives rise to disturbances of motor function, of which the most familiar is *parkinsonism. Others are *chorea, *dystonia, and *athetosis.

BASAL METABOLIC RATE (BMR) is the minimum rate of energy expenditure required by the body under resting (basal) conditions in order to maintain essential functions.

BASCH, SAMUEL SIEGFRIED KARL RITTER VON (1837–1905). Austrian physician and pathologist. He devised the earliest *sphygmomanometer (1881).

BASE. A substance that liberates hydroxyl *ions in solution, accepts *protons, and combines with an *acid to form a salt and water only. Bases, which turn red litmus-paper blue, include oxides and hydroxides of metals, and ammonia.

BASEDOW, KARL ADOLPH VON (1799–1854). German physician. In 1840 he gave a good description of *thyrotoxicosis, which he treated with *iodine.

BASEMENT MEMBRANE. A delicate extracellular membrane consisting of mucopolysaccharide and fine fibrous protein which underlies most animal *epithelium, and constitutes the outer layer (outside the plasma membrane) of the double membrane of many structures, such as the skeletal muscle fibre.

BASOPHIL. Any cell with an affinity for basic stains. When otherwise unqualified, 'basophil' means a *leucocyte whose large basophilic granules contain *heparin and vasoactive amines, and which is important in the inflammatory response. See also ALLERGY.

BASTIAN, HENRY CHARLTON (1837–1915). British neurologist. He described sensory *aphasia in 1869. His *Brain as an organ of mind* (1880) was widely acclaimed. He never surrendered his belief in spontaneous generation.

BASTIANELLI, GUISEPPE (1862–1959). Italian surgeon. He described preoperative skin *disinfection with a 1:1000 benzene solution of iodine followed by a 50 per cent tincture of iodine.

BATEMAN, THOMAS (1778–1821). British pioneer dermatologist. He wrote *Synopsis of cutaneous diseases according to the arrangement of Dr Willan* (1813).

BATHING. See BALNEOTHERAPY; MINERAL SPRINGS; SWIMMING.

BATS AS CARRIERS OF DISEASE. In some parts of the world bats provide an animal reservoir of *rabies infection, and transmission to humans may occur from bat bites; transmission by inhalation of aerosolized virus in bat-infested caves is also recorded. Bites from vampire bats are said to be more likely to cause the rarer paralytic form, 'dumb' rabies.

BATTERED BABY SYNDROME describes the clinical state of an infant injured by an adult, usually a parent or step-parent. The child shows multiple contusions and fractures, sometimes with evidence of intracranial (subdural) bleeding. It is not always immediately obvious that the lesions are traumatic or have been wilfully inflicted. It is now more often called non-accidental injury of childhood.

BATTLE EXHAUSTION is disabling physical and or emotional fatigue associated with active military service. Many names have been applied to this psychiatric syndrome and its variants, including combat neurosis, combat fatigue, *shell-shock, effort syndrome, disordered action of the heart, irritable heart, *da Costa's syndrome, etc.

BAYLISS, SIR WILLIAM MADDOCK (1860–1924). British physiologist. His researches were upon enzyme action and the innervation of the heart and intestines. He wrote *The nature of enzyme action* (1908), *Principles of general physiology* (1915), and *The vasomotor system* (1923).

BCG. See BACILLE CALMETTE–GUERIN.

BEAN, WILLIAM BENNETT (1909–89). American physician. Chairman, Department of Medicine, University of Iowa, 1948–69; Sir William Osler Professor of Medicine, 1969–74. Professor Emeritus 1980–89. Editor-in-Chief, *Archives of Internal Medicine*. Medical historian and prolific writer.

BEAT KNEE is a chronic inflammatory condition of the subcutaneous prepatellar *bursa near the knee joint occurring in miners.

BEAUMONT, WILLIAM (1785–1853). American military surgeon and student of gastric digestion. As a military surgeon, while stationed at a fort in Michigan (1820-25) he cared for a patient named Alexis St Martin, who had an abdominal gunshot wound resulting in a permanent gastric *fistula. Beaumont took advantage of the opportunity to make a series of observations on the digestion of food in the stomach. His work was summarized in a book describing more than 200 experiments on St Martin. See also ARMED FORCES OF THE USA; MEDICAL SERVICES; GASTROENTEROLOGY.

BECQUEREL, ANTOINE HENRI (1852–1908). French physicist who demonstrated the *radioactivity

of *uranium salts (1896). He suggested the possibility of *radiotherapy after sustaining an accidental burn from carrying *radium in his pocket. In 1903 he shared the *Nobel prize for physics with Marie and Pierre *Curie.

BEDBUG. *Cimex lectularius*, a blood-feeding pest, once common in neglected households but scarce since the advent of efficient insecticides, at least in the civilized world. A related species, *Cimex columbarius*, preys on pigeons in dovecotes; other species occur in the tropics. Itching is the chief consequence of bedbug bites.

BEDDOES, THOMAS LOVELL (1803–49). British physician and poet. He trained at Göttingen and practised in Europe, living in Zurich. His best-known works were *The bride's tragedy* (1822), a play, and *Death's jestbook and the fool's tragedy* (1850), published posthumously.

BEDLAM. A madhouse or lunatic asylum, now commonly used figuratively (with lower-case b) to describe a state of general uproar. The word derives from the Hospital of St Mary of Bethlehem (later *Bethlem Royal Hospital), which was founded in London in 1247 as a priory. It later became a hospital, and in 1402 was used specifically for the mentally ill. Originally in Bishopsgate, it was rebuilt in 1676 near London Wall, where inmates were exposed to public view, and the name of bedlam was then applied.

BEDSORE. An area of *necrosis involving the skin and the underlying tissues, also known as pressure sore or decubitus *ulcer. It occurs particularly over body prominences, and is due to prolonged compression of these areas by the body weight in patients immobilized in bed whose position is not altered at regular intervals. Prevention depends upon dedicated nursing and the use of protective applications and dressings.

BED-WETTING is nocturnal enuresis, or involuntary discharge of urine during sleep, defined as occurring in children over the age of 3 years. Bed-wetting is a common and troublesome sleep disorder, occurring mainly in boys between the ages of 4 and 14 years. Many causal factors have been suggested, such as physical conditions, psychological factors, depth of sleep, failure of arousal, and constitution. Conditioning techniques and drugs, including tricyclic antidepressants, have proved effective in treatment in some cases.

BEHAVIOURISM is a system of psychology based purely on objective study and analysis of behaviour in animals and man, without reference to factors such as will, choice, consciousness, imagination, and personal experience. See also PSYCHOLOGY.

BEHRING, EMIL ADOLF VON (1854–1917). German microbiologist and serologist. In 1889 he became one of *Koch's assistants at the Institute for Hygiene in Berlin. With *Kitasato he described *tetanus *antitoxin in 1890, and later that of *diphtheria. Thereafter he developed passive and active *immunization against tetanus and diphtheria. In 1901 he was the first Nobel prize-winner in medicine or physiology.

BEJEL is a form of non-venereal or endemic *syphilis similar to *yaws, occurring particularly in Bedouin Arabs in the Middle East; the infection is usually acquired in early childhood. The causative organism is morphologically indistinguishable from that of syphilis, *Treponema pallidum*, and the diagnosis is made largely on epidemiological grounds. *Penicillin is effective as in syphilis.

BEKESEY, GEORG VON (1899–1972). Hungarian-Swedish physicist. A pioneer in auditory physiology and psychoacoustics, he won the *Nobel prize for medicine and physiology in 1961.

BEL. A unit for comparing levels of power, equal to 10 *decibels; most often used to express sound intensities.

BELL, SIR CHARLES (1774–1842). British surgeon and neuroanatomist. A brilliant anatomical draughtsman, he distinguished motor from sensory nerves (1811) and described the *long thoracic nerve (Bell's nerve) and facial palsy (*Bell's palsy).

BELLADONNA is the poisonous plant known also as deadly nightshade (*Atropa belladonna*) which contains the *alkaloid *atropine.

BELLEVUE HOSPITAL in New York began as a six-bed infirmary in 1736 in a Public Workhouse and House of Correction. It became one of the foremost hospitals of the world, offering a vast range of services, being a public hospital for New York City. It has been an integral part of the New York University School of Medicine since 1968. It is famed for its emergency services, and started the first American hospital-based ambulance service (1809). For the USA it was the first place for many advances, among them anatomy dissection (1750), lying-in wards (1799), a school of nursing (1873), and caesarean section (1877). It was there that cardiac *catheterization began, and this won a Nobel prize for D. Richards and André Cournand. See also HOSPITALS IN THE USA.

BELL–MAGENDIE LAW. The rule that anterior spinal roots carry motor fibres, and posterior roots sensory fibres (See NEUROMUSCULAR DISEASE).

BELL'S PALSY is sudden paralysis of the muscles on one side of the face, due to blocked conduction in the *facial nerve on that side; the resultant facial appearance is characteristic. The cause is unknown; a viral aetiology is suspected but is only rarely established. Complete recovery within a few weeks is usual, although not invariable.

BENCE JONES, HENRY (1814–73). British physician and chemist. In 1848, he described 'albumose' ('Bence Jones protein') in the urine of patients with multiple myeloma (see MYELOMA).

BENDS is a symptom of *decompression sickness (also called caisson disease).

BENEVOLENT SOCIETIES are those formed for any caring or charitable purpose, which may be registered under the UK Friendly Societies Act 1974. A benevolent society is generally subject to the same rules and enjoys the same privileges as a *friendly society. It may not, for example, divide its funds among its members.

BENIGN describes *neoplasms that do not display malignancy, that is invasiveness, remote spread (*metastasis), and *anaplasia. Benign tumours, usually encapsulated, may compress or displace neighbouring structures but do not invade and destroy them.

BENNETT, JOHN HUGHES (1812–75). British physician. An early *histologist, he was the first to describe *leukaemia in the UK as *Cases of hypertrophy of the liver and spleen in which death took place from suppuration of the blood* (1845).

BENZENE (C_6H_6) is a colourless liquid aromatic *hydrocarbon found in coal-tar. It is used as a solvent and in manufacturing many organic chemicals. It is toxic and leukaemogenic (see ONCOLOGY).

BENZODIAZEPINES are now the most commonly employed group of drugs for *hypnotic and *sedative purposes, and as minor tranquillizers (anxiolytics). Among the advantages they have over the *barbiturates, which they have supplanted, are less frequent and less potent side-effects, and a much wider safety margin in the event of overdosage. Once thought unlikely to induce dependence, it is now known that this may follow prolonged use, and withdrawal symptoms may then be severe. Some commonly used compounds are listed in PHARMACOLOGY and under TRANQUILLIZERS; see also SLEEP.

BENZOIN, Gum Benjamin, a natural brown aromatic resin obtained from certain trees, is a constituent of Friar's Balsam (compound benzoin tincture), formerly popular as an inhalant in *respiratory infections.

BENZPYRENE ($C_{20}H_{12}$) is a yellow crystalline polycyclic *hydrocarbon found in small quantities in coal-tar. It is carcinogenic, and is one of the most harmful constituents of tobacco smoke (see SMOKING).

BEREAVEMENT. See GRIEF.

BERGER, HANS (1873–1941). German psychiatrist. He made original observations on the changes in electrical potential which could be recorded through the intact skull and which led to the development of *electroencephalography.

BERGMANN, ERNST VON (1836–1907). German surgeon. An early *neurosurgeon, he published an important work, *Die chirurgische Behandlung der Hirnkrankheiten* (1888). He introduced steam sterilization in 1886 and devised a full aseptic routine in 1891.

BERIBERI is a condition due to deficiency of *vitamin B$_1$, (*thiamine or aneurin). The word is of Sinhalese origin, meaning 'great weakness'. Thiamine plays a vital role in energy metabolism; it is an essential dietary constituent, as the body is unable either to synthesize or store it. Thiamine need is roughly related to energy (i.e. *carbohydrate) intake. It is widely distributed in the diet, the richest sources being the seed germs of cereals and pulses. In rice-eating communities, beriberi occurs when polished rice is the staple diet; in Western countries, the condition is almost confined to chronic alcoholics, who have a large energy intake in the form of alcohol but little or no normal food.

The chief features are numbness and muscle weakness due to *polyneuropathy, and 'high-output' heart failure with *oedema. In 'dry' beriberi the former predominate, in 'wet' beriberi the latter. There may also be cerebral manifestations, with marked memory disturbances (*Wernicke's encephalopathy).

BERNADETTE, of Lourdes (1844–79). Born in Lourdes, France, the eldest of nine children from a poor family Soubirous, she was a frail child who suffered from asthma. Between February and July 1858 she had visions of the Virgin Mary, who spoke to her in the Massabielle grotto. Despite hostile opposition in 1862 the Pope declared the visions to have been authentic. She became a nun in 1866. Lourdes is now a place of pilgrimage, with up to three million visiting the shrine of Our Lady of Lourdes each year, among them about 60 000 sick and maimed. Many cures are claimed, but are difficult to substantiate scientifically. Bernadette was canonized in 1933.

BERNARD, CLAUDE (1813–78). French physiologist. The son of a vine-grower in St Julien, Rhône, he started work as a pharmacist's assistant in Lyons, and in his leisure time wrote two plays.

One of the greatest physiologists of the 19th century, he was the founder of experimental medicine. His views were mechanistic, and all life to him was a matter of physiochemical reaction. His three most important achievements were: proof that the liver could synthesize *glucose (1857), demonstration of the digestive activity of the *pancreatic secretion (1849–56), and the discovery of the *vasomotor nerves (1858). He also showed that 'piqure' of the floor of the fourth *cerebral ventricle in dogs caused *glycosuria (1849). He investigated the paralysing effect of *curare, and developed the concept of internal secretion (i.e. *hormones). On his death in 1878 he received a public funeral, the first French scientist to be so honoured.

BERRY, GEORGE PACKER (1898–1985). American physician, bacteriologist, medical educator. Dean, Harvard Medical School, 1949–65. President, Association of American Medical Colleges, 1951–52. Recipient, Flexner Award, Association of American Medical Colleges.

BERT, PAUL (1833–96). French physiologist. His renown as a physiologist rests on his appreciation of the importance of the partial pressure of the blood gases and on his book *La pression barometrique* (1878).

BERTHOLD, ARNOLD ADOLPH (1804–61). German physiologist. He showed that if a cock's *testicles were transplanted into its abdominal cavity it retained its secondary sexual characteristics including a normally developed comb. This observation showed that the testicle produced a *hormone, and was a landmark in *endocrinology.

BERYLLIOSIS is an occupational *pneumoconiosis due to inhalation of dust containing the toxic metallic element beryllium. Chronic berylliosis is associated with diffuse pulmonary disease that resembles *sarcoidosis. An acute form also occurs and has a significant mortality.

BESNIER, ERNEST HENRI (1831–1909). French dermatologist. He founded the first laboratory for dermatological histopathology at the Hôpital S. Louis. His name is often attached to *sarcoidosis (sarcoid of Besnier–Boeck) of which he published an early account. His textbook, *La pratique dermatologique* (1900), was outstandingly successful.

BEST, CHARLES HERBERT (1899–1978). Canadian physiologist. While still in medical school he collaborated with Frederick *Banting in experiments leading to the isolation of *insulin. The *Nobel prize was awarded for this work, to Banting and to Macleod (head of the department in which the research was done). Banting shared his award with Best. Later in his career Best conducted other successful pieces of research: discovery of histaminase (an enzyme which degrades *histamine), recognition of *choline as a dietary factor, and purification of *heparin.

BESTIALITY is sexual perversion involving the substitution of an animal for a human partner.

BETA-BLOCKERS are drugs, such as *propranolol, which cause selective beta-adrenergic blockade. See ADRENERGIC BLOCKADE.

BETA-RAYS are formed of a stream of beta particles, i.e. of either *electrons or *positrons, emitted by *radioactive disintegration of an unstable nucleus. Beta-rays are of greater penetrating power than *alpha-rays.

BETATRON. A machine for accelerating a continuous beam of *electrons to high speeds with the electric field produced by a changing magnetic flux. A continuous source of *gamma-rays can be produced by arranging for the fast electrons to strike a metal target.

BETHLEM ROYAL HOSPITAL AND THE MAUDS-LEY HOSPITAL, LONDON, have served the mentally ill over several centuries. The Royal Hospital was founded in 1247 by Simon Fitzmary, alderman of the City of London. He gave his lands in the City to the church of St Mary of Bethlehem to found a priory. The name was contracted to Bethlem, and a corruption of it became *bedlam. By the 14th century, it had become a hospice, caring for the sick, wayfarers, and pilgrims. By 1403 it is known that six of the inmates were mentally ill. In 1547 it was incorporated as a royal foundation for the reception of the mentally ill. The old hospital at Bishopsgate in the City was vacated in 1676 for a new building on London Wall. It was then that the inmates were exposed to public view for entertainment, and the name of bedlam was applied. However, as public opinion and that of the medical profession changed, the care of the mentally ill became more humane. The fabric of the City hospital decayed rapidly, and it was moved to Southwark. In 1815, an unusual feature was the provision of accommodation for Criminal Lunatics, as they were then called. This function of caring for the criminally insane was transferred to Broadmoor in 1863–4. The hospital finally moved to Beckenham in Kent, on the outskirts of London, when buildings were opened in 1930. In 1948, with the start of the NHS, the hospital joined with the Maudsley.

The Maudsley Hospital was founded by Henry Maudsley, a Yorkshireman who, after qualifying in medicine, became superintendent of the Manchester Royal Lunatic Asylum. In 1907 he offered £30 000 ($45 000) to the London County Council to set up a new hospital for the mentally ill. A site in Denmark Hill was bought in 1911, and building began in 1913. It finally became a mental hospital in 1923. Chairs were established as early as 1936 and the psychiatric school became part of the University of London in 1924. The Second World War led to evacuation, but in 1948 the Maudsley Hospital and the Bethlem Royal Hospital joined to create the academic Institute of Psychiatry which was established on a site near the Maudsley in Denmark Hill.

BETHUNE, NORMAN (1890–1939). Chest surgeon and blood transfusion pioneer. On the outbreak of the Spanish Civil War, Bethune took a motorized service of refrigerated blood to the front. The Japanese invasion of China in 1937 so angered him that he joined the 8th Route Army and became, by the time of his death in November 1939, a legend to the people of China.

BETZ CELL. Large pyramidal nerve cell found in the motor areas of the *cerebral cortex. The Betz cells are the cell bodies of many 'upper motor neurones', the axons of which form the corticospinal (pyramidal) tracts. They are concerned with initiating voluntary movement.

BEVAN, ANEURIN (1897–1960). British politician. In the Labour Government of 1945 he was made Minister of Health and Housing and it became his duty to see the *National Health Service Act (1946) on to the statute-book. In his negotiations with the medical profession he proved more flexible and patient than had been anticipated, and a successful conclusion was reached in 2 years. In January 1951 he was moved to the Ministry of Labour and resigned soon afterwards when prescription charges were introduced.

BEVERIDGE, SIR WILLIAM, 1st Baron Beveridge (1879–1963). British civil servant and social reformer. When he sought government employment at the outbreak of the Second World War he was offered chairmanship of a committee enquiring into the co-ordination of the social services, which was not expected to report until after the war. Within 18 months he had produced the *'Beveridge Report' for a complete social service. It met with a cool reception from government, but in 4 days 70 000 copies were sold and public acclaim forced its acceptance as the basis of a *National Health Service.

BEVERIDGE REPORT. Basic provision for social security in the UK evolved from the proposals made by Beveridge in 1942 (*Social insurance and allied services*. Report by Sir William Beveridge, Cmd. 6404, HMSO, November 1942). Three systems of benefit were recommended: social insurance payable on a contractual basis; social assistance payable on a test of need; and children's allowances payable to all without contract or test of need.

The first, and central, proposal was a universal comprehensive insurance scheme covering the whole population and providing for 'interruption and destruction of earning power and for special expenditure arising at birth, marriage or death'. Benefits would be paid without test of need in return for contributions made jointly by the insured person, the state, and, where appropriate, the employer. The second and third proposals provided for those whose need was not fully met by social insurance (requiring proof of need), and for flat-rate children's allowances payable irrespective of parental income. Most of these recommendations were implemented by July 1948.

BEZOAR. A concretion made of hair or other material found in the stomach or intestines of animals and occasionally of man. The name derives from the Arabic for 'antidote to poison', a quality which the objects were supposed to possess; the original (highly prized) was the *lapis bezoar orientale* obtained from the wild goat of Persia.

In man, 'bezoar' refers to a hair-ball found in the stomach, consisting either of hair (trichobezoar) or of vegetable or fruit fibre (phytobezoar). It may produce abdominal discomfort, pain, vomiting, or bleeding. *Barium meal examination reveals a filling defect; it may be examined with a *gastroscope, through which it may sometimes be broken up and dispersed. Alternative methods are enzymatic digestion and surgery.

BEZOLD, FRIEDRICH (1842–1908). The first surgeon to give a clear account of the surgical pathology of mastoiditis.

BICARBONATE. Any acid salt of carbonic acid (H_2CO_3), that is one in which one hydrogen atom has been replaced by a metal and which therefore contains the *anion HCO_3^-. When otherwise unqualified, 'bicarbonate' is taken to mean sodium bicarbonate (sodium hydrogen carbonate), which is in common use in oral preparations as a soluble *antacid with a rapid but transitory action and as an intravenous infusion to combat metabolic *acidosis.

BICHAT, MARIE FRANCOIS XAVIER (1771–1802). French anatomist and surgeon. He was the creator of descriptive anatomy. Bichat finally exploded the theory of humours by stressing the importance of the tissues, being the first to use this word in its modern sense. He believed that pathological changes affected them rather than whole organs.

BIER, AUGUST KARL GUSTAV (1861–1949). German surgeon. The leading surgeon of his time in Germany, he was the first in Europe to use spinal *anaesthesia (1899).

BIGELOW, JACOB (1786–1879). American physician. A member of a distinguished medical family, he practised in Boston. His most influential contribution was a treatise on the self-limiting nature of many diseases,

especially those now known to be caused by infection. This publication soon reduced the widespread therapeutic practices of bleeding, sweating, and purging of patients with fever.

BIGNAMI, AMICO (1862–1929). Italian physician. He showed that the *malaria parasite reproduces through the *Anopheles* mosquito, establishing an important link in its life cycle.

BILE. In Galenic medicine, two of the four *humours. In modern physiology it is the viscous dark-yellow alkaline secretion of the *liver in vertebrates; it is of chief importance in the digestion of *fats and the absorption of the fat-soluble *vitamins A, D, and K. Its major constituents are: *cholesterol, bile salts (formed from cholesterol in the liver, they have the property of emulsifying fats), bile pigments (*bilirubin and *biliverdin, degradation products of *haemoglobin), other waste products, and *electrolytes. Bile is secreted into the *duodenum via the common *bile duct after storage between meals in the *gall bladder, in which it is concentrated by reabsorption of water.

BILE DUCT, or common bile duct, is formed by the union of the *cystic duct from the *gall bladder with the common hepatic duct (itself formed by the union of ducts from the right and left lobes of the *liver); it discharges *bile into the *duodenum.

BILHARZ, THEODOR (1825–62). German anatomist. He accompanied *Griesinger to Egypt in 1850 and became professor of descriptive anatomy at the medical school of the Kasr-el-Aini hospital in 1856. During his dissections he noted an undescribed trematode which he named *Distomum haematobium*; it was renamed *Bilharzia haematobium* in 1856 and 2 years later was given its current name *Schistosoma haematobium*. It causes schistosomiasis or *bilharziasis.

BILHARZIASIS, now more usually called schistosomiasis, is due to infestation with one of three species of *flukes (parasitic trematode worms) of the genus *Schistosoma*, namely *S. haematobium*, *S. mansoni*, and *S. japonicum*. The first was discovered by Theodor *Bilharz.

The disease is endemic in over 70 countries across the world, and is believed to affect more than 200 million people. It occurs when low standards of sanitation allow the voiding of urine or faeces into fresh water where certain species of freshwater *snails are present to act as intermediate hosts to the parasites. The adult worms (male and female) are about 3 cm long and inhabit the veins draining the pelvic viscera, notably the bladder and lower bowel, the females' eggs being excreted in the urine and faeces. These release mobile forms which invade the snail, where further forms (cercariae) develop which are able to penetrate the intact skin of man, especially after bathing in infested water; here they develop into adults, completing the life cycle. The infestation causes chronic ill-health, chiefly due to anaemia, and a variety of specific, often serious, complications.

Control of the disease may be directed towards treating the infestation in man (*chemotherapy is effective), to snail control (use of molluscicides), to improving personal hygiene and sanitation, or to a combination of all three.

BILIRUBIN is the chief pigment of *bile, formed mainly from the breakdown of *haemoglobin. After formation it is transported in the plasma bound to the *albumin fraction of plasma protein (in which form it cannot be excreted in the urine) and reaches the *liver; here it is combined with glucuronic acid to form bilirubin mono- and di-glucuronides, which are water soluble and which are then excreted in the bile. Elevation of bilirubin in the blood causes *jaundice. If this is accompanied by dark coloration of the urine (biliuria), the excess bilirubin must be of the water-soluble form that has passed through the liver and has been reabsorbed as a result of biliary-tract obstruction (obstructive jaundice). If not, it is due to excessive breakdown of haemoglobin (haemolytic or 'acholuric' jaundice).

BILIVERDIN is one of the *bile pigments, an intermediate product in the breakdown of haemoglobin to *bilirubin.

BILLINGS, JOHN SHAW (1839–1913). American military surgeon and librarian. He directed the compilation of the *Index Catalogue* of the library of the surgeon-general's office, and was a founder of the *Index Medicus* (see MEDICAL BOOKS AND LIBRARIES). He was a major planner of the *Johns Hopkins Hospital and Medical School.

BILLROTH, CHRISTIAN ALBERT THEODOR (1829–94). German surgeon. Billroth was the first European surgeon to adopt *antisepsis and became the pioneer of *abdominal surgery. He was the first to resect the stomach (1881), the oesophagus (1872), the pancreas (1884), and the larynx (1873) for cancer. He founded a training school for nurses in Vienna. A lover of music, he was a close friend of Brahms, who dedicated two string quartets to him. His last paper was entitled 'Wer ist musikalisch?'.

BILLS OF MORTALITY were weekly official returns of the number of deaths that, from 1592 onwards, were published by the London Company of Parish Clerks for 109 districts in and around London. Although these statistics are inaccurate, they are of value in indicating broad epidemiological trends (see EPIDEMIOLOGY)

during the following two centuries, until the first year of death registration in 1837. They illustrate, for example, the gradual rise in *smallpox deaths throughout the 17th century, and the subsequent fall, with epidemics in 1681, 1685, and 1694–5.

BINET, ALFRED (1857–1911). French psychologist. With *Simon he devised a method of assessing mental age and *intelligence quotients (Binet–Simon test, 1905–8).

BIOASSAY. Measurement of the strength or concentration of a drug or other biologically active substance by comparing its effect on an organism, organ, or tissue with that of a standard preparation.

BIOAVAILABILITY is the extent to which a drug becomes available to the body tissues in a pharmacologically active form following administration.

BIOCHEMISTRY. Biochemistry is a pervasive subject, which provides an approach to understanding the diverse activities of all living organisms. This description is limited to basic principles and to some examples relevant to medicine.

Introduction
Chemistry defines the structure of substances and their properties through their content of a finite number of elements, composed in turn of indivisible units or atoms which are themselves made up of protons (positively charged), electrons (negatively charged), and neutrons (electrically neutral). Elements differ according to the numbers of protons and electrons (equal) and neutrons contained within their constituent atoms. Biochemistry is a method of understanding the structure and function of living organisms in terms of their chemistry.

Cells
In animals the *cell is the unit of life. It is bounded by a *membrane composed of phospholipids (fatty molecules bearing a charge). These align as a double layer, with the charged ends lying in the extracellular fluid and the intracellular cytosol (both water-based fluids) and the fatty ends buried internally. Within the cell are various organelles (functional compartments also bounded by membranes), e.g. nuclei (containing genetic information in deoxyribonucleic acid–DNA), mitochondria (see later), and lysosomes (digestive particles).

Bioenergetics and energy transduction
It is important to an understanding of bioenergetics and energy transduction to appreciate that some atoms have a propensity to lose electrons or to acquire them, resulting in the formation of positively or negatively charged

*ions. Water, which is composed of hydrogen and oxygen, (H_2O) dissociates weakly into protons (H^+) and hydroxyl ions (OH^-). If positively or negatively charged ions are separated, e.g. by an impermeable layer or membrane, then a potential difference will be created, which is an energized state capable of doing work.

Living organisms can transduce energy, and most life as we know it depends ultimately upon the transduction of solar energy. Plants and photosynthetic microorganisms capture light from the sun in a pigment (*chlorophyll) contained within particles termed chloroplasts, and use the energy to synthesize sugars and starch from atmospheric carbon dioxide and water. From sugars are synthesized fats and, with nitrogen, *amino acids for protein synthesis, the nitrogenous bases for *DNA and * RNA (ribonucleic acid) synthesis, and other essential organic molecules. Energy transfer is effected through a compound (ATP) utilized ubiquitously in the transfer of chemical energy. ATP stands for adenosine triphosphate, the transferable energy being contained in the bond linking the two terminal phosphates. It is formed by the reaction adenosine diphosphate (ADP) + phosphate + energy → ATP, and utilized by a variety of energy-requiring processes which reverse this reaction.

Animals (and plants in the dark) derive energy from the breakdown of foodstuffs (synthesized by *photosynthesis), mainly by oxidation (cell respiration) in particles termed mitochondria. Both in photosynthesis and in mitochondrial respiration the energy is initially captured by separation of protons and electrons. In photosynthesis, the light-driven reaction splits water (H_2O) into protons, electrons, and oxygen. In further reactions independent of light, the recombination of protons and electrons to form hydrogen drives the synthesis of ATP, which in turn drives the reaction of hydrogen (in combination with a carrier, NADP) with carbon dioxide to form sugars. In mitochondrial respiration, hydrogen atoms released during the degradation of sugars or fats are held in combination with a carrier (NAD or NADP) and split into protons (H^+) and electrons, the latter being captured by electron transport proteins. The transduction of light energy to ATP in photosynthesis and the transfer of chemical energy from nutrients to ATP in mitochondrial respiration depends critically upon membranes which are impermeable to (provide a barrier to) protons and which contain the electron-transport proteins. The flow of electrons (e) is coupled to the ejection of protons (derived mainly from water) and to the creation of a proton gradient. Proton flow down the gradient is coupled to the synthesis of ATP at specific locations in the membrane where an ATP synthase protein is inserted. Electron transport terminates with the formation of water. This is illustrated in Fig. 1.

In most animal cells, ATP synthesis is almost wholly based on reactions requiring oxygen. A few reactions can generate ATP in the absence of oxygen, but the rate is never fast enough to generate more than a small fraction of the requirement. This explains why delivery of oxygen to most tissues is essential for life.

Forms of energy transduction effected in living organisms by the breakdown of ATP to ADP and phosphate include the generation of electricity (electric eels), the emission of light (fireflies), mechanical work (muscles), sound (muscles plus vocal cords), and the storage of information (brain). Thus, in generating electricity ATP effects the separation of positive and negatively charged ions in membranes, thereby creating an electrical potential; in generating light ATP activates a chemiluminescent protein (luciferase—named after Lucifer); in muscle contraction ATP effects the sliding of two proteins (*actin and *myosin) over one another.

Metabolism

The chemical reactions that take place in the body are known collectively as metabolism. Connected sequences of reactions are known as metabolic pathways; an example is the breakdown of the sugar, glucose, to carbon dioxide and water, which involves a total of 19 reactions in two cell compartments and generates 38 ATP molecules. The reactions of metabolism are not spontaneous, and each reaction requires a catalyst or *enzyme. Enzyme-catalysed reactions result in chemical change, and lead to the formation of a new chemical substance. Yet other reactions in metabolism result in vectorial change, i.e. the transfer of a substance, unchanged, across a membrane separating two compartments (e.g. the transfer of a glucose molecule from the blood *plasma into a muscle cell). Such vectorial change requires a catalyst, known as a transporter which is located in the membrane, and, in effect, each transporter creates a channel through which small molecules may pass. Enzymes and transporters are proteins, and the nature of *proteins and their relation to *genes and *genetics is discussed below.

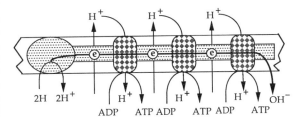

Fig. 1 Schematic representation of energy transduction in mitochondrial respiration. The flow of electrons ⓔ from hydrogen (H) to oxygen (O) is coupled to the synthesis of protons (H^+), and the return of protons is coupled to the synthesis of ATP. The precise number of protons pumped per molecule of ATP synthesized is still a matter for dispute.

▭ electron-transport proteins; ▦ ATP synthase.

Some metabolic pathways (catabolic) degrade molecules with the formation of ATP (degradation of sugars, fats, and amino acids). Others (anabolic) result in biosynthesis, e.g. glucose from dietary amino acids, glycogen and starch from glucose, fat (triacylglycerol) from glucose, amino acids from glucose and ammonia and proteins from amino acids.

It is self-evident that the many reactions of metabolism in living organisms require co-ordination and control. Cellular control mechanisms that underly the regulation of metabolism, growth, and development, and of defence against a hostile environment, are discussed below.

Some organisms (animals in particular) cannot synthesize all of the molecules needed for metabolism, and some are necessarily obtained from food. In man these include about one third of the 21 amino acids found in proteins (so called essential amino acids), some polyunsaturated *fatty acids (essential fatty acids), and the *vitamins—small molecules usually required for the synthesis of so-called coenzymes (NAD and NADP, which transport hydrogen in cell respiration, are coenzymes). Nutritional requirements in man thus have their biochemical basis in the needs for overall daily energy metabolism (joules or calories) and for small molecules that the body cannot synthesize.

Proteins

Proteins are composed of amino acids, linked together by *peptide bonds. Individual amino acids are bipolar and contain a basic group (amino group), an acidic group (carboxyl group), and a side-chain or group attached to a carbon atom. Peptide bonds are formed by reaction of the carboxyl group of one amino acid with the amino group of the next, with the elimination of water. These chains of amino acids (peptides) can vary in length in individual proteins from approximately 10 to 4000. Twenty-one different amino acids are found in proteins, and each individual protein has a unique and invariant sequence of amino acids within the peptide chain(s) (some proteins contain more than one peptide chain). This unique sequence is referred to as the primary structure. The synthesis of proteins requires mechanisms that achieve the primary structure and terminate synthesis.

The backbone of a peptide is composed of the peptide bonds, which tend to assume spontaneously a helical (coiled) configuration (secondary structure). Projecting from this helical chain are the side-groups of the individual amino acids. Some amino acids have polar side-groups (positively or negatively charged), others are uncharged and hydrophobic (dislike water). In aqueous solution—the natural environment except for membranes—the helical peptide chain may fold (imagine crushing a coiled spring into a ball) so that the hydrophobic side-chains are at the centre and the charged ones at the exterior, yielding globular proteins. This so-called tertiary structure is sometimes reinforced by struts (disulphide bridges), which are also used to join polypeptide chains together. In general, the folding involved in secondary and tertiary structure occurs spontaneously, and is determined by the primary structure. Some peptides require assistance in folding because of a propensity to aggregate, and this is effected by other proteins known as chaperonins (cf. chaperone). Proteins to be inserted into membranes (e.g. transporters) have hydrophobic regions that span the lipid (oily) layer of the membrane, and more polar regions of the peptide may project from one or both faces of the membrane.

Some proteins undergo structural modification after synthesis. This may include addition of further chemical groups (e.g. sugars), the formation of disulphide bridges, the cleavage of closed loops to give two chains, and the association of different peptides to form multi-subunit proteins.

Proteins have many functions; mention has already been made of enzymes and transporters, which catalyse the reactions of metabolism, and contractile proteins, respectively. There are structural proteins (generally so-called fibrous proteins), notably in skin, in the tendons of muscles, and in bones. In blood there are transport proteins, which convey, for example, oxygen, metals such as iron, and nutrients such as fats and *cholesterol in the bloodstream. Some proteins have other molecules, essential to their function, bound to them. Thus *haemoglobin, which carries oxygen, is composed of a protein (globin) and a haem (a particular form of organically bound iron which carries oxygen). In electron-transport proteins, haem iron transports electrons, i.e. the function of haem is determined by the protein to which it is attached.

Enzymes catalyse reactions by combining with their substrates (a term for the reacting chemicals). Certain regions of the protein molecule (often in a cleft formed by tertiary structure) constitute the substrate-binding site(s). Substrates bind, the reaction is effected by their interaction with neighbouring groups, and the products of the reaction dissociate. It is possible to interfere with the action of enzymes (or transporters) by use of inhibitors. These may be structural analogues of the substrate, which block the substrate-binding site(s), or they may bind elsewhere and alter the tertiary structure of the enzyme, thus nullifying its catalytic activity. Enzyme (or transporter) inhibition is of practical significance because many drugs and poisons are inhibitors of enzymes or transporters.

Genes and protein synthesis

The primary structure of a protein is encoded in the *gene for that protein. Genes are the functional units of chromosomes composed of DNA, located in the cell nucleus. DNA is a linear polymer of four types of nucleotide, each of which consists of a sugar (deoxyribose), one of four bases (Adenine, Guanine, Cytosine, or Thymine), and phosphate. DNA is double-stranded, the chains are helical and complementary, and held together by the pairing of bases on the inside (G with C, A with T) (complementary base-pairing). A sequence of three nucleotides (triplet) codes for an amino acid or for a 'start' or 'stop' signal, and is known as a codon. There are four bases and hence a total of 64 possible triplet codons but only 21 amino acids plus 'start' and 'stop'. The genetic code is said to be degenerate because there can be more than one codon for an individual amino acid, 'start', or 'stop'. DNA replication in cell division is accurate because of base-pairing with the template strand. Each strand of DNA (chromosome) contains many genes and much intervening DNA.

For protein synthesis a gene is transcribed on to an RNA molecule (messenger RNA; mRNA). This differs from DNA in that ribose replaces deoxyribose and uracil replaces thymine. mRNA is single-stranded, individual mRNAs are limited to a single gene, and multiple copies may be transcribed from the single gene within a cell. The mRNA is then edited (portions—introns—are removed) and the mature mRNA leaves the nucleus and passes to a *ribosome (a specific type of intracellular organelle) composed of ribosomal RNA (rRNA) and containing the enzymes necessary for peptide bond synthesis.

The amino acids are reacted with another form of RNA (transfer RNA; tRNA) to form aminoacyl tRNA. Each tRNA is specific for a particular amino acid and carries its own code (an anticodon) which enables it to bind to the correct codon on mRNA. The aminoacyl tRNAs are presented two at a time, thus allowing for formation of a peptide bond, following which the penultimate tRNA dissociates and the next one engages. The mRNA is thus translated from end to end (from start to stop codons) and the newly formed peptide is extruded from the ribosome and eventually released. Some proteins are destined to enter intracellular organelles. Such trafficking is coded for by a terminal amino acid sequence (leader sequence) excised following entry. Cells have a full complement of genes, but only a selection of genes is transcribed in particular cell types.

*Mutations arise when the sequence of bases in DNA is altered (e.g. by irradiation). Mutations are harmful (i.e. they lead to disease) when they lead to malfunction in a vital protein. Two examples are sickle-cell *anaemia (haemoglobin mutation) and *haemophilia (mutation in a blood-clotting protein).

Cell control mechanisms
In humans, individual cells demonstrate autoregulation. They are capable, for example, of adjusting the relative rates of oxidation of alternative fuels (e.g. glucose or fat) according to supply; and of adjusting the overall rate of oxidations, and hence of ATP synthesis, according to the rate of ATP breakdown.

For most enzymes, control of rate is determined by substrate concentration. But certain key enzymes

(usually one or two per metabolic pathway) act as pacemakers and these may have regulator sites in addition to substrate-binding sites. Regulator sites modify enzyme activity (increase or decrease) when key metabolites (effectors) are bound. Thus the enzyme phosphofructokinase, which regulates the rate of glucose breakdown in muscle, is inhibited by ATP and activated by ADP and by other products formed when ATP is broken down to furnish energy for muscle contraction. This type of regulation is termed allosteric. Other enzymes are regulated by interconversion, e.g. by reversible phosphorylation. This process involves two regulatory enzymes, a kinase and a phosphatase. The kinase phosphorylates (adds phosphate from ATP to) the enzyme, the phosphatase dephosphorylates it. An example is provided by the enzyme glycogen phosphorylase which breaks down glycogen (a storage form of glucose) in liver and muscle. Glycogen phosphorylase is more active when phosphorylated, i.e. action of the kinase increases activity and action of the phosphatase decreases it. Kinases and phosphatases usually act on several enzymes, thus allowing simultaneous changes, i.e. programming. Enzyme concentration also determines enzyme activity, and the concentration of a particular enzyme can be altered through a change in the rate of gene transcription (i.e. of mRNA production). This is known as enzyme induction or repression and is effected through a region of the gene (the promoter) which regulates transcription.

In humans and other animals the metabolic activities of different tissues are co-ordinated by *hormones. These usually bind to specific proteins (*receptors) located on the external face of the cell membrane, and modify the activities of intracellular enzymes by reversible phosphorylation or an altered rate of gene transcription. One well-established mechanism, linking the receptor binding of a hormone to the ensuing changes in intracellular enzyme activities, involves the formation and release of a second messenger (cyclic AMP) at the intracellular surface of the cell membrance (Fig. 2). This may activate a protein kinase and/or alter the rate of gene transcription, and thereby modify the activities of enzymes in metabolic pathways. Not all hormones act in this way. The steroid hormones enter cells and are conveyed to the nucleus, where they may interact directly with the promoter regions of certain genes.

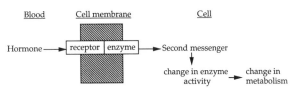

Fig. 2 Schematic representation of hormone action through a cell membrane receptor and a second messenger system.

Defence mechanisms

Animals possess specialized cells (*leucocytes, *macrophages, *lymphocytes) that are capable of killing invading *bacteria or *viruses. One mechanism involves specific enzymes that generate oxygen free-radicals, capable of damaging vital cell constituents. By achieving a high concentration in the vicinity of the virus or bacterium (or following ingestion) damage is done to the parasite while minimizing damage to host tissues. Yet other specialized cells (lymphocytes) may recognize foreign proteins (*antigens) through cell-surface receptors, and put in train the synthesis of *antibodies. These are proteins capable of combining specifically with the surface proteins of bacteria or viruses, or the toxins produced by them. Once bound, they may neutralize toxins or they may lead to the destruction of bacteria by a number of mechanisms. The diverse specificity of antibodies involves variations in the primary structure of a particular region of the antibody molecule. A number of mechanisms allow the bodily complement of lymphocytes to generate variation in the structure of antibody genes. Once the synthesis of an antibody against a particular antigen is effected, such antibody-producing cells (clones) are retained and can proliferate to produce further antibody if the antigen is encountered again.

This brief account has dealt with four of the major themes in biochemistry, namely the transduction and transformation of energy in living organisms; the relationship between protein structure and biological activity as exemplified by enzymes, transporters, and antibodies; the storage of structural information in genes and its translation into protein structure during protein synthesis; and cellular control and defence mechanisms.

PHILIP RANDLE

BIOENGINEERING. See BIOMEDICAL ENGINEERING.

BIOFEEDBACK is a technique whereby information about a physiological variable (such as arterial pressure or heart rate) is immediately relayed to the individual on whom the measurement is being made; the objective is to train the individual in the voluntary control of the function being measured.

BIOLOGY is the scientific study of living organisms; its two main branches are botany and zoology. Further subdivisions include cytology, histology, morphology, physiology, embryology, ecology, genetics, and microbiology. Related subjects include biochemistry, biophysics, and biometry.

BIOMEDICAL ENGINEERING is the application of engineering techniques to a wide range of biological and medical problems, from the manipulation of cellular and subcellular biological systems to the provision of physical aids for the disabled (see also PHYSICS, MEDICAL; REHABILITATION).

BIOMETRY. The science of applying statistical methods to the analysis of biological data; quantitative measurement of biological facts, especially with respect to variation (see STATISTICS).

BIOPHYSICS is a branch of biology that seeks to apply the laws of physics to the explanation of biological phenomena.

BIOPSY is the removal of tissue from the living body for diagnostic examination. It is sometimes also used to describe the tissue specimen itself.

BIOTECHNOLOGY. The technological exploitation of biological discoveries.

BIOTIN is a water-soluble *vitamin, usually considered as part of the *vitamin B complex, but also known as vitamin H. It functions as a *coenzyme concerned in carboxylation and decarboxylation, and is required for many metabolic processes, including normal energy formation and storage. It is widely distributed in all foodstuffs, and spontaneous deficiency probably does not occur in man.

BIRD-FANCIER'S LUNG is a form of *hypersensitivity *pneumonitis associated with *allergy to bird excreta, also known as 'pigeon-breeder's lung', etc. It is often misdiagnosed as bronchitis if no occupational history is taken. Recurrent attacks may lead to pulmonary *fibrosis.

BIRDS AS CARRIERS OF DISEASE. While birds have their own diseases analogous to those of man (e.g. avian malaria, tuberculosis) which they transmit to each other, they rarely pass them on to man. An exception is ornithosis, a viral *pneumonia which can be transmitted to man by pigeons, ducks, poultry, etc.; it was once called *psittacosis because it was thought to be exclusively a disease of parrots. Birds may provide a reservoir for certain *insect-borne viruses which can affect man when bitten by the same insects, such as West Nile fever and several varieties of *encephalitis.

BIRTH CANAL. The canal formed by the dilated female genital organs during *labour, through which the fetus passes during delivery; it consists of the *cervix uteri, the *vagina, and the *vulva.

BIRTH CONTROL is usually a euphemism for *contraception, although the term properly includes methods of population limitation such as *abortion, *infanticide, and 'moral restraint'.

BIRTH MARKS. Visible congenital marks; *naevi.

BIRTH RATE. The proportion of births to population, normally expressed as the number of live births per 1000 persons per year. The average world rate during 1970–75 was 31.8; for Europe and North America, respectively, 16.1 and 16.5.

BIRTHS AND DEATHS REGISTRATION ACTS, 1874 AND 1953. The 1874 Act made registration of births compulsory for the first time. The 1953 Act was the definitive enactment covering all aspects of the registration of births and deaths in UK. See LAW AND MEDICINE IN THE UK.

BISCHOFF, THEODOR LUDWIG WILHELM, (1807–82). German anatomist and physiologist. He was interested in embryology and reproduction, describing the development of the rabbit and clarifying the process of fertilization in the doe. In physiology he was an early student of *metabolism and the first to show that the blood contained free *oxygen and *carbon dioxide. He was violently opposed to women entering medicine.

BISEXUALITY is, strictly, the *hermaphrodite condition. More commonly used to denote facultative *homosexuality or one who has sexual intercourse with both sexes and thereby is at increased risk of acquiring *HIV infection.

BISMUTH is a white, crystalline metallic element (symbol Bi, atomic number 83, relative atomic mass 208.98), various compounds of which have found uses in medicine. Examples are: bismuth aluminate, subnitrate, etc., employed for their weak *antacid action; bismuth subgallate, used as a mild astringent in suppositories; and bismuth chelate (tripotassium dicitratobismuthate) used to coat the surface of peptic ulcers and promote healing.

BITE, INSECT. Biting members of the class Insecta include representatives of the orders Hemiptera (e.g. bugs, lice), Diptera (e.g. flies, mosquitoes), Siphonaptera (e.g. fleas), and Hymenoptera (e.g. bees, wasps, ants). While in many, the bites they inflict cause only local irritation, more serious consequences may follow the injection of venom by species such as bees and wasps, including severe and occasionally fatal allergic reactions (see ANAPHYLAXIS). Furthermore, insect bites are responsible for transmitting several important infectious and parasitic diseases, including *malaria, *plague, *onchocerciasis, *filariasis, *trypanosomiasis, *leishmaniasis, *typhus, and about 100 known virus infections, such as *yellow fever (see ARBOVIRUS; INSECTS AS VECTORS OF DISEASE; and under the names of individual insect species). Arthropod bites of medical importance are also caused by non-insect species, notably arachnids (e.g. *ticks, *mites, *spiders, and *scorpions).

BITTNER, JOHN JOSEPH (1904–61). American biologist. His best-known work was in the discovery of a factor in the milk of mice which can transmit a tendency to mammary cancer in the offspring. This factor behaved like a *virus, and its description added weight to the hypothesis that some neoplasms are caused by viruses.

BIZZOZERO, GIULIO CESARE (1846–1901). Italian histologist. He served as a medical officer in Garibaldi's army. He studied the microscopic appearance of the *lymph nodes, gave the *reticulocyte its name, and showed that *platelets were normal elements of blood (1882).

BLACK, GREENE VARDIMAN (1836–1915). American dentist. He advanced techniques of conservative dentistry by drilling out cavities caused by *caries so that the shape held fillings in place, and by making a porcelain crown for front teeth which was screwed into a root cavity filled with gold.

BLACK, JOSEPH (1728–99). British physician and chemist. A pioneer of chemistry, he was the first to make detailed gravimetric studies of a reversible chemical reaction. He showed that chalk when heated lost something, and that the resulting quicklime when slaked gained something. This 'something' was a gas which he called 'fixed air' (carbon dioxide), also present in expired air. He introduced also the notion of 'latent heat.'

BLACK BOX. Any self-contained portable unit of electronic equipment or any mysterious box with undefined contents sometimes used by practitioners of so-called 'fringe medicine'.

BLACK DEATH is the popular name for the bubonic/pneumonic *plague pandemic which devastated Europe in the middle of the 14th century and recurred at intervals until the pandemic of 1664–45, after which it virtually disappeared from northern and western Europe. 'Black Death' is the appellation introduced by the historian Elizabeth Markham in 1823; earlier names included 'Oriental Plague', 'Great Pestilence', and 'Great Mortality'. Although textbooks mostly explain the epithet in terms of *cyanosis, *purpura, and *gangrene, from the context, Mrs Markham was clearly using 'black' in the sense of 'disastrous'.

BLACKOUT. Sudden temporary loss of *consciousness. It is also used in other senses, e.g. to mean the temporary blindness without loss of consciousness experienced by aviators subject to extreme acceleration stress.

BLACKWATER FEVER is a dangerous complication of falciparum *malaria, characterized by massive intravascular haemolysis with haemoglobinuria, jaundice, and anaemia, leading in some cases to oliguric renal failure associated with acute tubular necrosis. The pathogenesis is incompletely understood, but it usually occurs in subjects previously infected with *Plasmodium falciparum*, and *hypersensitivity is thought to be involved.

BLACKWELL, ELIZABETH (1821–1910). Anglo-American physician. Born in Bristol, she emigrated to New York with her parents in 1832 and, after her father died in 1839, supported herself by teaching. Her interest in educating women was aroused and she decided to become a doctor. Her attempts to enter a medical school were unavailing until finally she was accepted by the University of Geneva in New York State, from which she graduated MD in 1849. In 1850 she returned to Europe, visiting England and France. In Paris, while attending a school for midwives she acquired a purulent *ophthalmia and lost the sight of an eye. In London she attended lectures at *St Bartholomew's Hospital with the permission of James *Paget. She then opened a dispensary for women in New York. In 1859, again in England, she became the first woman to be admitted to the British *Medical Register. In 1875 she became professor of gynaecology and obstetrics at the London School of Medicine for Women. Elizabeth Blackwell was a pioneer in the cause of women's education. She was the first British woman to qualify in medicine (see also WOMEN IN MEDICINE).

BLACK WIDOW SPIDER. A venomous *spider of the genus *Latrodectus* (*L. mactans*) which can bite and evenomate man, causing severe symptoms and occasionally death.

BLADDER. See URINARY BLADDER.

BLALOCK, ALFRED (1899–1964). American surgeon. His best-known work was in devising surgical methods of treating *congenital abnormalities of the heart and great vessels.

BLANE, SIR GILBERT, Bt (1749–1834). British physician. Blane sailed to the West Indies as physician to Admiral Rodney in 1779 and acquitted himself so well that he was made physician to the fleet. He did much to improve hygiene and discipline in the navy and introduced lemon juice as a preventive against *scurvy. He wrote *Observations on diseases of seamen* (1785).

BLASTOMYCOSIS. 'North American blastomycosis' is a *fungal infection, primarily of the lungs, which may spread elsewhere in the body, particularly to the skin. It is due to the fungus *Blastomyces dermatitidis*. The pathogenesis of the condition is poorly understood, and diagnosis may be difficult unless the organism is suspected on epidemiological grounds and specifically sought. 'South American blastomycosis' has similar features but a different geographical distribution; it is caused by another fungus, *Paracoccidioides brasiliensis*, and is also known as paracoccidioidomycosis. The most effective treatment of both conditions is with *amphotericin B or ketoconazole.

BLEEDING TIME primarily measures *platelet function: one method is to stab the earlobe with a needle and blot off the drop of blood which appears every 30 seconds until oozing ceases. The normal value is between 4 and 5 minutes. The time may extend to 9 minutes or more when the platelets are deficient in quantity or quality.

BLENNORRHOEA (BLENHORRHEA) is a free discharge of *mucus, sometimes used synonymously with *gonorrhoea.

BLEPHARITIS is any inflammatory condition of the eyelids.

BLEPHAROSPASM is recurrent spasmodic closure of the eyelids.

BLEULER, EUGEN (1857–1939). Swiss psychiatrist. He is best known for his studies of *schizophrenia. He introduced this term instead of *dementia praecox, which it was previously called.

BLINDNESS. Lack of sightedness, from whatever cause. See OPHTHALMOLOGY.

BLISTER. A localized epidermal swelling containing clear fluid, i.e. a *vesicle or *bulla.

BLOOD is the fluid tissue present in the circulatory system of higher animals. Like other tissues, it consists of formed elements (blood cells) in an unorganized ground substance (*plasma), the special feature being that the ground substance is a liquid in which the formed elements are suspended. See HAEMATOLOGY.

BLOOD ALCOHOL. Since *ethanol diffuses throughout total body water (about 40 litres in an adult male of average weight), each alcoholic drink of average social quantity (containing about 10 g of ethanol) raises the blood alcohol by about 25 mg/dl; a peak level is reached about 1 hour after ingestion and is maintained for about 2 hours. Thereafter, the level declines as elimination by hepatic metabolism and excretion occurs at a fairly constant rate of 10 g/hour. In the UK, the Road Traffic Act of 1967 prescribed 80 mg/dl as the maximum permissible blood alcohol level for being in charge of a motor vehicle but the levels are lower in other countries.

BLOOD BANK. A store of donated blood for use in *blood transfusion. (See HAEMATOLOGY.)

BLOOD CULTURE. The culture of micro-organisms from specimens of blood to determine the presence and nature of *bacteriaemia.

BLOOD GAS ANALYSIS is determination by various means of blood concentrations of *oxygen, *carbon dioxide, *hydrogen ions, and *haemoglobin. Additional values, either calculated or measured directly, include the partial pressures of oxygen (pO_2) and carbon dioxide (pCO_2) and the percentage saturation of haemoglobin with oxygen.

BLOOD GROUPS. See GENETICS; HAEMATOLOGY.

BLOOD LETTING is the therapeutic removal of a quantity of blood (*phlebotomy or *venesection); once a panacea, it is now used only in a few specific conditions; these include *polycythaemia, *haemochromatosis, one type of *porphyria, and occasionally *heart failure with circulatory overload.

BLOOD PRESSURE, when otherwise unqualified, is taken to mean arterial pressure. This is still normally recorded in millimetres of mercury (mmHg) rather than *SI units (kilopascals or kPa); the systolic pressure (i.e. during cardiac *systole) is written first, followed by the diastolic (*diastole), thus: 120/80 mmHg. See also KOROTKOFF SOUNDS.

BLOOD SUBSTITUTES. When the only fully adequate substitute, i.e. compatible whole blood itself, is not available, blood loss must be countered by using blood substitutes (fluid and *electrolyte solutions, appropriate when blood volume is contracted for other reasons, are of only temporary benefit after *haemorrhage as the fluid is rapidly lost into the tissues). Substances in use are those of large molecular weight which will remain in the circulation for long periods. They include blood derivatives, such as *plasma and *albumin and solutions of *dextran. Dextran is a *polysaccharide of high molecular weight which takes several weeks to be metabolized. Although it expands blood volume, it does not replace the lost oxygen-carrying capacity of the blood. Another 'plasma expander' in current use is based on gelatin. Both are likely to be replaced in the future by substances at present under development, which are also able to carry *oxygen.

BLOOD SUGAR is the level of *glucose in the circulating blood, the normal fasting value of which is in the range 3.5 to 5.2 mmol/l. See also GLUCOSE TOLERANCE TEST.

BLOOD TRANSFUSION. See HAEMATOLOGY.

BLUE BABIES are infants born with cyanotic *congenital heart disease, i.e. with developmental defects of the heart and/or great vessels, allowing deoxygenated venous blood to short-circuit the lungs and to pass directly into the left side of the heart and arterial circulation, causing visible blueness (*cyanosis) of skin and mucous membranes.

BLUNDELL, JAMES (1790–1877). British obstetrician. He was the first ever to give a transfusion of human blood on 22 December 1818.

BMR. See BASAL METABOLIC RATE.

BOARD OF CONTROL, THE, succeeded the Commissioners who had been appointed in the UK under the *Lunacy Act of 1890. Under the *Mental Deficiency Act of 1913, the paid Commissioners in Lunacy became Commissioners of the Board. The *National Health Service Act of 1946 stripped the Board of most of its powers, transferring them to the Minister of Health. These related to the licensing of houses, the registration of hospitals, the approval of nursing homes and other places receiving mentally ill and mentally handicapped patients. The Board was abolished in 1960 and its remaining powers relating to visitation and inspection of institutions, etc. were later vested in the Mental Health Act Commission (see MENTAL HEALTH ACTS).

BODLEY SCOTT, SIR RONALD (1906–82). English physician. His published papers indicate that his interest in *haematology began in 1933 and he subsequently published extensively on the reticuloses and haemolytic states, and with A. H. T. Robb-Smith described histiocytic medullary reticulosis in 1939. After military service in the Middle East in the Second World War, he was elected physician to St Bartholomew's Hospital and developed his research interests in *leukaemia and *lymphoma. At times seeming somewhat shy and reserved, he nevertheless possessed a rich vein of kindness and humility and an astringent wit, and was a notable figure in British medicine. As the preface to this volume makes clear, Sir Ronald (with Paul Beeson) originally conceived the idea of the first *Oxford Companion to Medicine* and the planning of the book was well advanced under his guidance and leadership at the time of his sudden and untimely death in 1982.

BODY LOUSE. *Pediculus humanus humanus* (also known as *Pediculus humanus corporis*), is a surface *parasite of man, which flourishes under conditions of overcrowding and poor hygiene. As well as causing skin irritation and local reaction, it is a vector of some forms of *typhus and of the treponemal infection *relapsing fever.

BODY-SNATCHERS. Before the *Anatomy Act of 1832, the demand for bodies for anatomical dissection led to the growth of professional gangs of 'body-snatchers', or 'resurrectionists' as they were also known.

These groups, who worked during early winter evenings when they were least likely to be observed, could extract a body from a recent grave within an hour and leave no trace. It was a lucrative trade, which continued for some time even after the 1832 Act had regulated the supply of bodies for dissection. The first instance on record was in 1777. The body of Mrs Jane Sainsbury was taken from the burial ground near Gray's Inn Lane. The criminals were convicted and imprisoned for 6 months. See also ANATOMY.

BOERHAAVE, HERMAN (1668–1738). Dutch physician. His method of bedside teaching drew students to Leiden from all over Europe. He lectured in Latin and revived the Hippocratic approach, founding the *eclectic school. His textbooks, translated into all the European languages, circulated throughout the civilized world. His case report of a man who died from rupture of the oesophagus, *Atrosis nec descripti prius morbi historia* (1724), was the first presented in modern form with history followed by physical examination, diagnosis, course, and autopsy. The modern medical curriculum, with its sequence of natural science, anatomy, physiology, and pathology, is derived from him. His pupils spread his doctrine throughout Europe; both the Edinburgh and the old Vienna schools owed much to him. His *Aphorismi* (1709) and his *Elementia chemiae* (1732) are his best-known works.

BOHR, CHRISTIAN (1855–1911). Danish physician. He was the first to establish the Sans-shape of the *oxygen dissociation curve of *haemoglobin in 1904, and the influence of *carbon dioxide on it. He was the father of Niels Bohr, a founder of modern atomic physics.

BOILS, are acute staphylococcal *abscesses of the skin and subcutaneous tissues; the medical term is furuncles. They are common in normal subjects, but especially so at puberty and in persons with poor hygiene or oily skin. The *staphylococci gain access via hair follicles. Local factors such as irritation, and general conditions like *diabetes favour infection. The usual course is over 4 or 5 days, during which time the centre of the lesion becomes *necrotic and forms *pus, changing from red to yellow in the process. Spontaneous drainage to the exterior is usual and healing follows. A 'blind boil' is one that fails to discharge, and regresses to become a persistent indolent *nodule. An aggregate of connecting furuncles is a *carbuncle.

BOLOGNA, UNIVERSITY OF, was founded in the late 11th century and became famous for the study of law. Medicine was introduced by *Alderotti in the 13th century. In the medieval period it attracted medical students from all over Europe; among the more famous were Guy de *Chauliac, *Vesalius, *Paracelsus, *Valsalva, and *Morgagni, some of whom taught there.

BONE MARROW is the tissue that occupies the cavities of bones, of major importance in blood cell formation.

BONE MARROW TRANSPLANTATION was introduced in 1964 for treatment of some immunodeficiencies and blood disease, among them *aplastic anaemia and some varieties of *leukaemia in children. The object of the grafting is to correct marrow failure in immunodeficiency or aplastic anaemia, and in leukaemia to replace diseased with healthy marrow. The first step is to destroy the malignant or defective marrow, in the past with X-rays, but nowadays increasingly with a variety of other chemotherapeutic and immunosuppressant agents. With no functioning marrow there is no production of white cells and red cells. The patient becomes vulnerable to any infection, however slight, since the white cells are normally important in fighting it. There is also severe anaemia because of shortage of red cells. It is important to find a donor whose marrow is immunologically compatible with that of the patient; this can be difficult, just as it may be in all grafting procedures (see TRANSPLANTATION). Marrow is infused into the patient in the hope that some of the immature stem cells which produce both red and white cells will settle in and repopulate the recipient's marrow. The infused cells are transported to all organs of the body, but it is hoped that they will flourish in the sort of environment to which they are accustomed without being rejected. The procedure is becoming increasingly successful, giving increased expectation of life to sufferers, especially children. Graft-versus-host disease and infection are still troublesome complications, but methods are improving steadily and the number of disorders treatable by this method is increasing.

BONE SCANNING uses scanning techniques (see NUCLEAR MEDICINE SCANNERS) after administering an appropriate *radioisotope to detect abnormal lesions of bone, particularly those due to *metastases of malignant *tumours.

BONE-SETTER. An unqualified practitioner who specializes in the treatment of bone *dislocations and *fractures. See also OSTEOPATHY.

BORBORYGMI are rumbling noises which arise from the intestinal movement of gas and liquid.

BORDET, JULES JEAN BAPTISTE VINCENT (1870–1961). Belgian microbiologist. His early work was on *bacteriolysis and *haemolysis and he demonstrated the specificity of *agglutinins and *precipitins. In Brussels his researches were into what he called 'alexin', now known as complement (see IMMUNOLOGY). He proved the diagnostic value of *complement fixation tests. An unexpected by-product of his work was isolation of the whooping cough (*pertussis) bacillus now known as *Bordetella pertussis* (bacillus of Bordet and Gengou). In 1919 he was awarded the *Nobel prize in medicine for his work on lysis by complement.

BORDEU, THEOPHILE DE (1722–76). French physician. He wrote on lead colic (see LEAD POISONING) and speculated that the effects of *castration were due to loss of an internal secretion from the *testes. His patients included Louis XV, Mme du Barry, and the Duchesse de Bourbon.

BORELLI, GIOVANNI ALFONSO (1608–79). Italian mathematician. He attempted to explain muscular action in purely mechanical terms in his posthumous work *De motu animalium* (1680).

BORGOGNONI, TEODORICO (Theodoric of Lucca) (*c*. 1205–98). Italian surgeon. For 33 years he taught medicine and surgery at the University of Bologna. He completed his progressive and original work *Chirurgia* in 1266 (first printed in 1498), in which he deplored *suppuration and advocated inhalation of vapours from sponges soaked in hypnotic drugs (soporific sponges) to allay the pain of surgery.

BORNHOLM DISEASE, also known as *pleurodynia, is a benign self-limiting *virus infection giving acute chest (occasionally abdominal) pain and fever, often occurring in epidemics. It may be mistaken for more serious conditions, e.g. pulmonary *embolism, *pneumonia, *coronary thrombosis, etc. Viruses of the *Coxsackie B group are the usual cause. The name is that of a Danish island where an epidemic was described in 1934.

BORODIN, ALEXANDER PORFIRYEVICH (1833–87). Russian biochemist and composer. Borodin was the illegitimate son of the wife of an army doctor and an Imeretian prince. He became a physiological chemist and his method of estimating *urea was widely used. *Prince Igor* and the B Minor Symphony are his best-known compositions. He supported careers in medicine for women.

BORRELIA BERGDORFERI. The causal agent of Lyme disease (see RHEUMATOLOGY).

BOSTOCK, JOHN (1773–1846). English physician. His principal contribution was to demonstrate that in patients with *renal disease the serum contained excess *urea and was deficient in *albumin, while the urine was of low specific gravity. Bostock also described *hay fever, drawing on his own experience as a sufferer.

BOTALLO, LEONARDO (?1519–88). Italian anatomist and surgeon. He gave the first account of *hay fever (1565) and his name is attached to the *ductus arteriosus and the *foramen ovale. His patients included Charles IX (1560) and Catherine de *Medici.

BOTANY is the scientific study of plants.

BOTULISM is a severe and often fatal form of *food poisoning due to a potent *neurotoxin (botulinum) pre-formed in contaminated canned or bottled food by the anaerobic bacterium *Clostridium botulinum*. The condition is very rare in the UK. The toxin (one of the most potent poisons known to man) is thermolabile and is destroyed if the food is re-cooked for 10 minutes at 90 °C. Botulinum toxin injected directly into muscle is proving to be an effective treatment for *dystonia, spasmodic *torticollis, and some other movement disorders.

BOUGIE. A cylindrical instrument of varying calibre used chiefly to dilate constricted passages, e.g. the lower oesophagus in *achalasia, or the *urethra in postgonorrhoeal *stricture.

BOUILLAUD, JEAN BAPTISTE (1796–1881). French physician. He noted the association of *aphasia with lesions of the frontal lobes (1825) and heart disease with *rheumatic fever (1836).

BOWDITCH, HENRY PICKERING (1840–1911). American physiologist. He showed that *nerve fibres do not seem to be subject to fatigue, and this has been referred to as Bowditch's law.

BOWDLER, THOMAS (1754–1825). British physician and editor. He devoted his life to charitable works. In 1818 he published the *Family Shakespeare* from which all matter was omitted which could not 'with propriety be read aloud in a family'. The verb to 'bowdlerize' was first used in its current sense in 1836.

BOWEL is a synonym for *intestine.

BOVINE SPONGIFORM ENCEPHALOPATHY (BSE) is a slowly progressive and ultimately fatal neurological disorder of adult cattle. It was given this name because of the spongy appearance of brain tissue, known technically as grey matter vacuolation, when sections are examined under the microscope. It was first identified in the UK in 1986, but may have occurred as early as 1985. It belongs to a group of progressive, degenerative, and fatal diseases of the central nervous system, caused by unconventional transmissible agents, usually called prions but also termed 'slow viruses'. Similar diseases include *scrapie in sheep and goats, transmissible mink encephalopathy, and *kuru and *Creutzfeldt–Jakob disease in man. The disease initially produces signs of apprehension, anxiety, and fear in affected animals, followed by behavioural, gait, and postural abnormalities with, eventually, recumbency and death, usually within 6 months. The available evidence strongly suggests that the condition was due to the consumption of animal foodstuffs derived from the carcases of scrapie-infected sheep in which the process of rendering had been inadequate to destroy the agent. Since 1986 a policy of slaughtering all affected animals has been followed in the UK. A Working Party, established jointly by the Ministry of Agriculture, Fisheries and Food and the Department of Health, recommended also that milk from such cows should not be used for human consumption and that ruminant-based protein should no longer be used in ruminant rations. It seems likely that the scrapie agent, although transmissible to cattle, is not pathogenic to man, as meat and offal derived from sheep have been consumed by humans for many years and there is no epidemiological evidence that Creutzfeldt–Jakob disease has ever been acquired from such a source. Thus it is highly improbable that the consumption of meat or meat products from cattle carrying the agent will prove pathogenic to man. Nevertheless, research is continuing and the question of a potential risk to humans is still under review.

Reference
Department of Health, Ministry of Agriculture, Fisheries and Food. (1989). *Report of the Working Party on Bovine Spongiform Encephalopathy.*

BOW LEGS. A deformity of the legs, known as genu varum, in which bowing causes an abnormally wide gap between the knees (cf. *knock knees).

BOWMAN, SIR WILLIAM, BT (1816–92). British anatomist and ophthalmologist. He described *Bowman's capsule, which invests the renal glomerulus.

BOWMAN'S CAPSULE is the glomerular capsule, comprising a dilatation of each *renal tubule at its commencement surrounding the *glomerulus. It consists of a double layer of *epithelium (capsular and glomerular epithelium).

BOXING. Although boxing is a sport favoured and supported by many, an increasing tide of medical and lay opinion takes the view that a so-called sport whose primary objective is to injure one's opponent, and if possible to render him unconscious, is becoming unacceptable in civilized society. Professional boxing has been banned by law in Sweden, Norway, and Iceland. Despite increasingly stringent medical supervision, including the use of *electroencephalography, brain *scanning, and ophthalmological examination, deaths continue to occur as a result of brain damage sustained in the ring, while post-traumatic encephalopathy (the 'punch-drunk' syndrome) continues to occur. Even amateur boxing, with its shorter bouts, the use of headguards, and even more careful medical supervision, is not without risks.

As reports from the Royal College of Physicians of London, the British Medical Association, and other medical organizations across the world have made clear, any severe blow to the head, however caused,

not only produces *concussion, due to jarring of the brain within the rigid skull cage, but almost inevitably results in the death of a small number of brain cells. Neuropathological studies have confirmed that some nerve fibres within the brain may be divided. Recurrent insults give rise to cerebral atrophy, enlargement of the cerebral ventricles, and cavitation of the septum pellucidum (which separates the two lateral ventricles). These changes are associated with progressive deterioration of the intellect (*dementia), a slow, shuffling gait, and other features resembling those of *Parkinson's disease. While many other sports carry a significant risk of physical injury, and while a similar post-traumatic encephalopathy is well-recognized to occur, for example, in steeplechase jockeys after repeated head injuries due to falls, the primary aim of most other sports, unlike boxing and martial arts, is not to inflict injury upon one's opponent. There seems little doubt that increasing concern about the unacceptable consequences of boxing will ultimately result in the professional sport, at least, being banned by law in many countries. The last attempt to achieve a ban in the UK, by Lord Taylor of Gryfe, who introduced a bill into the House of Lords in early 1992, was unsuccessful. Also see SPORT AND MEDICINE.

BOYD, SIR JOHN SMITH KNOX (1891–1981). British bacteriologist. In 1929 he became assistant director of hygiene in the *Royal Army Medical Corps India where he isolated the strain of *dysentery bacillus called *Shigella boydii*. He proved the preventive value of *tetanus toxoid. He left the army in 1946 when appointed director of the Wellcome Laboratory for Tropical Medicine.

BOYD, WILLIAM (1885–1979). British/Canadian pathologist, author, and lecturer. After wartime service in a field ambulance, he was appointed professor of pathology at the University of Manitoba, Winnipeg, where he served for 22 years. He became professor of pathology at the University of Toronto in 1937, where he remained for 14 years. In 'retirement' he became professor at the new medical faculty in Vancouver. Having written special pathology texts for surgeons (1925) and internists (1931) he produced his readable *Textbook of pathology: introduction to medicine* in 1932. At the age of 85 he edited its eighth edition. With Dr Maude *Abbott he revived the profession's interest in museums; there are four in North America which bear his name, as does the Academy of Medicine Library in Toronto.

BOYD ORR, JOHN, 1st Baron Boyd Orr of Brechin Mearns (1880–1971). British physiologist and nutritionist. He became director-general of the Food and Agriculture Organization of the United Nations (1946–47) and acted as Chancellor of Glasgow University from 1946 until his death. He made notable contributions to the study of *malnutrition and specific dietary deficiencies. He wrote many books on the science of *nutrition and on economic policy including *The national food supply and its influence on public health* (1934) and *Food—the foundation of world unity* (1948). In 1949 he was awarded the *Nobel Peace Prize for advocating a world food policy based on human needs rather than trade interests.

BOYLE, ROBERT (1627–91). Anglo-Irish scientist. Boyle made many contributions to science, the most famous still being known as *Boyle's law. He helped to overthrow the Aristotelian idea of the division of the world into the elements of earth, air, fire, and water. He believed that it is made up of particles, with powers of motion and varying organizations. This portended current views of the nature of the world. His outstanding work was *The skeptical chymist* (1661). He was a prominent member of the *Royal Society.

BOYLE'S LAW is one of the fundamental laws governing the behaviour of gases; it states that at constant temperature, the volume (V) of a gas varies inversely with the pressure (P) exerted on it, and that the product PV therefore remains constant.

BOYLSTON, ZABDIEL (1679–1766). American physician. He was the first physician in America to employ *smallpox inoculation, and as a result was much persecuted.

BRACE. An *orthopaedic or *orthodontic appliance for supporting or correcting the alignment of bony structures or the teeth.

BRACHIAL PLEXUS. A network of *nerves derived from the lowest four cervical and the first thoracic spinal nerves, the branches of which supply the arm and shoulder girdle. It is situated partly in the neck and partly in the axilla, and is susceptible to traction injury in certain road accidents, especially those involving motor-cyclists.

BRADYCARDIA is an abnormally slow rate of heart beat (usually taken as 60 per minute or less).

BRADYKINESIA is abnormal slowness or paucity of muscle movements.

BRAILLE is the system of embossed printing in which alpha-numeric characters are represented by different combinations of six raised dots. It was perfected in 1834 by the Frenchman Louis Braille, a teacher of the blind, and adopted as standard in the UK by the British and Foreign Blind Association in 1869–70. See OPHTHALMOLOGY.

BRAIN, SIR WALTER RUSSELL, Bt, 1st Baron Brain (1895–1966). British neurologist. He was president of the Royal College of Physicians of London from 1950 to 1957. Brain was a cultured physician and a skilled clinical neurologist who possessed considerable diplomatic skill. His main clinical interests were in aphasia and in the neurological syndromes that accompany some forms of malignant disease.

BRAIN. See ANATOMY; NEUROLOGY; NEUROSCIENCE.

BRAIN (STEM) DEATH. During the second half of the 20th century major advances in *resuscitation technology began to confront doctors with problems of a new kind. Through the skilled and judicious use of artificial *ventilation, of drugs capable of maintaining a collapsing *blood pressure, of alimentation via the intravenous route, and of elimination of the waste products of *metabolism by *dialysis, it became possible to maintain a circulation in bodies whose brains were irreversibly dead. This inevitably led to a profound re-evaluation of what was meant by death. Whether they liked it or not, doctors were forced to confront some basic philosophical issues.

A consensus gradually emerged that death could be perceived as irreversible loss of the capacity to be conscious, combined with irreversible loss of the capacity to breathe spontaneously, and hence to maintain a spontaneous heart beat. This concept was not really radically new. It was basically a secularized reformulation (in the language of modern *neurophysiology) of much older concepts of death. 'Irreversible loss of the capacity for consciousness' was the same as 'departure of the (conscious) soul from the body'. And 'irreversible loss of the capacity to breathe spontaneously' was what many older writers meant by 'loss of the breath of life'.

Most people die because their circulation stops, and doctors can't get it going again. If the circulation resumes within a matter of seconds, the patient will, at worse, have suffered a fainting attack. If the circulation is restored only within 3 or 4 minutes the patient will have suffered severe anoxic brain damage, for anoxia (oxygen deprivation) of this severity not only stops the machine, it wrecks the machinery. The cerebral hemispheres (the part of the brain subserving all perceptive, cognitive, and affective functions) will have been irreversibly damaged, whereas the brainstem (the part of the brain subserving vegetative functions—which is less vulnerable to anoxia) will have been spared. If the heart stops for longer periods, both the cerebral hemispheres and the brainstem will have died, and the patient will be dead according to classic criteria.

Major intracranial catastrophes can also irreversibly destroy the brainstem. When certain parts of the upper brainstem are destroyed, the individual is rendered unconscious, for these parts 'activate' the cerebral hemispheres, generating, as it were, the 'capacity for consciousness'. When the brainstem is destroyed, spontaneous respiration, which is 'driven' by cells in the lower part of the brainstem, will also cease. But if such patients are put on ventilators (and the heart is thereby supplied with oxygenated blood) cardiac function can, for a while, be maintained. This is because the heart beat (unlike breathing) is not 'driven' by the nervous system. Anyone who has seen an isolated frog's heart beating in a jar will be familiar with this phenomenon.

Hence there is only one kind of death (brainstem death), although there are several ways of dying: the brainstem can die because the circulation has ceased for sufficiently long, or it can be destroyed as a result of a primary intracranial catastrophe.

The clinical state which was to become known as 'brain death' was first described by two French neurologists in 1958. They called it 'coma dépassé' (literally a state beyond coma). Affected individuals not only failed to relate to the external environment, they could not even maintain homeostasis (a stable internal environment).

Over the next decade doctors working in *intensive care units became increasingly familiar with the condition, and standard criteria for its diagnosis were set up in many countries. It was established that such patients had a 'blocked cerebral circulation'. No blood could enter the head because the intracranial pressure had been lastingly higher than the systolic arterial pressure. Brain death was described by some as 'physiological decapitation'. It was also proved unequivocally that even if ventilation was maintained in such patients, no individual ever regained consciousness. All patients, moreover, developed asystole (cessation of the heart beat) within a relatively short time.

Diagnosis

The diagnosis of brainstem death is straightforward, despite the very stringent criteria adopted for its identification. Before brainstem death can be diagnosed, certain preconditions have to be fulfilled. If the patient fulfils these preconditions, certain clinical tests are then applied.

(a) Preconditions

1. The patient has to be deeply unconscious, on a ventilator, in an intensive care unit. The diagnosis of brainstem death cannot be made at the roadside, in accident and emergency departments, on patients dying at home, or in the general wards of a hospital.
2. The cause of the coma must be known without a shred of doubt. Patients in coma of unknown cause can never be diagnosed as brainstem dead. The cause of the coma must be 'irremediable', 'structural' brain damage. The determination of the 'irremediable' nature of the brain damage is not based on theoretical grounds, but is painstakingly established, after the application of all potentially useful therapeutic measures.
3. Conditions such as drug intoxication, hypothermia, or profound metabolic upset (which are capable of

causing a reversible disturbance of brainstem function) have to be strictly excluded.

Only after the patient has been through these very tight 'filters' is he or she deemed to be a suitable candidate to be tested for irreversible loss of brainstem function.

(b) Tests. These assess the integrity of the brainstem reflexes and the capacity for spontaneous respiration. The doctors performing the tests have to provide unambiguous answers to the following questions:

1. Do the pupils constrict when a bright light is shone into them?
2. Does the patient blink when his/her cornea is touched?
3. Is there grimacing in response to firm supraorbital pressure or to painful stimuli applied to other parts of the body?
4. Is there any movement of the eyes in response to the irrigation of the eardrums with ice-cold water?
5. Is there any coughing or gagging when a catheter is passed down the airway?

These tests assess function at various levels of the brainstem (in a 'slice by slice' manner), the responses mutually reinforcing one another.

Finally, if all the tests have given negative responses, the doctors then assess whether the individual can breathe spontaneously. After proper preoxygenation, the patient is disconnected from the ventilator. Disconnection is maintained for a period sufficient to allow endogenously produced *carbon dioxide to build up to a level (50 mmHg) which would stimulate the respiratory centre in the brainstem if it still contained live nerve cells. If respiration does not begin spontaneously, this gives final confirmation of the diagnosis of brainstem death.

The tests have to be performed by two doctors of appropriate seniority, who are experienced in the management of such cases. The doctors may be *neurologists, *neurosurgeons, *anaesthetists, or intensive care specialists. The relevant tests are always repeated after a short period, to document the fact that the abnormal state has persisted for a period several times longer than nerve cells can survive deprivation of their blood supply.

The diagnosis of brainstem death is made in a systematic and unhurried manner. No haste is involved. The potential recipient of organs may be anxious to receive the organs of a brainstem dead donor. However, the doctors looking after the potential donor remain totally committed to his or her case. Transplant surgeons are not involved in the diagnosis of brainstem death.

The diagnosis of death on neurological (as distinct from cardiological) grounds is now accepted practice in nearly all countries of the world. It has formal legal sanction in many countries. In others it is based on codes elaborated by the highest medical authorities. The British code is based on the recommendations of the Conference of Medical Royal Colleges and their faculties in the UK, a body which meets periodically to assess national and international developments in this subject.

C. PALLIS

BRAIN SCAN. Radiological examination of the brain with *computerized axial tomographic, *magnetic resonance scanning, or following the intravenous injection of *radioisotopes (radioisotope scanning or gamma-encephalography). Echoencephalography is scanning with ultrasonic waves.

BRAINSTEM. The part of the brain connecting the *cerebral hemispheres with the *spinal cord, comprising, from above downwards, the *mid-brain, the *pons, and the *medulla oblongata.

BRAN is the non-absorbable residue (husk) of wheat, barley, and other grains (see FIBRE, DIETARY).

BREECH DELIVERY. Delivery of an infant when its buttocks present in labour. See also OBSTETRICS.

BRETONNEAU, PIERRE FIDELE (1771–1862). French physician. He noted the intestinal lesions of *typhoid fever (1820) and foretold that it would prove different from *typhus (1828). He distinguished *diphtheria from *scarlet fever (1826), and was the first to carry out *tracheostomy in *croup (1825).

BREUER, JOSEF (1842–1925). Austrian physician. He undertook research into the reflex control of *respiration with *Hering (*Hering–Breuer reflex, 1868) and into the functions of the *labyrinth. With Sigmund *Freud he devised the 'cathartic' treatment of *neurosis, but the two fell out and after 1896 they never spoke to each other again.

BRIDGES, ROBERT SEYMOUR (1844–1930). British physician and poet. He always intended to retire from practice at the age of 40, but in 1881 a severe attack of pneumonia led him to do so when 37. Thereafter he devoted himself wholly to poetry; he had already written much verse in the preceding nine years. In 1913 he was made Poet Laureate and in 1929 received the Order of Merit. In his last year, aged 85, he published his most renowned work *The testament of beauty*.

BRIGHT, RICHARD (1789–1858). British physician. He was an unimpressive lecturer but his genius lay in correlating clinical observations with post-mortem appearances. In his *Reports of medical cases* (1827) he established the association of *oedema and *albuminuria with *nephritis (Bright's disease).

BRIGHT'S DISEASE. An obsolete synonym for acute glomerulonephritis. See NEPHROLOGY.

BRILL'S DISEASE is recrudescent *typhus, also known as Brill–Zinsser disease.

BRISSAUD, EDOUARD (1852–1909). French neurologist. He was probably the first to suggest that *gigantism was the result of *acromegaly during the period of growth (1895).

BRISTOL ROYAL INFIRMARY in south-west England, is the oldest charity hospital founded outside London. It began in 1736 after public subscriptions in order to minister to the sick poor. Like similar institutions, it soon became inadequate so a new building was raised in 1784, completed in 1814, and still remains in use. Further expansion began in 1966 and now the BRI offers a full range of medical and surgical specialties, and is a major health resource for the city, and the south-west region. It is a main base for clinical teaching of students at Bristol University.

BRITISH ANTI-LEWISITE, or BAL, is an alternative name for dimercaprol (2,3-dimercaptopropanol, $C_3H_8OS_2$). It is a chelating agent, i.e. a chemical that forms tight complexes with lead and other heavy metals, and is used to treat poisoning with *lead, *mercury, *arsenic, *gold, and *bismuth. It is given intramuscularly in oil. Lewisite was a lethal arsenic-containing war gas, named after an American chemist, W. Lee Lewis (1879–1943).

BRITISH ASSOCIATION FOR THE ADVANCEMENT OF SCIENCE. Founded in 1831, the British Association for the Advancement of Science (BAAS) exists to promote interest in and understanding of the concepts, language, methods, and application of science. It holds conferences, meetings, and study groups; provides an information service; organizes visits and excursions; and publishes an annual report and two quarterly periodicals. It has 17 scientific sections and one for young persons known as the British Association for Young Scientists. An important achievement of BAAS is the publicizing of scientific events and progress through its annual meetings, the proceedings of which are extensively reported in the lay press.

BRITISH MEDICAL ASSOCIATION. See MEDICAL COLLEGES, ETC. OF THE UK; MEDICAL SOCIETIES.

BRITISH MEDICAL JOURNAL. See MEDICAL JOURNALS.

BRITISH PHARMACEUTICAL CODEX is a book of authoritative guidance to those prescribing and dispensing medicines 'throughout the British Empire', produced by the Council of the Royal *Pharmaceutical Society and first published in 1907. Revised and extended editions appeared at intervals until 1979, when the title was changed to *The Pharmaceutical Codex*. The book supplements the information in the *British Pharmacopoeia* by providing data on actions, uses, undesirable effects, etc. of pharmacopoeial substances and preparations, and by providing formulae and standards for a range of materials not included in the *Pharmacopoeia*. See also PHARMACY AND PHARMACISTS.

BRITISH PHARMACOPOEIA. The *British Pharmacopoeia (BP)* provides approved names and standards for the quality of substances, preparations, and other articles used in medicine and pharmacy, together with information on action, use, dose, solubility, storage, and labelling.

The first *pharmacopoeia to be officially used throughout England was published by the Royal College of Physicians of London in 1618 (the *London Pharmacopoeia*). The appearance of rival works from the Edinburgh and Dublin Colleges led Parliament to provide, in the *Medical Act of 1858, for the publication of the first *British Pharmacopoeia*. The *BP* was compiled by the *General Medical Council until 1970, when the copyright was assigned to the Crown by the *Medicines Act. This Act set up a British Pharmacopoeia Commission charged with the responsibility of preparing new editions and amendments to them, under the authority of the Health Minister. The *BP* excludes substances used in veterinary medicine and surgery, which are the subject of a separate compendium. Drugs recognized by the *British Pharmacopoeia* have 'BP' after their names. See also PHARMACY AND PHARMACISTS.

BROAD STREET PUMP. See CHOLERA; SNOW, JOHN.

BROCA, PAUL (1824–80). French surgeon and anthropologist. He was a pioneer of *orthopaedics as well as *neurosurgery. In 1861 he showed that the left inferior frontal cerebral convolution (Broca's gyrus) was related to speech. He was one of the first to localize and *trephine for *brain abscess.

BROCK, SIR RUSSELL CLAUDE, Lord Brock of Wimbledon (1903–80). British surgeon. He was almost the first, and certainly the most prominent, British surgeon to concern himself with *cardiac surgery, and rapidly reached a dominating position in this specialty.

BRODIE, SIR BENJAMIN COLLINS, Bt (1783–1862). British surgeon and physiologist. He became president of the Royal College of Surgeons of England in 1844, president of the Royal Society in 1858, and first president of the *General Medical Council in 1858. His most important publication was *On the pathology and surgery of diseases of the joints* (1819).

BROMIDE. A salt of hydrobromic acid (HBr). Bromides depress the *central nervous system and were once widely used as *sedatives and *tranquillizers. They are now obsolescent.

BROMOCRIPTINE (an *ergot derivative) is a stimulant of *dopamine-sensitive receptors in the brain, and inhibits the release of *prolactin and *growth hormone by the *pituitary gland. It is therefore used in preventing and suppressing *lactation, in treating *galactorrhoea in both men and women, and in *acromegaly. It has also proved helpful in treating cyclical breast and menstrual disorders (e.g. menstrual and premenstrual *migraine). Because of its dopamine-like (agonist) effect, bromocriptine may be used as an alternative to *levodopa in the control of *parkinsonism.

BROMPTON HOSPITAL, named after the district of London in which it is situated, is renowned for its work in diseases of the chest. It began in Chelsea as a Hospital for Consumption (*tuberculosis); a London solicitor (Sir) Philip Rose found that no other London hospital would take patients with the disease. It soon needed to expand, and the foundation stone was laid at Brompton in 1844 by the Prince Consort for a larger hospital than that of the original 20 beds. In 1947 the Institute of Diseases of the Chest was developed as part of the Postgraduate Medical Federation of the University of London. An amalgamation of the Brompton with the London Chest Hospital took place in 1948, and later (1971) these were joined by the National Heart Hospital under a single Board of Governors.

BRONCHIAL (OR BRONCHOGENIC) CARCINOMA. *Carcinoma arising from the epithelium of the bronchial tract (see BRONCHUS); it is the commonest lung cancer.

BRONCHIECTASIS is a condition of chronic and recurrent bronchopulmonary *suppurative infection, associated with permanent abnormal dilatation of part of the bronchial tree.

BRONCHIOLITIS. Inflammation of the bronchioles (see BRONCHUS).

BRONCHITIS is inflammation of the *bronchi, the larger air passages of the lung. The term covers a wide variety of acute and chronic conditions, chronic bronchitis being a major cause of cardiopulmonary disability. See also CHEST MEDICINE.

BRONCHODILATOR. Any agent that dilates the passages of the bronchial tree, particularly one that relieves *bronchospasm.

BRONCHOGRAPHY is the radiographic visualization of the bronchial tree after introduction of *radiopaque contrast material into a bronchus.

BRONCHOPNEUMONIA is a form of *pneumonia, i.e. inflammation of the *parenchyma of the lung, associated with infection and inflammation of the smaller bronchi and bronchioles. The condition, often a secondary occurrence in the course of some other disease, tends to be patchy and multifocal within the lung.

BRONCHOSCOPY is endoscopic examination (see ENDOSCOPY) of the tracheobronchial tree.

BRONCHOSPASM is tonic contraction of the smooth muscle in the bronchial walls, causing increased respiratory resistance, particularly to expiration. See ASTHMA.

BRONCHUS. Any of the larger air-passages of the lungs, which begin at the bifurcation of the *trachea (or windpipe) into left and right main bronchi, and further subdivide into smaller passages to supply the various pulmonary segments. The bronchi are lined with mucous membrane; their walls consist of cartilage, smooth muscle, and fibrous tissue. The smallest air tubes, which complete the connection to the air sacs or *alveoli, are termed bronchioles and unlike the bronchi proper, have no cartilage in their walls.

BRONK, DETLEV WULF (1897–1975). American physiologist. He carried out noteworthy studies on action currents in *nerve fibres. He was president of *Johns Hopkins University (1949–53), of the US *National Academy of Sciences (1950–62), and later of Rockefeller University. He exerted great influence on developments in American science.

BRONZED DIABETES. See HAEMOCHROMATOSIS.

BROUSSAIS, FRANCOIS JOSEPH VICTOR (1772–1838). French physician. He condemned all the old medical theories. He believed that all disease was based on *gastroenteritis and that all vital functions depended upon inflammation or irritation: if inflammation was moderate, health resulted; if feeble, debility; if excessive, disease. He prescribed *leeches in huge numbers, up to 100 per patient, to allay the inflammation.

BROWN, JOHN (1735–88). British physician. In *Elementa medicinae* (1780) he described the 'Brunonian system', holding that all tissues were 'excitable' and that life was the result of stimuli acting upon them. Disease, he maintained, could be constitutional or local and due either to excessive (sthenic) or insufficient (asthenic) stimulation. The treatment was to prescribe opium for the first and alcohol for the second. His doctrine aroused great interest on the Continent, but little in his own country.

BROWN, JOHN (1810–82). British physician and essayist. He was noted particularly for his *Horae subsectivae* (3 vols, 1858–82) and *Rab and his friends* (1859).

BROWNE, SIR THOMAS (1605–82). British physician and author. Practising first in Oxford and later near Halifax, he settled in Norwich in 1636. He was greatly honoured and respected in his lifetime as a saintly and profound scholar. His *Religio medici*, distinguished for its elegance and its profundity, is one of the greatest of medical classics. Two surreptitious and anonymous editions appeared before the authorized, also anonymous, edition (1643); it was placed on the *Index expurgatorius* by the Vatican. Browne also wrote *Pseudodoxia epidemica* (1648) and *Hydrotaphia and the Garden of Cyrus* (1658); *A letter to a friend* (1690) and *Christian morals* (1716) were published posthumously.

BROWN FAT is a special form of pigmented *adipose tissue capable of rapid liberation of energy; it is prominent in the newborn of many species, including man, and in hibernating mammals. It appears to be important in the maintenance of body temperature immediately after birth and on waking from hibernation.

BROWNLEE, JOHN (1868–1927). British epidemiologist. Appointed first director of the statistical department of the *Medical Research Council in 1914, he made important contributions to the epidemiology of *tuberculosis and *measles.

BROWN-SEQUARD, CHARLES EDOUARD (1817–94). Mauritian physician. Trained in Paris, he roamed the world, practising at different times in Philadelphia, New York, Virginia, London, Boston, and Paris. A single-minded research worker, he described the results of hemisection of the *spinal cord (Brown-Séquard syndrome, 1849), elucidated the function of the *adrenal glands, and attempted rejuvenation with 'testicular fluid' from guinea-pigs (see SEXUALITY AND MEDICINE).

BRUCE, SIR DAVID (1855–1931). British bacteriologist. He was commissioned in the Army Medical Service in 1883. He was posted to Malta where he identified the cause of Malta fever; the organism is now known as *Brucella melitensis*, the disease as *brucellosis. After being assistant professor of pathology at Netley, he was sent to Africa to investigate the cause of *tsetse fever in cattle. He identified the organism now known as *Trypanosoma brucei* (See TRYPANOSOMIASIS).

BRUCELLOSIS is a generalized infection caused by one of several species of a genus of bacteria called *Brucella* (after Sir David *Bruce), usually acquired by man as a result of contact with animals. In the UK the commonest infection is with *Brucella abortus*, and is also known as undulant or abortus fever; infection is common in cattle, in which it causes abortion, and results in man from contact with cows or their milk. In the USA, *B. suis* (from pigs) is called hog-slaughterer's disease, and other varieties of brucellosis are caused by *B. melitensis* (sheep and goats) and *B. canis* (dogs). Undulant fever is an *influenza-like illness which may be prolonged if not treated. It usually responds to *antibiotics.

BRUISING is patchy blue discoloration of the skin following injury. A bruise, or contusion, is due to extravasation of blood into skin and subcutaneous tissues; as it resolves, the formation of *bile pigments adds a yellowish hue.

BRUIT. A sound or murmur heard on *auscultation over the heart, peripheral blood vessels, or highly vascularized organ (such as the thyroid gland in *thyrotoxicosis), due to blood turbulence.

BRUNSCHWIG, HIERONYMUS, (otherwise Brunswyck or Braunschweig) (?1450–?1533). Alsatian surgeon. He published one of the first books on the treatment of wounds, *Buch der Wund-artsney* (1497), as well as a handbook of pharmacy, *Liber de arte distillandi* (1500).

BRUNTON, SIR THOMAS LAUDER, Bt (1844–1916). British physician. He was the first clinical pharmacologist and pioneered a scientific approach to treatment. He showed the value of *amyl nitrite in *angina when still a house physician (1867). His most important publication was *Textbook of pharmacology and therapeutics* (1885).

BSE. See BOVINE SPONGIFORM ENCEPHALOPATHY.

BUBO. A swelling in the groin or armpits due to enlarged *lymph nodes. See PLAGUE.

BUDD, WILLIAM (1811–80). British physician and epidemiologist. He worked out the method of spread of *typhoid fever by studies in his own practice, and in 1866 showed that the *cholera epidemic in Bristol could be controlled by hygienic measures.

BUG is a term broadly applied to any species of *insect belonging to the Hemiptera, of which there are more than 1600 British species and 50 000 world-wide. They are characterized by the adaptation of the mouth parts to sucking, usually the sap of plants but in a few cases blood. Those of medical importance include *Cimex lectularius*, *Cimex hemipterus*, and the reduviid bugs which transmit American *trypanosomiasis.

BULBAR PARALYSIS is any form of paralysis affecting the muscles of the lips, tongue, mouth, pharynx, and larynx, usually due to pathological changes affecting the motor nerve nuclei in the *medulla oblongata of the *brainstem, but sometimes due to disease involving the relevant motor cranial nerves or muscles. See also MOTOR NEURONE DISEASE; NEUROMUSCULAR DISEASE; POLIOMYELITIS.

BULIMIA. Persistent and severe increase in appetite with increased hunger. Bulimia nervosa is part of the syndrome of *anorexia nervosa, referring to those patients (about one-third) in whom fasting is periodically interrupted by 'binge' eating followed by self-induced vomiting.

BULLA. A large vesicle or *blister.

BUNDLE OF HIS. Part of the specialized conducting system of the *myocardium, also known as the atrioventricular bundle. It orginates in the *atrioventricular node and then runs in the interatrial septum down to the interventricular septum, where it divides into right and left bundle branches. It conducts the cardiac excitation impulse, distributing it via the two branches to the subendocardial *Purkinje network of both ventricles.

BUNION. An enlarged and deformed knuckle joint of the great toe (first metatarsophalangeal joint) with overlying bursitis (see BURSA).

BURKE, WILLIAM (1792–1829). Irish labourer and murderer. He murdered inmates of William Hare's lodging house in Edinburgh to provide subjects for Robert *Knox's anatomy classes. He was hanged in Edinburgh in 1829. His accomplice *Hare turned King's evidence and was freed in the same year (see also ANATOMY).

BURKITT'S LYMPHOMA is an undifferentiated malignant B-lymphocytic *lymphoma found in children in Africa and New Guinea, where its geographical distribution follows closely that of *malaria. A viral aetiology is probable and the *Epstein–Barr virus (similar to, or identical with, that thought to cause *glandular fever) has been isolated from many cases. It occurs almost exclusively in children, and most frequently presents as a tumour of the jaw or as an abdominal mass. The response to cytotoxic drugs such as *methotrexate or *cyclophosphamide can be dramatic; relapses, however, are common.

BURNET, SIR FRANK MACFARLANE (1899–1985). Australian immunologist and experimental virologist. He was awarded the Nobel prize in physiology and medicine in 1960 for elaboration of the clonal selection theory of *antibody formation. He was director, of the Walter and Eliza Hall Institute, 1944–65, president of the Australian Academy of Science, 1965–69.

BURNS are lesions of the skin and mucous membranes caused by injury from heat, other forms of radiation, and corrosive fluids. Burns are graded into three degrees of severity: first-degree burns are those showing redness or *erythema only; second-degree burns also show *vesicles or blisters; and in third-degree burns the whole thickness of the skin is destroyed.

BURSA. A bursa is a closed synovial sac located at an anatomical site of friction, i.e. between skin, tendons, bones, and muscles. A bursa may become inflamed through trauma or infection (bursitis). Bursitis also occurs in diseases involving joint synovial membranes, such as *gout and *rheumatoid arthritis.

BURSITIS. See BURSA.

BURULI ULCER. Granulomatous ulceration on the leg or forearm due to a *mycobacterium (*Mycobacterium ulcerans*), often requiring surgical excision and skin grafting. Buruli ulcer occurs in Australia, New Guinea, and the Nile district of Uganda (whence it derives its name). The epidemiology is unknown, but it is possibly associated with flooding of rivers.

BUTAZOLIDINE® is a proprietary name for *phenylbutazone.

BYPASS. An additional or alternative channel which diverts fluid (blood, intestinal contents, etc.) around an obstruction or away from a particular area, short-circuiting it. It is usually a temporary (e.g. cardiopulmonary bypass) or permanent surgical expedient (e.g. femoropopliteal bypass, coronary bypass, jejunoileal bypass, etc.).

CABOT, RICHARD CLARKE (1868–1939). American physician and sociologist. He discovered 'ring bodies' in the *erythrocytes of some patients with *anaemia. He inaugurated the *clinicopathological conference as a teaching exercise at the Massachusetts General Hospital. He became increasingly concerned with ethical and social aspects of medical practice, and introduced the first social service department in an American hospital.

CACHEXIA. Extreme wasting of the body; emaciation.

CADAVER. A dead body.

CADMIUM. A soft, silvery-white, metallic element (symbol Cd, atomic number 48, relative atomic mass 112.40) which, in nature, occurs together with zinc. Cadmium has widespread industrial uses, for example in electroplating, in manufacturing fusible alloys, control rods for nuclear reactors, storage batteries, red and yellow pigments, etc. Chronic occupational exposure to the metal or its salts in aerosol or dust form damages several body systems, notably the lungs (in which emphysema has been shown to occur), the olfactory nerve (anosmia), and the kidneys (albuminuria, glycosuria, aminoaciduria). Acute exposure to cadmium fumes is highly irritant to the lungs, causing dyspnoea, bronchospasm, haemoptysis, and, in severe cases, pulmonary oedema. Oral ingestion causes acute gastroenteritis. Unlike zinc, it has no known physiological role.

CADUCEUS. The wand carried by an ancient Greek or Roman herald, in particular the fabled wand carried by Hermes (or Mercury) as the messenger of the gods; the latter is usually represented with two serpents twined round it. Because Hermes could induce sleep with it, it was called by Milton 'his opiate rod' (*Paradise Lost*, xi, 133). The use of a white caduceus by Roman officers when they went to treat for peace led to its being regarded as a symbol both of office and of eloquence. It was later adopted as a symbol of medicine by many organizations.

CAECOSTOMY (CECOSTOMY). A surgically created artificial opening connecting the *caecum to the abdominal surface.

CAECUM (CECUM). The first part of the large *intestine, situated in the right lower quadrant of the *abdomen, which forms a pouch-like cavity connecting the terminal *ileum to the ascending *colon and the vermiform *appendix.

CAESAREAN (CESAREAN) SECTION is the delivery of a fetus by transabdominal and transuterine surgical incision. Roman law enforced this procedure in the event of a mother's death. See also OBSTETRICS.

CAFFEINE is a weak *central nervous system *stimulant consumed almost universally in *tea, *coffee, and most 'cola' drinks. It is also an ingredient of many proprietary *analgesic preparations. Although often under suspicion, ill-effects from the long-term consumption of caffeine have not been clearly established.

CAIRNS, SIR HUGH WILLIAM BELL (1896–1952). British neurosurgeon, born in Australia. He studied medicine at Adelaide, and was a Rhodes scholar at Oxford, before becoming a house surgeon at the London hospital. In 1926–27 he was awarded a Rockefeller travelling fellowship to study neurosurgery in Boston with Harvey *Cushing. He returned to the UK and by 1932 had established a neurosurgical unit at the London. Five years later, he went back to Oxford as professor of surgery. With the advent of war in 1939, Cairns devoted himself to providing a neurosurgical service for the army. He made important contributions to the treatment of military head injuries (see NEUROSURGERY), organizing a special hospital which occupied St Hugh's College in 1940–45. His work also involved the creation of mobile army surgical units, the provision of crash helmets for army motor-cyclists, and the early field trials of penicillin.

CAISSON DISEASE is a synonym for *decompression sickness; a caisson is a chamber in which compressed-air work is carried out.

CAIUS, JOHN (1510–73). British physician. He practised briefly in Cambridge, Norwich, and Shrewsbury, recording his experiences in *A boke or counsell against the disease commonly called the sweate or sweating sickness* (1552). In 1552 he moved to London and was elected president of the Royal College of Physicians for the years 1555–60, 1562, 1563, and 1571. He presented the president's insignia to the College and strenuously upheld its rights to prevent surgeons from prescribing drugs. At the command of Henry VIII he was the first to teach anatomy publicly at the Barber-Surgeons' Hall. Caius was the most learned classicist of his generation in Europe. In 1557 Philip of Spain and Queen Mary granted Caius letters patent to refound Gonville Hall at Cambridge as Gonville and Caius College. He was a munificent benefactor of this foundation and Master from 1558 to 1573.

CALAMINE is a topical skin preparation consisting of *zinc oxide with 0.5 per cent ferric oxide in various bases, used in conditions where the intention is to relieve itching. It is mildly *astringent.

CALAMUS SCRIPTORIUS is an anatomical term for part of the floor of the fourth *cerebral ventricle.

CALCANEUM is the heel-bone, also known as the calcaneus or os calcis. It provides the insertion for the *Achilles tendon.

CALCIFEROL is either of two *vitamin D compounds, ergocalciferol (vitamin D₂) or cholecalciferol (vitamin D₃), used in treating *rickets.

CALCIFICATION. Abnormal deposition of *calcium in organs and tissues is of two general types. The first occurs in any dead or injured tissue because of local biochemical changes favouring the precipitation of calcium salts. In this case, whole-body calcium metabolism is normal.

The second type is metastatic calcification, where the deposits occur in essentially normal tissues. The usual cause is a raised blood calcium level (*hypercalcaemia) due to *hyperparathyroidism, hypervitaminosis D, or bone demineralization caused by extensive *metastatic deposits in the bones (usually deriving from breast carcinoma).

CALCINOSIS is deposition of *calcium salts in various tissues of the body.

CALCITONIN, also called thyrocalcitonin, is a *hormone of vertebrates, secreted in mammals by the parafollicular cells of the *thyroid gland and in other vertebrates by a separate gland developed from gill pouches. It is secreted in response to *hypercalcaemia, and opposes the action of *parathyroid hormone. Thus it inhibits bone resorption, and lowers plasma levels of

*calcium and *phosphate. It is of value in the treatment of *Paget's disease of bone and of hypercalcaemia.

CALCIUM is a metallic element (symbol Ca, atomic number 20, relative atomic mass 40.08) of central physiological importance as a major component of the skeleton, as a factor in the control of blood *coagulation, and in the electrochemical processes involved in cellular *excitation and the functioning of nerves and muscles, including cardiac muscle. Calcium is an essential component of the human diet, the recommended daily allowance being about 1 g. Among the factors influencing calcium metabolism are the *parathyroids, *calcitonin secretion by the *thyroid gland, and dietary intake of *vitamin D (see OSTEOMALACIA; RICKETS).

CALCIUM ANTAGONISTS. A group of drugs, more properly called calcium-channel blockers, which have a variety of important actions on the cardiovascular system. The three principal agents are chemically unrelated: they are verapamil (introduced in 1967), nifedipine (1977), and diltiazem (1984). Their common action is to inhibit the influx of calcium (induced by *depolarization) into myocardial and smooth muscle cells through specialized 'slow' channels in the cell membrane. Their haemodynamic effects include depression of cardiac contraction, peripheral vasodilatation, and augmentation both of normal myocardial perfusion and of that through narrowed coronary arteries. They are of established value in the treatment of *angina pectoris, of *hypertension and of various cardiac arrhythmias, but should not be used in cardiac failure or in combination with beta-blockers.

CALCULUS. Any abnormal concretion or stone formed within a hollow organ or tract by precipitation from fluids and secretions. Common sites of calculus formation are the biliary tract (see GALLSTONE), the urinary tract, and the *salivary glands.

CALF LYMPH is the material formerly used to induce infection with *vaccinia, for prophylactic *immunization against *smallpox.

CALLIPERS, or 'calipers', are instruments used to measure thickness or calibre, resembling compasses (e.g. to measure skinfold thickness in the assessment of obesity). In the singular, 'caliper' denotes a metal splint for supporting a diseased or fractured leg, which by taking the weight off the foot helps the patient to walk.

CALLUS is the hard bony tissue formed at the site of a *fracture during the process of healing, the precursor of new bone.

CALMETTE, LEON CHARLES ALBERT (1863–1933). French microbiologist. In 1917 he was appointed assistant director of the Paris *Pasteur Institute, succeeding *Metchnikoff. Here he developed with *Guérin the protective vaccine against *tuberculosis (*Bacille Calmette–Guérin (BCG)) which was first used for inoculating children in 1924.

CALOMEL is mercurous chloride (Hg_2Cl_2), formerly used as a *purgative, in teething powders, and in treating *syphilis, but now discarded as it shares the toxicity of most *mercury compounds. See also PINK DISEASE.

CALORIE REQUIREMENTS IN HEALTH. Since the introduction of the Système International d'Unites (*SI units), the familiar 'calorie', or more accurately 'kilocalorie' (kcal), has been officially replaced by the 'megajoule' (MJ) and *energy values are so expressed here, with the old units in parentheses, thus: 1 MJ (239 kcal).

Energy is required to maintain body *metabolism, for physical activity, and in children and pregnant women for growth; energy needs vary according to these factors. They also vary between individuals (because of differing metabolic 'efficiency'); and, except during pregnancy and lactation, requirements are generally lower in women. A full statement of normal requirements therefore involves specification of body weight, age, sex, and level of activity (there is a five- or six-fold variation between sleep and heavy work). Average daily values for moderately active men and women of average weight (65 kg and 55 kg, respectively) are:

men	12.6 MJ (3000 kcal)
women	9.2 MJ (2200 kcal)

For the second half of pregnancy, add 1.5 MJ (350 kcal) and for lactation, 2.3 MJ (550 kcal). Over 50 years of age subtract 10 per cent; over 70, 30 per cent. Normal ranges are about ±10 per cent of these values.

CALORIMETER. Any instrument that measures heat transfer, that is *energy production or consumption. In indirect calorimetry energy consumption is calculated from respiratory gas exchange.

CALVARIUM. The vault of the *skull.

CALYX. Any cup-shaped structure.

CAMPHOR is a white crystalline organic solid (formula $C_{10}H_{16}O$) with a characteristic odour, derived from the wood of the camphor tree (*Cinnamomum camphora*); it has some industrial uses. In medicine it found a place as a mild antipruritic in topical preparations, and as an ingredient of camphorated tinctures and oils.

CAMPION, THOMAS (?1567–1620). British physician, barrister, poet, and musician. He practised in London, but largely occupied his time in writing masques, songs, and music, in all of which he became a recognized authority.

CANADA, THE ROYAL COLLEGE OF PHYSICIANS AND SURGEONS OF. See ROYAL COLLEGE OF PHYSICIANS AND SURGEONS OF CANADA.

CANADA BALSAM is an oleoresin and obtained from the balsam fir *Abies balsamea* and used as a mounting medium for histological preparations.

CANCER is any malignant neoplasm, i.e. an uncontrolled new growth of cells exhibiting invasiveness and remote spread (metastasis). See ONCOLOGY.

CANCEROPHOBIA is a morbid fear of *cancer, and/or an unwarranted belief by the patient that he or she is suffering from cancer.

CANCER RESEARCH CAMPAIGN. A non-governmental charitable organization for the support of cancer research in the UK, founded in 1923. The Cancer Research Campaign (CRC) is wholly dependent on gifts, donations, bequests, and other voluntary sources for its income. It is estimated that it funds over one-third of cancer-related research in the UK in several hundred projects through grants to universities, medical schools, hospitals, and research institutes. In terms of income and expenditure, the CRC is the largest British charity concerned with medical research. Its aims are 'to attack and defeat the disease of cancer in all its forms, and to promote its cure, by research into its causes, distribution, symptoms, pathology and treatment'. See also FOUNDATIONS, ETC. IN THE UK.

CANDIDA is a genus of fungi found normally on skin and mucous membranes; occasionally it causes superficial infections (candidiasis or moniliasis) particularly of warm, moist areas. *Thrush of the mouth or vagina is an example. Systemic candidiasis occurs only as an opportunistic infection, i.e. one that develops when there is a pre-existing deficiency of the body's *immune system.

CANNABIS is a general term for products of the hemp plants *Cannabis indica* and *Cannabis sativa* which contain the active principle tetrahydrocannabinol and compounds closely related to it. Synonyms include: marijuana, hashish, bhang, ganja, pot, etc. See SUBSTANCE ABUSE.

CANNIBALISM is the consumption of the flesh of one's own species. In Papua New Guinea it was the means of transmission of the slow virus-like agent of *kuru.

CANNON, WALTER BRADFORD (1871–1945). American physiologist. He carried out early studies of the upper gastrointestinal tract in animals and man using *fluoroscopy with bismuth suspensions as contrast medium. He studied the phenomena of *shock, and popularized the concept of the action of *adrenaline in stress reactions—'fight or flight'.

CANNULA. A tube or stout hollow needle, usually employed with a *trocar, used for insertion into a blood vessel or body cavity; after insertion, the trocar is withdrawn to allow flow of fluid through the cannula.

CANTHARIDES is made from the dried Spanish fly (*Lytta vesicatoria*). Its active principle is a powerfully irritant substance called cantharidin. It was once used on the skin as a blistering agent (vesicant). Its irritant action on the genitourinary tract when taken internally explains its traditional use as an *aphrodisiac. It is highly toxic.

CAPGRAS SYNDROME is a mental disturbance, described in 1923 by the French psychiatrist Jean Marie Joseph Capgras (1873–1950), in which the patient misidentifies a familiar person (e.g. spouse) as an impostor and persists in this delusional belief despite recognition of features, clothes, etc. It is sometimes termed the 'illusion of false recognition', and is an uncommon result of paranoid *schizophrenia, although it has also been observed in organic disorders and *affective psychoses.

CAPILLARY. The smallest vessel of the blood circulatory system. Capillaries are fine hair-like channels forming a vast network throughout the tissues of the body, connecting the arterial and the venous sides of the circulation. Their walls act as semipermeable membranes, allowing free exchange of respiratory gases, fluids, nutrients, waste products, etc. between the blood and tissue spaces, but normally retaining the blood cells and larger molecules, such as those of *proteins.

CAPSULE. Any fibrous and/or membranous covering enclosing an anatomical structure; also, a small soluble container of a single dose of a medicinal substance intended to be swallowed.

CARBACHOL is a synthetic drug with actions similar to, but more prolonged than, those of *acetylcholine. It is therefore used when 'cholinergic' or 'parasympathomimetic' effects are required. See PARASYMPATHETIC NERVOUS SYSTEM.

CARBIMAZOLE is a drug that blocks the synthesis of *thyroid hormone, widely used in the treatment of hyperthyroidism (*thyrotoxicosis).

CARBOHYDRATE. Any of a large group of organic compounds made up exclusively of carbon, *hydrogen, and *oxygen and having the general formula $C_x(H_2O)_y$. They include the simpler *sugars (monosaccharides and disaccharides) and more complex *polysaccharides such as *starch, *cellulose, and *glycogen. They play a central role in the *metabolism of all living organisms; starch is the principal form of energy storage in plants, and glycogen in animals. They provide the major energy component of human food. Their ultimate metabolic fate is combustion to *carbon dioxide and water with release of energy (17.2 kilojoules or 4.1 kilocalories per gram of carbohydrate).

CARBOLIC ACID. See PHENOL.

CARBON DIOXIDE (CO_2), once called carbonic acid gas, is normally present in the atmosphere in a concentration of about 0.03 per cent; it is colourless, odourless, and tasteless. It provides carbon for plant *photosynthesis and is the end product of *respiration in animals. It plays a central role in many physiological processes, such as the control of breathing and maintenance of the *acid–base equilibrium.

CARBONIC ANHYDRASE. An *enzyme that catalyses the formation and dissociation of carbonic acid from and into *carbon dioxide and water. Carbonic anhydrase, which contains *zinc, is notably present in *erythrocytes and in the cells lining the *renal tubules. See also ACETAZOLAMIDE.

CARBON MONOXIDE (CO) is a colourless and almost odourless, highly poisonous gas produced by incomplete combustion of carbonaceous fuels; it is present in exhaust fumes, coal gas, and many types of smoke. It has a high affinity for *haemoglobin, with which it combines irreversibly to form the bright red compound, carboxyhaemoglobin. The resultant displacement of oxygen causes death from *asphyxia, without the *cyanosis seen in other forms of tissue *hypoxia.

CARBON TETRACHLORIDE (CCl_4) is a heavy, colourless, volatile liquid employed as an industrial solvent and for some other non-medical purposes, e.g. in fire extinguishers, as a pesticide against wasps, etc. Because of its toxicity, it is no longer used in dry-cleaning. It was formerly used in medicine as an *anthelminthic. It is highly toxic, particularly to the liver, kidneys, and central nervous system.

CARBOXYHAEMOGLOBIN. See CARBON MONOXIDE.

CARBUNCLE. An aggregation of connecting furuncles or *boils.

CARCINOGEN. Any agent that causes *cancer.

CARCINOGENESIS. The process of *cancer induction.

CARCINOID SYNDROME. See ARGENTAFFINOMA.

CARCINOMA. A malignant *neoplasm (new growth) arising from epithelial cells, which spreads by invading neighbouring structures and tissues and which may give rise to satellite growths (*metastases) at a distance, groups of malignant cells having been conveyed there in body fluids.

CARDANO, GIROLAMO (1501–76). Italian Renaissance polymath. Cardano's many written works embrace medicine, mathematics, physics, philosophy, religion, music, geology, and the theory of games, but his fame now rests chiefly on his contributions to mathematics, especially algebra (e.g. 'Cardano's rule' for the solution of third-degree equations), although for many years he was also a successful practising physician.

CARDIAC describes anything pertaining to the *heart or the upper portion of the *stomach.

CARDIAC ARREST is sudden cessation of the heartbeat, due either to ventricular *fibrillation or ventricular standstill (*asystole). Consciousness is lost several seconds after the circulation is halted, and irreversible brain damage can occur in as little as 3 minutes. If an effective circulation is reinstated within this time, and can be maintained, complete recovery is possible. See RESUSCITATION.

CARDIAC ASTHMA is paroxysmal breathing difficulty due to episodic failure of the left side of the heart, with consequent congestion and oedema of the lungs. Paroxysmal nocturnal *dyspnoea, related to lying down and characteristic of left-sided heart lesions, such as *aortic incompetence and arterial *hypertension, is an example. See also ORTHOPNOEA.

CARDIAC CATHETERIZATION. The introduction of a radiopaque *catheter into a peripheral vein (or artery when the left side of the heart is catheterized) followed by its advancement under fluoroscopic control until the tip lies in a chamber of the heart. Although the manoeuvre was first performed in 1929, the technique has been fully exploited only during the past 30 years. It is now a routine and invaluable adjunct in the diagnosis of heart disease and haemodynamic studies. See CARDIOLOGY; FORSSMAN.

CARDIAC GLYCOSIDES are a group of glycosides (naturally occurring compounds of a sugar and a hydroxy-substance) found in certain plants (notably *Digitalis* and *Strophanthus*). They have important and specific effects on the heart; they increase the force of systolic contraction and the mechanical efficiency of the failing *myocardium; they inhibit atrioventricular conduction; and they enhance the inherent 'automaticity' of cardiac tissue. These actions are valuable in treating heart failure and managing certain *arrhythmias.

See also CARDIOLOGY; DIGITALIS; PHARMACOLOGY; HERBAL REMEDIES.

CARDIAC MURMUR. Cardiac murmurs are adventitious noises generated by the heart's action, recurring with each beat, and heard by *auscultation over the precordium. They are of varying intensity, duration, pitch, and quality; occasionally, they may be loud enough to be heard without a *stethoscope. Murmurs result from disturbances of normal flow pattern (turbulence) within the cavities of the heart and great vessels. Cardiac murmurs are broadly classified according to their timing into systolic and diastolic, respectively, accompanying the contraction and relaxation phases of the cardiac cycle. Diastolic murmurs almost invariably indicate organic heart disease; systolic murmurs may or may not do so.

CARDIAC OUTPUT is the minute volume of the heart, that is the amount of blood pumped by the heart in a minute. It is equal to the product of the *stroke volume and the heart rate.

CARDIAC SURGEON. See CARDIOTHORACIC SURGERY.

CARDIAC TAMPONADE is compression of the heart, interfering with effective cardiac function, due to the accumulation of fluid under pressure within the surrounding pericardial sac. Tamponade is not solely dependent on the volume of the *effusion, being most likely when fluid accumulates rapidly (e.g. bleeding into the *pericardium following cardiac rupture) or within a pericardial sac rendered unduly rigid by previous *inflammation and *fibrosis. Cardiac action may remain unhampered by even massive effusions when these form gradually, as the pericardium is normally distensible.

CARDIOGRAM, when otherwise unqualified, is synonymous with electrocardiogram or ECG. See ELECTROCARDIOGRAPHY.

CARDIOLOGIST. A physician specializing in diseases of the heart.

CARDIOLOGY
Congenital heart disease
About 8 in 1000 babies are born with a congenital heart abnormality. In some cases, it is associated with such other severe abnormalities that life is unsustainable. In many others it is trivial or self-correcting. However, some 4000 babies born each year in the UK have abnormalities that require surgical treatment. Most cases are unexplained; a small proportion are due to gene defects, such as *Down's syndrome, or to drugs such as *thalidomide or *warfarin. Children of parents with congenital heart disease have a 1–2 per cent risk of inheriting such an anomaly. There are many types, which are not all easy to classify but which broadly fall into one of three categories: abnormal communications;

obstructive *lesions; and the displacement or absence of chambers, vessels, or *valves.

Abnormal communications

These include atrial and ventricular *septal defects ('holes in the heart') and persistence of the *ductus arteriosus (joining the *aorta to the pulmonary artery). In each of these conditions, there is usually a large shunt of blood from the left side of the circulation to the right. In most cases, this is well tolerated until adolescence or early adult life, but then heart failure ensues. Infective *endocarditis is an important complication of ventricular septal defect and persistent ductus, but is rare in atrial defects. Surgical correction in early childhood is appropriate for most of these anomalies, but small ventricular septal defects may close spontaneously. Surgery is unsuccessful if the defects are associated with severe pulmonary hypertension.

Obstructive lesions

These include *coarctation of the aorta, *pulmonary stenosis, and *aortic *stenosis. Coarctation is associated with upper limb *hypertension and may be complicated by rupture of the aorta or of an intracranial *aneurysm, leading to *subarachnoid haemorrhage. The hypertension may lead to cardiac failure. The coarctation should be resected in childhood. Congenital pulmonary stenosis is often mild and then requires no treatment; more severe cases lead to right heart failure and are best treated at an early age by balloon dilatation or surgery. Congenital aortic stenosis can present in infancy but is much more commonly discovered incidentally during physical examination during childhood. As with other forms of aortic stenosis, *angina, *syncope, and *heart failure may eventually develop, or sudden death may supervene. It is treated by surgical or balloon valvotomy or by valve replacement.

Another rare but important obstructive lesion is the hypoplastic left heart syndrome. This may involve mitral or aortic *atresia and usually causes death within days of birth.

Combined obstructive lesions and abnormal communications

The commonest of these is *Fallot's tetralogy—the combination of pulmonary stenosis, ventricular septal defect, dextroposition of the aorta, and right ventricular hypertrophy. It is the most frequent cause of *cyanosis in children over the age of 3 years; without surgery it leads to death within the first few years of life in most cases. It is now usually corrected by resection of the stenosis and closure of the septal defect.

Displacement lesions

The most important of these is transposition of the great arteries, in which the aorta arises from the right ventricle and the pulmonary artery from the left. Life cannot be sustained unless there is a communication, such as a patent *foramen ovale or a septal defect, between the two circulations. A variety of procedures have been devised to reroute the circulation, but where possible it is best to carry out a 'switch' operation, the surgeon detaching the aorta and pulmonary artery from their origins, and connecting them each to the appropriate ventricle.

Coronary heart disease

Coronary heart disease is the commonest cause of death in both men and women in the Western World. In 1991, 171 179 (26 per cent) of the 646 181 deaths in the UK were attributed to coronary heart disease. Under the age of 65, it is predominantly a male disease, with 21 000 men dying of this cause in 1991 compared with 6300 women. However, it is a common disorder of elderly women in whom it causes a substantial degree of disability due to angina and heart failure. There have been remarkable changes in the numbers of deaths attributed to coronary disease in different countries in the past 50 years. In the USA there was a rapid increase in coronary deaths over a period from the 1930s to the 1960s; since then the death rates have virtually halved. Similar findings have been reported from Australia and a number of other countries. In the UK the peak was reached in the late seventies, with a substantial fall subsequently, particularly in the younger age groups.

Pathology

The fundamental lesion of atherosclerotic coronary disease is the fibrolipid *plaque. This probably starts as a 'fatty streak' which may progress to the fully developed lesion. This is variably composed of lipid and smooth muscle cells and their products, such as fibrous *protein and complex *carbohydrates. In some plaques, fatty material predominates, with a large pool of *cholesterol and its esters; such fatty plaques may be separated from the *lumen by only a thin fibrous cap, which is prone to rupture. Other plaques are solid and mainly composed of smooth muscle cells and connective tissue. Calcification may be superimposed. Plaques are most often located at the bends and branches of arteries. Plaques may gradually encroach upon the arterial lumen, becoming haemodynamically important when the lumen diameter is reduced to less than 50 per cent. The fibrous cap is prone to rupture; exposure of the contents of the plaque to the blood triggers *platelet adhesion and *fibrin deposition. If the lumen is occluded by clot, a myocardial infarction will ensue. If the lesion is less severe, the artery may not occlude, but the process may lead to further narrowing.

The aetiology and prevention of atherosclerotic coronary disease

The ultimate causes of coronary disease remain uncertain, but epidemiological studies have identified a number of risk factors. Most important of these are cigarette *smoking, hyperlipidaemia, and hypertension.

Other associations are a family history of coronary disease at a relatively young age, high fibrinogen levels, physical inactivity, *diabetes, insulin resistance, and obesity. It seems logical to correct these risk factors, where possible, but proof of the benefit of doing so has yet to be established. Strong circumstantial evidence supports the view that stopping smoking reduces the risk progressively over the succeeding years.

Trials in which the cholesterol level has been lowered either by drugs or by diet have shown a diminution in the number of cardiac events such as myocardial infarction and cardiac death, but have not shown a reduction in total death. This is probably because the trials have not been large enough to show such an effect, or because they have produced only slight falls in the cholesterol, but the possibility also exists that lowering cholesterol may have adverse effects. Trials of antihypertensive drugs have produced minor reductions in cardiac events.

Angina pectoris

The syndrome of angina pectoris was first described by William *Heberden in 1768, and his description has not been bettered:

There is a disorder of the breast marked with strong and peculiar symptoms, considerable for the kind of danger belonging to it, and not extremely rare which deserves to be mentioned more at length. The seat of it, and the sense of strangling, and anxiety with which it is attended, may make it not improperly called angina pectoris.

They who are afflicted by it, are seized while they are walking (more especially if it be uphill, and soon after eating) with a painful and most disagreeable sensation in the breast, which seems as if it were to extinguish life, if it were to increase or continue; but the moment they stand still, all this uneasiness vanishes . . . The pain is sometimes situated in the upper part, sometimes in the middle and sometimes at the bottom of the os sterni, and often more inclined to the left than to the right side. It likewise very frequently extends from the breast to the middle of the arm.

Heberden recognized the four essential features of angina—its location, character, relationship to exertion, and duration—but he did not associate it with the heart—this was left to *Jenner and Parry a few years later.

Angina is due to myocardial *ischaemia; in the vast majority of cases it results from coronary atherosclerosis, but it may be due to aortic stenosis, *cardiomyopathy, and a number of other disorders, including coronary spasm. *Atheroma is liable to cause angina on exercise when the diameter of a coronary artery is narrowed to less than 50 per cent. The diagnosis may be made with confidence on history alone if all the four main characteristics are present; when the symptoms are less typical, further diagnostic methods are needed. The resting *electrocardiogram (ECG) is often normal; it is important to recognize that a normal ECG does not negate the diagnosis. Most patients with angina will have ST depression on an exercise test, particularly if they are exercised until they develop pain. Nuclear imaging with thallium will usually demonstrate that there is a transient defect in perfusion of the myocardium during an episode of angina. *Coronary angiography is seldom required for diagnosis but is essential for delineating the location and severity of coronary stenoses if angioplasty or coronary bypass surgery is contemplated (see also CARDIOTHORACIC SURGERY).

The symptoms of angina can usually be prevented or treated effectively by one or more of the three classes of drug available for this purpose: nitrates, *beta-blockers, and *calcium antagonists. Nitrates were introduced by Lauder Brunton more than a century ago but retain their place in management. Sublingual glyceryl trinitrate is standard therapy for an attack, but it is particularly effective if given prophylactically when an attack is anticipated. Long-acting nitrates, such as isosorbide dinitrate, or mononitrate, are also of value, but are often reserved for patients who do not respond to beta-blockers alone. For many physicians, beta-blockers are the mainstay of anginal prevention, partly because of their effectiveness, but also because it is believed that they reduce the risk of myocardial infarction and death. Disadvantages are the side-effects, including tiredness, lethargy, and cold extremities. Calcium antagonists are also effective in preventing angina. Some—the dihydropyridines such as nifedipine—are general vasodilators which cause a *tachycardia. They are often best combined with a beta-blocker. Others, such as verapamil and diltiazem, tend to slow the heart and are better not administered with a beta-blocker, but combine well with nitrates.

If drugs fail to control symptoms, alternative strategies of treatment include percutaneous transluminal coronary angioplasty (PTCA) and coronary artery bypass graft (CABG) surgery. In angioplasty, an inelastic balloon is mounted close to the tip of a specially designed cardiac catheter. The catheter is guided into the affected artery and the balloon inflated at the site of the stenosis or stenoses. In most cases this technique is effective in reducing the degree of stenosis and in relieving angina. Initially, when introduced by Gruntzig in 1977, angioplasty was applied only to a proximal stenosis in a single artery, but with increasing experience and better apparatus, more distal stenoses and several arteries may be treated. The technique may seriously damage the artery, causing dissection or occlusion, and lead to a myocardial infarction. Because of these risks, which occur in 1–5 per cent of patients, it is customary to arrange for immediate coronary surgery if these complications occur. Coronary angioplasty is immediately effective in some 80–90 per cent of patients identified as being suitable for the procedure, but in some 25 per cent of these, restenosis occurs within the next 6 months. Symptoms do not necessarily recur, in spite of this, but if they do, a repeat angioplasty is often successful. Additional procedures, such as laser angioplasty, stenting, and atherectomy are still experimental and have not, as yet, been shown to be superior to angioplasty, except in some isolated cases.

Coronary bypass graft surgery (see also CARDIO-THORACIC SURGERY) has proved extremely successful in relieving the symptoms of angina in a high proportion of patients. As originally practised, a saphenous vein is removed from the leg and used to bypass narrowed segments of arteries. Grafts may be inserted into any or all of the major coronary arteries or their larger branches. Some grafts occlude shortly after surgery, but most remain open for at least 5–10 years; after this they may be gradually narrowed by atherosclerosis. For this reason, there is an increasing tendency to graft one or both internal mammary arteries as an alternative, as they do not seem as prone to late closure. The mortality of coronary bypass surgery in the good risk patient is about 1–3 per cent but it may be substantially higher if the left ventricle has been seriously damaged by previous infarction. Surgery abolishes symptoms in at least 50 per cent of patients, and greatly relieves it in 30–40 per cent more. It also reduces the risk of death in high risk patients, such as those with stenosis of the left main coronary artery or if three-vessel disease is accompanied by severe ischaemia.

Unstable angina

Angina is said to be unstable if it has recently developed for the first time or when pre-existing angina worsens for no apparent reason. It is believed that unstable angina is usually the result of plaque rupture upon which platelet thrombus becomes superimposed. Its importance lies in the high risk (about 20 per cent) of progressing to myocardial infarction over a period of days or weeks. Clinical trials have shown that it is best treated by a combination of drugs. These include both *aspirin and *heparin to prevent further thrombosis, and an intensive anti-ischaemic regimen. It is customary to use nitrates (intravenously if symptoms continue) together with beta-blockers and calcium antagonists. If medical treatment fails to control symptoms, early recourse is made to angioplasty or surgery.

Vasospastic (Prinzmetal's or variant) angina

Prinzmetal described a form of angina in which episodes of severe angina develop apparently spontaneously; during the attacks the ST segment of the electrocardiogram is strikingly elevated. Coronary angiography has shown that these attacks are due to intense coronary vasoconstriction (vasospasm). Although it can complicate coronary atherosclerosis, in most cases the angiogram is normal between episodes.

Myocardial infarction

Myocardial infarction occurs when there has been occlusion of a coronary artery. This is usually the consequence of plaque rupture, followed by platelet and fibrin thrombosis. The most characteristic clinical feature is intense central chest pain, but other symptoms are common and may predominate, especially in the elderly. These include syncope, *dyspnoea, fatigue, nausea, and vomiting. The pain usually starts abruptly and may last for several hours, but it can be of a stuttering nature, waxing and waning over a similar period. The infarction is often preceded by episodes of unstable angina.

The greatest risk obtains during the first hours after the event, with ventricular fibrillation being the most frequent cause of death at this time. For this reason, a high proportion of patients die suddenly outside hospital, often with little or no warning. The risk of death remains high over the first two days, due to *arrhythmias, cardiac rupture, cardiac failure, and shock. Most of these complications relate to the amount of muscle damaged in the infarction.

The mortality in patients who reach hospital used to be in the region of 30 per cent but today when all available measures are undertaken it averages about 10 per cent. It is very dependent upon age, with mortality in the region of 3 per cent in those under 50, and not rising steeply until after the age of 70. The diagnosis of myocardial infarction is usually suspected on the history, but requires confirmation by ECG and cardiac enzyme tests.

There are three major aspects to the treatment of myocardial infarction, apart from general management: the relief of symptoms, cardiopulmonary resuscitation, and the use of drugs to prevent or reverse thrombosis. General management includes bed rest initially, followed by a gradual increase in activity over the following days. Patients are nowadays usually admitted to a coronary (or cardiac) care unit (CCU) for a day or two, so that they can be closely monitored clinically and electrocardiographically during this critical period. Discharge from hospital for the uncomplicated case is at about the end of one week, at which time the patient is fully ambulant.

Pain relief usually requires the use of opiates, sometimes in large doses. Cardiopulmonary resuscitation (see below) is needed only if cardiac arrest supervenes. Antithrombotic therapy includes thrombolytic drugs, antiplatelet drugs, and *anticoagulants. Large clinical trials have demonstrated that thrombolytic drugs (such as streptokinase) reduce the mortality of in-hospital myocardial infarction by some 25 per cent. These drugs are most effective when given soon after the onset of symptoms, and are largely ineffective once 12 hours has elapsed. They should be avoided in those who are in danger from haemorrhage, such as those who have recently had surgery or a *stroke, who have a *peptic ulcer, or a bleeding diathesis. With these exceptions, thrombolytic therapy is now regarded as routine for those who have recently sustained a myocardial infarction. Streptokinase is the drug most commonly used, but it has the disadvantage that it may produce allergic reactions or *hypotension. Furthermore, because it causes *antibody production, it should not be re-administered during the succeeding year, or even longer. When re-administration is necessary because of reinfarction, an alternative, such as the genetically engineered but much more expensive alteplase, should be used.

Oral aspirin, given soon after the onset of the event, has also been found to reduce mortality in myocardial infarction; thrombolytics and aspirin are additive in their effects. Heparin is also commonly used; it protects against re-occlusion of the affected coronary artery, but increases the risk of haemorrhage.

Other forms of therapy are used selectively. Cardiac failure, especially pulmonary *oedema, is a common complication of myocardial infarction. Immediate treatment is with oxygen, diuretics, and nitrates, which are often given intravenously. Cardiogenic *shock is a much-dreaded complication, which affects perhaps 5 per cent of patients and is associated with a 50–80 per cent mortality. Treatment is largely ineffectual, but oxygen and inotropic drugs, such as dopamine and dobutamine, are employed. Beta-blockers are sometimes used in the acute phase, particularly if there is hypertension or continuing chest pain. Antiarrhythmic drugs may be necessary for ventricular or supraventricular tachycardias.

After the acute event is over, further active management is necessary to improve the rate of return to normality and to prevent recurrent infarction or death, which are common in the succeeding months. *Rehabilitation programmes are beneficial in overcoming the frequent problems of anxiety and depression in the convalescent period; they may also accelerate physical recovery and reduce subsequent mortality. Beta-blockers are now used routinely in post-myocardial infarction patients, unless there are contraindications, or the patient is considered to be at such low risk that their side-effects might outweigh the benefits. Aspirin, which will normally have been introduced in the acute illness, is continued indefinitely. *Angiotensin-converting enzyme (ACE) inhibitors are prescribed if there is cardiac failure, or if it is thought to be imminent.

Valvar heart disease

Rheumatic fever and its sequelae are now uncommon in the UK, and will remain so except in the immigrant population. The once common conditions of *mitral stenosis and regurgitation, and aortic regurgitation, are now relatively rare, but calcific aortic stenosis is an important condition in the elderly, and its prevalence may well increase as the population ages. Surgery for valvar heart disease of all kinds is, for the most part, very effective. Artificial prostheses (mechanical valves) are widely used because of their overall reliability and durability, in spite of the fact that their use requires the administration of anticoagulants. Heterografts and homografts (*allografts) have the advantage that they do not require anticoagulant administration but they often start to deteriorate after about 7 years. Balloon valvoplasty is also proving satisfactory in mitral and pulmonary stenosis, but is of limited value in aortic stenosis.

Cardiomyopathy and specific heart muscle diseases

The cardiomyopathies are disorders of heart muscle that are not due to coronary atherosclerosis, congenital or valvar heart disease, or to hypertension. Some cardiologists limit the term 'cardiomyopathy' to disease which is primarily in the myocardium and of unknown origin, describing those forms of myocardial disease which are secondary to disorders such as connective tissue or neuromuscular diseases as 'specific heart muscle disease.' Cardiomyopathy presents in one of three distinctive clinical forms—dilated, hypertrophic, and restrictive.

Dilated cardiomyopathy

Often, no cause can be found but it is probable that in many cases it is the late result of a viral infection. Other identifiable causes include *AIDS, *alcohol, and anthracyclines. The ventricles contract very poorly and dilate progressively. The clinical picture is one of cardiac failure with dyspnoea and oedema, which may be of abrupt or insidious onset. The diagnosis is largely based on the exclusion of other causes of heart failure, such as coronary disease or *hyperthyroidism. The prognosis is poor in most cases, although if a cause (such as alcoholism) can be identified, the condition may be reversible. Treatment is as for other types of heart failure. Cardiac transplantation is life-saving if the symptoms are severe and life expectancy short.

Hypertrophic cardiomyopathy

In this condition, there is massive hypertrophy of the ventricles, especially the interventricular septum. The non-compliant chambers impair diastolic filling and the septum may obstruct the outflow tract of the left ventricle, giving rise to 'subaortic stenosis'. It is frequently familial; in about half the affected individuals, inheritance is as a single autosomal dominant trait. Symptoms include breathlessness, angina, and syncope, and there is a considerable risk of sudden death due to arrhythmias. The condition may be suspected on physical signs and the ECG, but echocardiography provides the definitive diagnosis. Treatment with drugs is of limited value, as is surgery for resecting part of the septum.

Restrictive and infiltrative cardiomyopathies

These forms of cardiomyopathy are relatively rare. Their main feature is stiffness of the ventricular walls, which leads to impaired diastolic filling. There are a number of causes, including *sarcoid, *amyloid, and the hypereosinophilic syndrome. The clinical picture resembles that of pericardial constriction, from which the differentiation may be difficult. The presence of the relevant diseases elsewhere and examination of the heart by *echocardiography and *CT scanning may be helpful, as may cardiac *biopsy.

Arrhythmias and conduction disorders

Arrhythmias and conduction disorders are a major cause of disability and death. Ventricular fibrillation is the commonest immediate cause of death. It is usually a consequence of ischaemic heart disease, but can result from any of the other major forms of heart disease, as well as from drugs, electrolyte disorders, electrocution, and drowning. It is seldom self-terminating, usually requiring electrical defibrillation for its correction. Implantable defibrillators are coming into increasing use for patients who are considered to be at high risk of sudden death, but are very expensive.

Ventricular tachycardia is most frequently a complication of cardiomyopathy or ischaemic heart disease. Attacks may last from seconds to hours, but most instances are self-terminating. The symptoms resulting from it include palpitation, angina, breathlessness, and syncope. It can be treated or prevented by a variety of drugs, such as quinidine, lignocaine, mexiletine, and amiodarone.

Ventricular ectopic beats are common in normal individuals, but more so in those with cardiac disease. In general, they produce few symptoms apart from palpitation, and are better left untreated. Some forms are associated with a liability to progression to more serious arrhythmias, and may justify the use of antiarrhythmic drugs.

Several classes of drug are now used in the prevention of ventricular arrhythmias, but they are all potentially dangerous because they themselves can provoke arrhythmias. Amiodarone rarely causes arrhythmias but has serious non-cardiac side-effects, including *thyroid disorders and pneumonitis.

Atrial fibrillation is usually a complication of rheumatic heart disease, cardiomyopathy, ischaemic heart disease, or hyperthyroidism. It often precipitates the patient into cardiac failure, but is also hazardous because of the risk of thromboembolism. It may be paroxysmal, but usually eventually becomes established unless there is a precipitating factor, such as acute myocardial infarction or hyperthyroidism, which can be treated. It can be controlled by *digitalis therapy, but may require electrical cardioversion by direct-current countershock. Anticoagulants are needed to prevent emboli if the arrhythmia is persistent.

Paroxysmal tachycardias are common, and may result from disorders in the function of any part of the heart, or from an anomalous pathway of conduction, as in the Wolff–Parkinson–White syndrome. In this latter condition, impulses can bypass the normal conduction pathway of the bundle of His, and a re-entrant circuit may be set up. Drugs may control the paroxysms, but alternative forms of treatment include antitachycardia *pacemakers and interventions in which an abnormal pathway or tissue can be rendered inactive by electrical or radiofrequency ablation.

Heart block and the sick sinus syndrome are responsible for severe bradycardias or asystole (cessation of the heart beat), which can cause syncope or sudden death. In most cases, the only satisfactory treatment is the use of an implantable pacemaker. These are now very reliable and last for many years. Earlier models paced the ventricles only at a fixed rate, but increasingly more sophisticated devices are used which either involve both atria and ventricles or respond to physical activity with increases in rate.

Heart failure

In clinical terms, heart failure is a syndrome of symptoms and signs which are attributable to impaired cardiac performance. These are associated with inadequate perfusion or congestion of tissues and organs. Many of the features are the consequence of the body's inappropriate responses to the cardiac disorder, and include excessive activation of the *sympathetic and *renin–angiotensin systems. Symptoms include dyspnoea, fatigue, and peripheral oedema. Heart failure is an end stage of almost any type of heart disease. It is becoming increasingly common because of the ageing population. Management depends essentially on the prevention or control of the underlying condition. The prognosis is poor, most patients with severe symptoms dying within a year or two.

Apart from correction or amelioration of the underlying condition, treatment is directed at improving the function of the heart and increasing the excretion of water and sodium. The latter is achieved by *diuretics, but the most effective treatment is with the use of angiotensin-converting enzyme (ACE) inhibitors. These have been shown not only to relieve symptoms but to improve prognosis. If medical treatment fails, cardiac *transplantation may be indicated. This procedure has proved most effective in extending the life of patients with heart failure and greatly improving their quality of life. Survival at 1 year is now about 90 per cent and at 5 years more than 50 per cent. Its application is seriously limited by a shortage of donors.

Diagnostic techniques

Most cases of cardiac disease can be diagnosed on the basis of a careful history and physical examination, supplemented by the traditional techniques of electrocardiography and *chest X-ray, but several other methods of investigation play an important part in defining the precise nature and severity of the disorder.

Echocardiography and Doppler ultrasound

Echocardiography exploits the phenomenon that when an ultrasonic beam encounters a boundary between structures of different acoustic densities, some of the waves are reflected and can be detected by a probe. Although it is customary to place the ultrasonic probe on the chest wall, better definition can be obtained if a probe is inserted into the *oesophagus (transoesophageal echocardiography). Echocardiography can demonstrate the structure and function of the heart, and plays an important role in the diagnosis of congenital anomalies, valvar heart disease, and ventricular hypertrophy. The principles of Doppler ultrasound have been used particularly in the investigation of congenital and valvar heart disease, in which characteristic patterns of blood flow can be identified.

Nuclear cardiology

Nuclear imaging techniques are of value in two main contexts in heart disease: the demonstration of abnormalities of myocardial perfusion and the study of left ventricular function. Certain radiopharmaceuticals (such as thallium-201) are distributed in the myocardium in proportion to the myocardial blood flow. Thallium imaging has proved to be of particular value in detecting transient ischaemia in patients with suspected angina pectoris. If the isotope is injected at the time of pain during an exercise test, a localized defect will be observed, which will disappear after a period of rest. A myocardial infarction produces a persistent perfusion defect in the affected area.

In radionuclide ventriculography, red cells are labelled with an isotope such as technetium. Images can be obtained of the left ventricular chamber throughout the cardiac cycle (by using the ECG to 'gate' the images). This allows evaluation of various aspects of ventricular function.

Magnetic resonance imaging and computerized tomography

These techniques are beginning to play an important role in cardiology, particularly in conditions such as congenital heart disease and aortic dissection.

Cardiac catheterization and angiocardiography

This involves the introduction of a radiopaque *catheter into a peripheral artery or vein, and advancing the tip into the great vessels and heart itself. This allows the measurement of pressures within the heart; injection of radiopaque medium permits visualization of the chambers of the heart and great vessels (angiocardiography). The procedure, which is performed under local *anaesthesia, produces slight discomfort and entails some risk, including cardiac arrest and death in about 1 in 1000 patients. Until the development of high-quality echocardiography, it was used extensively in the investigation of congenital and valvar heart disease, but is now employed relatively little for this purpose. Coronary angiography, in which radiopaque contrast medium is selectively injected into the coronary arteries, is an essential prerequisite for angioplasty and coronary artery bypass surgery.

DESMOND JULIAN

CARDIOMYOPATHY is any disease affecting primarily the *myocardium, particularly one of unknown or doubtful aetiology.

CARDIOSPASM is synonymous with *achalasia of the cardia.

CARDIOTHORACIC SURGERY
History

Cardiothoracic surgery is a relatively new endeavour in the overall discipline of *surgery, owing to the difficulties encountered upon entering the thoracic cavity surgically. The problem of ventilation with a collapsed lung (*pneumothorax), and the technical difficulties of working on a beating heart are only two of a number of such obstacles. Indeed, as little as 90 years ago, the famous German surgeon *Billroth stated that 'the surgeon who should attempt to suture a wound of the heart would lose the respect of his colleagues'. Nevertheless, in 1897 Rehn was able to repair successfully a tear of the heart ventricle. In 1913 Doyen unsuccessfully attempted the first internal heart surgery, attempting a closed repair of *pulmonary valve *stenosis. This same operation was later successfully developed by Brock and Sellors in London in 1948. Prior to this, Souttar carried out the first successful operation on an intracardiac structure, successfully opening a stenotic *mitral valve in 1925 by performing a closed mitral commissurotomy. Harken and Bailey in the United States satisfactorily completed the first of a series of closed mitral valvotomies in 1948. The first half of the 20th century was marked by other significant milestones in cardiac surgery, including the first resection of a ventricular *aneurysm by *Sauerbruch in 1931 in Germany, the first closure or ligation of a patent *ductus arteriosus by Gross at Harvard in 1938, and the first resection of a thoracic aortic *coarctation by Crafoord in Stockholm in 1945.

The modern era of cardiac surgery was ushered in by two significant advances. The first was the development of the *Blalock–Taussig shunt, using the subclavian artery to direct oxygenated arterial blood into the pulmonary circuit via the pulmonary artery. This revolutionized the care of cyanotic congenital '*blue baby' heart disease. The second critical development was the conception and refinement over a 20-year period of the *heart–lung machine by John Gibbon, culminating in the use of this remarkable machine, capable of taking over the function of the heart and lungs, for the successful repair of an atrial septal defect in 1953. The subsequent 30 years marked the accelerating use of the heart–lung machine to address and correct acquired and congenital heart defects, leading to the current era of cardiothoracic surgery.

The recent history of lung surgery follows a somewhat similar course. Intrathoracic surgery, as indicated above, was limited until the development in 1904 by Sauerbruch and Breslau of positive-pressure ventilation that allowed for lung resection without lung collapse. The first *pneumonectomy, or resection of a lung, utilizing modern techniques was successfully undertaken by Reinhoff, in 1933, on a child at the Johns Hopkins Hospital. The first successful resection of the oesophagus was completed by Torek in New York in 1913. In 1933 Ohsawa and Seou performed the first oesophageal resection, with the re-establishment of gastro-oesophageal continuity.

Heart valve replacement

The surgical correction of *valvular disease, as indicated above, figured predominantly in the early era of open-heart surgery. Replacement of heart valves with mechanical valves was first successfully accomplished in 1961 by Starr in Portland, Oregon, using a ball-and-cage device. Subsequently, various forms of tilting disc valves were developed and introduced clinically. Currently, the St Jude tilting disc valve is the most widely used mechanical heart valve in the world, yielding excellent durability and haemodynamic function. The St Jude and similar mechanical *prostheses use pyrolite carbon, a strong and durable material with low potential for clot formation. The expected failure rate for the current generation of mechanical valvular prostheses is far less than 1 per cent/year. The rate of infection for these prosthetic valves is approximately 0.2 per cent/year. Unfortunately, the prosthetic heart valves do require thinning of the blood, anticoagulation, with oral *anticoagulant agents to allow proper function. Despite this precaution, the risk of clotting complications of the valve, or embolism of clots from the valve, is approximately 1–2 per cent/year, and the complications of bleeding secondary to the use of these oral anticoagulants is also approximately 1 per cent/year. Because of these complications, an alternative substitute after resection of abnormal valves is a bioprosthesis. In general, these valves are harvested from pigs and then sewn on to cloth struts to allow for surgical insertion. These porcine valves are preserved in glutaraldehyde and, in general, do not require anticoagulation: however, the expected durability of these valves is 10 to 13 years, at which point patients require re-operation and valve replacement. Ross in London and Barrett-Boyes in Australia have pioneered work in the use of transplanted human cadaveric valves in the form of homografts as an alternative valve substitute, with good results.

In recent years, an increasing effort has been made to repair and not replace diseased valves. This is most applicable to the mitral valve, which can either be opened by incising between the leaflets, performing an open commissurotomy, placing a ring around a leaking valve, called an annuloplasty, or actually repairing torn portions of the mitral valve leaflets (valvuloplasty). Intermediate to long-term results with these procedures are encouraging. Significant freedom from the complications associated with valve replacement is a major advantage of the valve repair procedures when appropriately applied.

Coronary artery grafting bypass (coronary bypass)

Inadequate blood supply to the heart due to atherosclerotic obstruction of the *coronary arteries causes chest pressure or pain called *angina pectoris, which was first described in 1768. Another hundred years passed before the association between coronary artery obstruction and angina was recognized, and still another hundred years before the modern era of coronary bypass surgery arrived. The clinical feasibility of *saphenous vein bypass grafting, the current technique of surgical relief of coronary obstruction, was established in the 1960s by Johnson in Milwaukee and Favaloro at the Cleveland Clinic. The first use of the internal mammary artery (IMA) in humans dates to the Vineberg procedure, reported in 1946. The first direct IMA to coronary graft was reported in 1967 by Kolessov in the Soviet Union and subsequently carried out in the United States.

The potential objectives of coronary bypass surgery include: (1) the relief of low blood flow to the heart (*ischaemia); (2) the relief of anginal symptoms; (3) the prolongation of survival; (4) the prevention of myocardial infarction; (5) the preservation of cardiac function; and (6) improvement in exercise tolerance. Trials of medical versus surgical management for coronary artery disease were performed in the early 1970s with the initial growth in expertise in performing coronary bypass surgery. These studies showed that surgery provided better relief of angina and improvement in functional capacity and a reduction in the incidence of fatal myocardial infarction, but no difference in the incidence of late, non-fatal myocardial infarctions. These studies also demonstrated that patients with obstruction of the left main coronary artery, or significant obstructions of three major coronary arteries and left ventricular dysfunction, enjoyed a significant survival advantage with surgical versus medical treatment.

Current symptomatic indications for coronary bypass surgery include unstable angina that is unresponsive to standard medical therapy and must be treated with intravenous medications, or that has been increasing in severity, or that occurs at rest. Similarly, severe exertional angina that is unresponsive to medical therapy is also an indication for surgical intervention. Angina that persists after *myocardial infarction is a further indication, as are ischaemia or haemodynamic instability following an unsuccessful percutaneous *angioplasty, or following acute myocardial infarction. Cardiogenic shock complicating myocardial infarction, or mechanical complications of a myocardial infarction such as mitral regurgitation or acute ventricular septal defect, may be further indications. In general, each of these clinical indications needs to be correlated with appropriate anatomical or physiological abnormalities. These include a greater than 50 per cent blockage of the left main coronary artery, a greater than 50 per cent obstruction of all three major coronary arteries (three-vessel disease) with impaired left ventricular function, or three-vessel disease with normal left ventricular function but inducible ischaemia on physiological testing. Two-vessel disease with significant proximal blockage of the left anterior descending coronary artery, severely depressed left ventricular function with evidence of reversable ischemia, or less commonly, coronary artery disease associated with life-threatening ventricular *dysrhythmias are other surgical indications. Coronary stenoses not normally indicated for surgery may be bypassed concomitant with other indicated procedures, such as repair of aortic or mitral valvular disease.

The recent advent of percutaneous transluminal coronary angioplasty (PTCA) has generally usurped any role of bypass surgery for one- and two-vessel disease, but the consensus is that coronary bypass surgery remains the indicated treatment for three-vessel disease. Angioplasty has an associated 30 per cent restenosis rate at 6 months and approximately a 1–2 per cent acute failure rate. Emergency coronary bypass surgery in the setting of failed angioplasty carries approximately a 10 per cent mortality, compared with approximately 1–2 per cent mortality in an elective setting. Therefore, PTCA should be undertaken with the understanding that an almost tenfold increase in mortality exists in the event of emergency coronary bypass surgery.

The overall risk of death following elective coronary bypass surgery is approximately 1–2 per cent for patients with stable angina, 3 per cent for patients with unstable angina, 5–10 per cent for postinfarction angina or failed PTCA, and 30 per cent for cardiogenic shock. Independent predictors of increased risk include: (1) reoperation; (2) urgent or emergency surgery; (3) older age, especially in an emergency or urgent setting; (4) left ventricular dysfunction, especially with an ejection fraction less than 25 per cent; (5) female gender; and (6) a small body surface area, probably correlating with the technical difficulties of working with smaller coronary arteries.

Surgery is performed by placing the patient on cardiopulmonary bypass. That requires insertion of a cannula, or tube, into the right atrium to carry the blood away from the heart into a heart–lung machine which oxygenates the blood and removes carbon dioxide. The blood is then returned to the systemic circulation by way of a second cannula inserted into the aorta. Access to the heart is obtained by splitting the breast bone, a median sternotomy. After instituting cardiopulmonary bypass, a clamp is placed across the aorta eliminating blood flow to the heart. Because this creates an ischaemic condition, preservation of heart function is obtained by arresting the heart's function with a cold potassium (cardioplegic) solution maintained at 4 °C. Such conditions decrease the heart's oxygen consumption by 95 per cent or more, allowing a period of blood-free surgery on a still, non-beating heart. With these conditions, the coronary arteries can be incised beyond the areas of obstruction and a saphenous vein or internal mammary artery sutured to the coronary artery beyond the level of obstruction. After completing these anastomoses, the cross-clamp is removed from the aorta. The heart is allowed to reperfuse and start beating, and at this point the proximal portions of the bypass grafts are sewn to the aorta, in this manner receiving a source of blood flow. During the period of cross-clamping the patient is also cooled systemically to approximately 28 °C by a heat exchanger included in the cardiopulmonary bypass circuit. This systemic cooling helps prevent rewarming of the heart from blood flowing around it and allows for maintenance of lower systemic pressures and red blood cell levels.

The results of cardiopulmonary bypass surgery from data published from large studies in the 1970s and more recent data are quite favourable. For patients with three-vessel disease and an ejection fraction between 35 per cent and 50 per cent, the large United States CASS study indicated a significant ten-year survival rate difference of 75 per cent for surgical treatment compared with 58 per cent for medical treatment. Patency of the saphenous veins at 10 years is approximately 50 per cent. The internal mammary artery, on the other hand, enjoys a patency of approximately 95 per cent at 10 years. The long-term occlusion of these bypass grafts is due to accelerated *atherosclerosis and results in a reoperation rate of approximately 17 per cent at 12 years.

Congenital heart disease

Congenital heart disease can most simplistically be broken down into two types, cyanotic 'blue baby' disease on the one hand, and acyanotic heart disease on the other. Cyanotic patients generally have inadequate pulmonary blood flow and are approached surgically by increasing blood flow to the pulmonary circuit, through either a bypass or shunt technique. Acyanotic patients generally have problems of heart failure because excessive blood flow is recirculated to one portion of the heart due to a short-circuiting of the normal flow patterns through a hole in the heart (atrial or ventricular septal defect) or an abnormal or anomalous connection of the major vessels (e.g. transposition of the great arteries). Many congenital heart diseases are associated with a combination of these two classes of abnormality.

Almost all congenital heart defects are currently amenable to either complete early correction, with or without cardiopulmonary bypass, or early palliation, for example by the creation of a temporary shunt to increase blood flow to the lungs, with later definitive treatment. As technical abilities improve, it is increasingly possible to reconstruct the heart to resemble normal *anatomy. Mortality rates for even the most complex of congenital heart operations are now approaching less than 5 per cent. Long-term survival data following these operations are only recently becoming available, since many of these procedures are less than 20 years old, but generally seem to be quite favourable.

Pacemakers and automatic implantable cardioverter defibrillator devices (AICD)

The ability to maintain the heart's normal heartbeat with external electrical stimulation has existed for some 30 years. This pacemaker capability requires placement of a wire, or lead, through one of the large veins into the right ventricle of the heart. Occasionally, the lead must be placed through a chest incision directly on to the outside surface of the heart. The lead is connected to a generator unit the size of a woman's powder compact, which contains a battery and the microcircuitry capable of interpreting and processing the impulses received and transmitted to the lead. The pacemaker generator has a life expectancy of 5–10 years, at which time it must be replaced. Dual chamber units are currently available that are capable of sensing the patient's own rhythm with a second lead placed in the atrium, and transmitting this impulse to the ventricle, allowing maintenance of this internal rhythm. The pacemakers available today are extremely sophisticated devices, capable of external reprogramming and of sensing the patient's motion or activity and increasing the heart rate based upon the activity levels.

Until recently, malignant abnormal rhythms originating in the cardiac ventricles, known as ventricular tachycardia and *ventricular fibrillation, were commonly associated with sudden death, and were treatable only by medication. However, the ability to apply an external countershock to reset the electrical rhythm of the heart has existed for many years. The automatic implantable cardioverter *defibrillator (AICD) device, which can sense these abnormal rhythms and internally apply a countershock, has recently gained wide clinical use. These AICDs are also becoming more sophisticated and miniaturized and the most advanced units can be implanted using internal lead systems similar to those applied for pacemakers.

Current advances and future horizons in cardiac surgery

The past 10 years have again seen an explosive advance in innovations in cardiac surgery, resulting in operations on more seriously ill patients with improved outcomes. The introduction of *immunosuppression agents, most notably *cyclosporin, has allowed the resurgence of cardiac as well as lung and other organ *transplantation. Early and intermediate survival following cardiac transplantation is now approximately 80 per cent. The introduction of mechanical assist devices, most notably the intra-aortic balloon pump, which can mechanically assist the heart's pumping function, has allowed survival of patients with severely compromised heart function. Ever more sophisticated monitoring devices, including the transoesophageal *echocardiogram, allows continuous on-line visualization of the heart and measurement of its pumping function, even with a closed chest. New pharmacological agents can improve myocardial function and decrease such complications of open-heart surgery as bleeding disorders induced by the cardiopulmonary bypass circuit.

Thoracic (non-cardiac) surgery

Non-cardiac thoracic surgery was nearly synonymous with surgery for *tuberculosis in the middle of this century. The advent of antituberculous chemotherapy nearly extinguished the working knowledge of this type of surgery among thoracic surgeons. However, the recent resurgence of tuberculosis, mostly related to the epidemic of *AIDS, has refocused attention on pulmonary surgery for tuberculosis and other infections. The remainder of pulmonary surgery consists primarily of pulmonary resection for lung *cancer and other neoplasms. Advances in this area rely predominately on changes in *chemotherapy and/or *radiation therapy, and multimodality treatment of these diseases in a synergistic approach to eradicating tumour, rather than advances in surgical technique. Resection of the oesophagus for cancer has been modified in similar ways, although the Japanese have recently advocated wide lymph node dissection for oesophageal cancer because of the predilection of this tumour to metastasize widely even at an early stage. Skinner, in New York, has been a strong advocate, with some improvement in results, for radical, wide, *en-bloc* resections of oesophageal cancer. Finally, Onringer, in Michigan, has advocated the feasibility of resecting the oesophagus without a thoracic incision. Perhaps one of the greatest advances in treatment of both of these neoplasms is the rigorous application of a tumour-staging system and advances in careful, appropriate staging of these tumours with refinement in *computerized tomography (CT), *magnetic resonance imaging (MRI), and *ultrasound technology. These advances have allowed for accurate prognosis and a better approach to treatment.

Benign thoracic conditions

Benign diseases of the thorax requiring surgical intervention predominantly involve the oesophagus. These include either oesophageal stricture or reflux refractory to medical treatment or associated with inflammatory changes in the oesophageal mucosa. A variety of surgical techniques exist as approaches to these problems. In general, they should be referred to well-practised oesophageal surgeons, as the subtleties of these techniques can have significant impact in terms of outcome.

Recently, much attention has been directed toward the approach to Barrett's disease of the oesophagus, which is now widely accepted as a precancerous condition. More aggressive surveillance and possibly resection on patients with this condition is now becoming widely accepted. Lung transplant surgery has also enjoyed recent successes with the advent of the new generation of immunosuppressive agents, similar to that seen with cardiac transplants. Most recently, the attempt to use *gene therapy in the treatment of *cystic fibrosis, previously a significant indication for lung transplantation, gives hope of eradicating this cause of significant non-neoplastic injury to the lung.

Finally, the past 5 years have seen the explosive growth of video-assisted thoracic surgery and thoracoscopic surgery. These techniques avoid the significant morbidity of the thoracic incision, which frequently requires excision or division of ribs to allow adequate intercostal exposure. Treatment of *pleural effusions, *pneumothorax (collapsed lung), open lung biopsies and even lung resections, lobectomies, and oesophageal operations using this technique have recently been reported. It is too early to determine whether thoracoscopy will be an appropriate treatment in lung resection of neoplastic growth; however, this reinterest in an old technique seems to be revolutionizing thoracic surgery.

TODD ROSENGART
O. WAYNE ISOM

CARIES. *Necrosis and decay of bone or teeth, for example *spinal caries, *dental caries.

CARMINATIVE means having the property of relieving gastric *flatulence or of generally 'soothing' the stomach.

CARNEGIE, ANDREW (1835–1919). Philanthropist. Carnegie was born in Scotland and emigrated to the USA in 1848. He established a trust to aid education in Scottish universities. His Carnegie Corporation of New York (1911) was liberally endowed for the furtherance of civilization.

CARNEGIE INSTITUTION, Washington, DC. See RESEARCH INSTITUTES.

CAROTENE is an orange-yellow unsaturated *hydrocarbon ($C_{40}H_{56}$) widely distributed in plants (e.g. carrots, tomatoes, many flowers, fungi, etc.) and present also in dairy products and egg yolk. It is a pro-vitamin, which can be converted into *vitamin A by the liver. An excessive dietary intake may lead to an increased concentration in the blood (carotenaemia) sufficient to cause yellowness of the skin resembling *jaundice.

CAROTID is the name of the two great *arteries, on either side of the neck, which supply blood to the head. The name derives from *Galen, and the fact that compression of these vessels led to *carus*, a profound sleep.

CAROTID SINUS. A dilated portion of the *carotid artery adjacent to its division into external and internal branches, the wall of which contains *baroceptors sensitive to changes in arterial pressure. Nerve fibres from these receptors run in the *glossopharyngeal (ninth cranial) nerve back to central *vagal nuclei to induce reflex changes in heart rate. External manual pressure over the carotid sinus (simulating a rise in arterial pressure) causes a reflex *bradycardia; undue pressure, or an abnormally sensitive carotid sinus due to degenerative changes in the arterial wall, may cause 'carotid sinus *syncope'.

CARPHOLOGY is random plucking at the bedclothes (literally 'straw-gathering'), also known as floccillation.

It has been recognized since the time of *Galen as a sign of grave illness, particularly of exhausting fevers like *typhoid. See, for example, Mistress Quickly's account of the death of Falstaff in Shakespeare's *Henry V* (II. iii).

CARPOPEDAL SPASM is flexion of the wrists and plantar-flexion of the feet, due to abnormal neuromuscular irritability, typical of *tetany.

CARPUS. The eight small carpal bones of the wrist.

CARREL, ALEXIS (1873–1955). French surgeon and physiologist. His early work was on the development of methods of suturing blood vessels, for which he was awarded a *Nobel prize in 1912. During the First World War he investigated the prevention and treatment of wound infections by employing a continuous drip of sodium hypochlorite solutions. Afterwards he studied methods of culturing living tissues. In the late 1930s he collaborated with Charles Lindbergh in attempts to devise an artificial cardiac pump.

CARRIER. A person who harbours pathogenic microorganisms and can transmit infection to others, though he or she is healthy and without clinical symptoms. *Streptococcal, *staphylococcal, *diphtheria, *typhoid, and many other infections can be transmitted by symptomless carriers (see INFECTIOUS DISEASES). The term is also used to denote the clinically unaffected carrier of a gene responsible for a genetic disorder (see GENETICS).

CARRIÓN, DANIEL ALCIDES (1850–85). Peruvian physician. Carrión inoculated himself with material from *Oroya fever, which occurs on the western slopes of the Andes in some narrow valleys. The disease is now known to be caused by *Bartonella bacilliformis*. This is the only member of the genus known to cause disease in man, although other species affect animals. Essentially the disease is a virulent *septicaemia; a variant is verruca peruviana, where nodules appear in the skin. Carrión died of the disease shortly after infecting himself.

CARTILAGE is the tough, firm, animal skeletal tissue known as gristle. There are several varieties (elastic, fibrous, hyaline) but it basically consists of rounded cells scattered in a resilient *polysaccharide-containing matrix with numerous *collagen fibres (fine in hyaline cartilage, thicker in fibrous cartilage); in adults it has no blood vessels. Cartilage is important as a supporting and shock-absorbing material, and is also the main precursor tissue of bone and part of the body's growth mechanism.

CARUNCLE. Any small fleshy protuberance.

CASCARA is an extract of the bark of a California buckthorn (*Rhamnus purshiana*) widely used as a *laxative because it contains irritant anthracene compounds. Its full name is 'cascara sagrada' (sacred bark).

CASE. An instance of a particular disease or condition. Purists object to use of the word as synonymous with 'patient', although this usage is common.

CAS-EVAC is the proprietary name in Sweden and Canada of a *cascara mixture sold elsewhere as Cascara Evacuant. The term is also used in military medicine (see ARMED FORCES OF THE USA; DEFENCE MEDICAL SERVICES (UK)) to indicate casualty evacuation by air.

CASONI, TOMASO (1850–1925). Italian physician. Casoni described a diagnostic test for *hydatid disease. The worm forms cysts containing a clear fluid in various organs. If a little of this fluid is injected into the skin, a white papule develops; this increases in those infected by the disease but disappears in those who are not. A negative response, however, does not exclude the possibility of present or past infection.

CASSAVA is a starchy root vegetable cultivated for food in parts of tropical America, the Caribbean, and Africa. It is used to make soups, flour, and bread, and in some communities provides the major dietary source of energy. Tapioca is a product of cassava. If it contains a moderate excess of *cyanide, it may cause tropical ataxic *neuropathy.

CASSIA is a genus of shrubs from which senna is obtained. See LAXATIVES.

CAST. A mould formed by aggregation or precipitation of material or cells in a renal tubule and excreted in the *urine in that shape. Occasional hyaline casts are seen in normal urine.

CASTELLANI, ALDO (1877–1971). Italian tropical physician. In 1902 he demonstrated *trypanosomes in the *cerebrospinal fluid of patients with sleeping sickness, the cause of which was then unknown. During 12 years in Ceylon, he identified the causal agent of *yaws, *Treponema pertenue*. He took a special interest in fungal disorders of the skin, and devised the paint that bears his name.

CASTOR OIL is a stimulant obtained from seeds of the castor oil plant *Ricinus communis*.

CASTRATION is the removal or destruction of the male *gonads. The term is sometimes also used to indicate removal of, or destruction of, the female *ovaries.

CASUALTY. An accidental wound, injury, or death; or a person who is injured or killed in an accident or incident of warfare.

CASUALTY EVACUATION is the removal of *casualties from a battle zone (or scene of peacetime disaster) to reception areas, casualty clearing stations, field hospitals, base hospitals, etc. according to medical and surgical need and to the dictates of the military situation. Casualty evacuation by air (*Cas-Evac) is now all-important.

CASUALTY SURGERY is accident and emergency (A&E) surgery. (See SURGERY OF TRAUMA.)

CAT (OR CT). See COMPUTERIZED AXIAL TOMOGRAPHY.

CATABOLISM is any metabolic process in which complex organic molecules are converted into simpler ones, with the liberation of energy. The reverse process is termed '*anabolism'.

CATALEPSY is a state of total and trance-like unresponsiveness, so that patients or their limbs tend to remain in whatever position they are placed (a sign also known as *flexibilitas cerea* or waxy flexibility).

CATAPLEXY. Abrupt attacks of muscle weakness and atonia (causing falling or 'giving way at the knees') and usually occurring in response to such emotions as fear, anger, surprise, and mirth. It is generally associated with *narcolepsy.

CATARACT. Opacity of the crystalline lens of the eye (see OPHTHALMOLOGY).

CATARRH. is any inflammatory condition of a *mucous membrane accompanied by a copious discharge of *mucus.

CATATONIA is one clinical variety of *schizophrenia, first described as 'tension insanity' by Kahlbann in 1874. It is 'that condition in which the patient sits quietly or completely mute and motionless, immovable, with a staring countenance, the eyes fixed on a distant point and apparently completely without volition, without any reaction to sensory impressions, sometimes with a full-fledged *flexibilitas cerea* as in *catalepsy'.

CATECHOLAMINE refers to any of a group of chemically congeneric compounds derived from the *amino acid *tyrosine and exemplified by *adrenaline (epinephrine) and *noradrenaline (norepinephrine). Their physiological effects resemble those of stimulation of the *sympathetic nervous system.

CATGUT is surgical *ligature material derived from sheep intestine by suitable chemical treatment and sterilization. It is slowly absorbed in the body, and is thus well suited to its purpose.

CATHARSIS is synonymous with *purgation. The word is also used in psychiatry in the transferred sense of *abreaction.

CATHETER. A flexible tubular instrument for introduction into an organ or body cavity (e.g. to drain the *urinary bladder). Catheters are of all varieties and sizes, depending on their purpose. Some, notably cardiac catheters, are radiopaque so that they can be placed under radiographic control.

CATHODE. A negative *electrode. A cathode ray is a stream of *electrons emitted from a cathode when an electrical discharge takes place in a vacuum tube.

CATION. An *ion carrying a positive electric charge.

CATS AS CARRIERS OF DISEASE. Only rarely do domestic cats transmit diseases to man. Flea-bite dermatitis and the fungal infection *ringworm are perhaps the most familiar. *Cat-scratch fever is a benign, self-limiting condition affecting regional lymph-nodes; and cats are often implicated in the transmission of *toxoplasmosis. Among other conditions of which cats are occasionally known as putative transmitters are *rabies, *toxocariasis, *leptospirosis, *tularaemia, *yersiniosis, and *salmonellosis.

CAT-SCRATCH FEVER is a benign, subacute, self-limiting, regional *lymphadenitis, the agent of which has not been identified.

CAUDA EQUINA. The collection of spinal roots that occupy the spinal canal below the termination of the *spinal cord at the level of the first lumbar vertebra; so called because of its fancied resemblance to a horse's tail.

CAUSALGIA is a severe pain of burning quality, exacerbated by touch, which follows injury of a major nerve of the extremities. The precise mechanism of the pain is not known, but it is accompanied by autonomic changes and can, in the absence of treatment, lead to muscle *atrophy and joint *fixation. It is often relieved by sympathectomy.

CAUTERIZATION is the burning or searing of tissue by application of (originally) a branding iron or (now) any other heated metal instrument, or the similar destruction of tissue by application of a caustic substance. The electric cautery is commonly used in modern surgery.

CAUTERY. Originally a branding-iron, now any device employed for *cauterization.

CAVELL, EDITH (1865–1915). British nurse. Edith Cavell was matron of a Red Cross hospital in Brussels during the First World War when Belgium was conquered by the Germans. With others, and using the hospital as a base, she helped about 200 Allied military to escape capture by the invaders. When caught she confessed, and was tried and shot. This caused an outcry throughout the neutral and combatant countries opposed to Germany.

CAVITY. Any hollow space, or potential space, within the body; a destructive lesion produced by *dental caries.

CELL AND CELL BIOLOGY. The term 'cell' was first used by the microscopist *Hooke in 1665 to describe the structures he saw in thin slices of cork. Although he was not seeing cells but the spaces where cells had been during the life of the tree, in the following years other microscopists made observations that supported his idea of living matter being composed of small structural units. Even so, more than 150 years passed before the accumulated observations on cells were brought together into a general 'cell theory', usually attributed to *Schleiden and *Schwann in 1838. According to this theory, the cell is the smallest component of life that can exist independently. All living organisms are composed of cells and, as concluded by *Virchow in 1855, cells can only arise from pre-existing cells.

Cells vary enormously in size and shape, which may explain why scientists took so long to recognize their fundamental role in life. The smallest *micro-organisms, such as *mycoplasmas, are less than one micron (μm) (less than one-thousandth of a millimetre) in diameter, whereas the ostrich egg has a diameter of several centimetres; skeletal muscle cells are long and thin but red blood cells are biconcave discs; plant cells have rigid thick walls but cells such as the amoeba can change their shape from one moment to the next. Nevertheless, it has been possible to classify living organisms according to the characteristics of the cells of which they are composed and the way in which they are organized.

The first large division is into cells such as *bacteria which have no well-defined *nucleus (prokaryotes) and organisms composed of cells with nuclei and clearly defined *chromosomes (eukaryotes). Eukaryotes may be single-celled or multicellular organisms and most can be classified as either animals or plants; an important difference is that most plants are capable of *photosynthesis. Single-celled animals (protozoa) include the *malaria parasite, *trypanosomes, and amoebae; single-celled plants include *Euglena* and yeasts. A few organisms are difficult to classify as animals or plants, and there are also organisms that can exist during different stages of their life cycles either as single-celled or multicellular organisms. Multicellular organisms develop from one cell (a fertilized egg), which differentiates into many different cell types. The number of cells in a multicellular organism varies greatly from one organism to another; the average human comprises approximately 100 million million cells.

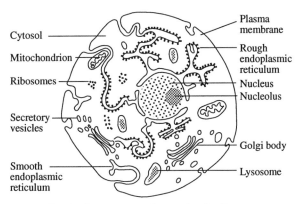

Cytosol

Mitochondrion

Ribosomes

Secretory
vesicles

Smooth
endoplasmic
reticulum

Plasma
membrane

Rough
endoplasmic
reticulum

Nucleus

Nucleolus

Golgi body

Lysosome

Fig. 1 The basic structure of an animal cell.

Cell structure

The detailed knowledge we have today about the structure and function of cells is largely due to the development of the electron *microscope in the 1940s, and the availability of an increasingly wide range of biochemical and tissue culture techniques.

All cells are surrounded by a thin lipid *membrane (Fig. 1). This is a very selective barrier, allowing some substances to pass across it and excluding others in order to maintain a relatively constant internal environment. Some of the many different types of *proteins embedded in the cell membrane play an active role in transporting substances across the membrane, by acting as pumps or catalysts. Some act as *receptors, detecting changes in the external environment and initiating appropriate responses from the cell; others provide a mechanism for cells to interact and communicate. In plant cells the cell membrane is surrounded by a cell wall, a thick, cellulose-containing structure which provides protection for the cell and forms the rigid skeleton of the plant.

Little detailed structure can be seen in the cells of prokaryotes, but in eukaryotic cells many different subcellular structures ('organelles') have been identified. Just as the different organs of the human body work together to maintain the body, so the different organelles of a cell each have their own characteristic activities but work together to maintain the cell. What remains inside the cell when the organelles have been removed is the gel-like* cytoplasm.

The largest organelle in a eukaryotic cell is the nucleus, which is surrounded by a double membrane and contains the genetic material, *deoxyribonucleic acid (DNA). Through the information contained in a coded form within its chemical structure, DNA determines the specific morphological and biochemical characteristics of each type of cell and controls its metabolic activities. Although the same genetic information is generally present in each cell of an organism, only a proportion of it is used (expressed) in any given type of cell. Genetic

information is expressed in the form of proteins, and the specialized functions of different cell types are, to a large extent, determined by their protein complement. When a cell divides, the DNA carried in chromosomes in its nucleus is copied and passed on to each daughter cell, thus ensuring that the next generation of cells has all the information needed to function correctly.

Within the nucleus, DNA is combined with histones and other structural proteins to form chromatin, seen in a microscope as a dark, diffuse material. The first visual indication that a cell is about to divide is when the chromatin condenses to form rod-like chromosomes. A constant number of chromosomes is formed in the cells of each species. The somatic cells of humans (i.e. not sperm or egg) are described as diploid because they contain two complete sets of chromosomes. There are 23 pairs of chromosomes in each cell, 22 pairs of somatic chromosomes (one of each pair derived from each parent) and one pair of sex chromosomes, either two Xs in the female or an X and Y in the male.

Each nucleus also contains one or more nucleoli. The main function of a *nucleolus is to manufacture the precursors of *ribosomes. In the electron microscope ribosomes appear as small, dense particles either free in the cytoplasm or attached to the membranes of the endoplasmic reticulum (see below). Ribosomes are the sites where proteins are synthesized.

The structure of proteins is determined by the 50 000–100 000 or so *genes (units of genetic information) contained within the structure of DNA. When a protein is to be synthesized, the information in the corresponding gene is copied into a molecule of *messenger RNA (mRNA) which then moves into the cytoplasm, where it associates with ribosomes. Amino acids, the building blocks of proteins, are lined up on the mRNA in the correct order and joined together to form the protein. Each amino acid reaches the site of protein synthesis attached to a molecule of transfer RNA (tRNA) which acts like an adaptor, ensuring that the sequence of amino acids in the protein is that specified by the genetic instructions passed on from DNA to mRNA.

The endoplasmic reticulum is an intricate system of membranes that spreads throughout the cytoplasm. Part of it is studded with ribosomes and is called rough endoplasmic reticulum because of its appearance in the electron microscope. Proteins synthesized on these ribosomes move to the smooth endoplasmic reticulum (areas without ribosomes), the Golgi apparatus, and then the cell membrane for secretion. On the way the proteins often have carbohydrates added, turning them into glycoproteins.

The Golgi apparatus consists of a stack of curved, flattened sacs surrounded by many interconnecting tubules and vesicles. Proteins reach one side of the apparatus inside vesicles which bud off from the surface of the endoplasmic reticulum. Similarly, vesicles bud off from the other side of the Golgi apparatus to carry the proteins to the cell membrane, where the vesicles and membrane fuse and the proteins are secreted into the extracellular fluid.

Running through the cytoplasm is the cytoskeleton, an intricate network of solid fibres and hollow tubes. The cytoskeleton does the same job for the cell as scaffolding does on a building site. It determines the basic shape of the cell and provides a framework that allows materials to be moved from one place to another. Unlike the poles and girders of scaffolding, however, the three main components of the cytoskeleton—microtubules, actin filaments, and intermediate filaments—are not permanent static structures. They are themselves assembled from subunits and can be taken apart rapidly and then reassembled in a different way as part of the processes of providing cells with shape and form, moving cells, or moving and organizing things within cells. Microtubules occur as single tubules or as precisely arranged groups of tubules in structures such as cilia (used for moving material past the cell surface), flagella (used for cell locomotion), and the mitotic spindle formed during cell division.

Cells generate energy by oxidizing fuel molecules derived from the diet. *Mitochondria (the 'power stations' of the cell) are the main sites of oxidation. Each mitochondrion is a sausage-shaped organelle surrounded by a double membrane, and most of the activities concerned with the energy metabolism of the cell and the synthesis of *adenosine triphosphate (ATP) occur on the highly folded inner membrane or in the region within it. Plant cells, but not animal cells, also have *chlorophyll-containing organelles called chloroplasts, which can capture light energy and perform the basic reactions of photosynthesis.

Lysosomes are a collection of small vesicles which form the cell's digestive system. The *enzymes inside them can degrade any material which the cell needs to digest—whether derived from the cell itself or from its surroundings. In the process of *phagocytosis, particulate material is taken into the cell in vacuoles formed by invagination of the cell membrane. The vacuoles fuse with the lysosomes, exposing their contents to the digestive enzymes. The process of pinocytosis, in which fluid is engulfed, is essentially similar.

Another organelle about the same size as the lysosome is the peroxisome. Peroxisomes contain enzymes involved in special oxidation processes, during which peroxides are formed.

Inheritance

The body continually needs to make new cells in order to grow or to replace cells that have become worn out or lost through the ravages of day-to-day existence. The replacement process goes on in many tissues, but the main sites are those where the cells are in direct contact with the external or internal environment, such as the skin or the lining of the intestine. New cells are formed when existing cells divide, and it is estimated that about 100 000 000 000 (10^{11}) cells in the body (about 0.002 per cent of the total) divide each day. During cell division (*mitosis) (Fig. 2) the genetic material in the nucleus, contained within the DNA of the chromosomes, is first duplicated so that identical sets of information are passed on to each of the two daughter cells.

The period between cell divisions is called interphase. The onset of prophase is signalled by the chromatin condensing to form chromosomes. The centromere region of each chromosome then divides, separating the chromosome into two daughter chromatids. During early and late metaphase the membrane of the nucleus is lost and the chromatids attach to the centre of a framework of microtubules (the mitotic spindle) which extends across the cell. During anaphase the chromatids move outwards towards the ends of the spindle. Finally, during telophase, they complete their journey, the spindle breaks down, and a nuclear membrane is formed around each new set of chromosomes, which begin to decondense into chromatin. The cytoplasm between the two nuclei then constricts, dividing the parent cell into two.

The daughter cells formed during mitosis have the same total number of chromosomes as the parent cell. In contrast, in meiosis, which occurs during the maturation of the sex cells, the number of chromosomes is halved (as the chromosomes divide once but the cells divide twice) so the gametes—the spermatozoa and ova—are haploid, i.e. they only have a single set of chromosomes. In addition, during the formation of the *gametes, a process of crossing-over (exchanging of parts) occurs, ensuring a mixing of the genetic information passed on to the progeny.

Cell differentiation

The different organs of the body contain different types of cells—nerve cells are typical of the brain, leucocytes and erythrocytes of the blood, and so on. All these cells are derived from a single fertilized egg by mitosis, and most contain exactly the same genetic information. Hence the development of differences among cells (cell differentiation) must require a differential use of the genetic information they contain. The mechanism of cell differentiation is not yet understood, but it is thought that in early development there are some crucial cell divisions, during each of which at least one of the daughter cells becomes different from its parent. Over many cell divisions divergences accumulate and the process of change becomes irreversible. What has become a liver cell can then no longer regress to a common precursor which could redifferentiate as a nerve cell, for example.

In addition to fully differentiated cells, many tissues of the body contain stem cells, precursor cells which are not fully differentiated. These can divide to produce more stem cells but can also give rise to progeny which can differentiate. Stem cells in the bone marrow, for example, give rise to granulocytes (white blood cells), *macrophages, and erythrocytes (red blood cells).

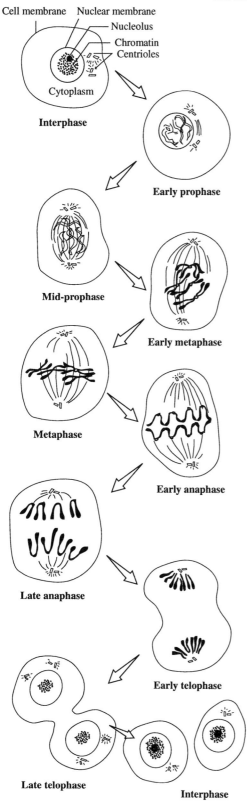

Cell membrane   Nuclear membrane
Nucleolus
Chromatin
Centrioles
Cytoplasm

Interphase

Early prophase

Mid-prophase

Early metaphase

Metaphase

Early anaphase

Late anaphase

Early telophase

Late telophase

Interphase

The growth process

If the process of cell division proceeded unchecked, a single cell would rapidly grow into an unacceptably large mass of tissue, one cell becoming two, two become four, and so on. In fact, the growth of tissues is carefully and accurately regulated in response to the specific needs of the body.

The formation of new cells, which accounts for growth, depends on the synthesis of DNA, RNA, and proteins. Many of the molecular mechanisms regulating growth affect the synthesis of these substances during the different phases of the cell's life cycle. The life cycle of a eukaryotic cell has four consecutive phases, designated G_1, S, G_2, and M. DNA is synthesized during the S phase, RNA and protein during G_1, S, and G_2. During the M phase (mitosis), RNA synthesis stops and protein synthesis is reduced. Cell division takes place after each full cycle is complete.

Cell growth and differentiation are regulated by growth factors which bind to specific receptors on the cell surface. Chemical signals are generated inside the cell, increasing the production of DNA, RNA, or proteins and leading to an increased rate of mitosis.

Malignant transformation

If the delicate control of growth breaks down, cells will continue to divide even though there is no need for further cells of that type. Even if the controls in only one cell break down, that cell can multiply to form an unwanted mass of cells (a *tumour). The different forms of *cancer develop as a result of a series of genetic '*mutations' which increase the rate of growth and independence of cells, and change them from being normal to malignant.

The transformation of normal cells to malignant, cancerous cells can be brought about by mutagenic chemicals, ionizing *radiation, or certain *viruses. Such transformed cells show several differences from normal ones, with the overall characteristic of growing continuously and chaotically without regard for their neighbours. The abnormal characteristics of transformed cells are passed on to succeeding generations of cells.

Tumour cells synthesize and release large amounts of growth-stimulating factors. Some of these can make normal cells malignant; others stimulate the growth of the cells that produced them, which may be important in establishing and maintaining their malignancy.

The cancer-forming viruses transform cells by adding cancer-causing genes (oncogenes) to the DNA of the infected cells, or by causing oncogenes that are already present but latent to become active. The oncogenes act by producing proteins that enhance cell proliferation and growth.

LIZ EVANS
WALTER BODMER

Fig. 2 The stages of cell division.

CELLULITIS is diffuse spreading *inflammation of the connective tissues, often of *streptococcal origin.

CELLULOSE is the basic structural component of cell walls in higher plants and some fungi. It is a complex long-chain *polysaccharide, made up of about 30 000 *glucose units, which is non-digestible and non-absorbable by man, although it is by herbivorous animals. See also FIBRE, DIETARY.

CELSIUS. The degree Celsius or centigrade (°C) temperature scale was originally devised by Anders *Celsius (1701–44) and based on the melting point of ice (0 °C) and the boiling point of water (100 °C). The unit (and therefore expressions of temperature difference) is identical to the kelvin (K), the *SI unit of temperature; the relation between the two is given by: K=°C + 273.15.

CELSIUS, ANDERS (1701–44). Swedish mathematician and astronomer. A thermometer scale of 100 degrees had been in use for some years; Celsius' contribution was to fix two 'constant degrees', the freezing and boiling points of water, and to divide the zone between into 100 degrees. This was called the Swedish scale until 1800, since when it has been known as the Celsius or centigrade scale.

CELSUS, AULUS CORNELIUS (*fl.* AD 25). Roman writer. Celsus, a contemporary of the emperor Tiberius and a member of a noble family, was not medically trained. He compiled an encyclopaedia, of which only the eight books dealing with medicine, *De re medicina*, survive. They were largely translations drawn from many sources. Written in elegant Latin, they describe operative methods, paediatrics and dentistry, and give graphic descriptions of disease. His were the first medical works to be printed, in 1478.

CENSUS. An official enumeration of the population of a country or district with recording of statistics relating to it. See OFFICE OF POPULATION, CENSUSES AND SURVEYS (OPCS).

CENTIGRADE. See CELSIUS.

CENTRAL MIDWIVES' BOARD. A body created in the UK by the first Midwives Act of 1902, which came into operation on 1 April 1910. The Board was required to keep a Roll of certified midwives and to regulate the conditions of their certification and practice. It was at first nominally responsible to the *Privy Council, but in 1919 control of the Board was taken over by the new *Ministry of Health. See also MIDWIVES ACT 1951.

CENTRAL NERVOUS SYSTEM. That part of the nervous system consisting of the *brain and *spinal cord, contained within the *cranium and the *vertebral column, respectively.

CENTRE. A known or putative collection of *nerve cells within the *central nervous system in which control of a particular function resides.

CENTRIFUGE. An instrument which, by means of rapid rotation, applies centrifugal force to samples placed within it, allowing their separation into components according to density.

CEPHALOSPORINS are *antibiotics related to the *penicillins but relatively penicillinase-resistant. The newer cephalosporins are used mainly against Gram-negative organisms. The chief indications for their use are: enterobacterial infections of the urinary and biliary tracts, *gonorrhoea, severe infections with *Haemophilus influenzae* (usually in childhood), and Gram-negative bacillary *meningitis. See also ANTI-INFECTIVE DRUGS.

CEREBELLAR TONSILS. Rounded projections from the inferior surfaces of the cerebellar hemispheres.

CEREBELLUM. That part of the *brain concerned chiefly with the adjustment and co-ordination of movement and with muscle tone and balance. It lies in the posterior cranial fossa behind the brainstem, with which it connects by three pairs of peduncles; it consists of two hemispheres and a central vermis.

CEREBRAL ABSCESS is an *abscess in the substance of the brain. It may be due to local spread of a suppurative infection (particularly in the *middle ear or the *paranasal sinuses); to blood-borne (metastatic) infection from elsewhere in the body (there are particular associations with cyanotic *congenital heart disease and with chronic suppurative pulmonary infections such as *bronchiectasis and *empyema); or it may complicate head injury. The usual clinical presentation is that of an intracranial space-occupying lesion, with focal neurological signs; indications of the pyogenic illness are not always obvious.

CEREBRAL ATROPHY is *atrophy of the cerebral hemispheres.

CEREBRAL BLOOD FLOW. As measured by applying the *Fick principle in which the uptake of a gas (e.g. nitrous oxide) by the brain is determined from the difference between its concentration in arterial and mixed cerebral venous blood samples, cerebral blood flow (CBF) is expressed as volume per 100 g of brain tissue per minute, the value being an average for the brain as a whole. Alternative methods are available for assessing regional differences in flow within the brain.

CEREBRAL COMPRESSION is the compression of brain tissue as a result of increased intracranial pressure, cerebral oedema, tumour, haemorrhage, abscess or other infection, or skull fracture.

CEREBRAL CORTEX. The grey matter which forms the outermost layer of the two *cerebral hemispheres.

CEREBRAL HAEMORRHAGE (HEMORRHAGE). One of the common causes of *stroke or cerebrovascular accident. Major intracerebral haemorrhage leads to sudden impairment of brain function, with acute headache, dizziness, partial or complete loss of consciousness, *hemiplegia, *aphasia, sensory disturbances, and other manifestations depending on the site of bleeding within the brain. Blood often appears in the *cerebrospinal fluid when haemorrhage extends into the *cerebral ventricles or *subarachnoid space. In patients who recover, there is likely to be a greater or lesser degree of permanent neurological deficit as a result of brain tissue destruction. The usual antecedents are *hypertension (present in at least two-thirds of patients) and weakening of arterial walls by *atherosclerosis.

CEREBRAL HEMISPHERES. The right and left halves of the *cerebrum, the largest structures of the *central nervous system. Among other important components, the hemispheres have the cerebral cortex as their outermost layer and enclose the lateral ventricles. See also BRAIN.

CEREBRAL PALSY is any paralysis or other dysfunction due to perinatal damage to the motor areas of the brain. See SPASTIC DIPLEGIA.

CEREBRAL PEDUNCLE. One of the main structures of the *midbrain; essentially the two peduncles are the stalks joining the midbrain to the *cerebral hemispheres.

CEREBRAL THROMBOSIS. *Thrombosis due to *atherosclerosis in arteries (either extracranial or intracranial) supplying the brain accounts for most *strokes, the carotid, middle cerebral, and vertebral arteries being common sites. The extent and duration of interference with cerebral function depend on the area of resultant *ischaemia and/or *infarction of brain tissue, which varies with the size and position of the vessel occluded and the availability of *collateral (anastomotic) blood supply. The clinical manifestations of major cerebral infarction closely resemble those of *cerebral haemorrhage, but cerebral thrombosis also causes many minor and temporary syndromes of cerebral dysfunction.

CEREBRAL TUMOUR normally means intracranial *tumour, that is a *neoplasm within the cranial cavity, whether originating in the brain itself or in its neighbouring structures (*meninges, *cranial nerves, blood vessels, skull bones, and *pituitary and *pineal glands) or resulting from the *metastatic spread of malignant tumours elsewhere in the body (such as primary neoplasms of the lung, breast, kidney, etc.).

The major clinical manifestations of brain tumours are those due to their space-occupying effect (raised intracranial pressure and cerebral compression) together with neurological disturbances which vary with the site of the lesion; unless removed, they are likely to be fatal because of the space-occupying effect, regardless of whether their pathological classification is malignant or benign. That distinction is further blurred by the fact that primary malignant brain tumours rarely metastasize to extracranial sites.

CEREBRAL VENTRICLE. Any of the four cavities within the brain which are continuous with each other, with the central canal of the *spinal cord, and with the *subarachnoid space; and through which *cerebrospinal fluid circulates. They are known as the right and left lateral ventricles, the third ventricle, and the fourth ventricle.

CEREBROSPINAL FEVER. See MENINGOCOCCAL MENINGITIS.

CEREBROSPINAL FLUID (CSF) is the fluid that circulates within the cavity formed by the *cerebral ventricles, the *subarachnoid space, and the central canal of the *spinal cord. Total CSF volume averages 80–120 ml, the fluid being formed by the *choroid plexus and reabsorbed into the venous blood via the *arachnoid *villi. Normal CSF is a clear, colourless fluid with a cell count of not more than $0.005 \times 10^9/l$ (5/mm³) and a *protein concentration averaging 0.24 g/l (range 0.16–0.33 g/l). The pressure, with the subject recumbent, varies between 0.60 and 1.8 kPa (4.5–13.5 mmHg). Examination of the CSF is of diagnostic value in many conditions. A sample is normally obtained by inserting a suitable needle through an intervertebral space (L4–5) into the lumbar subarachnoid space, measuring the pressure, and then withdrawing a sample (*lumbar puncture).

CEREBROVASCULAR ACCIDENT is synonymous with *stroke.

CEREBRUM is a term applied either to the *brain as a whole, or to its uppermost portion made up of the two *cerebral hemispheres connected by the corpus callosum, excluding the *brainstem and *cerebellum.

CERTIFICATION is attestation, usually written, to facts within the knowledge of the responsible person or persons. In medicine it was once widely used in relation to the *certification of insanity, and less often in relation to other diseases. Medical certificates are still used by employers or for claiming sickness benefit, for example.

CERTIFICATION OF INSANITY. Legal protection for the mentally disordered exists in most countries, although detailed provision varies. In England and Wales, the *Mental Health Act of 1959 abolished 'certification' of such patients, and allowed them to be admitted into any hospital. Under the Act, special powers for compulsory admission when necessary may be used, either for observation up to 28 days (Section 25) or for longer periods subject to renewal after 1 year and every 2 years thereafter (Section 26). In either case, application must be made either by the patient's nearest relative, or by the Mental Welfare Officer (employed by the local authority), supported by the medical recommendations of two doctors. In urgent cases, application for detention for up to 72 hours may be made by any relative, or by the Mental Welfare Officer, supported by only one medical recommendation (Section 29). Patients' rights are protected by Mental Health Review Tribunals with legal, medical, and lay members to consider applications for discharge or reclassification of patients detained under Section 26. See also PSYCHIATRY.

CERVICAL SMEAR. An exfoliative cytological staining procedure for examining the uterine *cervix, particularly in the detection and diagnosis of malignant and premalignant conditions. Sometimes called the *Papanicolaou test, cervical smear examination is often used in 'screening' normal women in order to detect carcinoma of the cervix at the earliest and most curable stage.

CERVIX UTERI. The neck of the womb or *uterus, the narrow terminal portion which projects into the *vagina.

CESTODE. *Tapeworm.

CHADWICK, SIR EDWIN (1800–90). British civil servant, barrister, and sanitary reformer. He was a pioneer of sanitary reform whose persistence was not always universally acceptable. He urged registration of the causes of death and competitive examinations for entry to the Civil Service.

CHAGAS, CARLOS RIBEIRO JUSTINIANO (1879–1934). Brazilian physician. Almost by chance he discovered a previously unknown *trypanosome, now known as *Trypanosoma cruzi*, which was causing a hitherto unrecognized illness in children. He is unique in that he described the causal agent, the clinical picture, the insect vector (reduviid bugs), the host, and the epidemiology of what is now called Chagas' disease (South American *trypanosomiasis).

CHAGAS' DISEASE. See CHAGAS; TRYPANOSOMIASIS.

CHAIN, SIR ERNST BORIS (1906–79). Anglo-Russian biochemist. His most important work was carried out with *Florey and led to the isolation and purification of *penicillin. For this he, Florey, and *Fleming were awarded the *Nobel prize in 1945. In 1948 a professorial chair was created for him at the Instituto Superiore di Sanita in Rome. He returned to London in 1961 as professor of biochemistry at Imperial College. He was knighted in 1969. Chain was also an accomplished pianist and gave a recital with his son at Wigmore Hall in 1975.

CHALAZION. A small firm nodule on the eyelid due to chronic inflammation of a *sebaceous gland.

CHAMBERLAYNE, WILLIAM (1619–89). British physician and poet. His best-known works are *Love's victory, a tragi-comedy* (1658) and *Pharonnida, an heroick poem* (1659).

CHAMBERLEN. The Chamberlen family made up a dynasty of obstetricians founded by a French protestant émigré William Chamberlen who settled in Southampton, England, in 1569. His son PETER CHAMBERLEN THE ELDER (d. 1631) trained in Paris and was probably the first to use the short obstetrical forceps, zealously guarded as a family secret for over a hundred years. He moved to London in 1596, became a *barber-surgeon and *accoucheur to the queens of James I and Charles I. He was prosecuted by the Royal College of Physicians of London for prescribing, escaping imprisonment only through the intercession of the Archbishop of Canterbury with the president.

Peter the Elder's brother, PETER CHAMBERLEN THE YOUNGER (1572–1626), was a barber-surgeon and licensed by the Bishop of London to practise *midwifery.

Peter the Younger's son, also PETER CHAMBERLEN (1601–83), trained at Cambridge and Padua. He lectured on anatomy to the barber-surgeons and became physician to the king. Arguments with the RCP over the incorporation of midwives under his presidency led to his being deprived of his fellowship in 1649.

Peter's eldest son, HUGH CHAMBERLEN THE ELDER (?1632–?) trained under *Mauriceau in Paris and translated his textbook. He is thought to have sold the family secret to the Dutch obstetrician, Hendrik van Roonhuysen, in 1692.

Hugh's brother, PAUL CHAMBERLEN (1635–1717), practised as a midwife, but was better known for his '*anodyne necklace'.

HUGH CHAMBERLEN THE YOUNGER (1664–1728), son of Hugh Chamberlen the Elder, studied at Leiden. He practised with success as an obstetrician in London.

CHAMPETIER DE RIBES. See RIBES.

CHAMPNEYS, SIR FRANCIS HENRY, Bt (1848–1930). British obstetrician. He was a strong supporter of the *Midwives Act of 1902 and became the first chairman of the *Central Midwives' Board. Champneys was the first to use Listerian methods in obstetrics and did much to regularize the position of midwives. He was an authority on and composer of church music.

CHANCRE is the primary lesion of *syphilis, occurring at the site of infection, which is usually, though not invariably, the genital region. It begins as a small, hard painless lump any time between 1 and 12 weeks after exposure, and then usually breaks down to become an ulcer with a raised hard border. Regional nodes are enlarged. Healing takes place after some weeks, leaving a small scar.

CHANCROID, also known as 'soft chancre' or 'soft sore' is an infection acquired by venereal contact and usually, apart from inguinal *lymphadenopathy, localized to the genital region. The lesion is macular at first, then pustular, and finally ulcerated. The causal organism is the Gram-negative bacillus *Haemophilus ducreyi*; most infections respond well to *sulphonamides or *tetracycline. Chancroid is much commoner in tropical countries than in Europe and the USA. See SEXUALLY TRANSMITTED DISEASES.

CHAPIN, CHARLES VALUE. See PUBLIC HEALTH IN THE USA.

CHAPLAIN, HOSPITAL. A priest attached to a hospital on a full-time or part-time basis whose main function is the pastoral care of those hospital patients subscribing to his or her faith, although the ministry may extend also to members of staff. Large hospitals may have several chaplains of different denominations. Although it is usual for chaplains to be employed and paid by the hospital, they are authorized or licensed by the appropriate religious authority; and they remain largely independent of formal hospital hierarchies.

CHARCOT, JEAN MARTIN (1825–93). French neurologist. At the Salpêtrière, he created the greatest neurological clinic of the day; he attracted pupils destined to become leaders in this field; and he set about classifying diseases of the nervous system. His innumerable, original observations were not limited to neurology. He described the Charcot–Leyden crystals of asthmatic sputum (1853); the 'lightning pains' of *tabes dorsalis (1866); the scanning speech, intention tremor, and nystagmus of *multiple sclerosis (Charcot's triad, 1866); neuropathic *arthropathy (Charcot's joints, 1868); the recurrent fever of obstructive *cholangitis (Charcot's intermittent hepatic fever, 1877); and familial peroneal muscular atrophy (Charcot–Marie–Tooth's syndrome, 1886). He also made use of *hypnosis in treating hysterics. He left a record of his observations in *Leçons sur les maladies du système nerveux faites à la Salpêtrière* (5 vols, 1872–87). He was an authority on art as well as being an accomplished painter himself.

CHARING CROSS HOSPITAL AND MEDICAL SCHOOL. Founded together in 1818 by Benjamin Golding, Charing Cross Hospital and Medical School comprise one of London's major medical teaching institutions, with a current annual intake of about 120 undergraduate students. For 150 years the hospital and school occupied a central London site close to the present Charing Cross railway station, a mansion in Villiers Street having first been acquired (1823) and organized as a General Infirmary and Dispensary. It was replaced not long afterwards (1834) by a larger building on the same site. Eventually the hospital and medical school transferred to a new building in 1973, retaining the Charing Cross name.

In 1984, in accordance with the general policy of the University of London on the reorganization of medical education a merger was arranged between the Charing Cross Medical School and the Westminister Medical School.

CHARITE HOSPITAL, BERLIN. The Charité Hospital, now the teaching hospital of the Humboldt University of Berlin has a long and distinguished history dating from the beginning of the 18th century. The original structure was demolished and replaced in 1797, and there followed a series of reconstructions, renovations, and additions to the buildings which took place at intervals throughout the 19th century and into the present century. The Charité established itself as the leading centre of medical science in the German-speaking world, and one of the most important in Europe, positions it continued to occupy until the advent of the Nazi regime in the 1930s. A selection of the great names of medicine associated with the Charité during this period includes Johannes *Mueller; Emil *Dubois-Reymond; Rudolf *Virchow; Albrecht von *Graefe; Wilhelm *Griesinger; Robert *Koch; Ludwig *Traube; August *Bier; Ferdinand *Sauerbruch; Friedrich *Krause; and a number of others only little less deserving of mention. A modern reconstruction with the provision of new buildings took place during 1976–82.

CHARITIES ACT 1960. The UK Charities Act of 1960 repealed most earlier legislation relating to charities (including medical charities), and now contains almost all the statutory provisions. In addition, it introduced a number of reforms. Restrictions on the holding of land by charities were abolished; a public central register of all charities was established; and co-operation between charities and the state welfare service was facilitated. Under the Act, the Charity Commissioners have power to advise, assist, and control charities.

CHARLATAN. A pretender to medical skill or knowledge, a medical impostor, a quack.

CHARMS are magical formulae, often verses, which when said or sung are supposed to ward off evil, or bring good luck. When worn in written form about the person, a charm is called an amulet.

CHARNLEY, SIR JOHN (1911–82). English surgeon. Although best known for his pioneering contributions to operations for replacement of the hip joint, Charnley had already contributed notably to *orthopaedic surgery in his work on compression arthrodesis, and with his book on *The closed treatment of common fractures* (1950). For his work on *hip replacement, he supplemented his surgical skill by meticulous studies on engineering, on materials science, and on the control of infection during surgical operations.

CHAUFFARD, ANATOLE MARIE EMILE (1855–1932). French physician. He was one of the earlier physicians to combine clinical and laboratory interests. He published one of the first complete accounts of *haemochromatosis and described juvenile *rheumatoid arthritis (Chauffard–Still–Felty syndrome, 1896) and familial spherocytosis (congenital acholuric *jaundice of Chauffard and Minkowski, 1900).

CHAULIAC, GUY DE (c. 1300–68). French surgeon. De Chauliac was the most eminent surgeon of the 14th century, and a writer of great learning. His book *Chirurgia magna*, written in 1363, was first printed in 1498 and was regarded as authoritative for at least a century afterwards. In it he advocated early excision of cancer, the treatment of fractures with slings and traction, and operations for *hernia and *cataract. He had many distinguished patients, including Jean of Luxemburg, the blind king of Bohemia (1336), Pope Clement VI (1342) at Avignon, and his successors Innocent VI and Urban V.

CHEIROPRAXIS. See CHIROPRACTIC.

CHEKHOV, ANTON PAVLOVICH (1860–1904). Russian writer and physician. He started writing when a student and practised medicine only during the *cholera epidemic of 1892–93. His best-known plays are *The Seagull* (1896), *Uncle Vanya* (1899), and *The Cherry Orchard* (1904) (also see MEDICAL TRUANTS).

CHELATING AGENT. A chemical agent that forms a closed ring of atoms engulfing a central polyvalent metal ion. Such agents have the property of 'locking up' (sequestering) unwanted metal ions; for example they are added to shampoos to soften water by sequestering ferric, calcium, and magnesium ions. Chelating agents are of therapeutic value in treating *poisoning with heavy metals; examples are *dimercaprol, *penicillamine, and sodium calcium edetate, all of which promote, for example, the elimination of lead and are useful in *lead poisoning.

CHEMICAL PATHOLOGY is a term, now somewhat *démodé*, broadly equivalent to 'clinical *chemistry'.

CHEMICAL WARFARE, as exemplified by the use of poisonous gases or fumes, has a long history extending from the pre-Christian era through the Middle Ages to modern times. In the First World War, Germany was the first to use poison gas, in the Ypres salient on 22 April 1915, when an attack was launched with a mixture of *chlorine and *phosgene; from then on gas was employed by both sides, *mustard gas being the most dangerous. At the Washington Conference in 1922 the great powers agreed to prohibit the use of asphyxiating and poisonous gas warfare and none was employed in the Second World War. Gas was used by the Americans in 1965 against the North Vietnamese, but this was mainly of the non-lethal variety employed by the police of many countries in riot control. However the defoliant Agent Orange was also used there.

Newer and more potent forms of chemical warfare (e.g. the group of *anticholinesterase substances or '*nerve gases') are now known, and more will undoubtedly be discovered.

CHEMISTRY, CLINICAL
Introduction and history
Virtually all diseases in the human result in chemical changes within the cells of the body, and as a result there is frequently a change in the chemical composition of body fluids, particularly blood and urine. Such fluids can be collected and chemically analysed to ascertain whether changes show a particular disease state. The analyses usually involve quantitative measurement to ascertain the concentration of particular substances. The chemical analysis of body fluids is the province of the clinical chemist, who has a central role in modern *medical practice.

Observing chemical change in urine in disease has a long history. *Hippocrates taught the importance of observing the physical appearance of urine in terms of colour, consistency, and sediment. A Hindu, Ayus Veda, first reported, in AD 500, that urine from diabetics attracted insects because of its glucose ('sugar') content.

Although the term 'clinical chemistry' is now accepted internationally, different terms have been used since the 19th century—physiological chemistry, clinical *biochemistry, and, uniquely in the UK and some former colonies, chemical *pathology. These terms reflect the sources of some of the disciplines that have contributed to modern clinical chemistry practice: chemistry, *physiology, biochemistry, and pathology.

The specialty is predominantly practised within a laboratory providing a service to hospital patients, either as an autonomous laboratory or as a part of the hospital's pathology laboratory. The subject's beginnings were the result of *physicians in various parts of the world recruiting chemists to perform quantitative chemical analyses on blood and urine. Such services were not available in the conventional pathology laboratory, which specialized particularly in histopathology (*pathology) and *microbiology.

An early and classical example of such recruitment was that of Donald Van *Slyke by Dr Rufus *Cole, a physician at the Hospital of the Rockefeller Institute in New York in 1914. The clinical staff of the hospital obviously considered that chemical analysis of patients' fluids was potentially of importance in diagnosis and the monitoring of treatment. They did not direct Van Slyke's studies, but his reading of *physiology and medical textbooks indicated that there were many common clinical conditions, such as kidney disease and *diabetes, which resulted in excess acid in the blood. The acids responsible were different in the two conditions, but both resulted in a lowering of the bicarbonate concentration in the blood, which was known to preserve the organism from excess acid production by neutralization of the acid. Van Slyke devised elegant methods for measuring bicarbonate in blood. The methods were then used in the diagnosis and monitoring of treatment, helping in understanding the metabolic processes of these two common disease conditions, and preventing death in many patients.

Van Slyke's work up to 1920, and also the work of Folin and Wu in the USA, produced a number of analytical methods with considerable potential in aiding clinical *diagnosis and treatment, but there were few individuals in clinical laboratories capable of exploiting them. A strong stimulus was required. This was provided by the discovery of *insulin as an effective treatment for lowering the blood glucose ('sugar') level in diabetics. This treatment involved measurement of the patient's blood glucose, which led physicians to recruit chemists to the earliest established clinical chemistry laboratories. In the UK the first quantitative measurement of blood glucose was carried out in the laboratory of the Manchester Royal Infirmary in October 1921. Thus the wide practice of clinical chemistry began. Clinical chemistry laboratories were established in Edinburgh, Manchester, London, and Birmingham in the UK, many others in the USA and Europe.

By the 1930s the number and different types of analyses performed had increased twentyfold. The first textbooks on the subject began to appear in the 1930s. By the start of the Second World War the establishment of clinical chemistry laboratories, and the recruitment of clinical chemists, had become widespread. The types of analysis performed had increased to approximately 40 and involved analyses to aid in the diagnosis and treatment of *thyroid disease, diabetes, *renal disease, vomiting and diarrhoea, *gout, bone disease, *gastric ulceration, bleeding in the alimentary canal, *liver disease, *meningitis, and *pancreatic disease. Estimation of the blood level of *sulphonamide drugs in *monitoring the treatment of infection was also introduced.

The subject did not progress significantly during the war years.

By the 1950s the development of the subject was taking place in university departments and the larger hospitals in the USA, Scandinavia, UK, Holland, and Australia; Germany was recovering from its wartime problems. The number of hospitals with clinical chemistry laboratories grew steadily. Particularly in the USA, private laboratories, not necessarily attached to a hospital, became established, and some were considerable commercial undertakings. Throughout the next two decades expenditure on health care grew dramatically as it paralleled the general increase in the standard of living, encompassing dramatic developments in clinical science. Clinical chemistry played an integral part in such developments. Medical conditions were identified in scientific terms and treated on the basis of a better understanding of the chemical basis of the disease state. Better methods for the investigation of such common conditions as diabetes, renal, bone, liver, and endocrine diseases were devised, leading to better treatment and monitoring of such conditions. There was also a considerable increase in the understanding of inherited diseases, such as *cystic fibrosis.

During the past 40 years emphasis has been on the devising of new methods of chemical analysis, based upon clinical need but with the equally important driving force of technological innovation, particularly in terms of new apparatus.

The following is a description of the principal technological innovations with which clinical chemistry has been involved or has instigated.

Photoelectric colorimetry
Even up to the present time, many clinical chemistry techniques involve combining the analyte that is to be determined with a reagent that produces colour, the amount of colour being proportional to the concentration of the analyte. In the early days the colour was read by eye, now sophisticated photoelectric *colorimeters are used. Many methods are highly sensitive, involving the use of as little as 10 microlitres (μl) of blood serum, thus making such tests possible in paediatric practice.

Flame photometry
This technique enables the concentration of sodium and potassium *ions in body fluids to be determined in a matter of minutes. It replaced techniques that took several hours. Such a technological innovation had a dramatic effect on the treatment of acute dehydration by diarrhoea and vomiting, particularly in young children.

Chromatography
Chromatographic techniques, initially introduced in the late 1940s, allow the separation of substances present in biological fluids, so that they can be specifically identified. This technique has been of particular benefit

in the investigation and treatment of *inborn errors of metabolism.

Radioimmunoassay

In 1953 Yalow and Berson, in the USA, introduced a technique which revolutionized a considerable area of clinical chemistry, and as a result had a dramatic effect on clinical medicine. Using the well-known reaction between a *protein (*antigen) and its *antibody, and by labelling either the protein or the antibody with radioactive iodine, they were able to measure antigen or antibody concentration. With further developments and modifications the technique has become an integral part of clinical medicine, including research endeavour, throughout the world.

Blood gas analysis

The introduction in 1960 of the Astrup technique for blood gas analysis was an important milestone in the discipline of clinical chemistry. This development took place in the Clinical Chemistry Department of the Rigshospitalet, Copenhagen. Following a catastrophic outbreak of *poliomyelitis in that city in 1953, Poul Astrup and his colleagues recognized that laboratory methods of assessment of patients on respirators were poor. They combined with the Radiometer Company to produce the Radiometer Astrup Microequipment for blood acid–base measurement. Using this apparatus complete acid–base assessment of patients, from fingerprick quantities of blood was made possible—an outstanding development. The technique has importance in a wide variety of diseases, including diabetic coma, renal and gastrointestinal disease, pulmonary disease, and the monitoring of patients during *anaesthesia.

Automation

Probably the most outstanding contribution to clinical chemistry over the last 40 years, in relation to its efficiency and managerial organization, and its ability to deal with workloads which doubled every 5 years, was the invention by Leonard Skeggs (a clinical chemist from Cleveland, USA) of the continuous-flow analyser. This was marketed by the Technicon Corporation of New York as the AutoAnalyzer and is in use to this day in a variety of forms throughout the world. Before its introduction in my laboratory in 1960 it would take a technician about 4 hours to carry out 30 serum *creatinine determinations, a test of renal function. The work was demanding and labour-intensive. The first AutoAnalyzer could perform these analyses in 1 hour. Each specimen was loaded into the apparatus, specimen and reagents were carried through plastic tubes to a colorimeter, and the level of creatinine in each specimen was recorded as a peak on a flow chart. Little use of technical labour was combined with better results in terms of accuracy and precision. Gradually during the 1960s virtually all the commonly used clinical chemistry determinations could be analysed on AutoAnalyzers.

More recently a number of automatic clinical chemistry analysers have been introduced by companies such as Hitachi and Toshiba. Automatic analysis is now an integral part of clinical chemistry practice.

Computers

Finance departments were the first to use computers in the provision of health care, but in the mid-1960s clinical chemists began to realize that the fast output of analytical results resulted in a log-jam of data, which could be solved only by the use of the digital computer. Computers to collect, record, report, and store patient results are now an integral part of even the smallest clinical chemistry laboratory.

The present-day clinical chemistry laboratory

In summary, the role of a clinical chemistry laboratory based in a hospital, the commonest situation, is as follows. Following history taking and clinical examinations, the clinicians looking after patients request the laboratory to carry out analyses on patients' specimens. The type of analysis requested is based upon the clinician's requirement to aid his clinical assessment and judgement by quantitative chemical analysis. The specimen is collected either by a doctor, nurse, or specially trained personnel, and dispatched to the laboratory with the clinician's request for analysis. The results are then communicated to the clinician who originally requested them.

Sometimes under special circumstances the laboratory staff advise the clinician on which tests are most appropriate for a particular patient or disease state, and may also help in interpretation.

Quality assurance

Clinical chemistry laboratories have a four-decade history of the use of quality assurance techniques, and thus clinical chemistry has been in the forefront of what are now described as techniques of audit, assessing excellence in professional practice.

Techniques of internal quality control based upon industrial quality control techniques are now commonplace in clinical chemistry laboratories. In addition, virtually all clinical chemistry laboratories are subjected to external quality assessment. They receive specimens with concentrations of analytes unknown to them and, after performing analyses on such specimens, the results are returned to a central agency. They are judged on their performance. Such techniques were pioneered in the USA; in at least two states performance had to be shown to be satisfactory if a laboratory was to continue to practise.

In the UK the present scheme was introduced in 1969, sponsored by the Department of Health; surveys are conducted every 2 weeks throughout the year, involving over 500 laboratories. The surveys are made by the Wolfson Research Laboratories in Birmingham and the

Department of Clinical Chemistry, Edinburgh Royal Infirmary. This scheme is not involved in any legislation regarding the licensing of laboratories, but represents an educational process to inform laboratories concerning the quality of their performance compared with that of others. The provision of information is meant to help those laboratories not performing well to perform better. Laboratories that do not perform satisfactorily are reported to a panel of four professional clinical chemists, who then try to help the poorly performing laboratory to improve its quality assurance.

Types of staff employed
This varies from country to country but, in general, involves graduate staff, both medically and scientifically qualified, and technicians. Medical graduates usually follow an undergraduate medical training followed by postgraduate training in clinical chemistry; this may involve a training period lasting 8 years. Science graduates enter with a degree in chemistry, biochemistry, or biological sciences and usually a Ph.D. followed by a training period lasting 5 years. Technicians, sometimes called technologists or, in the UK, medical laboratory scientific officers (MLSO), may enter without a degree but are subjected to at least 6 years of formal training.

Professional organizations
The international body responsible for the subject is the International Federation of Clinical Chemistry; it was formed in 1952 and has about 50 national member organizations. Many countries have national associations for clinical chemistry. Their objectives are frequently to represent the discipline professionally and also to organize scientific communication and collaboration.

The American Association of Clinical Chemists was founded in 1950 and has approximately 5000 members. The UK Association of Clinical Biochemists was founded in 1953 and has over 1500 members.

The examining body for medical doctors and scientists in the UK is the Royal College of Pathologists. For medical laboratory scientific officers it is the Institute of Biomedical Science (formerly called the Institute of Medical Laboratory Scientists).

T. P. WHITEHEAD

CHEMORECEPTORS are sensory end-organs responsive to chemical stimuli. The chemoreceptors include those responsible for *taste and *smell perception as well as those within the circulation which respond to changes in *blood gas tensions and *hydrogen ion concentration.

CHEMOTAXIS. The locomotor movement of an organism or cell in response to a directional chemical stimulus, i.e. either towards or away from its concentration gradient. An example is the movement of *polymorph leucocytes towards bacteria in response to

substances released by the reaction between the bacteria and *complement, part of the *inflammatory reaction.

CHEMOTHERAPY is treatment, particularly of infections and malignant disease, with chemical agents selectively directed against invading organisms or abnormal cells. See ANTIMETABOLITES; ANTINEOPLASTIC CHEMOTHERAPY; INFECTIOUS DISEASES; PHARMACOLOGY; SULPHONAMIDES.

CHERNOBYL. The purpose of the radioactivity in a nuclear power station is to heat water. As in coal-fired power stations, the steam that results drives turbines which produce electricity. On 26 April 1986, there was a serious accident in the nuclear power station 10 miles from the city of Chernobyl, then part of the Soviet Union. Owing to failure to observe safety regulations (Western experts also blame the reactor design) the normal chain reaction in the radioactive core of one of the four reactors was insufficiently controlled. As a result, steam pressure rose to dangerous levels: there were several explosions and a fire that took several hours to put out, and large amounts of radioactive material were scattered over a wide area and into the atmosphere (later descending in a very dilute and relatively harmless form as fallout and in rain all over the world).

At the reactor there were two instant deaths and 29 later ones—mostly firefighters who were very close to the escaping radiation for an hour or more. In addition, about 150 others at the reactor site suffered *radiation effects of varying severity. Contrary to first reports, there were no deaths or injuries (or radiation effects) among the 50 000 people living in the town of Pripyat near the power station, but very large numbers of people over a wider area were exposed to dilute radiation of varying amounts (International Atomic Energy Agency 1991).

At first it was felt that the radiation levels to which the local population were exposed were not high enough to justify the disruption and hardship of mass evacuation. But then it was feared that there could be further releases of radioactivity and, in view of this—and because of strong public fears—it was decided 48 hours later that the local population should be evacuated. Finally, about 135 000 people were evacuated and rehoused outside a 30 km exclusion zone. This decision does not mean that it is actually dangerous (in the sense that most people use the word) to be inside this zone. The remaining reactors continue to produce electricity and the risk to the workforce is small. In addition, the sensible and humane decision has been taken to allow some old people to return to their homes.

In an accident of this kind, those very close for any appreciable length of time may be in great danger, due mainly to radiation burns and impairment of the ability of the bone marrow to maintain a normal supply of blood cells. The actual risk depends on the amount (more correctly, the concentration) of the radiation, the time exposed, the type of radiation, and many other factors needing expert assessment. Only a short distance away (a few hundred yards or less) the now much less concentrated radiation carries for each individual little or no risk of any immediate harm, but a small risk to future health.

This risk is of three main kinds, which should be neither exaggerated nor minimized (Brewin 1992). First, each exposed person is very slightly more likely to get some kind of cancer in later life than they would have been if there had been no accident. One way to get this into some kind of perspective is to compare it with the tobacco risk, both risks having been well studied for many years. There are three main differences:

1. The size of the dilute radiation risk is likely to be considerably less than the risk of even very modest cigarette smoking.
2. Unlike tobacco-related *cancers, where most are unlikely to be cured, at least one-half of radiation-induced cancers will be curable.
3. Unlike the effect of cigarette smoking, even the worst possible estimated effect of the Chernobyl accident will be too small to have any detectable effect on national or international cancer *mortality *statistics.

The second kind of risk is theoretically that of a slight increase in the normal incidence of birth defects due to genetic abnormalities, as a result of radiation to the testicles of future fathers or to the ovaries of future mothers. This has not occurred in the children or the grandchildren of survivors of the 1945 nuclear bombing of Japan, but it remains a theoretical risk. A second cause of birth defects, radiation of the unborn child in early pregnancy, occurred in Japan, but did not occur after Chernobyl, presumably because of the much lower dose received by the local population as a result of the Chernobyl accident. Occasional media stories and photos of individual cases of birth defects are unhelpful, since such cases can be found in any community. As with cancer, or any other ill effect, only a true numerical comparison can say whether or not there has been any increase in the normal incidence of birth defects.

As regards the general health of those living near the reactor at the time of the accident this is unlikely to show any radiation effects. The amount of radiation is too small. Several independent international bodies have confirmed this. For example, several years after the accident, when comparisons were made with similar populations (exposed to far less radiation), no differences were found in general health (nor in the amount of cancer, nor in the number or birth defects). A possible exception needing further evaluation is the preliminary report (Baverstock *et al.* 1992) of a significant increase in cancer of the *thyroid in children, one child having died (most cases of thyroid cancer in children do not cause ill-health or death).

What can be done to minimize harm to exposed populations after such an accident from nuclear power or nuclear weapons? The exposure is of three main types: from skin contact, from breathing, and from food or drink. Where there is radioactive material in the air those who don't need to be out of doors can reduce what is probably only a small risk still further by staying indoors as much as possible in the first few days. Secondly, if there is radioactive iodine in the fallout, iodine tablets taken as soon as possible will reduce the amount of radiation taken up by the thyroid gland. This is because the thyroid gland is virtually the only part of the body that needs iodine and if it has enough normal iodine for its needs, the radioactive iodine is unwanted and is excreted in the urine.

The combined effects of mass relocation of populations (to protect them from small risks) and of fears for the future have caused great distress and hardship. The international advisory committee commented 5 years after the accident that in its view both the relocation of populations and the food restrictions after this tragic accident should have been less extensive. But intense public anxiety remains, and it is not easy to balance all the conflicting dangers and fears.

THURSTAN BREWIN

References

Baverstock, K., Egloff, B., Pinchera, A., Ruchti, C., and Williams, D. (1992). Thyroid cancer after Chernobyl (letter). *Nature*, **359**, 21–2.

Brewin, T. B. (1992). Excessive fear of dilute radiation. *Journal of the Royal Society of Medicine*, **85**, 311–13.

International Atomic Energy Agency (1991). *The International Chernobyl Project. Assessment of radiological consequence and evaluation of protective measures*. International Atomic Energy Agency, Vienna.

CHESELDEN, WILLIAM (1688–1752). British surgeon and anatomist. He devised his celebrated lateral operation for *stone in 1729. He wrote *Anatomy of the human body (1713)* and *Osteographia (1733)*.

CHEST MEDICINE. Chest medicine today is a dynamic, popular, and growing subspecialty, strongly orientated towards pulmonary physiology and critical (*intensive) care. Chest physicians, sometimes called pulmonologists, are also unavoidably concerned with lung diseases causally related to *smoking—lung cancer, chronic *bronchitis, and *emphysema. Their other major interests consist in *occupational and *environmental problems, including urban air *pollution, *hypersensitivity phenomena involving the lung, the diagnosis of obscure lung diseases, and the evaluation of respiratory impairment and disability (see CLINICAL INVESTIGATION).

The origins of chest medicine, however, were different. *Tuberculosis, especially of the lungs, provided the stimulus: early on, the diagnosis and treatment of *pneumonia, lung *abscess, emphysema, and *bronchiectasis were more the responsibility of general physicans than of tuberculosis specialists (Keers 1978).

Tuberculosis

Tuberculosis has been a major cause of illness and death in man and in animals since earliest recorded history. However, the disease did not become the responsibility of a special group of physicians until awareness of its transmissibility was well established. *Villemin produced tuberculosis in animals by *inoculating them with cheesy material from the lungs of humans who had died of the disease. This was in 1868, 14 years before *Koch's stunning discovery in 1882 that tiny micro-organisms found in the cheesy material caused tuberculosis.

The diagnosis of lung disease was greatly enhanced by three other discoveries: (1) *percussion by *Auenbrugger in 1761; (2) the *stethoscope by *Laënnec in 1824; and (3) the *X-ray by *Roentgen in 1895. None of these had immediate widespread impact, however. Auenbrugger's *Inventum novum* was not translated from Latin until 1824; Laennec's stethoscope was not broadly accepted for at least two or three generations; and it was not until 1910-15 that chest X-rays (radiographs) came into relatively common use (see RADIOLOGY). Even then, reluctance to accept X-ray observations was common: at the 1918 meeting of the US National Tuberculosis Association, leading authorities maintained that 'annular shadows' seen on the chest X-rays could not be cavities as the characteristic physical signs of cavitation could not be elicited in the overlying area of the chest; they were regarded initially as interlobar pockets of *pneumothorax.

Before Laënnec died of tuberculosis at the age of 42, he made a painstaking and remarkably accurate correlation of post-mortem findings with the symptoms, clinical course, and the physical findings of various lung diseases, including emphysema, a study initiated by Bayle (1774–1816).

Hermann Brehmer believed that fresh air was beneficial for tuberculosis, and created in 1826 the first hospital or *sanatorium exclusively for the care of the disease; it was located in Görbersdorf in the mountains of southern Germany. Peter Dettweiler in 1876 made further progress by adding rest to the fresh-air regimen promulgated by Brehmer.

Meanwhile, in 1841 in England, the Hospital for Consumption was founded in a London suburb by remodelling an existing building. A new building was added in 1846, another in 1854; this institution later became the *Brompton Hospital (Bishop 1967). Presumably the Brompton did not care for much except tuberculosis until its rural affiliate, Frimley Tuberculosis Sanatorium, was built in 1904. Without doubt, the Brompton became the world's first general chest hospital.

The world's first out-patient tuberculosis *clinic was started in Edinburgh in 1887 by Sir Robert *Philip. In addition, together with Rist in France, he reorganized the International Union Against Tuberculosis in 1922.

The migration—and later banishment—of tuberculosis from cities to the mountains was prompted by realization of the infectious nature of the disease; general awareness of this fact took at least two or three generations after Koch's discovery in 1882. For some time thereafter, tuberculosis patients were regarded virtually as lepers.

Edward L. *Trudeau founded the first US tuberculosis sanatorium in the Adirondack mountains in 1884, and he began laboratory research on the disease in Saranac Lake, NY, at the same time.

*Artificial pneumothorax was first used to treat pulmonary tuberculosis by Forlanini in Italy in 1894; it was also introduced independently by an American surgeon, John B. *Murphy, in 1898. *Thoracoplasty, the most effective method for treating the condition before *chemotherapy, was systematized and made practical by *Sauerbruch and others in the early 1900s. Lung *resection for tuberculosis, which reached its zenith under chemotherapeutic coverage in the late 1950s and early 1960s, was introduced by *Tuffier in 1891.

Chemotherapy

Three unrelated discoveries accounted in different ways for the metamorphosis of tuberculosis treatment into modern chest medicine: (1) effective antituberculosis chemotherapy, begun with the discovery of *streptomycin by *Waksman in 1944 and of *para-aminosalicylic acid (PAS) by Lehmann in 1946; (2) the *spirometer by *Hutchinson at the Brompton in 1846; and (3) the cigarette early in the 20th century.

While streptomycin and PAS provided a promising start, *isoniazid, introduced in 1952, was a major breakthrough (Fig. 1). It had been synthesized many years before, but its remarkable antituberculous properties came to light much later. It took a few years to learn how to derive maximum benefit from streptomycin, PAS, and isoniazid, and from other 'wonder' drugs later discovered. Effective chemotherapy has greatly simplified and shortened the treatment of tuberculosis, has reduced its incidence, and has even threatened to put many lung physicians and surgeons out of work.

After more than 70 years, the *spirometer was rediscovered in the early 20th century: this led to the science of modern pulmonary physiology and thus improved diagnosis, therapy, and understanding of complex pulmonary problems. The rigid *bronchoscope was introduced. Meanwhile, radiology was expanding and its quality and technique were improving steadily. Bronchograms (see BRONCHOGRAPHY) and body section films (planigrams; tomograms (see TOMOGRAPHY)) also added greatly to diagnosis.

The greatest impetus to chest medicine was when the tobacco companies made it much easier, cheaper, and socially acceptable to smoke, by inventing the cigarette; cigarettes soon overtook cigars, chewing tobacco, and

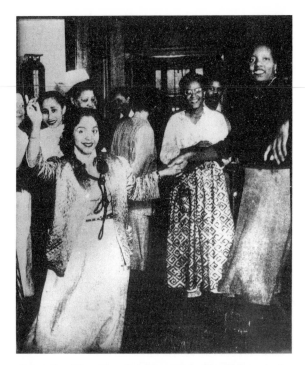

Fig. 1 Sea View Hospital, New York City. Tuberculosis patients dancing in a ward, happy with the results of their isoniazid treatment. (Reproduced from *Life* magazine, 3 March 1952)

snuff. Cigarettes were in common use by men by the 1920s: the adverse effects first became manifest 20–30 years later, in the 1940s and 1950s. The same process is now occurring in women.

The institution best prepared to switch into modern pulmonology in the UK was the Brompton and its affiliated Institute of Diseases of the Chest, now the Cardiothoracic Institute. In the US the way was led by *Bellevue Hospital in New York City, where James Alexander Miller established a tuberculosis service in 1903. These institutions deserve major credit for the evolution of chest medicine to its present status, the first under the leadership of J. Guyett Scadding and the latter under J. Burns Amberson. During this period, needle, *lymph node, and open lung *biopsies enabled us to identify various new diseases and treat them more effectively.

The gradual definition of truly effective antituberculosis chemotherapy required considerable, often cooperative, clinical research. One of the first controlled studies, by Amberson and associates at Bellevue Hospital, clearly established that *gold therapy (sanocrysin) was totally ineffective against tuberculosis. Beginning in the 1950s, dozens of clinical trials of various drug regimens were carried out. One of the earliest, by the British *Medical Research Council, showed conclusively that isoniazid and streptomycin together were far more effective (due to less drug resistance) when

streptomycin was given daily instead of twice weekly. Other agencies in the UK, in Europe, in the USA (US Public Health Service, US Veterans Administration—Armed Forces), and later India (the Tuberculosis Chemotherapy Centre in Madras), all performed highly productive co-operative studies of chemotherapy regimens. Lung surgery, especially resection, expanded when it became clear that chemotherapy prevented postsurgical tuberculous complications. And surgical cases benefited greatly from preoperative physiological evaluation. But in due course, it became clear that preoperative chemotherapy was so effective that surgery was seldom necessary.

Advances in *microbiology, especially the new-found ability (beginning in the 1930s) to culture *mycobacteria from *sputum, resected tissue, and other sources, enabled microbiologists to identify several mycobacterial diseases other than typical tuberculosis (Runyon 1959).

Thus, physicians specializing in treating tuberculosis became interested in the rapidly developing radiology, microbiology, physiology, pathology, anatomy, and other methods of studying the lungs in health and disease between 1900 and 1960. *Empyema, lung abscess, and bronchiectasis, all complications of pneumonia before the advent of sulfapyridine (1938), *penicillin (1941), and other antipneumonia chemotherapy, occurred far less often, to be replaced by a virtual epidemic of lung cancer, chronic bronchitis, and emphysema.

Chronic bronchitis

Not many years ago—at least in the USA—chronic bronchitis was not considered a distinct disease; it was regarded simply as a symptom—i.e. any chronic cough resulting from many causes. But, following British work, it was found in the USA in the late 1950s that chronic bronchitis is a major disease capable of causing disability and premature death (Mitchell 1961).

Carcinoma of the lung

This condition is also one with which chest physicians are concerned in relation to diagnosis and management. However, surgical treatment is the province of the *cardiothoracic surgeon, and other treatment is usually supervised by the radiotherapist and/or oncologist.

Asthma

Bronchial *asthma is an important disease which, like tuberculosis, has always been with us. For centuries it was treated by general physicians, and only became a concern, and then a responsibility, of the chest physician, after tuberculosis was controlled. Other reasons for this development include expanding knowledge of *immunology, frequent confusion of asthma with chronic bronchitis and emphysema, and the many tuberculosis physicians with less and less to do.

Immunology had its origin with Koch's demonstration of tuberculin hypersensitivity in 1890, and von *Pirquet's observation in 1905 that the introduction of a foreign substance, such as an infectious agent, into animal tissue could alter its capacity to react to subsequent applications of the same material. Gerald Webb (1871–1948), a leading tuberculosis specialist in his day, was a founder and the first President of the American Association of Immunologists. Today, many obscure lung diseases are either known or suspected to be due to *hypersensitivity. Thus hypersensitivity lung diseases and asthma constitute an important part of modern chest medicine.

Chest medicine as a specialty

The American Board of Internal Medicine, created in 1936, added a 'Pulmonary Disease' subspecialty board in 1940. Diplomates of the parent Board seeking certification were fewer than a dozen per year for the first 10–15 years. However, interest accelerated to the point where 750–1000 candidates per year sought certification in 1980, 1981, and 1982; some 65–75 per cent of candidates are currently being certified.

The National Heart Act was passed by the US Congress in 1948. *National Institutes of Health funds for research and training in lung disease became available. Responding to pressure from the American Thoracic Society and the American College of Chest Physicians, the National Heart Institute became the National Heart and Lung (and soon thereafter also, Blood) Institute in 1969.

The new US specialty of chest medicine was found to be short of manpower. In 1973 five of the 102 US medical schools had no faculty members concerned with chest disease training or research, 12 had only one full-time equivalent (FTE), 15 had only two, and 70 had fewer than five; it was estimated that 4327 pulmonologists were needed, whereas fewer than 2000 were available in 1973.

A review of the origin and development of some of the societies and the most widely circulated journals throws light on the early days of chest medicine. In the USA, the *American Review of Tuberculosis* began in 1917; *Pulmonary Disease* was added to its title in 1955, and it became the *American Review of Respiratory Disease* in 1959. After a few years of heated discussion, the American 'Trudeau' Society changed its name to the American Thoracic Society in 1960, to reflect the changes in the interests and work of its members.

The American College of Chest Physicians and its journal *Diseases of the Chest* (changed to *Chest* in 1970) were founded in 1935. The *British Journal of Tuberculosis* was founded in 1907, added *Diseases of the Chest* to its title in 1943, and became the *British Journal of Diseases of the Chest* in 1959.

In the UK, the journal *Thorax* was established many years ago and the history of the Thoracic Society and British Thoracic Association, later amalgamated to form the British Thoracic Society, was summarized in *Thorax* by J.G. Scadding in 1983. The *Canadian Lung Association Bulletin* was founded in 1927. The *Acta Tuberculosea Scandinavica* was founded in 1925; it became the

Acta Tuberculosea et Pneumonologica in 1961 and the *Scandinavian* (later *European*) *Journal of Respiratory Disease* in 1979. *Respiration* (Basel) was founded in 1944. The *Revue de Tuberculose et de Pneumologie* was founded in 1893; it became the *Revue Française des Maladies Respiratoires* in 1897; this French journal was clearly the oldest concerned with both tuberculosis and general chest medicine.

US pulmonary training programmes became popular in the 1970s. By 1981, the manpower situation in the USA had changed remarkably: a study by the US Department of Health and Human Services revealed not only that shortages had been corrected, but a surplus (the largest for all medical subspecialties) of more than 3500 might exist by 1990 if no changes occurred.

Pulmonary physiology

The history of clinical pulmonary physiology is closely intertwined with the specialty of chest medicine. Hutchinson's spirometer was not employed in clinical medicine until the 1940s. Practical pulmonary physiology was greatly enhanced by the introduction of many new techniques such as the *pH meter for blood, the 'Riley bubble' method of measuring oxygen and carbon dioxide, *cardiac (pulmonary artery) catheterization, and the body *plethysmograph. Investigators in Scandinavia and on the Continent were working in those same areas independently at the same time.

The new information provided by the measurement of arterial blood gases (ABG) helped in the development of treatment for several, then poorly understood, conditions (e.g. adult *respiratory distress syndrome (ARDS; see below), chronic *cor pulmonale (heart failure due to lung disease), acute and chronic *respiratory failure, and hypoxaemic erythraemia (increased number of circulating red blood cells resulting from oxygen lack). These developments played a vital role in founding modern critical respiratory care.

Assisted respiration

The evolution of artificial *respirators added a new dimension to pulmonary medicine. The Drinker type tank respirator and *cuirass were developed to deal with the respiratory paralysis resulting from *poliomyelitis. By the early 1960s, these instruments had fallen into almost total disuse because of effective vaccination against poliomyelitis and the introduction of new superior respirators. First came intermittent positive pressure breathing (IPPB), and by the late 1960s, the volume ventilator. The tank respirator and the cuirass applied alternately positive and negative pressure to the chest, thus replacing breathing muscles. IPPB applies positive pressure up to a preset level through the mouth when the user inhales, and shuts off during exhalation. The volume ventilator forces a preset volume of air into the user's lungs, utilizing whatever pressure is required. These increasingly sophisticated machines require special knowledge and expertise and, together with chest *physiotherapy, have generated the new technological support specialty of respiratory therapy.

ARDS is a newly defined disease, which has been seldom recognized and poorly understood for a long time. Other names for it include congestive atelectasis, adult hyaline membrane disease, traumatic wet lung, and shock lung. In its fully developed state, it can be treated by supporting ventilation with a volume ventilator and using positive end-expiratory pressure (PEEP). This has resulted in approximately a 50 per cent chance of survival in patients who previously had had virtually none.

Other recent advances
Other major advances include ventilation and perfusion lung *scans, *computerized axial tomography (CT or CAT scanning), pleural and lung biopsies by means of specially designed needles inserted through the chest wall, flexible *fibre-optic bronchoscopy with brush biopsy, pulmonary *angiograms, mediastinoscopy (instrumental visual examination of the mediastinum) and sophisticated pulmonary function tests, including tests of small *airway function and *exercise tolerance.

Pulmonology has evolved into one of the most popular subspecialties of internal medicine. It is still concerned with tuberculosis but to this have been added many important problems including chronic obstructive pulmonary disease or chronic bronchitis and emphysema (COPD), lung cancer (more than 120 000 new cases in the USA in 1982), environmental and occupational lung diseases (especially those due to coal, silica (*silicosis), asbestos (*asbestosis), beryllium (*berylliosis), cotton), asthma, various chronic pneumonias including those due to *hypersensitivity reactions, idiopathic pulmonary fibrosis (or, in the UK, cryptogenic fibrosing alveolitis; progressive fibrosis of the small air sacs or alveoli of the lung, of unknown cause), lung damage due to urban air pollution, and ARDS.

I conclude that chest medicine began world-wide with efforts to systematize the treatment of tuberculosis in the mid-1800s. It evolved into the general chest subspecialty it is today in the 1950s and 1960s in the USA; however, it seems that this evolution took place some years earlier in the UK, and in Europe, especially in France.

The pulmonologist, aided by a host of special tests and skills, is now indispensable in medicine.

(the late) R. S. MITCHELL

References
Bishop, P. J. (1967). The Brompton Hospital and its first medical report. *Tubercle*, **48**, 344.
Keers, R. Y. (1978). *Pulmonary tuberculosis. A journey down the centuries*. Baillière Tindall, London.
Mitchell, R. S. (1961). A summary of the 3rd conference on emphysema. *American Review of Respiratory Diseases*, **83**, 402, 563.
Runyon, E. H. (1959). Anonymous bacteria in pulmonary disease. *Medical Clinics of North America*, **43**, 273.

Further reading
Ashbaugh, D. G. *et al*. (1967). Acute respiratory distress in adults. *Lancet*, **ii**, 319.
British Medical Research Council (1955). Various combinations of isoniazid with streptomycin or with P.A.S. in the treatment of pulmonary tuberculosis. *British Medical Journal*, **i**, 435.
Comroe, J. J. Jr. *et. al*. (1971). *The lung: clinical physiology and pulmonary function tests*, (2nd edn). Year Book Publishers, Chicago.
Forssmann, W. (1929). Die Sondierung des rechten Herzens. *Berlin Klinische Wochenschrift*, **8**, 2085.
Koch, R. (1882). Die Aetiologie der Tuberkulose. *Deutsche Med. Wochenschrift*, **16**, 221.
Laennec, R. T. H. (1819). *De l'ausculation médicate ou traité du diagnostic des maladies des poumons et du coeur*. Paris (English translation, 1827).
Roentgen, W. C. (1895). Ueber eine neue Art von Strahlen. *Sitzungsber. Phys-Med. Gesell., Würzburg*, **137**, 132.
Scadding, J. G. (1977). Chest medicine: a specialty in search of an identity. *Canadian Lung Association Bulletin*, **56**, 3.
Schatz, A., Bugie, E., and Waksman, S. A. (1944). Streptomycin, a substance exhibiting antibiotic activities against gram-positive and gram-negative bacteria. *Proceedings of the Society of Experimental Biology and Medicine*, **55**, 66.
Villemin, J. A. (1868). *Etudes sur la tuberculose; preuves rationelles et expérimentales de sa specificité et de son inoculabilité*. Ballière, Paris.
von Pirquet, C. (1907). Der diagnostisch Wert der Kutanen Tuberkulin reacktion beider Tuberkulose des Kindesalters auf grund von 100 sektionen. *Wiener Klinische Wochenschrift*, **20**, 1123.

CHEST PHYSICIAN. A physician specializing in diseases of the lungs and respiratory tract. See CHEST MEDICINE.

CHEYNE, JOHN (1777–1836). British physician. Cheyne practised in Leith and Dublin. He was the first to write in English on paediatrics, publishing *Essays on the diseases of children* in 1801-2.

CHEYNE–STOKES RESPIRATION is a form of periodic breathing in which there is a cyclical waxing and waning of depth of respiration. Breaths become successively deeper until they reach a maximum, then successively shallower until total *apnoea supervenes; the apnoeic period may last for as long as half a minute before breathing gradually picks up again, as if the patient were 'remembering to breathe' (Hippocrates). Cheyne–Stokes breathing occurs in *coma due to many causes, indicating central nervous system depression. Though usually a result of severe illness, it is sometimes observed in acute alcohol intoxication and even exceptionally in deep normal sleep.

CHIARI, HANS (1851–1916). Austrian pathologist. Chiari described with Arnold a malformation of the hindbrain in which there is a downward projection of the *cerebellar tonsils which extend through the *foramen magnum near the origin of the *spinal cord. If this is unsuspected at *lumbar puncture, sudden impaction of the tonsils in the foramen may cause sudden death. He also described with Frommel a disorder following childbirth in which menstrual periods are suppressed and lactation persists a long time. Eventually, in the 1970s, this was found to be due to excessive secretion of *prolactin from the anterior lobe of the *pituitary gland.

CHIASM is an anatomical term denoting an intersection or *decussation, particularly that of the *optic nerves.

CHICKENPOX, also called varicella, is a contagious *exanthem affecting mainly children and caused by the varicella-zoster (V-Z) virus (see HERPES ZOSTER). A maculo-vesicular *rash appears in crops over a few days after an incubation period of about 3 weeks, chiefly on the trunk and face, accompanied by variable fever and malaise. The infection usually resolves without serious incident, although *encephalitis is a rare complication. The condition may be much more severe in immuno-deficient patients, including newborn infants of infected mothers. Second attacks of clinical varicella are unusual, although reactivation of the latent virus may cause *herpes zoster.

CHILBLAIN. Localized redness and swelling of the extremities, often accompanied by itching and pain, and associated with recurrent exposure to cold when inadequately protected by gloves, stockings, etc. Also known as 'pernio'.

CHILDBIRTH. See OBSTETRICS.

CHILD WELFARE. After the UK Parliament intervened in 1802 to protect the moral and physical welfare of children employed in factories, and with the growing 19th century disapprobation of the exploitation of many young persons, several statutory instruments were promulgated to protect the welfare, needs, and interests of British citizens under the age of 18. Chief among these were the Education Act of 1870; the Children and Young Persons Act of 1933, dealing *inter alia* with prevention of cruelty and exposure to moral danger, employment, and court proceedings; the Children Act of 1948, providing for the care and welfare of children deprived of a normal home life; the Children and Young Persons (Harmful Publications) Act of 1955; the Children and Young Persons Act of 1963, covering employment in film, television, and theatre; and the Children and Young Persons Act of 1969, concerning the provision of care facilities and introducing more stringent safeguards for the private *fostering of children.

CHILL. Any sensation of coldness that causes shivering. It may be due to inadequate protection against a low environmental temperature; or to a rising body temperature in *fever, when it is termed a *rigor.

CHIMERA. An organism containing genetically distinct cell lines derived from different *zygotes (cf. *mosaicism, in which different cell *genotypes are derived from a single zygote).

CHINESE RESTAURANT SYNDROME. Symptoms appearing a few minutes after a meal, attributed to the food additive monosodium glutamate. They are due to vasodilatation and include headache, facial flushing, and a sense of pressure in the chest.

CHIROPODY is a *profession supplementary to medicine concerned with care of the feet and the diagnosis and treatment of minor foot disorders. It is now termed 'podiatry' in the USA.

CHIROPRACTIC is a profession concerned with the diagnosis, treatment, and prevention of biomechanical disorders of the musculoskeletal system, particularly those involving the spine. Like osteopathy, it is not an alternative to conventional medicine, but is a complementary discipline which offers patients an additional treatment option for conditions affecting the structure and function of the body which are biomechanical in origin and which are likely to respond to manual methods of treatment. A variety of gentle and specific manual techniques are used. Diagnostic procedures include detailed history-taking, orthodox clinical examination, and the judicious use of *radiographs and laboratory tests, as well as specialized procedures to assess spinal biomechanics. Long-established in the United States and in many parts of continental Europe, the profession has now achieved statutory recognition and regulation in the UK.

CHIRURGERY is *surgery; literally, 'hand work'.

CHISHOLM, GEORGE BROCK (1896–1970). Canadian psychiatrist. At San Francisco in 1945 he was chairman of the drafting committee whose work led to the creation of the World Health Organization. He served as its director-general for its first five formative years. His army years as a major-general and his practical experience as a psychiatrist enabled him to found and develop a strong organization.

CHLAMYDIA. A genus of coccoid Gram-negative micro-organisms generally now regarded as *bacteria but resembling *viruses in their inability to replicate except within cells, i.e. they are obligate intracellular parasites. *Chlamydia* is responsible for a variety of infections in both man and animals, the two species of human importance being *C. trachomatis* and *C. psittaci.* Human chlamydial infections include *trachoma, inclusion *conjunctivitis, *swimming pool conjunctivitis, some cases of *non-specific urethritis, *lymphogranuloma venereum, *psittacosis, and pelvic inflammation in women.

CHLOASMA. A patchy brown discoloration of the skin often seen in normal *pregnancy (chloasma gravidarum or chloasma uterinum).

CHLORAL HYDRATE is a long-established *hypnotic and *sedative drug ($C_2H_3Cl_3O_2$) which continues to be of limited value, particularly in treating insomnia in the elderly.

CHLORAMPHENICOL is an *antibiotic with a wide spectrum of antibacterial and antirickettsial activity. Its application is limited by the fact that in rare instances it causes fatal depression of the bone marrow. Hence it is reserved for certain specific indications, notably *typhoid fever, *Haemophilus meningitis, and some other severe infections where safer alternative drugs prove ineffective. See also ANTI-INFECTIVE AGENTS.

CHLORHEXIDINE is a chemical agent used in many preparations for local *disinfection of skin and mucous membranes. It is effective against many Gram-negative and Gram-positive bacteria, although some species of *Pseudomonas and *Proteus are relatively resistant. It is ineffective against *viruses, *fungi, *spores, and *acid-fast bacteria.

CHLORINE is a greenish-yellow poisonous gaseous element (symbol Cl, atomic number 17, relative atomic mass 35.453). It is powerfully irritant and destructive to lung tissue when inhaled. It was the first poison gas to be used in modern *chemical warfare (Ypres, 1915). In solution it is used as a disinfectant and bleaching agent. Its compounds are ubiquitous in nature, e.g. sodium chloride in common salt, rock salt, sea water, and physiological fluids. It is a constituent of many organic compounds.

CHLOROFORM ($CHCl_3$) is a sweetish clear volatile liquid also known as trichloromethane and formerly used as an inhalational anaesthetic. It was introduced as an obstetric *analgesic in 1847 by James Young *Simpson of Edinburgh. Strong moral and religious opposition was eventually overcome, to a large extent by the administration of chloroform to Queen Victoria by John *Snow at the birth of her eighth child, Prince Leopold (1853). Thereafter obstetric analgesia became known as 'chloroform à la reine' and opposition faded. It has now been superseded by other, safer anaesthetics (see ANAESTHESIA).

CHLOROMA is a rare manifestation of acute myeloid *leukaemia, in which leukaemic infiltrates form *tumours (chloromas, or granulocytic sarcomas) which have a green colour when sectioned. The colour is due to the presence in high concentration of the enzyme myeloperoxidase.

CHLOROPHYLL is the green pigment (which has several chemical variants) found in all algae and higher plants. It has the fundamental property of absorbing energy from light, *carbon dioxide from the atmosphere, and water from the environment to synthesize *carbohydrates. This process is *photosynthesis, the first link in the 'food chain'. Chlorophyll preparations are used in some topical and atmospheric deodorants.

CHLOROQUINE, a derivative of *quinoline, was introduced in 1946 as an antimalarial drug and remains one of the most valuable agents available for the suppression and treatment of *malaria. It is also useful against some other protozoal infections, notably *amoebiasis. It has also been found useful in some patients with *rheumatoid arthritis and related disorders, such as *lupus erythematosus, but its value in these conditions is limited by side-effects, which can include corneal opacities and irreversible retinal damage.

CHLOROSIS is a term describing the green complexion said to have been characteristic of *iron deficiency *anaemia in young women during the 19th century, but rarely, if ever, observed today.

CHLORPROMAZINE, a *phenothiazine derivative introduced in 1952, was one of the first major *tranquillizers, used also as an antiemetic agent. Proprietary names include Largactil® and Thorazine®.

CHOLANGIOGRAPHY is radiographic visualization of the biliary tract (*bile duct) after introducing an appropriate *radiopaque medium. Various techniques are available, including oral or intravenous administration, retrograde injection via an *endoscope introduced through the *duodenum, and transhepatic cholangiography, in which a needle is inserted percutaneously into an intrahepatic duct in the centre of the *liver.

CHOLANGITIS is inflammation of the *bile duct system, and is usually associated with *gallstones.

CHOLECYSTECTOMY is surgical removal of the *gall bladder.

CHOLECYSTITIS is inflammation of the *gall bladder.

CHOLECYSTOGRAPHY is radiographic examination of the *gall bladder, opacified by the oral administration of a *radiopaque substance which is concentrated in the bile.

CHOLERA is an epidemic diarrhoeal disease characterized by devastating intestinal loss of fluid and *electrolytes, the replacement of which constitutes the vital element in treatment. It is now predominantly a disease of Latin America and Asia, particularly of the Indian subcontinent, although in the 19th century there were several world pandemics. It occurs only in man, there being no animal reservoir, and spreads mainly by (faecally contaminated) drinking water. The causative organism, *Vibrio cholerae* or comma bacillus, elaborates an *enterotoxin which promotes the secretion of electrolytes into the *bowel lumen. *Immunization against cholera, although still widely offered to travellers to endemic areas, is of little value.

CHOLESTEROL ($C_{27}H_{45}OH$) is a *steroid alcohol, of white waxy appearance, present in the tissues of all animals but not higher plants. It is abundant in the human diet (except of *vegans), notably in egg yolk, butter, cheese, and liver and is synthesized by the human *liver. It has many physiological roles: as a precursor of *bile salts, of *myelin, of steroid *hormones, and other compounds; and as a component of many tissues. Pathologically, it is a principal constituent of many *gallstones and of *atheroma deposits in arteries. Elevation of the *serum cholesterol is among the established 'risk factors' associated with *atherosclerosis and cardiovascular disease, but there is no firm agreement as to the nature of the relationship.

CHOLINE is an organic *base, an important dietary constituent because of its physiological role in *lipid and *nerve metabolism (e.g. in forming *acetylcholine). It is usually classified with the *vitamin B complex, but is not a true vitamin for man (although it is for cockroaches and some mammals) as it can be synthesized by the human body. Choline is widely distributed in animal food products (especially egg yolk and fats) as well as in some of vegetable origin.

CHOLINESTERASE. See ACETYLCHOLINE.

CHONDROMALACIA PATELLAE is a degenerative condition of the patellar (knee cap) cartilage, usually occurring in young adults and sometimes following injury. It may be painful but is often painless and can cause intermittent *effusions into the knee joints. The cartilage on the posterior aspect of the patella becomes roughened.

CHOREA, derived from the Greek for 'dance', is a condition characterized by involuntary repetitive jerky movements affecting all parts of the body but most noticeable in the limbs, face, and tongue. Chorea may be a manifestation of several disorders but when the term is unqualified it implies that variety which occurs in children in the course of acute *rheumatic fever (also known as *Sydenham's chorea, chorea minor, or St Vitus' Dance); the sufferers may merely be regarded by those around them as restless, fidgety, and clumsy. There are also various hereditary choreas, of which the best known is *Huntington's chorea, a tragically progressive genetically determined disease in which choreic movements become increasingly severe and intellect and personality gradually deteriorate.

CHORIOCARCINOMA is a malignant *tumour of the *trophoblast arising from a hitherto normal pregnancy, an aborted pregnancy, or a *hydatidiform mole; also known as trophoblastoma, chorioepithelioma, etc.

CHORION. The outermost membrane of the developing *embryo, derived from the *trophoblast and a lining layer of primitive *connective tissue. It develops the branching projections known as chorionic villi and gives rise to the embryonic side of the *placenta.

CHORIONIC CELL BIOPSY. It is now possible to remove cells from the chorion through the vagina and cervix from about 8 weeks of pregnancy onwards and to examine these in order to sex the fetus and to determine whether or not it is carrying a gene responsible for a variety of inherited diseases. This method of antenatal diagnosis, while it carries a small risk of inducing abortion, is safer than *amniocentesis and can be carried out several weeks earlier during pregnancy. See also GENETICS.

CHORIONIC GONADOTROPHIN is the *gonadotrophin secreted by the *placenta and found in large quantities in the urine of pregnant women, whence it may be extracted for use in the treatment of *hypogonadism and *infertility associated with failure of ovulation. Estimation of this hormone in the urine is the basis of most tests for early pregnancy.

CHOROID. The middle of the three concentric layers forming the coat of the eyeball. It is pigmented, and consists almost entirely of blood vessels. Together with the *iris and the ciliary body, it makes up the uveal tract. See OPHTHALMOLOGY.

CHOROIDITIS is inflammation of the *choroid. See OPHTHALMOLOGY.

CHOROID PLEXUS. Small projections of blood vessels from the *pia mater into the *cerebral ventricles which secrete the *cerebrospinal fluid.

CHRISTADELPHIAN. A member of a religious sect believing in conditional immortality, founded in 1833 by Dr John Thomas of Brooklyn (1805–71). Adherents are sometimes called Thomasites.

CHRISTIAN, HENRY ASBURY (1876–1951). American physician. He was the first chief of medicine at the Peter Bent Brigham Hospital when that opened in 1910. His clinical interests were broad, reflecting his early experience in pathology, with special attention to renal and cardiovascular diseases. His name appears in the eponymic titles of two disorders: *Hand–Schuller–Christian disease and *Weber–Christian disease.

CHRISTIAN AID is a division of the British Council of Churches. It is mainly the overseas agency of the Council, responding to calls on its expertise and money by helping refugees and victims of natural disaster and famine with shelter and medical care. Although Christian in origin and outlook it aims to serve all, irrespective of race, nationality, religion, or political belief.

CHRISTIAN SCIENCE is a religious doctrine which maintains, among other beliefs, that physical healing as well as spiritual salvation is the proper concern of religion and that when man recognizes his status as the image and likeness of God, pain, sorrow, and death will be overcome. Accordingly, conventional therapeutic medicine is rejected. The movement was founded in the USA by Mary Baker *Eddy, who in 1875 published *Science and health with key to the scriptures*; this remains the textbook of Christian Science, which is now a worldwide denomination with several hundred churches in the UK and several thousands elsewhere.

CHRISTMAS DISEASE is a genetic disorder of blood *coagulation, closely resembling *haemophilia and often called 'haemophilia B'. Like haemophilia A, it is inherited as an X-linked recessive trait. It is due to a deficiency of coagulation factor IX (Christmas factor, or plasma thromboplastin component). The authors of the original description (1952) proposed the name 'Christmas disease' after the surname of the first patient examined in detail and the report was published in the Christmas number of the *British Medical Journal*.

CHROMAFFINOMA. A benign or malignant *tumour of chromaffin cells (i.e. staining strongly with chrome salts) which causes excessive secretion of *catecholamines; synonymous with *phaeochromocytoma.

CHROMATIC ABERRATION is formation by a *lens of an image fringed by a spectrum of colours, since the refractive index of glass varies for light of different colours. Lenses constructed so as to correct for chromatic aberration are termed 'achromatic' or 'apochromatic'.

CHROMATIN is the nucleoprotein material of *chromosomes, forming that part of the cell nucleus which stains strongly with basic dyes. See CELL AND CELL BIOLOGY.

CHROMATOGRAPHY is a method of chemical analysis by which the components of a mixture are separated, identified, and sometimes quantified. The basic principle is the movement of the mixture (termed the mobile phase; it may be a gas or a liquid) in contact with a selectively absorbent stationary phase (a solid, or a liquid supported on a solid). The particular technique is identified by the terminology, thus: gas–liquid chromatography; gas–solid chromatography; column chromatography (mobile phase liquid, stationary phase a column of solid); thin-layer chromatography (stationary phase a thin layer of solid on a plate); paper chromatography (filter-paper used as stationary phase); etc. After separation, the separated components of the mobile phase are either visualized on the stationary phase or removed by elution and quantified. See also CHEMISTRY, CLINICAL.

CHROMOSOME. A chromosome is a thread-shaped structure, consisting largely of *deoxyribonucleic acid (DNA) and *protein. Chromosomes are found in the nucleus of every animal and plant *cell (bacteria and viruses have similar structures which consist of DNA, or sometimes *ribonucleic acid (RNA) only). Chromosomes occur in pairs, and there may be from one to over 100 pairs per nucleus according to species; man has 23 pairs, so that normal somatic human nucleated cells have 46 chromosomes in the paired (or diploid) state. Germ cells or gametes (i.e. *ova and *spermatozoa) have only one member of each pair (the haploid state). Chromosomes consist of linear arrays of segments of DNA known as *genes, each of which is the hereditary determinant of a single *polypeptide. Chromosomes are usually visible only in microscopic preparations during cell division (*mitosis), when they contract by coiling into short thick rods a few micrometres long. See also GENETIC CODE; GENETICS.

CHRONICALLY SICK AND DISABLED PERSONS ACT 1970. A UK enactment which made wide-ranging legislative provision for the welfare of the chronically sick and disabled. The 29 sections of the Act cover such matters as: the duty of local authorities to provide practical assistance in the home; the duty of housing authorities to make special provision for the chronically sick and disabled; access to, and facilities at, premises open to the public; the provision of public sanitary conveniences; the provision of appropriate signs; access to, and facilities at, university and school buildings; representation of those with experience of the needs of the chronically sick and disabled on various national and local advisory committees; the employment of disabled persons; the separation of younger from older patients in long-term hospital care; chiropody services; the use of invalid carriages on the highway; the provision of badges for display on motor vehicles; the laying of an annual report before Parliament; special educational treatment for the deaf and blind, for children with autism and other forms of early childhood psychosis and for those with dyslexia; and other related matters.

CHRONIC ILLNESS. A long-continued or permanently established illness.

CHVOSTEK, FRANTISEK (1835–84). Austrian surgeon. He described twitching of the facial muscles in latent *tetany when the *facial nerve is tapped (Chvostek's sign, 1878).

CHYLE is *lymph containing emulsified fat (chylomicrons) derived from digested food in the intestine via the intestinal lacteals. It passes into the *thoracic duct and on into the venous circulation.

CHYLOUS VESSELS are *lymph vessels containing *chyle draining the small intestine, also called lacteals because of the milky white appearance conferred on them by the chylomicrons.

CIBA FOUNDATION. An independent foundation well known in both European and North American medical and scientific circles for organizing and financing high-quality limited-invitation colloquia and for publishing the ensuing discussions. Meetings are held in the Foundation's Regency house in Portland Place, London. It also provides limited research funding. It is endowed by the Ciba–Geigy Aktiengesellschaft, the international chemical industries and pharmaceuticals group, but is independent in its activities.

CICATRIX. A *scar; scar tissue.

CILIARY ACTION is the undulant motion of fine hair-like processes (cilia) projecting from the surface of some epithelial cells such as those lining the respiratory passages. This sweeping action propels fluid, mucus, and particulate matter along the passages.

CIMETIDINE is one of the *H_2 receptor antagonists, pharmacological agents which block the effects of histamine on H_2 receptors (unlike conventional *antihistamine drugs, which are H_1 receptor antagonists). They are potent inhibitors of gastric acid secretion and are therefore used in treating *peptic ulcer, *reflux oesophagitis, and the *Zollinger–Ellison syndrome. Cimetidine may cause some adverse side-effects, and treatment is often limited to courses of 4 to 6 weeks at a time, but some patients take a small dose indefinitely.

CIMEX HEMIPTERUS is a *bedbug infesting man in the tropics.

CIMEX LECTULARIUS is the common *bedbug of temperate countries.

CINCHONA is a genus of evergreen trees native to the Andes but cultivated elsewhere because of the value of their bark (cinchona bark, Jesuit's bark, peruvian bark, etc.), which is the source of the pharmacologically important quinoline group of *alkaloids. These have several actions, the two most important being antimalarial (e.g. *quinine) and antiarrhythmic (e.g. *quinidine).

CIRCADIAN RHYTHM. A biological *rhythm with a frequency of about 24 hours.

CIRCLE OF WILLIS. The major arterial *anastomosis at the base of the brain formed by the internal carotid arteries, the anterior and posterior cerebral arteries, the anterior communicating artery, and the posterior communicating arteries.

CIRCULATION. The entire system within which blood circulates, i.e. the heart and blood vessels.

CIRCUMCISION is removal of the *prepuce or foreskin in the male. Although said to be the oldest and commonest of all surgical operations, only rarely is it justified on medical grounds. It is usually performed in the newborn male as a religious ritual. Female circumcision (removal of the clitoris) is regarded as unethical by Western society but is still performed as a ritual in some African communities.

CIRRHOSIS OF THE LIVER. A group of conditions characterized by extensive destruction of *liver tissue and replacement *fibrosis. There are several causes and corresponding pathological types, one of which is related to the prolonged excessive consumption of *alcohol.

CITRATED CALCIUM CARBIDE. See ABSTEM®.

CLAIRVOYANCE is *extrasensory perception.

CLASSIFICATION is commonly defined as the act of arranging things in classes according to common characteristics. In medicine and other sciences it usually presupposes a defined method or scheme designed to provide knowledge in some specific area. It can be regarded as an attempt to discover order in the world and is thus of vital importance in the sciences. Indeed, it has been said that the beginning of science is classification.

One of the earlier attempts was *Aristotle's Ladder of Nature, but in medicine the 18th century saw the vogue for systems and classifications reach its height, a predictable development in the Age of Reason. Perhaps the main impetus derived from *Linnaeus, whose *Philosophica botanica* (1751) established the binomial nomenclature in botany, which he later extended to the animal kingdom in the 10th edition of his *Systema naturae* (1758). Each natural object was given a generic and a specific name, although more than 200 years later the terms 'genus' and 'species' have yet to be precisely defined. In his *Genera morborum* (1763) he assayed a classification of diseases on the same principle and his method was followed by Boissier de Sauvage. William *Cullen and his pupil John *Brown (1735–88) both published nosological systems, but the most ambitious was the *Nosographie philosophique* (1789) of Philippe *Pinel.

Linnaeus was the ultimate authority on botany and

natural history until the work of de Candolle and *Cuvier in the early 19th century, but his rigid method was clearly inapplicable to medicine. Only in dermatology were there persistent efforts to classify in the publications of *Willan, *Bateman, and *Alibert.

It soon emerged that a logical all-inclusive classification of all human diseases was unattainable, although some system of nomenclature was essential, even if never completely satisfying or exhaustive. The reasons are numerous and obvious. The difficulty in defining a 'disease' is one barrier; it is largely an abstract notion. Aetiology is no foundation, because the cause of many diseases is unknown. Morbid anatomy is not a sure basis, for many grave mental diseases are unaccompanied by organic changes. The *Royal College of Physicians attempted to remedy this deficiency and published its *Nomenclature of diseases*, of which eight editions appeared between 1869 and 1960. It has been replaced by the *World Health Organization's (WHO) *International classification of diseases* and its *International classification of causes of death*. There is still little agreement on the names by which diseases should be known, and the Council for International Organizations of Medical Sciences has published a further *Nomenclature of diseases*.

The fact that *diagnosis is no more than an act of classification underlines the relevance of this topic to medicine. The diagnostic process consists of placing the sick person in a class containing others with illness of a similar pattern. Inseparable from this subject are attempts to introduce new systems and schemes of nomenclature into the medical sciences. For many centuries anatomical terminology was confused (see ANATOMY). In 1887 the subject was raised at an international anatomical congress by W. *His and a commission was formed to make recommendations for a logical terminology. The body reported to a meeting in Basel and its scheme was adopted in 1895. The new terminology became known as Basel Nomina Anatomica (BNA). In 1928 the Anatomical Society of Great Britain and Ireland appointed a committee to consider modifications to the BNA; its recommendations were adopted in 1933 and the modified scheme was called the Birmingham Revision (BR). At the 5th International Congress of Anatomists held in Oxford in 1950 a committee made further recommendations adopted unanimously at the 6th Congress in Paris in 1955. This nomenclature is now recognized as the Paris Nomina Anatomica (PNA).

(the late) R. BODLEY SCOTT

CLAUDICATION. A limp, limping, or lameness. But see INTERMITTENT CLAUDICATION.

CLAUSTROPHOBIA is morbid fear of confined spaces.

CLEAN AIR ACTS 1956–68. Efforts to abate *atmospheric pollution, dating back many centuries, were intensified after the 'smog' experiences in the USA and UK in 1948 and 1952. In the UK, legislation to control the nuisance resulted; the Clean Air Acts of 1956 and 1968 were passed, and in 1970 a standing Royal Commission on Environmental Pollution was created. Local authorities were made responsible for the control and prevention of atmospheric pollution, and were empowered to establish 'smokeless zones' in which only smokeless fuels may be used. They were able to give grants towards the cost of installing smokeless appliances, and were authorized to take action against owners or occupiers of premises discharging black smoke into the air. Similar enactments have been introduced in the USA and other countries, especially in cities and regions subject to 'smog', such as Los Angeles.

CLEARANCE TESTS measure the efficiency with which a tissue or organ, usually the *kidney, removes a particular substance from the *plasma. It is the ratio of the rate of excretion of the substance to its plasma concentration, that is UV/Pt, where U and P are the respective urinary and plasma concentrations of the substance in mmol/l, V is the volume of urine in ml, and t is the time in minutes, the clearance, or C, thus being expressed in ml/min. It is the hypothetical volume of plasma which would be totally cleared of the substance each minute at the observed rate of excretion. Where a substance is completely cleared from plasma on passing through the organ, or almost so, then the value of C provides an estimate of total plasma flow. This is true, for example, of low concentrations of para-aminohippuric acid, renal clearance of which provides an estimate of total renal plasma flow. Similarly, clearance of inulin, wholly cleared by glomerular filtration and not subject to tubular reabsorption, is used to measure glomerular filtration rate.

CLEFT PALATE is a congenital deformity of the *palate; the two halves fail to fuse completely in the midline during embryonic development. The result is a palatal groove or complete fissure, often associated with a *hare lip. There is a strong causal genetic component. Surgical repair is usually successful.

CLEIDOCRANIAL DYSOSTOSIS is a genetically transmitted (dominant) disorder characterized by defective and delayed ossification of the clavicle and skull bones. Partial or complete absence of the clavicles enables the patient to bring the shoulders together in front of the chest. Other congenital defects may also be present, particularly of the central nervous system.

CLERGYMAN'S THROAT is weakness and hoarseness of the voice, sometimes with pain on speaking, associated with overuse of the voice and faulty voice production. The condition may be aggravated by upper *respiratory tract infection.

CLIMACTERIC describes any critical period of human life, particularly one associated with bodily changes; it is applied especially to the *menopause in women.

CLIMATE (AND DISEASE). See ENVIRONMENT AND DISEASE; TROPICAL MEDICINE; ECOLOGY IN RELATION TO MEDICINE; HEAT AS A CAUSE OF DISEASE; FROSTBITE; etc.

CLINIC. An establishment or part of an establishment set aside for the examination and treatment of patients; a session in which this takes place, or in which students receive clinical instruction.

CLINICAL CHEMISTRY. See CHEMISTRY, CLINICAL.

CLINICAL INVESTIGATION
Introduction
Most *diagnoses are made following a detailed history and examination. Clinical investigations may yield further diagnoses or confirm the clinical suspicion. Clinical investigations can also help monitor the response to therapy or disease progression. Further investigations can help delineate the structure of organs or measure their function. For example, if a patient complains of breathlessness, the physician may request a chest *X-ray to assess the structure and breathing tests to assess the function of the lungs. More detailed views of the lung can be viewed under the *microscope and a diagnosis made. Nowadays many non-invasive tests have replaced previous means of making diagnoses.

Cardiology
Assessing structure
(a) Radiological. The chest X-ray remains a valuable simple method of assessing cardiac size. In cardiac failure the heart size is often increased and pulmonary *oedema (fluid in the lungs) may be visible. Where there is concern regarding the patency of the coronary arteries, more detailed radiological techniques (coronary *angiography) are used. Under local anaesthetic a fine tube is inserted into the femoral artery at the top of the leg and fed up to the heart and manoeuvred into the origin of the coronary arteries. By injecting a contrast medium (a special radiopaque dye), the structure of the arteries can be visualized and any blockages or narrowings will be demonstrated. Small narrowings can be treated during the procedure by inflating tiny balloons wedged in the narrowed portion of the artery; this is helpful for treating many cases of angina. This technique is known as angioplasty.

Other blood vessels can be examined in a similar way. For example, narrowing of a renal artery can lead to *hypertension, the diagnosis can be confirmed by renal angiography. It is often possible during the procedure to open up a narrowing in the artery, thus combining investigation and treatment.

(b) Ultrasound (see also ULTRASONICS IN MEDICINE). Ultrasound of the heart, echocardiography, can yield vital information regarding heart structure and function. A probe is gently held on the chest, over the heart, and by directing the probe in different directions the size of the heart and the four chambers can be accurately measured. This technique is particularly useful when a heart *murmur has been heard. The four heart *valves can be visualized by echocardiography and the extent of valvular damage can be assessed. Leaking or narrow valves can be demonstrated and this is very useful when surgery is considered. If a pericardial effusion (fluid around the heart) is present the heart may be enlarged on the X-ray but with echocardiography the cardiologist can rapidly differentiate between a pericardial effusion and other causes of a large heart.

Ultrasonic techniques are also useful in determining flow in arteries and veins. This is known as the Doppler method and is particularly useful for assessing flow through the *carotid arteries to the brain.

Ultrasound examination is also used if an abdominal aortic *aneurysm is suspected. Aneurysms are bulges that can develop in arteries and which are likely to rupture if above a certain size. They can be corrected by surgery, but the operation is a fairly major procedure. With ultrasound the size of the aneurysm can be carefully measured and monitored.

Assessing function
(a) The electrocardiogram. The *electrocardiogram (ECG) gives a reading of the electrical activity of the heart. Leads are attached to the wrists, the ankles, and the chest. Analysis of the tracing can determine rhythm problems of the heart. If a patient suffers from *palpitations on an intermittent basis then the ECG may appear entirely normal. By carrying around a small tape-recorder device, the ECG can be monitored for 24 hours and computer analysis can determine the electrical nature of the palpitations so that therapy can be directed accordingly. If a person complains of severe chest pain and a heart attack is suspected, then the ECG changes may confirm the diagnosis. However, it may take several hours for the changes to develop. If *angina is suspected, the resting ECG may be completely normal and an exercise test is performed. The patient is connected to the ECG machine and begins to exercise, usually by walking on a treadmill, following a standard protocol. The patient's heart rate, blood pressure, and ECG are all carefully monitored. If, because of poor circulation within the coronary arteries, the heart muscle becomes compromised, classic changes will be evident on the ECG. If the ECG remains completely normal, then the diagnosis of angina will be re-evaluated.

(b) Blood tests. If coronary artery disease is suspected, the patient is routinely screened for hyperlipidaemia and *diabetes mellitus. Blood tests can also be useful to determine whether heart muscle damage has occurred, for example, following a heart attack.

Respiratory medicine (see also CHEST MEDICINE)
Assessing structure
(a) Chest X-ray. The chest X-ray will demonstrate most structural abnormalities affecting the lungs, and is usually more sensitive than examination. Fluid can be seen within or surrounding the lung. Pneumonia affecting a lobe of the lung is usually obvious, and most lung *cancers are seen on a simple chest X-ray. Certain conditions have classic appearances. *Tuberculosis, for example, classically affects the upper lobes and can cause cavitation. A patient who complains of a cough or fever and whose chest X-ray demonstrates cavitating lesions in the upper lobes of the lung will be isolated and screened for tuberculosis. Other conditions, for example, pulmonary thromboembolic disease (blood clots in the lung), may be suspected following the X-ray. Most information is derived from the simple P–A (Posterior–anterior) view and, if necessary, lateral views can be obtained, or a cross-sectional analysis of the lungs can be made using computerized tomography.

(b) Bronchoscopy. Bronchoscopy is usually performed using a flexible fibre-optic instrument inserted into the windpipe via the nose. The procedure is performed under light sedation with local *anaesthetic to damp down the cough reflex. A detailed view is obtained of the bronchial tree and this test is particularly useful for diagnosing lung cancer. Tiny biopsies can be taken from suspicious-looking lesions. Samples of secretions can also be taken during the procedure and this can help to diagnose some types of pneumonia. Samples can be taken further out into the lungs (transbronchial lung biopsies).

Assessing function
(a) Respiratory function tests. Some patients may complain of breathlessness and yet have normal looking chest X-rays. It would seem that the structure of their lungs is relatively normal but the function is in some way impaired. An example would be *asthma where the chest X-ray is usually normal but the patient complains of breathlessness and a troublesome cough. Asthma is one type of 'obstructive' lung disease and expiration is often impaired. A simple way of measuring this is by estimating the peak of flow. The patient simply blows hard into a small meter and the reading is given in liters/minute. The physician can then compare the value with the normal expected for the age and sex of the patient. Some patients with asthma monitor their own peak flow at home. With asthma the peak flow is usually lowest early in the morning and assessing the response to treatment over a period of 24 hours can be very helpful. More detailed respiratory function testing is available at the hospital, and it is possible to determine gas transfer and degrees of air-trapping within the lung. One of the simplest tests is the forced vital capacity (FVC). The patient is asked to take a big breath and then to exhale as fast and hard as possible. Eighty per cent of the FVC is normally exhaled in the first second and the term to describe this is 'forced expiratory volume' or FEV_1 with the '1' standing for 1 second. Asthma is often aggravated by exercise, so the tests may be repeated after a period of gentle exercise and a deterioration in the FEV_1 would be indicative of asthma.

(b) Blood gases. In cases of severe lung disease requiring hospital admission, measurements of the arterial *oxygen and *carbon dioxide levels can be very useful. A blood sample is taken, usually from the arm (radial artery at the wrist or brachial at the elbow) and can be rapidly analysed. If a very ill patient has a low level of oxygen (*hypoxia) and fails to improve, ventilatory support (assisted *ventilation) may be considered—the arterial oxygen level helps to determine the concentration of oxygen that should be administered to the patient.

*Nephrology
Assessing structure
The size and shape of the kidneys can be determined by ultrasound examination. If there is a blockage in the system with, perhaps, a *stone stuck in one of the ureters, the back pressure may cause expansion of the pelvis of the kidney; this should be apparent on ultrasound examination. Most kidney stones, unlike *gallstones, show up on plain X-rays of the abdomen.

The intravenous urogram (IVU) is an X-ray examination of the kidneys and bladder. An injection of a contrast medium is given intravenously and the structure of both kidneys becomes apparent on the X-ray. If nephritis, or other types of kidney disease are suspected then a small sample biopsy of the kidney can be taken with a needle, under local anaesthetic, and sent to the laboratory for analysis. The inside of the bladder can be examined by *cystoscopy, which is performed under general anaesthetic. Small samples of the bladder wall can be taken for analysis and stones can be removed.

Assessing kidney function
(a) Urine tests. Much can be learned from simple urine tests. 'Dip stick' testing with specially coated plastic strips can help detect the presence of blood or excess protein in the urine. The presence of either would suggest a problem within the urinary tract. Microscopy may demonstrate cells or clumps of cells, which may point to *nephritis (inflammation of the kidney). Urine collection over 24 hours can accurately monitor protein loss and give other information regarding kidney function. Significant protein loss suggests that the filtering system is damaged within the kidney. This can occur with glomerulonephritis and other kidney diseases.

(b) Blood tests. If renal failure develops, there is a build-up of waste products in the body. The level of serum creatinine gives an indication of renal function; it will be elevated in renal failure. The body pH may fall with renal failure and the level of potassium can rise—at times to dangerous levels. The blood tests help determine whether haemodialysis is required.

(c) Other tests. Intravenous injection of a *radioisotope is also useful for assessing renal function; the level of function of the two kidneys can be compared on the final scan.

*Gastroenterology
Assessing structure
(a) Upper GI tract. *Barium meal examinations have now been virtually replaced by endoscopic examination of the *oesophagus, *stomach, and *duodenum. Under light sedation the endoscope is swallowed and *ulcers can be visualized. Endoscopy, in addition to being more sensitive than traditional X-ray examination of the stomach, etc. enables biopsies to be taken and lesions to be treated. If a patient complains of vomiting blood, for example, and an ulcer is found and still appears to be bleeding, application of a heated probe or injection of adrenaline into the ulcer base can help stop the bleeding.

(b) Small intestine. Barium studies are still useful in determining the presence of lesions of the small intestine. In a 'barium meal and follow-through' some barium is swallowed and its progress monitored by X-ray screening, with 'stills' taken for later, reference. A faster method is a 'small bowel enema' when a tube is passed via the nose into the duodenum and the contrast medium instilled via the tube. The progress of the barium can again be timed and monitored by X-rays.

(c) Large intestine. The barium *enema is the radiological method of assessing the large bowel. After suitable preparation, contrast is instilled via the rectum and followed along the length of the colon. Lesions such as *tumours or *polyps can be identified by this method.

The rectum can also be visualized by a short tube, the sigmoidoscope. Fibre-optic examination of the entire large bowel (colonoscopy) can be time-consuming, but has the advantage that specimens can be taken for later analysis, and it is often possible to remove polyps during the procedure.

Hepatology (see also GASTROENTEROLOGY)
Assessing structure
(a) Radiological techniques. Ultrasound examination of the liver is simple and useful. An obstruction in the biliary tract such as a gallstone may cause expansion of the biliary tree as the back pressure builds up. The stone and the resulting expansion, or dilatation, of the system may be visible on ultrasound examination. Some tumours may also show up on ultrasound but a much more detailed image can be obtained following computerized tomographic scanning. The biliary tree can be visualized by endoscopic techniques. Dye is injected into the common bile duct and the pancreatic duct; this is known as endoscopic retrograde cholangio-pancreatography (ERCP). Any small stones lodged within the biliary system can be removed during the procedure.

(b) Biopsy. Under light sedation and local anaesthesia a needle is inserted through the chest wall into the liver and a tiny sample of liver can be obtained for microscopic analysis, which is usually diagnostic.

Assessing function
(a) Blood tests. The liver has many functions. These include functioning as a filter to remove bacteria entering the body from the intestine; dealing with waste products from the body's metabolism; synthesizing new proteins, etc. If the liver malfunctions, there may be an increase in the incidence of septicaemia (infection of the blood) and in the blood concentration of the waste products (elevation of bilirubin), and evidence of the impaired production of new proteins (reduced serum albumin and clotting factors).

*Neurology
Assessing structure
(a) Radiological techniques. *Computerized tomographic (CT) scanning is the main X-ray technique used to visualize the brain. Cross-sectional images can be built up on the computer to provide a detailed image of the brain. Brain tumours, unless very small, can be diagnosed and cerebral haemorrhages can be seen. This is a useful test if a brain tumour is suspected or if brain damage is suspected following *trauma. More invasive imaging can demonstrate the arterial system (angiography) within the brain.

*Magnetic resonance imaging (MRI) is also known as nuclear magnetic resonance (NMR). Cross-sectional images of the brain and spinal cord can be built up, similar to those produced by CT scanning, but the computer data are generated by strong magnetic fields rather than X-rays. MRI is more time consuming than CT scanning and some patients are unable to tolerate lying still for long enough. MRI is more sensitive than CT at detecting conditions such as *multiple sclerosis and is better for imaging the brainstem and spinal cord.

Assessing function
(a) The electroencephalogram (EEG). The EEG gives a reading of the electrical activity within the brain (See Figs 1–4). This is particularly useful in assessing patients with possible *epilepsy. Leads are applied to different

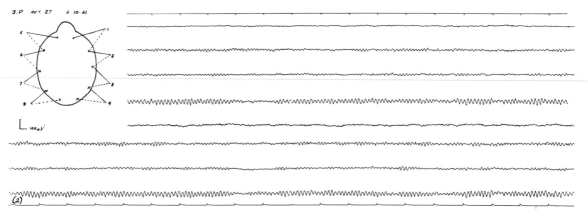

Fig. 1 An eight-channel EEG recording demonstrating rhythmical activity at 8–12 Hz in the posterior region of the head on both sides. The activity is much more evident when the eyes are shut, as here, and almost disappears when they are open; it is the normal alpha rhythm. (Reproduced by kind permission of D. D. Barwick.)

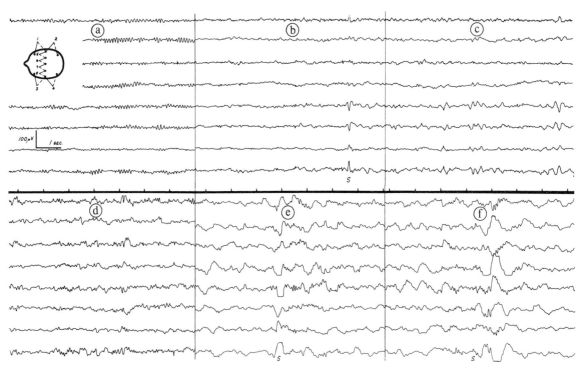

Fig. 2 Serial EEG recordings demonstrating the stages of drowsiness and sleep in a normal man aged 20 years. (a) Early drowsiness; the EEG shows a normal alpha rhythm. (b) Light (stage 1) sleep; the record is of low voltage with mixed frequencies, and a sharp wave is seen at the vertex in response to a sound stimulus at S. (c) Light sleep with dominant slow activity in the theta range at about 5 Hz. (d) Stage 2 sleep; the record shows increasing slow activity and so-called sleep spindles begin to appear. (e) and (f) Stages 3 and 4 of sleep; the record shows increasing irregular delta activity and so-called K complexes are seen in response to the sound stimulus at S. (Reproduced by courtesy from Kiloh, L. G., McComas, A. J., Osselton, J. W., and Upton, A. R. M. (1981) *Clinical electroencephalography*, (4th edn), London.)

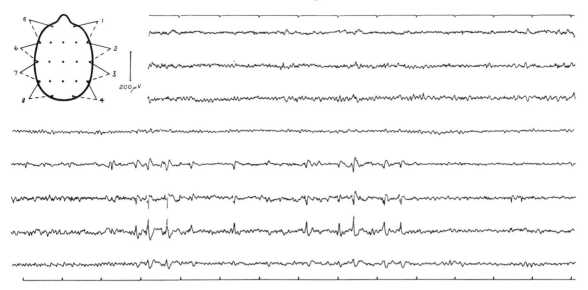

Fig. 3 A recording demonstrating focal spike discharges arising in the left mid-temporal region against a background of almost normal activity. This appearance, seen in an EEG recording between attacks, is the so-called interseizure pattern characteristic of temporal lobe (complex partial) epilepsy, occurring in a 30-year-old man. (Reproduced by courtesy from Kiloh, L. G., McComas, A. J., Osselton, J. W., and Upton, A. R. M. (1981) *Clinical electroencephalography*, (4th edn), London.)

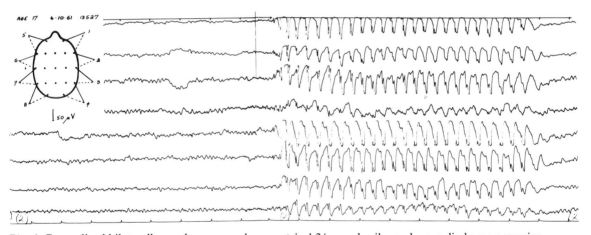

Fig. 4 Generalized bilaterally synchronous and symmetrical 3/second spike-and-wave discharge occurring spontaneously in a girl aged 17 years and associated with a clinical attack of petit mal (an absence seizure). (Reproduced by kind permission of D. D. Barwick.)

sites on the scalp and a series of readings are obtained on a long printout. The patient's response to various stimuli can be assessed. Hyperventilation may be performed and the response to patterns of lights (visual evoked response) or sound (auditory evoked responses) can give added information.

(b) The electromyogram (EMG). EMG is performed by recording electrically from a muscle, using a fine needle or surface electrode and interpreting the electrical activity at rest and during contraction. Clues to many types of muscle disease can be obtained in this way.

(c) Nerve conduction studies. Stimulating peripheral nerves with electrical currents and monitoring the passage of the impulse along the nerve can give considerable information regarding the extent and type of injury or disease suffered by a nerve. The nerve (sensory or motor) is stimulated by electrodes on the skin and the conduction velocity is measured in metres/second.

(d) Lumbar puncture. Lumbar puncture is performed under local anaesthetic with the patient curled up on his or her side. A fine needle is introduced between the lower vertebrae (below the level of the spinal cord). A small sample of the *cerebrospinal fluid (CSF) is taken for analysis. Normally the CSF is 'gin clear'. The presence of many white blood cells will give a milky appearance to the CSF; this is typical of bacterial meningitis. Haemorrhage within the brain may cause blood staining of the CSF. Within a few hours of haemorrhage the altered blood within the fluid becomes yellowish in colour. Detailed *biochemical, *microbiological, and cytological analyses can be performed on the CSF.

(e) *Haematology

Blood tests. Blood tests are inevitably the mainstay of haematological investigation. An automated counter can give a rapid printout of the *haemoglobin level, the white cell (*leucocyte) count, and *platelet count. Further information can be obtained by examining a thin film of the blood under the microscope. Abnormal blood cells may suggest a diagnosis of *leukaemia.

Marrow examination. A sample of bone marrow can be taken, under local anaesthesia, from a back portion of the pelvis. Examination of the marrow may help determine the cause of *anaemia or of other blood diseases.

Other tests. The haematologist can arrange further tests to determine the rate of destruction of blood cells by the spleen or estimate the level of vitamin absorption in order to explain certain types of anaemia.

*Rheumatology

Assessing structure

X-rays of joints give valuable information to the rheumatologist, and the pattern of joint damage can help point to certain diagnoses. *Rheumatoid arthritis, for example, characteristically damages certain small joints of the hands. In complicated joint problems MRI scanning is useful, but it is currently too time-consuming and expensive to be performed as a routine. With *arthroscopy it is possible to visualize the inside of the knee, for example.

Blood tests

Blood tests are very helpful in diagnosing and monitoring certain rheumatological conditions. The presence of autoantibodies in the blood may suggest certain *autoimmune types of joint disorders and if the blood uric acid level is high this would suggest *gout as the cause of the painful swollen joints. For estimating the *erythrocyte sedimentation rate (ESR) some blood is instilled into a thin glass or plastic tube, and the rate of the sedimentation of the red cells measured at the end of an hour. Diseases with high levels of *inflammation, such as rheumatoid arthritis, are often associated with a high ESR and the response to therapy can be estimated from serial ESR estimations.

Endocrinology

Blood tests

Blood tests enable the endocrinologist to estimate levels of hormones and establish diagnosis. High levels of thyroid hormones are found in hyperthyroidism (an overactive thyroid). Patients with diabetes mellitus can now monitor their own level of blood sugar at home with a simple finger-prick test. This enables them to adjust their diet and insulin doses themselves, and is much more accurate than urine testing.

JANICE MAIN
HOWARD C. THOMAS

CLINICAL MEDICAL OFFICER. See PUBLIC HEALTH MEDICINE IN THE UK.

CLINICAL PATHOLOGY is the application of laboratory methods to clinical problems.

CLINICAL PHARMACOLOGY is that branch of *pharmacology dealing with the actions and uses of drugs in patients.

CLINICAL PSYCHOLOGY is the application of the techniques of *psychology to clinical problems, e.g. by psychometric testing and the assessment of intellectual capacity, mental state, emotional adjustment, etc.

CLINICAL RESPONSIBILITY is responsibility for the care and management of patients.

CLINICAL TRAINING AND METHOD is part of the education needed by medical students and doctors. Its intention is to show how to gather relevant information about a patient and his or her disease and to analyse it for diagnosis, prognosis, and treatment. Such training is an apprenticeship, the student working with patients under the guidance of a teacher. For centuries diagnosis by physicians was made by talking to the patient and casting an eye over him or her, i.e. inspection. Surgeons were more accustomed to handling the bodies of their patients. Now the fundamentals of the clinical methods are those of history-taking, mental and physical examination, and special tests. The history relates the symptoms which the patient describes. This is allowed to emerge as far as possible in the patient's own way, but training is needed in how to elucidate these symptoms more accurately. This has to be done by direct questioning, being careful, however, not to lead the patient's answers. The patient expresses himself in one way and the doctor has to translate what he or she is told into the medical idiom so as to understand and ultimately interpret the symptoms as indicating a disorder of bodily functioning. For every system, too, there are symptoms which might be present but which may not be mentioned. For example, a person with abdominal pain must be asked about digestion, vomiting, heartburn, relationship of pain to meals, and about defecation, constipation, and diarrhoea. And since so many functions are interrelated there may have to be direct questions about (say) the urinary system and the genital system in all abdominal conditions. Indeed some enquiry has usually to be made about every system in the body. There have to be general questions about weight (going up or down), appetite, and sleep. All this may be very confusing to the patient who may go to the doctor complaining of earache but then is asked about matters to do with the chest and abdomen, and about walking and gait, later having the feet examined! From an uninformed position this may seem odd, but it is the duty of clinical training to remind the student and doctor of interrelated phenomena so that the patient and the disorder are fully and properly assessed.

As the history proceeds some preliminary assessment is made of the patient's appearance and behaviour, voice, expression, understanding of words, and also of any evidence of anxiety, fear, or depression. Apart from their importance in understanding the patient, these may determine how he or she is finally told of the doctor's diagnosis, prognosis, and proposed treatment. Thereafter the full physical examination is carried out, unless the condition for which the patient consults is obvious and relatively circumscribed, without influence on other parts. The pulse is felt not only for its intrinsic value, but because it establishes a tactile relationship between patient and doctor in a professional way. There is then a definite procedure, almost a drill, for examining each system and part of the body. It is this systematic process which clinical training tries to inculcate. Such a system is the foundation of clinical method and is particularly needed when diagnosis is in doubt, so that all appropriate information is garnered.

The examination often, indeed usually, includes the use of bedside instruments such as the ophthalmoscope, otoscope, nasal specula, tongue depressors, stethoscope, tendon hammer, thermometer, rubber gloves and finger stalls, and vaginal and anal specula.

Subsequently, where indicated, special tests may be requested from experts in radiology, haematology, microbiology, chemical pathology, and morbid anatomy. It is part of clinical training to understand and interpret reports from these specialists in the light of the history and examination, so that as complete a picture as possible may be built up about the patient and the ailment. The investigations available have increased greatly in scope and complexity. Only those regarded

by the clinician as essential in order to clarify diagnosis and management should be employed, and they should be planned to give the maximum possible information with the minimum of risk. Such planning is invariably dependent upon the information derived clinically and the importance of *communication skills in the doctor–patient relationship must not be overlooked.

A basic programme of clinical training is necessary for all doctors to help them establish a base of knowledge and skill upon which more specialized training, combined with the fruits of increasing experience, is then superimposed; this varies considerably in its content and duration depending upon the specialty in which the doctor ultimately intends to practise (see POSTGRADUATE AND CONTINUING MEDICAL EDUCATION).

CLINICAL TRIALS OF TREATMENT. One of the most exciting advances of medicine in the 20th century has been the development of the randomized controlled trial (RCT). Before it was adopted as the gold standard of therapeutic evaluation, physicians reported their successes, and, less often, their failures, in single case reports or uncontrolled series of patients. When the new treatment was *penicillin for lobar *pneumonia, *vitamin B_{12} for *pernicious anaemia, or *insulin for diabetic coma, the effect was so dramatic that control patients were entirely unnecessary. But those dramatic events occur only once in about every 10 000 instances. By far the majority of evaluations are concerned with small increments of efficacy or small decreases in toxicity. In those cases it is extremely important that the patients undergoing the experimental and control treatments be as similar as possible; that desirable state of affairs can only be achieved by assigning the patients to their treatment groups at random. Employing historical or simultaneous non-randomized controls has been shown many times to be misleading.

The vain search for randomization substitutes
However, because of the common misconception that randomized control trials (RCTs) are too expensive (it costs very little to randomize; the extra costs come from the expenses of delivering exemplary care, especially the costs of recording accurately what is done and measuring the results, all essential parts of good medical care) continuous efforts are made to find a substitute for randomization. Such efforts can be looked at in an open-minded way, but I predict that they will be found wanting. The chances of discovering, without a control group, a dramatic cure of a previously incurable state are now practically nil. Most of the 'slam-bang' discoveries have been made. Instead we now must document small improvements in efficacy, or small decreases in toxicity. To distinguish such improvements as real and not the result of various biases or chance requires that the patients be as similar as possible at the start of therapy. That requires randomized assignment to treatment groups.

Importance of maintaining high quality of RCTs

The randomization process must be truly 'blinded' so that the investigator selecting a patient for the study cannot suspect or know which treatment is being given next and thus bias the study by selectively admitting patients for particular treatments.

'Blinding' of therapies is less important, but helpful when possible. 'Blinding' of the dropout, or withdrawal, process is necessary to keep from obviating the original advantages of randomization. This most important goal is best accomplished when the therapies are double-blind. 'Blinding' of the investigators as to the trends in relative efficacy and toxicity is most important to avoid bias in the selection of patients to be randomized or who ask to drop out. This requires that an impartial board or committee follow the data and make decisions about stopping or modifying the study.

Ethics of randomization

When it is not known whether a new therapy is better or worse than the standard, it is more ethical to randomize the patients than to give one or other of the therapies as if the knowledge of relative efficacy or toxicity were available. In other words, decision-making in medical practice based on ignorance is unethical. Convincing medical practitioners, members of institutional review boards (IRBs) and those responsible for health policy decisions (third parties) of this obvious point has been a most difficult challenge. The fallacy we must overcome is typified by the operating principles of the IRBs and the third parties, who determine which medical intervention will be allowed or paid for, and which not. Interventions that are approved by the so-called clinical experts do not require peer review or detailed informed consent, while efforts to determine whether the dogma are correct do. Physicians are allowed to do almost anything to patients that they think might be helpful, as long as they do not try to learn from the experience by calling it research. Those responsible for treatment policies make it extremely difficult to document the efficacy of what we do in a reliable manner.

These false principles have led to the current popularity of 'outcomes research', a big mistake of the nineties. It is believed by those appropriating money to and supervising health care that one can learn what doctors should be doing by computerized measurement of what they are doing. We are in great danger of adopting a policy of 'regression to the mediocre'.

The uncontrolled pilot trial is counterproductive and therefore less ethical because it so often leads to three unreliable conclusions:

(1) the new treatment is so *effective* that it would be unethical to assign patients randomly to a control group in the future;

(2) the new treatment is so *ineffective* that it would be unethical to assign patients randomly to that treatment in the future;

(3) the new treatment is so similar to the old that it would be a waste of time to do a properly controlled trial in the future.

All three of these outcomes could result from the selection of the patients to be treated, rather than the treatments per se.

Therefore it is most important, for ethical as well as scientific reasons, that randomization begins as soon as possible, as one purpose of a trial is to detect the effects of a new treatment on patients who need treatment. Hence the principle that I have advocated for many years, and to which I finally seem to be winning some converts: *randomize the first patient.*

Meta-analysis of randomized control trials

The advent of meta-analysis (M-A), an increasingly used method of combining data from multiple different trials, has revolutionized the world of therapeutic evaluations. The development of procedural, computer, and statistical methods for finding RCTs, extracting and combining their data, and drawing conclusions that could not be drawn from individual studies has resulted in the following dramatic changes in the way we should do things:

1. We should no longer worry about sample size when we plan new studies. Small studies can be combined to reach meaningful conclusions.

2. We should register and publish all RCTs, no matter how small or inconclusive.

3. In designing and executing RCTs we should be aware of the certainty that the meta-analyst will want to consider subgroup responses. Individual RCTs are rarely large enough to facilitate conclusions about average effects in average patients. They are never large enough to allow conclusions to be drawn from multiple end-points in multiple kinds of patients. We should keep this in mind when we design RCTs.

However, we must remember that meta-analysis is retrospective research, and is thus subject to all of the biases of studies that are not truly prospective. Literature searches may be incomplete. Publication bias must be worried about, although the tendency to publish most large studies makes it relatively unimportant. The most potent source of a biased conclusion is the acceptance or rejection of an RCT which comes to a different conclusion from the one desired by the meta-analyst. Although an M-A protocol is essential, its initial definition of acceptance and rejection is rarely absolute. In clinical medicine as in most other fields, observer variability in decision-making is common, and observer bias flourishes in a medium of observer variability. To minimize and measure these sources of error, we are convinced that observers must be 'blinded' to the source and outcome of an RCT when they make inclusion decisions and extract the data. In addition, all decisions must be made independently in duplicate and settled in conference while the investigators are still blinded. At present that is the only way we can reliably minimize and measure errors and biases.

Cumulative meta-analyses

The production of RCTs is a continuing process, and meta-analyses must be updated. This need has led to our development of the method of *cumulative meta-analysis*, a process by which a new meta-analysis is performed each time a new RCT is accessed. The impact of the new study on the pooled estimate can then be examined and one can determine the year when a new treatment could be shown to be effective. Trends in

the control rate and in treatment differences, smoothed out by cumulation, may be helpful in making treatment policy decisions. Finally, the software used to analyse repeated RCTs may be programmed to rearrange the order of the RCTS, by publication date, by an arbitrary score for quality, by control rate, by mean age, or by any other factors deemed important in understanding a large number of RCTs. Figure 1 illustrates a classical and a cumulative (by date of publication) meta-analysis of the effects of streptokinase in the treatment of acute *myocardial infarction. Figure 2 illustrates the slowness with which clinical experts have responded to the results of the RCTs, as a result of many factors, such as their being unable to keep up with the clinical trial literature

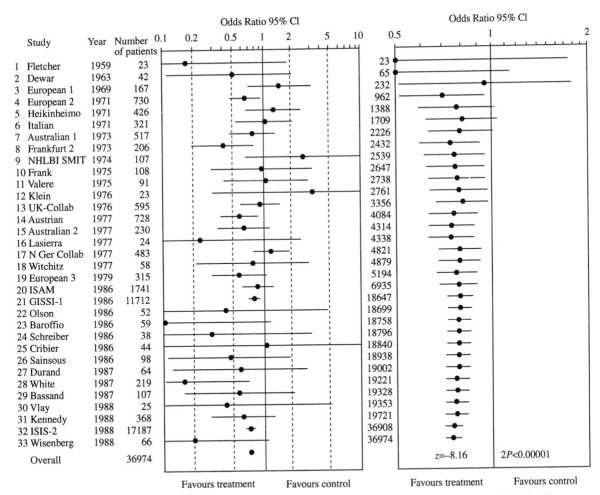

Fig. 1 Classical (left) and cumulative (right) meta-analyses of the 33 randomized control trials (RCTs) of streptokinase of patients with myocardial infarction. (Reproduced by kind permission of the editors and publishers of the *Journal of the American Medical Association*.)

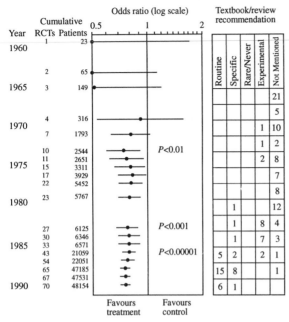

Year	Cumulative RCTs	Patients	Odds ratio (log scale)	Routine	Specific	Rare/Never	Experimental	Not Mentioned
1960	1	23						
	2	65						
1965	3	149						
	4	316						21
1970	7	1793						5
	10	2544	P<0.01			1		10
1975	11	2651					1	2
	15	3311					2	8
	17	3929						7
	22	5452						8
1980	23	5767			1			12
	27	6125	P<0.001		1		8	4
	30	6346			1		7	3
1985	33	6571						
	43	21059	P<0.00001	5	2		2	1
	54	22051						
	65	47185		15	8			1
	67	47531						
1990	70	48154		6	1			

Favours treatment — Favours control

Fig. 1 Cumulative meta-analyses (left) of RCTs of streptokinase treatment of patients with acute myocardial infarction; the studies were added annually instead of individually. On the right is a tabulation of the published recommendations of respected cardiologists as to whether the drug should be used routinely (all patients without a contraindication), for specific use (selected patients only), rarely or never, if they regard it as being still experimental, and finally the number of textbook chapters or review articles published in the years in question on the management of patients with acute myocardial infarction that do not mention use of the drug.

and not as yet accepting the importance of cumulative meta-analysis.

Finally, the advent of cumulative meta-analysis illustrates the importance of abandoning the testing of the null hypothesis (frequentism) in favour of a Bayesian approach to information accumulated by clinical trials. This is best illustrated by the fact that classic bio-statisticians insist that accepted *P* values need to be adjusted by the multiple-look aspects of meta-analysis. The data indicate that this theory may well be wrong, and suggest that the whole basis of statistical inference from clinical trials needs to be re-examined. If the rate of type one errors (see STATISTICS) were to be increased by looking at the data in multiple meta-analyses, we should be able to document this by the cumulative meta-analysis technique. In over 100 instances we have

seen none in which a result that is positive at the *P* = 0.05 level (see STATISTICS) is later reversed so that no treatment effect is apparent. We see fluctuations around a given level of significance that result from changes in the mean point estimates and 95 per cent confidence intervals, but studies with a positive trend seem to become more positive as the numbers increase, and studies without an early positive trend tend later not to show an effect. We need a lot more experience in accumulating completed trials before we can make reliable conclusions about a system of accepting early results that might replace the classic one, but we must start thinking about the exciting ideas represented by cumulative meta-analyses.

For instance, we should stop acting as if there are no prior clinical trial results to be considered when we undertake an RCT. Actually the pharmaceutical industry should be the first to agree that testing the null hypothesis is silly whenever a new RCT is started after a number have been completed. In the future our sample size calculations have got to include the results of past RCTs. These can be adjusted according to ideas about quality or other fine points of the past RCTs, but we should stop acting as if the past studies did not exist. We should replace 'testing the null hypothesis' with 'testing the validity of the probability statement resulting from meta-analysis of all preceding trials'.

Summary in the form of recommendations

1. *Randomize the first patient when a clinical outcome is to be measured.*
2. *Register all clinical trials at inception and annually.*
3. *Correct the double standard of requiring peer review and informed consent for all randomized control trials (RCTs), but not for poor research or use of unproven therapies.*
4. *Also correct the double standard that third parties have created of reimbursing institutions for the use of procedures established by testimony and uncontrolled experiences, but requiring that RCTs be paid for out of scarce research funds.*
5. *Before starting a new trial perform a meta-analysis of all pertinent published trials.*
6. *In basing sample size estimates on desired alpha, beta, and difference, include credible data from past similar trials.*
7. *Do not worry about power. Meta-analysis of available small trials is a more modern way of handling the problem.*
8. *Whenever possible, include economic data in early trials.*
9. *Publish all completed trials.*
10. *Remember that the most important determinant of a reliable RCT is proper 'blinding' of the randomization process so that investigators entering patients into the trial have no way of determining which treatment is being given next.*

THOMAS C. CHALMERS

CLINICOPATHOLOGICAL CONFERENCE. A case conference (see CABOT) at which presentation and discussion of the clinical features and diagnosis precede description of the pathological findings, the latter often based on *autopsy examination.

CLIOQUINOL is a chemical antibacterial agent (iodochlorhydroxyquinoline) known also under the proprietary names Vioform® or Enterovioform®; its use is now restricted to topical application. It formerly enjoyed a vogue as an antidiarrhoeal remedy, but was withdrawn after being implicated in the causation of *subacute myelo-optic neuropathy.

CLONE. A group of cells or organisms which are genetically identical having descended from a single cell or organism which has reproduced asexually and without mutations.

CLOQUET, JULES GERMAIN (1790–1883). French anatomist and surgeon. In an investigation of *inguinal hernia he found a *lymph node, more or less constantly present under the inguinal ligament. This node was later found to be important in the surgery of cancer of the external genitalia, as the disease often spreads to it. He used *hypnotism as an aid to relief of pain in surgical operations, and also used *acupuncture. He published *Anatomie de l'homme* (5 vols, 1821–31).

CLOSTRIDIUM is a genus of *anaerobic, *spore-forming *bacilli widely distributed in nature and found particularly in soil. Some species are dangerously pathogenic for man if conditions favour their multiplication; they include the agents of *tetanus, *botulism, and *gas-gangrene.

CLOT. A coagulum of *blood or *lymph. See HAEMATOLOGY.

CLOVER, JOSEPH (1825–82). British *anaesthetist. Clover advocated the use of *nitrous oxide as an induction agent in about 1870, some time after it had been used as a dental anaesthetic in the USA by *Wells. After the initial induction with nitrous oxide, he continued the anaesthetic with *ether. This was an important step towards safer anaesthetic administration. He invented an inhaler (*Clover's apparatus) which was used for the administration of ether until well into the 20th century. He also invented a *chloroform bag.

CLOVER'S APPARATUS was the first piece of equipment to provide a convenient means of regulating the amount of *ether vapour inhaled during general *anaesthesia. It was described in 1877 by Joseph *Clover under the name of the Portable Regulating Ether Inhaler. In later years the design was substantially modified.

CLUBBING OF THE FINGERS is caused by thickening of the soft tissues, particularly at the base of the nail, with longitudinal convexity of the nail itself. Finger clubbing, especially in association with hypertrophic *pulmonary osteoarthropathy, often signifies serious disease of the heart or lungs, notably *bronchial carcinoma (of which it may be the first sign) or chronic lung sepsis (*abscess, *empyema, *bronchiectasis). Finger clubbing alone, without osteoarthropathy, occurs in cyanotic *congenital heart disease, *infective endocarditis, pulmonary arteriovenous malformations and some diseases of the liver and intestine (e.g. *Crohn's disease, *ulcerative colitis, some types of *liver *cirrhosis). Occasionally it occurs without apparent cause, and may be genetically determined.

CLYSTER. *Enema.

COAGULATION is *clot formation, resulting in an insoluble complex of *fibrin. See HAEMATOLOGY.

COARCTATION is any abnormal constriction or narrowing. The term usually denotes a congenital abnormality of the *aorta obstructing the arterial circulation to the lower half of the body but sparing that to the head, neck, and arms so that *blood pressure in the arms is high. The condition can be corrected by surgical excision and *anastomosis.

COCAINE ($C_{17}H_{23}O_4$) is an *alkaloid, first isolated by Niemann in 1860 from the leaves of a Peruvian shrub *Erythroxelon coca* and introduced into clinical practice by *Freud and Köller in 1884 (see LOCAL ANAESTHESIA). It is a powerfully addictive central nervous *stimulant and *euphoriant (see SUBSTANCE ABUSE) and its medical use is now confined to combination mixtures with *morphine or diamorphine for relief of intractable pain in terminal malignancy. As a local anaesthetic it has been superseded by newer compounds except in topical preparations for surface anaesthesia of the nose, throat, larynx, and eye.

COCCIDIOIDOMYCOSIS is a *fungal infection, endemic in parts of south-western USA, Central and South America caused by the diphasic fungus *Coccidioides immitis*. It usually causes a mild upper *respiratory infection with complete recovery, but chronic and disseminated variants with features like those of *tuberculosis may also occur. Like other fungal infections, it can be dangerous in patients with immunodeficiency.

COCCUS (pl. cocci) is a spherical *bacterium (from the Greek *kokkos* meaning a berry). Varieties include the *streptococcus (growing in chains), *staphylococcus (growing in bunches or clumps), *diplococcus (growing in pairs), *meningococcus (causing *meningitis), and *gonococcus (causing *gonorrhoea).

COCCYDYNIA is pain in the *coccyx.

COCCYX. The terminal portion of the *spine, a small triangular bone made up of four fused vestigial vertebral bodies. It is analogous to the tail of animals.

COCHLEA. A snail-shaped structure situated in the inner ear, containing the essential organ of hearing (organ of *Corti) which converts sound into nervous impulses for transmission to the brain. (See OTORHINO-LARYNGOLOGY).

COCHRANE, ARCHIBALD (ARCHIE) LEMAN (1909–88). British physician and epidemiologist. Between 1946 and 1960 he made major contributions to the aetiology and epidemiology of *pneumoconiosis in Wales before becoming director of the MRC Epidemiology Unit in Cardiff, David Davies Professor at the Welsh National School of Medicine, and, later, first president of the *Faculty of Community Medicine. He is remembered particularly for his application and promotion of randomized controlled *clinical trials.

CODE, in biomedical terminology, is now often used to signify the chemical storage of information, as in *genetic code.

CODEINE ($C_{18}H_{21}NO_3.H_2O$) is one of the *opium *alkaloids, also known as methylmorphine. Being less addictive than *morphine and hence less liable to abuse, codeine is widely prescribed, especially in mixtures, as an *analgesic (often in combination with *aspirin or *paracetamol), as an antitussive agent, and in antidiarrhoeal preparations.

CODE OF HAMMURABI. Hammurabi, the founder of the first Babylonian empire, laid down a legal code c.2100 BC which was discovered at Susa in 1902. Clauses 215–23 relate to medicine, laying down the fees appropriate to various services. Number 221, for example, reads: 'If a physician set a broken bone for a man, or cure his diseased bowels, the patient shall give five shekels to the physician.' The Code also set penalties for an unsuccessful outcome; in the case of loss of life or of an eye, the doctor was to have his hands cut off if the patient was a nobleman, or to render value for value if a slave.

CODEX. Formerly a collection of recipes for the preparation of medicines, the usage is preserved in the title of the *British Pharmaceutical Codex, now the *Pharmaceutical Codex*. See PHARMACY AND PHARMACISTS.

COD LIVER OIL is a rich source of the fat-soluble *vitamins A and D, long popular (in the UK since the end of the 18th century) as a dietary supplement.

COELIAC (CELIAC) DISEASE is a syndrome, usually beginning in early childhood after weaning, associated with *malabsorption of foodstuffs and due to abnormal sensitivity of the intestinal mucosa to dietary *gluten. The main features are those of undernutrition with abdominal symptoms and the frequent passage of bulky, pale, frothy, and offensive stools *(steatorrhoea). The condition (also called non-tropical *sprue or gluten-sensitive enteropathy) is of unknown aetiology but seems to have a genetic component. See GASTROENTEROLOGY.

COENZYME. A non-protein substance that is essential to the catalytic action of an *enzyme, e.g. by acting as a temporary carrier of an intermediate product in a chemical reaction. The coenzyme (sometimes known more broadly as a cofactor, coferment, or accessory factor) is not itself consumed by the reaction. Many *vitamins act as coenzymes.

COFFEE. The pharmacological effect of coffee is due mostly, if not entirely, to its *caffeine content, by virtue of which it acts as a mild central nervous system *stimulant. More serious charges than that of causing *insomnia have been levelled against coffee-drinking (associations with *coronary heart disease and with pancreatic *carcinoma have, for example, been mooted) but none has been satisfactorily proved.

COGNITION is a term covering knowledge or the act of knowing in all its modalities (perceiving, remembering, imagining, etc.). It is distinguished from two other components of consciousness, namely affection (emotion) and conation (willing).

COHEN OF BIRKENHEAD, HENRY (1st BARON) (1900–77). British physician. A brilliant clinician and teacher, deeply involved in the advisory machinery leading to the establishment of the *National Health Service. He was a notable president of the British Medical Association in 1951 and of the *General Medical Council from 1961 to 1974.

COHNHEIM, JULIUS FRIEDRICH (1839–84). German pathologist. An early experimental pathologist, his monographs on *inflammation and *suppuration, proving the *diapedesis of *leucocytes, disproved Virchow's (1873) theories on the behaviour of white blood cells. In 1877 he suggested the origin of *tumours in 'embryonic rests' and devised the 'frozen section' technique as well as using silver and gold impregnation stains. He successfully transmitted *tuberculosis by inoculating infective material into the anterior chamber of a rabbit's eye.

COITUS. Sexual intercourse.

COITUS INTERRUPTUS is sexual intercourse in which withdrawal takes place before male *ejaculation, the intention being to avoid female insemination and *conception. Tension and anxiety are attributed to its use as a method of *birth control, and the reported failure rate is high.

COLCHICINE ($C_{22}H_{25}NO_6$) is an *alkaloid obtained from plants of the genus *Colchicum*, particularly the root of *C. autumnale*, the meadow saffron or autumn crocus (or, in the country, 'naked ladies'). It is a specific remedy against *gout, a property known since ancient times. In cell preparations, it prevents *mitosis from proceeding beyond *metaphase by disrupting *microtubules.

COLD. Viral inflammation of the *mucous membranes of the nasopharyngeal passages. Person-to-person transmission readily occurs by droplet infection, and protective immunity following an attack is limited by the many different *viruses involved. No specific remedy exists for this common and annoying affliction. The prevention and, where necessary, treatment of secondary bacterial infection are particularly important in patients with pre-existing heart and lung disease.

COLD ABSCESS. An *abscess which develops slowly and without signs of acute *inflammation, usually due to *tuberculosis.

COLD SORES. The facial eruption caused by the *herpes simplex virus.

COLE, RUFUS (1876–1966). American physician. At the New York Rockefeller Institute he developed and implemented his ideas for a clinical research centre in which a few diseases were studied intensively in scientific laboratories located close to the patient care area. This is regarded as the forerunner of a modern clinical research centre. Cole collaborated in work which led to development of antisera effective in treating the commoner *pneumococcal infections.

COLEY, WILLIAM BRADLEY (1862–1936). American surgeon. He observed regression of an apparently inoperable *sarcoma in a patient who had an attack of facial *erysipelas. Coley therefore tried to induce erysipelas in other patients with advanced malignant diseases, and eventually employed a suspension of streptococci and prodigiosis bacilli—'Coley's toxin'. He later reported several instances of five-year survival in patients so treated. However, reactions to the toxin were severe and the results unpredictable, so that the treatment lost favour.

COLIC is cramp-like spasmodic abdominal pain associated with intermittent contraction of smooth muscle in the wall of the large intestine, the biliary tract (biliary colic), or the urinary and urethral tract (renal colic).

COLITIS is inflammation of the *colon. See also ULCERATIVE COLITIS.

COLLAGEN is a fibrous *protein, which forms the intercellular fibres of vertebrate *connective tissue (the 'white fibres') and is a major constituent of skin, tendon, ligament, cartilage, and bone. On boiling, it yields gelatin. Collagen fibres have a high tensile strength but, unlike *elastin fibres, little reversible extensibility. The basic molecular *polypeptide protocollagen contains an *amino acid, hydroxyproline, rare in other tissues. It is arranged in the form of a left-handed helix, with three such spirals wrapped round each other to form a right-handed superhelix.

COLLAGENOSIS is any disease of *collagen. It is often used synonymously with 'connective tissue disorder', a term for a heterogeneous group of conditions of uncertain (but probably *autoimmune) aetiology, including *rheumatoid arthritis, systemic *lupus erythematosus, *scleroderma, *dermatomyositis, *polyarteritis nodosa, etc.

COLLAPSE. Circulatory failure, or extreme prostration from some other cause.

COLLAPSE THERAPY is treatment of pulmonary *tuberculosis with *artificial pneumothorax.

COLLATERAL. Used chiefly with reference to tissue and organ *perfusion, to mean blood circulation through lateral or secondary channels, which can allow perfusion to continue when flow in the main vessels is obstructed. In arterial occlusion due to *thrombosis or *embolism, the availability of such a circulation to bypass the obstruction may prevent *infarction, or at least limit its extent.

COLLES, ABRAHAM (1773–1843). Anglo-Irish surgeon. He described Colles's *fracture in 1814; Colles's law was the erroneous statement that a healthy woman becomes immune to *syphilis if she gives birth to a syphilitic infant.

COLLIP, JAMES BERTRAM (1892–1965). Canadian biochemist. He developed a method for extracting substantial quantities of insulin from bovine pancreatic tissue. Later, when the *Nobel prize was awarded to Banting and Macleod for the discovery of insulin, Macleod shared his monetary award with Collip (and Banting shared his with Best). At *McGill University in 1927 he also carried out important early studies on *parathyroid hormone.

COLLODION is a solution of cellulose nitrates (guncotton) in a mixture of *alcohol and *ether. Collodions are painted on the skin and allowed to dry, when they form a flexible occlusive film useful in sealing minor cuts and wounds. They have also been used to hold a dissolved drug in contact with the skin for a long period.

COLLOID. A substance that disperses into particles much larger than atoms or molecules (for example, smoke particles in air). In a colloidal solution, the solvent is called the dispersion medium and the dissolved substance the disperse phase. A colloidal solution differs from a true solution in particle size, which prevents the solute from passing through a semipermeable membrane; nor does the solute depress the freezing point of the solvent. Common examples are aqueous solutions of *starch and *albumin.

COLOBOMA is congenital absence of part of the eye, usually of a sector of the iris, conferring a keyhole appearance on the *pupil.

COLOMBO, MATTEO REALDO (?1516–59). Italian anatomist. In his posthumously published *De re anatomica* (1559) he described the pulmonary circulation. It is uncertain whether this was plagiarized from *Servetus or possibly from *Ibn al-Nafis, although it seems likely that he understood its physiological significance better than either.

COLON. That part of the large *intestine which extends between the *caecum and the *rectum, comprising ascending, transverse, descending, and pelvic (or sigmoid) portions.

COLONOSCOPY is the endoscopic examination of the *colon. The flexible *fibre-optic *endoscope allows visualization of the internal surface of the colon along its entire length.

COLORIMETER is any instrument for measuring intensity of colour. Colorimetric analysis is part of many biochemical methods.

COLOSTOMY. An artificial opening of the *colon on to the *abdominal surface, surgically created so as to bypass the distal part of the colon and the *rectum and to divert intestinal contents into a receptacle fitted for the purpose.

COLOSTRUM is the *mammary secretion produced during the first few days after *parturition, before the production of *milk proper. It is a yellowish fluid particularly rich in *protein, including *antibodies; it contains less *fat and *carbohydrate than milk.

COLOUR (COLOR) BLINDNESS. Defective colour vision is a genetically determined condition, usually inherited as a sex-linked (*X-linked) recessive character. It is common in males (about 8 per cent of the population), much less so in females (about 0.5 per cent). Many complex variants of colour 'blindness' have been described, of which the commonest is failure to perceive red or green, or the difference between them; subjects with this condition are sometimes termed dichromats. Trichromats, i.e. those with normal vision, also include some individuals with either weak red vision or weak green vision. Monochromats, i.e. those with total colour blindness, are very rare, as are dichromats with defective blue-violet perception. In patients with minimal lesions of the visual pathways, field defects for colour can often be demonstrated when the visual fields for white objects are still complete. Many subjects are unaware of their defective colour vision, differentiating colours by their brightness (intensity). The disability is rarely a handicap, except in those whose occupations require them to recognize colour signals.

COLOUR (COLOR) VISION is the ability to perceive the complete colour spectrum conferred by differential stimulation of receptors sensitive to the three primary colours. See also COLOUR BLINDNESS.

COLPORRHAPHY. Surgical repair of prolapse of the *vaginal wall.

COLPOSCOPY. The *Concise Oxford Dictionary* defines *cancer as 'a malignant growth or *tumour that tends to spread and reproduce itself (*invasion*). It corrodes the part concerned and generally ends in death'. Cancer of the cervix (neck of the womb) fulfils these criteria, and screening for cervical cancer is based on the theory that cancer is preceded by a long period, up to 20 years, of a *pre-invasive* state, and, during this time, treatment of the pre-invasive condition, sometimes known as 'carcinoma *in situ*' (CIS) or cervical intraepithelial neoplasia (CIN) prevents the subsequent onset of frank cancer—a theory that is *generally* accepted.

Fortunately, the pre-invasive disease can be identified by *screening procedures—but first a word about the condition. Generally, cancer of the cervix originates in the most superficial layer of the *skin, 'the epidermis'— a millimetre or so in thickness. The pre-invasive state is confined to this layer and is eventually recognized by changes in cell structure and pattern. Because these cells 'flake off', or desquamate, when mature, such cellular changes can be recognized by scraping the surface (a cervical smear) and examining the cells under a microscope. This test, routinely performed every 3–5 years, forms the basis of the screening procedure.

However, examination of the smears alone gives little or no information as to the exact source or extent of the change. Colposcopy, magnified examination of the skin surface of the cervix, fulfils that function.

Colposcopy is undertaken with patients positioned as for cervical smear examination and should cause little or no discomfort. Usually manual vaginal examination is first carried out. The neck of the womb is visualized after insertion of the *speculum or 'telescope' and then illuminated by an outside light source: it is generally prepared by cleansing with a weak salt solution and inspected for obvious abnormalities.

First undertaken in the 1920s, the procedure has been greatly improved by the use of fibre-optic light transmission. Modern optics have made an ongoing contribution, so that the field can now be magnified 4–40 times. Moreover, abnormal or 'pre-invasive' tissue has certain biochemical and physical characteristics that enable it to be identified by preliminary treatment— thus swabbing the cervix with 3 or 5 per cent acetic acid results in whitening of abnormal tissue by coagulation of *mucus within the cells, where it is found in higher concentrations. Abnormal tissue thus identified can be subjected to precise pathological scrutiny by taking a tiny *biopsy—again, a procedure that should be without discomfort. Based on those findings, treatment can be individualized for each patient. Colposcopy and colposcopically directed biopsy are thus a means to an end—the precise treatment of specific conditions.

For example, pre-invasive cancer (CIN) is both a cellular change (changes within the cells) and a change in their general pattern. Thus within the superficial layer of skin (the epidermis) cells are 'layered'—upright at the base, flattened at the surface—a process known as 'maturation'. In pre-invasive disease this differentiation is lost, the cells assuming a rounded similarity. For descriptive purposes, such a change confined to the deepest layer (the most minor degree of change) is termed 'CIN1', – but the presence of changes throughout the layers (the most severe) is called 'CIN3'.

Details of cellular change are outside the scope of this article; suffice it to say that CIN1 may be managed by observation only and has a significant chance of spontaneous resolution, whereas CIN3 has about a one-third chance of progression to cancer and should be completely removed. Differences in cellular patterns give 'clues' by their colposcopic appearance—CIN being more likely the larger the relative area of disease, being thicker and whiter and often producing a 'mosaic'-type pattern. None the less, precision can be achieved only by biopsy.

Certain developments over the past few years have combined to make the appearance more obvious to the patient—television documentaries in particular. Attempts to limit inconvenience by treatment at the first visit, based on colposcopic appearance, have yet to be confirmed as the most appropriate means of diagnosis and treatment.

In addition to diagnosis, colposcopy is the means by which precise, local treatment may be undertaken— usually by *laser or *diathermy under local *anaesthesia in out-patient departments. Again, this is a painless procedure. In summary, colposcopy is an optical means of precise definition of pre-invasive disease of the neck of the womb, allowing local treatment, thus preventing subsequent development of cancer. Such treatment should aim to leave the cervix normal in its function and is largely successful in this, and its therapeutic, aim.

S. C. SIMMONS

COMA is a state of complete *unconsciousness, in which the patient fails to respond to arousal stimuli,

even when vigorous or painful (cf. *stupor, in which vigorous stimuli elicit some response).

COMMENSAL describes an organism which 'eats at the same table' as another of a different species, but which confers on the latter neither benefit nor harm. The *bacteria that normally inhabit the human *intestine are commensals.

COMMITTEE ON SAFETY OF MEDICINES. A body established by the UK Health Ministers in 1972 under the *Medicines Act 1968. It is now a part of the Medicines Control Agency under the Department of Health. It has two main functions: to give advice with respect to safety, quality, and efficacy in relation to human use of any substance or article (not being an instrument, apparatus, or appliance) to which any provision of the Act is applicable; and to promote the collection and investigation of information relating to adverse reactions for the purpose of enabling such advice to be given. The Committee, the membership of which is drawn predominantly from academic medicine, advises on the issue of Clinical Trial Certificates and of Product Licences; without the latter, a drug cannot be marketed in the UK. In the event of serious adverse reactions, they may also ask that a drug already on the market be withdrawn. As the terms of reference indicate, the Committee is advisory, and Ministers retain executive responsibility.

COMMON COLD. See COLD.

COMMON COLD RESEARCH UNIT. An establishment of the *Medical Research Council housed in a small isolated hospital in Wiltshire (the Harvard Hospital, built by *Harvard Medical School during the Second World War for medical research and subsequently donated to the British government). From 1946 a programme of research into the common *cold and related infections was carried out there, with the assistance of volunteers who spent (in pairs) two weeks under conditions of strict isolation. The unit was closed in 1990.

COMMUNICABLE DISEASE. See *INFECTIOUS DISEASES.

COMMUNICATION BETWEEN DOCTORS AND PATIENTS
Introduction
Doctors have always needed to communicate satisfactorily with patients. Until the 19th century treatments were largely ineffectual, and doctors' reputations and livelihood depended upon their 'bedside manner'. When diagnoses became soundly based, coming to depend on the understanding of the pathological basis of disease, and as, in this century, treatments became powerfully effective, good communication, albeit wrongly, seemed less necessary to good

doctoring. The advent of the UK *National Health Service demoted it even more. The 'bedside manner' became less important, except in private practice.

'Doctor knows best' was the order of the day, but as patients became better educated and more knowledgeable about both health and disease, the slogan became unsustainable, especially since patients now properly expect to have a large say in decisions about their treatment. Other factors have played a part: a non-élitist culture, the growth of consumerism, patients' organizations developing as pressure groups, and, within the hierarchy of medicine, the relative rise of other health professionals, often perceived as more approachable and caring. Doctors are now, rightly, being challenged to explain more, to inform better, and to be more appreciative and concerned about their patients. Patients insist on being treated as individuals, rather than repositories of organs. The great majority of complaints about doctors arise from them not explaining things fully.

Good communicating ability should equip the doctor to meet these new challenges. Yet we should keep its importance in perspective. Better the doctor who is thorough in history-taking, examining, investigating, diagnosing, and treating, than one who is all kindness and sympathy. But he or she should be wise and skilful in both; rigour and caring must not stand as contraries. They should be side by side and effectively interact.

The necessary skills have been studied, and we know they may be learned. Medical schools now place an emphasis on teaching them. This is timely. We know that patients retain little of what their doctors have told them; we know that medical students and doctors could still be better trained. Spread of instruction will not produce doctors who all communicate similarly. Personalities of both doctors and patients are involved and so individual approaches must develop. Each doctor will communicate in his or her own way, indeed, ways, since different patients and different situations warrant different techniques.

Purposes

Medical communication serves three main purposes. It permits *interchange of information* between doctor and patient. It is concerned with *the engagement of feelings*, which enhances the therapeutic benefit of the doctor–patient relationship by fostering trust and confidence in the doctor's abilities and permitting reassurance. Thirdly, it assists in obtaining *compliance*. The good doctor aims to secure the patient's agreement with the recommended course of action. The patient has the right to demur, but where there has been good interchange of information, including what choices the patient should make, and where trust exists, such refusals are infrequent, because the patient and the doctor are in concert about how to proceed.

A consultation between doctor and patient has something of the characteristics of classical drama. Act one is the *exposition*. The patient tells the story, urged on by the doctor. Act two is *development*. The doctor questions further and the patient responds; the examination takes place and any investigations; twists and turns are explored. Dominating these proceedings, a crucial shift takes place, moving from the patient's *complaint* to the doctor's *diagnosis*. The doctor can now construe the problem in terms of *pathology, where his or her medical training best functions. So we move to the final act, *resolution*, by discussion and treatment. Without resolution there is no sense of satisfaction. When the situation has been properly resolved in this way both doctor and patient have the feeling that all has turned out well. But this will not be achieved unless information has passed from the doctor to the patient about what is wrong, how serious it may be and what has to be done about it. Every stage of the drama requires good communication.

Some techniques and their underlying principles

Friendship is not necessary to good medical communication. Indeed, a certain distance should be maintained. It helps the doctor to maintain what *Osler called *aequanimitas*, or imperturbability, so that he or she may proffer advice (and get it accepted) that may be hard for the patient, such as stopping a long-cherished habit, like smoking, undergoing a mutilating operation, or quitting a too strenuous job when there is not much chance of getting another.

Doctors and patients are not equals in the setting of the consultation. Patients are not normal people but people weakened by their condition, and in that state they need their doctor to be firm, dependable, rock-like. This does not mean that doctors should appear hard; it does mean that they can be utterly depended upon. The doctor should not share the patient's uncertainty. He or she must always know what to do next, even if it is only to seek a further opinion or to wait and see.

All patients should be welcomed at the start of the consultation. This helps to put a patient at ease. However, if this cannot be achieved, the doctor should make plain an awareness of the unease. 'Only connect' was E. M. Forster's advice. It is not enough. The doctor has to connect with concern.

Patients do not relax if they perceive that their doctor is in a hurry; anyway, attempts to cut a patient short generally fail. For their part, patients should respect that the doctor has other patients to see and consider what their own obligations are. In facilitating good communication there are tasks for the patient as well as for the doctor. It is worthwhile considering beforehand what you want to tell the doctor so that you can be reasonably concise. The doctor will almost certainly want to know when the condition began; you do not assist by dating it from when the cat had kittens. Yet such responses are common.

The doctor must listen attentively. The consultation time belongs to the patient. When the patient stops talking the doctor may become actively questioning.

Yet it may produce more useful information for him or her just to pause. If the patient has stopped because to go on would be painful, he or she should be encouraged to do so. 'I plied him with the spur of silence', Max Beerbohm wrote, and Michael Balint taught that 'if you ask questions all you get is answers'. The doctor has the choice of questioning, prompting, and saying nothing. It is a hard skill to get it right, as also to know when to employ 'closed' questions requiring specific answers, and when to use 'open' questions that leave the patient free to direct the course.

Doctors must learn to overcome a patient's embarrassment when talking about certain symptoms, as describing their drinking habits, or detailing their social situations. Embarrassment is certainly a hindrance to the consultation. One technique is to forbid it outright; to indicate that 'we have business to do together; embarrassment gets in the way; therefore we had both better grit our teeth and get on with it'. This works. The doctor is being straightforward and the patient will follow suit. If the embarrassment is due to a third party being present, a student or a relative, they may be asked to leave. If, on the contrary, it is due to the absence of a third party during a physical examination, a chaperone should be summoned.

Embarrassment is natural; not so shame. It stems from deeper intrapsychic forces and will be enhanced if the patient senses that the doctor is being judgmental or critical. That was not the reason for consulting. The doctor may show disapproval of a behaviour on health grounds but not on moral grounds. Although the doctor is a person with his own moral standards he is not such a person when dealing with a patient.

Nor should a patient's complaint ever be regarded as trivial and hence treated dismissively. It is not for the doctor to decide this. Patients always have a reason for visiting the doctor. It may be openly expressed in the complaint. Often it is hidden and it may be that he or she draws comfort or emotional sustenance from the doctor's presence. It may not be necessary to bring this out during the consultation, but the doctor performs a number of roles and should not disdain that one. The doctor may neither be flippant nor mocking. Also, questions must not be asked just to gratify curiosity; indeed the knowledge that this will not be done encourages the patient to supply information of a very personal kind in response to questions of a relevance that is obscure. It must be that the doctor has a good reason for asking. Nor may the doctor indicate that he considers a patient to be foolish. Ignorant, possibly, and seeking to have that ignorance dispelled, but not stupid. The relationship is lost if the patient feels that the doctor thinks that.

Touching a patient can be a most important means of cementing the relationship; the doctor should, however, only use this means of communication where it feels both natural and appropriate to convey feelings of sympathy.

Patients are often very sensitive (a reputation for perspicacity can be gained by telling a patient 'I can see that you are a very sensitive person', for so we all view ourselves) and some doctors are crassly insensitive, having no idea how unkindly they may be handling some of their patients. Patients are often humiliated. One ready way to do this is by talking callously about them, as though they were not there, to students. The presence of students may, however, be turned to good account if they have been properly introduced to the patient. The illness or the treatment can be explained to the student with the intention that the patient listen so that he may feel that nothing has been concealed from him.

When giving information to a patient the doctor must employ appropriate language. If technical terms are to be used, 'it goes by the name of'—which some patients like—they must be explained. Yet quite complex explanations about the illness or the treatment may be necessary. 'Everything should be made as simple as possible', Einstein is reported as saying, 'but not more simple'. Repetition is often necessary or the patient may be asked to repeat the information to the doctor, or, if there is a relative at hand, to tell him or her while the doctor listens. Above all, the patient should be encouraged to ask questions if he or she has not followed anything. The doctor can give the patient a written account to take away; there are explanatory leaflets for most conditions, often prepared by concerned sufferers with medical help.

How much to tell the patient, especially in the matter of *prognosis, calls for much judgement, but the patient generally indicates if wanting to know more. It is always easier to add information than to retract it. Doctors differ about whether there may be some circumstances in which to lie to a patient. An extreme case is whether to reply honestly to a 10-year-old child with *leukaemia, where all possible treatments have failed and who seeks reassurance that he is not going to die. If you would lie in those circumstances, you concede that it is a matter of degree. The cardinal rule should be never to extinguish hope. Yet there are very few circumstances where the doctor need consider lying.

A patient may be given information by more than one person and care should be taken that they all agree on the message.

Some special situations

When the patient is a child, much of the give and take of information goes on between the doctor and mother, but you may observe that the child is keenly taking it all in. Children need to sum up this stranger, the doctor, if they are to give their trust, and the time spent in taking the history is useful. If the mother reports her difficulties with the child, the doctor must always be aware that the latter is the patient, and be prepared to see things from his or her perspective. If the examination or the treatment will hurt, the telling of this should be directly to the child, who, if properly informed, may well prove more stoical than the mother.

Much sensitivity is required with adolescent patients. During the time of teenage rebelliousness there must be no doubt in the patient's mind whose side the doctor is on. Certainly the patient should at some time be seen alone or with a neutral chaperone.

Handicapped patients also demand extra sensitivity. They do not want to find the doctor exhibiting the same critical, pitying, or humiliating approaches that they are used to from the public. Complete straightforwardness is called for. It is a bad mistake to regard the person who is deaf, incoordinated, or has speech difficulties as stupid.

Ethnic, cultural, and religious differences between patient and doctor may create problems, but these should be quickly resolved by bringing them into the open and indicating that they have to be got over. Language or pronunciation barriers call for an interpreter. Hospitals maintain lists of staff who can speak a variety of languages. Patients from ethnic minorities, and patients treated by doctors from ethnic minorities, are often somewhat on their guard. Once they find complete acceptance then the confidence developed is all the greater.

Gender difference between doctor and patient can lead to problems. Male doctors, including *obstetricians, are often curiously insensitive to the feelings of women patients in respect of physical examination, and particularly about being demonstrated, when pregnant, to students. Some male doctors have a lot to learn about this and the sooner they do, the better. Conversely, women doctors still encounter some resistance, even some cheek, from male patients. Ignoring it is the best policy.

Teaching communication skills
Firm evidence now exists that such skills may be imparted by teaching, and that, once learned, they persist. Medical students are increasingly receiving instruction. *General practitioners, also, have set about acquiring them, though not many hospital doctors. The most potent teaching tool is the video-recorder. Technology has provided Burns' much wished power 'to see oursels as others see us'. For a doctor or a student, to watch an interview played back is a chastening lesson. It can be with a real patient or with an actor trained to play the patient role. The doctor or student is often more appalled than he or she need be, and it is the role of the teacher to indicate to him or her, as they observe their errors of commission or omission, how the communication should have gone. An actor interviewee may well conduct this teaching. If the interview has been with a patient, then comments from that source can assist the learning experience.

Conclusion
There are three lessons to be learned from studying doctor–patient communication. First, the doctor who considers only the illness and not the patient fails the patient. Secondly, the doctor who is genuinely concerned about a patient will make few mistakes and they will all be rectifiable. Thirdly, both patients and doctors could improve their communication skills.

NEIL KESSEL

COMMUNITY CARE. See SOCIAL WORK AND MEDICINE.

COMMUNITY HEALTH COUNCILS (CHCs) were set up under the *National Health Service (Reorganization) Act 1973 to represent the 'consumer interest'. There is a CHC in each NHS health district, giving 195 Councils in England and 22 in Wales. Local Health Councils (LHCs) perform the same function in Scotland. They are required to assess the adequacy of local health services from the users' viewpoint. They have a right to basic information about planning and operation of services, to be consulted about substantial future developments, to visit NHS hospitals and institutions, and to have access to the District Health Authority (DHA) and its senior officers. Each CHC issues an annual report, and the DHA is required to publish replies recording action taken on issues raised. CHCs normally have between 18 and 24 members, of whom at least one-half are appointed by the local authority and at least one-third by voluntary organizations with an interest in the NHS; the remainder are appointed by the Regional Health Authority on the basis of special knowledge and experience. See also NATIONAL HEALTH SERVICE.

COMMUNITY MEDICINE. See PUBLIC HEALTH.

COMMUNITY NURSING. See NURSING IN THE UK; NURSING IN THE USA AND CANADA.

COMMUNITY PHYSICIAN. The term was formerly used in England and Wales (not Scotland) for a specialist in *community medicine. The community physician replaced the former *medical officer of health but the traditional term 'Public Health' has now been revived in the UK.

COMPANY OF BARBER-SURGEONS. See BARBER-SURGEONS, COMPANY OF.

COMPARATIVE ANATOMY is the study of the structure of lower animals in relation to each other and to man.

COMPARATIVE MEDICINE is the study of medicine with reference to species other than man.

COMPATIBILITY. See BLOOD TRANSFUSION; HLA.

COMPENSATION NEUROSIS is a *neurosis following industrial injury or other episode where there is a question of indemnification for a real or presumed disability, and where the issue of possible financial compensation is thought to play a part in the genesis of the neurotic illness.

COMPLEMENT is a series of 15 or more thermolabile enzymatic *proteins found in body fluids, which when activated are important in the body's defences against *micro-organisms. The three main functions of complement are the promotion of *inflammation, *phagocytosis, and *lysis. Activation of the components occurs in a cascading sequence, initiated either by binding of specific *antibody (IgG or IgM) to surface *antigens (the 'classical' pathway) or release of various *polysaccharides and IgA aggregates (the 'alternative' pathway). See also IMMUNOLOGY.

COMPLEMENTARY (ALTERNATIVE) MEDICINE
Matters of definition

'Complementary medicine' is a term of comparatively recent origin and of growing currency, which is used to denote a number of systems of medicine which were previously described as '*alternative medicine', or even as 'fringe medicine'. This change in nomenclature is not trivial, for it expresses a welcome recognition that in matters as complex as the pursuit of health or the treatment of disease there is room for diverse approaches, which may complement one another, depending on the nature of the problem and on the physical and psychological 'make-up' of the actual or potential patient.

There are two particular reasons why it is difficult to give a clear positive definition of complementary medicine. First, it is far from being a single entity, comprising as it does many systems, ranging from long-established and well-recognized disciplines such as *homoeopathy and *osteopathy, through less interventive systems such as aromatherapy and psionic medicine, to systems which may be closer to cults than to therapies, such as *herbalism or transcendental meditation. Fulder (1984) lists 73 different 'therapies in complementary medicine'.

The second reason that makes definition elusive stems from the hidden question both in 'complementary' and in 'alternative' medicine—'complementary to what? alternative to what?' The 'medicine', which is the object of these questions, is no easier to define than its complement or alternative, for it is equally diverse and equally, or more reluctant, to stand still with a view to be defined. It is sometimes called 'scientific' or 'orthodox'—but a great deal of effective medicine is not based on 'hard science', and 'orthodox' implies a fixity of belief which is alien to what should be an open discipline. However, if we were to describe it as the medicine that is currently taught in medical schools and practised in surgeries and clinics, that may convey what is meant. There is perhaps no completely satisfactory adjective to distinguish this form of medicine from the systems that are the specific subject of this article; but I shall call it 'mainstream medicine', to indicate only that it is what most doctors practise for most of their time.

A paradox of therapy

Particularly over the past half-century, mainstream medicine has been dramatically extended in its effective scope, both for the prevention of illness and for its treatment; yet it has never been so generally criticized, both in words by ethicists and publicists, and in action by patients and doctors who turn, even as a first choice, to other methods. There are a number of possible explanations for this. To the extent that mainstream medicine is science-based, professional, and paternalistic, it may suffer in esteem from a fairly general mistrust of experts, and particularly of scientific experts; from suspicion that professional men, and even women, may depart from their obligation to put the interests of their patients before their own; and from fears that the autonomy of the patients may be threatened by arrogance or paternalism. Through lack of time or lack of appropriate skill, doctors can make mistakes, both in what they do and in what they say, or fail to say; and it is the mistakes which attract gossip and journalistic attention.

These are matters of attitude, in itself an important determinant of what people do; but I believe that a more fundamental cause of the growing recourse to systems other than mainstream medicine may lie in a quite reasonable general incomprehension of what John Ryle called the 'natural history of disease', in relation to what medicine can (and cannot) do. That part of medicine which is science-based is relevant to the actual *cure* of only a small part of human illness and misery; but it can also contribute materially to the *relief* of suffering; and *reassurance* following competent assessment and investigation is a further benefit, little though it can figure in a calculus of 'outcomes'. These are worthwhile benefits, but they still leave a vast burden of chronic or fatal acute illness, for which science-based medicine is not synonymous with mainstream medicine, but only a part of it. Assessment, understanding, comfort, and talking to patients and relatives remain as obligations for doctors, and for nurses; but time may be short, other preoccupations compelling, or there may be a lack of rapport with particular individuals. It would be truly arrogant to suggest that these vital components of therapy are the exclusive prerogative of mainstream medicine; and it is perhaps here that other systems can be truly 'complementary'. I must in honesty enter one caveat—although mainstream medical intervention is critical in only a minority of episodes of illness, in those particular episodes it is critical indeed; and I would plead that at least in acute illness, and possibly in any illness, 'complementary' medicine should also be 'subsequent' to an assessment of the clinical situation by competent 'orthodox' means.

Examples of complementary medicine

A sympathetic observer, searching for 'a common bond' to unite these diverse therapies, finds it in the claim, 'They all attempt, in varying degrees, to recruit the self-healing capacities of the body' (Fulder 1984). He adds that 'symptoms are used as tools or guides to the nature of the patient's upset or imbalance'. These criteria may be useful in linking the diverse forms of complementary therapy; but they do not serve, as is implied, to distinguish them from mainstream medicine. Recognition of the *vis medicatrix naturae* goes back to classical times; and natural recuperative powers benefit patients, without respect to the system by which they are treated. Mainstream diagnostic medicine also relies heavily on the analysis of symptoms—as Robert Platt was wont to put it, 'If you listen to the patient, he will tell you what is wrong with him'.

It would clearly not be possible even to annotate all the forms of complementary treatment; this account will be limited to a few of those that enjoy wide currency; are legally permitted in a number of countries or states; and have recognized training programmes, codes of practice, and registers of qualified practitioners. Within these criteria, it would not be for me to say whether all complementary therapies are equal (although I suspect they may be, in the good sense of giving time and support to patients); or whether in the Orwellian phrase, some may be more equal than others. I shall conceal my judgement on the latter point by rigid adherence to alphabetical order.

*Acupuncture

This part of traditional Chinese medicine has caught the public imagination, and has become widely practised in the West, by doctors as well as by other therapists. Its origins go back for several millenia, but it has developed over the centuries (it would have been something of an indictment, had it not); and the recent discovery of the *endorphins affords a possible physiological basis for its well-attested success in the relief of pain, and even in the induction of *anaesthesia during surgery. Although *pain relief is the aspect of Chinese traditional medicine which is closest to Western medicine, it is only a small part of the whole, being supplemented by exercises and herbal remedies, and also forming part of an elaborate system of promoting health and treating a gamut of disease states. Acupuncture points arranged along meridians are accorded specificity for particular purposes, both in pain relief and in general therapy. These points may be stimulated not only by actual needling, but also by electrical stimulation or by burning a small cone of dried mugwort (*Artemisia vulgaris*) over the prescribed point—the technique of *moxibustion*. For the relief of pain, acupuncture is quite commonly used both in family practice and in pain clinics; and it is also available as part of general health maintenance by traditional methods. In their consideration of acupuncture, a Working Party of the British Medical Association (BMA) gave the cautious advice, after noting the risks of infection or of mechanical injury, that 'the practice of acupuncture should conform to the same ethical and technical standards as does medical practice'(British Medical Association 1986).

*Chiropractic

This system originated in the USA in the 1890s. Its founder, D. D. Palmer, an experienced manipulator of the *spine, formed the view that misaligned or maladjusted vertebrae impinged on nerves, thus interfering with what he termed 'innate intelligence', an entity necessary for the health of the structures supplied by the damaged nerves. He stated that 'a subluxed vertebra is the cause of 95% of all diseases', a claim which, coming some years after the work of Pasteur, may be seen as an overstatement. Modern chiropractic does not claim that degree of universality, and concentrates on the treatment of musculoskeletal disorders, in which it enjoys considerable success. It is established and legally recognized in the USA in many states of the Union, in France, Scandinavia, and now in the UK. The British Chiropractors Association defines chiropractic as 'an independent branch of medicine concerned with the diagnosis and treatment of mechanical disorders of *joints, particularly spinal joints, and their effects on the nervous system'. Chiropractic diagnosis includes the use of X-rays, but treatment is by manipulation, without recourse to 'drugs' or surgery. Patients whose problem, even if it be a musculoskeletal condition, is not adjudged to be due to spinal displacement, are customarily referred to doctors, and there are now no formal barriers to such referral.

*Homoeopathy (homeopathy)

While it can scarcely compare in antiquity with Chinese, or for that matter Indian, traditional medicine, homoeopathy is the longest-established of the systems of complementary medicine to have arisen in Europe. It is also notable for the high proportion of its practitioners who have a registrable medical qualification, and are thus in a position to exercise true 'complementarity' in their own practice, having recourse, for example, to surgery in appropriate circumstances. The founder of homoeopathic medicine, Samuel Hahnemann, was legitimately discontented with the rigorous measures that made up 18th century orthodox therapeutics, and he had made the chance observation that *quinine in ordinary doses given to normal people mimicked the symptoms of *malaria, for which quinine was a remedy in common use. Combining these two perceptions, he arrived at a system of therapy based on agents which, when given to normal people, simulated the symptoms of particular diseases, for which these agents were then given in very small amounts. The principles that 'like cures like', and that medicines should be carefully prepared in small dosage, have remained central to both medical and lay homoeopathy. Development has taken place in such details as the appropriate dilution, and the alternation of shaking the solution (succussion) with further dilution. Hahnemann believed that succussion was critical in increasing the activity or 'potency' of medicines, which could then act more strongly on the miasmata of chronic disease; these latter views are now more influential among homoeopathic therapists who have not taken a medical qualification.

*Osteopathy

Since both disciplines make extensive use of spinal manipulation, there is a prima facie likeness between osteopathy and chiropractic. However, although they share a belief in the importance of spinal displacements, the 'father' of osteopathy, Andrew Still, stressed pressure on arteries, partially occluding blood flow, in contrast to the chiropractic emphasis on pressure on nerves, impeding the flow of impulses. Together with homoeopathy, which has long-standing associations with registered medical practitioners, osteopathy is perhaps the one among the complementary disciplines now receiving full professional recognition, with formal registration of qualified osteopathic practitioners, a recognized curriculum, and provision for continuing supplementary education. A Working Party of the King Edward's Hospital Fund suggested in 1991 that statutory regulation and registration of mainstream osteopathic practitioners was both feasible and desirable. Although osteopathy embraces different schools and techniques, there is sufficient common ground to make registration appropriate and an Osteopath's Act is now (1993) on the UK Statute Book.

Legal and ethical aspects

It is neither criminal nor unethical to undertake the treatment of patients at their own request without being medically qualified, subject to certain provisos. The main legal proviso is that the person giving treatment must not falsely claim or imply that he is medically qualified. In the event of harm resulting which is reasonably attributable to the treatment given, an unqualified practitioner might be more vulnerable to a claim for damages, since he would lack both a defence that he had conformed to an agreed standard of practice, and the services of an experienced professional defence organization. For many years, alternative forms of treatment were considered so unethical that a doctor associating professionally with their practitioners ran the risk of disapproval by his colleagues, and formal censure by professional regulatory bodies. As medicine itself

has become more self-confident, and as it has become apparent that, for whatever reason, countless patients have derived both comfort and objective benefits from alternative forms of treatment, these attitudes have changed—a change that will be greatly encouraged by moves towards regulation and registration of those practising these various techniques. The term 'complementary' is itself an indication that this change is under way. As an ethical safeguard for patients, registration should require adherence to a code of practice, which will ensure primacy for the interests of the patient, adherence to confidentiality of clinical information, and openness of communication and conduct—in other words, the hallmarks of professional status.

DOUGLAS BLACK

References
Fulder, S. (1984). *The handbook of complementary medicine*. Coronet Books, Hodder & Stoughton, London.
British Medical Association (1986). *Alternative medicine*, Report of the Board of Science and Education. Chameleon Press, London.

COMPLEMENT FIXATION is inactivation of *complement occurring when an *antibody reacts with its homologous *antigen. As the presence of complement can be detected by the *haemolysis of sensitized red blood cells added to the medium, complement fixation is used as an indicator in various immunological tests (e.g. *Kahn test).

COMPLEX. Any substance or compound formed by the combination of simpler substances; in *Jungian psychology, a group of repressed emotional factors.

COMPLIANCE is the extent to which a patient obeys the advice of his doctor, particularly with respect to the taking of medicines.

COMPOUND. Any chemical made up of more than one element, the elements being united in definite proportions by mass.

COMPULSION is an irresistible urge towards a particular form of behaviour, regardless of considerations of logic or social acceptability.

COMPUTERIZED AXIAL TOMOGRAPHY, often abbreviated to CAT or CT, is a method by which an *X-ray image of a cross-section of the body or head at any particular depth is reconstructed electronically and displayed. See RADIOLOGY; SCANNERS; TOMOGRAPHY.

COMPUTERS are electronic devices which accept data, apply logical processes, and supply the results of these processes. See COMPUTERS IN MEDICINE.

COMPUTERS IN MEDICINE
Clinical computing
A clinical computer application is one that is directly involved in support for the care of the patient, as opposed to administration of that care, the management of hospitals, or the control of finances.

This definition encompasses a truly huge number and diversity of computer systems, which are only loosely related. Although the number and sophistication of medical computing applications have increased markedly in the past decade, the field is very far from mature: we await the emergence of an intellectual framework which unites and structures the amorphous discipline which has come to be known as 'medical informatics'. For the present we can investigate the different strands of the computing domain that could be pulled together under this heading.

Three application providers
In each subsector of medical computing we find represented (at least) three distinct groups of application 'provider'. These are the academic, the commercial, and the user.

There is a healthy amount of academic research in all areas of medical computing. Most of this is conducted as part of general research into computer science, with medicine being one of a number of domains of application, but recently the UK universities have started to recognize 'medical informatics' as an academic discipline or subdiscipline in its own right. This trend follows the continental example—notably that of Germany and The Netherlands—where medical informatics is represented by whole departments in universities. The applications that result from the academic sector are rarely used by large numbers of practising clinicians (although there are notable exceptions); however, lessons learned in their development are disseminated through the computing community, potentially influencing the design of those computer systems that are used more widely.

In general, computer applications that are widely used by clinicians today are produced by commercial 'software houses', of which there are a great number in the medical sector. The application types that are developed tend to be those with which the computing community has most experience: database systems and image-processing systems (sold with the imaging devices). The flow of ideas from academia to industry is at best haphazard: in order to improve this communication, and to help industry capitalize on the advanced developments coming from the universities, the Commission of the European Communities set up the AIM I and II (advanced informatics in medicine) programmes, whose goals were to stimulate joint academic and industrial research and development of sophisticated medical computing applications (Noothoven van Goor and Cristensen 1992).

There is a third sort of application provider—the user.

In many hospitals and *general practitioner (GP) practices a plethora of small-scale computer programs have been written by the very people who intend to use them. In many other cases although the eventual users have not actually programmed the computer him or herself, they nevertheless have carried out the design and paid or persuaded another to implement that design. While most of these are small database systems that are used for a relatively short period of time, some are quite sophisticated and have become accepted and used by users other than the designer/programmer. They tend to share the feature that they are well suited to the task for which they were designed. One of the most difficult problems in medical, or any form of, computing is providing the user with a system that actually does what he or she requires of it: if the application has been designed or programmed by the user, then this problem is unlikely to arise.

Bearing in mind this distinction between system 'providers', we can investigate the different sorts of medical application that are being developed or are commonly in use.

Patient record systems
The most common form of medical computing application is the medical record system. This is generally a means of storing and presenting some of the information that would normally be stored in the patient's paper records. Advantages of keeping some of this information in a computerized database are:

1. Instant access to the record. There is no need to fetch the record from a central store, which takes time, especially if the record is currently being used by someone else.
2. Greater legibility of the record. It is generally significantly easier to read machine-printed text than that which is hand-written.
3. Structured presentation of the record. Some medical records can accumulate hundreds of pages. A computerized medical record system can sift through this vast array of data and present details most relevant to the condition at hand. Similarly, important observations and abnormalities can be flagged for attention (by presenting those results in a different colour for example).
4. Integrity of the record. Through the use of range checking and other forms of data validation programs, infeasible observations and impossible results entered by accident can be rejected then and there, meaning that the information in the medical record is of greater quality than a paper-based system.
5. Support of aggregated reports. Computers can analyse databases in a number of ways: data need not just be looked at relating to the individual patient. Results can be extracted for a group of patients, or a group of clinicians, or a geographical area, meaning

that the user of the system can get a much better idea of what is 'going on' with respect to his or her patients.

There are disadvantages associated with the automated record, which is why they are still relatively rare.

1. High initial investment. The costs associated with purchasing a medical record system, necessary computer equipment, and training is much greater than the very cheap paper alternative.
2. Tedious data capture. Clinicians often feel that the effort associated with entering patient information into a computer system outweighs any benefits that accrue from the data. This problem can be ameliorated to a great extent through the use of 'friendly' user-interfaces.
3. Inflexible storage and communication. Once a medical record system is built, unless it is designed very carefully, it can be very difficult to change the way it works. This is a problem, given the constantly changing nature of medical care. Similarly, the information stored in one department's computer system might not be in a form which can be understood by the system in another department. Neither of these problems occur with the paper record.

Some commercial medical record systems are used widely; in particular there are a few GP systems that are used in hundreds of practices across the UK. In hospitals, medical record systems tend to be designed and used locally—tailored to the way a particular group of clinicians practise medicine. These are fairly common, partly because modern database programming languages (so-called fourth-generation languages) greatly facilitate the production of useful applications. There is a great deal of interest in creating standards that will help different database systems communicate with each other: so far only very simple standards have been adopted by the international standards organizations. Examples of basic standards are ICD-9, OPCS, and Read codes. More ambitious attempts to standardize the structure of clinical information (such as the GALEN project (1993) and the NHS Common Basic Specification[3] (NHS Management Executive 1992)) have not yet been widely adopted.

Image processing
Many modern imaging instruments, such as CT (*computerized tomography) scanners, ultrasound scanners, and MRI (*magnetic resonance imaging) depend on computers to process and present their findings to *radiologists. Recently there has been a move to dispense with 'paper-based' records for all manner of radiological investigations. The benefits of computerized storage that have been described for medical record systems would equally apply to *radiology records. Although there is not such a problem with data entry, the problems of standardization and high initial

investment remain, with a new one: that of storage space. The amount of information contained within a typical X-ray photograph is huge: it has been estimated (Greenes and Brinkley 1990) that the storage of all the images produced by a medium-sized radiology unit over a year would be in the order of 10^{12} 'bytes'—a typical 'personal computer' would be able to store 1/10 000th of this. Computer applications that attempt to provide this integrated image storage and presentation function are generically called PACS (picture archiving and communication systems).

Decision support systems
The term 'decision support system' (DSS) encompasses 'Rule-based systems', 'knowledge-based systems', and 'expert systems'. These systems have in common the fact that they manipulate and present medical data so as to help clinicians make sound, informed decisions. The simplest DSSs merely select which data from a given set are most important for the clinician, and present the data in such a way as to guide the decision-making process. Most medical record systems fulfil this function.

More advanced DSSs will not only present the medical data, but will derive potential 'decisions' from the data. Some DSSs will ask about the presence and nature of a range of symptoms in a subject, and deduce from this possible diagnoses (an example of this is Internist (Miller *et al.* 1982)). Other DSSs will take the patient's diagnoses, medical history, and existing drug regimen and suggest treatment that might be prescribed (examples of these are MYCIN (Shortliffe 1976) and EDCP/Diabeta (Williams 1989)). Each of these systems has to be able to work with incomplete data, and must be capable of dealing with and reflecting the uncertainty inherent in clinical decision-making. Because of these problems, medical DSSs tend to be adept at manipulating probabilities: early systems exploited Bayes' theorem and more recently causal probabilistic reasoning has been harnessed (as in, for example, MUNIN (Andreassen *et al.* 1987)).

Advanced decision-support systems (i.e. more sophisticated than mere data presentation systems), or knowledge-based systems, have tended to be the domain of academics, and have only rarely been adopted by the clinical community at large. One of the reasons for this is their inevitable specialization. Knowledge-based systems enable users to gain access to a depth of medical knowledge that they themselves do not possess. The way that medicine is structured in the UK, generalists see patients with a wide variety of conditions, meaning that the number of times that a specialist system would be used would be relatively small: too small, perhaps, for the expense of purchase and training to be justified. On the other hand, a clinician who sees a lot of patients with a particular condition will probably be a specialist already and so will not have need of the 'expert' system. There are exceptions to this observation: for example the system of de Dombal *et al.* (1972) is used in a number of UK accident and emergency departments. It is also expected that, as financial pressures on GPs increase, the long-term cost savings associated with decision-support systems (not requesting inappropriate tests, fewer referrals to specialists) will encourage them to invest in such systems, at least for relatively common conditions such as *diabetes and *hypertension. An alternative approach would be to develop decision-support systems that could help in a wide number of conditions and diseases: an expert system where the expertise has come from a large and varied team of experts. As might be expected, this approach is fraught with difficulties of a philosophical as well as practical nature. However, significant progress in this area has been made in recent years as, for example, in the LEMMA project of the European Community's AIM programme (Fox *et al.* 1992).

There remains a paradox, however; although de Dombal and colleagues have clearly shown the benefit of computer support for managing the acute abdomen with relatively junior doctors working in accident and emergency department, there has been little or no encouragement from the *National Health Service (NHS) to extend its use; one has to wonder why not?

Metabolic modelling
One area where computers have been of great assistance for clinicians is in the area of research; especially in the form of computerized mathematical modelling. One of the missions of natural science is to understand natural phenomena in terms of underlying models and theories; clinical medicine is no different. Some aspects of biological systems can be understood in terms of simple equations, but many can be reasonably modelled only by composing together a number of smaller, simpler sub-systems. When this happens, the models can become 'non-linear,' and difficult to solve and analyse mathematically. Computers are useful in these as experimental test-beds: a computer can be so programmed that it mimics the behaviour of the model, starting from a number of different initial conditions, and its resulting state can be compared with the findings in real patients to see if the model is a good one. This is a branch of the scientific method, facilitated by computer. There are a number of mathematical modelling approaches that can be supported through the use of a computer; these include compartmental modelling, using partial differential equations; causal probabilistic modelling, using Bayesian networks; and stochastic modelling, using statistical techniques. Examples of the sort of work that has been carried out in this area can be found in Carson *et al.* (1983).

Patient-centred computing
One last area of clinical computing that often gets neglected is the application that is used by patients themselves. Although the patient would not normally be thought of as a clinician, he or she is a very important 'provider of care'. Some 'patient-oriented' computer applications are intended to be used in the clinic, worked by the patient: these include patient education systems by which a patient can learn about the nature and management of his or her condition. Other patient-operated systems are intended to be used at home; although these still tend to be experimental, the rapid reduction in cost of computer equipment, coupled with the great wish many patients have to manage their own illness, mean that we will surely see more of these in the future.

Computer-aided learning
With increasing pressure on teacher/student ratios, and the improved availability of suitable computer hardware and software, computer-aided (or assisted) learning is beginning to come to the attention of medical schools and those who plan the curriculum. There are still very few areas where suitable software has been developed and tested, but there is considerable interest, and the availability of 'multi-media' (combination of computer software with video disc and other media) and 'virtual reality' means that we can look forward to some new and interesting approaches to teaching and learning.

Computers in medical administration and management
The potential of computers for better patient care and improved health service administration and resource utilization was clearly recognized in the mid-1960s, but much developmental work has been necessary, and useful and acceptable systems only began to be available in the late 1980s. The complexity of health care has been largely responsible for this over-long gestation period, but too many systems have failed because they were not well enough designed or tested and did not satisfy the real needs of the users. The introduction of 'new technology' has caused anxiety amongst the users as they perceived it as a potential threat to their jobs. The general change in computer-culture across the country has now made it easier to introduce computer systems in health care without such anxieties prevailing, but care is still needed to ensure that systems are seen as being really useful in supporting health care rather than simply reducing manpower.

Software developed in the 1970s and early 1980s was often insufficiently advanced to provide the flexibility and rapid response required by the user. Modification of the software to overcome problems and make the system more closely fit its environment was time-consuming and expensive. Communication between systems and machines was always difficult and often impossible. The result has been a number of separate computer systems, each fulfilling a particular job but with little or no integration between the systems. The tremendous advances that have occurred in computer software, combined with the adoption of industry standards and an 'open systems' philosophy have altered the scene entirely. It is now much easier to share databases and to tailor systems to match local needs and to include new data items without a complete re-write of the system. Despite improvements in technical issues such as these, information issues still hinder communication and integration. Datasets designed for management (such as the Körner dataset) are of little clinical use, and although it is often said that 'management information should be a by-product of patient care', this is rarely the case. There is still a great deal of unnecessary 'redundancy' in data collection and storage, with identical data being held on different systems.

Political issues regarding the appropriateness of holding confidential clinical information at a corporate hospital-wide level remain to be solved, as do those regarding the sharing of such data between hospital and general practice and the building and holding of 'Registers' of people with certain diseases (such as diabetes mellitus) where health care may be shared between a number of providers. The introduction of the 'purchaser-provider split' and contracts for health care means that confidential clinical information may be needed to support a claim for payment. The European Community is developing a directive on 'data protection' which appears to make it very difficult, if not impossible, to use personal data in such a way without specific permission from the subject on each and every occasion. Unless these and similar related issues can be sensibly overcome, we are moving from the era where it was nearly impossible to communicate between systems for technical reasons to an era where the communication problems are equally difficult but are influenced by political/ethical considerations.

The introduction of the current *National Health Service (NHS) reforms with the creation of the 'purchaser–provider split' has introduced a new need for better information on 'resource management' and 'audit', and has opened a new perspective on accounting within the service. Computer systems previously developed for patient administration, for example, no longer fulfil the needs of the new contracting processes. Keeping track of resource usage within hospitals and between departments has become of major importance as the emphasis of hospital management has shifted from simply facilitating the operation of the hospital to supporting contracting and accounting.

In hospitals

Most hospitals are now developing and implementing a computer strategy of their own to suit new business plans, contracting arrangements, and clinical services. Successful integrated hospital information systems supporting all these functions are few and far between, and failures are both common and expensive. Most hospitals have a number of discrete departmental systems, each of which fulfils a specific role but rarely communicates effectively with other systems. The result is redundancy of data: similar data being entered and held (often in

a slightly different form) on a number of distinct databases. Lack of data and software compatibility accounts for this inefficient and unsatisfactory state of affairs. Attempts to overcome this involve, on the one hand, attempts to fit the whole operation and administration of a hospital into a single system and, on the other hand, the development of a relational database 'view', where information is generated by bringing together data from many sources, perhaps distributed on a network. This pool of data exists on a network, distributed through many machines (servers). These data can be added, updated, and retrieved by programs (clients) elsewhere on the network. In principle all the data relating to a patient can be brought together in a single displayed or printed report.

In order for this to be achieved, technical standards of data storage and handling need to exist and be followed strictly. Until recently, there was little in common between computer systems made by different manufacturers, meaning that communication of data was very difficult. The development of 'industry standards' (such as the UNIX operating system, relational database structures, and structured query language (SQL), and 'open systems architecture' has made such an approach possible and cost-effective.

Thus the backbone of a hospital information system would be a local area network (LAN) extending throughout the site, to which is linked a number of computer terminals and systems. Typically, the terminals are personal computers, each with considerable local processing power in their own right. There will be a number of computer systems connected to the network and each of these can be accessed from any of the terminals. The personal computer can act in one of two modes: it might be a 'dumb terminal', acting as a window on to a remote powerful computer that both stores and processes the data of interest; or it might act as an intelligent 'client' that itself processes data that it collects from central 'server' machines.

Examples of discrete hospital systems fulfilling specific functions include:

(1) laboratory information systems (e.g. *microbiology, *haematology);
(2) clinical information systems (e.g. diabetes, medical record, audit);
(3) decision support systems (e.g. acute abdomen diagnosis and management);
(4) nursing systems (e.g. care plans, rostering, dependency);
(5) pharmacy systems (e.g. stock control, drug interaction);
(6) case-mix;
(7) in-patient and out-patient management (e.g. appointments, admissions);
(8) contract management;
(9) personnel systems;
(10) payroll.

Linkage of these to a network facilitates access from sites across the hospital. The observance of common technical standards by all of these different systems is a necessary but not sufficient condition for successful 'systems integration'.

Once the technical problems have been solved, we need to address more conceptual issues: what information should be communicated, how should it be structured, what does it mean, with whom should it be communicated? These are not technical questions and, as such, solutions are much harder to find. Some of these (essentially informatics) questions are global to the whole NHS and are being tackled on that basis. For example, it is important that the same terms are used by different health-care providers if they are talking about the same thing, and terminological standardization is being tackled by the Centre for Coding and Classification, part of the Information Management Group of the NHS (Chisholm 1990). Other informatics issues will be local and specific to each hospital. Even were these informatics issues to be successfully addressed, we would still have to consider the organizational and political difficulties attendant on introducing a large information system into an extremely socially complex organization such as a hospital. All these issues combine to render the successful implementation of integrated hospital systems extremely problematic, and indeed we find that such hospital information support systems (HISS) are very rare, and those that do exist are modest in scope.

In general practice

Computers are becoming commonplace in general practice. There is, however, a plethora of different systems and no clear 'market leader'. The consequence is that, although they may well provide specific support for a given practice, communication with outside agencies (e.g. local hospital, laboratories, Family Health Service Authority (FHSA)) is difficult or impossible. With the introduction of new contracts for GPs, new functions are needed to support the business as well as medical objectives of the practice. The very nature of general practice means that the systems have to be able to cope with the breadth of medicine, and cannot address the detail of disease-specific need. The function that most GP systems support include:

(1) practice register (e.g. age/sex, disease);
(2) *immunization and *vaccination;
(3) *screening (e.g. cervical *cytology);
(4) repeat prescribing;
(5) case notes;
(6) letter and report writing, word processing;
(7) practice accounts.

Pilot developments exist in the area of 'decision support' where 'knowledge-based' systems containing expert knowledge in the form of computer programs which interact with the 'medical records' to focus the knowledge on the particular needs of a given patient.

Thus standards of 'good medical practice' can be applied to the management of conditions such as hypertension and diabetes mellitus. Such systems vary in complexity from those which simply apply fixed protocols to the management of a given patient to those where the protocol of care for a given patient is derived from a knowledge-base (e.g. set of 'rules'), resulting in a 'care-plan' more specifically tailored to the individual needs of that individual. There appear to be great opportunities for focusing the reams of medical knowledge that often sit on dust-covered shelves on the practice of medicine. Such systems offer the potential for improved uniformity and availability of 'good health care' by underpinning the application of standards of good practice.

JEREMY HOLLAND
PETER SÖNKSEN

References

Andreassen, S., Woldbye, M., Falck, B., and Andersen S. K. (1987). MUNNIN–a causal probabilistic network for interpretation of electromyographic findings. In *10th International Joint Conference on Artificial Intelligence*, Milan, pp. 366–72. Kaufman.

Carson, E., Cobelli, E., and Finkelstein, l. (1983). *The mathematical modelling of metabolic and endocrine systems*. New York.

Chisholm, J. (1990). The read code classification. *British Medical Journal*, **300**, 1992.

de Dombal F., Leaper, J., Staniland, J., McCann, A., and Horrocks, J. (1972). Computer aided diagnosis of abdominal pain. *British Medical Journal*, **ii**, 9–13.

Fox, J. *et al.* (1992). LEMMA: methods and architectures for logic engineering in medicine. In *Advances in medical informatics; results of the AIM exploratory* action, (ed. J. Noothoven van goor and J. Christensen). IOS Press, Amsterdam.

Greenes, A. and Brinkley J. (1990). Radiology systems. *Medical informatics*, (ed. E. Shortliffe and L. Perreault). Addison-Wesley, Reading, Massachusetts.

Information Management Group, NHS Management Executive (1992). *Common basic specification generic model*, Vols I and II. NHS Management Executive, Leeds.

Miller, R., Pople, H., and Myers, J., (1982). Internist–I, an experimental computer based diagnostic consultant for general internal medicine. *New England Journal of Medicine*, **307**, 468–76.

Noothoven van Goor, J. and Christensen, J. (1992) *Advances in medical informatics: results of the AIM exploratory action*. IOS Press, Amsterdam.

Shortliffe, E. (1976). *Computer-based medical consultations: MYCIN*,. Elsevier-North Holland, New York.

The GALEN Project Consortium (Rector, A. *et al*). (1993). GALEN; generalised architecture for language encyclopaedias and nomenclature in medicine. In *Commission of the European Communities DG XIII 1993* Annual Technical Report on RTD: Health Care, Brussels.

Williams, C. D., *et al.* (1989). *A technical and operational evaluation of a rule-based co-operative system for decision making in diabetic care*, DHSS Report, London.

CONCEPTION. The fertilization of an *ovum by a *spermatozoon and the implantation of the resulting *zygote.

CONCRETION. A solid mass formed by aggregation or cohesion, such as a *calculus.

CONCUSSION is jolting of the *brain due to a blow on the head, resulting in temporary disturbance of consciousness. Repeated concussion may result in permanent brain damage.

CONDITIONED REFLEX. A *reflex response which, through experience or training, has been induced to follow a stimulus not naturally associated with it.

CONDITIONING is the training process by which a response comes to be elicited by a stimulus other than that normally associated with it.

CONDOM. *Contraceptive *sheath.

CONDUCTION is transmission of energy change along or through a body, particularly the transmission of a nervous impulse along a *nerve fibre.

CONDYLE. A rounded protuberance on a bone.

CONDYLOMA. A wart-like growth in the anal or genital region. Small condylomata are due to *virus infection, often of venereal origin (*condyloma acuminata*). Larger, flat-topped condylomata occur in secondary *syphilis (*condylomalata*).

CONFABULATION is a manifestation of severe *amnesia for recent events, whereby the patient gives detailed and convincing but totally fictitious accounts of his activities. It is characteristic of *Korsakoff's syndrome.

CONFIDENTIALITY. See PROFESSIONAL CONFIDENCE.

CONFUSION is the clouding of intellectual functions, with disturbances of perception, recognition, recollection, and reasoning.

CONGENITAL ABNORMALITIES. The incidence of children with at least one major *malformation apparent at or soon after birth, stillbirths included, is about 1.5 per cent. If children are observed for a year, and some minor malformations are included, the incidence rises to 4 or 5 per cent. The commonest major congenital abnormalities are: *talipes, *congenital heart disease, *spina bifida, *anencephaly, *cleft lip and palate, *Down's syndrome (mongolism), *hydrocephalus, and *congenital hip dislocation.

Most congenital abnormalities are due to a combination of genetic and environmental factors; in the above list, only Down's syndrome is completely genetically determined, although many rarer syndromes are associated with *chromosome or *gene mutations. Many environmental agents can be shown experimentally to cause congenital abnormalities, and include dietary factors, hormones, chemical agents including drugs, physical agents such as radiation, and infection. *Thalidomide and *rubella (German measles) are examples of agents known to be important in man.

CONGENITAL DEFORMITY is a malformation present at birth; the name does not imply that the defect is genetic (i.e. *inherited). The incidence of such malformations is about 5 per cent of all live births, including trivial defects such as webbing of the toes, accessory nipples, etc.

CONGENITAL DISABILITIES CIVIL LIABILITY ACT 1976. This Act ensures that children born in the UK with a disability have a remedy in damages in certain cases where it can be proved that their disability is attributable to a wrongful act committed by any person, other than the mother, against the parent before their birth.

CONGENITAL HEART DISEASE. Congenital cardiac defects are fairly common, being present in about one out of every 300 children born alive. Most can be corrected or alleviated by cardiac surgery (see CARDIOTHORACIC SURGERY).

CONGENITAL HIP DISLOCATION is a developmental deformity of the *hip joint, commoner in girls, occurring with a frequency of 0.2–0.3 per cent of all births. If detected at or soon after birth, treatment by *splinting gives excellent results, but if untreated the condition causes permanent disability and an unsightly waddling gait. Careful examination of the hips is therefore essential in the routine examination of newborn infants.

CONGENITAL MALFORMATION. See CONGENITAL ABNORMALITIES; CONGENITAL DEFORMITY.

CONGENITAL SYPHILIS is transmitted by an infected mother to the fetus across the *placenta. Congenital *syphilis is a tragedy, now fortunately rare, and is preventable by routine serological testing during antenatal care and adequate treatment of maternal syphilis when diagnosed.

CONGESTION is accumulation of blood in a part, organ, or tissue.

CONJUNCTIVITIS. *Inflammation of the conjunctiva, the delicate membrane which covers much of the exposed part of the eyeball. See OPHTHALMOLOGY.

CONNECTIVE TISSUE is a broad term embracing the supporting cells and non-cellular components of tissues and organs, that is tissue other than the *parenchyma. Examples are *fibrous tissue, *elastic tissue, *collagen, and *neuroglia.

CONNECTIVE TISSUE DISEASES. See COLLA-GENOSIS.

CONN'S SYNDROME. Primary aldosteronism, i.e. increased secretion of *aldosterone by the *adrenal cortex not secondary to a known extra-adrenal stimulus. The usual cause is an aldosterone-secreting *adenoma of the cortex. The features of Conn's syndrome result from excessive aldosterone secretion, causing sodium and water retention and potassium excretion; they are *hypervolaemia, *hypertension, and *hypokalaemia. Conn's syndrome is an uncommon (about 1 per cent) but important, and potentially curable, cause of hypertension.

CONOLLY, JOHN (1794–1866). British physician. After indifferent success in practice and as professor of practical medicine at University College, London, he became resident physician at the Middlesex Asylum, Hanwell. Here he was one of the first to abolish all mechanical restraints of the insane. He was one of the founders of the British Medical Association.

CONSANGUINITY is blood relationship, that is having descent from a common ancestor.

CONSCIOUSNESS. The mind's awareness of its existence; the waking state.

CONSILIA is an archaic term for professional opinions or consultations. It was applied to letters written by physicians in the 15th, 16th, and 17th centuries, describing the symptoms and therapy of diseases, and was used by the Royal College of Physicians of London to describe a meeting of physicians.

CONSTITUTION. The totality of an individual's mental and physical characteristics, inherited and acquired.

CONSTRICTIVE PERICARDITIS is a form of *pericarditis in which chronic inflammation renders the *pericardium rigid and unyielding, interfering with cardiac action and particularly with diastolic expansion of the chambers of the right side. The cardinal manifestations are those of systemic venous congestion (often out of proportion to *dyspnoea as the pulmonary circulation is relatively protected) with a low cardiac output; *pulsus paradoxus is usually present. Chest X-ray often demonstrates pericardial calcification. Treatment is by surgical resection of the fibrosed or calcified pericardial tissue. Tuberculosis was once the commonest cause, but other aetiologies are now more likely (e.g. viral, bacterial, neoplastic, traumatic); only a few patients have previously suffered from acute pericarditis.

CONSULTANT. A specialist in a branch of medicine, qualified to give advice or services; in the UK, a doctor working in the highest career grade of the hospital service.

CONSULTATION means seeking advice, by a patient from a doctor, or one doctor from another.

CONSULTING PRACTICE. The practice of a doctor to whom patients are referred by other doctors, and who is not consulted directly by patients.

CONSUMPTION is an obsolescent term for pulmonary *tuberculosis.

CONTACT LENSES are small glass or plastic lenses worn inside the eyelids in contact with the *cornea and *conjunctiva for correcting refractive errors of the eye. They replace conventional spectacles. See also OPHTHALMOLOGY.

CONTAGION is the transmission of *infectious disease from one person to another by direct contact.

CONTRACEPTION is the prevention of *conception or impregnation by a variety of means, including: periodic abstinence (rhythm method); control of *ejaculation (*coitus interruptus); the use of spermicidal chemicals in jellies, creams, or pessaries; mechanical *occlusion (*condom or occlusive *pessary such as cap or diaphragm); prevention of implantation (*intra-uterine device in the form of coil, spiral, or loop); surgical *sterilization of man or woman (*vasectomy, ligature of *Fallopian tubes); or the use of synthetic *hormones (a *progestogen alone, or a combination of an *oestrogen and a progestogen) to control the female reproductive cycle. The latter is not only widely acceptable but is also, short of sterilization, the most effective method of fertility control. Oestrogen-containing oral contraceptives carry a small risk of thromboembolic and cardiovascular complications, which increases with oestrogen content, cigarette-*smoking, age, *obesity, *diabetes mellitus, *hypertension, and hyperlipidaemia.

Birth control has a long history, dating back to early civilizations. The outstanding pioneers in the early part of the 20th century were Mrs Margaret *Sanger in the US and Dr Marie *Stopes in the UK.

CONTRACEPTIVE PILL, MALE. So far, no hormonal or other pharmacological method of controlling male fertility has been developed to the point of clinical usefulness, although it is likely that this will not be long delayed. In 1984 it was noted that 19-nortestosterone, an effective *androgen which also acts as a *progestogen and which has been used for many years as an *anabolic steroid, may be able to produce the desired combination of effects (suppression of spermatogenesis with maintenance of androgenic action). Different compounds are now being developed but none has yet been licensed for clinical use in the UK.

CONTRACT PRACTICE. In the UK most doctors work for and within the *National Health Service; their contract is not with their patients but with hospital authorities or, in the case of general practitioners, with Family Health Service Committees. Where doctors work solely on a private basis the arrangement is a personal contract between doctor and patient and is termed 'contract practice'.

CONTRACTURE is inability fully to extend a joint or joints due to pathological changes in the surrounding tissues or in the joint itself.

CONTRALATERAL. On the opposite side.

CONTROL. In *clinical trials of treatment, 'control' designates a group of patients who remain untreated (or treated with drugs or methods accepted as the best hitherto available) who are then compared with another group of patients given the experimental treatment.

CONTROL OF POLLUTION ACT 1974. This UK Act extended existing statutory provisions dealing with certain aspects of public health and pollution control. It related particularly to: waste on land, refuse collection, and depositing of poisonous waste; pollution of water; noise pollution, including that arising from construction sites, and the creation of noise abatement zones; and pollution of the atmosphere. The Act also increased existing penalties for a large number of pollution offences.

CONVALESCENCE is the gradual recovery of health and strength after illness.

CONVALESCENT HOMES are intermediate-care hospitals or nursing homes for the reception and supervision of patients recovering from illnesses and surgical operations who are not yet considered fit enough to return home.

CONVULSION. Violent spasmodic involuntary contraction of large muscle groups such as occurs for example in *epilepsy.

COOLEY, THOMAS BENTON (1871–1945). American paediatrician. Cooley described a form of *anaemia occurring in children of parents who emanate from the Mediterranean region, and which is thus of genetic origin. The anaemia is severe, with enlargement of the *spleen and a characteristic appearance of the face which is caused by the activity of the bone marrow thickening the facial and cheek bones. In recent years it has been recognized as a constituent of the genetically determined *haemoglobinopathies and is classed as beta-*thalassaemia major.

COOPER, SIR ASTLEY PASTON, BT (1768–1841). British surgeon, FRS (1802). Cooper was a tireless dissector and expert anatomist but, although immensely successful in practice, he was not possessed of great originality of mind or dexterity of hand.

CO-ORDINATION is the physiological mechanism whereby the activity of a number of muscles is simultaneously and sequentially controlled to produce a particular motor action.

COPERNICUS, NICOLAUS (1473–1543). Polish astronomer, whose fundamental contribution to scientific thought changed for ever man's view of the universe. The copernican or heliocentric theory of astronomy proposed a daily motion of the Earth around its own axis and a yearly motion around a stationary Sun, replacing the Ptolemaic or geocentric idea of the heavens which had hitherto held sway. He received his medical training in Padua (1497–1503); in addition to his command of theology, mathematics, law, and astronomy, he mastered all the medical knowledge of his day. Following his return to Poland to settle in Frauenberg (where his financial security was assured by a cathedral canonry) he undertook medical practice among the poor and needy of that city.

COPROLALIA is the compulsive or obsessive use in speech of words relating to *faeces.

COPROPHAGIA is the eating of *faeces.

CORAM, THOMAS (?1668–1751). British philanthropist. He was instrumental in establishing the Foundling Hospital in London in 1745.

CORDUS, VALERIUS (or Cordes) (1515–44). German botanist. His *Dispensatorium* (1535) was the first adequate *pharmacopoeia to be published.

CORI, CARL FERDINAND (1896–1984). American medical biochemist. Most of his scientific work, carried out in collaboration with his wife Gerta (see CORI, GERTA THERESA), was concerned with the metabolism of *carbohydrates, in particular the 'Cori cycle' whereby the liver storage compound *glycogen is converted successively into blood glucose, muscle glycogen, and lactic acid, with the release of energy. The first intermediate in this enzymic process, the activated compound glucose 1-phosphate, is sometimes termed the 'Cori ester'; the enzyme responsible for its reversible production from glycogen, polysaccharide phosphorylase, was isolated and purified by the Coris in 1943, enabling them to achieve the *in vitro* synthesis of glycogen. Further studies elucidated the influence of hormones such as *insulin and *adrenaline on the various steps in the cycle, and the mode of action of the enzymes concerned. In 1947 he was awarded the *Nobel prize in medicine jointly with his wife Gerta and Bernardo A. *Houssay for their work on carbohydrate metabolism.

CORI, GERTA THERESA (née Radnitz) (1896–1957). American medical biochemist. Her scientific achievements are inseparable from those of her husband, and she shared with him and Bernado A. *Houssay the 1947 *Nobel prize for medicine.

CORIUM. The dermis or 'true skin'. See SKIN.

CORNEA. The transparent avascular layer of tissue forming the front part of the fibrous coat of the eye, through which the *iris and the *pupil are visible. The lack of blood vessels accounts for the fact that the cornea can be grafted without the recipient becoming immunized against it. See also OPHTHALMOLOGY; TRANSPLANTATION.

CORONARY BYPASS is the surgical relief of obstructive disease of the coronary arteries by creating one or more additional channels connecting the aorta to a point or points beyond the sites of obstruction; a saphenous vein homograft, an internal mammary artery, or a suitable prosthetic material is employed. The full descriptive term 'aortocoronary bypass graft' is preferable. See CARDIOTHORACIC SURGERY.

CORONARY HEART DISEASE is a general term, synonymous with 'ischaemic heart disease', embracing all cardiac disorders resulting from impairment of the coronary arterial circulation by *atherosclerosis. It includes *angina pectoris, *coronary thrombosis, various *arrhythmias, *heart block, and *heart failure. Coronary heart disease is a major cause of death and disability in Western countries, accounting for about half of the total mortality. Many regard it as the outstanding problem of *preventive medicine. See also ATHEROSCLEROSIS.

CORONARY THROMBOSIS is thrombotic obstruction of a coronary artery occurring on the basis of preexisting *atherosclerosis, and giving rise to *infarction of the *myocardium. It is a common cause of sudden death. The terms 'coronary thrombosis', 'myocardial infarction', and 'heart attack' are virtually synonymous.

CORONERS. The office of coroner, in whatever country it exists today, is derived from the ancient English office, and in whatever country, its purpose can be expressed in the words of the Coroners Act of 1887 which substantially repeated the words of the ordinance of 1194 which is thought to have created the office:

Where a coroner is informed that the dead body of a person is lying within his jurisdiction and there is reasonable cause to suspect that the person has died a violent or unnatural death, or has died in prison . . . the coroner . . . shall as soon as practicable, issue his warrant for summoning not less than 12 and not more than 23 good and lawful men . . . to enquire as jurors touching the death of such person as aforesaid.

The jury is now discretionary in many such inquests and has been reduced in number. In most countries there has been added to the ancient duty that of enquiring into deaths the cause of which has not been ascertained or cannot be certified by an attending medical practitioner. In such cases, if the coroner is satisfied that the deceased died a natural death he may certify the death for the purpose of registration without holding an inquest or even an *autopsy.

In the UK, English coroner law applies only to England and Wales. The coroner is unknown in Scotland and the investigation of unnatural and suspicious deaths is the duty of the Procurator-Fiscal—the public prosecutor for the area.

In Ireland, the entire country was under British rule until 1920, when it was partitioned into Northern Ireland (under British rule, but with its own Parliament) and the Irish Free State, which soon became a republic. There was a coroner system under British rule, and it has been continued both in Northern Ireland and the Republic since 1920. Although subject to local legislation in their respective territories (not since 1972 in Northern Ireland when its Parliament was dissolved), the systems in both cases remain similar to those applying in England and Wales.

In the USA, Canada, Australia, and New Zealand the coroner system was imported by early colonists. In America colonization started in the 17th century, and the system the colonists introduced was the one that then obtained in England. It has now been replaced in many states by the medical examiner system, although a coroner system still obtains in some, but differs in many respects from that in England and Wales.

In Canada, Australia, and New Zealand, colonization occurred in the 19th century, and workable and satisfactory systems (for the period) were established which have been enabled by local legislation to keep pace with developing social demands, and which do not differ greatly from those in England and Wales; their purpose remains the same. See also FORENSIC MEDICINE; LAW AND MEDICINE; PATHOLOGY.

COR PULMONALE is the common term for pulmonary heart disease, meaning hypertrophy and eventual failure of the right side of the heart due to the strain of forcing blood through a pulmonary vascular system which has become distorted and obstructed by longstanding lung disease, usually chronic *bronchitis and *emphysema.

CORPUS CALLOSUM. The bridge of white matter connecting the two *cerebral hemispheres.

CORPUS LUTEUM. The yellowish body formed from an *ovarian follicle after ovulation occurs in the middle of each menstrual cycle; it secretes *progesterone, which prepares the *endometrium for implantation of the fertilized *ovum. If pregnancy supervenes, the corpus luteum enlarges, persists and continues to secrete progesterone; if not, it atrophies and the prepared endometrium is shed (*menstruation).

CORRIGAN, SIR DOMINIC, Bt (1802–80). Irish physician. He is often credited with first describing the characteristic pulse of *aortic incompetence ('Corrigan's pulse'), but the description in an article by *Vieussens in 1715 antedated his by more than a century.

CORROSIVE SUBLIMATE is mercuric chloride ($HgCl_2$), a highly poisonous white crystalline soluble salt.

CORSET. A closely fitting reinforced inner body garment sometimes prescribed medically as a support for the spine, or for a sagging abdominal wall.

CORTI, ALFONSO GIACOMO GASPARE (1822–76). Italian anatomist. In 1851 he published a minutely detailed account of the microscopic anatomy of the *cochlea, and his name is attached to several of its structures.

CORTICOSTEROIDS are *steroids secreted by the *adrenal cortex, and their synthetic analogues. They are of two main groups, whose actions overlap: the first group, the *glucocorticoids* (e.g. *cortisone, cortisol or *hydrocortisone, *prednisone, prednisolone) act predominantly on carbohydrate, fat, and protein metabolism; the second group, the *mineralocorticoids* (e.g. *aldosterone, 11-deoxycorticosterone (DOC)) have as their main function the maintenance of fluid and electrolyte balance. The glucocorticoids have many uses in medicine apart from their obvious

role in hormone replacement therapy, being widely employed as *antineoplastic, anti-inflammatory, and *immunosuppressant agents.

CORTICOTROPHIN is one of the *peptide *hormones secreted by the anterior lobe of the *pituitary gland, the action of which is to stimulate the cortex of the *adrenal gland to release *corticosteroids. Corticotrophin is also known as adrenocorticotrophic hormone (ACTH). The use of corticotrophin as an alternative to corticosteroids is now less important than its role in the assessment of *adrenocortical function.

CORTISOL. See HYDROCORTISONE.

CORTISONE was the first *glucocorticoid used in medicine, when *Hench in 1949 described its dramatic effect in patients with *rheumatoid arthritis. It is not biologically active and exerts its pharmacological effects by metabolic conversion to cortisol (*hydrocortisone). See also CORTICOSTEROIDS.

CORVISART DES MAREST, BARON JEAN NICHOLAS (1755–1821). French physician. He became personal physician to Napoleon and often accompanied him on campaigns. He did much to popularize percussion, translating *Auenbrugger's book on the subject in 1808. He published one of the first accounts of heart disease, *Essai sur les maladies et les lésions organiques du coeur et des gros vaisseaux* (1806).

CORYZA is a running nose due to *catarrhal inflammation of the nasal mucous membrane, such as that which occurs in the initial states of a *cold.

COS (now Kos), is an island in the Dodecanese, near the shores of Turkey, north of Rhodes. An early site of 'temple-healing' (see TEMPLE MEDICINE) is found in Asklepieia, dedicated to *Aesculapius. Cos was also the birthplace of *Hippocrates *c*.560 BC.

COSMETIC SURGERY is surgery intended to improve or to alter the patient's appearance.

COT DEATH. See SUDDEN INFANT DEATH SYNDROME.

COTTAGE HOSPITALS. See HOSPITALS IN THE UK.

COTTON, NATHANIEL (1705–85). British physician and poet. He trained at Leiden, but returned to England to practise in St Albans, where he maintained a private asylum, Collegium Insanorum. Cotton published anonymously much moralistic verse and prose.

COUE, EMILE (1857–1926). French pharmacist and amateur psychologist. Coué studied pharmacy in Paris and later bought a retail pharmacy in Troyes, where he remained until 1910. He interested himself in *hypnotism and developed the notion of '*autosuggestion'. He acquired international renown with his maxim 'every day in every way I am getting better and better.'

COUGH. Forcible expulsion of air from the lungs and air passages with a characteristic noise: a cough is initiated by an expiratory effort against a closed *glottis and completed when the glottis is abruptly opened, releasing air under pressure together with any matter present in the air passages. Coughing may be voluntary or reflexly induced.

COUMARIN is a generic term for a group of oral *anticoagulants derived from the vegetable product coumarin, found in various plants (sweet clover, tonka bean, etc.) or synthesized. *Warfarin is an example. The coumarin drugs inhibit the hepatic synthesis of the *vitamin-K-dependent coagulation factors.

COUNTER-IRRITATION is the principle, of dubious validity, of alleviating deep-seated pain by inflaming the skin with hot or irritant applications (e.g. hot-water bottles and linaments).

COURNAND, ANDRÉ FREDERIC (1895–1988). French/American cardiovascular and respiratory physiologist. He won the *Nobel prize in physiology and medicine (with D. W. Richards and W. Forssmann) in 1956 for the development of cardiac catheterization.

COURVOISIER, LUDWIG (1843–1918). French surgeon. Courvoisier is remembered for his law which states that if a *stone obstructs the bile passages the *gall bladder is less likely to distend than when the blockage is due to a tumour or some other cause. Courvoisier's sign is when the gall bladder is distended due to some abnormality other than a stone and can be felt.

COWLEY, ABRAHAM (1618–67). British physician and poet. Cowley never practised, but was involved in founding the *Royal Society. His poems were highly regarded, particularly 'On the Death of Mr William Harvey'.

COWPOX is a mild eruptive condition of cows, usually confined to the udder and teats, and occasionally transmitted to man by contact. With material from a cowpox lesion on the hand of a milkmaid, Edward *Jenner in 1796 inoculated a boy and subsequently showed that he was immune to *smallpox infection. Although the *vaccinia virus used nowadays is thought to have been originally derived from the cowpox virus, the contemporary strains of the two are biologically distinct.

COXSACKIE VIRUS. A group of small *ribonucleic acid (RNA) *viruses belonging to the *enterovirus genus and responsible for several human infections. Most are asymptomatic or cause only a non-specific *influenza-like illness; occasionally these viruses are implicated in more serious infections of the central nervous system, heart, and lungs. Two subgroups, A and B, are recognized on the basis of their effects when inoculated into mice and their ability to grow in tissue culture. Coxsackie B virus is the usual cause of *Bornholm disease. The name of the virus derives from a small town in New York State where the group was first identified and separated from other major enterovirus groups (polioviruses and *echoviruses).

CRABBE, GEORGE (1754–1832). British physician, poet, and clergyman. Highly regarded as a poet in his lifetime, his best-known works are *The library* (1781) and *The village* (1783). (See also MEDICAL TRUANTS.)

CRAB LOUSE. A species of human *louse (*Phthirus pubis* or *Pediculus pubis*) which infests the hair of the pubic and perineal regions but may also be found in hair elsewhere on the body, excluding the scalp. The usual transmission is by sexual intercourse. The crab louse is not known to be a *vector of disease.

CRACKED POT SOUND is a physical sign once thought to suggest pulmonary cavitation: the characteristic sound is elicited by percussing the chest wall, thus expelling air from a large cavity into a small bronchus. A somewhat similar sound may be elicited by tapping the thin skull of an infant with severe *hydrocephalus.

CRAMP is sustained painful involuntary contraction of *muscle.

CRANIAL NERVES are the 12 pairs of nerves which arise from the *brain and are analogous to the 31 arising from the *spinal cord. They are identified by Roman numerals, as follows: I (olfactory); II (optic); III (oculomotor); IV (trochlear); V (trigeminal, which has ophthalmic, maxillary, and mandibular sensory divisions and a motor division); VI (abducens); VII (facial); VIII (auditory or vestibulocochlear); IX (glossopharyngeal); X (vagus); XI (accessory); and XII (hypoglossal).

CRANIOMETRY is measurement of the dimensions of the skull.

CRANIOSCOPY. Visual inspection of the head.

CRANIUM. The *skull.

C-REACTIVE PROTEIN. An abnormal *globulin, the appearance of which in the circulation is a non-specific indicator of an inflammatory process.

CREATININE. A nitrogenous end-product of muscle metabolism, the production of which is related to total muscle mass and is therefore fairly constant within a given individual. Creatinine is freely filtered by the renal *glomeruli, so that its renal *clearance rate provides an approximate measurement of glomerular filtration rate without the need to administer an exogenous indicator substance. As its concentration is readily measured in plasma and urine, the plasma level and clearance rate of endogenous creatinine are useful indicators of *renal function, particularly when sequential observations are made in the same patient.

CREDE, KARL SIEGMUND FRANZ (1819–92). German obstetrician. He is remembered for his method of expressing the *placenta by abdominal pressure (Credé's manoeuvre, 1854) and for popularizing the prophylaxis of gonococcal *ophthalmia in the newborn by instilling silver nitrate eyedrops.

CREMATION. The modern cremation movement in Great Britain was pioneered by Sir Henry Thompson Bart, FRCS, Surgeon to Queen Victoria. His interest in cremation was aroused following a visit to the Vienna Exhibition in 1873, where a model of Professor Brunetti's cremating apparatus was exhibited. Sir Henry had been so impressed that he wrote a paper entitled '*The treatment of the body after death*', which was published in the *Contemporary Review* for January 1874. His main reason for supporting cremation was that 'it was becoming a necessary sanitary precaution against the propagation of disease among a population daily growing larger in relation to the area it occupied'.

Encouraged by the reception of his article, Sir Henry called a meeting of a number of his friends at his house at 35 Wimpole Street on 13 January 1874, when the following declaration was drawn-up and signed by those present, representing the realms of art, science, literature, and medicine, 'We, the undersigned, disapprove the present custom of burying the dead, and we desire to substitute some mode which shall rapidly resolve the body into its component elements, by a process which cannot offend the living, and shall render the remains perfectly innocuous. Until some better method is devised, we desire to adopt that usually known as cremation.'

By this simple act, The Cremation Society of Great Britain or, as it was then known, The Cremation Society of England, came into being.

The Society raised funds to build a crematorium at Woking, Surrey. However, the Home Secretary refused to allow the cremation of human remains. It was not until the celebrated trial of Dr William Price in 1883 that cremation was pronounced legal. The eccentric Dr Price was arrested attempting to cremate the body of his five-month-old son. He was tried at Cardiff Assizes, and the result of the trial announced in February 1884 that 'cremation is legal provided no nuisance is caused in the process to others' was the breakthrough the Society had been waiting for.

Following this decision, the Society carried out the first human cremation at Woking on 26 March 1885. Mrs. J. Pickersgill, a well-known figure in literary and scientific circles, was cremated and was the first of three cremations to be carried out that year at the crematorium. Woking was established through the efforts of private enterprise, and it was not until 1901 that the first municipal crematorium was opened in Hull.

In 1902, owing to the efforts of Sir Charles Cameron, who succeeded Sir Henry Thompson as the Society's President, an Act of Parliament, 'For the Regulation of burning of human remains, and to enable burial authorities to establish crematoria', was passed. Thus, cremation had achieved a form of governmental regulation and thereby became officially recognized in the highest quarters. The new Act of Parliament gave powers to the Home Secretary to make Regulations, which were published as statutory Rules and Orders in March 1903. The Act made provision for the completion of medical certificates, and continues to form the basis of present-day legislation, although this has been under review by the Home Office for several years.

By the end of 1934, there were 28 crematoria and 8337 cremations had been carried out. Since the inception of the movement, this increase, in terms of modern experience, may not seem spectacular, but its growth over the period had been steady and pointed clearly in the direction of the growing acceptance of the principle of cremation. The foundations laid by the pioneers were proving capable of bearing a growing superstructure, the limits of whose height and breadth were as yet unknown.

The year 1946, which brought peace following the Second World War, also witnessed a rise in the annual figure of cremations in Great Britain to 50 000. However, a period of intense frustration followed the end of the war. Local authorities, concerned with the many social demands being made upon land resources, hoped cremation might make a substantial contribution to the solution, and so they were disappointed by the refusal of the Minister of Health, Mr Aneurin Bevan, to approve their plans, owing to the severe restrictions on building activities imposed by the Treasury. The Society submitted a memorandum to the Minister impressing on him that there were insufficient crematoria to meet the growing demand. This achieved some measure of success; this was the beginning of a post-war policy of encouraging local authorities to provide crematoria where the need was proved, and, where possible, to combine with neighbouring local authorities to provide these services.

The post-war deadlock was eventually broken in 1954. By this time, the Minister had recognized the need for a national plan for crematoria. The steady rate of growth during the 1950s quickened into a period of rapid expansion from 1960 onwards. The number of crematoria increased from 58 in 1950 to 203 in 1968 when, for the first time, the cremation rate exceeded 50 per cent.

Table 1 Cremation in the UK

Year	Number of crematoria in UK	Number of deaths	Number of cremations	%
1885	1	597 357	3	–
1905	13	594 567	604	0.10
1925	16	538 348	2 701	0.50
1945	58	550 763	42 963	7.80
1965	184	612 247	271 130	44.28
1985	222	654 701	443 687	67.77
1992	226	622 410	437 000	70.21
1993	227	644 768*	453 045*	70.26*

* Provisional

The International Cremation Federation, of which The Cremation Society of Great Britain was a founder member, had for many years fought for the repeal of the canons forbidding Roman Catholics to adopt cremation. The Federation appealed to all prelates to support its request at the Council of Churches in Rome and, eventually, in July 1963, the Pope pronounced it legal within the Church to seek cremation without incurring any penalties. However, it was not until 1966 that the ban was lifted on Roman Catholic priests conducting services in crematoria.

Preference for cremation continued steadily to rise (Table 1) and, by the early 1990s, had reached a rate of approximately 70 per cent in the Great Britain, the second highest in the world next to Japan, with over 14 million cremations having been carried out since the movement's inception. This represents a saving in land-space estimated to be equivalent to an area the size of the City of Bath or ten times the area of the City of London.

With greater awareness by society of the need to safeguard the environment, 1990 saw the introduction of the Environmental Protection Act 1990, destined to have far-reaching consequences for the cremation movement. Although crematoria were recognized as not being significant polluters, regulations were introduced to control and measure their emissions. The effect was to require all crematoria to upgrade or replace their equipment, thus requiring substantial capital expenditure which would ultimately be passed on to the public. Nevertheless, cremation will still remain cheaper than burial in the vast majority of cases, and crematoria will also have a tangible means of showing that they are not harming the environment. Cremation will also continue to be the most preferred and hygienic form of disposal of the dead, thus fulfilling the aspirations of the original pioneers of the movement beyond, one would suspect, their wildest expectations.

ROGER N. ARBER

CREPITATION is a fine crackling sound or sensation, such as may be heard for example on *auscultation of the lungs during *respiration when there is fluid in the alveolar air spaces, or may be felt by the palpating fingers when there are bubbles of air in the subcutaneous tissues.

CREPITUS is used interchangeably with *crepitation and has the same meaning, but is reserved by some to denote the grating sensation produced when fractured bony surfaces are moved against each other.

CRETINISM is a condition of *thyroid gland deficiency present from birth or early infancy. Thyroid hormone is necessary for normal development, particularly of the brain and skeleton, so that untreated cretinism presents a picture of *mental handicap, *dwarfism, and other developmental defects, in addition to the manifestations of hypothyroidism which characterize *myxoedema in the adult. Early diagnosis and treatment may not be able wholly to reverse the effects that thyroid deficiency in the *uterus has on fetal development.

CREUTZFELDT–JAKOB DISEASE is a rare form of rapidly progressive *dementia, usually beginning in middle age and often causing death within a year. The mental deterioration is often accompanied by neurological disturbances and characteristic electroencephalographic changes. There is evidence that Creutzfeldt–Jakob disease is due, like *kuru, to a transmissible agent, a prion similar to other 'slow viruses' which cause spongiform encephalopathies in animals. Cases of transmission by corneal transplant and to a neurosurgeon operating upon the brain of an affected individual have been described.

CRI DU CHAT SYNDROME is a form of severe mental handicap associated with *microcephaly, widely separated eyes, and a characteristic cry, said to resemble that of a cat. The condition is due to a specific *chromosomal aberration, namely *deletion of the short arm of chromosome 5.

CRILE, GEORGE WASHINGTON (1864–1943) American surgeon. He made some early contributions to concepts of surgical *shock, and pioneered the use of regional nerve block for certain kinds of surgery. Later his main interest was in the surgery of the *thyroid.

CRIMINAL PROCEDURE (INSANITY) ACT 1964. The four major provisions of this UK Act were: amendment of the form of the special verdict required by the Trial of Lunatics Act 1883, the new wording being 'a special verdict that the accused is not guilty by reason of insanity'; amendment of the procedure for determining unfitness to plead; conferment of further powers on courts for making orders for admission to hospital;

and empowerment of the prosecution to put forward evidence of *insanity or diminished responsiblity.

CRIPPEN, HAWLEY HARVEY (1862–1910). Crippen is notorious as the doctor who murdered his wife and dismembered her, burying her remains in the basement of his London house. He fled by ship with his mistress, Ethel Le Neve. He was apprehended because the vessel on which he chose to travel was equipped with the new wireless telegraphy. The police were able to radio the master and the police in the USA, who arrested him as he landed. Two facts make him interesting: he was the first person to be caught by radio; and he belongs to the rare group of doctors known to have committed murder.

CRISIS. The turning-point of an illness, formerly used particularly in respect of *fevers: an abrupt fall in temperature was termed 'resolution by crisis', as compared with the more gradual return to normal levels of 'resolution by lysis'.

CROHN, BURRILL B. (1874–1983). American surgeon. His special interest was inflammatory diseases of the bowel, and in particular a disorder which he described with Ginzburg and Oppenheimer in 1932 under the designation 'regional ileitis'. This chiefly affects the terminal part of the small intestine, but also occurs in the colon. It is now usually referred to as *Crohn's disease.

CROHN'S DISEASE is a chronic inflammatory *bowel disease, also known as regional ileitis or regional enteritis, the aetiology of which is unknown. It has a predilection for the terminal *ileum, but any part of the intestine may be affected. Clinical manifestations are various and troublesome; they include chronic ill-health, abdominal pain, diarrhoea, weight loss, intestinal obstruction, and sometimes *fistula formation. The condition is persistent, and treatment is often somewhat difficult and unsatisfactory.

CRONIN, ARCHIBALD JOSEPH (1896–1981). British physician and novelist. He was in general practice in South Wales and later in London until 1930, when he retired to write novels, usually with a medical theme. His two most successful were *Hatter's castle* (1931) and *The citadel* (1937).

CROSS-INFECTION is infection transmitted from one hospital patient to another.

CROUP is a hoarse croaking and ringing *cough characteristic of *laryngeal inflammation and partial obstruction, occurring particularly in children.

CRUELTY TO ANIMALS ACT 1876. A UK enactment which allowed experiments to be made on living animals for the advancement of science, subject to prescribed restrictions. The Act, which applied only to vertebrates (mammals, reptiles, birds, fishes, and amphibians) continued to govern animal experimentation in the UK until it was superseded by the Animals (Scientific Procedures) Act (1986). This makes it an offence to carry out any scientific 'procedure' except under licence. Procedures are defined as anything carried out for a scientific purpose that may cause 'pain, suffering, distress or lasting harm' to protected animals. The Act regulates all experimental or other scientific procedures on animals through a system of personal and project licensing operated by the Home Office. This covers animal use in research, regulatory (e.g. safety and toxicity) testing, production, and other scientific uses. The award of licences and certificates and other relevant matters are ultimately subject to the authority of the Secretary of State at the Home Office, who is advised by an Animal Procedures Committee, an independent statutory body which is required to lay an annual report before Parliament. That Committee consists of a chairman, appointed by the Secretary of State, and not less than 12 other members, including at least eight medical or veterinary practitioners or biological scientists, at least one lawyer, and representatives of animal welfare organizations.

CRUSH SYNDROME is a condition resulting from acute and extensive injury to *muscle (as in some war casualties) with release into the circulation of its pigment *myoglobin and damage to the kidneys (lower nephron *nephrosis). Renal insufficiency causes *oliguria and *azotaemia, and there is myoglobinuria (myoglobin in the urine).

CRUTCH. A support with a cross-piece for the armpit or elbow and another for the hand, designed to take the weight of the body off the leg while walking.

CRUVEILHIER, JEAN (1791–1874). French morbid anatomist. He was one of the founders of *morbid anatomy. He gave the first account of *multiple sclerosis in 1835 and described the Cruveilhier–Baumgarten syndrome of persistent or recanalized para-umbilical veins in *portal hypertension.

CRYOSURGERY is surgery using special instruments that lower temperature, producing intense localized coldness and local tissue destruction.

CRYOTHERAPY is the application of low temperatures in medical and surgical treatment.

CRYPTOCOCCOSIS is infection with the *fungus *Cryptococcus neoformans*, usually involving the lungs but sometimes spreading throughout the body, particularly to the *brain and *meninges. Cryptococcosis (also known as torulosis), like other fungal infections, is a particular hazard in patients whose immune defences have been weakened by disease or *immunosuppressive drugs.

C.T. Computerized tomography. See RADIOLOGY; SCANNERS; TOMOGRAPHY.

CUIRASS, originally meaning a breastplate made of leather, is used in medicine to denote a covering for the chest, as in 'cuirass *respirator', a device for applying intermittent positive external pressure. 'Carcinoma en cuirasse' denotes a form of malignant *neoplasm in which there is diffuse infiltration by the growth of the skin over the chest.

CULDOSCOPY is the inspection of the female pelvic organs with an *endoscope introduced through the roof of the posterior part of the *vagina.

CULEX is a widely distributed genus of biting *mosquitoes, important both because of their nuisance value and because many species are vectors of infectious and parasitic diseases, such as the *arbovirus encephalitides and *filariasis.

CULLEN, WILLIAM (1710–90). British physician. Cullen had little originality, but he enjoyed a great reputation as a clear, systematic, and inspiring teacher. His later years were clouded by the virulent attacks of John *Brown whom he had earlier supported and encouraged.

CULPEPER, NICHOLAS (1616–54). British astrologer. He incurred the wrath of the Royal Colleges of Physicians of London by publishing an unofficial translation of their *pharmacopoeia in 1649 as *A physical directory or a translation of the London Dispensatory*. This and *The English physician* (1653) enjoyed immense sales.

CULTURAL SHOCK is the emotional experience associated with abrupt transition from one set of societal values to another.

CULTURE is the maintenance of cells, tissues, or organs in artificial conditions which allow them to live, develop, or reproduce.

CUPPING is the application of suction to the body surface to promote bleeding, the device employed being known as a cupping-glass. It is now obsolete.

CURARE is a generic term for various extracts of tropical plants originally used as arrow poisons to paralyse quarry. The active *alkaloids, such as tubocurarine, block the action of *acetylcholine at neuromuscular junctions by competitive inhibition, that is by occupying the *receptor sites on the motor end-plate which normally combine with acetylcholine. Muscle relaxant

drugs of the curare type have found important applications in medicine, notably in the treatment of *tetanus and as an adjunct to general *anaesthesia.

CURETTE. A spoon- or scoop-shaped surgical instrument employed in removing material from the wall of a cavity (especially the uterus) or other surface.

CURIE, MARIE SKLODOWSKA (1876–1934). Franco-Polish physicist. In 1895 she married Pierre Curie the physicist. She and her husband, together with Henri *Becquerel, were awarded the *Nobel prize for physics in 1903 for discovering *radioactivity. In 1893 they had isolated two new elements from pitchblende, *radium and polonium. For this she received the Nobel prize for chemistry in 1911.

CURIE, PIERRE (1859–1906). French physicist. Curie married Marie in 1895, and with her and *Becquerel won the *Nobel prize for physics in 1903 for their discovery of *radioactivity. He discovered piezo-electricity and made contributions to magnetism and other fields of physics. He described the three radioactive emanations of *radium, later designated as α, β, and γ, that is alpha, beta, and gamma particles and rays. In 1906 he was run over by a dray in Paris and killed. His daughter, Irène, born in 1897, married Fréedéric Joliot, and together these two advanced the work begun by the Curies.

CUSHING, HARVEY WILLIAMS (1869–1939). American neurosurgeon and physiologist. He began his academic career at *Johns Hopkins, where he became interested in *neurosurgery. In 1912, he became first chief of surgery at the Peter Bent Brigham Hospital. He carried out many craniotomies to remove *brain tumours, usually under local anaesthesia. He observed changes in body appearance associated with *pituitary tumours (*Cushing's syndrome), and also noted that removal of the pituitary led to atrophy of the genitals. As author of the classic biography of William *Osler, he shared Osler's interest in medical history. His own historical collection was bequeathed to Yale University, where he worked during retirement.

CUSHING'S SYNDROME is the complex of symptoms and signs which results from the effects of excessive *corticosteroid activity, whether these come from primary overactivity of the *adrenal cortex itself, from overstimulation by excess *corticotrophin secretion by the anterior *pituitary gland, or from exogenous administration of corticosteroids. Its manifestations include: a characteristic type of *obesity; purplish *striae of the skin; *hypertension; *osteoporosis; *amenorrhoea or *impotence; muscular weakness; and *diabetes mellitus.

CUSHNY, ARTHUR ROBERTSON (1866–1926). British pharmacologist. Cushny was the earliest British experimental pharmacologist and his researches on *digitalis, the secretion of urine, and the pharmacology of optical isomers were of great value. His book, *The secretion of urine* (1917), was rapidly accepted as the ultimate authority on the subject, and his *Textbook of pharmacology and therapeutics* (1899) went to eight editions in his lifetime.

CUVIER, GEORGES LEOPOLD CHRETIEN FREDERIC DAGOBERT, Baron Cuvier (1769–1832). French naturalist, zoologist, comparative anatomist, palaeontologist, educationalist, and scientific administrator, generally regarded as the founder of palaeontology. His most famous work was *Règne animal distribué d'après son organisation (1817)*, which gave an account of the whole animal kingdom, both living and fossil. Alternative anatomical nomenclature perpetuates his name in association with the common cardinal veins (ducts of Cuvier) and the ductus venosus (canal of Cuvier).

CYANIDE. Any salt of hydrocyanic acid (HCN) containing the ion CN^-. All cyanides are highly poisonous; they interfere with oxygen uptake by cells by combining with cytochrome oxidase, an enzyme necessary for cellular oxygen transport. The fatal dose of cyanide is about 250 mg, as compared with about 50 mg for hydrocyanic (prussic) acid.

CYANOCOBALAMIN is vitamin B_{12}, a water-soluble *vitamin essential for the normal development of *erythrocytes. Lack of this vitamin, which is usually due to impaired absorption rather than to dietary insufficiency, causes *pernicious anaemia. See also HAEMATOLOGY.

CYANOSIS is blueness of the skin and mucous membranes due to an increased concentration of reduced *haemoglobin in the superficial capillary circulation.

CYBERNETICS is the study of communication and control systems in organisms and machines.

CYCLIC AMP. Cyclic adenosine 3′,5′-monophosphate, or cAMP, is the intracellular mediator or 'messenger' compound involved in the action of many *hormones and *catecholamine *neurotransmitters. It is produced by the action of adenyl cyclase, a membrane-bound *enzyme, on *adenosine triphosphate (ATP).

CYCLOPHOSPHAMIDE is an *alkylating agent of value in a wide range of malignancies, and as an *immunosuppressant.

CYCLOSPORIN is an *immunosuppressive agent, effective in preventing *transplant rejection.

CYCLOTHYMIA is a tendency to mood swings, with alternating periods of elation and depression. When this exceeds the normal bounds of mood change, it constitutes *manic-depressive psychosis. See also PSYCHIATRY.

CYCLOTRON. An apparatus for accelerating charged particles of atomic magnitudes by imparting to them energies of several million electronvolts. The charged particles are subjected to an oscillating electric field while held in spiral orbit by a constant magnetic field (see RADIOTHERAPY).

CYPROTERONE. A synthetic anti-androgenic steroid, which inhibits spermatogenesis and causes reversible male infertility. In men, it has been used in the treatment of severe hypersexuality and sexual deviation, and in the treatment of disseminated *prostatic cancer. In women, cyproterone combined with an *oestrogen (in several repeated courses of 21 days from the fifth day of the menstrual cycle followed by an interval of 7 days) is effective in some cases of severe *acne refractory to other forms of treatment; such a regimen is also *contraceptive. The same treatment can benefit female *hirsutism.

CYST. Any hollow formation, particularly one containing fluid ('cyst' is derived from the Greek word for 'bladder').

CYSTIC DUCT. The duct of the *gall bladder, which connects it with the common *bile duct.

CYSTICERCOSIS is infestation with the intermediate or larval form of *Taenia solium*, the pig tapeworm (see *TAENIA).*

CYSTIC FIBROSIS is a severe genetic disorder characterized by abnormal (viscid) *mucus production by glands throughout the body, affecting particularly the lungs, *pancreas, and gastrointestinal tract. A rise in the concentration of sodium and chloride in the sweat is a valuable diagnostic feature. Cystic fibrosis is inherited as an autosomal recessive trait; hence both parents are normally unaffected but carry the gene (as heterozygotes) and one-quarter of their children are likely to be born with the disease. Recent localization and isolation of the causal gene have raised the prospect of gene therapy (see GENETICS).

CYSTIC MEDIAL NECROSIS is a pathological condition affecting the medial layer of the aorta, predisposing to the development of aortic *dissecting aneurysm; it is characterized by degeneration of elastic and muscle fibres, with cyst formation.

CYSTINURIA is a genetic disorder in which the *epithelial transport of certain *amino acids including cystine is defective. Their excretion in the urine may cause urinary *calculi, which are responsible for the main clinical manifestations of the disease.

CYSTITIS is inflammation of the *urinary bladder.

CYSTOSCOPY is the inspection of the interior of the *urinary bladder with an *endoscope.

CYTARABINE is one of the *antimetabolite group of drugs. It acts by interfering with *pyrimidine synthesis and is used to induce or maintain remission in acute *leukaemias. It has also been used as an antiviral agent. It can cause severe bone marrow depression.

CYTOCHEMISTRY involves the study of the chemical behaviour of cells.

CYTOGENETICS is the study of *chromosomes.

CYTOKINE. A chemical substance that promotes cell division. See ONCOLOGY.

CYTOLOGY is the study of *cells.

CYTOLYTIC. Describing or pertaining to an agent that causes dissolution of cells.

CYTOMEGALOVIRUS. A genus of viruses which with the *Herpesvirus* genus, comprises the family Herpetoviridae. *Cytomegalovirus* (CMV) is so-called because it has a cytopathic effect associated with the production of giant cells containing intranuclear and cytoplasmic inclusion bodies. Infection is widespread in the human population and usually passes unnoticed. But, like *toxoplasmosis, the virus causes serious damage in two susceptible groups: fetuses, transplacentally infected, who may be born with severe central nervous system defects (such as microcephaly, mental handicap, deafness, blindness, quadriplegia, etc.) or other congenital abnormalities; and patients whose immune system has been depressed by immunosuppressive therapy or for other reasons, who may develop hepatitis, haemolytic anaemia, polyneuritis, encephalitis, or other syndromes. CMV is also sometimes incriminated as the cause of an illness resembling *infectious mononucleosis in previously well adults; a condition called post-transfusion mononucleosis comes into this category. CMV infection is often termed 'cytomegalic inclusion disease' because of the histological finding of typical giant cells.

CYTOPLASM. All the *protoplasm of a cell excluding the *nucleus. It contains the various *organelles responsible for cellular metabolic activities. See CELL AND CELL BIOLOGY.

CYTOTOXIC. Describing or pertaining to an agent which poisons or damages cells.

DA COSTA, JACOB MENDEZ (1833–1900). American physician. He was one of the original members of the Association of American Physicians. During the American Civil War he described a disorder in young soldiers characterized by *palpitations and symptoms suggestive of *neurasthenia. This came to be called 'irritable heart', or Da Costa's syndrome. In some of the patients he mentioned an abnormal heart sound, a 'systolic click', now thought to be caused by billowing of a mitral valve leaflet.

DA COSTA'S SYNDROME. One of a variety of synonyms for cardiac neurosis (e.g. soldier's heart, effort syndrome, neurocirculatory asthenia, etc.). See CARDIOLOGY.

DACRYOCYSTITIS is inflammation of the lacrimal (tear) sac.

DACTINOMYCIN is a cytotoxic antibiotic, also known as *actinomycin D.

DALE, SIR HENRY HALLETT (1875–1968). British physiologist and pharmacologist. After some years working with Paul *Ehrlich, Dale joined the Wellcome Research Laboratories in 1904. Over a period of 10 years he established his reputation as an experimental pharmacologist. In 1914 he was made director of the department of biochemistry and pharmacology of the projected *National Institute for Medical Research which was finally established in 1920; in 1928 Dale became its director. From 1938 to 1960 he was chairman of the *Wellcome Trust and from 1940 to 1945 president of the Royal Society. In 1936 he shared the *Nobel prize in medicine with Otto *Loewi for work on the chemical transmission of nerve impulses.

Dale's research was mainly in experimental pharmacology. In his early years he showed that *ergotoxin would reverse the hypertensive effect of *adrenaline (1906) and established the oxytocic effect of posterior *pituitary extract (1909). From 1914 to 1929 he worked on the active constituents in *ergot and then on *histamine and *acetylcholine. In much of his research he was associated with *Barger and they were the first to use the term *sympathomimetic'.

DALTON, JOHN (1766–1844). English chemist. He was one of the founders of modern chemistry, and so of its application to medicine. He developed the chemical theory of Definite Proportions, usually called the Atomic Theory. Being colour-blind, he attended court to receive a Royal Society prize from George IV in the scarlet robes of an honorary DCL, unaware of the extent to which they deviated from his customary Quaker's garb. He realized, however, that he had unusual colour vision and made detailed observations which he reported to the Manchester Literary and Philosophical Society in 1794. This report aroused much interest in daltonism, as *colour-blindness was known for many years.

DANA, CHARLES LOOMIS (1852–1935). New York neurosurgeon. He described an operation to divide the posterior spinal nerve roots to relieve pain, *spasticity, and *athetosis.

DANDRUFF consists of dry scaly flakes shed from the skin of the scalp which tend to collect in hair and to be removed by brushing and combing; its basis is the essentially normal phenomenon of shedding dead epidermal cells from the *skin, but it is more noticeable in those with the greasy skin characteristic of *seborrhoea.

DANDY, WALTER EDWARD (1886–1946). American neurosurgeon. He developed diagnostic methods for localizing tumours by injection of air into the cerebral ventricles or into the spinal subarachnoid space (*pneumoencephalography). He was among the first to localize and remove *prolapsed intervertebral discs.

DANGEROUS DRUGS ACTS 1965, 1967. In the UK the 1965 Act restricted the importation, exportation, production, sale, cultivation, and use of raw *opium, coca leaves, *poppy-straw, *cannabis, cannabis resin, preparations of cannabis resin (Part I), prepared opium (Part II), and a number of other drugs listed in the schedule (Part III). It also specified certain offences, powers of search and arrest, and penalties. The 1967 Act introduced further measures to control drug addiction. They included: notification by medical practitioners of persons addicted; restriction of the prescription and supply of addictive drugs to those authorized by the Secretary of State; investigation of contraventions; requirements for safe custody and record-keeping in respect of specified drugs; and conferment of powers on the police to search and obtain evidence. The maximum penalty in relation to this and the principal act of 1965 was increased to 10 years' imprisonment. See SUBSTANCE ABUSE.

DARWIN, CHARLES ROBERT (1809–82). English naturalist. The grandson of Erasmus *Darwin. Henslow, professor of Botany at Cambridge, procured for him the post of naturalist to the *Beagle*. The observations which he made on that voyage, and his subsequent reflections, led him to believe in evolution of the species through the mechanism of natural selection acting on spontaneous variations. This theory was matured during long years of semi-invalidism at Downe, perhaps the most striking instance of 'creative malady' described by Sir George *Pickering; and it was given to the world, partly because of similar ideas communicated to him by A. R. Wallace, and certainly without precipitancy, in November 1859, in his book *The origin of species*.

DARWIN, ERASMUS (1731–1802). British physician and writer. He was a friend of Samuel Johnson and a member of the Lunar Society of Birmingham, which also counted Josiah Wedgwood, Joseph *Priestley, and James Watt as members. He was the grandfather of Charles *Darwin and Francis *Galton. His publications were *The loves of the plants* (1789) and *Zoonomia* (1794).

DAUNORUBICIN. A *cytotoxic antibiotic.

DA VINCI, see LEONARDO.

DAVY, SIR HUMPHRY (1778–1829). Born in Penzance, England, Davy intended to be a doctor, but soon turned to science. He gave lectures at the Royal Institution in London and in 1802 became professor of chemistry. His *Elements in agricultural chemistry* was published in 1813. His great interest in electrolysis, especially as a form of chemical analysis, led him to discover sodium and potassium, and later the alkaline-earth metals, magnesium, calcium, strontium, and barium, as well as boron. He helped Michael *Faraday in his early career. Davy is popularly known for his invention of a safety lamp for miners, which helped prevent explosions of firedamp (mainly methane gas) and air.

DAWSON, SIR BERTRAND EDWARD, 1st Viscount Dawson of Penn (1864–1945). British physician. He was chairman of the Consultative Council on Medical and Allied Services, the report of which (the

Dawson Report) foreshadowed the National Health Service. Dawson was a medical statesman and courtier who played an important part in planning the *Ministry of Health and the *Emergency Medical Service.

DAWSON REPORT, 1920. The interim (and in the event the only) report of the Council on Medical and Allied Services, set up under the chairmanship of Sir Bertrand *Dawson (later Lord Dawson of Penn) shortly after the return to power of Lloyd George's coalition government in 1918. The intention was to make recommendations fulfilling the election promise that a general health service would replace the *Poor Laws in medical care. The Council's 1920 report, a discussion document, was revolutionary and far seeing; it introduced the concept of *health centres, emphasized the importance of *preventive medicine and its integration with therapeutics, and accorded a central role in the reorganized system to the family practitioner. Though generally well received, the Council's work was overtaken by other urgent matters pressing upon the new *Ministry of Health (notably a financial crisis in the voluntary hospitals), and a final report was never published.

DAY HOSPITAL. A hospital where patients receive day care only, continuing to live in their own homes; this arrangement is often usefully employed, for example, in treating psychiatric illness. See also GERIATRIC MEDICINE; PSYCHIATRY.

DDT. See DICHLORO-DIPHENYL-TRICHLOROETHANE.

DEAF MUTISM is congenital total deafness with failure to acquire the faculty of speech.

DEAFNESS is partial or complete loss of the sense of hearing. See OTORHINOLARNYGOLOGY.

DEATH, DYING, AND THE HOSPICE MOVE-MENT. Attitudes to death and dying have changed over the centuries. The early Middle Ages saw a dying person as part of the community with a central part to play in familiar rituals. The later Middle Ages brought an intense concentration on the individual facing judgement and a righting of the great imbalance between the virtuous but poor and the sinful rich and powerful. The Victorian era introduced a new concentration on death beds, tombs, and the mourning family. A far more abrupt change has occurred in the 20th century (perhaps after the holocaust of the First World War) when death became a forbidden subject, a new taboo. The tendency not to tell a dying person the truth, the likelihood of an impersonal death in hospital or nursing home, and the inability of society to allow any display of emotion in public (other than in the *media) have made dying and *bereavement intensely lonely experiences. The old acceptance of destiny has gone, and a new sense of outrage that modern advances cannot finally halt the inevitable creates a very negative climate among dying people and their families. The challenges of their care are thus more demanding as well as more rewarding if they are truly faced and people are to find any meaning in the situation.

Such care was considered an essential part of the *family doctor's commitment, yet it has rarely had the attention in *medical education that it warrants. The needs of the dying in hospital may be crowded out of the attention of those responding to the urgent demands of acute care. Although a great deal has been learned, and much published, during the past three decades, the attitudes and skills of the *hospice and *palliative care movement are only slowly spreading through the general field, in both hospital and the community.

On making decisions

Doctors are committed to giving appropriate care to their patients, not to every treatment that may be technically possible. The prolongation of life should not in itself constitute the exclusive aim of *medical practice, which must be concerned equally with the relief of suffering. These two aims must be balanced as the doctor and the whole multidisciplinary team aim to act in a patient's best interests. Many interventions in themselves serve only to increase suffering without a balance of benefit. Such decisions are not easy, especially where a patient is no longer competent to discuss and make an informed choice as to which treatments he wishes. If he is already unconscious, a document previously drawn up, preferably with a designated proxy, may help the clinician in making judgement in this situation.

The doctor may not embark on any conduct with the primary intention of causing a patient's death, and if a terminally ill patient expresses a desire to commit *suicide a doctor may not in law facilitate the suicide. Nor can he respond to suggestions from a family to end life, although he does not have to continue futile treatment. In no country so far has physician-assisted suicide been made legally possible, although the situation in The Netherlands is that if certain guidelines are adhered to there will be no prosecution. There is evidence, however, that these guidelines are frequently not observed, and also some disquieting reports suggesting both social and individual pressure. In no way should such action be confused with appropriate palliative care, and doctors in this fast-developing field have been careful to emphasize this fact.

Skilled control of the physical, social, and emotional problems of far-advanced and terminal disease does not necessarily have to wait until all other treatment ceases, but may indeed make it more effective. When the clinician is involved with active treatment such as *chemotherapy, with the control of *pain and other symptoms, and with support to both patient and family, it will be easier to recognize diminishing returns in the former and to discontinue it without any member of

the family or of the caring team feeling that now no treatment is being given. To accept a situation where treatment is directed to the relief of symptoms and the alleviation of general distress will no longer mean an implicit 'there is nothing more that we can do' but an explicit 'everything possible is being done'. This should in no way be termed 'passive *euthanasia', and nothing would undermine such good practice more than any form of legalized direct and intended killing. A 'right to die' could all too easily become a 'duty to die' and discourage the development of this important branch of medicine.

The evolution of hospice and palliative care

Hospices 'for the dying' were founded in France in 1842 and, with no connection, in 1879 in Ireland. Mme Jeanne Garnier and the Irish Sisters of Charity both took the early Christian word which, from the 4th century onwards, had meant hospitality for the sick and destitute, and for pilgrims and travellers. They had no particular connection with dying. Several homes with different titles—Catholic, Jewish, and Protestant—were founded on both sides of the Atlantic during some 20 years at the turn of the 20th century. Caring for only a fraction of those in need, they had a very limited impact upon *general practice, which by the 1950s was becoming increasingly able to lengthen the time between the diagnosis of malignancy and the patient's death. The modern hospice movement grew out of the need to address better long-term control of pain and other symptoms, together with concern for the patient as a person and for his family at such a time.

Unusually effective pain control with the regular giving of oral opioids was observed by the author in St Luke's Hospital (founded in 1893 as a home for the dying poor) from 1948 onwards; it was introduced and developed from 1958 in St Joseph's Hospice (founded 1905). The decade between was spent in medical training, but also saw the introduction of many of the *drugs that were to be used in the increasingly effective control of symptoms. To the basic principle of giving *analgesic drugs regularly to prevent pain occurring, rather than to allow a patient to suffer before receiving relief, could be added an ever-more-sophisticated analysis of often complex problems with increasingly effective specific adjuvant treatments. With such an approach, patients were able to remain alert and often surprisingly active, and to be free to address all the other pressures of a mortal illness. Opportunity was given for a deepening of family communication and relationships, and to attend to unfinished business of all kinds. Possibilities of more ready access to the truth of the situation opened up as confidence in relief to the end developed. This, in turn, gave greater control to the patient and more choice as to where he spent his last days.

When St Christopher's Hospice opened in 1967, as the first modern hospice dedicated to research and education as well as to care, it set out to lay the scientific foundations for practice in this field that could be interpreted in the home as well as in other settings, and could become a part of medical, nursing, and other teaching. In 1969 it pioneered both a hospice home-care team, complementary to the local primary care teams in the community, and drug studies in pain control. Systematic bereavement support began in 1971, and a study centre opened in 1973 to accommodate the increasing number of visitors, both from this country and from overseas. Many of these set out to interpret the basic hospice principles in their different cultures and settings. A Hospice Information Service grew from these demands and today is in contact with a widespread network among nearly 60 countries, supplies information packs (contributed by members) about many different developments in the field, newsletters, and regularly updated UK and overseas directories.

Professionals from North America came on sabbaticals to St Christopher's in the early 1970s, and, in 1974, established a home-care team with no back-up beds in New Haven and a similar consulting hospital team in New York. The following year the Palliative Care Unit and Service was established in Montreal. These three different patterns have developed world-wide, while in the UK both independent and NHS units and home care and hospital teams have proliferated. Government support has gradually increased, but nearly all capital and well over 50 per cent of funding comes from public support. Hospices are major fund raisers in the voluntary sector.

Various professional associations and national and international organizations now set guidelines and standards. In the UK the title 'The National Council for Hospice and Specialist Palliative Care Services' illustrates the different names that have been chosen. It is becoming the accepted single voice for a movement that is now a recognized medical specialty with recognized principles.

Principles of terminal care

Maximizing potential
Until death a patient should be enabled to live at his own maximum potential, performing to the limit of his physical activity and mental capacity, with control and independence wherever possible. He should be recognized as the unique person he is and helped to live as part of his family and in other relationships with some awareness from those around of his hopes and expectations and of what has deepest meaning for him.

Place of choice
Patients should end their lives in the place most appropriate for them and their families, and where possible have choices in the matter. If the patient is given some insight into the serious nature of his disease, this will help him to make realistic decisions.

The patient and family as the unit of care
When a person is dying, his family find themselves in a crisis situation, with the joys and regrets of the past, the demands of the present, and the fears of the future all brought into stark focus. If this time is to be fully used, there needs to be some degree of shared awareness of the true situation. In general, sharing is more creative than deception.

Bereavement follow-up
The family has to recover. A bereavement follow-up service will identify and support those in special need, working in co-operation with the family doctor and any local services that can be involved.

Competent symptom control
The patient and his family will not use the time left to them to the full unless there is good control of pain and all the other symptoms that may arise. All doctors and nurses should be aware of the development of these skills, and special units have a responsibility to initiate research and disseminate such knowledge. Once good symptom control is achieved it is then easier to become aware of the mental and social aspects of suffering.

An experienced clinical team
A multidisciplinary medical approach is as important in the later stages of the management of disease as in the earlier phases. A group of consultants in a hospice unit or team may act merely as a resource while the patient remains in the care of his family doctor or of the clinicians who were involved with his initial treatment. A team may, however, take over his management completely, particularly if there is some special need, such as intractable physical distress or complex family problems.

Supportive team nursing
The particular character of the *nursing of dying patients includes the time given to do things at the patient's pace, to listen to the fears that are often revealed first to the helper in an intimate situation, to offer tenderness, understanding, and humour alongside practical deftness, and to greet and include the family both as cared for and as carers.

An interprofessional team
Teams are particularly needed by those who are grappling with emotional as well as with practical demands. *Psychiatrists, *social workers, and *chaplains have frequently been involved as support. Volunteers may have an important role, but must receive sensitive selection, training, and support.

Home care
A *home-care programme must be developed according to local circumstances, and be integrated with the family practices of the area and any local beds that may be

available. Skilled support and confidence in their ability may enable a family to keep a patient at home, often confounding all predictions. Even so, some people who have said they would like to die in their own homes need in-patient care, if only for the last few days.

Methodical recording and analysis
The evaluation and monitoring of clinical experience help in the establishment of soundly based practice. Research into the common clinical syndromes of dying patients, in pharmacology, therapeutics, and psycho-social studies, is needed to define and refine practice and attitudes.

Teaching in all aspects of terminal care
Teaching in this field is much in demand by students and graduates of all the disciplines concerned, as it has only a meagre place—if any—in general curricula. Although much of the future development must be more closely integrated with general teaching centres, the special units are likely to maintain their role of stimulating initial interest and organizing courses.

Support for staff
All members of staff will at times become drained by the work, and need both formal and informal support.

Efficiency is very comforting, and competence in administrative detail gives security to patients, families, and staff. It eases the liaison with outside contacts that is so essential for the small specialized team, and supports those who are managing such work among other pressures.

The search for meaning
The work will at times cause pain and bewilderment to all members of the staff. Those who commit themselves to remaining near the suffering of dependence and parting find they are impelled to develop a basic philosophy, part individual and part corporate. This grows out of the work undertaken together, as members find that they each have to search, often painfully, for some meaning in the most adverse circumstances, and gain enough freedom from their own anxieties to listen to another's questions of distress.

This search for meaning can create a climate in which patients and families can reach out in trust towards what they see as true and find acceptance of what is happening to them. We can, in some respects, reach back into the ways of coming to terms with death of the past. The values which the hospice movement tries to establish, alongside its commitment to excellence in practice, have something akin to the earlier assurance of community, the affirmation of the individual person, and the concern for the bereaved family. These values should be considered wherever a patient may be dying.

CICELY SAUNDERS

Note. In this article, the use of 'he' denoted 'he or she'; 'him' included 'her', and so on.

Further reading
Saunders, C. and Sykes, n. (1993). *The management of terminal malignant disease*, (3rd edn). Edward Arnold, London.
Stoddard, S. (1992). *The hospice movement – a better way of caring for the dying*, (2nd edn). Random House, New York.

DEBRE, ROBERT (1882–1978). French paediatrician. He described a form of *rickets to which his name is attached along with that of *Fanconi and de Toni. His son Michel became de Gaulle's prime minister. Debré was much concerned with social problems, including those of the underdeveloped world. He was a pioneer in the understanding of tuberculous *meningitis and its treatment with BCG (*bacille Calmette–Guérin).

DECEREBRATE RIGIDITY is a posture of fixed extensor rigidity of the trunk and limbs which ensues in experimental animals when the *brainstem is transected below the midbrain and *lower motor neurone activity is released from cerebral influence. A similar state may occur in man as a result of lesions of the brainstem.

DECIBEL is the unit used to measure the comparative intensity of two vibrations (frequency of sound). If I_1 and I_2 are two intensities, then their relative intensity is $10 \log_{10} (I_1/I_2)$ decibels. Usually I_1 is a reference intensity (the intensity of the weakest sound of the same frequency that the ear can detect); 50 dB then corresponds to human speech while 120 dB is the pain threshold.

DECLINE. A period of an illness during which the patient's condition deteriorates.

DECOMPENSATION is failure of an organ or system to compensate for a functional overload imposed by disease, used especially for the heart. 'Cardiac decompensation' implies a stage of disease in which compensatory mechanisms (such as *myocardial *hypertrophy) can no longer overcome the extra work load imposed, for example by a *stenotic aortic *valve, and symptoms therefore arise.

DECOMPRESSION SICKNESS is an unpleasant and often dangerous condition due to a rapid fall in ambient (environmental) pressure, which results in unreactive gases, chiefly nitrogen, coming out of solution in the blood and body fluids and forming bubbles. This is manifested by joint pain (the 'bends'), chest pain, breathlessness, and in severe cases spinal cord *infarction. Unless the situation is promptly reversed by recompression, the bubbles being forced back into solution, irreversible changes (e.g. *paraplegia) become established, or death may ensue. Very gradual decompression avoids the condition, as nitrogen is then released slowly enough from the blood to be eliminated by the lungs.

Decompression sickness ('*caisson disease') occurs in workers in compressed air (e.g. in tunnel construction and in deep-sea diving) if they return too rapidly to normal atmospheric pressure. Necessary decompression times (calculated according to time spent at particular pressures) must be observed rigorously. It may also occur in aviators experiencing subatmospheric pressures after rapid ascent to high altitude (see AEROSPACE MEDICINE). Treatment consists of immediate recompression in a compression chamber, followed by gradual decompression according to the schedules. Decompression sickness is a medical emergency. (See also ENVIRONMENT AND DISEASE.)

DECUBITUS is the manner or posture of lying in bed; a *bedsore may be called a decubitus ulcer.

DECUSSATION. A crossing in the form of the letter X, used particularly of *nerve fibres, tracts, etc. in the nervous system.

DEEPING, GEORGE WARWICK (1877–1950). English doctor. Deeping practised for a while before becoming a novelist and writer. His best-known work is *Sorrell and son* (1925).

DEFECATION. The evacuation of *faeces.

DEFENCE MEDICAL SERVICES (UK)
History
There can be few cultures in history where fighting men have neither expected nor received some form of medical and surgical support. But this support has been largely dependent on the scientific knowledge of the time, the resources made available, and the attitudes of commanders in the field.

Although the Romans supported their combatants with medical men, and surgeons accompanied King Henry V's army at Agincourt, it was not until the middle of the 18th century that a medical advance greatly increased the effectiveness of fighting men, and this was at sea. The results of Dr James *Lind's controlled clinical trial of remedies for *scurvy while serving on HMS *Salisbury* in 1747, when finally recognized by the Board of Admiralty many years later and applied to the Fleet, made possible the blockade of the French and Spanish ports during the Napoleonic wars.

Those wars also saw the development of mobile stretchers in the Grand Army of France, the improvement in treatment of casualties, and the beginnings of a separation of practice between the army, with its land battles, and the navy, where most of its fighting was at sea. James *McGrigor, one of the most enlightened of the doctors to be associated with the wars against Napoleon, was the first to organize an evacuation chain for casualties, during the Peninsular Campaign of 1808–14.

In the 19th century, developments in surgery and in the understanding of the causes of *infectious disease made a significant difference to the management of the sick and wounded in the armed forces. It required, however, disasters of considerable magnitude before the public came to appreciate the neglect of medical support to their armies in the field, and the consequences of that neglect. The Crimean War (1854–56) is particularly memorable for both military and medical incompetence. Florence *Nightingale was the driving force behind the improvements in medical organization, and the elevation of the status of *nursing which followed that campaign. In Northern Italy, the battle of Solferino (1859), in which the carnage was particularly severe and the wounded were scandalously neglected, resulted in the foundation of the *Red Cross, which was to have such an important role in future conflicts.

While the naval service had had a medical structure since Tudor times, and naval surgeons were granted warrants by the Navy Board in conjunction with the Barber-Surgeons, the doctors in the army had no military status and were members of the Army Medical Department as civilians until the end of the century. Naval surgeons had been granted warrant rank and uniform in 1805, but neither the army nor the navy was anxious to give professional men appropriate recognition. As a result of pressure from the medical profession, itself increasing in social status as the century wore on, the Royal Army Medical Corps (RAMC) was formed in 1898.

The new Corps was severely tested within a year, when the South African War broke out; military disasters and high casualty rates in a country with poor communications brought the new organization to breaking point. *Typhoid fever killed many more men than did the enemy. It is to the great credit of the RAMC and its leadership during the few years of peace that remained, that the lessons of the South African War were well learned and a proper structure was devised capable of supporting the British Army in the bloodbath of the First World War. The Queen Alexandra's Imperial Military Nursing Service was formed in 1902, a medical stores depot was established, field *hygiene became an important area of study and practice, and a comprehensive plan was evolved for the collection and evacuation of casualties from the front.

By 1914 the medical support for the army and the navy had some common factors and some important differences. Doctors and nurses had achieved the recognition of officer status, belonged to their parent service in every way, and were recruited from their civilian professions to maintain, in uniform, the standards to which they had been trained. Training in military medicine and skills, as well as in clinical practice, in both services was recognized as an essential part of preparation for war. The navy, however, fought its actions at sea and casualties could not be evacuated until the ship returned to port, where base hospitals had been built in Portsmouth (1746), Plymouth (1752), and Chatham (1827). They lived or died on board, and the ships' surgeons had to do the best they could. Hospital ships were not an option in a fleet action and only served to support naval bases or operations at a distance from the home country. The army now appreciated that, particularly in a European war, casualties could, and should, be sent to the rear as quickly as possible so that definitive procedures could be carried out in an atmosphere conducive to success.

The catastrophe that befell Europe in 1914 therefore found the medical services small in size but comparatively well prepared, although neither the politicians nor the commanders had any idea of how devastating or prolonged the conflict was to be. In common with their parent arms, the medical services underwent rapid expansion, the RAMC rising to a total of 167 000 officers and men in an army of nearly 4 million. The magnitude of the land battle, particularly on the Western front, dwarfed the problems of the naval service. The casualty evacuation plan, although modified by experience, proved its worth. The clinical advances, particularly in the management of *trauma, were remarkable. The correct procedures for the surgical management of severely damaged tissue by debridement and delayed primary suture, the better management of chest and abdominal wounds, and the use of intravenous fluids in surgical *shock were all developed during these terrible 4 years. Yet other conditions were less well understood. Trench *immersion foot was intractable in the conditions of wet and cold that prevailed on the Western front. The stress of manning the front line under heavy fire, in appalling conditions, for long periods without rest or sleep produced manifestations that were often labelled either cowardice or 'shell shock'. The generals had little idea of what conditions at the front were like and the public at home heard only from those relatives who survived to get home on leave or for convalescence.

The Royal Flying Corps, formed in 1912, soon began to find its own special medical problems as aircraft were able to fly higher and faster, so that *altitude sickness, the requirement for oxygen, and other problems of flight required expert attention. A Special Medical Board with two RAMC officers and two civilian consultants was established in 1916 to oversee these and other problems. In 1918, the Royal Air Force was formed, with the medical services reorganized and given RAF ranks in the following year. The medical problems of the RAF were clearly distinct from those of the other two services, and were concentrated around the special physiological circumstances of flight; research into aviation *physiology (see AEROSPACE MEDICINE) was an essential part of the role of the RAF medical services, and has so remained.

The inevitable run-down of the services following the end of the First World War resulted in a diminution of the skills that had been learned during the conflict. However, the RAF established its own hospitals after the war, at Halton (1919), Cranwell, and Uxbridge. The air transport of casualties was an obvious development to be explored, and this was first achieved in Somaliland in 1919, after which air transport became

an acceptable method, which was much improved by 1939.

Between the two world wars, the armed forces were involved in peace-keeping or minor skirmishes throughout the British Empire, but the inevitable drift into peace-time inertia was a problem for all three services, exacerbated by the economic problems affecting all of Europe. The medical services suffered from a severe shortage of recruits, and there were few incentives to follow a military career; it was not until rearmament began that numbers rose. Two major developments occurred shortly before the Second World War which were to have a profound effect on the care of war casualties. The first of these, *blood transfusion, became available in time for the RAMC to set up the Army Blood Transfusion Service before the outbreak of war. The effects of the second, the development of *sulphonamides, followed in 1943 by *penicillin and the other *antibiotics, were only apparent during the war, but in the long term were to have a profound influence on *morbidity and *mortality in war.

Military planners have always tended to assume that the next war will resemble the last. Contrary to expectations, the Second World War proved to be a global conflict of rapid movement, with a dramatic rise in the value of air power, and with deadly new weaponry which brought it to its close and which presented the world with terrifying new problems in maintaining the peace. The concept of a land evacuation chain stood the test of time; advances in surgery, the arrival of antibiotics, and blood transfusion resulted in a remarkable reduction in the mortality from gunshot wounds and other trauma. In South-East Asia, recognition that *malaria would disable far more men than would the enemy resulted in a comprehensive anti-malarial campaign, which ultimately contributed to victory in that theatre. A better, but still incomplete, understanding of psychological reactions to the stresses of war enabled many more men to be returned to their units without serious long-term disabilities.

The character of the war at sea was changed by the advent of air power, shown in the Far East to be particularly effective and capable of surprise when carrier-based, and was notable for a sustained submarine campaign against merchant shipping. Survival among those torpedoed and cast adrift in lifeboats was the subject of much study by the Royal Naval Physiological Research Committee set up by the *Medical Research Council. The committee also examined the problems of diving and *decompression sickness, living and working in submarines, and the problems of *motion sickness, and it continues its excellent work up to the present day.

The aftermath of the 1939–45 war was dominated by the advent of nuclear weapons and by the rise of the Soviet Union as an aggressive and confrontational military power. The Korean War, and later the American involvement in Vietnam, were usually seen as conflicts between the forces of communism and the West; it was in the latter war that real medical advances were made.

The overwhelming superiority of American air power in Vietnam allowed a comprehensive system of air evacuation for casualties in forward units, together with early and adequate blood transfusion and surgery within the first 6 hours, which resulted in a significant reduction in morbidity and mortality. This experience provided lessons that are still valid today, but it must be remembered that the superiority of American air power and the ready availability of helicopter transport were peculiar to Vietnam and may not be reproducible in future conflicts.

The South Atlantic Campaign of 1982 presented new and exceptional challenges to the medical services. There were great difficulties involved with a task force operating 8000 miles from its home base, having as its objective the landing of soldiers and marines on hostile territory under limited air cover. Added to these were the problems of evacuating casualties from the battle area, providing emergency surgery, and returning them to the UK, while keeping the medical services adequately supplied (medical supplies being in competition with the requirements of the fighting arms). The essential solution was to provide a hospital ship (the passenger liner *Uganda*, taken up from trade) operating in close co-operation with the land forces, who themselves were supported by a Field Ambulance and the Medical Squadron of 3 Commando Brigade. Evacuation of casualties from the front line was by helicopter on an 'opportunity basis' when possible, initially to a casualty clearing station at the original bridgehead, and thence to the hospital ship. Casualties from damaged and sinking ships were also readily transferred because of the proximity of other vessels in the narrow waters about the Falkland Islands, although the nature of those casualties, with burns and smoke inhalation predominating, were essentially unchanged from those in earlier maritime conflicts. Evacuation of casualties who had been rendered stable in the hospital ship was by Royal Naval survey vessels, temporarily converted to 'ambulance ship' roles and plying between the scene of conflict and South America, whence the Royal Air Force provided an efficient air evacuation service to the home base.

The South Atlantic campaign was perhaps the first in which co-operation among all three services was both essential and demonstrably effective. It was noteworthy in that few planners had given thought to mounting such an operation beforehand, and that the whole task force and its support were put together at great speed. Although considerable risks were taken, the operation was remarkably successful. The use of helicopter evacuation of casualties demonstrated their pivotal role in future conflicts. The use of 'ambulance ships' was a necessary feature of a seaborne operation far from the home base and allowed the hospital ship, with its comprehensive surgical facilities, to remain off shore and within easy reach of operations. As might have been expected, the shorter the time elapsing between wounding and resuscitation, the greater the chance of survival. Thus we may note that current thinking, much influenced by this experience, suggests that the essentials of successful medical support are; *resuscitation of casualties as close as possible to the point of wounding; early stabilization and blood transfusion; rapid evacuation; and definitive treatment at a hospital base facility, preferably in the home country.

The operation to remove the Iraqis from Kuwait in 1991 resulted in very few casualties among British servicemen, but the experiences of that campaign reinforced these concepts, now very much in the minds of medical planners. They also underlined the importance of inter-service co-operation at every level, of the ready availability of reserve forces, and of the essential part that good communications, command, and control will play in any future conflict. The greatest success of this operation, however, was *preventive medicine and its application to the maintenance of the fighting efficiency of the troops. These factors are now regarded as highly relevant to medical support in the future, as the dangers of a world conflict and world-wide nuclear war recede, but other problems, notably that of chemical warfare in the Third World, remain serious threats.

The central control of the medical services

After the First World War, the medical departments of the three services were located in London, with single-service staffs, each controlled by a director-general who reported to his single-service Board. These arrangements persisted until 1963 when the first serious attempts were made to centralize the professional control of the armed forces by giving increased powers to the Chief of Defence Staff at the expense of the Single Service Chiefs. Subsequently, a series of reports were commissioned by Ministers to review the overall structure, and particularly the top management of the medical services, but it was not until the Yellowlees Report of 1984 that a unified medical headquarters was insisted upon by the then Secretary of State. This concept, while realistically creating a surgeon-general with overall responsibilities, raised serious problems. The scheme, based on integrated single- and tri-service functions at Ministry of Defence level, virtually abolished single-service staffs and at first expected the surgeon-general to continue to manage his single service, while at the same time being responsible for developing tri-service policy. With the passage of time this scheme was seen to be unworkable, and it has subsequently evolved by stages to allow the surgeon-general to concentrate on his task of unifying the policies and activities of the medical services, while the essential management of front-line support, recruiting, and training remains with the single-service heads. Further progress along the road of tri-service unification could be achieved only if it were carried out across the armed forces as a whole, and the Canadian experience has shown that such an arrangement does not work. The surgeon-general's position is now well established and the holder of that office is considerably more effective than the original Yellowlees concept would have allowed.

Postgraduate education, training, and research

The ability to attract high-quality men and women to the medical services now depends more on professional opportunities and training than on financial reward, and much attention has been paid to these in recent years. As the services faced the end of conscription (which ceased in 1962), it became apparent that young medical officers had to be encouraged to obtain higher degrees and qualifications to ensure their professional credibility, and secondments to the *National Health Service (NHS) for this purpose became common. As the medical profession began to organize regular training programmes, chiefly through the *Royal Colleges, so it became necessary for the services to fulfil civilian training requirements, and all service medical officers now expect, and receive, the same postgraduate education as their civilian counterparts, which is necessary to enable them to be accredited as consultants or recognized as *general practitioner trainers.

Training with special relevance to the tasks of the single service to which the medical officer belongs has long been considered essential. For that purpose the Royal Army Medical College at Millbank was built before 1914 and was particularly successful in both training and research in tropical medicine.

The naval medical school, originally established at Haslar in 1881, was moved to Greenwich in 1912 and finally to Alverstoke after the Second World War. With the increasing complexity of maritime medicine, particularly since the advent of the nuclear submarine with its extended range and ability to remain submerged for very long periods, the medical school was reorganized as a centre for research and specialist training in 1969, becoming the Institute of Naval Medicine.

The Royal Air Force established a physiological laboratory at Farnborough in 1938, which became the Institute of Aviation Medicine and has been a centre of outstanding research into the problems of aircrew and for the training of Royal Air Force personnel in this complex subspecialty of *occupational medicine.

These separate establishments are, however, expensive to maintain, and there are frequent calls to replace them with a single centre for training and research. Their disparate roles make this a very expensive alternative to the existing arrangements.

The increasing complexity of medicine has meant that supporting technicians must be equally well trained. *Radiographers, laboratory *technicians, and *physiotherapists must attain appropriate civilian standards both to ensure the highest standards within the services and to provide them with an adequate career which

they can continue into civilian life. The services have carried out the greater part of this training themselves, but much of this is now done on a tri-service basis or in civilian establishments.

The nursing services

From the earliest times, naval nursing had been carried out on board on an '*ad hoc*' basis by the 'loblolly boys' who were seamen or marines of good character, but in 1853 sick-berth staff were provided for all seagoing ships and the Sick Berth Branch, with a proper career structure, was formed in 1884 as a result of the recommendations of the Hoskins Committee, which also proposed the formation of a female nursing service. This was established in 1885 and became the Queen Alexandra's Royal Naval Nursing Service. We have also seen how the Queen Alexandra's Royal Army Nursing Corps (renamed from the Imperial Military Nursing Service in 1948) evolved from the rough and ready arrangements that preceded Florence Nightingale and her reforming zeal. The Corps soon acquired military ranks, nurses also being recruited to the other ranks, and a training centre of its own. The Princess Mary's Royal Air Force Nursing Service became an integral part of the RAF in 1950, and finally assumed RAF officers' ranks in 1980. All three nursing services have trained their own nurses during the past 30 years, but this is becoming more difficult with the increasing complexity of nurse training in the civilian profession, with which service training must equate. It seems likely that nurse training will, in future, be done only in combined civil–military nursing schools. The administration of the nursing services has followed the medical model, with a Director of Defence Nursing Services.

The dental services

Although comparatively late on the scene, *dentistry in the armed forces has been in advance of its civilian counterpart in both quality and effectiveness. The captive military population has always had regular dental checks and this has resulted in a high standard of dental fitness, vital to those servicemen committed to conflict. In addition to their dental role in war, they have also been integrated into the order of battle as resuscitation officers and as general assistants to both surgeons and *anaesthetists, but at present there remains pressure to replace service dentists by civilians.

Service hospitals

The nature of medical support to the Royal Navy required the establishment of naval hospitals at base ports at an early stage, and three major naval hospitals founded in the 18th century continued until recent times, at Chatham (which finally closed in 1960), at Haslar, and at Plymouth. Since the Second World War, the army has been obliged to close the military hospitals in England at Netley, on Southampton Water, and at Millbank, where the closure of the Queen Alexandra

Military Hospital was followed by a new building at Woolwich, the Queen Elizabeth Military Hospital, to replace the old Royal Herbert Hospital. In addition to this new hospital in London, the Victorian building of the Cambridge Military Hospital, with its maternity unit at the adjoining Princess Louise Hospital, and the Duchess of Kent Military Hospital at Catterick continue to serve the British Army and its dependents in the home base. The Royal Air Force began with the advantage of being able to plan its hospital programme unhindered by historical considerations, and built major hospitals at Halton (1919), Wroughton, and Ely, although smaller ones were also built and later closed, as has Ely. In addition to the home hospitals, all three services maintained hospitals abroad, consistent with their commitments, but these have now (1993) shrunk to a small, and reducing, number in Germany, and hospitals in Gibraltar, Cyprus, Hong Kong, Belize, and the Falkland Islands.

The fate of the hospitals abroad is dependent on government policy with regard to the places in which they are sited; the hospitals in Hong Kong and Gibraltar are already identified for closure, and those in Germany face reduction to two in the near future, and possibly one only in the longer term.

Since the advent of the NHS, it is often asked why service hospitals are required at home. They are expensive to run and frequently sited in ancient buildings, many of which are listed, and most of which require major refurbishment. Against these obvious disadvantages may be set certain major benefits. They can provide rapidity of treatment, particularly for surgery, which allows men and women to return to duty as quickly as possible, and in which their families can be treated as a priority. They provide facilities available to the NHS in places where they are much needed for the civil population. They provide opportunities for training that are not readily available in the NHS because of its need to restrict numbers in training to match requirements, and because of the services' need to train personnel for their military role. Finally, they provide buildings from which medical personnel, actively engaged in their professional work, can be readily deployed as units to the scene of operations. The advantages of deploying men and women who have worked and trained together as a comprehensive group with a pre-defined war role should be obvious. Nevertheless, there are at present too many service hospitals in the UK for the current size of the armed forces and plans are now well advanced to retain only some three or four of the existing hospitals. Others, in areas where there remains a significant population of servicemen and their dependents, are likely to be closed but replaced by Military District Hospital Units (MDHU), which would be attached to existing district general hospitals in the NHS.

It also seems likely that, with a decreasing patient base overall, the services attempt to cover too many specializations at present. All specialist disciplines require

extensive, and expensive, training, and some of these currently available within the services could be dealt with in the civilian sector. Others, deemed necessary 'in house' because of the military implications, could be provided in one tri-service centre.

The reserve forces

Since the sea-fencibles and the militia at the end of the 18th century, the reserve forces have played a significant part in the history of the nation. During previous major conflicts, the professional soldiers and sailors were rapidly diluted by a large influx of reservists, whose great contribution was that they arrived already trained for war. As the size of the regular forces continues to be reduced at a rate faster than that of the nation's commitments, so the need for vigorous and well-trained reserve forces becomes more important. An inherent difficulty lies in the reluctance of employers to release reservists for training and, more particularly, for operational purposes. Reservists must be free to go to war when summoned, their jobs must be protected for the duration of hostilities, and during their period of recall they must serve on the same basis as regulars. Above all, politicians must have the will to use reservists; they demonstrated a reluctance to do so during the Gulf War.

The Territorial Army remains the largest of the three reserve forces with a continuing major role in any future conflict of any magnitude, and it is seriously examining its structure to meet changing operational demands in the future. The medical branch of the Royal Naval Reserve is now directing its training towards the support of amphibious operations and the evacuation of casualties by sea, while the RAF Reserve is giving the same attention to casualty evacuation by air.

Looking ahead

Medical support to operations is always dependent on the operational plan, and emerging operational concepts must dictate future medical planning. What then must the medical services be prepared for in the future?

National defence at home and defending our national interests abroad must remain the first priority. A major war in Europe is increasingly unlikely, but can never be discounted. But we are certain to be increasingly involved in multinational operations to keep the peace under the aegis of the United Nations, NATO, or the Western European Union. At the time of writing, British Forces are engaged in many operations around the world, including the former territory of Yugoslavia and in Cyprus. Certain operations will always be medically led from the start; an RAMC Field Ambulance was the first major unit into the Balkans after the breakup of Yugoslavia.

Peace-keeping is one thing, war is another. The United Kingdom is unlikely to fight a war of any size without allies, and planning must be carried out with them, continuing to address all the problems of standardization of equipment and procedures that have bedeviled the North Atlantic Treaty Organization (NATO) for 40 years.

Counter-terrorism presents special problems, and there is likely to be a role for the services in responding rapidly to major natural disasters and in humanitarian aid if political suspicions and difficulties can be overcome.

In addition, because advances in technology now allow the media to bring instant war into the sitting room, the services have to consider the public's concerns with an immediacy that was never there before, and this particularly applies to anything to do with medical support. Casualty reporting has to be immediate, explanations fulsome, and the confusion of war minimized.

These dramatic changes since the Second World War mean that a number of basic concepts which have been immutable for 80 years are being challenged. First among these is the extent to which the single-service medical services should continue to operate independently. As has been seen, the trend is towards much greater integration and co-operation, and this trend must continue, if necessary at the expense of tradition and custom. However, dedicated single-service medical support for operational units must remain the aim. The role of service hospitals continues to be scrutinized. The structure of the land evacuation chain and the units that comprise it, including field ambulances, field hospitals and forward surgical teams, are being reviewed. The training requirements for medical personnel, to meet the changing face of warfare, are being constantly questioned.

The armed forces are now smaller than they have been for many years. Some may judge the world to be a safer place of late, but that is doubtful. The argument between those who advocate the defence of the country as a first priority and those who believe that money is better spent on health and social welfare will continue for the foreseeable future. But military men and women, and their families, have higher expectations of their medical support than ever before, and will not lightly go into battle without the very best that can be provided by their country. Nor should they.

G. J. MILTON-THOMPSON

DEFENESTRATION. See FENESTRATION.

DEFIBRILLATION is the termination of atrial or ventricular *fibrillation by applying an electric shock to the heart, encouraging the subsequent resumption of co-ordinated contractions.

DEFICIENCY. Partial lack or complete absence of something, for example of a dietary component.

DEFORMITY. Malformation or distortion of part of the body, congenital or acquired.

DEGENERATION is pathological change in a tissue or structure, causing it to depart from its healthy, specialized, fully functional state.

DEGLUTITION is the act of swallowing or the ability to swallow.

DEHYDRATION. Loss or removal of water; the condition resulting from excessive water loss.

DEJA VU is the illusion that a new experience has happened before.

DEJERINE, AUGUSTA (née Klumpke) (1859–1927). Franco-American neurologist. An American living in Geneva with her family, she learned from a magazine in 1877 that Madeleine Brès had become an MD (Paris). Stimulated by this example she determined to train in medicine and, against strong opposition, was admitted as an extern in 1882 and an intern in 1885. In 1888 she graduated MD and married Joseph *Dejerine, thereafter devoting herself to working with her husband in neurology. She described with her husband the paralysis resulting from damage to the lower part of the *brachial plexus (Dejerine–Klumpke paralysis, 1885).

DEJERINE, JOSEPH JULES (1849–1917). French neurologist. In 1888 he married Augusta Klumpke, with whom he published *L'anatomie des centres nerveux* (1895–1901). His main studies were on *tabes dorsalis, *myotonia congenita, facioscapulohumeral *muscular dystrophy, and *motor neurone disease. His name is attached to 11 syndromes.

DELETION is the loss of part of a *chromosome. See also GENETICS.

DELIRIUM is a state of acute and severe *confusion. There is mental excitement, with *illusions, *delusions, and *hallucinations, and physical restlessness. Delirium is characteristic of severe toxic and febrile states and may follow withdrawal of drugs or alcohol in those addicted.

DELIRIUM TREMENS is an acute episode of profound mental and physical disturbance associated with severe and prolonged *addiction to alcohol (*alcoholism) and usually following acute alcohol withdrawal.

DELIVERY is the process of childbirth, in particular the second and third stages of *labour, during which the infant and the *placenta are expelled from the *uterus. See also OBSTETRICS.

DELPECH, JACQUES MATHIEU (1777–1832). French surgeon. Delpech was a brilliant technician with an interest in *orthopaedics, of which he was the first exponent in France. He founded an orthopaedic clinic in Montpellier and published *De l'orthomorphie* (1816). He was the first to undertake subcutaneous Achilles *tenotomy. In 1832 he was shot dead by a patient who believed his operation for *varicocele had prevented his advantageous marriage.

DELUSION. A false opinion or belief, contrary to fact and unassailable by evidence or reason. It is usual to exclude from this definition articles of religious faith or other beliefs shared by persons of similar culture, tribe, etc.

DEMENTIA is deterioration of intellectual function associated with pathological changes in the brain (cf. AMENTIA).

DEMENTIA PARALYTICA. Synonym for *general paralysis of the insane.

DEMENTIA PRAECOX. An outmoded term for *schizophrenia, first used by the Belgian psychiatrist B. A. Morel in 1857 (*démence précoce*) and later by E. *Kraepelin.

DEMOGRAPHY is the numerical study of human populations. See also EPIDEMIOLOGY.

DEMYELINATION is loss of the *myelin sheath of *nerve fibres. Patchy demyelination is characteristic of some diseases of the central nervous system, notably *multiple sclerosis. Demyelination of peripheral nerves occurs in some varieties of *polyneuropathy. See NEUROMUSCULAR DISEASE.

DENDRITE. One of the short branching processes extending out from the body of a nerve cell (*neurone), which act as *receptors for impulses.

DENERVATION is deprivation of the nerve supply to an organ, or tissue.

DENGUE is an *influenza-like *virus infection of tropical and subtropical regions. The virus is transmitted by biting *mosquitoes of the genus *Aëdes*, most commonly *A. aegypti*. Although the condition may be unpleasant, it is self-limiting, and complete recovery is the rule; a maculopapular rash appears about the fourth day and fades after a day or two. Occasionally dengue viruses (there are four types) cause a more severe haemorrhagic fever.

DENTAL CARIES is the common form of tooth decay, widespread in most Western societies, particularly where the *fluorine content of the water supply is low. The process involves disintegration first of the outer enamel of the tooth then of the *dentine, with eventual destruction of the whole tooth; it is generally held to

be due to acids formed by the action of bacteria in the mouth on dietary carbohydrate. See also DENTISTRY.

DENTAL HYGIENIST. A member of a profession supplementary to dentistry, trained in the care of the mouth, gums, and teeth, and the prophylaxis of *dental caries and *periodontal disease. See also DENTISTRY.

DENTAL NURSE. A dentist's assistant or receptionist, or a person combining these functions.

DENTAL SERVICE. In the UK dental services are provided as part of the National Health Service under the *National Health Services Acts 1946 and 1977. There is a large private sector, and many dentists practise both within and outside the state service. See also DENTISTRY.

DENTAL SURGERY is a synonym for dentistry, of US origin but now current in all English-speaking countries; alternatively, it means the premises where dentistry is practised.

DENTINE is the main substance of *teeth. It resembles bone but is denser and contains no cells or blood vessels, although it is penetrated by cell processes from connective tissue cells (odontoblasts) in the pulp cavity of the tooth. Ivory is dentine.

DENTIST. A qualified and registered practitioner of *dentistry, broadly defined as oral medicine and surgery with major emphasis on the diagnosis and treatment, including prosthetics, of conditions of the *teeth and gums.

DENTISTRY IN THE UK AND USA
Dentistry in the UK. Introduction
The provision of dental care in the UK can be traced back as far as the time of the Roman occupation (55 BC–AD 410). Emperor Claudius arrived in Britain in AD 43 and was accompanied by his surgeon, Scribonius Largus, who, in addition to his surgical duties, also treated dental ailments. A small instrument similar to the volsella, referred to by Celsus (30 BC) and found amongst archaeological discoveries of that age, is believed to have been brought to Britain by Largus.

There is little reliable evidence of any development of the practice of dentistry until the 14th century, although it is known that the druids attempted to treat dental problems by incantation and magic. Religious orders, specifically established for the healing of sick priests and monks, included amongst their skills the ability to extract teeth.

Early general practitioners of dentistry were barbers and charlatans who, dressed in picturesque clothes and with musical accompaniment to drown the anguished cries of their victims, succeeded in earning lucrative incomes. In the larger cities it was also possible to find a physician or a surgeon to undertake extractions.

In 1300 the Company of Masters of Barbery and Surgery was formed in the City of London, comprising two groups, one of which included the tooth-drawers. They were held in scant respect, largely because of their paucity of training and crude methods of operating. In 1540 a new Company was founded under a Royal Charter granted by Henry VIII which united the Guild of Surgeons and the Company of Masters of Barbery and Surgeons, to become the Company of *Barber-Surgeons of London. The company certainly did much to raise the standards of surgery, but specifically excluded 'the drawing of teeth' from its constraints of practice.

After its dissolution in 1745 by an Act of Parliament, there emerged the Company of Surgeons, which in 1800 became the *Royal College of Surgeons of London, and, in 1843, of England. It is to this College that dentistry in the UK owes the pattern of its evolution from a trade to a profession.

At this time there were no dental schools and no qualifying degrees or diplomas; anyone could practise dentistry, and many did so as itinerant tooth-drawers, advertising widely and garishly. However, an increasing number of physicians and surgeons undertook apprentice training with a practising dentist and thus became sufficiently skilled to practise.

By the end of the 18th century, a number of the London teaching hospitals provided courses of lectures on dentistry, the most notable being that at Guy's by James Fox and that at St George's by John *Hunter and William Rae. Nevertheless, dentistry in Britain was falling behind. Already, in France L'Ecole Dentaire had been founded in 1699, and in the US the Baltimore College of Dental Surgery was founded in 1839.

Trade to a profession

By the middle of the 19th century there was a general awareness in the UK of the urgent need to raise the status of dental practice. Early pressure to persuade the Royal College of Surgeons to establish a diploma in dental surgery failed, on the grounds that it would be contrary to the College Charter.

Meanwhile, in 1859, the first dental hospital was opened in Soho Square, London, mainly by members of the newly founded Odontological Society of London. Associated with this hospital, in 1860 the first dental school was opened and named The London School of Dental Surgery. Soon afterwards the Metropolitan School of Dental Science and the National Dental Hospital were founded, from which it became possible to be awarded a diploma—the MCDE. Bona fide dentists could be awarded the diploma '*sine curriculo*'.

Stimulated by continuing pressure, both the Royal College of Surgeons and the government acceded to the demands of the profession, and in 1858 the Medical Bill was successfully laid before Parliament, empowering the Royal College of Surgeons to establish a diploma course, hold professional examinations, and award the

Licence in Dental Surgery (LDS RCS Eng). The first examinations were held in 1860, and soon afterwards similar diplomas began to be awarded by the Royal Colleges in Glasgow, Edinburgh, and Dublin.

Despite the availability of formal teaching leading to a professional qualification, there was still no control over unqualified practice. Even after the passing of the Dentists Act of 1878, which established the Dentists Register, anyone could practise dentistry provided he did not call himself a dentist or dental surgeon.

In 1879 the British Dental Association was founded (it was incorporated in 1880), its primary concern being to enforce the new Act, to eliminate unregistered practice, to encourage high standards of professional conduct and education, and to promote research.

It took 43 years to remedy the defects of the 1878 Act. The Dentists Act of 1921 required everyone who practised dentistry to be registered annually, although it did allow people who 'had been in reputable practice' and who did not possess a formal dental or medical qualification to register, provided they satisfied the requirements of the Dental Board of the United Kingdom and were of good 'personal character'. It is only quite recently that the last of the so-called '1921 men' left the register.

The Dental Board was under the authority of the *General Medical Council, and was charged with maintenance of the Register, regulating professional discipline, the educational standards of the schools, dental health education, and the financial welfare of the schools and students. The 1957 Dentists Act consolidated all previous Acts and, at the same time, authorized the founding of the *General Dental Council, which established the independence of the dental profession and finally completed the transformation of dentistry 'from a trade to a profession'.

Dental education
Dental schools
The book by Pierre Fauchard, *Le chirurgien dentiste, ou traité des dents*, published in 1728, heralded the birth of dentistry as a clinical science. In two 900-page volumes, the book covered all aspects of dentistry, including oral *anatomy and *physiology, oral *pathology, *surgery, *orthodontics, and *prosthetics. Several books by UK authors appeared, notably by Blake, Fox, Bell, and Swell, all of which were based upon lecture courses given in their teaching hospitals. The most notable of all was that by John Hunter, surgeon to St George's Hospital, who in 1771 published his work *The natural history of the human teeth*. Not only did this book report Hunter's anatomical and pathological findings, but it also described his scientific investigations. Clearly, he was steeped in the discipline of science, and the quality of his observations and interpretations is attested by the frequency of references to his work today, some 200 years later.

By the end of the 19th century nine dental schools

had been established in the UK, three being in London. The remaining seven were founded after 1900, the last being the Dental School of the Welsh National School of Medicine in Cardiff, which was opened in 1965. In addition, soon after the Second World War, the Postgraduate Dental Institute was opened at the Eastman Dental Hospital in London.

However, having greatly benefited during the postwar years, the dental schools of the UK, like those in the USA and elsewhere in the world, began to find themselves in difficulties. Reductions in university funding resulted in less money being available to maintain or replace ageing buildings; changing patterns of dental disease, mainly the decline in dental caries prevalence, led to questions being asked concerning the number of schools needed and the number of dental students required to qualify each year. The eventual outcome was the merger in 1983 of the Royal and Guy's Dental Schools, the closure in 1991 of University College Dental School, and the closure in 1994 of the Edinburgh Dental School and its conversion into a postgraduate centre for Scotland.

Teachers
Up until the end of the Second World War the vast majority of the clinical teaching of dental students was undertaken by part-time teachers, who spent the major part of their working life in their practices. Their contribution was mainly concerned with the practical skills of conservative dentistry, prosthetic dentistry, and surgery. Much of the treatment provided in the dental hospitals with which the schools were associated comprised treating the ravages of oral *sepsis brought on by neglect. Students became highly skilled in the techniques of extracting teeth under general and local *anaesthesia, and in the administration of short-lasting, primitive anaesthetics, using nitrous oxide and oxygen. Such has been the improvement in dental health that students today do not acquire these skills to a similar extent.

Teaching of the preclinical subjects of anatomy, physiology, and *biochemistry was usually given with the medical students, as was the teaching in pathology and bacteriology.

The introduction of the *National Health Service in 1948 had a profound effect on dental education. It took over the financing and administration of the dental hospitals, refurbishing them with modern equipment and providing adequate staff, who became fully integrated into the NHS career structure. The NHS also set targets for the number of dentists required to provide the treatment needs of the community. These targets were accepted by the universities, of which the dental schools had become part, and, through the University Grants Committee, whose Dental Sub-Committee made quinquennial visits to the schools, funding was allocated to implement approved developments. In these 'halcyon' years there were large and rapid increases in the numbers of full-time academic staff, the establishment of

chairs, formation of new departments, and the development of research. Over a period of 35 years, all the dental schools but one were rebuilt and expanded, the exception being The Royal, which merged with Guy's.

These rapidly introduced changes created serious problems, in that there were very few people available with a background appropriate for senior academic appointments. However, the situation was largely overcome, certainly in the longer term, through the establishment by the Nuffield Foundation of a series of fellowships and scholarships, which enabled young dental graduates to return to the university to gain a scientific education, and dental students to intercalate a B.Sc. degree. The success of this scheme can be judged by the number of recipients of these awards who hold, or have held, chairs and other senior academic appointments, and by the international acclaim of their research contributions.

Sadly, the financial constraints now being imposed on universities are making academic dentistry a much less attractive career. Posts are being 'frozen', promotion is more difficult, and funding for research, the life-blood of academia, is severely restricted.

Advances in dental practice
The years since the end of the Second World War have seen tremendous changes in the patterns of dental education and practice. In simple terms, these changes have evolved as a result of research, mainly conducted in the dental schools of the world, and the change in attitudes towards dental health of the public. These advances have extended across the whole spectrum of dentistry and have included the development of equipment, instruments, techniques, and treatment procedures.

Dental practice has not been unaffected by major advances in pharmacology. Drugs are now available which, while not used for the treatment of dental ills, can profoundly influence patterns of dental treatment. Such drugs include *anticoagulants and the *corticosteroids. Furthermore, the availability of a range of new anaesthetic agents has rendered the simple 'gas and air' anaesthetic obsolete, and has largely taken dental anaesthetics out of the hands of the dentist into those of the specialist anaesthetist.

Major advances have occurred in the treatment of inflammatory diseases of the gums. Whereas hitherto, 'pyorrhoea alveolaris' was regarded as untreatable other than by extraction of teeth, much can now be done to control the progress of the disease and to prevent its onset.

The prevalence of dental decay has declined dramatically in the Western world over the past 15–20 years. Despite the considerable increase in knowledge of the cause and natural history of this disease, the precise reason for the fall in prevalence is not clear. Decay is of multifactorial origin, and its prevalence is influenced by dietary factors, oral hygiene, fluorides, and others as yet unknown. What can be said is that oral hygiene has generally improved, and that the use of fluoride-containing toothpastes has increased.

In the field of restorative dental surgery, there have been several relatively recent major advances. The first is concerned with the development of local anaesthesia. Modern vasoconstrictor-containing anaesthetic agents have been developed, which enable procedures to be carried out on teeth entirely free of pain. Furthermore, in a small minority of patients the anxiety of a procedure can be controlled by the use of intravenously administered drugs.

As recently as 40 years ago, students were taught conservative dental surgery using a treadle-powered drill to prepare cavities. However, they soon graduated to the electrically powered drill, to which were fitted steel burs which, after little use, became blunt, especially when being used to cut undiseased enamel. This problem was overcome to a large extent by the arrival of the tungsten carbide bur in the early 1950s. In the 1960s came the airturbine drill, which was virtually vibration-free and extremely fast. Indeed, compared with previous powered rotary instruments, the airturbine was likened to 'cutting butter with a hot knife'. The disadvantages of the airturbine were the irritating high frequency noise which it generated and the intense heat generated at the cutting site. The high-frequency noise has been reduced somewhat, and the heat generated is controlled by the use of a water spray built into the handpiece. Adequate illumination has always been a problem in cavity preparation, but recently airturbine handpieces have been fitted with an in-built fibre-optic light, which bathes the operating site with an intense localized light.

There have been important advances in materials used in the conservation of teeth. The traditional filling materials have been much improved; the gold materials have been alloyed to provide greater dimensional stability and easier handling, and the silver–tin alloys have been modified to provide quicker setting times, greater strength, and easier handling. New non-metallic materials of the same colour as natural teeth are now available, but their durability would seem to fall considerably below that of the older metallic materials.

Perhaps the most important advance has been the philosophical change in the approach to cavity preparation. Hitherto, with almost sacramental dogma, cavities were prepared following principles enunciated by G. V. Black at the beginning of the century; implicitly these principles involved the considerable loss of valuable sound tooth tissue in order to prevent recurrence of disease. This 'extension for prevention' policy has now largely been abandoned and, as a result, cavities are smaller, teeth become less likely to fracture, and fillings are kept well clear of gum margins, thus contributing to the prevention of periodontal disease.

Another important advance has been the development of endodontics, which is concerned with the treatment of diseased root canal and pulp chamber tissues.

Improved materials and instruments, and development of clinical and technical skills, together with a greater understanding of the biology of the root canal and associated structures, encourage the not unreasonable statement that 'no tooth need be extracted'.

There have been equally important advances in prosthetic dentistry, not only in the field of materials science, which includes use of the new metallic alloys and plastic denture materials, but, even more importantly, there has developed a much greater understanding of the physiological principles of mastication and orofacial muscular activity. These advances have exerted a profound effect on the design of *dentures, especially partial dentures which are supported by remaining teeth rather than soft tissues, with minimal, if any, hazard to the teeth themselves or supporting tissues.

Orthodontic practice has been greatly influenced by the increased understanding of the growth patterns of the facial skeleton. This work has been dependent largely on computer analysis of considerable volumes of radiographically derived numerical data. Use of fixed appliances has become more widespread as a result of the availability of new highly adhesive materials. The scope of orthodontic care has been greatly increased and its results can be predicted with accuracy.

In the UK, dentistry has evolved in very close relationship with medicine and enjoys equal status as a sister profession. This relationship is particularly strong in the specialties of oral medicine and surgery, in which most, but by no means all, practitioners are qualified in both dentistry and medicine. Both subjects are regarded as mainly 'postgraduate' and owe their development to the explosion in understanding of *virology, *immunology, *microbiology, and *pharmacology. Many of the soft-tissue diseases of the mouth, hitherto treated by purely empirical procedures, can now be tackled rationally and with prospects of success. Oral surgeons now venture far beyond the removal of unerupted wisdom teeth, enucleation of cysts, and the dental aspects of the management of *fractures of the facial skeleton. They now undertake full care of patients with *malignant disease, correction of congenital and hereditary facial defects, and repair of disfigurement following *trauma. They work in close collaboration with the oncologist, the plastic surgeon, and anaesthetist. A very interesting new development in the field of oral surgery is implantology, made possible by the availability of biologically inert materials such as titanium. This technique provides a means of replacing individual teeth or groups of teeth permanently, and of providing dentures which are retained by implanted supports and thus are not dependent on the traditional retention forces of cohesion and adhesion.

Postgraduate education and research

Since the end of the Second World War there has been a major growth of postgraduate education in the UK, a vitally necessary activity in view of the pace of advance of dental practice. Gone is the old attitude that once qualified there is nothing further to learn. Indeed, dental schools now teach that graduation is merely a stage in the learning process.

Many practitioners keep up to date by attending courses organized by the British Dental Association and the learned societies, such as the *Royal Society of Medicine and the Odonto-Chirurgical Society of Edinburgh. However, a major advance has been the establishment of postgraduate qualifications at the universities and Royal Colleges. General practitioners have a wide range of available, clinically based courses, either part- or full-time, leading to an M.Sc. degree. Others are attracted to the Membership in General Dental Practice of the Royal College of Surgeons of England. As further encouragement, that College has just established a separate faculty for general practitioners.

Those planning a career in the hospital service, or an academic post in clinical dentistry, need to obtain a Fellowship in Dental Surgery of one of the Royal Colleges of Surgeons. This diploma ranks as equivalent to the FRCS and has a pass rate of about 30 per cent. Originally the fellowship was directed towards oral surgery, but its scope has been extended to encompass a wide variety of clinical subjects.

Orthodontics with oral surgery was recognized as a specialty in the NHS from its outset in 1948. The early consultants were appointed on the basis of long and wide experience, but it was necessary to provide a recognized career structure, including specialist training and appropriate qualifications. The Diploma in Orthodontics was established by the Royal College of Surgeons of England in 1953, and in 1988 this became the Membership in Orthodontics. This diploma had been preceded some years previously by the Diploma in Dental Orthopaedics of the Royal Faculty of Physicians and Surgeons of Glasgow (later to become the Royal College of Physicians and Surgeons). Orthodontists aspiring to consultant status usually additionally obtain the FDS diploma.

Other postgraduate clinical qualifications include the Diploma in Restorative Dentistry of the Royal College of Surgeons of Edinburgh, and the Diploma in Public Health of the English Royal College. The University of Birmingham offers a mastership in Community Dental Health and that of Dundee, a Diploma in Public Dentistry.

There is a great demand for *postgraduate education, especially amongst younger practitioners, indicating a clear need for courses of all kinds. This need and desire will, to some extent, be met when the Edinburgh School assumes fully its new role as the Postgraduate Institute for Scotland.

In the UK, dental research has been carried out since the 18th century. The early work was deductive and based upon meticulous observation, painstaking recording, and imaginative observation. Such workers included John Hunter; Sir John Tomes and his son,

Charles; J. Kilian Clarke, who identified the role of *Streptococcus mutans* in the initiation of the caries process; Warwick James; and E. W. Fish. During the 1930s research methods became more experimental in nature, with R. V. Bradlaw's classical work on the innervation of dentine, Arthur Bullied's and J. D. King's studies on the *bacteriology of periodontal disease, and May Mellanby's studies on the relationship between *nutrition and *caries. The years after the Second World War saw a tremendous surge forward in dental research, which resulted from the creation of full-time academic posts, the training in research methods which Nuffield fellowships and scholarships ensured, and the attraction to dental academia of a number of non-dentally qualified basic scientists.

This forward thrust was part of an international escalation of activity, in which the International Association for Dental Research has played a vital co-ordinating role. The British division of this federal organization is the senior non-American division; it was formed in 1931 with six members and now has a membership of some 700.

Apart from research carried out in the university dental schools, important work was conducted in the Department of Dental Science of the Royal College of Surgeons and the *Medical Research Council Dental unit at Bristol. Sadly, recent financial constraints have seriously jeopardized the future stability of these units.

The need for research on commercially produced dental health products has led to the development of closer working relationships between academic departments and industrial companies. An example of such a collaboration is the development and clinical testing of the fluoride-containing dentifrices.

Despite the financial restrictions, dental research in the UK, as in the USA and elsewhere, is flourishing and there is every sign that this will continue.

Career prospects

The young dental graduate, on qualification, has a considerable choice in the kind of career he can follow. The majority, of course, take up NHS general practice, although an increasing number do carry out part of their work under private contract. A number of practitioners, especially in London, the major cities, and in the south-east of England confine their practice entirely to private work. Indeed, some have chosen to restrict their practice to a particular specialization, orthodontics and periodontics being notable examples.

Careers in hospital dentistry have been mentioned above, but in addition to obtaining the appropriate qualifications, it is necessary to climb the 'hospital ladder', beginning as a house officer and progressing through the training grades over an 8 year minimum period to reach the career post status of consultant. At present there are three consultant specialties, namely oral surgery, orthodontics, and restorative dentistry.

University teaching attracts a number of graduates,

especially those with an interest in scientific matters. Some enter preclinical departments and make invaluable contributions, both as teachers and as research workers in anatomy, physiology, and biochemistry in relation to dentistry. Others become clinical teachers, who not only need to obtain research degrees but the clinical qualifications comparable with those of the hospital consultant. Indeed, the *pons asinorum* of academic dentistry is obtaining an honorary consultant contract.

Another avenue followed by graduates is that of community service, which over the past 40 years has been transformed from the 'Cinderella' of dentistry to a vibrant and thriving branch of practice with its own career structure.

Finally, each year the Royal Navy, the Army, and the Royal Air Force recruit a number of young dental graduates who undertake, in the first instance, to serve for a period of 5 years. A number of these are selected for permanent, full-career commissions.

The years after the Second World War have seen the development of the 'dental team', which comprises dental nurses, *hygienists, *technicians, and practice administrators. This development has involved training programmes for nurses and hygienists, leading to recognized professional qualifications. Courses for hygienists are held at many of the dental schools and last for 1 year; nurses may also attend courses at dental schools, but they are also available at colleges of further education in many of the cities and towns throughout the country. Technicians may also be trained at the dental schools, but many enter training as apprentices in a practice and attend day-release courses at colleges of further education.

Dentistry in the USA

There can be no doubt that dentistry has developed along very similar lines in the UK and the USA. The courses at the dental schools are almost identical, although the US student is, on average, 3 or 4 years older than his UK colleague, as often he or she will have obtained a science degree before entering the dental course.

The history of dentistry in the USA and the UK has many common features, in that the early US practitioners were barber-surgeons and itinerant operators who advertised their forthcoming visits to the cities and towns and their willingness to attend to dental problems. Both countries had medical practitioners with some training in dental matters, who operated in the larger population centres in their permanent practices.

The first dental school was chartered in the USA in 1840, when the Baltimore College of Dentistry was established with an initial programme leading to the DDS degree. As this college was not part of a university, it was not until 1867, when the Harvard School of Dentistry was established, that university status was given to dentistry. The first state university to have a dental school was the University of Michigan, which

from the outset prescribed academic admission requirements. Additional schools began to appear, and by 1884 there were 21, some of which had very short histories whereas others subsequently became world-renowned centres of excellence. By 1983 there were 60 schools accredited by the Commission of Dental Accreditation of the American Dental Association. Since that year a number have closed, basically for fiscal reasons.

Whereas the UK dental graduate is required simply to register his qualification with the General Dental Council, who will issue a licence to practise, the US graduate has to present himself for a further State Board Examination, which he is required to pass before he can practise in a particular state. In this way the number of dentists working in any state can be controlled. This is especially relevant in the more attractive states, such as Florida and California. Moves are being made to establish a form of national dental licensing, and it can reasonably be expected that such a system will be in operation within the next decade.

In the US, specialist practice has been carried out for many years, and presently there are eight recognized specialties. These are oral pathology, endodontics, periodontology, oral surgery, othodontics, public health dentistry, paedodontics, and advanced general practice. To carry out such specialist practice the dentist is required to undergo 2–4 years of theoretical and clinical training at an approved institution, pass the prescribed examination, and be certified by the appropriate specialist board.

At the present time there are in the US about 125 000 practising dentists, most of whom are in general practice, with some 16 000 in specialist practice.

US practitioners appreciated the value of dental hygienists decades before their colleagues in the UK. Indeed, by the early 1920s hygienist training had been established in New York City, Boston, and Rochester, NY. By 1980 the Commission on Dental Accreditation had recognized 200 hygienist training programmes, which were producing in excess of 5000 new hygienists per year. As in the UK, there is a considerable annual wastage of hygienists, who give up work for family and other reasons.

Research in the US has developed along lines very similar to that in the UK, although on a much larger scale. The establishment in 1921 of the International Association for Dental Research (IADR), a US initiative, has had a profound world influence. From the very outset, the founders of the association visualized the development of a federation of nationally based divisions and sections throughout the world. The British division was established in 1931; it was followed in 1934 by the Johannesburg Section. However, the major expansion of the Association occurred after the Second World War and today IADR members are to be found in some 80 countries. International meetings are held annually, every third one being held outside the North American continent. At the 1992 meeting held in

Glasgow there were some 3500 registrants and almost 2000 research presentations. The IADR publishes the *Journal of Dental Research*, which each year publishes about 150 papers plus the abstracts of communications given at the annual international meeting and the division and section meetings. Thus, by means of its scientific meetings at national and international levels, and its publication of papers and abstracts, the IADR is fulfilling a most valuable role in the co-ordination of research and in the dissemination of new knowledge.

It would be impossible to describe the many important research advances made in the many centres of excellence in the USA. However, the contribution made to the prevention of dental decay by means of fluorides must be mentioned. Studies leading to our present fund of knowledge and understanding have continued relentlessly for almost a century, beginning with the simple but far-reaching observations of Dr Fredrick McKay, a newly qualified dentist, practising in Colorado Springs; through the epidemiological work of H. Trendley Dean in the 1930s, and the first community fluoridation studies in the Middle West by F.A. Arnold; to the more recent work on the mode of action of fluorides and the topical delivery of fluoride by means of dentifrices.

The bulk of this work was funded by the US Government through the National Institute of Dental Research and the five regional institutes; the dental schools, notably the Forsyth Dental Center in Boston and the Eastman Dental Center in Rochester, NY; and by the oral health-care industry.

Conclusions

The past century and a half has seen dentistry change from a trade to a profession, and the past 50 years have seen that profession undergo even further far-reaching changes. New materials have been introduced, new instruments and new operative techniques have evolved, pain during treatment can now be almost completely eliminated, and gum diseases are largely treatable. The most important change, however, is the change in attitude of the public towards dental health. There is now an overwhelming desire to retain the natural dentition for life, a state that can now be accepted as a practical possibility.

What will happen during the next 50 years is by no means predictable, but there can be no doubt that patterns of practice will change as new techniques and new materials emerge. What can be forecast with confidence is that dentistry will remain an exciting, interesting, and satisfying profession, which will continue to attract to its ranks young men and women of high intelligence and practical skills.

M. N. NAYLOR

DENTISTS ACT 1957. This enactment consolidated earlier UK legislation relating to dentists and other dental workers. The main provisions dealt with the constitution and duties of the General Dental Council and the following matters: education; examinations; qualification for registration; registration of Commonwealth and foreign practitioners; use by registered dentists of titles and descriptions; the dentists' register and procedure for registration; disciplinary procedures; exemption from jury service and other duties; and restrictions on carrying on the practice and business of dentistry.

DENTITION. The *teeth considered as a set or complement, that is, their number, type, and arrangement; alternatively, the process of tooth development, growth, and extrusion.

DENYS, JEAN BAPTISTE (?1640–1704). French physician. He became a member of a scientific group called the 'Montmort Academy' who interested themselves in the work of *Lower and others on blood transfusions. Denys, and another, were appointed to study the problem. In 1667 after experiments with dogs and calves he transfused 12 oz (340 g) of lamb's blood into a young man, who improved greatly. Later he had two fatalities, a Swedish traveller, Baron Bunde, and Antoine Mauroy, who was deranged. Denys was accused by Mauroy's wife of murder, although it is possible that she poisoned her husband. In 1668 he was cleared of this charge but the court forbade further transfusions unless sanctioned by the Faculty of Medicine.

DEOXYRIBONUCLEIC ACID is usually abbreviated to DNA. Its structure (see Fig. 1) was elucidated, using X-ray diffraction, by M. H. F. Wilkins, F. H. C. Crick, and J. D. Watson in 1953, a discovery for which they later received the *Nobel prize. It is composed of linear molecules found in *chromosomes and some *viruses, consisting of two interwound helical chains of polynucleotides (a nucleotide consists of a pentose sugar, a phosphate group, and a nitrogenous base derived from either *purine or *pyrimidine). In DNA the sugar of each nucleotide is 2-deoxy-D-ribose and the base is one of the following four: adenine, cytosine, guanine, or thymine (cf. *ribonucleic acid (RNA), in which uracil replaces thymine). The order of the bases determines the *genetic code, each sequence (triplet) of three bases coding for one *amino acid. Complementary base pairs (i.e. the bases opposite each other on the two helical chains) are linked by hydrogen bonds. DNA carries genetic information for all organisms except the RNA viruses. Each of the 46 chromosomes in human body cells consists of two strands of DNA, containing up to 100 000 nucleotides. Along each strand, about 1500 bases, on average, form a *gene. See also BIOCHEMISTRY; CELL AND CELL BIOLOGY; GENETICS.

DEPARTMENT OF HEALTH AND SOCIAL SECURITY (DHSS). The department of UK government which was formerly responsible for health and the social

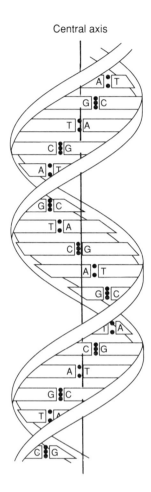

Central axis

Fig. 1 The structure of DNA. The diagram is a model of the Watson–Crick DNA double helix. The two bands represent sugar–phosphate backbones of the two strands, which run in opposite directions. The vertical line represents the central axis round which the strands wind. The position of four nucleotide bases, C, A, T, and G, is shown, together with the hydrogen bonds (●) which link them together. (From Weatherall, D. J. (1985). *The new genetics and clinical practice*, (2nd edn). Oxford University Press.)

services in England, succeeding the former *Ministry of Health. The DHSS effectively formed the top tier of the *National Health Service structure in England and operated as a civil service department with its own internal medical and other professional staff. In 1991 it was divided into two departments, of Health and Social Security. The Department of Health, headed by a Secretary of State, is responsible for overall policy-making, planning, and financial control within the health service, and is directly accountable to Parliament. The health services for Scotland, Wales, and Northern Ireland are operated independently under the authority of their separate Secretaries of State. With the DH, the departments concerned are jointly known as the Health Departments. See also GOVERNMENT AND MEDICINE IN THE UK; NATIONAL HEALTH SERVICE.

DEPARTMENTS OF MEDICAL ILLUSTRATION within medical schools or hospitals specialize in the photography of clinical, anatomical, and pathological problems,and in the preparation of other visual material for texts, lectures, etc. See also ILLUSTRATION AND PHOTOGRAPHY IN MEDICINE.

DEPERSONALIZATION is an abnormal mental state characterized by a subjective loss of identity; the patient seems to himself to be remote from his own body and not responsible for its words and actions. It occurs in various mental illnesses, but may also be experienced by normal subjects under certain conditions; for example, prolonged sleep deprivation. The term was introduced by Dugas in 1898.

DEPILATORY. Any preparation or procedure for removing hair.

DEPOLARIZATION. Living cells carry a positive charge on their surface because of unequal ionic concentrations on either side of the cell membrane, and are thus said to be polarized. In tissues capable of being stimulated or excited, like *nerve and *muscle, the polarity is temporarily lost during excitation, as positively charged sodium ions flood into the cell. This loss or reversal of polarity is termed depolarization. Persistent depolarization occurs if cell metabolism is compromised, for example by injury or *anoxia.

DEPOSIT. Any accumulation of solid material in a particular location.

DEPRESSION is abnormal lowering of mood manifest as sadness, melancholy, and dejection, often accompanied by *psychomotor retardation and depression of many other functions such as appetite, *libido, ability to sleep normally, and so on. Although the manifestations resemble those of *grief, endogenous depressive illness by definition, unlike reactive depression, has no obvious external cause. See also CYCLOTHYMIA; MANIC-DEPRESSIVE PSYCHOSIS; PSYCHIATRY.

DERMATITIS is any skin condition involving inflammation; when unqualified, it is a non-specific term covering a variety of skin disorders. See also DERMATOLOGY.

DERMATOGLYPHICS. See FINGERPRINT.

DERMATOGRAPHIA is the eliciting of a *weal when the skin is firmly stroked with a blunt instrument (also known as dermographism). It is a form of *urticaria, but can be demonstrated in a small minority of otherwise normal subjects.

DERMATOLOGIST. A physician who specializes in skin diseases. See DERMATOLOGY.

DERMATOLOGY comprises all that is known about skin, in health and in disease. It is a vast field of knowledge since the skin around us is the one organ on which each of us makes daily observations. Whether it be the infant bemused by his rosy fingers, the adolescent bewitched by *acne, or the aged bemoaning the loss of hair, everyone has an interest in the skin. For here is a canvas on which portraits appear, not only of ageing but also of the spectre of disease.

For centuries the skin was observed for signs of *smallpox, *syphilis, *leprosy, and *pellagra. Despite their unparalleled opportunity to observe these external diseases, physicians, surgeons, philosophers, and charlatans had little to offer in the way of understanding or treatment. But, it was from the ever-branching paths of specialization that knowledge was to come. Robert *Willan in England (1757–1812) was the first to publish and classify the portraits of skin disease. Further systemization came from Jean Louis *Alibert (1768–1837) in Paris, as he taught his disciples to view each dermatosis as a specific branch off a dermatological tree. The third great centre was in Vienna, where Ferdinand von *Hebra (1816–1880) represented the full flowering of the new discipline of dermatology.

Description and classification represented the major achievement of this fledgling specialty, and today over 8000 specific skin diseases are identifiable. Yet, during the 19th century some causes of these diseases were discovered. In 1831, David Gruby was the first to show that *fungi can cause disease, and, in 1834, François Renucci demonstrated that *scabies was due to a mite, medically confirming what the poor people of Paris had known in the 16th century when they picked these barely visible mites from their burrows in the outer skin. More insight was provided by the brave volunteers for experimental induction of disease, such as smallpox. Likewise, allergic contact dermatitis and drug eruptions made their entry on to the stage of diseases with a known aetiology.

Not until the *microscope and the *biopsy, i.e. a surgical sample, were commonly employed did knowledge make a quantum leap. Then the *pathologist could see the skin in all its structural and cellular detail, and study the derangements. At the same time, the new science of *bacteriology provided understanding of infectious disease, such as *impetigo and *boils. By 1906 the *spirochaete had been spotted as the cause of syphilis, and in 1910 the magic bullet of Ehrlich had been found on the 606th trial of arsenical antimicrobial compounds. Dermatology continued to grow in wisdom as each new basic science was brought to bear on its mysteries. Thus, it was a great advance forward when, in 1914, Joseph *Goldberger showed pellagra to be due to a simple nutritional deficiency. However, the missing vitamin, nicotinic acid, was not isolated until the 1930s.

Today, *biochemistry, *pharmacology, *cell *physiology, *immunology, *genetics, *electron microscopy, *internal medicine, and *molecular biology have each brought great treasures of knowledge to dermatology, in both diagnosis and therapy. We no longer look on the skin as a mere covering sheath. It is a dynamic organ, shimmering with countless biochemical syntheses and intercellular messages.

The invisible part of this most visible organ, skin, has become visible to the eye of the microscopist with his stains, his *immunofluorescence, his electron beams. It has become visible to the biochemist and molecular biologist with their *DNA probes, their PCR (*polymerase chain reactions), and their *chromosomal spreads, and it has become visible to the biologist with its intercellular messengers and mediators of inflammation (*cytokines) all performing in his tissue culture of skin cells.

With all of this, the diagnostic grasp of skin disease has grown. Whereas Willan in 1800 could cite but a few constellations of disease, the modern dermatologist can cite thousands. Not only does he have the landmarks of morphology, the insight of an informed history, but he also has the wealth of laboratory data. The blood may tell of hair loss due to *anaemia, of phrynoderma due to vitamin A deficiency, or of *ulcers due to lack of zinc. The urine may point to the hand eruption due to *porphyria cutanea tarda or of the flushing from a carcinoid tumour. The X-ray may disclose the lung *cancer responsible for *dermatomyositis or the foreign body responsible for pain. The *CT scan may disclose the pancreatic tumour responsible for necrolytic migratory *erythema.

Nor are the other laboratory areas lacking in diagnostic prowess. The microbiologist may discern the precise cause of a dystrophic nail to be *Trichophyton rubrum*. Or a culture of a biopsy specimen may disclose the skin disease to be sporotrichosis, or even an atypical mycobacterial infection from a swimming-pool abrasion. The viral culture can make the diagnosis of a type 1 or type 2 *herpes simplex. But the most important diagnostic tool remains the biopsy, i.e. excision of a tiny representative sample of the diseased skin. Here the pathologist can see a cellular basis for diagnosis. He sees the cell separation of *pemphigus, the cellular infiltrates of metabolic disease, and, most importantly, the uncontrolled cell growth of malignancy, such as the *T-cell *lymphomas. His tools include immunofluorescence for *antibodies, specific stains for chemicals, and electron microscopy for *viruses.

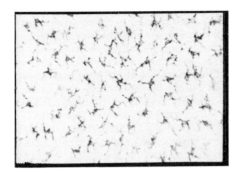

Fig. 1 Langerhans cells (surface view of these cells in the upper epidermis). They form the outermost immune defense system of the skin against contact allergens, such as poison ivy, primrose, and nickel.

The diagnostic grasp is further strengthened by challenge of the patient. Such challenge may range from environmental inhalants to foods, from toothpaste to drugs. Or the challenge may be local, i.e. exposure of an area of skin to a chemical from work or a hobby which may be causing an allergic *dermatitis. Supplementary diagnostic insight may be provided by actual injection of material into the skin, such as *tuberculin, hormones, or other chemicals.

Likewise, exposing patches of skin to sunlight or *ultraviolet light is of great value in diagnosing *photosensitivity. Such tests include the prior application of possible photosensitizing chemicals.

Nor has therapy of skin disease lagged. From the early conquest of smallpox by *vaccination we have come to see syphilis almost eradicated by *penicillin, leprosy subdued by dapsone, and cancer of the skin totally excised by Mohs' surgery. We have witnessed lymphomas of the skin, such as Alibert's dreaded *mycosis fungoides, treated with topical nitrogen mustard and systemic chemotherapy. Precancerous lesions in the form of sunlight-induced actinic keratosis are now destroyed by the simple application of 5-fluorouracil cream for a few weeks.

Relief is brought to photosensitive patients with antimalarial drugs (*chloroquine) and to the poison-ivy sufferer with *cortisone derivatives, both topically and systemically. Indeed, the discovery in 1950 of the universal anti-inflammatory action of cortisone has been of benefit to countless millions with dermatitis of all kinds.

Pharmaceutical research has accomplished much more for dermatological therapy. By combing 1500 derivatives of vitamin A, one (isotretinoin) was found to be dramatically effective in treating the scarring type of cystic acne. It acts, to a large degree, by suppressing *sebum formation. An analogue, retinoic acid, is similarly helpful in the topical treatment of comedone acne. Much excitement was created when it was discovered serendipitously that its long-term topical use can also erase wrinkles in many cases. Most recently, an ointment

containing an analogue of the sunlight vitamin (D_3, calcipotriol) has proved effective in treating *psoriasis, long known to respond to ultraviolet light. It is truly sunlight in a salve. And the usefulness of ultraviolet light therapy has now been extended to the treatment of certain skin conditions by simply irradiating the patient's blood flowing through a bypass outside the body.

Perhaps the greatest boon to dermatology has been the parade of antimicrobial agents for bacterial disease, beginning in 1937 with sulphanilamide and proceeding through penicillin and *tetracycline to the modern wide-spectrum compounds such as erythromycin, cephalosporins, and quinolones. Even greater fire power is provided by the *antibiotics that have to be given intravenously.

The skin diseases due to fungi felt the first blow when oral griseofulvin was introduced in 1959. This was followed by ketoconazole, which provided killing power for fungi, including yeast. *Thrush, *candidiasis, and *paronychia became diminished fears, as did the yeast-driven seborrhoeic dermatitis. Even in a shampoo, ketoconazole has given real relief to those suffering from dandruff. More recently, three additional oral compounds, fluconazole, itraconazole, and terbinafine, have been introduced. Fungal infections of the toe-nail (Fig. 2), present for a lifetime, have disappeared under their influence.

In the field of antiviral agents, *acyclovir is a wonder drug specifically engineered and synthesized to inhibit the herpes simplex virus responsible for cold sores (herpes simplex). In high dosage it is also effective against shingles (*herpes zoster) (Fig. 3) caused by the varicella (*chickenpox) virus. All should be aware of the need for immediate oral treatment to avert years of postherpetic pain in the older patient. It is understandably

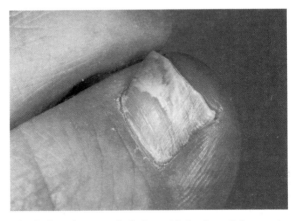

Fig. 2 Onychomycosis (a fungal infection of the great toe-nail). Clearing of the proximal plate was achieved by oral fluconazole for 8 weeks.

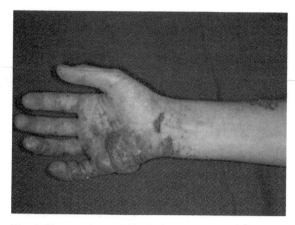

Fig. 3 Herpes zoster (shingles). Prompt treatment with oral acyclovir can prevent the chronic pain which otherwise accompanies this blistering eruption due to the virus of chickenpox.

an effective treatment also for *chickenpox, caused by the same virus as shingles.

Surgery for skin lesions has had its measure of advances in precision removal of just the lesion, in sophisticated plastic patterned excisions, and in Mohs' technique for histological tracking of the furthest reaches of skin cancer during the actual operation. Axillary *hyperhidrosis has been eliminated by excision of the affected skin. The newest surgical techniques include liposuction for skin contour control, and the

use of *lasers for treating a variety of skin growths as well as for removal of tattoos. Most remarkable has been the essentially scarless elimination of the superficial, yet disfiguring, *haemangioma, called *port wine stain.

Indeed, nowhere has there been greater impact of technology on clinical dermatology than in the field of the laser. Scarcely 30 years ago, the CO_2 laser was introduced as an optical-beam scalpel, permitting bloodless surgery. Today, the pulsed-dye laser, with its precision yellow beam of 585 nm wavelength, allows truly selective destruction of the fine blood vessels of vascular birthmarks (Fig. 4). With pulses of 450 msec, the thermal destruction is limited to the oxyhaemoglobin within the vessel, and scarring is avoided. Similarly, selective photothermolysis of another mode is used in destroying pigmented lesions such as moles, age spots, or tattoos. Here, lasers, such as the Q-switched ruby laser, are used, which emit a red light (694 nm) in ultrashort bursts of 40 nsec, targeting only the undesirable pigment. Before the remarkable specificity of the modern lasers, one could only excise or destroy the entire affected area of skin, with subsequent scarring.

Cutaneous *melanoma has become the most serious surgical problem of the skin. It has increased in the USA almost threefold in the last four decades. A major risk factor is ultraviolet radiation, but others include easily sunburned skin, a family history of melanomas, and the presence of melanoma precursors, i.e. dysplastic and congenital *naevi (Fig. 5). The public must be aware of these and monitor their skin for early detection of melanomas. Early detection and removal lead to high cure rates, whereas metastatic disease is virtually incurable. Australia, a land of sunshine and melanomas, has taken the lead in educating the public as to the need for sun-protective creams and clothing, surveillance, and surgery of suspects. Only in this way can cancer of the

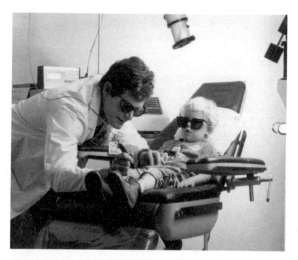

Fig. 4 Laser therapy. Selective elimination of vascular birthmarks and tattoos can be achieved with tunable dye laser therapy and Q-switched ruby lasers therapy, respectively. (Photograph courtesy of University of Massachusetts Medical Center.)

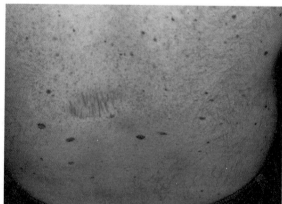

Fig. 5 Dysplastic naevi (moles). These multiple, irregular moles are a family trait which predispose to the development of malignant melanoma, cured in this patient by prompt excision (note the scar).

skin and the fatal malignant melanomas be averted. Such behaviour also affords the cosmetic benefit of reduction in the wrinkles of photoageing.

Just as syphilis was best recognized by dermatologists aware of the *chancre and the secondary syphilitic rash, today the HIV immunodeficiency disease, *AIDS, may make its first appearance on the canvas of the skin, and thereby be recognized by skin specialists. It may appear as an innocent red spot, a whitening of the sides of the tongue, or a dismayingly severe display of warts (*verrucas), *molluscum contagiosum, or bacterial infection.

A similar display of recalcitrant viral, bacterial, and yeast infections of the skin is seen in patients with transplanted organs. Thus, 77 per cent of renal *transplant patients develop warts; these and the swarm of other infections result from the patient's general immunity having been intentionally suppressed by drugs to prevent organ rejection. Seeing these patients, as well as the rare individual born with an immune deficiency, makes one aware that cutaneous health bespeaks the continuous presence of an effective cellular and humoral immunity of white cells and cytokines.

With the growing awareness of AIDS has come greater interest in the other sexually transmitted diseases. Pride of place goes to syphilis, transmitted by the spirochaete. Even more common are the contagious viral diseases, herpes simplex, warts, and molluscum contagiosum. Genital wart infections are of major concern because of their frequency, and because certain types are associated with genital and cervical carcinoma. Although warts do not greatly differ in clinical appearance, at least 66 different types of the human papillomavirus have been isolated from warts. This typing, based on DNA hybridization techniques, reveals that type 16 is associated with squamous cell *carcinoma. Type 16 and type 18, as well as an assortment of other specific wart virus types, are being found commonly in cervical neoplasia, but their role remains unclear.

The skin, at times, is a window to other internal disease. We may see the cutaneous metastasis of internal tumours, the flush of systemic *lupus erythematosus, the pyoderma gangrenosum of *ulcerative colitis. We can look for the seborrhoeic eruption of histiocytosis, the yellow nails of pulmonary disease, and the thickened skin of *systemic sclerosis. No less does the skin tell us of genetic disorders. From the abnormal fingerprints to the congenital ichthyoses, from the blisters of epidermolysis bullosa to the photosensitivity of xeroderma pigmentosum, one can sense the daunting gene disorders.

With greater knowledge of the nature of skin disease has come awareness that an identifiable disease does not necessarily bespeak a single cause. Hives (*urticaria) can have almost as many causes as there are patients suffering from them. Indeed, many skin diseases are morphologically unique and recognizable clinically such as erythema multiforme, lichen planus, or contact dermatitis. Yet, they are but reaction patterns asking for detective work to discern the cause in any given patient. To this end, a complete history of all that comes into or around the patient is essential. The focus is on drugs, 'bugs', and foods, any of which may be responsible for any of the patient's cutaneous disease. In addition, there should be a careful medical review, since some skin changes herald systemic disease such as *diabetes mellitus, renal disease, or cancer. The search is a serious one, since elimination of the cause may be the only cure.

Great as the advances of dermatology have been therapeutically, the future holds a continuing challenge. There is still no specific drug to combat *itch. There is no systemic antiviral drug to treat the common wart. Nor do we yet have a 'magic bullet' for psoriasis. Somewhere, in some laboratory, in some clinic, in some researcher's mind, the answers are to be found. We must continue to seek for them if we are to restore the beauty of that original masterpiece, human skin.

W. B. SHELLEY

Further reading

Champion, R. H., Burton, J. L., and Ebling, F. J. G. (ed.) (1992). *Rook/Wilkinson/Ebling textbook of dermatology*, (5th edn), 4 Vols. Blackwell Scientific Publications, London.

DuVivier, A. (1993). *Atlas of clinical dermatology*, 2nd edn. W. B. Saunders, Philadelphia.

Parish, L. C. and Lask, G. P. (ed.) (1991). *Aesthetic dermatology*. McGraw-Hill, New York.

Schoen, L. A. and Lazar, P. (1990). *The look you like: medical answers to 400 questions on skin and hair care*. Marcel Dekker, New York.

Shelley, W. B. and Shelley, E. D. (1992). *Advanced dermatologic diagnosis*. W. B. Saunders, Philadelphia.

DERMATOME. The segment of skin supplied with sensory fibres by a specified spinal *nerve.

DERMATOMYOSITIS is an *autoimmune disorder, which is usually grouped with the *connective tissue disorders, in which there is inflammation and weakness of *muscles, particularly those of the limb girdles, combined with a rash. When a similar condition occurs without skin changes, the condition is called *polymyositis. Some patients prove to be suffering from an underlying malignant *neoplasm, the commonest being *carcinoma of the breast or lung. No cause can be found in the remainder, but it is now clear that humoral and T-cell-mediated immunity are involved in the pathogenesis. The condition is serious, with an overall mortality rate which was in the past up to 50 per cent, but corticosteroid and immunosuppressive drugs are effective in treatment and, in patients who survive, recovery may be complete. See also NEUROMUSCULAR DISEASE.

DERMATOSIS is a general term for any disorder affecting the *skin.

DERMIS is the corium or 'true skin'. See SKIN.

DERMOID is an abbreviation of dermoid *cyst, a cystic growth derived from displaced elements of *ectoderm, containing *keratin and hair and occasionally other ectodermal structures such as teeth and nerve tissue. It may occur anywhere, especially in the *ovary. It is not usually malignant.

DESCARTES, RENE (1596–1650). French philosopher. Descartes's book *De homine* (posthumous, 1664) is described as the first textbook of physiology. He took a mechanistic view of the human body which was, he held, controlled by the mind acting through the *pineal. His book was written from a theoretical standpoint but he postulated the *reflex arc, nervous co-ordination of muscular action, and changes in the form of the *lens on ocular accommodation.

DESENSITIZATION is the treatment of *allergy by injecting gradually increasing amounts of the responsible allergen.

DESQUAMATION is shedding of the outer layer of the *skin, as in 'peeling'.

DETECTION, in *genetics, is diagnosis of the clinically inapparent heterozygous carrier state in *recessive disorders; it is also diagnosis of other subclinical or preclinical disease by *screening.

DETERMINISM is the doctrine that all phenomena and events result from antecedent causes and can therefore never be said to occur by chance. Applied to human motivation, this philosophy denies the concept of free will.

DETOXIFICATION is the elimination of poison from the body, or its neutralization. It is applied also to the supervised withdrawal of drugs or alcohol from an addict.

DEUTERANOMALY is a minor defect of *colour vision in which perception of green is weaker than normal ('green-weakness').

DEVENTER, HENDRIK VAN (1651–1724). Dutch obstetrician. He made influential contributions to his subject, particularly on the anatomy of the female *pelvis. He recognized *disproportion and suggested that the pelvic bones might separate during labour. He introduced a classification of variations in pelvic shape and size. One commonly used pelvic measurement, the oblique diameter of the pelvis (the distance between one sacroiliac joint and the contralateral iliopubic eminence) is sometimes known as Deventer's diameter. See also OBSTETRICS.

DEVONSHIRE COLIC is *colic due to *lead poisoning.

DEXAMPHETAMINE. See AMPHETAMINE.

DEXTRAN. See BLOOD SUBSTITUTES.

DEXTROCARDIA is a congenital anomaly in which the position of the heart is reversed, so that it lies on the right side of the chest; the abdominal viscera are usually also transposed, when the condition is known as situs inversus. Dextrocardia is obvious on physical examination of the chest, on radiography, or from the *electrocardiogram. If no other cardiac defects are present, it is completely innocent.

DEXTROSE. See GLUCOSE.

DIABETES INSIPIDUS is a disorder characterized by excessive excretion of water (polyuria), accompanied by great thirst (polydipsia), due to deficiency of the *antidiuretic hormone (ADH) normally secreted by the neurohypophysis of the *pituitary gland. In some patients the condition follows damage to the base of the brain by *trauma, *tumour, or other identifiable lesions such as *tuberculosis; a few cases are familial; and in the remainder no cause is obvious. The polyuria can be controlled by regular administration of ADH preparations, such as *vasopressin.

DIABETES MELLITUS is a common disorder which has been known since antiquity. A treatment was described in the Ebers papyrus, it was named *madhumea* (honey-urine disease) in India in the 6th century AD, and a graphic clinical description survives from Arateus of Cappadocia (AD 130–200), in which he states 'Diabetes is an awkward affection melting down the flesh and limbs into the urine . . . The patients never stop making water . . . Life is short and painful . . . They are affected with nausea, restlessness and a burning thirst and at no distant term they expire.'

Little further attention was paid until the 17th and 18th centuries, when various dietary therapies were propounded and it was established, first, that there was glucose in the urine, and then, through Matthew Dobson in 1771, that there was excess sugar in the blood. The possible role of the *pancreas was shown experimentally by von Mehring and Minkowski in the 1880s, and led to major efforts to extract the active principle, *insulin, which was finally achieved by *Banting and *Best in 1921.

It was obvious by this stage that diabetes existed in different degrees of severity, with younger people wasting away, with severe *hyperglycaemia and an accumulation of ketoacids (acetoacetate and 3-hydroxybutyrate) in the blood, and dying relatively rapidly in the pre-insulin era. In older people the disease was more benign, occurring often in overweight people, and controlled with sugar-free diets, although such individuals were more prone to infections and often had symptoms of thirst and polyuria. It was concluded that this was just a milder form of the disease but that the cause was the same, i.e. a deficiency of insulin due to damage to the β cells of the islets of Langerhans in the pancreas. However, in the 1970s, it was shown that the young-onset type was an *autoimmune disease associated with particular so-called *HLA types, specifically DR3 and DR4. In such patients, *antibodies to the pancreas, 'islet-cell antibodies', could be demonstrated in more than 80 per cent of caucasian patients at diagnosis. Most recently, antibodies to a specific enzyme, glutamic acid decarboxylase (GAD), have also been shown. This type became known as insulin-dependent diabetes mellitus (IDDM) and is marked by total or near-total lack of insulin. By contrast, the other type of diabetes was shown to be associated with lack of effectiveness of insulin, 'insulin resistance', with insulin present, but not enough to overcome the resistance. This is known as non-insulin-dependent diabetes mellitus (NIDDM).

Previously, diabetes was considered to be a disease of the developed world. IDDM is indeed predominantly a disorder of those of northern European origin (Europids) with a pronounced north–south gradient. Incidence figures approach 30 per 100 000 per year in northern Scandinavia, falling to less than 10 per 100 000 per year in southern Europe. Accurate data are sparse in the Third World, but estimates of 1 to 5 per 100 000 are probably reasonable. Figures are, however, rising. NIDDM by contrast is commoner, comprising 80–85 per cent of all diabetes, affecting 2–8 per cent of the adult population in developed nations, 1–2 per cent in the poorest countries of the Third World, but with an explosive increase in rapidly developing groups, e.g. 10–15 per cent in Mauritius, and more than 25 per cent in Nauru and some Amerindian groups. This increase is associated with ageing, obesity, physical inactivity, and urbanization, with some ethnic groups, e.g. those of Asian Indian origin, particularly susceptible. It is estimated that now there are between 100 and 200 million diabetic people world-wide.

Diabetes is a chronic disorder with major long-term sequelae. There is specific damage to small blood vessels of the eye (retinopathy), which can lead to blindness. Diabetes is one of the commonest causes of blindness in those under 65 years of age. There is also damage to kidneys (nephropathy) which can lead to *renal failure and the need for kidney *transplantation. The nervous system is also affected (*neuropathy) with diminished sensation in the feet a common manifestation. This can be associated with ulceration, *gangrene, and amputation. Blood vessel diseases (stroke, heart attacks, and peripheral vascular disease) are two to five times commoner in the diabetic than the non-diabetic population, and are the commonest cause of premature death in NIDDM. There is still much debate as to the precise cause of the specific complications, but there is accumulating evidence that the onset can be delayed or prevented by good control of blood glucose. This has less effect on large blood vessel disease, where attention to *cholesterol, other blood fats, and other risk factors may be more important.

Treatment of diabetes depends on the type and on the severity of the blood glucose disturbance. In the commoner NIDDM type, treatment by a change of diet is often sufficient. This requires avoidance of easily absorbed sugars and calorie restriction in the overweight. If this fails, then drugs can be used; sulphonylureas, which improve insulin secretion, or metformin, which decreases glucose production. Special foods are not needed: a 'healthy' diet which should be taken by the whole population is appropriate.

By contrast, IDDM patients are totally dependent upon insulin. This is given by subcutaneous injection, ideally once before each meal with a short-acting insulin, and at bedtime with an insulin which lasts overnight. Insulin was originally obtained from beef pancreas and subsequently from pigs. In the past 10 years, human insulin has been made by *genetic engineering and is now widely used.

The aims of treatment are to maintain day-to-day well-being, to keep blood glucose levels within near-normal limits, and to prevent or retard the development of the long-term complications. Patients measure their own blood (or, less ideally, urine) glucose and adjust their life-style and therapy accordingly. Unfortunately, giving insulin subcutaneously does not reproduce normality, and patients are at risk of *hypoglycaemia. Efforts to improve insulin delivery include the use of implanted pumps, and pancreas or pancreatic islet transplantation. So far none of these has gone beyond the experimental stage owing to technical problems. None the less, much can be achieved with sensible life-style modification and patient education directed at self-management.

K. G. M. M. ALBERTI

DIABETIC COMA. See DIABETES MELLITUS.

DIAGNOSIS is the basis of clinical practice: it is organized around the fact that most patients present to physicians with subjective complaints which are, for the most part, non-specific, appearing in the course of multiple disorders. *Diagnosis is the process of identifying the disease or other circumstances responsible for the patient's complaints, that is, his or her illness.*

Diagnosis is critical to *clinical practice because it allows categorization of clinical experience, recognition of patterns of presentation of various disorders, and orderly and sequential application of the clinical acts that follow, namely the application of management strategies and the formulation of prognoses.

The complexity of the diagnostic process derives from the extraordinarily varied modes of presentation of symptom-producing disorders, and is made more complex by the impact of the patient upon their expression. A variety of types of host resistance and psychosocial factors affect disease expressivity to a considerable degree, including, in fact, definition of what may be acceptably defined as illness in the culture from which the patient comes.

Diagnosis rests upon clinical observations of several types. The most time-honoured, and still the most productive, are the medical history and the *physical examination, in which clinical data are gathered from the patient at the time of the initial or subsequent encounters. Despite the extraordinary panoply of diagnostic technologies presently available, some 88 per cent of diagnoses in primary care have been demonstrated to be established by the end of a brief history and some portion of the physical examination (Crombie 1963; Sackett and Rennie 1992); in another study, 56 per cent of patients in a general medical *clinic had been assigned correct diagnoses by the end of the history-taking, and this figure rose to 73 per cent by the end of the physical examination (Sandler 1980). The accuracy and yield of these basic clinical procedures depend on the sophistication and meticulousness with which they are carried out. When they are done well, they are extraordinarily powerful, not only offering reliable diagnostic information, as noted above, but often providing reliable insights into the probable generic nature of the patient's disorder, the organ or organ system involved, the physiological derangements that have resulted, the pace of the process as well as its extent or degree, and a view of the urgency of the situation and its probable outcome.

The diagnostic process is, ultimately, an exercise in the reduction of uncertainty (Bolinger and Ahlers 1975). The clinician begins with maximal diagnostic uncertainty and, through a process of hypothesis generation and deductive reasoning, attempts to reduce this to a minimum. Absolute diagnostic certainty is rarely achievable although clinicians generally tend to pursue it as though it were, or, more importantly, as if it were needed in order to intervene effectively on behalf of the patient. Kassirer (1989) has noted the costs and patient risks incurred when physicians pursue diagnostic certainty with inordinate zeal through excessive and often redundant testing. In general, the closer one approaches certainty in diagnosis the less is the likelihood that the information provided by a given additional test will add substantively to the clinical process.

Fundamentally, diagnosis involves two basic procedures, namely collecting the facts and analysing them. The deployment of technological diagnostic procedures should be based upon preliminary diagnostic formulations, usually derived from the history and physical examination. Each test procedure should, in effect, be performed to answer a specific diagnostic question. Thus, the ordering of large numbers of laboratory examinations in an unselective approach is inefficient

and costly, not infrequently exposing the patient to unnecessary risks not only from the test procedures themselves, but from the misguided therapeutic interventions that may follow from the diagnostic impressions they produce. Furthermore, such test ordering patterns suborn the diagnostic process, and expose it to levels of inaccuracy that need not burden it.

Beyond these considerations, tests must be selected with due understanding of, and appreciation for, their functional characteristics (Sackett and Rennie 1992), namely sensitivity, specificity, and positive and negative predictive values.

In analysing the facts bearing on a diagnosis, a systematic approach is essential. In general, this involves assigning clinical weights, or orders of importance, to the various facts uncovered, and then assembling those that seem most likely to be relevant to the patient's disorder. After these have been assembled in groups or clinical patterns, the usual next step is the selection of a central feature or finding, or group of such features or findings, around which the diagnostic analysis can be oriented. The disorders that may cause these central features are next assembled and each candidate disorder is examined in terms of the specific features of the case at hand. In this way the most likely diagnosis, that is, the one that best explains the clinical features observed in the patient at hand, is selected.

Research in the diagnostic process has appeared increasingly in the clinical literature in recent years. Computer-based models have been constructed, clinical algorithms assembled, and the process of decision analysis introduced. The chief problems for the near future appear to revolve around the construction of a process which can, in a rational manner, incorporate new technological procedures and computer-based systems into an arrangement that retains and respects the diagnostic role of the clinician as well as the therapeutic potential of the physician's presence and advice.

JEREMIAH A. BARONDESS

References
Bolinger, R.E. and Ahlers, P. (1975). The science of "pattern recognition". *Journal of the American Medical Association,* **233**, 1289–90.
Crombie, D.L. (1963). Diagnostic process. *Journal of the College of General Practitioners,* **6**, 579–89.
Kassirer, J.P. (1989). Our stubborn quest for diagnostic certainty. *New England Journal of Medicine,* **320**, 1489–91.
Sackett, D.L. and Rennie, D. (1992). The science of the art of the clinical examination. *Journal of the American Medical Association,* **267**, 2650–2.
Sandler, G. (1980). The importance of the history in the medical clinic and the cost of unnecessary tests. *American Heart Journal,* **100**, 928–31.

DIALYSIS is the process of separating *colloids in solution from other dissolved substances (crystalloids) by selective diffusion through a semipermeable membrane. Such a membrane is slightly permeable to crystalloid molecules, which therefore diffuse through the membrane until their concentration is equal on the two sides; the larger molecules or groups of molecules in the colloidal state, on the other hand, will not. See also RENAL DIALYSIS

DIALYSIS DISEASE is a collective name for disorders arising during the treatment of chronic *renal failure by prolonged intermittent *renal dialysis, and is thought to be attributable to the method of treatment rather than to the primary kidney condition. These disorders include 'dialysis dementia', a serious encephalopathic syndrome due to excess *aluminium in the water supply; bone disease, due to disturbance of calcium metabolism; haemopoietic abnormalities; cardiovascular complications, including *hypertension; and psychiatric disorders.

DIAPEDESIS is the outward leakage of blood cells through vessel walls.

DIAPHORETIC describes agents or procedures that promote sweating.

DIAPHRAGM. The muscular partition separating the cavities of the thorax and abdomen; each half is called a hemidiaphragm. During inspiration the diaphragm contracts and descends; during expiration it relaxes and ascends. This term is also used to describe a contraceptive device used by the woman to prevent the entry of sperms into the uterus.

DIAPHYSIS. The main portion, or shaft, of a long bone. See also EPIPHYSIS.

DIARRHOEA (DIARRHEA) is an abnormal increase in the frequency and/or liquidity of the stools.

DIASTASIS is separation, particularly referring to bones normally adjacent to each other.

DIASTOLE is the rest period of the cardiac cycle, between cardiac contractions. During diastole, the two atrioventricular *valves (mitral and tricuspid) open and allow the *ventricles to fill with blood in preparation for the next contraction.

DIATHERMY is heating of tissues by passing through them a high-frequency electric current of high-frequency electromagnetic radiation ('short wave'). The technique can be employed to apply warmth to structures beneath the skin, like muscles and joints, or in surgery to cause heat coagulation and *necrosis by localized intense application.

DIATHESIS is a constitutional predisposition to develop a particular disease or group of diseases. Thus, 'allergic diathesis' means *atopy.

DIAZEPAM is one of the *benzodiazepine group of anxiolytic drugs ('minor *tranquillizers') widely known by one of its proprietary names, Valium.

DICHLORO-DIPHENYL-TRICHLORO-ETHANE ($C_{14}H_9Cl_5$), usually called DDT, is an effective insecticide once widely used to control insect-borne diseases; but its use is now banned in many countries because of its toxic effects and acquired insect resistance.

DICOUMAROL (DICOMAROL) is an oral *anticoagulant, now largely superseded in clinical practice by warfarin.

DIETARY REQUIREMENTS IN HEALTH. The healthy diet requires an energy content sufficient to meet energy expenditure (see CALORIE REQUIREMENTS IN HEALTH), together with at least minimal levels of *protein (including essential *amino acids), *vitamins, essential minerals (calcium, phosphorus, magnesium, iron, zinc, and iodine), essential *trace elements (copper, manganese, cobalt, fluorine, chromium, selenium, and molybdenum), *electrolytes (sodium, potassium, and chloride), and water. Minimum requirements vary with age, sex, size, physical activity, pregnancy, and lactation (see NUTRITION). In addition to the above, a small quantity of unsaturated fat is probably necessary for young children.

DIETETICS is that branch of the medical sciences concerned with the prescription and arrangement of diets. See also DIET IN TREATMENT.

DIET IN TREATMENT. Many medical conditions require therapeutic control of diet, the most obvious being *obesity, in which a reduced total energy intake is essential. Conversely, high energy diets are indicated where patients have become wasted as a result of *anorexia nervosa, *thyrotoxicosis, fever, gastrointestinal disorders, and many other causes. Other dietary restrictions commonly prescribed involve salt (fluid and water retention, e.g. in *heart failure or *hypertension), protein (liver failure; renal failure), saturated or animal fat (the various manifestations of *atherosclerosis), and carbohydrate (*diabetes mellitus). Restrictions may also be imposed by *allergies or *hypersensitivity (e.g. to *gluten in *coeliac disease) or by metabolic diseases (such as *gout and *phenylketonuria).

An equally long list could be made of conditions in which specific dietary supplements are required to compensate for previous deficiency or excessive loss of vitamins or other essential elements (e.g. vitamin C in *scurvy, thiamin in *beriberi and chronic *alcoholism, protein in protein-losing nephropathy).

Food–drug interactions, such as those that occur between *monoamine-oxidase inhibitors and certain foodstuffs, may also require dietary regulation. See also NUTRITION.

DIETITIAN. A health professional trained and qualified in *dietetics and skilled in the prescription and preparation of therapeutic diets. See also DIET IN TREATMENT; NUTRITION.

DIEULAFOY, GEORGES (1839–1911). French physician. He is remembered for his apparatus for aspirating *pleural effusions.

DIGESTION is the process by which the major food components—proteins, *fats, and complex *carbohydrates—are broken down into absorbable units. The process takes place principally in the small intestine, but begins in the mouth with mastication and salivation, and continues in the stomach with further mixing and the action of gastric juice, until digestion is completed in the small intestine by the pancreatic juice, *bile, and intestinal juice. The succession of *enzymes in these secretions results in an orderly chemical breakdown of food into *amino acids, *fatty acids, glycerol, and primary *sugars, which, along with minerals and vitamins are absorbed through the intestinal wall into the hepatic circulation.

DIGITALIS is the generic name for preparations of the leaf of the purple foxglove (*Digitalis purpurea*) and related plants, and for the active substances, *cardiac glycosides, which they contain. Digitalis is of great value in treating heart disease, particularly *heart failure and some cardiac *arrhythmias.

DIMERCAPROL is an alternative name for *British Anti-Lewisite.

DIOPTRE. Unit of refractive power of a lens. The power in dioptres is the reciprocal of the focal length of the lens in metres. Hence a lens of focal length 1 m has a power of 1 dioptre.

DIOSCORIDES (also known as Pedianos Dioscorides of Anazarbus) (*fl.* AD 50–70). Greek surgeon. Little is known of his life, although he was thought to have served as a medical officer in the Roman army. He compiled the first *herbal, in which he described 600 plants and 35 animal products. Although written in Greek it is usually known as *De materia medica*. It was regarded as authoritative for 1600 years and 90 of his drugs are still in use.

DIOXIN is a group of organic compounds (heterocyclic hydrocarbons) with possible *cancer-inducing and *teratogenic properties.

DIPHTHERIA is an acute and dangerous infectious disease, primarily of young children, affecting the nose, throat, and larynx and occasionally superficial wounds. The name derives from a characteristic grey necrotic false membrane which forms in these areas (*diphthera* was the skin of the goat on which Jove wrote the destiny of man), and which may produce symptoms and signs of obstruction.

The condition is due to the bacillus *Corynebacterium diphtheriae*, which produces a powerful *toxin. Although the infection remains local the toxin, carried in the circulation, may affect the heart, causing *myocarditis and *heart failure, and the peripheral nervous system, causing *polyneuropathy with variable paralysis, which may involve respiratory muscles and cause respiratory failure.

The incidence of the disease has been greatly reduced since the mid-1950s by prophylactic active *immunization; this is now normally carried out in the first year of life with diphtheria toxoid (modified toxin) combined in a triple vaccine with *tetanus and *pertussis vaccines. Treatment of the disease, now rare, is urgent. It includes *antitoxin administration, *penicillin, and sometimes *tracheostomy.

DIPHYLLOBOTHRIUM LATUM is the fish *tapeworm, the fully grown adult of which is the largest (up to 10 m) tapeworm known to infest man. It is acquired by eating inadequately cooked freshwater fish (including salmon, pike, and perch), particularly from the smaller lakes of the Nordic countries and parts of North America. The worm consumes *vitamin B_{12} and may cause *megaloblastic anaemia (see HAEMATOLOGY) in the host.

DIPLEGIA is double paralysis, that is of both arms or of both legs (e.g. *spastic diplegia).

DIPLOCOCCUS. A *coccus that occurs in pairs.

DIPLOPIA is double vision, that is the perception of two images of a single object.

DIPSOMANIA is a form of *alcoholism in which excessive drinking is confined to periodic bouts. This pattern is thought by some to be a reflection of an underlying *manic-depressive psychosis.

DISABILITY AND REHABILITATION, THE ROYAL ASSOCIATION FOR (RADAR) is especially aware of the plight of three million disabled people in the UK. It campaigns on their behalf, and provides information and advice on all forms of handicap. A *Directory for the disabled* shows a range of activities and concern with statutory services, benefits, and allowances: mechanical and other aids; housing and home modifications; education; further education; employment; mobility and transport; holidays in the UK and abroad; sports and leisure; sex and personal relationships; legislation; contact organizations; legal and advisory services.

DISABLED PERSONS EMPLOYMENT ACT 1944. This UK Act was designed to enable persons handicapped by disablement to secure employment or to work on their own account. It covered the definition of disablement; vocational training and industrial rehabilitation; and provision for employment, including the establishment of registers and employers' quotas.

DISC is usually taken to mean intervertebral disc, one of the tough flexible pads which separate adjacent vertebrae in the *spine. It consists of a soft centre, the nucleus pulposus, surrounded by a circular ring of fibrous tissue, the annulus fibrosus. See also PROLAPSED INTERVERTEBRAL DISC.

DISEASE. Any sickness, ailment, or departure from the generally accepted norm of good health; most often, a specific disorder or type of disorder, disorder of a specified part, organ, tissue, or function, or a disorder due to a specified agent.

DISINFECTION is the removal or destruction of pathogenic (disease-causing) micro-organisms (bacteria, viruses, etc).

DISINFESTATION is the removal or destruction of ectoparasites such as lice, or pests and vermin of any other sort.

DISK is an alternative spelling of *disc, usual in the USA (and formerly in the UK).

DISLOCATION is a displacement, especially that resulting in disarticulation, of a *joint.

DISORIENTATION is a state of *confusion characterized by impaired appreciation of time, place, and identity.

DISPENSARY. Premises where drugs and medicines are dispensed, or the department of a hospital responsible for the supply of drugs, fluids for infusion, etc. Formerly, a charitable establishment for the treatment of out-patients.

DISPROPORTION means in particular cephalopelvic disproportion, in which the fetal head is too large in relation to the size of the mother's *pelvis to allow normal *delivery.

DISSECTING ANEURYSM is the extravasation of blood through an intimal tear into the wall of an artery, most often the *aorta, producing a *haematoma within the medial layer of the wall; the collection of blood may track up and/or down the length of the aorta and along its major branches, including the carotid, subclavian, coronary, renal, and femoral arteries; it may re-enter the aorta at some other site or may rupture externally. The manifestations are severe chest pain, often radiating posteriorly or downwards, together with those due to partial or complete occlusion of the vessels named, for example *hemiplegia, *myocardial infarction. Arterial pulses are often impalpable or significantly unequal. *Aortic incompetence may occur if the aortic valve is involved in the dissection, or the lesion may track into the *pericardium, causing life-threatening cardiac *tamponade. Dissecting aneurysm is a dangerous condition with a high mortality rate. Known predisposing factors include *atherosclerosis, *hypertension, *Marfan's syndrome, and *cystic medial necrosis of the aorta.

DISSECTION is the separation of anatomical structures for purposes of demonstration and study, or to facilitate surgical procedures.

DISSEMINATED SCLEROSIS is a synonym for *multiple sclerosis.

DISSOCIATION is the reversible separation of the molecules of a compound under a particular set of conditions (e.g. electrolytic dissociation, whereby molecules are split into ions).

DISTRICT NURSE. Community nurse.

DISULFIRAM. Also known as Antabuse®, disulfiram inhibits the *oxidation of *acetaldehyde formed from the metabolism of *ethanol. When alcohol is drunk after taking disulfiram, large quantities of acetaldehyde accumulate in the body and very unpleasant symptoms result; they include flushing, throbbing headache, tachycardia, vomiting, and, with large doses of alcohol, *arrhythmias, *hypotension, and collapse. Disulfiram is used in the treatment of *alcoholism, so as to ensure abstinence. It occurs naturally in the fungus *Coprinus atramentarius* (see POISONOUS FUNGI).

DIURESIS is increased excretion of *urine.

DIURETIC. Any agent which increases the volume flow of *urine.

DIURNAL RHYTHM is the *rhythm of a diurnal as opposed to a nocturnal event or events; it is also sometimes used synonymously with *circadian rhythm.

DIVERTICULITIS is inflammation of one or more *diverticula of the *colon.

DIVERTICULUM. A blind sac-like dilatation of the wall of a larger cavity. Diverticula of the *colon caused by *herniation of the mucous and submucous intestinal layers through areas of weakness in the muscular wall are common in the second half of adult life; this condition (diverticulosis) is symptomless unless inflammation (diverticulitis) supervenes, causing manifestations similar to those of the irritable bowel or 'spastic colon' syndrome.

DIVING. The medical hazards of recreational diving are as for *swimming, with the additional danger of diving into shallow water and sustaining severe spinal injury, including that due to haematomyelia (bleeding into the spinal cord). Deep-sea diving requires ascent to the surface in properly graduated stages if *decompression sickness is to be avoided. At depth, the eardrums may be injured, while breathing of inappropriate gas mixtures can cause either nitrogen narcosis or oxygen poisoning (see ENVIRONMENT AND DISEASE).

DIZZINESS is any sensation of giddiness, unsteadiness, or lightness of the head, including the more specific *vertigo.

DNA. Abbreviation of *deoxyribonucleic acid.

DOCHEZ, ALPHONSE RAYMOND (1882–1964). American physician. He made some original observations on serological differentiation of *pneumococcal types, and showed that the specificity is a property of the *polysaccharide in the capsule; this he called the 'specific soluble substance'. This work was an important factor in developing immunochemistry. Later, at Columbia University, he devoted his attention to the aetiology of *scarlet fever and with Dick, of Chicago, demonstrated that the haemolytic *streptococcus containing erythrogenic toxin was responsible. His last major work was on the common cold: he transmitted this disease to primates and human volunteers with bacteria-free filtrates.

DOCTOR. The widest anglophone usage is as a courtesy title to indicate a licensed and qualified medical practitioner (be he graduate, diplomate, or licentiate). The two major exceptions to this rule are that in the UK the title is not accorded to surgeons, marking their separate descent from the barbering profession, whereas in the USA it is extended not only to surgeons but to dentists as well. The title is also used to identify holders of other university doctorates (of philosophy, etc.).

DOCTORS AS ATHLETES. Without claiming any special distinction for doctors as athletes, at least two 20th century physicians of eminence have also been outstanding athletic performers, namely Lord (Arthur) Porritt and Sir Roger Bannister. Arthur Porritt, running for his native New Zealand, came third in the historic 1924 100 yard race at the Paris Olympics, won by Harold Abrahams. He later became President of the Royal College of Surgeons of England and Governor-General of New Zealand as Sir Arthur Porritt before receiving a life peerage. Bannister, who in 1954 became the first man in the world to run a mile in less than four minutes, has expressed doubts as to whether similar achievements will be possible for doctors in the future; the training demands now inseparable from world-class athletic performance are so rigorous and time-consuming as to be incompatible with simultaneous medical education.

DOCTORS AS MISSIONARIES. Healing is central to many religions, and, from the beginning of history, religion and medicine have been closely related, sometimes indistinguishable: Christ sent his apostle 'to preach the kingdom of God and to heal the sick'. Healing was the proper concern of the early Church, Greek medicine being eschewed as a pagan art. The saints, like present-day physicians, became highly specialized—St Sebastian and later St Roch for *plague, St Lazarus for *leprosy, St Vitus for *epilepsy, St Blaise for throat diseases, St Anthony for *ergotism, and so on.

Today, when most (but not all) religions leave healing of the sick to doctors, religion and medicine continue to be combined in the medical missionary, i.e. a missionary who is medically qualified and who combines medical practice with the propagation of his or her religious beliefs. Mission hospitals throughout the Third World, sometimes in remote and difficult areas, testify to the value of the health care provided by this group of doctors. (See also DOCTORS IN OTHER WALKS OF LIFE; MISSIONARIES, MEDICAL).

DOCTORS AS PATIENTS. Doctors do not generally unburden themselves about their health problems, partly because they have an understandable reticence, and partly because they are in the business of providing care. They do, however, have special difficulties both as patients when seeking or receiving medical aid, or as the consequence of hazards related to their profession.

In general terms, their attitude to illness was well summarized by Philip Rhodes (1986), who wrote:

'Doctors as patients are much like others, but they are sceptical and therefore do not consult other doctors much about minor physical illness. When they are ill there may be special problems of communication with their attendants, and these may be even greater when they are dying. They are subject to abuse of alcohol and of drugs, as well as to certain so-called "stress diseases" occasioned by the nature of their work. They respond to health education (in tobacco smoking) when the evidence is sure, but they please themselves about nostrums of various kinds where there is good reason to doubt, which is the stuff of their daily lives. They do not get carried away by extravagant claims, and they try to keep medicine in its proper place—neither too much nor too little, and preferably stay out of the hands of the doctors.'

Although both in terms of mortality and morbidity doctors enjoy a better standard of health and a longer lifespan than most, this is largely due to the benefits of their inheritance, in particular their stock, and because they are prosperous. The care they receive when seriously ill, unless they are unlucky (which is unusual), is excellent. None the less, there are three illnesses, *alcohol misuse, *drug abuse, and *mental illness, which cause special difficulties to themselves, their families, colleagues, and patients. It is the possible risk to the public which explains and justifies society's concern about doctors' health and the exceptional measures taken to help them. Although these issues are of world-wide importance, and all developed countries have developed mechanisms to deal with the problem, this article deals specifically with the UK, by way of example.

In the UK the formal procedures date from the *Merrison Enquiry of 1975, leading to the *Medical Act of 1978 which laid upon the profession, through the *General Medical Council (GMC), the responsibility of protecting the public from the consequences of doctors whose fitness to practise is seriously impaired by reason of a physical or mental condition (Merrison 1975). Invariably reference to these procedures results from a lack of insight or of the desire to get better.

The numbers so affected in the UK are small. In the 12 years since 1980 only 424 doctors have been referred to the GMC, and this from a profession numbering some 120 000 registered members. This may not reflect the true incidence, which could well be higher, but may indicate that, although there can be no grounds for complacency, the public is not being looked after by a population of addicts or mentally impaired doctors.

And in the UK how are these doctors managed? The first criterion is the acceptance that they are ill and need help. With this their problems acquire a respectability, which greatly facilitates management. Secondly, through a pragmatic application of the Medical Act, the GMC has been enabled to develop an informal mechanism for handling these doctors which, if they co-operate, minimizes the judicial factor and facilitates their treatment. And, finally, experience has shown that many of them can be so helped that they return to professional practice, with all this means for their self-respect, their happiness and well-being, and that of their families.

It should not be thought, however, that this is either an easy or a quick process. It needs a great effort by the patient, the recognition that he or she will always be at risk of relapse, and skilled and long-term help from a large team of caring individuals, including treating psychiatrists, employers, or colleagues, GMC officials, support groups such as the Doctors and Dentists Groups of *Alcoholics Anonymous (AA), and, most importantly, the family. A key factor for success is the discipline imposed by the threat of possible legal sanction by the GMC. These doctors require extended help over a long period, but many do get better (Lloyd 1990). Sadly there are also failures and tragedies.

Two major problems remain. The first relates to prevention and the second as to how to involve a profession in problems which most of its members prefer to ignore. The one affects the other.

Although the numbers with severe disability referred to the GMC are small, the history of their illness commonly extends back over many years and signs may, with hindsight, have been first apparent in their student days. Then, with the stresses of medical practice and the frailty of the individual concerned, a progressive deterioration of health, personality, and professional skills ensues. Of course there are many with substantial disability who never deteriorate to the extent that brings them to the attention of the authorities. But this does not mean that they neither require help, nor that patients may not be at risk. Clearly what is required is an approach which through earlier recognition and better local management, prevents continuing harm, both to the doctor and to the public. Progress in these respects has been achieved but more remains to be done.

Doctors do learn from experience. Their rejection of smoking has reduced the profession's death rate from cancer of the lung to well below that of other groups in the UK. There has been a similar lessening of death from cirrhosis of the liver, an indicator of the incidence of alcoholism, which suggests that in a country with increasing alcohol consumption, doctors have moderated their drinking habits. Although the incidence of suicide still remains high, especially in some groups of doctors and their spouses, the profession is beginning to show increased awareness of the consequences of stress and mental illness and is taking steps to ameliorate them.

Measures have also been developed which aim at earlier detection and better local management. Local medical committees, which represent family doctors, have not only statutory obligations but have been encouraged to develop informal local mechanisms to help sick doctors. In the hospitals the so-called 'three wise men' procedures have similarly evolved, and are well supported by Directors of *Public Health representing the employer. The National Counselling and Welfare Service for Sick Doctors provides confidential, nonthreatening, professional advice and access to treatment at the request of a sick doctor, the doctor's family, or a colleague. And the Doctors and Dentists Groups of AA provide moral support and encouragement, often over many years and on a daily basis. Fundamental to all this is the acceptance that these doctors are ill and require not only treatment but rehabilitation if their lives are not to be wasted and their families and their patients harmed.

Unfortunately, such evidence as we have suggests that the measures outlined are not as effective as they should be, and a recent GMC report stated that 'the profession could do very much more to tackle illness amongst it members at an earlier stage' (Kessel 1992). There are several possible reasons for this, and a number of difficulties to be overcome.

The Department of Health has seemed to have failed

in its responsibilities to its staff, whether they be doctors or domestics. The GMC is properly limited in what it can do by the Medical Act. It has, however, interpreted its obligations in an enlightened way, and much that has been achieved has resulted from the lead it has given to the profession. It sees that part of its role is that of a catalyst to effect change.

Doctors generally are not greatly interested in ill-health either among themselves, their families, or their colleagues, until it strikes, and unless the possible consequences can be serious. The explanation for this indifference is probably deeply rooted in the psyche of doctors but, whatever the cause, it has a profound effect both on the management of illness in the individual and in the provision of services. This is especially true of those illnesses which, to a layman, are those more socially unacceptable. Several suggestions have been made which are aimed at preventing illness or deterioration of illness; some of which, if imaginative, have either been ineffective or unacceptable to doctors.

Thus, where a doctor's own medical care and that of his family is concerned it is important that, like everyone else, he should be registered with a *family doctor, preferably not a friend or close colleague, to whom he should always go in the first instance for advice and treatment. In the past 10 years this has become accepted as good practice. None the less, when ill, many doctors still treat themselves or their families, order their investigations, and directly refer to a specialist colleague without consulting their *general practitioner (GP) (Richards 1989).

To overcome this problem, with its associated disadvantages, it has been suggested that doctors should lose their right within the *National Health Service (NHS) to prescribe or to order investigations either for themselves or their families. The belief is that if they had to use the standard NHS procedure they would insist upon a better service, which would be to the benefit of all users. The counter-argument is that it would be inconvenient to the doctor to introduce such a rule, as the present flexible mechanism relieves some pressure on GPs. A further problem is that doctors, especially the alcoholic or those with mental and marital problems, delay seeking medical advice. What is needed here to facilitate earlier recognition and referral is a system of health care which carries the confidence of the doctor's spouse and family. Ideally this should be the GP service but, if this cannot be upgraded in the profession's esteem, it has also been suggested that this need might be met by a preferential care system for doctors and their families. An improved Occupational Health Service might provide the answer, but such services within the NHS have been criticized as being among the poorest in the country. And, regrettably, not all occupational health physicians have the confidence of other doctors.

Some progress has been made. The National Counselling and Welfare Service for Sick Doctors, the informal and formal mechanisms in the GP and hospital services for those more seriously affected, where patients may be at risk, and the continuing tradition of special responsibility accepted by many doctors for sick colleagues and their families, have helped many at a time of great need. Still more needs to be done. It is encouraging that the two principal medical organizations, which not only represent but lead the UK profession, the GMC and the *British Medical Association (BMA), both show a continuing concern and are endeavouring to improve matters. These two bodies, together with the Department of Health, share the responsibility for providing proper and effective health care for doctors and their families; this is in the interest of both the profession and the public.

A. ALLIBONE

References
Kessel, W. I. N. (1992). *Annual Report of the Screener for Health*. Minutes of the General Medical Council.
Lloyd, G. (1990). Alcoholic doctors can recover. *British Medical Journal*, **300**, 728–800.
Merrison, A. W. (1975). *Report of the committee of inquiry into the regulation of the medical profession*, pp. 328–52. HMSO, London.
Rhodes, P. (1986). Doctors as patients. In *The Oxford companion to medicine*, pp. 315–18. Oxford University Press.
Richards, C. (1989). *The King Edward's Hospital Fund for London, Project Paper, No. 78*.

DOCTORS AS TRUANTS TO LITERATURE. In 1936, Lord Moynihan of Leeds (1865–1936), a famous surgeon, gave a Linacre lecture, published the same year and republished in 1983. He called his lecture: *Truants—the story of some who deserted medicine yet triumphed*. It is fascinating to realize how varied are the achievements of men—I am sure there will be more women truants in times to come—who started their careers as doctors. There have been politicians and musicians, philosophers and philanthropists, scientists and botanists, bibliophiles and missionaries, true polymaths, and famous sportsmen. But in no field are the doctors as many as in literature.

There are doctor-authors to be found in every country and culture, and there seem always to have been doctor-authors—Lord Moynihan went as far back as Imhotep, physician to Pharaoh Zoser, more than 2000 years BC, whom he called 'the true father of medicine'.

Why is it that doctors, more than members of any other learned profession, write all sorts of books, fiction and poetry, drama and detective stories, humour and cookery books?

There are obvious similarities between the tasks of a doctor and those of an author. Edmund Pellegrino writes that 'both medicine and literature are ways of looking at man and both are, at heart, moral enterprises.' He continues, 'medicine and literature are linked, too, because they both tell the story of what they see'—all doctors are trained to take and write down the patient's history. Further, 'language, the stuff of literature, is also the means of *communication between the patient and the physician. Both medicine and literature probe, although from radically different perspectives, the same subject: the truths that are revealed—and concealed—in man' (E. R. Peschel).

Many authors have confirmed that their medical training was a great help to them in their work as authors. Anton Chekhov wrote

My study of medicine significantly broadened the scope of my observations and enriched me with knowledge whose value for me as a writer only a doctor can appreciate. It also served as a guiding influence; my intimacy with medicine probably helped me to avoid many mistakes. My familiarity with the natural sciences and scientific methods has always kept me on my guard; I have tried whenever possible to take scientific data into account.

The same testimony has been given to me by several contemporary doctor-authors.

Jean Bernard, famous French doctor-author, member of the French Academy, who started composing poetry when a prisoner of war, divided doctor-authors into three categories, namely:

(1) those who start out as working physicians but, at a specific time, abandon medicine to become full-time authors (e.g. T. Smollett, W. Somerset Maugham, A. Conan Doyle);

(2) those who throughout their lives work both as doctors and as writers, but keep the two professions apart (e.g. Anton Chekhov, William Carlos Williams); and

(3) those whose literary work is filled with, and based entirely upon, their medical experiences.

British doctor-authors (in alphabetical order)

Aikin, John (1747–1822).

Akenside, Mark (1721–70). Physician and bibliophile, physician to St Thomas Hospital, London and to George III's Queen. At the age of 17 he wrote a philosophical poem, *The pleasures of imagination*. Although he continued to write, his later years were more concerned with medicine than poetry. Because of his arrogance he became the target of Tobias Smollett's satire in *Peregrine Pickle*.

Arbuthnot, John (1667–1735). Physician to Queen Anne. It has been said that he is remembered only as the recipient of Alexander Pope's *An epistle to Dr Arbuthnot*, but that seems a spiteful and unfair judgment. He wrote *Of the laws of chance* and later, encouraged by Jonathan Swift, a satire, *The history of John Bull*, in which he created John Bull as representing England.

Beddoes, Thomas Lovell (1803–49).

Bell, Josephine (?).

Blackmore, Sir Richard (?1650–1729).

Bridges, Robert (1844–1930). The first and only doctor to be made Poet Laureate, he served in London hospitals but retired after an attack of pneumonia at the age of 37 to devote himself exclusively to poetry, which he did for more than 45 years. His last work, *The testament of beauty*, is regarded as his most renowned.

Brown, John (1810–82).

Browne, Sir Thomas (1605–82). He was educated in Oxford, studied medicine at Montpellier, Padua, and Leiden, and returned to Oxford to practise. Later he moved to Halifax and, in 1636, to Norwich, where he stayed until his death in 1682. His *magnum opus*, *Religio medici*, an elegant and deep work, was first published in a pirate edition in 1642 and only later in a version authorized by the author. It was placed on the *Index expurgatorius* by the Vatican, thus being forbidden reading for Catholics. He also wrote *Pseudodoxia epidemica* (1648), generally called *Vulgar errors*, a great work in seven books, in which he discussed the complete knowledge of the time and, with the help of his own experiments and logic, exposed many of the common superstitions and errors of folklore.

Campion, Thomas (1567–1620).

Chamberlayne, William (1619–89).

Cowley, Abraham (1618–67).

Crabbe, George (1754–1832). '. . . Of all "truants" probably professionally the most incompetent' (Lord Moynihan)—he was ordained as a priest and became curate of Aldeburgh. He was saved from relative obscurity by Benjamin Britten, who based the story of his opera *Peter Grimes* on Crabbe's *The borough*.

Cronin, Archibald Joseph (1896–1981). At one time, he was said to be the most read author in the world. He wrote many successful novels from his own experiences as a doctor in the mining districts of Wales: *Hatter's castle*, *The stars look down*, *The citadel*, etc. In later years he wrote an extremely popular series for television, *Dr Finlay's case book*.

Darwin, Erasmus (1731–1802).

Deeping, George Warwick (1877–1950).

Denton, William (1605–91).

Dover, Thomas (1660–1742).

Doyle, Sir Arthur Conan (1859–1930). He practised for some time in Southsea, but in 1890, when he moved to London, he abandoned medicine and became a full-time author. He created Sherlock Holmes and Dr Watson and their abode in 221b Baker Street. The first Sherlock Holmes story, *A study in scarlet*, appeared in 1887. Doyle also wrote some famous historical novels (*Micah Clarke* and *The White Company*) and short stories during his early career (*Doctors–tales from medical life*), and early science fiction—a series of books figuring the mad Professor Challenger.

Freeman, Robert Austin (1862–1943).

Garth, Sir Samuel (1661–1719). During the times of, and after, the plague, he fought against the apothecaries, who wanted to dispense medicines on their own, and supported the Royal College of Physicians, which organized the first dispensary for the poor in 1699. The fight continued, and it was not until Garth had published his famous *The dispensary* that the antagonism between doctors and apothecaries ceased. *The dispensary* is a burlesque poem in Homerian style, ridiculing the disputants who, at the time, could easily be identified.

Gilbert, William (1540–1603).

Gogarty, Oliver Joseph St John (1870–1957). He was a close friend of James Joyce, who portrayed him as Buck Mulligan in *Ulysses*. A senator in the Irish Parliament; an ear, nose, and throat (ENT) surgeon; and bon vivant, he practised in London but moved to New York, where he died. He wrote several novels, and his poems, including the moving *Non dolet*, were included by his friend W. B. Yeats in the *Oxford anthology of modern poetry*.

Goldsmith, Oliver (1730–74). Perhaps never a qualified doctor? He wrote *The vicar of Wakefield*, of which Lord Moynihan said that 'it will be read as long as the English language exists', and which includes the lines which begin:

> When lovely woman stoops to folly
> And finds too late that men betray

He also wrote *She stoops to conquer*, a stage comedy in a different vein.

Grainger, James (?1721–60).

Hamilton, Sir David (1663–1721).

Harington, Sir John (1561–1612).

Harvey, Gabriel (1545–1630).

Hoadley, Benjamin (1706–57).

Hooker, Joseph Dalton (1817–1911).

Keats, John (1795–1821). He studied medicine at Guy's Hospital, qualified and worked a short time as a doctor, but soon abandoned medicine for poetry. He died from tuberculosis at the age of 25. His first volume of poetry was published in 1817; in 1818 came *Endymion* ('A thing of beauty is a joy for ever'), followed by such famous poems as *Hyperion*, *Ode to a nightingale*, and *Ode on a Grecian urn*. Tennyson regarded Keats as the greatest poet of the 19th century.

Keynes, Sir Geoffrey Langdon (1887–1982).

Knowles, James Sheridan (1784–1862).

Lever, Charles James (1806–72).

Locke, John (1621–1704).

Lodge, Thomas (1558–1625).

McCrae, John (1872–1918).

Maugham, William Somerset (1874–1965). During his long life he became immensely popular, first as a playwright—in 1908 he had four plays running simultaneously in London—later as an author of novels, and especially short stories. His first novel, *Liza of Lambeth*, is set in the London slum where Maugham, for a short period, worked as an obstetric clerk. He soon abandoned medicine, but later paid his tribute to it when in *The summing up*, he wrote, 'I do not know a better training for a writer than to spend some years in the medical profession.' His most famous novel is *Of human bondage*, an autobiographical story with several similarities to Marcel Proust's *Remembrance of things past*. Other well-known novels are *Cakes and ale*, *The moon and sixpence*, and the later *The razor's edge*.

Mavor, Osborne Henry (1888–1951). He studied and practised medicine, and for a short time was professor of medicine in Glasgow. For the rest of his life he was a very successful playwright and wrote more than 40 plays under the pseudonym James Bridie, the best known being *Tobias and the angel* (1930), *The anatomist* (1931), and *Daphne Laureola* (1949).

Moir, David Macbeth (1798–1851).

Moore, John (1729–1802).

Ross, Sir Ronald (1857–1932).

Smiles, Samuel (1812–1904).

Smollett, Tobias (1721–71). A ship's surgeon and author, he is regarded, together with Richardson, Fielding, and Sterne as an originator of the English novel. He studied in Glasgow and obtained a post as a surgeon's mate during the mismanaged expedition to Cartagena in 1741, later to be described in his first novel. In 1744 he was back in London with a practice in Downing Street and, in 1748, he published his first book, *The adventures of Roderick Random*, based upon his experiences in the navy. He continued in medicine and in 1750 obtained his MD at Aberdeen. The next year saw the appearance of his new novel, *Peregrine Pickle*. He spent some time in Bath and criticized the Bath waters—Bath plays an important role in his last novel, *The expedition of Humphrey Clinker* (1771). Before that he had edited the *Critical Review*, published several other novels, and his *Travels through France and Italy*, regarded as overcritical of all he saw. Smollett's travels appeared in the shadow of Sterne's *A sentimental journey*, in which Sterne ridiculed Smollett as 'Smellfungus'. Smollett also wrote *A complete history of England* (1757–58), which brought him much criticism but also, for the first time, financial security.

The novels that can be read today are *The adventures of Roderick Random* and *The expedition of Humphrey Clinker*. In *Roderick Random*, Smollett was the first novelist 'to draw from the Navy his most notable characters and his liveliest scenes' (H. W. Hodges). We find here the first description of the food and drink on board naval ships:

our provision consisted of putrid salt beef and salt pork, which though neither fish nor flesh, savoured of both; bread, every biscuit whereof, like a piece of clock-work, moved by its own internal impulse, occasioned by the myriads of insects that dwelt within it

and to drink what the sailors styled 'The Necessity'; 'three half-quarters of rum, diluted with a certain quantity of water'—the 'grog', after the admiral 'Old Grog', so named on account of his fondness for a clock which was made of grogram. *The expedition of Humphrey Clinker* is an epistolary, letters between a travelling gentleman, Mr Bramble, and his physician, a charming story of travels in 18th century England. The very first letter begins, 'Doctor, the pills are good for nothing—

I might as well swallow snowballs to cool my veins.' Smollett's reputation sank during the 19th and early 20th centuries but now stands high.

Stables, William (Gordon) (1840–1910).

Stacpole, Henry de Vere (1863–1951). He is remembered for his romance *The blue lagoon* (1908).

Treves, Sir Frederick (1853–1923).

Vaughan, Henry (1622–95).

Warren, Samuel (1807–77).

Wilde, Sir William (1815–76).

Wolcot, John (1738–1819). Writing under the pseudonym Peter Pindar, he was known for his satirical verse and pamphlets.

Young, Francis Brett (1884–1954). He practised in Devon and served during the First World War in East Africa. He published several novels from the West Midlands and from his African experiences, the best known being *Portrait of Claire* and *My brother Jonathan*.

Young, Thomas (1773–1829).

Non-British doctor-authors
Only a few names are quoted from some of the large language areas, but there are doctor-authors to be found in every country and language.

Germany/Austria
Benn, Gottfried (1886–1956). He is regarded as perhaps the leading poet of 20th century Germany. He studied medicine in Berlin, in 1912 both graduated and published his first collection of poems, *Morgue*, which made him one of the most important representatives of German expressionism. For a short period he was captured by Nazi ideas, an aberration that cost him dearly, and it was only after the Second World War that he was again accepted in the literary world and could publish his poems. Almost until his death in 1956 he continued a modest practice among the poor and destitute in Berlin. Many of his most famous poems were written during this second active period of his life, poems of solitude and suffering; life only gave emptiness and:

> To live is to build bridges
> over waters disappearing

Büchner, George (1813–37).

Döblin, Alfred (1878–1957). A Jewish doctor who himself became an anti-Semite, he lived and worked in the eastern part of Berlin and wrote many novels, the best known being *Berlin Alexanderplatz*, which was made into a famous film by R.W. Fassbinder.

Hoffmann, Heinrich (1809–74). A German physician who made important contributions to psychiatry, he wrote the immortal *Struwwelpeter* (*Schock-Head Peter*, 1847), which, in 1939, when counting stopped, had seen 593 editions and had been translated into most languages.

Scheffler, Johannes (Angelus Silesius) (1624–77).

Schiller, Johann Christoph Friedrich von (1759–1805).

Schnitzler, Arthur (1862–1931).

France
Céline, Louis Ferdinand (1894–1961). He was said to 'crash' into literature with his two novels, *Voyage au bout de la nuit* (1932) and *Mort à credit* (1936), both with a doctor as the main character and with much autobiographical material. Céline wrote about people at the bottom of society and lived close to them himself, regarding men to be 'disgusting, shocking and absurd!' In his novels, Céline, for the first time, created a modern French written language.

Duhamel, Georges (1884–1966).

Rabelais, François (?1494–1553). He became a Franciscan monk and later got his MD in Montpellier in 1530, becoming one of the leading physicians in France. He and his books were several times condemned by the Catholic Church, and Rabelais had to live outside France for long periods. Eventually he was given absolution and could return to France where he ended his days, not as a doctor but as a priest, as vicar of Meudon in Paris.

For many centuries he was thought of only as a jester, but in the 18th century he was rediscovered, and today he is regarded as one of the greatest names in world literature, with an important influence on such authors as Swift, Sterne, and Joyce.

His great work is the story of the giants *Gargantua and Pantagruel*, in five volumes, all with different titles, published between 1532 and 1564. The first tells of the cloister Thélème, with its monastic rule of 'Do as you like', a message which should be seen in context with Rabelais's fight against the rigid ideas of the sophistry of the time. Rabelais is a snorting joker, he snorts from zest for life and happiness, he jokes with everything and everybody. He fills his work with urine and excrements, with anatomy and medicine, with obscenities, with words—he is said to have invented 600 new French words—but his work never gives offence, it leads to laughter.

Sue, Eugene (1804–57).

USA
Holmes, Oliver Wendell (1809–94). He was professor of anatomy and physiology at Harvard University and author of novels, poems, and essays. Holmes is famous especially for his *Autocrat of the breakfast-table* (1857–58), essays notable for their kindly humour and width of erudition.

Percy, Walker (1916–90). MD, philosopher, linguist, and author, he published several philosophical works until he realized that nobody read him. He then started writing a series of novels, e.g. *The moviegoer*, *The last gentleman*, and *The Thanatos syndrome* (1987), but yet had difficulties in reaching the wide readership he

Doctors in literature

deserves. Percy wrote much of a deep anxiety, of an 'everydayness' which damages life, with people passing each other without meeting.

Williams, William Carlos (1883–1963). He was a man in whom medicine and literature had formed a creative symbiosis—he worked his whole life as a practising physician amongst the poor in New Jersey and wrote whenever he found time. He was primarily a poet—the patients and their lives were his teacher, they inspired him and filled his poems. His fame came late; he was awarded the Pulitzer prize posthumously, at a time when his poetry was published in England for the first time. His most ambitious work was *Paterson*, a long, free verse apotheosis to a suburban industrial city.

Russia

Bulgakov, Mikhail (1891–1940). A Russian prose writer and dramatist, he started his career in medicine, but after the revolution abandoned medicine and became a journalist and author. For long periods he was forbidden to publish, and his plays were banned by the Russian authorities. He tried to emigrate but was never given a passport. His most famous work is *The Master and Margarita* (written between 1928 and 1940 but not published until 1966–67); others are *The heart of a dog* and *The White Guard*. During his lifetime, when his novels could not be published in Russia, he was famous for his plays, especially *The days of the Turbins*, performed more than 1000 times.

Chekhov, Anton (1860–1904). When only a schoolboy, he had to take responsibility for his mother and siblings, and he started to write short stories. He studied medicine in Moscow and opened a practice. Later he moved to a country house outside the city, where he practised medicine among the poor peasants for many years with wide responsibilities: 'my district compasses 25 villages, four factories and a monastery'. He contracted tuberculosis at an early age and by the age of 25 complained of coughing and blood spitting. He denied his tuberculosis for at least another 12 years, 'I am still far from tuberculosis!', until at the age of 37 he had a major haemorrhage and had to admit that he was ill. He moved to the Crimea but frequently travelled to Moscow, where he married the famous actress Olga Knipper, only a few years before his premature death in 1904, when only 44 years old.

Chekhov wrote about 700 short stories, many, in fact, with the format of a short novel. During his younger days he wrote small comic pieces, the major short stories were written between 1885 and 1895, and the major plays thereafter. Some of the most famous short stories are *Ward No. 6*, *The steppe*, *The black monk*, and *The lady with the little dog*. The cavalcade of plays began with *The seagull* (1895), the first performance of which, in St Petersburg, was a complete disaster due to the actors' misunderstanding of the play. The new production in 1898 in Moscow started the triumphant, and still ongoing, march over the world's stages of *The seagull*, followed by *Uncle Vanya* (1900), *Three sisters* (1901), and *The cherry orchard* (1904).

Anton Chekhov often paid tribute to his medical studies and training as being important for his authorship, 'There is no doubt in my mind that my study of medicine has had serious impact on my literary activities.' There are, however, remarkably few traces of medicine in his short stories. The opposite could be said of the plays. In all except *The cherry orchard*, doctors, often described as being both incompetent and alcoholic, played important roles with critical comments about what was being enacted on stage.

The principal characteristic in Chekhov's writing lies in his deep understanding of human nature, in his humour, empathy, and compassion. The plays demonstrate that a non-happening may also be genuinely dramatic.

Why does an author write?

Primo Levi in his book *L'altrui mestiere* (*Others' professions*) has given nine answers: because it is necessary, to entertain, to teach, to improve the world, to spread ideas, to get rid of anxiety, to become famous, to get rich, or by habit. Are there other reasons specific for doctors which make them abandon knife and stethoscope for the pen, or, today, for the word processor? Many have answered that writing is necessary and that it is great fun. Some say it is escapism, helping them from becoming burnt-out. Jean Bernard wrote to survive. It seems that doctors like to write, although for many it does not come easily. Chekhov once wrote that 'The fire in me burns with an even, lethargic flame; it never flares up or roars!' The US surgeon Richard Selzer says that he writes slowly, only a few pages per day and Oliver Sacks said: 'A deadline might create a dead man!'

In his everyday work the doctor-author lives an exciting story—but there is a danger: if the doctor becomes too artistically sensitive, he might lose the cool objectivity necessary for most doctors' decisions. This is an important reason why some doctor-authors abandon medicine.

In 1735 Alexander Pope, in his famous *An epistle to Dr Arbuthnot*, gave this answer:

> Why did I write? What sin to use unknown
> Dipt me in Ink, my Parent's, or my own?
> As yet a child, nor yet a Fool to Fame,
> I lisp'd in Numbers, for the Numbers came.
> I left no Calling for this idle trade,
> No Duty broke, no Father dis-obey'd.
> The Muse but serv'd to ease some Friend, not Wife
> To help me thro' this long Disease, my life.

LARS ERIK BÖTTIGER

DOCTORS IN LITERATURE. Doctors appear in so many novels and plays that a short account must be selective and personal, limited in this case largely to the classics. They seldom play a major part, except for an occasional hero or villain. Singling out doctors for special attention does not mean that they are in any way unique; a medical qualification may in fact be irrelevant. Nevertheless, their portrayal in fiction does provide an opportunity to learn how lay people view doctors; naive medical readers will no doubt be shocked by the amount of ill-feeling. Through the ages the behaviour of doctors has been imaginatively dissected—and on the whole found wanting.

Professionalism

Fictional works by medically qualified writers, however partisan, might be expected to give some idea of life and work as a doctor. Medical and surgical practice in the 18th century, for example, is documented with coarse realism by Tobias Smollett, *surgeon's mate and unsuccessful *physician, in *The adventures of Roderick Random* (1748) and *The expedition of Humphrey Clinker* (1771). There are many doctors in his books, not always sympathetically drawn.

There are also many doctors in Arthur Conan Doyle's writings, but he tends to accept their professional qualities without comment. However, he did write *Round the red lamp* (1894), 15 short stories of medical life, 'to make doctors something more than marionettes'. One of his strongly held beliefs was in the importance of the healing touch, 'that magnetic thing which defies explanation or analysis.' He compared the energetic and up-to-date young doctor unfavourably to the wise old physician (not for the last time in fiction): 'I thought of his cold, critical attitude, of his endless questions, of his tests and his tappings. I wanted something more soothing—more genial.' It would surely be unfair to cite Dr Watson as an example of an inept doctor—his role was as a sidekick rather than a physician—but the problem-solving skills of Sherlock Holmes could be recommended to doctors.

Francis Brett Young's *My brother Jonathan* (1928) and other less readable medical novels, and A.J. Cronin's *The citadel* (1937) convey a romantic, black-and-white view of medical practice; their books were best sellers in their time but their appeal has not lasted. More substantial is *The Pasquier chronicles* (1933–41) by another doctor, Georges Duhamel. The hero in this epic tale is a doctor and biologist (read scientist) who is involved in the social and philosophical issues of a society in crisis, and not surprisingly reflects the increasing rift between science and humanism.

Of the few uncomplicatedly sympathetic portraits of doctors by non-medical writers, the best is Honoré de Balzac's 'beloved' Dr Bénassis in *The country doctor* (1833). Walter Scott's Dr Adam Hartley in *The surgeon's daughter* (1828) is decent, competent, and incorruptible, as upright as his teacher, Gideon Gray ('there is no harder worker in all Scotland and none more poorly requited'). One of Emile Zola's last novels, *Dr Pascal* (1893) provides an idealized image of the humane, hard-working, broad-minded physician, who is not interested in making money.

Dr Tertius Lydgate in George Eliot's *Middlemarch* (1871–72) is the best-known example of the traditional English physician. He 'was convinced that the medical profession offered the most direct alliance between intellectual conquest and social good. He cared not only for "cases" but for each individual'—sentiments that have a modern ring. He was a good man, idealistic and ambitious, but emotional entanglements led to his downfall, condemning (*sic*) him to successful and fashionable practice instead of an independent life of research which he so much desired.

A further opportunity to show the doctor in a good light arises when he is confronted by disaster. Young Dr Turnhall in *Two years ago* (1857), the last of Charles Kingsley's social novels, at first upsets the local villagers by his prediction of a *cholera outbreak, but when the *epidemic strikes he is rapidly accepted because of his courage and dedication. By contrast, Dr Stockman in Ibsen's *An enemy of the people* is reviled and ostracized by the community for attributing an epidemic to deficiencies in the local water supply. Dr Rieux in Camus's celebrated novel, *The *plague* (1947), sometimes inhuman and ruthless in the eyes of his patients, is a dedicated and concerned doctor, capable of facing up to his powerlessness and frustration in the face of the epidemic. An arrogant exterior may hide the humility and compassion of the best doctors.

Not unexpectedly, few women doctors are portrayed in early fiction. An exception is Dr Rhoda Gale in Charles Reade's *A woman hater* (1877), who is competent and efficient but somewhat lacking in feminine qualities. Alexander Solzhenitsyn (*Cancer ward* 1970) does not have a very high opinion of women doctors.

Mixed views

Ambivalent attitudes towards doctors are displayed by Shakespeare and Dickens. Shakespeare's views of doctors have to be considered in the context of their time, when much treatment was undertaken by quacks, such as the contemptible Dr Pinch (*The comedy of errors*, 1594). On the whole, proper doctors are treated with respect: the physician who treated Lear (*King Lear*, 1608) is humane and considerate; the Scottish doctor called to the unhinged Lady Macbeth (*Macbeth*, 1606) admits that the illness is beyond his competence, and is thought none the worse for saying so.

The dedicated physician, Lord Cerimon (*Pericles*, 1609), is repeatedly praised: 'Your honour has through Ephesus pour'd forth/Your charity, and hundreds call themselves/ Your creatures who by you have been restor'd' and 'Reverend Sir, /The Gods can have no mortal officer/More like a God than you'. But he is responsible for restoring Pericles's wife, Thaisa, to life, and so might be considered a special case.

Less certainty exists about more conventional doctoring. Mistress Quickly (*The merry wives of Windsor*, 1602) describes the French Dr Caius, for whom she works, 'that calls himself doctor of physic', as a fool and physician. Pericles complains 'Thou speak'st like a physician, Helicanus/who minister'st a potion unto me/ That would'st tremble to receive thyself'. And there is the well-known sentiment in *Timon of Athens* (1623 Folio): 'Trust not the physician,/His antidotes are poison, and he slays/More than you rob, takes wealth and lives together.'

Compared with the unflattering way in which Dickens treated lawyers, doctors come off lightly. Although numerous, none plays a major role in his novels. They are often gently ridiculed; none is learned or high-principled. Sir Parker Peps (*Dombey and son*, 1848) is 'one of the Court physicians, and a man of immense reputation for assisting at the increase of great families'. Mr Jobling (*Martin Chuzzlewit*, 1843) is an unscrupulous knave 'who had a habit of sucking his lips and saying "Ah". . . which inspired great confidence'. Dr Slammer (*Pickwick papers*, 1837–39) is small, fat, and irascible. Others exhibit more admirable qualities. Dr Jeddler (*The battle of life*, 1844) 'looked on the world as a gigantic joke' although he was kind and generous. Dr Bayham Badger (*Bleak house*, 1852–52), a fashionable and ambitious general practitioner, is rather a fool but generally sound, and Dr Alan Woodcourt, the young ship's surgeon in the same novel, is tender-hearted but sensible. Mr Chillip (*David Copperfield*, 1849–50) is a kind and amiable village practitioner.

None of Dickens's doctors is particularly memorable, in stark contrast to the hilarious descriptions of the medical students in *Pickwick papers*: Benjamin Allen, 'he presented altogether a rather mildewy appearance' and Bob Sawyer. And his graphic exposure of the dangerous activities of Sairey Gamp and Betsy Prig alerted society to the scandal of untrained *nurses.

The sins of doctors
Doctors are accused of every sin, including murder (Herman Melville, *White-jacket*, 1850; Frank Danby, *Dr Phillips. A Maida Vale idyll*, 1887; Hjalmar Söderberg, *Dr Glas*, 1900). The prize for the most decadent goes to the central character, Dr Bardamu, in L.-F. Céline's astonishing first novel, *Journey to the end of the night* (1932). He is a seedy and ignorant individual who shares the degradation of the society in which he works. Any high-mindedness is destroyed by the nightmare of the city and its denizens. Céline had been an idealistic doctor, and it is arguable that by denigrating the medical profession he was reflecting his own disillusionment. But the greatness of the novel lies in its profound despair at the sordidness of the human condition, from which no one—least of all doctors—can escape.

The three doctors in Anton Chekhov's plays (*The seagull*, 1895; *Uncle Vanya*, 1900; and *Three sisters*, 1901) share all the worst characteristics: cynicism, indecision, incompetence, and little knowledge of medicine; two of them are *alcoholic. Dr Astrov in *Uncle Vanya* 'knows as much about medicine as I know about astronomy'. Chekhov, 'I look upon medicine as my

lawful wife',. . . seems to be warning that the basic human instincts are a constant threat to the passionate involvement of the dedicated physician. Dr Plair (Graham Greene, *The honorary consul*, 1973) is profoundly cynical (as are so many of Greene's characters), but he is redeemed by his devotion to medicine.

Scarcely concealed contempt for the hubris, pedantry, and certainty of doctors is widespread. 'There are worse occupations in this world than feeling a woman's pulse' (Laurence Sterne, *A sentimental journey*, 1768). Dr Slop in *The life and origins of Tristram Shandy* (1760), by the same author, is a figure of fun, perhaps in order to exorcise the unpleasantness of medical treatment at the time. Love of money is a popular theme. Chaucer's doctor of physic in *The Canterbury tales* (*c.* 1387)—a man of importance, serious, sober, and moral, 'who knew the cause of every malady'—appreciated gold 'in special', not for the money, of course, but for its use as a cordial in therapy.

Amusing descriptions of the sleight of hand with which doctors receive and dispose of their fee are given by Ivan Turgenev in *The district doctor* (1852) and by Marcel Proust in *A la recherche du temps perdu* (1913–26). Anthony Trollope's *Dr Thorne* (1858), who scandalizes his colleagues by offering change when paid for consultations, is firmly put in his place; 'The true physician should hardly be aware that the last friendly grasp of the hand had been made more precious by the touch of gold.' Perhaps financial transactions removed the awe and fear by reducing the doctor to the status of tradesman, or worse, 'We are angels when we come to cure, devils when we ask for payment' (Walter Scott, *The abbott*, 1831). That people might feel better for paying is not considered.

Some of the more scathing opinions of doctors have come from writers who suffered from chronic ill-health. Jean Molière, who had repeated *haemoptyses from *tuberculosis while acting, complained in his play *Le malade imaginaire* (1673), 'Why does he need four doctors—is not one enough to kill a patient?' and berated the medical profession, 'Your best knowledge is pure nonsense/Vain and impudent doctors,/With your fine Latin words you cannot cure/The suffering that is driving me to despair.'

Bernard Shaw's hatred of doctors was based on his own suffering at their hands. *The doctor's dilemma* (1906), although not one of his best plays, is well known for the undignified behaviour of its doctors and its polemical preface. The latter is a comprehensive criticism of the medical establishment, 'The tragedy of illness at present is that it delivers you helplessly into the hands of a profession which you deeply distrust.' 'Let no one suppose that the words doctor and patient can disguise from the parties the fact that they are employer and employee.' 'It is simply unscientific to allege or believe that doctors do not under existing circumstances perform unnecessary operations and manufacture and prolong lucrative diseases.'

Marcel Proust, surrounded by doctors who could do little for his asthma, was highly sceptical, 'The mistakes made by doctors are innumerable'. In *A la recherche du temps perdu* he writes, 'For each ailment that doctors cure with medications (as I am told they occasionally succeed in doing) they produce ten others in healthy individuals by inoculating them with that pathogenic agent a thousand times more virulent than all the *microbes—the idea that they are ill.' He dissected his physicians with the same intensity as he did his other characters, and found them wanting: narrow-minded and consumed by self-interest, unconcerned with any deeper meaning to life other than the physical ills they could not cure. The renowned specialist, Dr Cottard, is self-important and ineffectual, 'an imbecile'. And yet fear of illness causes Proust in the end to concede: 'To believe in medicine would be the supreme madness, if not to believe in it were not an even greater one, for from this heaping of mistakes have come out in the long run some verities'.

Doctors, and particularly specialists, as portrayed in *The doctor's dilemma* and in the ridiculous figure of Sir Roderick Glossop, brain *surgeon, in P.G. Wodehouse's novels, are arrogant, snobbish, and patronizing. Dr Raste, the *general practitioner in Arnold Bennett's *Riceyman steps* (1923) had 'the pompous solemnity of a little man conscious of rectitude'; 'often spoke more loudly than he need—the result of imposing himself on the resistant stupidity of the proletariat'; and 'had a general preference for not being quite sure; he liked to postpone judgement'.

Despotic, callous, and unsympathetic attitudes are displayed by Dr Tyrrell in Somerset Maugham's *Of human bondage* (1915), by the extremely unpleasant medical superintendent, Hofrat Behrens in Thomas Mann's *The magic mountain* (1924), and by the boorish medical hierarchy in A.E. Ellis's *The rack* (1958). The last two are powerful accounts of the claustrophobic effect of *sanatorium treatment of tuberculosis; both can be recommended for their many examples of patient–doctor non-communication.

A recurrent complaint is that doctors have no time to talk to patients: they 'never tell you anything outright' and 'no one stops for a moment to say a few words' (*Cancer ward*). It is only fair to add that the staff themselves recognize their failure. Bedside manners leave much to be desired: doctors are insensitive and insincere, they have 'a healthy man's jovial condescension' (*Of human bondage*) towards ill people, and are poorly equipped to deal with serious illness and dying. Leo Tolstoy's harrowing novella, *The death of Ivan Ilyich* (1884), is an indictment of the confusion and false optimism of doctors faced with an illness they cannot diagnose, 'the doctors couldn't say what was the matter—at least they could, but each said something different'.

Rivalries among doctors do not improve their image. Examples can be found in *Middlemarch* between Dr Lydgate and the general practitioners; in *The doctor's dilemma*; in Virginia Woolf's *Mrs Dalloway* between Sir William Bradshaw and Dr Holmes; in *My brother Jonathan*, with its two doctor brothers—one dedicated and the other worldly wise and bored; and in *The rack*, where the doctors squabble over private patients. Anthony Trollope's *Dr Thorne* (1858) brings down the wrath of the self-elected leader of the profession (appropriately called Dr Fillgrave) for doing his own prescribing and collecting money. William Thackeray in *The history of Pendennis* (1848–50) contrasts Dr Firmin ('among the meanest scoundrels in fiction'— Squire Sprigge) who, although 'only a doctor', becomes a *consultant through the help of fashionable friends and a good marriage, with the kindly and professional Dr Goodenough, based on John Elliotson, professor of medicine at University College Hospital, to whom the work is dedicated. Dr Raste (*Riceyman steps*) is made to voice the age-old professional antagonism, 'I'm not a *specialist. He uttered the phrase with a peculiar intonation, not entirely condemning specialists, putting them in their place, regarding them very critically and rather condescendingly, as befitting one whose field of work and knowledge was the whole boundless realm of human pathology.'

Many of the failings of doctors exposed by writers of fiction continue to thrive; so much for the belief that artistic endeavour can change the world.

A. PATON

Further reading
Cousins, N. (ed.) (1982). *The physician in literature*. Saunders, Philadelphia.

Peschel, E. R. (ed.) (1980). *Medicine and literature*. Neale Watson, New York.

Posen, S. (1992). The portrayal of the physician in non-medical literature. *Journal of the Royal Society of Medicine*, **85**, 5–7, 66–8, 314–17, 520–3, 659–62

Posen, S. (1993). The portrayal of the physician in non-medical literature. *Journal of the Royal Society of Medicine*, **86**, 67–8, 128–9, 345–8, 410–12, 582–6.

Rousseau, G. S. (1981). Literature and medicine: the state of the field. *Isis*, **72**, 406–24.

Trautmann, J. and Pollard, C. (1975). *Literature and medicine. Topics, titles and notes*. Pennsylvania State University, Pennsylvania.

DOCTORS IN OTHER WALKS OF LIFE (MEDICAL TRUANTS). The idea seems to have emerged that doctors are a unique profession in deserting their calling for another. Some have even justified this in expansive terms, 'It has always been one of the salient characteristics of medical men in all countries, and at all times,' wrote Lord Moynihan in his *Truants*, 'that they have ardently followed other pursuits than that of their own profession . . . They have developed what the Greeks called *parergon*—work by the side of work.' The special relevance of medical experience to authors is discussed above (see DOCTORS AS TRUANTS

TO LITERATURE), and echoes Somerset Maugham's conclusion of the importance of medical training for a lesson about life, as well as giving an elementary knowledge of science and scientific method.

Nevertheless, we have no data to show whether medicine really has had proportionately more truants than others—the law, for instance, where 90 per cent of barristers are said never to make a satisfactory, permanent living, or Holy Orders, which can show some bizarre final occupations for some of its members. What follows, then, is an account, without any special claim, of the more distinguished or interesting truants from medicine, drawn largely from Dr Alec Cooke's contribution to the first edition of this book, Lord Moynihan's *Truants*, and 'Outside medicine', a series of articles published some years ago in the *British Medical Journal*.

Scientists
Berzelius, Joseph (1779–1848). Swedish chemist; made important contributions to theory and nomenclature.

*Black, Joseph (1728–99). Scottish chemist; discovered concepts of latent heat and specific heat.

*Boyle, Robert (1627–91). English chemist, a founder of the Royal Society; formulated Boyle's Law.

*Brown, Robert (1773–1858). Scottish botanist; discovered brownian motion.

*Copernicus, Nicolaus (1473–1543). Polish mathematician and astronomer; showed that the Earth and other planets revolve round the sun.

Flett, Sir John Smith (1869–1947). Scottish director of the Geological Survey of Great Britain and of the Museum of Practical Geology.

Forel, Auguste (1848–1931). Swiss authority on ants.

*Galvani, Luigi (1737–98). Italian expert on electricity.

*Gerard, John (1545–1612). English botanist; wrote *The herball*.

*Genser, Conrad (1515–65). Swiss professor of botany, natural history (and Greek).

*Gilbert, William (1540–1603). English pioneer on magnetism.

*Grew, Nehemiah (1641–1712). English botanist; first to recognize the existence of male and female sexes in the plant kingdom.

*Henry, Augustine (1857–1930). English botanist, having many genera and species named after him.

Hill, John (1716–75). English botanist; wrote *The vegetable system*.

*Hooker, Sir Joseph Dalton (1817–1911). English botanist, Director of Kew Gardens, and president of the *Royal Society.

Hutton, James (1726–97). Scottish geologist; emphasized the importance of volcanic action for the formation of rocks.

*Huxley, Thomas Henry (1825–95). English naturalist, who contributed fundamentally to the study of evolution; president of the Royal Society.

*Jenner, Edward (1749–1823). English naturalist; wrote in detail about the life and habits of the cuckoo.

Linnaeus, Carl (1707–78) (see LINNE). Swedish botanist, who introduced the modern system of biological nomenclature.

Lister, Martin (1638–1712). Scottish naturalist; expert on spiders and shells.

Mantell, Gideon Algernon (1790–1852). English geologist; his extensive collection of fossils was sold to the British Museum.

*Muffett, Thomas (1553–1604). English naturalist; wrote *Insects, or lesser living creatures*.

*Owen, Sir Richard (1804–92). English zoologist and president of the Royal Society.

*Petty, Sir William (1623–87). English founder of the Royal Society, and polymath; creator of economic science.

*Prout, William (1785–1850). English chemist; propounded the hypothesis that the atomic weights of all elements are exact multiples of either the atomic weight of hydrogen or half that of hydrogen (Prout's law).

Scarburgh, Sir Charles (1615–93). English mathematician; wrote a treatise on trigonometry.

*Sloane, Sir Hans (1660–1753). Irish botanist and collector, who refounded Chelsea Physic Garden; president of the Royal Society.

Stensen, Nicholas (1638–86). Danish geologist; distinguished between rocks containing fossils and those predating this period.

Thompson, Sir Henry (1820–1904). English astronomer, with his own observatory; he donated much apparatus to the Greenwich Observatory.

Thompson, John Vaughan (1779–1847). English marine biologist, who made important studies on barnacles, crabs, and other crustaceans.

Tyson, Edward (1650–1708). English zoologist, who published accounts of dissections of numerous different animals.

Ward, Nathaniel Bagshaw (1791–1868). English botanist; inventor of the wardian case.

*Wollaston, William Hyde (1766–1828). English chemist; invented the reflecting goniometer, enabling the exact measurement of crystals.

Woodward, John (1665–1728). British geologist; created the first geological museum, at the University of Cambridge.

The Church and humanists
*Barnardo, Thomas John (1845–1905). English instigator of the Custody of Children Act and founder of refuges for homeless children.

Chance, Frank (1826–97). Englishman, on the committee that prepared the *Revised version of the New Testament*.

Cogan, Thomas (1736–1818). English founder of the Royal Humane Society.

*Grenfell, Sir Wilfred Thomason (1865–1940). Scottish missionary who established local services in Labrador.

Hicks, John (1840–99). English Bishop of Bloemfontein.

Legg, John Wickham (1843–1921). English expert on the liturgy.

*Lettsom, John Coakley (1744–1815). English Quaker prison reformer; freed his slaves on his West Indian estates.

*Livingstone, David (1813–73). Scottish missionary in Africa; prominent in antislavery movement.

Petrus, Julianus (1215–77). Italian priest, who became Pope John XXI in 1276.

Secker, Thomas (1693–1768). English divine; successively Bishop of Bristol, Bishop of Oxford, Dean of St Paul's, and Archbishop of Canterbury.

*Schweitzer, Albert (1875–1965). Alsatian missionary (musician and philosopher) in the Congo.

Bibliophiles

Askew, Anthony (1722–72). The sale of his books and manuscripts took 27 days, the principal purchasers being the British Museum and the kings of England and France.

Bernard, Francis (1627–98). English linguist and scholar; his library contained 50 000 volumes.

*Keynes, Sir Geoffrey (1896–1985). English book collector and bibliographer of Berkeley, Blake, Hazlitt, Harvey, etc. After his death part of his collection passed to the Cambridge University Library.

Maty, Matthew (1718–76). Dutch–Huguenot Principal Librarian of the British Museum.

Mead, Sir Richard (1673–1754). English collector of books, manuscripts, statuaries, coins, gems, and drawings—said to be the largest collection of its time.

Morton, Charles (1716–99). English Principal Librarian of the British Museum.

*Osler, Sir William (1849–1919). Canadian scholar whose library after his death passed to McGill University, where it forms an important part of the university library.

Williams, Sir John (1840–1926). Founder of the National Library of Wales.

Linguists

Brown, Edward Granville (1862–1926). An expert in Islamic languages and professor of Persian at Cambridge University.

Good, John Mason (1764–1827). He knew 13 languages.

Latham, Robert Gordon (1812–88). Professor of English language and literature at University College, London, and an authority on the Scandinavian languages.

Leared, Arthur (1822–79). Wrote a book in Icelandic.

Macalister, Sir Donald (1854–1934). A Scotsman who spoke more than a dozen European and Eastern languages; while he was principal and vice-chancellor of Glasgow University it was said that the university had

no foreign visitors with whom MacAlister could not converse in their native tongues.

*Young, Thomas (1773–1829). An English polymath who helped to decipher the Rosetta Stone.

Zamenhof, Louis (1859–1917). The Russian who invented Esperanto.

The law and politics

*Addison, Sir Christopher (later Lord) (1869–1951). English member of Parliament: successively Minister for Munitions, Minister for Reconstruction, and (first) Minister of Health.

Bickersteth, Henry (later Lord Langdale) (1783–1851). English Master of the Rolls.

Clemenceau, Georges Benjamin (1841–1929). French Prime Minister and Minister of war.

Crosby, Sir Thomas (1842–1929). English Lord Mayor of London.

Elliott, Walter (1888–1958). Scottish politician; successively Minister for Agriculture, Secretary of State for Scotland, and Minister of Health.

Fernando, Sir Hilariose Marcus (?–1936). Sri Lankan statesman; Director of the State Mortgage Bank.

Finch, Sir John (1626–82). English ambassador to Turkey.

Finlay, Robert (later Viscount Finlay) (1842–1929). Scotsman; the only doctor to be appointed Lord Chancellor.

Foster, Walter Balthasar (later Lord Likeston) (1840–1913). Irish Member of Parliament, and Parliamentary Secretary to the Local Government Board.

*Huggins, Geoffrey (later Viscount Malvern) (1883–1971). English Prime Minister of the Federation of Rhodesia and Nyasaland.

*Jameson, Sir Leander Starr (1853–1917). English Prime Minister of Cape Colony; earlier led the Jameson Raid into the Transvaal.

Knighton, Sir William (1776–1836). English private secretary and keeper of the Privy Purse to the Prince Regent.

Marat, Jean Paul (1743–93). French revolutionary, stabbed to death in his bath by Charlotte Corday.

*Summerskill, Edith (later Baroness) (1901–80). English Minister of National Insurance.

*Sun Yat-Sen (1866–1925). Chinese revolutionary; first President of the Chinese Republic.

Tanner, Charles (1850–1901). Irish nationalist politician.

*Tupper, Sir Charles (1821–1915). Canadian High Commissioner in London and subsequently Prime Minister of Canada.

Wood, Leonard (1860–1927). US general who became successively governor of Santiago, Cuba, Moro, and the Philippines.

Philosophy

Bridges, John Henry (1832–1906). English authority on Comte and the editor of Roger Bacon's *Opus major*.

*James, William (1842–1910). US professor of philosophy at Harvard.

*Locke, John (1632–1704). English philosopher founder of political economy.

*Maimonides (1135–1204). Noted Jewish theologian and philosopher.

The arts

*Borodin, Alexander Porfiryevich (1833–87). Russian army officer and composer.

Cathcart, George Clark (1860–1951). English sponsor of the Promenade Concerts.

Haden, Sir Francis Seymour (1818–1910). English founder and President of the Royal Society of Painter Etchers.

Knowles, James Sheridan (1784–1862). Irish actor and playwright; colleague of Kean, Macready, and Kemble.

Neel, Louis Boyd (1905–81). English musicologist, conductor, and founder of an orchestra.

Tonks, Henry (1862–1937). English Slade professor of fine art at London University; among his pupils were Augustus John and William Orpen.

Wall, John (1708–76). English founder of the Royal Worcester Porcelain Factory.

*Wyndham, Sir Charles (1837–1919). English actor-manager.

Miscellanea

Birkbeck, George (1776–1841). English founder of the London Mechanics Institute, subsequently Birkbeck College.

*Caius, John (1510–73). English co-founder of Gonville and Caius College, Cambridge.

Gann, Thomas (1867–1938). English expert on Mayan archaeology.

*Gibbons, William (1649–1728). English introducer of mahogany into the UK.

*Grace, William Gilbert (1848–1915). The most celebrated of all English cricketers.

*Longstaff, Tom George (1875–1964). English Himalayan climber and member of the second Everest expedition in 1922; president of the Alpine Club.

*Moore, Francis (1657–1715). English originator of *Old Moore's almanac.*

*Park, Mungo (1771–1806). Scottish explorer of the Niger River.

Pim, Joshua (1870–1945). Irish tennis singles champion at Wimbledon 1893 and 1894, and doubles champion in 1890 and 1893.

*Stallard, Hyla Bristow (1901–73). English international and Olympic athlete.

Stokes, Lennard (1856–1933). English rugby player; secured Rectory field for the Blackheath Club.

In conclusion, some medical students who for various reasons did not qualify in medicine, but attained distinction in other walks of life, may be mentioned:

Berlioz, Hector (1803–69). Composer.

Brecht, Bertolt (1898–1956). Dramatist.

*Darwin, Charles Robert (1809–82). Zoologist, botanist, and geologist.

*Davy, Sir Humphry (1778–1829). Chemist.

Foucault, Jean Bernard (1819–68). Physicist who determined the speed of light.

*Galilei, Galileo (1564–1642). Physicist and astronomer.

*Galton, Sir Francis (1822–1911). Writer on anthropology, heredity, and eugenics.

Goethe, Johann Wolfgang (1749–1832). Poet, dramatist, and philosopher.

Leech, John (1817–64) . Caricaturist and cartoonist.

Smith, Sydney (1771–1845). Dean of St Paul's and a noted wit.

Thompson, Francis (1859–1907). Poet.

S. LOCK

Reference
Monro, T. K. (1951) *The physician as man of letters, science and action*, (2nd edn). Edinburgh and London.

Further reading
Moynihan, Lord (1936). *Truants*. Cambridge.
Munk, W. (1878–1968). *Roll of the Royal College of Physicians of London*. Vols i–v. London.
Smith, A. W. and Stearn, W. T. (1972). *A gardener's dictionary of plant names*, London.

DOCTORS WHO HAVE EXPERIMENTED UPON THEMSELVES, see SELF-EXPERIMENTATION.

DODDS, SIR EDWARD CHARLES, Bt (1899–1973). British clinical biochemist. When appointed to the Courtauld chair of biochemistry at the *Middlesex Hospital in 1925 he was the youngest professor in the university of London and became the leading clinical biochemist in the country. His researches on the *oestrogens were particularly noteworthy: he first synthesized diethylstilboestrol in 1938, and *aldosterone was discovered in his laboratory in 1952.

DOGMATIST. An adherent of the school of medical thought which grew up after the death of *Hippocrates; its chief characteristic was the assumption of a priori principles not derived from observation, investigation, or inductive reasoning.

DOGS AS CARRIERS OF DISEASE. The dog can only rarely be incriminated as the transmitter of human disease. The encephalomyelitis of *rabies is the most serious threat, from which the UK is protected by its stringent *quarantine laws; apart from Australasia and Japan, the distribution of rabies is world-wide, being particularly prevalent in Asia. *Hydatid disease occurs wherever a close association is found between dog, sheep, and man. The *helminth *Toxocara canis* is a common parasite of dogs, and may endanger young children through the ingestion of ova which have been excreted in the faeces; this is particularly likely to occur in toddlers playing with soil in public parks where dogs are exercised. Serious human infestation (larva migrans) is rare, but occasional tragic complications ensue, particularly endophthalmitis, retinal detachment, and blindness. Other known canine *zoonoses include *ringworm, *leptospirosis, and *salmonellosis.

DOMAGK, GERHARD (1895–1964). German experimental pathologist and chemotherapist. He undertook a systematic search for bactericidal agents and, in 1932, found that *Prontosil ® red controlled *streptococcal infection in mice. It was rapidly shown by French workers that this effect was not due to the dyestuff but to the *sulphonamide group which was split off from it in the body. It was the start of *antibacterial chemotherapy. In 1939 he was awarded the *Nobel prize for this discovery but the Nazis forbade him to accept. In 1947 he received the medal, but not the prize.

DOMINANCE is the expression of a genetic characteristic in a *heterozygote.

DOMINANCE, CEREBRAL. Dominance of one *cerebral hemisphere over the other is usually assessed by hand preference; on this criterion the great majority (96 per cent in some series) of individuals have left hemispheric dominance, i.e. they are right-handed, the remainder being either left-handed or of mixed handedness. In most people, including many left-handers, the left hemisphere controls speech and related functions; but there is a raised probability of right- or bilateral-hemisphere speech representation among left-handers. Most left-handers are, however, neurologically and cognitively normal. There is no evidence that atypical speech representation is in any way detrimental to normal development. (See also LANGUAGE, COGNITION, AND HIGHER CEREBRAL FUNCTION.)

DONDERS, FRANCISCUS CORNELIUS (1818–89). Dutch ophthalmologist. He undertook much fundamental research on the eye but was best known for separating the errors of refraction from those of accommodation. His major work *The anomalies of refraction and accommodation* (1864) was first published in English.

DONOR. In *transplantation or *transfusion, the donor is the organism from which the transplanted organ or tissue has been removed.

DOPAMINE is a naturally occurring monoamine which acts as an excitatory *neurotransmitter, notably in the *basal ganglia. Dopamine is formed by the decarboxylation of dopa (dihydroxyphenylalanine) and is an intermediate in the synthesis of the *catecholamines *adrenaline and *noradrenaline, and of *melanin.

DOSE. The quantity of a medicine (or the amount of radiation) to be administered to a patient at one time. In radiation physics the 'absorbed dose' is the energy imparted by ionizing radiation to unit mass of irradiated matter; it is measured in *rads (0.01 joule per kilogram) or in grays (Gy: 1 Gy = 10 rad).

DOSIMETRY is the measurement of an absorbed *dose of ionizing radiation.

DOUGLAS, JAMES (1800–86). Canadian psychiatrist. In 1832 he witnessed the arrival by ship of Asiatic *cholera to Quebec city, something he knew well from India. In 1845 Douglas and two other physicians, angered by the government's neglect of the 'insane', made a contract to look after their hospitalization. They acted under pressure from the governor-general, who was appalled at the previous inhumane treatment. Douglas devoted the remaining years of his life to the mentally ill in Quebec.

DOUGLAS, POUCH OF. See POUCH OF DOUGLAS.

DOVER, THOMAS (1660–1742). British physician and privateer. While training in London, Dover lodged with Thomas *Sydenham and in 1682 started practice in Bristol. In 1708 he sailed on a privateering voyage, during which a Spanish ship was captured. In February of the following year he discovered on Juan Fernandez Alexander Selkirk, the castaway who inspired Defoe's Robinson Crusoe. He later practised unsuccessfully in London. He was the author of *The ancient physician's legacy to his country* (1733), which contains the original prescription for 'Dover's Powder': opium, ipecacuanha, liquorice, saltpetre, and tartar vitroleus in equal quantities. The powder was once a favoured prescription for the alleviation of cough, pain, etc.

DOWN'S SYNDROME, also called trisomy 21 or mongolism, is a congenital disorder characterized by mental retardation and a variety of physical abnormalities, including the well-known facial appearance which gives the condition its common, but now outmoded, alternative name. It was described in 1866 by John Langdon Haydon Down. Although associated with a chromosomal abnormality (usually trisomy 21, i.e. an additional *chromosome in this position, making a total complement of 47 instead of the normal 46), the parents in most instances are genetically normal, the anomaly resulting from non-disjunction during the process of germ-cell formation. This type is commoner in children of older mothers, the risk rising from 1 per cent below the age of 40 to about 4 per cent at age 45. Less commonly, Down's syndrome results from other mechanisms, such as chromosomal translocation (see GENETICS), in which case it may be inherited from either parent and the risk of recurrence is relatively high (theoretically 25 per cent although actually rather less, probably as a result of countervailing selection processes). In all instances, of course, identical twins will each have the condition. For purposes of genetic counselling it is essential to distinguish the non-disjunction cases from the others. Prenatal diagnosis of Down's syndrome is one of the major reasons and justifications for *amniocentesis.

DOYLE, SIR ARTHUR CONAN (1859–1930). British physician and author. After unsuccessful practice in Southsea, Hampshire, Doyle turned to writing. His most successful novels were those recounting the adventures of Sherlock Holmes, an amateur detective, whose character was said to be founded on that of Joseph *Bell, Doyle's distinguished teacher of surgery in Edinburgh. The first of these stories was *A study in scarlet* (1887). His later years were devoted to spiritualism. (See also DOCTORS AS TRUANTS TO LITERATURE).

DRAINAGE is any procedure for allowing or facilitating the escape of fluid, pus, secretions, or effusions from a wound or body cavity.

DRAKE, DANIEL (1785–1852). American physician. Drake practised and taught clinical medicine in Lexington, Kentucky, and Cincinnati, Ohio. He travelled extensively in the Mississippi valley, acquiring information about epidemics of *malaria and other diseases indigenous there. He is regarded as one of the few contributors to medical knowledge in America during the first half of the 19th century.

DRAUGHT. A dose of liquid medicine (i.e. a potion).

DREAMS are the manifestation of partial, often irrational, *consciousness during sleep. They consist of a succession of images and emotions and may be accompanied by motor activity; they may or may not have a relationship to the events of waking life. Their occurrence is promoted by certain drugs, notably the *benzodiazepines, widely used as *sedatives and *hypnotics. In *psychoanalysis the study of dream content and patterns is valued as a method of examining subconscious thought processes. See also SLEEP.

DRESSING. Any protective covering for a wound, skin infection, etc.

DRINKER, CECIL KENT (1887–1956). American physiologist. He carried out extensive studies of pulmonary function and lymphatic circulation in the lungs. Later, with his brother Philip, he developed the Drinker *respirator, or '*iron lung', used in management of patients with *poliomyelitis who had respiratory paralysis. He also studied oxygen toxicity and *decompression sickness in divers and submarine personnel.

DRIP. Any *infusion (usually intravenous), the rate of which is controlled by observing and adjusting the frequency of drops in a drip-chamber.

DROPSY is an abnormal accumulation of fluid in the tissue spaces, that is *oedema.

DROWNING is death by submersion. The lungs fill with water, or else the *glottis reflexly closes to prevent this; in either case gas exchange ceases and death from *asphyxia ensues.

DRUG ADDICTION. See SUBSTANCE ABUSE.

DRUG REGULATION. In the UK the misuse of drugs is controlled by the Misuse of Drugs Act 1971, which came into operation in 1973. It consolidates and extends previous legislation and regulates the export, import, production, supply, and possession of dangerous or potentially harmful drugs. It is largely restrictive in its terms, the general effect being to render unlawful all activities involving the drugs controlled under the Act, except as provided in the regulations specified. The drugs subject to control are listed in Schedule 2 of the Act, and the term 'controlled drug' means any substance or product so listed. In the USA similar functions are fulfilled by the Federal *Food and Drug Administration.

DRUGS. A drug is any substance, organic or inorganic, used for medicinal purposes. Each drug may have several different names. In addition to its chemical designation, it will have an approved name, known as its generic or non-proprietary name, agreed in the UK by the *British Pharmacopoeia Commission. It is also likely to have at least one, and possibly several, proprietary names given by its manufacturers. Approved names may be followed by an indication of the drug's status, e.g. BP (*British Pharmacopoeia*), USP (*United States Pharmacopoeia*), BPC (*British Pharmaceutical Codex*), BNF (*British National Formulary*).

DRUGS PREVENTION OF MISUSE ACT 1964. This UK Act penalized the possession and restricted the importation of drugs of certain kinds. Those listed include: β-aminopropylbenzene, β-aminoisopropylbenzene, and most synthetic compounds derived from these; chlorphentermine; pemoline; *lysergamide, and N-alkyl derivatives of lysergamide; dimethyltryptamine; and *mescaline.

DRUNKEN DRIVING. Alcohol is a common cause, probably the main cause, of road accidents, which are a major cause of death and disability in young and relatively young people. Accordingly, most civilized countries have laws relating to drinking and driving.

In the UK, the Road Traffic Act of 1972 made it an offence to drive, to attempt to drive, or to be in charge of a motor vehicle while unfit to drive through drink or drugs, or while having a blood alcohol concentration of more than 80 mg/100 ml. Later legislation introduced breath analysis as the definitive test for alcohol, the legal upper limit being 35 μg per 100 ml of breath. The offence carries a penalty of up to 4 months' imprisonment or a fine of up to £100, or both, on a summary conviction, or up to 2 years' imprisonment and a fine on conviction or indictment. Except where there are special reasons, the person convicted must also be disqualified from holding a driving licence for a period not less than 12 months. Failure to provide a specimen for testing of blood alcohol concentration will also result in disqualification. Police are empowered to administer breath tests for alcohol to drivers whom they have reasonable cause to suspect of driving under the influence of alcohol, or who have committed a traffic offence, or who are involved in a traffic accident. They are not, so far, empowered to administer such tests totally at random. See also FORENSIC MEDICINE.

The legal limits for blood alcohol levels allowable in many Scandinavian countries are much lower, and in some instances a mandatory prison sentence is imposed. In the USA the laws vary greatly among different states.

DUBOIS-REYMOND, EMIL HEINRICH (1818–96). German physiologist. He was the first to show the existence of a resting current in nerve (1845) and to suggest that nerve impulses might be transmitted chemically (1877).

DUBOS, RENE JULES (1901–81). American microbiologist. In 1928 he began a lifelong association with the Rockefeller Institute (later Rockefeller University). In the department headed by O.T. Avery, he used his experience with soil organisms to find species capable of degrading *pneumococcal *polysaccharides. This goal was achieved, but the products were too toxic for therapeutic use; nevertheless the results encouraged others who developed such important products as *penicillin and *streptomycin. Dubos later discovered a bacterium antagonistic to other Gram-positive pathogenic cocci, and isolated two active substances: gramicidin and tyrothricin. Again these were too toxic for systemic use, but they could be used topically to treat surface infections. In the latter half of his career Dubos became a respected and effective philosopher and interpreter of biomedical subjects, writing several widely read books including: *The bacterial cell; So human an animal; Mirage of health; Choices that make us human; Pasteur; Free lance of science*; and *Man adapting*.

DUCHENNE, GUILLAUME BENJAMIN AMAND (1806–75). French neurologist. His name is associated with one form of *muscular dystrophy, the Duchenne type; Aran–Duchenne disease (progressive muscular atrophy) (see also NEUROMUSCULAR DISEASE); progressive bulbar palsy; lesions of the upper part of the

*brachial plexus (Erb–Duchenne palsy); and the distinction of central from peripheral facial paralysis.

DUCREY, AUGOSTO (1860–1940). Italian dermatologist. Ducrey discovered the bacillus named after him, *Haemophilus ducreyi*, which causes the sexually transmitted disease, *chancroid or soft sore.

DUCT. Any tube-like structure for the passage of fluid.

DUCTLESS. Having no duct. It is used of the endocrine *glands, the secretions of which pass directly into the circulation. See also ENDOCRINOLOGY.

DUCTUS ARTERIOSUS is a blood vessel which connects the *pulmonary artery to the *aorta and is an important component of the fetal circulation, allowing the cardiac output to bypass the, as yet non-functioning, lungs. At birth it closes, diverting blood from the right ventricle through the pulmonary circulation for oxygenation. Its abnormal persistence is known as patent ductus arteriosus and is one of the commoner forms of *congenital heart disease; when it occurs, some of the blood in the aorta is shunted back into the pulmonary artery, where the pressure is normally much lower, causing recirculation through the lungs.

DUKE-ELDER, SIR WILLIAM STEWART (1898–1978). British ophthalmologist. His chief contribution to medicine was his editorship of the *System of ophthalmology* (19 vols, 1958–76). He was largely instrumental in founding the Institute of Ophthalmology of London University in 1948, and was its first director.

DULLNESS. Impaired resonance on *percussion.

DUNANT, JEAN HENRI (1828–1910). Swiss humanitarian. After witnessing the battle of Solferino in 1859, where there were nearly 40 000 casualties, Dunant published *Un souvenir de Solferino* (1862). In this he proposed the formation of a voluntary relief society which later became the International *Red Cross. In furthering his aims he so neglected his business that he was made bankrupt in 1867 and lived in penury until 1895 when 'rediscovered' by a journalist. Thereafter he received many honours, an annuity, and in 1901 the first *Nobel peace prize.

DUNCAN, JAMES MATTHEWS (1826–90). British obstetrician. Duncan became an assistant to Sir James *Simpson in Edinburgh and co-operated in the experimental inhalation of *chloroform.

DUNLOP, SIR DERRICK MELVILLE (1902–80). Scottish physician. In 1963 he was invited by the Government to form the Committee on Safety of Drugs, becoming its first chairman and moving to the same post in the *Medicines Commission when it was established in 1969. He was largely responsible in the UK for the smooth introduction of effective measures to control medicines.

DUODENAL ULCER. See PEPTIC ULCER.

DUODENUM. The first part of the small *intestine (about 12 cm long), connecting the *stomach to the remainder of the intestine.

DUPUYTREN, BARON GUILLAUME (1777–1835). French surgeon and pathological anatomist. He stressed the importance of pathological anatomy and endowed a chair in this subject in Paris. He described a *fracture of the lower end of the fibula (1819), *congenital hip dislocation (1826), and his *contracture of the palmar fascia (1831) (see below).

DUPUYTREN'S CONTRACTURE is a form of *fibrosis which thickens and shortens the palmar fascia (the fibrous sheet underneath the skin of the palm of the hand), producing a flexion deformity of the fingers (usually most marked in the little and ring fingers) so that they cannot be completely straightened. The condition occurs particularly in older men, and can be improved by surgery.

DURA MATER. The outermost and the strongest layer of the *meninges, the three membranes enveloping the brain and spinal cord.

DUST DISEASE. See PNEUMOCONIOSIS.

DWARFISM, or smallness, is shortness of stature that is less than the third percentile for children of the same age and racial origin. There are many causes. It may be secondary to many general disorders when they occur in childhood before growth is complete, for example those associated with *malnutrition, *malabsorption, low cardiac output, *hypoxia, and *renal failure. Hormonal disturbances may be responsible, such as *hypothyroidism, *hypoparathyroidism, or *gonadal dysgenesis; or precocious puberty can cause premature fusion of the *epiphyses. Smallness may be due to primary skeletal abnormalities, particularly *achondroplasia, but also *rickets, *osteogenesis imperfecta, and *kyphoscoliosis from various causes.

The most important group for diagnosis and treatment are those resulting from failure of normal action of human pituitary *growth hormone (HGH). This may be due to panhypopituitarism, an iatrogenic cause of which is prolonged corticosteroid treatment for rheumatoid arthritis or asthma. Or the deficiency may be selective for HGH, which results in the pure or 'perfect' dwarf. Except in those where end-organ unresponsiveness is responsible (as in African pygmies) the logical and effective treatment is administration of HGH

itself, provided it is begun early enough, i.e. before the epiphyses have fused.

DYING DECLARATION. A declaration made by a person on his or her deathbed; it is legally admissible as evidence in a prosecution for homicide.

DYNAMOMETER. Any instrument for measuring power. In medicine, it is an instrument for measuring the force of muscular contraction, particularly of the hand grip.

DYSARTHRIA is difficult or unclear speech because of impaired functioning of the muscles involved in articulation.

DYSAUTONOMIA is a *recessive genetic condition, also known as the Riley–Day syndrome. The main features are: absence of tears, pyrexia, blotching of the skin, sweating attacks, insensitivity to pain, and defective growth. There appears to be a generalized defect of autonomic and sensory nerve fibres. The term is also sometimes used to identify any disorder of the *autonomic nervous system.

DYSCHONDROPLASIA is a rare congenital disorder of *cartilage growth, also known as Ollier's disease or multiple enchondromatosis. There is inappropriate and uncontrolled growth of cartilage cells, mostly within the shafts of long bones, giving rise to bowing and deformities, usually more marked on one side.

DYSCRASIA was originally any disordered condition of the body, but is now used almost exclusively in the phrase 'blood dyscrasia', to mean a pathological condition affecting the *blood cells.

DYSENTERY is inflammation and irritation of the large *intestine, giving rise to bloody *diarrhoea. The word is now used mainly for two types of intestinal infection: bacillary dysentery, due to bacilli of the genus *Shigella, and amoebic dysentery due to the protozoan *Entamoeba histolytica.

DYSFUNCTION is any impairment of function of a part, organ, tissue, or system.

DYSGENESIS is impairment of development.

DYSKINESIA is impairment of voluntary muscular movement. The term is often used to identify spontaneous involuntary movements due to disease of the *basal ganglia or to drugs such as *phenothiazines.

DYSLEXIA is word-blindness: that is, difficulty in reading or spelling not explicable by low intelligence and assumed to be associated with a specific central defect.

See also LANGUAGE, COGNITION, AND HIGHER CEREBRAL FUNCTION.

DYSMENORRHOEA (DYSMENORRHEA). Painful *menstruation.

DYSOSTOSIS is impairment of normal *ossification in fetal *cartilage, a cause of *dwarfism.

DYSPEPSIA is any form of *indigestion.

DYSPHAGIA. Difficulty in swallowing.

DYSPHASIA is impairment of language function due to brain damage (usually left-sided) causing defective speech, comprehension of speech, reading, and writing. See also LANGUAGE, COGNITION, AND HIGHER CEREBRAL FUNCTION.

DYSPHONIA is impairment of voice production (phonation), as for example in *clergyman's throat (dysphonia clericorum). Spasmodic dysphonia is a focal form of *dystonia affecting the vocal cords.

DYSPLASIA is disordered development or growth.

DYSPNOEA (DYSPNEA). Difficult or disordered breathing; shortness of breath.

DYSRHYTHMIA is synonymous with *arrhythmia.

DYSTONIA is a movement disorder, believed to result from dysfunction of the *basal ganglia of the *brain, characterized by involuntary muscular spasms which induce abnormal movements or postures. It may affect one part of the body, such as the muscles around the eyes (*blepharospasm) or those of a hand, foot, or the neck (focal dystonia, including *writers' cramp and spasmodic *torticollis); many parts of the body (segmental or multifocal dystonia); one arm and leg on the same side (hemidystonia); or the whole body (generalized dystonia).

DYSTROPHY is an abnormal nutritional state of tissue, or wasting; it is used particularly in respect of the so-called 'muscular dystrophies.'

DYSURIA is pain and/or difficulty in passing *urine.

EAR, NOSE, AND THROAT STUDIES. See OTO-RHINOLARYNGOLOGY.

EBERS PAPYRUS. The best preserved of the four principal medical papyri in existence (the others being known as the Berlin, the Hearst, and the *Edwin Smith papyri). It was found between the legs of a mummy in a tomb near Luxor, advertised for sale, and acquired by Professor Ebers in 1872. The papyrus (dated about 1550 BC) describes the elaborate *pharmacopoeia possessed by the ancient Egyptians, listing such preparations as pills, pastilles, snuffs, gargles, inhalations, ointments, poultices, bandages, suppositories, and enemata.

EBOLA DISEASE is one of the two varieties of African haemorrhagic fever or *Marburg disease, caused by a virus immunologically distinct from the Marburg virus. It is a severe (mortality rates of up to 90 per cent) fever with major haemorrhagic manifestations. The causative agent is a large, rod-shaped *ribonucleic acid (RNA) *virus.

EBSTEIN, WILHELM (1836–1912). German physician. He described diabetic nephropathy in 1881. His name is associated with the periodic fever sometimes seen in *Hodgkin's disease (Pel–Ebstein fever, 1887) and a congenital anomaly of the tricuspid valve (Ebstein's anomaly, 1866).

ECCHYMOSIS. Bluish irregular patch of discoloration due to the subcutaneous *extravasation of blood; a bruise.

ECCRINE describes glands that discharge their secretion through a duct, as opposed to *ductless or *endocrine glands; an equivalent term is exocrine. 'Eccrine' refers particularly to the sweat glands.

ECG is an abbreviation for electrocardiogram. See ELECTROCARDIOGRAPHY.

ECHINOCOCCUS is a genus of small *tapeworms, a species of which, *Echinococcus granulosus*, causes *hydatid disease.

ECHOCARDIOGRAPHY is examination of the structures and movements of the heart with reflected pulsed ultrasound. As a non-invasive investigation employing non-ionizing energy, it has become established as a useful additional method of evaluating heart disease. It is of particular value in *pericardial effusion, in mitral valve lesions, and in hypertrophic obstructive *cardiomyopathy. See also CARDIOLOGY; ULTRASONICS.

ECHOENCEPHALOGRAM. The record obtained by echoencephalography, the examination of brain structures with reflected pulsed ultrasound. Since the introduction of *computerized axial tomography, this method has been used less often (see also RADIOLOGY).

ECHOLALIA is habitual repetition by the patient of words and phrases spoken to him. It may be a developmental phenomenon in speech acquisition and in handicapped patients, having no particular significance. But in a person of normal intelligence, it is sometimes thought to suggest *schizophrenia. It is also characteristic of *Gilles de la Tourette syndrome.

ECHOPRAXIS is the meaningless automatic imitation by a patient of gestures and movements made by others.

ECHOVIRUS. *E*nteric *c*ytopathic *h*uman *o*rphan *virus*. Members of the *enterovirus group are associated with upper respiratory tract, gastrointestinal, and aseptic meningeal infections. 'Orphan' reflects the fact that at first no pathogenic role could be assigned to echoviruses.

ECLAMPSIA. *Encephalopathy complicating severe *toxaemia of pregnancy.

ECOLOGY IN RELATION TO MEDICINE. The relationship between environment and disease is largely dealt with elsewhere (see, for example, ENVIRONMENT AND MEDICINE I,II; OCCUPATIONAL MEDICINE). There remain several human maladies associated with specific natural ecosystems, mostly occurring in the relatively uncontrolled environments of the Third World and mostly due to *parasites. *Malaria is an obvious example, requiring the presence of the anopheline mosquito and of the natural conditions necessary for it to breed. *Onchocerciasis or 'river-blindness', another tragically burdensome disease, can be transmitted only in the vicinity of 'white' (i.e. rapidly moving) water, where the black fly (*Simulium damnosum*) breeds and transmits the infective larvae of *Onchocerca volvulus* to man. Schistosomiasis or *bilharziasis requires the presence of certain freshwater snails as intermediate hosts. And there are many other examples.

Sometimes disease may be controlled by controlling the environment, as witness the disappearance of malaria and leprosy from Europe in recent centuries, and the deliberate eradication of malaria from other areas in modern times. But interference with ecology may have the opposite effect of introducing hitherto non-existent diseases; this may occur, for instance, with schistosomiasis and the creation of large man-made lakes for hydroelectric schemes.

ECONOMICS, MEDICAL. See HEALTH-CARE ECONOMICS.

ECT. See ELECTROCONVULSIVE THERAPY.

ECTASIA. Dilatation or expansion, as of an organ or blood vessel or part of it.

ECTODERM. The outermost of the three germinal layers of the *embryo, from which are derived the skin and its various appendages, the nervous system, and the special sense organs.

ECTOMORPH. One of the three constitutional types in W.H. Sheldon's (1940) classification (the others being *endomorph and *mesomorph). The ectomorph is lean and cerebral, as a result of a supposed predominance of those tissues and organs derived from *ectoderm.

ECTOPIA is abnormal development of an organ or structure outside its usual location (e.g. ectopia cordis—heart outside the thorax; ectopia lentis—displacement of the ocular lens; etc.).

ECTOPIC BEATS are premature cardiac contractions initiated by an ectopic focus, that is by an area of *myocardium other than the normal *pacemaker in the *sinoatrial node of the right atrium. The term is virtually synonymous with *extrasystole, except that ectopic (or premature) beats are followed by a 'compensatory' pause before normal cardiac rhythm resumes, so that the total number of beats is unchanged; whereas a 'true' extrasystole is an interpolated additional beat. The distinction is not important clinically.

ECTOPIC PREGNANCY is pregnancy arising from implantation of the fertilized *ovum somewhere other than in the *endometrium, often in the *fallopian tube. Such an extrauterine pregnancy is usually short-lived, but may cause an acute abdominal emergency by rupturing the tube.

ECTROPION is the eversion of a margin or edge, usually of an eyelid.

ECZEMA is inflammation of the *skin. The term, by itself devoid of precise diagnostic significance, is most often used to mean *atopic *dermatitis.

EDDY, MARY BAKER (1821–1910). Mary Eddy was the discoverer and founder of *Christian Science. In childhood she suffered much invalidism, but was able to marry and have one child. From 1866 until about 1875, while partially incapacitated by a severe spinal illness,' she studied the New Testament extensively; this led to her formulation of Christian Science, the basic teaching of which is that God, Spirit, and His perfect spiritual creation are the only ultimate realities, and that the ills of mankind can be overcome through an understanding reliance on God's spiritual law by means of prayer. Her first book, *Science and health*, was published in 1875. It was revised several times and the later versions were called *Science and health with key to the scriptures*. She held many public meetings, attracting followers to her gospel, and eventually established the Christian Science Church.

EDEMA. See OEDEMA.

EDINBURGH ROYAL INFIRMARY was opened in 1729 as the first voluntary hospital in Scotland, and to help in the teaching of medical students from the university's newly created faculty of medicine (1726). The original infirmary had four beds. It later moved several times before becoming the great institution it is today. Early on it had maternity beds, and later a Lying-in Hospital which ultimately developed into the Edinburgh Royal Maternity and Simpson Memorial Hospital, opened in 1879, which was finally merged with the Royal Infirmary in 1939 as the Simpson Memorial Maternity Pavilion. A training school for nurses began in 1872, based on the teachings of Florence *Nightingale, who advised the infirmary at the start.

The roll of great names associated with the infirmary is enormous. Among them in medicine are *Cullen, *Argyll Robertson, and the *Monros. Those who qualified but did not practise in Edinburgh include *Bright, *Hodgkin, *Addison, *Corrigan, and *Colles. Others were Conan *Doyle, creator of Sherlock Holmes, who modelled his detective on the Edinburgh surgeon, Joseph Bell. In surgery were *Syme, *Lister, Spence, Fraser, Yarmouth, and Dott, and in obstetrics the Hamiltons, *Simpson, Matthew *Duncan, Croom, Milne Murray,

Freeland Barbour, Ballantyne, Haig Ferguson, and R.W. Johnstone.

EDITORS, MEDICAL. See MEDICAL JOURNALS.

EDRIDGE-GREEN, FREDERICK WILLIAM (1863–1953). He devised the sensitive methods currently used for the testing of *colour vision. He published *The physiology of vision* (1920).

EDWIN SMITH PAPYRUS. One of the four principal medical papyri in existence (see EBERS PAPYRUS). It was discovered in 1862 at Thebes by Edwin Smith, an American Egyptologist and bequeathed by him to the New York Academy of Medicine. It records 48 case histories classified according to the organ affected, and describes various injuries affecting males.

EEG. See ELECTROENCEPHALOGRAM.

EFFUSION. A collection of fluid within the body (e.g. pleural effusion: in the *pleural cavity).

EGAS MONIZ, ANTONIO CAETANO DE (1874–1955). Portuguese neurosurgeon, he was the first to carry out cerebral *angiography (1927) and frontal *leucotomy (1935). A man of many and varied talents, he wrote an operetta and was a distinguished historian and literary critic. He was elected to parliament in 1908, and became Foreign Minister in 1918. A political quarrel in 1919 led to a duel and his retirement from politics. He was awarded the *Nobel prize for medicine in 1949.

EGO. The conscious self. Freudian *psychology further elaborates this definition.

EHRLICH, PAUL (1854–1915). German haematologist, immunologist, and pharmacologist. Ehrlich's earliest interest was in *haematology. He learned histological staining methods from his cousin Carl *Weigert and applied these to the *leucocytes, developing the tri-acid stain and differentiating the various white cells (1879). He introduced the fuchsin stain for the *tubercle bacillus and the diazo test for *bile (1883). In 1896 he undertook the standardization of *antitoxin and, while accepting *Bordet's views on *bacteriolysis, introduced the terms 'amboceptor' and '*complement'. In 1899 he announced his 'side-chain theory' and subsequently sought for specific chemotherapeutic remedies for infectious diseases in his pursuit of the '*therapia sterilisans magna.' In 1910 he introduced the organic arsenical salvarsan (606; arsphenamine), the first drug with any pretensions to specificity in treating *syphilis. In 1908 he shared the *Nobel prize with *Metchnikoff for work on immunity.

EIJKMAN, CHRISTIAAN (1858–1930). Dutch physician. After training in bacteriology, Eijkman was sent to the Dutch East Indies to investigate *beriberi, then so widespread that an epidemic due to infection was suspected. He noted a beriberi-like syndrome in fowls which was cured when the diet was changed from polished to unpolished rice (1888). He showed that there was a factor in rice polishings which protected against beriberi in man. He shared the *Nobel prize with Gowland *Hopkins in 1929 for his work on accessory food factors (*vitamins).

EINTHOVEN, WILLEM (1860–1927). Dutch physiologist. Einthoven was professor of physiology at Leiden and devoted his life to studying electrical changes in the heart. In 1895 he devised the sensitive string galvanometer and subsequently recorded and worked out the characteristics of the human *electrocardiogram. He was awarded the *Nobel prize for this work in 1924.

EISELSBERG, ANTON FREIHERR VON (1860–1939). Austrian surgeon. He showed that removal of the *parathyroid glands during thyroidectomy caused *tetany (1890) and attempted their transplantation (1892).

EISENMENGER'S SYNDROME, COMPLEX, REACTION. The term Eisenmenger's syndrome refers to a form of *congenital heart disease in which pulmonary hypertension is present from early life and causes a reversed (right-to-left) shunt of blood, regardless of the level (aortopulmonary, atrial, atrioventricular, ventricular) at which the shunt takes place; the syndrome accounts for about 7 per cent of adult congenital heart disease. Eisenmenger's complex is the particular case in which the shunt occurs through a *ventricular septal defect. When pulmonary hypertension develops in later life (after puberty) as a pulmonary vascular reaction to increased blood flow through the lungs (due usually to a left-to-right shunt through an atrial septal defect), the term Eisenmenger reaction (or acquired Eisenmenger syndrome) is used.

EJACULATION is the emission of *semen which is the normal accompaniment of male *orgasm.

ELASTIC TISSUE is *connective tissue in which fibres of *elastin predominate.

ELASTIN is a *protein with elastic properties, fibres of which form the basic constituent of elastic tissue.

ELASTOSIS is any pathological condition affecting elastic fibres.

ELECTRICITY is fundamental in many bodily functions. Indeed, Galvani in the 1780s might be said to be the discoverer of electrical phenomena. He noted that a frog suspended from a metal railing twitched whenever a leg came into contact with the upright support. Now it is known that electrical currents of small power accompany nerve impulses, muscular contractions, the beating of the heart, and many other functions. Diagnostically these are found summated in *electroencephalography, in *electromyography, and *electrocardiography, from which impairment of function may be identified and its nature sometimes deduced.

ELECTRIC SHOCK. The first fatality due to electrocution was reported in 1879; since then electricity has been, and continues to be, a significant cause of death and injury, particularly from burns (approximately 1000 deaths annually in the USA). Although most serious cases involve electricity workers, many also occur in domestic settings, where minor and even fatal shocks are all too frequent.

The extent and severity of electrical injury vary with the intensity of the current and its path of flow through the body. The former is greater the higher the potential difference (voltage) between the points concerned and lower the greater the resistance offered. Skin and bone have high resistance, whereas blood, muscle, and nerve are good conductors, conductivity being roughly proportional to water content—hence the danger of skin moisture, and of electrical appliances in the bathroom. Even small currents can cause fatal cardiac ventricular *arrhythmias on passing through the heart. Cardiac and respiratory arrest can also result from high-voltage injury to the medullary centres of the brain. Another important variable is duration of current flow; alternating current is more dangerous than direct, partly because the tetanic muscle contractions it induces tend to prolong contact.

ELECTROCARDIOGRAPHY is the recording of the galvanometric deflections which accompany the cardiac cycle, the resultant record being termed the electrocardiogram or ECG. Since this may be done from *electrodes placed on the body surface, the technique is reliable, relatively cheap, and portable. Since its introduction by *Einthoven in the early 20th century it has become one of the most frequently performed investigations in modern medicine (see CARDIOLOGY). It is also one of the most useful, being essential in all forms of heart disease and often very helpful in conditions not primarily related to the heart, such as endocrine and metabolic disorders. It is 95 per cent accurate in diagnosing *myocardial infarction, and promptly elucidates most cardiac *arrhythmias. Interpreting electrocardiograms is not difficult to learn and several computer programs are now available for their automatic analysis.

ELECTROCONVULSIVE THERAPY (ECT) passes an electric current through the brain and induces temporary loss of consciousness accompanied by generalized epileptiform convulsions. Present practice is to administer a light general anaesthetic and a muscle relaxant drug before ECT. The major indication is *depressive illness refractory to treatment with drugs. See also PSYCHIATRY.

ELECTROCUTION is death caused by an *electric shock, or execution by means of electricity.

ELECTRODE. A conductor through which an electric current enters or leaves a medium or a vacuum; the positive electrode is the *anode*, the negative electrode the *cathode*.

ELECTRODIAGNOSIS is any diagnostic method employing electrical or electronic apparatus.

ELECTROENCEPHALOGRAPHY (EEG) records the electrical activity of the brain. See also CLINICAL INVESTIGATION.

ELECTROLYTE. A compound that in solution dissociates into *ions; the solution is then able to conduct electricity. Strong electrolytes are those which are completely dissociated, weak electrolytes those which dissociate only to a limited degree.

ELECTROMYOGRAPHY (EMG) records the electrical activity of *muscle. See also CLINICAL INVESTIGATION.

ELECTRON. The negatively charged elementary particle which is the planetary constituent of all atoms; the number of orbiting electrons determines the physical and chemical properties of an element apart from mass and radioactivity.

ELECTRONICS was once easy to define as the study of movement of free *electrons in a vacuum. Now it includes the movement of electrons in all materials and is a branch of electrical engineering making major contributions to developing computers, microchips, and vast numbers of instruments, many used in medicine. Virtually all investigative, diagnostic, and even therapeutic machines now use electronic theory and practice. Chemical, haematological, and other laboratories rely on them. Data are processed by them. Small electronic devices are inserted into the body, for example as a capsule to be swallowed which then transmits impulses to a recorder giving information about contractions of the alimentary canal. This is one form of telemetry. Cardiac *pacemakers are placed in the heart to control its rate of beating. More and more devices will surely be invented with the co-operation of doctors, scientists, technologists, and engineers. These small instruments can give information without a risk of potential harm resulting from serious invasion of the body. An outstanding recent example of this is the CT (*computerized tomography) scanner, which takes multiple images of the body that are then assembled by a computer to give diagnostic images. Outlines of many parts of the body are thus obtained, especially of the head and brain.

ELECTRON MICROSCOPY employs a beam of *electrons instead of a beam of light to illuminate the object under study. *Resolution is limited by the wavelength of the illumination; the short wavelength of electrons enables magnifications of up to 200 000 times to be achieved.

ELECTRONYSTAGMOGRAPHY is a method of recording eye movements such as *nystagmus electrically whether they occur spontaneously or are induced by optokinetic or caloric stimulation.

ELECTRO-OCULOGRAPHY. Recording and interpretation of electrical potentials generated by eye movements.

ELECTROPHORESIS is the migration of the electrically charged solute particles present in a colloidal solution towards the *electrode with opposite charge when two electrodes are placed in the solution and a potential difference is applied to them. It is a technique widely employed in biochemical analysis, for example in the separation and study of *plasma proteins.

ELECTROPLEXY is a synonym for *electroconvulsive therapy.

ELECTROTHERAPY is the direct use of electrical energy in medical treatment. The first book on this subject, by Kratzenstein, appeared in 1745, the same year as the invention of the Leyden jar; and by 1830 *Duchenne was treating patients with *faradic (interrupted) current. Direct electrotherapy is used nowadays to produce muscular contractions as an aid to muscular re-education and for passive exercise in certain neurological conditions. High voltages are applied briefly in treating cardiac ventricular fibrillation (see CARDIOLOGY). Repetitive stimulation of the heart is the function of cardiac *pacemakers, employed in cases of *heart block where the intrinsic heart rate is too slow. Repetitive stimulation of the phrenic nerve, diaphragm, and abdominal wall muscles has similarly been employed as a form of *artificial respiration. Iontophoresis (or *ionotherapy) is a method of introducing ionized drugs (e.g. alkaloids such as histamine, local anaesthetics) through the skin by applying an electric charge. Other current research concerns the stimulation of growth and repair processes by electrical energy, including the treatment of non-united fractures, and the use of electricity to control incontinence and sexual dysfunction.

ECT (*electroconvulsive therapy) is used in psychiatric treatment, chiefly of depression.

ELEPHANTIASIS is brawny swelling of the skin and subcutaneous tissue due to chronic lymphatic obstruction by filarial worms (see FILARIASIS). The legs and genitalia are often involved, producing the striking elephantine appearance.

'ELEPHANT MAN'. Joseph Merrick (1860–90), a severely deformed sufferer from multiple *neurofibromatosis (von Recklinghausen's disease), was exhibited as a freak ('the Elephant Man') in sideshows at fairs in England and Belgium. He was rescued from this sad life by Sir Frederick *Treves, in 1886; Treves arranged his admission as a permanent resident in the *London Hospital until his death in 1890. The story of Merrick aroused public interest and Merrick was the subject of a well-known essay by Treves himself, recently retold in a popular book (M. Howell and P. Ford (1980), *The true history of the Elephant Man*, London) from which a play and film were made.

ELIXIR. A liquid mixture of drugs with syrup and alcohol or chloroform water.

ELLIOTSON, JOHN (1791–1868). British physician who was one of the founders of and first physicians to, *University College Hospital. Elliotson was an outstanding clinical teacher and an early 'stethoscopist', but he became obsessed with *mesmerism and *phrenology and, because his views were unacceptable, resigned his hospital appointments in 1838. He died 30 years later in penury.

ELLIS, HENRY HAVELOCK (1859–1939). British physician: Ellis was a pioneer in the scientific study of sex (see SEXUALITY AND MEDICINE). His researches were embodied in his *Studies in the psychology of sex* (6 vols, 1897–1910). He also produced popular editions of literary classics.

EMACIATION. Extreme wasting; *cachexia.

EMASCULATION. *Castration of the male; the removal of masculine characteristics.

EMBALMING is the chemical preservation of dead bodies.

EMBOLISM is the *occlusion of an *artery by a *thrombus, air bubble, fat globule, or other material which has travelled to the point of blockage from elsewhere through the blood stream.

EMBOLUS. A mass of material which has travelled from elsewhere through the bloodstream to occlude an artery (e.g. a thrombus, a fragment of cancerous or other tissue, a fat globule, an air bubble, etc.).

EMBRYO. A developing organism. In man the term is used for the stages between 2 and 8 weeks after *conception; before then the embryo is a fertilized ovum (*zygote); afterwards a *fetus.

EMBRYOLOGY is the science of study of the formation and development of the *embryo.

EMERGENCY SURGERY. See SURGERY OF TRAUMA.

EMETIC. Any drug, substance, or procedure that induces *vomiting. With the possible exception of pharyngeal stimulation and the administration of an *ipecacuanha mixture, attempts at removing ingested poisons with emetics (e.g. sodium chloride, mustard, copper sulphate, and apomorphine) are unreliable and dangerous.

EMETINE is a naturally occurring *alkaloid formerly used in the treatment of *amoebiasis. It is toxic, particularly to the heart, and has now largely been replaced by *metronidazole.

EMI SCAN is now an outmoded term: the first *computerized tomography (CT) scanners were made by the British firm EMI.

EMOTION is the basic mental process of feeling, also known as affect, as distinct from the processes of knowing (cognition) and willing (conation).

EMPEDOCLES of Acrages (now Agrigentum) (*c.* 492–*c.* 432 BC). He held that there were four elements: earth, water, fire, and air. These were eternal and unchanging. Nothing was ever created nor destroyed, only transmuted. Health was due to a balance of the elements, disease to an imbalance. He believed that the blood ebbed and flowed through the vessels. He died by throwing himself into the crater of Mount Etna.

EMPHYSEMA is distension of tissue with air. In pulmonary emphysema, the lungs are permanently and irreversibly over-inflated, the air sacs being both distended and formed into larger units by partial destruction of their walls. Subcutaneous (or 'surgical') emphysema is air in the subcutaneous tissues following trauma or surgical operation.

EMPIRICISM was one of the post-Hippocratic schools of medical thought and practice. Unlike the *Dogmatists, with whom they were coeval, the Empiricists rejected theory and based their system on observation and experiment. Symptomatology and therapeutics

were the two major components of their approach, the later being further subdivided into pharmacology, surgery, and dietetics. However, empiricism later became synonymous with ignorance, unscientific thought, and quackery.

EMPLOYER'S LIABILITY (DEFECTIVE EQUIPMENT) ACT 1969. This Act imposes 'strict liability' on UK employers. Under it, if an employee is killed or suffers personal injury as a result of a defect in equipment provided by the employer, then the latter is deemed to have been negligent regardless of where the fault actually lies. The plaintiff employee, or next of kin, recovers damages from the employer, whether or not the employer is indemnified by the supplier, installer, or maintainer of the equipment.

EMPYEMA is a collection of *pus in a body cavity, unless otherwise stated the *pleural cavity.

ENCEPHALINS. See ENKEPHALINS.

ENCEPHALITIS, or inflammation of the brain, results from severe central nervous system infections, especially by certain viruses. Type 1 *herpes simplex virus is the commonest cause of endemic fatal encephalitis in adults, and has a mortality rate of about 70 per cent; encephalitis in the newborn is usually due to type 2 herpes simplex associated with maternal genital herpes infection. The commonest variety of mild encephalitis is due to *mumps, but many other organisms may be responsible, including *enteroviruses (*polioviruses, *Coxsackieviruses, and *echoviruses), arthropod-borne or *arboviruses (about 30 geographically named types), and *adenoviruses (including *rabies). Encephalitis was a rare complication of *smallpox vaccination and may still follow childhood infections such as *measles. Clinically, encephalitis is suggested when, to the characteristic headache, fever, and neck stiffness of *meningitis are added progressive depression of consciousness and focal neurological signs.

ENCEPHALITIS LETHARGICA ('sleeping sickness') occurred in a world-wide *pandemic, especially in Europe, in the 1920s; it was presumed to be due to a virus, but no organism was ever isolated. It was often fatal, caused a typical reversal of sleep rhythm with nocturnal wakefulness and daytime sleepiness, and was often followed in survivors by post-encephalitic *parkinsonism.

ENCEPHALOMYELITIS is any inflammatory condition affecting both the brain and spinal cord.

ENCEPHALOPATHY is any degenerative or other non-inflammatory pathological condition of the brain, acute or chronic.

ENCYCLOPAEDIAS OF MEDICINE. Historical pride of place must go to the famous *Naturalis historica* of Pliny the Elder (AD 23–79), dealing with man and healing as well as other parts of natural science. Pliny claimed that it contained 20 000 facts culled from 200 authors. It was, moreover, an encyclopaedia in the true and original sense, i.e. a work arranged for systematic study rather than occasional reference, as are the alphabetical encyclopaedias of today. Although the feat has sometimes been attempted in the past (e.g. *Cyclopaedia of practical medicine* (1834–5), no modern work exists with full claim to the title, although many large and definitive textbooks are available for such subdivisions of the whole as internal medicine, surgery, paediatrics, and so on. Some of the general English language encyclopaedias (e.g. *Britannica, Chambers', Everyman*) include some coverage of most medical topics and major biographies. Perhaps closest come the important medical dictionaries (Dorland, Black, Stedman, Taber, Butterworth, Blakiston, Churchill, Wiley) and the *British Pharmaceutical Codex*.

ENDARTERECTOMY is surgical removal of the diseased inner layer (*intima) of an artery.

ENDEMIC. Continuously prevalent in some degree in a community or region.

ENDOCARDITIS is *inflammation of part of the endothelial lining membrane (endocardium) of the heart, particularly of that overlying one or more of the heart *valves.

ENDOCARDIUM. The *endothelial membrane lining the chambers of the heart.

ENDOCRINE GLANDS are ductless and release *hormones directly into the blood or other extracellular fluids. The major endocrine glands are the *pituitary, the *thyroid, the *parathyroids, the *adrenals, the *pancreas, and the *gonads (ovaries and testes).

ENDOCRINOLOGIST. A physician specializing in disorders of hormone production by the *endocrine glands.

ENDOCRINOLOGY is the study of the regulation and function of the endocrine glands and the action of *hormones. The word 'endocrine' derives from the Greek and was first used in 1913 to describe glands which secrete substances into the blood, unlike the 'exocrine' glands, which release their products through a duct. The concept of 'internal secretion' had been developed earlier, and the term 'hormone' for 'chemical messengers' or effectors was introduced in 1905. The major endocrine glands each produce one or more unique hormones, whose synthesis, structure, and mode of action

have been largely defined. The boundaries of endocrinology, however, have been greatly extended with the discovery that many tissues other than the endocrine glands secrete their own hormones and growth factors, which may have 'autocrine' (self-regulatory), 'paracrine' (regulating effects in the vicinity of the producer cells), or endocrine roles. Furthermore, disordered function of the immune system is now known to cause some of the most common endocrine diseases.

Endocrinology arose from clinical and later experimental observation. The physical and emotional effects of castration in the male had long been recognized, and in the 19th century the manifestations of a number of diseases which are now known to be endocrine were described. In 1871, *Fagge attributed *cretinism to congenital absence of the thyroid gland, in 1873 *Gull described a similar but acquired disease in adults, and in 1883 *Kocher described the same clinical picture after surgical removal of the gland. *Semon suggested that all these conditions were the result of the loss of thyroid function, and in 1891 Murray reported successful treatment with thyroid extract. Many studies of the effects of removal of apparently functionless glands led to definition of the endocrine system. These were followed by efforts to isolate and purify the active compounds, to define their chemical structure and mode of action.

Hormones can be divided broadly into three categories, namely 'peptides' (small proteins), 'steroids' (derivatives of cholesterol), and 'amines'. All are synthesized in specialized cells, where they are stored until released in a controlled fashion. The hormones are not in solution in blood but are loosely bound to specific transport proteins; a fraction is 'free' and it is this free hormone which is active. A further complexity is that some hormones (e.g. *thyroxine and *testosterone) are secreted as inactive prohormones and subsequently converted to the active form. Hormones may have a single target organ or may affect many different tissues. Peptide hormones do not enter their target cells but combine with specific receptors on the cell surface; this act of combination transfers the message into the *cell and initiates a variety of processes, often ending in modulation of *gene activity. Steroid hormones and the major amine hormone thyroxine enter cells and bind to individual receptor proteins, the resulting complex interacting with the *DNA of specific genes in the cell nucleus.

Hormone secretion is closely regulated. At its simplest there may be a direct connection with what is to be controlled (e.g. parathyroid hormone acts to increase the concentration of calcium in the blood, but its secretion is inhibited by calcium and normally an equilibrium is maintained). The most complex hormonal regulatory systems are integrated by the *hypothalamus in the brain, mediated by the pituitary gland, and given effect through the thyroid, adrenals, and gonads. Both the size and hormone output of the latter glands are determined by individual hormones (thyroid-stimulating hormone,

TSH; adrenocorticotrophic hormone, ACTH; luteinizing hormone, LH; and follicle-stimulating hormone, FSH) produced by specific cells in the anterior pituitary gland. The hypothalamus regulates the secretion of the pituitary hormones by producing its own stimulatory or inhibitory hormones, which it releases into small blood vessels linking it directly to the anterior pituitary. The hormones of the thyroid, adrenals, and gonads can themselves inhibit the effects of hypothalamic hormones on the pituitary and the release of the hypothalamic hormones by the hypothalamus itself. The whole operates as a negative feedback control system, but the hypothalamus is also able to impose rhythmicity (e.g. circadian) and to integrate environmental influences.

The hypothalamus

The hypothalamus is not only an important regulatory centre but produces a range of small peptide-releasing and release-inhibiting hormones, which control the anterior pituitary. Two hormones, arginine vasopressin (AVP) and oxytocin, are made in the hypothalamus and are transported through nerve *axons to the posterior pituitary, where they are stored until released. AVP acts on the kidney to conserve water; its release is associated with thirst and may be induced by falls in blood pressure. Oxytocin is released during *parturition, when it causes uterine contraction, and by suckling, when it causes milk ejection.

Tumours and other destructive lesions of the hypothalamus can cause a variety of endocrine disorders, mostly because of secondary failure of anterior and posterior pituitary function. AVP deficiency results in production of large volumes of urine, a condition known as *diabetes insipidus, and is treated with a synthetic analogue.

The pituitary gland

The pituitary gland is divided into two anatomically distinct parts, anterior and posterior. The gland is anatomically and functionally connected to the *hypothalamus of the brain. Another important anatomical relation is to the *optic chiasm, which lies immediately above; *tumours of the pituitary gland expanding upwards may cause visual-field defects. The posterior pituitary is essentially an outgrowth of the hypothalamus. The anterior pituitary comprises different cell types which produce six peptide hormones: FSH, LH, TSH, and ACTH, which have already been mentioned, and also growth hormone (GH) and prolactin.

Growth hormone induces production of another growth factor, insulin-like growth factor I (IGF-I), from the liver, and both are essential for growth. GH secretion is controlled by hypothalamic growth hormone-releasing hormone (GHRH), although the hypothalamus also produces a hormone which inhibits secretion of both growth hormone and many other hormones (somatostatin). Growth hormone deficiency is a rare cause of growth failure; it is most often due to inability to produce GHRH, but may be due to hypothalamic or pituitary tumours. Growth hormone deficiency is treated by injections of genetically engineered GH. Excess production of GH and IGF-I before puberty results in *gigantism, and, after puberty, in *acromegaly. Patients with acromegaly characteristically have coarse features, large hands and feet, thick greasy skin, and enlargement of the viscera. Gigantism and acromegaly are due to benign tumours of GH-producing cells; the treatment is surgical although drugs and *radiotherapy may ameliorate the condition.

Prolactin promotes lactation. It has no known function in men or in women other than in the *puerperium. The secretion of prolactin is unusual in that its secretion is persistently suppressed by the hypothalamus; therefore while hypothalamic disease results in general pituitary failure it is associated with an increase in prolactin output. Increased prolactin secretion may cause inappropriate lactation (galactorrhoea) and can interfere with the regulation of LH and FSH secretion, producing *amenorrhoea and infertility in women and decreased libido in men. Small prolactin-secreting tumours are relatively common and may be treated with drugs or surgery.

Adrenocorticotrophic hormone (ACTH), which regulates the adrenal cortex, is a peptide of 37 amino acids cleaved out of a larger peptide molecule, part of which also affects the pigment cells of the skin. ACTH over-production may result in pigmentation, while suppression results in a failure to tan on exposure to sunlight. Excess production of ACTH by small pituitary tumours over-stimulates the adrenal cortex, leading to excess secretion of glucocorticoid steroids and is one cause of *Cushing's syndrome (see below). Treatment is by surgery, radiotherapy, or drugs. ACTH deficiency is usually part of general pituitary failure and is treated by giving adrenal steroids.

The gonadotrophins, LH and FSH, and TSH are chemically similar. Pituitary tumours secreting TSH and causing thyrotoxicosis (see below) are very rare. Tumours secreting fragments of gonadotrophins are not uncommon but are usually 'functionless', being unaccompanied by distinct hormonal syndromes, although they may enlarge to cause pituitary failure (*hypopituitarism) through compression of the pituitary gland within its bony confines at the base of the skull. Other causes of hypopituitarism are *thrombosis of its blood supply following post-partum haemorrhage (*Sheehan's syndrome), adjacent tumours of the brain, and autoimmunity.

The thyroid gland

The thyroid gland lies in the neck across the front of the trachea. It produces the prohormone thyroxine and its active derivative triiodothyronine which regulates the level of metabolic activity in many tissues. Thyroxine contains four atoms of the trace element iodine and the thyroid gland has the capability to capture iodide from the blood. Dietary deficiency of iodine results in a failure of thyroid hormone synthesis, with consequent increase in TSH leading to enlargement of the thyroid gland (*goitre). Moreover iodine deficiency in the fetus impairs brain development, causing mental retardation (*cretinism); world-wide iodine deficiency is one of the major public health issues with an estimated 200 million people affected. Disorders of the thyroid gland make up a large part of the practice of clinical endocrinology; they are more common in women than in men, and in England about 4 per cent of women will develop a disorder of thyroid hormone production and 10 per cent will have an enlargement of the gland. In many patients in England thyroid disease, often with goitre, is the result of an *autoimmune process, causing antibody-mediated tissue damage or alteration in function by the generation of antibodies which can combine with the TSH receptor to stimulate the gland. Elsewhere in Europe nodular development secondary to iodine deficiency is common. Benign and malignant tumours of the thyroid are not rare. Any thyroid swelling is regarded as suspicious until its nature is defined; some require excision. Most thyroid cancers are curable by surgery with or without treatment with radioactive iodine.

Thyrotoxicosis is the clinical state induced by overproduction of triiodothyronine, resulting in increased metabolism in most tissues, while hypothyroidism is the converse situation. Thyrotoxicosis, which is often episodic, may be treated with drugs to control thyroid hormone production or, if persistent, by destruction (with radioactive iodine) or removal of part of the gland (surgery). Hypothyroidism is simply treated by giving thyroxine which can be converted in peripheral tissues of the body to the active triiodothyronine.

The adrenal glands

The adrenal glands lie atop each kidney and consist of two parts: an outer cortex and inner medulla. The adrenal cortex produces steroid hormones: cortisol, which affects carbohydrate and protein metabolism and reduces inflammation, and aldosterone, which increases sodium transfer across membranes, particularly in the kidney. The size of the adrenals and cortisol secretion are both determined by ACTH from the pituitary, whereas aldosterone secretion is regulated by the separate renin–angiotensin system. An excess exposure to cortisol causes Cushing's syndrome, characterized by obesity, plethoric moon-face, thin skin, muscle weakness, and fatigue. This picture is most often due to administration of large doses of steroids for therapeutic purposes, but may result from ACTH-producing tumours or tumours of the adrenal cortex. Overproduction of aldosterone (*Conn's syndrome) causes high blood pressure or weakness, and may be due to a tumour or over-development of the secreting cells. Treatment of these conditions is determined by definition of the cause. Destruction of the adrenal cortex

(by autoimmunity, infection, or tumour deposits) causes *Addison's disease, which is usually insidious with non-specific symptoms of fatigue, anorexia, and weight loss, with skin pigmentation due to excess ACTH synthesis. The disorder is treated by administration of appropriate amounts of often synthetic steroids. The adrenal medulla is a specialized part of the *autonomic nervous system and releases *catecholamines (adrenaline and noradrenaline) in response to stress. Catecholamine-secreting tumours (phaeochromocytoma) are a rare cause of hypertension or paroxysmal headaches or palpitations; most arise from the adrenal medulla.

The gonads: ovaries and testes

The gonads, ovaries and testes, are endocrine glands producing sex hormones as well as, respectively, ova and spermatozoa. The hormones, oestrogen in the female and testosterone in the male, are steroids which largely determine the physical and emotional changes at puberty and maintain the secondary sexual characteristics (such as breast development and body shape in women, and beard growth and musculature in men) and libido throughout adult life. The production of both is determined by the hypothalamic–pituitary system. Pulsatile release of gonadotrophin-releasing hormone from the hypothalamus regulates the differential secretion of LH and FSH.

The ovulatory cycle in women reflects a complex sequence of hormonal events: at the outset FSH stimulation progressively increases oestrogen production, initially from several but later from one dominant ovarian follicle; the latter grows rapidly towards mid-cycle, producing a rise in oestrogen which triggers a sudden surge in LH secretion which is followed, 36 hours later, by ovulation (release of an ovum from the dominant follicle); the follicle then forms the corpus luteum which produces progesterone, another steroid, as well as oestrogen; the corpus luteum has a limited life of 10 days, at the end of which progesterone and oestrogen production fall, which is the signal for initiation of the next cycle. If the ovum is fertilized, the conceptus produces human chorionic gonadotrophin, a hormone similar in structure to LH and FSH, which maintains the corpus luteum and progesterone production necessary for continuation of the pregnancy. Oestrogen and progesterone both prepare the uterus during the cycle for implantation of the fertilized ovum; if this does not occur the late-cycle fall in these hormones results in spasm of the uterine blood vessels, necrosis of the tissue lining the uterus, and menstruation. Infertility may be due to failure of any component of this sequence. Treatment of infertility in the woman requires precise definition of the cause. The modern practice of reproductive endocrinology often involves the hormonal manipulation of the sequence. The female menopause occurs when the supply of potential follicles is exhausted, with consequential fall in oestrogen production.

In the adult male, testosterone is produced in the

*Leydig cells of the testis, under the stimulus of LH. The production of spermatozoa is controlled by testosterone and FSH, and is a continuing process.

In both men and women sexual development and fertility may be abnormal because of chromosomal abnormalities (commonly loss of an *X chromosome in a woman, resulting in *Turner's syndrome; or in a man the presence of an additional X chromosome, causing *Klinefelter's syndrome), failure of embryonic gonadal development, and genetically determined resistance of tissues to particular hormones, or abnormal synthesis of hormones. These various conditions, most of which are rare, may not be obvious at birth and may become apparent only because growth or puberty, or both, are delayed.

The parathyroid glands
There are four parathyroid glands, which lie behind the thyroid. They produce parathyroid hormone (PTH), a peptide hormone which interacts with vitamin D to control the level of calcium in the blood. PTH liberates calcium from bone and increases the retention of calcium by the kidney. The secretion of PTH is inhibited by a rise in calcium in the blood. Vitamin D, although present in food, is mostly produced in the skin when exposed to sunlight, and is now regarded as another steroid hormone. Ingested or produced vitamin D is inactive, but it is processed first in the liver and then in the kidney (under the influence of PTH) to the active steroid, which increases calcium absorption from the gut and is essential for normal bone formation. Lack of vitamin D causes rickets in children or softening of the bones (*osteomalacia) in adults. Excess PTH or vitamin D results in a rise in calcium in the blood, which may cause non-specific symptoms. Small PTH-secreting tumours arising in one of the four glands are not uncommon; they can be excised surgically.

The endocrine *pancreas
The endocrine pancreas comprises clumps of cells (islets of *Langerhans) distributed throughout the exocrine gland. The islets comprise specialized cells producing the hormones *insulin, *glucagon, and somatostatin. The former two hormones are concerned with carbohydrate metabolism and are discussed under *diabetes mellitus. Somatostatin is also found in the central nervous system and is a representative of an expanding class of small peptide hormones involved in the regulation of gastrointestinal function, which also act as transmitter substances in the nervous system.

Although hormones are generally produced by specialized cells, their genes are present in all tissues. Malignant transformation of a cell may result in the expression of such a gene and the unregulated production of a hormone from an unusual site. Syndromes of 'ectopic hormone production' are well recognized (e.g. oat cell carcinomas of the lung producing either ACTH or AVP). Interestingly, the high blood calcium associated with some cancers may be due to the activation of a gene product, parathyroid hormone-related peptide, which is not normally expressed.

R. L. HIMSWORTH

ENDODERM. The innermost of the three germinal layers of the *embryo, from which are derived most of the alimentary tract, the lungs and respiratory tract, and the bladder and urethra.

ENDODONTIST. See DENTISTRY IN THE UK AND USA.

ENDOMETRIOSIS is a condition in which fragments of tissue resembling the uterine mucous lining (endometrium), and subject to the same variations in phase with the menstrual cycle, occur in other organs and tissues, giving *dysmenorrhoea and other symptoms. See also GYNAECOLOGY.

ENDOMETRIUM. The mucous membrane lining the cavity of the *uterus. Its thickness and vascularity vary with the phase of the menstrual cycle, and it is partially shed at *menstruation, along with some blood.

ENDOMORPH. One of the three constitutional types in W.H. Sheldon's (1940) classification (the others being *ectomorph and *mesomorph). There is a supposed predominance of tissues derived from *endoderm, leading to a soft roundness of the body with prominence of the digestive organs and truncal *adipose tissue.

ENDOMYOCARDIAL FIBROSIS. A form of *cardiomyopathy of unknown aetiology first described in Uganda, in which there is invasion of the endocardium and the inner part of the myocardium by fibrous tissue. The function of one or both ventricles is impaired, and there is often overlying mural thrombosis. The condition is rare in temperate countries, but is now established to be the cause of a significant proportion of cases of heart failure occurring in tropical Africa, America, and Asia.

ENDOPLASMIC RETICULUM. An internal system of membranes found in most cells on ultrastructural examination. Part of the endoplasmic reticulum, known as the granular reticulum, or ergastoplasm, bears large numbers of *ribosomes. See also CELL AND CELL BIOLOGY.

ENDORPHINS are a class of naturally occurring *polypeptide substances produced within the body which combine with opiate *receptors and raise the threshold to pain; they are also referred to as natural opiates or opioid peptides, and include the two pentapeptide compounds known as methionine enkephalin and leucine enkephalin. The endorphins may be relevant to *acupuncture *analgesia.

ENDOSCOPY is examination of part of the interior of the body by visual inspection through an instrument (endoscope) designed for the particular cavity or region under investigation. Modern endoscopes are flexible internally illuminated optical tubes, the design and range of which have been greatly extended by the development of *fibre-optics.

ENDOTHELIUM. The layer of cells lining the interior of the blood vascular system, the lymphatic system, and the serous membranes.

ENDOTOXIN is a toxic material liberated by disintegrating bacterial cells (as opposed to an *exotoxin, which is secreted by intact bacteria). Endotoxins are lipopolysaccharides found particularly in Gram-negative *bacteria and are potent pyrogens (i.e. cause fever).

ENDOTRACHEAL TUBE. A tube, often surrounded by an inflatable cuff, inserted into the *trachea to maintain a clear *airway in situations where this might otherwise become obstructed (e.g. general *anaesthesia and other unconscious states), and to allow artificial ventilation.

END-PLATE. A specialized structure forming the junction between a motor nerve fibre and a muscle fibre, through which the nerve impulses stimulate the muscle fibre by the release of *acetylcholine. See also NEUROMUSCULAR DISEASE.

ENEMA. A liquid injected into the rectum. It is most often used to empty the bowels of faeces.

ENERGY, the capacity for work, properly expressed in terms of the derived *SI unit, the joule (defined as the work done when a force of one newton acts over a distance of one metre). In practice, the calorie, the unit of heat (the amount of heat required to raise the temperature of one gram of water through one degree Celsius), is still used in physiology and medicine to express energy values, the unit employed being the larger calorie or kilocalorie (equal to 1000 calories). The calorie is equivalent to 4.1868 joules. The convenient SI replacement unit for the kilocalorie is the megajoule (MJ), equivalent to 239 kilocalories. See also CALORIE REQUIREMENTS IN HEALTH; ENERGY REQUIREMENTS.

ENERGY REQUIREMENTS. Energy requirements are increased when the metabolic rate is raised (e.g. fever, *thyrotoxicosis, *neoplasia, hyperkinetic cardiac states, etc.) and reduced when it is lowered, as in *myxoedema and with advancing age. See also CALORIE REQUIREMENTS IN HEALTH.

ENGLISH SWEAT was a mysterious illness, also called sweating sickness, which appeared in 1485 and caused a number of *epidemics with a high mortality rate over the next 100 years, after which it seems to have disappeared. It was possibly a form of *influenza.

ENKEPHALINS. Two pentapeptide compounds, methionine enkephalin and leucine enkephalin, belonging to the group of naturally occurring opioid substances called *endorphins and found in various parts of the central and peripheral nervous system as well as in some other body tissues such as the adrenal medulla and gastrointestinal tract. The precise physiological role of the enkephalins is not fully elucidated, but they are thought to act as *neurotransmitters involved in processing painful and perhaps other sensory stimuli.

ENOPHTHALMOS is a sinking in or retraction of the eyeball into the orbit.

ENTAMOEBA HISTOLYTICA is a protozoan parasite which causes human *amoebiasis.

ENTERIC FEVER is an alternative name for *typhoid and *paratyphoid fevers.

ENTERITIS is a non-specific term embracing any condition involving *inflammation or irritation of part of the *intestine. See also CROHN'S DISEASE.

ENTEROTOXIN is an unsatisfactory term, since it is used in both possible senses: for a bacterial toxin originating in the intestine and causing *toxaemia; and for a substance which is toxic to intestinal cells, particularly that responsible for staphylococcal *food poisoning.

ENTEROVIOFORM® is a proprietary name for *clioquinol, formerly used as an antidiarrhoeal agent. See also SUBACUTE MYELO-OPTIC NEUROPATHY.

ENTEROVIRUS is a genus of small *ribonucleic acid (RNA) viruses pathogenic to man, whose entry is by the gastrointestinal tract. It includes the *poliovirus, *Coxsackievirus A and B, and the *echovirus groups, together with some more recently recognized members which fit into none of these three groups and are known simply as enterovirus (with a series number).

ENTROPION is inversion of an edge, usually of the eyelid.

ENURESIS. See BEDWETTING.

ENVIRONMENT AND MEDICINE I: PHYSICAL EFFECTS
Force and energy
The damage inflicted upon the body by physical forces is related to two factors: the total amount of energy supplied and the speed with which this energy is released. The human body has very limited capacities for absorbing or dissipating energy. The reason that fatalities in

motor accidents are so much greater at higher speeds is that the amount of energy produced is related to the square of the velocity. That is, twice the speed gives rise to four times the energy. This is even more marked when very high speeds are involved; the effect of a high-velocity bullet hitting a limb can be literally shattering, causing widespread tissue damage and fragmentation of bone, for which *amputation may be necessary. In the examples of other types of physical effect, given below, similar energy changes are the ultimate cause of damage, although not all changes are as severe or as sudden as a car crash, and some disorders are due to the body's response or attempts at repair. By contrast, loss of energy from the body is the cause of cold injury.

Vibration

To some degree vibration may be involved in the production of motion-sickness, particularly when the whole body is affected, as it may be in fighter aircraft. When localized, for example to the hands of those using vibrating tools, it can lead to 'white fingers' (*Raynaud's syndrome). This condition is due to spasm of the smaller arteries of the fingers.

Motion-sickness

Seasickness is the best known form of motion-sickness but perhaps not the commonest, for many are affected by motion in cars or buses. The organs that detect motion, called the semicircular canals, are situated in the inner ear. Diseases affecting these organs, such as labyrinthitis or *Ménière's disease, may produce symptoms similar to those of seasickness, that is *vertigo, nausea, and vomiting. It is possible to become conditioned to motion. Most people will not be affected by seasickness after 3 days, but some are completely incapacitated and never seem to adapt. Drugs may control motion-sickness, but their testing suffers from the difficulty of giving a standardized dose of motion, and many have unpleasant side-effects, such as dryness of the mouth which makes swallowing difficult. Consequently, the effectiveness of motion-sickness remedies is to be judged largely by their reputation amongst users. When drugs are necessary they need to be taken before exposure to motion. This is easily managed when boarding a plane or ferry but not so easily in a shipwreck or sinking. Many ships now carry inflatable liferafts, which are more easily launched than rigid lifeboats but have the disadvantage that their motion in the sea is quite violent. Most occupants will suffer from severe motion-sickness and may be unable to help themselves. A recent development, which could be useful in these circumstances, is the administration of drugs through the skin by means of a small patch, rather like a sticking plaster.

Sound

Noise as a cause of *deafness has led to regulations designed to protect hearing, either by limiting exposure or by using ear protection. The use of ear-defenders when using a chainsaw is a sensible precaution and, incidentally, a good example of preventive medicine. However, not only chronic exposures cause damage. Temporary, or even permanent damage, may be caused to the sound-sensitive cells within the inner ear by the very loud sounds of explosions or gunfire.

Light

The direct effects of light upon the skin are *sunburn and the development of the pigment *melanin, which we recognize as a 'tan'. There are both good and bad things to be said about sunlight. Without it we may fail to develop sufficient vitamin D; this can cause rickets in the young or brittle bones in the old. Too much sun can lead to a type of skin tumour called a *melanoma. Lasers, which are particularly coherent beams of light, are used in eye surgery, as the heat which they give up on contact with tissue can be very finely controlled. Lasers have been used to reattach the retina, where this has become detached, and also to alter the curvature of the eyeball in those with excessive short sight.

X-rays and ionizing (nuclear) *radiation

These physical factors are of diagnostic and therapeutic value, as well as having potentially harmful effects. Their importance can be gauged by the fact that their use has produced the specialties of *Radiology and *Nuclear medicine. Small and harmless amounts of radiation exist in the environment; natural radiation is given off by certain rocks and minerals. An example is the radioactive gas, radon, which has been detected in houses built over granite-bearing rocks.

Heat and cold

Body temperature is relatively constant at about 37 °C (98.4 °F) and is actively controlled within a range of a few degrees. There is usually a balance between the heat produced in the body from food (metabolic heat production) and the heat lost from the body in different ways. This balance can be upset, either by additional heat energy from outside or by greatly increased heat loss. There is then a net gain or loss of heat. A gain in heat causes a rise in temperature (*hyperthermia), and a loss causes a fall in temperature (*hypothermia). Within narrow limits these can be offset by sweating or shivering, but body temperatures below 25 °C or above 43 °C are generally incompatible with survival. Terrestrial extremes of temperature range from about −88 °C to +57 °C and survival in such conditions depends almost entirely on adequate protection.

Extreme environments

Many regions of the world have climates that are, from the physiological point of view, intolerable; yet people live there. The way in which they achieve this is by cultural and behavioural adaptation. Shelter and clothing produce a microclimate which changes less than the outside conditions. This allows physiological mechanisms to operate within their tolerance limits. A practical difficulty in considering heat is that it arrives in so many different forms: direct radiation from the sun; hot winds, such as the sirocco; heat due to interference with sweating; and heat conducted through the soles of the shoes. Because of the difficulties of adding the effects of these different forms of heat, ventilation engineers and physiologists have had to use bioassay, that is, the study of the physiological disturbances produced when the proportions of the different types of heat are changed. Assessment of how hot the surroundings are is most simply done by measuring the difference between the ordinary shade temperature and comparing it with the wet-bulb temperature. The smaller the difference, the greater the humidity and the greater the discomfort.

Cold climates

In countries which regularly experience severe weather conditions, individuals learn how to avoid the more extreme forms of injury such as *frostbite, which usually occurs accidentally. Even in temperate climates many are affected by a less severe but equally dangerous form of cold, namely immersion in water. The temperature of sea water, even in summer, around the coast of Britain limits survival time to a few hours and the fresh water of ponds, rivers, and canals in winter is often colder than the sea. It was estimated that two-thirds of fatal naval casualties during the Second World War died of drowning or exposure. At 15 °C most unprotected survivors will die within 6 hours; the importance of finding them within this time is obvious. In polar waters survival times are much shorter, death normally occurring within the hour. Much thought has gone into providing some sort of insulation that can be put on quickly before entering the water, but more thought needs to be given to the entry itself. Jumping into water from only 10 m can be a painful and dangerous experience. Some of those who abandoned the SS *Lakonia* were injured leaving the ship, which may have further reduced their ability to survive in what are usually thought of as warm seas. A less common type of cold injury, which was well recognized in the First Word War, is trench or *immersion foot, now more commonly referred to as non-freezing cold injury. This is not like frostbite, in which tissues are damaged by being frozen. Cold, particularly wet cold, may affect the tissues directly by damaging nerve fibres. It may also damage blood vessels, causing constriction of small arteries and even clots within the vessels; treatment has to be empirical. Fortunately, many cases recover completely, but some have minor residual symptoms such as patches of numbness.

Electricity and magnetism

Lightning strikes, at potentials of thousands of volts, cause a small number of fatalities each year, but even electric currents at potentials of only 240 volts carry the risk of producing a fatal shock. There were 27 deaths in England and Wales from accidental *electrocution in 1990. Such accidents are particularly likely if the current passes across the body, when it may stop the heart from beating. Dry hands or gloves, and shoes with rubber soles protect. A residual current device (RCD) should be available for outside use of electricity, such as grass- or hedge-cutting. If such devices detect a fault, due to the leakage of current through the body to earth, they switch off the current, within milliseconds, preventing serious shock. Minor shocks may only cause superficial burns, particularly if the hands are dry. A number of investigations have failed to find definite evidence that living under powerlines affects one's health. Theoretically the magnetic fields caused by the flow of current within such cables could affect the weak electrical activities within human cells but, so far, it seems that they do not.

Low pressures

The air above the surface of the Earth is acted upon by the force of gravity, so that it is more dense at sea-level and less dense at altitude. The standard pressure, exerted by this mass of gas, usually referred to as atmospheric pressure, is 101.325 kPa (760 torr). The higher one climbs, the less is the barometric pressure, and at a height of 5800 m it is approximately halved. At the summit of Mount Everest (8847 m) the pressure is about one-third of an atmosphere. The gases that form the atmosphere are: nitrogen, 79.9 per cent; oxygen, 20.4 per cent; argon, 0.9 per cent; carbon dioxide, 0.03 per cent; and water vapour. If air is breathed at such an altitude the oxygen pressure is equivalent only to about 6.3 per cent of 1 atm. This dependence of oxygen pressure upon height is the reason for the pressurization of aircraft. Most civil aircraft are pressurized to give a cabin pressure equivalent to an altitude of 6000 ft (80 kPa). One sits at an altitude equivalent to that of Everest while breathing at the slightly reduced oxygen pressure of about 16 per cent of 1 atm. A potentially fatal complication of low oxygen levels in the inspired air is *pulmonary *oedema. This condition, which can attack climbers, particularly those not acclimatized to altitude, leads to increasing difficulty in breathing, due to the lungs filling with fluid.

High pressures

Speech

Divers and pressure-workers are both exposed to raised pressures, either in the sea or within, nominally, dry environments. One effect, which is noticeable at moderate pressures, is a distortion of the voice. This 'Donald Duck' sound is due to the alteration of density and hence the speed of transmission of sound within the vocal apparatus. In helium-diving, special devices have been developed to decode this distorted speech.

Narcosis

At depths of 100 m (330 ft) the nitrogen gas contained in air exerts an effect like that of a narcotic drug. This was first noticed as causing a number of persistent but ill-defined problems. Divers at these depths were unreliable, sometimes seemed to have *hallucinations, and often did not complete their tasks. The reason for this behaviour was discovered in 1936, and the solution was quite simple: this was to breathe a mixture of oxygen with some other gas which was not narcotic. It is now known that nitrogen, argon, krypton, xenon, and neon all have narcotic properties, whereas helium and hydrogen are much less narcotic, if at all.

Oxygen

Although essential to life, oxygen at raised pressures is poisonous to a wide range of organisms. For humans, this effect first occurs at about 2 atm. The toxicity shows itself as generalized *convulsions. Convulsions under water are particularly dangerous and have led to deaths. Prevention involves calculation and judgement. To avoid oxygen poisoning one must avoid breathing oxygen at pressures above 2 atm, but to avoid *asphyxia one must not breath less than about 10 per cent of 1 atm. When diving, the oxygen pressure depends on the total pressure, which itself depends on depth. Using a 20/80 oxygen/nitrogen mixture (air) therefore allows one to go to a limit of 100 m, for at this depth the oxygen pressure is 2 atm. If pure oxygen is used, this limit would be reached at a depth of 10 m. Diving over a range of depths obviously requires the use of more than one breathing mixture, which must consist of oxygen in combination with another gas or gases, usually helium or helium and nitrogen.

Decompression

Decompression means the removal of pressure. The reason why decompression causes illness is an indirect one, due to the fact that a raised pressure causes gases to dissolve in the blood and tissues of the body. When the pressure is reduced the gases come out of solution and form bubbles. These bubbles cause decompression sickness, also commonly called the 'bends'. The solubilities of respired gases vary over a wide range and are usually expressed as the number of millilitres (ml) dissolved in 1 ml of water under a pressure of 1 atm and at a defined temperature (the figures given are for 20 °C). The most soluble gas in air is carbon dioxide (0.88 ml) and the next most soluble is oxygen (0.031 ml) However, mechanisms exist in the body to transport and exchange these gases as part of the normal processes of respiration. There is no such mechanism for nitrogen, which has a solubility of 0.154 ml. The body does not, however, consist entirely of water and, significantly, the solubility of nitrogen is some five times greater in fat. At a pressure of 1 atm the human body has dissolved in it some 800 ml of nitrogen, sufficient to cause decompression sickness in aviators or in space-walkers. Prevention in these cases

involves washing-out the nitrogen dissolved in the body by breathing oxygen. This must be carried out prior to decompression.

This is by no means an exhaustive catalogue of physical effects but, within the constraints of space, it is intended to illustrate some general principles and to pick out examples, either of importance or of interest.

E. E. P. BARNARD

ENVIRONMENT AND MEDICINE II: POVERTY AND HEALTH—A GLOBAL PERSPECTIVE. The association between poverty and ill-health is most obviously seen in the Third World, where over 1 billion people live in absolute poverty. In 1960, the richest 20 per cent of the world's population had incomes 30 times greater than the poorest 20 per cent. In 1990, the difference had increased to 60-fold. Disparities can also be considerable within countries, the worst example being Brazil, where the richest 20 per cent have an income 26 times that of the poorest 20 per cent (United Nations Development Programme 1992).

The mechanisms of the relationship between poverty and disease are numerous. They include educational disadvantage; lack of provision of health care; inadequate *nutrition, clean water, and shelter; cultural beliefs about the causation of disease; and the deleterious effects of war and conflict on the infrastructure of society. Although income is an important factor in determining health, economic growth does not invariably lead to improvements in health. Many of the mechanisms linking economic growth and human development at the national level are missing at the international level. Income tax and expenditure policies on areas such as education and health within countries help to redistribute wealth and enhance well-being to deprived sectors of the population. Such mechanisms do not operate at an international level.

Recognition of the limitations of traditional economic measures of development, such as growth in gross national product (GNP), has led to the introduction of other indicators. For instance, the United Nations Development Programme introduced the Human Development Index (HDI) in 1990. It combines life expectancy, adult literacy, and the purchasing power to buy commodities for satisfying basic needs. The HDI ranks countries in relation to each other. Clearly, there are limitations in the use of a composite index such as this, but it has been useful in drawing attention to the need to consider development in more than purely economic terms. Modifications to the HDI include a gender-sensitive HDI, which takes into account disparities between the sexes, and an income distribution-adjusted HDI, which takes into account inequalities in income.

The World Summit for Children in 1990 was dominated by the recognition that 40 000 children were dying every day, largely from preventable causes. Fourteen million children under the age of 5 years die every year. The immediate causes of more than 60 per cent of deaths are *diarrhoeal disease, *measles, *tetanus, whooping cough (*pertussis), and *pneumonia. These are all conditions that can be prevented or treated at very low cost. Several countries with a relatively low GNP (under US$1500 per person per year; US$1.50 = £1) have succeeded in bringing their under-five mortality rates to relatively low levels (under 50 per thousand). These include China, Sri Lanka, and Thailand. The Summit set 22 specific targets to be achieved by the year 2000, including the elimination of neonatal tetanus, the provision of *family planning education and services to be made available to all couples who wish to have them, and a 95 per cent reduction in deaths from measles.

In some respects, there have been considerable advances in public health; for instance, the rate of immunization in children in the Third World has increased from 15 per cent just over 10 years ago to around 80 per cent by the end of 1990 (UNICEF 1991). Vaccines prevented over 2.5 million child deaths in the Third World in 1990. There has also been a rapid rise in the use of oral rehydration therapy. The technique was little used at the beginning of the 1980s but by the end of that decade it was being taught to nearly one-third of families in developing countries. By 1988, it was preventing 1 million deaths per year from *dehydration secondary to diarrhoea.

Some disparities between developed and developing countries, such as life expectancy, nutritional level, *infant mortality, child mortality, access to safe water, and adult literacy, have narrowed between 1960 and 1990. The gap in other indicators of human progress, such as enrolment in tertiary education, expenditure on research and development, mean years of school, and the number of scientists and technicians per thousand is increasing. In general, the least developed countries are tending to improve their level of development at a lower rate than the rest of the developing world.

Several factors are responsible for the continued gap between rich and poor countries. One factor is the level of international debt. In 1983–89, for instance, there was a net transfer of US$242 billion from indebted developing countries to creditors. The total external debt of Third World countries has increased by a factor of 13 in the last 20 years. The debt of sub-Saharan Africa is currently around US$150 billion (equivalent to 100 per cent of its gross national product), although currently many African countries are paying back very little. It has also been suggested that the lack of market opportunities for developing countries costs them at least US$500 billion a year. Against this, overseas development assistance (ODA) runs only at US$ 54 billion a year, the equivalent of around 0.35 per cent of the combined GNP of industrial countries. This is well below the UN target of 0.7 per cent. Only a quarter of the aid goes to 10 countries which have about 25 per cent of the world's most impoverished people. Countries that spend more than 4 per cent of GNP on military activities receive about twice as much aid per capita as countries which spend less on military matters. Expenditure on crucial aspects of human development forms a small proportion of ODA. For example, basic education, primary health care, provision of safe water, family planning, and nutrition are allocated only 6.5 per cent of ODA.

There is concern that food production will not keep pace with population growth. Grain production on a per capita basis is likely to decline in the 1990s.

There has been a tendency over the past decade for growth in income to be slower in countries with faster population growth. The medium projection of the United Nations predicts a population of 10 billion in 2050, and a plateau of just over 11.6 billion in 2150. The next 40 years will see the fastest growth in human numbers ever recorded. Around 97 per cent of the increase will be in today's developing countries. Voluntary policies and programmes can be highly effective in encouraging reductions in *fertility. For example, in 1965 a typical Thai woman had 6.3 children, and in 1987 only 2.2. The importance of education of women has been shown by examples such as Kerala in India, where the female literacy rate of 66 per cent is almost double that of any other state in India. It has the lowest infant mortality in the country and a fertility rate of only 2.3 children per woman, with a prevalence of contraceptive use three times the national rate. The state government has given priority to spending on education and health and has distributed spending in an equitable manner.

In addition, it is of course important to expand the delivery of contraceptive services using a range of techniques to permit individual choice. To reach the medium population projection, the number of couples practising contraception will have to rise from 381 million in 1990 to at least 567 million by the year 2000. This will involve doubling the resources to population activities from 4.5 billion to 9 billion US dollars annually. This is a modest sum and amounts to about four days' world-wide military expenditure.

Poverty and health in 'developed' countries

There is much evidence that health inequalities exist between occupational classes in developed countries. For instance, in the UK, a working group under the leadership of Sir Douglas Black completed a review on inequalities of health in 1980. The report received a negative reception from the then Secretary of State, Patrick (now Lord) Jenkin. There was an attempt to minimize the impact of the report by the government, which refused to consider additional expenditure recommended by the group. Nevertheless, it stimulated a great deal of discussion and research over the ensuing years. It concluded that the poor health experienced by the lower occupational groups was noticeable at all ages. If mortality rates of occupational class I (professional workers and members of their families) had been experienced by classes IV and V (partly skilled and unskilled manual workers and their families), 75 000 deaths of people aged under 75 years, including nearly 10 000 children, would have been avoided. The report noted that the gap in mortality rates had increased within the 20 years up to the early 1970s.

In the case of infant mortality, a threefold increase in the mortality rates for children of skilled manual workers compared with children of professionals is particularly due to marked disparities in deaths from accidents and respiratory disease. Between the ages of 1 and 14 years, the differences between social classes narrow but are still in evidence. Again, accidents show the sharpest gradient in mortality, but differences in infective and parasitic diseases and disease of the respiratory system are also clearly evident. Among adults, the social class difference is particularly large for those in their 20s and 30s. Marked gradients are seen for accidents, *poisoning, and violence (particularly in males). Marked gradients are seen in both sexes in diseases of the respiratory system and lesser gradients in diseases of the circulatory, digestive, and genitourinary systems.

A major study of over 17 000 civil servants in Whitehall showed that men in the lowest employment grade had three times the mortality rate than those in the highest grade from *coronary heart disease and from a range of other causes. A number of risk factors for coronary heart disease, such as *smoking, *obesity, physical inactivity, and *blood pressure were more common in the lower grades. However, these factors explained only part of the observed difference in mortality (Marmot *et al.* 1984).

Influences in early environment are suggested by the association of short stature with an increased risk of coronary heart disease. Recently, a number of studies undertaken in Southampton by Barker and colleagues (1989) have indicated that factors operating *in utero* and early life may increase cardiovascular risk. For instance, they have shown that among men born 70 years previously, those who had lower birth weights and weights at 1 year had higher death rates from coronary heart disease. Since low birth weight is commoner amongst women from lower social classes, this may be a mechanism by which deprivation has an impact on health in the long term.

Local environmental influences, including the quality of housing, may have an impact on health. Work environment is also perceived differently between different grades. Jobs that provide little opportunity to learn and develop skills, and in which there is little opportunity to exert any control over working conditions, may be associated with an increased risk of cardiovascular disease. Exposure to noxious agents and injury at work may be higher amongst unskilled workers.

Other studies have investigated morbidity or general health status. These are important indicators of inequality because people are now living longer, and degenerative diseases take a long period to become evident. The annual General Household Survey (Office of Populations, Censuses and Surveys) asks people about both chronic and acute sickness. The social class gradient is most pronounced for long-standing illness which limits activity, particularly in the age-group 45–64 years. Self-reported disease and psychosocial ill-health (including inability to sleep and to concentrate, etc.) are also more likely amongst individuals from lower social classes. Other measures of relative social deprivation also relate to health. These include educational level, housing type, and income.

International studies suggest that mortality differentials between social classes are found in a range of European countries. It is difficult to compare the magnitude of social class differentials between countries because of the problems of standardizing measures. A study comparing mortality differentials according to educational level in Hungary, Finland, England and Wales, Denmark, Sweden, and Norway showed that a greater number of years of education was associated with lower mortality amongst males in all these countries. The association was somewhat less consistent for women. For all of these countries, except Hungary, changes between the early and late 1970s were studied. An increase in the inequalities over this period was noticeable only in the case of England and Wales.

In the UK, the gap between rich and poor is now greater than at any time since official records began in 1886. The number of people living on less than half the average income—the European community's definition of poverty—increased by a factor of more than two from 1979–88. Depending on the definition, between 20 and 25 per cent of children were living below the poverty line in 1988.

Four types of explanation for health inequalities were mentioned in the Black report: artefactual, selection, cultural or behavioural, and materialist. An artefactual relationship might occur, for instance, if social class were to be recorded differently on death certificates than at the census. Also, if the size of lower class groups were to decrease, it could be argued that these might contain a greater proportion of individuals at high risk of premature death. If unhealthy people moved down the social scale, this might explain in terms of selection the association between poor health and socio-economic status. There has been a great deal of research on behavioural components of the social gradient in health, and, clearly, cigarette smoking is responsible for part of the gradient. It seems unlikely that life-style is the whole explanation of differences, because the gradient in mortality seems to be higher for many causes, including areas not thought to be related to 'life-style'. The Black report described as materialist those explanations for socio-economic differences in health which involved differences in exposure to hazards to which poor individuals were more likely to come into contact because of the current distribution of wealth. These might include occupational exposures, physical and chemical hazards, poor-quality housing, and exposure to environmental factors operating *in utero* or early life. It seems likely that behavioural and materialist explanations are both relevant to the understanding of socio-economic differences in health. Differential access to health care probably explains only a small part of the social-class gradient in health.

Differentials in health can be seen at all socio-economic levels, including in the advantaged groups, such that, for instance, in the UK, non-manual home owners with two cars have lower mortality rates than those with only one car.

Unemployment has been associated with poor health in a number of studies. After adjusting for social class, Moser and colleagues (1987) found an excess mortality of 20–30 per cent among the unemployed, which did not seem to be a consequence only of health-related selection for unemployment. Raised standardized mortality ratios were noted for *suicide, lung *cancer, and *ischaemic heart disease. The mortality of wives of unemployed men was also higher than that of other married women. Studies of the health effects of unemployment in Calne, Wiltshire, by Beale and Nethercott (1988) showed an overall increase in morbidity, which did not seem to be explained by lower symptom tolerance. They suggested that unemployment led to chronic ill-health, and a recorded increase in consultations for cardiovascular disorders and other chronic complaints, which may have been in part psychosomatic.

Indices of deprivation have been developed. They have been used for a number of purposes, including (in the case of the underprivileged area score) the calculation of supplementary payments to *general practitioners who work in areas of deprivation in the UK, in an attempt to compensate for increased workload. The commonly used indices include a number of variables ranging from 4 to 11. All of them include unemployment, and most include overcrowding. There has been considerable criticism of the underprivileged area score as a measure of excess workload for primary care related to deprivation, but there is currently no consensus as to the optimum method.

A number of potential interventions might be effective in reducing socio-economic inequalities in health. These might include a reduction in the gap between the highest-and lowest-paid groups. Targets could be set for the reduction of social class gradients in mortality and morbidity. Strategies aimed at infants and children, including greater support of disadvantaged mothers and emphasis on improved educational opportunity, deserve emphasis. Clearly, it is also important to ensure that facilities for health care in poor areas are funded at a level that takes into account the greater needs of the population. Taxation policies could do more to discourage smoking and excessive drinking. Likewise, health promotion initiatives to reduce risk factors, such as smoking, poor diet, and physical activity, are useful. However, Sir Donald Acheson, former chief medical officer, has pointed out that 'there is a limit to the extent to which such improvements are likely to occur in the absence of a wider strategy to change the circumstances in which these risks arise by reducing deprivation and improving physical environment'.

Global environmental change and health

It has become apparent over recent years that a number of major changes are occurring in the world's environment which have potentially major implications for human health. In 1990, the United Nations Intergovernmental Panel on Climate Change produced a major report (Houghton *et al.* 1990). The 'best guess' of the scientists on the panel was of a realized 1 °C rise in temperature above the current average by 2025, assuming that emissions continue to grow at the current rate. The realized rise in temperature at a given time accounts for only 60–80 per cent of the final rise, because the thermal inertia of the ocean acts as a buffer, slowing temperature rise. By the end of the 21st century, they estimated a potential rise of around 3 °C, the upper estimate being 5 °C. Carbon dioxide accounts for about half of the total of greenhouse gas emissions. If no steps are taken to limit emissions, the IPCC predicted that by 2030, the effective carbon dioxide concentrations in the atmosphere will be twice those that prevailed in pre-industrial times. Global warming is also occurring at a time when stratospheric *ozone depletion is underway, caused by increased chlorine loading of the atmosphere to a level of more than six times the naturally occurring amounts. Chlorine loading is due to stable man-made compounds such as chlorofluorocarbons (CFCs), halons (used in fire extinguishers), methylchloroform, and carbon tetrachloride. This has led to the presence of an ozone hole over Antarctica during winter and spring, accompanied by increased levels of ultraviolet B radiation (UVB). Over the northern hemisphere, ozone levels have also fallen, although not, so far, to the same degree as in Antarctica. Increased *ultraviolet radiation leads to the formation of increased amounts of ozone in the troposphere (lower atmosphere), particularly from complex reactions involving car exhaust emissions. This tends to reduce elevations in ground level UVB exposure, but has significant effects on lung function, potentiating the effect of allergens and other pollutants.

The greenhouse effect is likely to have a number of implications for health. These can be considered as primary (direct effects of temperature on health), secondary (due to the effect of temperature rise and changes in rainfall patterns on crop and allergen production, water supply, and *insect vectors) and tertiary (the effect of factors such as changes in availability of food and water on societal stability, the economy, and the likelihood of conflict).

A number of studies have shown that death rates, particularly from cardiovascular disease in elderly people, rise after periods of high temperature. On the other hand, death rates also increase during cold spells. Therefore, the net effect of a rise in temperature on death rates is likely to vary between countries and regions, depending on the current balance between winter and summer deaths. In the UK, deaths tend to be higher in winter months.

Climate change may affect the distribution of a number of vector-borne diseases. The situation could be quite complex because a number of factors are involved, including rainfall and counter measures adopted by society. One of the major diseases to be affected could be *malaria. Early effects might be seen particularly at the boundaries of an area where malaria is endemic. For example, in Africa, the limits of malaria transmission tend to be defined by altitude, which reflects underlying temperature. An increase in temperature due to global warming could lead to a movement of malaria up slopes. A rise in sea-level, which is predicted to occur due to global warming, will lead to an increase in salt-water species of mosquito, and contamination by salt-water of inland water might, in turn, lead to a reduction in fresh-water species. Five of the numerous mosquito-borne diseases have been considered to be potential risks to the United States following a climate change, including malaria, *dengue fever, and *yellow fever. In the case of Australia, there may be an extension of the area to which the *virus causing Murray Valley *encephalitis will extend, and there could be an increased incidence of epidemic *polyarthritis caused by the Ross River virus.

Extensive algal blooms have been reported from around the world over the past couple of years, probably as a result of increased atmospheric CO_2, deposition of nitrates from sewage, and perhaps in response to warming. Algae and plankton may provide a reservoir for cholera. It has been suggested that the recent Latin American cholera epidemic may have been caused in this way.

Although estimates of the degree of sea-level rise have recently been revised slightly downward, there are still grounds for considerable concern because the 10 countries most vulnerable to sea-level rise include Bangladesh, Egypt, Pakistan, Indonesia, and Thailand, all of which have large, relatively poor populations. In the 1970s, for instance, floods caused the deaths of 300 000 people in Bangladesh.

A major area for concern is the degree to which climate change will affect food production and rainfall. Although models of climate change are not sufficiently well developed to predict with much confidence regional changes in climate, there may be a reduction of rainfall at the middle latitudes, particularly in the centre of continents. This could affect grain harvests and cause drought. This is of particular concern because increases in world population are already outstripping gains in grain production. Increases in ground-level ozone and in ultraviolet radiation may also have a deleterious impact on crops. Thus, climate change could add to difficulties in providing sufficient food, particularly for Third World populations. Although around 9000 km³ of water are available for human exploitation, local availability of

water varies widely. Nearly 75 per cent of the water is used for agricultural purposes. Decreases in rainfall in some areas, and rises in sea-level leading to increased salinization of fresh water in others, could threaten supplies in some parts of the world.

Climate may also affect respiratory diseases. Acute *bronchitis and *bronchiolitis are more common in winter, as is *pneumonia. *Asthma and *hayfever tend to peak in the summer months, with a second peak of asthma in the autumn. Hospital admissions for asthma tend to be more common in the last quarter of the year, perhaps related to viral infections. Climate change could affect the level of *allergens such as pollen in the atmosphere.

In the case of stratospheric ozone depletion and the resulting increase in ultraviolet radiation, there are a number of concerns for human health, particularly the potential for an increase in skin cancers and perhaps in cataracts. The United Nations Environmental Programme has estimated that a sustained 10 per cent depletion in stratospheric ozone would result in 300 000 additional cases of non-melanoma skin cancer, 4500 *melanomas, and 1.75 million cases of *cataract per year. There are a number of different types of skin cancer, the more common being basal cell and squamous cell *carcinomas, whose incidence is related to sunlight exposure. The more dangerous malignant melanoma is rarer, but increasing rapidly. It is thought to be caused by brief episodes of high exposure, especially in childhood. Fair-skinned people are at particular risk, as are those with large numbers of naevi. The recent increase is thought to be due to changes in life-style, particularly spending holidays in sunny areas and sunbathing. The highest risk in the world is in Queensland, Australia. Melanoma has a much better prognosis if it is caught early, and for that reason there have been a number of campaigns to increase public knowledge.

In order to reduce the impact of climate change, major changes in government policy will be required, particularly the reduction of emissions of greenhouse gases, and thus the use of fossil fuels, as well as reforestation. In the case of ozone depleting substances, the UK government has recently agreed to bring forward the date of phaseout to the end of 1995, but some believe this could be brought forward further and that CFC replacements, which also have some ozone-depleting potential, should be included in the ban.

ANDREW HAINES

References

Barker, D. J. P., Winter, P. D., Osmond, C., Margetts, B., and Simmonds, S.J. (1989). Weight in infancy and death from ischaemic heart disease. *Lancet*, **ii**, 577–80.

Beale, N. and Nethercott, S. (1988). The nature of employment morbidity. 1. Recognition. 2. Description. *Journal of the Royal College of General Practitioners*, **38**, 200–2.

Houghton, J. T., Jenkins, G. J., and Ephraums, J. J., (ed.) (1990). *Climate change. The IPCC scientific assessment*. Cambridge University Press, Cambridge.

Marmot, M. G., Shipley, M. J., and Rose, G. (1984). Inequalities in death – specific explanations of a general pattern? Occasional Survey. *Lancet*, **i**, 1003–6.

Moser, K. A., Goldblatt, P. O., Fox, A. J., and Jones, D. R. (1987). Unemployment and mortality; comparison of the 1971 and 81 longitudinal study census samples. *British Medical Journal*, **294**, 86–90.

ENZOOTIC. Descriptive of an infection which is continuously prevalent in an animal community, although it may not cause obvious morbidity or may affect few members of the community at any one time (cf. *endemic).

ENZYMES are *protein catalysts, i.e. substances which accelerate chemical reactions without themselves being used up in the process. Many are specific to the substance on which they act, called the substrate. Each enzyme requires optimum conditions to carry out its function, notably with respect to pH, temperature, the presence of accessory factors (coenzymes), and the absence of specific inhibiting substances. Enzymes are involved in all the metabolic processes upon which life depends and, since they determine the characteristics of cells, play an important role in *heredity.

An enzyme is usually named by attaching the suffix-*ase* to either its substrate (e.g. *amylase) or its type of action (e.g. dehydrogenase), except where a few older names (e.g. *pepsin, trypsin) have been retained. See also BIOCHEMISTRY.

EOSINOPHIL. A type of *leucocyte (white blood cell) containing large refractile granules which stain readily with the rose-coloured dye eosin. Eosinophils, which normally account for between 1 and 3 per cent of the total white blood cell population, are *phagocytic and perhaps also *cytotoxic for some larger parasites, including worms. They may also play a part in regulating *inflammation.

EOSINOPHILIA is an increase in the number of circulating *eosinophils in the blood.

EPENDYMA. The membrane lining the ventricles of the brain and the central canal of the spinal cord.

EPENDYMOMA. A tumour of the brain or spinal cord arising from cells of the *ependyma.

EPHEDRINE is a naturally occurring *alkaloid adopted from indigenous Chinese medicine in 1928. It is sympathomimetic, i.e. its actions mimic the effects of stimulating the *sympathetic nervous system. Because it is effective by mouth, it is a useful if somewhat outmoded addition to Western therapeutics, for example as a nasal decongestant or a bronchodilator in asthma.

EPICONDYLE. A bony protuberance above a *condyle.

EPIDAURUS (Epidhavros) is a town on the north-east coast of the Peloponnese in Greece. Here was the principal temple of the god of medicine, *Aesculapius, whom Milton refers to as 'the God in Epidaurus' (*Paradise Lost*, ix, 506). Patients who slept in the temple were cured during the night or had the method of cure revealed to them in a dream. See TEMPLE MEDICINE.

EPIDEMIC. An outbreak of disease such that for a limited period a significantly greater number of persons in a community or region suffer from it than is normally the case. Thus an epidemic is a temporary increase in *prevalence. Its extent and duration are determined by the interaction of such variables as the nature and infectivity of the causal agent, its mode of transmission, the degree of pre-existing and newly acquired immunity, etc. See also EPIDEMIOLOGY.

EPIDEMIOLOGY
Definition
Why do diseases occur? How can we measure and explain their rise and fall? Why do some people become sick while others remain healthy? How effective are our efforts to prevent and control common diseases? Such questions are as much a part of medicine as the familiar task of diagnosing and treating sick individuals. They constitute the domain of epidemiology, the branch of medicine concerned with describing and explaining the occurrence of disease in populations.

A disease starts with an interaction between the individual and some external influence, such as *infection, *diet, or chemical exposure. Clinical research is concerned with the evolution of the process once that interaction has occurred: its subject of study is the already sick patient. Epidemiology studies that initiating interaction and all those environmental and personal characteristics which may explain its occurrence. Being concerned with contrasts between the sick and the healthy, it must study the population as a whole and its *environment. This is its identifying characteristic.

Whereas clinical investigation provides the scientific basis for the care of patients, epidemiology provides the scientific basis for the care of communities—that is, for *public health policy and prevention. Its methods are concerned with disease rates and unbiased comparisons of groups, rather than with accuracy in individual cases.

History
There have long been two views of the origins of disease. The first supposes that something within the individual goes wrong: perhaps by chance, a mechanism fails. On this view one looks for the causes of disease within the individual by analysing the malfunction of bodily mechanisms. On the other viewpoint one looks for factors external to the individual, with which the body has been unable to cope. In fact, few diseases can be

understood by either of these approaches alone. Conditions such as *achondroplasia (dwarfism), in which an internal *genetic defect explains everything, are rare. Equally rare are conditions where everyone is equally susceptible to an external agent. Most diseases are initiated by an external agent, but the effects are greatly modified according to the individual's constitution.

The environment impinges on the individual principally by the mouth (food and water), the respiratory tract (air and its pollutants), the skin, and the mind. These identify the kinds of exposure which epidemiology may need to measure. The importance of genetic and other constitutional factors is in determining susceptibility to these external agents.

*Contagion or *miasma?

There have also long been two views of the nature of the environmental influence on disease. One, the contagion theory, supposes that there are specific agents which produce specific diseases. The other, the miasma theory, supposes that an unhealthy environment has a more general debilitating effect. Thus *malaria ('bad air condition') was attributed to the unpleasant emanations from swamps; and many would still hold that a bad environment is, in a general manner, 'bad for health'.

The contagion theory originated in the behaviour of *epidemics, where contact seemed enough to cause disease, regardless of the local environment. This led to attempts to control disease by isolation:

The leper in whom the plague is, his clothes shall be rent, and his head bare, and he shall cry, Unclean, unclean . . . He shall dwell alone; without the camp shall his dwelling be. (Leviticus 13:45–6)

The contagion theory was unable to explain cases which arose apparently *de novo*, with no recognized contact, and for centuries, too, it lacked any explanation of the mechanism by which disease moved from person to person. Occasionally there were suspicions of the existence of invisible *micro-organisms. In 1557 Girolamo Cardano wrote that 'the seeds of disease are minute animals, capable of reproducing their kind'; but his opinion was more than 300 years before its time, and it was not accepted. The general view was that if something could not be seen then it did not exist.

The advent of the microscope brought the possibility of identifying a mechanism for contact-spread. In 1658 Kircher claimed to have seen micro-organisms in blood from cases of bubonic *plague, and no less a man than William *Harvey agreed with him. However, it now seems that what he was looking at were not germs but red blood cells, and a demonstration of the existence of germs had to wait for *Pasteur in the late 19th century.

Agostino Bassi, an Italian lawyer, demonstrated in 1816 that muscardine, a disease of silkworms, could be acquired only by contact with other affected silkworms, and he then identified a *fungus as the transmitting agent.

In the UK a pioneer of the new thinking was William *Budd, a rural general practitioner in North Tawton, Devonshire. He was dubious of the miasmatists' theory of *typhoid, and he wrote of his village:

Much there was offensive to the nose, but (typhoid) fever there was none . . . Privies, pigstyes, and dungheaps continued, year after year, to exhale ill odours, without any specific effect on the public health . . . I ascertained by an enquiry conducted with the most scrupulous care . . . that for ten years there had been but a single case.

On 11 July 1839 the situation in North Tawton suddenly changed, and in the next 4 months Budd saw 80 cases of typhoid fever. In three instances where individuals left the village he observed that new outbreaks began among their contacts in previously unaffected areas. He concluded that typhoid fever is a 'contagious or self-propagating fever' and that 'the contagious matter is cast off, chiefly, in the discharges from the diseased intestine'. The typhoid *bacillus was not identified until 1880, illustrating how epidemiological methods may identify sources of disease and point to appropriate control measures even when the mechanisms have not been elucidated.

During the middle of the 19th century the *contagium vivum* theory was widely adopted as the best explanation of infectious diseases, although for non-infectious illness the miasmatic theory survived.

Numbers—not impressions

Scientific epidemiology began with the marriage, halfway through the 19th century, of medical concern for the environment with the new skills of medical *statistics, particularly as that subject was being taught in Paris by Pierre Louis; his students became the epidemiological leaders in the UK and the USA.

A quantitative approach to the description of disease outbreaks had begun much earlier with the publication in 1563 of the London *Bills of Mortality, which recorded deaths from the plague. In that year a total of 17 404 plague deaths were recorded in London and adjacent parishes, forming 85 per cent of all burials.

When the *Royal Society of London was formed in 1662, one of its patrons was a wealthy tradesman, John Graunt. In the same year he published his *Natural and political observations upon the Bills of Mortality*, in which he calculated the first 'life table', estimating the probability of an individual's survival to successive ages; he identified the excess of male births and the seasonal and urban–rural differences in *mortality, and he proposed a comparison of mortality tables between different countries. He was the first analytical demographer.

In 1836 the Registration Act provided for detailed annual reports on all deaths in England and Wales, and this enabled the brilliant William *Farr to set up the world's first national system of vital statistics.

If the origin of modern epidemiology were to be given

a date it would be 1850, the birth year of the 'London Epidemiological Society'. The founders were a group of the leading physicians of the day who had become convinced that mass diseases could not be controlled by treatment alone: they therefore sought to prevent disease by controlling its underlying causes. Their methods of enquiry were quantitative and objective, depending largely on the newly developed skills of medical and vital statistics.

During the 20th century mass *infectious diseases have declined in Western countries, their place as the leading causes of death being taken by chronic diseases, particularly *cardiovascular diseases and *cancers. By this time American research had become active and well-endowed, and its contribution to chronic disease epidemiology has been large. It is exemplified by the Framingham Heart Study. In 1948 all the adults in this small town in Massachusetts were invited to the first of a series of medical examinations, and for the next 30 years a record was kept of all cardiovascular illnesses. From this study originated our recognition of the 'coronary risk factors'—traits that mark susceptibility to a disease which may not become evident until decades later.

More recently the techniques of epidemiology have been increasingly applied to clinical practice, so as to evaluate the natural history and outcome of illnesses, and the performance of diagnostic tests and treatments. 'Clinical epidemiology' has helped to bridge the gap between epidemiology and mainstream medicine; more significantly, *medical journals now publish an increasing number of papers on population-related research, written by clinicians. Recognition of the limitations of treatment in the advanced stages of chronic disease is stimulating interest in the causes, natural history, and prevention of disease. Once again, as when the London Epidemiological Society was formed in 1850, the best clinicians are involved not only with treatment but also with the causes and control of contemporary mass diseases.

Methods

Cases

To measure the burden of disease in a population usually requires the counting of cases, implying that for any given disease everyone is either a case or not a case. This assumption works well enough in clinical practice, since management decisions are also dichotomous ('treat' or 'not treat'); and also only the severer cases go to hospital, thus heightening the separation of 'cases' and 'not cases'.

This simple concept breaks down when it is applied in the population, where most diseases come in all sizes. An infection may be fatal in one person and symptomless in another. Cancer is a process, ranging from minor microscopic deviations up to a fatal illness, with all degrees in between, and the possibility of arrest at any but the late stages. *Blood pressure in a population

shows a continuous distribution and any definition of *hypertension is arbitrary; and similarly with heart disease, *diabetes, and almost all other acquired diseases. The real question is not 'Has he got it?' but 'How much of it has he got?'

The definition of a case is arbitrary, and it must be related to the purpose in hand. There are no universal solutions, and in epidemiology one must look for *ad hoc* answers based on rigorous application of general principles to particular situations.

Comparison of disease in different groups calls for careful standardization of case definitions and methods of ascertainment. Even then, identically defined case groups may differ if they come from different sources: a *general practitioner, a general hospital, and a special hospital will each see cases of differing average severity. Comparisons between hospitals, countries, or time periods can be misleading. The credibility of epidemiology rests on bias-free comparisons and a good report must show evidence that the methods were valid.

Rates

A description of cases becomes epidemiological only when it is related to the population in which those cases arose. This yields a rate, which is the hallmark of epidemiological data. The denominator of a rate is known as the 'at-risk population'. It might be the residents of a region, employees of a factory, or a general practitioner's list, or a representative sample of such a group; but it could not be volunteers, or any other ill-defined group.

Inferences are often extended beyond the actual study population. For example, a trial of hypertension treatment in one population may be used to guide treatment in another. The all-important question of whether findings may be generalized in this way is a matter of judgement, not statistics.

Sources of information

Much information about the health of populations is available from libraries, but this relates mostly to mortality. The quality of death certificates leaves much to be desired, and interpreting mortality data is not for amateurs. They have been a valuable means of identifying international and regional inequalities in health, and the comings and goings of disease; but startling differences can sometimes reflect only the vagaries of medical practice and diagnostic habits.

Systematic information on *morbidity (the burden of ill-health) is meagre. Hospital discharge data yield some intriguing observations, such as that the Welsh are more than twice as likely as East Anglians to be admitted to hospital for *gallstones; but it is hard to know if this reflects differences in incidence or in medical care. Thus, for example, the USA has twice as many surgeons in relation to its population as Britain and—not surprisingly—twice as many operations.

Epidemiological research starts in the library, but vital statistical information is often too superficial or unreliable to provide the answers. A survey is then necessary. Sometimes this can be a simple affair, as when a general practitioner questions a sample of patients on his list in order to determine their *smoking habits. Others are alarmingly big. Surveys, in fact, are only feasible for studying the commoner diseases. For example, in order to find enough cases of *multiple sclerosis it would be necessary to do neurological examinations on hundreds of thousands of people.

Types of epidemiological study

Studies can be descriptive (measuring the burden of a disease and its distribution in a population) or analytical (analysing and seeking to explain its occurrence). They can also be divided according to their design into cross-sectional studies (which describe disease at a particular point in time) and longitudinal or prospective studies (describing its evolution over a period).

The measure of disease from a cross-sectional study is the *prevalence rate, which is the proportion of a defined group having the condition at one point in time. This is appropriate in relatively stable conditions, but it would be unsuitable as a measure of an acute condition such as influenza.

In a longitudinal study the frequency of a condition is measured by its *incidence rate, which is the proportion of a defined group developing a condition within a stated period. Mortality rates, birth rates, and notification rates are all examples of incidence rates.

A problem commonly arises when comparing groups of different age structure, since the incidence of most diseases depends greatly on age. This can be solved either by comparing a series of age-specific rates, or by a technique of standardization such as the standardized mortality ratio (SMR), where a value of 100 represents the average experience of the reference population. Thus the SMR for lung cancer among publicans in England and Wales is 224; this means that relative to the country as a whole their risk of death from lung cancer is 2.24 times as great, after allowing for differences in age.

Risk and causation

A longitudinal study may show that exposure to some factor is associated with an increased incidence of a particular outcome (e.g. maternal age is a risk factor for a *Down's syndrome birth). A risk factor is a predictor: it may be a cause, or it may be just a coincidental association.

The risk to exposed individuals is an inadequate guide to public health policy, because it ignores the prevalence of exposure. A risk may be serious to the individual concerned; but if only a few individuals are affected then the total problem is small. To an older mother the risk of a Down's syndrome birth is sizeable, which is the basis for screening policy. However, about three-quarters of all Down's syndrome pregnancies occur in mothers who are under the age of 35. Exposure of many people to a small risk commonly causes more trouble than exposure of a small number to a high risk.

An aetiological hypothesis can be tested by a case-control study, where the analysis involves comparing the frequency of exposure in cases and controls. Although one of the commonest kinds of epidemiological study, it is potentially the most misleading. The control group may be inappropriate; bias can creep into the comparison of exposure frequencies; or an association (such as that between *ulcerative colitis and psychological problems) may have arisen because the disease caused the problem, not vice versa.

Observational studies identify associations but they do not prove causation. If A and B are found to be associated, then A may have caused B, B may have caused A, or C may have caused both (in which case C is known as a confounding factor: it provides an alternative explanation of an association). If a confounding factor has been identified and measured, then its effect may be calculated, but not otherwise: you cannot exclude the explanation you have not considered! The task of epidemiology is to provide and weigh the evidence on causality, but recognizing that it must always fall short of proof.

Epidemiology and the public health

Epidemiology provides the scientific basis for the diagnosis and treatment of populations, that is, for identifying and measuring their health problems and then formulating appropriate public health policies. However, as in the clinical sphere, the evidence does not of itself make the decisions. Epidemiology can provide the balance-sheet for public health decision-taking, in which so far as possible each benefit and cost is defined and quantified; but each item is measured in different units (years of life, disability, *pain; resources and economic costs; and so on). The policy decision requires a judgement on the appropriate weight to be assigned to each. Data do not make decisions.

Epidemiology has played an integral part in most of the historical public health successes. At first these were mainly in the control of major infectious diseases: diarrhoeal diseases, *smallpox, *diphtheria, *poliomyelitis, and *measles among others. More recently there have been at least partial successes in some of the mass non-infectious diseases, including chronic *bronchitis, lung cancer (in men), and dental *caries. For some other cancers, and for coronary heart disease, research has identified factors that need to be controlled, but implementation is still unsatisfactory. For many other diseases the aetiology still remains to be unravelled.

The tasks to which epidemiology now needs to be applied differ from those of the past. The approach and methods, however, are universally appropriate and the subject will always remain an integral part of medicine.

(The late) GEOFFREY ROSE

Further reading
Cochrane, A. L. (1972). *Effectiveness and efficiency. Random reflections on health services.* Nuffield Provincial Hospitals Trust, London.
Lilienfeld, A. M. and Lilienfeld, D. E. (1980). *Foundations of epidemiology*, (2nd edn). Oxford University Press, New York and Oxford.
Rose, G. (1992). *The strategy of preventive medicine.* Oxford University Press, Oxford.
Rose, G. and Barker D. J. P. (1986). *Epidemiology for the uninitiated*, (2nd edn). British Medical Journal, London.

EPIDERMIS. The outer layer of the *skin.

EPIDERMOPHYTOSIS is a superficial *fungal infection of the *skin. See also TINEA.

EPIDIDYMIS. A coiled tubular structure attached to the back of the *testicle, connecting it to the *vas deferens. Its function is the storage and maturation of *spermatozoa before their discharge.

EPIGASTRIUM. That part of the abdominal wall overlying the *stomach: the upper central area, in the angle made by the two sides of the rib cage.

EPIGLOTTIS. The hinged cartilaginous flap behind the tongue which during swallowing, drops down to close the *glottis, so preventing food or drink from entering the *airway leading to the lungs.

EPILEPSY is a periodic disorder characterized by outbursts of excessive activity in part of the brain, which in the fully developed form (major epilepsy or grand mal) spread to involve the whole cerebrum. The classic manifestations are loss of consciousness and generalized convulsions, the body at first going into extensor rigidity (the tonic phase) and then into a series of jerking movements (the clonic phase). When these have subsided, there may be a period of apparent sleep before consciousness, sometimes clouded or confused, returns. Attacks of grand mal are often preceded by some form of premonitory *aura, the nature of which is thought to indicate the region in which the irritable cerebral focus resides. Minor or partial expressions of epilepsy and psychomotor and autonomic epilepsy 'equivalents' can occur as well as major attacks, or be the sole manifestations. About two-thirds of all cases of epilepsy are 'idiopathic', that is no structural or metabolic cause can be determined. In modern terminology, the principal types of epileptic attack are tonic–clonic (major) seizures, absence seizures of childhood (also called petit

mal), and partial seizures of many different types. A large variety of effective *anticonvulsant drugs is available to treat the many different variants.

EPILOIA. See TUBEROUS SCLEROSIS.

EPINEPHRINE. See ADRENALINE.

EPIPHYSIS. The separately ossified end of a growing *bone. During growth, a cartilaginous plate (the epiphyseal cartilage) intervenes between the epiphysis and the main shaft (diaphysis) of the bone. When growth ceases, there is bony union between the two, and the cartilage disappears.

EPISIOTOMY is a surgical incision of the *perineum and *vagina performed during *labour to enlarge the outlet of the *birth canal and prevent spontaneous tearing of these tissues.

EPISPADIAS is congenital absence of all or part of the upper *urethral wall, occurring more commonly in males, when the urethral opening may be anywhere on the dorsum of the penis. Epispadias may be associated with urinary incontinence but many surgical methods are available for partial or complete repair.

EPISTAXIS is bleeding from the nose.

EPITHELIOMA. Any tumour derived from *epithelium.

EPITHELIUM is the general name given to the firmly adherent sheet of cells of epidermal origin covering the body surface, both external and internal, comprising the *skin and *mucous membrane (mucosa) lining tubes and cavities. (The term excludes the *endothelium lining the vascular system, embryonically derived from mesoderm.)

EPONYM. The name of a person used as part of the name of a disease, syndrome, anatomical feature, etc. (e.g. *Bright's disease, *Pott's fracture). The doctor, or doctors, associated with an original description or invention are the most frequent to be so honoured, but a few diseases are named after patients (e.g. *Christmas disease) or places (e.g. *Marburg disease).

EPSOM SALTS. Hydrated magnesium sulphate (Mg SO$_4$.7H$_2$O), a white crystalline soluble salt used as a *laxative, particularly for rapid bowel evacuation. Magnesium sulphate paste was also used formerly as a local application to assist drainage of boils and carbuncles. The mineral springs at Epsom, Surrey, were a popular source of medicinal magnesium sulphate.

EPSTEIN–BARR VIRUS is a large enveloped *deoxyribonucleic acid (DNA) virus of the genus *Herpesvirus* (like herpes simplex virus (HSV) and varicella-zoster virus (V-ZV): see HERPES SIMPLEX). Epstein–Barr (EB) virus can cause several infections most notably *infectious mononucleosis. There is also an association with *Burkitt's lymphoma and nasopharyngeal *carcinoma.

ERASISTRATUS, of Chios (b. *c*.304 BC). Greek anatomist and physiologist. He studied in Athens, later in Cos, and finally in Alexandria, renouncing practice to undertake research in the museum. He wrote extensively, but none of his work survives. He dissected the human body and is alleged to have carried out vivisection on prisoners. He has been regarded as the founder of physiology. A *pneumatist, he believed the arteries and veins came from the heart and divided repeatedly. The veins, he claimed, contained blood, the arteries pneuma, and the nerves a special 'psychic' pneuma. He regarded the heart as a bellows and appreciated the difference between motor and sensory nerves.

ERB, WILHELM HEINRICH (1840–1921). German neurologist. He was interested in the electrical reactions of muscle and *electrotherapy (1868). He described the knee-jerk (1875); brachial palsy (Erb–Duchenne paralysis, 1874); syphilitic spinal paralysis (Erb's progressive paraplegia, 1875); *myasthenia gravis (Erb–Goldflam disease, 1878); showed that *tabes dorsalis was due to *syphilis (1879); and classified the *myopathies (1891).

ERETHISM is abnormal sensitivity or arousability, particularly of the sexual organs; it is used more specifically of the psychiatric manifestations of chronic *mercury poisoning ('mad as a hatter').

ERGOMETRINE is an *alkaloid of *ergot, also known as ergonovine; it has a particularly powerful stimulant effect on the muscle of the pregnant *uterus. Its major therapeutic use is in control of post-partum *haemorrhage, but it was also once used in treating *migraine (see ERGOTAMINE).

ERGONOMICS is the study of man in his working environment, and particularly of the principles governing the efficient use of human energy. See also OCCUPATIONAL MEDICINE.

ERGOT is a parasitic *fungus, *Claviceps purpurea*, which infests various grasses, including rye and wheat. It contains several *alkaloids, which are powerful stimulants of smooth muscle; some have been used in medicine, notably *ergometrine (ergonovine), used to stimulate uterine contractions, and *ergotamine, used in treating migraine. Ingestion of rye bread made with contaminated grain or medical overdosage may cause *ergotism.

ERGOTAMINE is any *alkaloid of *ergot ($C_{33}H_{35}O_5N_5$), an effective agent in the treatment of many patients with *migraine, because of its powerful constricting effect on vascular smooth muscle.

ERGOTISM is acute or chronic poisoning with *ergot *alkaloids, either from eating food made from contaminated grain, or from excessive and prolonged medicinal use of *ergotamine. The manifestations are mostly attributable to the stimulation of involuntary muscle; especially widespread constriction of blood vessels. They include headache, vomiting, diarrhoea, abdominal cramps, *paraesthesiae, *convulsions, and dry *gangrene of the extremities.

ERGOTOXIN, a derivative of *ergot, is a mixture of three *alkaloids (ergocornine, ergocristine, and ergocryptine). It was formerly used as an *oxytocic and in the treatment of *migraine, but has been replaced by the less toxic alkaloids *ergometrine and *ergotamine, respectively.

ERLANGER, JOSEPH (1874–1965). American physiologist. He collaborated with Herbert S. *Gasser in studies of nerve conduction, developing the cathode ray oscillograph as an instrument for measurements. For this work they received the *Nobel prize in 1944.

EROGENOUS ZONES are parts of the body which, when stimulated, arouse sexual pleasure and accompanying physiological changes. Such zones are said to vary between individuals, but usually include the lips, tongue, breasts, genitals, and sometimes the anus.

EROTICISM. Sexual excitement; a sexually excitable temperament.

ERYSIPELAS is a potentially severe *streptococcal infection of the skin and subcutaneous tissues, most often affecting the face, accompanied by fever and systemic symptoms. Its characteristic feature is bright redness of the affected area with a sharply demarcated edge. Its frequency and danger were markedly reduced by antibacterial *chemotherapy.

ERYSIPELOID. A bacterial infection of animals, including various farm animals, poultry, and fish; in pigs it is called 'swine erysipelas'. The causative organism is a Gram-positive bacillus, *Erysipelothrix rhusiopathiae*. Infection in man is almost invariably occupational, and takes place through a cut or abrasion on the hand or arm; it manifests as a localized area of purplish erythema, sometimes with regional lymph node involvement. Spontaneous resolution is usual, but the organism is also sensitive to many antibiotics. Septicaemia with endocarditis is a rare complication.

ERYTHEMA is redness of the *skin associated with increased skin *capillary blood flow.

ERYTHEMA MULTIFORME. A skin condition associated with widespread erythematous, bullous, and purpuric lesions, often involving mucocutaneous junctions. Erythema multiforme may follow virus (especially *herpes simplex) or other (for example *mycoplasmal) infections, may occur as a reaction to certain drugs (notably long-acting *sulphonamide preparations and *barbiturates), or may arise without obvious antecedent cause. It ranges in severity from a minor skin eruption to a severe and dangerous illness, with extensive skin necrosis, lesions of the eyes, mouth, and genitalia, and involvement of other systems and organs, such as the kidneys, lungs, and gastrointestinal tract (erythema multiforme major or Stevens–Johnson syndrome).

ERYTHROCYANOSIS. A bluish redness of the legs and feet, often with swelling and sometimes painful, seen most often in young women in cold weather.

ERYTHROCYTE. Red blood cell or corpuscle. In the mature form normally present in blood, the erythrocyte is a biconcave non-nucleated discoid cell about 8 micrometres (μm) in diameter and about 2 μm thick. A litre of blood contains about 5×10^{12} erythrocytes. See also HAEMATOLOGY.

ERYTHRODERMA is extensive and persistent redness of the *skin occurring in various skin disorders, particularly exfoliative dermatitis.

ERYTHROMELALGIA is redness and pain in the limbs, characteristically paroxysmal and affecting predominantly the feet.

ERYTHROMYCIN is an *antibiotic isolated from *Streptomyces erythreus*, introduced in 1952. It has a wide spectrum of antibacterial activity, broadly similar to that of *penicillin. See also ANTIBACTERIAL AGENTS.

ERYTHROPOIESIS is the formation and development of *erythrocytes.

ERYTHROPOIETIN is a protein *hormone produced by the juxtaglomerular cells of the kidney, which stimulates the production of *erythrocytes by the *bone marrow. It is secreted in response to a fall in renal oxygen tension. It is now used to treat the *anaemia of renal failure, especially in patients undergoing *dialysis.

ESCHAR. A slough of dead tissue.

ESCHERICHIA COLI is a Gram-negative *bacillus which normally inhabits the large *intestine, often simply termed 'coliform bacillus'(and formerly known as *Bacillus coli*). Under certain conditions some strains are pathogenic, particularly when transferred to other sites, such as the urinary tract. *E. coli* is widely employed as an experimental system in *genetic engineering.

ESERINE is an *alkaloid, also known as physostigmine, obtained from the Calabar bean. It is an *anticholinesterase agent, employed in medicine, particularly ophthalmology, for its cholinergic effects. See also ACETYLCHOLINE.

ESMARCH, JOHANNES FRIEDRICH AUGUST VON (1823–1908). German military surgeon. He devised the 'first field dressing' (1869) and the rubber bandage for rendering a limb bloodless before amputation (Esmarch's bandage, 1873).

ESOPHAGUS. See OESAPHAGUS.

ESOPHORIA is a latent convergent *squint, i.e. one which appears when visual stimuli are eliminated, when the affected eye deviates towards the midline.

ESQUEMELING, JOHN (*fl. c.* 1680). French surgeon. As a Protestant, he was not allowed to practise in France because of his religion. He went to the West Indies, had sporadic apprenticeships with surgeons, and eventually joined the thriving buccaneers as a surgeon. In 1678 he first published in Dutch what became an English work *Buccaneers of America*, which ran to many editions. It is one of the few accounts of buccaneering by one who took part, and has been a source of many romances. It was published in paperback as late as 1967.

ETHAMBUTOL is an antituberculous drug, usually given with other drugs, such as *rifampicin and/or *isoniazid. It may also be used with isoniazid to prevent *tuberculosis in susceptible close contacts.

ETHANOL (C_2H_5OH), also known as ethyl alcohol, spirits of wine, or simply alcohol, is produced by fermentation of sugars. It is a colourless, volatile inflammable liquid with many applications in medicine: e.g. as a solvent, antiseptic, and tincture. The pharmacological effects of alcohol itself, chiefly central nervous system depression and peripheral *vasodilatation, occasionally find legitimate application in therapeutics, but are mostly employed socially and recreationally. Hence the medical importance of alcohol relates to its roles as a drug of addiction and as a general tissue poison. See also ALCOHOLICS ANONYMOUS; ALCOHOLISM; DELIRIUM TREMENS; KORSAKOFF'S SYNDROME; PROHIBITION; SPIRITS; SUBSTANCE ABUSE; WINE.

ETHER. Diethyl ether ($C_2H_5OC_2H_5$), also known as *anaesthetic ether in UK usage. Ether is now rarely used as an anaesthetic agent because of its inflammability and irritant effect on the respiratory tract. It is unsuitable for induction and often causes nausea and vomiting. The term ether is also employed in a generic chemical sense to mean any compound formed by the condensation of two alcohol molecules and having the general formula R-O-R.

ETHICAL ISSUES IN MODERN HEALTH CARE

Since its earliest beginnings, medical practice has rested on a solid foundation of principles and values designed to promote and protect patients in their relationships with their doctors. Not surprisingly, therefore, both patients and doctors have long enjoyed an instinctive feel for a relationship built upon mutual confidence and trust. Yet recently, this apparently stable relationship has shown signs of becoming destabilized because of scientific discoveries and technological innovations, and the revolution in social attitudes and behaviour which these have spawned. So, for example, within the past 20 years we have found ourselves able to replace organs, introduce life through surrogate motherhood, prolong life artificially using life-support systems, engage in genetic engineering with potentially dramatic effects, and assemble data about people and their illnesses on a scale hitherto unimaginable.

For the same reasons, medicine has become progressively demystified, thus stripping away the aura which, traditionally, patients have associated with their image of the healing physician. Medical care is beginning to share the features of other technical services in a consumer society which seeks to assess quality in terms of value for money and effectiveness. The duty of care placed upon the individual doctor is thus no longer the only focus. We think also in terms of human rights, the benefits that medicine can confer on society as well as the individual, the quality of life as well as the length of survival, equality of access to health services, and of the ever more daunting task of determining priorities when the capacity of medical science to improve and extend our lives exceeds our ability to pay for everything possible. Thus, today doctors and other health professionals, law makers, and indeed the whole of society, have become consciously absorbed in confronting one major ethical dilemma after another, as these are thrown up through the new possibilities in life created year after year by the cascade of scientific advance.

Here we summarize the main approaches which academic moralists use today when analysing specific problems. We then describe three of the ethical 'hotspots' in medicine concerned with confidentiality, conflicting rights, and rationing in health care, to try to illustrate the possible effects that may result by adopting differing lines of reasoning.

Basic principles

Doctors, because of their professional knowledge and skills, are uniquely placed to make decisions about patients which can affect their quality of life and at times their very survival. They are thus in a position of relative power in their relationship with their patients. The purpose of medical ethics is to ensure that doctors use their knowledge to benefit patients, that they do not abuse their power, and that they practise within a framework of values determined by society itself.

Medical practice is founded on four general moral principles. First, doctors have an obligation to respect their patients' autonomy, particularly their right to make choices in accordance with their own values and convictions. Secondly, the general principle of non-maleficence—the avoidance of harm—is of special significance in medicine because society allows doctors some tolerance, provided that the total effect of their actions results in greater overall benefit for their patients. The third principle, beneficence (doing good), is recognized as a fundamental commitment for doctors. And the fourth principle, justice, requires doctors to act justly and fairly with their patients.

These four principles, baldly stated, are of themselves insufficient to inform medical practice; indeed at times they are contradictory. So, each society has to balance and interpret them in accordance with its own cultural, religious, and secular values, which is why medical ethics is a relatively dynamic discipline.

Analysing ethical problems: three approaches

Against this background, there are three distinctive and potentially conflicting approaches when deciding what course of action to take with ethical problems. These are the duty- and right-based approaches, and utilitarianism (O'Neill 1991; Botros 1992).

(a) The duty-based approach. This approach is the most familiar to health professionals. It originates in very general obligations such as, for example, the requirement not to kill or to cause harm. These obligations are usually adapted and codified by professional organizations and institutions, to be expressed as guidelines or rules of conduct which individual practitioners are expected to follow. Varying degrees of tolerance may be permitted where the guidance does not fit the circumstances of every individual case; but in any departures from the rule the practitioner is held accountable and is required to justify any actions taken.

For doctors following this approach the key question is 'What is the right thing to do?'. Duty-based ethics are therefore concerned with doctors' actions rather than with the results of such action. It therefore relies for its effectiveness on its appeal to the doctor's sense of conscience, placing on him or her the obligation to discharge a moral duty because that is what the rules say.

Most doctors adopt a duty-based approach to problem-solving, precisely because they are members of a profession with a history and tradition of ethically based actions which are inculcated from the moment they are admitted. Typically, therefore, doctors understand implicitly that they should not kill their patients, or steal from them, or lie to them, or cheat them. More explicitly, their professional guidance (such as the guidance published by the UK *General Medical Council) will exhort them, for example, to have regard for 'their patients' best medical interests'. Other specific rules of professional conduct may govern some specific situations, for example, the conduct of medical research involving human subjects, when to disclose clinical information about a patient to a third party, or how to investigate a child in whom there is a suspicion of abuse. In other words, the doctor's duty of care, and therefore what action should be taken, is made quite clear.

The great strength of the duty-based approach is the sense of security the rules give practitioners in the decisions they have to make in their everyday work. But conflicts may arise nevertheless, some of which are more easily reconciled than others. For example, given the moral imperative not to lie to the patient, how does a doctor then justify lying to a patient when, for other reasons, he or she judges deception to be in the patient's best interest? Or again, given the general duty not to kill, but also to relieve suffering, how should the doctor act in a situation where a treatment conferring some immediate benefit will nevertheless shorten life? Sometimes these conflicts are reflected in different sets of professional guidance, adding to the doctor's difficulty in deciding what best to do.

Lastly, there are some circumstances where the duty-based approach will conflict absolutely with other approaches. For example, a doctor's duty to sustain life may bring him or her in direct conflict with colleagues who, following a rights-based approach, would hold that a terminally ill patient has a right to be helped to commit suicide.

(b) The rights-based approach. Rights-based moralists hold that the autonomy of the individual patient is paramount; individuals therefore have the absolute right to determine their own destiny, even in circumstances where others may judge that the proposed action may be against the patient's best interests. The rights-based moralist would therefore argue that the duty-based doctor, adhering conscientiously to professional guidance, would nevertheless be acting against a patient—and therefore doing wrong—if the patient's wishes were expressly to the contrary. Exponents of the rights-based approach are not interested primarily in the actions of the doctor, but rather in how those actions impinge upon the patient. So, the rights-based moralist would ask 'Has the doctor wronged the patient as a result of the action taken?', rather than 'Has the doctor done the right thing?'

Doctors following a rights-based approach would say that the autonomy of patients must take moral precedence over prohibitions against harming them, or over duties (actions) to benefit them. So, for example, the rights-based moralist would argue that the doctor who deliberately concealed a feasible treatment option from a patient would wrong that person even if the very action of that concealment could be held to benefit the patient. Similarly, the rights-based doctor who acquiesced in a terminal patient's request for *euthanasia would be

said not to have wronged the patient even though the duty-based ethicist would condemn the doctor's action as wrong.

The self-evident strength of the rights-based approach is that it underlines the inviolable rights of the individual. However, it has obvious limitations. For example, the unborn child, or the senile or comatose patient, can only ever be passive beneficiaries since they cannot determine their own destiny. In practical terms their rights therefore have to be protected by others, but this, of itself, contradicts the principle of self-determined destiny.

Moreover, as people increasingly see themselves as consumers of health care and entitled to the same standing they have in other service sectors, the concept of rights is becoming much broader. In a message to the United States Congress in 1962, President John. F. Kennedy identified four rights of consumers: the right to choose, the right to be heard, the right to safety, and the right to be informed. The incorporation of these values into a traditional rights-based approach to resolving ethical problems would widen its scope considerably. With initiatives like the Patients' Charter in the British *National Health Service (NHS) and the growth of health consumerism in other industrialized countries, this is a likely eventuality.

(c) Utilitarianism. Both duty-based and the rights-based moralists are primarily concerned with the individual patient. The utilitarianist, by contrast, will externalize a problem to take account of wider aspects. Utilitarianism started as a reform movement in 19th century England, in which philosophy was related to its social context. Its principal exponents were Jeremy Bentham (1748–1831) and John Stuart Mill (1806–1873) who popularized it as the 'Greatest Happiness Principle'. Utilitarianism is thus a school of philosophical thought which weighs actions in terms of their potential consequences. An action is right if it promotes good consequences ('happiness') and wrong if it promotes bad consequences ('unhappiness').

For the utilitarianist there is an overall judgement to be made in terms of more benefit or less harm, and the practitioner following this line of thinking will be prepared to break the rules of the duty-based approach and to abandon the rights of the individual provided that the general results justify such action. In practice, utilitarians rarely reject completely the moral importance of following rules or respecting rights. Rather, they find a way of accommodating these within a general framework which appears to present issues for the individual in terms of limiting widespread harm or of promoting the total good.

Leaving aside the problem of defining and measuring 'good', utilitarians can resolve conflicts by ranking all possible courses of action in terms of the total amount of good each would produce, and weighing these against the total amount of harm that might result. The problem for utilitarians is that, in attempting to maximize total good, they are, by definition, prepared deliberately and knowingly to impose burdens on one person for the benefit of others. For many doctors, with their duty-based approach to care, this burden may be unacceptable. Moreover, some feel uncomfortable with judging all actions in consequentialist terms; yet, for the utilitarian thinker the reasons or motives for an action are not relevant.

Perhaps the contrast between the utilitarian approach and others may best be illustrated by considering the situation of an infant born with severely disabling and totally incurable congenital handicap. Here, the utilitarian doctor would list the benefits to be gained by not keeping that child alive, including, in particular, relief for the child in not having to live with a compromised quality of life, and benefit to the community in not having to bear the huge costs of sustaining that individual life, so positively releasing resources for others. In determining the steps to be taken in a child's management, utilitarian doctors would thus bear the widest potential consequences of their proposed action in mind, and would act accordingly. Under these circumstances the utilitarianist could decide deliberately to sedate the child in order to end its life. Such an approach would conflict with duty-based professional rules which would require the doctor not to kill the patient, and also conflict with the rights-based approach since the child could be wronged, notwithstanding problems of autonomy and choice in a child who is also handicapped.

Using the framework

In considering the three approaches described above, one may seem instinctively preferable. In practice, the three doctrines are seldom applied as inflexibly and absolutely as their definitions imply. The actions taken by doctors, other health professionals, and health-policy makers will depend on the particular issue, and on the judgements made in individual cases. There is no easy reconciliation between these three approaches in many situations. Some of these paradoxes and conflicts may be seen in the examples that follow, because they reflect the real-life tensions of decision-making in contemporary medical practice.

Confidentiality

The duty of doctors to preserve secrets has been accepted since the time of Hippocrates in the 5th century BC and has been widely regarded as a cornerstone of medical ethics ever since. Why is confidentiality so important? Is it an unbreakable rule, and if not, on what basis may doctors decide to release information about patients?

Patients expect doctors not to disclose information about them without their consent but, as Hippocrates and other early scholars indicated, they have no absolute right to confidentiality. In English law, there is no general statutory duty of confidentiality. Indeed, for instance, there are some circumstances in which the law requires doctors to disclose information, notifying authorities of certain *infectious diseases or informing the Home Office of patients who are addicted to controlled drugs. In contemporary society confidentiality is usually regarded as an ethical matter rather than as a question of legal principle, and complaints that doctors have improperly disclosed information are usually dealt with by a professional body. The medical profession itself accepts that there are some circumstances in which doctors may be justified in disclosing information without authority to do so from the patient—for example, where a failure to reveal information would put the patient or someone else at risk of death or serious harm.

Confidentiality is justified on two main counts. For some, its primary purpose is to enable patients to control the use made of information about themselves; it is thus seen as part of patients' autonomy. In this context information is deemed to belong to the patient, with doctors having no intrinsic right to it. For others the purpose is pragmatic. Without the reassurance that information will not be disclosed, patients may feel inhibited from telling the doctor vital information about their lives or symptoms. Confidentiality is thus seen as one of the essential elements in building trust between patient and doctor, a trust which is a prerequisite for effective diagnosis and treatment. This trust is also central to the views of those who see maintaining confidentiality as a duty placed on doctors. An unauthorized disclosure of information would be seen in this context as the abuse of trust which patients necessarily place in doctors. These different perspectives reflect the 'rights-based', utilitarian, and 'duty-based' approaches to medical ethics discussed earlier.

In practice, doctors are unlikely to hold a consistently 'rights-based' or 'duty-based' approach, although one particular approach may dominate their thinking. Doctors have to make decisions about when to keep or disclose confidential information as part of their routine practice; for example, they must decide whether to tell close relatives information which the patient has not revealed, or may not even know. Less frequently, they will have to consider whether to act against a patient's wishes as when, for example, they may decide to inform the licensing authority of a patient's medical unsuitability to hold a driving licence. In all cases they are likely to consider a number of factors, weighing patients' right to autonomy against the needs of the wider community, and the duty to preserve a patient's trust against the protection of another individual. None the less, confidentiality is widely regarded as the norm, and disclosure of information without the patient's consent is an exception which must always be justified. Decisions of this kind may often be resolved into evaluating the benefits of two conflicting 'goods', as illustrated below.

Consider the case of a patient who is *HIV positive,

but who refuses to inform his or her sexual partner. In such a case the doctor would run a palpable risk of losing the patient's trust by revealing this information at a very difficult time for that patient. Making a direct intervention in the patient's life, which may irreparably damage the relationship between the patient and his or her partner, would disregard entirely the patient's right to control personal information and override the patient's right to autonomy. The disclosure could not be said to benefit the patient in the doctor's care, and the doctor would therefore have to decide whether his or her primary responsibility was to the patient, or to another unknown person or persons. To remain silent may put another person at unnecessary risk of contracting a fatal disease. Thus the doctor must choose between the competing and incompatible rights of patients and other individuals.

Conflicting rights: the abused child
In 1987, national attention in Britain was drawn to events in Cleveland, where children had been admitted to hospital with a diagnosis of suspected sexual abuse. Subsequently, many of the children were removed from their homes and parents, and placed in care.

Prior to this, although the problem of sexual abuse was familiar to professionals who cared for children, it was less widely recognized as a major problem by practitioners outside this specialist field. Certainly, it was not something which the general public believed to be a commonplace occurrence, nor a major issue for society. Thus, informed speculation at the time about the nature of any crisis involving child sexual abuse would surely have forecast a tragedy involving a single case of the type which has, all too frequently, occurred when children have been physically assaulted.

Instead, the Cleveland affair raised different issues. First, there was the power of professionals to take decisions which involved the care of children and whether this was too great. Secondly, the question as to what rights parents should have in such circumstances, independent of the rights of the individual child, was brought into sharp focus.

The *paediatricians who made the initial diagnosis decided to deal with the cases on the basis of what seemed to be three fundamental assumptions. Firstly, that the presence of certain physical signs, in the absence of any other clinical explanation for them, should raise the strong suspicion that sexual abuse had been perpetrated on a child. They relied particularly on anal signs which were considered highly indicative of sexual abuse. Secondly, the subsequent investigation, in particular the so-called 'disclosure interview', was the gold standard upon which the diagnosis should be determined. Thirdly, that the management of intrafamilial sexual abuse should rely heavily on the principle that a child suspected of being abused had to be removed from the family because only then would he or she be free of the 'control' of the potentially abusing adult.

This does not seem an unreasonable approach for a doctor, in following the explicit and implicit rules governing duty to a patient. This was especially so at the time of the Cleveland crisis, because extant child protection guidance was imprecise on the question of sexual abuse but tended to follow the parallel of physical abuse, where good practice was to intervene early to protect the child when there was a risk of further harm.

This duty-based approach, coupled with a focus on the right of a child to be protected from harm, led to large numbers of children being removed from their families often for long periods. Yet, in some cases, further investigation would reveal that they had not, in fact, been sexually abused at all; this led some parents who were feeling humiliated, to complain angrily that their rights had been abused by the investigating professionals. So, to rely solely on a rights-based approach in such circumstances would be fraught with difficulties. In addition to the issues concerning the specific rights of children and parents, there is the added complication that many young children cannot be regarded as autonomous in deciding the appropriateness of various alternative courses of action. Furthermore, there are all the complexities of family dynamics and relationships to consider, and the long-term consequences—in terms of benefit and harm—of disturbing these.

Could the utilitarian perspective have provided a better basis for justifying events in Cleveland at that time? It would be absurd to argue that the cases of individual children should be handled in a way which deliberately subordinated their interests in order to engineer a greater good. Nevertheless, greater good may well have emerged from the Cleveland affair. Had the children and families not been dealt with in the way in which they were, there would have been no controversy. There would then have been no judicial inquiry whose findings and recommendations led to new child protection guidance and training of staff. The inquiry's conclusions also influenced the drafting of sections of the Children Act 1989, which aimed to improve the rigour and quality of the handling of child abuse, as well as establishing parental rights. Without the controversy, the public and the caring professions would not have been as well informed as they are now about the problem of sexual abuse of children. Thus, as a consequence of the events in Cleveland, this type of child abuse is probably better recognized, better managed, and more children and families in need are helped in more appropriate ways.

This example of child abuse illustrates the complexity of the conflicting ethical issues underlying the choice of the proper approach to problems which involve not just symptoms and signs but human feelings and emotions as well as social and legal considerations.

Rationing health resources fairly
The health services generally use huge resources compared to other services and industries. In Britain, for

example, the NHS spends some £35 (US $52.5) billion each year in providing health care to the population. Despite the size of such budgets, most health care systems in the world are undergoing funding crises of one sort of another, as the resources available to supply health care are being rapidly outstripped by the scale of the need and demand for it. Consequently, health-policy makers are preoccupied with the difficult task of deciding how the money available is to be allocated against competing priorities.

Prioritizing

In theory at least, the starting point for making choices is diverse; for example, priority might be given to using life-saving resources where they will produce most benefit; alternatively, they might be used to confer benefit on people in greatest need. The concept of deploying resources in such a way that they provide maximum benefit is close to the utilitarian approach described earlier.

The practical difficulties of application are formidable. There is little consensus on how health should be defined, other than in very general terms, and there are problems of measurement and of the availability of valid data. Moreover, there are relatively few data routinely available about the effectiveness of different forms of treatment, or on how to assess good and bad outcomes of care for patients treated in the same way. Thus, a strategy of distribution of health resources based upon maximum benefit falls down if there is no agreed way of measuring the potential benefits themselves. One recent attempt to overcome this difficulty is the concept devised by health economists of quality adjusted life years (QUALYs). The QUALY takes a year of healthy life expectancy to have the value one. A year of unhealthy life expectancy is scored less than one, the precise value being lower the worse the quality of life of the person concerned. Costs of particular treatments can then be expressed per QUALY to allow a standard basis for comparison of the benefits of different health investments: for example, kidney *transplantation as against *hip joint replacement. Resource decisions can then be based upon which services give the best cost per QUALY ratio.

Other explicit forms of prioritization have been tried. For example, in the USA the *Oregon state legislature has involved the general public in the process. Following discussion within the local community, five health care values were identified as most important to the citizens of Oregon: autonomy and dignity; prevention of disease; access and justice; cost control; allocation for fairness. Later, on the basis of the community's views and expert testimony, lists were compiled of over 700 treatments which were placed in priority order. The State legislature then decided what the basic health care package for its citizens should be, compiled from the list of prioritized services identified. Those involved with the Oregon initiative see this approach as fairer, more open, and more honest than the pre-existing system, which they saw as based on the hypocritical postulate that the State should aim to provide 'everything for everybody' (Crawshaw 1991).

Although approaches like QUALYs or the Oregon experiment are claimed by their adherents to be inherently fairer than the status quo, they have not been implemented widely. This is partly because the utilitarian approach they reflect conflicts with both the duty-based and the rights-based approaches to health care. Thus, for example, doctors see their duty of care—and therefore their priority for care—as directed to the patient before them at any particular time, and not for hypothetical future patients nor for the patients of others. Similarly, although a citizen might say in a general discussion on priorities that, for example, kidney transplants should be limited to a certain number each year in order to fund, say, more chiropody for the housebound elderly, he is likely to see things more in terms of personal rights and entitlements when a close relative actually develops renal failure.

For doctors, times are changing nevertheless. Although most doctors still abhor the notion of rationing affecting the care of their individual patient, many are now involved in decisions about the allocation of resources to particular services. Many also take part in discussions about the effectiveness of different interventions and in the management of their own budgets at the operational level. If rationing is necessary, arguably the person closest to the point of decision-making is the best one to decide.

Inequalities in health and health-care provision

The need for health care differs greatly between different groups in society. For example, in general, older people have poorer health than the young, and therefore have a greater need for care. Similarly, in the UK, as in most countries, health inequalities are related to other social inequalities. People who are socially and materially deprived have an increased risk of ill-health. This is true for many conditions ranging from tooth decay to heart disease and *cancer; and it results in increased sickness absence, restriction of activity, perinatal mortality, and premature death. The causes of these are well known, although the exact part played by each is hard to tell with accuracy: material deprivation, social status, stress, and behaviour, both unhealthy and healthy, are all known to be important.

Most health services show inequalities in provision; for example, there are marked disparities in access to all kinds of health care. The problem is compounded by the fact that many disadvantaged communities have the fewest health professionals, because the living and working conditions are preferable in better-off areas. Yet the less congenial, more disadvantaged areas are the very ones where, arguably, health services are most needed; this paradox has been called the 'inverse care law'. However, physical accessibility to care is not the only barrier which the disadvantaged face. Services are sometimes provided inappropriately by staff who cannot communicate effectively with people from a different background.

Finally, the debate about how best to use health resources centres increasingly on the design of the health-care system itself. In recent years, the so-called managed-market system has been proposed as the best model. Others argue that a free market is inappropriate for health care because poor people may not be able to afford the help they need. A fundamental decision for any health-care system is therefore whether equity is to be one of its fundamental values or whether it will accept a degree of inequity in return for other presumed benefits.

The desire by British society for a fair distribution of health care and a reduction in inequalities in health was an important part of the NHS at its foundation. The desire for equality, including elements of altruism as well as social justice, remains a popular goal today. However, it must be recognized that there is potential for conflict between equality and efficiency in health services. A more equal distribution of resources might not produce the most health improvement for the population as a whole.

Conclusion

Medical ethics is not an exclusive domain of the health professional. It should not be the subject of dry academic discourse amongst doctors. Ethical and moral dilemmas, some old, some new, and all challenging, are everyday occurrences. Often they are described in media accounts and become the subject of public concern and discussion. Issues such as when a comatose patient's life support system should be switched off, whether a doctor should give contraceptive advice to a teenager without her parent's knowledge or consent, or whether a woman should be allowed to be paid to carry the child of an infertile couple, are all matters about which the man and woman in the street will have opinions. It is the role of the caring professions, society, and sometimes government to ensure that these and similar issues are properly addressed.

DONALD IRVINE
LIAM DONALDSON

Acknowledgement. We thank Ms Jane O'Brien (GMC) for her most helpful contribution.

References

Botros, S. (1992). Ethics in medical research – uncovering the conflicting approaches. In *Manual for research ethics committees*, (Section 4), (compiled by C. Gilbert Foster). Kings College, London.

Crawshaw, R. (1991). Oregon sets priorities in health care. *Bulletin of Medical Ethics*, **69**, 32–5.

O'Neill, O. (1991). Introducing ethics: some current positions. *Bulletin of Medical Ethics*, **73**, 18–21.

ETHICS (OF EXPERIMENTATION). See CLINICAL TRIALS OF TREATMENT; EXPERIMENTAL METHOD; VETERINARY MEDICINE IN RELATION TO HUMAN MEDICINE.

ETHIONAMIDE is an antituberculous drug, administered in combination with one or more other drugs. Nausea can be a limiting side-effect.

ETHMOID. A small cuboidal bone forming part of the *cranium, centrally placed between the orbits at the root of the nose. It is pierced by the nerves that carry olfactory impulses to the brain, accounting for its name, which means sieve-like.

ETHOLOGY is the branch of biology concerned with animal behaviour.

ETHYL ALCOHOL. See ETHANOL.

ETHYL CHLORIDE (C_2H_5Cl) is a highly volatile liquid used as a spray-on cooling agent for the skin to induce *local anaesthesia.

ETIOLOGY. See AETIOLOGY.

ETIQUETTE, MEDICAL, is the unwritten code of honour governing relations between members of the medical profession, and their personal conduct.

EUGENICS is a science which has the objective of improving the inherited characteristics of humans by controlling *genetic transmission.

EUKARYOTES are unicellular or multicellular organisms, animal or plant, whose cells contain genetic material borne on *chromosomes within a distinct *nucleus separated from the *cytoplasm by a nuclear membrane; they undergo nuclear division by *mitosis. All organisms are eukaryotic except blue-green algae and *bacteria, which are *prokaryotes. See also CELL AND CELL BIOLOGY.

EUNUCH. A castrated male. When *castration has occurred before puberty, a eunuch is devoid of *secondary sexual characteristics.

EUPHORIA. Mood elevation characterized by a sense of well-being, cheerfulness, and optimism independent of objective circumstances, associated with mental disorder (for example in *mania, *general paralysis of the insane, and *multiple sclerosis) or drug intoxication (for example with the *amphetamines, *cocaine, and to a lesser extent with *ethanol).

EUSTACHIAN TUBE. The mucosa-lined passage in the *temporal bone which connects the cavity of the *middle ear with the *nasopharynx.

EUSTACHIO, BARTOLOMEO (1524–74). Italian anatomist. He described the *Eustachian tubes in *De auditus organis* (1562); wrote useful works on the kidney and the teeth; and discovered the suprarenals (adrenals), the thoracic duct, and the abducens nerve.

EUTHANASIA. In modern usage, euthanasia generally means 'mercy killing' although the literal 'easy death' remains implicit. Compulsory euthanasia, e.g. for the old, the incurably ill, the mentally disordered, the criminal, the genetically imperfect, and so on, is a concept abhorrent to most human beings, although one which is arguably still accepted in states which have retained the death penalty for particular crimes.

However, a substantial body of reasoned and sincere opinion supports the legalization of some form of voluntary euthanasia; in the UK during the past 50 years no fewer than three Bills with this intent have been presented to Parliament. None were successful, if only because of the risk of abuse; the balance of opinion favours the conclusion of the *World Medical Association (1950) that voluntary euthanasia must always be medically unethical (see SUICIDE). Nevertheless, voluntary euthanasia, with specific safeguards, is now accepted in The Netherlands. In the UK, a House of Lords Select Committee chaired by one of us (JW) decided (in 1994) to recommend no change in the present law under which deliberate euthanasia or assisted suicide, even at the explicit request of the patient, are criminal offences; the Committee did, however, recommend advance directives ('living wills') which would ask doctors to refrain from prolonging life unnecessarily by artificial means.

Reference
Report of the Select Committee on medical ethics (1994.) HL Paper 21–1. HMSO, London.

EVISCERATION. Removal or exteriorization of the abdominal viscera; disembowelling.

EVOKED RESPONSE. See CLINICAL INVESTIGATION.

EVOLUTION. Development according to natural laws and by means of natural processes; differentiation into species from common ancestors. See NATURAL SELECTION.

EVULSION. Extraction with force; tearing out.

EWING, JAMES (1866–1943). American pathologist. His major interest was in the pathology of *neoplastic diseases, and his textbook on pathology of *tumours was a standard reference work. His name is attached to a form of malignant bone tumour. He was especially interested in the effects of X-rays and radium on neoplastic lesions.

EXANTHEMA. One of a group of infectious fevers characterized by a rash or skin eruption (exanthem), such as *measles, *chickenpox, etc. See also INFECTIOUS DISEASES.

EXCIPIENT. An inert substance mixed with a medicinal compound to act as a vehicle and facilitate administration.

EXCISION. Surgical removal; cutting out.

EXCITABILITY is the property possessed by specialized tissues like *nerve and *muscle, the cells of which are capable of being stimulated, that is of passing from the resting to the excited state. See also DEPOLARIZATION.

EXCITATION. See DEPOLARIZATION.

EXCRETION is the elimination of waste matter from the body, the principal organs of excretion being the kidneys, liver, lungs, bowel, and skin.

EXERCITATIO ANATOMICA DE MOTU CORDIS ET SANGUINIS IN ANIMALIBUS. William *Harvey originally communicated his preliminary views on the circulation of the blood in the lectures he gave as Lumleian Lecturer in Anatomy to the Royal College of Physicians of London, on 16, 17, and 18 April 1616. Twelve years later, at the age of 50, he published his definitive exposition of the subject in this classic work; its title is usually shortened to *De motu cordis*. In full, it reads in English as follows: *Movement of the heart and blood in animals: an anatomical essay* by William Harvey, Englishman, Physician to the King, and Professor of Anatomy in the College of Physicians of London (Frankfurt: William Fitzer, 1628).

Thus did Harvey destroy the false Galenic concept of the circulation which had held sway for over fourteen centuries, and he laid the foundation for all future studies of the cardiovascular system.

EXFOLIATION. *Desquamation, particularly in flakes or layers, usually referring to the skin.

EXHAUSTION is a state of extreme fatigue, with no further energy reserves available.

EXHIBITIONISM is public genital exposure, usually with intent to shock or alarm and so to gain sexual gratification. It occurs almost exclusively in men and may be powerfully compulsive.

EXOCRINE describes a gland which releases its secretion by a duct, rather than directly into the blood circulation as with *endocrine or *ductless glands.

EXOPHTHALMIC GOITRE is a synonym for Graves disease. See THYROTOXICOSIS.

EXOPHTHALMOS is forward displacement of the eyeball.

EXORCISM is the act of exorcizing or expelling an evil spirit by adjuration, by performing certain rites, or by repeating certain formulae. It is part of religion, not medicine.

EXOSTOSIS. A small bony projection from a bone surface.

EXOTOXIN. A toxic substance secreted by intact *bacteria (as opposed to *endotoxins, which are liberated when bacteria disintegrate). Exotoxins are heat-labile *proteins, and can be extremely poisonous. See, for example, BOTULISM.

EXPECTATION OF LIFE is average future life, one of the derived values in conventional *life tables, of which the observed data are recorded deaths and the census of population classified according to age. Expectation of life (symbol $\overset{\circ}{e}$) is calculated by dividing the number of survivors to year of age x into the total number of years lived by that cohort from age x until all have died. For example, the life table of US white females (1949–51) showed 294 attaining the age of 100 and having a total number of years to live of 566. The expectation of life for this group at that age was therefore $e_x = 1.92$ years. (The calculation assumes that the deaths in each year are uniformly distributed over that year.) This figure is hypothetical, like all other values in a life table except the mortality rates observed during the specific calendar period. See also EPIDEMIOLOGY.

EXPECTORANT. Any medicinal agent which promotes the ejection by coughing of material accumulated in the air passages. Most expectorants are mild irritants which stimulate the secretion of *mucus.

EXPECTORATION is ejection by coughing of *mucus, *exudate, and other material from the air passages.

EXPERIMENTAL METHOD. Despite the success of Harvey and his successors such as Richard *Lower and Stephen *Hales, the importance of deliberate experiment for medicine did not begin to reap its full harvest until around the middle of the 19th century. It is doubtful if it could have progressed far until chemistry and physics had advanced sufficiently and there was the simple practical difficulty that an experiment on any living mammalian creature was liable both to cause pain and to cause infection or other complications—obstacles not shared by the vastly simpler physical or chemical experiment. One might, indeed, point to three moments of acceleration in biomedical experimental

research: first around the 1870s, when *anaesthesia and *antisepsis together for the first time allowed humane animal experimentation. This was associated also with the birth of the Physiological Society, later to bud off the Biochemical, Medical Research, and British Pharmacological Societies. Next, around 1935, when industrial chemistry was now ready for the demands of the pharmaceutical industry, came *Domagk's discovery of a simple *chemotherapy for *streptococcal infection (see Holmstedt and Liljestrand 1963), together with the growth of knowledge about chemical transmission of nervous activity (involving the very simple chemical *acetylcholine). These, with similar work, and the simplicity of the molecules involved, jointly sparked off a therapeutic revolution. Third was the period after the Second World War, when enormous advances in electronic technology, in new materials (the significance of plastics for medicine would itself be an interesting study), in the use of radioactive substances, and in a wide variety of chemical techniques, vastly increased the precision and sensitivity of methods available to the experimenter.

'Clinical science'
There was one other experimental development, especially important for medicine, namely that of deliberate experiment in man and with patients. There has always been an element of experiment in medicine, especially in therapeutics, simply because there was so much to learn. But we owe particularly to Sir Thomas *Lewis, physician at *University College Hospital, London, a clear and forceful articulation of the characteristic and fruitful way in which scientific observations can be made in the clinical environment, on volunteers or on patients, experiments which satisfy the most rigorous scientific demands.

Today, clinical research has been transformed, as were the preclinical sciences, by advances in technology. As one tracks back from the drug or procedure concerned, one sees in turn the contribution of clinician, epidemiologist, chemist, biochemist, anatomist, physiologist, and pharmacologist; of clinic and laboratory; of human, animal, and inanimate experimental material. To believe that any one discipline alone carries the credit is an illusion, a result of looking, not at the whole historical development, but at a snapshot at a single time.

To illustrate this, the following sections will review, in turn, examples of experimental work that has been important for medicine, drawn, in turn, from physics and chemistry, from work with animals, and from human or clinical studies.

Some contributions from physics and chemistry
The most famous, most dramatic, and most rapidly adopted gift from physics to medicine is probably the experimental work that led to *Roentgen's discovery of *X-rays. Today, a considerable amount of related purely

physical research is supported in a medical environment, such as: working out on models how to focus therapeutic radiation at a required point; development of the 'whole-body' counter, together with a suitable isotope, as a way of discovering the total body content of ions such as sodium; developing increasingly sensitive methods of measuring radiation dose; and analysing the way in which radiations of various types and energy transfer that energy to water or to other molecules. The whole field of radiological protection requires much physical experiment.

The physicist and physical chemist have been equally important in developing the *computerized tomography (CT) scanner, electron-spin and *nuclear magnetic resonance (ESR and NMR) techniques, and *mass spectrometry. The CT and the NMR-based scanners have offered major new advances beyond the normal X-ray in the non-invasive visualization of internal body structures; and in more specialized ways, both ESR and NMR techniques, once developed, offer delicate ways of assessing the chemical state in biological structures of significant molecules. The impact of mass spectrometry on the quantitation of substances in the body has been astonishing: combined with gas–liquid *chromatography, it has lowered the limits of detection of many elements by 10^3 or 10^6, as well as offering means of determining the complete chemical structure of novel substances from quantities of a few micrograms.

The triumphs of X-ray crystallography in establishing the structure of *haemoglobin, the *deoxyribonucleic acid (DNA) helix, and the α-helix and β-sheets of *protein structure are well known. Such work continues and, combined with high-resolution *electron microscopy and *freeze-fracturing, a new world of molecular detail is opening up to medical research that compels new conceptual approaches. But there are many other contributions. The design of new prostheses, and of power units for operating them where muscle power is inadequate; the development of metals and plastics (for implantation within the body) which will not corrode or provoke tissue reactions; the use of *ultrasonics for non-invasive monitoring of fetal development, or for detecting bubble formation in the early stages of *decompression sickness; miniaturization of electronic equipment to allow recording and telemetric transmission of biological data from a freely moving human or animal; electromagnetic flowmeters of shape and size suitable for small blood vessels; *fibre-optical devices to aid *endoscopy or operative techniques at deep sites; and quite modest, but none the less important, contributions to the design of anaesthetic equipment to minimize airway resistance, flammability, liability to produce static electricity, or for reliability in producing a known concentration of anaesthetic. One may guess that there is hardly any branch of physics which has not offered some field for medical exploitation. Equally, the debt that drug development owes to synthetic chemistry is enormous, matched only perhaps by the insight that

flows from knowledge of the detailed chemical structure of biological molecules. As one example of the latter one may cite the *glycoproteins: for many years these were regarded as molecules of rather specialized interest only to biochemists, then they were recognized as including the *blood group proteins, and are now seen as providing a means, through the many glycoside permutations available, of specific cell recognition (see IMMUNOLOGY).

Animal experiment in medical research

Deliberate experiments on living animals have been made at least since the time of *Galen; but there was neither systematic work nor a sustained debate on the issues involved until the birth of modern physiology in the 19th century. The debate goes back at least to 1831, when Marshall *Hall faced the criticisms that his experiments were both cruel and fruitless. His own ideas, now almost entirely forgotten, are really remarkable, for their astonishing modernity, expressed in his proposal (Hall 1831) for the formation of a Physiological Society.

Most of the issues discussed today were already there in principle: 'alternatives', definite scientific objectives, avoidance of unnecessary repetition, the minimizing of suffering, proper record-keeping, openness to criticism, publication.

One may wonder what has happened in the interim, and it is worth noting some major changes. An obvious one is that standards of health and well-being, in both man and animals, have risen enormously since 1830. What would now be regarded as intolerable suffering was then an everyday affair and accepted as part of life. Although cruelty has always evoked revulsion, the level of acceptable suffering in a world where humans were cut for stone or had a limb amputated without anaesthesia, would be different from today. Equally, today expectations of what medicine can achieve have risen dramatically. Thus any debate about animal experiment today takes place against a changing background, with more being demanded in health and well-being and less being tolerated of pain and suffering. To meet these points, there has also been an immense change in experimental technology. The discoveries of anaesthesia and antiseptics were probably the key developments, allowing at last the possibility of humane experimentation. But technical developments since then have allowed far more scientific information to be obtained, more precisely, with much greater sensitivity, in the study of bodily processes. The use of plastics alone has transformed many procedures from the severe to the nearly trivial, as in the collecting of *lymph from an animal's *thoracic duct via a fine plastic tube carried through its skin. At the same time, the care of animals has improved, with greater knowledge of their housing and nutritional needs, diseases, and general husbandry. With healthy animals, fewer experiments are wasted and more information is obtained from them.

A second great change is in the scale of animal experiment, as a result, one can suppose, both of the enhanced ability to measure bodily processes, and of its great success. Instead of a few thousand experiments a year, there are now over 3 million, many of them conducted in the research laboratories of pharmaceutical companies as well as in universities and research institutes.

The third important development is the growth of regulatory bodies. The *thalidomide tragedy gave rise in the UK to the *Dunlop Committee and then to the Committee on Safety of Medicines, to ensure, as far as possible, that the new drugs developed by the pharmaceutical industry should be as safe as possible. This also entails, of course, whether by guidance or specific instruction, the requirement of satisfying an appropriate range of animal tests both for efficacy and for toxicity. The pharmaceutical industry, which wishes to sell its products internationally, now faces similar requirements imposed by different bodies all over the world. There have been similar developments in other fields, such as those relating to food additives, insecticides, and agricultural products, in order to protect both consumer and worker; and the far-reaching *Health and Safety at Work legislation requires testing of any chemical substance—whether the final product or some intermediate—to which humans may be exposed in their work place (see OCCUPATIONAL MEDICINE). All this increases greatly the number of experiments to be done. As a result, those developing substances for use in any of these ways find themselves caught between the conflicting demands of public safety and 'consumerism' on the one hand, and animal welfare on the other.

There is now a considerable literature about various aspects of animal experiment, and no more can be done here than to indicate the main issues and conclusions that seem to be emerging. It is sometimes questioned whether, if man is so different, animal experiment can be relevant to his problems. But man and other vertebrates are built on the same pattern—heart, lungs, kidneys, liver, endocrine glands or organs, and central nervous system. Thus a great deal can be learnt from one vertebrate species that is applicable to another, and it is only when one comes to the higher functions, or to specific differences in 'way of life' or sexual cycle, that comparisons become more remote. Man is something of a genetic hybrid compared with most laboratory animals, and the specific differences between animals may yield 'models' to match genetic differences in man; so the guinea-pig shares with man his need for *vitamin C, as some dogs show a *haemophiliac condition like that of man. It is for the skill of the experimenter to choose that animal most appropriate to the problem (in man or animals) that he wishes to study.

Alternatives

It has been suggested that a great many, if not all, animal experiments could be replaced, without serious loss, by non-animal methods, using computer models, quantum mechanical design of new chemical entities, tissue culture, or much lower organisms. But this now reveals an unawareness of how biomedical science has developed. To begin to study some physiological, pathological, or pharmacological response, one almost always needs to start with the whole animal. But once the 'target' organ or tissue is identified, one can move to perfused or isolated preparations. Then one may be able to focus down further on to particular cells, or even parts of cells, and ultimately to pure enzymes or other macromolecules. Many of the 'alternatives' proposed have already been introduced by the animal experimenters themselves, as a natural development of their work of analysis. Tissue culture is already 80 years old. Equally, the use of models for teaching or analysing functions, like the use of the relationship between chemical structure and pharmacological action to predict new activity, are a century old.

Toxicity testing

This has come to assume increasing importance. Man steadily invents, and is exposed to, new materials and new processes, all of them carrying possible new hazards. Along with this, the public increasingly demands absolute safety, e.g. of medicines, or in the industrial environment. It backs up this demand with increasingly ready litigation. Most medical research asks 'What effects are produced if . . .?' or 'How are these effects mediated?' But toxicity testing presents a new challenge, that of testing for a 'negative', i.e. a lack of harmful action, so as to allow a responsible authority to give an assurance of safety to an increasingly litigious public.

Here, modern *genetics clarifies the problem. Humans carry around 100 000 *genes. The demand for safety means that a new substance must not have an unwanted effect on any of these genes or their products. It is immediately obvious that whole-animal testing will be obligatory. Only then is the whole range of the genome exposed *in active form*. A selection of gene products, expressed, for instance, in an isolated tissue or cell culture, will not be 'enough'. Furthermore, only in the whole organism are the new liabilities to toxicity, of which we still know nothing, displayed.

One help, however, is the recognition of what have been called 'housekeeping' genes; it is these that mediate the familiar biochemical processes common to most living cells. Effects on these can be readily identified on so-called 'alternative' preparations. Extensive toxicological work in each area of study (carcinogenicity, allergy, irritancy, teratology) now points to procedures which begin with screening on a series of simple systems; these may lead at once to rejection of a material; and if it goes forward to animal work, information has usually been gained on actions, doses, and the like, so that the animal testing can be made more precise and less demanding.

Another important development, due to the British Toxicology Society, is the increasing replacement of the notorious LD_{50} test with a 'fixed-dose' procedure. This involves a simple, interesting, and important conceptual change: instead of finding the dose which produces a particular effect, lethality, so that death is a necessary end-point, the new test seeks to identify the first significant toxic effect resulting from a range of doses. As soon as these are located, the experiment can stop. It has already much reduced animal use and suffering.

The benefits from animal experiment
The benefits to which animal experiment has contributed fall under two headings: benefits to knowledge, and benefits to practice. The first of these becomes so much taken for granted, that to remark on it almost seems like a defence of mere wanton curiosity. But the importance of the understanding that has been won of the way the human or animal body works in health and disease can be made more vivid by supposing that all we had learnt by experimental work in, say, the last two millennia were lost (Garrison 1929). We would not now distinguish nerves from tendons, or know that arteries did not contain air; or that our kidneys secrete urine; or that blood was not just another body fluid like sweat or urine, but was constantly circulated to support all the body's activities; or that the pink pulp inside our skulls was the seat of perception, intelligence, memory, and emotion. Our attitude to ourselves, and our fellows, would be quite different, with unlimited scope for magical thinking. Our attitude to animals, too, which owes so much to experimental work, would itself be different. Had animal experiment been prevented, it would have meant the perpetuation of avoidable ignorance for 2000 years. Perhaps that is the essential point; one may sometimes feel there is an excess of 'knowledge'; yet men do not willingly accept what could then be implied—that we should accept continuing ignorance.

If one turns to benefits for practice, some caution is needed. In the wake of some major advance, the medical scientist sometimes claims too much. Yet the history of vaunted remedies now abandoned, the lessons of the *placebo response and the *clinical trial, and the obvious importance for human welfare of the great secular changes in population pressure and personal wealth, require one to look for some really objective evidence for the achievements of scientific medicine. Figure 1 gives a conspectus of some of the therapeutic discoveries, to all of which animal experiment contributed, arranged by the date of their first introduction. There is little there that anyone would wish, today, to be without.

Some special points need attention by those wishing to facilitate new advances. The beautiful study by Comroe and Dripps (1977) of the history of advances in respiratory and cardiovascular medicine showed how variable was the lag between a first discovery and its practical application, ranging from less than a year for X-rays or *ether anaesthesia to 250 years for *blood transfusion. Perhaps the significant figure is the median

of the lag-times they record: about 25 years. Impatience does not pay in medical research. Another feature, very familiar to the research worker, is the unexpectedness of many discoveries. Experiment, by its very nature, implies that there is something not yet known. Some experimental outcomes are readily envisaged at least as possibilities; but it is generally true that the more original a discovery, the less predictable it is. There are therefore great difficulties in commissioning a particular research outcome. Finally, one can make two comments about experimental work: first, that a limited body of work can lead to an almost unlimited benefit; *polio vaccine does not have to be discovered again and its usefulness reaches far into the future. That introduces a sort of 'multiplier' into the discussion. Secondly, of all the variegated suffering in the world, the vast bulk of it is useless, or useful at best as a training ground for endurance and courage. It seems that it is only the suffering inflicted in experimental work, or in the medical or veterinary practice based on it, that promises less suffering in the future.

Benefits to animals
A great deal of *veterinary medicine is the same as that for humans. The same anaesthetics, antiseptics, *antibiotics, *tranquillizers, *hormones, and *analgesics are used; and a comparison of the *British Pharmacopoeia (Veterinary)* with the **British Pharmacopoeia* shows that half the former comes from the latter; the rest is for various specifically animal diseases. For the latter, some achievements have been dramatic. Sir Leonard *Rogers calculated, in 1937, that over 100 million animals had been saved by inoculation against *anthrax and *rinderpest, and a similar number from swine erysipelas in Germany, since the vaccines were discovered. Distemper is another example, now almost abolished, yet once killing dogs by the hundreds of thousands. A recent example is the successful *chemotherapy of the African 'East Coast fever', due to *Theileria parva* that has been killing half a million cattle a year. Man is often seen as 'exploiting' animals; but the achievements of veterinary medicine allow a higher view than this.

Legislation and the control of experiment
As to legislation, the UK has been a pioneer, and its 1876 *Cruelty to Animals Act, criticized as it was, provided almost the only hard evidence available as to the pattern of modern experimental work. The new legislation which has superseded it (see ANIMALS (SCIENTIFIC PROCEDURES) ACT 1986) has preserved its leading features: that experiments may be done to advance knowledge as well as for specifically identified benefit; that the number of experiments done be recorded and returned under suitable categories; that there should be an independent inspectorate, expert in the field, and unifying practice; that there should be an independent advisory committee; and that the personal responsibility

for proper conduct of an experiment always remains with the individual actually doing the experiment.

The annual return of experiments done is of particular value in discussions of animal experiment. A total of over 3 million experiments seems very large at first sight, although expressed as one experiment per head of population every 10 years, its impact is different. The returns make clear, however, the main distribution of the work. First, animals are used less often as one moves up the scale of development: about 58 per cent of experiments are done on mice, 22 per cent on rats, falling to 0.3 per cent on dogs, 0.17 per cent on cats, 0.13 per cent on primates, and 0.01 per cent on equidae.

A small proportion, 4 per cent, of analytic experiments are done wholly under anaesthesia, and it is for experiments of this type that cats and dogs are chiefly used. Around 80 per cent are done without anaesthetic, and these must not involve any procedure more severe than simple inoculation or superficial venesection. A further 16 per cent are done where some more severe procedure is done under anaesthesia, the animal recovers from the anaesthetic, and the experimental observations are made subsequently. Both types of experiment are subject to the 'pain condition', requiring, *inter alia*, that any animal suffering severe pain which is likely to endure must forthwith be painlessly killed. Severe

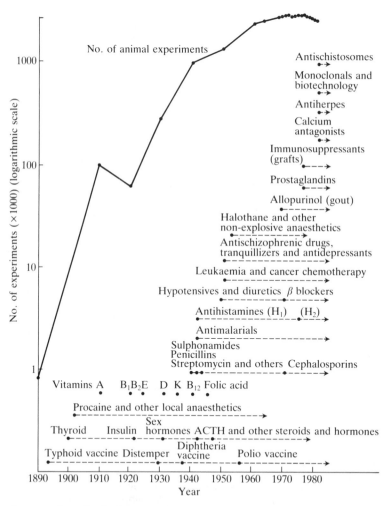

Fig. 1. Animal experiment and medical advance. The approximate date of introduction of an advance is marked with a black dot. Broken lines indicate continued development. The growth of animal experiment since 1890 is also shown using a logarithmic (proportional) scale of the total number of experiments performed in the UK. The numbers are plotted at wide intervals of time until 1970, after which yearly figures are given. (Reproduced from Paton, W.D.M. (1984), *Man and mouse: animals in medical research*, Oxford University Press, Oxford and New York.)

pain is, in fact, very rare, both because experimenters are as humane as anyone else, and because it constitutes in itself a major physiological disturbance, distorting any observations made. The fields of work may be analysed in various ways: thus around 67 per cent of the experiments are concerned with diagnosis of disease, selection of products (which precedes work specifically done for regulatory bodies), work done for registration, or batch control, under the *Medicines Act or its overseas equivalent, or for the *Health and Safety at Work Act, the Agricultural Poisonous Substances Act, or the *Food and Drugs Act. Among specific areas, studies of infection and immunology account for 37 per cent of all experiments, of neoplasia for 4 per cent, toxicity testing in various aspects 15 per cent, use of aversive stimuli 0.9 per cent, application of substances to the eye 0.45 per cent, and the whole field of hazards and safety evaluation 4.8 per cent (of which cosmetics and toiletries contribute less than a tenth). In weighing such figures one needs to consider, too, the pattern and frequency of the diseases to which they relate: infection, cancer, psychological disorder, eye disease, and skin disorder and blemish.

Experiment on man and clinical research
In a rough way, one can recognize three areas: (1) empirical clinical trial in the course of medical treatment; (2) self-experiment; and (3) deliberate trial or experiment on subjects not for their immediate specific benefit but to gain knowledge.

Empirical trial
Empirical trial must be as old as human history, and to this day 'clinical experience' remains a powerful resource. It tends to make the experimental scientist feel uncomfortable, as does any observation that cannot be precisely replicated. Yet its strength lies in its very unselectivity of clinical material; *all* is grist to the clinical mill, so that it is one of the best sources of the unexpected. Indeed, the latest approach to the avoidance of adverse reactions is precisely to try systematically to collect as early as possible the 'one-off' reactions to drugs that occur in general practice. The recognition of the interaction of *monoamine-oxidase inhibitors with other drugs and with amines in the food is only one of the examples where a single 'uncontrolled' clinical observation was the source of an important advance. The post-marketing surveillance of *adverse reactions is essentially an attempt to apply *Pasteur's dictum generally, and to encourage the practitioner to prepare his mind for, and to report, the unexpected reactions that chance offers him. In favourable circumstances, too, the responses of a single patient can yield fully convincing results: as when the response to substance (drug or foodstuff), to its withdrawal, and then to re-challenge, allows the clear recognition of an allergen or of some genetic biochemical deficiency. The single patient with

chronic pain may, in the same way, allow one to discover not only the potency, but also the duration of action and side-effects of different analgesics.

Self-experiment
Self-experiment has some importance in the debate on animal experiment, when it is suggested that the scientist should use himself rather than animals for his purposes. The scale of self-experiment is underestimated. The journals of clinical pharmacology contain very many papers in which the investigators and their colleagues are themselves the subjects. Those experiments point to an area where human study offers a unique advantage, namely, that the subject's testimony can be used, for instance in respect of sleep, memory, mood, cognitive capacity, or pain sensation.

Work on the circulation is another field of fruitful self-experiment, studying the postural and other cardiovascular reflexes, and of great importance for the treatment of cardiovascular disease, shock, and hypertension. J. B. S. Haldane and his colleagues ushered in extensive respiratory experiment, exploiting the capacity of the investigator himself to perform complex respiratory manoeuvres, to throw light on the regulation of respiration. Similar studies have been made on the control of voluntary movement and of visual reflexes and eye movement. Such experiments continue to this day.

A special area is that of 'personnel research', work catalysed especially in the Second World War, to ensure man's safety in adverse conditions in air, under the water, on the surface of the water, or in heat and cold.

Finally, one must recall work in tropical medicine. Humans have volunteered to be infected with *yellow fever, *poliomyelitis, *malaria, and infectious disease, as well as undertaking the less hazardous but hardly appetizing ingestion of *roundworms and threadworms. A remarkable recent example was that of Ralph Lainson and his colleagues in work on *leishmaniasis in South America. To identify the vector (*sandflies) of the disease, they used themselves (at night, stripped to the waist) as bait, identified the specimens concerned, mapped out their natural occurrence, learnt how they became carriers, and produced an infection by a deliberately infected sandfly—a truly remarkable study of the subtle adaptation between the various species of organism, insect, and animal.

Experiment on other human subjects
Finally we come to deliberate trial on subjects other than the investigator, where the primary objective is not the subject's own benefit, but a more general gain. A landmark in this field is the paper, still worth reading, by Sir Austin Bradford Hill and his colleagues, on the first clinical trial of streptomycin published in 1948 (Hill 1962). They were confronted with a drug already proved to be active against tuberculosis *in vitro* and *in vivo* in

the guinea-pig; it was in short supply; encouraging, but inconclusive, clinical reports had appeared; and not long before there had been the depressing example of *gold therapy in tuberculosis for which exaggerated claims had persisted for over 15 years. The question was how to use the amount of drug available to best advantage, in a rigorously controlled investigation (Hill 1962).

The result was a study, followed by others, which proved beyond doubt that streptomycin was effective; but it did more, when other dosage and other drugs were later tested by a similar technique, in allowing decisive information to be obtained about the development of resistant organisms and about toxicity. As a trial, the results were perhaps less instantly dramatic than, say, Mary Walker's demonstration of the effect of the *anticholinesterase eserine in *myasthenia, or the effect of *sulphonamides in *puerperal fever. But this modestly written paper constituted a landmark in the introduction of scientific cogency into therapeutic medicine (see also CLINICAL TRIALS).

Conclusions

One may end this account by noticing three developments. First comes the growth of clinical experiment. A good deal of what has been surveyed has been conceptually fairly simple: the effect of a drug, or of some physiological stress, or of some infecting organism. But if we return to Sir Thomas Lewis's 'clinical science', we recognize there an explicitly *analytical* process. Thus in his classic book on *The blood vessels of the human skin and their responses* (1927), we find not only a description of the characteristic response to skin injury, with its *erythema, *weal, and flare, but recognition, from the characteristics of the flare, that nerves are indeed involved but that the spinal cord is not, and (using the clinical material available) that sensory, not sympathetic, nerves are involved. It is this deeper study of clinical material, exemplified also by Beeson's work on pyrogens, or by many endocrinological studies, that, together with advancing technology, gives experimental clinical research such promise today. Its great advantages lie in the possibility of the subject's co-operation, the availability of testimony, the fact that man is so genetically variable, the sheer range of clinical material, and the direct relevance of the outcome to human disease.

Secondly, there is a sense in which animal and human research are drawing together. In everyday life, one takes for granted sporadic discomforts. Similarly, in the life of a pet, there are casual discomforts. One of the striking things that emerges from advances in experience and technology is the greatly reduced pain and suffering involved in both clinical and experimental procedures. For the writer, it seems that there is now a realistic goal that can be aimed at: that the suffering of experiment, animal or man, can be reduced to that of everyday life. In a world of free interacting organisms, one cannot hope for more.

Thirdly, the impact of *molecular biology and genetics opens an extraordinary, and largely unpredictable, future. The *polymerase chain reaction (PCR) promises to allow us in time to make as much as we wish of any bodily constituent. Work on macromolecule assembly will allow new structures to be created (make your own receptor or ion channel!). Artificial *mutations will produce new biological products. Of the whole genome, with its 100 000 genes, only a few thousand have been identified, and hence have become available for experimental study. What do the remaining tens of thousands of genes hold in store?

(The late) W. D. M. PATON

References

Beeson, P. B. (1980). How to foster the gain of knowledge about disease. *Perspectives in biology and medicine* Winter, Part II.

Comroe, J. H. and Dripps, R. D. (1977). *The top ten clinical advances in cardiovascular-pulmonary medicine and surgery 1945–1975, Washington, DC.*

Garrison. F.H. (1929). *An introduction to history of medicine.* Saunders, Philadelphia and London.

Hall. M. (1831). *A critical and experimental essay on the circulation of the blood.* London. (Reprinted 1847 in *Lancet*, i, 58–60, 135, 161).

Hill, Sir A. B. (1962). *Statistical methods in clinical and preventive medicine.* Oxford University Press, New York.

Holmstedt, B. and Lljestrand, G. (1963). *Readings in pharmacology.* Pergamon, Oxford and London.

Lewis, T. (1927). *The blood vessels of the human skin and their responses.* Shaw, London.

Paton, W. D. M. (1984). *Man and mouse: animals in medical research.* Oxford University Press, Oxford and New York.

Rogers, Sir L. (1937). *The truth about vivisection.* Churchill, London.

EXPERIMENTATION (ANIMALS AND MAN). See CLINICAL TRIALS; EXPERIMENTAL METHOD; VETERINARY MEDICINE.

EXPERT EVIDENCE. See MEDICAL EVIDENCE.

EXPERT WITNESS. See MEDICAL EVIDENCE.

EXPOSITION. See COMMUNICATION BETWEEN DOCTORS AND PATIENTS.

EXSANGUINATION. Severe loss of blood.

EXTEROCEPTORS are sensory *receptors which receive stimuli from the immediate external environment, particularly those in the skin responsible for the sensations of touch, heat, and pain.

EXTRAPYRAMIDAL SYSTEM is a collective term for those structures (nuclei and tracts) involved in the central nervous control of motor function other than the pyramidal tracts and their connections; the *basal ganglia (see PARKINSONISM) are major components of the system.

EXTRASENSORY PERCEPTION (often abbreviated to ESP) is knowledge of, or a response to, an external object, thought, or event which has not been obtained through any of the five known senses. Anecdotal evidence seeming to demonstrate such perception abounds, but rigorous supporting scientific data are lacking. The subject remains a matter of legitimate debate among experimental psychologists. Telepathy, clairvoyance, precognition, and psychokinesis are four modalities of this phenomenon.

EXTRASYSTOLE. An extra or interpolated cardiac contraction occurring independently of, and in addition to, the normal cardiac rhythm, due to discharge of an irritable focus somewhere in the *myocardium other than the *sinoatrial node pacemaker; also termed 'ectopic beat' or 'premature beat'. Isolated extrasystoles are not uncommon in otherwise healthy individuals.

EXTRAVASATION is the escape or seepage of blood from a vessel into the tissues.

EXUDATE. A mixture of fluid, *protein, *cells, and cell debris derived from the blood as part of an inflammatory response (see INFLAMMATION).

EYE. The special sense organ adapted to receive visual stimuli and transmit them to the brain in the form of nervous impulses from which images can be constructed. See also OPHTHALMOLOGY.

F

FABRICIUS AB AQUAPENDENTE, HIERONY-MUS (1537–1619). Italian anatomist. Fabricius directed his attention to *embryology in his *De formatio foetu* (1600) and named the hen's *ovary as ovarium, the site of egg production, for the first time. He described the *placenta in detail. In 1603 in *De venarum ostiolis* he described the valves of the veins; he must have taught his pupil William *Harvey about them as they were crucial in Harvey's demonstration of the circulation of the blood. Fabricius was also the first to show changes in pupillary size in response to light and the use of the *larynx in speech.

FABRY, WILHELM (Fabricius Hildanus) (1560–1634). The leading German surgeon of his time, he is sometimes described as the 'father of German surgery'; he was the first to amputate above the gangrenous area. He devised a *tourniquet and was skilled in operations on the eye and for stone.

FACET. A small flat smooth articular surface of a bone.

FACIAL HEMIATROPHY is wasting of one half of the face, a condition of unknown aetiology also known as Romberg's disease.

FACIAL NERVE. The seventh *cranial nerve, which carries predominantly motor fibres to the facial muscles (see BELL'S PALSY); it also carries sensory fibres for taste from the anterior part of the tongue in the chorda tympani, and parasympathetic fibres to the *salivary and *lacrimal glands. Small branches carry the motor supply to the stapedius muscle of the *middle ear and relay skin sensation around the external auditory meatus.

FACIES. Apart from its restricted anatomical use, the word facies (pronounced fay-sheez) is used to denote the whole facial appearance of a patient, especially when suggestive of a particular disorder. A characteristic facies is often said to be present in *acromegaly, *thyrotoxicosis, *myxoedema, acute *glomerulonephritis, *Down's syndrome, *tabes dorsalis, *myasthenia gravis, *parkinsonism, *Addison's disease, chronic *alcoholism, *mitral stenosis, congenital *syphilis, *Cushing's syndrome, *cretinism, facioscapulohumeral *muscular dystrophy, *adenoidal hyperplasia, *Wilson's disease, *polycythaemia, *pernicious anaemia, *lupus erythematosus, *scleroderma, lepromatous *leprosy, *Paget's disease, *eunuchoidism, and a number of childhood *exanthemata (e.g. *measles) and other diseases associated with skin manifestations, including abnormal *pigmentation. This catalogue is not exhaustive.

FACTOR. An agent, usually a chemical substance such as a *hormone, *enzyme, or dietary component, which plays a significant role in a physiological or pathological process, the nature or end-result of which is often indicated by an adjectival description (e.g. antihaemophilic factor, thyrotropin-releasing factor, pellagra-preventing factor, nerve growth factor, etc.). Occasionally, and less helpfully, the identification may be an *eponym (e.g. Castle's factor, later shown to be the intrinsic factor that is missing in *pernicious anaemia) or merely a serial letter or number.

FACTORY ACTS. The first legislation in the UK designed to protect factory workers concerned young people in cotton mills, and dates from the first decade of the 19th century. From 1819 onwards, several Acts of Parliament and statutory regulations, again mostly concentrated on the textile industries, dealt with various aspects of factory work, including safety, work hours and meal times, and employment of women and children.

Following a Royal Commission set up in 1876, comprehensive legislation was attempted in the Factory and Workshop Act of 1878. A second effort was made in the Factories and Workshops Act of 1901, which remained the principal law until repealed by the Factories Act of 1936, itself to be replaced by the Factories Act of 1961. The last of these, with some amendments, remains in force.

Each successive piece of legislation was followed by the revelation of deficiencies requiring new regulations to be made under enabling clauses or new legislation. The 1961 Act was no exception, chiefly because of new and unpredicted occupational hazards. Accordingly, in

1970 another Royal Commission (under Lord Robens) was appointed to consider accidents and other dangers in places of employment, and related matters. As a result, all regulations on occupational safety and health are now made under powers identified and explained in the *Health and Safety at Work Act 1974.

FACULTIES. See MEDICAL COLLEGES, ETC. OF THE UK; MEDICAL COLLEGES, ETC. IN NORTH AMERICA; MEDICAL EDUCATION, POSTGRADUATE.

FACULTY. A particular ability, especially mental ability.

FAECES are excrement discharged from the alimentary canal through the anus. They form in the *colon and consist largely of undigested food (in which *cellulose and other non-absorbable *carbohydrates predominate), a mass of *bacteria, shed intestinal cells, *mucus, water, *bile pigment (responsible for the colour), and other secretions.

FAHRENHEIT, GABRIEL DANIEL (1686–1736). German physicist. He conceived (*c.* 1720) the idea of using mercury in a *thermometer in place of alcohol because it neither boiled nor froze at temperatures ordinarily encountered.

FAHRENHEIT TEMPERATURE SCALE. The temperature scale devised by *Fahrenheit is still in fairly wide non-scientific use. On this scale the melting point of ice is 32° and the boiling point of water 212° (at standard atmospheric pressure). Fahrenheit devised this scale by dividing the interval between the temperature of a mixture of ice and water and that of the normal human body into 64 parts and assigning a value of 32 to the former. 0° was the lowest temperature encountered in Danzig in the winter of 1719. To convert a temperature value in degrees Fahrenheit to degrees Celsius (or centigrade), subtract 32 from it and multiply the remainder by 5/9 (or 0.56).

FAINT. Sudden temporary loss of consciousness due to transient reduction in blood supply to the brain; synonymous with *syncope.

FAIRLEY, SIR NEIL HAMILTON (1891–1966). Australian physician. He did original work on schistosomiasis (*bilharziasis), for the diagnosis of which he devised an *antigen which was used for decades. He was a professor in Bombay, and from 1929 to 1939 was on the staff of the Hospital for Tropical Diseases in London. His work on intravascular *haemolysis and on the *anaemia of *malaria won him the Fellowship of the Royal Society in 1942. He joined the Australian Medical Corps at the outbreak of the Second World War, and his work on the protection of troops serving in heavily malarious areas, first with *mepacrine and then with *proguanil,

was critical in the success of the Pacific and Burmese campaigns.

FAITH HEALING. See COMPLEMENTARY (ALTERNATIVE) MEDICINE.

FALLEN ARCH. The normal longitudinal arch of the foot, higher on the inner side, extends between the two areas of the sole which take the weight of the body, namely the heads of the metatarsals (the long foot bones) and the *calcaneum. This arch is maintained by the strong *ligaments of the sole, whose integrity is, in turn, dependent on the action of the foot muscles, especially those of the big toe. Muscular weakness, often combined with mechanical overload due to prolonged standing or obesity, stretches the ligament (causing aching in the sole) and eventually permanently weakens it; the longitudinal arch is then reduced or disappears, and the condition called *pes planus* (fallen arch, or flat foot) is established.

FALLING SICKNESS was formerly a common designation for *epilepsy.

FALLOPIAN TUBE. The uterine tube, a paired slender hollow structure which leads from the region of each *ovary to the upper part of the cavity of the *uterus and acts as a conduit for shed *ova.

FALLOPIO, GABRIELLE (otherwise Fallope or Fallopius) (1523–62). Italian anatomist and surgeon. In his *Observationes anatomicae* (1562) he corrected some of the faults in Vesalius' *Fabrica* and described the *Fallopian aqueduct and tubes still known by his name, although the latter were well known and accurately defined by *Herophilus in the 4th century BC.

FALLOT, ETIENNE LOUIS ARTHUR (1850–1911). French physician. Fallot discovered a relatively common *congenital abnormality of the heart and great vessels with four associated defects—hence named *Fallot's tetralogy.

FALLOT'S TETRALOGY is a relatively common form of cyanotic *congenital heart disease, in which the following four anatomical abnormalities occur: pulmonary valve *stenosis, *hypertrophy of the right ventricular wall, ventricular septal defect ('hole in the heart'), and rightwards displacement of the *aorta so that it arises partly from the right ventricular cavity instead of exclusively from the left. The anomaly can be corrected surgically (see CARDIOTHORACIC SURGERY).

FAMILIAL DISEASE. Genetically transmitted disease in which the abnormal *gene is *recessive, so that neither parent is affected (being *heterozygous and carrying only one abnormal gene) but their children, who inherit two abnormal genes (one-quarter on average), develop the condition. Of the unaffected children, two-thirds will be heterozygous carriers of the gene.

FAMILY DOCTOR SERVICE OR FAMILY PHYSICIAN. See PRIMARY MEDICAL CARE.

FAMILY PLANNING is a euphemism for *contraception, although a full definition must also embrace other methods of limiting family size, such as *abortion, celibacy, and legal sanctions.

FAMINE is protracted starvation of a community, which if sufficiently prolonged causes deaths from protein-energy *malnutrition itself and from the ravages of intercurrent infectious disease. It may follow failure of a community's staple crop, as in the great Irish potato famine of the 1840s, or other natural disasters; or it may be man-made, as when it occurs during war as a result of inefficient politico-economic systems with inadequate food distribution. Famine continues in spite of 20th century civilization (e.g. in Bangladesh and many parts of Africa). In famine relief, energy foods must have first priority, with additional *protein for children.

FANCONI, GUIDO (1892–1979). Swiss paediatrician. *Fanconi's anaemia and the *Fanconi syndrome are named after him. He was the first to describe *cystic fibrosis of the pancreas. By analytical *epidemiology he showed that the virus of *poliomyelitis was transmitted not by droplet but by the intestinal route, so changing the form of public health measures in this disease. He predicted accurately that *Down's syndrome was due to a *chromosomal abnormality, 20 years before *trisomy 21 was discovered.

FANCONI'S ANAEMIA is a rare, recessively inherited form of aplastic *anaemia described by *Fanconi in 1927 but unrelated to Fanconi's syndrome. *Bone marrow failure develops usually between the ages of 5 and 10 years, and there are often associated abnormalities of the skeletal and renal systems, together with patchy melanotic skin pigmentation. Both patients and unaffected relatives show an increased incidence of malignant disease. The prognosis is poor.

FANCONI'S SYNDROME is characterized by signs of proximal renal tubular dysfunction, with aminoaciduria, glycosuria, hyperphosphataemia, and excessive loss of water and bicarbonate, presenting with renal tubular *acidosis and *rickets or *osteomalacia. It may occur as a pure genetically determined disorder or in association with other inherited conditions. Or it may develop in relation to acquired diseases, such as *amyloidosis, *multiple myeloma, and *Sjögren's syndrome. It may also follow renal *transplantation, poisoning with heavy metals, or administration of drugs.

FARADAY, MICHAEL (1791–1867). English physicist. He made notable chemical discoveries before turning to his work on electromagnetism, which laid the foundation for both the generation and the application of electrical power. Apart from the obvious practical applications of *electricity in medicine, the principles established by Faraday are also basic to understanding conduction in nerves and across membranes. Faraday himself suffered from nervous illness.

FARADISM, or faradization, is the therapeutic application of a faradic (i.e. induced) electrical current.

FARCY is the chronic cutaneous and lymphatic form of *glanders.

FARMER'S LUNG is a pulmonary disorder, both episodic and chronic, due to occupational exposure to fungal *spores contained in the dust of mouldy hay. The condition is an *allergic response to the spores of *Micropolyspora faeni* and *Thermoactinomyces vulgaris*, and is also classified as a form of 'extrinsic allergic alveolitis' or *hypersensitivity pneumonitis'.

FARR, WILLIAM (1807–83). British physician and pioneer British medical statistician; he compiled life tables, tables of causes of death, and vital statistics (see EPIDEMIOLOGY).

FASCIA consists of bands or sheets of fibrous *connective tissue, enclosing muscles, groups of muscles, and other organs.

FASCICULATION. Spontaneous twitching of small groups of muscle fibres (each group representing a fasciculus, or bundle, of fibres). It may be benign but can also be due to denervation. It is widespread and prominent in *motor neurone disease (see NEUROMUSCULAR DISEASE).

FASCIOLIASIS is infestation with *Fasciola hepatica*, the liver *fluke, common world-wide in sheep and cattle, occasional in man. The condition is acquired from eating encysted forms of the parasite attached to water plants such as water-cress. Serious liver disease can occasionally result.

FAT. Any of the simple *lipids, that is triglycerides of glycerol and *fatty acids, particularly oleic, palmitic, and stearic acids. Fat is contained in the cells of *adipose tissue, where it is the principal *energy store of the body (0.038 MJ/g). It accounts for about 20 per cent of body weight (average build) and in a person of normal weight (70 kg) stores about 530 MJ. In prolonged starvation, 95 per cent of energy requirements are met by combustion of free fatty acids and *ketones from this reserve. Fat also provides a physiological packing material with shock-absorbing and thermal insulating properties. It can be synthesized within the body and is not an essential component of the diet, although the fat-soluble *vitamins and traces of *polyunsaturated fatty acids such as linoleic acid are.

FATAL ACCIDENTS ACT 1976. The law concerning recovery of compensation by dependants for fatal injuries suffered at work is governed in the UK by the Fatal Accidents Act of 1976. Briefly it provides that if death results from a wrongful act, fault, or neglect which would have entitled the injured person, had he not died, to recover damages, the person who would have been liable is still liable; any action in respect of that liability shall be for the benefit of the dependants of the deceased person. The Act defines dependants as either spouses or blood relatives, excluding, for example, mistresses, friends, and servants. 'Injury' includes disease (e.g. scrotal cancer, *mesothelioma) and mental or physical impairment, even when the fatal nature of the disorder is not manifest until years later. Compensation is purely financial and based on the deceased's earning capacity, there being no component in respect of grief, emotional suffering, etc.

FATIGUE. See SLEEP.

FATTY ACIDS are monobasic organic acids having the general formula R.COOH, where R is a group of hydrogen and carbon atoms. See also LIPIDS.

FAUCES. The passage between the mouth and the pharynx, containing the *tonsils.

FAUCHARD, PIERRE (1678–1761). French dental surgeon, regarded as the founder of dentistry in France. He was one of the first to crown teeth, to make dentures, and to deal effectively with caries. He gave the first description of *pyorrhoea alveolaris. He published *Le chirurgien dentiste ou traité de dents* (2 vols, 1728), the first dental textbook.

FAVISM is a form of *glucose 6-phosphate dehydrogenase (G6PD) deficiency found in people of Mediterranean origin in whom severe haemolytic red blood cell destruction occurs after eating the Italian broad bean *Vicia faba*. Like other variants of G6PD deficiency, it is inherited as an *X-linked recessive trait (see GENETICS); and patients are also sensitive to a wide range of oxidant drugs (including antimalarials, antibacterials, *anthelminthics, *analgesics, and *sulphonamides).

FAVRE, MAURICE (1876–1954). French physician. He classified the *reticuloendothelioses. His name is eponymously attached, with that of Nicolas, to the venereal disease known as *lymphogranuloma venereum.

FEEDBACK. See HOMEOSTASIS.

FEE-SPLITTING is clandestine payment by a specialist, usually a surgeon, of part of his fee to the doctor who referred the patient. This practice, although not necessarily illegal, is unethical. The American College of Surgeons withdraws membership from those who are proved to have done this.

FELDSCHER. A semi-trained medical orderly responsible for primary care in the comprehensive health service established in Tsarist Russia in 1862. Feldschers were failed students of Peter the Great's medical school in Moscow. Their role has been compared to that of the *barefoot doctors of China.

FELON. A small *abscess or *boil, particularly a *whitlow underneath a finger or toe nail.

FEMINIZATION is the appearance in a male of female *secondary sexual characteristics.

FEMORAL TRIANGLE. The anatomical area at the top of the thigh bounded by the inguinal ligament (upper), sartorius muscle (lateral), and adductor longus muscle (medial).

FEMUR. The thigh bone, the largest and longest in the body, extending from the hip to the knee joints.

FENESTRATION is an operation for the improvement of hearing in *otosclerosis, now largely superseded by more effective procedures. It consisted of making a 'window' in the *labyrinth of the ear. See also OTORHINOLARYNGOLOGY.

FENFLURAMINE is one of the *anorectic drugs used as a short-term adjunct in the treatment of *obesity; it is also known as Ponderax®.

FERMENTATION is the *anaerobic decomposition by micro-organisms of organic substances into simpler compounds, particularly of sugar into *ethanol and *carbon dioxide by *yeasts, the process used in manufacturing bread, beer, and wine:

$$C_6H_{12}O_6 \rightarrow 2C_2H_5OH + 2CO_2$$

The *enzyme concerned is yeast zymase.

FERNEL, JEAN FRANCOIS (1497–1558). French physician and philosopher, who played a considerable part in breaking down the dogma of *Galen (see PHYSIOLOGY). His *Universa medica* (1554), the first 'modern' textbook of medicine, was the standard work for 100 years.

FERRIER, SIR DAVID (1843–1928). British neurologist, who established the localization of function in the *cerebral hemispheres by electrical stimulation. He was the author of *The functions of the brain* (1876).

FERTILITY, or fecundity, is the ability to reproduce. In strict demographic usage a distinction is drawn: fecundity means ability to have children, whereas fertility relates to the actual number of children produced.

FERTILITY CONTROL. *Birth control.

FERTILITY DRUG. Any drug administered to induce *ovulation and *pregnancy in patients with anovulatory *infertility. Clomiphene (Clomid®) is an anti-oestrogen which, by inhibiting the negative feedback effect of gonadal *steroids on the *hypothalamus, stimulates pituitary release of *gonadotrophin. Or gonadotrophin itself may be administered. Hyperstimulation may lead to multiple ovulation and multiple pregnancy.

FERTILIZATION, *IN VITRO*, that is allowing union between male and female *gametes (*ova and *spermatozoa) to take place under laboratory conditions outside the body, has been widely and successfully practised for many years in many animal species, including farm animals and subhuman primates. The *zygote is allowed partially to develop in the culture medium, and pregnancy is induced by its introduction into the oviduct or *uterus (depending on the stage of development) of a female. The whole process is known as *in vitro* fertilization and *embryo transfer. No increase in fetal or neonatal defects has been noted.

More recently the technique has been introduced into clinical practice. Preovulatory ova or oocytes are obtained by *laparoscopy or other methods. Many pregnancies have been established and successfully taken to term in patients with infertility due, for example, to *Fallopian tube blockage, resulting in 'test-tube babies'. This is now well-established as a method of treatment of certain types of male, as well as of female, subfertility.

The use of *in vitro* fertilization alone, that is without intent to implant the embryo, as a research method of studying the earliest stages of human development raised several ethical misgivings as did embryo research and preimplantation embryo biopsy for diagnosis of genetic disease. Following the passage in the UK of the Human Fertilization and Embryology Act in 1990 all such procedures are now licensed under the rigorous control and statutory authority of a formal licensing body.

FESTINATION is the characteristic hurrying or shuffling gait of *parkinsonism.

FETAL ALCOHOL SYNDROME. A rare syndrome of impaired fetal growth and development associated with a high maternal intake of *ethanol during pregnancy. The fetus is most vulnerable to the deleterious effects of alcohol at, and immediately following, conception, before the mother knows she is pregnant. Features of the syndrome include growth retardation, microcephaly, mental handicap, and a characteristic combination of craniofacial deformities. Other malformations, such as *neural tube defects, may also occur.

FETISHISM is a sexual deviation, almost exclusive to males, in which erotic feelings are aroused by inanimate objects, such as articles of clothing, excreta, etc.

FETOSCOPY is examination of the fetus with an *endoscope inserted into the uterus as a method of *antenatal diagnosis.

FETUS. The offspring of a viviparous animal while in the *uterus. In man, the term is conventionally used during the period from 8 weeks after conception until *delivery; before then it is an *embryo, afterwards an infant.

FEVER is a rise in body temperature above normal (37 °C when measured orally); it is also termed pyrexia.

FEVER HOSPITALS. *Isolation hospitals.

FIBIGER, JOHANNES ANDREAS GRIB (1867–1928). Danish experimental pathologist. In 1913 he showed that a *nematode was associated with *carcinoma of the stomach in rats. The tumour was produced if the larval stage of the parasite was fed to rats by giving them the intermediate host, the cockroach. His discovery stimulated much experimental cancer research. He was awarded the *Nobel prize for medicine in 1926.

FIBRE, DIETARY. Fibre is the alimentary residue of vegetable food, consisting of the fibrous and viscous *polysaccharides which give plants their structure and form; these are not digested in the small intestine and pass unchanged into the large intestine where they are fermented to a variable extent. The polysaccharides concerned are *cellulose, hemicellulose, lignins, pectins, gums, and mucilages. See also GASTROENTEROLOGY; NUTRITION.

FIBRE-OPTICS is the development and application of image transmission along flexible transparent fibres made of glass or plastic. See ENDOSCOPY.

FIBRIL. A small thread-like structure or filament.

FIBRILLATION is the uncoordinated electrical and/or mechanical activity of individual muscle fibres. See ATRIAL FIBRILLATION; NEUROMUSCULAR DISEASE; VENTRICULAR FIBRILLATION.

FIBRIN is an insoluble protein precipitated from the blood in a fibre network during clotting, which provides the basic structure of the clot (*thrombus). It is formed from the soluble blood protein fibrinogen (coagulation factor I) by the action of an enzyme, *thrombin. Thrombin is derived from a precursor protein *prothrombin (factor II).

FIBRINOGEN. Coagulation factor I. See FIBRIN.

FIBRINOLYSIS is the enzymatic degradation of *fibrin. The protease concerned is plasmin, formed from a normally circulating precursor plasminogen under a variety of circumstances which result in the release of 'activator' substances.

FIBROADENOMA. An *adenoma containing fibrous tissue: a benign *tumour often occurring in the breast.

FIBROBLAST. The chief cell of *connective tissue, of elongated and somewhat irregular shape, terminating at either end in *cytoplasmic processes and possessing an oval *nucleus.

FIBROID is the common name for a benign *tumour (leiomyoma or fibromyoma) derived from smooth muscle, found most often in the *uterus. Fibroids are often multiple and may grow large, producing symptoms and signs because of their space-occupying effect. They can readily be removed surgically. See also OBSTETRICS AND GYNAECOLOGY.

FIBROMYOMA. See FIBROID.

FIBROSARCOMA. A *sarcoma of *connective tissue originating from fibroblasts.

FIBROSIS is abnormal proliferation of fibrous tissue.

FIBROSITIS. A diagnostic category lacking precision, equivalent to such labels as 'non-articular *rheumatism', 'muscular rheumatism' and, more recently, 'fibromyalgia'. The symptoms are episodic pain and stiffness, particularly in the neck, shoulder, and back; localized tenderness, sometimes with palpable subcutaneous nodules, may be found on examination of these areas.

FIBROUS TISSUE is undifferentiated *connective tissue, in which *fibroblasts predominate.

FICK METHOD AND PRINCIPLE. A well-established method introduced by the German physiologist A. E. Fick (1829–1901) for estimating *cardiac output, involving measurement of oxygen consumption by the subject (normally about 250 ml/min); of arterial oxygen content (about 200 ml/l); and of pulmonary arterial (mixed venous) oxygen content measured in a blood sample obtained by cardiac catheterization (about 150 ml/l). Pulmonary blood flow (normally equal to cardiac output) is then calculated in l/min by dividing the oxygen uptake by the pulmonary arteriovenous oxygen difference; an average value is 5 litres/min (i.e. 250/50). The

Fick principle can be applied to blood flow through any organ or tissue where the uptake or release of a substance by the organ is known or can be measured, and the arteriovenous concentration difference of that substance across the organ can also be measured.

FIELD HOSPITALS are temporary and mobile hospitals established near a battle.

FILAMENT. Any very thin, thread-like structure.

FILARIASIS is a term loosely applied to human infestation with several species of thread-like *nematode worms transmitted by biting insects, mostly in the tropics. Some cause no or only minor symptoms. Those of medical importance include: *Wuchereria bancrofti* and *Brugia malayi*, which cause *elephantiasis (lymphatic filariasis) and are transmitted by mosquitoes; *Onchocerca volvulus*, which causes *onchocerciasis (river blindness) and is transmitted by blackflies; and *Loa loa*, which causes transient subcutaneous swellings known as Calabar swellings (loiasis) and is transmitted by deerflies of the genus *Chrysops*.

FILATOV, NIL FEODOROVICH (1847–1902). Russian paediatrician. Filatov described a variety of contagious fever with desquamation of the skin, and also the spots in the mouth in early *measles, more usually known by the name Koplik.

FILLING. Material employed to occlude a tooth cavity, such as gold, *amalgam, and various synthetic compounds.

FINGERPRINT. A visual record, made usually by ink impression on paper, of the cutaneous ridge patterns on the palmar surface of the terminal phalanx of each finger. Apart from the familiar use of fingerprints for identification by the police, the study of cutaneous ridge patterns (dermatoglyphs) is of interest to both anthropologists and geneticists. Abnormal fingerprint patterns may be found in *cystic fibrosis and in some other diseases.

FINLAND, MAXWELL (1902–87). US physician long associated with the Thorndike laboratory at the Boston City Hospital, he made basic contributions to the study of infectious diseases and their treatment.

FINSEN, NIELS RYBERG (1860–1904). Danish physician. Finsen proved that rays of short wavelength were responsible for the bactericidal power of sunlight, and developed a method of treating *lupus vulgaris by ultraviolet light. From the age of 23 he was an invalid, but directed from his bed the Light Institute which he founded in Copenhagen in 1896. He received the *Nobel prize for medicine in 1903.

FINSEN LAMP. A source of ultraviolet radiation formerly used to treat *lupus vulgaris; its basis was a carbon arc lamp of high amperage.

FIROR, WARFIELD M. (1896–1988). He was a student and intern under William Stewart Halsted, and remained at Johns Hopkins for his surgical career. He was a quintessential teacher, a brilliant scholar, and an outstanding investigator. He studied intestinal obstruction, canine empyema, and hepatic physiology.

FIRST AID is the immediate assistance to accident victims and the acutely ill, to be administered by anyone present before professional attention becomes available. Among many simple measures which may be helpful, those of life-saving importance are arrest of haemorrhage, relief of airways obstruction, pulmonary ventilation by mouth-to-mouth insufflation, and circulatory maintenance by external cardiac compression.

FISCHER, EMIL HERMANN (1852–1919). German biochemist. His vast range of researches included the hydrazines, the *purines, the *amino acids, and the *proteins. He synthesized veronal (1904) and most of the *sugars and *polypeptides. He was awarded the *Nobel prize for chemistry in 1902.

FISHBEIN, MORRIS (1889–1976). American physician and editor. Following residency training in pathology, Fishbein turned to medical publishing work, as assistant editor of the *Journal of the American Medical Association* (see MEDICAL JOURNALS). He became editor of that publication in 1925, and during the next quarter of a century not only guided its progress but helped to sponsor several specialty journals of the *American Medical Association (AMA). He personally led the campaign of the AMA against quacks, and, to a considerable extent was the spokesman of the AMA.

FISHER, SIR RONALD AYLMER (1890–1962). British statistician and geneticist. He devised the techniques of design and analysis of experiments and unravelled the genetics of the *rhesus blood groups.

FISSURE. An anatomical groove or cleft; or a longitudinal *ulcer, particularly in the anal region.

FISSURE OF ROLANDO. The central sulcus of the *brain, the deep fissure in each cerebral hemisphere separating the frontal from the parietal lobe.

FISSURE OF SYLVIUS. The lateral cerebral sulcus, the deep cleft at the side of the *brain separating the temporal from the frontal and parietal lobes. It is also called the sylvian fissure.

FISTULA. An abnormal passage between an internal structure and the body surface, or between two internal structures. The term is applied to channels created surgically as well as those arising as a result of a pathological process.

FISTULA-IN-ANO. A *fistula joining the anal canal to the body surface near the anal orifice.

FIT. An attack or paroxysm, especially one accompanied by convulsions, as in major *epilepsy.

FITZ, REGINALD HEBER (1843–1913). American physician. He is often credited with being the first to advocate surgical treatment for acute appendicitis.

FIXATION is a term with various medical connotations, depending on context. These include: the holding of a visual image in focus; the utilization of *complement; the process of fixing histological and other specimens by chemical action; in psychiatry, a mental obsession or (in Freudian psychology) arrested emotional development; in surgery, mechanical immobilization of a part or parts.

FIXATIVE. Any chemical compound used in the fixation of histological, anatomical, or pathological specimens (e.g. formaldehyde). See PATHOLOGY.

FLAGELLATION is a sexual deviation involving whipping. See MASOCHISM; SADISM.

FLAP. An *autograft of skin and other tissue which retains its original blood supply during the process of grafting.

FLAT FOOT. *Fallen arch or *pes planus*.

FLATULENCE. Air or gas in the intestinal tract. See WIND.

FLATUS. See WIND.

FLEAS are active, wingless, haematophagous (blood-feeding) *insects which parasitize man and many animal hosts. They belong to the order *Siphonaptera* and comprise many genera and species. Those of chief medical importance are responsible for the transmission of bubonic *plague and murine *typhus, and for causing flea-bite *dermatitis.

FLEMING, SIR ALEXANDER (1881–1955). British bacteriologist. In 1922 he discovered *lysozyme, the 'natural antibiotic' present in many body fluids. In 1928 he isolated *penicillin, the product of a mould, *Penicillium notatum*, and showed that it had a profound bacteriostatic effect in the laboratory. He made no efforts to apply it clinically. In 1945 with Howard *Florey and Ernst *Chain he was awarded the *Nobel prize for medicine in recognition of this discovery.

FLEMMING, WALTHER (1843–1905). German anatomist and cytologist. He first used the word '*chromatin' (1879) and described the longitudinal splitting of *chromosomes in *mitosis (1880). The classic description of *cell division is to be found in his book *Zellsubstanz, kern and Zelltheilung* (1882).

FLETCHER, SIR WALTER MORLEY (1873–1934). British physiologist and medical administrator. In 1914 when the Medical Research Committee (see MEDICAL RESEARCH COUNCIL) was formed he became the first secretary and proved a brilliant administrator.

FLEXNER, ABRAHAM (1866–1959). American educationalist. Flexner was famous for his study of American and Canadian medical schools, and was the brother of Simon *Flexner. He wrote a book that was highly critical of American colleges, and contrasted them unfavourably with German universities. This book attracted the attention of Henry S. Pritchett of the *Carnegie Foundation for the Advancement of Teaching, and he persuaded Flexner, in 1908, to undertake a study of medical education in North America. The resulting *Flexner Report* was published in 1910 and had a great influence on modern medical education.

FLEXNER, SIMON (1863–1964). American microbiologist and research institute administrator. While serving on a special commission in the Philippines he discovered a strain of *dysentery bacillus which was long known by his name. He later became the first director of the newly formed *Rockefeller Institute in New York City, a post which he retained until 1935. There he attracted a group of able biomedical investigators, and provided conditions for them to work effectively. In addition he continued to carry on his own research on such problems as *poliomyelitis and the production of an effective antimeningococcal serum.

FLEXNER REPORTS. In 1908 Abraham *Flexner was asked to report on the state of medical education in North America. Initially he spent some time observing the system at the *Johns Hopkins medical school, which he chose as a model; he then set out to visit about 160 'medical schools' in the USA and Canada. The *Flexner Report*, published in 1910, was harshly critical in pointing out specific deficiencies, both educational and financial, in many schools, emphasizing inadequate laboratories and libraries for the students; it urged the importance of close affiliation with a university. This provoked a sensational reaction, and within a few years many private schools he had described were obliged to close. The general scheme he advocated—

beginning with a strong foundation in basic science, then studying clinical medicine in an atmosphere of critical thinking, with incorporation of the medical school in a university if possible—was widely accepted not only in North America but also in British and European medical schools, a report on which he published in 1912.

FLIES. A general term for winged insects, but usually restricted to the two-winged flies (order Diptera). Dipterous flies may transmit infections and parasitic diseases (e.g. the *sandfly transmits *leishmaniasis and sandfly fever, the blackfly is the vector of *onchocerciasis, and the *tsetse fly of *trypanosomiasis) and are directly responsible for myiasis or infestation by *maggots.

FLINT, AUSTIN (1812–86). American clinician, remembered for description of the 'Austin Flint' *murmur, a presystolic murmur at the cardiac apex heard in patients with insufficiency of the aortic valve (*aortic incompetence).

FLOATERS are spots in front of the eyes, also known as *muscae volitantes*, due to small mobile opacities in the *vitreous humour.

'FLOPPY INFANT' SYNDROME is a self-explanatory descriptive term covering a number of infantile neurological, *neuromuscular, and myopathic disorders, of which the common denominator is muscular *hypotonia with muscle weakness. Sometimes no underlying cause can be demonstrated, and the hypotonia gradually improves; such cases have been labelled benign congenital or infantile hypotonia.

FLOREY, HOWARD WALTER. Baron Florey of Adelaide and Marston (life peer) (1898–1968). Australian experimental pathologist. His early interest was in the bacteriolytic agent *lysozyme and he recruited the assistance of the biochemist Ernst *Chain, who drew Florey's attention to Fleming's paper on the inhibitory effect of a product of *Penicillium notatum* on bacterial growth. Investigation of this substance, *penicillin, began in 1938 and by 1940 they were able to show that it protected mice infected with virulent *streptococci. Clinical trials were undertaken in 1941 and the value of penicillin was triumphantly established. Florey's part in this was recognized by a knighthood in 1944 and the award of the *Nobel prize, together with Chain and Fleming, in 1945. In 1960 he became President of the Royal Society and in 1962 Provost of Queen's College, Oxford. He was made a life peer in 1965 and received the Order of Merit the same year.

FLOURENS, PIERRE JEAN MARIE (1794–1867). French comparative anatomist. He identified the 'respiratory centre' in the *medulla oblongata in 1837 and showed the effects of removal of the *cerebrum and the *cerebellum in pigeons as well as those of lesions of the *semicircular canals. He did not believe in the cerebral localization of function and effectively destroyed the theories of *Gall and the *phrenologists.

FLOYER, SIR JOHN (1649–1734). British physician. In 1707 he introduced the 'Physician's Pulse Watch' to run exactly for one minute and made many original observations on the *pulse frequency. He was a powerful advocate of cold baths and described the morbid anatomy of *emphysema of the lungs in a broken-winded mare.

FLUDD, ROBERT (1574–1637). British physician, alchemist, and writer. He was the author of *Philosophia moysaica* (1638) and many incomprehensible mystical works.

FLUKES are flatworms of the class Trematoda; the term 'fluke' derives from a resemblance to a miniature plaice or flounder. Flukes parasitize man and animals, with predilections for various organs or tissues; the main types involve blood (*bilharziasis or schistosomiasis), liver (*fascioliasis), intestine, and lung (*paragonimiasis). They all require at least one intermediate host, sometimes two; the first of these is always a mollusc.

FLUORESCEIN is a dark-red, crystalline, organic compound ($C_{20}H_{13}O_5$), resorcinolphthalein which dissolves in alkaline solutions to give a liquid of intense green fluorescence. It is widely used as an indicator and dye in medical and biological techniques.

FLUORIDATION is the addition of a minute quantity of a fluoride (usually one part per million of fluoride ion) to drinking water in order to protect growing children against *caries. See DENTISTRY.

FLUORINE is a yellowish-green, gaseous element, resembling *chlorine, but more reactive (symbol F, atomic number 9, relative atomic mass 18.998). Exposure to high concentrations of fluorine or its salts causes the syndrome of *fluorosis, but minute quantities stimulate bone formation and are incorporated into the normal structure of bone and teeth. The beneficial effect of *fluoridation of drinking water in preventing *caries in the teeth of growing children is well established.

FLUOROSCOPY. See RADIOSCOPY.

FLUOROSIS is fluorine toxicity characterized by mottling of dental enamel and by skeletal changes.

FLUOROURACIL is an *antimetabolite drug used to treat certain *cancers, particularly of the breast, gastrointestinal tract, and skin. It acts by blocking an *enzyme essential for *pyrimidine synthesis.

FLUSH. Temporary increase in blood flow through an area of skin.

FLUX. An excessive flow or discharge of material.

FLYING DOCTOR SERVICES. A number of services providing medical and surgical assistance to remote areas by light aircraft, sometimes piloted by the doctors themselves, now operate in various parts of the world. Such services were pioneered in Australia, the idea having been originally conceived in 1912 by the Revd John Flynn, superintendent of the Presbyterian Australian Inland Mission. The first operation of what became the Royal Flying Doctor Service of Australia began in Cloncurry, Queensland, in May 1928; the free service now covers most of Australia and Tasmania. Other services operate in Canada (the Saskatchewan Air Ambulance Service), in Newfoundland (the International Grenfell Association), in East Africa (the African Medical and Research Foundation), and elsewhere.

FOCAL SEPSIS is any isolated pocket of bacterial infection (e.g. around the teeth); it was once thought to be important in causing some chronic disorders of otherwise unknown aetiology (e.g. *rheumatoid arthritis).

FOCUS. The site of origin of a process, for example, epileptic focus, focus of infection, etc.

FOLIC ACID is a poorly water-soluble vitamin forming part of the *vitamin B complex, also known as pteroylglutamic acid. It is widely distributed in many foodstuffs, green leaves being particularly rich sources. In the body folic acid functions as a *coenzyme necessary for synthesis of *nucleic acids; in its absence, there is a failure of normal red blood cell formation, leading to *megaloblastic anaemia. Deficiency, or relative deficiency, of folic acid can arise in several ways: decreased intake when the diet is poor, particularly if vegetables are lacking, and in patients with chronic alcoholism; impaired intestinal absorption in conditions such as *coeliac disease and *sprue, and *malabsorption induced by some anticonvulsant drugs (e.g. *phenytoin); increased requirement, as in megaloblastic anaemia of pregnancy and in *thyrotoxicosis; impaired utilization due to the administration of folic acid antagonist drugs (e.g. *methotrexate); and impaired storage of folate in extensive liver disease.

FOLIE A DEUX is the occurrence of the same mental symptoms (usually one or more *delusions) in two closely associated people. Sisters living together are most often affected, but it also occurs in husband and wife, mother and daughter, etc.

FOLIN, OTTO (1867–1934). Swedish/American biochemist. He was a pioneer of *colorimetric micromethods of blood and urine analysis, which made practicable immense developments in clinical chemistry. Folin also contributed to the understanding of nitrogen metabolism, and showed that *proteins were broken down to *amino acids before being absorbed.

FOLLICLE-STIMULATING HORMONE, often abbreviated to FSH, is one of the gonadotrophic hormones of the anterior *pituitary; it stimulates the growth of *Graafian follicles in women and of *spermatozoa in men.

FOLLICULITIS. Inflammation of a hair follicle.

FOMENTATION is the application of heat to the surface of the body, usually with a hot cloth which has been placed in boiling water and then wrung out. It may be covered with a thermal insulating material such as oilskin. Its purpose is *vasodilatation, thus assisting superficial *staphylococcal infections to 'point' and drain. The increase in local blood flow is also held to be soothing.

FOMITES are substances or articles (toys, clothes, books, etc.) capable of transmitting infection.

FOOD comprises a mixture of *fats, *proteins, and *carbohydrates, together with water, minerals, *vitamins, and non-absorbable elements such as *cellulose and *fibre, which when consumed maintains life and growth, that is provides *energy, and builds and repairs tissue. See also NUTRITION.

FOOD ADDITIVES are chemical agents added to food as preservatives, flavouring, colouring, or nutritional items. See FOOD AND DRUGS ACTS 1955, 1970, 1976.

FOOD ALLERGY. *Allergens in food provoke reactions analogous to those that occur in other sites, modified by the content of the gastrointestinal tract (see ALLERGY; ANAPHYLAXIS). How and why some individuals acquire hypersensitivity to some food proteins usually remains a mystery, but allergy to bovine milk protein may be associated with lack of breast feeding in infancy. The possible relationship between food allergy and some gastrointestinal disorders of unknown aetiology, such as *ulcerative colitis, is speculative. See also NUTRITION.

FOOD AND DRUG ACT 1906. President Theodore Roosevelt signed the US Pure Food and Drug Act into law in 1906, one of many bills relating to food and medicines to be brought before Congress at the beginning of the 20th century. The main thrust of the Act was to make it illegal to manufacture or introduce an adulterated or misbranded food or drug anywhere in the USA. Its provisions were repealed and replaced by, or transferred to, later legislation, notably President Franklin D. Roosevelt's Food, Drug and Cosmetic Act of 1938.

FOOD AND DRUG ADMINISTRATION of the USA (FDA) began just after the Second World War, when the first edition of the 'Requirements of the United States Food, Drug and Cosmetic Act' was subtitled. 'A Guide for Foreign Manufacturers and Shippers'. This outlined legal requirements for importers. The FDA now enforces the laws enacted by US Congress concerning foods, drugs, and cosmetics. Before marketing it is necessary to obtain prior approval of new drugs from the FDA, which exercises stringent control on imports. If a drug is marketed and proves dangerous, there are powers of recall of stocks wherever they may be. Manufacturers of drugs in the USA must be registered with the FDA. The objective is to ensure the wholesomeness of food and the safety and efficacy of drugs available to the public. The remit covers not only these but also labelling, directions as to use, appropriate warnings of adverse effects, advertising, and the prohibition of misleading statements. Drug manufacture and containers have to conform to prescribed standards. Biological products, cosmetics, animal products, medical devices, and electronic devices are also subject to FDA control. It is an excellent safeguard for the US consumer, although, as with any bureaucratic machine, it is sometimes pilloried for being overcautious and making errors, and for taking too long to reach decisions.

FOOD AND DRUGS ACTS 1955, 1970, 1976. The UK Food and Drugs Act of 1955 incorporated all previous relevant legislation regarding these substances and added some new provisions. The first major step was taken by the Sale of Foods and Drugs Act of 1875, which covered the addition of injurious ingredients and prevented the sale of products not of the proper nature, substance, and quality. The practice of adulteration by addition (e.g. water to milk, sand to sugar, dried leaves to tea) or subtraction (e.g. cream from milk) became illegal. Various subsequent amendments and regulations—for example, the Public Health (Preservatives in Food) Regulations of 1925, which prohibited all except natural preservatives and small amounts of benzoic acid and sulphur dioxide in particular named foodstuffs—culminated in the Sale of Food and Drugs Act of 1928, and 10 years later in the first Food and Drugs Act of 1938. Requirements relating to premises where food was handled were added and powers were created to make regulations in respect of standards and labelling. The 1955 Act consolidated the foregoing, extending control of colouring agents and preservatives and recognizing the importance of micro-organisms in food-borne illness. A 1970 Act later authorized the treatment of milk (*pasteurization) by the application of steam. The 1976 (Control of Food Premises) Act introduced stringent new regulations to prevent the sale of food (cooked or uncooked) from dangerously unhygienic premises.

FOOD CHAIN. The chain of organisms existing in any biological community through which energy is transferred, the links usually being three or four and each link eating the preceding one. The first link (sometimes called energy level or trophic level) is occupied by green plants and is the producer level (T1); all subsequent links are consumer levels, herbivores being primary consumers (T2), smaller and larger carnivores being secondary consumers (T3 and T4, respectively). At each trophic level much energy is lost by *respiration.

FOOD IDIOSYNCRASY is hypersensitivity to particular items of diet not due to their intrinsic toxic qualities and not explicable on an immunological basis. See NUTRITION.

FOOD POISONING, when not a manifestation of food *allergy, is due to contamination with either toxic chemicals or with *bacteria.

Chemical poisoning may result from accidental contamination of food, or from eating *poisonous plants (laburnum, foxglove, deadly nightshade, certain *fungi) or animals (certain fish and shellfish which have been invaded by dinoflagellates). Two food additives, monosodium glutamate and sodium nitrite, may each cause occasional mild disturbances (the *Chinese Restaurant Syndrome is thought to be due to the former).

But most cases of food poisoning are due to bacteria. A typical, short, sharp illness of rapid onset is usually caused by a toxin elaborated by *Staphylococcus aureus* in foods (e.g. cream cakes) which have been at room temperature for some hours. Another, much more serious, 'toxic' type of food poisoning is *botulism. Other bacteria cause disease by multiplying within the body; of these the commonest is the *Salmonella group, producing many disorders ranging from mild *gastroenteritis to *enteric (typhoid) fever. Other examples include *Shigella* *dysentery and *cholera.

FOOD VALUES. See NUTRITION.

FORAMEN. An anatomical passage or opening.

FORAMEN MAGNUM. The large hole in the occipital bone at the base of the skull through which the *brainstem passes from the cranial cavity to become continuous with the *spinal cord.

FORAMEN OF MONRO. The communication between the third and the lateral *cerebral ventricles.

FORAMEN OVALE. The valvular aperture in the interatrial septum which provides an internal communication between the right and left sides of the fetal heart up to the moment of birth. The rise in left atrial pressure then causes it to close, preventing further flow. A pathological increase in right atrial pressure in postnatal life may re-establish patency of the foramen, allowing a right-to-left interatrial shunt. There is another foramen ovale in the bone of the base of the skull, through which passes the mandibular division of the *trigeminal nerve.

FORCEPS, ARTERY. Surgical forceps, of which many designs exist, used to clamp blood vessels and hold them occluded until a catch on the forceps is released.

FORCEPS, OBSTETRIC. Instruments designed to engage the head of the fetus during childbirth and assist in its extraction. See OBSTETRICS.

FORCEPS, SURGICAL. Instruments for grasping, holding, or compressing, designed for particular surgical applications.

FORENSIC MEDICINE. The description of 'forensic medicine' covers a wide spectrum of professional interests and, in fact, deals with any aspect of medicine which has an interface with the law. (See also LAW AND MEDICINE IN THE UK; LAW AND MEDICINE IN THE USA.)

The practice of clinical medicine itself gives rise to a legion of legal problems; foremost amongst these is medical malpractice and negligence. There is also a wide field of *ethical and legislative matters, intertwined with a veritable jungle of administrative regulations which impinges on every aspect of the practice of medicine. The disposal of the dead, drug safety and regulations, consent, professional secrecy, disciplinary procedures, *transplantation, compensation, reports, certificates, and a host of other matters confront doctors during their daily practice.

Many subspecialties contribute to forensic medicine, the major division being between those that are 'clinical', that is they deal with the living patient, and those that are 'pathological', concerning the dead body— although a number, such as forensic *serology and *toxicology, span both groups.

Forensic pathology

Historically, the oldest section of forensic medicine— forensic pathology—is certainly the one that gains most public attention, almost solely because of its central role in the investigation of homicide, although forensic pathology has a far wider range of interests than murder. Certain types of death attract legal investigation, whether they occur in a jurisdiction with a *coroner, under a Procurator-Fiscal system as in Scotland, or a Medical Examiner system which is increasingly used throughout the USA.

The coroner system

Central to the work of the forensic pathologist in Britain is the coroner system (excluding Scotland, which has a somewhat similar Procurator-Fiscal system).

The coroner was established in AD 1194, as part of the fund-raising activities following the massive ransom required for King Richard I. The original wide fiscal duties have contracted down to a responsibility for the investigation of sudden deaths, although determinations on treasure trove remain a legacy from medieval times.

The modern coroner—who was introduced into many parts of the world, including the USA, during the British Imperial period—is usually a lawyer, but may be a doctor, some of whom also have a legal qualification. He is employed by local government, but functions under the Coroner's Acts and Rules laid down by Parliament. His basic function is to investigate all deaths that cannot be satisfactorily certified by physicians in the usual way. These include deaths:

1. where no doctor was in attendance during the last illness or within 14 days before death;
2. where the cause of death is unknown or the body unidentified;
3. due to industrial *poisoning, violence, neglect, *abortion, drugs, or *alcohol;
4. during surgical operation or before recovery from anaesthetic; or
5. during police or prison custody.

Over a quarter of the 600 000 deaths recorded annually in England and Wales are reported to coroners, and, in the majority of cases, the coroner will request an autopsy.

About 80 per cent of such cases are due to natural disease, where deaths can be disposed of by the coroner by simple documentation, but the remainder, which prove to be unnatural, must be the subject of a coroner's inquest.

An inquest is a public court inquiry (in certain circumstances with a jury of at least eight persons), to determine by means of a 'verdict' or 'finding', precisely 'where, when, and by what means' a person came to his or her death. Accidents and *suicides form the greater part of inquests, but medical mishaps, drug or drink deaths, industrial diseases, and a range of less common conditions are also dealt with.

Where death is due to criminal action, the coroner adjourns the inquest until any criminal proceedings are completed. If no suspect is charged, then an inquest is likely to return a verdict of 'unlawful killing'. In recent years, the coroner has lost his power either to commit a person for trial or to impute criminal or civil liability, so that his jurisdiction is now confined to a fact-finding inquiry, which, however, may be used as the basis for further action in other courts.

The forensic pathologist

When a death thought to be caused by murder or manslaughter is discovered by the law enforcement agencies, the forensic pathologist is usually called in at an early stage. Where suspicious circumstances exist, the pathologist will be summoned to the scene of the death and will examine the body *in situ*, a most useful way of obtaining the best impression of what may have

occurred. Many such deaths turn out to be innocent, in that the pathologist can declare them to be caused by accident, suicide, or even arising from natural causes; but where obvious or suspected crime has occurred, meticulous investigation takes place at the locus of the death. The pathologist will relate the position of the body to any blood splashes, marks upon adjacent structures, and the immediate environment of the body in a way that he could never do several hours later in the mortuary. He will study the clothing, especially if it is soiled, disarranged, or damaged, and interpret this in the light of his later autopsy findings. The presence of trace evidence upon the body may be vital and, with his non-medical forensic science colleagues, he will retrieve and evaluate any foreign material upon the body, which might have been lost if the body had been transported from the scene before expert examination.

The detective officers wish to know the identity of the body and often, the best estimate of the time of death. The latter is extremely difficult, and much forensic medical research has been directed towards this problem. The body temperature falls after death from the normal 37 °C and, theoretically, back-calculations from the temperature of the corpse at the scene should give the number of hours since death. Unfortunately, so many variables distort this calculation that any hope of accuracy is vain. The initial temperature may be considerably higher or lower than 37 °C, due to fever, exposure, brain damage, etc. The physique, clothing, posture, age, and other intrinsic factors alter the rate of cooling, as do obvious environmental conditions such as air temperature, wind, rain, snow, and sun.

The identity of a body may also be an insoluble problem. Although most persons found dead are identified by relatives or friends, some victims of homicide may have been deliberately concealed to allow decomposition to render them unidentifiable. Sometimes mutilation or even dismemberment adds to the difficulties of identification, as does long immersion in water. Sometimes the body is partly or wholly skeletalized. The pathologist uses his anatomical and even anthropological skills to try to arrive at the correct identity. The following questions must be answered where possible. Is it human? Fragments or skeletal remnants may pose difficulties in this respect. If human, is it male or female? Depending on the state of preservation, anatomical difference in the organs and bones give the answer where obvious appearances cannot be relied upon. What is the age? In infants, children, and young adults the size and maturity of the bones can give accurate results, but in middle age and beyond only specialized techniques can get nearer than decades as units of estimation. What was the stature? Where intact, direct measurement is possible, although the corpse varies by several inches from the live height. Where only limbs or bones are available, anatomical formulae may allow approximate calculations to be made. The race may be vital, especially in these days of ethnic mobility.

The last, but vital, question is 'What is the personal identity?' All manner of features may assist, such as scars, old operations, deformities, tattoos, industrial stigmata (scars of industrial injury), head and beard hair, old *fractures seen on X-ray, *blood groups, teeth and dental work characteristics, signs of obvious pregnancy, old injuries, fingerprints, sinus patterns, etc.

Once the scene of death has been thoroughly examined by pathologist and forensic scientist, the body is removed to the mortuary and an *autopsy started. Many of the techniques mentioned above will be continued here, as the clothing is carefully removed and preserved for laboratory examination.

The pathologist makes a careful external examination of the body, which in cases of death by violence may be of more use in interpreting the nature of the trauma than the internal examination. However, it is the latter which more often reveals the exact mode of death. Any contributing factors, such as pre-existing natural disease, and the contribution of alcohol or drugs, are also evaluated. Blood and other body fluids and tissue samples are usually retained for analysis, and samples of tissues are commonly taken for later microscopic examination.

Modern advances in forensic techniques have added to the repertoire of the pathologist, who is no longer confined to mere inspection of morphological changes. Histochemical procedures may assist in determining whether wounds were caused before or after death, and similar techniques may determine whether a heart attack, too recent to be detected by the naked eye or by classic microscopical methods, may have contributed to death.

In a criminal death, the pathologist has to interpret wounds, head injuries, gunshot wounds, stabbing, and more rarely poisoning, before preparing a report, which will be used by the prosecution in any subsequent criminal trial. Frequently, a second autopsy will be conducted by another pathologist retained by the lawyers defending an accused person. This second pathologist, although he rarely discovers much to dispute in the physical findings, may well have a different interpretation of those facts and may give testimony in court as to his opinions upon the findings, if they benefit the defence.

Sudden and/or unexpected deaths

The pathologist seeks to discover the natural disease causing death and to exclude any unnatural process, including criminal action. About 80 per cent of English coroner's cases fall into this category. The autopsy reveals the true cause of death in all but a few occult conditions, and this assists the governmental agencies responsible for constructing mortality statistics in increasing greatly the accuracy of their tables, for it has been shown repeatedly that causes of death given by doctors without the benefit of autopsy are incorrect in about half of all cases, the error being substantial in a quarter. In Western countries, *coronary heart disease

and other degenerative conditions of the cardiovascular system account for the great majority of sudden deaths.

The most common cause of death in industrialized countries in males between the ages of 15 and 30 years is accident. Deaths due to road-traffic accidents now assume almost epidemic proportions in Europe and America, and are especially serious as they tend to involve healthy active people in the productive period of life. Forensic pathologists perform autopsies on the victims of traffic, domestic, and industrial accidents with several objects in mind. The cause of death and, more importantly, the mechanism of death is determined. Many accidents are unwitnessed or seen by persons with a confused recollection of the events. The pathologist's findings can help to reconstruct the accident, with consequent help to both the legal consequences and to preventive measures. For instance, the mandatory use of crash helmets for motor-cyclists and seat-belts for motorists arose substantially from the findings published by pathologists.

Domestic accidents are almost as common as road accidents, and again the autopsy may reveal hidden or unexpected causes from disease or toxic states in the victims of falls, electrocution, fires, etc. The legal consequences include criminal charges, civil actions for negligence, and substantial insurance claims.

In industrial situations, the legal consequences are even more likely, with relatives and trade unions naturally keen to obtain the maximum compensation both from national schemes, as in the scheduled industrial diseases, and from the employers, via negligence actions for both injuries and disease. Coal-worker's *pneumoconiosis from dust, asbestos and asbestos-related *cancer, heart disease allegedly brought on by exertion, and a host of other claims make the autopsy upon a presumed industrial death a most essential procedure.

Although public and medical attitudes have changed radically in recent years, suicide still carries a stigma. In Britain, changes in the law have made it no longer a crime to commit or attempt to commit suicide, and the coroner's procedure has been modified to make the investigation more discreet than hitherto, although undesirable publicity about what is basically a mental illness still occurs.

The task of the pathologist is to confirm the mode of death, to detect suicide where it is unsuspected or has been concealed, and to exclude criminal action. In addition, it must be separated from those masochistic exercises in males, which are accidental deaths, but which have been frequently mistaken for suicide in the past. The mechanism of death, especially if it be by an overdose of drugs or other poison, must be fully investigated. The prime function of the forensic pathologist here is to ensure that other modes of death are excluded so that an unwarranted verdict of self-destruction is not arrived at mistakenly. On some occasions this might wrongly invalidate a recent life insurance policy.

Death may be associated with medical treatment. When death takes place during, or soon after, a surgical operation or major medical procedure—or under an anaesthetic—the case is almost always the subject of a medicolegal investigation. A forensic autopsy, coupled with a full appraisal of the clinical history, is important not only in interpreting the chain of events, but may also assist in preventing similar tragedies in the future. Where allegations of medical, surgical, or anaesthetic malpractice are made, then the full autopsy findings are indispensable in getting at the truth. Similar importance attaches to deaths from untoward drug reactions and other mishaps in medical care, which these days all too readily lead to litigation by the relatives.

Deaths in custody, whether in police hands or in prison, tend to be emotive events, often leading to accusations of mistreatment or neglect by the custodians. A full investigation, of which the autopsy is an indispensable part, is necessary to allay—or occasionally to confirm—these allegations.

Deaths of infants are not medicolegal cases *per se*, but many proceed to forensic autopsies because of other factors. The most common cause of infant mortality after the first week of birth is the 'cot' or 'crib' death, more accurately known as the '*sudden infant death syndrome*'. Still little understood, it is probably due to immaturity of the respiratory control system, but a detailed autopsy is necessary to exclude other causes and to allay some of the self-recrimination that always attaches to the parents, who may think that death was due to smothering or some other untenable explanation.

Another less common cause of infant death is child abuse, the so-called '*battered baby syndrome*' and again the forensic medical investigation must exclude or confirm signs of repeated injury. *Stillbirths are often examined forensically to differentiate them from deliberate infanticides. Deaths of mothers after *abortion, now much rarer due to extensive birth control and medical terminations of pregnancy, must be investigated if there is any doubt that the miscarriage was due to anything other than natural causes.

Other conditions requiring the attention of the forensic pathologist include deaths from self-neglect: chronic alcoholism and drug abuse have increasingly come into this category in Western countries and have reached epidemic proportions in many large urban communities. In the UK a marked increase in both acute and chronic alcoholism has occurred in the past decade. Some 700 000 alcoholics are known to doctors, of whom a not insignificant number die from the metabolic effects of long-term drinking, as well as from accidents, fires, and intercurrent infections brought on by their condition. The pathologist is often faced with these deaths, as well as those of abusers of many drugs and, latterly, youthful '*glue sniffers', who may suffer sudden death from the effects of inhaling the fumes of organic solvents.

In all these problems, and many others, the forensic pathologist has a wide range of ancillary disciplines to call upon for specialist assistance.

Forensic odontology

A young offspring of forensic pathology is *odontology, the application of dental expertise to legal matters. The major contribution of the forensic *dentist is in the field of identification, either in individual cases or in the mass disaster, especially aircraft crashes. The dental expert carefully records all the dental data from an unknown corpse and compares this with the dental records made during life, which can give a positive identity as good as that given by fingerprints, as long as ante-mortem data are available. Much of the evidence for the identification of Adolf Hitler, Martin Bormann, Eva Braun, etc., was based upon dental characteristics.

Another task for the forensic odontologist is the matching of teeth and bite marks in assaults and murders. Marks upon the skin—and sometimes even on foodstuffs such as cheese or apples—can be matched with the dentition of a suspect, using tooth spacing, notching, and other characteristics.

Forensic toxicology

Again a long-standing partner of pathology, the science of the detection of poisons is a vital adjunct to the pathologist. Although homicidal poisoning has declined greatly in advanced countries—perhaps in large measure due to the efficiency of the toxicologists—the role of these specialists has increased greatly in relation to environmental, accidental, and self-poisoning. The experts in this field are now almost exclusively chemists rather than doctors, and the complexity of their analytical methods has developed explosively in line with the advances in scientific technology in general. However, the pathologist still has an interpretive role to play in fatal poisoning, as the actual laboratory findings on toxic levels in body tissues are often difficult to relate to the mechanism of death. A large proportion of the toxicologist's work now relates to therapeutic substances, and the distinction between medicinal administration and overdose may be difficult to evaluate.

Other disciplines that the forensic medical expert may need to call upon at times include anatomists and anthropologists, where skeletal remains need intensive study. Radiologists co-operate in these investigations on bones, and also have an important role in X-raying the victims of suspected child abuse and in searching for foreign objects at autopsy, especially firearm missiles and bomb fragments. Photography and video are also used extensively, for both teaching purposes and the recording of evidence; many pathologists are themselves proficient photographers, and many forensic scientists are expert document examiners, skilled, for example, in detecting forgery.

Even entomologists may be called upon where the time of death is a vital problem: the insect infestation of decaying corpses may be used to get some idea of the time since death by an expert study of the various maturation stages of certain fly maggots. Similarly, biologists may assist in identifying the source of diatoms and may even help with the rate of growth of moulds or vegetation where these have invaded decomposed bodies.

Thus a wide variety of specialist skills may be recruited by the forensic pathologist when the occasion demands. Once again, we see that almost any scientific activity can have an interface with the law.

Forensic medicine and the living person

One further very important aspect of forensic medicine needs to be mentioned, the activities of those doctors practising 'clinical forensic medicine'. The examination of persons for purely legal purposes relates to such matters as sexual assaults, common physical assaults, child abuse, drunkenness (especially *drunken driving), and civil matters such as insurance and compensation examinations.

In the UK, the doctors responsible for assisting the police and courts with the criminal side of this work are the 'forensic physicians', or 'police surgeons', who are *general practitioners who carry out this task under a specific contract with their local police forces.

Until 1983, the most frequent task of the police surgeon was to take blood samples from motorists suspected of driving with more than the permitted level (80 mg/100 ml) of alcohol in their blood. New legislation then introduced breath analysis as the definitive test for alcohol: this newer technique is carried out by trained police officers, so blood sampling by doctors is much less frequent.

The police surgeon also examines women and girls complaining of rape and other sexual assaults, and often also examines the alleged perpetrator. Other victims and offenders arrested by the police, in any sort of assault, may be examined by these doctors. They are often the first doctors at a scene of a suspicious death, before the forensic pathologist arrives.

The other important forensic practitioner is the forensic psychiatrist. Again, most are not exclusively medico-legal in their activities, unless in one of the few academic posts that exist in this specialty or in those attached to the *prison service. The majority are clinical psychiatrists in hospital or private practice, who take a special interest in legal matters. As their name suggests, they examine offenders with a view to establishing whether there is any mental abnormality which might either make them unfit to stand trial or to cause the court to take account of their mental state when passing sentence. The concept of 'diminished responsibility', usually relating to murder offenders, may reduce the sentence or substitute for a prison sentence confinement in a mental institution. The work of the forensic psychiatrist is difficult, onerous, and often very controversial.

B. KNIGHT

Further reading

Helpern, M. and Knight, B. (1979). *Autopsy*. Harrap, London and New York.

Kind, S. S. (ed.) (1972). *Science against crime*. Aldus, London.

Knight, B. (1991). *Forensic pathology*. Edward Arnold, London.

Knight, B. (1992). *Simpson's forensic medicine*, (10th edn). Edward Arnold, London.

Knight, B. (1992). *Legal aspects of medical practice*, (5th edn). Churchill Livingstone, Edinburgh and London.

Picton, B. (1971). *Murder, suicide or accident?* Robert Hale, London.

Thorwald, J. (1965). *The century of the detective*. Harcourt, Brace & World, New York.

FORME FRUSTE is an atypical, partial, or abortive expression of a disease or condition.

FORMULA. A specification, usually in symbols and/or numerals.

FORMULARY. A collection of formulas or prescriptions.

FORSSMAN, WERNER (1904–79). German surgeon. His place in medical history is due to his demonstration in 1929 that a radiopaque *catheter can be inserted into a superficial arm vein and passed from there until its tip enters the right atrium of the heart. Forssman, whose purpose was to find a method of injecting drugs directly into the heart, carried out this first cardiac catheterization on himself, subsequently confirming the position of the catheter by taking an X-ray of his chest. Many years were to elapse before this now standard procedure was fully exploited, but the pioneer experiment received eventual recognition when Forssman shared the 1956 *Nobel prize with André Frederic *Cournand and Dickinson Woodruff *Richards.

FOSSA. An anatomical term for a depression or hollow in a bone, body surface, or other tissues.

FOSTER, SIR MICHAEL (1836–1907). British physiologist. He founded the *Journal of Physiology* in 1878 and was the author of the influential *Textbook of physiology* (1876).

FOSTERING is the rearing of offspring by other than the natural parents.

FOTHERGILL, JOHN (1712–80). British physician. Fothergill was a Quaker who practised in London with great success and developed a botanical garden at Upton, Essex, 'second only to Kew'. He described 'putrid sore throat', which was either *diphtheria or malignant *scarlatina, in 1748 and trigeminal neuralgia (*tic douloureux) in 1773. Fothergill co-operated with Benjamin *Franklin in attempts to reconcile the American colonies and Great Britain.

FOUNDATIONS AND CHARITIES IN CANADA.

For years the mainstay of medical research in Canada has been the Medical Research Council, which was an outgrowth of the country's Wartime National Research Council. The influence of leaders such as Sir Frederick *Banting, Wilder *Penfield, and Ray Farquharson was evident in the peacetime developments which followed. Gradually, private foundations have entered the health field, providing a complementary source of much-needed funds. Thus, since *The Oxford companion to medicine* was published, most large hospitals in Canada have developed their own foundations which, with local variations, support medical research and education, nursing, and sometimes veterinary projects.

Another recent tendency has brought large community foundations into the picture as well. A good example is the Vancouver Foundation, which now administers more than 490 separate 'trusts', with a combined endowment of approximately CAN$400 (US$300, £200) million. Some of these trusts, such as the Blue Cross residual funds, after health insurance became universal in Canada, tend to be channelled selectively into health projects, including medical research. Substantial capital funds, from similar sources in Alberta and Manitoba, have been devoted to health research and promotion. In Ontario, two large foundations have been set up to dispense annual grants in the health field from funds derived from physician-sponsored pre-paid medical care plans prior to 1970. The largest, Physicians Services Incorporated Foundation, with assets of CAN$50 (US$38, £25) million, has contributed to medical research, health care research, the biomedical sciences, and medical education in Ontario.

The Associated Medical Services Foundation, also in Ontario, has pioneered a unique role in establishing a professorship in the *history of medicine in each of that province's five medical schools. In addition, its Jason Hannah Institute for the history of medicine has assisted in the publication of research work in that field across Canada.

There has been a growing emphasis by disease-related societies on research into specific illnesses, such as *cancer, *Parkinson's disease, *Alzheimer's, *muscular dystrophy, *arthritis, *cystic fibrosis, heart disease, *epilepsy, and others.

Family foundations continue their interest in the medical field, e.g. the Websters, the Molsons, the Birks, and the Bronfmans in Montreal. The McLaughlin foundation continues its clearly defined role in postgraduate medical fellowships. The Blackburn and the Ivey foundations continue to serve the University of Western Ontario in London in an exemplary way.

Understandably, some of the larger foundations have clauses in their charters requiring that funds be granted to specific institutions. Thus, the Max Bell fund, directed by the Oxford-trained dean of Canadian foundation executives, Donald Rickerd, is required to give, annually, 30 per cent of its grants to McGill University in Montreal, half of that sum to go to the Faculty of Medicine. The J. P. Bickell trustees are required to give to the superb Hospital for Sick Children in Toronto, one-half of their annual net income.

Some foundations have innovative provisions, such as the Banting Foundation. Sir Frederick wanted its objectives to include medical research fellowships to undergraduate or 'summer' students, as well as to postgraduates.

Others are limited to specific areas of Canada, by the donors or their successors. However, a recent large foundation, the Geoffrey Wood (1988), provides for Canada-wide support for medical research and for universities.

Medical libraries rarely receive the foundation support which their catalytic role in medical research deserves. This cannot be said of the Woodward Biomedical Library at the University of British Columbia in Vancouver. It has become, thanks to its benefactor, the late P. A. Woodward, a world-class establishment. Surrounded by medical research laboratories, its resources play a key role in the life of Canada's second largest university. Its history of medicine and science collection is second only to that of the *Osler Library at McGill.

Research funds continue to be available to Canadian medical faculties from senior American foundations such as Rockefeller, Macy, Kellogg, Kresge, Howard Hughes, and others. Changes in emphasis have taken a veteran supporter into other fields, in the case of the Donner Canadian Foundation, but its trustees greatly influenced medical research in Canada for several decades.

In summary, medically interested foundations in Canada are maturing, and a tendency to accept a division of labour is becoming evident. The value of smaller foundations, in filling special niches, is becoming increasingly evident. It might be added, parenthetically, that some slightly frustrated executives in foundations spend more time in explaining what they will *not* support than what they will. That is to be expected in a developing field where ready funds are hard to trace and pin down. With governmental deficits abroad in the land, there is likely to be increased reliance on privately husbanded funds for medical research, education, and patient care.

W. C. GIBSON

FOUNDATIONS AND CHARITIES SUPPORTING MEDICAL CARE IN THE UK.

Charity is a very old concept in English law, stemming ultimately from the

Christian doctrine of *caritas*—loving one's neighbour and expressing that love in practical ways. Like most English law, however, it has primarily been shaped by cases. What precisely it is can be quite elusive and can rapidly become extremely complicated (Gladstone 1982). Although first stated with any comprehensiveness in a statute of 1601, the recognition of charitable activity, for the benefit of others, was already well developed in the Middle Ages. It included the relief of poverty, the advancement of education, the advancement of religion, the provision of medical and social care, and a variety of other public purposes.

Hospitals in the Middle Ages were essentially charitable, in that they were run for the benefit of others and charged little or nothing. Prior to the Reformation, they were run by religious orders. They looked after the poor—wealthy people were sick at home—and the emphasis was on care rather than cure. Only in the 19th century did hospitals other than charitable foundations become common, some of the new hospitals being funded by local government (often in conjunction with workhouses) and others being private ventures.

Thus, in Britain, health-related charities are as old as hospitals themselves. Specifically, the oldest surviving foundation is *St Bartholomew's Hospital at Smithfield. Others, such as *St Thomas's or the Royal Bethlehem are medieval foundations, but with a break at the Reformation, when the assets of their parent orders were sequestered.

The 19th century, when Britain was the richest country in the world, was a boom period for charitable bequests, particularly for hospitals, and most of the more prestigious institutions date from this time. Their geographical distribution was uneven, with a disproportionate number in the main cities. Until the 20th century they tended not to charge patients for their services. Senior medical staff were unpaid, but their hospital appointment lent prestige to their private practice.

From around 1900 onwards—considerably later in the psychiatric hospitals—hospital practice began to be transformed by advances in medicine. Somewhere in the early years of the 20th century the moment came when, on balance, medical therapies were more likely to do net good than net harm. The voluntary, charitable hospitals were at the forefront of these developments. They largely left the job of caring for chronic patients to the municipal (local government) hospitals and concentrated their attention on the active treatment of acute illness. Their clientele changed from the poor to anyone suffering from acute, treatable illness, or accident. While all this was a matter for justifiable pride, it brought serious, chronic financing problems with it. Charitable income (from endowments, donations, and bequests) always tended to lag behind expenditure.

The death blow to the old system was struck by the Second World War, following the depression of the 1930s. By the end of the war, the voluntary hospitals needed rebuilding, repair, and re-equipment on a massive scale, which simply could not be provided from the old sources. Moreover, a social revolution was about to transform Britain, aiming at a fairer society, public ownership, and an end to poverty. The *National Health Service was born. Virtually (but not quite) all the old voluntary hospitals were nationalized, and central government took over sole responsibility for their financing. It seemed as though there was virtually no place left for charity in British medicine (Prochaska 1992).

Or was there? In fact there was. The most obvious was in *medical research*. Indeed, *The Oxford companion to medicine* restricted the UK entry on foundations entirely to medical research. Secondly, in time a large and diverse crop of new *voluntary organizations* was born (joining older, surviving charities like Dr Barnardo's and the Macmillan Foundation) to reach the parts not adequately reached by state services. This has included a wide range of patient/condition-based groups, which often combine some fund-raising for research with other activities, the whole *hospice movement, and a diverse range of charities delivering services at the local level. Often these organizations depend on a mix of governmental and charitable funding, along with some element of charges. Finally, there is some continuity—and even now some revival—of the *older hospital charities*, along with a large new crop of *NHS-linked charitable fund-raising* activities. The latter is a controversial development. There are fears that it will siphon off public donations from established voluntary bodies to shore up state services. Undoubtedly there needs to be clarification of the principles that ought to guide public-sector bodies like health authorities in their fund-raising activities, and there should be close scrutiny of how they spend the charitable monies raised.

To take each of these types of charitable activity in turn.

Medical research

In the field of medical research in Britain, it would be hard to overstate the importance of charities. There are more than 1000 charities supporting some type of medical research, with a combined contribution of some £320 ($480) million in 1992–93, compared with a figure for the Government's *Medical Research Council (MRC) of around £250 ($375) million for the same year (Association of Medical Research Charities; MRC 1993). Thus, in total, the medical research charities outweigh the MRC in financial importance, and their income may well rise faster than that of the Council. However, it is also worth recognizing that industry's contribution to medical research for the same period is estimated at some £1.2 ($1.8) billion, and that the total from all sources exceeded £2 ($3) billion (Research for Health 1993; note that these figures are for England only, whereas those given by the AMRC and MRC are for the UK).

Table 1 Summary of hospice and palliative care services in the UK and Ireland

In-patient units	Units	Beds
Independent or voluntary hospice units	123	1937
NHS/Cancer Relief Macmillan Fund (joint or separate funding)	50	573
Marie Curie Cancer Care Centres	11	318
Sue Ryder Homes	9	165
Total	193	2993

The number of beds per hospice unit ranges from 2 to 62.
Source: *1993 Hospice Directory*.

A full list of the 1992–93 expenditures on medical research of the charities that are members of the Association of Medical Research Charities (AMRC) is shown in the succeeding article on FOUNDATIONS, CHARITIES, AND GRANT-MAKING BODIES SUPPORTING MEDICAL RESEARCH IN THE UK. (The AMRC estimates that its members account for some 85 per cent of the registered charitable total.) These charities vary enormously in size, from the *Wellcome Trust at the top, to many that are small. The top five accounted for three-quarters of the AMRC total.

Most of the medical research charities are disease- or condition-specific, as the right-hand column of Table 2 in the succeeding article indicates—although there are important exceptions, most notably Wellcome. Targeting a condition is a major factor in their foundation and in their continuing public appeal. Typically their administration is small, and at least as much concerned with fund-raising as with spending. In general they have to limit the length of time for which they will commit funds to any one project or programme, and their style is responsive. In other words, they receive proposals from researchers in their field of interest and judge them on a competitive basis. They rely heavily on peer review, as does the MRC, and virtually all of them have advisory panels of distinguished medical scientists to help them oversee their research spending.

No other country in the world is relatively so dependent on charities to underpin the financing of medical research.

Voluntary organizations
Whereas the medical research charities collectively have great wealth to dispense, this is not true at all of the very large number of charities set up to deliver a service or to promote understanding of a disease or condition. There are literally thousands of them, with new formations every year, and with a substantial failure rate. Generally they are heavily dependent on the efforts of volunteers and of small numbers of staff, and live from hand to mouth financially. While not all of them are heroes and

heroines, let alone saints, the quality of their work is often remarkable.

Any typology is almost bound to oversimplify the range and diversity. I simply select three examples.

The first are organizations like Age Concern, MIND, Mencap, the Muscular Dystrophy Group, the Terrence Higgins Trust, the Royal National Institutes for the Blind and for the Deaf, and SANE—all national charities designed to help a particular group of people who have a health-related problem or disability. One person or a small group generally lies behind their foundation. A new health problem (such as the health of Somali refugees in Britain) or the recognition that an old problem has been seriously neglected (incontinence, for example) may lead to the formation of a new organization. Initially it will be underfinanced, fragile, and struggling for recognition. If it survives and prospers, it will establish a niche for itself and its own particular style of working. This may (as with MIND and Mencap) involve networks of local groups, or it may be quite centralized. Part of its function may be to raise money for medical research, but it will also have wider roles concerned with shaping public opinion and national policy, and with support to patients and carers.

The second category to which I wish to call attention are essentially local charities, delivering care on the ground to groups of people who have special needs. Charities in the field of homelessness are an example, such as Centrepoint, The London Connection, St Mungo's, Thomas Coram. Some of these are old (Coram dates back to the 18th century) and some new, but they stem from the ancient tradition of doing something practical for the weakest members of society who are one's true neighbours. Nowadays they rely heavily on public-sector funding, as well as on public charity. Often they are in no sense an alternative to mainstream public services but are the principal providers.

My third category is perhaps simply a special example of my second, in the form of the hospice movement. As Table 1 indicates, there are now just under 200 hospices in the UK and Ireland, with a combined count of 3000 beds. There are also 400 home-care teams and 200 day-hospices with beds. This is now a world-wide movement and it has ancient roots—clearly a modern hospice can claim to be firmly in the tradition of the medieval hospital. But in its modern form it is the creation of Dame Cicely Saunders, who registered St Christopher's Hospice as a charity in 1961 and opened it in 1967 in Sydenham, South London. She can properly claim to have revolutionized professional and public expectations about the care of people who are dying, starting with those who have cancer. The gold standard has been set by the voluntary hospice movement in terms of pain control, talking and listening on a basis of humility, and recognizing that death is not merely physical, but spiritual. It would be difficult to find a more powerful

Table 2 Voluntary income of charities (including government fees) 1990–91

	£m*	Percentage share
Public donations	3900	47
Companies	400	5
Trusts	600	7
Central government		
Fees	2200	27
Grants	500	6
Local government		
Fees	200	2
Grants	450	5
Total	8250	100

Source: R. Hazell, Nuffield Foundation. *£1 = US$1.50.

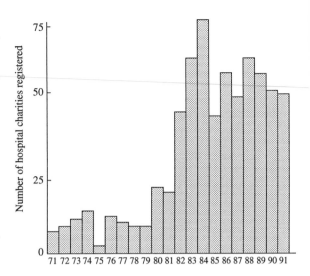

Fig. 1 Rate of registration of independent appeals for hospitals (Charity Commission Code 435). (from Lattimer and Holly 1992.)

example of the contemporary influence of charities. Yet it also has to be said that most hospices, like most other modern charities, are in a fragile position financially. It is easier to raise the initial money to build them, than to keep them running. Not unreasonably, the public and charitable foundations expect the government and the NHS to pay a substantial part of the running costs. The general assumption is that 50 per cent governmental and 50 per cent charitable funding would be a reasonable target, but actually that is hard to achieve year after year, both in terms of continual fundraising from the public and in being confident that the public sector will maintain its contribution.

What stands out from any summary of this kind is the diversity, the financial fragility, and yet the immense energy and creativeness of the voluntary sector in Britain today. The overall funding of the sector is summarized in Table 2. Of course, one must bear in mind that health is only one strand (although an important one) in this total. Many human problems do not, in any case, neatly separate between health and other sectors. Homelessness is an example. For homeless people, health is not the main issue except when they happen to be gravely ill, yet all homelessness has serious health implications.

Hospital charities old and new

As already noted, many of Britain's best-known hospitals were charitable foundations until they were absorbed into the National Health Service in 1948. At that date there was considerable controversy about what would happen to their assets. In the event, their operating assets (land, buildings, equipment) were transferred to the Minister of Health, but any

investments that they held were retained as separate charitable funds to be used for the purposes for which they were originally given. Forty-five years and a number of reorganizations later, that basically remains the position. In 1990–91 the Directory of Social Change estimated that the money held in trusts by NHS authorities and special trustees amounted to £693 million (£1 = US$1.50), producing an annual income of £220 million (Lattimer and Holly 1992). Allowing for major fund-raising appeals, such as the Wishing Well appeal at *Great Ormond Street and the Royal Marsden appeal, the Directory of Social Change estimated the charitable income of the NHS at that time at £370 million a year—appreciably more than the combined expenditure of the medical research charities, then put at £265 million.

In addition, there are a small number of hospitals that were not absorbed into the National Health Service and still function as independent charities; King Edward VII Hospital for Officers (Sister Agnes' Foundation) is the best known.

While a large number of UK grant-making charities include medicine and health in their objective, there are two medium-sized foundations that are specific to health, namely King Edward's Hospital Fund for London (generally known as The King's Fund) and the Nuffield Provincial Hospitals Trust. Between them they command assets of some £150 million (1992–93). Each in its own way has considerable influence on health policy in the UK, on health services research, and on the way in which the National Health Service is run.

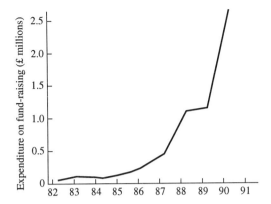

Fig. 2 Health Authority fundraising expenses paid from trust funds (from Lattimer and Holly 1992).

The inter-relationship between charity and the NHS has waxed and waned over the years—or more accurately, it waned in the first 25 years and is now waxing. It looks likely to be quite an important dilemma for the future, along with broader questions about the public/private mix in health care.

Aneurin Bevan, founder of the NHS, was firmly against reliance on voluntary funding. In his speech in the House of Commons (30 April 1945), in moving that the NHS Bill be read a second time, he said, 'It is repugnant to a civilized community for hospitals to have to rely upon private charity. I have always felt a shudder of repulsion when I have seen nurses and sisters who ought to be at their work, and students who ought to be at theirs, going about the streets collecting money for their hospitals' (Webster 1991).

For many years Bevan's was the dominant view. NHS staff were forbidden to solicit patients for contributions towards the cost of their care, or for donations towards the work of the NHS. For years a feature of NHS charitable funds was that they raised virtually no new money and yet did not spend their income. But by now Bevan must be turning in his grave. The number of new hospital charities registered suddenly jumped in the 1980s (Fig. 1), as did health authority expenditure on fund raising (Fig. 2). As the Directory of Social Change has argued, these changes raise some intriguing issues. For example, how does one define the boundary between what ought to be funded by the Exchequer and the proper role of charity? How does one reassure donors that they are doing more than saving money for the Chancellor? Is the majority of the money raised simply diverted from hard-pressed voluntary bodies, which are chronically underfunded, into NHS bank accounts? How can one protect such organizations from unfair competition in fund raising by the NHS, if the latter can deploy sophisticated experts to plan and manage its public campaigns, meeting the costs out of public funds?

Can we really expect members and officers whose main business is running a public service, answerable to parliament through ministers, to be able at the same time to discharge their duties as charitable trustees?

These are good questions which require answers. Nevertheless, it seems clear that it will be difficult to return to a situation whereby they do not arise. Philanthrophy has a continuing place in health care and medical research in Britain, and a place which seems less likely to diminish than to grow.

ROBERT J. MAXWELL

References
Association of Medical Research Charities, 29–35 Farringdon Road, London ECIM 3JB. The Association publishes its handbook annually, containing details of its members and affiliates. It is the best source of up-to-date information on charitable activity in this field in Britain.
Gladstone, F. (1982). *Charity law and social justice*. Bedford Square Press/NCVO, London.
Lattimer, M. and Holly, K. (1992). *Charity and NHS reform*. Directory of Social Change, London.
MRC (1993). *Medical Research Council Annual Report 1991–92*. MRC, 20 Park Crescent, London WIN 4AL.
Prochaska, F. (1992). *Philanthropy and the hospitals* of *London*. Clarendon Press, Oxford.
Department of Health (1993). *Research for health*. Department of Health, London.
Webster, C. (ed.) (1991). *Aneurin Bevan on the National Health Service*. Wellcome Unit for the History of Medicine, Oxford.

FOUNDATIONS, CHARITIES, AND GRANT-MAKING BODIES SUPPORTING MEDICAL RESEARCH IN THE UK (with a brief note on Europe). Medical research is undertaken in the UK in universities, hospitals, and in *Medical Research Council (MRC) units and privately funded research institutions. The universities receive the bulk of their support from the government through the Higher Education Funding Council for England (HEFCE) financed by the Department for Education. Parallel bodies have been set up for Wales and Scotland in consultation with the Welsh Office and the Scottish Office Education Department, i.e. the Higher Education Funding Council for Wales and the Scottish Higher Education Funding Council. In Northern Ireland the Department of Education (Northern Ireland) will be responsible for funding research). The hospitals are funded through the *National Health Service (NHS), which is the responsibility of the *Department of Health. The Medical Research Council, which receives an annual grant from the office of Science and Technology (created in 1992 as a branch of the Cabinet Office), finances the *National Institute for Medical Research at Mill Hill, Hampstead; the Clinical Research Centre, which moves to the *Royal Postgraduate Medical School in December 1994; and 47 research units. There are also many institutes supported by charitable funds, such as, for example, the *Imperial Cancer Research

Fund (ICRF) Laboratories, the Kennedy Institute of Rheumatology, and the Wellcome Trust/CRC Institute of Developmental Biology and Cancer in Cambridge.

Following a report on *Priorities in medical research* (1988) by a House of Lords Select Committee on Science and Technology, a new Department of Health Research Directorate, has been created. This organization has responsibility for research supported through the Department of Health.

In some NHS hospitals, private endowments remaining from the days when the hospitals were charitable institutions, are now used for the welfare of patients as well as for the support of research. In addition, there are many welfare services provided from charitable funds for individuals with various ailments (see SELF-HELP ORGANIZATIONS). Thus, while the institutions providing the basic structure of medicine in the UK receive their support from the government through various channels, these institutions also receive supplementary income, mainly for the support of research and welfare, from private sources. This situation has largely developed since the Second World War; when the NHS was established (1948), the universities received increasing government support, and the MRC (founded 1913) began to respond to the exponential growth of science.

With the diminished requirement for support for health and welfare from private sources, those who wished to help the sick transferred their assistance to medical research and the care of the grossly disabled and underprivileged. Since this article is concerned with the support of medicine over and above the basic support of the NHS and the universities, its scope is limited to a description of the MRC and the medical research and welfare charities. The contribution of innumerable individual and corporate benefactors to the care of the sick, although substantial, is not described.

The universities and the NHS

The support of medical research provided by the government through the universities and NHS is still very considerable, since university staff are expected to devote a proportion of their time to research, and the staff of hospitals, especially those attached to medical schools, also undertake a substantial amount of research. In addition, the universities provide the facilities for research, and the government pays a large proportion of the fees of students. This support is very difficult to quantify. An idea of its scope can be obtained from *Current research in Britain: biological sciences (1991)*, British Library Board.

On top of this base the MRC and the private charities, trusts, and foundation provide support for the development of research. This system, called the dual-support system, is the basis for the funding of major activities in university research. However, since the abolition of the 'binary line' which distinguished the long-established universities from the polytechnics, all of which are now

Table 1 The divisions, laboratories, and units funded by the Medical Research Council

National Institute for Medical Research
  Divisions
    Physical Biochemistry
    Biological Services
    Immunology
    Neurophysiology and Neuropharmacology
    Parasitology
    Virology
  Laboratories
    Cellular Immunology
    Computing
    Developmental Biochemistry
    Developmental Biology
    Eukaryotic Molecular Genetics
    Embryogenesis
    Gene Structure and Expression
    Leprosy and Mycobacterial Research
    Lipid and General Chemistry
    Mathematical Biology
    Molecular Immunology
    Molecular Structure
    Neurobiology
    Protein Structure
    Yeast Genetics

Clinical Research Centre
  Divisions
    Biochemical Genetics Research Group
    Division of Clinical Sciences
    Bone Diseases Research Group
    Dermatology Research Group
    Haemostasis Research Group
    Nutrition Research Group
    Section of Comparative Biology
    Section of Computing Services
    Electron Microscopy Support Group
    Endocytosis Research Group
    Section of Glycoconjugates
    High Pressure Neurological Syndrome Research Group
    Immune Response and Immunopathology Research Group
    Immune Deficiency Research Group
    Antigen Presentation Research Group
    Section of Medical Physics
    Section of Medical Statistics
    Microbial Pathogenicity Research Group
    Section of Molecular Rheumatology
    Division of Psychiatry
    Division of Sexually Transmitted Diseases
    Section of Surgical Research
    Transplantation Biology Section
    Vascular Biology Team

Table 1 (*cont.*)

Research Units
   Anatomical Neuropharmacology
   Applied Psychology
   Biochemical and Clinical Magnetic Resonance
   Biostatistics
   Blood Group
   Blood Pressure
   Brain Metabolism
   Cell Mutation
   Cellular Immunology
   Child Psychiatry
   Clinical Oncology and Radiotherapeutics
   Clinical Pharmacology
   Clinical Sciences Centre
   Cognitive Development
   Collaborative Centre
   Cyclotron
   Dental Research
   Dunn Nutrition
   Environmental Epidemiology
   Epidemiology (South Wales)
   Epidemiology and Medical Care
   Experimental Embryology and Teratology
   Human Biochemical Genetics
   Human Genetics
   Human Movement and Balance
   Institute of Hearing Research
   Immunochemistry
   Leukaemia
   MRC Laboratories, The Gambia
   MRC Laboratories, Jamaica
   Medical Sociology
   Laboratory of Molecular Biology
   Molecular Haematology
   Molecular Immunopathology
   Molecular Medicine Group
   Muscle and Cell Motility
   Neurochemical Pathology
   Neuropathogenesis
   Protein Function and Design
   Protein Phosphorylation
   Radiobiology
   Reproductive Biology
   Social and Applied Psychology
   Social and Community Psychiatry
   Toxicology
   Tuberculosis and Related Infections
   Virology
Interdisciplinary Research Centres
   Brain and Behaviour Research
   Brain Repair
   Cell Biology
   Mechanisms of Human Toxicology
   Protein Engineering
   Institute of Molecular Medicine

universities, much of the funding providing research infrastructure money has been taken away from the universities and transferred to the research councils, including the MRC, on the advice of the Advisory Board for the Research Councils (ABRC), so that the dual-support system is under threat. It is even possible that charities, like commercial organizations, may in future be required to pay overheads on research grants.

Medical Research Council
The MRC had a budget of £227 (US$340) million per annum for 1991–2, of which it allocated about £78 (US$112) million to university research under the dual-support system, and about £132 (US$198) million per annum for the support of its own full-time staff, who work either in its institutes or its units of varying size, which are usually located in or in relation to the universities (MRC 1992). An idea of its range of interests is given by the list of its units and divisions (Table 1). It is responsible to Parliament and publishes an annual handbook and report which gives fuller information.

Private funds
The private funds are referred to as charitable funds because they are, for the most part, distributed by organizations that are registered under the Charities Act administered through the Charity Commission. The British concept of charity goes back to the time of Queen Elizabeth I and is very difficult to define. It is concerned with the support of activities in the fields of education, health, welfare, and the care of the under-privileged. To be registered as a charity an organization has to be recognized by the Charity Commissioners as falling under the definition of a charity, as evolved through the centuries. Such recognition confers considerable privileges, such as Corporation Tax relief. In addition, the Inland Revenue, if it approves the donations of the charity, provides substantial tax relief. The charities have various titles. The Foundations are, for the most part, the result of the establishment of a charity by one man (e.g. Wolfson), but may be called Trusts if they were founded under a will settlement (e.g. Wellcome). The collecting charities, which receive their income from individual donations, collections, subscriptions, and legacies, may be called Funds (Imperial Cancer), Foundations (British Heart), Campaigns (Cancer Research), etc. Whatever their source of funds, they are usually distributed on the advice of expert committees to support medical research and the welfare of the sick. The 46 major medical research charities (AMRC 1992) together spend about £230 (US$345) million annually on biomedical research. The research charities are listed in Table 2 with their biomedical research expenditure for 1992–3. As can be seen in Table 2, some of these charities have been created

Table 2 Expenditure on medical research in the UK by AMRC members and affiliated charities 1992–93

Charity	Expenditure*	Subjects
Wellcome Trust	£77 231 000	Human and veterinary medicine, history of medicine
Imperial Cancer Research Fund	£49 932 000	Cancer
Cancer Research Campaign	£44 199 000	Cancer
British Heart Foundation	£20 943 697	Cardiovascular diseases
Arthritis and Rheumatism Council	£11 800 000	Rheumatic diseases
Leukaemia Research Fund	£9 053 201	Leukaemia
Yorkshire Cancer Research Campaign	£4 845 158	Cancer
Multiple Sclerosis Society	£4 700 000	Multiple sclerosis
Ludwig Institute for Cancer Research	£4 490 000	Cancer
Action Research	£3 500 000	Crippling disease
British Diabetic Association	£2 631 780	Diabetes and related subjects
Muscular Dystrophy Group	£1 931 117	Muscular dystrophy and allied neuromuscular diseases
Sir Jules Thorn Charitable Trust	£1 874 000	Medical research
National Asthma Campaign	£1 829 009	Asthma
Cystic Fibrosis Research Trust	£1 644 300	Cystic fibrosis
Scottish Hospital Endowments Research Trust	£1 500 000	General
Marie Curie Research Institute	£1 490 000	Cancer
North of England Cancer Research Campaign	£1 400 000	Cancer
Ciba Foundation	£1 380 519	Medical and clinical research
William Harvey Research Institute	£1 161 720	Medical research
Parkinson's Disease Society	£1 143 683	Parkinson's disease
Birthright	£1 100 000	Healthier babies and healthier women
British Lung Foundation	£1 044 141	Diseases of the chest and lungs
National Kidney Research Fund	£1 010 000	Kidney diseases
The Stroke Association	£959 247	Respiratory diseases and stroke
Wessex Medical Trust	£925 854	Medical research
Tenovus Cancer Fund	£924 664	Cancer and leukaemia
Motor Neurone Disease Association	£900 000	Motor neurone disease
Mental Health Foundation	£834 680	Mental disorders and handicap
Leverhulme Trust	£823 700	Medicine and health
Lister Institute of Preventive Medicine	£762 000	Medical research
Brain Research Trust	£721 436	Neurological diseases
Wishbone Trust	£630 000	Bone and joint surgery
Guide Dogs for the Blind Association	£540 000	Ophthalmology
Sub-total	£259 855 906	

*£1 = US$1.50.

for the support of research into and cure of specific diseases, whereas others are more general. Table 3 gives an idea of the topics that these funds support. Approximately 45 per cent of the support is for cancer research, and this is the main source of income for this topic in the UK.

The programmes of the charities are geared to their particular interests, while the MRC covers a much broader field. The charities are able to fulfil purposes such as the provision of laboratories, major equipment, and university chairs for special purposes, which are not readily available through the university financial system. In addition they can arrange programmes for support of research overseas, for example in the tropics, Commonwealth, and Europe.

It is appropriate to mention the particular example of the *Wellcome Trust because of its projected great size. Until 1986 this Trust owned the pharmaceutical company, the Wellcome Foundation Ltd. Since then, in 1986 and 1992, 60 per cent of the shareholding has been sold. As a consequence of these sales, the Wellcome Trust, now the Wellcome Trust Ltd, has an income of £220 million per annum projected for 1992–93. This income is of a similar order to that of the Medical Research Council. The policy for spending these large private funds will have a considerable impact on the support of medical

Table 2 (*cont.*)

Charity	Expenditure	Subjects
Nuffield Foundation	£499 670	Science, medicine, social science, and ageing
Spastics Society	£450 000	Cerebral palsy
Research into Ageing	£400 000	Ageing
Liver Research Unit Trust	£389 205	Liver disease
Foundation for the Study of Infant Deaths	£386 026	Infant deaths
Cancer and Leukaemia in Childhood Trust	£380 000	Oncology
Iris Fund for Prevention of Blindness	£342 140	Blindness
International Spinal Research Trust	£320 000	Paralysis
Beit Memorial Fellowships for Medical Research	£302 825	Medicine
Restoration of Appearance and Function Trust	£295 000	Restorative surgery
DEBRA	£280 600	Genetics
Royal National Institute for the Blind	£265 000	Prevention of blindness
British Retinitis Pigmentosa Society	£254 927	Retinitis pigmentosa
Bradford's War on Cancer Campaign	£250 000	Oncology
Hearing Research Trust	£240 000	Hearing
British Digestive Foundation	£225 000	Gastroenterology
Blond Mcindoe Centre	£219 480	Transplantation immunology and causes of rejection
Smith and Nephew Foundation	£217 000	Medicine and surgery
Friedreich's Ataxia Group	£200 000	Neurology
Children's Liver Disease Foundation	£166 662	Hepatology
Living Again	£143 461	Severely disabling physical and nervous diseases and brain damage
British Council for Prevention of Blindness	£134 354	Ophthalmology
Bardhan Research & Education Trust	£120 750	Gastrointestinal diseases
Barnwood House Trust	£106 000	General
TFC Frost Charitable Trust	£100 000	Ophthalmology
REMEDI	£68 000	Rehabilitation, aid to medical self-help groups
Psoriasis Association	£66 555	Dermatology
Tuberous Sclerosis Association	£65 000	Neurology
Migraine Trust	£56 542	Migraine
National Back Pain Association	£46 117	Back pain and allied conditions
Primary Immunodeficiency Association	£40 000	Immunology
National Eczema Society	£38 237	Dermatology
Brain Damage Research Trust	£35 000	Neurology
Mason Medical Research Foundation	£35 000	General
Association for Spina Bifida and Hydrocephalus	£31 363	Spina bifida and hydrocephalus
Royal Surgical Aid Society	£23 000	Surgery
Little Foundation	£4 454	Prenatal neuro-development diseases
Sub-total for charities less than £0.5m	£7 180 525	
Total AMRC charities expenditure	£266 791 184	

research in the UK in the coming years. The change in the balance of support away from government to private sources will undoubtedly be the subject of lively debate.

Support for medical research in Europe

Support varies greatly from country to country and is undergoing major change because of the changing political situation, especially in Eastern Europe. The concept of charity is not recognized in Europe in the same form as in Britain, but there are major organizations called *Fondation*, *Stiftung*, *Stichting*, *Fondazione*, which provide private funds. The bulk of funds, however, come from government sources operating through various departments. The chief executives of some of the major foundations meet regularly in an organization called the Hague Club which was founded in 1971 (The Hague Club 1991). Arrangements are available through organizations in Britain and Europe to

Table 3 Topics of research supported by charities, 1991

Topic	Annual expenditure (£000)*
Cancer	100 637
Nervous diseases	12 000
General	67 334
Chest and heart	22 848
Tropical medicine	1 950
Arthritis and rheumatism	15 768
Mental health	770
Diabetes and cystic fibrosis	3 977
Kidney diseases	1 000
Digestive diseases	270
Ageing	448

Source: The Association of Medical Research Charities.
*£1 = US$1.50

exchange research workers. The European Community in Brussels has been developing a considerable involvement and should always be borne in mind when considering ways in which research might be funded.

Conclusions

These various organizations provide between them a very considerable supplementary (and in the case of cancer, primary) support for research in the UK and Europe. The variety of interests embraced by these organizations provides a considerable range of opinion in considering proposals. It can therefore be said that, in the UK at any rate, any good idea has a chance of catching a sympathetic ear. By contrast, this is not the case in many countries in Europe, for example Italy, where it is very difficult to develop a research career in medicine. The disadvantages of the support of research through the grants system is that their temporary nature tends to encourage short-term projects and provides an initial opportunity but relatively few long-term posts for research workers. The MRC's and the Wellcome Trust's career posts provide some solution to this requirement, as do some university positions. The recent cut-back in university funds is, however, having a severe effect on the availability of such posts (since when posts are frozen or disestablished those involved primarily in research are often the first to go, in order to preserve those more concerned with teaching); this is discouraging new entrants into medical research.

P. O. WILLIAMS

References

AMRC (1992). *The Association of Medical Research Charities handbook*. AMRC, London. (Also annual reports of individual charities named in the *Handbook*.)
British Library Board (1991). *Current research in British biological sciences*, 2 Vols, (6th edn) British Library Board, London.
Commission of the European Community (1992). *EC research funding: a guide for applicants*, (3rd edn). Commission of the European Community, Brussels.
Medical Research Council (1992). *Medical Research Council handbook 1992–1993*. MRC, London.
Priorities in medical research, Select Committee on Science and Technology (1988). Vol. I. HMSO, London.
The Hague Club (1991). *European foundation profiles*. The Hague.

FOUNDATIONS IN THE USA: THEIR ROLE IN MEDICINE AND HEALTH
Introduction

The concept of philanthropy is by no means of recent origin. Indeed, the antecedents of modern philanthropic foundations may be found in antiquity, and for centuries individuals and organizations have had charitable inclinations and concern for the well-being of society. Until recent times, religious bodies were the predominant source of philanthropic gifts, often to schools, hospitals, almshouses, or other local charities.

Despite this long history, however, the philanthropic foundation as we know it is a relatively modern entity, and is, to a large degree, a predominantly American development. In fact, American philanthropic foundations are, in large measure, a phenomenon of the 20th century, although they had their roots in the second half of the 19th century. In 1867 George Peabody established what was probably the first American private foundation; the Peabody Fund was endowed in the amount of $2 (£1.3) million, and its income was directed primarily toward the improvement of education in the southern United States. A similar objective was identified for the Slater Fund, organized in 1882. By 1890 18 private foundations had been established, but only one had a capital of more than $10 (£6.7) million.

Since 1900, more than 3300 private foundations have been formed, with a dramatic increase in the rate of their establishment since the First World War. Between 1950 and 1959, 1272 new foundations came into being. During the 20th century, the number of foundations with assets of over $100 (£67) million has increased from seven in the second decade to almost 60 in 1993. The Ford Foundation, currently the nation's largest, has assets of more than $6.3 ($4.2) billion. The assets of the John D. and Catherine T. MacArthur Foundations exceed $3.1 billion, and the two largest of the medically orientated foundations, Robert Wood Johnson and W. K. Kellogg, have assets of $4.0 (£2.7) billion and $5.3 (£3.5) billion, respectively. In addition, in the past 25 years, many large corporations have established charitable foundations. Under an earlier law, corporate foundations were able to allocate up to 5 per cent of their profits for charitable purposes on a tax-free basis; after 1 January 1982, the limit was increased to 10 per cent. Although many corporate foundations make significant gifts, few if any approach even the 5 per cent figure.

The regulation of foundations

Throughout most of the history of philanthropy in the US, federal laws governing private foundations were relatively lax, particularly in respect to the amount of charitable contributions they were expected to make in any given year. Although most of the major foundations followed a policy of expending current income and, in some cases, of using principal as well, the trustees of some foundations simply expanded principal by paying out relatively little income. Despite the many benefactions of major foundations, the organizations were not, and are still not, without their critics, many of whom object to their tax advantages, and particularly to those situations where a foundation's holdings are used to control a business in which the foundation's trustees are involved as owners or managers. In the 1960s these issues occupied the attention of Congressman Wright Patman of Texas. Under his direction, extensive studies were made of foundation operations in general, and their business relationships in particular. Patman's studies did uncover abuses by a relatively small number of foundations, and as a result, after extensive hearings, Congress passed legislation in 1969 that mandated an annual payout by private foundations of more than 5 per cent of their assets or the whole of their investment income. Rigid regulations regarding the business holdings of foundations were also established, and the potential for abuse was greatly reduced.

No responsible individual could argue with the implementation of measures to prevent abuses of the privilege to establish and operate tax-exempt foundations, and most foundation officers and trustees supported a payout requirement. The necessity of expending all income, however, irrespective of its magnitude, produced a serious problem, particularly because the advent of high inflation rates adversely affected the 'buying power' of foundation grants.

As a result of a vigorous effort on the part of the Council on Foundations, the body representing the large majority of private, community, and corporate foundations, as well as prospective donees and interested citizens, Congress in 1979 removed the requirement for foundations to pay out investment income if it exceeded 5 per cent of the assets. Income over the 5 per cent level may be added to the capital and thus help maintain the foundation's buying power.

Foundations in the 20th century

The example set by the small number of foundations established in the 19th century, and a growing concern, on the part of men of great wealth, with problems of importance to the nation, led after 1900 to the establishment of a number of large private foundations by such public-spirited men as Andrew *Carnegie, John D. *Rockefeller, Julius Rosenwald, Edward Harkness, and James B. Duke. Their foundations represented unique and valuable avenues for private support of various fields of human endeavour; for the most part general

education, medical education, medical research, and health care were the beneficiaries. Because the founders availed themselves of the counsel of far-sighted men like Frederick C. Gates and Abraham *Flexner, their grants were innovative and their contributions significant.

For example, one of Carnegie's chief benefactions took the form of general libraries, which served the populace in many cities and towns. Equally important, the Carnegie libraries established the importance of the community library, so that today most cities and towns, both large and small, provide a public library for their citizens. In like manner, Carnegie's support of Flexner's epochal study of American medical education in 1908–10, which not only documented the inferior nature of the process as it then was structured but also set out a blueprint for its upgrading, had far-reaching results. In the decade following the publication of the *Flexner Report, Rockefeller, through his General Education Board, provided the financial support that enabled a number of universities, including Johns Hopkins, Western Reserve, and Washington University, to implement Flexner's recommendations and to develop outstanding academic medical centres dedicated to excellence in medical education, research, and patient care.

In 1918 the Commonwealth Fund, created by the Harkness family, began its notable history in medicine and health. Among its early programmes was one that aided in the development of new disciplines, particularly child psychiatry. Commonwealth funding for construction of hospitals in rural areas, which previously lacked adequate hospital beds, was another important contribution. The latter programme was the model for the federal government's Hill–Burton legislation in 1946, which greatly expanded hospital facilities in many underserved areas. The foregoing examples emphasize two key roles that foundations have played—and should continue to play—if they are to serve most effectively:

(1) support of preliminary studies and pilot projects identifying new approaches to existing needs; and
(2) the provision of grants to enable verification of new approaches, so that, if successful, they can be reproduced on a wide scale and benefit society as a whole.

Replication of new methods, techniques, or other innovative programmes may, and often does, involve such large sums of money that foundations cannot take on that responsibility; inevitably, government, with its greater resources, must become involved after a model programme has been created and its effectiveness validated. The rural hospital effort initiated by the Commonwealth Fund and then greatly expanded through the federal Hill–Burton programme is an excellent example of this sequence. An even more impressive illustration can be seen in the remarkable expansion of biomedical research in the USA after the Second World War. At the turn of the century, the biomedical research effort was, by today's standards, minuscule, and, in fact, continued to be so for the next several decades. The establishment of the Rockefeller Institute for Medical Research (now Rockefeller University) was a key development in the advancement of medical research, in that it emphasized the importance of support for basic and clinical investigation in the medical sciences. Support of a small number of carefully selected investigators in a few medical schools in the 1920s and 1930s, much of it provided by the Rockefeller Foundation and the Commonwealth Fund, further demonstrated the importance of providing able individuals with support over a long enough time to enable them systematically to explore a problem and ultimately to produce the new knowledge essential to medical progress.

The impact of the Second World War
During the Second World War, to meet medical needs generated on the battlefield, the government initiated major efforts to obtain adequate amounts of penicillin and blood substitutes for the treatment of the wounded. These efforts, involving the participation of industry and based on the application of knowledge previously derived from fundamental research, led to realization on the part of the public and its elected representatives that greater sums of money to ensure funding of research in the biomedical field was in the nation's best interests. Without the ready example set earlier by several foundations, the government's massive support through the *National Institutes of Health (NIH), which saw more than a tenfold increase in research funding over a period of 20 years, would almost certainly not have occurred as early as it did.

In the face of the extremely large government investment in research after the Second World War, most foundations decreased their participation in biomedical research, feeling that their resources were so dwarfed by those of the federal government that they could have little impact. Instead, foundation attention was to a large degree directed to new areas where philanthropic participation promised to enhance progress. For example, in the medical area, the need for medical school curricular reform, resulting from the growth in the body of knowledge, was made possible primarily by large grants from the Commonwealth Fund. As academic medical centres expanded, foundation initiatives, notably those of the John and Mary R. Markle Foundation, responded to the need for more academically orientated physicians by providing support for promising young men and women pointing toward academic careers. Just as the NIH fellowship awards, which were a prominent feature of the expansion of research support by the government, were based to a large extent on the example of the much smaller but pioneering fellowship programmes (e.g. the National Research Council Fellowships in the Medical Sciences) sponsored by the Rockefeller Foundation and the Commonwealth Fund, so did the Markle Scholar Awards constitute a model for

the career development awards established in the 1960s by the NIH. Later, grants from a group of foundations (the Alfred P. Sloan Foundation and the Josiah Macy, Jr Foundation, in particular), stimulated medical schools to increase opportunities for minority students. In the late 1960s and the early 1970s, health-care delivery became a major focus for the Commonwealth Fund, the Carnegie Corporation, the Rockefeller Foundation, and the Robert Wood Johnson Foundation. A noteworthy development of the period, and one that has been maintained, was the joint participation in large projects by groups of foundations. For example, a co-operative effort of the Carnegie Corporation and the Commonwealth Fund, which explored the need for training programmes to prepare able young men and women to work in new areas within the expanded health-care field, was the antecedent of the major Clinical Scholars Program of the Robert Wood Johnson Foundation.

Recent foundation initiatives
As medical science progressed rapidly and became a topic of increasing interest to the public, a dramatic shift in the public's attitude toward medical care resulted, best expressed by the now time-worn cliché that medical care came to be considered as a right rather than a privilege. As a result, the health-care delivery system rapidly became overtaxed, not only in terms of available personnel but also in terms of its cost. New technology brought new benefits, but also enhanced the complexity and cost of health care. The development of life support devices introduced new and vexing ethical problems. Major foundations concerned with medicine and health found a broad menu of problems calling for solution, and provided funding for studies addressing these problems. In addition, small, local, private foundations, community foundations in various major cities, corporate foundations, and particularly the voluntary health organizations have been active in their support for medicine.

Among the foundation-supported projects that have had an important impact on health and medical care are those that have:

(1) expanded the availability of health professionals, e.g. physicians, nurse practitioners, and physician assistants;
(2) increased the number of ethnic minorities and women in the health field;
(3) supported alternative approaches to health-care delivery, such as prepaid care and *hospices (modelled on those in the UK, notably St Christopher's);
(4) explored difficult questions in medical *ethics, such as the definition of death and the allocation of limited resources in the face of excessive demands;
(5) analysed and subsequently defined rational and effective health policies for the nation;
(6) attempted to define effective methods of *health education, to enable the individual to use medical

resources intelligently and more cost effectively; and

(7) recognized the problems related to an ageing population, and supported efforts to provide comprehensive care to this growing segment of society in an efficient, effective, and compassionate manner.

The voluntary health organizations

Voluntary health organizations have provided substantial support for the health field. At least two had their origins early in the 20th century, e.g. the *Tuberculosis Society (now the American Lung Association) in 1904 and the American *Cancer Society in 1913. Along with the American Heart Association, the Tuberculosis Society, and the American Cancer Society were the prototypes of many comparable associations, all of which depend in large measure for their resources on annual fund drives. In their early years, these organizations directed their funds primarily toward patient education and patient care, but as the medical research enterprise began to grow, some voluntary agencies allocated funds to support laboratory and clinical investigation.

The Tuberculosis Society and the National Polio Foundation elected not to close their doors when their respective objectives were achieved. After the introduction of effective antituberculosis agents changed dramatically, and for the better, the prognosis of tuberculous infections, the Tuberculosis Society became the American Lung Association and has since used its funds for the prevention and treatment of pulmonary diseases such as emphysema. In like manner, the National Polio Foundation, founded in 1938 by the late president Franklin D. Roosevelt, a victim of the disease, raised large sums of money through annual drives called the March of Dimes. When the Salk and Sabin vaccines were developed in the 1950s and poliomyelitis became preventable, the Polio Foundation changed its name to the March of Dimes Birth Defects Foundation and adopted as its new purpose the prevention of congenital and hereditary abnormalities—a far broader and more difficult goal.

In the past three decades a large number of other voluntary agencies, almost without exception concerned with a single disease entity such as *diabetes, or a group of diseases of similar nature such as *leukaemia, have come into being. To name only some, there are now groups whose purpose is to combat *muscular dystrophy, *multiple sclerosis, *leukaemia, *cerebral palsy, *retinitis pigmentosa, renal infections, diabetes, and *cystic fibrosis. Perhaps the most recent major entry in the field is the *Alzheimer's Disease Foundation, created in response to the increasing recognition of this serious neurological problem, which has in turn reflected the steady increase in the proportion of the population aged over 65.

Support of basic medical research

Historically, as noted above, foundation support of research, although tiny by today's standards, was a major factor in pointing to the importance of laboratory investigation in leading to medical progress. Indeed, in 1940, philanthropy provided almost four times as much money for biomedical research as did the federal government. After the Second World War, as the programmes of the National Institutes of Health (NIH) expanded, the situation changed dramatically, so that by 1950 NIH funding of research was almost twice that of philanthropic organizations, and federal funding now dwarfs that of private foundations. As already noted, the availability of, and increase in, massive federal funding during the period from 1950 on, led many foundations to discontinue, or at least minimize, grants for basic research, on the basis that they would at best have minimal impact.

However, in recent years two philanthropic organizations have been vigorous supporters of basic medical research, namely, the Howard Hughes Medical Institute, whose assets of over $7.5 (£5) billion make it far and away the largest entity of its kind, and the Lucille P. Markey Charitable Trust.

The Howard Hughes Medical Institute, which is classified as a medical research organization rather than as a private foundation, provides almost $300 (£200) million annually for basic research in leading academic medical centres. Its investigators are paid directly by Hughes, rather than by the institutions in which they hold academic positions, and they work in laboratory space leased by Hughes. In recent years Hughes has also made awards to colleges and medical schools to support students interested in ultimately pursuing research.

The Markey Charitable Trust, because its donor specified that it should exist for only 15 years, has expended interest and principal from the original bequest of about $300 (£200) million, and, as a result, has been able to award approximately $50 (£33) million annually:

(1) to enable outstanding young men and women, both Ph.Ds and MDs, or MD/Ph.Ds, to enhance their development for productive careers in research; and

(2) to support established scientists to pursue exciting new ideas to the point where federal funding can be attracted.

The future

The challenges before the medically oriented foundations are demanding indeed. Despite the substantial collective resources held by the foundations of the USA, even the largest among them can only address a small segment of the problems needing solution. A significant advantage of the private foundation, and of the community and corporate foundation, is flexibility. Innovative approaches carry a degree of risk as well as of promise, and private organizations are less vulnerable than government in being in the vanguard of the attack on difficult problems. Since foundations are, in a real sense, comparable to venture capital firms in the investment sector, they do take risks, and they must be aware of their exposure to failure, even when their grantees are highly competent and dedicated. But the overall contributions of the medically orientated foundations in the USA have been impressive and in many instances seminal, and they will continue to have an exciting role in the decades that lie ahead.

ROBERT J. GLASER

Further reading

Fosdick, R. B. (1952). *The story of the Rockefeller Foundation*. Rockefeller Foundation, New York.

Glaser, R. J. (1992). The impact of philanthropy on medicine and health. *Perspectives in Biology and Medicine*, **36**, 46–56.

Harvey, A. M. and Abrams, S. L. (1986). *For the welfare of mankind: The Commonwealth Fund and American medicine*. The Johns Hopkins University Press, New York.

FOUNDLING HOSPITALS were established in many countries, especially in the 18th century, to receive children abandoned by their parents. This was commonplace in an age of poverty and deprivation when many families were too large. Babies were left in maternity hospitals and the mothers could not be traced or were vagrants. Thousands of children were left in the streets to fend for themselves or became 'objects of charity', and the mortality among them was appallingly high. One of the more famous was The Foundling Hospital of London founded in 1739 by the sea captain Thomas *Coram, whose heart was wrung by the plight of these unfortunates.

FOURNIER, JEAN ALFRED (1832–1914). French venereologist. His life was devoted to studying *syphilis, and his many publications covered its clinical, pathological, preventive, therapeutic, and social aspects.

FOVEA is an anatomical term for a small pit.

FOWLER'S POSITION is a position in bed in which the patient lies on his back with the head elevated and the knees drawn up, so that the *pelvis is the lowest part of the body.

FOX, SIR THEODORE FORTESCUE (1899–1989). Editor of the *Lancet* from 1944 to 1964. An outstanding interpreter for the general reader of breakthroughs in medical research, from 1944 to 1948 he also played a crucial part in persuading the British medical profession to enter the *National Health Service. See MEDICAL JOURNALS.

FOX, WILLIAM TILBURY (1836–79). British dermatologist. A pioneer in his subject, he was the author of a well-known work, *A treatise on skin diseases* (1864).

FRACASTORO, GIROLAMO (*c*.1478–1553). Italian physician. He is best known for his narrative poem *Syphilus sive morbus Gallicus* (1530), which gave the disease of *syphilis its name. He was also a pioneer in epidemiology and formulated the doctrine of *contagion, holding that disease might be transmitted by contact, by *fomites (a word he introduced), or at a distance by *seminaria*. This anticipated the discovery of bacteria. His views are set out in *De contagione et contagionis morbis et curatione* (1546). He gave an excellent description of *typhus.

FRACTURES. A fracture is a break, rupture, or discontinuity, usually of a bone. A pathological fracture is one that occurs in bone already weakened by an existing pathological process such as *osteomalacia, *metastatic cancer, *tuberculosis, etc. A compound (or open) fracture is one complicated by an associated skin wound. A simple fracture, as its name implies, is a simple break; a comminuted fracture is one in which a part of the damaged bone is broken into fragments; and a 'greenstick' fracture is seen in immature bones in children when the break in a long bone is only partial and the unbroken portion of the shaft of the bone bends.

FRAGILITAS OSSIUM. See OSTEOGENESIS IMPERFECTA.

FRANCIS, WILLIAM W. (1878–1959). Osler librarian at *McGill University. From 1922 to 1929, working with his colleagues Dr Archie Mailoch, and Reg Hill of the Bodleian Library, he was the chief cataloguer in editing and seeing through the Oxford University Press the *Bibliotheca Osleriana*. He accompanied the 7000 rare volumes to McGill University and was the internationally revered presiding genius and encourager of students in the Osler Library until his death.

FRANK, JOHANNES PETER (1745–1821). German physician. He first distinguished *diabetes insipidus from *diabetes mellitus (1794). He published in six volumes a *System einer vollständigen medicinischen Polizei* (1779–1817) which covered the whole of *public health, hygiene, and community medicine.

FRAUD AND MISCONDUCT IN MEDICAL RESEARCH.

On 26 March 1974 Dr William Summerlin, an *immunologist at the Sloan-Kettering Institute, New York, used a black felt-tip pen to darken a transplanted skin patch in two white mice. His hope was to show that he had overcome the normal difficulties of rejection of a foreign *transplant by its recipient. Thus, by incubating the tissue for some time in a nutrient solution, he alleged that he could remove the substances that prevented the *graft from being accepted. Nevertheless, after

Summerlin had demonstrated this work at a formal departmental meeting, the deception was discovered by a laboratory technician, and, when confronted by Dr Robert Good, the distinguished head of the institute, he confessed. A subsequent inquiry censured not only Summerlin but also Good for not providing sound experimental planning and guidance.

At the time, Summerlin's behaviour was perceived as an aberration—so much so that he was sent on prolonged sick leave with full salary. To be sure, earlier cases had been reported, such as the Piltdown Man hoax and Sir Cyril Burt's work on the inheritance of *intelligence quotients, but the nature of some of these was still controversial. Nevertheless, from this time onwards it became clear that a certain amount of fraud was an inevitable concomitant of scientific research.

In many ways, therefore, with the Summerlin case, 1974 may be seen as a watershed, with the continual revelation of fresh cases ever since (particularly, but not exclusively, in the USA), so that a number of features are now much clearer. Thus at the time of writing I know of the following number of definite cases: Australia, 5 (including none other than William McBride, one of the first to describe the teratogenic effects of *thalidomide); UK, 11; USA, 30; Switzerland, 1. Undoubtedly cases have occurred elsewhere, but these have not been officially investigated.

Background to research misconduct

Of those reported cases, there seem to have been two principal backgrounds to the fraud. On the one hand were doctors without much research experience: some family doctors in the UK and some hospital physicians in the USA. Usually their research was part of a multicentre drug trial, and the motive for the fraud was greed. Several hundreds of pounds may be paid for each patient entered into such a study—hence the temptation to invent patients and data.

On the other hand, there were energetic, middle-grade research workers working flat out in a prestigious research institution under a distinguished, but often remote, head of department. Their yearly number of publications (articles and conference abstracts) was often excessive and the peer pressure to produce positive results intense. Thus the research tended to be in 'hot' topics—*molecular *biology, *cancer, *cardiology—with the rewards not money but prestige, promotion, and prizes. And others in the department, including the bosses, were caught up in the deception by accepting 'gift' or 'honorary' authorship (putting their names on a paper for which they could take no responsibility).

Other causal factors

There have been three other causal factors in these cases of fraud. First, the 'Messianic complex', an inner conviction of the righteousness of one's view on a theory of the cause of, say, cancer or *schizophrenia, to such an extent that no experimental proof is necessary and invention of the supporting data will save time as well as humanity. This probably explains McBride's fraudulent work. He was convinced that Debendox®, an effective antiemetic for vomiting in pregnancy, produced *fetal deformities, despite the lack of any evidence for this in human beings. Moreover, he failed to find that similar drugs produced deformities in studies in rabbits, so that he then falsified his results to produce a paper concluding that they did—and subsequently testified to this effect in an American lawsuit against the drug. Secondly, and rarely, the research worker has suffered from frank *mental illness; and, thirdly, in rather more instances there has been a criminal element in the fraudster's make-up.

Nobody has any idea of the true prevalence of fraud, and whether this differs among the various scientific disciplines, estimates having varied a thousandfold or more. Expert peer review of papers submitted to journals for publication has been largely ineffective in detecting cases, most of which have come to light through 'whistleblowers', usually close colleagues. And most authorities now agree that a better collective term for the phenomenon is 'scientific misconduct', which can cover the whole spectrum from minor to major lapses.

Spectrum of misconduct

This spectrum of research misconduct is wide. It ranges from 'sloppy' science and inappropriate authorship, through self-delusion and bias, and failure to declare a conflict of interest, to the three most serious forms, which are as follows.

Piracy

Piracy is the deliberate exploitation of other people's ideas without their permission. An example was given by Sir Peter *Medawar in his book *Advice to a young scientist* of a research worker who would hang around the common rooms of university institutes eavesdropping on conversations, whereupon he would rapidly set up the research himself and publish his results before the originator could do so.

Plagiarism

Plagiarism is (probably overall the commonest type), copying ideas, data, or text without permission or acknowledgment. A famous example is of E.A.K. Alsabti, an Iraqi immunologist, who worked at various research centres in the UK and USA. While working at the M.D. Anderson Hospital in Houston, Texas, Alsabti picked up a paper written by Daniel Wierda and addressed to Dr Jeffrey Gottlieb at that hospital seeking a referee's opinion upon its suitability for publication in the *European Journal of Cancer*. By then, however, Gottlieb had been dead for 2 years, but Alsabti removed Wierda's name from the paper, added his own, and the names of two fictitious authors, and submitted it to the *Japanese Journal of Medical Science and Biology* which published it rapidly—well before the appearance of Wierda's original article.

Wierda protested to the editor of the Japanese journal, who formally retracted the paper, and articles about the case appeared in various journals, one of which led to Alsabti's dismissal from an internal medicine residency programme (and subsequently from at least two others elsewhere). A subsequent inquiry showed that he had plagiarized some 60 articles: most of them he then published in obscure journals, of which many were later retracted.

Fraud

Fraud is deliberate deception, usually involving the invention of data. One of the earliest and most publicized cases was that of John Darsee, a Harvard research worker. In 1981 he was seen to falsify data during a laboratory study; his overall head of department, the distinguished cardiologist Eugene Braunwald, decided that this was a single bizarre act, allowed him to continue to work under close supervision, but terminated his fellowship from the National Institutes of Health (NIH). Six months later, however, it became clear that Darsee's data in a multicentre study of treatments to protect the damaged heart muscle after a myocardial *infarction were different from those at three other research units taking part.

Harvard Medical School set up a committee of investigation, as did the NIH and Emory University, where Darsee had also worked. It emerged that he had committed an extensive series of frauds, originating during his undergraduate days at Notre Dame University and continuing at Emory and Harvard. These included reports of non-existent patients or collaborators, and invented data, as in the multicentre trial. There were also procedures and results that, on reflection, were virtually impossible to achieve: drawing blood from the tail vein of a rat weekly for all of its 90-week lifespan, and obtaining blood specimens in all 43 members of a family on two consecutive days after an overnight fast twice a year, as well as complete sets of 24-hour urine specimens (including that for a 2-year-old child). In all, Darsee published over 100 articles and abstracts, many of them in prestigious journals and with distinguished co-authors; many of these had to be retracted.

Darsee's case has attracted a lot of attention, partly because it was the first major publicized case of true fraud that was not a isolated blemish on the face of science; not mad—rather, bad; partly, because it concerned prestigious institutions, co-authors, and journals; partly, because of the charismatic personality of the central figure; partly, because it initiated the whole debate about the rights and wrongs of authorship, data retention, supervision of juniors, and the management of suspected cases of fraud; and, finally, partly because it shifted the whole climate of feeling of trust to thinking the unthinkable—the possibility that things might not be as they seemed.

Reaction of the scientific community

Initially, as the Darsee case showed, the scientific community reacted to any disclosure of scientific misconduct with disbelief and shock. Nevertheless, from the early 1980s a series of reports recommended preventive and corrective measures—initially from the USA, then from Australia, the UK, and Denmark (which has only recently reported some cases). Most of these have three underlying principles. First, the onus rests on the university or hospital department concerned and not on outside organizations (including medical and surgical journals), which have neither the resources nor the skills to investigate allegations. Secondly, the inquiry should be done in stages so that the proceedings may be stopped if they disclose no reason for further action. Thirdly, 'due process' should prevail, including strict confidentiality to protect both the 'whistleblower' and the suspected culprit.

At every step those involved must follow procedures designed to ensure full confidentiality and natural justice. If a finding of serious medical misconduct is upheld, then several bodies need to be informed: the licensing authority (the *GMC in the UK); the employing authorities; grant-giving bodies; and editors of journals—who should be told whether articles that they have published have been classified as valid, questionable, or fraudulent. If, however, the integrity of the researcher is vindicated by the investigation (the third stage of the procedure, after the initial screening and inquiry), then he or she should be offered the opportunity of having an appropriate public statement released.

Perhaps even more important, however, is the prevention of the early stages of scientific misconduct, by the elimination of sloppy science. The exemplary guidelines drawn up by the Harvard Medical School include close supervision of new investigators, each supervisor being responsible for only a few research workers and holding regular discussions in the laboratory; the prolonged retention of data by the unit; and the establishment of a policy on authorship, which eschews gift authorship. And Harvard has gone even further by recommending that candidates for promotion should be allowed to list only a very limited number of articles in their curricula vitae—for example, 10 in an application for a full professorship.

Despite all these recommendations, academic bodies were slow to implement them, and after a series of such cases where the 'whistleblowers' often seemed to be more penalized than the perpetrator, the US Congress lost patience. In 1989 the National Institutes of Health set up two bodies—the Office of Scientific Integrity (OSI) and the Office of Scientific Integrity Review (OSIR). The first of these was to be concerned with monitoring investigations and promoting high standards of research; the second to oversee the operation of OSI.

Neither had an easy time, and in 1991 a new body, the Office of Research Integrity was established. Nevertheless, as with action taken by other official bodies, their very existence is a tribute to the concern that medical science has shown in dealing with this small but definite blemish in its midst. We may have to accept that a little research misconduct is inevitable, but at least we are now trying both to prevent it and to deal with the established cases.

STEPHEN LOCK

FRATRICIDE. Homicide of a brother.

FREEZE FRACTURE is a specialized technique for preparing tissue for examination by *electron microscopy.

FREY TEST. An intradermal test (now mainly of historical interest) for *lymphogranuloma venereum, in which antigenic material was injected intracutaneously; a positive result was a raised red papule of at least 8 mm diameter appearing within 48 to 72 hours. The causal organism is *Chlamydia trachomatis*; the test has largely been abandoned because of false positive and negative reactions.

FREMITUS. Palpable vibrations, that is a *thrill; a noise which can be felt as well as heard when a hand is placed on the body surface.

FREUD, ANNA (1895–1982). Austrian psychiatrist. Anna Freud was born in Vienna, the youngest daughter of Sigmund *Freud. She extended her father's work in *psychoanalysis to children and adolescents and therefore contributed to education and the development of psychiatry in these age-groups. When Austria was annexed by Nazi Germany she fled with her father to London, and cared for him until he died. She continued her work in a clinic which she founded in London. She wrote several books, notably *Normality and pathology in childhood* (1968).

FREUD, SIGMUND (1856–1939). Austrian psychiatrist. In 1891 he became interested in *aphasia, but shortly afterwards started to develop his ideas on *psychoanalysis with *Breuer. They split in 1895 and never spoke to one another again because of Breuer's disapproval of Freud's views.

Subsequently he occupied himself with the study of the determinants of human thought and behaviour, and by 1907 regular meetings were being held at Freud's house. The group included *Jung, *Adler, *Bleuler, and Sandor Ferenczi; they founded the International Psychoanalytical Association, which was based in Nuremberg. The first three named above seceded because they could not accept Freud's intellectual dominance. The authoritarian character of the

movement tended to alienate European opinion. When it was proscribed by the Nazis as a Jewish doctrine many of its disciples fled to the USA, while Freud came to the UK in 1939 just before he died. For these reasons Freud's views were less influential in Europe than in the USA, where they dominated psychiatry until 1960. See also PSYCHIATRY; PSYCHOLOGY.

FREYER, SIR PETER JOHNSTON (1851–1921). Irish surgeon. He devised and developed the operation of suprapubic *prostatectomy.

FRICTION is the sound or sensation of rubbing produced by the relative movement of inflamed serous surfaces in contact with each other (e.g. pleural friction, pericardial friction).

FRIEDREICH, NIKOLAUS (1826–82). German physician. He is remembered for his descriptions of *hereditary ataxia (Friedreich's ataxia (1863, 1876)) and *paramyoclonus multiplex (1881).

FRIEDREICH'S ATAXIA. See HEREDITARY ATAXIA.

FRIENDLY SOCIETIES are legally recognized voluntary associations in the UK which raise funds by subscription or contribution to provide relief and assistance in old age, sickness, or other hardship to its members or their surviving dependants. Friendly societies, the functions of which are similar to some of those performed by the medieval guilds, began to be founded in the 17th century and were widely established by the 18th century. Legislation has existed since 1793 regulating their activities to ensure good management and the protection of their assets. A Registry of Friendly Societies was established in 1875; registration confers certain legal privileges; and there is a legal officer, the Chief Registrar of Friendly Societies, who exercises a supervisory function. Their method of operation remains unchanged; they receive regular small sums from their members, which they accumulate and invest, and with which they subsequently meet members' claims. In the USA, fraternal insurance organizations provide the equivalent of British friendly societies. Trade unions are not friendly societies, although they have overlapping functions, and are governed by separate legislation.

FRIGIDITY is lack of sexual interest or responsiveness in the woman, analogous to male *impotence.

FROSTBITE is the condition resulting from freezing of the extremities; in mild, reversible cases it affects only superficial tissues, in more severe instances freezing causes subsequent *necrosis of deeper structures, including blood vessels and muscles. *Prophylaxis is crucial.

FROZEN SHOULDER. Severe pain and immobility of the shoulder joint, often accompanied by painful swelling of the hand (shoulder–hand syndrome). Frozen shoulder, or pericapsulitis, may develop some weeks after a *coronary thrombosis, but may also complicate other acute illnesses (e.g. *stroke) and injuries to the arm; it may also develop spontaneously. Reflex sympathetic stimulation is thought to be involved, hence the alternative name, reflex sympathetic dystrophy.

FRUCTOSE ($C_6H_{12}O_6$) is a simple hexose monosaccharide, also known as laevulose or fruit sugar. Together with *glucose, it makes up the molecule of the disaccharide sucrose or cane *sugar. Fructose, which occurs naturally in many fruits, is converted into glucose in the liver.

FRUSEMIDE, Furosemide (US) or Lasix®, is a powerful *diuretic which acts by inhibiting resorption in the ascending limb of the loop of Henle in the kidney, causing a copious increase in excretion of sodium, chloride, and water. Potassium depletion may follow. Frusemide is chemically related to the *sulphonamides, and may be given intravenously as well as by mouth.

FSH. See FOLLICLE-STIMULATING HORMONE.

FUGUE. An episode of disturbed behaviour in which a patient wanders about in a state of clouded consciousness and performs actions for which he is subsequently *amnesic. It is generally regarded as a hysterical 'flight from reality' but may also be a post-epileptic phenomenon.

FULGURATION is the destruction of tissue, often of malignant *tumours, with electric sparks.

FULMINANT describes pathological conditions that develop suddenly and are of great severity.

FULTON, JOHN FARQUHAR (1899–1960). American physiologist and medical historian. He was the author of *Neurophysiology*, a much-used textbook. He wrote biographies of Robert *Boyle and Harvey *Cushing. With Cushing and *Klebs he founded the Yale library of medical history.

FUMIGATION is disinfection with gas or fumes, such as formaldehyde vapour or sulphur dioxide.

FUNCTIONAL is often used to describe symptoms that have no discernible organic or structural cause and are considered to be psychogenic.

FUNDUS. The rounded bottom of a hollow organ, the part furthest away from the opening. The fundus of the eye, for example, is the interior of the back of the eye as seen on *ophthalmoscopic examination.

FUNGAL DISEASES. Diseases due to infection with *fungi are known collectively as mycoses, the commonest being those involving the skin or mucous membranes; (see CANDIDA; TINEA.) Infection of other organs, particularly the lungs, and disseminated infection, occur less often but are more dangerous (see ASPERGILLOSIS; BLASTOMYCOSIS; COCCIDIOIDOMYCOSIS; CRYPTOCOCCOSIS; HISTOPLASMOSIS; PHYCOMYCOSIS; SPOROTRICHOSIS; etc.). Severe mycoses occur increasingly as *opportunistic infections in *immunosuppressed patients.

FUNGI form a separate division of the plant kingdom in that, unlike bacteria and viruses, they are *eukaryotic; they differ from other plants in lacking chlorophyll and are thus obliged to exist as saprophytes or parasites on other plants and animals. Fungi are sometimes classified as a separate kingdom. They range from the simple unicellular forms known as *yeasts to many more complex organisms based on a mycelial structure and exhibiting both sexual and asexual modes of reproduction (mildews, moulds, rusts, toadstools, mushrooms, etc.). Apart from their importance in industry, baking, brewing, and agriculture, they are of specific medical interest in three ways: as a major source of *antibiotics (see FUNGI AS SOURCE OF DRUGS); as an occasional cause of serious poisoning (see POISONOUS FUNGI); and as agents of human disease, either by direct infection (see FUNGAL DISEASES) or because of their allergenic properties (see e.g. FARMER'S LUNG).

FUNGI AS CAUSE OF POISONING. See POISONOUS FUNGI.

FUNGI AS SOURCE OF DRUGS. Much the most important group of drugs derived from fungi are the *antibiotics. The *penicillin group, for example, derivatives of 6-amino-penicillinic acid, are obtained naturally or semisynthetically from the moulds *Penicillium* and *Aspergillus*; the original penicillin G was derived from *Penicillium notatum*. *Streptomyces* species have provided *streptomycin, *neomycin, the *tetracyclines, and others; *Cephalosporium* species the *cephalosporins and so on. *Yeast extract is a valuable source of B *vitamins. A number of other fungal species contain pharmacologically active substances: examples are *Amanita pantherina* (*atropine), *Amanita muscaria* (*muscarine), and *Coprinus atramentarius* (*disulfiram). Certain 'mushrooms' are consumed illicitly because of their *hallucinogenic properties, for example *Psilocybe mexicana* which contains psilocybin and related compounds.

FUROR. A pathological rage.

FURUNCLE. A *boil.

GABA. See GAMMA-AMINOBUTYRIC ACID.

GADDESDEN, JOHN OF (?1280–1361). British physician and priest, thought to have been the original of Chaucer's 'Doctor of Phisyk'. He was the author of *Rosa medicinae* or *Rosa anglica* (1314), described as a 'farrago of Arab views and rustic superstitions'.

GAG. To retch; also a device for keeping the jaws separated during surgical procedures.

GAIT. The manner of walking; it is often of diagnostic significance.

GALACTORRHOEA (GALACTORRHEA) is excessive or inappropriate secretion of milk.

GALACTOSAEMIA (GALACTOSEMIA) is an *inborn error of metabolism affecting the metabolism of *galactose, a normal constituent of human milk. Unless galactose is eliminated from the diet such infants may die within a few days of birth. Survivors are mentally retarded and develop *cataracts and liver *cirrhosis. It is inherited as an autosomal *recessive trait.

GALACTOSE is a hexose *sugar which with *glucose makes up lactose or milk sugar; it is thus a normal constituent of human milk. It differs from glucose only in the position of the hydrogen and hydroxyl groups on one carbon atom, but cannot be utilized by the body except after hepatic conversion into glucose. Absence of the necessary enzyme causes *galactosaemia.

GALEN (AD ?131–201). Greek physician of *Pergamum. He became physician to the Emperor Commodus in 180 and to the Emperor Septimus Severus in 193. Much of his fine library was destroyed by fire in 192. It is not known where he died.

Galen has been described as a 'prolix disputatious vainglorious windbag'. Undoubtedly he was a talented man of great industry and an astute diagnostician who followed *Hippocrates in medicine and *Aristotle in science. His anatomy was based on his dissection of animals such as apes, oxen, and pigs. He is thought never to have dissected a human body, which explains why many of his descriptions were incorrect. His physiology and pathology were derived from *Erasistratus. He held that food was absorbed and converted into blood in the liver, whence it entered the right ventricle by way of the vena cava and some passed through pores in the septum to the left ventricle. His theory was that in the liver the blood was imbued with natural spirits, in the left ventricle with vital spirits; in the brain these were converted to animal spirits; the organism was pervaded by and under the control of a '*pneuma'. Galen's views were strictly *teleological and based on humoralist doctrine. His philosophy was rigidly *determinist. He wrote extensively on all aspects of medicine and acquired such authority that no one dared to question his anatomical views until *Vesalius, or his physiological views until *Harvey.

GALENICAL. A medicinal substance of vegetable origin; a herbal 'simple'.

GALILEI, GALILEO (1564–1642). Italian scientist. As a result of his observation of sunspots through the recently invented telescope, Galileo became convinced of planetary, including terrestrial, movement round the sun, as suggested by *Copernicus, in contrast to the prevalent view that the earth was fixed. He also founded the science of mechanics; he emphasized the importance of mathematical analysis of natural phenomena; and the was one of the founders of *experimental method.

GALL, FRANZ JOSEPH (1758–1828). Austrian physician, who, with J. C. Spurzheim, devised the pseudoscience of *cranioscopy, later called *phrenology. They claimed that the brain consisted of 27 (later increased to 37) organs responsible for traits of character and revealed by palpable protuberances on the surface of the skull.

GALL BLADDER. A muscular sac attached to the under surface of the liver and communicating through the *cystic duct with the common *bile duct and thence with the *duodenum. It stores and concentrates the *bile.

GALLOP RHYTHM. Triple or quadruple (instead of the normal double) rhythm on auscultation of the heart, due to the addition of a third (ventricular filling) sound and/or a fourth (atrial) sound. Gallop rhythm is usually pathological, and in adults invariably so; it is suggestive of myocardial failure.

GALLSTONE. A *calculus precipitated from *bile found in the *gall bladder or *bile duct. The commonest variety is composed mostly of *cholesterol; less usual are gallstones derived from bile pigments. Gallstones may be symptomless, or may give rise to abdominal pain, indigestion, and obstructive *jaundice.

GALTON, SIR FRANCIS (1822–1911). British eugenist, who was for a short time a medical student. He interested himself in heredity and 'improving the race'. He initiated the study of *eugenics and was responsible for developing *anthropometry and *biometrics. He described the individuality of *fingerprints in 1893.

GALVANI, LUIGI (1737–98). Italian physician. He noted that chance contact with the iron of a balustrade from which frogs' legs were suspended by copper hooks caused muscular spasm. He believed he had found a new kind of 'animal electricity' and was never convinced that contact of the two metals in a moist environment generated the current.

GALVANISM is the therapeutic application of electricity in the form of direct current.

GALVANOMETER. An instrument for detecting, measuring, or comparing small electric currents.

GAMBLE, JAMES (1883–1959). American paediatrician. In 1915 he focused his investigations on children who were being treated for *epilepsy with dietary induction of starvation *ketosis. In them he demonstrated the role of ammonia production by the kidney in neutralizing excess quantities of acid. In portraying his results he developed the 'Gamblegram', a bar graph showing various proportions of electrolytes and unidentified acid or base. This work was of fundamental importance in subsequent studies of acid–base changes.

GAMETE. A male or female germ cell, that is a spermatozoon or ovum. Gametes are haploid, having only half the number of *chromosomes possessed by somatic cells. Male and female gametes unite to form a zygote.

GAMMA-AMINOBUTYRIC ACID is a naturally occurring *amino acid of plants and animals, usually abbreviated to GABA. In the brain it is an inhibitory *neurotransmitter, being secreted by neurones in the *basal ganglia and *limbic system. Abnormal depletion or malfunction of GABA appears to be associated with severe movement disorders such as *Huntington's chorea. Some have suggested that GABA functions as a natural anticonvulsive agent.

GAMMA CAMERA. An electrical instrument that produces cathode-ray tube images of *gamma ray emissions from radionuclides or from substances labelled with radionuclides used as tracers in *nuclear medicine.

The gamma camera has some advantages over conventional scanning equipment. It can be operated at any angle, whereas most scanners are limited to the horizontal plane. It allows rapid measurement of the distribution of radioactivity in bodily organs and tissues after the ingestion or injection of tracer substances, and serial exposures can be used to study changing patterns.

GAMMA-RAYS are electromagnetic *radiation of the same nature as *X-rays but of shorter wavelength (10^{-10} to 10^{-13}m). They are emitted (in units called photons) by the nuclei of radioactive atoms during decay. See also BETATRON.

GANGLION. A structure containing a collection of nerve cell bodies, situated outside the central nervous system; or, a cystic swelling arising from a tendon sheath.

GANGRENE is the death and *putrefaction (enzymic and bacterial decomposition) of a mass of tissue, associated with obstruction of arterial blood supply.

GANSER SYNDROME, also known as 'the syndrome of approximate answers', was described by S. J. M. Ganser in prisoners awaiting trial, and said to occur also in epileptics and in various types of mental disorder. The patient gives perversely wrong answers to simple questions, and his actions may be similarly perverse (e.g. trying to write with the wrong end of a pencil). It seems to be an expression of a wish to appear irresponsible in a situation which would be solved or mitigated by irresponsibility. It is regarded by some as a form of *hysteria rather than frank *malingering.

GAOL FEVER is a name for epidemic *typhus, due to the organism *Rickettsia prowazekii* and transmitted by the human *body louse (*Pediculus humanus humanus*).

GARGOYLISM. See HURLER'S SYNDROME.

GARLAND, JOSEPH (1893–1973). American paediatrician, and editor of the *New England Journal of Medicine* from 1947 to 1967. During the period of his editorship the journal grew in stature and in circulation (see MEDICAL JOURNALS). The feature 'Case records of the Massachusetts General Hospital' was established in 1923. During his editorship the features 'Doctors afield', and 'By the London post' were inaugurated, and toward the end of his stewardship 'Seminars in medicine of the Beth Israel Hospital' and 'Physiology for physicians' were added. After retirement he wrote his autobiography, *A time for remembering*.

GARRISON, FIELDING HUDSON (1870–1935). American librarian and medical historian. In 1891 he began his long service in the Army Medical Library, Washington, where he remained until 1922 (see MEDICAL LIBRARIES). He published his largest work *Introduction to the history of medicine* in 1913. He took a leading part in preparation of the *Index catalogue of the Surgeon General's library*, as well as the *Index medicus*, and the *Quarterly cumulative index medicus*.

GARROD, SIR ALFRED BARING (1819–1907). British physician. His chief interest lay in chemical aspects of medicine, and he first described the excess of uric acid in the blood of patients with *gout. Garrod was the first to make a clear distinction between *osteoarthritis and *rheumatoid arthritis in his book *Gout and rheumatoid gout* (1859).

GARROD, SIR ARCHIBALD EDWARD (1857–1936). British physician. He was the son of Sir Alfred *Garrod and in 1919 became the first full-time professor and director of the new medical unit at St Bartholomew's. This was the first such chair in the University of London. A year later he followed *Osler as regius professor of medicine at Oxford. His interests, which had been purely clinical in his early years, later became biochemical, and he wrote the classic work *The inborn errors of metabolism* (1909).

GARTH, SIR SAMUEL (1661–1719). British physician, chiefly noted for his strenuous support of the Royal College of Physicians' plan for free dispensaries for the needy, which he defended with vigour and some wit in a poem 'The Dispensary' (1699).

GAS. The physical state of a gas (the gaseous state) is such that it always occupies the whole of the space in which it is contained. In a perfect gas the component molecules would move freely, but in a real gas they are subject to small intermolecular forces (van der Waals' forces).

GAS CHAMBER. A device for judicial or mass execution, usually using hydrocyanic acid gas.

GAS GANGRENE is a dangerous complication of extensive wounds, particularly when contaminated with soil, due to anaerobic infection with toxin-elaborating *Clostridia (of several species but notably *C. perfringens*). The condition, which causes muscle *necrosis and gas formation locally together with systemic *toxaemia and *shock, is also known as clostridial myonecrosis.

GASKELL, WALTER HOLBROOK (1847–1914). British physiologist. He published fundamental work on the innervation of the heart and viscera and wrote *The involuntary nervous system* published in 1916 (posthumously).

GASSER, HERBERT SPENCER (1888–1963). American physiologist. His best-known scientific work was with *Erlanger in St Louis, making use of the cathode ray oscillograph in studies of nerve impulse conduction. For this they received the *Nobel prize in 1944.

GASTRECTOMY is surgical excision of the *stomach, in whole or in part.

GASTRIC FISTULA. An abnormal communication between the *stomach and the body surface.

GASTRIC JUICE is the secretion of the glands in the wall of the *stomach. The major components are *mucus, the digestive enzyme *pepsin, *hydrochloric acid, and a protein which promotes absorption of *vitamin B_{12}, called 'intrinsic factor'.

GASTRIC LAVAGE is irrigation of the *stomach, usually with a large bore tube and dilute saline solution. Although a traditional emergency measure in cases of poisoning, it is now thought to be of doubtful efficacy; if performed, prior endotracheal *intubation with a cuffed tube is advisable.

GASTRIC ULCER. See PEPTIC ULCER.

GASTRIN is a *polypeptide *hormone released by glands in the pyloric (lower) part of the *stomach in response to *protein foods; it is a powerful stimulant of acid and *pepsin secretion from the rest of the stomach, and, less strongly, induces pancreatic secretion and gall bladder contraction.

GASTRITIS. Inflammation of the *stomach.

GASTROENTERITIS is inflammation of the *stomach and *intestine, the diagnosis usually associated with the familiar syndrome of diarrhoea and vomiting. Self-limiting viral infections with this presentation are common ('gastric flu').

GASTROENTEROLOGIST. A physician specializing in diseases of the gastrointestinal system, including the liver.

GASTROENTEROLOGY is literally the study of the stomach and intestines, but effectively covers the whole alimentary tract from mouth to anus (Fig. 1), with the adjacent organs of the pancreas, and liver and gall bladder (hepatology). These organs receive, digest, and process food for the absorption into, and nutrition of, the body.

In the mouth, food is chewed by the teeth and gums

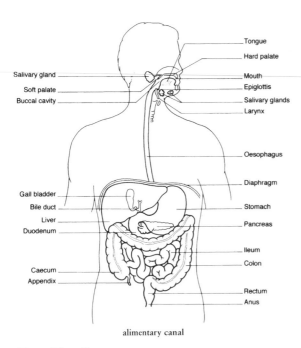

Tongue
Hard palate
Salivary gland
Mouth
Soft palate
Epiglottis
Buccal cavity
Salivary glands
Larynx

Oesophagus

Diaphragm

Gall bladder
Bile duct
Stomach
Liver
Pancreas
Duodenum

Ileum
Colon
Caecum
Appendix

Rectum
Anus

alimentary canal

Fig. 1 The alimentary tract.

(see DENTISTRY). Mineral and *vitamin B deficiencies may inflame the mouth (stomatitis), lips (cheilosis), and tongue (glossitis). Glossitis is caused by deficiency of iron, riboflavin, nicotinic acid (pellagra), and vitamin B_{12}. A furred tongue is common, especially in smokers, and harmless.

Food is moistened by the salivary glands (parotid, submandibular, and sublingual). The masticated food stimulates the taste buds to start reflex secretion of saliva. About 1 litre/day of this mildly alkaline fluid cleans and protects the mouth and begins digestion with its enzymes amylase (digesting starch) and lipase (digesting fat). Protective mucus lubricates the food, aiding swallowing. The mouth absorbs certain drugs, for example glyceryl trinitrate, which relieves *angina pectoris. Inflammation of the mouth and tongue may lead to *carcinoma, which is more common in smokers.

The mouth, pharynx, and oesophagus
The tongue pushes the food up to the palate and down to the back of the throat (pharynx) which then opens. The food then enters the gullet (oesophagus). The larynx at the top of the windpipe (trachea) prevents food going down the wrong way into the lungs. Peristaltic waves of contraction move the food down into the stomach, while the sphincter valves at the upper and lower ends of the oesophagus relax in turn. Disturbances of muscular contraction (motility) cause spasm, pain, and difficulty in swallowing (dysphagia). Tests include

radiography (barium swallow), measurements of acidity and motility, *endoscopy, biopsies, and *cytology.

A weak lower sphincter allows gastric acid to pass up (reflux) and inflame the oesophagus (oesophagitis) with heartburn. If the upper sphincter relaxes, acid may enter the mouth, as may swallowed saliva (water brash). An inflamed oesophagus may narrow (*stricture) with dysphagia. Causes of reflux include pregnancy, obesity, smoking, and a weak diaphragm (hiatus hernia). Treatments include reducing weight, barrier-blocking drugs to prevent reflux, and antisecretory drugs to reduce the acidity of the refluxate. Operations can prevent reflux, and dilate strictures. Swallowed air distends the oesophagus, and relaxation of the upper sphincter allows belching. A belch can be suppressed, voluntarily and temporarily.

Oesophageal carcinoma is common and related to smoking and food *carcinogens. This *cancer is treated by operation or *radiotherapy. Inoperable strictures can be dilated endoscopically and kept open by tubes (stents) or by laser treatment.

The stomach and duodenum
The stomach receives, stores, and partly digests food before pumping it on. The top of the stomach (the body) receives food and drink and lubricates it with mucus. The parietal cells of the body secrete 1–2 litres/day of hydrochloric acid to kill microbes in food and to help iron absorption. Acid converts pepsinogens into pepsin *enzymes to start the digestion of protein. Lipase begins fat digestion. Parietal cells also make *intrinsic factor which, combined with dietary *vitamin B_{12} (extrinsic factor), is absorbed in the ileum. Gastric secretion is stimulated by the thought, sight, taste, and chewing of food, via the nervous system; there are also local stimulant physicochemical effects of food in the stomach and duodenum.

Food entering the lower stomach (the antrum) stimulates the *hormone gastrin, which releases *histamine from the body; this, together with the nervous stimuli, excites acid and pepsin secretion. The antrum then pumps partly digested food through the exit valve (pylorus) into the duodenum, where the acid is neutralized by alkali, from the lining cells, and pancreatic juice.

These secretions are excited by two duodenal hormones. Secretin is carried by the blood to the pancreas to release sodium bicarbonate. Cholecystokinin-pancreozymin (CCK-PZ) both contracts the *gall bladder to squirt its bile into the duodenum, and releases pancreatic digestive enzymes.

The stomach may become inflamed (gastritis). In autoimmune *pernicious anaemia, vitamin B_{12} is not absorbed: treatment is by regular injections (see HAEMATOLOGY). The commonest gastritis is an infection, usually in childhood, by the *bacterium *Helicobacter pylori*. This inflammation usually causes no symptoms, but it may worsen, from superficial to atrophic gastritis, to gastric atrophy and ulceration, and even to carcinoma. *H.pylori*, together with excess gastric acid inflaming the duodenum, may cause duodenal erosions and ulcers.

An *ulcer in the stomach is a break in the lining (mucosa), as in the skin or mouth. An erosion is a superficial ulcer. Gastric ulcer and duodenal erosions and ulcers may cause indigestion. Tests include radiography (barium meal) and endoscopy (gastroduodenoscopy), with biopsies, cultures, and gastric secretion measurements. Ulcers cause not only pain but also complications. Ulcers bleed, with blood vomited (haematemesis) or passing downwards, digested, blackened, and defaecated (melaena). Continued bleeding from erosions or ulcers is an emergency, requiring transfusion and even operation if the bleeding is not stopped by endoscopy with injections, cautery, or laser treatment. Ulcers may erode through the wall and penetrate a neighbouring organ, or perforate into the peritoneal cavity, with *peritonitis usually needing surgical repair. Ulcers shrink when they heal and such contraction can partly block the stomach exit (*pyloric stenosis), needing operation.

Ulcer pain may be relieved by antacids. Relief is temporary, so ulcers should be healed. Mucosal defences can be strengthened by not smoking and by administration of bismuth, carbenoxolone, and sucralfate. Acidity can be reduced by frequent antacids, but it is better to reduce acid production. Histamine receptor blockers (cimetidine, ranitidine) reduce the stimulant effect of histamine on the parietal cell. Omeprazole stops the chemical synthesis of acid by the enzyme $H^+K^+ATPase$.

The longer and the more powerful the treatment, the quicker ulcers heal. They usually return when treatment is stopped, so that some patients need continuous (maintenance) acid inhibitors. Many doctors now try to prevent recurrence by eradicating *H.pylori* with 1 or 2 weeks of antibacterial drugs. Some doctors use such an on–off regimen to heal ulcers and keep them healed.

The brainstem has a vomiting centre stimulated by emotions, nauseating smells or drugs, pregnancy, and abnormal motions (seasickness). Nausea means feeling sick. With vomiting the abdominal muscles contract and expel the contents of the stomach, and even of the intestine, upwards through the relaxed sphincters of the oesophagus and out through the mouth.

The small intestine and pancreas

The small intestine (duodenum, jejunum, and ileum) can be imaged by barium radiography or a long endoscope, and can be biopsied. The jejunal mucosa is lined by circular folds which slow the movement of the food and increase the surface for absorption. Tiny finger-like villi have brush borders of minute microvilli for further digestion and absorption of food. Fat is broken into fatty acids and monoglycerides, which form tiny droplets (micelles). These enter the cell, pass into the *lymph and then the blood. Proteins are split into smaller *peptides and *amino acids, to be absorbed into the blood.

Starches are broken into sugars (maltose, sucrose, and lactose) which are digested by enzymes (maltase, sucrase, and lactase) into glucose, fructose, and galactose, and absorbed. Lactase may be absent (alactasia—especially in the East where milk is not a staple food), in which case milk products cannot be digested and can produce pain and *diarrhoea.

Coeliac disease is an intolerance of the protein part of wheat germ (gluten). Patients develop malabsorption of fat and vitamins, and need a strict, lifelong gluten-free diet. Tropical sprue has similar features but is due to altered gut bacteria and usually responds to antibiotics.

The commonest *inflammation of the small intestine is Crohn's disease. This can thicken, ulcerate, and narrow any part of the gut (regional enteritis) with pain, malabsorption, weakness, and *anaemia. Crohn's is treated by anti-inflammatory drugs, may need operation, and can recur in the other parts of the intestine.

Gastroenteritis means inflammation of the stomach and intestine. This is used to describe an acute illness of diarrhoea, often with vomiting and abdominal discomfort; it is sometimes referred to as 'food poisoning' or gastric flu. The illness may start within hours of eating the food or fluid responsible, and important factors include inadequate refrigeration, food prepared in advance, poor human hygiene, inadequate cooking or holding temperature and reheating. Most gastroenteritis is bacterial (*Campylobacter jejuni*, *Salmonella*, *Shigella*, *Coliforms*), some is viral, and other pathogens include parasites (*Entamoeba*, *Cryptosporidium*, *Giardia*, worms) and *fungi (certain mushrooms). Gastroenteritis is preventable by high standards of public and personal hygiene. Healthy adults recover quickly and oral rehydration or antibiotics are not usually necessary except in parasitic infections, which may require specific *chemotherapy.

The pancreas lies within the duodenal loop. It is both an *endocrine organ (see DIABETES) and helps digest food by producing alkali and enzymes: trypsin/chymotrypsin (protein), lipase (fat), and amylase (starches).

With pancreatic diseases, food is not fully digested, there is malabsorption and faeces are fatty, pale, bulky, offensive, floating, and difficult to flush (steatorrhoea). This can be helped by taking large and frequent quantities of pancreatic extracts. Abnormalities of the pancreas can also be detected in the blood and urine, and by imaging. The pancreas may be involved in *cystic fibrosis (mucoviscidosis) (see PAEDIATRICS).

Inflammation (pancreatitis) is usually caused by excess alcohol or by biliary stones. Acute pancreatitis presents with severe pain and vomiting; abdominal and cardiorespiratory complications may prove fatal. Survivors can recover completely or have recurrences. The incidence of chronic pancreatitis is usually proportional to the alcohol consumption of a particular population. Recurrent chronic continuous pain may require operation. Pancreatic carcinoma is becoming more common, perhaps because of alcohol and tobacco use. Operations are difficult, dangerous, and rarely curative.

The liver and gall bladder

The liver is the body's biggest organ, a chemical factory receiving from the portal vein the products of digestion from the intestine. These it processes into the various chemicals needed by different parts of the body, which pass out of the liver along the hepatic veins to the heart and general circulation. The liver also makes *bile, stored by the gall bladder until delivered via the bile duct to the duodenum to help digest fat.

Red blood cells survive for only 4 months, and then their *haemoglobin is turned by the liver into bile. In *jaundice the eyes, skin, and urine turn yellow from excess bilirubin in the blood, due to increased destruction of the blood cells (haemolysis), liver damage (hepatic), or blockage of the bile ducts (obstructive).

Stones in the gall bladder are becoming more common, possibly owing to richer diets. Stones may be symptomless or may produce acute and recurrent attacks of pain, acute inflammation (cholecystitis), or blockage of the bile ducts. When stones cause symptoms they should be removed (cholecystectomy), at *laparoscopy or *laparotomy. Some stones can be dissolved by tablets, and others may be shattered by external ultrasound waves (lithotripsy).

Imaging is by ultrasound (*ultrasonics) or endoscopic retrograde cholangiopancreatography (ERCP). ERCP can be interventional, widening the valve where the bile duct enters the duodenum (sphincterotomy), removing stones, or dilating inoperable strictures with little tubes (stents).

Viruses can infect the liver. *Hepatitis A is transmitted faeco-orally, either person-to-person or from food or drink. Immunoglobulin gives temporary passive immunization. Travellers to the Third World should consider active immunization by injections.

Hepatitis B is transmitted parenterally (by routes other than the gastrointestinal tract), especially by blood-to-blood contact (including shared needles and transfusion of blood or its products), sexual intercourse, or from mother to fetus. Fever, loss of appetite, nausea, and vomiting may be followed by the production of dark urine, pale stools, and cholestatic jaundice. Death from hepatic failure is rare (1 per cent), but up to 10 per cent of patients may become chronic *carriers of the virus and develop chronic hepatitis, *cirrhosis, or even liver cancer. Those with risky work (health care) or practices (sexual, parenteral drug abusers) need active immunization, and booster doses if immunity wanes.

Other hepatitis viruses include blood-transmitted hepatitis C (once called non-A non-B), D (delta), and E. Chronic viral hepatitis responds to *interferon. The liver may also be infected by *amoebae, various *worms, *flukes, and bacteria.

The liver may be chronically inflamed (chronic active hepatitis) by autoimmunity (see IMMUNOLOGY).

Treatment is anti-inflammatory (*corticosteroids) and immunosuppressive (*azathioprine).

Alcohol inflames and destroys the liver in proportion to the length and quantity of consumption. Early alcoholic liver damage is symptomless. Alcoholic fatty liver may present acutely. The later stages are alcoholic hepatitis and then cirrhosis. Alcohol damage to the liver, as to any other part of the body, can be prevented by personal, cultural, or governmental action, and, in the early stages, liver damage may be halted or reversed by permanent abstinence.

Cirrhosis is chronic and irreversible. Causes include alcohol and inflammation from the biliary tree, either secondary to obstruction or primary (probably autoimmune). Rarely, iron (*haemochromatosis) or copper (Wilson's disease) is deposited. In all forms of cirrhosis the liver fibroses (hardens) and blocks bile ducts (jaundice) or veins (portal *hypertension), with bleeding in little veins (varices) in the gut, especially in the lower oesophagus. The spleen may enlarge (splenomegaly) with increased destruction of the red, white, and platelet blood cells (hypersplenism). Portal hypertension can increase fluid in the abdomen (*ascites), particularly with disturbed liver chemistry, which can also upset the hormonal balance and damage the brain (*encephalopathy, *coma). Acute exacerbations may be treated successfully, but the cirrhosis persists and may turn malignant (primary liver cell cancer). The liver is also a common site for secondary tumours.

Drugs, industrial chemicals, and plant products can damage the liver acutely and chronically. Most life-threatening, severe acute and chronic liver damage cannot be cured medically. Liver *transplantation is sometimes indicated, and can be successful.

The large intestine

After the digestion and absorption of much of the food in the small intestine, the liquid faeces pass through the ileo-caecal valve into the colon, up through the ascending, across the transverse, down the descending and into the sigmoid colon, finally to be expelled from the rectum through the anus. The colon absorbs salts and water from the faeces to produce solid stools. Disturbed motility from diet, drugs, and emotion can alter the consistency and frequency of bowel action (usually not more than thrice a day, not less than twice per week). By 'constipation' patients mean either hard, small, infrequent faeces or straining at stools. 'Diarrhoea' may be used for frequent or loose watery stools or both.

Motility disturbances occur anywhere in the alimentary tract (irritable gut), especially the colon. Most people may have occasional abdominal pain, with or without constipation and/or diarrhoea. Some people complain to their doctors and become patients with the irritable bowel syndrome. Other bodily activities may be disturbed by fatigue and stress. Dysmotility produces bloating (abdominal distension from wind) and pain from bowel spasm. Pain is occasionally severe inside the anus (proctalgia fugax).

Doctors disagree whether irritable bowel syndrome is related to personality traits, stress, or depression, or whether there is an underlying disturbance of nervous control. Treatments therefore are varied, such as a high-fibre diet to deal with constipation and diarrhoea, and antispasmodic drugs for pain. Patients have been helped by explanation, antidepressants, hypnosis, and self-help groups.

The colon can be inflamed by Crohn's disease (see above) and also by idiopathic proctocolitis (*ulcerative colitis) where there is bloody diarrhoea, possibly severe, fulminant, and lethal. Fortunately most cases are mild initially, usually in the rectum (proctitis). Over the years it may spread upwards to some or all of the colon (total proctocolitis) and persists throughout life, with bouts and remissions. The cause is unknown, possibly autoimmune. Attacks usually respond rapidly to corticosteroids, given topically (*suppositories, *enemas), as tablets, or by injection in emergency. Patients in remission are reminded that their disease is chronic and potentially lifelong and are all advised to take maintenance tablets permanently (usually containing 5-amino-salicylic acid). They should be checked regularly, both for compliance and because of the risk of malignant transformation in long-standing total colitis. In patients with unresponsive colitis, with chronic disease responding poorly to treatment, and with premalignant changes, removal of the whole bowel (proctocolectomy) is recommended. The ileal contents are then either brought out through an artificial opening in the abdominal wall (ileostomy) or connected by an ileal pouch to the anus.

A diverticulum is a little outpouching of the lining of the bowel through its wall. These diverticula are common in the colon, especially the sigmoid colon, particularly in developed countries lacking cereal fibre in the diet. There may be no symptoms, abdominal pain, or constipation and/or diarrhoea. The diverticula may become inflamed (*diverticulitis), requiring admission to hospital, antibiotics, and even an operation, especially if the colon bleeds or perforates.

Polyps are little tumours, some of which become malignant, especially in familial polyposis. Colorectal carcinoma is among the commonest cancer, with familial and dietary factors. Patients should see their doctors if there is rectal bleeding or change in bowel habit. The bowel can be examined digitally, by endoscopes (proctoscope, sigmoidoscope, colonoscope with biopsies), or by barium enema radiography. Early diagnosis of early cancer leads to cure by colectomy. It is usually possible, after excising part of the colon, or rectum, to allow normal defecation. Only rarely is it necessary nowadays to bring out the colon as an opening on the abdominal wall (colostomy). Screening systems are under trial to detect early colorectal cancer, especially in those with a family history.

The anal canal is about 4 cm long with two sphincters. When the rectum is distended by faeces the internal sphincter relaxes to allow faeces to pass downward at a suitable time and place. One then consciously relaxes the normally contracted external sphincter and defecation follows. Experts in this area (proctologists) can now study the electrical and muscular control of this region and help and advise on dealing with constipation and incontinence. Internal piles (haemorrhoids) are enlarged veins inside the anal canal, associated with straining at stool and constipation, and may pop out (prolapse) and bleed. These can be treated successfully by proctological surgeons, who can also treat prolapse, tears (fissures), and discharging tracts (fistulas).

J. H. BARON

Advice
The British Digestive Foundation, 3 St Andrews Place, London NW1 4LB (071 486 0341) recommends books, booklets, and self-help societies in gastroenterology. It welcomes donations for research and education in this field.

GASTROENTEROSTOMY. A surgically created *anastomosis between the *stomach and (small) *intestine.

GASTROSCOPE. An *endoscope used for inspecting the interior of the stomach.

GASTROSTOMY. A surgically created artificial opening from the cavity of the *stomach to the exterior.

GAUCHER'S DISEASE. Three principal diseases causing abnormal accumulation of glycosphingolipids are identified by this name, all of autosomal recessive inheritance and associated with glucocerebroside deficiency. Type I, the commonest, causes enlargement of the *liver and *spleen, anaemia, and often bony lesions, beginning either in infancy or in late adult life. Type II, confined to infants, causes severe neurological manifestations as well as hepatosplenomegaly, usually with death in the first year of life. In type III, which is rare, signs of both visceral and neuronal involvement develop in childhood or early adult life.

GEE, SAMUEL JONES (1839–1911). British physician. With Thomas *Barlow he described the cervical *opisthotonos of infants (1878) and *coeliac disease (1888). He was the author of a small handbook, *Auscultation and percussion* (1870), which ran to six editions.

GEIGER COUNTER. An instrument, also known as a Geiger–Müller counter, for the detection of ionizing *radiations, and capable of registering individual particles or *photons. It has some limitations but has proved a widely useful method for measuring high-energy *beta particle emissions.

GEL is a colloidal solution that has set to a jelly, the viscosity being so great that it has the elasticity of a solid.

These attributes are due to a mesh-like structure of the disperse phase, through which the dispersion medium circulates.

GENE. A linear segment of *deoxyribonucleic acid (DNA) forming part of a *chromosome, on average about 1500 bases in length. Genes are the basic units of heredity, controlling the manufacture of individual *polypeptides and hence of the individual inherited characteristics of an organism. See also GENETICS.

GENERAL BOARD OF HEALTH. Following the first *Public Health Act of 1848, a General Board of Health was appointed in England to control local authorities. Its members were Lord Shaftesbury, Sir Edwin *Chadwick, and Dr Southwood Smith; its medical officer was Sir John *Simon, *medical officer of health to the City of London. The Board attacked many abuses in public health, but vested interests and political opposition resulted in its abolition 10 years later.

GENERAL DENTAL COUNCIL. See DENTISTRY; DENTISTS ACT 1957; GENERAL MEDICAL COUNCIL.

GENERALIST. One whose knowledge and skills are not restricted to a particular field; a general physician or internist.

GENERAL MEDICAL COUNCIL was established by the Medical Act of 1858, after 18 years of parliamentary debate, during which no fewer than 17 attempts had been made, amid increasing public concern, to secure Parliament's approval for a bill to regulate the medical profession. The Council's central purpose is, and always has been, to protect the public by overseeing *medical education and keeping a register of qualified medical practitioners.

The need for a regulatory body with statutory powers had long been recognized. Before 1858, 19 separate licensing bodies conferred professional titles on the basis of very different tests of varying standards. Most of the titles had no more than a local value, so that, for example, an Edinburgh practitioner might be unable to practise in London, or even in Glasgow. Graduates of the University of London were prohibited by law from practising in London, and could be prosecuted by the Royal College of Physicians for doing so. The essential purposes of the 1858 Act were to secure a radical improvement in the overall quality of medical education, and to work towards the establishment of a common standard which would be accepted throughout the UK.

The purpose of the Act itself was stated in its preamble, 'It is expedient that persons requiring medical aid should be enabled to distinguish qualified from unqualified practitioners'. Estimates based on the census returns of 1841 suggested that, of the 15 000 people then practising medicine in England, nearly 5000 were unqualified. The wide divergences in standards of medical education meant that, even among qualified practitioners, competence could not be guaranteed, and the compilation and publication of a definitive register was therefore an urgent priority.

One small section of the 1858 Act concerned the matter for which the Council is now best known to the public. This authorized the Council to erase from the register the names of those practitioners who had been convicted of a criminal offence in a Court of Law or had been judged by the Council 'after due inquiry to be guilty of infamous conduct in any professional respect'. The provision appears to have attracted little notice at the time, and it would have come as a surprise to those who set up the Council to know that, 135 years later, the public would be aware of the GMC chiefly as a body concerned with professional ethics and discipline.

In addition to its main functions, the Council was also given the duty of publishing a 'pharmacopoeia'—an official publication listing drugs and directions for their use. This was a complex task and an initial attempt was unsatisfactory, but the first edition of the *British Pharmacopoeia* was published in 1867 and was well received. This publication continued to be the concern of the Council until responsibility for it was transferred to the Secretary of State and the *Medicines Commission under the *Medicines Act 1968.

Until 1921, when the Dental Board of the United Kingdom was founded, the Council was also responsible for registering dentists, and continued to exercise certain functions in respect of dentists until the creation of the *General Dental Council in 1957.

The Council was called into existence to serve the public interest in the specific ways outlined above. It was not formed to be a professional parliament or a union for protecting the profession's interests, and this distinction has been borne in mind by the Council throughout its existence.

The constitution of the Council

The first Council had 24 members, representing the English, Irish, and Scottish Universities, the *Royal Colleges, the *Society of Apothecaries of London and the Apothecaries' Hall in Dublin, together with six doctors appointed by the Queen on the advice of her Privy Council. Sir Benjamin *Brodie, at that time the most distinguished member of the profession and its undisputed head, was selected from outside the ranks of the appointed members to be their President. The Council was a distinguished group, 14 of its members being included in the *Dictionary of national biography*.

Five new members, directly elected by the profession in a postal ballot, were added under the Medical Act 1886 and the Council increased gradually in size until, under the Medical Act of 1950, there were 47 members: 11 directly elected, 28 appointed by the licensing bodies, and eight (by now including three lay people) nominated by the Crown.

Radical change was brought about by the *Medical Act 1978, following an independent inquiry chaired by Dr A. W. (later Sir Alec) Merrison. The most significant of the changes was the requirement that the majority of Council members should henceforth be elected by the medical profession which, through the payment of fees for registration and for the retention of doctors' names on the register, has always provided the overwhelming proportion of the Council's income. At present the Council has 102 members: 54 *elected* by the profession by post using the 'single transferable vote' method; 35 *appointed* by universities with a medical school and by the Royal Colleges and Faculties and the Society kof Apothecaries; and 13 lay people *nominated* by the Crown. Proposals at present under consideration would provide for a significant increase in the proportion of lay people in the Council's membership.

The principle of self-regulation
The Council is based on the principle that a profession can be regulated most effectively if the regulatory mechanism is controlled by the profession itself, if it is financially independent of the state, and if it has the backing of the law. As such, the Council has been a model for similar Medical Councils in a number of other countries and for several regulatory bodies in the health-care professions in the United Kingdom. The regulation of a number of other professions is similarly based on the keeping of a central register.

The Merrison Committee, comprehensively reviewing the Council's work in 1975, made the following comments:

An instructive way of looking at regulation is to see it as a contract between public and profession, by which the public go to the profession for medical treatment because the profession has made sure it will provide satisfactory treatment. Such a contract has the characteristic of all freely made contracts – mutual advantage.

. . . Looked at from this point of view one could as well argue that the performance of the contract should be enforced by a regulating body of laymen as of doctors. It is the case that the medical profession has been regulated by a predominantly professional body for well over a century, and evidently a lay regulating body would labour under a substantial disadvantage. It is the essence of a professional skill that it deals with matters unfamiliar to the layman, and it follows that only those in the profession are in a position to judge many of the matters of standards of professional competence and conduct which will be involved.

We are in no doubt that the community will indeed be best served by a professional regulating body. At so many points . . . it is on the self-respect of the medical profession that the public must rely for high standards of medicine. That is the essential argument for a predominantly professional regulating body and why we recommend a predominantly professional GMC.

The working of the Council
The Council elects a President and Treasurers from among its members, and its administration is under the direction of a *Registrar. The staff are organized into divisions which serve the Council's various functions. General elections of elected members take place every 5 years, and the other members serve for periods of up to 5 years at a time, at the discretion of their appointing and nominating bodies. Members can serve for successive periods, until their seventieth birthday.

Much of the Council's work is, inevitably, carried out through committees which exist to consider policy questions and determine certain cases in pursuit of the Council's education, registration, and fitness to practise functions. The committee chairmen, with other members of the Council, form the President's Advisory Committee which advises the President on matters relating to the Council's functions, and in particular on constitutional or policy matters. The Council meets in full session three times a year, usually in public, in order to receive reports from the committees and determine matters of policy.

The *Medical register
The register is at the heart of the Council's work. By making public a definitive list of those qualified to practise medicine it effectively sets a boundary for the profession, enabling the public, or those who act on their behalf, to distinguish the qualified from the unqualified—as envisaged by the original Act of 1858. Other publications, such as the *Medical directory*, provide lists of doctors but these are neither comprehensive nor validated in the same way as the register.

The preparation of the first register was a complicated process and inevitably some cases were contentious. The July 1859 edition contained nearly 15 000 names, all of which had to be carefully scrutinized. Many of the applicants could produce little by way of documentation, some made claims of dubious honesty, and a few attempted outright fraud. Registration did, however, produce immediate results in conferring legitimacy on those who could rightly claim to be trained and experienced medical practitioners, and in disposing of the claims of those who could not demonstrate that they fulfilled the necessary requirements.

The published *Medical register* is in regular use among health authorities, Registrars of Births and Deaths, and others, including pharmacists and funeral directors, all of whom may have reason to confirm the validity of a doctor's registration. It is also made available through libraries and can be purchased by any interested individual. The register itself is kept by the Council on a card index and a computer database. At present the main list of the register contains some 148 000 names.

Medical education
The register would be of little value if entry to it were not controlled through the maintenance of high standards of medical education, and the education of medical students as they progress through the successive stages of their training has always been one

of the Council's main preoccupations. The Council's educational responsibilities do not cease once a doctor has gained primary qualifications and been granted registration; the Education Committee has a statutory duty to undertake 'the general function of promoting high standards of medical education and of co-ordinating all stages of medical education'. Thus, the Council is concerned with the continuum of medical education, up to and beyond the point where a doctor is judged fit to take unsupervised clinical responsibility for patients, recognizing the essential unity of all stages of medical education.

In its early years, the Council used its influence to ensure that the universities and other licensing bodies required their students to receive a sound general education before admission, and the Council retains a responsibility for such academic requirements. Initially, when the Council was given the very general task of ensuring proper undergraduate medical education, it was possible for a doctor to become registered on the basis of a qualification obtained either in medicine or in surgery. In 1886 Parliament decided that the compulsory qualifying examination should lead concurrently to 'sufficiency' of knowledge in medicine, surgery, and midwifery, and gave the Council power to inspect the examinations. It was not until 1950 that the Council was given power to visit courses of instruction in medical schools, and only in 1978 was it statutorily charged with promoting high standards rather than simply ensuring sufficiency.

The Council's educational responsibilities have been exercised mainly through visitations, inspection of examinations, and the periodic issue of recommendations on basic medical education, on general clinical training and, most recently, on the training of specialists. Although the Education Committee has power to recommend to the Privy Council that a registrable qualification is no longer of a sufficiently high standard to confer the right to registration, the Committee and the Council have always preferred to reach an agreed position rather than use that power. The Council has recently been engaged in detailed discussions with the medical schools which will, it is hoped, lead to revised recommendations on the undergraduate curriculum designed to bring about radical change in the character of basic medical education, putting the emphasis on the learning experience rather than on factual instruction.

Registration of UK and EU qualifications

Those granted primary medical qualifications in the UK have been obliged since 1953 to gain 12 months' supervised experience in medicine and surgery before being granted full registration. In order to enable them to practise, under supervision, during this *'pre-registration' year they are granted provisional registration by the Council. Once pre-registration training has been satisfactorily completed, doctors may proceed to full registration, enabling them to practise in the UK without restriction. Full registration has also been available, as of right, since June 1977 to nationals of an EU country who hold qualifications granted in a member state.

Registration of overseas qualified doctors

The Council first became concerned with the registration of doctors who had qualified overseas following the Act of 1886, which established reciprocal arrangements between the UK and the British Empire. Similar arrangements were later extended to Italy, Japan, and Belgium but all reciprocity ended in 1980 when, on the Council's own recommendation, the emphasis was placed on the maintenance of standards in this country rather than on the willingness of two countries to grant mutual privileges to each other's doctors.

Various types of registration are now granted to doctors who have qualified outside the EU. It is open to the Council to recognize, for *full registration*, qualifications granted in any country overseas if it remains satisfied that those qualifications are of a standard equivalent to that of medical degrees granted in the UK. The Council currently recognizes for this purpose certain qualifications granted in Australia, Hong Kong, Malaysia, New Zealand, Singapore, South Africa, and the West Indies. Doctors holding one of these qualifications may apply for full registration or, if they have not yet completed a pre-registration year, for provisional registration. The Council can also give *temporary full registration* to distinguished doctors who come to the UK temporarily as visiting professors or to provide some special service.

Most doctors who come to this country with an overseas qualification receive *limited registration*, which enables them to work under supervision in hospitals. In order to obtain limited registration, doctors have to hold a qualification accepted by the Council for that purpose—over 800 qualifications are accepted in that way—and must show that they have been offered a suitable appointment in the UK. The Council must also be satisfied that the doctor can meet its requirements with regard to character, experience, knowledge, and skill, and is sufficiently competent in the English language. Before limited registration is granted, applicants must, unless exempt under specific arrangements, meet the requirements of the Professional and Linguistic Assessments Board (PLAB) which conducts tests of linguistic ability and professional knowledge. Growing numbers of doctors are now sponsored for exemption from the PLAB test to undergo specific training programmes in this country. Their sponsors are required to provide the Council with assurances as to their professional standards and proficiency in English.

When the Council has been satisfied on all these points, limited registration is granted for a specific period and a specific range of medical practice. Further grants of limited registration can be made, up to a maximum aggregate of 5 years. Doctors with limited registration can apply for full registration if they can show that they have sufficient knowledge, skill, and experience, and in judging such applications the Council requires high standards in the interests of the public.

The Council has recently reviewed the manner in which doctors who qualified overseas are granted registration enabling them to practise in the UK, and is seeking a change in the law to replace the present arrangements with a single form of 'training registration'.

Standards of professional conduct

The definition and maintenance of high standards among doctors are, it will be apparent from the above, fundamental to the work of the General Medical Council. The little-noticed provision in the 1858 Act, giving the Council power to remove from the register the names of any doctors judged unworthy to remain on it, gave the Council a clear disciplinary function from the outset. As case law began to accumulate,the Council found itself, indirectly at first but later by means of formal notices, issuing warnings to the profession about certain forms of behaviour that might give rise to disciplinary action. These were consolidated in 1914 into a single Warning Notice, which was supplemented in later years, but it was only when the Merrison Committee was conducting its enquiry that serious attention began to be paid to the need for doctors to receive not just warnings about inappropriate behaviour but positive advice on standards of professional conduct.

The Merrison Committee formed a clear view of the Council's potential role, not as a 'lawmaker' for doctors, but as a centre for public debate on questions of both professional conduct and medical ethics, and under the Medical Act 1978 the Council was given a general power to provide 'in such manner as the Council think fit, advice for members of the medical profession on standards of professional conduct or on medical ethics'. In response to this new duty the Council set up a committee now known as the *Standards Committee*, whose remit is to keep under review the Council's general guidance to the profession on a wide range of subjects. That guidance is published in a booklet entitled *Professional conduct and discipline; fitness to practise* (generally known as the 'blue booklet'), which is issued regularly to the whole profession and to all new entrants. It is not a code of conduct but rather a statement of ethical principle and a guide to the Council's fitness to practise functions. The Standards Committee has made it its task to define the principles that underlie good professional conduct, to apply those principles to new situations as the circumstances of medical practice change, and, where necessary, to make recommendations to the Council for revised guidance to doctors. The Committee aims to provide positive guidance which is of relevance and value to doctors in their daily work, and particularly in their relationships with professional colleagues and patients.

In recent years the Committee has played a significant part in the development of definitive advice to the medical profession on the ethical principles that should be applied to the handling of cases of *HIV infection and *AIDS. It has also brought the Council's general guidance on professional *confidentiality up to date and helped the Council to develop a less restrictive, more positive approach to advertising by doctors and the provision to the public of information about their services.

Fitness to practise

The Council's functions in relation to the fitness to practise of doctors are carried out by three statutory committees, elected from among the Council members. The Preliminary Proceedings and Professional Conduct Committees deal with criminal convictions of doctors and allegations of serious professional misconduct. The Health Committee deals with cases where a doctor's fitness to practise may be seriously impaired by reason of a physical or mental condition.

Professional conduct

The disciplinary functions of the Council continue to be those that attract the greatest public attention, largely because of the publicity which inevitably attends some cases where an allegation of serious professional misconduct has been made. The number of doctors who become the subject of disciplinary action is, however, extremely small by comparison with the number of doctors on the register at any one time.

The Act of 1858 established the Council as the first statutory professional tribunal of its kind. The Council's disciplinary powers have been developed in certain respects, and the terminology describing them has changed, but its essential jurisdiction over a doctor's registration remains the same as it has been since 1858. However, changing social attitudes, and developments in medical practice, do, rightly, influence the attitude of the Council towards certain types of conviction and misconduct, and this is reflected in the fact that allegations made against a doctor are not judged against an unchanging code but are assessed by a panel composed chiefly of the doctor's professional peers. The point was recognized by Lord Justice Lopes as long ago as 1894 when defining the phrase, then current in the legislation governing the Council, 'infamous conduct in a professional respect':

If a medical man in the pursuit of his profession has done something with regard to it which will be reasonably regarded as disgraceful or dishonourable by his professional brethren of good repute and competency, then it is open to the General Medical Council, if that be shown, to say that he has been guilty of infamous conduct in a professional respect.

Another important guideline is provided by the words 'in the pursuit of his profession'. Any action by the Council that may result from a disciplinary inquiry will depend not only on the seriousness of the offence but on the extent to which the allegation depends on matters bearing directly on the doctor's practice of medicine. Again, this involves detailed peer assessment but an increasingly significant part has been played in all stages of the Council's disciplinary work by its lay members, whose task is to represent the public interest by bringing to the Council their own expertise from outside the medical profession.

When the Council learns that a doctor has been convicted of a criminal offence, or a complaint is received about a doctor's professional conduct, the information is first studied by one or more *preliminary screeners* appointed from among the Council members. Three of these, who are medically qualified, share the initial screening and two others, who are lay members, are also consulted about any case where the medical screeners consider that no action should be taken by the Council.

It is the task of the nine medical and two lay members of the *Preliminary Proceedings Committee*, who meet in private, to decide on the basis of documents on each case whether the matter should be referred to the Professional Conduct or Health Committees for inquiry. Sometimes the Preliminary Proceedings Committee adjourns a case for further inquiries, for example into a doctor's state of health. The Committee may also decide to conclude the matter with a letter of advice or warning to the doctor. Complainants are always notified of the action taken.

The *Professional Conduct Committee* normally sits in public, in panels of 11 members, including two lay members. Its procedure is akin to that of a criminal court and the same rules of evidence apply. A legal assessor—usually a QC—advises on questions of law. Witnesses may be subpoenaed and evidence is given on oath. Most cases heard by the Committee concern allegations that a doctor has disregarded professional responsibilities towards patients, or has abused their trust in some other way.

The Professional Conduct Committee must decide whether a charge or charges against a doctor are proved and, if so, what action should be taken in relation to the doctor's registration. Where a charge is found proved the Committee may:

(1) conclude the case with a warning, or
(2) postpone its determination, or
(3) direct that the doctor's registration shall (for a period of up to 3 years) be conditional on compliance with certain requirements, or
(4) direct the suspension of the doctor's registration (for up to 12 months), or
(5) direct the erasure of the doctor's name from the register (this remains in force indefinitely but the doctor can later apply for restoration).

The doctor has 28 days in which to appeal, to the Judicial Committee of the Privy Council, against a direction made by the Committee, and in the meantime the direction does not take effect, but where the public interest requires it the Committee may direct immediate suspension so that the doctor is prevented from practising during the appeal period.

Although the total number of cases considered by the Committee has remained broadly constant, in recent years its hearings have become increasingly lengthy and complex, so that its overall workload has shown a steady increase.

Detailed statistics about the types and numbers of cases considered by the Committee are published in the Council's annual reports, together with accounts of some specific cases illustrating particular aspects of professional conduct to which the Council wishes to draw attention.

The health procedures

The Council's health procedures, introduced in 1980, have enabled action to be taken in over 400 cases where a question has arisen concerning a doctor's state of health. The procedures, which are voluntary in their basis and therapeutic in their intent, are designed to aid the rehabilitation of sick doctors while securing the protection of the public. They have achieved those aims in many cases, and have been successful in generally raising awareness, among doctors and their employers, of the need to offer effective support to sick colleagues.

Before these procedures came into effect the Council could do nothing in the case of a sick doctor unless there was reason to take action through the disciplinary machinery, which was not suited to cases of this kind. The procedures do not supersede local arrangements which exist to offer help to a doctor who may be ill; rather, the Council has always intended the existence of its Health Committee, with power to impose suspension or conditional registration, to strengthen the hand of local colleagues seeking to offer advice to sick doctors, and to make that advice more acceptable to the doctors themselves. The Council's procedures serve to provide an effective means of handling cases where local action is either inappropriate or unsuccessful.

Evidence raising a question about a doctor's health usually comes to the Council from concerned colleagues, but may also come from a health authority, the police, pharmacists or, occasionally, patients. Sometimes doctors originally referred for disciplinary action are transferred to the health procedures if it appears that an illness may be the underlying cause of the problem. A *preliminary screener* of health cases, who is a medical member of the Council and usually a psychiatrist, considers the information in all such cases and must decide if it raises the question whether the doctor's fitness to practise is 'seriously impaired by reason of a physical or mental condition'. About two-thirds of cases require action by the Council, and almost invariably a mental condition—a psychiatric illness or some form of addiction—is identified.

Where the screener decides to take action, the doctor is invited to be medically examined, usually in the local area, by at least two doctors. The examiners report to the screener who, if the examiners consider the sick doctor's fitness to practise to be seriously impaired, invites the doctor to follow their recommendations. This always involves continuing medical supervision, and usually there are recommendations concerning future management and certain limitations on practice designed to protect the public. If the doctor co-operates with this procedure, medical supervision is arranged and the screener sees regular reports on the doctor's progress. Where good progress is maintained the limitations on practice are gradually removed until the doctor is able to return to unrestricted practice without supervision.

Only where a doctor does not co-operate with the screener, or accepts recommendations and later ceases to comply with them, or suffers a serious deterioration in health, does the *Health Committee* become involved. About a quarter of all cases take this course. The Committee, composed of 12 Council members including a lay member, meets in private and is advised by specialist medical assessors and a legal assessor. Its procedures are governed by legal rules, but its hearings are not adversarial. Witnesses may be called, but the principal evidence usually comprises written medical reports. If the Committee finds the doctor's fitness to practise seriously impaired, it may impose conditions on registration for up to 3 years, or suspend registration for up to 12 months. The Committee does not have the power of erasure. Cases are reviewed on a regular basis until the Committee is satisfied that the doctor may safely resume practice without restriction.

The Council's duty to protect patients is paramount, but the aim of the health procedures is to secure the complete rehabilitation of the doctor. To that end, the Health Committee continues to seek ways to provide more general support for the doctors who appear before it. The Council has been financing a pilot scheme, lasting 2 years from spring 1992, under which experienced doctors were appointed as 'liaison advisers' to advise and help sick doctors under the Council's care. The aim is to help such doctors to overcome the many professional, social, and personal problems which are consequent upon their illnesses. The Council has also recently supported the establishment of a research project to look at ways in which the various local mechanisms, which are intended to deal with the problems of sick doctors, could be made more effective.

Standards of professional performance

The procedures described above cover situations where a doctor's professional conduct or state of health raise doubt as to whether his or her registration should continue without restriction. The procedures are carefully defined by law and, in conduct cases, require charges to be brought which relate to specific, closely defined allegations. These must be specific as to time and place, and capable of being tested in the same way as a charge in a criminal court. This method is not, however, suited to the broader assessment of a doctor's standard of professional performance which may be required when allegations are made suggesting that a pattern of serious deficiency of knowledge, skills, or attitudes is putting patients at risk. The Council has long felt concern about its lack of powers to deal with a number of cases of this kind, which cannot be effectively handled within the present legal framework. It has therefore devised new procedures, outside the scope of the existing legislation, whose primary aim would be to protect the public by preventing potential risk where a doctor's standard of performance is seriously deficient. The proposal is for a remedial procedure based on a thorough local assessment of the doctor's performance. In a successful case, the doctor's standard of performance would be raised by means of peer assessment which identified areas of serious deficiency, followed by remedial education and training in the relevant areas, and reassessment after training. Government Ministers have expressed their support for the Council's proposals and the Council hopes to secure the necessary powers as soon as parliamentary time can be made available.

Conclusion

The General Medical Council is the statutory body responsible for the regulation of the medical profession in the UK, but it is only one of the many bodies that have played a major role in the functioning of that profession and the maintenance of its standards. The Privy Council, the universities, the Royal Colleges, and the various professional associations have, through their members, ensured that throughout the whole of its life the Council has had people, from within the Council and outside it, of the highest quality to serve upon it. On its list of members is represented a wide spectrum of expertise and opinion which, together with the unflagging industry and ability of successive generations of officers and staff, has enabled the Council to carry out its increasingly demanding duties in the interests of the public.

R. KILPATRICK

Acknowledgement
I am grateful to the staff of the Council, and in particular to Alan Kershaw, for help in compiling this entry.

Further reading
Annual Reports of the General Medical Council.
GMC (1980). *Recommendations on basic medical education.* GMC Education Committee, February.
GMC (1987). *Recommendations on the training of specialists.* GMC Education Committee, October.
GMC (1991). *Constitution and functions.* GMC, London.
GMC (1992). *Recommendations on general clinical training.* GMC Education Committee, February.
GMC (1993). *Professional conduct and discipline: fitness to practise.* GMC, London
Heseltine, M. (1949). The early history of the General Medical Council (1858–1886). *The Medical Press,* 7 September, CCXXXII, No. 5757.

Medical Act 1983. HMSO, London.

Pyke-Lees, W. (1958). *Centenary of the General Medical Council 1858–1958.* London.

Report of the Committee of Inquiry into the Regulation of the Medical Profession (1975). Cmnd. 6018, April 1975, London.

GENERAL OPHTHALMIC SERVICES (UK) are the responsibility of the Family Health Services Authority, which is the part of the UK *National Health Service (NHS) responsible for primary care. Ophthalmic medical practitioners and ophthalmic *opticians test sight and prescribe glasses within the service. A patient requiring ophthalmic attention within the service for the first time must obtain a certificate from his doctor stating that he needs a sight test. He is then free to choose where he is tested. There is a routine charge of £15.00 for sight testing. However, certain people are exempt from this charge:

(1) those partially sighted or blind;
(2) those under 16 years of age;
(3) those under 19 years of age in full-time education;
(4) those over 40 years old with a family history of glaucoma;
(5) those with diabetes mellitus;
(6) those on low income, such as those on income support or family credit; and
(7) those with complex prescriptions, such as high myopes, *aphakics, or *astigmatics.

In addition, financial help for the purchase of spectacles is available in the form of vouchers. Groups qualifying for vouchers include:

(1) those under 16 years of age;
(2) full-time students under 19 years of age;
(3) those receiving income support, or anyone in the family on income support;
(4) those receiving family credit; and
(5) people who fill in an AG1 form, i.e. those who think they may be entitled because of low income but are not on income support.

Certain hospital services are also free of charge. These include:

(1) visual aid devices on loan;
(2) special contact lenses to those receiving income support, etc.;
(3) cosmetic lenses;
(4) artificial eyes;
(5) visual fields and refraction;
(6) binocular visual testing by orthoptists;
(7) optometry visits for handicapped adults.

P. HASSETT

GENERAL MEDICAL PRACTICE. See PRIMARY MEDICAL CARE.

GENERAL NURSING COUNCIL was set up to control the profession of nursing by the Nurses Registration Act 1919. In 1983 it was superseded by the United Kingdom Central Council for Nursing, Midwifery and Health Visiting, under the Nurses, Midwives and Health Visitors' Act of 1979. See NURSES ACTS 1943–49; NURSING IN THE UK.

GENERAL PARALYSIS OF THE INSANE is chronic syphilitic inflammation of the brain, developing in the later stages of untreated *syphilis. The characteristic manifestations are progressive *dementia with personality deterioration, sometimes featuring *delusions of grandeur, accompanied by generalized weakness of upper motor neurone type. They develop between 10 and 20 years after the primary infection. In the absence of antisyphilitic treatment the patient progresses to a state of hopeless insanity. Early treatment with *penicillin can result in complete recovery.

GENERAL PARESIS is a synonym for *general paralysis of the insane.

GENERAL PRACTITIONER. A doctor providing *primary medical care.

GENERIC is used to denote the non-proprietary, unbranded name of a drug or pharmaceutical preparation. See PHARMACEUTICAL INDUSTRY.

GENETIC CODE. The relationship between the nucleotide sequences along *chromosomes and the *proteins which the body synthesizes and which determine its inherited characteristics. See DEOXYRIBONUCLEIC ACID; GENE; GENETICS.

GENETIC COUNSELLING is the provision of expert advice by clinical geneticists or other clinicians to prospective parents.

GENETIC ENGINEERING. This term is used to describe the manipulation of DNA (*deoxyribonucleic acid) by any method not involving animal breeding. It is based on a number of techniques derived from recombinant DNA technology. It is possible to fractionate DNA using a family of enzymes, derived from bacteria, called restriction endonucleases, or restriction enzymes. After digestion of DNA with restriction enzymes the resulting fragments can be inserted into an appropriate vector, that is another DNA molecule capable of replicating in a bacterial cell. The simplest cloning vector is a *plasmid, a simple DNA molecule that replicates in the cytoplasm of bacteria separately from the bacterial DNA. If fractionated DNA is mixed with plasmids that have been cut with restriction enzymes, and the mixture treated in a way that favours reassociation of DNA fragments, some of the pieces of 'foreign' DNA will be incorporated into plasmids. These are now recombinant molecules which can be inserted into bacteria, where they replicate independently from bacterial DNA. In this way, or using more sophisticated cloning vectors, it is possible to generate any fragment of DNA that is required. This procedure, which is also called gene cloning, is used to isolate genes for sequencing, for clinical studies, or for use as probes for genetic diagnosis.

Genetic engineering encompasses many other techniques. For example, it is possible to insert 'foreign' genes into cells, either directly or attached to a transport vector such as a *retrovirus. This form of genetic manipulation is used to study the function of genes in a new environment, to determine which parts of a gene are involved in its regulation, and, more practically, as an approach towards gene therapy. In the latter case the idea is to insert a normal gene into a cell to correct the action of a defective gene that causes disease.

Genetic engineering and recombinant DNA technology are also used to produce human *proteins in bacterial cells, *insulin, *erythropoietin, and *growth hormone for example, and for developing novel *vaccines and diagnostic agents.

There are many other potential uses for genetic engineering in medical practice. For example, it is possible to 'switch off' certain genes that may be involved in neoplastic transformation by inserting complementary sequences to the messenger RNA of the particular gene, so-called antisense technology (see MOLECULAR BIOLOGY). Genes can be inserted into fertilized eggs and may be expressed in various tissues of the offspring. The development of transgenic animals is used to study the control of particular genes and also to produce disease models, particularly in mice. The transgenic approach is also being used to insert human genes into larger animals for the production of therapeutic agents.

GENETIC MAPPING assigns individual *genes to particular *chromosomes and to particular chromosomal locations. See GENETICS.

GENETICS AND MEDICAL PRACTICE. Although genetics, the branch of science which encompasses the study of heredity, touches on every aspect of clinical practice, it is a relative newcomer to the medical sciences. Clinical genetics evolved after the Second World War and, despite its importance, it still forms only a small part of the curriculum of many medical schools. But because of enormous advances in the field in recent years it is likely to become a subject of prime importance in medical research and practice in the third millenium.

Historical outline

Until the middle of the 19th century thoughts about heredity were extremely confused. In essence, it was believed that a preformed embryo is encapsulated in the mother's ovum and that an ill-defined influence from the father galvanized things into activity. The 'preformation' theory was summarized by Bowler as follows, 'The theory of pre-existing germs held that all organisms grow from miniatures or "germs" created by God at the beginning of the universe, stored one within the other like a series of Russian dolls. The first woman, Eve, literally contained within her ovaries the whole of the rest of the human race, generations after generations of miniatures packed one inside the other, each waiting for an act of fertilisation to give it a chance to grow . . . The male semen merely provided the stimulus that triggered off the expansion of the outmost miniature.' It followed that if the germ defined an individual, their characteristics depended on what God had created, not on anything that had been transmitted from the parents. Even after the discovery of sperm, the preformation hypothesis was not abandoned and some held that an individual was preformed in the sperm, and only nurtured by the mother. The long struggle between ovists and spermists continued throughout the 18th century, and, although medical scientists started to recognize that disease might occur in successive generations of a family, a reasonable hypothesis on which to try to understand these observations had to wait for over 100 years.

Modern genetics was born in the 19th century. Its roots can be traced to two major developments, *cell theory and the discovery that the inheritance of certain genetic traits follows simple mathematical laws. In 1889 Walther *Flemming, a German anatomist, discovered that when cells are dividing it is possible to see thread-like structures which absorb colour from particular dyes. Flemming called these structures 'chromatin', and later they became known as *chromosomes. When a cell divides, by a process which later became known as *mitosis, chromosomes appear to divide, and identical copies are passed on to the next generation of cells. The notion that they might contain genetic information was developed by the German zoologist August Weismann. Although his ideas on how this process might occur were vague, he developed one critical concept. If the hereditary material from both parents resides in chromosomes, and is mixed in a fertilized egg, the egg ought to contain twice as much as the parental cells; in every succeeding generation it would double. Clearly this cannot happen. In 1887 Weismann reasoned that the only way round this conundrum is that during the process of cell division in eggs and sperm there is a reduction in the amount of hereditary material by half. This type of reduction division became known as *meiosis. These ideas were extended and developed by the American biologists Walter Sutton and Edmond Wilson, work which led to a clearer picture of how chromosomes are inherited. Except during the formation of *gametes, that is ova or sperm, cells divide by mitosis which is preceded by doubling of each pair of chromosomes. This ensures that the two daughter cells each acquire a set of chromosomes identical to the parental cell, a state which is called diploid. On the other hand, during gamete formation cell division occurs by meiosis, to give progeny with half the number of chromosomes (the haploid state); fertilization restores cells from the haploid to the diploid state.

The other major advance during the 19th century was the discovery by Gregor *Mendel that inheritance of certain factors follows two simple mathematical rules. Mendel spent most of his life working in the Augustinian monastery in Brno, where he combined his clerical duties with a passionate interest in science. He was stimulated to carry out his breeding experiments by observations on ornamental plants, for which he tried to breed new colour variants by artificial insemination. He selected the pea for his experiments and crossed varieties with differences in single characters such as colour (yellow or green) or the form of seed (round, or angular and wrinkled), and simply counted all the alternative types in the offspring of first-generation crosses, and crosses in later generations. Based on the results of these experiments Mendel formulated the concept of what later became known as the *gene, a unit of heredity which is passed from generation to generation in a way which follows two simple laws. First, genes segregate; members of the same pair of genes, or alleles, are never present in the same gamete (eggs or sperm) but always separate and are transmitted in different gametes. Secondly, genes assort independently; members of different pairs of genes move to gametes independently from each other. To put it in a nutshell, alleles segregate; non-alleles assort. Mendel's work had no immediate impact and was forgotten until it was rediscovered independently by several workers at the beginning of the 20th century.

The true significance of sexual reproduction and meiosis became apparent only during the early part of the 20th century, following a brilliant series of breeding experiments using the fruitfly *Drosophila* by Thomas Hunt *Morgan and his colleagues. When maternal and paternal chromosomes become closely wound round each other during meiosis it is possible for genes to pass from one to the other by a process called crossing-over, or recombination. Mendel's laws had only described the patterns of inheritance of individual genes, but Morgan's group in the USA and William Bateson in England realized that if two genes are on the same chromosome, and particularly if they are close together, they will tend to be inherited together. The genes are then said to be linked. The closer together a pair of genes are on the same chromosome the less chance they will have to cross over. Hence, Morgan reasoned, the number of crossovers is a measure of the distance between genes. These seminal ideas led to the production of maps of genes on chromosomes, work that involved many linkage studies and the application of complicated mathematical models for their analysis. From the work of Herman *Müller it became clear that genes can change their structure, that is undergo *mutation, and that this process may be speeded up under certain conditions, for example on exposure of cells to *radiation.

These studies in the USA were mirrored by equally important developments in England at about the same time. Here, for the first time, statistical methods were used to study the behaviour of genes in populations. The work of biometricians like Ronald *Fisher, J. B. S. *Haldane, and Karl *Pearson, as well as clearly distinguishing between simple Mendelian inheritance and more complex hereditary systems under the control of many different genes, paved the way for the amalgamation of Mendelism and Darwinism, which formed the basis for modern evolution theory.

Human genetics

Study of this topic was developed in England at the end of the 19th century. It was initiated by the ideas of Francis *Galton who was interested in improving the human species by selective breeding, work which was summarized in the first edition of his book *Hereditary genius*, first published in 1869. Although much of Galton's later thinking about genetics was confused, because, unlike Mendel, the traits in which he was most interested did not follow simple patterns of inheritance, he was the instigator of quantitative human genetics. And those who followed him, particularly Karl Pearson and Ronald Fisher, laid the foundations of quantitative genetics and, later, of population genetics. Biochemical genetics was also born at about this time through the work of Archibald *Garrod. In his book *Inborn errors of metabolism*, published in 1909, Garrod described several rare diseases which he thought were due to inherited defects in the body's chemical pathways. Because of doubts about the importance of Mendel's findings, Garrod did not immediately appreciate the true significance of his observations. However, he noted that there was a high incidence of parental consanguinity in some of his families and William Bateson pointed out to him that this is precisely what would be expected if the conditions that he was describing were inherited in a Mendelian recessive fashion. Garrod had, in effect, laid the basis for the understanding of the genetic basis of biochemical individuality, a concept he later expanded to encompass an explanation for individual susceptibility to common disease.

Human genetics flourished in England during the first half of the 20th century. When Francis Galton died in 1911, University College, London, was left sufficient money to establish the Galton Eugenics Professorship and Department of Applied Statistics, which included the Galton and Biometric Laboratories. Although much of its early work involved eugenics, that is the improvement of the population by selective breeding, it also established the scientific basis for human genetics. Work carried out at the Galton Laboratory, which became the mecca for workers in the field from all over the world in the period just before and just after the Second World War, placed human pedigree analysis on a firm statistical basis, established the first genetic linkages in man, and laid the basis for the study of genetic disease.

While human genetics was founded on a basis of pedigree linkage analysis, knowledge about the cellular and biochemical aspects of human heredity also advanced rapidly during the first half of the 20th century. Laborious studies of cultured cells gradually led to the conclusion that humans have 46 chromosomes; 22 pairs are called autosomes and the other pair constitute the sex chromosomes. The human sex chromosomes were called X and Y, terminology derived from earlier work on the chromosomes of *Hemiptera* by Edmond Wilson. Females have two X chromosomes while males have one X and one Y sex chromosome. By using cultured white blood cells it became easier to study human chromosomes, and the introduction of phytohaemagglutinin stimulation of mitosis in white cells, combined with treatment in hypotonic solution, greatly improved the quality of chromosome preparations and facilitated the analysis of their morphology and numbers. Another major advance in *cytogenetics was the discovery that when chromosome preparations are stained with quinacrine mustard or Giemsa they show alternative light and dark banding regions (Fig. 1). Chromosome banding was an invaluable advance for identifying individual human chromosomes, in both health and disease. The

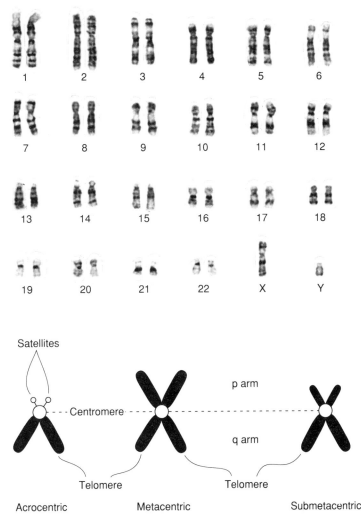

Fig. 1 Human chromosomes. (a) The normal human male karyotype. The chromosomes are identified by their size, banding patterns, and position of the centromere. Trypsin–Giemsa banding. (Kindly prepared by Dr J. Jonasson.) (b) The anatomy of human chromosomes. (Both diagrams are reproduced from Weatherall 1991).

first congenital defect found to be associated with an autosomal chromosome anomaly in man was *Down's syndrome; in 1959 Lejeune examined the chromosomes of nine mongoloid children and found that in each case there were 47 chromosomes. The discovery of many other human cytogenetic abnormalities followed.

Human biochemical genetics evolved in the post-war period and took a major step forward with the discovery by Linus Pauling and his colleagues that the *haemoglobin of patients with *sickle-cell anaemia migrates at a different rate in an electric field from normal haemoglobin. This suggested that sickle-cell disease results from a structural variant of haemoglobin. In subsequent years many human proteins were examined by electrophoresis and every one examined turned out to be polymorphic, that is there were genetically determined structural variants. In many cases these were harmless but others were associated with abnormal function or stability of the protein and hence with disease. In 1956 Vernon Ingram discovered that sickle-cell haemoglobin differs from normal haemoglobin by a single *amino acid substitution. In subsequent years other variant proteins were studied in the same way. Many single-gene disorders were found to be due to the synthesis of an abnormal enzyme or protein, and it was possible to relate the particular structural changes to abnormal function or stability.

The first gene to be assigned to a human chromosome was for colour blindness, found to be on the X chromosome by workers at Columbia University in 1911. Another 57 years were to pass before the first gene was assigned to anything but the X chromosome; a particular blood group was assigned to chromosome 1 by a team in *Johns Hopkins University in 1968. For the next 20 years progress was very slow in assigning human genes to chromosomes, largely because there were so few markers for linkage studies. By 1976 at least one gene had been assigned to each of the 23 autosomes, yet by 1987 at least 1215 genes had been assigned, 365 of which are known to be the site of mutations that cause disease. This remarkable period of progress stemmed from the use of new mapping techniques, first involving the fusion of human and animal cells, and later from advances in the recombinant DNA field.

When methods for fusing human and rodent cells were developed in the 1960s it was found that their chromosomes become mixed together and that subsequently many of them are lost from the now hybrid cell; human chromosomes are lost preferentially and in a random fashion. It is therefore possible to propagate hybrid cells containing specific human chromosomes. Using a variety of techniques to detect gene products it is possible to determine whether a particular gene resides on these chromosomes. But the other, and even more effective, way of mapping human genes had to wait for the technical developments of molecular biology.

From the mid-1960s the new techniques of molecular biology were applied to the study of human genetics.

Several of these methods have been central to the extraordinary developments which have occurred in this field over the past 20 years. From the seminal studies of Watson and Crick it became apparent that DNA consists of a double helix made up of two chains of nucleotide bases wrapped around each other (see MOLECULAR BIOLOGY). There are four bases, adenine (A), guanine (G), cytosine (C), and thymine (T). Because of their particular shapes, A always pairs with T, and C with G; the bases, and hence the chains or strands, are linked by relatively weak hydrogen bonds. It turned out that the two strands of DNA can be dissociated and reassociated *in vitro*, by heating and cooling for example. This reannealing reaction is highly specific, and under the right conditions will occur only between DNA strands that have identical or almost identical base sequences. Thus, to find a particular gene buried away in a large amount of DNA, a length of DNA with an identical sequence is constructed so that it will anneal to the gene but not to the rest of the DNA. This is the principle behind constructing gene probes to find genes of particular medical interest. Another major advance followed the discovery of a family of bacterial enzymes, called restriction endonucleases, or restriction enzymes, which cleave DNA at particular sequences of bases. Thus it was now possible to fractionate human DNA. This led to the development of human gene cloning. This is based on the principle of inserting pieces of human DNA into an appropriate vector, that is another DNA molecule capable of replicating in a bacterial cell. The first cloning vectors were plasmids, lengths of DNA that replicate in the cytoplasm of bacteria. If DNA is fractionated and the plasmid DNA is cut with the same enzyme, and the mixture treated in a way that favours reassociation of the DNA fragments, some of the pieces of human DNA will be incorporated into plasmids. These are then inserted into bacteria, where they replicate independently from the bacterial DNA. Thus it is possible to generate what are called 'gene libraries', that is fragments of DNA representing almost the complete human genome growing on bacterial plates. Genes that are being sought can be identified from particular colonies by hybridization with radioactively labelled gene probes. Once human genes could be grown in this way they could then be isolated, sequenced, and their structure determined. Subsequently a variety of ingenious cloning vectors were developed, some based on *bacteriophage, others on yeast.

Using these techniques it was possible to isolate genes from patients with a variety of single-gene disorders and to determine the precise molecular pathology. It was also possible to introduce human genes into different cell lines and to analyse both how they are controlled and how this may be defective in disease. And it was now feasible to persuade human genes to make their products in bacteria, hence opening up a completely new approach to the production of therapeutic agents.

But the technology of the molecular era had even

more important implications for the development of human genetics. In particular, it provided an opportunity for developing maps of the entire human genome. It is estimated that there are about 50 000–100 000 genes distributed among the 23 pairs of human chromosomes. In 1927 J. B. S. Haldane reasoned that if it were possible to map 50 or more inherited characters, that is to place them in the appropriate position on their chromosomes, they could be used as markers for predicting whether children would inherit genes for important diseases. The idea is beautifully simple. Suppose that we wish to follow the progress of a particular genetic trait through a family but have no way of identifying it. It is only necessary to find a gene that we can readily identify and which is linked to the gene for the trait that we are looking for. If the two are so close together that they always pass together through successive generations, we now have a 'handle' on the gene that we can't identify; if the marker gene is inherited so must the gene that is supposed to be linked to it. And, of course, if we know the chromosomal location of the marker gene, it follows that the gene that we cannot identify must be close to it on the same region of the particular chromosome. DNA technology has provided us with a vast array of linkage markers of this type.

Normal people vary considerably from one another in the structure of their DNA. Much of this variation reflects single base changes which can be identified by particular restriction enzymes and which give different length DNA fragments after digestion. These restriction fragment length polymorphisms (RFLPs) offer useful linkage markers. However, it turned out that there are regions of DNA, usually consisting of repetitive sequences, which vary considerably in their length between different individuals. These hypervariable regions, or minisatellite DNA, provide particularly polymorphic and informative linkage markers. And there are even more common and highly polymorphic repetitive regions of DNA called microsatellites. All this genetic variability in the structure of DNA has provided a rich source of markers, the existence of which has transformed modern human genetics.

Modern linkage analysis has led to the discovery of the genes involved in such important monogenic disease as Duchenne *muscular dystrophy, *cystic fibrosis, chronic granulomatous disease, and many others. By searching for segregation of these disorders with particular linkage markers it has been possible to identify the particular chromosome involved and then to pinpoint the position that is occupied by the mutant gene. Linkage studies of this type may land the geneticist many millions of bases away from the particular gene for which they are searching. However, by some ingenious developments in molecular biology it is possible to 'walk' or 'jump' along chromosomes and, with some luck, to identify the particular gene that is responsible for a disease.

Having found the mutant gene, the next step is to sequence it and hence to make an educated guess about the likely structure of its product based on its DNA sequence. This new approach, called reverse genetics or positional cloning, has led to the identification of the protein product of the genes involved in muscular dystrophy and cystic fibrosis and has already led to some understanding of their function and how this is affected by the mutations that cause these diseases.

These remarkable successes, together with other improvements in mapping technology, have spawned the Human Genome Project (HUGO). Essentially this involves generating both genetic and physical maps of the entire human genome. A genetic map will consist of linkage markers spread at convenient lengths along all the human chromosomes. In essence, it will be like a road atlas which shows the position of towns along roads. The physical map, on the other hand, will describe the details of the roads, that is the complete base sequence of the entire human genome. Current estimates suggest that these remarkable achievements may be completed by the end of the second decade of the 21st century.

Medical genetics

Medical genetics now touches on every aspect of clinical practice. Broadly speaking, its scope can be divided into the study of single-gene disorders, chromosomal abnormalities, the genetic component of common polygenic disease, and somatic cell genetics, that is acquired disorders of the genetic machinery of cells which may be passed on to their progeny. The latter is of particular importance in the *cancer field.

Single-gene disorders

In the clinical geneticists' bible, *Mendelian inheritance in man*, Victor McKusick lists over 4000 diseases which either definitely, or very likely, result from the action of a single mutant gene. These conditions can be inherited as autosomal recessive or dominant traits, or in a sex-linked fashion. Autosomal dominant disorders are passed on by affected individuals to half their offspring of either sex; recessive disorders occur only in those (statistically one in four) who have the same harmful gene on each chromosome of the pair (in other words, he or she is homozygous, the offspring of two heterozygous carriers who each have only a single harmful recessive gene). Because females have two X chromosomes, most diseases that are carried on the X chromosome behave as recessives in women; the action of the defective gene is compensated by its normal allele on the other X chromosome. However, these conditions may be expressed in males if their single X chromosome happens to be the one carrying the abnormal gene from their mother.

Using the techniques of molecular biology, it has been possible to characterize the different varieties of mutations that underlie single-gene disorders. Most of these conditions are heterogeneous. For example, the common genetic blood disease beta-thalassaemia has been shown to result from over 100 different mutations.

It appears that cystic fibrosis and Duchenne muscular dystrophy are equally heterogeneous at the molecular level. There are many different types of mutations. In some cases entire genes are removed, or deleted. In others, single base changes scramble the genetic code in various ways so that messenger RNA cannot be used as a template for synthesizing normal proteins. Many genetic diseases result from mutations which interfere with the splicing together of the messenger RNA exons after their introns have been removed (see MOLECULAR BIOLOGY). And yet others are caused by mutations that interfere with the processes of initiation or termination of protein synthesis on the messenger RNA template.

Many recessive single-gene disorders can now be identified in carriers, either by simple biochemical tests or by DNA analysis. Couples who are both carriers for recessive diseases have the option either not to have children, to adopt, or to take the risk of having an abnormal child. DNA technology offers another possibility. By removing a small piece of tissue from around the *fetus, a technique called *chorion villus sampling (Fig. 2), it is possible to analyse fetal DNA for many monogenic diseases and to offer termination of those pregnancies in which the fetus has received an abnormal gene from both parents. Although this approach was possible using amniotic fluid as a source of cells for biochemical or cytogenetic analysis, the DNA era has greatly increased the number of conditions that can be identified antenatally.

There is now great interest in the possibility of correcting genetic disorders by 'gene therapy'. Many approaches are being explored. The most popular is to insert the normal counterpart of the defective gene into a retrovirus which is able to transfer the human gene into a particular cell population and insert it into the genome. To be successful this technique requires knowledge of the major regulatory regions that have to be inserted together with the particular gene, an ability to define the appropriate cell population for treatment, and confidence about the safety of the procedure. Many difficulties remain, but this approach seems likely to be successful, at least for a limited number of monogenic diseases. Otherwise these conditions have to be treated rather unsatisfactorily by replacement therapy or other symptomatic approaches.

Cytogenetic disorders

Each of the 23 pairs of human chromosomes is either maternal or paternal in origin. Each chromosome can now be identified with certainty using banding techniques, and they are numbered sequentially from 1 to 22, and X and Y, from largest to smallest. When describing chromosomal pathology, cytogeneticists refer to the appearance of the chromosome during a phase of mitosis called metaphase, during which the chromosome is in a particularly compact state and can be examined easily under the light microscope. Each chromosome appears to be composed of two halves, called sister chromatids. The chromatid halves are separated from each other along their lengths except at one point, called the centromere, where they are joined (see Fig. 1). The centromere divides chromosomes into two unequal regions, which are called short and long arms, p and q for short. The total number of chromosomes per cell is described by an Arabic number and, if relevant, the sex chromosome constitution is indicated by one X and/or Y for each sex chromosome. Thus the normal male chromosome constitution, or karyotype, is written 46,XY, and a normal female 46,XX. If there is an extra chromosome, its number is preceded by plus, if one is missing by minus. For example, trisomy 21 is written 47,+21. Extra material on a chromosome arm is indicated by plus; for example, 14q+ means that there is extra material on the long arm of chromosome 14. Similarly, a deletion is indicated by a − sign.

The frequency of chromosomal abnormalities at birth is approximately 5–6/1000. Of these, about 2/1000 are due to variation in the number of sex chromosomes, 1.7/1000 to variation in numbers of autosomal chromosomes, and 1.9/1000 are major chromosomal rearrangements. These anomalies account for 60 or more different clinical disorders. Among the more common and best defined are mongolism or Down's syndrome (trisomy 21), Edwards' syndrome (trisomy 18), *Klinefelter's syndrome (sex chromosomes XXY), and *Turner's syndrome (XO, that is a sex monosomic disorder). Trisomies usually result from fertilization of gametes carrying two copies of a particular chromosome; in the case of Down's syndrome the gamete carries two copies of chromosome 21. Such abnormal gametes result when homologous pairs of chromosomes fail to separate at the anaphase stage of the first or second division of meiosis, a phenomenon called non-dysjunction.

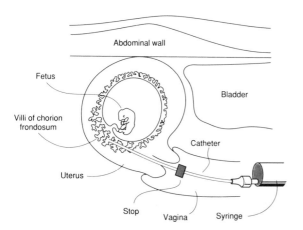

Fig. 2 The principle of chorion villus sampling to obtain trophoblast tissue for fetal DNA analysis (reproduced from Weatherall (1991), by kind permission of the author).

Diagnostic cytogenetics is usually confined to the analysis of children with congenital anomalies or mental retardation and their families. However, it is also used widely in prenatal (*antenatal) diagnosis programmes for the identification of Down's syndrome, particularly in mothers at high risk. Cytogenetic analysis can be carried out after chorion villus sampling or on cells from amniotic fluid obtained later in pregnancy. Cytogenetics also has important applications in other fields, particularly in the diagnosis of different forms of cancer which are associated with particular cytogenetic changes. Many of these advances are being facilitated by the development of better techniques for chromosome analysis, particularly improvements in *in situ* hybridization and fluorescent microscopy.

Genetic factors in common diseases; multifactorial inheritance

It has been known for a long time that many common diseases, including heart disease, *hypertension, *diabetes, the major *psychoses, *autoimmune disease, and others, have an important genetic component. However, epidemiological studies have shown that these conditions may all be precipitated by a variety of environmental agents. Thus their aetiology reflects a complex interaction between nurture and nature. These diseases rarely follow a Mendelian pattern of inheritance, and susceptibility or resistance is thought to reflect the action of several different genes.

One approach to estimating the importance of the genetic component is to study their occurrence, or concordance, in monozygotic compared with dizygotic twins. Twin concordance rates for some common diseases are shown in Table 1. It is clear that late onset, insulin-resistant diabetes (type 2 diabetes) is, for all intents and purposes, a genetic disease, whereas the genetic component in ischaemic heart disease is relatively small. Using linkage analysis together with DNA polymorphisms, a great deal of progress has been made in recent years in determining some of the genes involved in these polygenic systems. For example, it is now clear that early onset diabetes (type 1 diabetes) is associated with particular polymorphisms of the class 2 genes of the *HLA-DR system and of another locus which appears to be close to the insulin gene. Several different enzyme variants have been found in families with type 2 diabetes of unusually early onset. And polymorphisms or structural changes of several different families of genes, including those for the low-density lipoprotein receptor and various lipoproteins, have been found to be associated with an increased likelihood of developing coronary artery disease. The long-term objective of work in this field is to define the important genes involved in susceptibility or resistance to these diseases, in order to learn more about their underlying cause and to be able to define high-risk individuals so that suitable preventative measures may be established early in life.

Somatic cell genetics and cancer

Although a few forms of cancer can be traced through families in a way that suggests the action of a single gene, in most cases this is not possible. However, it is now apparent that many forms of cancer result from mutations of *oncogenes, that is genes that are involved in the normal regulation of cell proliferation, maturation, and differentiation. Oncogenes can be abnormally activated in a variety of ways, including point mutations, amplification, and translocation on to different chromosomes. It is also clear that some cancers result from the inheritance of recessive genes, the action of which may become unmasked by a variety of mechanisms, all of which have in common the inactivation of the normal partner which somehow is able to suppress the action of its abnormal allele. Although loss of anti-oncogene activity of this type was originally thought to be restricted to some rare childhood tumours, it is now clear that it occurs in many common cancers, including those of lung, breast, bowel, and bone.

It is currently believed that the generation of cancer involves at least two genetic events, and often many. For

Table 1 Twin concordance for some common diseases

Condition	Concordance (per cent)	
	Monozygotic	Dizygotic
Cleft lip±cleft palate	35	5
Cleft palate alone	26	6
Spina bifida	6	3
Pyloric stenosis	15	2
Congenital dislocation of the hip	41	3
Talipes equinovarus	32	3
Hypertension	30	10
Diabetes mellitus (insulin-dependent)	50	5
Diabetes mellitus (insulin-independent)	100	10
Ischaemic heart disease	19	8
Cancer	17	11
Epilepsy	37	10
Schizophrenia	60	10
Manic depression	70	15
Mental retardation	60	3
Leprosy	60	20
Tuberculosis	51	22
Atopic disease	50	4
Hyperthyroidism	47	3
Psoriasis	61	13
Gallstones	27	6
Sarcoidosis	50	8
Senile dementia	42	5
Multiple sclerosis	20	6

Modified from Connor and Ferguson-Smith (1987).

example, colon cancer seems to involve the interaction of mutations in at least six different oncogenes. This new branch of genetics promises to yield valuable advances in both the diagnosis and management of cancer.

Diagnostics and therapeutics
Recombinant DNA technology offers many possibilities for diagnosis and treatment. The development of gene probes against micro-organisms promises to transform diagnostic *microbiology. Similar techniques are finding wide application in diagnostic *pathology and *forensic medicine. For example, using the hypervariable region gene probes that were mentioned earlier in this section, it turns out that every human being has a unique pattern, or DNA fingerprint (Fig. 3). Despite early technical setbacks, DNA fingerprinting is now used widely in forensic medicine. DNA is relatively stable and can be extracted from many different sources, even bones that have been buried for thousands of years.

Recombinant DNA technology is also playing a major role in the *pharmaceutical industry. Recombinant human proteins such as erythropoietin, growth hormone, and insulin are already in clinical use. It has also been possible to produce a wide variety of different growth factors and lymphokines. For example, several human haemopoietic growth factors are already

being used in clinical practice for treating patients with bone marrow failure. Recombinant DNA technology is also being used to produce vaccines and to 'humanize' monoclonal antibodies for therapeutic purposes.

Broader issues in human biology
Molecular genetics is providing invaluable information throughout the whole of human biological research. Molecular approaches to population genetics are telling us how genes have become disseminated throughout populations and why particular genetic diseases are so common in some racial groups. Because our evolutionary history is written in our DNA the comparison of DNA sequences, between different human populations and between humans and their nearest evolutionary ancestors, is providing important information about our place in the evolutionary tree and about how human populations have evolved and diverged. As this work develops it may have important implications for clinical medicine, in particular with respect to genetic susceptibility or resistance to important environmental factors that are responsible for some of the major killer diseases of rich societies.

Human molecular genetics is also making important contributions to the understanding of development. It is helping to characterize some of the important genes involved in different stages of human development and the complex mechanisms whereby genes are regulated at various stages. Again, this work promises to have important medical applications for the understanding of developmental abnormalities. Finally, molecular and cell biology, combined with new approaches to human genetics, are starting to make some inroads into the problems of ageing and behaviour.

Genetics is likely to be one of the major areas of development in the medical sciences in the next millenium and promises to lead the way towards an understanding of many of our intractable killer diseases.

D. WEATHERALL

Further reading
Bowler, P. J. (1989). *The mendelian revolution*. Johns Hopkins University Press, Baltimore.
Geleherter, T. D. and Collins, F. S. (1990). *Principles of medical genetics*. Williams and Wilkins, Baltimore.
Lewin, B. (1994). *Genes V*. Oxford University Press, Oxford.
Singerm, M. and Berg, P. (1991). *Genes and genomes*. University Science Books, Mill Valley, California and Blackwell Scientific Publications, Oxford.
Weatherall, D. J. (1991). *The new genetics and clinical practice*, (3rd edn). Oxford University Press.

GENGOU, **OCTAVE** (1875–1957). Belgian bacteriologist and serologist. With Jules *Bordet he demonstrated the fixation of *complement in *antigen–antibody reactions, an important observation in *serology. They also discovered the bacterial cause of *whooping cough, now known as *Haemophilus pertussis* but formerly as the Bordet–Gengou bacillus.

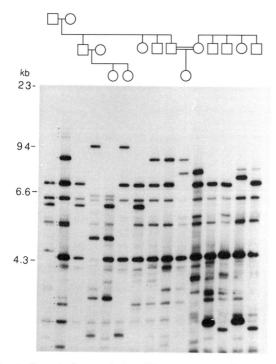

Fig. 3 Genetic fingerprinting. The patterns are from the individuals shown in the pedigree; each member is above his or her respective track.

GENITAL HERPES. See HERPES SIMPLEX.

GENITALIA. The organs of reproduction (often used synonymously with external genitalia).

GENITOURINARY DISEASE affects the urinary tract (*ureter, *bladder, *urethra) and/or the *genitalia. See also SEXUALLY TRANSMITTED DISEASE; UROLOGICAL SURGERY.

GENOME. The totality of the *genes in a complete haploid set of chromosomes. See GENETICS.

GENOTYPE. The genetic constitution of an individual, often as contrasted with *phenotype. See GENETICS.

GENTAMICIN is the most important of the *amino-glycoside group of *antibiotics, all of which are ineffective by mouth (except in intestinal infections), bactericidal, and active against both Gram-negative and Gram-positive organisms. They are ototoxic and nephrotoxic, and are best avoided in pregnancy. See ANTIBACTERIAL AGENTS.

GENTIAN is a bitter extract of the root of gentian plants, once an ingredient of many supposed tonics and appetite-stimulating mixtures.

GENU VALGUM, GENU VARUM, ETC. are deformities of the knee joint. Genu valgum is the deformity known as knock-knee and genu varum that known as bowleg.

GEOGRAPHICAL FACTORS IN DISEASE. See ENVIRONMENT AND DISEASE; EPIDEMIOLOGY; TROPICAL MEDICINE.

GERARD, JOHN (1545–1612). British herbalist. Gerard was master of the *Barber-Surgeons' Company in 1607, superintendent of Lord Burghley's gardens, and herbalist to James I. In 1597 he published his celebrated *Herball*.

GERHARD, WILLIAM WOOD (1809–72). American physician. During an epidemic of *typhus fever in Philadelphia he was able to call attention to clinical features which clearly differentiated it from typhoid fever: suffusion of the conjunctivae, petechial eruption, mildness of abdominal symptoms, and, in fatal cases, lack of swelling of Peyer's patches in the intestine. Typhoid and typhus were recognized as different diseases thereafter.

GERHARDT, CARL JAKOB CHRISTIAN ADOLF (1833–1902). German physician. In 1865 he devised the ferric chloride test for *ketone bodies (Gerhardt's test). In 1887 he diagnosed laryngeal carcinoma in Prince (later Emperor) Frederick.

GERIATRICIAN. A physician who specializes in the health, care, social welfare, and diseases of old people. 'Old' is usually taken to mean over the age of 65. See GERIATRIC MEDICINE.

GERIATRIC MEDICINE (GERIATRICS) is a specialty of medicine concerned with the care of old people. A related term, gerontology, was coined to designate the study of ageing, but it is etymologically incorrect as it implies study restricted to old men (γέρουτζ). The correct term for the study of age (γῆραζ) and ageing is geratology. Social gerontology is concerned with the social processes that impinge on ageing and contribute to its manifestations; biological gerontology deals with the nature and origins of the processes in the cell and the organism that cause senescence.

The nature of ageing

Ageing in the sense of senescence is a progressive loss of adaptability of an organism as time passes. As we grow older the homeostatic mechanisms on which survival depends become on average less sensitive, less accurate, slower, and less well-sustained. Sooner or later we encounter one of the everyday challenges of life to which we can no longer mount an adaptive response and we die. A rise in mortality rate with age is therefore the biological hallmark of ageing. In the human this rise begins around the age of 11 to 13 years and, apart from perturbations due to violent deaths in early adult life, it is continuous and close to exponential thereafter. Measures of the prevalence of chronic disease and disability and use of health services also show a broadly exponential and continuous relationship with age through adult life. There are no discontinuities in later life that could provide a biological justification for separating the elderly from the rest of the adult human race. Moreover, we age at different rates, so that interindividual variance increases with age. Although on average functional abilities decline with age, some individuals aged 80 will still be performing within the normal range for 30-year-old people. In terms of diagnosis and treatment it is important that the treatment of an older person should be devised on an assessment of his or her *physiology and not on the basis of age. Properly selected and cared for, older people can profit as well as younger from the interventions of modern medicine, such as *intensive care, *cardiac surgery, and renal *dialysis. Unhappily, owing to ageist prejudice they may be denied appropriate access to such services.

Medical implications of ageing

Four important characteristics of disease in later life can be identified. The longer we live the more time we have to accumulate diseases and disabilities, and *multiple *pathology* is common among old people who fall ill. The reductionist tradition of seeking a unifying diagnosis for a patient's manifold symptoms and signs may mislead a doctor encountering an old person who may be more likely to be suffering from two or three common diseases than from one rare one. Interactions between multiple diseases and their treatments are a further source of difficulty in the practice of geriatric medicine.

Because of loss of adaptability, diseases may have a cryptic, atypical, or *non-specific presentation*. Inflammatory responses are slower in many old people, so that a *pneumonia may present as a *delirium before signs are apparent in the chest or before the *leucocyte count and temperature have risen. Visceral pain sensation may also be reduced so that myocardial infarction (*coronary thrombosis) or perforation of an abdominal viscus may present as sudden collapse or disorientation without complaint of pain. Loss of adaptability also results in *rapid deterioration* of an older patient if correct treatment is not instituted. Furthermore there will be a *high incidence of secondary complications* of the disease and of its treatment, and for these to be recognized and dealt with promptly, intensive vigilance from medical and nursing staff is required. For all these reasons older people who fall ill need urgent access to the best of modern diagnostic and therapeutic facilities, and will, on average, need more investigations than do younger adults if a comparable precision of *diagnosis is to be obtained.

In addition to these four implications of ageing for acute care, age-associated loss of adaptability has implications for the further management of illness in older people, and for their return to life in their own homes. Most younger adults usually have sufficient functional reserve to recover spontaneously from illness; more old people will require a specific programme of *rehabilitation*. As a specific example, most women aged 80 in Western societies do not have enough muscle bulk or strength to rise from an armless chair without help from their arms or from another person. A few days of immobility because of a brief self-limiting illness such as *influenza may lead to further critical loss of strength, which renders the victim bed-bound unless *physiotherapy is provided to facilitate the recovery of strength and confidence.

Loss of adaptability also makes a person more *vulnerable to the environment*. Depressing, ambiguous, or frightening surroundings in hospital can demoralize or confuse an older person. At home there may be an 'ecological gap' between what old people can do and what their housing demands of them. They may not be able to get upstairs to the only toilet in the house, for example, or may not be able to use the telephone to call for any help they may need. Good-quality care needs to pay scrupulous attention to bridging such gaps, either by improving the patient's function (a therapeutic intervention) or reducing the demands of the environment (a prosthetic intervention). Such matters may make the difference between an old lady living happily in her own home and a withdrawn and miserable resident of an institution.

The bridging of such ecological gaps requires a multidisciplinary approach to their assessment, and a detailed knowledge of the facilities available in hospital and community. Specialist geriatric teams have a core membership (in alphabetical order) of doctor, nurse, *occupational therapist, physiotherapist, and *social worker, and this team should be involved in preparing vulnerable old people for discharge from hospital. The multidisciplinary team and the knowledge leading to appropriate and cost-efficient *use of complex community resources* are among the particular characteristics of geriatric medicine as a service specialty.

Components of human ageing

The investigation of human ageing usually starts by identifying and measuring differences between young and old people, but not all such differences are due to ageing. *True ageing* comprises changes that have actually occurred to individuals as they have grown older but other differences, although frequently mistaken for ageing, are due to other factors. Because of *selective survival* people who reach old age will be different from those who died in middle age. This has been demonstrated for some *genetic factors, and selective survival is probably also associated with life-style and personality factors.

If ageing is characterized by loss of adaptability, it can be assessed biologically only by presenting the same challenge to individuals and measuring their responses. *Differential challenge* refers to the fact that society is organized in such a way that older people tend to be offered more severe challenges than face the young, and then their poor outcome is attributed to age. Thus 20 years ago it was clear that old people in Britain became *hypothermic not only because of age-associated changes in metabolism, but also because, for various reasons, they were living in colder houses than younger adults. Nowadays the most gross examples of differential challenge are found in the health services, where old people are on average offered worse treatment and care than are the young. This has been documented in the USA in comparisons of the time spent by doctors in taking a history from patients of different ages and in the quality of treatment offered to younger and older *cancer patients. In Britain older patients have been shown to have poorer access to *nephrology care, to cardiological investigation and surgery, and to *coronary care and thrombolytic therapy.

Cohort effects are most prominent in the field of mental functioning, in societies which, like our own, have been changing rapidly over the past century. Intelligence takes different forms in different cultures and the society for which older people were educated was very different from that in which the young are now being brought up. In longitudinal studies, where we are tested against our own former selves rather than against other people younger than ourselves, it is found that mental function declines less and later than appears in cross-sectional studies.

True ageing is caused by an interaction between *intrinsic* (genetic) effects and *extrinsic* (environmental and life-style) factors. Single *genes with a powerful effect on lifespan have been identified in some experimental animals, but in man lifespan and ageing rate seem to be polygenically determined. The most widely accepted theory is that the intrinsic ageing rate is largely determined by the effectiveness of the body's systems for detection and repair of environmentally induced damage to cells and their components. Although the intrinsic rate of ageing in man has slowed during his evolution, T. B. L. Kirkwood has demonstrated that the process of natural selection will not produce repair and detection mechanisms sufficiently accurate to prevent senescence totally.

The significance of extrinsic influences on ageing lies in the scope for prevention and reversibility. Some life-style and environmental factors may have an irreversible impact in early life. The effect of childhood calcium intake on bone mass may prove to be one example. The work of D. J. P. Barker and colleagues suggests that the lifetime susceptibility to some diseases with a significant effect on longevity may be determined partly before birth through dietary and life-style influences acting on pregnant women. In contrast, evidence is accumulating of the benefits of life-style change in middle life and old age, both in terms of recovering lost function and in retarding further deterioration. Courses of physical exercise by old people can improve muscle strength, for example, and giving up smoking can reduce coronary heart disease risk even in late life. Among several age-associated changes or diseases thought at one time to be due to intrinsic ageing but now known to have significant extrinsic determinants are vascular disease, high *blood pressure, loss of muscle bulk and strength, *osteoporosis and fractures, high tone *deafness, and the majority of cancers.

Demography of ageing

The numbers and proportions of older people are increasing in both the developed and developing world. Already more than half of the world's population of people aged over 65 live in developing countries. The *World Health Organization (WHO) has a Global Programme concerned with ageing, and some international charities and agencies are directing attention to the plight of older people in developing countries. During economic development, agrarian cultures break down and traditional forms of family support for old people may be disrupted by industrialization, migration of young families to urban centres, and changes in cultural values and responsibilities. Economic development rarely includes provision for health and social services to replace the traditional structures which it destroys.

Two processes lead to the ageing of populations. The first is the so-called *demographic transition*. When a nation reaches a certain stage of economic development its infant and child mortality rates start to fall steeply, but it usually takes another 20 or 30 years for fertility and mean family size to fall commensurately. A bolus of unprecedented survivors from childhood is therefore released into the population, eventually to become old. At a later stage of economic development mortality rates in middle age and later will also fall, thus increasing the numbers of survivors into old age. This latter change is now well established in the UK and other developed countries. It is unclear whether it represents a general improvement in health so that the new survivors into old age will be fitter than their predecessors, or an increased survival of people with chronic illness and disability so that older people are becoming less fit. Probably both effects are operating but affecting different diseases, so leading to changes in the causes and pattern of disability in later life without major alteration in the overall numbers of people affected.

Declines in mortality in middle age are producing increasing numbers of people in contemporary Europe who fall into the category of the Third Age. The Third Age citizen is one who has completed his or her main career and has perhaps raised a family, but from the age of 55 or so has 20 or more years of potentially enjoyable life ahead. There is increasing concern about a lack of social planning, including appropriate provision for the prevention and treatment of ill-health, for this large population group.

The history of geriatric medicine

The commonly expressed idea that old age and its associated diseases and disabilities are recent phenomena is a misapprehension. Several of the world's ancient texts refer to the infirmities of old age. As recognized by Dr John Smith FRCP in 1666, one of the most poignant allegorical descriptions of the disabilities of later life can be found in Chapter 12 of Ecclesiastes.

Early medical writers also noted accurately the common afflictions of old age, from which some hints of the epidemiology of age-associated disease and disability through the ages may be gleaned. *Hippocrates (460–370 BC) noted urinary difficulties, constipation, *apoplexy, *pruritus, *cataract, hardness of hearing, and joint pains as being common in later life. In his second book of rhetoric, *Aristotle offered some unflattering comments on the thinking and conversation of old men. He noted that, because they had often been disappointed in life, they tended to be pessimistic and cautious in expressing opinions and favoured expediency rather than honour. We can perhaps recognize here the conflict between the idealistic impetuosity of youth and the experienced caution of maturity that remains familiar today.

Because it is assumed that life expectancy at birth must have been low in ancient Greece, the old men of whom Aristotle wrote are sometimes presented as perhaps being only in their forties. This is to misunderstand the implications of life expectancy in undeveloped communities, where the carnage that reduces life expectancy takes place in infancy and childhood. Once past those early years, fitness may be high because of the intense natural selection the survivors have been through. Longevity in the presence of the presumed low life expectancy at birth is actually well documented in classical Greece. Sophocles died at 91, Euripides at 78, Plato at 81, Isocrates at 98, and all were still active. Agesilaus, King of Sparta, died in his eighties on the way back from commanding an active military campaign in Egypt.

Patterns of survival in the Roman Empire may have been different owing to the intensive urbanization of life, the frequency of epidemic diseases, and, possibly, endemic lead poisoning due to the use of lead acetate as a sweetening agent in cooking. Cicero considered that old age began at 46, but this might have reflected the age at which a rich Roman was able to retire, rather than an age at which faculties began to fail. At the time of the Emperor Tiberius, *Celsus presented a description of the diseases of old age very similar to, and perhaps derived from, that of Hippocrates, but he added some useful observations on *stroke, raising the possibility that this may have been a common affliction in Imperial Rome. *Aretaeus the Cappadocian, writing in the second century, described an irreversible dotage as a calamity of old age; this may be one of the earliest descriptions of senile *dementia.

In his *Canon of medicine*, *Avicenna, physician to the Caliphs of Baghdad (980–1036) noted four ages of man, the period of growth, the prime, a period of elderly decline, and finally decrepit old age. Avicenna's recommendations for elderly people, emphasizing a well-chosen diet and the benefits of a temperate and well-ordered life, were later extolled by several writers, including Maimonides in the 12th century, Luigi Cornaro in the 16th, and George Cheyne in the 18th.

Francis Bacon set out a programme for observational research linking longevity with environmental and lifestyle factors that would give him an excellent claim to the intellectual fatherhood both of modern *epidemiology and geratology. An empirical approach to the clinical medicine of old age did not emerge, however, until the 19th century. *Charcot's lectures on the 'Diseases of old age', translated into English by William Tuke in 1881, provided a detailed, albeit nosologically flawed description of some of the common diseases of later life. G. M. Humphry published in 1889 a survey of 900 people aged over 80; this was the first essay on the social circumstances of older people in the general population.

The American physician I. L. Nascher (1863–1944) coined the term 'geriatrics' in his seminal textbook *Geriatrics: the diseases of old age and their treatment*, published in 1914. He considered that there was an analogy to be drawn between geriatrics and *paediatrics. There is some social justification for this view in the vulnerability of ill old people and their frequent need for help from family members and others. The biological analogy is dubious since there are few, if any, diseases that only older people suffer from that correspond to the *inborn errors of metabolism, and for example, *Kawasaki disease or *Reye's syndrome that are exclusive to the practice of paediatrics. Nascher also established the tradition of attempting to distinguish between physiological and pathological ageing, which had the unfortunate consequence of offering doctors a rationale for disclaiming responsibility for any problems of their aged patients that are not classified as pathological.

The origins of geriatrics as a medical specialty accepting global responsibility for the physical, mental, and social well-being of older people lie with the pioneer work of Marjorie Warren at the West Middlesex Hospital in the late 1930s. She noted that many elderly patients consigned to the long-stay wards were capable of a better life if offered proper medical diagnosis and rehabilitation. When the *National Health Service was established in the UK, responsibility for the old workhouse hospitals in which most of the long-stay patients were confined fell upon the same health authorities as those involved with the traditionally more privileged charity hospitals which had previously concerned themselves with the acute and curable illnesses of the middle classes and 'deserving poor'. With support and encouragement from medical officers in the *Department of Health, the specialty of geriatrics was created in order to discharge this new responsibility. Unfortunately, despite the skill and dedication of some of its founding figures, the new specialty was for many years regarded as one to which only those doctors who had failed to make careers for themselves in more desirable specialties would be recruited. Forty years on, with more than 800 consultants and over 150 training posts, geriatrics has won its spurs as the second largest adult medical specialty in Britain.

There are now several different approaches to providing geriatric services in Britain, and the specialty is more usefully defined in terms of the responsibilities it accepts rather than the specific duties it undertakes. Geriatric medicine remains largely a hospital-based specialty, but with close links with community agencies. Three main models of geriatric service now exist in the UK. In the *traditional model* of service, geriatric departments largely restrict their activities to those patients specifically referred to them for assessment, rehabilitation, and long-stay care. In the *age-defined model*, geriatric departments provide all medical services for patients above a specified age referred to hospital. In the *integrated model*, physicians with special responsibility for the elderly provide specialist expertise in the care of older people in the context, for acute care, of multidisciplinary teams of consultants working with the same nursing and junior medical staff. In all three models, geriatric services offer rehabilitation, day hospital, out-patient services, home visiting, and some long-stay care in addition to acute care. Respite care is also provided in which elderly patients can be admitted on scheduled or occasional short-term stays to help in supporting informal carers.

Geriatrics is a recognized specialty in only four countries of the European Community (UK, Irish Republic, Spain, and The Netherlands) and the British approach to incorporating the specialty into health services has not been replicated elsewhere, except in some centres in Australia and New Zealand. In North America the emphasis has been on geriatric assessment units or teams taking selected older patients from other specialties largely for rehabilitation and resettlement in the community. In contrast to the British services, which have never been adequately evaluated, North American models have been subjected to randomized controlled trials, clearly demonstrating their efficacy in terms of cost-effective improvements in survival and functional abilities.

In recent years public and political interest in ageing has focused increasingly on the preventive and *public health aspects of control of disease and disability in later life. At the same time, improved technology is making many specialist medical and surgical interventions more appropriate for frailer patients. *Primary care is also becoming more sensitive to the needs of older people. All these factors may reduce the role of the conventionally trained British geriatrician. It seems likely that if this happens the specialty will continue to discharge its mission of special responsibility for older people through generalist secondary care, in tertiary care rehabilitation, or even to some extent within the remit of other specialties such as *cardiology, *anaesthetics, or *gastroenterology.

Academic developments

The first journal concerned with the medicine of old age appeared in Germany in the 1930s, and there is now a considerable number of specialist journals in the field. The Gerontological Society of America was founded in 1945, dedicated to fostering research on all aspects of ageing to inform public policy. The British Geriatrics Society was founded in the 1950s and many countries have national societies dedicated to geratology or geriatrics. The International Association of Gerontology provides an umbrella organization within which workers from the clinical, sociological, and biological fields can meet simultaneously every 4 years. Professorial chairs in geriatric medicine are now found at most medical schools in Britain, and many in Italy, and are increasing in numbers in North America. In Europe, chairs are also established in the Nordic countries, the Irish Republic, Switzerland, The Netherlands, and Spain. Chairs have also been established in Australia, New Zealand, and a few other countries.

In the early 1940s the US National Institutes of Health established a gerontology unit in Baltimore; it became the Gerontology Research Center in 1966. For 35 years from 1941 its research programme was directed by Nathan W. Shock. In 1974 the National Institute on Ageing was established under the directorship of Dr R. N. Butler whose influential book *Why survive? Growing old in America* had stimulated great public and political concern about the inadequacies of medical and social provision for the growing numbers of aged people in the electorate of the USA. The Institute provides dedicated funding to intramural and extramural research in all aspects of ageing. Ageing as a field of specific scientific endeavour has received little dedicated funding in other countries. In England geratological research flourished for a time with *Medical Research Council (MRC) funding. Dr Alex Comfort published the first edition of his unique review of the field *The biology of senescence* in 1956, and stimulated a series of symposia on ageing under the auspices of the CIBA Foundation. Also in the 1950s A. T. Welford in Cambridge directed a unit concerned with the *psychology of ageing. Withdrawal of MRC support led to Britain's loss of both these pioneer workers in ageing; Alex Comfort went to California, A.T. Welford to Australia.

There are five main lines of development in geratological research. *Nosological research* has identified and classified diseases of later life. Early work demonstrated that some diseases thought to be rare in elderly people, *motor neurone disease for example, were merely being underdiagnosed. More recently apparently unitary diagnoses, such as senile dementia, are being shown to be heterogeneous, subsuming a range of disorders which may carry different prognoses and respond differently to treatment. *Health services research* has examined and compared different modes of delivery of care to older people. *Clinical research* has ranged from descriptive studies of the physiology of later life, through drug trials, to enzymological studies of ageing tissues in animals and man. Research in the basic *cellular processes* of ageing has accelerated enormously as a result of the newer techniques of *molecular medicine. The recent identification of single gene mutations with a significant effect on lengthening lifespan in experimental animals offers particular promise for unravelling the metabolic processes determining lifespan.

The fifth tradition of geratological research is that of *theoretical biology*. Theoretical aspects of the biology of ageing have been addressed by a distinguished succession of scientists. Some of the predictions of theory can now be put to experimental tests, using large colonies of short-lived laboratory species such as the fruit-fly *Drosophila* and the nematode *Caenorhabditis*.

The future

The immediate future of the medicine of old age will be dominated by the provision of appropriate care for the increasing numbers of elderly people in the world. 'Appropriate' in this context must include the ability of the recipient to benefit (clinically appropriate) and the availability of resources (economically appropriate). As technology advances, more health interventions will become less challenging physiologically and therefore clinically appropriate for more old and frail people. Economic constraints will mean that ethical questions relating to the use of age as a criterion in health care rationing will have to be debated. In the longer term, further ethical problems may arise if prolongation of maximum lifespan becomes possible through genetic manipulation. It is likely that the central issue will be seen not as the virtue inherent in life prolongation itself, but rather what benefits the intervention brings through the prevention of age-associated disabilities.

J. GRIMLEY EVANS

Further reading
Butler, R. N. (1975). *Why survive? Being old in America*. Harper and Row, New York.
Comfort, A. (1979). *The biology of senescence*, (3rd edn). Churchill Livingstone, Edinburgh.
Finch, C. E. (1990). *Longevity, senescence and the genome*. University of Chicago Press, Chicago.
Grimley Evans, J. and Williams, T. F. (1992). *The Oxford textbook of geriatric medicine*. Oxford University Press.
Kane, R. L., Grimley Evans, J., and Macfadyen, D. (eds) (1990). *Improving the health of older people; a world view*. Oxford University Press.

GERONTOLOGY is the scientific study of *ageing and the biological processes involved therein. It is to be distinguished from *geriatrics, which is that branch of medicine concerned with diseases of older patients and the care of the aged.

GERONTOPHOBIA. A morbid dislike of old people; alternatively, a dread of growing old.

GESNER, KONRAD (1516–65). Swiss physician and botanist. He was a pioneer of bibliography, publishing *Bibliotheca universalis* (20 vols, 1545–49). He was the first to describe the canary and wrote *Historia plantarum* (1541) and *Historia animalium* (4 vols, 1551–58). His great work *Opera botanica* was never completed although he drew nearly 1500 plates for it.

GESTALTISM, or gestalt psychology, is a school of *psychology concerned with perception, which developed from about 1914 as a reaction against traditional association psychology. The central tenet is that building up images by piece-by-piece association is not the only basis of perceptual processes, but that patterns, configurations, and forms ('gestalt' is German for 'form') can be recognized as integrated entities on the basis of previous experience. When presented by a trick drawing, which can be recognized either as a vase or as two separate human profiles, the image that is immediately perceived is determined by such experience.

GESTATION is the development of the fertilized *ovum in viviparous animals during the period between conception and birth. Calculated from the beginning of the last menstrual period rather than the date of conception, the average duration of gestation in the human is 40 weeks.

GIANT CELLS are large cells formed by the fusion of several *macrophages, characteristic of foreign-body *granuloma reactions.

GIANTS, in medicine, are those whose height exceeds 2.0 m (80 in), or children who exceed the mean height for their age by three standard deviations or more. They either represent the extreme end of the normal distribution curve, or are suffering from an endocrine abnormality, usually pituitary *gigantism. To judge from the list of those exhibited in London during the 19th century and therefore presumably authentic, giants rarely exceed 2.44 m (8ft) in height (Chang Woo-Goo, the Chinese giant from Fychon, who was exhibited in 1865 and again in 1889, was 2.49 m (8ft 2 in)). Reports of greater stature are of course legion, for example Goliath at 6 cubits and a span was 3.40 m (11 ft 3 in) (but only if the cubit is accepted as 0.53 m (21 in) and a span 0.23 m (9 in)); and Eleazer, sent to Rome by Vitellius, was over 3.66 m (12ft, 7 cubits).

In Greek mythology giants were the sons of Ge who heaped Ossia on Pelion in order to scale the walls of Heaven and dethrone Zeus; with the aid of Hercules they were defeated and entombed under Mount Etna. In Scandinavian mythology giants were evil beings dwelling in Jotunheim and able to control their stature at will. The giants of nursery mythology (e.g. Galligantus, Blunderbore, Bellygan) were little better.

GIARDIA LAMBLIA is a flagellated *protozoan of low to moderate pathogenicity, formerly thought to be a harmless intestinal *commensal but now recognized as a cause of *diarrhoea, abdominal pain or discomfort, flatulence, and *malabsorption when heavy infection of the small intestine occurs. Light infections are probably asymptomatic. Giardiasis is one of the infections which may complicate immune deficiency syndromes. It should also be considered in the differential diagnosis of traveller's diarrhoea, particularly where symptoms do not develop until several weeks after the patient has returned home. It is sensitive to *metronidazole.

GIBBON, JOHN HEYSHAM Jr (1903–74). American surgeon. He designed a *heart–lung apparatus which was used successfully in open-heart surgery (see CARDIOTHORACIC SURGERY).

GIBBUS. A hunchback, humpback, or crookback; forward angulation of the spine (*kyphosis).

GIDDINESS is synonymous with *dizziness.

GIEMSA, BERTHOLD GUSTAV CARL (1867–1948). German pharmacist. He worked in the Institut für Schiffs- und Tropenkrankheiten in Hamburg and introduced his modification of *Romanowsky's stain for blood cells in 1890.

GIGANTISM. Stature over 2.0 m (80 in) is taken as pathological (see GIANTS). The usual cause is hypersecretion of *pituitary growth hormone beginning in childhood, before the *epiphyses of the long bones have fused. The other manifestations are those of *acromegaly.

GILBERT, THE ENGLISHMAN (Gilbertus Anglicus) (*fl.* 1250). A British physician who studied and practised abroad. Gilbert is known chiefly on account of his book *Compendium medicinae* or *Lilium medicinae*, the contents of which were mostly borrowed from the Arabs but did include some records of his own experiences.

GILBERT, WILLIAM (1540–1603). British physician and physicist. His interest in magnetism led to the publication in 1600 of his major treatise on the subject, *De magnete, magneticisque corporibus, et de magno magnete tellure*. Perhaps his outstanding contribution was the hypothesis that the properties of the lodestone were related to the fact that the Earth itself also acted as a magnet. He also dispelled the confusion then existing between static electricity and magnetism by carefully distinguishing the attractive qualities of rubbed amber (the amber effect) from those of the lodestone. He was also the first Englishman to espouse the Copernican view of the universe.

GILLES DE LA TOURETTE SYNDROME is a severe form of multiple *tic, in which convulsive vocal sounds, including *coprolalia, accompany the motor spasms. It now seems that the syndrome (also known as *maladie des tics* or convulsive tic) has an organic basis due to a disorder of dopaminergic neurones; it is often relieved by phenothiazine drugs such as *haloperidol.

GILLIES, SIR HAROLD DELF (1882–1960). Anglo-New Zealand plastic surgeon. As an officer in the Royal Army Medical Corps Gillies organized a unit for facial injuries in the First World War and later became the acknowledged 'father of plastic surgery'.

GINGIVITIS is inflammation of the gums.

GLAND. Any specialized structure which elaborates and secretes or excretes chemical substances, the action or function of which takes place elsewhere than in the gland itself. The primary classification of glands is into *exocrine and endocrine (*ductless).

GLANDERS is a bacterial infection of horses, asses, and mules, occasionally transmitted to domestic animals and man. Human infection is rare, and now virtually unknown in Europe and the USA; it is, however, very dangerous, untreated glanders carrying a mortality rate reported to be over 90 per cent. The disease may affect the skin or lungs and is accompanied by severe general symptoms. The causative organism, *Pseudomonas mallei*, is an aerobic, non-motile, Gram-negative *bacillus. It is susceptible to *sulphonamides and also to *antibiotics. See VETERINARY MEDICINE.

GLANDULAR FEVER. See INFECTIOUS MONONUCLEOSIS.

GLAUBER, JOHANN RUDOLPH (1604–70). German physician and chemist. He discovered a number of salts, including sodium sulphate, *sal mirabile* or *Glauber's salt.

GLAUBER'S SALT is hydrated sodium sulphate ($Na_2SO_4.10H_2O$), also known as saltcake; it is employed in the manufacture of soap, detergents, and dyes, and was formerly used as a *purgative.

GLAUCOMA is increased intraocular pressure, usually of unknown cause, when it may occur in more than one family member; it is less often due to identifiable pathological changes (e.g. *iritis) obstructing the reabsorption of aqueous humour in the angle between the *iris and *cornea (the filtration angle). Pharmacological or surgical treatment is essential if normal vision is to be preserved. In the minority of cases where glaucoma develops acutely, relief is urgently required. See OPHTHALMOLOGY.

GLEET. A mucoid *urethral discharge, most often due to *gonorrhoea.

GLIA is synonymous with *neuroglia.

GLIOMA. One of a group of tumours of the central nervous system derived from *neuroglia.

GLIOSIS is proliferation of *neuroglial elements in areas of damage to nervous tissue, analogous to *fibrosis outside the nervous system.

GLISSON, FRANCIS (1597–1677). British physician. He published *De rachitide* (1650) and *Anatomia hepatis* (1654). In the latter he describes the *integument of the liver, now known as Glisson's capsule.

GLOBIN is the *protein (polypeptide) moiety of *haemoglobin and similar molecules, such as *myoglobin.

GLOBULIN comprises a large class of *proteins lacking a prosthetic group, soluble in dilute saline solutions but not in water; they are widely distributed in plants and animals. Those in the circulating *blood may be divided into *immunoglobulins and non-immune globulins, the former synthesized by *lymphocytes and *plasma cells, the latter by the *liver. The non-immune globulins have various functions, including the binding and transport of lipids, steroids, non-functioning haemoglobin, copper, and iron; *prothrombin, the coagulation factor, is a globulin.

GLOBUS HYSTERICUS. The mistaken belief that there is a lump in the throat, giving rise to a sensation of choking or difficulty in swallowing.

GLOMERULONEPHRITIS is inflammation of the renal *glomeruli, formerly known as *Bright's disease. See NEPHROLOGY.

GLOMERULUS. A small bulb of blood *capillaries covered by thin epithelium projecting into the capsule of each *renal tubule in the vertebrate. The human kidney contains about a million such units. See NEPHROLOGY.

GLOMUS. Any of a number of small anatomical structures consisting chiefly of a rich plexus of blood vessels with an abundant nerve supply. They have either a *chemoreceptor or an arteriovenous *anastomotic function.

GLOSSITIS is inflammation of the tongue.

GLOSSOPHARYNGEAL NERVE. The ninth cranial nerve arises from the *medulla oblongata and leaves the skull through the jugular foramen with the tenth (*vagus) nerve. It is a mixed nerve, supplying motor fibres to the *pharynx and sensory (taste) fibres to the back of the tongue, the *fauces, the *nasopharynx, and the ear; it also carries parasympathetic fibres to the *parotid gland, and afferent fibres from the *chemoreceptors and *baroceptors of the *carotid sinus and body.

GLOSSOPHARYNGEAL NEURALGIA is a condition closely resembling trigeminal neuralgia (see TIC DOULOUREUX) but occurring within the sensory distribution of the *glossopharyngeal nerve.

GLOTTIS. The opening of the *larynx, comprising the vocal cords and the space between them.

GLUCAGON is a *polypeptide *hormone stored in and released by the alpha cells of the *islets of Langerhans. It raises the blood sugar by stimulating the hepatic breakdown of *glycogen (glycogenolysis); its action thus opposes that of *insulin. Several factors may promote the secretion of glucagon: they include pituitary *growth hormone, *hypoglycaemia, starvation and other forms of stress (e.g. trauma, exercise), and some dietary *amino acids (arginine, alanine).

GLUCOCORTICOID. Any of the group of *corticosteroids which act predominantly on carbohydrate, fat, and protein metabolism, i.e. cortisol and its analogues.

GLUCOSE is the simple hexose *sugar (monosaccharide), $C_6H_{12}O_6$, the end-product of metabolic breakdown of the higher *carbohydrates and the body's major source of energy; its combustion to carbon dioxide and water provides 17.2 kJ/g. It is also known as dextrose.

GLUCOSE 6-PHOSPHATE DEHYDROGENASE (G6PD) is an *enzyme which catalyses the dehydrogenation of glucose 6-phosphate to 6-phosphogluconolactone, initiating the pentose phosphate pathway of *carbohydrate metabolism. *X-linked deficiency of this enzyme can render the individual liable to develop *haemolytic anaemia (see FAVISM), and in many countries it is associated with resistance to malarial infection.

GLUCOSE TOLERANCE TEST. A method of assessing the adequacy of *insulin secretion by the *pancreas. A glucose load is administered (100 g by mouth) to the fasting patient and the blood sugar is measured at half-hourly intervals. Normal function is indicated (assuming normal alimentary absorption) if the fasting level is less than 5.2 mmol/l (94 mg/dl), the half-hour peak less than 10 mmol/l (180 mg/dl), and the fasting level is restored within 2–2.5 hours.

GLUE-SNIFFING is commonest among adolescents in the USA and in the UK. The solvent usually concerned is toluene, cheaply available in model-aeroplane glue, but other industrial solvents are also employed, including *acetone, *benzene, diethyl *ether, hexane, and ethyl acetate. One method is to squeeze the glue on to a piece of cloth and inhale the vapour from a plastic bag. The resultant intoxication is said to be not unlike that produced by alcohol. Excitement, uninhibited and aggressive behaviour, *dysarthria, *ataxia, sleepiness, stupor, and nausea and vomiting may all occur, followed by a hangover. *Polyneuropathy is a serious complication. Opinion seems to differ as to whether glue-sniffing is truly *addictive. Almost all chronic glue-sniffers appear to be young people with considerable pre-existing personality difficulties.

GLUTATHIONE is a naturally occurring tripeptide which functions in the body as a respiratory *coenzyme. Its use has been suggested in treating conditions such as alcoholism, cirrhosis of the liver, skin disorders, and certain types of poisoning but there is no evidence that it is efficacious.

GLUTEN is the *protein of wheat flour, of which it comprises 8 to 15 per cent. It is important in the pathogenesis of *coeliac disease and non-tropical *sprue.

GLYCERYL TRINITRATE, also known as nitroglycerin or trinitrin, is a well-established agent for the prophylaxis and treatment of *angina pectoris. Like *amyl nitrite, it is a powerful smooth muscle relaxant and peripheral vasodilator. It is usually administered in tablets, which, to be effective, must be dissolved under the tongue and not swallowed. It is also important that they are freshly dispensed.

GLYCOGEN is 'animal starch', the carbohydrate storage substance of animals and fungi. Stored mainly in the liver and muscles, it is a *polysaccharide made up of large numbers of *glucose molecules.

GLYCOPROTEIN. A class of complex *proteins containing *carbohydrate groups (e.g. mucoproteins).

GLYCOSURIA is *glucose in the urine.

GNATHOSTOMA is a genus of *roundworms normally parasitic in wild felines and canines, the intermediate hosts of which are fish. Man is occasionally infected by eating raw fish, the syndrome associated with this infestation being that of 'wandering swellings' beneath the skin. It occurs in the East, notably India, Thailand, and China.

GNOSIS. Knowledge; cognition; an acquired skill involving the recognition of sensory information.

GNOTOBIOTICS is the study of germ-free animals and the techniques involved in rearing laboratory animals entirely free from micro-organisms or whose microflora can be precisely specified.

GOATS AS CARRIERS OF DISEASE. Malta fever is an unpleasant form of *brucellosis acquired by drinking goat's milk, and was common when goat's milk was widely consumed in Mediterranean countries. It can cause lifelong ill-health with recurrent and debilitating fever. Napoleon Bonaparte probably suffered from it. The causative organism is *Brucella melitensis*.

Another condition which may be transmitted by drinking goat's milk, especially in the former USSR, is Central European encephalitis, also known as biphasic meningoencephalitis. However, the causative virus is more often transmitted by tick bites.

Goats are occasionally responsible for other diseases. A superficial fungal *tinea infection, that due to *Trichophyton verrucosum*, affecting mainly the scalp and beard areas of skin, can be acquired from goats as well as from some other animals. Goats do, or at one time did, provide a reservoir of infection for the parasite *Schistosoma japonicum* (see BILHARZIA). The liver *fluke, *Fasciola hepatica*, can infect goats and there are some other *helminth infestations which can be passed from goats to man.

GODLEE, SIR RICKMAN JOHN, Bt (1849–1925). British surgeon. On 25 November 1884 he was the first to remove successfully a *cerebral tumour.

GOGARTY, OLIVER JOSEPH ST JOHN (1878–1957). Irish otolaryngologist, writer, wit, and bon vivant His wit was often directed against specific persons and he lost popularity because of his capacity 'to detect flaws without a compensatory restraint in publishing them'. His best-known book was *As I was going down Sackville Street* (1937). He was also the origin of stately, plump Buck Mulligan, in *Ulysses*, the novel written by his friend James Joyce.

GOITRE (GOITER) is enlargement of the *thyroid gland, usually visible and palpable, and moving upwards on swallowing. The enlargement may be symmetrical or asymmetrical, diffuse or nodular, soft or firm to hard; increased vascularity is indicated by a systolic or continuous *bruit on auscultation over the lobes. In *thyrotoxicosis, enlargement tends to be smooth, diffuse, and vascular (*Graves disease) or nodular (toxic nodular goitre); in *Hashimoto's disease (autoimmune thyroiditis) and thyroid *carcinoma, the consistency is firm or hard, the more so with carcinoma. Most goitres, however, are 'simple', that is, associated with none of these conditions. In many, if not all, thyroid enlargement results from stimulation of the gland by the *thyroid-stimulating hormone (TSH) of the anterior *pituitary. Both *iodine deficiency and iodine excess produce goitre via this mechanism as may ingestion of several chemical *goitrogens. Goitrogens act by inhibiting either the trapping of iodine by the thyroid gland or its subsequent synthesis to thyroid hormone. As well as drugs used to treat hyperthyroidism (*carbimazole, *thiouracil, perchlorate), they include cyanates, *lithium, cobalt, resorcinol, *para-aminosalicylic acid, and vegetables of the genus *Brassica* ('cabbage goitre'). Slight goitre can be physiological, particularly in young women.

GOITROGEN. Any substance causing enlargement of the thyroid gland, that is which produces *goitre.

GOLD has been used in treating *rheumatoid arthritis since 1929. Gold salts have an action on *collagen and *synovial membrane, but how they work remains uncertain. Gold is said to be the best treatment for arresting progression of the arthritis, particularly in early cases. It can, however, have serious side-effects, particularly on the kidneys, liver, brain, and blood, and its use requires skill and experience.

GOLDBERGER, JOSEPH (1874–1929). American public health officer. Goldberger studied many infectious diseases in Cuba and in the southern USA. He became interested in *pellagra and showed it to be a nutritional deficiency in people whose dietary staples were pork fat and hominy. Later the specific nature of the deficiency was shown to be lack of *niacin (nicotinic acid or nicotinamide). See also EPIDEMIOLOGY.

GOLDBLATT, HARRY (1891–1977). American experimental pathologist. He helped to develop the Autotechnicon apparatus for fixing and staining tissues for histological study. He is best known for showing that clamping the renal artery in dogs results in *hypertension.

GOLDSMITH, OLIVER (1730?–74). Anglo-Irish physician and writer. He practised in Southwark in 1756 and in 1758 was examined for the post of naval surgeon at Surgeons' Hall, but found 'not qualifyd'. In 1761 he met Samuel Johnson and later became a member of 'the Club'. He made another attempt at practice in 1765, but with no more success. David Garrick said of him 'he wrote like an angel, but talked like poor Poll'. His most renowned works were *The vicar of Wakefield* (1766), *The deserted village* (1770), and *She stoops to conquer* (1773).

GOLFER'S ELBOW is inflammation of the muscle tendons around the medial *epicondyle of the elbow.

GOLGI, CAMILLO (1843–1926). Italian pathologist. His work was mainly on the histology and pathology of the central nervous system. He broke fresh ground with the silver impregnation methods he devised in 1873. He described the intracellular *Golgi apparatus and the nerve endings in muscle known as the *Golgi organs. In 1886 he showed that *malarial rigor coincided with the parasite's sporulation, and in 1889 differentiated the quartan and tertian parasites. He shared the *Nobel prize for medicine with *Ramon y Cajal in 1906.

GOLGI APPARATUS is a complex intracellular structure (*organelle) forming part of the internal membrane system connected with the *endoplasmic reticulum, from which secretory *vacuoles containing newly synthesized compounds bud off and migrate to the cell surface. Although the function of the Golgi apparatus (also known as the Golgi body, Golgi network, or Golgi complex) is not fully understood, it seems to be concerned with secretion and with linking *carbohydrate groups to *protein molecules in the formation of *glycoproteins. See CELL AND CELL BIOLOGY.

GOLGI ORGANS are sensory *receptors found in mammalian tendons, also known as Golgi tendon organs, Golgi corpuscles, or Golgi tendon spindles. They are stimulated by muscle tension.

GONADOTROPHIN is one of the *hormones controlling *gonadal function; it is secreted by the anterior *pituitary and by the *placenta.

GONADS. *Gamete-producing organs. In humans they are the *ovary (female) and *testis (male), producing respectively *ova and *spermatozoa. In humans, as in other vertebrates, the gonads also secrete sex *hormones.

GONIOMETER. An instrument for measuring angles, for example in determining the limits of flexion and extension of a joint.

GONOCOCCUS is the causative organism of *gonorrhoea, *Neisseria gonorrhoeae*, a Gram-negative aerobic *diplococcus.

GONORRHOEA (GONORRHEA) is one of the commonest of sexually transmitted diseases (STD), caused by infection with the gonococcus (*Neisseria gonorrhoeae*). The infection is primarily urethral in men, and urethral and/or endocervical in women; the main symptom is a purulent urethral discharge, though in women the initial infection often passes unnoticed. Many complications can result from untreated gonorrhoea; they include urethral stricture (men), pelvic inflammatory disease (women), and sterility (both sexes). Remote complications also occur, such as *dermatitis, *arthritis, *endocarditis, etc. See also SEXUALLY TRANSMITTED DISEASE.

GOODENOUGH REPORT. The report, published in May 1944, of an interdepartmental committee set up by the British government under the chairmanship of Sir William Goodenough 2 years earlier to enquire into the organization and future of medical education in the UK. Its recommendations laid down guidelines which British medical education has followed since then. See MEDICAL EDUCATION, UNDERGRADUATE.

GOODPASTURE, ERNEST WILLIAM (1886–1960). American pathologist and microbiologist. He became interested in viral infections of man, and was among the first to use the chick embryo for isolation and propagation of viruses. He also described a syndrome of human disease, probably immunogenic, in which there is *vasculitis in the small blood vessels of the kidneys and the lungs. This is still called Goodpasture's syndrome.

GORGAS, WILLIAM CRAWFORD (1854–1920). American military surgeon. In Cuba, after the Walter *Reed group had shown that *yellow fever is transmitted by mosquitoes, Gorgas instituted mosquito control measures and almost eradicated the disease in the Havana region. He then moved to Panama and, employing the same methods, reduced the mosquito population so that construction of the Panama Canal could be completed.

GORGET. A channel-shaped surgical instrument used in *lithotomy.

GOUGEROT, HENRI (1881–1955). Parisian dermatologist. He made contributions to the understanding of *lupus, *syphilis, and *leprosy, as well as *allergy. He delineated *sporotrichosis with Beurmann. He was the doyen of *dermatology in France, and syndromes of rosettes in polymorphs, purpura, and multiple skin nodules were named after him.

GOUT is an acute or chronic crystalline joint disease associated with increased *uric acid in the blood. It is one of the most ancient and most respectable of diseases, its clinical features having been well-known for at least two and a half millennia. A most important contribution of modern medical science has been to control the excess of uric acid with drugs designed to limit its production (the xanthine oxidase inhibitor *allopurinol) and to promote its excretion (uricosuric compounds such as *probenecid).

GOVERNMENT AND MEDICINE IN THE UK
Introduction
The first involvement of government in medicine in the UK was the introduction of measures to stop the spread of *infectious disease, particularly plague, through *quarantine. Henry VIII introduced a system for the quarantine of travellers from overseas and in 1543 Queen Elizabeth I issued *plague orders for the quarantine of ships. This was about two centuries later than in Mediterranean countries, where Venice was the chief port of entry for the Far East. Since then, there has been a gradual involvement of government in all aspects of medicine–population-based *public health, provision of personal curative and preventative care, financing of health care, education and regulation of health care workers, and medical research. These are dealt with separately below.

The development of population-based public health took place in a haphazard way as medical knowledge and capacity to intervene successfully developed and the financial costs of health-care delivery grew. A major milestone was the 1948 *National Health Service (NHS) Act, in which government accepted responsibility for the provision of a comprehensive preventive and curative service for the whole population, funded primarily through central taxation. Since then this aspect of government's involvement has dominated the relationship with medicine. This involvement has been considerable and often traumatic as the capacity of modern medicine to do more for an increasingly ageing population produced enormous cost pressures.

The health care delivery system was changed frequently, with *general practice being restructured in the 1960s and again in the late 1980s. The hospital and community health service were restructured in 1974, 1982, and 1992. Initially, development of the NHS was seen as non-political with broad agreement between the political parties on the need for change. Royal Commissions were the way to deal with problems. This consensus was broken by the Conservative government under Mrs Thatcher in the late 1980's.

Driven by public and professional disquiet in the apparent inability of the hospital system to meet the demands on it, the government set up a review into the financing and delivery of health care. This was conducted in private. It recommended the continuation of central taxation as the financing mechanism, but recommended sweeping changes in the delivery system. They are described in detail below, but in essence, separated the purchase of care from the delivery of care and sought to improve the efficiency of the delivery by introducing competition between hospitals and other providers of care, including the private sector. It provided widespread debate both within the health-care profession, the major political parties, and, to a lesser extent, the public. At the present time the government continues to refine the reforms and has yet to get agreement of the other political parties to support the way forward.

Government and public health
A series of quarantine Acts and Orders in Council directed against plague in the 17th and 18th centuries set the scene for the major public health interventions of the 19th century. The impetus was to tackle communicable disease, this time cholera. The first Public Health Act was passed in 1848 and was quickly followed by a period of major government involvement in sanitary reform, with government giving local bodies powers to act against private interests opposed to that reform. This included the appointment of *Medical Officers of Health, such as Duncan in Liverpool and Simon in London.

Much of this work was undertaken on the basis of completely erroneous beliefs about the causes and methods of the spread of communicable diseases. However, as knowledge developed, so too did government's involvement, discharging its responsibilities through local authorities. This expanded to personal preventive services when in 1918 local authorities were given responsibility for maternal and child health and school health services.

Local authorities continued to be responsible for public health until 1974. They were responsible for enforcing population-based measures such as food hygiene and environmental health regulations and personal preventive programmes such as the above-mentioned maternal and child health services and *tuberculosis control programmes.

In 1974 there was a major reorganization of public health, with local authorities retaining responsibility for broad-based public health measures relating to food hygiene and environmental health while personal preventive programmes become the responsibility of the NHS. This was not such a clear-cut split as the legislators had hoped for. It led to a period of considerable confusion, with the medical responsibilities and knowledge for infectious disease control lying with health authorities and the operational responsibilities lying with local authorities.

The present position is that government accepts that it has a responsibility for the health of the population. It discharges this partly through legislation covering the environment, safety, and infectious disease control. It ensures that local mechanisms are in place to enact that legislation–primarily local government authorities and health authorities. The latter are also responsible for individual- and population-based preventive health programmes.

The multidisciplinary nature of preventive health programmes is recognized at a central level with an interministry cabinet-level committee having responsibility for co-ordinating policy. The *Department of Health is the lead ministry. In 1992 it produced a major policy document, *The nation's health,* which set out a strategy and targets for reducing mortality and morbidity through preventive measures.

Inevitably there is debate between the responsibility of government and the responsibilities (and rights) of the individual. It is less of a problem with infectious disease control where there seems general acceptance that legislation is necessary to prevent unnecessary spread of infection. However, accident prevention and chronic disease prevention through legislation are more contentious.

The introduction of legislation making the wearing of seatbelts compulsory was contentious. Likewise the role of the government in reducing tobacco consumption. However, there would appear to be a general consensus at present that governments have responsibility for reducing unnecessary mortality and morbidity through accidents and chronic disease as well as infectious disease, and that public health interventions at national and local level, backed by legislation where necessary, must take place.

Government and personal health services

The involvement of government in personal curative health care is relatively recent. It started as a network of last-resort medical care under the Poor Law in the latter half of the nineteenth century (also see HOSPITALS IN THE UK). Other hospital care developed either based on descendants of monastic institutions or as new voluntary hospitals supported by charitable funds. These hospitals deliberately avoided the care of patients for whom local government hospitals were responsible–the elderly with chronic disease, the mentally ill and mentally handicapped, and those with infectious disease.

The government's first major involvement in the general provision of health care was the *National Health Insurance scheme of 1911 which provided general practitioner care for low-paid workers only–not their dependents.

In 1920 a committee under the chairmanship of the king's physician Lord *Dawson produced a report, *Future provision of medical and allied services.* It proposed a system of domiciliary care and primary-care centres staffed by *primary-care doctors, *dentists, *nurses, *pharmacists, *midwives, and *health visitors. This would be backed by specialists based in secondary-care services, supported in turn by the teaching centres. Although this was not acted upon immediately, it produced the framework on which the NHS was built in 1948.

Between 1920 and the Second World War the counties and the cities developed their own acute hospital services alongside the voluntary. It was obvious that some services were best provided to populations of millions rather than thousands, and the concept of regionalization for specialist services gradually developed. This was accelerated by preparation for the Second World War, during which emergency medical services were organized on a regional basis and funded by central government. This gradual involvement of government in personal health services culminated in 1948 in the NHS. This was not, as is commonly thought, an abrupt decision forced through by a post-war Labour government, but the logical conclusion of the gradual development referred to above, and had been discussed widely both by health professions and politicians.

The NHS Act (1946) which came into effect on 5 July 1948 set out provision for a health service, free at point of access, funded through general taxation. It became 'the duty of the Minister of Health to promote the establishment in England and Wales of a comprehensive health service designed to secure improvement in the physical and mental health of the people and the prevention, diagnosis and treatment of illness and for that purpose to provide or secure the effective provision of a service in accordance with the provisions of the Act. Services so provided shall be free of charge, except where any provision of the Act expressly provides for the making and recovery of charges'.

From 1948 to 1974 the NHS consisted of three branches brought together only at government level–a public health service run by local authorities, hospital and specialist services, and a framework for general practice provided by general practitioners. Certain functions were retained at a national level, such as the secure psychiatric hospitals and the Public Health Laboratory services. The hospital and specialist services were administered by a structured system of regional boards and hospital management committees, with regions defined on the principle that each region would have at least one medical school and associated teaching hospital to act as a focus for teaching research and tertiary care. The teaching hospitals and the London postgraduate hospitals were run by *Boards of Governors dealing directly with the *Ministry of Health. General practitioner services were run by *executive councils based on local authority boundaries. They contracted with the independent general practitioners to provide services for lists of patients on a capitation basis with relatively few item-of-service payments. There was relatively little planning or management in this area, apart from a Medical Practices Committee at national level which controlled the distribution of general practitioners geographically.

From 1968 to 1974 there was considerable debate and consultation on the structure for health and social services. Centrally the responsibilities for health and social services were brought together in a Department of Health and Social Service, local authorities took on responsibility for social services and new health authorities took on responsibility for public health services as well as hospital and community health services. A complex managerial system consisting of 14 Regional Health Authorities (RHA) and 90 Area Health Authorities was drawn up, with many of the Area Health Authorities being subdivided into districts. The Boards of Governors of teaching hospitals were wound up. Regions were accountable to the Secretary of State, as were the chairmen of the Area Health Authorities but not the authorities themselves. The latter were accountable as a corporate body to the RHA. However, there was no line of accountability of officers. In England and Wales, general practitioner services became managed by Family Practitioner Services accountable to the Area Health Authorities, but in Scotland and Northern Ireland they became the responsibility of the new health boards. In Northern Ireland the health boards also took on responsibility for social services. Elsewhere formal committees (Joint Consultative Committees) were set up to collaborate with the matching local authorities. *Community Health Councils were introduced as statutory bodies with a right to be consulted as representing the consumer. Committees of health-care professionals were also set up–again with a statutory right to be consulted. On top of these structures was set up a formal standardized planning structure.

The proposals on which these changes were based evolved under both Labour and Conservative governments and were finally enacted under the 1974–76 Labour administration. They proved to be costly and complex and excessively bureaucratic. A Royal Commission was set up and sat from 1976 to 1979. It resulted in a further reorganization in 1982 aimed at simplifying the NHS management structure below regional level. In England, Area Health Authorities were abolished and replaced by 192 district Health Authorities directly accountable to the regions. The reorganization in Scotland, Northern Ireland, and Wales was simpler but brought into place a similar pattern of management to that in England.

This structure persisted for the nest 10 years with only minor modifications. However, in 1985 an enquiry undertaken for the Secretary of State by Sir Roy Griffiths introduced the concept of general management at all levels in regions and districts. At the centre, a management board, chaired by a chief executive, part of, but at arms length from the Department of Health (DH) (now a separate department from Social Security) was set up, along with s supervisory board chaired by the Secretary of State.

In the latter part of the 1980s a review of the NHS took place. This was carried out in private by the Conservative government. It examined both the financing and the delivery of health care in the UK, as well as the government's role in health. It took place against a background of considerable tension in the NHS and concern, particularly from the professionals working within it, that there were insufficient resources to meet the demands placed upon it. In particular, it was felt that there was insufficient growth in the funding of the health services to meet the demands of new technology and an increasingly elderly population.

The conclusions of the review were that the health service should continue to be free at time of access and funded in the main through central taxation but that there should be fundamental changes in the way that the service was managed.

The solution was to split the service into two sections–purchasers and providers. District Health Authorities (DHAs) were allocated budgets based on their population and were charged with responsibility for purchasing health care for their populations. Hospitals and community health services competed to provide the service for the DHAs and their funding depended on their ability to attract contracts from these purchasing authorities. There was thus in effect an internal market in health care.

On the purchasing side of the health service, the DHAs were initially responsible to the Regional Health Authorities, but in 1994 the latter were to be replaced by eight Regional offices of the NHS Management Board, which remained an 'arms-length' division of the DH.

DHAs merged to form larger purchasing authorities, and in many ways areas formed purchasing alliances with the local Family Health Services Authorities (FHSAs), who continued to have responsibility for managing the independent family practitioners. The latter were encouraged (for practices with 10 000 patients of more) to take part in the purchasing process by becoming 'fund holders'–being delegated a proportion of the DHA's budget to allow them to buy certain services, primarily elective surgery and community nursing–for their own patients.

On the providing side of the system, hospitals and community services were encouraged to become self-managed NHS Trusts. In essence, they became free-standing public sector businesses with a board of non-executive and executive officers with a chairman appointed by, and accountable to, the Secretary of State. These NHS Trusts own their own assets, follow commercial financing principles, and employ their own staff. They rely entirely on the internal market for funding. In addition, the small private sector in the UK is allowed to compete with the NHS Trusts for contracts with DHAs.

The aim of the reforms was to bring modern managerial practices into what remains a publicly owned and managed service. It relies heavily on the principle that competition between the providers will increase efficiency and lower costs.

The changes came into effect on the 1 April 1992. They were the subject of enormous debate both by the health-care professionals and by the public at large and politicians. They were opposed by the two major opposition parties, and by the *British Medical Association. Health-care professionals were split, with most managers supporting the changes and doctors and nurses unsure or against. In practice, the complexity and radical nature of the reforms meant that many did not understand them. The reforms have gone ahead however, but remain the subject of considerable debate as to their effectiveness. They are also the subject of considerable international interest. Most countries are examining their health services, in terms both of how they finance them and how they deliver them. The problems they face are similar—cost pressures due to new technology and ageing populations, and a rapidly changing delivery system where in-patient care is being replaced by out-patient domiciliary care. The latter, in particular, causes both difficulties and opportunities in dealing with surplus hospital capacity. Many are coming up with solutions similar to those put in place in the UK—separating the roles of provision and purchasing of health care; introducing private-sector management disciplines while retaining a publicly owned delivery system; decentralizing power and responsibility. Whatever solutions they or the UK government introduce, the one guarantee is that they will not be the complete answer. Governments will always be required by their populations to ensure that a system for health care is in place. The increased demands of the complexity of health care and the pace of change mean that they will not always be able to meet that requirement. They will therefore continue to adjust the system. At least they will be seen to be doing something.

A. D. M. GRANT

GOVERNMENT AND MEDICINE IN THE USA. The USA differs from other industrialized countries in the structure of its health-care system and the responsibilities of government with regard to the population. More resources are devoted to health care in the USA than in any other nation, representing the greatest share of gross domestic product (GDP) among industrialized countries (Table 1). The USA also has wider availability of expensive new medical technologies than anywhere else in the world. Despite these features, however, Americans suffer serious problems with access to health services. The USA is the only industrialized country with a large uninsured population. Medical costs have risen sharply in recent years (Table 2), contributing to a shift in the public's attitude toward the health-care system. Whereas at present, government in the USA plays a smaller role with regard to health care than in any European country, this scenario may change in the 1990s as attitudes toward government involvement in the health care system continue to shift.

Development of the health-care system
The present limited role of government in the American health-care system has been shaped by historical circumstances. Health policy in the USA occurs in

Table 1 USA versus selected countries, 1990

	USA	UK	Canada	West Germany
Health expenditures as a percentage of GDP	12.1	6.2	9.3	8.1
Per capita health spending (in US dollars)	2566	972	1770	1486
Infant mortality (percentage of live births)	0.91	0.79	0.68	0.75
Availability of magnetic resonance imaging units (number per million people)	3.7	–	0.5	0.9
Percentage of public satisfied with the current health care system	10	27	56	41

Table 2 Annual compound growth in real per capita health spending (GDP deflator), 1980–90

	USA	UK	Canada	Germany	France	Japan
Percentage	4.4	3.1	4.3	1.5	3.3	3.7

the context of broader public policy, and shifts in the national mood result in parallel changes in the perceived responsibilities of American government. The development of government's role in the health-care system has been a response to such shifts in public concerns.

Since the Second World War, four major swings in broad public concerns have occurred, each affecting perceptions of government responsibilities. The first— the 'national defence surge'—occurred in response to publicly perceived external threats from the USSR during the 1940s. Public anxiety grew out of events such as the Berlin blockade, the Korean War, and the launching of Sputnik. The second stage—the 'human welfare surge' of the 1960s—was a response to that decade's civil rights movement and concerns over dignity and equality for all citizens. The third shift—the 're-industrialization surge' of the late 1970s—was a response to perceived threats to the American standard of living from sustained inflation, increasing unemployment, and declining industrial productivity. A weakening economy and rekindled concerns about the national defence capacity came to overshadow interest in human welfare programmes.

In the 1990s, the USA is entering a fourth phase— the 'post-Cold War phase'—with increased attention devoted to domestic issues. The breakup of the USSR and other socialist countries, as well as perceived economic competition from abroad, have placed strong emphasis on America's position in the new world order. In 1992, President Clinton was elected on a platform comprising domestic economic and social concerns. These broad shifts in the public mood, grounded in historical circumstances, are the context within which American health policy has developed.

The debate over national health insurance in the USA has paralleled these shifts in public concerns. At the end of the Second World War, interest in some form of governmentally sponsored national health insurance was at a peak. Legislative activity in national health care had been delayed by the war, but by the late 1940s a myriad of proposals were introduced into the Congress. At the same time, however, political horizons in the USA underwent a change. In response to perceived Soviet threats to the security of the West, new public leadership emerged. These individuals were committed to major increases in defence spending, and to resisting the incursion into American life of what were then seen as Soviet-like economic and social policies, including governmental economic planning, nationalization of industry, and the 'cradle-to-grave' welfare state. In this

new environment, the nation's practising physicians, hospitals, and insurers were able to resist the move towards compulsory government health insurance and to gain support for a voluntary private approach.

This retreat from some form of national health insurance did not, however, prevent the USA from gradually adopting national policies supporting health insurance. Over the next 25 years, the USA adopted a programme of tax subsidies for employees with private insurance, and three public-sector programmes for the unemployed and retired:

(1) compulsory health insurance for the aged (Medicare);
(2) a non-contributory, federal/state insurance programme for the poor (Medicaid); and
(3) a system of over 1000 governmentally subsidized community health centres located in low-income, medically underserved communities.

In so doing, the USA created a two-track health-care system: private *health insurance for the employed and their families, and public insurance for the unemployed and the retired. This is the system in which medicine is practised in the USA today, and which is subject to attack under a Clinton presidency.

Political traditions and the role of government

The changes described above took place within the context of strong political traditions concerning the responsibilities of government. The result is that, unlike in the UK, the role of government in the USA in the direct provision of health services is limited.

In the post-war period, the USA has differed from much of Western Europe in its resistance to government assuming larger responsibilities for economic planning, and owning and operating key sectors of the economy (airlines, utilities, defence industries, etc.). Few aspects of American life are more characteristically American than the nation's array of voluntary community service organizations, including colleges, health agencies, welfare societies, volunteer fire squads, etc. This practice of attending to community needs through private–public partnerships profoundly shaped the USA's framework for financing and delivering medical care, and has served to limit the direct responsibility of government at all levels. The historical commitment to pluralism and non-governmental ownership has meant that government assumes responsibility for providing services directly only when the private sector is unable to carry the burden. Today the American public has begun to see its health-care system as falling into this latter category.

Uncontrolled costs

The major impetus for changing government's role in health care comes from the USA's total inability to control costs. In contrast to overall improvements in the nation's health care, the problem of rising costs has worsened. The nation's medical bill grew from 6 per cent of the country's gross domestic product (GDP) in 1965 to 12 per cent in 1990; this figure is projected to reach 18 per cent by the year 2000. Real per capita health spending has quadrupled since 1965. When the great expansion of health insurance occurred in the 1960s, few foresaw that simply changing the way that individuals paid for their health care would result in such phenomenal growth in the costs of health services. In an effort to stem this ever-increasing expenditure, government has gradually increased its intervention in day-to-day medical practice and hospital operations.

To control rising health-care costs, government initially called for voluntary restraints by hospitals and physicians. Private agencies were asked to define and plan on a voluntary basis for their community's health needs, particularly to avoid expensive duplication of health-care facilities. Unfortunately, this approach proved largely ineffective. Americans began to move away from their traditional assumption that medicine could be self-regulating, and towards the belief that there was need for more government involvement.

As a result, the USA developed a series of interventions by which the government, without taking over the ownership and operation of the major health-care institutions, started to have a more direct regulatory role in the provision of medical care. It instituted limits on the proliferation of costly capital equipment and facilities, and limits on the use of hospitals, or 'utilization control'. This form of intervention was developed in response to the growing belief that current forms of health insurance encouraged expensive overhospitalization. Once again, however, these efforts proved unable to limit substantially the rate of growth of expenditures.

By the 1970s, America's economy suffered from high levels of inflation and an unemployment rate higher than any since the Great Depression. In response, government undertook wage and price controls, giving it unprecedented authority, including the ability to determine the prices that could be charged by private hospitals and individual physicians. The results of this intervention were dramatic: for the first time in 25 years, hospital and medical care price increases fell below those for the overall cost of living. When federal limitations were lifted in 1975, however, medical care prices jumped back up to one-and-a-half times the overall increase in the cost of living.

Starting in the 1970s, the nature of government's intervention in medicine began to change with the move to reindustrialize the economy. A growing interest in improving the economy's performance through 'deregulation' led to similar proposals for medicine. It was reasoned that without regulation, health-care costs could be contained through the introduction of market-place incentives into the delivery of medical care through the establishment of competing health-care plans in communities. These organizations could take many different forms, but their common characteristic would be the provision of comprehensive medical service by means of a defined set of physicians and hospitals to a voluntarily enrolled population paying a prospective per capita fee. Individuals would choose among these comprehensive care entities, known as health maintenance organizations (HMOs), through insurance plans on the basis of better service or lower premiums.

Additional government measures were instituted in the 1980s with the goal of containing the rise of health-care costs. In 1983 Congress enacted a new prospective payment system for hospitals, replacing cost-based reimbursement for patient care. The new system introduced a predetermined payment schedule for each of approximately 475 diagnosis-related groups (DRGs), which were sets of diagnoses into which patients in hospital could be classified. Hospitals are paid the predetermined fee associated with each DRG regardless of the actual costs of treating a particular patient.

A second fundamental reform occurred in 1989 with the introduction of the resource-based relative value scale (RBRVS). This measure established a new payment schedule for physician services, using a methodology which compares the time and skill level of each physician service or procedure with other services or procedures physicians provide. RBRVS was intended to reduce payment disparities between primary care physicians such as family doctors, and medical specialists such as surgeons. Both the prospective payment system and the RBRVS were developed for government to use in paying for health-care services through public programmes, although private insurance companies have now begun to imitate these measures.

Health-care reform in the 1990s

Despite the efforts outlined above, the USA's health-care system has become an area of great public concern with regard to the need for reform. By 1990, HMOs enrolled just 15 per cent of the American population, and additional cost-control efforts have failed to contain the pace of medical inflation. Additionally, an estimated 37 million Americans are without health insurance at any given time, while benefits are being cut back for many of those with coverage. There is a sense among the public and among politicians that the policies of recent years have been insufficient to deal with the country's medical problems, and that fundamental reform of the health-care system is required.

During the presidential election of 1992, the debate

over reform of the health care system gained national stature. While it remains unclear which types of changes will be implemented, two major proposals are under consideration. Each holds a dramatically different view of the nature of government intervention into the medical care system.

Managed competition

Proponents of this approach advocate the adoption of extensive competitive market reforms to reduce health-care spending, on the same reasoning as deregulation and increased competitive activity for the airline, trucking, banking, and long-distance telephone industries. Supporters believe that once government planning and price-setting in these other industries ended, prices dropped and the quality of products and services improved. Thus, they believe that government needs to revamp completely its policies to encourage more competition in health care, as it did in these other industries. In particular, the federal government would provide substantial financial incentives through the tax system to individuals and businesses to enrol in less costly health plans, such as HMOs or other managed care plans. Individuals could still choose to enrol in more costly plans, but they would pay considerably higher taxes and premiums as a result.

Single-payer and all-payer systems

In a single-payer system payments to providers are made by a single entity. An alternative approach is to have multiple insurers that pay all physicians and hospitals at the same rate (an all-payer system). Under these proposals, payments to physicians and hospitals are determined either through negotiations between payers and providers (as is done in Germany and Canada) or unilaterally by a single agency (as is done by the federal Medicare programme). Most health-care decisions and priority setting would take place within the context of a spending limit or budget for almost all private and public expenditures for health care.

At present it is unclear which direction reform of the USA's health-care system will take. A great number of 'hybrid' proposals exist in addition to the two outlined above, and the lengthy process of policy-making and legislating health-care reform is just beginning as the country enters its new phase of concern over domestic issues.

The organization of governmental responsibilities

Since the Second World War, incremental shifts in America's health policies have led to the development of a highly complex system of intergovernmental relationships, with multiple sources of funding and many points of decision-making. Within this system public sector health responsibilities are shared between four units of government:

(1) the federal government in Washington;
(2) 50 state governments;
(3) 100 major city governments (such as New York City); and
(4) over 3000 county governments (subdivisions of states),

The division of responsibilities between these levels is not precise, with many overlapping health activities. This reflects various historical factors rather than a deliberate assignment of responsibilities among the four units of government. Most important among these has been the financial capacity of state or local governments to respond adequately to one or another serious health-care problem.

The federal government has emerged as the largest of the various units of government, expending almost two-thirds of the nation's public health-care outlays. The Department of Health and Human Services (DHHS), formerly the Department of Health, Education, and Welfare (DHEW), is the major health agency of the federal government, and has a budget second only to that of the Department of Defense. It consists of four major operating agencies: the *Public Health Service, the Health Care Financing Administration, the Social Security Administration, and the Office of Human Development Services. The first two of these agencies relate primarily to health concerns, while the second two are primarily concerned with welfare problems. The general organization of this cabinet-level department is shown in Fig. 1.

The Public Health Service within the Department of Health and Human Services consists of six agencies: the Alcohol, Drug Abuse and Mental Health Administration (responsible for research and demonstration programmes on the treatment of these health problems); the Centers for Disease Control (responsible for programmes for the prevention and control of infectious disease); the Food and Drug Administration (the principal focus for regulating the safety of foods, drugs, medical devices, and radiation-emitting equipment); the Health Resources Administration (responsible for the support of health professional education, health-care facility construction, and health planning); the Agency for Health Care Policy and Research (the focal point for research on the quality, appropriateness, and effectiveness of health-care services); and the National Institutes of Health (the locus for federal support of biomedical research).

The Health Care Financing Administration is the agency responsible for managing the large Medicare and Medicaid programmes. These two public insurance programmes account for approximately three-quarters of all federal government health outlays.

In addition to the Department of Health and Human Services, the Department of Defense and the Veterans Administration are important direct providers of federal health-care services. The Defense Department operates an extensive world-wide system of medical facilities to provide care to 2.1 million active duty and 1.4 million retired military personnel and their dependants. The Veterans Administration provides care through the largest single system in the USA (172 hospitals, 226 out-patient departments, and 95 nursing homes) to veterans who have military-service-connected disabilities, who are aged 65 years and over, and who are unable to pay for the cost of services elsewhere.

Although the federal government is the largest supporter of public sector health programmes, the primary legal basis for governmental actions to protect health in the USA rests largely with the 50 individual states. The nature of state government health activities varies greatly from jurisdiction to jurisdiction in relation to each state's political history, economic conditions, and major health problems. In general, state governments assume some responsibility for six major types of functions, usually organized around a state-level Department of Public Health:

1. The monitoring and control of potentially serious state-wide problems resulting from *communicable diseases, inadequate sanitation, the quality of water and food supplies, air pollution, disposal of hazardous chemical wastes, etc.
2. The maintenance of a basic quality control standard for all health professionals and health-care institutions within the state. This responsibility includes licensing, recertification, and enforcement of minimal standards of practice for most types of health care professionals—physicians, nurses, dentists, etc. This role also includes licensing of various health facilities, including hospitals, nursing homes, emergency rooms, etc.
3. The direct delivery of medical services provided from the state level directly to individuals, agencies, or institutions. These tend to include institutional services for long-term conditions such as *tuberculosis, *mental illness, *mental retardation (handicap), and ambulatory care services for communicable

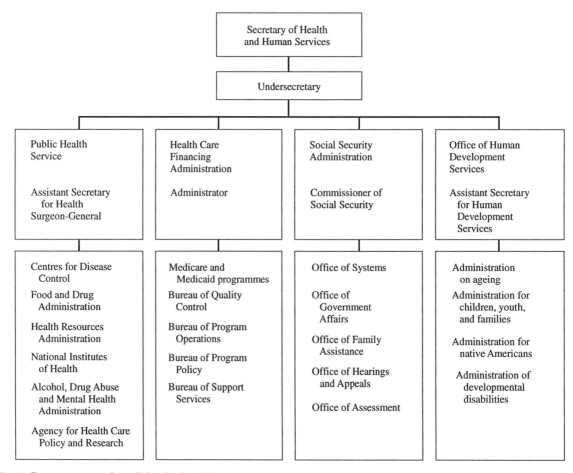

Fig. 1 Government and medicine in the USA.

diseases (e.g. venereal disease, tuberculosis), plus a variety of services related to disease prevention and health promotion, such as maternal and child health, school health, and *family planning services, etc.

4. The Medicaid programme for the poor is jointly administered by individual states and the federal government, and varies considerably between jurisdictions. It is usually the largest single health programme administered by state governments.

5. The management of a system of state-wide health planning serves to co-ordinate the decisions made about health resources in a state—for example, it is responsible for reviewing the need for major capital expenditures proposed by individual hospitals and nursing homes.

6. The final function involves state-sponsored universities. These state public institutions operate the majority of the nation's medical and dental schools and their related major teaching hospitals.

The remaining part of the US inter-governmental health system involves local governments. With few exceptions, all areas of the USA are served by local governmental health departments—either county- or city-sponsored. These agencies share in the local implementation of three of the five primary state government responsibilities and often receive substantial support from the federal government. The three are:

(1) the provision of community-wide public health activities (e.g. immunizations, etc.);

(2) the direct delivery of special services, such as maternal and child health, alcohol and family planning services, to residents of their jurisdictions; and

(3) local health planning activities.

In addition, many county or city governments maintain one or more free-care public hospitals, nursing homes, and health centres, for use by patients unable to pay for the full costs of their health care.

Over the years the responsibilities of the various units of government for the provision of personal health services have constantly developed and changed in response to the movements and pressures of the American communities in which they have functioned. The degree of change, the relative emphasis upon the various problems of medical care, and the division of health responsibilities between the different levels of government have varied quite directly with the intensity of general social economic ferment. In this regard, the role of government in medicine has not been uniquely different from that in other areas of American life.

ROBERT J. BLENDON
TRACEY STELZER HYAMS

GOWERS, SIR WILLIAM RICHARD (1845–1915). British neurologist. He devised a *haemoglobinometer in 1878 and described Gowers' tract of the *spinal cord in 1880. His two best-known publications were *Epilepsy*

(1881) and *A manual of diseases of the nervous system* (1886).

GRAAF, REGNIER DE (1641–73). Dutch physiologist and physician. In 1672 he described the maturing ovarian vesicle containing the ovum (*Graafian follicle) although he did not identify its contents.

GRAAFIAN FOLLICLES are maturing ovarian follicles. See OVULATION.

GRACE, WILLIAM GILBERT (1848–1915). British physician and cricketer. He practised in Bristol from 1879 to 1899. He was the most celebrated of all cricketers and a legend in his own time. He played first-class cricket from 1865 until 1908, scored 54 869 runs, and took 2876 wickets; he made 126 centuries and his highest score was 400 not out in 1876.

GRAEFE, FRIEDRICH WILHELM ERNST AL-BRECHT VON (1828–70). German ophthalmologist. Regarded as the founder of modern *ophthalmology, von Graefe attracted innumerable postgraduates to his clinic. He established the *Archiv für Ophthalmologie* in 1854 and founded the German Ophthalmological Society in 1868. He introduced *iridectomy in *glaucoma (1855) and operation for *cataract by linear extraction (1867). He described the '*lid lag' in *exophthalmos (von Graefe's sign) and many of the opthalmoscopic appearances in disease, including *papilloedema in cerebral tumour. He died of pulmonary *tuberculosis at the age of 42.

GRAFT. Any transplanted organ or tissue. See also ALLOGRAFT.

GRAFT REJECTION is usually classified into three types: immediate, due to blood group mismatch or *major histocompatibility complex (MHC) mismatch; acute (weeks to months), due to *antibody or T-*lymphocyte responses to MHC antigens; and chronic (months to years), usually due to *immune complex deposition. See also IMMUNOLOGY; TRANSPLANTATION.

GRAFT-VERSUS-HOST DISEASE (GVH) is a reaction by transfused or transplanted T-*lymphocytes against host *antigens. It is a major complication of bone marrow transplantation, causing lesions of the skin, joints, and heart, and sometimes *haemolytic anaemia.

GRAHAM, EVARTS AMBROSE (1883–1957). American surgeon. With Warren H. Cole he developed *cholecystography. Later his interest shifted to thoracic surgery. He performed the first total *pneumonectomy, and was among the first to call attention to the association of tobacco smoking with lung cancer.

GRAHAM, JAMES (1745–94). British quack doctor. He studied medicine in Edinburgh, but probably never qualified. He set up a Temple of Health and Hymen, first in the Adelphi and later in Pall Mall where Emma Lyon (later Lady Hamilton) held court as Goddess of Health. A fee of 50 guineas allowed use of the Celestial Bed for the treatment of infertility. In 1782 his property was seized for debt and he moved to Edinburgh where he eventually died insane and in penury. See MEDICAL CULTS AND QUACKERY.

GRAM, HANS CHRISTIAN JOACHIM (1853–1938). Danish physician. He worked with Friedländer in Berlin and in 1884 published his well-known staining method, *Gram's stain.

GRAM'S STAIN is an empirical method of staining, and hence of classifying, bacteria introduced by H. C. J. *Gram. According to their reaction to the staining sequence (crystal violet, iodine solution, decolorization by *ethanol, counterstaining), bacteria are either Gram-positive (not decolorized) or Gram-negative (decolorized and counterstained). See also MICROBIOLOGY.

GRAND MAL. Major *epilepsy.

GRANULATION is part of the process of tissue repair after damage by trauma or infection; small nodules form, composed of vascular tissue, developing fibrous tissue and inflammatory cells.

GRANULATION TISSUE. See GRANULATION.

GRANULOCYTE. One of the two main groups of *leucocytes (white blood cells), the other being non-granular leucocytes (lymphocytes and monocytes). Granulocytes are subdivided into *neutrophils, *eosinophils, and *basophils, according to the staining reaction of the granules in their cytoplasm. They are also termed polymorphonuclear leucocytes because of their lobate nuclei.

GRANULOMA. A mass of *granulation tissue.

GRAVES, ROBERT JAMES (1796–1853). Irish physician. He was an acute clinical observer, and described *exophthalmic goitre in 1835; he asked that his epitaph be 'he fed fevers'. His *Clinical lectures on the practice of medicine* (1848) earned him a European reputation.

GRAVES DISEASE is the commonest cause of *thyrotoxicosis. See ENDOCRINOLOGY.

GRAY, HENRY (?1825–61). British surgeon and anatomist. He published *Anatomy, descriptive and surgical* (1858), with illustrations by H. V. Carter drawn from Gray's fresh dissections. This was the standard British textbook on *anatomy for over a century and is still in print.

GREAT ORMOND STREET, is the site in London of the Hospital for Sick Children, often referred to as GOS. The hospital was founded in 1852 by Charles *West and Henry *Bence Jones in No. 49, the former home of (Sir) Richard *Mead, physician to Queen Anne. Before this there was very little provision for ill children in London and the UK. Its work rapidly expanded and premises next door were bought, and now there are several hospitals within the group. Early support came from Queen Victoria, Lord Shaftesbury, and Charles Dickens. Sir James Barrie donated the copyright of *Peter Pan* to the Hospital. In 1946 it became the headquarters of the Institute of Child Health of the University of London, devoted to research and teaching, mainly of postgraduates from all over the world.

GREAT WINDMILL STREET SCHOOL. The two best-known of the private medical schools of London in the 18th century were located in Great Windmill Street and Leicester Square. Both were associated with John and William *Hunter. William Hunter had bought 16 Great Windmill Street and, after rebuilding it, began a course of lectures there in 1767. Beginning as an anatomy school, it later expanded into chemistry, surgery, and medicine. Other famous doctors connected with it included Matthew *Baillie, Sir Charles *Bell, and Peter Mark *Roget. The school, sometimes claimed to be the ancestor of the *Middlesex Hospital Medical School, ceased to exist in about 1833. It was the first medical school in London.

GREENWOOD, MAJOR (1880–1949). British epidemiologist. In 1917 he became director of the division of medical statistics in the newly established *Ministry of Health and in 1928 the first professor of epidemiology at the *London School of Hygiene and Tropical Medicine. He was a pioneer in introducing *statistics to medicine and published important works on epidemics, infectious diseases, and experimental epidemiology.

GRENFELL, SIR WILFRED THOMASON (1865–1940). In 1892 he was selected to be the pioneer physician to the fishing villages of Newfoundland's Labrador coast. His work was overwhelming in volume, and in 1900 a hospital ship was added to his armamentarium. Over the years hundreds of Canadian, American, and British doctors and nurses aided him in his work. See also MISSIONARIES, MEDICAL, etc.

GRIEF in the medical context is a deep sense of sorrow and suffering usually occasioned by bereavement, to which it is a normal though painful emotional response. Psychiatrists recognize several components of this state: somatic manifestations, including weakness and sighing respiration; abnormal behaviour patterns, such as lethargy and aimless activity; guilt feelings with regard to the deceased person; outbursts of hostility towards others; preoccupation with an idealized image of the dead person, and sometimes identification with that image. The duration of grief and of its outward expression varies with religious belief, race, and culture, but its excessive prolongation must be considered morbid. It may develop into overt *depressive illness.

GRIESINGER, WILHELM (1817–68). German psychiatrist. His early researches were in pathology and included the identification of the *hookworm as the cause of 'tropical chlorosis'. He took a rigidly organic view of psychiatry, believing all mental disorder was due to structural disease of the brain. He defined clearly the psychiatric syndromes, and his book *Die Pathologie und Therapie der psychischen Krankheiten* (1845) exerted great influence on psychiatric thought.

GRIPPE. *Influenza.

GRISEOFULVIN is an antifungal *antibiotic effective by mouth. It becomes selectively concentrated in *keratin, and is useful for widespread or intractable fungus infections of the skin and nails. It is not active when applied locally.

GROMMET is the term applied to a plastic ventilation tube inserted into the *tympanic membrane.

GROSS, ROBERT E. (1905–88). American surgeon. A trailblazing paediatric surgeon, he contributed early studies on the surgery of aortic coarctation and grafting. His texts on abdominal surgery of infants and children were classics. In 1947 he was named the William E. Ladd Professor of Child Surgery at the Harvard Medical School and Surgeon-in-Chief at the Children's Hospital. Twenty years later he became Cardiovascular Surgeon-in-Chief.

GROSS, SAMUEL DAVID (1805–84). American surgeon. In 1859 the first edition of his encyclopaedic *System of surgery* appeared; this was regarded as the standard American work for the next 30 years. In 1869 he made an important address before the *American Medical Association advocating the training of nurses in the pattern developed by Florence *Nightingale; this furthered the development of that profession in America.

GROUP PRACTICE. See PRIMARY MEDICAL CARE.

GROUP THERAPY is collective *psychotherapy of a group of individuals.

GROWTH HORMONE is one of the *hormones secreted by the anterior lobe of the *pituitary gland, also known as somatotrophin. See also ACROMEGALY; DWARFISM; GIGANTISM.

GRUMBLING APPENDIX. A colloquial term for recurrent subacute *appendicitis.

GUANETHIDINE is a drug sometimes used in the treatment of *hypertension, also known as Ismelin®.

GUERIN, CAMILLE (1872–1961). French bacteriologist. With *Calmette, Guérin produced the first anti-tuberculosis vaccine, called *Bacille Calmette–Guérin (BCG). It is still used to immunize children, especially babies and infants at risk of being exposed to *tuberculosis.

GUIDI, GUIDO (1508–69). Distinguished Italian physician, surgeon, and anatomist. Author of *Chirurgia* (1544), considered to be one of the most beautiful scientific books of the Renaissance and of *Anatomia* (c. 1560), the original of which is preserved in Cosimo I de Medici's library. They were not, however, published until after his death, and then only in an unsatisfactory version prepared by his son, so that evaluation of Guidi senior's true merits as an anatomist still awaits detailed analysis of the original work. But it seems certain that his description of certain structures, notably of the cranial bones, the vertebrae, and the intervertebral discs, were superior to any available hitherto. His latinized name (Vidius Vidius) has been preserved in the alternative designation of the pterygoid canal of the sphenoid bone and the structures it contains (vidian canal, nerve, artery). Guidi is also noted because he was an early performer of experiments on living animals, while as a physician he was credited with the description of a new childhood disease (chickenpox).

GUILLAIN–BARRE SYNDROME. An acute or subacute, predominantly motor, *demyelinating *polyneuropathy which leads to progressive muscular weakness and may culminate in paralysis of all four limbs and of the muscles of respiration, requiring assisted ventilation. A rising protein concentration in the *cerebrospinal fluid is a characteristic finding. Eventual recovery is the rule, although there are occasional recurrences and some patients show residual muscular weakness. The aetiology of this alarming condition, which affects both young and old adults, is not certain; in many cases there has been an infective illness of some sort, often a viral infection, during the weeks preceding the onset of the paralysis and a delayed hypersensitivity reaction of an autoimmune nature is probable. G. Guillain (1876–1961) and A. Barré (1880–1967) were French neurologists. See NEUROMUSCULAR DISEASE.

GUILLOTIN, JOSEPH IGNACE (1738–1814). French physician. He was a member of the commission investigating *Mesmer. After the Revolution he became the deputy for Paris in the Estates General and was involved in administration. He suggested that it would be more humane to use some kind of machine rather than an axe for judicial decapitation. His idea was well received and Dr Louis, secretary of the Academy of Surgery was ordered to design an instrument (see GUILLOTINE). It was first used to execute Pelletier, a highwayman, on 25 April 1792. Guillotin was the founder of the *Académie de Médecine.

GUILLOTINE The modern history of the familiar French instrument of judicial execution begins with Dr *Guillotin, who in 1789 proposed two reforms in respect of capital punishment: first that the act should be carried out swiftly and painlessly for both the rich and the poor, and secondly that this should be achieved by means of a machine. The ideas were adopted in 1791, and a German called Schmidt supplied a guillotine for each of the *départements* of France, experiments having first been made with dead bodies from hospitals. In fact, though under different names, similar devices had been employed in other parts of Europe for many centuries, including Scotland, England, Germany, and Italy. In Italy, from the 13th century, it went under the name of *Mannaia* and was used for the execution of criminals of noble birth.

GUILT. Feelings of guilt, imagined, exaggerated, or justified, are thought by many psychiatrists to be a significant element producing mental and emotional disorders, including *anxiety states, *depression, *delusions of persecution, and obsessive/compulsive disorders.

GUINEA-PIGS, or cavies, are a genus of small rodents native to South America but now domesticated worldwide. As experimental animals guinea-pigs have many advantages. They are vegetarian, docile and easy to handle, and very consistent in their weight within a strain and age-group. They are susceptible to infections, including human and bovine *tuberculosis, and are therefore used in many bacteriological studies. They provide a laboratory model for *anaphylaxis, and are widely employed in *immunology. Much nutritional research has also used guinea-pigs, which are, for example, wholly dependent on exogenous *vitamin C.

GUINEA WORM. A *nematode *parasite, also known as the Medina worm or *Dracunculus medinensis*, which infests man in parts of West Africa, the Middle East, Asia, the Caribbean, and South America. The female of the species (the male dies after copulation) burrows in the subcutaneous and tissue spaces, reaching lengths up to more than a metre, producing an ulcer where one end comes into contact with the skin surface. Through this ulcer, larval forms are discharged when contact is made with water. The larvae enter and develop in the intermediate host, the freshwater crustacean *Cyclops* (water flea). Human infestation occurs when water containing infected water fleas is swallowed; the larvae penetrate the duodenal wall and continue to develop in the tissue spaces. Treatment is with *anthelminthics (particularly niridazole or thiabendazole) and/or surgery, but the time-honoured method of extracting the worm by gradually winding it out on a stick over several days is often still employed.

GULL, SIR WILLIAM WITHEY, BT (1816–90). British physician. He was the first to describe *anorexia nervosa, *paroxysmal haemoglobinuria (1866), and *myxoedema (1873).

GULLSTRAND, ALLVAR (1862–1930). Swedish ophthalmologist. His work led to better understanding and treatment of *astigmatism. He was the inventor of the *slit lamp (1902) and was awarded the *Nobel prize in 1911.

GUM. Any of a large class of *polysaccharides exuded from plants, which harden on drying; soluble in water but not in alcohol or ether.

GUMMA. A *granulomatous mass, single or multiple, occurring as a late complication of *syphilis. Gummata develop between 1 and 10 years after the primary infection, and may be situated anywhere in the body, superficially or deep.

GUNSHOT WOUNDS are the characteristically peppered, usually extensive, wounds caused by the multiple lead pellets from a shotgun cartridge. They are clinically and radiologically unmistakeable. Attempts to remove pellets lodged in or near vital structures may be inadvisable. The term is also used for wounds caused by single missiles such as bullets fired from rifles, handguns, or automatic weapons of all kinds.

GUT. *Intestine.

GUTHRIE, GEORGE JAMES (1785–1856). British military surgeon and ophthalmologist. He founded the Royal Westminster Ophthalmic Hospital in 1816 and became surgeon to the *Westminster Hospital in 1827. He published *On gun shot wounds of the extremities* (1815).

GUTTMANN, SIR LUDWIG (1899–1980). Anglo-German neurologist. An *émigré* from Germany, for years he was research assistant in the department of surgery at Oxford and in 1944 was asked by the government to establish a National Spinal Injuries Centre at the *Stoke Mandeville Hospital, Buckinghamshire. The hospital, and he as its director, rapidly gained world-wide renown.

GUY, THOMAS (c. 1644–1724). English philanthropist. Born in Southwark, London, Guy was a bookseller who made a fortune, which he used to found *Guy's Hospital in his native borough. This he did after being made a governor of *St Thomas's Hospital, also then in Southwark, in 1704. The two hospitals existed side by side until early in the 19th century when St Thomas's moved to Westminster to make way for the London Bridge railway station.

GUY'S HOSPITAL, London, was founded in 1721 by Thomas *Guy. Guy died before his hospital could be finished but left money in his will for its completion. It opened in 1725 and was incorporated by Act of Parliament in the same year. The building of 1725 has been restored and remains on site, although it is no longer used for patients. There has been extensive expansion in the past 20 years. The Medical School was originally established in combination with that of St Thomas's but a famous row of 1836 split them apart, with rioting by the two groups of students, for the Guy's school had been founded in 1825. In the 1980s the two separate schools combined once more as a new union within the University of London. See also HOSPITALS IN THE UK.

GYMNASTIC THERAPY is remedial physical exercises undertaken as part of *physiotherapy. Remedial gymnasts are a small profession, separate from physiotherapists, of those who specialize in this form of treatment.

GYNAECOLOGIST (GYNECOLOGIST). A specialist in diseases of the female reproductive organs.

GYNAECOLOGY (GYNECOLOGY). See OBSTETRICS AND GYNAECOLOGY.

GYNAECOMASTIA (GYNECOMASTIA) Enlargement of the male breasts, a main feature of *feminization.

GYRUS. One of the convoluted ridges of the *cerebral cortex.

H

HABITUATION connotes psychological dependence on continued taking of a drug, as distinct from physical addiction. The distinction is regarded by some as dubious. See ADDICTION; SUBSTANCE ABUSE.

HABITUS is the bodily constitution or physique, particularly by reference to external appearance; sometimes it is used to indicate apparent disposition to disease, for example 'apoplectic habitus'.

HAECKEL, ERNST HEINRICH PHILIPP AUGUST (1834–1919). German physician and zoologist. He was an enthusiastic supporter of Darwinism and in his *Generelle Morphologie der Organismen* (1866) stressed his belief that 'ontogeny recapitulates phylogeny'. His attempts to apply evolutionary doctrine to philosophy and religion entailed denial of the immortality of the soul, free will, and a personal god, and evoked a storm of hostile criticism.

HAEM (HEME) is an iron-containing organic compound (an iron protoporphyrin) which in combination with *globin forms *haemoglobin, conferring both its red colour and its oxygen-carrying power.

HAEMAGGLUTINATION (HEMAGGLUTINATION). Agglutination of *red blood cells.

HAEMANGIOMA (HEMANGIOMA). A benign growth of blood vessels.

HAEMATEMESIS (HEMATEMESIS) is vomiting of blood.

HAEMATOLOGIST (HEMATOLOGIST). A physician or a pathologist specializing in diseases of the blood.

HAEMATOLOGY AND BLOOD TRANSFUSION
Introduction

The blood or haemopoietic system in humans consists of several interconnected compartments—the peripheral *blood, the *bone marrow, and the *lymph-node system. The circulating blood, consisting of some 5 litres in a man, almost 10 per cent less in a woman, comprises a fluid component (the *plasma), making up some 55 per cent of the total blood volume. The plasma contains the three basic cell types; the *erythrocytes (red cells), the *leucocytes (white cells), and the thrombocytes (*platelets).

The erythrocytes, or red cells, are largely concerned with oxygen transport, the leucocytes, or white cells, play various parts in defence against infection and tissue injury, while the thrombocytes, or platelets, are immediately involved in maintaining the integrity of blood vessels and prevention of blood loss. Although all the red cells appear virtually identical under the microscope, two main types of white cells can readily be distinguished; these are the granulocytes and the lymphocytes. In the granulocytes the *cell cytoplasm is packed with enzyme-containing granules, which are essential for the cells' capacity to kill bacteria. The lymphocytes are members of the immune system and are involved in defence against infection, particularly viral infection.

Given the large volume of blood which has to be maintained throughout life and the short lifespan of most white cells and platelets (2–5 days) and the survival of red cells (120 days), it is essential that there is a highly efficient factory for production of these cells. This factory is the bone marrow. The compact packaging in nature does not allow wasted space and while embryologically the haemopoietic system is in the liver, the cells which are destined to provide all the blood throughout life migrate to the bone marrow early in fetal life. At birth, because of low oxygen tension in the womb, every bone in the human body contains bone marrow. Thereafter the marrow space begins to contract, although in overall terms as growth occurs the total amount of marrow increases, such that in a man this weighs some 6 kg. A closer look at the bone marrow reveals that this is an extremely complex anatomical structure, with highly intricate relationships between the various different cell types which have to mature from a common ancestor to provide the cells in the blood described above. It is hardly surprising with such complexity and high turnover that mistakes and problems arise and give rise to a substantial number of blood diseases.

In conjunction with the peripheral blood and bone marrow there are also organs normally thought of as part of the immune system (the system of defence against infection, see IMMUNOLOGY). This system consists of the *spleen, thymus, and lymph nodes. These lymphoid organs act as sites where lymphocytes (white cells) can perform their immune functions and reproduce. The interrelationship between the bone marrow and these lymphoid organs helps to maintain the balance of the appropriate numbers of cells in the immune system. In addition, the spleen performs an additional function—removing from the circulation blood cells that are no longer functioning adequately. The cells are broken down and the products can then be reused.

Haematology is the term given to the discipline of investigation and treatment of blood disorders, to include disorders of the bone marrow, the peripheral blood cells, lymph nodes, and spleen.

Anaemia

Blood is a tissue that has always fascinated man, being regarded as the essence of life. The humoral theory of disease was probably based on the Ancients' observation of shed blood in various disease states. In the 17th century William *Harvey considered that 'Blood acts above all the powers of the elements and is endowed with notable virtues and is also the instrument of the omnipotent creator. No man can sufficiently extol its admirable and divine faculties.' Harvey also felt the blood to be 'The fountain of life and the seat of the soul'. In 1669 *Lower noted that the change from the dark blue of venous to the bright red of arterial blood was due to 'imbibing air in its passage through the lungs'. In 1790 Antoine Laurent *Lavoisier discovered *oxygen and proved that it was the constituent in air responsible for the change of blood colour. In 1852 von Liebig showed oxygen combined with a substance in the red cell. *Hoppe-Seyler isolated the substance a few years later and named it haemoglobin. Van *Leeuwenhoek, a draper of Delft, first observed human red cells in 1674, but the detailed analysis of all other blood elements and development of staining techniques had to wait until the mid-19th century and studies by Paul Ell in 1840 and *Osler in 1874. The origin of the cells remained a matter of debate until 1868, when Neumann showed that they developed from parent cells in the bone marrow.

The 20th century has seen a rapid development of understanding and sophistication in defining normal and abnormal red cells, white cells, and platelets. Anaemia is the term given to a state where a person has a reduced number of red blood cells in the peripheral blood circulation and hence a reduced amount of the oxygen-carrying pigment, haemoglobin.

Hereditary anaemias

For red cells to work accurately, all the constituent parts of the proteins that make up the structure have to be in perfect working order. If even one subunit is out of place, the function can be distorted. Some of the common blood disorders are hereditary disorders in which one single amino acid may be out of place, and this prevents oxygen being carried accurately. A common example of this is *thalassaemia, prevalent in many Mediterranean areas. The result of the disorder is that the person cannot maintain the red blood cells at appropriate levels and if the defect is complete with an abnormal haemoglobin derived from each parent, long-term survival of such individuals is not possible. Such hereditary blood disorders can now be treated in a dramatic way with a bone marrow transplant from a family member who is either not affected or less severely affected. Increasing numbers of such life-saving operations are now carried out. Nevertheless, most people with haemoglobinopathy defects do not have life-threatening problems but remain chronically anaemic throughout life.

Acquired anaemia

Within modern Western countries in the 20th century, the commonest cause of anaemia relates to deficiency of iron. This can be caused by a decrease of iron in the diet or, more commonly, by a chronic loss of blood, often from the gastrointestinal tract, for example due to ulcers or more commonly, in women, due to heavy menstrual loss. The physician can often easily ascertain which mechanism is operative and correct the problem by treating the underlying cause of blood loss and replacing the deficiency with orally absorbed iron preparations. There is sadly a widespread view that all anaemia must be iron-deficient and it is terribly important to ensure the correct diagnosis before starting long-term iron administration. Iron given for some hereditary causes of anaemia can actually cause damage by producing iron overload.

*Vitamin B_{12} and *folic acid are critical in the development of the nuclear *DNA proteins in cells throughout the body. If absent, either singly or together, a large number of tissues suffer the consequences. As the marrow has a continuous turnover of cells, the deficiency of these vitamins may present first as anaemia. The predominant cause of vitamin B_{12} deficiency is an inability to absorb the vitamin from the diet because of the lack of a cofactor normally present in the lining of the stomach. This anaemia is called *pernicious anaemia, as before the discovery of B_{12} this was fatal. Currently, treatment of B_{12} deficiency is straightforward, but the vitamin B_{12} needs to be given by subcutaneous or intramuscular injections at regular intervals throughout life. Folic acid deficiency occurs in people who have a poor diet, in people who have bowel problems and *malabsorption, or, occasionally, in pregnancy. The pregnant women who are at risk are those who have low folic acid stores prior to the pregnancy and overt deficiency occurs due to the extra demand for the vitamin from the developing baby. Folic acid deficiencies are usually easily treated by providing the vitamin in tablet form.

There are two other major mechanisms causing

anaemia. First, there is the rapid breakdown of blood cells while still in the circulation. This kind of anaemia is called haemolytic (lysis anaemia) and relates to an increased fragility of the red blood cells. Again, some red blood cell diseases causing such fragility can be inherited but others are acquired, often when the body produces a protein which attaches to the red cells and shortens their survival. This form of anaemia can arise spontaneously or be induced by drugs.

The other main cause of anaemia is a large group of disorders in which the bone marrow develops a disease which impairs its function, and there is simply an imbalance between normal destruction and reduced production. Bone marrow function has to fall below 20 per cent before this becomes a major clinical problem. Diseases in this category are predominantly tumours of the bone marrow such as leukaemia (discussed below).

Bleeding problems

In the 17th century, Malpighi and Borelli came to the conclusion that the dense sponge-work which made up a blood clot was formed from the fluid part of the blood. It was not until late in the 18th century that Hewson and John Hunter firmly established that clots were formed from the 'coagulable lymph'. In 1845 Buchanan showed that the change was brought about by a series of enzymes, and by 1900 the view was accepted that the soluble substance in blood called fibrinogen was converted into the solid-fibrin clot by an enzyme, thrombin. It is now evident that the whole process that causes clotting has to be balanced by an equally complex process in which clotting is prevented, unless a vessel is damaged. These opposing forces of clotting and clot lysis are in a very delicate balance and, once again, can be disturbed if the individual inherits a defect of a factor within the clotting cascade or acquires a defect that allows clots to develop.

Hereditary clotting problems

The classic and well-known hereditary clotting problem is *haemophilia, which is split into two types: haemophilia A (classical haemophilia) and haemophilia B (*Christmas disease). It was through Queen Victoria that several European royal families came to be affected with haemophilia A. The first clinical account was written by John Otto from Philadelphia in 1803. Since that time we have come to understand the genetic nature of the disorder in which the defect is passed on via the X (sex) *chromosome to male offspring of female carriers (X-linked inheritance). Females rarely suffer from the disease because they are protected by a normal gene copy on the normal X chromosome. There is a 50 per cent chance of male offspring inheriting the abnormal X chromosome and developing the disease. Daughters similarly have a 50 per cent chance of inheriting the abnormal X chromosome and becoming a carrier. The other 50 per cent of males and all females will be normal. The biological defect is absence, or marked reduction,

of factor VIII, a particularly important clotting factor in the clotting cascade. Treatment of the condition is by replacement of factor VIII, which presently has to be obtained from blood products donated by other people (see blood transfusion, below). Replacement factors became available from blood plasma in the late 1950s and became much more sophisticated in the 1970s and 1980s, when large amounts of donated plasma from blood transfusion services throughout the world were made into concentrated factor VIII products. This allowed enormous freedom for individuals with the disease. Sadly, much plasma became contaminated with the *AIDS virus (HIV), usually when donors were paid to give blood. Once HIV-infected blood had become incorporated in the plasma chain, large numbers of haemophiliacs within the UK and in the USA became infected. Presently all plasma products obtained through the UK Blood Transfusion Service (and similar services elsewhere) are stringently checked for a series of viruses, including HIV, and plasma is treated appropriately to prevent transmission of any form of known virus particle.

It will soon be possible to produce coagulation factor replacement treatment by more artifical means, possibly in the future replacing the dependence on human products.

Platelet defects

The small cells in the circulating blood, platelets, produced in the bone marrow, are a critical first defence against minor injury to vessels. In fact, very minor abrasions do not require clotting factor involvement at all but simply induce platelets to stick together at the point of injury and plug the defect. Self-evidently, therefore, one needs to have an adequate number of circulating blood platelets. This can sometimes be interrupted when there is destruction of platelets by an immune process caused by the body and directed at the surface of the platelet (as in thrombocytopenic *purpura). A more problematic cause of the fall of platelet counts occurs once again when there is a bone marrow disease such as leukaemia, where platelet production is substantially impaired.

Blood transfusion

14th November 1666

At the meeting of Gresham College to-night, there was a pretty experiment of the blood of one dog let out, till he died, into the body of another on one side while all his own ran out the other side. The first died upon the place, and the other very well and likely to do well. This did give occasion to many pretty wishes, as of the blood of a Quaker to be let into an Archbishop an' such like; but may if it takes be of might us to man's health for the mending of bad blood by borrowing from a better body.

In 1875 Laudois found that when the red cells of one animal were mixed with the serum from another of a different species the cells clumped together. In 1900

*Landsteiner showed that similar clumping took place when human red cells were mixed with some, but not all, sera from other humans. He proved conclusively that human sera contains 'naturally occurring' antibodies active against the surface of red blood cells. It subsequently transpired that the red cell had a number of chemicals (*antibodies) on the surface which gave a distinctive pattern, and that this blood group in an individual was inherited. The commonest known blood groups are the A, B, and O groups and the *rhesus group, and all these and others have to be taken into account when blood transfusions from one person to another take place, in order to avoid incompatibilities.

The era of modern blood transfusion came of age during the Second World War, when technologies for typing blood, collecting blood in large volumes, and providing a very good consistent product were all improved dramatically. Within the UK there is a voluntary blood transfusion system, in which in each of the 17 Health Authority Districts there is a Regional Blood Transfusion Service. The role of the service is to collect blood from voluntary donors living in the geographical area in order to:

(1) provide a product for transfusion of red blood cells for individuals who bleed or require the product for operation;
(2) provide blood platelet transfusions separated from the whole blood; and
(3) provide plasma, which can then be subfractionated into various blood components used in medicine, including the production of factor VIII for haemophilia.

Blood product safety

The past decade has brought to attention more than ever before the issue of transmissible agents in biological fluids such as blood. In essence, the tragedy of the HIV virus and other viruses, such as *hepatitis virus, have made all concerned within the blood transfusion industry highly motivated to ensure the safety of the product. It remains true that in a voluntary blood transfusion system the vast majority of blood donations are safe, and the overall system within the UK requires continued support of the voluntary donor approach.

Malignant blood disorders and marrow transplantation

A haematologist or haematological physician in practice will spend a great deal of his or her time dealing with individuals suffering from blood malignancies. Within the Northern Region of England some 500 new cases per annum from a population of 3 million will occur. When people think of blood cancers they automatically think of acute leukaemia, and most regard acute leukaemia as being commonest in children. In fact, the commonest form of blood tumour is lymph-node *cancer, (*Hodgkin's disease and non-Hodgkin's *lymphoma), accounting for some 200–250 cases out of a case load

of 500. Acute leukaemia will account for some 100–120 cases, only one-fifth of which will occur in children below the age of 15. Contrary to popular opinion, most acute leukaemia occurs in individuals over the age of 50.

Childhood leukaemia

Four to six per cent of blood cancers will occur in children under 15. The commonest form of tumour is acute lymphoblastic leukaemia, and because this disease arises from a group of cells in the bone marrow, spreading throughout the bone marrow, all the blood cells will be reduced, causing a lack of red cells, normal white cells, and blood platelets. Hence patients will develop anaemia with a bleeding tendency and predisposition to infection. The past 20 years have seen marvellous improvements in the management of childhood leukaemia, with the introduction of combination cytotoxic *chemotherapy, and it is now possible in 1993 to predict that 70 per cent of children will be cured using chemotherapy alone. For individuals in particular poor-risk groups it is now appropriate to do marrow transplants, transferring marrow from one person to another early on, and it is hoped that this will improve the outlook for such individuals.

Adult leukaemia

Once an individual is aged over 15, the outlook after conventional treatment with cytotoxic drugs is not so satisfactory. There is, in fact, a deterioration of outcome with advancing age of the subject. Thus, in patients over 60, accepted conventional cytotoxic chemotherapy will not cure the patient, though it may control the disease for a while. Even in the age-groups between 15 and 50 years, outcome on conventional treatment is unsatisfactory, so that it is now accepted in Western countries that a bone marrow transplant, either from a matched family member or using the individual's own recycled bone marrow, will be used to enhance the chance of sustained remission or cure.

Lymph-node cancer (Hodgkin's disease and non-Hodgkin's lymphoma)

In cancer medicine many of the early advances were seen in treating blood cancers because of their intrinsic sensitivity to anticancer drugs. Hodgkin's disease, a tumour that arises in cells within the lymph nodes and spleen, has been largely conquered with combinations of anticancer drugs over the past 15–20 years. In 1960 only 5–10 per cent of patients would survive 5 years from the diagnosis of Hodgkin's disease. In 1993 60 per cent of them will survive 10 years.

Patients with non-Hodgkin's lymphoma, the more common form of lymph-node cancer, tend to have a poor outlook with conventional chemotherapy and radiotherapy, and various forms of marrow transplant have been introduced to treat them. Presently the biology of these tumours is rapidly being unravelled with further understanding of the involvement of chromosome defects and how these translate into tumour activity. The next 5–10 years will see undoubted improvements and evolution of more biologically orientated treatments.

Bone marrow transplantation

The ability to replace an individual's bone marrow after using high-dose anticancer drugs and high doses of radiation, has made a substantial impact on the treatment of malignant blood disorders. Nevertheless, there is a general perception that once an individual has found a suitable donor for a bone marrow transplant that the problems are solved. This is far from the case, and bone marrow transplants, even in fully matched donors, pose huge biological and clinical problems since the bone marrow can attack the body into which it has been placed, causing *graft-versus-host disease. Even after a successful transplant it remains possible in a substantial proportion of patients that the underlying malignant disease may return. Thus, investigating the complications of marrow transplantation and more efficient ways to eradicate the underlying malignant diseases must continue. The use of this technology to allow additional treatments to be given for non-haematological cancers, such as breast cancer or testicular cancer, is being investigated.

Bone marrow donor panels

The vast majority of transplants are performed between members of the same family who have the same tissue type. It is crucial that such typing is very accurate otherwise major complications may occur. For patients who do not have an appropriate family donor, the possibility of a transplant did not exist until recently. Surges of enthusiasm by relatives of individuals requiring transplants have brought about the existence of large voluntary donor panel organizations. Within such organizations members of the public agree to have their tissue type assessed. The data relating to the tissue type are then computerized and throughout the UK, Europe, and the USA there are many such databases. It is hoped that having such large numbers of potential donors will allow any given individual to find an appropriate donor.

Sadly the situation is complicated, and even when tissue typing in a test tube is satisfactory, major complications can often occur as a result of such transplants. In 1992 they are still few and somewhat tentative. The best results of transplants in matched, unrelated donor situations occur in children. All patients nevertheless suffer some complications and it remains to be seen whether such transplants will represent a major step forward in the treatment of leukaemia.

S. PROCTOR

HAEMATOMA (HEMATOMA). A swelling due to *haemorrhage into an organ or tissue.

HAEMATOMYELIA (HEMATOMYELIA) is *haemorrhage into the substance of the *spinal cord, sometimes due to trauma. In addition to signs of interference with motor tracts, dissociated sensory loss like that of *syringomyelia may occur.

HAEMATURIA (HEMATURIA) is the presence of blood in the urine.

HAEMOCHROMATOSIS (HEMOCHROMATOSIS), also known as bronzed diabetes or iron storage disease, is a condition due to excessive absorption and storage of *iron. Deposition of iron compounds in various organs and tissues leads to fibrotic changes and functional impairment. The classic features are skin *pigmentation (due to *melanin and *haemosiderin), *cirrhosis of the liver with hepatomegaly, *diabetes mellitus, *hypogonadism, and cardiac *arrhythmias and *heart failure. Idiopathic haemochromatosis is due to an autosomal *recessive gene. *Haemosiderosis with similar effects can occur if massive overconsumption of iron overcomes the physiological mechanism limiting iron absorption, or as a result of repeated blood transfusions.

HAEMOCYTOLOGY (HEMOCYTOLOGY) is the study of blood cells and their disorders.

HAEMOCYTOMETER (HEMOCYTOMETER). An apparatus in which blood cells are counted.

HAEMODIALYSIS (HEMODIALYSIS). See NEPHROLOGY.

HAEMODILUTION (HEMODILUTION) is a decrease in the concentration of circulating *red blood cells. It occurs, for example, soon after an acute episode of bleeding, when the *plasma volume is restored by redistribution of tissue fluid but sufficient time has not elapsed for the loss of red blood cells to be made good.

HAEMODYNAMICS (HEMODYNAMICS) is the science of the movement of *blood.

HAEMOGLOBIN (HEMOGLOBIN) is the oxygen-carrying respiratory pigment contained in red blood cells and giving them their colour. Haemoglobin is a complex spheroidal molecule (molecular weight 64 458 daltons) consisting of *globin, a protein, and the iron-containing compound *haem. Its precise structure was elucidated in 1960. It is made up of two pairs of identical coiled *polypeptide chains, with haem groups bound to each of the four; each haem group takes up and releases one molecule of *oxygen. The chains differ in their component *amino acids, and are of four main types (alpha, beta, gamma, and delta); normal adult haemoglobin (HbA) consists of a pair of alpha chains (141 amino acids each) and a pair of beta chains (146 amino acids each). Before birth fetal haemoglobin (HbF) predominates;

this is made up of two alpha chains and two gamma chains, and operates more effectively at low oxygen tensions. Many abnormal variants of haemoglobin have been described, depending on variation in this basic protein structure.

Haemoglobin confers on blood the capacity to carry about 60 times the amount of oxygen that could be transported in physical solution alone. The total blood volume (about 5 litres) carries about 1 litre of oxygen. In a normal adult at rest, one-quarter of this is released in the tissues each minute and simultaneously replenished by passage through the lungs. See HAEMATOLOGY; RESPIRATION.

HAEMOGLOBINOMETER (HEMOGLOBINOMETER).
Any of various types of instrument for measuring the *haemoglobin concentration of blood.

HAEMOGLOBINOPATHY (HEMOGLOBINOPATHY)
is any of a group of conditions in which there is a genetically determined defect of the protein part (*globin) of the *haemoglobin molecule. An important example is *sickle-cell disease.

HAEMOGLOBINURIA (HEMOGLOBINURIA) is
the excretion of free *haemoglobin in the urine.

HAEMOLYSIS (HEMOLYSIS) is the lysis or dissolution of *red blood cells, liberating their *haemoglobin into the surrounding medium, normally *plasma.

HAEMOLYTIC ANAEMIA (HEMOLYTIC ANEMIA)
is *anaemia due to excessive or premature *haemolysis of *erythrocytes. See HAEMATOLOGY.

HAEMOLYTIC (HEMOLYTIC) DISEASE OF THE NEWBORN,
formerly known as erythroblastosis fetalis, is a condition in which maternal *antibody causes haemolytic destruction of fetal *red blood cells, resulting in the birth of a child with varying degrees of *anaemia, *jaundice, *oedema, and *prematurity. The usual, although not invariable, cause is *rhesus incompatibility (see GENETICS; HAEMATOLOGY; OBSTETRICS), an Rh-negative mother having been immunized by a previous Rh-positive pregnancy (or by a *blood transfusion). Such immunization can now be prevented by the use of anti-D Rh antibody to destroy Rh-positive cells which escape into the maternal circulation at the birth of the first Rh-positive child.

HAEMOPHILIA (HEMOPHILIA) is a genetically
determined bleeding disorder, due to deficiency of coagulation factor VIII, sometimes known as anti-haemophilic globulin (see HAEMATOLOGY). Haemophilia is the classic example of an X-linked recessive trait; hence the condition occurs only in males, who are hemizygous, and is transmitted only through *heterozygous females (see GENETICS). Females are not affected except in the unlikely case of a *homozygote resulting from the union of a haemophiliac with a female carrier. The condition is characterized by repeated spontaneous or traumatic haemorrhages, and is similar to the usually milder *Christmas disease, due to factor IX deficiency, which is sometimes called haemophilia B.

HAEMOPHILUS (HEMOPHILUS) is an important
genus of Gram-negative *bacilli, species of which cause a variety of human infections; they require blood constituents for growth, and are frequent inhabitants of the upper respiratory tract. *Haemophilus influenzae*, as well as being involved in other types of infection, is an important cause of bacterial *meningitis. The agent of *chancroid (*Haemophilus ducreyi*) belongs to this genus; that of *whooping cough was formerly regarded as belonging to it but has been reclassified as *Bordetella pertussis*.

HAEMOPTYSIS (HEMOPTYSIS). Coughing up of
blood.

HAEMORRHAGE (HEMORRHAGE) is the escape
of *blood from the cardiovascular system.

HAEMORRHAGE, POST-PARTUM. Excessive bleeding from the *uterus following childbirth and separation of the *placenta from the uterine wall.

HAEMORRHOIDS (HEMORRHOIDS). Dilatation
and varicosity of *veins of the superior rectal and inferior (anal) haemorrhoidal plexuses. The pathological changes in the vessels are similar to those in *varicose veins elsewhere. Haemorrhoids, or piles, produce various symptoms, chiefly discomfort, pain, and bleeding. Internal piles (i.e. of the superior plexus) may *prolapse, and external piles (inferior plexus) may become *thrombosed. They can be treated, either by injection or surgery.

HAEMOSIDEROSIS (HEMOSIDEROSIS) is a localized or a general increase in body *iron in an insoluble storage form called haemosiderin. It is characteristic of *haemolytic anaemia.

HAEMOSTASIS (HEMOSTASIS) is arrest of *haemorrhage, whether as a result of normal physiological mechanisms or by surgical or pharmacological intervention.

HAEMOSTATIC (HEMOSTATIC). Any agent which
assists the arrest of bleeding.

HAFFKINE, WALDEMAR MORDECAI WOLFE
(1860–1930). Russian bacteriologist. He developed a *cholera *vaccine which was shown by field trials in India in 1893 to reduce mortality by 70 per cent. In 1896 a *plague vaccine was turned down by the Indian and Russian governments. In 1902 his plague vaccine

was shown to have considerable protective activity and to reduce mortality sixfold. A commission of inquiry exonerated Haffkine when several patients receiving his plague vaccine developed *tetanus.

HAGEDORN, WERNER (1831–94). German surgeon. He devised a surgical needle flattened from side to side, with a straight cutting edge and large eye.

HAHNEMANN, CHRISTIAN FRIEDRICH SAMUEL (1755–1843). German physician and founder of *homoeopathy*. He practised with little success at first, supporting himself by translation of foreign works. Unhappy at contemporary methods of treatment, he founded his doctrine of homoeopathy on an observation that *quinine could cause symptoms similar to those of *malaria. From this he concluded that diseases could be cured by drugs which caused symptoms similar to their own—*similia similibus curantur*. He expounded his views in *Organon der rationalen Heilkunde* (1810). In 1811 he was permitted to lecture on homoeopathy by the faculty in Leipzig but fell foul of the *apothecaries because he insisted on dispensing his own medicines. After Prince Schwartzenberg died while under his care in 1819 his writings and his medicine were publicly burned, and in 1821 he moved to Coethen. Later he moved to Paris, where he pursued a lucrative homoeopathic practice until his death.

HAIR consists of slender filaments of dense *keratin made up of cornefied *epidermal cells enclosing a variable amount of pigment. Each filament arises from a depression in the skin known as a hair follicle and is associated with a *sebaceous gland. Active cell division takes place within the follicle at the base of the hair. In moulting animals there is a synchronous alternation between growing and resting (shedding) phases; human hair shows a similar but asynchronous alternation. Body hair distribution is largely controlled by sex hormones and therefore has diagnostic significance in *endocrinological disorders.

HALDANE, JOHN BURDON SANDERSON (1892–1964). British physiologist, biochemist, and geneticist who applied mathematical analysis to genetic problems, was involved in research on evolution, and pioneered methods of measuring linkage between genes.

HALDANE, JOHN SCOTT (1860–1936). British physiologist. He was the leading respiratory physiologist of his time and carried out practical research into the causes of explosions and death in mines (1906), war gases (1914–18), and deep-sea diving. In 1911 he led an expedition to *Pike's Peak, Colorado, to study the effects of atmosphere on breathing. He published an important work, *Respiration*, in 1922.

HALES, STEPHEN (1677–1761). British physiologist and cleric. He carried out much experimental work,

being the first to estimate arterial *blood pressure in animals and blood flow in *capillaries. He studied plant physiology and devised methods for the artificial ventilation of ships and prisons.

HALF-LIFE is a measure of the rate of decay of the *radioactivity of a radioactive *isotope. The half-life is the time taken for the activity to be reduced by one-half, that is for one-half of the atoms present to disintegrate. The value is constant for a given isotope, and varies between isotopes from less than a millionth of a second to more than a million years.

The *biological half-life* is the rate of removal of a substance by biological processes such as *excretion or *metabolism. The *effective half-life* is the actual rate of disappearance of radioactivity of a labelled substance introduced into a biological system, i.e. the rate due to radioactive decay and biological removal combined.

HALFORD, SIR HENRY Bt (1766–1844). British physician. His term of office as president of the Royal College of Physicians of London extended from 1820 until his death in 1844 and remains a record.

HALITOSIS. Bad breath.

HALL, MARSHALL (1790–1857). British physician and physiologist. His views on the importance of reflex mechanisms in various involuntary activities were widely acclaimed abroad, but for some time derided in the UK. He was one of the founders of the British Medical Association.

HALLENBECK, GEORGE A. (1915–88). American surgeon. He had a lengthy career at the Mayo Clinic. He was deeply concerned with the pathophysiological origins of disease, and made important contributions to the understanding of gastrointestinal physiology and early studies in renal and hepatic transplantation. In 1969 he moved to the University of Alabama in Birmingham, and later built up the Department of Surgery at Scripps Clinic in California.

HALLER, ALBRECHT VON (1708–77). Swiss physician, anatomist, and physiologist. Haller ranks as a polymath. A reformer of medical education, he founded a botanical garden at Göttingen and wrote extensively on botany. He was the first of the great medical bibliographers, and wrote poems and three romantic novels. He was an anatomist and embryologist of distinction, but his fame rests chiefly on his eminence as a physiologist. His researches covered the mechanics and the control of breathing, the role of bile in the digestion of fat, the irritability of muscle, the automatism of the heart, and the formation of bone. His *Elementa physiologiae corporis humani* (8 vols, 1757–66) is one of the classics of physiology.

HALLUCINATION is seeing or hearing objects or sounds which do not exist. Hallucinations may also be tactile, gustatory, or olfactory.

HALLUCINOGEN. A drug which induces *hallucinations. Hallucinogens include *cannabis, *mescaline, and *lysergide (LSD).

HALOPERIDOL is a potent antipsychotic drug used in the treatment of *schizophrenia, *mania, and acute behavioural disturbances. It is a *dopamine antagonist. Its side-effects may be limiting, particularly those due to disturbances of the *extrapyramidal nervous system.

HALOTHANE is widely used for inhalational general *anaesthesia. Halothane is $CF_3CHBrCl$, a colourless non-flammable volatile liquid, also known as Fluothane®.

HALSTED, WILLIAM STEWART (1852–1922). American surgeon. He pioneered the use of *cocaine injections for *local anaesthesia, but himself became addicted to the drug, necessitating long struggles to rid himself of the habit. He nevertheless developed a famous school of surgery, devising a radical *mastectomy operation, and emphasizing the importance of gentle handling of living tissues. He introduced the use of rubber gloves in surgery to reduce the risk of infection.

HAMARTOMA. A benign *tumour due to excessive growth of one cellular element in otherwise normal tissue. Many hamartomas contain vascular tissue.

HAND–SCHÜLLER–CHRISTIAN DISEASE is a rare condition causing multifocal eosinophilic granulomata; its chief features are multiple lesions of flat (membranous) bones, *exophthalmos, and *diabetes insipidus.

HANGING is death due to suspension by the neck. In judicial hanging, death results from compression of the medulla oblongata owing to immediate dislocation at the upper end of the cervical spine.

HANGNAIL. A torn shred of skin beside a finger-nail.

HAPTEN is a substance which elicits an immune response only when combined with a carrier *protein.

HAPTOGLOBIN. Any of a number of serum *globulins able to form a stable compound with free *haemoglobin.

HARA-KIRI, or *Seppuku* (sometimes incorrectly called *hari-kari*), is a method of voluntary or obligatory *suicide which was prevalent in the Middle Ages among the Japanese samurai class. A samurai might opt for *hara-kiri* rather than capture and disgrace in war, or

might be allowed this honourable option in place of public execution of the death penalty. It requires the subject to be clad in a formal white kimono and, using a dagger in his right hand while squatting upright, to open his abdomen from left to right and upwards; he then cuts the carotids or stabs himself in the throat or, if there is a witness present, the suicide must instead be beheaded immediately after the disembowelling.

HARD SORE. The *chancre of primary *syphilis.

HARE, WILLIAM (*fl.* 1827). Hare was the Irish lodging-house keeper in Edinburgh who co-operated with William *Burke in murdering his lodgers to provide anatomical specimens. He turned King's evidence and was freed in 1829.

HARE LIP. A congenital groove or cleft in the upper lip, which may be associated with a similarly *cleft palate, due to failure of developmental fusion of the two sides.

HARINGTON, SIR JOHN (1561–1612). British courtier, and wit, who was the godson of Elizabeth I, and he installed a water closet in her palace at Richmond. He described it in terms 'more Rabelasian than mechanical' in the *Metamorphosis of Ajax* (1596) (A jakes=a privy) and was banished from Court. He published an English versification of the *Regimen sanitatis Salernitanum* (1607).

HARRISON, ROSS GRANVILLE (1870–1959). American biologist. He is credited with inventing *tissue culture, and employed it with success in showing that *nerve fibres form within *nerve cells and migrate outward from them.

HART, ERNEST (1836–98). English medical editor and publicist. He worked for the *Lancet*, but in 1866 became editor of the *British Medical Journal*, a post which he retained until shortly before his death in January 1898. Over this period, he gradually gave up his ophthalmic practice, but turned his attention to public issues—the improvement of poor law hospitals, diseases carried by water and milk, smoke abatement, the medical education of women, and medical life insurance. See MEDICAL JOURNALS.

HARVARD UNIVERSITY was founded in 1636 in Cambridge, Massachusetts, USA, and is the oldest such institution in the USA. At its inception it was Harvard College for men, named after a Puritan minister who left his books and half his estate to the college. Radcliffe College for women, now part of the university, began in 1879, being named after Ann Radcliffe who founded the first scholarship in 1643. The Harvard Medical School started in a basement in 1782 with a faculty of three and a few students. There is now a faculty (full- and part-time) of almost 4000. The first teaching hospital of the school was the *Massachusetts General Hospital, which opened to patients in 1821 and was in Boston on the other side of the Charles River from Cambridge. The faculties of medicine, dentistry, public health, and business administration of Harvard are now in Boston. The school has many other hospitals affiliated to it.

Harvard University, through its graduates, has contributed greatly to American culture and scholarship. Its medical school is of high international renown, with many past members of staff making contributions of lasting value to medicine and science. They included among very many others Oliver Wendell *Holmes, Edward Reynolds (eye surgeon), John Collins *Warren (ether), Henry Jacob *Bigelow, the *Cabots (internal medicine and surgery), Harvey *Cushing (neurosurgery), and William Bosworth Castle (haematology). Nobel prizewinners have included George *Minot and William Murphy (1934) for work on pernicious anaemia; Fritz Lipmann (1953) for discovery of an important coenzyme; John Enders, Thomas Weller, and Frederick Robbins for work on polio viruses; Baruj Benacerraf (1979) for studies in genetics, and David Hubel and Torsten Weisel for neuroscience (1981).

HARVEY, WILLIAM (1578–1657). British physician and the discoverer of the circulation of the blood.

William Harvey's discovery of the circulation of the blood marks the birth of scientific medicine, and *De motu cordis* remains a milestone in scientific literature, not only for its conclusions, but for the manner in which they were reached. Harvey showed that the heart acted as a pump, that the pulse wave was due to the heart's contraction expelling blood into the arteries, and that the blood passed from the right ventricle, through the lungs to the left ventricle, and thence to the arteries, to return by way of the veins to the right ventricle. He deduced the existence of the capillaries linking arteries and veins, although in the absence of the microscope he could not see them. He argued that the structure of the valves in the heart and veins could be explained only by the passage of blood in one direction, and that the effects of ligating arteries and veins proved its movement to be centrifugal in the first and centripetal in the second. Finally, a simple calculation showed that the volume of blood expelled by the left ventricle could only be accommodated by assuming its circulation. The clarity of his arguments, his meticulous observations, and the conviction carried by his experiments set the pattern for scientific papers for all time.

HASHIMOTO'S DISEASE is *autoimmune *thyroiditis, a common cause of diffuse firm enlargement of the thyroid gland, particularly in women. Although at the outset it may be associated with transient *thyrotoxicosis, it often leads on to *myxoedema.

HASHISH is a preparation of *cannabis.

HASTINGS, SIR CHARLES (1794–1866). British physician. In 1828 he founded the *Midland Medical and Surgical Reporter* and in 1832 the Provincial Medical & Surgical Association. His journal adopted this name in 1840 and 'British' was substituted for 'Provincial' in 1856. The two thus became the British Medical Association and the *British Medical Journal*. See also MEDICAL COLLEGES, ETC. OF THE UK; MEDICAL JOURNALS.

HAUSTUS. A medicinal draught.

HAYEM, GEORGES (1841–1933). French physician. He devised a counting chamber and developed routine methods of enumerating the blood cells. He described the *platelets and was the first to count them accurately. Many of his laboratory methods are still in use. He separated acquired *haemolytic anaemia (Hayem–Widal, 1898) from the familial type. He won popular acclaim by his work in the Paris *cholera epidemic of 1880 when he showed the value of intravenous saline. His two books laid the foundations of modern haematology: *Du sang et de ses altérations anatomiques* (1889) and *Leçons sur les maladies du sang* (1900).

HAY FEVER is seasonal allergic *rhinitis. See ALLERGY.

HEAD, SIR HENRY (1861–1940). British neurologist. He carried out experimental studies on the return of sensation after a cutaneous nerve in his forearm had been divided and sutured. From these he described 'epicritic' and 'protopathic' sensibility. His classic work *Aphasia and kindred disorders of speech* was published in 1926.

HEADACHE. Any persistent pain in the head; also termed cephalgia, or, when confined to one side, hemicrania.

HEALTH AND SAFETY AT WORK ACT 1974. This UK Act was largely based on the recommendations of the Robens Committee, the Committee on Health and Safety at Work, which reported in 1972 (Cmnd. 5034). In summary, it was an Act designed to safeguard the health, safety, and welfare of persons at work; to protect others against risks to health or safety in connection with the activities of persons at work; to control the keeping and use and to prevent the unlawful acquisition, possession, and use of dangerous substances; and to control certain emissions into the atmosphere. It imposed requirements on the employment medical advisory service and amended the law relating to building regulations. As well as providing one comprehensive and integrated system of law in relation to these matters, the Act established a Health and Safety Commission and Executive to administer its provisions.

HEALTH ASSURANCE. In Western Europe and North America health care is commonly financed by insurance schemes (see HEALTH CARE SYSTEMS, ETC).

In the UK, the publicly financed *National Health Service is responsible for the vast majority of health care, although private insurance schemes provide a small but growing minority with medical care outside the Service. The Royal Commission on the National Health Service, which reported in 1979, examined the relative merits of the two financial systems (Ch. 21, paras 14–23), but were not convinced that the claimed advantages of insurance finance, 'would outweigh their undoubted disadvantages in terms of equity and administrative costs' (Ch. 22, para. 74).

HEALTH-CARE ECONOMICS
Introduction
During the past decade there has been increased questioning of medical practice and vigorous efforts to control the expansion of health-care costs. Economists have been drawn increasingly into the policy debate and the analysis of the efficiency of clinical practice. What is the nature of health economics? What contribution can economists make to the more efficient use of scarce resources in health-care systems world-wide?

The nature of economics
There are two certainties in life: death and the scarcity of resources. All decision-makers, public and private, have to make choices about how to allocate scarce resources amongst competing activities. It is not possible to meet all demands in the UK *National Health Service (NHS) and, as a consequence, decision-makers have to decide, implicitly or explicitly, who will live and who will die, and who will live in pain and discomfort and who will be treated.

A decision to treat one patient deprives another patient, often outside the health-care system, of care from which he or she might benefit. Thus every allocation or 'rationing' decision involves an opportunity cost: the value of the best alternative way of using resources which are foregone when a treatment decision is made.

The practice of economics involves the valuation of the costs (what is given up) and the benefits of unavoidable choices. If resource allocation is efficient in health care, it is necessary to demonstrate that interventions are provided at least cost and produce benefits which are the most highly valued by society. The economist is not concerned with maximizing 'health gains' (that is the preserve of the doctor). The economist is not concerned with minimizing cost; if he was he would spend nothing, like accountants sometimes appear to wish to do. The economist is concerned with valuing costs and benefits and informing decision-makers, clinical and non-clinical, about which interventions give 'the biggest bang for the buck'.

Only if practice is efficient is it ethical. If practitioners are inefficient, they deprive patients of care from which they could benefit. Such practice is unethical and can be avoided only by multidisciplinary research to identify efficient health-care practices and appropriate incentives to ensure that decision-makers behave in a cost-effective manner.

The nature of health economics
Over 50 years ago John Maynard Keynes argued that economics was a way of thinking rather than a body of well-established facts, i.e. it is like medicine. The economic way of thinking makes explicit the decision-making processes and analyses the costs and benefits of alternative choices in an open framework. Three important areas in which these techniques can be used are: in the economic evaluation of treatment options, the economic analysis of behaviour of decision-makers (e.g. doctors), and the economics of the determinants of health.

Economic evaluation of treatment options
There are well-established principles to inform the design and execution of good economic studies (e.g. Drummond *et al.* 1987). Economic evaluation is concerned with *comparing* the *effects* (outcomes) and *costs* of a treatment with its next best alternative. This comparison of costs and outcomes can be carried out using one of five techniques (Table 1).

There are two types of costing analysis: disease or social costs and cost minimization. The identification of the costs to society of a particular disease (e.g. *diabetes, *schizophrenia, or *alcohol use) is of limited use. It informs decision-makers about the total cost but does not help them identify which intervention reduces those social costs to the maximum extent at least cost.

The other type of costing study is cost minimization. This technique is useful if the outcomes are identical; then the costs of the alternative treatment 'routes' can be identified, valued, and measured. This technique is of limited use if the outcomes of treatments are not identical.

Cost-benefit analysis (CBA) involves the identification, measurement, and valuation of all the costs and benefits of the competing (or alternative) treatments in terms of money. In health care, benefits are valued by using willingness-to-pay techniques which are complex and controversial.

This complexity has resulted in most economic evaluation using cost-utility or cost-effectiveness techniques. Cost-effectiveness analysis (CEA) involves the costing of the alternatives and the measurement of the outcomes of the alternatives in terms of some common unit (e.g. life years saved, or reduction in units of blood pressure). This is a useful technique for informing choices within therapeutic categories where the outcome measure is common. It is of little use in informing resource allocation across therapeutic categories where the outcome measures differ.

To overcome this deficiency in CEA, cost-utility

Table 1 Types of economic evaluation

	Cost measurement	Outcome measurement: what?	Outcome measurement: how valued?
Disease costing	Money	Omitted	None
Cost minimization	Money	Assumed identical	None
Cost-benefit analysis	Money	All effects produced by the alternatives	Money
Cost-effective analysis	Money	Single common specific variable achieved to varying extents	Common units (e.g. life years)
Cost-utility analysis	Money	Effects of the competing therapies and achieved to differing levels	QALYs or HYEs

Derived from Drummond *et al.* (1987).
Abbreviations: HYEs, (healthy year equivalents); QALYs (quality-adjusted life years) are global outcome measures.

analysis was developed in the 1980s. This technique involves the costing of the alternative interventions and the valuation of their benefits in terms of a common outcome measure (e.g. quality-adjusted life years, or QALYs). This facilitates the creation of 'league tables' to inform purchasers' choices.

In evaluating any study, there are eight issues of particular importance which have to be addressed (Table 2). Of these, cost and outcome measurement and valuation are of central importance. The quality of life aspects of outcome measurement raise difficult issues in the choice of appropriate descriptors of social, psychological, and physical well-being, of valuation and of validity. There is no adequate single 'gold standard' measurement and many incomplete contenders for this title (see Spilker *et al.* 1990 for a review of these issues).

Table 2 Questions to be asked of all economic evaluations

1. Are the research question and the trial design clearly identified and feasible?
2. Are both the experimental and control (comparator) arms of the trial well-described?
3. Are all relevant costs of different decision-making groups (e.g. the patient, his or her carers, the hospital, the health-care system) and society identified, quantified, and valued?
4. Are all the relevant effects (outcomes measured in terms of enhancements in the length and quality of life) of the competing therapies identified, quantified, and valued?
5. Is the sample appropriate and sufficient in size to ensure statistical power for costs and effects?
6. Are marginal (incremental) costs and effects identified?
7. Are costs and effects discounted (to take account of time preference) appropriately?
8. Are the results subjected to sensitivity analysis?

The practice of economic evaluation is crude and evolving rapidly: the 'technology' is like that used in clinical trials 30 years ago. It is essential to identify and agree on practice guidelines so that performance can be appraised. This is particularly important because some countries (e.g. Australia) now require the pharmaceutical industry to produce economic evaluations when they apply for reimbursement acceptance in the government health-care system.

Much of the clinical trial literature in the recent past has measured limited 'end-points' (physiological rather than related to survival and its quality) and have ignored costs. Such an approach does not inform choice, is of little use, and must be replaced by trials which incorporate appropriate economic measurements in their design and execution.

The economic analysis of behaviour
The practice of economic evaluation will produce results that inform the decision-makers' quest for efficient practice. Sir Robert Walpole argued that every man has his price. Aneurin Bevan quashed medical opposition to the NHS reforms by 'filling their mouths with gold'. Both Walpole and Bevan knew that behaviour can be manipulated by the use of monetary and non-monetary incentives.

The method of remuneration affects doctors' behaviour. Payment on the basis of fee per item of service, as in the UK *general practice contract, induces higher levels of activity and facilitates the achievement of ambitious *immunization, *vaccination, and *cytology targets. Capitation fees, particularly if list sizes are limited, may induce shorter consultation times. A salaried system of payment, as with UK hospital doctors, may induce consultants to demand junior assistants so that unattractive, routine jobs can be delegated and consultants can enjoy private practice, research, or leisure. Such observations are superficial and the literature on the effects of pay on physician behaviour is limited.

The price of doctor labour affects its use and the way it is combined with other labour (skill mix) and capital. Health care is produced by combining doctor time, nurse time, bed time, ancillary time, drugs, and other inputs. It may be possible to reduce costs and improve the outcomes of the care process by altering the input mix, and such changes may be achieved by manipulating price (pay) signals. Again the literature is limited; however, it has been shown that aides could be substituted for some doctors in ambulatory care, and US hospital efficiency could be increased by increasing the employment of doctors.

The behaviour of consumers as well as providers can be changed by manipulating prices. US experiments have shown that small changes in prices can be used to reduce utilization with perhaps only small effects on patient health (Manning *et al.* 1987).

Provider and consumer incentives can have significant effects on behaviour. Both groups can be seen to adjust their behaviour to changing prices and this has induced some economists to conclude that the only way to pay doctors is to change the system regularly. Only with such changes can perverse behaviours be minimized.

The determinants of health
Much of health-care practice is still poorly evaluated (Fuchs 1984) and only 10 or 20 per cent of it is founded on good science. The *health education–health promotion literature is equally unscientific: it is often motivated by human 'wish lists' which bear no relation to the costs and benefits of competing policies.

Any society wishing to improve health would invest in policies to reduce tobacco consumption (Godfrey and Maynard 1988). Unfortunately industrial lobbies are powerful, and governments are reluctant to lose the votes of their supporters. Initiatives such as 'Health of the Nation' reflect these realities and make policies such as the banning of tobacco advertising difficult, even though they appear efficient.

'Adequate' exercise, 'controlled' alcohol use, 'good' nutritional habits, and other behaviours influence health, but the benefits and costs of investing in such policies are poorly evaluated. Furthermore, investment in health promotion, unlike health care, is not supported by a powerful lobby and is opposed by powerful industries.

Conclusions
Economics is a way of thinking, and analysis by its practitioners facilitates understanding of how health-care systems work and whether interventions are efficient (Drummond and Maynard 1993). Economics has been described as the 'dismal science' as it focuses decision-makers' attention on the harsh realities of resource scarcities and the inevitability of death. The challenge to those who allocate society's scarce resources in health-care systems is how to allocate limited resources to avoid morbidity and death to the maximum extent possible. To meet this challenge, doctors and economists must learn to co-operate so that the knowledge base is increased by good science, and patients receive more and better health services from budgets which are inevitably limited.

ALAN MAYNARD

References
Drummond, M. F., Stoddart, G., and Torrance, G. (1987). *Methods for economic evaluation of health care programmes.* Oxford University Press, Oxford.

Drummond, M. F. and Maynard A. (eds) (1993). *Purchasing and providing cost effective health care.* Churchill Livingstone, Edinburgh.

Fuchs, V. (1984). Rationing health care. *New England Journal of Medicine*, **311**, 24, 1572–3.

Godfrey, C. and Maynard, A. (1988). Economic aspects of tobacco use and taxation policy. *British Medical Journal*, **297**, 339–43.

Manning, W. G., Newhouse, J., Duan, N., Keeler, E. B. Leibowitz, A., and Marquis, S. M. (1987). Health insurance and the demand for health care: evidence from a randomised experiment. *American Economic Review*, **77** (3), 212–38.

Spilker, B., Molinek, F. R., Johnston, K. A., Simpson, R. L., and Tilson, H. H. (1990). Quality of life bibliography and indexes. *Medical Care*, **28** (2), Supplement 1990.

HEALTH-CARE SYSTEMS AND THEIR FINANCING. Health-care financing is, at root, neither about health nor about financing but about a society's values and its power structure. The financial arrangements and levels of funding reflect the values of each society, particularly the interlocking sets of concepts that shape policy within the broader cultural character of that society. Each country, for example, has a distinct sense these days of how much money should be spent to relieve what kinds of ills, pains, and anxieties (Payer 1988). Each invests to a greater or lesser extent in technology and engineering to repair the flaws of nature, to stay the hand of death.

At the beginning of the 1990s, leaders in London, Bonn, and Washington DC sounded surprisingly alike in their grave concern over the threat posed by escalating medical costs to their nations' economic future. Yet the level of spending and rate of growth differed widely. The British were spending only 6 per cent of GNP (gross national product) and not providing a wide array of medically indicated services, especially for the elderly and for children. At the other extreme, the USA was spending 12 per cent of GNP and providing a large number of unnecessary services to insured patients, while not providing some of the services needed by 37 million without insurance. Yet the British (and the Germans in between) took their health cost crisis more seriously than did the Americans and pushed through fundamental changes. Consistent with our thesis, these changes in structure and financing reflected new values. These included a shift from hospital-based to ambulatory (out-patient) and home-based services, and from professionally orientated payment schemes to market-orientated ones. Meantime, the Americans spent one-third of all their economic growth on medical interventions.

Societies vary in what they mean by 'health care', and that meaning changes over time. Usually, the term comes down to little more than medical services, but the implications of 'health care' deserve reflection. For the arrangements of the entire society have more to do with health status than do medical services. The amount of stratification and poverty built into the economy; the degree of discrimination against groups by ethnicity, religious faith, sex, or age; the extent to which workers earn so little they cannot house and feed their families well; the range of environmental hazards; and the degree of educational deprivation profoundly affect health status. What self-deceptions, then, occur when we talk about the financing of health-care systems but really mean just medical services? As the reality of services catches up with their billing, 'health care', a paradigm shift from cure to comfort and functioning is taking place. The latter incorporates the former (since cure ends discomfort and disability completely) but goes much further. The reorganization and financing of services are following suit.

Besides broadening their mandate within what might traditionally be considered medical matters, health-care systems and their finances have taken on a wide range of social and personal problems, such as alcohol and drug abuse (see SUBSTANCE ABUSE), sexual dysfunctions (see SEXUALITY AND MEDICINE), manifestations of stress, and the problems of ageing (Conrad and Schneider 1992). Critics charge that social problems are being 'medicalized'. Those involved often prefer to medicalize a problem than to treat it as a crime or a personal failing. Medicalization also diverts attention from economic, political, or organizational causes of illness by focusing on individual patients, one by one. A prime example are states that profit from cigarette and alcohol taxes, even as they spend large sums on the medical consequences. Poverty, industrial hazards, and pollution (see ENVIRONMENT AND MEDICINE) are other examples where political and industrial leaders prefer to focus on the consequent illnesses. Since physicians are trained to concentrate on the patient, they find this approach quite compatible. No one has examined the clinical and societal implications of these choices more than Howard Waitzkin (1983, 1991).

Even within the confines of medical services, financial

arrangements reflect boundaries of inclusion and exclusion. Hospital-based specialty services and *primary care are always included. Nursing homes are included in some systems and not considered part of medicine in others. Home health care has been excluded until recently, but now the potential for less costly and more humane care of people with chronic problems in their homes, and the invaluable services of carers (often the adult children of old parents), are beginning to receive financial and staff support in a number of countries. Systems are ambivalent about prevention. Should it be paid for, or is it its own reward? How many preventive measures are cost effective, or is cost effectiveness not the issue? In some quarters, prevention has become the latest fashion. As Lowell Levin, professor of *public health at Yale University, says, 'Medicine has finally discovered a rationale for limitless service—health!'

Values and culture shape the internal workings of health-care finance as well. In a number of countries, for example, people have to spend all they have saved over a lifetime on long-term care before they are finally picked up as wards of the state in a welfare safety net. Yet if they suddenly become acutely ill, no expense will be spared to rescue them from death and restore them to a state of semi-illness so that they can continue to pay for long-term care out of their savings. A visitor from a 'primitive' tribe would be hard-pressed to understand such 'advanced' health-care financing. We, in turn, might be hard-pressed to explain. Thus, both the level and internal structure of health-care financing (which is largely sick-care financing without the candour) reflect the values and social arrangements of each society.

Money in

Discussions of health-care financing often get confused because people jump back and forth across this simple distinction. The ways and effects of how a payment system collects money are quite distinct from the ways and effects of how providers are paid. In some arrangements, there are overlapping sets of money in/money out.

Two major and two minor forms of collecting money prevail (Glaser 1991). Governments collect taxes, usually at the state or federal level, and usually by income or by sales (value added) tax. Usually they are not earmarked for health care, which then makes the size of the budget a telling barometer of how much political leaders value medical services against transportation, the military, and other demands. In the nations of the former Soviet Union, for example, the paltry amount allocated to health care from general taxes is the major reason why they are moving now to health insurance, the second major form of collecting money. Mandatory health insurance is, of course, a form of earmarked tax. Outside the USA, premiums almost always reflect income but not health condition, since the purpose of health insurance is to share the costs of the ill across a large population of people who are not ill. In some cases, people with chronic conditions may be asked to contribute a supplement. Only in the USA are groups and individuals routinely charged by their health status and risks, regardless of income (Light 1992). Only in the USA do insurers exclude coverage for specific risks (exclusion clauses) or refuse to write a policy at all for high-risk individuals or groups.

Virtually all health-insurance plans pay as they go, but a third, minor way to collect money is prepaid savings. Here, the policy holder deposits contributions into his or her own account and draws against them in the future. This arrangement only makes sense for predictable costs known well ahead of time. It is common for pensions, and may be adopted for old-age long-term care. Finally, charitable contributions are a minor source of funds for medical expenses, although they play a larger role in capital investments. Also to be considered, uncollected but important, are the personal savings of potential patients.

The holders of money collected may be governments, non-profit institutions, or commercial enterprises. The last are rare outside the USA, and profit motives seem to distort the social goals of health insurance. Specifically, commercial insurers aim to cover as few high-risk people as possible and to pay out as few of the claims as possible. In the USA, this has led to a plethora of techniques to do both, prompting one author to formulate 'the inverse coverage law' (Light 1992). It holds that the more one needs health insurance, the less coverage one will be given and the more one will pay for it.

Confusion often arises because different parties have two contradictory concepts in mind when they use the word 'insurance'. Commercial insurance theory holds that the more closely one calibrates premium and coverage to risk, the more fair and efficient the insurance is. Actuarial fairness holds it to be unfair for those at lower risk to support those at higher risk. Social insurance theory, on the other hand, is based on social solidarity and holds that the costs of health care should be borne by everyone in a community or society, regardless of risk. A determining reality is that half of medical costs today go to the care of only 5 per cent of the population, and about 70 per cent go to about 10 per cent of the population. The costs of medicine even vary greatly among high-risk groups, such as people over 75 years of age or pack-a-day smokers. From the perspective of social insurance, the end-point of calibrating premium and coverage to risk would be no insurance at all.

Money out

Doctors, hospitals, and other providers or facilities can get paid in a number of ways, starting with direct pay from patients. Out-of-pocket cash does not play a major role except in the USA, where one-quarter of its extraordinarily high medical bills are paid from patients' savings, an average that ranges from less than 5 per cent of some hospital services to 100 per cent of *plastic surgery, extensive *psychotherapy, and many home-*nursing services. Oddly enough, it is in the USA

that influential policy leaders (mainly from business and the right wing of government) say that the nation's spiralling costs are due to patients paying for so little of their care that they do not exercise restraint and market discipline. The ability of patients to do either is in fact severely limited.

A second, related way in which providers get paid is from patients who then receive reimbursement from their insurance fund. This method prevails in the USA, where its private, voluntary health-insurance system was created by hospitals and doctors in the 1930s to help reduce their unpaid bills without interfering with the doctor–patient relationship. Passive reimbursement of fees has encouraged providers to charge more and more. It has also encouraged insurers to obfuscate the claims process so that many patients never get the money due to them. Claims adjusters have reported that they have lists of over 140 reasons for rejecting a patient's claim for reimbursement, about half of them forms of harassment. A third of the patients whose claims are rejected give up trying to understand the forms and the process. The staff of the US Senate Permanent Subcommittee on Investigations found that a major non-profit insurance company circulated large numbers of patients' claims from office to office in order to delay their payment.

More common in other health-care systems is direct payment from the insurer to the provider. This, in turn, can be structured in different ways. Providers can be paid according to a fee schedule. A recent variation of this might be called a problem schedule, where the provider receives a fixed amount for all costs involved in solving a problem rather than a fixed amount for each procedure done. This limits the payer's outlay and motivates providers to figure out how to solve medical problems for less cost. It has revolutionized hospital care, prompting hospitals to work up patients before they are admitted and discharge them earlier to a less costly recovery unit or with the support of home health care. Known as diagnosis-related groups, or DRGs, the system clusters the thousands of medical problems into several hundred groups and then calculates the average cost for treating them. Many complex problems surround this system, and other more simple systems attempt to accomplish the same goals.

Besides fee and problem schedules, providers may contract with payers for a book of business, and these contracts can be written in several ways, particularly in terms of how the risk of cost overruns are shared between the payer and the provider. Providers may also receive a capitation payment, that is, a fixed amount for each person (not patient) who signs up with their practice. Here, the 'provider' may range from a *general practitioner, who receives a capitation for everyone in his or her practice panel, to a vertically integrated health-care delivery system such as an HMO (health maintenance organization). A capitation payment takes us full circle to an annual premium, and indeed HMOs are provider–insurers in one. If an HMO has 25 000 enrollees at $1000 (£667) per annum capitation fee each, it is, in effect, a $25 (£17) million mini-insurance company. Thus, following the discussion above, an HMO can pay its doctors by fee, by contract, by capitation, by salary, or by combinations of these.

All of these kinds of payment carry with them incentives, disincentives, and opportunities for abuse. Any kind of lump sum (DRGs, contracts, salaries, capitation) can result in underservice or lower quality. Any kind of fee for item of service can occasion overservice to generate more fees.

The roles of government

Governments can, and do, play a variety of roles in health-care systems and their financing. These roles depend on national values, the power of élites, and the perceived need for intervention. One role is to ensure quality, at least through licensure laws and often through certifications, inspections, and quality-reviewing practices. A second role is to set rules for coverage or to provide coverage directly. Generally, statutory coverage began with the working class for basic medical services and expanded from there to nearly everyone and nearly every kind of medical service. In some societies, the affluent are free to choose their coverage, while in others, universal coverage leaves only supplemental insurance as an option.

A third role arises when governments provide health insurance or services themselves. In health-care systems where the government has largely set rules and monitored services, this role has increasingly involved them as payers and heightened their concern about medical costs. Increasingly, controlling costs has led governments more deeply into the heart of medicine—determining which treatments are most effective and at what cost. The USA is probably leading this effort. Its Congress has established a large programme in outcomes research with its own budget, and increasingly, its oversight agency issues clinical guidelines for areas of medicine.

The dynamics of health-care financing

We best understand the patterns of how money is collected, providers paid, and governments behave through models of health-care systems and their dynamics. No system perfectly fits a given model; rather the models highlight certain features or central tendencies so that the character of different systems becomes clearer (Light 1993).

Most societies and their governments aim to have a health-care system that keeps people as healthy and vital as possible, at minimum cost. Historically, they emphasized free services to the working class, not only to restore their productivity, but also to quell anger towards industrialists who forced them to work

Table 1 The societal or state model of a health-care system

Inherent values and goals	To strengthen the state via a healthy, vigorous population To minimize illness and maximize self-care To minimize the cost of medical services to the state To provide good, accessible care to all sectors of the population
Image of the individual	A member of society; thus the responsibility of the state, but also responsible for staying healthy
Power	Centred on the governance structure of the society Secondary power to medical associations
Organization	A national, integrated system, administratively centralized and decentralized Organized around the epidemiological patterns of illness Organized around primary care Relatively egalitarian services and recruitment patterns Strong ties with health programmes in other social institutions
Key institutions	The Ministry of Health (or its equivalent) and its delegated system of authorities
Division of labour	Proportionately fewer doctors and more nurses, etc. Proportionately fewer specialists, reflecting epidemiology More teamwork, more delegation
Finance and cost	All care free or nearly free Taxes, premiums, or a mix Costs relatively low Doctors' share relatively low
Medical education	A state system, free, with extensive continuing education

in hazardous conditions and support for socialist parties, by medicalizing their problems (Engel 1844; Rimlinger 1971). This might be called the societal or state model of health care (Table 1). It implies that finances are provided as centrally and cheaply as possible, through existing taxes, as Bismarck wanted to do in his version of the world's first national scheme for health insurance. The societal or state model implies a national health service, which Bismarck also sought but was not granted as the workers' sickness funds lobbied successfully to be the vehicle for his scheme. Thus, the societal or state model exemplifies central funding and nationally integrated services that are an extension of *public health; such a scheme was introduced in the UK in 1948. Citizens' health, then, is a governmental responsibility, although citizens have the complementary obligation to maintain their health. Such a system centres on primary care and wide accessibility through central planning of clinics and hospitals. *Occupational medicine, public health campaigns, and health education are examples of links with other aspects of social life. The medical profession has little or modest power, and doctors receive low or modest incomes. Many less-affluent countries have health-care systems that approximate to this model.

The medical profession has pressed wherever it can for a quite different model of medical services. This model centres on the goals of providing the best clinical medicine for every sick patient, by enhancing the autonomy and power of the medical profession and by developing scientific medicine to its highest level. This implies a system of fees paid to private practitioners, ideally a private system of direct pay and insurance that reimburses patients, so that the doctor–patient relationship is not invaded by third parties (Table 2). As medical leaders in the USA cried, in their successful campaigns to eliminate insurance schemes early in the 20th century, 'No middlemen!'

The professional model of medical services is obviously decentralized and not co-ordinated for public health or other purposes. It has little to do with worksites, schools, or other institutions. Patients are regarded as private citizens who live as they wish and seek medical services when they want. Doctors choose their specialty and where they want to practise. As a result, one gets far more specialists than problems needing their attention, and geographical maldistributions as doctors choose the more affluent sections of metropolitan areas. Medical schools and professional societies form its centre, constantly promoting new clinical advances and training more specialists. Doctors are well paid, and the system as a whole costs a good deal more than the societal model.

Needless to say, most national 'health-care' systems have become heavily influenced by professional priorities. Some might even say that the medical profession has captured or co-opted national systems to its goals.

Table 2 The professional model of a health-care system

Inherent values and goals	*To provide the best possible clinical care to every sick patient* (who can pay and who lives near where a doctor has chosen to practise) To develop scientific medicine to its highest level To protect the autonomy of physicians and services To increase the power and wealth of the profession To increase the prestige of the profession
Image of the individual	A private person who chooses how to live and when to use the medical system
Power	Centres on the medical profession, and uses state powers to enhance its own
Key institutions	Professional associations Autonomous physicians and hospitals
Organization	A loose federation of private practices and hospitals Centred on doctors' preferences of specialty and location Emphasizes acute, hi-tech interventions Weak ties with other social institutions as peripheral to medicine
Division of labour	Proportionately more doctors, more specialists Proportionately more individual clinical work by physicians; less delegation
Finance and costs	Private payments by individual or through passive reimbursement by insurance plans Costs about twice the percentage of GNP of the societal model Doctors' share greater than in the societal model
Medical education	Private, autonomous schools with tuition Disparate, voluntary continuing education

Professional capture, however, has had unanticipated consequences which stem from both excesses and neglects inherent in the professional model. Specialization builds on itself and generates a complex, costly division of labour. Together with autonomy, specialization leads to a fragmentation of services, patient complaints of depersonalized and arrogant treatment, more *malpractice suits, and rapidly escalating costs. The professional model also creates protected, non-competitive markets in which *pharmaceutical and equipment corporations thrive. A large medical–industrial complex grows up around the organizational and financial protections of the doctor–patient relationship. These corporations prosper by providing specialists with ever-improved tools, machines, and chemicals by which to provide the best clinical treatment to every sick patient. Of particular importance for the industry and the professional model are improved diagnostics, because the more they find, the more there is to treat. William Kissick, a professor of medicine and management at the University of Pennsylvania, has formulated a law of professionalized health care: 'A healthy patient is an insufficiently diagnosed patient.'

The dynamics of professional capture and the ironies of success have a great deal to do with the repeated cost crises experienced by advanced health-care systems since the 1970s. In the 1980s and 1990s, these crises were often seen as due to the entrenched inefficiencies of highly bureaucratized systems. What the systems needed, declared policy advisers, was a good dose of competition to shake out inefficiencies and make services responsive to patients. Finances needed to be restructured so that providers would compete on efficiency and quality for contracts.

This common policy analysis of the 1980s overlooked the degree to which professionalism, rather than socialist or governmental bureaucracy, was the problem. For beyond Oliver Williamson's analysis of hierarchy as the central alternative to markets is professionalism.

Table 3 The buyers' revolt: axes of change in the 1980s

Dimensions	From provider-driven	To buyer-driven
Ideological	Sacred trust in doctors	Distrust of doctors' values, decisions, even competence
Economic	*Carte blanche* to do what seems best: power to set fees; incentives to specialize, develop techniques Informal array of cross subsidizations for teaching, research, charity care, community services	Fixed prepayment or contract with accountability for decisions and their efficacy Elimination of 'cost shifting'; pay only for services contracted
Political	Extensive legal and administrative power to define and carry out professional work without competition, and to shape the organization and economics of medicine	Minimal legal and administrative power to do professional work but not to shape the organization and economics of services
Clinical	Exclusive control of clinical decision-making Emphasis on state-of-the-art specialized interventions; lack of interest in prevention, primary care, and chronic care	Close monitoring of clinical decisions, their cost and their efficacy Emphasis on prevention, primary care, and functioning; minimize high-tech. and specialized interventions
Technical	Political and economic incentives to develop new technologies in protected markets	Political and economic disincentives to develop new technologies
Organizational	Cottage industry	Corporate industry
Potential disruptions and dislocations	Overtreatment Iatrogenesis High cost Unnecessary treatment Fragmentation Depersonalization	Undertreatment Cuts in services Obstructed access Reduced quality Swamped in paperwork

Ideally, the professional carries out all the functions of markets in a single, integrated moment. He/she identifies what is needed, selects the best product at the best price, and completes the transaction. Many of the 'inefficiencies' of national systems, however, stem from entrenched professional privilege. So does the lack of accountability. Of particular relevance is research that has documented extensive variations in clinical treatments and costs for the same medical problems, without clear evidence that any one is more effective than the other. In short, the unanticipated problems of professional capture have exposed the medical profession's own weaknesses in service and accountability. Governments, employers, and insurers (depending on who the payers are in a given system) have moved from concern, to hand-wringing, to revolt.

The buyers' revolt
The revolt of the 1980s and 1990s centres on payers transforming themselves into active buyers, and that transformation in turn centres on a collapse of the sacred trust in which doctors have been held (Table 3). The buyers want accountability—exactly how much things cost and the relative benefits of alternative treatments. Clinically and financially, the buyers' drive for cost-effectiveness leads towards performance-based contracts. The byword is competition, although what buyers mean is monopsony competition (a monopoly buyer), in which one or a few dominant buyers make doctors and hospitals compete on their terms. One might call it buyer-dictated competition.

Given that the misdiagnosed problems have less to do with substituting markets for governmental regulation and bureaucracy than with substituting markets for professional entrenchment, the problem is that competition can easily play into the hands of the doctors and backfire as a strategy to increase efficiency or moderate medical expenditures. Doctors hold most of the cards. They are the consumer's (i.e. the patient's) principal agent as well as the seller of services to the buyer. In many places outside large cities, there are not so many competitors to choose from. This does not mean there is no market, as some aver, but rather that there is a monopoly market in which the provider can dictate terms.

Medical work often has a contingent, emergent quality as doctors try to figure out what the problem is, see what happens when they try one treatment, and then go on to try something else (Table 4). This means there often is no clear service product or package, analogous to a half-hour massage or a week's stay at a resort. Pricing is very difficult, and the vagaries of illness can result in large profits or large losses for the contracting providers (Table 5). The costs of gathering accurate information on costs and quality, and of monitoring contract performance are very high. The managerial superstructure not only grows larger than the old bureaucracy but is much more highly paid. The opportunities for 'sweetheart' contracts to

Table 4 Basic imperfections in medical markets (market failure?)

The problem is that many aspects of clinical medicine do not meet the basic criteria for markets. Here are ten reasons why:

1. Often the 'product' is difficult to define because it is emergent and contingent on what happens as the patient is being treated.
2. Property rights are fuzzy.
3. The seller/providers decide what is to be bought and are the buyers' as well as the consumer/patients' agent. Moreover, patients often want it that way, with passion.
4. The seller/providers control much of the information the buyer(s) need to 'shop', and they can easily manipulate it.
5. Information on products (however they are defined), quality (however it is defined), and price is very costly to gather and analyse. It is complex and hard to understand.
6. Shopping is complex, time-consuming, and costly, even if information is good. Most customers do not shop often.
7. People do *not* want to shop or buy; medical services are something most people avoid until they can avoid them no longer. By that time they are sick, or in pain, or injured.
8. The basic principles of expected utility theory are rarely satisfied. One does not have full information on costs, risks, and benefits of all alternatives, with all being borne by the buyer.
9. Many markets outside large cities offer little choice to buyers. This does not mean there is 'no market,' as some aver, but rather that there are monopoly markets where the seller/providers can impose monopoly prices if they want to.
10. Medical markets often do not 'clear'. Losing providers and institutions continue to work at half capacity, more inefficient than ever and probably at lower quality. While they produce a long-term costly drag on the budget, the 'winners' are swamped with a volume they cannot handle, resulting perhaps in a loss of quality and efficiency.

friends, the siphoning of money, and other corruptions are numerous. In general, competition in murky areas like health care requires more regulation than before the system was 'deregulated', because actors are encouraged to 'win', and because there is more opportunity for mischief. It may well be that competition in areas of social activity where the basic prerequisites for competition are not met increases inefficiency for the system as a whole. At the same time, out of the thousands of new arrangements, there will always be stellar successes of innovation and efficiency, and these will be paraded to show that competition does indeed work.

Doctors and other providers control most of the information that buyers and the market need for competition to take place; yet competition rewards them for not sharing that information or distorting what is shared. There are several easier ways to benefit from competition than becoming more efficient (Light 1990). In fact, efficiency is the hardest way and the least rewarding (Table 6). In the mature 'competitive' health-care markets in the USA, doctors, hospitals, and other sellers can, and do, use all the classic techniques that monopolies used near the turn of the 20th century, such as collusion, tying relations, and price fixing. They also corner markets, differentiate products, generate brand loyalty, substitute less or cheaper service, emphasize patient-pleasing service amenities, and avoid money-losing patients or shunt them off to another part of the system. All of these strategies increase profits rather quickly. At the end of a decade of the most intense effort to contain costs through provider competition, the USA learned that costs in constant dollars had risen faster than ever.

Just as winning in competitive health care may have little to do with efficiency or greater health gain, so losing may have little to do with inefficiency or poor clinical performance (Light 1991). Moreover, losers in medicine rarely collapse and disappear. Instead, half-empty hospitals and clinics limp along for years, sometimes decades, dragging along their fixed costs and high operating expenses. Closing down losers quickly, or turning them around, is vital if society is to benefit from competition. Ironically, competition may produce more losers than potentially existed before, because initially many competitors invest and expand in the hope or confidence that they will beat the others. This was evident, for example, in the business plans of British hospitals applying for greater independence through self-governing trust status. The Treasury quickly realized that if they all borrowed money and chased their ambitions, overall costs would rise significantly. In response, the Treasury greatly reduced their borrowing privileges, and the hospitals cried foul. To the extent that the Treasury was right, it was recognizing a well-kept secret about markets that advocates rarely discuss.

Finally, competition produces some disturbing side-effects. A commercial ethos replaces a service ethos, and doctors learn quickly how to think like entrepreneurs. Distrust is very costly; trust very cheap. People with profitable and unprofitable health problems find themselves pitted against one another. Generally, those with fewer and/or crisply definable and treatable problems are profitable, and those with more and/or chronic problems are not. Patients with these problems are more likely to be poorer. Important services that lose money and require cross-subsidies from other services fall out, like clinical teaching, clinical *research, *emergency or urgent care, *mental health services, and services to those with a wide variety of chronic conditions. Who will pay for them? No sensible buyer. At best, they become the grudging object of what now seems like extra funding from the government, even though they were paid for as a matter of routine before competition began.

All of these problems and costs of competition imply that if it is to be used in health care, it must be carefully

Table 5 Imperfect markets vs perfect markets

Ideal of perfect markets	Actual hazards of imperfect markets
Transaction and market costs zero	Large transaction and market costs
Many buyers and sellers	Few buyers and/or sellers; market capture
Nature, quality, effectiveness, and price of products or service known; no market failure	Nature, quality, effectiveness, and/or price of products or service incompletely known and variable; some market failure.
Power, rules, hierarchy do not exist	Power, rules, hierarchies found everywhere
Manipulations, gaming, cost shifting unknown	Manipulations, gaming, cost shifting prevalent; induced market failure
Losers collapse, disappear	Losers stay around; system carries their inefficiencies
Maximum efficiency	Maximum inefficiencies?
Responsive to customers	'Responsive' to customers; induced demand, product or service dilution or substitution, misleading information

Table 6 Alternative responses to competition (Why bother becoming efficient?)

Economist's terms	Professional's alias	Personal rewards
Collusion	Colleagueship, friendship, loyalty	Its own reward Avoid hard feelings, isolation Avoid losing money, or make money
Product differentiation	Specialization	More interesting work, prestige, income
Market segmentation	Serving those who can pay Specialization	More interesting, work, prestige, income
Market expansion	Quality Comprehensive care Meeting untapped needs	More income, work satisfaction
Cost shifting	Appropriate referral	Dispense with patient's problems and payment problems
Data manipulation	Serving the patient, the hospital, or clinic	'Beat them at their own game' More income
Product substitution or service dilution	Making compromises to a stingy payer	More income but feels awful
Manipulate demand (more or less, whichever pays)	Serving the patient within the capacity of the system to pay	Doing one's best More income than otherwise
Efficiency	Coercive upheaval Compromising quality	More income but disruptive Hard work Creates enemies Reduces professional power

Source: D. W. Light (1990).

targeted to where it can do good. This is possible but not easy (Saltman and von Otter 1992).

The return of community-based health care?
At the same time that political fashion for competition and privatization is spurring several health-care systems towards reforms that have already been shown to be complex and costly, another trend in organization and finance is arising from rather different values. This trend, led by the European office of the *World Health Organization (WHO), begins with the recognition that most costly medical problems start in the environment, in the economy, and in personal living (WHO 1987, 1991). It aims to allocate health-care resources around primary care and according to needs in the community.

Health, the central concern of society and the state, has returned to centre stage. Health promotion, prevention, and health education are making a comeback, with a new emphasis on how to manage the large number of costly chronic conditions that accompany an ageing society. Primary care and community-based programmes become the first line of defence; hospitals are being moved from the centre of the system to the hi-tech backup for general and specialist services in the community. The position of medical schools within the model raises many questions; for society still wants and needs their capacity to find new solutions to medical problems, even as it wants a delivery system based on prevention and primary care.

Needs-based purchasing by local health authorities is one thrust of the British reforms, and community-orientated primary care is making a comeback in the USA. This emerging trend differs from budget caps and other financial controls by restructuring current systems that centre on hospitals and specialty care so that they centre on the needs of citizens. Such reforms usually involve combining budgets and putting them on a capitated basis, so that the incentives are aligned with health status and health gain. They may even allow us to rediscover an early 20th century model of community-based care, where subscribers elected a board, hired a manager, discovered what the men, women, and children needed in the way of health education, prevention, improved working and local conditions, support services, and medical services. Then again, the medical–industrial complex is one of the great clinical and economic successes of modern times. Its influences on policy and finance are wide and deep.

DONALD W. LIGHT

References

Conrad, P. and Schneider, J. W. (1992). *Deviance and medicalization: from badness to sickness*, (expanded edn). Temple University Press, Philadelphia.

Engel, F. (1844). *The condition of the working class in England in 1844*. Progress publ., Moscow 1973.

Glaser, W. A. (1991). *Health insurance in practice: international variations in financing, benefits, and problems*. Jossey-Bass, San Francisco.

Light, D. W. (1990). Bending the rules. *The Health Service Journal*, **100** (5222), 1513–15. Second in a five-part series on the NHS reforms and competition.

Light, D. W. (1991). Embedded inefficiencies in health care. *Lancet*, **338**, 102–4.

Light, D. W. (1992). The practice and ethics of risk-rated health insurance. *Journal of the American Medical Association*, **267**, 2503–8.

Light, D. W. (1993). Comparing health care systems. In *The sociology of health and illness: critical perspectives* (3rd edn), (ed. P. Conrad and R. Kern). St. Martin's Press, New York.

Payer, L. (1988). *Medicine and culture: varieties of treatment in the United States, England, West Germany, and France*. Penguin, London.

Rimlinger, G. V. (1971). *Welfare policy and industrialization in Europe, America and Russia*. John Wiley, New York.

Saltman, R. B. and von Otter, C. (1992). *Planned markets and public competition: strategic reform in Northern European health systems*. Open University Press, Buckingham.

Waitzkin, H. (1983). *The second sickness: contradictions of capitalist health care*. Free Press, New York.

Waitzkin, H. (1991). *The politics of medical encounters: how patients and doctors deal with social problems*. Yale University Press, New Haven, Conn.

World Health Organization (1987). *Revised list of indicators and procedures for monitoring progress towards health for all in the European regions 1987–88*. Regional office for Europe, Copenhagen. World Health Organization (1991). *Healthy cities project: a project becomes a movement*. Regional office for Europe, Copenhagen.

HEALTH CENTRES. Under Section 21 of the UK *National Health Service Act 1946

it shall be the duty of every local health authority to provide, equip and maintain to the satisfaction of the Minister premises, which shall be called 'health centres', at which facilities shall be available for all or any of the following purposes—(a) general medical services; (b) general dental services; (c) pharmaceutical services; (d) any of the services which the local authority are required or empowered to provide; (e) services of specialists or other services provided for out-patients under Part II of the act.

The imperative words (e.g. 'shall') used in the Act did not specify time and circumstances, and did not confer an absolute duty. If general medical services are already adequate, then there is no 'duty to provide'; if, however, they are not, then the section imposes a definite duty on the authority to make appropriate provisions.

In addition to general practitioner (GP) and community nursing services, health centres usually provide antenatal, preschool, and school health services,

immunization, and vaccination (see PRIMARY MEDICAL CARE; PUBLIC HEALTH MEDICINE IN THE UK). They may also have facilities for health education, family planning, speech therapy, chiropody, audiology, dental services, ophthalmic services, and supporting social work services. They represent a departure from the traditional pattern of *general medical practice.

HEALTH DEPARTMENTS. A collective term for the several UK government departments responsible for health matters respectively in England, Scotland, Wales, and Northern Ireland. See DEPARTMENT OF HEALTH.

HEALTH EDUCATION (of the general public or of special groups such as school children) is aimed at influencing behaviour in such a way as to assist in promoting health and preventing disease.

HEALTH EDUCATION COUNCIL. The Council was set up in the UK in 1968 as a quasi-autonomous body under the authority of the then Secretary of State for Health and Social Services, registered as a charity, and incorporated under the Companies Acts. It covered England, Wales, and Northern Ireland. The Council comprised a chairman and 19 other members appointed by the Secretary of State from the fields of health, education, local government, the media, and business. It had important advisory and executive functions in relation to health education in the UK other than Scotland. It was replaced by a Health Education Authority with revised membership and powers in 1987; it has four executive and nine non-executive directors.

HEALTH FOODS are articles of food on sale to the public, often from dedicated retail outlets, which by virtue of their ingredients or method of manufacture are claimed to be 'healthier' than their conventional equivalents. In some cases, this view is supported by a significant body of medical opinion (e.g. foods with a high content of dietary *fibre or of *polyunsaturated fatty acids); in many others, a scientific foundation is less secure. However, certain articles of diet were promoted as health foods well in advance of their acquiring scientific respectability (e.g. raw carrots, garlic oil capsules, and wholemeal bread).

HEALTH, NATIONAL BOARD OF. A US body established by Congress in 1879 in the wake of the 1878 epidemic of *yellow fever in the southern states, aimed particularly at establishing uniform *quarantine procedures. It was dissolved 4 years later.

HEALTH SERVICE COMMISSIONER. See OMBUDSMAN.

HEALTH SERVICES AND PUBLIC HEALTH ACT 1968. This UK Act amended the *National Health

Service Act 1946 and the National Health Service (Scotland) Act 1947; it amended local authorities' services under the National Assistance Act 1948, the law relating to notifiable diseases and food poisoning, the Nurseries and Child-minders Regulation Act 1948, and the law relating to food and drugs. It allowed assistance to be given to certain voluntary organizations and enabled the Minister of Health and Secretary of State to purchase goods for supply to certain authorities.

HEALTH VISITORS. A health visitor is defined in the UK National Health Service (NHS) (Qualifications of Health Visitors) Regulations 1972 as 'a person employed by a local health authority to visit people in their homes or elsewhere for the purpose of giving advice as to the care of young children, persons suffering from illness, and expectant or nursing mothers, and as to the measures necessary to prevent the spread of infection'. In order to become a health visitor the individual must first be a registered general nurse who then acquires a specific post-registration qualification. The local health authority is required by Section 24 of the NHS Act 1946 to provide health visitors for these purposes.

HEARING. The capacity for sound perception. See OTORHINOLARYNGOLOGY.

HEARING AIDS are electronic devices which amplify sound and improve hearing in patients with some types of deafness. See OTORHINOLARYNGOLOGY.

HEART. The heart is the muscular pump which maintains circulation of the blood, situated in the thorax to the left of the midline. The right and left sides are separate functional units, each comprising a filling chamber, or atrium, and a much thicker and more muscular ventricle. The right side receives deoxygenated venous blood returning from the tissues and pumps it into the lungs via the *pulmonary arteries. From here, after oxygenation by pulmonary ventilation, it returns to the left side and is pumped by the left ventricle back into the tissues via the *aorta and the *arteries.

HEART ATTACK is a term commonly denoting *coronary thrombosis or cardiac infarction.

HEART BLOCK. Any condition in which a pathological process interferes with the origin or spread of the wave of excitation accompanying each normal contraction of the *heart. Heart block is classified according to the level within the specialized cardiac conducting system at which it occurs, usually readily apparent on *electrocardiography. Many types cause slowness of the pulse (bradycardia) or even temporary cessation of the heart beat (cardiac arrest). See CARDIOLOGY; STOKES–ADAMS SYNDROME.

HEARTBURN is an unpleasant burning sensation deep in the throat or behind the sternum (breast bone). It is often, if not always, associated with reflux of some of the acid contents of the *stomach back into the lower end of the *oesophagus.

HEART FAILURE is any condition in which the pumping function of the *heart, or of part of it, has become inadequate to its task.

HEART–LUNG MACHINE. An apparatus for pumping and oxygenating blood outside the body (extracorporeal oxygenator) bypassing the heart and lungs (cardiopulmonary *bypass); the object is to allow the cardiac surgeon to operate on a dry non-beating heart. See CARDIOTHORACIC SURGERY.

HEART SOUNDS. Sounds generated by the heart's action and heard on *auscultation over the left side of the chest. The first of two prominent sounds is due to closure of the atrioventricular (mitral and tricuspid) valves and marks the beginning of ventricular contraction. The second sound, sharper and shorter, is due to closure of the aortic and pulmonary valves and marks the onset of ventricular relaxation. A much softer and lower-frequency third sound may be detected in children and young adults shortly after the second sound, associated with the early rapid filling phase of ventricular relaxation. See PHYSIOLOGY; VALVES, CARDIAC.

HEART TRANSPLANT is an operation in which the heart of a human donor is transplanted into a patient deemed to have irreversible heart disease and otherwise negligible chances of survival, the transplant being connected to the recipient's circulation and taking over the functions of the diseased heart (which may or may not itself be removed). The donor is usually a young person in whom the heart is expected to be healthy and in whom irreversible *brain death has been established. Most donors are the victims of road accidents, or have suffered a *subarachnoid haemorrhage. See CARDIOTHORACIC SURGERY; TRANSPLANTATION.

HEAT AS CAUSE OF DISEASE. The consequences of exposure to abnormally high ambient temperatures range from mild to very serious, and are influenced by several factors, such as age, obesity, clothing, acclimatization, physical exercise, atmospheric humidity, and duration of exposure. Heatstroke (heat hyperpyrexia, hyperthermia) in its fully developed form has three cardinal features: cerebral dysfunction, which may include *coma and *convulsions; a hot and dry (anhidrotic) skin; and oral and rectal temperatures above 41 °C (106 °F). It is a medical emergency.

Heat exhaustion is a less serious condition developing usually over several days and associated with body depletion of water, salt, or both. Thirst, giddiness, fatigue, pyrexia, and *oliguria are characteristic, with the addition of muscular cramps when there is salt deficiency.

Heat *syncope is acute giddiness or loss of consciousness while exercising in the heat, due to widespread peripheral vasodilatation and blood pooling. The subject recovers on lying down. Prickly heat (miliaria rubra) is an itchy rash due to obstruction of the ducts of the sweat glands and escape of sweat into the epidermis. It is associated with prolonged heat load. See also ENVIRONMENT AND DISEASE.

HEAT EXHAUSTION. See HEAT AS CAUSE OF DISEASE.

HEATSTROKE. See HEAT AS CAUSE OF DISEASE.

HEBEPHRENIA is an outmoded term for one clinical variety of *schizophrenia. It was described by Hecker in 1871 as a progressive disease of puberty and adolescence (hence the name) in which there is a 'succession or changing appearance of various forms (*melancholia, *mania, and *confusion)' and a 'very quick termination in a psychic enfeeblement'.

HEBERDEN, WILLIAM, the elder (1710–1801). British physician. A scholarly and successful physician, he was the first to describe *angina pectoris in *Some account of a disorder of the breast* (1768).

HEBERDEN, WILLIAM, the younger (1767–1845). British physician, son of William *Heberden the elder. He took a particular interest in rheumatic diseases.

HEBRA, FERDINAND RITTER VON (1816–80). Austrian dermatologist. He discounted the humoral theory and believed that most skin diseases had local causes and required external medication. He established the parasitic cause of many such diseases and devised a classification based on histopathological changes. He described many dermatoses, published a successful textbook, and was widely acclaimed as a teacher. See also DERMATOLOGY.

HEIDENHAIN, RUDOLPH PETER HEINRICH (1834–97). German physiologist. He became interested in the glands and the nature of secretion, holding this to be due to intracellular activity and not, as widely believed, mechanical. From this he moved to investigating the urine and concluded, in opposition to *Ludwig, that the renal tubules had a secretory function.

HEIGHT. Vertical measurement, or tallness. The normal upper limit in man is about 2.0 m (80 in) but a few normal individuals are taller. See GIANTS.

HELIOTHERAPY is the treatment of disease by exposure to sunshine.

HELMCKEN, JOHN SEBASTIAN (1824–1920). British/Canadian surgeon. The year 1850 found him as surgeon in the Hudson's Bay Company fort at Victoria, British Columbia. He was elected to the parliament of Vancouver Island and was named speaker by the other members—three physicians and three laymen. It was said that he was the leading physician between San Francisco and the North Pole, and from Asia to the Rocky Mountains. He led the movement in 1870 which, a year later, brought British Columbia into the Canadian confederation.

HELMHOLTZ, HERMAN LUDWIG FERDINAND VON (1821–94). German physiologist and physicist. With his former fellows *Dubois-Reymond and Brücke he founded the 'New Physiology'. In 1847 he published one of the most important scientific papers of the century, *Über die Erhaltung der Kraft*, which did much to establish the first law of thermodynamics. Although von Helmholtz is now best remembered for his invention of the *ophthalmoscope (1851) he exerted immense influence on science in the 19th century, converting German universities into institutions for organized research. He published a classic handbook of physiological optics (1856–66) and modified *Young's theory of *colour vision.

HELMINTH. Any parasitic worm. Many helminths are important agents of disease in man. For their general classification see WORMS, and for further classification see FLUKES; NEMATODES; TAPEWORM; and under the names of individual worms and their diseases.

HELMINTHIASIS is infestation with parasitic worms. See BILHARZIA; CYSTICERCOSIS; FASCIOLIASIS; FILARIASIS; HOOKWORM; HYDATID; TAPEWORM; THREADWORM.

HELMONT, JOHANNES (John) BAPTISTA VAN (1579–1644). Flemish physician and alchemist. He was a follower of *Paracelsus, and a founder of the *iatrochemical school and of the modern ontological concept of disease. He held that every bodily process was controlled by an *archaeus* or *blas* and was due to a special ferment for which he invented the term 'gas'. All *blas* were presided over by an '*anima sensitiva motivaque*' or soul. He discovered *carbon monoxide, *carbon dioxide, and sulphur dioxide. He showed that the stomach contained acid. He was a believer in weapon salve, spontaneous generation, and the transmutation of metals.

HELP THE AGED was founded in the UK in 1961 and launched a housing scheme for the elderly, moving them out of slums and into sheltered homes where care and help in emergencies is available. The grouping of such homes also combats loneliness. Help the Aged has extended its interests into the conversion of flats and other accommodation. It helps, too, with rehabilitation and the work of day centres which the elderly attend. Dissemination of information about its affairs and about all matters of interest in *gerontology is another valuable activity and its activities have also extended internationally.

HEMATOLOGY, HEMOGLOBIN, etc. See HAEMATOLOGY, etc.

HEMIANOPIA is loss of half of the field of vision.

HEMIATROPHY is unilateral *atrophy (of the whole body or of a part, e.g. the face).

HEMIBALLISMUS is forceful involuntary movement of the limbs affecting one side of the body, often of the arm more than the leg and described as flinging. The usual cause is a stroke involving the contralateral subthalamic nucleus or its connections in an elderly individual.

HEMICRANIA is unilateral headache (the Greek version of the French *migraine).

HEMIPARESIS. See HEMIPLEGIA.

HEMIPLEGIA is paralysis, hemiparesis weakness, of one side of the body, a common result of a *stroke.

HEMLOCK is a *poisonous plant, *Conium maculatum*, containing the *alkaloid coniine. Hemlock is a tall white-flowered umbellifer with purple-spotted stems common in damp woods and by ditches. It is believed to have been the poison by which Socrates was put to death.

HENBANE is a *poisonous plant, *Hyoscyamus niger*, containing the anticholinergic *alkaloids *hyoscyamine and *hyoscine (scopolamine). Henbane, which belongs to the nightshade family, is an evil-smelling poisonous weed with dull, creamy, bell-shaped flowers.

HENCH, PHILIP SHOWALTER (1896–1965). American physician. Having become convinced that the course of *rheumatoid arthritis is potentially reversible, he obtained some of the first available adrenal *glucocorticoid (*cortisone) and tried its effect in patients with rheumatoid arthritis. The immediate results were spectacular, and this soon led to the wide use of cortisone in treatment of many inflammatory states, especially those thought to be immunogenic. In 1950, with *Kendall and Reichstein, a Swiss biochemist, Hench received the *Nobel prize for medicine for work on cortisone.

HENLE, FRIEDRICH GUSTAV JACOB (1809–85). German anatomist and pathologist. He is remembered for describing the loop of the *nephron (loop of Henle). He believed disease was often due to an external cause (*miasma) acting on the body, but his major work was a histological study of *epithelia.

HENOCH, EDUARD HEINRICH (1820–1910). German paediatrician. One of the pioneers of his specialty in Germany, his *Pathologie und Therapie der Kinderkrankheiten* (1865) was the standard textbook of the time. He described anaphylactoid purpura (*Henoch–Schönlein purpura, 1874).

HENOCH–SCHÖNLEIN PURPURA is a form of vascular *purpura occurring mainly in young children, sometimes known as allergic or anaphylactoid purpura.

HEPARIN, a naturally occurring, sulphur-containing complex *polysaccharide, is found in many tissues, especially the liver and the lung, and in *mast cells. It is a local *hormone which acts both as an *anticoagulant and, in conjunction with lipase, as an agent for clearing fat from the blood. Its powerful anticoagulant action is used in treatment, but preparations have to be injected.

HEPATITIS is inflammation of the liver. A number of viruses may be responsible:

Hepatitis A
(infective hepatitis). Transmitted by the faecal/oral route from contamination of foodstuffs by untreated sewage or poor hygiene. It has a 28-50 day incubation period. Acute illness in adults is very rarely fatal.

Hepatitis B
(serum hepatitis). Transmitted from all body fluids by poor surgical sterilization procedures, close contact, blood contamination: infection at birth, needle sharing (drug *addiction), sexual contact. It has a 50–150 day incubation period. It is an acute illness, resolving or causing chronic hepatitis for many years.

Hepatitis C
(non-A, non-B). Transmitted in untreated blood and blood products. Inadequate sterile procedures may increase the infection risk; 30–150 day incubation; >50 per cent of those infected go on to develop chronic hepatitis.

Hepatitis D
(delta agent). Transmission is the same as with hepatitis B. It is only able to infect in the presence of hepatitis B virus, and is associated with an increased risk of severe infection from Hepatitis B.

Hepatitis E
(epidemic hepatitis). Transmitted by faecal/oral route. It probably carries the same environmental risks as

hepatitis A. It has a 20–45 day incubation and is an acute resolving illness, with a 20 per cent mortality in pregnancy.

Other viruses able to cause hepatitis are those of *yellow fever, *infectious mononucleosis (Epstein–Barr virus), *herpes simplex, *cytomegalovirus, and *rubella (the last two particularly in the newborn). Hepatitis may also be caused by *Coxiella burnetii* (*Q fever) and *leptospirosis (Weil's disease, haemorrhagic jaundice, canicola fever, swineherd's disease). A wide variety of drugs and chemicals including alcohol, may cause jaundice.

HEPATOLOGIST. A physician specializing in diseases of the *liver.

HEPATOSCOPY is visual inspection of the liver surface by *laparoscopy. This technique, which also enables *biopsy specimens to be taken, is of great value in the diagnosis of liver disease, particularly of primary and metastatic *carcinoma. With experience, about 70 per cent of the liver surface can be examined by hepatoscopy. The *staging of *Hodgkin's disease, and the differential diagnosis of *jaundice are among the situations where hepatoscopy can also help.

HERBALISM is a system of fringe medicine based on remedies of plant origin. See COMPLEMENTARY (ALTERNATIVE) MEDICINE.

HERBALS are treatises intended to enable the user to identify and employ plants for medicinal purposes. Among the earliest manuscript herbals the best-known and the most influential was that of Dioscorides (1st century, AD), which was described 1600 years after it was written as 'the foundation and grounde-work of all that hath been since delivered'. Thereafter herbals continued to be published (e.g. by Pierandrea Mattioli (1501–77)). until the development of printing and wood engraving in the 16th century allowed the reproduction of fine and detailed representation of plants by the great German and Italian botanists. The British contribution was small, resting on such works as that of William Turner (d. 1568) and *Gerard's *Herball* (1597). Subsequently herbals became increasingly botanical in purpose, moving away from medicine and therapeutic application although many drugs in use today (e.g. *digoxin) are of botanical origin. See also PHARMACOLOGY; MEDICAL BOOKS AND LIBRARIES.

HERBS. Botanically, herbs are vascular non-woody plants, that is leafy plants with no persistent parts above the ground; alternatively they are plants used in medicine or cookery. A herb in the second sense need not be a herb in the first, but usually is.

HEREDITARY ATAXIA is a term covering a group of inherited central nervous system (CNS) disorders characterized by *ataxia, most of which are transmitted as autosomal *recessive defects, some being associated with specific *enzyme deficiencies. Some, too, show autosomal dominant or X-linked inheritance (see GENETICS). The best known example is *Friedreich's ataxia, which usually begins in late childhood and in which progressive CNS degeneration is most marked in the lateral and posterior columns of the spinal cord.

HEREDITARY HAEMORRHAGIC (HEMORRHAGIC) TELANGIECTASIA is a genetic (autosomal *dominant) disorder characterized by multiple patches of *telangiectasia on the skin and mucous membranes, especially inside the nose, mouth, and gastrointestinal tract and on the hands and feet. Recurrent bleeding from the lesions (e.g. *epistaxis) and iron-deficiency *anaemia are common consequences. The condition is also known as the Osler–Rendu–Weber syndrome.

HEREDITY. The transmission of characteristics from parent to offspring; the genetic make-up of an individual. See GENETICS.

HERING, KARL EWALD KONSTANTIN (1834–1918). German physiologist. Early in his career he studied the reflexes from the lungs with *Breuer, but later interested himself in sensory physiology, especially visual. He proposed a theory of *colour vision contrary to the Young–Helmholtz view. He enunciated the law of specific nerve energies, holding that each sensory nerve gives rise only to its own specific sensation.

HERING–BREUER REFLEX. A *reflex, mediated through the *vagus nerves, which operates to limit the depth of normal breathing.

HERMAPHRODITE. A plant or animal which carries both male and female gamete-producing organs (*gonads). The word derives from the fable of Hermaphroditos, son of Hermes and Aphrodite, with whom the nymph Salmacis was so much in love that she prayed for total union with him; her prayer was answered, and the two became one body (Ovid, *Metamorphoses*, iv. 347). Ironically, although he was an unwilling partner, his name designates the male:female state. True human hermaphroditism is very rare; the diagnosis depends on confirming the presence of both oocyte-containing ovarian tissue and sperm-containing testicular tissue in the same patient. *Pseudohermaphroditism, where *phenotype and *genotype are of opposite gender, is commoner.

HERNIA. Any abnormal protrusion of one anatomical structure or part of it, through another. The commonest variety is herniation of part of the *intestine through a weakness in the abdominal wall ('rupture').

HERNIATION. See HERNIA.

HEROIN, or diamorphine, is the di-acetyl derivative of *morphine. It is a powerful narcotic and analgesic, and extremely addictive. In some countries its medical use is proscribed altogether; in others, including the UK but not the USA, physicians find it of value in certain well-defined situations, such as the relief of severe pain in terminal malignant disease. See SUBSTANCE ABUSE.

HEROPHILUS (*fl.* 4th century BC). Megarian anatomist and physiologist. He was probably the first to dissect the human body in public and is suspected of having undertaken human vivisection of prisoners. His anatomical investigations of the brain, the eye, the nerves, and the vascular system were of great importance. He distinguished the *cerebrum from the *cerebellum and the *arteries from the *veins. He described the *meninges, the fourth *cerebral ventricle, the *thyroid, and the *salivary glands. He understood the function of the *nerves. He is remembered in the torcula Herophili; he named the *calamus scriptorius and the *duodenum.

HERPES SIMPLEX. The herpes simplex virus (HSV) causes a wide variety of human disorders, ranging from the familiar recurrent 'cold sore' around the lips to *encephalitis, which kills about half of its victims and leaves the remainder with various degrees of permanent cerebral incapacity.

Modern taxonomy recognizes two types of HSV (also known as *Herpesvirus hominis*) distinguished as 1 and 2.

HSV infection is either primary or recurrent. Most infections of the lips, mouth, pharynx, eye, and central nervous system are due to HSV type 1. Genital and neonatal infections are usually caused by type 2.

Herpetic infection occurs because the virus remains in sensory *ganglia supplying the skin and mucous membrane of the affected sites rather than the sites themselves.

HERPESVIRUS is a genus of large enveloped *deoxyribonucleic acid (DNA) viruses belonging to the family Herpetoviridae. See HERPES SIMPLEX.

HERPES ZOSTER, or shingles, like *chickenpox, is an acute infectious disease caused by the varicella–zoster (V–Z) virus. It is due to reactivation of the virus latent in sensory nerve *ganglia following a previous infection, usually of chickenpox. The resultant ganglionitis causes pain in the skin followed by virus multiplication in the same area, with the production of crops of characteristic skin lesions. Later scarring occurs, as reassertion of immunity terminates the overt disease. Typically the rash is unilateral, and most commonly over the trunk.

When in the ophthalmic distribution of the *trigeminal nerve, *corneal scarring may be a serious complication. Persistent pain (post-herpetic *neuralgia) may be a problem, especially in elderly patients. It can be very severe, and has been known to lead to suicide.

HERRICK, JAMES BRYAN (1861–1954). American physician. In 1910 he wrote the first description of the appearance of red blood cells in *sickle-cell anaemia. In 1912 he described clearly the clinical manifestations of sudden occlusion of a coronary artery (*myocardial infarction).

HERTZ is the derived *SI unit of frequency, equal to one cycle per second (symbol Hz). The name commemorated is that of the German physicist, Heinrich R. Hertz (1857–94).

HERXHEIMER, KARL (1861–1942). The leading German dermatologist of his day, he described the aggravation of a *syphilitic lesion with pyrexia which may occur shortly after treatment (Jarisch–Herxheimer reaction, 1895).

HESSELBACH, FRANZ KASPAR (1759–1816). German surgeon and anatomist. His name is attached to several anatomical structures but the best-known is the area bounded by the lateral margin of the rectus abdominis muscle, the inferior epigastric vessels, and the *inguinal ligament (Hesselbach's triangle).

HETEROLOGOUS. Different; having a different origin, different relations, or different components (*cf.* HOMOLOGOUS).

HETEROZYGOTE. Having different alleles at a particular genetic locus. See GENETICS.

HEVESY, GEORG CHARLES DE (1885–1966) Hungarian chemist. His seminal work in chemistry and radiochemistry resulted in the discovery of the new element hafnium in 1923; but his major discoveries related to the use of radioactive tracer substances in the study of chemical processes in living organisms, which led to his receiving the *Nobel prize for chemistry in 1943 and the Copley medal of the Royal Society in 1949. He is recognized as the founder of *nuclear medicine.

HEWSON, WILLIAM (1739–74). British surgeon and anatomist. He died at the age of 35 from a dissection wound. Hewson has been called the 'father of British haematology' and his researches on coagulation of the blood, the blood cells, and the lymphatic system were of great importance. They were published in *An* *experimental inquiry into the properties of the blood* (1771).

HEY, WILLIAM (1736–1819). British surgeon. He was one of the founders of the Leeds General Infirmary. He was a skilled operator and devised several surgical instruments. 'Hey's amputation' entails disarticulation through the tarso-metatarsal joint.

HIATUS HERNIA is herniation of part of the *stomach through the oesophageal hiatus of the *diaphragm into the *thorax. It is often associated with reflux of acid gastric contents into the lower part of the *oesophagus, and it is this which gives rise to the most frequent symptom, *heartburn, particularly when the patient lies flat in bed.

HICCUP. Spasmodic contraction of the *diaphragm, either isolated or occurring in short-lived repetitive bursts. There is usually no obvious cause, but hiccups are sometimes due to a pathological process irritating the diaphragm. Occasionally attacks are sufficiently prolonged and distressing to warrant active treatment, for example by crushing one of the *phrenic nerves to paralyse the diaphragm on one side.

HICKMAN, HENRY HILL (1800–30). British physician. Hickman experimented on animals with *carbon dioxide and *nitrous oxide, showing that they induced insensitivity to pain. He thought that this would be useful in surgery but was dismissed as a crank, and died at an early age.

HIGHMORE, NATHANIEL (1613–65). British physician. He described the *maxillary sinus ('antrum of Highmore') in his *Corporis humani disquisitio anatomica* (1651).

HILTON, JOHN (1804–78). English surgeon. His lectures to the *Royal College of Surgeons of England were collected and published under the title *On rest and pain*; in them, he emphasized the importance of rest in orthopaedic care. He was responsible for formulating Hilton's law, which states that the nerve trunk which supplies the interior of a joint also supplies the muscles responsible for moving that joint and the skin overlying their insertions. His name is also remembered in alternative anatomical nomenclature in connection with the pectinate or anocutaneous line (Hilton's white line), the laryngeal saccule (Hilton's sac), and the aryepiglottic muscle (Hilton's muscle).

HIP JOINT. The joint formed by the rounded upper end (head) of the *femur and the socket (acetabulum) of the hip bone.

HIPPOCAMPUS. An elongated eminence in the temporal lobes of the *cerebrum, related to the floor of the lateral *cerebral ventricles, part of which is also known as Ammon's horn.

HIPPOCRATES (460–*c.* 370 BC). Greek physician. Born in *Cos, the son of a physician, Hippocrates travelled and practised in Thrace, Thessaly, and Macedonia. He is mentioned by Plato in one of the early dialogues and by *Aristotle. There is so little known of him that some scholars deny his existence and speak of him as 'a name lacking any accessible historical reality'.

The corpus of 60 medical works known as the Hippocratic collection contains many contemporary with the Hippocratic school and some which are not. It may well have been the library of Cos. They are, however, all imbued with what has come to be regarded as the Hippocratic spirit. It is generally believed that Hippocrates himself wrote *Prognostics* and *Joints*. The *Hippocratic oath, although accurately reflecting the Hippocratic ethic, came much later.

Hippocrates set medicine free of the shackles of religion and philosophy and systematized the disorderly accumulation of knowledge at Cos and Cnidos. He was the first to record case histories, the first to base his practice on bedside observation, and the first to provide the physician with moral inspiration and ethical standards. Although his views on pathology were later discarded, his vivid disease pictures often allow a diagnosis to be made 2000 years after they were written.

HIPPOCRATIC FACIES. The facial appearance of impending death was described by *Hippocrates (*Prognostics*) as 'a sharp nose, hollow eyes, collapsed temples; the ears cold, contracted and their lobes turned out; the skin about the forehead being rough, distended and parched; the colour of the whole face being green, black, livid or lead-coloured'. This description was movingly echoed by Mistress Quickly in her account of Falstaff's death (*Henry V*, II. iii): '. . . for after I saw him fumble with the sheets, and play with flowers, and smile upon his fingers' ends, I knew there was but one way; for his nose was as sharp as a pen . . .'.

HIPPOCRATIC OATH. The Hippocratic oath is the best-known of the Hippocratic writings (see HIPPOCRATES), the original authorship of which is uncertain. The spirit of the oath transcends its archaisms and has continued to inspire the ethics of the medical profession. It reads as follows:

I swear by Apollo the physician, by Aesculapius, Hygeia, and Panacea, and I take to witness all the gods, all the goddesses, to keep according to my ability and my judgement the following Oath:

To consider dear to me as my parents him who taught me this art; to live in common with him and if necessary to share my goods with him; to look upon his children as my own brothers, to teach them this art if they so desire without fee or written promise; to impart to my sons and the sons of the master who taught me and the disciples who have enrolled themselves and have agreed to the rules of the profession, but to these alone, the precepts and the instruction. I will prescribe regimen for the good of my patients according to my ability and my judgement and never do harm to anyone. To please no one will I prescribe a deadly drug, nor give advice which may cause his death. Nor will I give a woman a pessary to procure abortion. But I will preserve the purity of my life and my art. I will not cut for stone, even for patients in whom the disease is manifest; I will leave this operation to be performed by practitioners (specialists in this art). In every house where I come I will enter only for the good of my patients, keeping myself far from all intentional ill-doing and all seduction, and especially from the pleasures of love with women or with men be they free or slaves. All that may come to my knowledge in the exercise of my profession or outside of my profession or in daily commerce with men, which ought not to be spread abroad, I will keep secret and will never reveal. If I keep this oath faithfully, may I enjoy my life and practise my art, respected by all men and in all times; but if I swerve from it or violate it, may the reverse be my lot.

HIP REPLACEMENT is an operation frequently undertaken in older patients disabled by *osteoarthrosis of the hip, in which the joint is totally replaced by an artificial ball-and-socket device. See ORTHOPAEDIC SURGERY.

HIRSCHSPRUNG'S DISEASE. See MEGACOLON.

HIRSUTISM is an abnormal degree of hairiness (in either sex).

HIRUDO MEDICINALIS, the medicinal *leech, is one of the 11 freshwater species found in the UK. Like the others, it is a blood-sucking worm-like aquatic animal with a sucker at each end capable of a powerful grip, and it secretes the anticoagulant hirudin. It is, however, the only one of the 11 capable of piercing the human skin. It was formerly extensively employed as a method of *blood-letting, but in recent years its use has been confined to *ophthalmology.

HIS, WILHELM, Sr (1831–1904). Swiss anatomist. He was a leading histologist whose most important work was on histogenesis, especially of nervous and lymphatic tissues. He showed that the *axon was an outgrowth from the primitive nerve cell and that the *neuroglia was of ectodermal origin.

HIS, WILHELM, Jr (1863–1934). German physician. He described the collection of specialized fibres in the heart which convey the impulse from the *atrioventricular node to the ventricles (*bundle of His, 1893). He wrote an account of Vollaynian fever as seen on the Russian front in the First World War; known on the

Western Front as *trench fever, it proved to be due to a *rickettsia.

HISTAMINE, $C_5H_9N_3$, is a substance universally present in tissues and secreted by *mast cells and *basophils. Acting as a local *hormone, it is responsible for a variety of functions: these include increasing the calibre and permeability of *capillaries; contraction of most smooth muscle, including that of the *bronchial tree; stimulation of acid and *pepsin secretion by the stomach; and acceleration of heart rate. The first two of these four are inhibited by conventional *antihistamine drugs and are said to be mediated by H_1 receptors; the second two are not, and are assumed to act through different (H_2) receptors (see H_2 RECEPTOR ANTAGONISTS).

HISTIOCYTE. The resting tissue form of the *cell otherwise known as a *macrophage. It is a large mononuclear highly *phagocytic cell found in all connective tissue which is also the essential unit of the *reticuloendothelial system, removing particles from the blood and lymph.

HISTOCHEMISTRY. An extension of microscopical staining techniques which uses chemical reactions in order to identify particular compounds or types of compound in the tissues and structures under examination. See PATHOLOGY.

HISTOCOMPATIBILITY ANTIGENS. See HLA.

HISTOLOGY is the study of tissues, the microscopic branch of *anatomy.

HISTOPATHOLOGY. See PATHOLOGY.

HISTOPLASMOSIS is a fungus infection due to inhalation of the *spores of the yeast-like organism *Histoplasma capsulatum*. The infection ranges from the totally asymptomatic or a mild flu-like illness through acute and chronic pulmonary forms to a severe disseminated involvement primarily of the *reticuloendothelial system which may spread to the heart, central nervous system, gastrointestinal tract, and other organs. Severe infection is particularly likely to occur in immunocompromised patients and at the extremes of age. Histoplasmosis is common in many parts of the world, including the USA.

HISTORIOGRAPHY OF MEDICINE. Long before professional historians developed an active interest, medicine's past was of critical consequence for medical practitioners and professors alike, eager to recruit the dead to their causes, to commemorate exemplary figures, to inspire their students, and to construct an imposing pedigree for their art. Not least, past heroes long possessed present authority. For the humanist physicians of the 16th and 17th centuries, the treatises of medicine's founding fathers, notably *Hippocrates and *Galen, were absolutely canonical, living founts of wisdom, rather than mere objects of antiquarian curiosity.

The first significant attempt to construct a full narrative of medicine's evolution was *Histoire de la médecine d'ou l'on voit l'origine et le progrès de l'art* (1696) by Daniel Leclerc, professor of medicine in Geneva. A derivative English work soon followed: the *History of physick* (1725–26) by the London physician, John *Freind. Freind's survey of Graeco-Roman and medieval medicine was structured with half an eye to contemporary English debates concerning the medical applications of the Newtonian mechanical philosophy: the past could still settle current controversies.

In the history of medicine, as with political and diplomatic history, the Enlightenment—the age of Edward Gibbon—and, even more so, the 19th century mark the scholarly watershed. Historians began to insist that the past was a different country, truly distinct from the present. Study of long-dead doctors and their august tomes gradually ceased to be definitive of medical thinking itself, and turned into a scholarly passion or pastime in its own right. The first history of medicine in this 'modern' mode was Kurt Sprengel's *Versuch einer pragmatischen Geschichte der Arzneikunde* (1792), which strove to steer a middle course between pedantic antiquarianism and high-flown philosophical interpretations. German scholarship led the field in the 19th century. In his *Lehrbuch der Geschichte der Medizin und der Volkskrankheit* (1845), Heinrich Haeser produced the first professed textbook of medical history—a work that gave consideration to historical *epidemiology as well as to the history of doctors. The first periodical devoted exclusively to medical history, the German-language *Janus*, was founded in 1846—it lasted only 2 years—and the first chair in the history of medicine was created in Vienna in 1850.

Great attention began to be devoted to furnishing authoritative editions of key texts. Nineteenth-century scholarship produced many of the editions of the classic authors still in use. The works of Galen were edited in Leipzig between 1823 and 1833, while the French philological scholar, Emile Littré, edited Hippocrates between 1839 and 1861. From 1844, the *Sydenham Society in England dedicated itself to publishing a renowned series of translations of Greek, Latin, and Arabic medical classics. Alongside the creation of a canon of classical medical texts, book-collecting became a prestigious avocation. Sir William *Osler (b. 1849) built up a celebrated personal library, now preserved in Montreal, and, most spectacularly, Sir Henry *Wellcome (b. 1853) channelled profits from his pharmaceutical business into the assembling of an enormous collection of medical books, manuscripts, paintings, and artefacts, that was to form the core of the Wellcome Institute for the History of Medicine in London.

Amongst historians of medicine, the pivotal figure is Karl Sudhoff, who was professor of the history of medicine at Leipzig from 1905 to 1925 and director of the first institute of the history of medicine. Sudhoff set particular store by manuscript research. Under his direction, the first enduring journal of the history of medicine was set up (*Sudhoffs Archiv*) and essential reference works were compiled, notably the *Biographisches Lexikon der hervorragenden Arzte* by August Hirsch and Julius Pagel, which began publication in 1884 and took 50 years to complete.

Sudhoff's Leipzig institute became the envy of, and model for, medical historians the world over. His successor, the Swiss Henry Sigerist (1891–1957), broadened the intellectual vision of medical history, and, as a committed admirer of the Soviet Union, developed a more socially oriented view of medical history. In 1932 Sigerist was appointed head of the newly founded Institute for the History of Medicine at the Johns Hopkins University, Baltimore. From 1933 there appeared, under his guidance, the *Bulletin of the History of Medicine*, and the American Association for the History of Medicine was founded.

Until recently the bulk of writings in the history of medicine have been 'in-house': written by doctors, for doctors, and principally about doctors. This tendency to treat medical history as essentially the contributions of physicians and biomedical scientists to the progress of medical knowledge and practice has come under attack, especially in the present generation. It has been accused of being Whiggish, that is, of judging the past in the light of hindsight. Many historians of medicine nowadays stress the dangers of anachronism, and insist, by contrast, that earlier physicians and medical belief-systems must be understood on their own terms, rather than being evaluated in terms of their contribution to modern medicine. They also seek to widen the vision, and pay more attention than heretofore to the history of patients as well as practitioners, to lay wisdom and popular forms of healing, to medical institutions and the paramedical professions, and to the social and political ramifications of medical knowledge. Hopefully a fruitful dialogue will develop between the unique medical expertise of 'practitioners' history' and the wider visions of professional historians.

ROY PORTER

Further reading
Webster, C. (1983). The historiography of medicine. In *Information sources in the history of science and medicine*, (ed. P. Corsi and P. Weindling), pp. 29–43. Butterworth Scientific, London.

HISTORY OF MEDICINE. All societies possess medical beliefs: ideas of life and death, disease and cure, and systems of healing. To speak extremely schematically, the historical development of medicine may be seen in terms of a series of stages. The most elementary belief-systems the world over have attributed sickness to ill-will, to various modes of malevolent spirits, sorcery, witchcraft, and diabolical or divine intervention. Such ways of thinking still pervade the pre-literate tribal communities of Africa, South America, and the Pacific, and were influential in Christian Europe throughout the Middle Ages and the Reformation era. A few radical protestant sects continue to view sickness and recovery largely in providential and supernatural terms; healing shrines like *Lourdes remain popular within the Roman Catholic Church, and faith-healing retains a following.

In Europe from Graeco-Roman antiquity onwards, and also amongst the great Asian civilizations, the leading approach to sickness and healing replaced such transcendental explanations by positing a natural basis for disease and healing. Amongst educated lay people and physicians alike, the body became viewed as integral to a wider cosmic scheme of law-governed elements and regular processes. Greek medicine in particular underscored the microcosm/macrocosm relationship, the correlations between the healthy human body and the harmonies of external nature. From *Hippocrates in the 5th century BC through to *Galen in the 2nd century AD, 'humoral medicine' emphasized the analogies between the four elements of external nature (earth, air, fire, and water)and the four humours or fluids (blood, phlegm, choler or yellow bile, and black bile), whose balance determined bodily health. The humours found expression in the temperaments and complexions that marked an individual's constitution. The task of *hygiene was to maintain a balanced constitution; the role of medicine to restore such balance when disturbed. The medicine of antiquity, which was transmitted via Islam to the medieval West and remained powerful throughout the Renaissance era, paid great attention to general health maintenance, through regulation of diet, exercise, hygiene, and life-style. In the absence of detailed anatomical and physiological expertise, and without the benefit of a powerful artillery of cures and surgical skills, the ability to advance diagnoses and prognoses was highly valued, and an intimate physician–patient relationship was fostered. The teachings of antiquity, which remained authoritative to the 18th century and still form an undercurrent of medical folklore, were more successful in assisting people to cope with chronic conditions and in soothing lesser ailments than in conquering the life-threatening infections that became *endemic and *epidemic in the civilized world (*leprosy, *plague, *smallpox, *measles, and, later, the 'filth diseases' such as *typhus, associated with urban squalor).

This rather personal tradition of bedside medicine long remained popular in the West, as did its equivalents in China and India (Ayurvedic medicine). But in Europe it was gradually supplemented and challenged by the creation of a more 'scientific' mode of medicine, grounded, for the first time, upon precise and systematic anatomical and physiological investigation, epitomized from the 15th century by the dissection techniques that were to become central to medical education. Landmarks in this programme include the publication of *De humani corporis fabrica* (1543) by the Paduan professor, Andreas *Vesalius, the first momentous anatomical atlas and a work that challenged truths received since Galen; and William *Harvey's *De motu cordis* (1628) which, by experimentally demonstrating the circulation of the blood and the role of the heart as a pump, put physiological enquiry on the map. Post-Vesalian investigations immeasurably advanced knowledge of the structures and functions of the living organism. Further enquiries saw the unravelling of the *lymphatic system and the lacteals (*chylous vessels), and the 18th and 19th centuries yielded a finer grasp of the nervous system and the operation of the brain. With the aid of microscopes and the laboratory, 19th century investigators explored the nature of body tissues and pioneered cell biology; pathological anatomy came of age. Parallel improvements in organic chemistry led to an understanding of *respiration, *nutrition, the digestive system and deficiency diseases, and to such specialties as *endocrinology. The 20th century has been the age of *genetics and *molecular biology.

Most spectacularly, 19th century science made enormous leaps forward in the understanding of infectious diseases. For many centuries, rival epidemiological theories had attributed *fevers to miasmas (poisons in the air, exuded from rotting animal and vegetable material, the soil, and standing water) or to contagion (person-to-person contact), with little solid evidence to clinch the dispute. From the 1860s, the rise of *bacteriology, associated especially with Louis *Pasteur in France and Robert *Koch in Germany, established the role of micro-organic pathogens. Bacteriology led, in time, to dramatic new cures.

In the short run, however, the anatomically based scientific medicine emerging from Renaissance universities and the Scientific Revolution, contributed more to information than to health. Drugs from both the Old and New Worlds, notably *opium and Peruvian bark (*quinine) became more widely available, and mineral and metal-based pharmaceutical preparations enjoyed a great if dubious vogue (e.g. mercury for *syphilis). But it would be tendentious to speak of a true pharmacological revolution before the introduction of *sulphonamides and *antibiotics in the 20th century, and surgery could make only limited progress before the introduction of *anaesthetics and *antiseptic and *aseptic operating-room conditions from the mid-19th century. In short, biomedical understanding long outstripped dramatic breakthroughs in curative medicine, and many would argue that the retreat of the great lethal diseases (*diphtheria, *typhoid, tuberculosis, etc.) was due, in the first instance, more to urban improvements, superior nutrition, and *public health regulations than to curative medicine. Indeed, the one early striking instance of the conquest of disease—the introduction first of smallpox inoculation and then of vaccination—

came not through 'science' at all but through the alert embracing of a tenet of popular medical folklore.

From the Renaissance, medical practitioners increasingly organized themselves professionally, commonly in a hierarchy with physicians at the head, and surgeons and apothecaries nearer the foot, and with other sorts of healers marginalized or vilified (justly or not) as quacks. Practitioners' guilds, corporations, and colleges received royal approval, and medicine gradually became incorporated within the public domain, particularly in the German-speaking parts of Europe, where the notion of 'medical police' (preventive public health) gained official backing from the 18th century. The state inevitably played the leading role in the growth of military and naval medicine (see DEFENCE MEDICAL SERVICES), and later in *tropical medicine. The *hospital sphere, however, long remained largely the responsibility of the Church, especially in Roman Catholic parts of Europe, and of urban philanthropic initiatives. Gradually (some would say, belatedly) the state took responsibility for improving the health of the populations of the emergent industrial societies, through public health regulation and custody of the insane in the 19th century, and through national insurance and national health schemes in the 20th century, although these latter developments often met fierce opposition from a medical profession seeking to preserve its autonomy against encroaching state bureaucracies.

The latter half of the 20th century has witnessed the continued phenomenal progress of immensely capital-intensive and specialized scientific medicine. *Transplant surgery and biotechnology have captured the public imagination. Alongside, major chronic and psychosomatic disorders persist in the advanced world, and there is little sign that the basic health problems of the developing world are diminishing. This situation exemplifies and perpetuates a key facet and paradox of the history of medicine: the unresolved disequilibrium between the remarkable capacities of an increasingly powerful science-based biomedical tradition and, on the other hand, the wider and unfulfilled health requirements of economically impoverished and politically mismanaged societies.

ROY PORTER

HIV. Human immunodeficiency virus. See AIDS AND HIV.

HIVES. Nettlerash or *urticaria.

HLA (HUMAN LEUCOCYTE (HISTOCOMPATIBILITY) ANTIGENS) play a major role in cross-matching procedures and in determining whether or not an organ or tissue *transplant will be rejected by the host. They occur on the surface of all nucleated cells, the initials deriving from their first identification on human leucocytes (human leucocyte antigen) (see also IMMUNOLOGY). They are genetically determined by a region on chromosome 6, termed the major histocompatability complex or MHC. A number of genetic loci, each with multiple alleles (see GENETICS), are concerned and are designated by letters (HLA-A, HLA-B, and so on), while the actual antigen is identified by a number (e.g. HLA-B27).

Statistical associations between the presence of particular HLA antigens and particular diseases are being increasingly demonstrated; for example, there is a strong correlation between *ankylosing spondylitis and HLA-B27, and many other such correlations, although of varying strength, have been described.

HOADLEY, BENJAMIN (1706–57). British physician and playwright. Of his numerous plays the most successful was *The Suspicious Husband* (1747), in which David Garrick played.

HODGKIN, THOMAS (1798–1866). British physician. Hodgkin was a Quaker who was appointed curator of the museum at *Guy's Hospital, but was not elected to the post of physician because of an altercation with the hospital treasurer. He was a keen geographer and died of *dysentery on a journey with Sir Moses Montefiore in Palestine. He is buried at Jaffa. He described cases of enlarged spleen and lymph nodes (1832) subsequently called *Hodgkin's disease by Sir Samuel *Wilks.

HODGKIN'S DISEASE is a malignant disease of the lymphoid and reticuloendothelial systems which was described by Thomas *Hodgkin in 1832. See HAEMATOLOGY; ONCOLOGY.

HOFFMANN, HEINRICH (1809–74). German psychiatrist. He is now remembered for his minatory book for children *Struwwelpeter* (1847), which is still in circulation.

HOLISTIC MEDICINE is a doctrine of preventive and therapeutic medicine which emphasizes the importance of regarding the individual as a whole being integral with his social, cultural, and environmental context rather than as a patient with isolated malfunction of a particular system or organ. Although the term has recently become fashionable, the underlying philosophy is nothing new and has always been inseparable from good medical practice.

HOLLAND, PHILEMON (1552–1637). British physician and translator who was described by Fuller as the 'translator generall of his age'. His most popular works were Pliny's *Natural History* (1601), Plutarch's *Morals* (1603), and Camden's *Britannia* (1610).

HOLMES, SIR GORDON MORGAN (1876–1967). Anglo-Irish neurologist. His most outstanding work was on the physiology of the *cerebral visual cortex, the *thalamus, and the *cerebellum, but he was also a clinical neurologist of genius.

HOLMES, OLIVER WENDELL (1809–94). American physician and author. He is best remembered for poems including 'Old Ironsides' and other writings including *The autocrat of the breakfast-table* (1858), *The professor at the breakfast-table* (1860), and *The poet at the breakfast-table* (1872), but his medical treatise on the contagious nature of *puerperal fever was an important contribution, which aroused great interest and controversy.

HOLT, LUTHER EMMETT (1855–1924). American paediatrician. Holt was one of the first American physicians to limit his practice to diseases of children and was influential in establishing paediatrics as a special field of medical practice. His textbook *Diseases of infancy and childhood* went through many editions, and is looked upon as an American medical classic.

HOMATROPINE is an analogue of *atropine, with similar but weaker anticholinergic effects.

HOME, SIR EVERARD BT (1756–1832). British surgeon. As John Hunter's brother-in-law and executor, he destroyed all Hunter's notebooks and manuscripts in 1823 having used their contents in preparing papers he claimed as his own.

HOME NURSING. Under Section 25 of the UK National Health Service Act 1946, confirmed by a National Health Service Act 1977, the local authority must provide for home nursing, either by arrangement with voluntary organizations or by employing nurses themselves.

HOME OFFICE PATHOLOGIST. Forensic pathologist. See FORENSIC MEDICINE.

HOMEOPATHY. See HOMOEOPATHY.

HOMEOSTASIS is a physiological state of constancy, deviation from which is countered by the operation of one or more negative-feedback loops. For example, any tendency of tissue *carbon dioxide tension to rise is countered by an increase in pulmonary ventilation and its increased elimination; conversely, *hypoventilation cancels any tendency for pCO_2 to fall. Increased generation of heat within the body causes *vasodilatation and sweating, leading to increased heat loss, so that body temperature remains constant. *Thyroid hormone inhibits its trophic hormone, *thyroid-stimulating hormone (TSH), and so on. Countless such mechanisms constantly operate to maintain the *milieu intérieur* described by Claude *Bernard.

HOMES FOR THE AGED are private or charity-funded nursing-homes for old people.

HOMICIDE. The killing of man; murder or manslaughter. See FORENSIC MEDICINE.

HOMOEOPATHY is a system of medicine founded by Samuel *Hahnemann (1755–1843) based on the doctrine that diseases can be cured by administering minute doses of drugs which in larger amounts cause the symptoms of the particular disease being treated, that is the principle of *similia similibus curantur* (cf. *allopathy). See COMPLEMENTARY MEDICINE.

HOMOGRAFT. *Allograft.

HOMOLOGOUS. Similar; having a similar origin, similar relations or similar components (cf. *heterologous).

HOMO SAPIENS is the only surviving species of *Homo*, a genus of catarrhine primates (i.e. narrow nasal septum, menstrual cycle, no prehensile tail) which includes several extinct species (e.g. Neanderthal man). The anatomical distinctions between *Homo* and other catarrhine primates include: large brain; absence of brow ridges; chin prominence; small canine teeth; and reduced toe size, with the big toe not opposable to others.

HOMOSEXUAL. See HOMOSEXUALITY.

HOMOSEXUALITY, sexual inversion, in which sexual orientation is towards individuals of the same gender, is the condition of a significant proportion of humanity; of the total population, male and female, about 4 per cent are exclusively homosexual. Facultative homosexuality is much commoner; many men can become homosexual when restricted to male company for prolonged periods, for example at boarding school or during long sea voyages; and the same is true for some women. Kinsey found that as many as 37 per cent of all US males had experienced homosexual contact to the point of orgasm; the corresponding figure for women was 13 per cent. Some few individuals live a bisexual existence, maintaining heterosexual and homosexual relationships simultaneously.

Modern Western society on the whole treats its homosexual minority with tolerance. In the UK, for example, the stigma of criminality was removed in 1966 from homosexual acts when they take place in private between consenting adults over the age of 21 (the minimum age was changed to 18 in 1994). While such acts are biologically perverse, being non-procreative, it can be argued that so too are the vast majority of heterosexual acts. A distinctive feature of present-day male homosexuality, as opposed to that among females, is its organized and institutionalized character, manifest in pubs, clubs, magazines, and male prostitution.

Homosexuality has no discernible organic basis, and has been thought to be psychologically determined; in

*Freud's view, Oedipal mother-attachment played an important role. However, some evidence is emerging to suggest that the condition may be due to an autosomal recessive *gene.

Medically, homosexuality is important because of venereal disease (see SEXUALLY TRANSMITTED DISEASE); 30 per cent of all sexually transmitted disease in males occurs in homosexuals, among whom promiscuity is common. Recently the acquired immune deficiency syndrome (*AIDS) has been shown to be closely associated with homosexual contact, especially in men.

HOMOZYGOTE. Having identical alleles at a particular genetic locus. See GENETICS.

HOOKE, ROBERT (1635–1703). British experimental philosopher. He was an early microscopist, and the first to use the word '*cell' in its biological sense. He made fundamental and original observations on respiration and combustion; he designed a *hearing aid; and was responsible for the architectural plans of the Royal College of Physicians and Bethlem Hospital. His most important publication was *Micrographia* (1665).

HOOKER, SIR JOSEPH DALTON (1817–1911). British physician and botanist. In 1839 he accompanied Sir James Clark Ross on HMS *Erebus* to Tasmania and New Zealand, bringing back many botanical specimens. He travelled extensively in the Himalayas, Sikkim, Tibet, and Nepal. He succeeded his father as director of Kew Gardens in 1865.

HOOKWORM. See ANKYLOSTOMIASIS.

HOPKINS, SIR FREDERICK GOWLAND (1861–1947). British biochemist. Hopkins's researches were wide-ranging and of fundamental importance. He identified *tryptophan (1901), showed that *lactic acid was formed by muscular contraction (1906), established the role of *vitamins (1912), and identified *glutathione (1921). In 1929 he was awarded the *Nobel prize for medicine with Christiaan *Eijkman for his work on vitamins.

HOPPE-SEYLER, FELIX (1825–95). German biochemist. Most of his work was on *haemoglobin, which he named in 1862. He obtained it in crystalline form, described its functions, and studied its spectrum as well as those of the substances derived from it.

HORDER, SIR THOMAS JEEVES, Bt, 1st Baron Horder of Ashford (1871–1955). British physician. Horder was the leading British clinician of his age and made valuable observations on cerebrospinal *meningitis and bacterial *endocarditis. He was an early exponent of the value of clinical pathology and claimed to have taken 'the bench to the bedside'. He was a member of many government and other committees.

HORMONE. An organic chemical substance secreted by a cell or group of cells which diffuses in body fluids to act on other cells, nearby or remote. (The definition was formerly restricted to such substances transported by the blood to act on remote cells.) See ENDOCRINOLOGY.

HORSESHOE KIDNEY is the congenital fusion of corresponding poles of the two kidneys, usually without functional disturbance.

HORSLEY, SIR VICTOR ALEXANDER HADEN (1857–1916). British surgeon and experimental physiologist. He proved that *myxoedema was due to thyroid deficiency by excising a monkey's thyroid gland (1883), he carried out researches on the localization of function in the brain and spinal cord (1884), and he reported on *Pasteur's antirabies treatment (1886). In 1885 he was appointed surgeon to *University College Hospital and the following year to the *National Hospital for Nervous Diseases. In 1887 Horsley was the first to remove an accurately localized *spinal tumour.

HOSPICE. Originally meaning a house of rest and entertainment for travellers and pilgrims, particularly one owned and run by a religious order, in current usage the word 'hospice' has come to signify a hospital or nursing-home specializing in the care and management of terminal illness. See DEATH, DYING, AND THE HOSPICE MOVEMENT.

HOSPITAL SHIP. A troopship or other ship adapted for the transport of the sick and wounded.

HOSPITALS IN THE UK
Origins
For the origins of real hospital instinct, one has to look to the East in pre-Christian times. Sir Henry Burdett (1891), doyen of hospital administrators at the end of the 19th century summed it up thus:

Throughout all that vast region of the East which accepted the system of Buddha—a region extending even to America . . . there were hospitals based upon the principles of benevolence and charity only less sublime than those of Jesus of Nazareth . . . They were hospitals in our modern sense of the word.

'*Hospitium*', meaning a place for guests, had its meaning extended, probably during Roman times, also to mean 'needing shelter'. The Romans, however, concentrated their expertise on the needs of their soldiers in the field. Soldiers were judged to be too valuable to be cast out to die, and in a typical Roman camp the hospital would be placed near an outer wall, far from the busy centre.

Throughout the Middle Ages there were, in effect, only two types of hospitals, both dependent upon the Church. They were the monastic infirmaria which were mainly used only for the care of the sick monks and formed part of monastic institutions; and lazar houses (*lazarettes) which were important and numerous because of the prevalence of *leprosy at that time. This disease declined in the 15th century and from then lazar houses disappeared from the UK.

The typical monastic infirmary was unlike our own hospitals. A monk who was ill brought with him his own bed and bedding. The form of the building was usually a long hall with an altar at the east end, the beds being arranged in two rows with their backs to the side walls. The beautiful hospice at Beaune in central France and St Mary's Hospital at Chichester (now an almshouse) are good examples.

The emphasis placed by the Church upon charity meant that monasteries provided refuge and solace for the poor and for an assortment of supplicants. The open ward, itself adapted from the Roman concept, was the single architectural feature which later was taken over from the monasteries, adapted and refined, and finally mass-produced.

The infirmarer at the monasteries was not a doctor: he was one of the monks, and his duties were primarily administrative and religious. Such a monk would acquire some medical knowledge, and in the library of the larger monasteries there was probably one large textbook of medicine. From the information on the rolls of these monastic hospitals, it is clear that the main virtues were compassion and sympathy, and abbots were urged to provide delicate food and appropriate medicines.

During the Middle Ages there was great fear of fever, and partly because of this there were attempts to segregate fever patients. No treatment was possible, herbs were worn to ward off the dreaded disease, and the rich would tend to leave the cities for the country, thus taking the disease with them. Fever apart, financial support for hospitals continued to be forthcoming from private benefactors and from the Guilds. Almsgiving was considered a noble virtue and men of standing had their own almoners. Almoners of monasteries not only dispensed alms but visited the old and infirm in their homes.

In the 15th century, civic responsibilty for the poor increased. A Bill was promoted, unsuccessfully, in 1414 to provide for the state foundation and financing of hospitals, which were to be put under public administration. There was a still greater decline in the years following the dissolution of the monasteries by Henry VIII. During the 16th century, hospitals virtually became independent of the Church and responsibility was taken by the laity. The Poor Law of 1601 established the principle of public responsibility and formed the basis of the Poor Law administration until the 19th century. This did not preclude private enterprise and the many 'private' almshouses that still exist bear witness to this.

The foundation and growth of voluntary hospitals

Between 1700 and 1825, 154 new hospitals and dispensaries were founded. This was the age of philanthropy,

when the care of the sick was no longer seen as the sole prerogative of the Church. The growth of scientific medicine as we know it today began only at the end of this time and the new hospitals reflected in their rules the driving force of patronage and of discipline. For instance the *Addenbrooke's 'Hospital Rules' of 1767 laid down:

Persons who meet with sudden accidents requiring the immediate Help of Surgery are received at any hour of the day or night without any recommendation. All other patients are admitted on MONDAYS between the hours of ten and twelve; and they are desired to attend punctually before eleven o'clock, it having been found inconvenient to admit any who offer themselves after that hour . . . That no patients be admitted who are able to subsist themselves and pay for medicines.

The need for hospital accommodation during the 18th century was overwhelming and increased with the growth of the urban population in the new manufacturing towns. The years 1750 to 1850 have been described by G. M. Trevelyan (1946) and others as 'the age of enlightenment'. Be that as it may, that century saw the evolution of science as we now know it out of philosophy. The work of scientists such as *Jenner, *Smellie, and *Hunter, to mention only three, as well as the philanthropic ideas they generated, had a direct bearing upon the foundation of hospitals in the UK. The establishment of voluntary hospitals provided the physicians and surgeons with the opportunity of gaining experience and, as it were in return, they gave their services in the treatment of the sick poor.

Table 1 illustrates the enormous increase in the number of voluntary hospitals founded in the UK during the 19th century and especially in the second half of Queen Victoria's reign.

It can be safely said that whereas until the middle of the 19th century there was little that could be done in hospital which could not be done as well, and probably more safely done, in a well-built home, after that date hospitals became the best places for the sick. This realization, and its expression in buildings, which over 100 years later are still in active use (Fig. 1), have influenced the concept of hospital care until the present day. The conviction that there were no limits to man's capacity to conquer disease was based upon scientific discoveries which, at the time, were regarded by the layman as little short of miraculous.

Perhaps the most significant, certainly the most dramatic, change in hospital medical practice came with the introduction of first *ether, and then *chloroform, as *anaesthetic gases. The first recorded use was in the Massachusetts General Hospital in 1846 and in October of the same year a leg was amputated under ether in University College Hospital, London. With this development came the opportunity for new surgical techniques and more extensive operations as surgeons discovered that, relieved from the horror of the inflicted

Table 1 Dates of foundation of voluntary hospitals in the UK to 1900

	London	Provinces	Scotland	Total
To 1700	2	2	0	4
	St Thomas's (1106)	Rochester (1078)		
	St Bartholomew's (1123)	Windsor (1168)		
1700–50	9	11	2	22
1751–1800	2	26	7	35
1801–50	23	97	10	130
1851–1900	76	280	41	397

Source: *The hospital year book 1935*, pp. 237–40 (by courtesy of the Institute of Health Service Management).

pain, the use of anaesthetic agents allowed them more time.

Less dramatic perhaps, but surely even more significant, was the attack on wound *sepsis. *Lister was appointed regius professor of surgery at Glasgow in 1860 and by then had completed his seminal research on blood coagulation. In Glasgow he turned his attention to wound sepsis and by 1865 was successfully using carbolic acid (*phenol) in the treatment of compound bone fractures. From this he went on to lay down principles of antiseptic practice which revolutionized hospital surgical procedures. As if this was not enough, he then turned his attention to the improvement of *ligatures which had proved so frequently to be the cause of secondary *haemorrhage and wound breakdown.

The winds of change

In a chapter such as this, there is no space for details of the historical development of individual hospitals. (Short notes on many appear elsewhere in this book.) Histories of most of the major hospitals in the UK have been written; other less well-known hospitals have also been written about and a fascinating and informative body of knowledge exists and repays study.

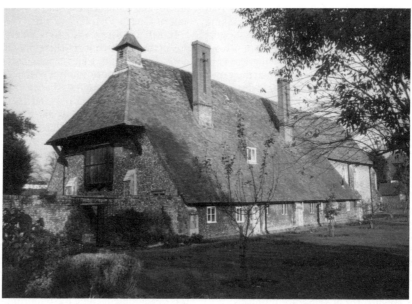

Fig. 1 St Mary's Hospital, Chichester, Sussex. Founded in the second half of the 12th century, the hospital is still in use as a home for elderly people. (Photograph by B. C. Gifford.)

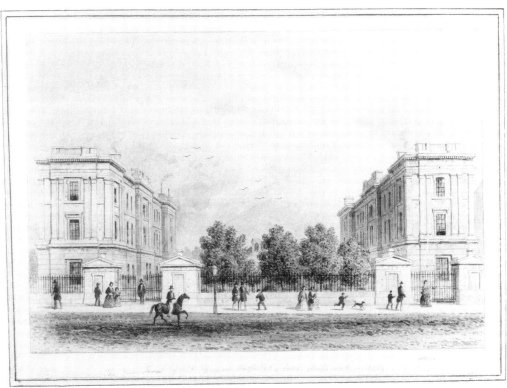

Fig. 2 St Thomas's Hospital, the new frontage in 1858. One of the oldest Foundations in the UK, St Thomas's moved in 1858 to its present site opposite the Houses of Parliament. (From a painting by T. H. Shepherd, copyright the British Museum.)

By the middle of the 19th century the way was clear for a rapid expansion of hospital work, freed as the doctors saw themselves to be from the handicaps of surgical pain, and of sepsis. *Dysentery, *leprosy, *typhoid, *malaria, the *plague, all were gradually conquered, and at the same time the range of surgery was vastly extended.

The research in the UK which produced these results was, in the main, based in the major hospitals of London and the university towns of England, Scotland, and Ireland (see, for example, Figs 2 and 3).

Associated with these scientific developments were changes in organization. 'Special' hospitals devoted to groups of patients with similar illnesses had existed for some time, the medical profession being divided about their value. Between 1840 and the end of the century the more esoteric ones had disappeared and names soon to become famous were established— 'Moorfields' in ophthalmology, The Royal National Orthopaedic, and 'Great Ormond Street for Children'.

The building of poor-law infirmaries was also a characteristic of Victorian times. These were the State 'hospitals' of the time, designed both for the housing of the destitute as well as for the care of the sick poor who had no other refuge. Conditions were frequently appalling. Pauperism was seen as a social evil and material help given to those unable to help themselves was seen as undesirable since it encouraged paupers to become dependent and not to help themselves.

The process of reform was slow and it was not until the end of the century that it could be said that poor-law infirmaries had become hospitals in the true sense of the word, a process made possible by legislative change which centralized their functions under the administration of metropolitan authorities.

Outside London and the big towns, 'cottage' hospitals, mostly staffed by general practitioners, were rapidly being established as the swing towards hospitals as places of safety and cure became entrenched. These small hospitals, sometimes having as few as 20 beds, provided an intimate and caring environment for the treatment of virtually all conditions except those requiring major surgery. To times well within living memory they were an integral part of the hospital scene from the 1860s until after the Second World War.

The 1914–18 war acted as a catalyst for change no

less than the Second World War. In 1920 a consultative committee of 15 doctors and five laymen under the chairmanship of the future Lord *Dawson of Penn produced a report which, in effect, was an outline of a future National Health Service. But not for the first, or last, time in history economic and social events intervened.

The depression of the 1920s, the effects of which extended well into the 1930s, produced an economic climate in which no new service could begin. The Cave Committee, and the Onslow Commission which followed, were set up to implement the Dawson Report's recommendations, and touched on one very sensitive matter—co-ordination between voluntary and public hospitals. But the debate on this which continued throughout the 1930s came to an abrupt end with the Munich crisis of 1938. At this time there was a generally held view (derived from experiences in the Spanish Civil War) that if war between Great Britain and Germany broke out, there would soon be heavy casualties as a result of aerial bombing. A hasty survey of all hospital beds throughout the country was made in 1938 and the Emergency Medical Service was organized shortly afterwards on the basis that voluntary and public hospitals would continue to run within a regional administrative structure, the Ministry of Health determining the functions and role of each hospital.

The Second World War (1939–1945)

For the first time staffs of voluntary and municipal hospitals found themselves working together in the peripheral hospitals. The workload fluctuated. In the early months of the war there was something of a mass exodus to the country; private practice dwindled and those senior medical staff of the teaching hospitals who did not find themselves in the armed forces were working in small, upgraded hospitals, often far away from their homes. After a few months, and until the severe bombing began in September 1940, the drift back began and local authorities opened up some of their closed beds. From then until the end of the war there was a fairly constant ebb and flow of the population.

With the advent of flying bombs, this decision was reversed, and in 14 days some 6000 patients from London were moved to hospitals in safer parts of the country. This had two consequences; first, that nursing and other staff went with their patients and many settled in their new homes and never returned to London; secondly, the speed of the transfer and efficiency with which it was carried out demonstrated what could be achieved nationally by an effective regional structure. By the end of the war some voluntary hospitals were able to remain open only because the Ministry of Health paid their debts.

Notwithstanding all this, planning continued and on 9

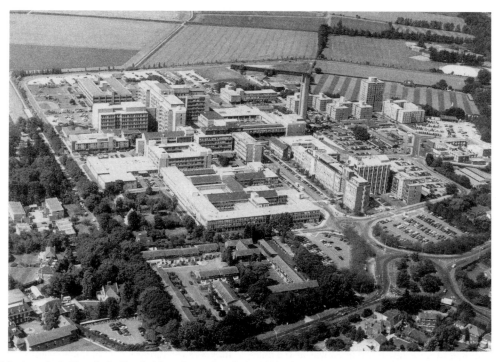

Fig. 3 Addenbrooke's Hospital, Cambridge, from the air in 1992. Opened as a hospital for the sick poor in 1766 near the centre of the city. Addenbrooke's moved to this 66 acre site in 1962. (Photograph by Martin Johns.)

October 1941 the Minister of Health said in the House of Commons: 'It is the objective of the Government as soon as may be after the war to ensure that by means of a comprehensive hospital service appropriate treatment shall be readily available to every person in need of it.'

The *National Health Service (1946–1968)

The years immediately following the Second World War witnessed a burst of social legislation without parallel in modern times. This legislation had been anticipated in part by the *Beveridge Report on social insurance and allied services, published in December 1942. It is a remarkable fact that in the middle of a war for survival, this report from a group of senior civil servants from the government departments involved in the administration of cash benefits and pensions should have caught the public imagination and become a best-seller.

The Ministry of Health appointed two 'surveyors' in 1941 to report on the state of all London hospitals and to make recommendations about their future management. In the provinces, the Nuffield Provincial Hospitals Trust (founded in 1939) undertook a co-ordinating role for the several parallel surveys being carried out. All this meant that serious thought was being given to such questions as the number of beds for a given population, and the ideal size of a teaching hospital.

The hospital surveys published in 1945 revealed that hospital facilities, in quality as well as in quantity, were far from satisfactory. When these deficiencies were quantified it became even clearer that 'the cost of the reforms needed would be on a scale which could only be found from the Exchequer'.

The National Health Service Act became law in November 1946 and as a result virtually all hospitals were taken over by the state. The voluntary hospital systems disappeared and local authorities had no further responsibilities for providing or maintaining hospitals. The remuneration and conditions of service of all employees were to be determined nationally, and ownership of all buildings and land vested in the state. The endowment funds of hospitals designated as medical teaching hospitals remained in the control of their new governing bodies; the endowment funds of all other transferred hospitals were taken into a central pool and used for the general benefit of all non-teaching hospitals. Hospitals were permitted to set aside separate accommodation for private patients. These patients were required to pay the full cost of their treatment and maintenance up to an approved maximum, and the accommodation had to be made available to non-paying patients if they needed it and if other accommodation was not available.

On 5 July 1948, when the 1946 Act came into effect, the hospital service was unique and self-sufficient. England and Wales were divided into 14 regions, each having within it a university medical school, and for each region a regional hospital board was appointed. Within the regions, hospitals were regrouped in accordance with plans prepared by the regional hospital boards and approved by the Minister of Health. The groupings were made to facilitate administration, and the boards appointed a hospital management committee to administer each one. Teaching hospitals were also grouped and each was administered by a board of governors. These boards, unlike hospital management committees, were accountable to the Minister of Health, and it soon became apparent that a good deal of effort would be needed to secure effective co-ordination and collaboration in practical matters of hospital administration—staffing, planning new services, and so forth—between the equally autonomous boards of governors and the regional hospital boards. This issue, of course, involved the responsibility of the Minister of Health, and in the words of Aneurin Bevan, his objective was 'to reconcile two normally conflicting interests, centralised financial responsibility and decentralised administration at the periphery'.

The years that followed saw a concentration of effort directed towards the hospital service. The serious reservations of the medical profession before 1948, although they did not evaporate, diminished substantially and rapidly. The King's Fund identified the need for trained administrators, and established experimental training courses for hospital administrators which were later developed into a national scheme.

These years witnessed an escalation in the capital spent on new and improved hospital buildings. The realization that some 20 years had elapsed without significant building having taken place brought home the fact that in many hospitals the boiler plants were in imminent danger of collapse. The replacement of these, and the building of out-patient departments in the place of the dreary waiting halls of the 1920s, were given a high priority. Hospital workloads shot up and still the feeling was present that a plateau could be reached, and ill-health, although not likely to be eradicated, would be controlled by the combination of state resources and medical skill.

Plans for whole new hospitals abounded; some, but not many, were completed. While new specialties such as *nuclear medicine and, later, *transplant surgery were growing, and existing specialties such as *radiotherapy, *neurosurgery, *gastroenterology, and *ophthalmic surgery were changing out of all recognition, so bureaucracy was also exercising a limiting and necessary function by rationalizing the provision of specialized hospital services.

The cost of this vast enterprise was being met from public funds and a growing awareness of the implications of uncontrolled medical growth was expressed. Improvements in the organization of patient services, such as the introduction of more efficient appointment arrangements in out-patient departments, and experiments in medical record-keeping, were matched by the growth of hospital work study departments and a more academic approach to management, conceived earlier as something in which success was more often due to intuition than intelligence.

Throughout the whole of this period the medical profession retained its position of dominance; the years also saw the growth of professionalism in the related disciplines. Most significant were the changes in outlook among nurses as their numbers grew and the managerial problems they faced became less amenable to the hierarchical structure which had remained virtually unaltered since it was first described by Florence *Nightingale. The growing awareness of these issues by the nursing profession gave rise to the setting up in 1963 of the Salmon Committee which was charged with the task of reorganizing the hospital nursing managerial structure.

Other health professionals became conscious of their indisputable places in treatment processes which increasingly were dependent upon teamwork. *Physiotherapists, *radiographers, *chiropodists, *occupational therapists, and *remedial gymnasts all developed professional associations—recognized by the Professions Supplementary to Medicine Act passed in 1960.

The barriers between teaching and non-teaching hospitals did not disappear but they became noticeably lower as the interdependence of hospitals became more marked. In other fields—*general medical practice, *public health, *health education—polarization seemed to intensify as the hospital service pursued its relentless course towards ever-increasing high-technology medicine. The public, in general, remained uninterested in the finer points, while the media were forever on the outlook for 'breakthrough' cures and *causes célèbres* of failure, which usually occurred in the long-stay institutions. On the whole the service was deemed successful and in 1968 the time seemed ripe to round off a few of the rough corners and remedy some of the more obvious organizational defects.

Reorganizations

The factors which, added together, supported the view that the National Health Service was due for change were the extravagant proliferation of separate bodies responsible for parts of the service and also the growing awareness that the development of community (as against institutional) facilities had been neglected; that 'consumer' interests were but poorly represented on the appointed bodies; and, finally, that even the immense resources of the state could not support the ever-increasing drain on money and expert staff.

The convoluted history of the first reorganization involving one Minister of Health and three Secretaries of State, which resulted in a change on 1 April 1974 in the reorganized service (changed by an Act passed by a Conservative government and put into effect by a Socialist one), is not all relevant in an article about hospitals. The unease of the medical profession, last experienced in the immediate post-war years, surfaced again and was given traumatic expression in the partial

strike by hospital medical staff in 1975 on the issue of the right to *private practice.

Large hospital building schemes declined in number and planning delays increased, but despite this the inexorable progress of high-technology medicine continued. Within 10 years transplant surgery had developed to the point that kidney transplantation was routine and the techniques for successful liver and heart *transplantation were understood. All this in hospitals which were also the base for ever-growing numbers of out-patients, for 'day' surgery, and for the successful *rehabilitation of those suffering from conditions or from the effects of accidents which, only a few years earlier would have rendered them chronically unfit and totally dependent for the rest of their lives.

In *psychiatry and in mental handicap the number of beds in hospitals diminished as the realization grew that community support backed up by occasional medical and nursing help produced a quality of life higher than that which could be achieved in a long-stay hospital ward.

As inflation exercised its insidious pressure and hospital costs rose, so (ironically perhaps) the numbers of private hospitals began to increase. Mainly providing surgical facilities, the private sector absorbed some of the growing numbers being added to NHS waiting lists. For patients who could afford the costs of medical insurance, the private sector offered opportunity to avoid the long delays which had become commonplace. The long wait between diagnosis and operative treatment, often amounting to years, became exacerbated by industrial disputes which forced hospitals to accept so-called emergency patients only, and which were a feature of the late 1970s and 1980s.

By 1980 informed opinion had moved away from the large concentrated hospital, and planning emphasis was on smaller units linked organizationally. A much closer linkage, too, was effected with community services as health authorities (reorganized again in 1982) were established with specific managerial responsibilities for all aspects of health care in the 250 or so districts in the UK

Approaching the 21st century

By the mid-1980s the word 'reorganization' had come to have negative implications as health-care professionals and lay people alike saw few if any tangible benefits from the upheavals of the organizational changes which had occurred since 1974. Successive governments had brought in new thoughts about the ways in which the National Health Service could be managed. All remained fundamentally within the framework of the original Act, but new boundary lines, new posts, new managerial techniques were all introduced by politicians with an enthusiasm which was rarely matched by those charged with the tasks of providing a service.

The Conservative administrations of first Margaret

Thatcher and then of John Major introduced new concepts with the idea that hospitals existed to provide services which were available to those who needed them as 'purchasers'. This has been further extended to include the proposal that hospitals may opt for 'Trust Status'—that is, a status which gives them independence in management while retaining them within the totality of the NHS. Thus such hospitals will be able to fix their staffing levels and remuneration rates for staff independently of regional or national control. This freedom, extending also to the determination of clinical quality, will, it is claimed, provide a freedom constrained only by local 'market' forces and an accountability which will be more realistic than anything known hitherto.

These radical changes to the National Health Service affect all parts of the service and go hand in hand with new provisions for general practitioners to hold and manage their own budgets. It will take time for the changes to take effect and, in the meantime, the business of caring for the sick continues in parallel with the training of so many types of carers, all essential to patient care.

Within living memory hospitals have changed from places providing custodial care for the sick poor to being the centre of the medical world, usually a vast complex of buildings housing specialized equipment and formidable skills. These years have seen a dramatic increase in the numbers of patients attending as out-patients and in the amount of day care provided. Reflecting these growth points have been the rising costs, attributable to increased use, inflation, and to the high costs of the medical advances that have been made and which so often have depended for their successful use on still more staff.

The crescendo of public criticism of hospital organization, dramatically but not always accurately reported by the media, has now become commonplace. The long waiting times for a hospital bed, the poor industrial relations, disparity of salaries, and disputes about priorities, all these are debated against the backcloth of the criticism that hospitals are pricing themselves out of existence.

But out of all this one can discern the resurrection of the original idea that the hospital could again become the focus of patient care at the centre of a network of community centres. The hospital embodies, in a unique way, centuries of scientific and humanitarian efforts; it produces an amalgam from often conflicting but basically complementary community and professional pressures. It should now actively seek out the role of catalyst and should monitor the quality of professional care provided—not only on its premises but in the larger community it serves.

W. G. CANNON

References

Trevelyan, G. M. (1946). *English social history*, (2nd edn). Longmans, London.

Further reading

Burdett, H. (1891). *Hospitals and asylums of the world*. Churchill, London.

Ives, A. G. L. (1948). *British hospitals*. London.

Pater, J. E. (1981). *The making of the National Health Service*. King Edward's Hospital Fund for London, London.

Rook, A., Carlton, M., and Cannon, W. G. (1991). *The history of Addenbrooke's Hospital*. Cambridge University Press.

HOSPITALS IN THE USA: THEIR DEVELOPMENT AND ORGANIZATION

Historical perspective

In the past 200 years the health-care system of the USA has undergone dramatic change. In early America the few hospitals that existed were almost exclusively in cities with over 30 000 residents, even though most Americans lived in rural areas. The first hospitals in the USA, almshouses, were facilities where the sick poor went for care. Here they were given more adequate food, shelter, and warmth than was possible in their homes, and were provided with such medical attention as was available. Those who were sick and had family to care for them remained at home. Little could be done for a patient in the hospital that could not be provided in the home without the stigma of having received charity care (Atwater 1989).

By the early 20th century, with the introduction of *aseptic techniques permitting safe abdominal *surgery, the hospital served all who needed a surgical procedure or trained nursing care. Between 1875 and 1925, the number of hospitals in the USA grew from just over 170 to about 7000, and the number of hospital beds increased from 35 000 to 860 000 (Rosner 1989). During this same period, hospitals, which had begun to develop in small rural towns throughout the country, were transformed into facilities that provided acute care and surgery using the expanding pools of medical and scientific knowledge and technology. The increasing number of hospitals in cities, which occurred in response to population gains, generally reflected the religious and ethnic make-up of the immigrant communities in which they were located, and also the economic and social conditions of these same areas (Rosner 1989).

The industrialization of the USA enhanced and expanded technology and scientific knowledge, both of which not only changed the practice of medicine but also *medical education. With the introduction of *antibiotics, expanding and advanced surgical techniques such as *cardiac surgery, and the development of renal dialysis, the very nature of medicine in the USA changed to an intervention-based practice. As the growth of technology began to spiral in the 1940s, 1950s, and 1960s, physicians frequently found themselves needing access to equipment and personnel available only in hospitals. Patient expectations changed, and increasingly the hospital became the focal point of the health-care delivery system. Between 1946 and 1982 the number of hospital admissions to all US hospitals increased from 15.7 million to a peak of 39.1 million. As the character of *medical practice began to change in response to cost-control measures, admissions declined to 33.8 million by 1990.

US hospitals: current organization

There are three types of hospitals in the USA: voluntary or not-for-profit, governmental, and proprietary or for-profit. Voluntary, public, and proprietary hospitals in the USA today face similar pressures but serve different constituencies. Many voluntary not-for-profit institutions, traditionally begun as religious or ethnic institutions, today are private institutions with missions that encompass both care of the poor and meeting community need, but balanced against the need to compete for paying patients to maintain revenues. Public or governmental institutions are operated by federal, state, or local governments and usually have a mission to serve all who seek care without regard to ability to pay. For this reason they primarily serve a poorer population with extensive social and health-care needs. In the case of federal hospitals the *Veterans Administration (VA) operates an autonomous health-care system (the largest public hospital system in the world) which serves US veterans and a limited number of family members insured through a special programme for veterans with total disabilities that are service-related. Investor-owned for-profit (proprietary) hospitals are institutions which are operated on a for-profit basis, often as part of hospital chains. They have a mandate from their investor/owner to make a return on investment no matter what constituency they serve.

The size and auspices of hospitals

The American Hospital Association indicates that, in 1990, there were 6649 hospitals in the USA. Of these, 337 were federal, 131 were non-federal, long-term or special care, and 5420 were non-federal, short-term general and other special care. It indicates that 5384 were community hospitals (defined as all hospitals except for those in the following categories: psychiatric facilities, federal facilities, and other special-care facilities). Of these, 3191 (59 per cent) were voluntary not-for-profit, 749 (14 per cent) were investor-owned, and 1444 (27 per cent) were operated by state or local governments. The federal government, through the VA, operated 337 hospitals with 98 000 beds providing nearly 1.8 million patient days and 58 527 million out-patient visits. In addition to community hospitals and the VA system, there were 757 psychiatric hospitals, of which approximately 17 per cent were not-for-profit institutions, 45 per cent proprietary, and 38 per cent governmental, either state or municipal. In addition, there were also a limited number of specialized facilities throughout the USA, including four hospitals, for respiratory diseases and 131 special long-term care facilities. Combined, this complex set of institutional providers operated 1.2 million in-patient beds, had an average daily census of

844 000 patients, and had nearly 34 million admissions in 1990.

Although the overall number of hospitals has remained relatively constant since 1950, the mix of facilities and services has changed dramatically. The number of VA hospitals has decreased by 19 per cent. The number of *psychiatric facilities has increased but the number of psychiatric beds has been reduced by nearly 75 per cent (these changes reflect the implementation of a national policy of deinstitutionalization of the mentally ill). Part of the reduction in psychiatric capacity resulted from a significant reduction in the number of state-operated long-term psychiatric hospitals, which were generally very large institutions, and a commensurate increase in the number of proprietary psychiatric facilities, usually smaller institutions with a shorter length of stay. There has been a 99 per cent reduction in the number of respiratory-care facilities (*tuberculosis hospitals). The number of voluntary not-for-profit hospitals increased by 11 per cent and the number of beds operated by voluntary not-for-profit hospitals doubled. The number of for-profit hospitals decreased by 39 per cent but the actual number of community hospital beds operated by proprietary firms in the USA increased by 140 per cent. In the past 20 years, the for-profit sector expanded its role in the health-care system by 77 per cent, increasing the proportion of community beds under proprietary auspices from 6.5 per cent of all community beds in 1972 to 11 per cent in 1990.

Since 1972 hospital occupancy rates have steadily declined and patients' lengths of stay have declined by nearly 10 per cent. The loss in patient activity has been partially offset by the growth in the out-patient sector. A greater proportion of diagnostic, treatment, and surgical procedures, which historically required in-patient admission, is being completed on an out-patient basis. In 1971 only 30.8 per cent of hospitals had organized out-patient departments as compared with 79.7 per cent in 1990. Over this period of time the number of out-patient visits to US hospitals increased from 181 million visits per year to more than 368 million. Overall hospital out-patient revenues as a percentage of total revenues have increased from 19 per cent in 1986 to 26 per cent in 1990, growing by nearly 45 per cent (*The comparative performance of US hospitals: the source book* 1991).

Hospital services

Today, US hospitals can best be described as facilities designed to provide advanced technology and skilled medical and *nursing care. Hospitals have become the place where only the sickest go for care as the use of technology has expanded. In their current role, however, US hospitals serve two primary constituencies: not only the sickest, most acutely ill, but also the medically disenfranchised, generally thought of as those without *health insurance or with *Medicaid. Voluntary and government hospitals, particularly those situated in inner cities, have increasingly become social institutions, particularly for the poor and underserved, returning to their archetypal role. These special populations present unique challenges to the facilities serving them. The homeless, *substance abusers, the deinstitutionalized mentally ill, and other low-income patients, as well as persons with *AIDS/HIV, increasingly rely on hospitals to meet social as well as medical needs, to serve as *family doctor and *social worker, and to provide tertiary medical services. Hospitals in the USA serve as major community employers, educators, and provide care to both the rich and the poor. In 1990 there were 927 000 community hospital beds in the USA, with an average daily census of 619 000 patients. During the same year nearly 3.5 million people were employed nationally in hospitals.

Increasingly, the intensity and range of services provided in US hospitals are expanding. The *Medicare case-mix index (a complexity of illness index based on relative resource consumption) of Medicare beneficiaries steadily increased between 1986 and 1989, and declined slightly between 1989 and 1990. The case mix of a hospital is an indication of the complexity and intensity of its patient mix. Larger hospitals in the USA tend to have higher case-mix indices. Not-for-profit and investor-owned hospitals serve a more complex mix of patients than government hospitals. This may be due to the high cost of advanced technology services which, as a result, are often not available at public institutions, or because many served by the public sector may more often seek only routine care at the government hospital site.

Growth of technology

The growth and increasing cost of technology are evidenced by recent trends in Medicare Part B expenditures (reimbursement for physician services under the Medicare programme) for specialized services and procedures, which grew at a rate of 12.3 per cent between 1985 and 1988. Certain components of these expenditures grew at even higher rates. A study examining these trends determined that the development of new technologies was the driving force behind the increases. The fastest growing categories were concentrated in services using *computerized axial tomography, *magnetic resonance imaging, and sonography. *Endoscopic procedures, for which a number of new applications have been developed, grew at a rate of more than 17 per cent (Berenson and Holahan 1992).

Hospital 'profit' margins

Overall, hospital 'profit' margins, the difference between total revenue and total expenses (including revenue from non-patient care sources), declined in the mid-1980s and increased in 1990. Urban hospitals had higher median 'profit' margins than rural facilities. In recent years the difference between rural and other

areas has declined. This may be due to increased Medicare payment rates for rural hospitals. Investor-owned hospitals experienced four consecutive years of decline in total profit margins, which stabilized in 1990. As of 1990 not-for-profit hospitals had a higher median total profit margin than did for-profit facilities (*The comparative performance of US hospitals: the source book* 1991). There may be a number of reasons why investor-owned facilities have lower margins, including lower case-mix indices, higher costs of depreciation, or lower occupancy rates. One study found that changes in Medicare payment had a greater effect on the profits of for-profit hospitals than they had on not-for-profit institutions (Hoerger 1991). A more complete study of the causes of the difference in profit margins among the three sectors needs to be completed in order to understand this issue fully.

Rural hospitals

Residents of rural communities in the USA face significant problems in obtaining health and hospital care. Between 1980 and 1987, 519 US hospitals closed or stopped providing in-patient care. Of these 364 were community hospitals; rural hospitals accounted for 163 (45 per cent) of those that closed. Rural hospital closures included a disproportionately high number of proprietary facilities which represent 8.2 per cent of all rural community hospital beds but 24.5 per cent of the rural hospitals that closed between 1980 and 1987 (DeFriese *et al.* 1992).

Additionally, a possible cause of many rural hospital closures is the problem of recruitment and retention of physicians in these communities. Without hospitals, rural communities are often unable to recruit physicians and 'without physicians to provide patient care and to produce the demand for inpatient care and ancillary services hospitals in many rural areas have been unable to survive' (DeFriese *et al.* 1992). The physician shortage in rural communities is a problem that many federal and state initiatives have attempted to address. The continuing disparity between physicians per 100 000 population in rural versus urban areas—192 per 100 000 in urban areas as contrasted with 41 per 100 000 in rural areas—demonstrates that the need continues unabated (Gesler *et al.* 1992).

The rural hospital crisis is a long-term problem. Between 1973 and 1983 rural US hospitals with fewer than 50 beds had a 35 per cent decrease in bed-days (Berenson and Holahan 1992), as compared with a 13.5 per cent decline for all US hospitals during this same period of time. In 1988 25 per cent of all rural hospitals had negative operating margins (DeFriese *et al.* 1992). Many involved in addressing rural health needs believe that changes in Medicare hospital reimbursement (Part A) have had a disproportionately unfavourable impact on rural hospitals. A number of reasons have been postulated. Rural facilities are less able to balance out the 'winners and losers' (admissions generating more or less revenue than expenses) under the Prospective Payment System (PPS) because of their smaller number of beds. Under the current Medicare reimbursement system, PPS, rural hospitals receive lower Medicare reimbursement rates than urban hospitals for the same services. Many of the rural counties which lost their single hospital provider are located near to, or contiguous with, larger metropolitan areas. Although these communities lost their sole institutional provider, there is access; those in need, however, must travel. These communities have become underserved rather than unserved.

Teaching hospitals

The role of the teaching hospital in US medical history has roots in the public hospital or early almshouses. These were the only hospitals in which physicians and students had access to patients who were required to participate in teaching as a condition of their hospital stay. In 1910, Abraham *Flexner issued a report to the Carnegie Foundation for the Advancement of Teaching, Bulletin No. 4, *Medical education in the United States and Canada*. This report, known as the *Flexner Report, made recommendations that led to the transformation of undergraduate medical education. Several other major studies of medical education, both undergraduate and graduate, that followed Flexner's also resulted in important changes in the training of physicians. 'Prior to World War II, most medical school graduates went into private practice following a one year internship' (Coggeshall 1965). As medical knowledge expanded, the specialization of medicine and medical training followed closely behind. After the Second World War residency training programmes, which train physicians in specific specialties, grew rapidly. Training increasingly took place at voluntary and public institutions.

The resulting 'teaching hospital' is an institution which has the care of patients as its primary goal, but in which patients are cared for in the teaching setting. In teaching hospitals resident physicians in training under the supervision of attending physicians provide patient care. It is a commonly held belief that the quality of patient care in teaching hospitals is superior because of the presence of residents and the availability of clinical research and new technologies; however, it has been suggested that there is an inherent conflict in teaching hospitals between patient-care responsibilities and educational goals. As previously noted, public hospitals were the original sites for medical education. Their relative importance as teaching hospitals began to decline in recent years. Yet even as recently as the mid-1980s 'almost one-half of the medical schools in the US had a predominant reliance on publicly owned institutions to carry out their mission of education, training and clinical research' (Friedman 1987). Today there are 1097 'teaching' hospitals that have one or more residency training programmes or 23 per cent of all community hospitals (*The comparative performance of US hospitals: the source book* 1991).

The growth of health-care expenditures: the role of hospitals

Health care is the fifth largest industry in the USA (US Department of Commerce 1992), growing from 5.3 per cent of the US gross national product (GNP) in 1960 to 9.2 per cent in 1980. By 1990, $666.2 billion were spent on the organization and delivery of health care in the USA, and health care expenditures had grown to 12.2 per cent of GNP. This represented an increase of nearly 800 per cent from 1970. At the same time, the gross national product increased by only 438 per cent. At the current rate of growth, health-care expenditures in the USA are projected to continue to spiral and to reach 1.6 trillion dollars or 16.4 per cent of GNP by 2000 (Sonnefeld *et al.* 1991).

The cost of providing care in US hospitals has escalated at an even greater rate, increasing by nearly 820 per cent over the past 20 years. Of total health-care expenditures, an estimated $256.0 billion, or 38 per cent, represent hospital expenditures. Some of this increase is due to the costs of technology, part is the result of population growth and utilization, and some results from rising manpower costs, including salaries and the spiralling costs of fringe benefits. Since 1986 the median salary and benefits expense per full-time equivalent employee has had an annual increase of 6.8 per cent as compared with an average annual increase in the consumer price index of 4.5 per cent. At the same time as costs per employee have risen, the number of employees per patient in hospital has increased as well, growing at an annual rate of 2 per cent (*The comparative performance of US hospitals: the source book* 1991). This steady increase may be the result of increasing case-mix complexity.

The union movement

The union movement and the growth of organized labour came late to health care because hospitals, the majority of which are not-for-profit institutions, were, until 1974, exempt from the National Labor Relations Act. A sentinel event in the unionization of health-care workers was the organization of Montefiore Hospital in New York City in 1958 by Local 1199, a national union representing pharmacists and drug-store employees. Although 1199 continually expanded in the numbers and types of employees it represented, as well as moving its influence beyond New York City, it was not until 1966, when the union successfully negotiated substantial increases in wages for its members at a number of New York City voluntary hospitals that the full strength of the union movement in hospital care began to grow. The costs of this important settlement, a significant addition to health-care costs, were largely borne by government through the Medicare and Medicaid programmes. This financial responsibility reflected a significant change and has been a continuing influence in the relationship between unions and hospitals. Beginning in the mid-1970s nurses joined the union movement. Part of the catalyst for this was increasing pressure on nurses, including increasing workloads and expanding roles and importance. In 1977, 1199 founded a division which represented nurses. Pressure from the labour movement caused the American Nurses Association to begin to serve as a trade union (Fink and Greenberg 1989).

Government expenditures for health care

The introduction of Medicare and Medicaid in 1965 provided new mechanisms of payment for health care for the elderly and the poor by shifting most of the economic responsibility to government. In 1960, prior to the introduction of Medicare or Medicaid, government spending (federal and state) on health care totalled $6.7 billion, or 24.7 per cent of total health-care expenditures. In 1990, public expenditures had grown to $282.6 billion or 42.4 per cent of total health-care expenditures. With this shift in financial responsibility came increasing governmental control of health care and health policy. For the past 15 years, both federal and state governments have developed far-reaching efforts directed at controlling cost, monitoring quality and utilization, and limiting growth of facilities and services. These efforts aimed at controlling costs and limiting the rate of growth in expenditures have not been effective.

Efforts to control the growth of health care and hospital costs

One of the earliest examples of federal efforts to control cost was the 1972 legislation which introduced Professional Standards Review Organizations (PSRO). The goal of the programme was controlling 'over-utilization' of health services by Medicare beneficiaries. The programme consisted of preadmission approval for a group of procedures and retrospective review of Medicare hospital stays. Days or full stays that were determined to be unnecessary were 'carved out' and Medicare payment was denied. A similar programme was implemented for Medicaid, and many private insurers began requiring prior approval for hospital admissions and concurrent review of hospital stays. In 1984, the Utilization and Quality Control Peer Review Organizations (PRO) programme replaced the PSRO programme. The PRO programme modified the focus of federal review to include quality of care with criteria-based appropriateness evaluation protocols. The quality review is completed as an addition to the monitoring of medical necessity of hospital admission or length of stay. The current focus of the PRO programme is on continuous monitoring of hospitalization. The PRO programme has been unpopular with hospitals and physicians as it is seen as intrusive and arbitrary. Although the quality of the organizations serving as PROs has varied as well, the efficacy of such reviews has steadily improved.

Another early effort at cost containment was the extension of certificate of need (CON) programmes to a national basis in 1975. The purpose of CON was to control the expansion of health facilities and technological services and therefore to control cost. To accomplish this, a network of state and regional agencies was established to be responsible for all health planning and resource development. In order to be eligible to receive capital reimbursement from Medicare and Medicaid, a provider was required, under the CON process, to obtain approval for the development, establishment, or expansion of services or facilities. The CON programme related only to hospitals and licensed facilities, but excluded physicians and other facilities in regard to major medical equipment. The programme was not effective nationally. Federal funding for the CON programme ended in 1986, although a limited number of states have retained the programme.

The most recent federal effort at cost containment was the 1983 introduction of the Prospective Payment System (PPS) for Medicare payment to hospitals. This system, which has now been extended to all payers in some states, uses diagnosis-related groups (DRGs) as the basis for hospital payment. Under this plan hospitals are paid a fixed payment which is based upon a patient's diagnosis. DRG payment rates were developed using a system which categorized all diagnoses into nearly 500 groupings. These groupings reflected the cost and length of stay of the average patient with particular diagnoses. If a patient were hospitalized for a shorter period of time, the hospital retained the savings. If a patient had a longer length of stay (within certain parameters) the hospital did not receive additional reimbursement. Hospital incentives regarding utilization and length of stay changed significantly under this system. Hospitals currently seek to increase the number of admissions while reducing lengths of stay. Although a prospective reimbursement system allows hospitals to project revenue and to plan expense levels accordingly, projecting the number of admissions and controlling length of stay are the challenges that hospital administrators must address. This payment system is meant to foster cost containment and to enhance facility management. The implementation of the DRG system has affected not only the management of hospitals but the delivery of medical care. Controlling length of stay became an essential objective for hospital administrators. Nationally, since the implementation of the DRG system in 1983, lengths of stay in community hospitals have decreased by less than one-half of a day to 7.2 days, decreasing by 5.6 per cent.

The medically uninsured: a growing problem for the USA

Despite the growth in health-care expenditures, approximately 25 per cent of the US population is without health insurance. More than 80 per cent of the uninsured are members of families where either one or both parents work. The majority of those who are employed but uninsured work for companies with fewer than 100 employees. As the cost of health insurance continues to rise and the nature of employment changes (increased service-based employment without health coverage), an increasing percentage of the population is uninsured. Many of those who are insured have limited access to needed health care because of the lack of personal resources to pay for care beyond the limits of coverage. Public hospitals throughout the country, as well as many voluntary institutions, have increasingly become the health-care safety net for these individuals and their families. Many of those who present at these hospitals, particularly in inner-city locations, increasingly seek routine non-emergency health care that would more appropriately be provided in a doctor's office or clinic setting. The National Association of Public Hospitals reports that in 1988, 30 per cent of in-patient days and 52 per cent of out-patient visits to its member facilities were by uninsured patients.

Conclusion

The hospital sector of the health-care delivery system in the USA has been, and continues to be, dynamic. The pressures faced by institutions and communities change as both the sources of funding and patients present new requirements. The current economic and political environment heralds continuing rapid change. This review has attempted to highlight only a limited view of the history of US hospitals and the current challenges to which they must respond.

HOLLY MICHAELS FISHER
THOMAS Q. MORRIS

General references
Except as otherwise noted all statistical information is from the following two references:

American Hospital Association (1991). *AHA hospital statistics: a comprehensive summary of U.S. hospitals 1991–92.*
Levit, K. R., Lazenby, H. C., Cowan, C. A., and Letsch, S. W. (1991). National health expenditures, 1990. *Health Care Financing Review*, **13**, 29–54.

Specific references
Atwater, E. C. (1989). Women, surgeons, and a worthy enterprise: the general hospital comes to Upper New York State. In *The American general hospital: communities and social contexts*, (ed. D. E. Long and J. Golden). Cornell University Press, Ithaca.
Berenson, R. and Holahan, J. (1992). Sources of growth in medicare physician expenditures. *Journal of the American Medical Association*, **267**, (5), 687–91.
Coggeshall, L. T. (1965). *Planning for medical progress through education.* A report submitted to the executive council of the Association of American Medical Colleges.
DeFriese, G. H., Wilson, G., Ricketts, T. C., and Whitener, L. (1992). Consumer choice and the national rural hospital crisis. In *Health in rural America* (ed. W. M. Gesler and T. C. Ricketts). Rutgers University Press.
Fink, L. and Greenberg, B. (1989). *Upheaval in the quiet zone: history of Hospital Workers' Union, Local 1199.* University of Illinois Press, Chicago.

Friedman, E. (1987). Problems plaguing public hospitals: uninsured patient transfers, tight funds, mismanagement, and misperception. *Journal of the American Medical Association,* **257** (14).
Gesler, W. M., Hartwell, S., Ricketts, T. C., and Rosenberg, M.W. (1992). Introduction to *Health in rural America.* Rutgers University Press.
Hoerger, T. J. (1991). Profit variability in for profit and not-for-profit hospitals. *Journal of Health Economics*, **10**, 259–89.
Rosner, D. (1989). Doing well or doing good. In *The American general hospital: communities and social contexts* (ed. D. E. Long and J. Golden). Cornell University Press, Ithaca.
Sonnenfeld S. T., Waldo, D. R., Lemieux, J. A. and McKusick D. R. (1991) Projections of national health expenditures through the year 2000. *Health Care Financing Review*, **13**, 1–27.
The comparative performance of US hospitals: the sourcebook (1991). Health Care Investment Analysis, Inc. and Deloitte & Touche.
US Department of Commerce (1992). *Statistical abstract of the United States 1992.* US Department of Commerce, Bureau of the Census.

HOST. Any organism infected or parasitized by another.

HOTEL DIEU, PARIS. A famous hospital in Paris, at one time regarded as the finest in the world. It is believed to date from between 641 and 691, although the first indisputable record is dated 829. It was founded by Landry, Bishop of Paris. See also MEDICINE IN FRANCE.

HOUSEMAID'S KNEE is the common name for prepatellar *bursitis, an occupational hazard of work involving frequent kneeling.

HOUSE MITES are the various species of the *arthropod genus *Dermatophagoides*, thought to be important in provoking asthma associated with house dust (particularly *D. pteronyssinus*).

HOUSE OFFICER. A doctor holding a *preregistration hospital appointment in medicine or surgery, the equivalent term in the USA being intern. See also POSTGRADUATE AND CONTINUING MEDICAL EDUCATION; RESIDENT HOUSE OFFICERS.

HOUSSAY, BERNARDO ALBERTO (1887–1971). Argentinian physiologist. He achieved renown for his researches in endocrine physiology and especially into the *pituitary and *carbohydrate metabolism. For these he shared the *Nobel prize in 1947 with C. F. and G. T. *Cori.

HOWARD, JOHN (1726–90). British sanitary and penal reformer. Howard's father left him well endowed and in 1773 he became high sheriff of Bedfordshire. Part of his duties involved visiting the local prison, where he was appalled by the conditions. He visited many other countries and their prisons, and found that all were insanitary, overcrowded, and disease-ridden. He correlated the incidence of gaol fever (*typhus) with the density of the prison population. In 1777 he published *The state of the prisons in England and Wales with preliminary observations and an account of some foreign prisons.* He advocated sanitary reforms, the regular whitewashing of walls, the making of smooth floors so that they could be washed, the isolation of the sick from the healthy, and the baking of clothes in ovens. This showed remarkable prescience in a time before the discovery of bacteria and the transmission of typhus infection by the *body louse. Bills were passed through Parliament as a result of his findings. He started the process of prison reform and his work had an effect on the design, cleanliness, and sanitation of hospitals. In 1789 he visited *lazarettes (hospitals for lepers and other sick poor) in Europe and died in 1790 of what was called camp fever, which may ironically have been typhus.

HOWELL, WILLIAM HENRY (1860–1945). American physiologist. He observed nuclear remnants in *red blood cells of patients with splenic dysfunction (called Howell–Jolly bodies). He also made important contributions to the understanding of blood *coagulation, and, with McLean, isolated an anticoagulant agent from tissues, which they named *heparin.

H$_2$ RECEPTOR ANTAGONISTS are drugs which, unlike the established *antihistamine agents, inhibit those effects of *histamine which are mediated by H$_2$ receptors, including histamine stimulation of gastric secretion. H$_2$ receptor antagonists, exemplified by the drugs *cimetidine and ranitidine, are potent inhibitors of gastric acid secretion and are used to treat *peptic ulcer.

HUA T'O (*fl.* 2nd century AD). One of the divinities of Chinese medicine. He was a surgeon who is said to have performed operations on the brain, chest, and abdomen after inducing sleep. He also practised *acupuncture and prescribed exercises.

HUFNAGEL, CHARLES A. (1915–89). American surgeon. With Robert Gross he conducted early studies on coarctation of the aorta. With David Hume he participated in performing the first kidney transplant, in 1947. He became professor of experimental surgery at Georgetown in 1950 and pioneered the development and placement of artificial valves in the surgical treatment of aortic regurgitation.

HUGGINS, GODFREY MARTIN (1883–1971). British/Rhodesian surgeon and politician. After his election to the Legislative Council in 1923, he became Prime Minister of Southern Rhodesia 1933–53, when the country became a self-governing colony. He helped bring about the Federation of Rhodesia and Nyasaland and was its first Prime Minister in 1953.

HUMAN LEUCOCYTE ANTIGEN. See HLA.

HUMAN TISSUE ACT 1961. The UK Human Tissue Act of 1961 authorizes donation of tissue from bodies for therapeutic purposes, for medical education, and for research. Section 1 (1) deals with donation in accordance with wishes expressed by the deceased. Section 1 (2) provides that the person in lawful possession of the body may authorize the removal of any part of it for such purposes provided he is satisfied that the deceased had expressed no objection and that the surviving spouse or relative has no objection. The removal must be effected by a fully registered medical practitioner, who must satisfy himself by personal examination that life is extinct. The 1961 Act is not to be construed as applying to post-mortem examinations directed to be made by a competent legal authority, for example for establishing or confirming the cause of death or for investigating the existence of abnormal conditions.

HUMERUS. The bone of the upper arm, which extends between the shoulder joint, where it articulates with the scapula or shoulder-blade, and the elbow joint, where it articulates with the radius and ulna, the two forearm bones.

HUMOURS. In medieval times the humours were four fluids supposedly secreted in the body and responsible for a person's character: these were blood, phlegm, choler (yellow bile), and melancholy (black bile). When blood was in preponderance, a man was sanguine or cheerful; phlegm, phlegmatic or calm; choler, choleric or quick-tempered; melancholy, melancholic.

HUNGER. A strong desire for food. See also HUNGER STRIKE; FAMINE; STARVATION.

HUNGER STRIKE. Wilful self-starvation by prolonged refusal of all food, usually by a prisoner hoping to gain release or as a protest against the conditions of his or her imprisonment; occasionally by others as a form of protest, generally political. 'Hunger strike' is something of a misnomer, since in total starvation the sensation of hunger disappears after a day or two. Duration of survival in subjects totally deprived of food is variable; the average is about 4 weeks, at which time body weight has been reduced by about half. Impending death is signalled by a marked drop in body temperature. Longer survival times are possible; for example, Terrence MacSwinney, Mayor of Cork, who was arrested in 1920 during the Irish Troubles, fasted for 74 days before dying in coma.

HUNT, DAME AGNES GWENDOLINE (1866–1948). British nurse. At the age of 10 years Agnes Hunt developed *osteomyelitis, which left her considerably disabled. Her mother's spartan upbringing, which forced her to lead a normal life, had profound influence on her later professional outlook. With great difficulty she became a nurse, and in 1900 opened a convalescent home for crippled children in Baschurch, Shropshire. In 1904 she was joined by Sir Robert *Jones and their aggressive approach revolutionized the treatment of cripples. In 1921 they moved to Oswestry, where they founded the Robert Jones and Agnes Hunt Orthopaedic Hospital.

HUNT, JAMES RAMSAY (1874–1937). American neurologist. He described *herpes zoster of the geniculate ganglion (the Ramsay Hunt syndrome).

HUNT, REID (1870–1948). American pharmacologist. He was the first to demonstrate the presence of thyroid hormone in the blood.

HUNTER, JOHN (1728–93). British surgeon. In 1771 he started his lectures on the theory and practice of surgery, the first attempt to give surgery a scientific basis. Hunter has been called the father of scientific surgery. He was an indefatigable worker, a brilliant investigator, and an original and stimulating thinker. He was, however, impatient, blunt, and unpolished. His lack of formal education made him a poor lecturer and a worse author. He read little and thus his research depended on his own original observations. He collected a vast range of specimens to illustrate health and disease in man and animals. These form the basis of his museum, which was accepted in 1800 by the Company of Surgeons (now the Royal College of Surgeons of England) with a subvention from the government.

Hunter's publications were numerous. The best known are: *Natural history of the human teeth* (1771); *On venereal disease* (1786), in which he claimed, on the strength of self-inoculation, that *syphilis and *gonorrhoea were the same disease; *Observations on certain parts of the animal oeconomy* (1786); *Treatise on the blood, inflammation and gun-shot wounds* (1794, published posthumously and seen through the press by *Home).

HUNTER, WILLIAM (1718–83). British anatomist and obstetrician and John *Hunter's elder brother. In 1768 he became the first professor of anatomy to the Royal Academy and 2 years later he founded the *Great Windmill Street Medical School, building a lecture theatre and a museum. The museum was left in the care of three trustees to pass, after 20 years, to the University of Glasgow. William Hunter was the leading teacher of anatomy and obstetrician in London; he published his celebrated work *The anatomy of the human gravid uterus* in 1774.

HUNTERIAN MUSEUM (OF GLASGOW). The museum was founded on collections of paintings, books, manuscripts, and coins made by William *Hunter, who built up one of the finest collections of coins in the world, as well as making massive contributions to obstetrics and anatomy.

HUNTERIAN MUSEUM (OF THE ROYAL COLLEGE OF SURGEONS OF ENGLAND). The museum is based on the remarkable collections of John *Hunter. In 1799 his whole collection of specimens was bought by the government and offered to the then Company of Surgeons, which received a Royal Charter the following year. He had built up his museum largely as a basis for his teaching of comparative anatomy, pathology, and surgery. In 1799 there were about 14 000 exhibits, including Charles O'Brien the famous Irish giant (about 8 ft tall), but this is trivial compared with the immense value of the series of specimens illustrating important themes of biology and surgery, which remain vital today. There are series of specimens on the comparative anatomy of living systems, on pathology and injury, and on reproduction. The museum is unique, and it was considerably extended in subsequent years, though a large part of it (mainly anatomical and osteological) was destroyed by bombing in 1941. Nevertheless enough remained for it still to be valuable to students of biology, anatomy, pathology, surgery, and history, who visit it in large numbers annually.

HUNTINGTON, GEORGE SUMNER (1850–1916). American physician. He joined his father in family practice in East Hampton, Long Island, New York, where his attention was drawn to a peculiar chronic neurological disorder that affected adult members of certain families. He moved to Pomeroy, Ohio, and wrote a description of the ailment he had observed in East Hampton; this description was published in *The Medical and Surgical Reporter of Philadelphia* in 1872, and this rare hereditary neurological disorder became known as *Huntington's chorea. The same familial disease has since been identified in many parts of the world. It is believed that the disease was introduced into the USA by a member of a Norfolk family who sailed on the *Mayflower*. Notably, it is now thought highly probable that some of the persons put to death for witchcraft after the trials in Salem, Massachusetts, suffered from this disease; their grotesque grimaces and postures caused others to think them bewitched.

HUNTINGTON'S CHOREA is a hereditary progressive neurological disorder characterized by *chorea and intellectual and emotional deterioration leading inevitably to *dementia. The disease is transmitted as an autosomal *dominant trait with complete penetrance (see GENETICS). The average age of onset is about 40 years. Hence tragically, the disease continues in the patient's offspring, of whom half will eventually be affected. The responsible *gene, associated with an abnormal repeat of three amino acids (cytosine, adenine, guanine—CAG) has now been located on *chromosome 4 (at 4p 16.3), making it possible to predict in many families which individuals at risk are likely to carry the gene, but such prediction causes sensitive ethical issues.

HURLER'S SYNDROME is one of a group of recessively inherited disorders known as the mucopolysaccharidoses. The syndrome (formerly called gargoylism) is due to a deficiency of the enzyme alpha-iduronidase. The main features, apart from the characteristic facial appearance, are mental retardation, dwarfism, widespread skeletal deformities, corneal opacities, deafness, visceral involvement, and cardiac anomalies; early death is usual.

HURST, SIR ARTHUR FREDERICK (1879–1944). British physician. Formerly Hertz, Hurst changed his name in 1916. At first he interested himself in neurology and during the First World War he treated many soldiers with '*shell shock' with success. Later he devoted himself to *gastroenterology and must be regarded as the founder of this specialty in the UK.

HUTCHINSON, SIR JONATHAN (1828–1913). British surgeon, ophthalmologist, and dermatologist. He was a medical polymath, making valuable clinical observations in surgery, venereology, dermatology, and ophthalmology. He has left many eponyms, of which *Hutchinson's triad of interstitial keratitis, notched teeth, and deafness in congenital *syphilis is the best known. He published the *Archives of surgery* (1889–99) in 10 volumes written by himself.

HUTCHINSON'S TRIAD is a combination of signs held by Sir Jonathan *Hutchinson to be *pathognomonic of congenital *syphilis. All are late manifestations of the condition, appearing later than the fourth year of life, and often not until adulthood. They are: interstitial *keratitis, often unilateral to begin with but eventually affecting both eyes and with associated *iridocyclitis; nerve deafness from involvement of the eighth cranial nerve in the internal ear, which may be progressive and eventually total; and a characteristic deformity of the upper central and other incisors of the permanent dentition, in which the teeth are widely gapped, tapered towards the cutting edge, and centrally notched (Hutchinson's teeth).

HUXHAM, JOHN (1692–1768). British physician. He described *diphtheria, but although he noted palatal palsy, he did not distinguish it from *scarlet fever. He wrote *On the malignant ulcerous sore throat* (1759).

HUXLEY, THOMAS HENRY (1825–95). British physician and biologist. His lectures and writings made him one of the most influential men of science of his time. He became a strong supporter of Darwinism and its leading interpreter.

HYALINE MEMBRANE DISEASE is one form of *respiratory distress syndrome of the newborn, in which affected infants, often premature, die within a few days of birth and are shown at autopsy to have eosinophilic hyaline material lining the alveoli and bronchioles, often with extensive *atelectasis. It is thought to be due to lack of pulmonary *surfactant resulting in failure to lower the surface tension within the lungs.

HYBRID. The offspring of a union between different races, species, genera, or varieties.

HYBRIDOMA. See MONOCLONAL ANTIBODIES.

HYDANTOIN is a crystalline base derived from allantoin. Diphenyl-hydantoin, or *phenytoin, is a drug with *anticonvulsant and myocardial depressant (antiarrhythmic) properties, also known as Epanutin® or Dilantin®.

HYDATID DISEASE is a condition which results from man acting as the intermediate host of a *tapeworm, *Echinococcus granulosus*, of which dogs and other canines are the main definitive hosts. Because sheep are the main intermediate hosts, hydatid disease tends to occur wherever dogs and sheep exist in close association with man, for example in sheep-rearing communities in rural areas, particularly in Australia, New Zealand, and Latin America, although it may occur sporadically anywhere, including Wales and the USA. The adult worm inhabits the upper jejunum of the dog, and the ova are excreted in the faeces. After ingestion by sheep, they lodge in the liver and lungs where they develop into cysts. The cycle is perpetuated by dogs feeding on sheep viscera. Human infection, often beginning in childhood, results from contamination with dog faeces (the ova can live for months in moist soil). Human hydatid disease is an unpleasant and dangerous condition, cysts in the liver and lungs sometimes reaching a great size. It is a classic cause of hepatomegaly. Surgery is often necessary, but can be hazardous, the dangers including *anaphylaxis and the induction of *metastases by 'daughter' cysts. The highest incidence in the world is in the Turkana people of Kenya, in whose society the dog plays an important and intimate role, for example, in child-minding.

HYDATIDIFORM MOLE. A mass of cysts occupying the uterine cavity resulting from the abnormal development of a fertilized *ovum.

HYDROCELE. A collection of fluid between the two layers of the tunica vaginalis, the serous membrane in which the *testis is enclosed.

HYDROCEPHALUS, 'water on the brain', is a condition in which there is an accumulation of *cerebrospinal fluid within the *cerebral ventricles, usually due to an obstruction to its circulation. There is dilatation of the ventricles and, in children in whom the cranial sutures have not yet fused, enlargement of the skull; cerebral atrophy and mental deterioration may result.

HYDROCHLORIC ACID is a solution of the pungent colourless gas hydrogen chloride (HCl) in water. It is of great physiological importance as a component of normal *gastric juice.

HYDROCORTISONE, also known as cortisol, is one of the *glucocorticoid *corticosteroids.

HYDROGEN ION CONCENTRATION. Since the hydrogen ion (H+) is the active constituent of all acids in the water system, the hydrogen ion concentration is useful as a measure of the acidity of a solution. It is the mass of hydrogen ions expressed in moles per litre (mol/l) of solution, but because of the wide range of values is more conveniently expressed as its negative logarithm to the base 10, that is the pH. The relationship between the two expressions is thus:

$$[H^+] = 10^{-pH} \text{ or } pH = -\log_{10} [H^+].$$

As pure water at ordinary temperatures dissociates slightly into hydrogen ions and hydroxyl ions ($H_2O = H^+ + OH^-$), the concentration of each type of ion being 10^{-7} mol/l, the pH of pure water is 7. Hydrogen ion concentration increases tenfold for each unit decrease in pH (and conversely for hydroxyl ions).

HYDRONEPHROSIS is dilatation of the pelvis and calyces of the kidney with consequent atrophy of renal tissue, due to obstruction to the flow of urine in the urinary tract.

HYDROPHOBIA is an alternative name for *rabies.

HYDROPS. *Dropsy.

HYDROTHERAPY, the 'water-cure' is a form of medical treatment originated by Vincenz Preissnitz at Gräfenberg in Germany in 1825 involving the external and internal application of water, also known as hydropathy. It is also any other form of treatment with water, for example *balneotherapy. See also COMPLEMENTARY (ALTERNATIVE) MEDICINE.

HYDROXYSTEROIDS are the excretion products of *corticosteroids.

HYGIENE is the science and practice of preserving health, in common usage often synonymous with 'cleanliness'. Hygieia, daughter of *Aesculapius and sister of Panacea, was the goddess of health.

HYGROMA. Any cyst or swelling, such as a *bursa, which is filled with fluid.

HYMEN. A membrane partly covering the external opening of the *vagina, usually intact in virgins.

HYOSCINE ($C_{17}H_{21}NO_4$) is an *anticholinergic alkaloid with similar effects to *atropine. Like atropine, it occurs in several solanaceous *poisonous plants; it is also known as scopolamine. It has a wide therapeutic application, being used particularly as an anti-emetic in *motion-sickness, for which it is still an effective drug; as a premedication agent in general *anaesthesia to minimize bronchial and salivary secretions; and as an antispasmodic in *dysmenorrhoea and gastrointestinal disorders.

HYOSCYAMINE is one of the *belladonna alkaloids, related to *atropine.

HYPERADRENALISM is overactivity of the *adrenal gland, particularly of the adrenal cortex. See ENDOCRINOLOGY.

HYPERAEMIA (HYPEREMIA) is an increase in blood flow through an organ, part, or area.

HYPERAESTHESIA (HYPERESTHESIA) is excessive sensitivity of sensory *receptors to stimuli.

HYPERBARIC MEDICINE is the treatment of disease, such as carbon monoxide poisoning, by exposure to atmospheric pressures greater than normal, and the study and treatment of conditions which may follow such exposure, for example *decompression sickness.

HYPERCALCAEMIA (HYPERCALCEMIA) is elevation of the serum *calcium concentration above the normal range (2.1–2.6 mmol/l).

HYPEREMESIS GRAVIDARUM is severe vomiting of *pregnancy, a form of pregnancy *toxaemia.

HYPERGLYCAEMIA (HYPERGLYCEMIA) is the elevation of the blood glucose concentration above the normal range, the upper limit of which is 5.2 mmol/l (or 94 mg/dl) in the fasting subject. See also DIABETES MELLITUS; GLUCOSE TOLERANCE TEST.

HYPERHIDROSIS. Excessive sweating.

HYPERKALAEMIA (HYPERKALEMIA) is elevation of the serum *potassium level above the normal range (3.4–5.4 mmol/l).

HYPERKERATOSIS is overgrowth of the horny layer (stratum corneum) of the *skin.

HYPERKINESIS is excessive motor activity, voluntary or otherwise. The term 'hyperkinetic syndrome' is applied to certain children who display overactivity, restlessness, fidgetiness, excitability, impulsiveness, distractability, short attention-span, learning difficulty, and aggression. The condition may or may not have an organic basis; if not, the features tend to disappear with increasing age. 'Hyperkinesis' is also used for several cardiovascular disorders, the common denominator of which is a persistently raised cardiac output (e.g. *thyrotoxicosis, wet *beriberi, arteriovenous *fistula).

HYPERMETROPIA is long-sightedness, in which the focusing power of the eye is not strong enough to focus near objects on the retina and they appear blurred, whereas distant objects are sharp. The defect is readily corrected by spectacles with appropriate (convex) lenses. See OPHTHALMOLOGY.

HYPERNATRAEMIA (HYPERNATREMIA) is elevation of the serum *sodium concentration above the normal range (135–146 mmol/l).

HYPERPARATHYROIDISM is increased activity of the *parathyroid glands. Primary hyperparathyroidism results either from an *adenoma of the gland secreting parathormone or from *hyperplasia of parathyroid tissue; it causes *hypercalcaemia and excessive mobilization of *calcium from bone; this may cause bone cysts or pathological *fractures. Secondary hyperparathyroidism occurs in response to conditions like *vitamin D deficiency and chronic renal disease, which tend to depress serum calcium levels.

HYPERPLASIA is an increase in the number of cells in a tissue (cf. *hypertrophy; *hypoplasia).

HYPERPYREXIA is extreme fever, defined as being present when the body temperature reaches 41 °C (106 °F) or above. It may be the upper limit of the body's response to infections and other challenges, but may also result from damage to the central nervous control mechanism, as in some cases of cerebral haemorrhage. In either instance hyperpyrexia may be a danger to life if allowed to continue, as is the case in heat stroke (see HEAT AS CAUSE OF DISEASE). 'Malignant hyperpyrexia', in which high fever is accompanied by widespread muscular rigidity, is a rare complication of general anaesthesia and is sometimes fatal. It is associated with a genetically determined metabolic abnormality of skeletal muscle.

HYPERSENSITIVITY is when an exaggerated and adverse response follows exposure of the patient to a particular foreign substance, the heightened sensitivity being the result of immunological 'memory' of previous contact with that substance. Hypersensitivity reactions are classified according to the nature and speed of response (immediate, delayed, or cell-mediated, complex-mediated, etc.). See ALLERGY; ANAPHYLAXIS; IMMUNOLOGY.

HYPERSOMNIA is abnormally long, deep, or frequent *sleep. Various conditions may underlie this phenomenon; they include *depression, *narcolepsy, the *Kleine–Levin syndrome, and the *Pickwickian (obesity-hypoventilation) syndrome.

HYPERTENSION. This is the term used to describe a higher than normal blood pressure on the arterial side of the circulation, which by virtue of its physical effects increases the risk of developing certain cardiovascular disorders, particularly *coronary artery disease, *stroke, *heart failure, and, to a much lesser degree, *kidney disease. Since blood flow is pulsatile, the pressure is conventionally assessed (in millimetres of mercury, mmHg) by recording both the peak (so-called systolic) pressure and the trough (diastolic) pressures in each measurement. Blood pressure is recorded then as systolic/diastolic pressure in mmHg.

Despite the familiarity of the term 'hypertension' to both lay and professional people, it is remarkably difficult to define. Blood pressure is a biological characteristic like height or weight with wide variations between people; nor is it constant from moment to moment in any individual. Direct intra-arterial blood pressure recordings over 24 hours show that the highest and lowest pressures over that period differ by as much as 100 per cent, being lowest at night and during sleep and highest on waking. Despite the obvious potential inaccuracy of assessing mean pressures over long periods of time by taking single measurements, albeit on repeated occasions, these so-called 'casual' blood pressure recordings correlate remarkably well in large population studies with survival and with the risk of later development of cardiovascular disease. The relationship between blood pressure and such risks is broadly linear and extends over the whole range of recorded pressures with no cut-off point to separate 'hypertension' from 'normotension'; but in this context it is very important to recognize that population studies are very imprecise in assessing the true risk in any particular *individual*.

Hypertension is then, as Sir George Pickering pointed out, a *quantitative* and not a *qualitative* concept—and not strictly therefore a disease. Although there are several conditions, mostly associated with kidney or *endocrine disease, which may cause hypertension, these account for only some 3–4 per cent of people diagnosed as hypertensive. In 97 per cent of such cases the high pressure is the consequence of *genetic (perhaps 30 per cent) and environmental (perhaps 70 per cent) factors and is called 'essential'.

There is a near normal distribution of blood pressure in populations, albeit with a 'tail' to the right, in a pattern resembling that of other variable biological characteristics. Although Platt once suggested a bimodal distribution of blood pressures, thereby perhaps implying single *gene inheritance, this view was disproved by Pickering in the 1960s. The current view is that arterial pressure is determined in any individual by a number of genes ('polygenic inheritance') reacting in a variable manner with several environmental factors. Among the latter are age, sex, 'stress' (difficult to measure), and *alcohol intake (an intake over 6 units per day is strongly associated with hypertension). An excess of dietary salt or a deficiency of potassium intake are widely quoted as causes, but the evidence is controversial. Obese subjects, particularly those with a high waist/hip ratio are more often hypertensive and resistance to insulin is common, though probably not causative. Higher arterial pressures are found in social classes 4 and 5 in both Europe and the USA. Epidemiological research has recently revealed an association between low birth weight and placental size and the development of raised blood pressure in middle age, suggesting that maternal *malnutrition may determine later susceptibility to hypertension. Blood pressure in affluent societies tends to rise with age in population studies but in developing countries, pressures do not rise and may even fall with age.

The evidence for polygenic inheritance of blood pressure depends on correlations between arterial pressures in family studies when observations have been made in parents and their children, in siblings, in identical and non-identical twins. There has been particular interest in examining differences in arterial pressures between parents and their natural or adopted children. A number of candidate genes are currently the subject of intensive research, but this problem presents much more difficulty than does research for the cause of single-gene disorders; the complexity of interaction between genes and environment makes for particular difficulty.

Given the lack of a cut-off point between 'normotension' and 'hypertension' how may hypertension be defined? The definition must be arbitrary; as good a definition as any holds that hypertension can be diagnosed when the risks of leaving the prevailing arterial pressure untreated are considered likely to outweigh the potential disadvantages of treatment designed to reduce it. The threshold pressure for diagnosis has therefore changed over the past 20 years as the pharmaceutical industry has improved the quality and effectiveness of antihypertensive drugs. A definition of hypertension in the USA requires pressures to exceed 140 mmHg systolic and 90 diastolic; WHO suggest a threshold of 160/95 and 160/100 is recommended by the British Hypertension Society. By the American definition some 33 per cent of Caucasian and 35 per cent of Negroid men of middle age in the USA are 'hypertensive'. The corresponding figure for a European definition is still high, at some 10–15 per cent of the middle-aged population.

These definitions imply that treatment can reduce both the *morbidity and *mortality of hypertension, and indeed this is the case. Several controlled trials have shown that the risk of stroke is reduced by some 40 per cent by lowering arterial pressure, but it is disappointing to find how much less has been the effect on coronary artery disease, which in middle age may be reduced only by some 7–14 per cent. The effect on coronary disease may be better in the elderly, and there is no doubt that treatment reduces the risk of heart failure substantially.

A particularly rapid rise of pressure over a short time, or a very high pressure *per se* may so damage terminal branches of the arterial tree that perfusion of kidney, heart, and brain is threatened. This very rare condition is still called 'malignant hypertension' (because mortality after 1 year was around 90 per cent before effective treatment became available). This used to be a major cause of kidney failure and is still a problem in some parts of the Third World, although it is now very rare in Europe and North America. Hypertension in the so-called 'benign' phase is, by contrast, unlikely to cause significant kidney dysfunction.

Blood pressure screening is now widely advocated. Undoubtedly, detection of those with high pressures receiving subsequent effective treatment will much reduce the risk of stroke and heart failure in these individuals, although prevention of myocardial infarction will be less effective; the latter, the most serious risk, is the one least effectively prevented. Another caveat is that people with untreated high arterial pressure almost always feel well, while a diagnosis of hypertension followed by treatment involves not only the side-effects of drugs but also the subtle ill-effects of being designated 'a patient'. Hence, measurements of arterial pressure should be done with particular care, and adequate measures must be taken to be sure that the high blood pressure is truly sustained and not a transient reaction to the doctor—so-called 'white-coat hypertension'.

The major difficulty remains of applying mass epidemiological data to the individual. When, and if, molecular biology can pin-point the true risk of a given pressure in an individual, as opposed to the crude population studies on which we now rely, this problem will become much easier.

J. LEDINGHAM

HYPERTHERMIA is treatment by inducing a high body temperature, either by external heating or by giving pyrogenic substances (cf. *hyperpyrexia).

HYPERTHYROIDISM is overactivity of the *thyroid gland. See THYROTOXICOSIS.

HYPERTRICHOSIS is excessive growth of hair.

HYPERTROPHY is an increase in size of an organ, tissue, or part as a result of increased size of its component cells (cf. *hyperplasia).

HYPERURICAEMIA (HYPERURICEMIA) is elevation of the concentration of *uric acid in the blood, important in the pathogenesis of urinary *calculi and *gout.

HYPERVENTILATION is abnormally deep and/or rapid breathing. See also ALKALOSIS.

HYPNAGOGIC HALLUCINATIONS are *hallucinations experienced by normal subjects in the drowsy state immediately before falling asleep. Similar hallucinations experienced on awakening are called hypnopompic. They resemble dreams.

HYPNOSIS. Induction of a state of abnormal suggestibility (see HYPNOTISTS). The technique is sometimes used for medical and dental anaesthesia or in the treatment of *hysteria or *neurosis. The term is less often used to identify the process of inducing sleep.

HYPNOTICS are drugs which induce sleep. Hypnotics are usually also *sedatives when given in lower dosage.

HYPNOTISM is the practice of inducing *hypnosis, a state of abnormal suggestibility. See HYPNOTISM ACT 1952; HYPNOTISTS.

HYPNOTISM ACT 1952. The UK Hypnotism Act of 1952, implemented on 1 April 1953, imposes certain regulations on the exhibition, demonstration, or performance of hypnotic phenomena in places licensed for public entertainment. Such exhibitions must have special authorization from the controlling authority, and are subject to any conditions which that authority wishes to impose. The Act also forbids performances involving the hypnosis of persons under the age of 21. The Act is not concerned with the use of hypnotic techniques other than for public entertainment.

HYPNOTISTS. Although the art of hypnotism, or of techniques allied to it, seems to have been practised since the earliest times, its introduction as a therapeutic technique is generally credited to the Austrian Franz Anton *Mesmer (1733–1815), who believed it to be based on a force he called 'animal magnetism'. Mesmer went to Paris in 1778 and gained considerable success with his treatment, which involved an impressive array of apparatus. His pupil, the Marquis de Puysegar, subsequently proved hypnotism to be equally effective without the paraphernalia of magnets, wires, and tubs of water. Bertrand championed the use of hypnotism in therapeutics, and it became well-established in 19th century France, schools being led by such distinguished names as *Richet and *Charcot. In England, Braid of Manchester discovered that a hypnotic trance could be induced by gazing at a bright object, and was the first to suggest the term 'hypnotism'. *Elliotson used the method as an anaesthetic in surgical operations but the discovery of chloroform in 1848 soon rendered it obsolete. In 1882 Gurney investigated the subject, following which the British Medical Association in 1892 pronounced favourably on the use of hypnotism in medicine. Present-day hypnotists are either hypnotherapists, medically qualified or otherwise, or entertainers, of whom there have been many. *Freud practised hypnotherapy before he developed the association methods of *psychoanalysis.

HYPOADRENALISM is diminished activity of the cortex of the *adrenal gland. See ADDISON'S DISEASE.

HYPOCALCAEMIA (HYPOCALCEMIA) is depression of the serum *calcium concentration below the normal range (2.1–2.6 mmol/l). See TETANY.

HYPOCHONDRIASIS is excessive preoccupation with the state of one's health.

HYPOGLYCAEMIA (HYPOGLYCEMIA). An abnormally low *blood sugar level, usually due to an excess of *insulin resulting either from an overdose in a diabetic patient or from an insulin-secreting tumour of the *pancreas (insulinoma). Other causes are rarer. The manifestations include hunger, sweating, irritability, confusion, and tremor; if unrelieved by the administration of glucose, these lead eventually to *convulsions, *coma, and death.

HYPOGONADISM is deficient *testicular function in the male, or deficient *ovarian function in the female.

HYPOKALAEMIA (HYPOKALEMIA) is depression of the serum *potassium below the normal range (3.5–5.4 mmol/l), sometimes termed hypopotassaemia. Low levels of serum potassium are associated with neuromuscular weakness and distinctive abnormalities on *electrocardiography.

HYPONATRAEMIA (HYPONATREMIA) is depression of the serum *sodium below the normal range (135–146 mmol/l).

HYPOPARATHYROIDISM. Deficient function of the *parathyroid glands, leading to absent or low levels of parathormone, *hypocalcaemia, *tetany, and hyperphosphataemia. The commonest cause is surgical, following operations on the parathyroids themselves, the *thyroid, or other neck structures in which the glands or their blood supply are removed or damaged. Idiopathic and genetic forms also occur.

HYPOPHYSIS. Synonym for *pituitary gland.

HYPOPITUITARISM is deficient function of the *pituitary gland, chiefly manifested by secondary deficiencies of its target endocrine organs (which may be selective), and by *diabetes insipidus when the posterior pituitary is involved. The causes include nonsecreting pituitary *tumours (especially chromophobe adenoma) and postpartum pituitary necrosis (Sheehan's syndrome) in addition to several less common conditions. In the prepubertal child, hypopituitarism usually results in *dwarfism and sexual *infantilism. See ENDOCRINOLOGY.

HYPOPLASIA is partial failure of development of a tissue or organ.

HYPOSPADIAS. A congenital abnormality in which the male *urethra fails to reach its normal termination at the end of the *penis, emptying instead through an opening beneath the penis or in the *perineum. See UROLOGICAL SURGERY.

HYPOSTASIS is circulatory stagnation in dependent organs, regions, or parts.

HYPOTENSION is a persistently low level of, or an acute drop in, arterial *blood pressure. Orthostatic or postural hypotension is a fall in arterial pressure on assuming the erect posture or on maintaining it for prolonged periods.

HYPOTHALAMUS is the region of the *brain below the third ventricle; it has many functions, being involved in control of the *autonomic nervous system, endocrine function, body temperature, sleep, appetite, water balance, emotion, and sexuality.

HYPOTHERMIA occurs when the body temperature falls to less than 35 °C (rectal measurement), either as a result of natural (environmental and pathological) causes or induced in order to facilitate certain surgical procedures. Accidental hypothermia, particularly in the elderly, is an important clinical diagnosis which may be missed if only a conventional clinical thermometer is used.

HYPOTHYROIDISM. See MYXOEDEMA.

HYPOTONIA is diminished tone in muscles.

HYPOVENTILATION is depressed breathing, with insufficient alveolar ventilation to maintain normal arterial blood gas tensions.

HYPOVOLAEMIA (HYPOVOLEMIA) is abnormally low circulating blood volume.

HYPOXIA is lack of oxygen supply.

HYRTL, JOSEPH (1810–94). Austrian anatomist. He published a famous textbook *Lehrbuch der Anatomie des Menschen mit Rücksicht auf physiologische Begrundung und pracktische Anwendung* in 1846.

HYSTERECTOMY is surgical removal of the *uterus. See GYNAECOLOGY.

HYSTERIA is a form of *psychoneurosis in which, according to *Freud, a repressed emotional conflict finds external expression in sensory and motor dysfunction, such as loss of sensation over parts of the body, temporary blindness, paralysis of limbs, loss or impairment of speech or hearing, or even convulsions, etc. Selective memory loss for personal events may also occur, including loss of personal identity, or an hysterical '*fugue' or *Ganser state. Occasionally the patient displays an incongruous lack of concern for his or her disability ('*la belle indifference*'). The term conversion hysteria is used to describe a situation in which a patient's inability to cope with reality is converted into a physical affliction, thereby becoming socially acceptable; the symptom is then said to carry a 'secondary gain', that is avoidance of the original problem causing the stress. In common usage, the adjective 'hysterical' is employed in respect of personality and behaviour traits which would more accurately be termed 'histrionic'.

I

IATROCHEMIST. An exponent of a school of thought existing in the 16th and 17th century that emphasized the underlying chemical nature of physiological and pathological phenomena.

IATROGENIC DISEASE. An 'iatrogenic' disorder is one resulting from the activities of the physician himself. It was originally used for psychogenic symptoms unwittingly induced by the medical attendant through suggestion, as with the mildly *hypertensive patient who develops headaches only after learning that his blood pressure is raised. The meaning now extends to include all conditions for which the doctor is responsible, for example adverse side-effects of drugs and unintended sequels of surgical operations.

IBN AL-NAFIS (1210–88). Arabian physician. Regarded by many as second only to *Avicenna, he wrote much, but only his *Compendium medicinae* remains. He concluded that the interventricular septum was solid and that blood passed by the pulmonary artery to the lungs and thence by the pulmonary vein to the left ventricle.

ICHTHYOSIS is any condition associated with the appearance of 'fish skin', that is skin which is dry, tough, and covered with scales. There are various types, some of which are inherited and present from an early age. Acquired ichthyosis should raise suspicion of underlying *malignant disease.

ICTERUS. Synonym for *jaundice.

ICTUS, the Latin word for 'blow, stroke, or thrust', was originally used in medicine to mean the beat of the *pulse and in the term *ictus solis* for *sunstroke. It is now a slightly archaic term for any sudden attack of illness, such as a *fit or a *stroke.

IDEA. An intellectual notion or concept.

IDEATION. The formation of ideas, or the ability of the mind to form ideas.

IDENTICAL TWINS are twins derived from a single fertilized *ovum and therefore possessing identical *genotypes; also known as uniovular or monozygotic twins (cf. fraternal or binovular *twins, resulting from the simultaneous fertilization of two ova). See also GENETICS.

IDEOLOGY has various senses, but present-day usage corresponds most closely to definition 4 of the *OED* (Supplement, vol. II): 'A systematic scheme of ideas, usually relating to politics or society, or to the conduct of a class or group, and regarded as justifying actions, especially one that is held implicitly or adopted as a whole and maintained regardless of the course of events.'

IDIOCY is an outmoded term for the severest grade of *mental handicap in which the adult mental age does not exceed 2 years and the *IQ 25.

IDOSYNCRASY refers to individual hypersensitivity to a drug, article of food, or other substance, not explicable on an immunological basis and not due to inherent toxicity of the substance concerned.

IDOXURIDINE is an antiviral agent effective against *herpes viruses but too toxic for systemic administration. It is used topically in the treatment of herpetic lesions of the skin, conjunctiva, and genitalia, and in *herpes zoster.

IGNIS SACER. *Erysipelas.

ILEITIS is inflammation of the *ileum. See also CROHN'S DISEASE.

ILEOCOLITIS is inflammation of the *ileum and *colon.

ILEOSTOMY. A surgically created opening of the ileum on to the abdominal surface.

ILEUM. The part of the small intestine between the *jejunum and the *caecum.

ILEUS. Intestinal obstruction from any cause, including that due to lack of intestinal motility.

ILLUSION. A misinterpreted *perception. An idea with no substance in fact or no rational basis.

ILLUSTRATION AND PHOTOGRAPHY IN MEDICINE. Examples of medical illustrations can be traced back to ancient Egypt and the earliest Arab manuscripts. The Egyptians produced what was probably the world's first surgical textbook around 1700 BC. While it contained no illustrations, it described in detail the treatment of 48 cases of battle wounds. The Egyptian tombs of the 25th century BC contain a number of sculptured relief illustrations of medical interest.

Aristotle, the founder of biological investigation, is reputed to have used drawings in his teaching. Towards the end of the 4th century BC, diagrams showing muscles, bones, nerves, arteries, and veins were produced by the early Greek anatomists. *Galen dominated medicine in the 2nd century AD. However, human dissection was considered unacceptable in Greece at that time and his books were based on dissection of monkeys and pigs. Medicine continued to be taught based on Galen's writings until the 14th century.

It was not until the 15th century and the work of *da Vinci that the scientific accuracy of human anatomical illustrations was assured. The illustrations, attributed to Calcar, in *Vesalius's famous anatomical text *De humani corporis fabrica* reached new levels of artistic excellence. Invention of the printing press in the 15th century made possible the efficient production of illustrated books, thus satisfying the needs of the growing numbers of universities.

Although the camera obscura was first described in 1589, it was over 100 years before it appeared in medical literature. In 1733 Cheselden's *Osteographia* depicted the artist van der Gutch working with the instrument. In the first half of the 19th century the work of Niécpe and Daguerre resulted in the camera obscura image being recorded chemically. The first medical application was reported 6 months later, in 1840, using the daguerrotype process to take photomicrographs of teeth and bones.

The first clinical photographs were taken in the late 1840s. By 1852 pre- and postoperative photographs were being used to assess patients' progress. Advances in optical devices enabled the examination of previously inaccessible parts of the body, e.g. the *larynx and *retina. Development of photographic apparatus kept pace, allowing the production of permanent records. Medical photography was well established in France by the 1880s, with most hospitals having photographers. Figure 1 shows an early example of clinical photography, taken in 1903. Not surprisingly, these developments were viewed with dismay by the art establishment. However, predictions about art's demise proved something of an overreaction and, as it transpired, totally unfounded.

The 20th century saw the introduction of a number of technical innovations, including roll-film cameras, synchronized sound on cine, and considerable improvements in black and white and colour processes. From the end of the Second World War illustration and photography became an accepted part of modern medical practice, with departments becoming established in major teaching hospitals and medical schools.

Nowadays medical illustration encompasses the use of a wide range of graphic, photographic, and electronic media which are used to record medical research and to present its results and achievements.

While the medical artist is still called upon to use traditional skills, there is much greater emphasis on computer technology. Digitizing tablets, optical disc drives, scanners, laser printers, slide writers, and a whole range of sophisticated software packages make up the tools of the trade. Illustrating medical textbooks, producing posters for presentations at scientific conferences, exhibition work, creating computer-generated slides, and desk-top publishing of leaflets and booklets are all commonplace activities. Gone are the days when the medical artist was primarily engaged in anatomical illustration. It has been claimed that the impact of computer technology will be greater than the invention of printing. It remains to be seen what the full implications of this rapidly developing technology will be, but, from the artist's point of view, the power to create and manipulate images is already at an unprecedented scale.

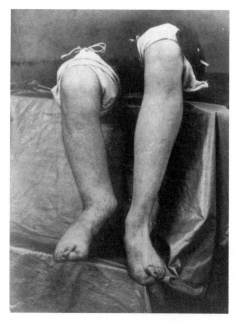

Fig. 1 An early clinical photograph (reproduced by kind permission of the University of Newcastle upon Tyne).

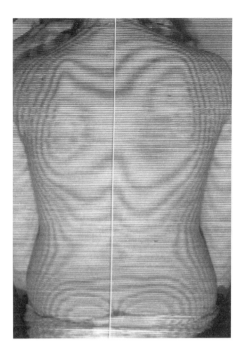

Fig. 2 Moiré topography (reproduced by kind permission of the University of Newcastle upon Tyne).

The medical photographer undertakes a wide range of clinical and non-clinical photography in a variety of locations, e.g. studio, ward, clinic, operating theatre, and post-mortem room. Essentially, photographs are required either for clinical records, research, teaching, or publication. Clinical photography involves recording the visible signs and various stages of a particular disease. Successful clinical photography, therefore, is very much dependent on matched photographs over time. A diagnosis is made by eliciting signs and symptoms. A good clinical photograph will pick up the signs in their best light, e.g. swelling and deformity, and will include a view showing the expression of the symptoms, e.g. a pained expression on the patient's face.

Photographs as an aid to research are used to provide objective records from which measurements are made, e.g. stereophotogrammetry. Other applications involve the use of invisible radiations, e.g. infra-red or ultraviolet, as an illustrative or diagnostic technique. Infra-red was used in medical work as early as 1906.

Potentially, any medical photograph is of value in teaching. A good-quality colour photograph may be used by a dermatologist to teach medical students about a particular skin condition. Nowadays clinical slide libraries are commonplace in medical schools. A series of slides or a video often provides an effective means of teaching a new surgical procedure. Sometimes a combination of photography and art is employed, with

drawings emphasizing features not clearly apparent in a photograph. Medical photographs produced in a medical school or teaching hospital are frequently required for publication in textbooks or medical journals. These may be of a clinical nature, but also include radiographs, scans, equipment, instruments, culture plates, specimens, photomicrographs, etc.

More specialized medical photographic techniques include moiré topography and fluorescein angiography. Moiré topography is an optical biostereometric method of depicting the three-dimensional shape of the human body. Essentially, shadow patterns are used, resembling the contour lines on a topographical map. The effect is created by positioning an object behind a grid of horizontal or vertical lines and illuminating it with a point source of light; the line shadows from the grid then conform to the object surface (Fig. 2). The technique is used in orthopaedics to evaluate *scoliosis (lateral curvature of the spine). Being entirely non-invasive, it is a particularly valuable screening method for the adolescent. While it does not replace X-rays, it can reduce *radiation exposure considerably.

Fluorescein *angiography of the eye, a procedure regularly undertaken by medical photographers, records blood circulation in the retina (Fig. 3). It is worth noting that this is a modern clinical investigation which would not have been possible without photography.

Much in the same way as the artist has adapted to the introduction of computer graphics technology, the

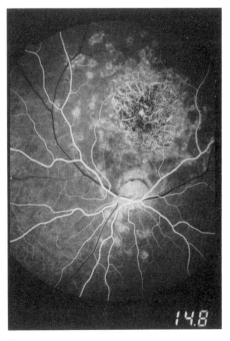

Fig. 3 Fluorescein angiography of the eye.

photographer is having to address digital imaging. The photographic process, with its dependence on silver, is still very much alive, and likely to remain so for many years to come. However, the impact of computers and electronic imaging is very apparent in modern medicine. Radiological imaging is no longer dependent on silver. Diagnostic procedures such as fluorescein angiography are now carried out on video, with individual frames being subjected to image enhancement, and hard copy produced via thermal printers. It is only a matter of time before electronic still cameras are used to record clinical material on disc. Eventually wards and clinics will have replay equipment to view those images. Digital imaging opens up new and exciting possibilities for communication. Hopefully medical illustrators will seize those opportunities and not repeat the artists' mistaken reaction to the arrival of photography.

More recently, with drives for greater efficiency in the public sector and large numbers of hospitals becoming trusts, a change in emphasis has occurred. There is increased demand for photography of a more general, non-medical nature. Graphics departments are now involved in producing promotional material and a whole range of patient information handouts and booklets.

The modern medical illustration department has a greater level of accountability than ever before. Internal trading, quality assurance, zero budgets, income generation, and the need to be competitive increasingly occupy the minds of managers and staff.

The specialist in any one particular area is slowly becoming a thing of the past. By necessity, medical illustrators are increasingly required to acquire a broader range of skills, encompassing more than one medium. In the rapidly changing world of medicine, flexibility and the establishment and maintenance of truly professional standards are the key to survival and success. All this, and the adoption of revolutionary technologies mentioned earlier, make for an exciting future.

K. G. MACLEAN

Further reading
Donald, G. (1986). The history of medical illustration. *Journal of Audiovisual Media in Medicine*, **9**, 44–9.
Koepfler, J. W. (1983). Moiré topography in medicine. *Journal of the Biological Photographic Association*, **51**, 3–10.
Ollerenshaw, R. (1961). Medical illustration in the past. In *Medical photography in practice* (ed. E. E. Linsson). Fountain Press, London.
Williams, A. R. (1984). *Medical photography study guide*. MTP Press, Lancaster, England.

IMAGE. The mental representation of a sensory *perception.

IMBECILITY is an outmoded term for *mental handicap, formerly categorized as the grade less severe than *idiocy, associated with an adult mental age of between 2 and 7 years, an *IQ between 25 and 50, and incapacity to manage personal affairs.

IMHOTEP (*fl.* 2980 BC) Egyptian physician and sage. Although Imhotep was previously believed to have been legendary, there is now no doubt that he was a historical personage who lived in the third dynasty during the reign of King Zoser (2980–2900 BC). He was priest, architect, and sage, but there is no contemporary evidence of his being a physician. Under the Ptolemies he acquired a great reputation for healing and was deified. Many miracles were wrought at his temples and he became the God of Medicine. The Greeks called him Imouthes and identified him with *Aesculapius.

IMMERSION FOOT is a form of cold injury, also called 'trench foot', resulting from prolonged immersion in cold water and encountered, for example, in survivors of accidents at sea. Intense *vasoconstriction results in anoxic tissue damage. On rescue the parts concerned are cold, numb, pulseless, and pale with peripheral *cyanosis. There follows a hyperaemic phase in which redness supervenes and in which pain may be intense; the limbs may be swollen, and the effects of trauma and infection become manifest. Some *anaesthesia may persist, occasionally indefinitely. In severe cases, *gangrene occurs. As well as sensory loss, abnormal temperature sensitivity can be a persistent sequel.

IMMUNE GLOBULIN. Synonymous with *immunoglobulin.

IMMUNE SYSTEM. The organs, cells, and molecules responsible for the recognition and disposal of foreign ('non-self') material which enters the body. See IMMUNOLOGY.

IMMUNITY is the recognition and disposal of foreign ('non-self') material that enters the body. See IMMUNOLOGY.

IMMUNIZATION is the acquisition of resistance by the *immune system to invasion of the body by particular foreign material. It may be active (deliberately induced to confer immunity against a specific disease), passive (conferring temporary immunity, say by the injection of immune serum or globulin), or natural (conferred by suffering from the illness concerned).

IMMUNOFLUORESCENCE is the use of specific *antibody labelled with a fluorescent dye (see FLUORESCEIN) to locate the homologous protein *antigen in tissue preparations. The technique may also be used in reverse, that is to locate antibody by means of labelled antigen.

IMMUNOGENETICS is the study of the genetic control of *immunity. See GENETICS; HLA; IMMUNOLOGY.

IMMUNOGLOBULINS. All *globulins with *antibody activity. (The term 'immunoglobulin' has replaced 'gammaglobulin' because not all antibodies have gamma mobility on electrophoresis.) The immunoglobulins are broadly classified into five groups on the basis of physical, antigenic, and functional variations, labelled respectively, M, G, A, E, and D. See IMMUNOLOGY.

IMMUNOLOGIST. A scientist specializing in the study of the *immune system and the relationship between immune phenomena and disease.

IMMUNOLOGY. The science of immunology originated in the common observation that people recovering from some *infectious diseases are protected from subsequent attacks. A child who has had *measles or *mumps, or the survivor of a *smallpox *epidemic, is unlikely to develop the disease a second time. There are three features of this 'immune response' which make it a unique biological phenomenon. It is, in the first place, an *acquired* response elicited by the initial exposure to the disease. Secondly, it *persists* in the form of an immunological memory, which can be recalled and reactivated months or years later. And finally, there is the extraordinary *specificity* of the reaction, as illustrated by the fact that an attack of smallpox protects against that disease, but not against *yellow fever. The investigation of this problem has occupied immunologists for more than a century.

In its early years immunology was essentially a practical science concerned with combating infectious diseases. It now covers a far wider field and encompasses all aspects of the body's ability to react to foreign or extraneous substances. There are many diseases caused by exaggerated or inappropriate immune responses, commonly known as *allergy or hypersensitivity, and a wide range of disorders, the *autoimmune diseases, in which the body reacts against itself. There are also diseases in which immunity is defective, of which *AIDS, due to infection with the HIV virus, is the most striking example. Immunology has also provided the rationale and the techniques for such notable medical advances as blood transfusion and organ *transplantation.

The earliest medical application of immunology was the introduction of *vaccination against smallpox by Edward *Jenner (1749–1823). He was a Gloucestershire physician who observed that dairy maids who developed *cow-pox were protected against smallpox. In 1796 he inoculated a young boy with fluid from a cow-pox pustule. A little pustule appeared at the site of injection and then disappeared. Some months later he injected him with material from a human smallpox case and was gratified to observe (as no doubt was the boy) that no disease developed. After some initial resistance, the practice of vaccination (L. *vacca*, cow) against smallpox became general, although the nature of the protection offered was not understood.

In the second half of the 19th century, as a result of the work of *Pasteur (1822–1895), *Koch (1843–1910), and others, it became apparent that infectious diseases were due to the invasion of the body by *micro-organisms, such as bacteria or viruses. It was also found possible to protect animals from infection by injecting them with altered or attenuated strains of the same organism. This was first observed by Pasteur in 1878, who noted that a culture of chicken *cholera, which had been left in the laboratory during the vacation, lost its virulence for chickens, and that animals inoculated with this culture were protected against the virulent strain. He immediately recognized the significance of this observation, and after confirming the phenomenon in *anthrax in animals, applied it to the prevention and treatment of human *rabies.

In some diseases it was found that if the animal recovered, its serum protected normal animals from infection. This suggested that immunity was due to a substance—a 'humoral factor'—in the blood. The most striking confirmation of this came from the studies of von *Behring (1854–1917) on *diphtheria and *tetanus. In both diseases the damage is done, not by the bacterium itself, but by *toxins produced by the organism and circulating in the blood. Von Behring showed that immunization with the toxin was sufficient to protect against the disease, and that this protection could be transferred to normal animals by injecting the serum. He proceeded to treat children with diphtheria by injecting serum from a horse immunized with diphtheria toxin. Von Behring recognized that the protective effect was due to substances circulating in the blood, and coined the term *antibody.

The humoral theory was almost immediately challenged by the observations of the Russian biologist *Metchnikoff (1845–1916) working in Paris. Observing primitive organisms under the microscope, he noted that some cells were capable of ingesting foreign particles and invading bacteria by a process that he termed *phagocytosis. He was able to show that similar cells capable of engulfing and destroying bacteria were present in the blood of vertebrates and that this process was enhanced in animals recovering from infection. He concluded that these cells were responsible for protective immunity and that the process was a cellular one. The controversy between the proponents of the cellular and humoral theories was a feature of early years of immunology, but as is so often the case, it turned out that both were correct and that immunity has both cellular and humoral components.

Antigens and antibodies

The ability to evoke an immune response is not peculiar to micro-organisms. Most foreign substances injected into the body will do so provided they are of sufficient molecular size. The most effective compounds are proteins and polysaccharides. Substances capable of eliciting an immune response are called *antigens* and the reactive molecules that appear in the serum as a result of immunization are referred to as *antibodies*. A remarkable feature of the reaction between antigen and antibody is its extraordinary specificity. The chemical nature of this specificity was first demonstrated in the elegant experiments of Karl *Landsteiner (1868–1943). He attached small molecules, of known constitution and structure, to large protein antigens and showed that the antibodies produced could distinguish subtle differences in chemical structure. He also demonstrated that the reaction was not with the whole molecule, but with small parts known as *antigenic determinants* or *epitopes*. One protein molecule might elicit antibody to a number of different determinants, each capable of reacting with different parts of the molecular surface. When antigen and antibody are mixed together in a test tube they combine, and the antigen–antibody complex may come out of solution in the form of a precipitate.

The antibodies circulating in the serum are extremely diverse. There are several classes, and in each class there are antibodies capable of reacting with a very large number of different antigenic determinants. The fundamental structure, however, is always the same (Fig. 1). They are protein molecules called immunoglobulins (Ig) which are made up of two sets of identical *polypeptide chains or sequences of *amino acids. There are two heavy (H) chains and two light (L) chains assembled into a Y-shaped structure. The two heavy chains make up the stem of the Y and continue into the arms linked to the two light chains. The latter are of two kinds, kappa and lambda. There are five main classes of immunoglobulin, each with its own characteristic H chain and biological properties. Each immunoglobulin molecule is bivalent and capable of reacting with two identical antigenic determinants. The reactive sites are at the ends of the two arms of the Y, and each determinant will, therefore, be in contact with portions of both the heavy and light chains. Each antibody has its own combining site, tailor-made to fit a particular determinant. The number of possible determinants, and

therefore, the number of different antibodies, is very large.

Generation of antibody diversity

Immunoglobulins are proteins, and like all proteins their synthesis is under genetic control. If each of the million or more antibodies that the animal can make required a separate gene, it would mean that a very large proportion of the genome would have to be taken up with this single task. This is highly improbable, so how is this degree of antigenic variation generated? The answer is that the diversity is not present in the genome of the sperm or ovum, as handed down by the parents, but arises in the lymphocytes of the embryo. In early embryonic development the lymphocytes proliferate at a furious rate. Many die and are eliminated. The chromosomal material in vertebrates, handed down from one generation to the next, contains several hundred genes devoted to the variable regions of the heavy and light chains of the immunoglobulin molecule. These code for the antigen-combining sites. In the early embryo the lymphocytes have a special propensity for rearranging these genes, producing a very large number of different combinations. There are also special regions of this part of the genome in lymphocytes, which have a very high mutation rate. These hypervariable regions are an additional source of variation. The combination of the two, gene rearrangement and somatic mutation, is thought to be sufficient to account for the enormous genetic diversity required to produce a million or more different antibodies.

The immune response

The entry of antigen into the body of vertebrates stimulates the production of immunoglobulins and specifically reactive cells. The latter have receptors on their surface analogous to the combining sites of antibodies, which enable them to react with antigens. Both the humoral and cellular responses are mediated by *lymphocytes. These cells originate in the *bone marrow and the *thymus gland and migrate to the blood, *lymph nodes, and *spleen. They also populate the lymphoid tissues of the alimentary tract and the lungs. For most of their life cycle they appear as small, featureless cells, 6 μm in diameter, containing small, round nuclei and very little cytoplasm. In this form they essentially function as repositories of genetic information. There are about 10^{12} lymphoid cells in the human body, and there is a rapid turnover rate, with 10^9 new lymphocytes being produced daily (Fig. 2). They are mobile cells which circulate between the blood, bone marrow, and lymphoid organs. They enter the tissues from the blood and drain back into the bloodstream via the lymphatic channels and lymph nodes. Lymphocytes also filter from the blood into the spleen and bone marrow. Like policemen on the beat, they are constantly on the move, ready to alert the immune defences to any intruder.

There are two classes of lymphocytes, T and B cells.

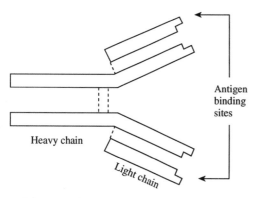

Fig. 1 Diagram of an antibody molecule, consisting of two heavy and two light chains.

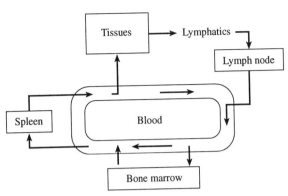

Fig. 2 The circulation of lymphocytes. Traffic through the tissues, lymph nodes, and spleen.

They are morphologically indistinguishable, but functionally distinct. The T or thymus-processed lymphocytes originate in the bone marrow and undergo a maturational development in the thymus gland in the neck. They or their progeny then re-enter the blood and populate the bone marrow and other lymphoid organs. When stimulated they produce the specifically sensitized cells, which generate cell-mediated immunity. The B lymphocytes are responsible for the humoral response and give rise to *plasma cells, which synthesize immunoglobulin. Like the T cells, they originate in the bone marrow. In birds they mature in the bursa of Fabricius, an organ associated with the lower bowel. In mammals, including man, this organ is absent and maturation occurs in the bone marrow itself. They are present in all lymphoid tissues (together with the T cells) and constitute 20 per cent of the lymphocytes in the peripheral blood.

The lymphoid tissues of the body are strategically placed to intercept invading organisms. They guard portals of entry, such as the alimentary and respiratory tracts, and are located in the draining lymph nodes and blood-filtering organs such as the spleen. In the lymphoid organs the lymphocytes are associated with *macrophages, large phagocytic cells which trap and process bacteria and other particulate *antigens. There are also 'antigen-presenting cells', which present the antigenic determinants to the lymphocytes in suitably stimulating form. The tissue macrophages form a network, found in many organs and referred to as the reticuloendothelial system. The system can be identified in animals by injecting a suspension of particulate carbon into the bloodstream. The carbon particles are rapidly removed from the blood and phagocytosed, staining the lymphoreticular system black.

In bacterial infections the organisms are trapped in the lymphoreticular tissue, phagocytosed by macrophages, and degraded. The processed antigenic determinants are then presented to the lymphocytes by the antigen-presenting cells. The effect is to stimulate B and T cells and cause them to divide and multiply. Early in embryonic life each lymphocyte acquires the capacity to respond to a particular determinant. From then on, the cell and all its progeny (the *clone) have the ability to react with that particular molecular configuration. There are a large number of potential antigens and the adult animal has cells capable of responding to every possible determinant. The number of lymphocytes reacting to any one determinant will, therefore, be small. However, on exposure to antigen these lymphocytes proliferate, producing a greatly expanded clone of cells, each capable of responding to that particular determinant. A mechanism of this kind was first suggested by the Australian microbiologist Macfarlane *Burnet and Jerne, a Swiss immunologist, in their clonal selection theory propounded in the 1950s.

B lymphocytes stimulated by antigen go on to form plasma cells (Fig. 3). These large cells, with increased cytoplasm, synthesize and secrete immunoglobulin. Each plasma cell produces antibody of one specificity, the same for all cells of the clone. Similarly, stimulated T lymphocytes proliferate and give rise to clones of specifically sensitized cells, capable of reacting with the antigen. There are several classes of T cells, each capable of responding to antigen in a different way. Some are able to destroy cells invaded by viruses ('cytotoxic T cells') others release substances ('lymphokines') which stimulate immune and inflammatory cells and generate a local inflammatory reaction. This reaction, known as delayed-type hypersensitivity, was discovered by Robert Koch in the 19th century, while investigating tuberculosis. It plays a very important role in many chronic inflammatory diseases. In addition to these cellular reactions, the T lymphocytes also assist in the production of antibody. They do not synthesize immunoglobulin themselves, but facilitate the process by providing an additional stimulus to the B cells ('helper function'). Collectively all these functions of the T lymphocyte are referred to as cell-mediated immunity.

Protective immunity

Most infectious agents encountered by the body do not penetrate the surface, but are prevented by a variety of physical and chemical barriers. These include the skin and epithelial lining of organs exposed to the exterior, such as the lungs and alimentary tract. These surfaces have a variety of specially designed protective substances. For example, lysozyme, an enzyme found in many secretions, is capable of breaking down the cell walls of many bacteria. If micro-organisms penetrate these barriers, they are faced by the phagocytic cells of the blood and lymphoreticular system. The macrophages and polymorphonuclear cells not only engulf bacteria, but are provided with an array of bactericidal mechanisms for destroying intracellular parasites. The serum, too, contains a formidable series of biochemical defences, including the *complement system.

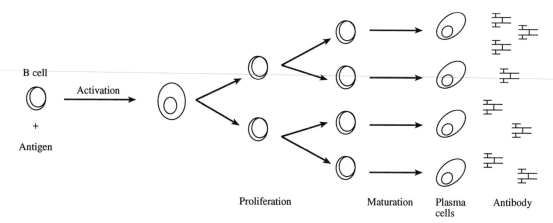

Fig. 3 Stimulation of B lymphocytes by antigen. The cells divide and proliferate to form an expanded clone. Mature B cells develop into plasma cells which synthesize antbody.

When activated, the latter triggers a complex series of enzymic reactions, the complement cascade, which amplify many of the protective devices of innate and acquired immunity. Among other things, it enhances phagocytosis and facilitates the destruction of bacteria and viruses. All these mechanisms of innate immunity, including phagocytosis and the complement cascade, are an integral part of the process of *inflammation—the body's reaction to injury.

Superimposed upon this *innate immunity* is a second system, tailored more precisely to the particular invading organism. This is the process of *acquired immunity*, in which the body responds by producing antibody and specifically sensitized T cells. Antibody subserves a variety of functions. For example, in bacterial infections it may coat the organisms and facilitate phagocytosis, or cause them to adhere and agglutinate, immobilizing them. It may also react with toxins and block their action, as shown by the therapeutic effect of antisera in diseases such as diphtheria. Most importantly, the combination of antibody and antigen may activate the complement system, which enhances many of the protective processes by several orders of magnitude.

Immunity to viruses is largely a T-cell function. This is because, unlike bacteria, viruses lurk inside living cells out of reach of antibody. The cytotoxic T lymphocyte travels through the tissues of the body in an unending search for abnormal cells. Viral infection is signalled by the appearance of foreign antigens at the cell surface. These are recognized by the T lymphocyte, which attacks the cell and destroys it, releasing the *virus into the extracellular space, where it can be acted upon by antibody.

After recovery from an infection the individual retains an 'immunological memory' of the antigens in the form of an expanded clone of cells capable of responding to those particular determinants. These 'memory' cells

enable the individual to respond to a subsequent infection swiftly and effectively.

The importance of the immune response in combating infection is illustrated by the fact that children born with inherited defects of the immune system succumb to a variety of infectious diseases. For instance, a child born without a thymus gland will fail to develop T lymphocytes. The resulting defect of cell-mediated immunity will render the infant susceptible to viral and fungal diseases. There are also children with B-cell defects who are unable to produce immunoglobulins and suffer repeated bacterial infections. If both T and B cells fail to develop normally, the consequences are even more serious. In the era before *antibiotics, few, if any, of these children survived into adult life. There are also immunodeficiency states which develop as a result of viral infections or the effects of drugs. The most important of these secondary immunodeficiencies is the acquired immune deficiency syndrome (AIDS) which follows infection with the HIV virus.

Allergy and hypersensitivity

When an immune response occurs in an exaggerated or inappropriate manner and results in tissue injury, this is referred to as allergy or hypersensitivity. The terms were originally coined to describe different phenomena, but time and usage have blurred the distinction and they are now used interchangeably. The discovery that immune reactions can damage tissue, as well as protect, was made in the unlikely ambience of a Mediterranean cruise. In 1901 the French physiologists *Richet and Poitier accompanied the Prince of Monaco on a cruise aboard his yacht. They were interested in the toxic properties of extracts of certain sea anemones and, while still aboard the yacht, demonstrated their toxicity to rabbits and ducks. On their return to France they began experiments on dogs, and observed, to their surprise, that the injection of small sublethal doses of the toxin did not protect the dogs from subsequent larger doses, but, on the contrary, rendered them more sensitive. A second injection of a minute and normally innocuous dose, would cause the dog to collapse and, in some cases, to die. They called this *anaphylaxis to distinguish it from 'phylaxis', or protection. It was subsequently shown that anaphylaxis could be produced in most vertebrate species with perfectly harmless proteins, such as egg albumin.

A mechanism of this kind, known as immediate-type hypersensitivity, underlies many allergic diseases, including such common disorders as *hay fever and bronchial *asthma. These diseases tend to occur in genetically susceptible individuals and are precipitated by exposure to environmental antigens, which may be inhalants, such as grass pollens or animal dander, or common articles of diet, such as milk or wheat proteins. Immediate-type hypersensitivity is due to a particular class of antibody, immunoglobulin E. This has the property of attaching itself to the surface membrane of *mast cells in the tissues. The cytoplasm of these cells is closely packed with granules containing potent chemical substances. If the subject is exposed to antigen, it will enter the tissues and combine with antibody at the mast cell surface. This triggers the disruption of the cytoplasmic granules, releasing pharmacologically active substances, which act on small blood vessels, smooth muscle, and mucus-secreting glands. The effect varies with the organ and the species. In man it produces hay fever in the nose and bronchial asthma in the lung. When the antigen is injected, the result may be explosive, inducing acute respiratory or circulatory failure. Anaphylactic shock of this kind may lead to collapse and even death in humans, after the injection of an apparently innocuous protein or following a bee sting.

Immediate-type hypersensitivity is only one of several allergic mechanisms. Tissue damage may result from the combination of antibody and antigen to form toxic complexes circulating in the blood. This may result in serious disease of the kidneys or the blood vessels, and is not infrequently due to viral antigens. This form of hypersensitivity is known as *serum sickness. A related type of injury due to insoluble immune complexes occurs in the tissues and is called the Arthus reaction. Finally, there is delayed-type hypersensitivity, in which tissue injury occurs as a by-product of cell-mediated reactions. A wide range of human diseases can now be ascribed to reactions of this kind.

Tolerance and autoimmunity

The immune system responds to foreign antigens and must, therefore, be able to distinguish them from the body's own constituents or 'self' components. The German chemist and pioneer immunologist Paul *Ehrlich first drew attention to this problem at the end of the 19th century. However, immunologists only began to address the matter seriously after the Second World War, when attempts were made to graft tissues and organs from one individual (or species) into another. They found that this was not possible, except in the case of identical twins. Transplanted skin, for example, survived perfectly well for a week or so, when it ceased to be viable and was rejected. The matter was investigated in genetically pure strains of rats and mice, where it was shown that the *rejection process was an immune response, mounted by the recipient of the graft to the donor tissue. Lymphocytes in the host become sensitized to antigens in the transplanted tissue, enter the graft and destroy it. It turns out that each individual of a species (apart from sets of identical twins) is genetically unique, and the differences are signalled by a system of antigens known as the major *histocompatibility complex (MHC). The most important of these, from the point of view of *transplantation, are the MHC class II antigens, which are present in all cells of the body. Elucidation of this problem made it possible to replace diseased organs, such as kidneys, by transplantation from healthy donors or even cadavers. Rejection in these cases is prevented by drugs that suppress the immune response, and donors are carefully selected by MHC testing to minimize the antigenic differences between the grafted tissues and the host.

In 1953 *Medawar and his colleagues showed that rejection of skin grafts in mice could be prevented if cells from the donor (or a genetically identical animal) were injected into the prospective recipient *in utero* or shortly after birth. This implied that the immune system would accept as 'self' any antigen to which it was exposed in fetal life. This state of unresponsiveness was called immune tolerance. Macfarlane Burnet and Fenner, in Australia, pointed out that this phenomenon, as well as the naturally occurring tolerance to 'self' components could be explained by supposing that lymphocytes reacting to antigens in the course of embryonic development were eliminated or rendered ineffective. Since the only antigens present in the fetus are 'self' components, this would lead to the elimination of autoreactive clones, leaving the mature immune system only able to respond to foreign antigens. We now know that 'clonal elimination' of this kind is only part of the story, and that immune tolerance is maintained by a highly complex mechanism, the details of which are only gradually being unravelled. An important element appears to be the MHC antigens in the tissues, which function as some kind of marker, allowing lymphocytes to recognize 'self' components.

An important advance in recent years has been the realization that immune tolerance may fail and give rise to diseases in which the body reacts against its own tissues. These *autoimmune diseases* may affect any organ in the body. The causes are largely unknown, although many of the diseases occur in genetically susceptible individuals and some are triggered by viral infections.

S. LEIBOWITZ

Further reading
Klein, J. (1991). *Immunology*. Blackwell, Oxford.
Roitt, I. M. (1994). *Essential immunology*, (8th edn). Blackwell, Oxford.

IMMUNOSUPPRESSION is the suppression by various agents of particular components of the *immune system, of value in the management of organ *transplantation and of certain disease states. Immunosuppression is usually non-specific (although not always: see e.g. HAEMOLYTIC DISEASE OF THE NEWBORN); it may therefore have dangerous unwanted effects, such as removal of the normal response to infection. See IMMUNOLOGY.

IMMUNOSUPPRESSIVE describes drugs (e.g. *azathioprine, *cyclophosphamide, *methotrexate, *mercaptopurine, *cyclosporin-A, *corticosteroids), biological agents (e.g. *antilymphocyte serum), or procedures (e.g. *X-irradiation, *plasmapheresis, *thoracic duct drainage) which depress all or part of the *immune system.

IMPERIAL CANCER RESEARCH FUND. An independent (i.e. non-governmental) British organization devoted to the raising of money from the public and its application to *cancer research. The Fund (abbreviation ICRF) has substantial research laboratories under its own direct control, and also provides grants to other research workers.

IMPETIGO is a superficial coccal infection of the *skin, primarily of the pilosebaceous follicles, characterized by formation of pustules and crusts. It occurs mainly in children.

IMPLANT. Any material inserted or grafted into the body, whether tissue or non-organic material. Examples are slow-release pellets containing drugs or hormones, and cardiac *pacemaker electrodes.

IMPOTENCE is the failure of the male to initiate, maintain, or complete sexual intercourse. See SEXUALITY AND MEDICINE.

IMPULSE. An impelling force, such as the cardiac impulse seen or felt over the precordium with each heart beat; a wave of excitation in nerve or other specialized conducting tissue; or a mental urge to act in a particular way.

INBORN ERRORS OF METABOLISM. Deoxyribonucleic acid (*DNA) is present in all living cells. It contains the information for cellular structure, organization, and function. *Genes are the units of heredity, composed of DNA, which form part of the *chromosomes. The genes code for particular *proteins which are important in controlling the structure and function of the body's cells. Frequent *mutations occur; that is, there is a stable alteration in DNA which can be passed from cell to progeny, unless the mutation causes death. Everyone carries defective genes but remains unaware of them. However, about 1 in 10 people will develop a genetic disorder at some time in their lives. Proteins are composed of *amino acids. As a consequence of a genetic mutation, a particular amino acid may be deleted, duplicated, substituted by another one, or otherwise changed. Already, more than 3000 disorders caused primarily by a single mutant gene and displaying *Mendelian inheritance have been discovered; they are referred to as inborn errors of metabolism. The term 'inborn errors of metabolism' was used first by the famous physician Archibald *Garrod in 1908. He published a second book in 1931 with the title *Inborn factors in disease*. This makes fascinating reading today and one is amazed at his foresight. At last *molecular biology and *genetics are elucidating the many problems that perplexed him.

Since the human *genome (all the DNA contained in a single set of chromosomes in a cell) is believed to contain 50 000–100 000 genes, since we are all different, and since our knowledge of disease at a molecular level is increasing so quickly, it is likely that many more disorders remain to be discovered. Already it is recognized that some disorders are multifactorial in their *aetiology: there may be predisposition to a particular disease which is modified by life-style and other environmental factors.

Inborn errors of metabolism, that is single gene disorders, may be inherited in one of three ways:

1. In recessive disorders both mother and father are carriers of the single abnormal gene and are healthy, but each of their offspring has a one in four chance of receiving the abnormal gene from both parents. This results in disease in the child; *cystic fibrosis is a well-known example of this. Such carriers are said to be heterozygous and the offspring who receive the double dose are homozygous.

2. In autosomal dominant inheritance the abnormal physical characteristic is manifest in the *heterozygote. An example of this is a metabolic disorder associated with extreme sensitivity to sunlight and the excretion of urine which becomes port-wine' coloured on standing (*porphyria variegata). It is not infrequent in White South Africans and all the affected cases have been traced back to one couple who married in 1688. Another example is brittle bone disease (*osteogenesis imperfecta). If the affected individual marries a normal person, then, on average, half their children will be affected.

3. In X-linked inheritance the abnormal gene is carried on the X chromosome (women have two X chromosomes and men have one X and one Y) Inheritance may be recessive or dominant. If it is recessive, the abnormal physical characteristic is only manifest in the woman if both X chromosomes are affected. In the man, since there is only one

X chromosome, he will always show the abnormal characteristic. *Haemophilia (the bleeding disease) and *Duchenne muscular dystrophy are good examples. If however the X-linked abnormal gene is dominant, the abnormal physical characteristic will be present in both men and women. An example is a form of *rickets which develops in spite of a normal intake of vitamin D in the diet and exposure to sunlight (vitamin-D-resistant rickets).

In practice, it may be very difficult to sort out the inheritance of an inborn error, and the account just given is somewhat simplified. The counselling of a patient, family, and extended family is very important, and, in many instances, specialist clinical geneticists may be necessary for this task.

In Western communities in which infectious diseases and lack of food are no longer problems, genetic disorders have assumed major importance. If the inborn errors of metabolism, disorders of chromosomes (e.g. *Down's syndrome), and structural malformations (e.g. neural tube defects such as *spina bifida) are added together, they account for over 50 per cent of all miscarriages, 25 per cent of perinatal deaths, and 25 per cent of severe handicaps. In some disorders the condition may not manifest itself until quite late in life (e.g. *Huntington's chorea). Many of the inherited metabolic disorders are rare, but there are so many of them that they make a significant contribution to morbidity and mortality.

It used to be thought that the mutation in each patient with a particular disorder, such as cystic fibrosis, was the same. As a result of developments in molecular biology it is now appreciated that there may be many different mutations in a gene, all producing the same disease but with different degrees of severity. For example, over 250 different mutations have already been described in cystic fibrosis.

Unfortunately, no treatment is known for many inborn errors of metabolism, but for some, treatment may be possible with varying degrees of success:

1. It may be possible to lower or remove the precursor that accumulates because of an inherited block in metabolism. An example of this is *phenylketonuria, for which all infants in Britain are tested, using a heel-prick sample of blood, soon after birth. The amino acid, phenylalanine, present in all protein foods (milk, meat, eggs, pulses, etc.) cannot be metabolized, but it is possible to treat the condition with a synthetic diet low in phenylalanine.
2. In some conditions a very high dose of a particular *vitamin may enable the defective *enzyme to function, e.g. large doses of *thiamine (a B vitamin) in some types of maple syrup urine disease. This name was given because the infant's urine smells of maple syrup; if untreated it is usually fatal.
3. It may be possible to provide a missing metabolite, for example in some types of *glycogen storage disease the patient cannot produce glucose properly and large amounts may be given day and night.

4. A drug may help in some conditions. For example in *gout, allopurinol prevents the excessive accumulation of uric acid.
5. In some conditions it is possible to avoid a substance which cannot be metabolized properly. For example, some infants are unable to metabolize lactose (milk sugar) which is present in breast, cow, and goat milk. Synthetic milk that does not contain milk sugar can be given instead.
6. It may be possible to replace the enzyme that is missing because the gene is defective. In some conditions this can be done with a *bone marrow transplant. In others, a liver transplant may be used, e.g. in *Wilson's disease in which copper accumulates in the liver and causes severe damage. New techniques involving *genetic engineering offer hope for the future, but are still very much in the experimental phase.

Phenylketonuria was mentioned above. In a normal individual the amino acid phenylalanine is converted to tyrosine by an enzyme in the liver. When the enzyme is defective this reaction cannot occur; phenylalanine rises to a high level in the blood, abnormal metabolites are produced, the brain tissue does not develop properly, and the production of *neurotransmitters (messages through the nervous system of the body) is impaired. As the apparently normal baby grows, it becomes apparent that he/she is not developing properly. If the condition is not diagnosed early and treated, severe permanent brain damage occurs. Treatment is with a synthetic *diet from which most of the phenylalanine has been removed. As this amino acid is essential for life, a small amount must be given with each feed or meal, and the amount has to be regulated carefully depending upon the blood level. The infant therefore receives a little breast or cow's milk, but mostly he/she is fed on synthetic milk. Later, the diet will be very different from a normal one. It will contain a synthetic substance to replace most of the usual protein and the child will have large helpings of vegetables and a special bread which does not contain phenylalanine. Synthetic diets like this have to be supplemented with vitamins and the essential elements (such as calcium, copper, zinc, and so on). It is probably necessary to continue the diet throughout life. Patients diagnosed early and treated do not become severely handicapped. They do tend to be hyperactive and have some educational difficulties, but they may hold normal jobs and, to the casual observer, be fine. Some neurological problems are now being seen in a few who have reached adult life. The reason is not known, but perhaps control of the diet has not been strict enough, or the diet may not be quite right because the knowledge to make it better is unknown, or perhaps some damage occurred in utero. With the application of molecular genetics demonstration of the nature of the mutations in patients may help to elucidate this problem.

For so many disorders there is no treatment at present, but prenatal diagnosis can be offered for some conditions if the parents desire it. This poses an ethical dilemma which only the individuals concerned can resolve. Some disorders, e.g. Duchenne muscular dystrophy, occur in males. It is possible to determine the sex of a fetus early in pregnancy and abort the males, if the involved individuals wish (see NEUROMUSCULAR DISEASE). Some conditions can be detected early in pregnancy by examining fluid or cells taken from the womb, e.g. some of the very severe brain disorders such as *Tay–Sachs disease in which abnormal fatty substances accumulate, and death is inevitable at varying ages from 2 years onwards, depending on the particular condition. The *carrier status for some disorders in eggs or sperm can be determined, and *in vitro* fertilization can assure that a fetus is unaffected.

Molecular genetics is developing fast and will have a major impact on our understanding of inborn errors of metabolism. Many applications will lead to better care of patients and their families, particularly because it will be easier to understand the pathological basis of these conditions. Research into cystic fibrosis is showing the way ahead. It is now known that the abnormal gene is on chromosome 7 and its many mutations have been demonstrated. Genotyping can be used to make an earlier diagnosis, screen the relatives for carrier status, and frequently assist in prenatal diagnosis. In addition, genetically engineered versions of naturally occurring enzymes are being made. One such is manufactured deoxyribonuclease, which is being tested in patients with cystic fibrosis to determine whether it will help to break down the thick secretions which damage the lungs in this disease.

Nature's experiment—the inborn errors of metabolism—are profoundly important in increasing our understanding of the pathogenesis of disease; with understanding comes treatment.

BARBARA CLAYTON

Further reading

Harris, H. (1963). *Garrod's inborn errors of metabolism.* Oxford University Press, London.

Sattelle, D. B. (1988). *Biotechnology in perspective.* Hobsons Publishing PLC, London. (This gives a good simple account of molecular biology.)

Scriver, C. R. and Childs, B. (1989). *Garrod's inborn factors in disease. Including an annotated facsimile reprint of* The inborn factors in disease *by Archibald E. Garrod.* Oxford Monographs on Medical Genetics, No. 16. Oxford University Press, Oxford.

Scriver, C. R., Beaudet, A. L., Sly, W. S., and Valle, D. (ed.) (1989). *The metabolic basis of inherited disease,* (6th ed.). McGraw-Hill, New York.

IN-BREEDING is reproduction by the mating of closely related individuals who therefore have similar *genetic constitutions. In-breeding of animals is often desirable, for example in the maintenance of genetically pure strains for laboratory purposes. In human populations in-breeding increases the incidence of disease due to harmful *recessive genes; in almost all societies union between closely consanguineous relatives is forbidden by custom, religion, or law.

INCEST is sexual intercourse between close relatives, particularly those of first degree, for example brother and sister, father and daughter, etc.

INCIDENCE. The frequency with which a given event occurs, for example the number of new cases of a particular disease occurring in a given population over a given period of time. It is important not to confuse incidence with *prevalence.

INCISION. A surgical cut; or the act of cutting.

INCOMPATIBILITY is a pharmacological, immunological, chemical, physical, psychological, or other mismatch.

INCOMPETENCE is the term employed for any defect of *valves in the cardiovascular system and elsewhere which fails to prevent retrograde flow.

INCONTINENCE, in a medical context, is failure to control the excretory functions of urination and defaecation. 'Double incontinence' implies loss of control of both. Incontinence may be due to defective *sphincter control in neurological disorders and in senility, but can also have local causes.

INCUBATION PERIOD is the clinically silent interval between invasion of the body by a disease agent and overt manifestations of the disease. (For another use of 'incubation', see TEMPLE MEDICINE).

INCUBATOR. An apparatus in which premature infants can be kept under optimal environmental conditions; or one which provides suitable conditions for the growth and development of micro-organisms, cells, tissues, organs, or embryos.

INDEX. One of various numerical values expressed as a ratio, proportion, or percentage: for example, the width of the heart expressed as a proportion of the width of the thorax on chest X-ray (cardiothoracic index); the cardiac output in $l/min/m^2$ of body surface (cardiac index); the length of the shorter arm of a mitotic *chromosome expressed as a proportion of the total length of the chromosome (centromeric index); the length of the upper arm expressed as a percentage of the length of the thigh (femorohumeral index); and so on. The term 'index case' means the first or original case, in *genetics synonymous with proband or propositus, in infectious disease *epidemiology, the case of the first patient to be detected in an epidemic.

INDEX FINGER. The forefinger, that is the second digit of the hand.

INDEX MEDICUS is a monthly catalogue of the world's important biomedical literature; titles of publications are indexed by subject and author. A cumulated index is published annually as the *Cumulated Index Medicus*. It is produced by the National Library of Medicine, Bethesda, Maryland, USA and is an essential source of reference for those wishing to search the biomedical literature. The *Index Medicus* dates from 1960, when it replaced the *Current List of Medical Literature*; the latter in turn had replaced the *Index-Catalogue of the Library of the Surgeon General's Office*, which was published from 1880 to 1950.

INDIAN HEMP, or *Cannabis sativa*, is the source of *cannabis (hashish, marijuana, pot, etc.). *C. indica* is a tropical variety.

INDIAN MEDICAL SERVICE, THE, (IMS) arose out of the activities of the East India Company, trading in India. The company came about under a charter granted to the Association of Merchant Adventurers in 1599 by Elizabeth I. By 1614 John *Woodall was appointed surgeon-general to the company, and his task was to provide competent surgeons and fit up their chests properly. These surgeons cared for those on board ships going out east, and also for those employed in India, especially in the trading stations set up there by the company. In 1764 the medical service had military and civil branches, as a navy and army were needed to protect the company's interests, especially from the French and Dutch. Hospitals were started and the medical officers practised in gaols and mental asylums, as well as supervising sanitation and public health. Early in the 19th century Acts were passed abolishing the monopoly of the company for trading in India and China. In 1857, after the Indian Mutiny, the British Government took over all activities of the East India Company. At first the medical services had three establishments in Bombay, Madras, and Bengal, which in 1897 were combined into the general IMS, still with military and civil divisions. The IMS has a long history of service in many fields, including medical education. In 1943 an Indian Army Medical Service took over the military branch. In 1947 the Dominions of India and Pakistan were founded and the days of the IMS run under British auspices were over.

INDIGESTION is an imprecise term embracing various symptoms which may be associated with food or eating, for example abdominal pain or discomfort, *heartburn, *flatulence, *nausea, *waterbrash, *vomiting, etc.

INDUCTION, meaning initiating or causing to occur, is used in various senses but especially with reference to general *anaesthesia, the onset of *labour, and the activity of *enzymes.

INDUCTOTHERMY. Heating the body, or part of it, by means of electrical induction.

INDURATION. Hardness; the process of becoming hard.

INDUSTRIAL HEALTH, MEDICINE, ETC. See OCCUPATIONAL MEDICINE.

INFANT FEEDING. Natural breast feeding has many advantages over artificial methods. They may be summarized as follows: it is easier; it is cheaper; it is safer (chiefly because of the great reduction in the risk of infection with enteropathogenic bacteria, but also because liability to other conditions is lessened, e.g. *kwashiorkor, iron-deficiency *anaemia, neonatal *tetany, *cot death, which is rare in breast-fed infants, infantile *eczema, cow-milk *allergy, *malabsorption, idiopathic *hypercalcaemia, and hyperosmolar ('*dehydration'); it is psychologically and emotionally beneficial to both mother and child; it is biochemically, nutritionally, and immunologically correct; and it provides some degree of physiological contraception for the mother, helping to ensure adequate family spacing. Contraindications to breast feeding exist, but are rare; in the infant, they are confined to severe physical malformation and certain *inborn errors of metabolism related to milk, such as *galactosaemia and alactasia. Social taboos militating against the maintenance of breast feeding for an adequate period (4–12 months in the Western world, often much longer in developing countries) are profoundly to be deplored.

INFANTICIDE is the killing of an infant, particularly the killing of a newborn infant by its mother, or the killing of newborn children as a societal practice, a primitive method of population control.

INFANTILISM is persistence of infantile characteristics into adult life, in particular failure to develop *secondary sex characteristics, sometimes accompanied by *dwarfism and *mental handicap.

INFANT LIFE PRESERVATION ACT 1929. This UK Act amended the law with regard to the destruction of children at or before birth. It provided that any person who by a wilful act intended to destroy the life of a child capable of being born alive or causes a child to die before it has an existence independent of its mother should be guilty of a felony (of child destruction), and should be liable on conviction to penal servitude for life. Evidence of 28 weeks' pregnancy or more was to be taken as proof that the child was capable of being born alive.

INFANT MORTALITY is measured by the number of deaths in the first year of life per 1000 live births.

INFANT WELFARE. See PAEDIATRICS.

INFARCTION is aseptic *necrosis which takes place in an area of tissue when the arterial blood supply to it becomes so little that cell life can no longer be sustained; it results from arterial *thrombosis, *embolism, or other obstructive disease occurring in the absence of available arterial supply from other (*collateral) vessels. The area of dead tissue is known as an infarct. An important example is *myocardial infarction in coronary arterial *atherosclerosis, the familiar and often fatal heart attack; another is cerebral infarction (a *stroke).

INFECTIONS. Conditions in which *micro-organisms invade and multiply in body tissues. See INFECTIOUS DISEASES; MICROBIOLOGY.

INFECTIOUS DISEASE HOSPITALS are special hospitals for the segregation, care, and management of patients suffering from communicable *infectious diseases. The need for such hospitals has largely been obviated by the development of *isolation units and *barrier nursing techniques in general hospitals, and by the greatly lessened hazard of many infectious diseases in an era of effective antibacterial therapy.

INFECTIOUS DISEASES

Definition

Infectious diseases are caused by living organisms. Most are referred to as *micro-organisms, as they can be visualized only with a microscope; the major groups of micro-organisms are the *viruses, *bacteria, and *fungi. There are three other groups, named *chlamydiae, *rickettsiae, and *mycoplasmas, which are intermediate between viruses and bacteria; they cause various infections, the commonest being pneumonia. Whereas bacteria, chlamydiae, rickettsiae, and mycoplasmas are unicellular organisms, viruses are not cells in the true sense—they rely upon the cells of their host (human or animal) for replication and propagation. Some infections are caused by larger multicellular organisms—the helminths or worms. The organisms causing infection range in size from tiny viruses, which can be seen only with the aid of an electron microscope, to worms which can be several centimetres long and therefore readily visible to the naked eye.

Terms synonymous with 'infectious diseases' include contagious diseases and communicable diseases. Not all infections are readily transmissible—some can originate within an individual's own body.

History

Infectious diseases are probably the oldest recognized diseases of man. Evidence of leprosy can be found on corpses from China and mummies from ancient Egypt dating from the 2nd century BC. *Plague, a bacterial infection transmitted by rat fleas, often referred to as 'The *Black Death', is frequently mentioned throughout history. Between 1348 and 1720 there were at least 10 plague *pandemics (see later) in Europe, which are claimed to have caused the deaths of approximately 25 million people. In the Great Plague of London in 1665 at least 70 000 were infected, many of whom died. *Smallpox, a lethal virus infection which has now been eradicated from the world, was described in India and China in pre-Christian times. The mummified head of the Pharaoh Rameses V, who died around 1160 BC, had lesions on the skin which were very similar to those left by smallpox. This infection has an additional place in history in that in the 18th century the English doctor Edward Jenner was the first to demonstrate that humans could be protected against infection by immunization. He inoculated a boy with fluid taken from lesions on the skin of a milkmaid infected with cowpox (a similar but much milder infection than smallpox). Jenner subsequently proved that the boy was immune to smallpox. This vaccine was eventually responsible for the total eradication of smallpox—the first time that a disease has been wiped out intentionally.

The invention of the microscope by Van *Leeuwenhoek in Holland in the 17th century allowed visualization of the larger bacteria for the first time. However, these were not identified and classified until two centuries later. The introduction of the electron microscope in the 20th century allowed the visualization of viruses.

Many factors influence national and international patterns of infectious diseases which are associated with war, malnutrition, and poverty. Hepatitis caused major problems for Allied troops during the North African campaign in the Second World War. In South-East Asia during the same war there were large outbreaks of *dysentery (a diarrhoeal disease) amongst both Japanese and Allied forces. It has been claimed that the availability of *sulphonamides (which cured dysentery) to the Allied forces but not to the Japanese prevented the invasion of Australia. Malnutrition and poverty go hand in hand with infection, leading to a decreased ability to withstand and overcome infection in association with a lack of preventative and treatment facilities.

During the 20th century there have been major changes in the pattern of infectious diseases in developed countries. The traditional contagions such as *diphtheria and *poliomyelitis have virtually disappeared from these countries, principally as a result of *immunization. Infections caused by bacteria have been controlled by antibiotics (see ANTI-INFECTIVE-AGENTS). While many infections have decreased, or even disappeared, in developed countries others have become more prominent. Examples include *food poisoning caused by *salmonellae, related mainly to the broiler-chicken industry, and infections in patients made particularly susceptible by modern medical and surgical techniques such as *cancer therapy and organ *transplantation. Travel by air has facilitated the importation into countries with temperate climates of infections such as *malaria normally encountered only in the tropics. The total number of travellers each year in the world is over 1 billion. Approximately 28 million people travel abroad from the UK each year, of whom nearly half a million visit Africa and a quarter of a million visit India. There were 50 000 cases of imported malaria diagnosed in Europe in 1991.

The ever-changing spectrum of infectious diseases is illustrated by the fact that whereas smallpox was eradicated from the world in 1978, several entirely new infections have been recognized in the past 20 years. These include food poisoning caused by a bacterium called Campylobacter, *legionnaire's disease, a type of pneumonia caused by another previously unknown bacterium, *Lyme disease, a bacterial (*spirochaetal) infection transmitted by a tick from deer to man, and the acquired immune deficiency syndrome (*AIDS) caused by the human immunodeficiency virus (HIV). Whereas the *legionella* bacillus usually originates in the environment (air-conditioning systems), *Campylobacter* is a common pathogen of animals. The best evidence available (not particularly strong) suggests that HIV is probably a variant of an animal (?monkey) virus. The interrelationship between man and animals in the context of infectious disease can be remarkably close. Infections contracted directly by man from animals are referred to as zoonoses; *anthrax, a serious skin infection contracted from infected cattle, and *rabies are examples.

Organisms causing infection

Table 1 gives details of the principal micro-organisms causing infection. These are bacteria, viruses, chlamydiae, rickettsiae, mycoplasmas, fungi, and *protozoa. The *helminths (or worms) include threadworms, roundworms, tapeworms, and worms causing certain tropical diseases such as *schistosomiasis. The size of organisms causing infection varies from 0.01 μm (viruses) to many centimetres (worms). Whereas viruses contain either DNA or RNA, the other micro-organisms incorporate both in their structure.

Source and transmission of infection

The source of an infectious disease can be another human, an insect, a bird or other animal, or, less commonly, an inanimate (non-living) source. Transmission of infection occurs by several routes. The most important of these are airborne spread, physical contact, inoculation (by needle or insect), or by food and drink. Certain infections e.g. German measles (*rubella) can be contracted through the placenta by the unborn *fetus from its mother.

Organisms enter the body either by inhalation into the lungs, ingestion (swallowing), or via direct contact (skin or mucous membranes). *Sexually transmitted diseases

Table 1 Micro-organisms

Type of microbe	Nucleic acids	Multiplication	Approx size (μm)	Visible by light microscope
Viruses (e.g. influenza, measles, HIV)	RNA or DNA	Virus induces host (human) cell to synthesize new viruses	0.01–0.3	No
Chlamydia (e.g. *C. trachomatis*, cause of trachoma which leads to blindness)	RNA + DNA	Multiply by binary fission	0.3	No
Rickettsiae (e.g. *R. prowazeki*, which causes typhus fever)	RNA + DNA	Multiply by binary fission	0.3	Sometimes just visible using special stains
Mycoplasmas (e.g. *M. pneumoniae*)	RNA + DNA	Multiply via elementary bodies	0.12–0.3	Sometimes just visible using special stains
Bacteria (e.g. *Salmonella*, *Legionella*)	RNA + DNA	Multiply by binary fission	0.5–0.8	Yes
Fungi (e.g. *Candida*)	RNA + DNA	Multiply by binary fission	Larger than bacteria (>5)	Yes
Protozoa (e.g. *Plasmodia*, causing malaria)	RNA + DNA	Depends on particular species	Larger than fungi	Yes

Table 2 Transmission of infection

By ingestion (food + drink)	By inhalation	By physical contact
food poisoning	measles, mumps, rubella	skin infection (e.g. impetigo)
Salmonella infection	influenza	sexually transmitted diseases
dysentery	*Legionella* infection	such as gonorrhoea, syphilis,
hepatitis A	meningococcal meningitis	and HIV infection
cholera	pneumonia	

By inoculation		From birds + other animals		Transplacental
				(mother to fetus)
By needle:	hepatitis B	Direct:	rabies (dogs)	rubella (German measles)
	HIV infection		psittacosis (birds)	toxoplasmosis
				Listeria infection
By insect:	malaria	Indirect:	worms (soil)	syphilis
	yellow fever		toxoplasmosis (cats'	HIV infection
			faeces in soil)	

are transmitted by contact between the mucous membranes of the genital tract. Table 2 illustrates the routes by which various infectious diseases are spread.

The incubation period of an infection is the time between a micro-organism entering the body and symptoms developing. This may vary from a few hours, as in certain types of food poisoning, to several years, as can occur in HIV infection.

The term '*epidemic' is used to denote a significant outbreak of infection in one area, while 'pandemic' is used to denote a particularly widespread outbreak, usually involving several countries or even continents.

Pathogenicity of micro-organisms
The term 'pathogenicity' refers to the mechanisms whereby micro-organisms cause infection. Certain organisms, such as the common *cold viruses, never penetrate below the surface of the mucous membrane (superficial lining) of the nose and throat, while others reach the deep tissues and bloodstream, causing potentially life-threatening *septicaemia (blood poisoning). Organisms may produce infection either on their own or with the aid of *toxins, substances which they themselves produce and which are released into the tissues and bloodstream. Examples of toxin-mediated diseases are provided by diphtheria and *tetanus, where the bacteria remain at the site of infection but their toxins circulate in the blood and cause serious effects on the heart and nervous system. The *cholera bacterium (*Vibrio cholerae*) causes its effects by producing a toxin which interferes with biochemical mechanisms in the lining of the bowel, leading to the release of large volumes of fluid and electrolytes, causing dehydration and, if untreated, often death.

Many organisms have a predilection for specific organs or tissues of the body. The *pneumococcus, as its name suggests, causes pneumonia, the *meningococcus causes *meningitis, and the *gonococcus, *gonorrhoea.

However, the pneumococcus can also cause meningitis and the other two organisms occasionally cause *arthritis.

Infection by one type of organism may reduce the body's defences to allow the invasion of another micro-organism. An example is the *influenza virus, which causes severe inflammation of the mucous membrane of the bronchi (tubes leading to the lungs) allowing *Staphylococcus aureus*, a bacterium which resides in the nose or throat in healthy people, to cause pneumonia.

The human body is divided into microbiologically 'clean' and 'dirty' areas. The 'dirty' areas are those that have contact with the outside world and include the skin and bowel. In health, almost all of the other organs and tissues in the body (e.g. heart, brain, muscles) are sterile (free from micro-organisms). Any breakdown in the body's defences against infection may allow organisms, usually bacteria, from the contaminated parts of the body to penetrate the clean areas. An example is provided by *peritonitis secondary to perforation of the large bowel.

Certain micro-organisms that are present in the body in health seldom cause infection. These are referred to as *commensal organisms as opposed to pathogenic organisms, which are the recognized causes of infection. Commensals such as *Staphylococcus epidermidis*, an organism present on the healthy skin, only cause infection when the body's defence systems are reduced by disease or treatment. A patient whose resistance to infection is significantly impaired is referred to as immunocompromised. An example is provided by a sufferer from *leukaemia who may have no normal white blood cells to combat infection, or a cancer patient who is being treated with *radiotherapy and/or cell-poisoning drugs which depress the immune system. AIDS patients are immunosuppressed because the human immunodeficiency virus (HIV) damages the immune system (see below).

The body's response to a micro-organism

The fact that a micro-organism has entered the human body does not necessarily mean that a disease process (infection) will result. The organism may be repelled on the surface of the body (skin or mucous membranes) by mechanical barriers or by natural chemical compounds. Should an organism overcome the superficial defences of the body and pass into the tissues, organs, or bloodstream, it is met there by a complex defence mechanism called the immune system (see IMMUNOLOGY). This has two major parts—the white blood cells (*polymorphs, *lymphocytes, and *macrophages) and various chemical components that interact with these blood cells. Whether or not an infection then results depends on the capacity of the body's defences to kill the organism.

Having entered the human body, a micro-organism may:

(1) be eliminated by the host defences without stimulating the immune system;

(2) be repelled by the defences (and at the same time causing a response by the immune system) without producing symptoms;

(3) cause an infection associated with signs and symptoms and, at the same time, stimulate the immune system.

The symptoms of an infection are not caused primarily by the micro-organism but by the reaction of the body's defence system. For example *fever, the commonest manifestation of an infectious disease, is produced by the release into the body of proteins known as *cytokines triggered by the infecting micro-organism. The intravenous injection of these substances can produce symptoms almost identical to those associated with influenza. Viruses stimulate host cells to produce *interferons, which have antiviral properties and can play a part in overcoming viral infections.

If the body's response to infection is exaggerated as a result of invasion by a particularly virulent organism (for example the meningococcus), an excessive and uncontrolled reaction may occur which can lead to bleeding, shock, and death. If the invading organism has stimulated the body's immune system, with or without symptoms developing, *immunity (resistance) to that micro-organism develops. This results from the organism leaving an 'imprint' on the memory of the immune system, enabling it to respond rapidly to any subsequent challenge by the same organism and thus preventing it from causing an infection. One of the mechanisms employed by the immune system to combat infection is the production of *antibodies against specific organisms. These are Y-shaped proteins produced by lymphocytes which bind to micro-organisms and either neutralize them or mark them out for destruction by cells of the immune system. While an immune response with antibody production occurs readily with organisms which invade the body, those that produce only surface infections, for example common cold viruses, do not stimulate lasting immunity. Other infections, such as influenza, may only stimulate immunity to one of the many subgroups of the organism and not to other members of the same group. This explains why an attack of influenza, unlike, for example measles which has only one strain of the virus and thus induces lifelong immunity to the infection, does not protect against future attacks by a different strain of the influenza virus. It also explains why the influenza vaccine recommended for one year may not protect against strains of the virus causing epidemics in future years.

Although most organisms are eradicated from the body once the infection has been overcome, in some instances the organism persists in the body for life. The *herpes simplex virus, which causes 'cold sores' around the mouth, and *Toxoplasma gondii* (*toxoplasmosis), a protozoal organism transmitted to man by healthy cats and by meat, are examples of 'persistent' organisms. Another is the varicella–zoster virus which causes *chickenpox in childhood and 'reactivates' in later life to produce shingles. *Immunosuppression, as in AIDS, may reactivate these 'persistent pathogens', which are common causes of death in patients suffering from AIDS.

Signs and symptoms of infection

Fever is the cardinal sign of infection. This is commonly associated with non-specific symptoms such as headache and aching in the muscles (myalgia). The signs and symptoms of specific infections vary according to the nature of the illness and the bodily system involved. Certain of the common infections of childhood, e.g. *measles, are associated with a rash, while food-poisoning organisms cause *diarrhoea. If the lungs are involved, the patient will have a cough and may be breathless. Meningitis produces severe headache and sometimes unconsciousness. Skin infection is associated with *abscess formation ('boils'); these contain *pus—a mixture of bacteria and dead white blood cells.

Treatment of infection

Infectious diseases can be treated by non-specific therapy and/or by specific therapy. Non-specific therapies include medications such as *aspirin given to relieve headache or reduce fever. Specific therapy depends on the use of antimicrobial agents. These have revolutionized the treatment of infectious diseases caused by bacteria. They have also had a significant effect on fungal and protozoal infections but, as yet, are relatively ineffective against viral diseases.

Antimicrobial therapy

At the beginning of the 20th century *Ehrlich, working in Germany, discovered a substance called Salvarsan®, a derivative of arsenic, which proved to have some efficacy in the treatment of bacterial infections, particularly *syphilis. However, it had unpleasant side-effects. At the time of his death in 1915 Ehrlich was searching for what he called a 'magic bullet', a substance that could destroy micro-organisms in the human body without causing harm to the cells of the body. His vision was rewarded when the *sulphonamides, developed from research into dyes, were discovered in the mid-1930s. These were followed by the first clinical use of *penicillin in 1941 and the subsequent discovery of many other *antibiotics. Antibiotics work either by killing micro-organisms or by inhibiting their growth by interfering with their basic constituents.

Although antibiotics have revolutionized the treatment of infectious diseases and saved many millions of lives, there are certain problems associated with their use. These are as follows.

1. Antibiotics are effective only against bacteria, fungi, and protozoa. There are relatively few antiviral agents, and those that are available, such as *acyclovir (used to treat shingles) or *zidovudine (also known as AZT or Retrovir®, used as a therapy for HIV infection), do not eradicate viruses from the body but only suppress the disease process. There are no antiviral drugs that are effective against common infections such as measles or a cold.

2. Many bacteria, and also some fungi and protozoa, which were previously sensitive to available antibiotics, have developed *resistance to them. Examples include staphylococci (which cause skin infections), *Escherichia coli* (the commonest cause of urinary-tract infections), and *Plasmodium falciparum* (the cause of the severe and potentially fatal form of malaria). The bacteria causing meningitis are, unfortunately, now developing resistance to penicillin. One of the most alarming aspects of bacterial resistance is the increase in resistance of the *tuberculosis bacterium (*Mycobacterium tuberculosis*) to antituberculous drugs, and there is an urgent need for new compounds to treat tuberculosis.

3. No antibiotics are totally free from side-effects, which can range from a mild rash to liver and kidney failure or, rarely, death from *anaphylaxis as with penicillin.

4. Antibiotics are expensive drugs which contribute to a major part of the drug bill in developed countries. In developing countries, because of their cost, many antibiotics are either not available or not freely available.

Prevention of infectious diseases

As with treatment, the prevention of infectious diseases can be considered under two headings: non-specific and specific.

Non-specific

Non-specific measures to prevent infection include food *hygiene, hand-washing, clean water supplies, and the provision of *isolation facilities. At one time individuals who had been in contact with a serious infection such as diphtheria or smallpox were isolated until the incubation time of the infection had expired. This procedure, known as *quarantine, is seldom used today.

Specific

Specific measures involve the use of *vaccines or, in certain infections, antimicrobial drugs. *Antiseptics and *disinfectants are also important in the prevention of infection.

There are several types of vaccine (Table 3). One type consists of bacteria or viruses which have been inactivated (killed), usually by a chemical process. Whooping cough (*pertussis) vaccine is an example. Another, exemplified by poliomyelitis vaccine, contains living micro-organisms, mainly viruses, whose virulence has been weakened to enable them to stimulate immunity without causing disease. A third form of vaccine, called a *toxoid, contains inactivated toxins, the chemical substances produced by bacteria such as diphtheria or tetanus. Vaccines mimic infections without causing disease and 'trick' the immune system into responding to them, thus producing immunity to the infection.

Table 3 Vaccines

Vaccines for childhood
  Measles
  Mumps
  Rubella
  Chickenpox*
  Diphtheria
  Tetanus
  Whooping cough
  Poliomyelitis
  Haemophilus influenzae type B
  BCG (tuberculosis)

Vaccines for travel
  Typhoid fever
  Hepatitis A
  Yellow fever
  (Cholera)†
  Rabies
  Japanese encephalitis

Other vaccines (for occupational or specific uses)
  Hepatitis B
  Pneumococcal
  Meningococcal‡
  Influenza
  Anthrax

* Not yet available in the UK.
† Not recommended as it is relatively ineffective.
‡ Not effective against the commonest strain (type B) of meningococcus in the UK.

Unlike the infectious diseases themselves, vaccines usually produce immunity of only limited duration, necessitating repeated doses (boosters). Those that contain inactivated organisms or toxins are generally very safe with few side-effects and can be given to all individuals. However, 'live' vaccines, although also generally safe, cannot be given during pregnancy as they may theoretically damage the fetus, or to the immunosuppressed, in whom they may cause clinical infection.

Vaccines take several weeks to provide protection against infectious diseases, as the immune system has to react and produce antibodies and other protective mechanisms. Immediate protection can be provided by the injection of pre-formed antibodies obtained from patients recovering from an infection (e.g. hepatitis B) or from pooled human blood donations (e.g. hepatitis A).

Antimicrobial drugs are employed in selected infections to prevent infection developing. The best-known example is the use of antimalarial drugs to prevent malaria in travellers to areas of the world where this infection occurs. Drugs used to prevent infections are called prophylactic agents.

Diagnosis of infection

Although some infectious diseases can be diagnosed by the clinician without recourse to ancillary aids, many require the use of a *microbiology laboratory for the identification of the infecting organism and the determination (if indicated) of its sensitivity to antimicrobial agents.

It may be possible for the microbiology laboratory to make an immediate diagnosis of the cause of an infection, by collecting a specimen such as *urine or *sputum and staining it with an appropriate dye (*Gram's stain is the commonest). The nature of the organism may be suggested in this way. However, in order to make a definitive diagnosis it is usually necessary for the specimen to be cultured in an incubator to allow the organism to grow; this can take 24 or even 48 hours. For tuberculosis it may be several weeks before the organism can be finally identified. Direct staining and culture are more appropriate for bacteria and fungi than for viruses or helminths. In many viral infections the diagnosis is made by examining the patient's blood for antibodies to the suspected micro-organism (e.g. HIV). These take a week or more to appear in the patient's blood. The diagnosis is therefore retrospective.

Various radiological techniques, e.g. chest X-rays or scans, may be helpful in confirming the diagnosis of infection. They are especially useful in localizing deep pockets of infection, such as abscesses.

Infection in developing countries

Most Third World countries are in the tropics or subtropics. In these countries infection is a most important cause of illness and death, especially in children. Of particular importance are the classic infectious diseases such as diphtheria and poliomyelitis, which have been eradicated from the developed world by the use of vaccines. The lack of clean water supplies in Third World countries results in the spread of many infections contracted from food and drink, such as hepatitis and dysentery. Tuberculosis is also a major cause of death in the Third World, where it is commonly associated with HIV infection and where resistance to antituberculous drugs is escalating.

It has been estimated that there are 15 million people in the world infected with HIV, of whom 3 million have developed AIDS and 1 million are children. The majority of the 15 million live in Third World countries.

Diseases peculiar to the tropics are found in Third World countries. These include malaria, *leprosy, and various worm infections, such as schistosomiasis (causing liver and bladder disease) and *filariasis (a cause of blindness). Malaria occurs in 100 countries and one-half of the population of the world is at risk of contracting it. There are 100 million cases diagnosed every year, of whom 1 million die. The burden of infection in these countries is exacerbated by *malnutrition, which leads to increased susceptibility to infection and a decreased ability to overcome it.

The future

As described above, the pattern of infection is ever-changing. It depends on a complex interaction between many factors involving humans, their animals, and the environment. On a world-wide basis AIDS is probably the biggest *public health hazard facing man at present. There is no reason to believe that other new infections will not appear in the future, probably caused by micro-organisms resistant to currently available antimicrobial agents. It has been suggested that if global warming becomes a reality then there may be a significant alteration in the balance of infection in different countries. For example, an increase in environmental temperatures in Europe might result in the migration northwards of insects, such as mosquitoes carrying malaria, at present resident only in tropical countries. In the UK we have already seen one effect of the recent drought when cattle invaded reservoirs with low water levels and contaminated them with a protozoal organism called *Cryptosporidium*, which then entered domestic water supplies.

Methods of animal rearing and food production are, at least in part, responsible for the increase in *Salmonella*, and possibly also *Listeria* infections. The use of sheep offal, including brains, to supplement cattle feeds has resulted in cattle contracting from sheep a transmissible agent known as a *prion (*pr* = protein; *i* = infectious) which has not yet been identified but is possibly a protein. This putative agent is thought to be the cause of a neurological disease in sheep called scrapie and, when acquired by cattle, produces *bovine spongiform encephalopathy (BSE), otherwise known as 'mad cow disease'. Other domestic animals, including goats and cats, have also contracted this infection and there is concern, although no evidence, that humans might acquire a similar disorder from eating beef, especially if contaminated with remnants of the cow's brain or spinal cord.

At the beginning of the 20th century, around 5 per cent of the population of the UK were aged 65 or over. By the end of the century this figure will have risen to over 20 per cent. As we control the classic childhood infectious diseases with vaccines, it is likely that infection will become a major problem in the geriatric age-group, particularly those who are crowded together in institutions, where outbreaks of *Salmonella* infection and influenza are common.

Modern medical and surgical practices, such as the treatment of cancer, organ transplantation, and the insertion of artificial heart valves and joints result in an increasing number of individuals who are especially at risk of infection, and these will increase significantly in the future.

In general, the laboratory confirmation of the diagnosis of infection is still relatively primitive, using methods introduced 100 years ago or more. This is likely to change in the near future with the introduction of new techniques, using immunological and molecular biological methods to provide rapid and early diagnosis of infection.

Penicillin was first introduced into clinical practice in 1941. Since then many new antibiotics have been introduced, but, possibly surprisingly, few are more active than penicillin, although penicillin's usefulness has decreased owing to increasing resistance of bacteria to it. There are pessimists who suggest that we will not discover any revolutionary new types of antibiotic, and there has certainly been a significant slowing down in the discovery of novel agents during the past 2 decades.

Attention is now being focused on finding new methods of treating infection, including the use of immunological agents, directed against specific parts of bacteria. An example is provided by a *monoclonal antibody which neutralizes the effect of the virulent toxin produced by the meningococcus. It is now possible to synthesize interferons in the laboratory and use them to treat certain viral infections, e.g. hepatitis B.

The pattern of infectious diseases will undoubtedly change as the result of the discovery and introduction of new vaccines. Major efforts are being mounted to find vaccines effective against HIV and malaria. Vaccine development is being revolutionized by *genetic engineering, which enables scientists to 'disable' pathogenic organisms, while retaining their ability to stimulate immunity to infection. There is, however, some concern that the protective effect of childhood vaccines might not last into middle and old age and, as a result, the childhood infections of today might become the geriatric infections of tomorrow.

                                                        A. M. GEDDES

INFECTIOUS DISEASES (NOTIFICATION) ACTS 1889, 1899. Shortly after the *Local Government Board was created in 1871, the forerunner of the present Department of Health, an effort was made to bring sanitary administration to all parts of the UK. One consequence was the introduction of compulsory notification of infectious diseases. The first to be made so notifiable was *cholera, under the *Public Health Act of 1875, after which notification was much more widely extended by the Notification of Diseases Acts of 1889 and 1899.

INFECTIOUS MONONUCLEOSIS, commonly called glandular fever, is an acute infectious disease primarily of young adults, causing fever, sore throat, generalized *lymphadenopathy, *splenomegaly, sometimes *hepatitis, atypical *lymphocytes in the blood, and producing high levels of sheep cell *agglutinins (known as heterophil *antibodies). Complications are uncommon but convalescence may be prolonged. The condition is due to the *Epstein–Barr virus, a member of the herpes group, which is also associated with *Burkitt's lymphoma.

INFECTIVE ENDOCARDITIS is a serious infection of the *endocardium overlying one or more of the heart *valves. Until the advent of *antibiotics the condition was invariably fatal within a few months. Formerly known as subacute bacterial endocarditis (SBE), it classically attacked valves already defective as a result of previous *rheumatic fever or *congenital heart disease, and the organism responsible was *Streptococcus viridans* in about 95 per cent of cases. More recently, the pattern has changed: a wider variety of microorganisms, including yeasts and moulds, is now encountered, and the formerly clear-cut distinction between acute and subacute forms of bacterial endocarditis is now less so. New categories of patient include the immunocompromised and intravenous drug abusers, many of whom do not seem to have pre-existing heart disease. Though classic SBE still occurs, the more general term 'infective endocarditis' is now preferred.

INFERTILITY is the condition of producing no or only few offspring.

INFESTATION is affliction by multicellular parasitic organisms, in many cases without invasion of skin or mucous membrane.

INFIBULATION is the practice of clamping or suturing the *labia majora or the *prepuce in order to prevent sexual intercourse.

INFILTRATION is the dissemination within a tissue or organ of another tissue, substance, or pathological change which is not normally present in it.

INFIRMARY. A hospital, or that part of a school, religious establishment, or other institution set aside as a sick-quarters. In the 18th century 'infirmary' was the common name for a public hospital, and in many provincial towns of the UK it is still retained. See HOSPITALS IN THE UK.

INFLAMMATION is the local tissue response to injury by *bacterial or other agents, consisting of dilatation of blood vessels, invasion of tissue by *leucocytes from the blood, and passage of fluid and proteins through capillary walls into the tissue. It is a protective mechanism (e.g. through leucocytes and *antibodies) against the invading micro-organisms, and attempts to confine them to the affected area. The cardinal clinical signs were described in the 1st century by *Celsus (as *rubor et tumor, cum calore et dolore* (redness, swelling, with heat and pain). To these *Virchow added a fifth, loss of function (*functio laesa*). The formation of *pus, or suppuration, is a later stage resulting from a concentration of leucocytes, bacteria, and their debris.

INFLUENZA is an acute viral illness occurring in sporadic epidemic and pandemic outbreaks. Pandemics, affecting many continents, have occurred at intervals varying from 8 to 18 years throughout the 20th century, and probably often before then. Epidemics occur annually in the winter months of temperate zones in many, but not usually the same, communities. Within a community, major cycles are usually of 2–4 years' duration. The clinical manifestations of influenza are familiar; it is characteristic that, despite the fact that the *epithelium of the respiratory tract is the site of primary infection, systemic symptoms, notably fever, *myalgia, and prostration, are out of proportion to those of local origin. Brief and self-limiting when uncomplicated, the disease can be deadly at the extremes of age and in those with pre-existing cardiorespiratory disorders because of secondary bacterial invasion of the lung (especially with *Streptococcus pneumoniae*, *Staphylococcus aureus*, and *Haemophilus influenzae*); the pandemic of 1918–19 is thought to have cost 15 million lives. Influenza is caused by three unrelated groups of orthomyxoviruses labelled A, B, and C; pandemics and major epidemics are due to group A. Within the group, however, there appears to be almost infinite *antigenic variation, probably as a result of genetic recombination, bedevilling both epidemiology and immunoprophylaxis. Vaccines of attenuated virus of an identified strain confer temporary immunity but are often of little value in a new epidemic.

INFRA-RED denotes that portion of the spectrum of electromagnetic radiation with wavelengths longer than those of visible light but shorter than those of radio waves, i.e. between about 0.8 and 1000 micrometres (10^{-6} m). Such radiation is sometimes called radiant heat or invisible heat radiation.

INFUSION. Intravenous administration of fluid other than blood, and by gravity rather than *injection.

INGELFINGER, FRANZ JOSEPH (1910–80). American physician and medical editor. He trained in gastroenterology at the University of Pennsylvania, and returned to Boston as chief of the section on the Boston University service at the Boston City Hospital. There, between 1942 and 1967 he trained a remarkably successful group of young physicians in this field, no fewer than 57 having worked under him. His special field of interest was in the pathology and physiology of the *oesophagus.

In 1967 Ingelfinger embarked on a new career—as editor of the *New England Journal of Medicine* (see MEDICAL JOURNALS). In the next decade its circulation rose from 100 000 to 170 000. He insisted on strict scientific review and evaluation of articles submitted for publication, but at the same time encouraged publication of amusing letters and recording of unusual medical syndromes. He promulgated what became known as 'the Ingelfinger rule', refusing to publish information that had been prereleased to the Press. This caused some resentment among science writers, but has generally been accepted and followed by other editors; also see MEDICINE AND THE MEDIA.

INGUINAL HERNIA is the commonest *hernia or rupture, in which the abdominal viscera protrude into the inguinal canal (the passage through which the *vas deferens, together with blood vessels and nerves, descends to the *testis).

INGUINAL LIGAMENT. The fibrous band marking the upper limit of the front of the thigh, formerly known as Poupart's ligament. It runs from the anterior superior spine of the iliac bone to the spine of the pubis.

INHALATION is a method of administering gases or drugs in gaseous, vapour, or aerosol form by drawing them into the lungs with inspired air. Inhalation is applicable to gaseous and volatile *anaesthetics, to volatile substances such as *amyl nitrite, and to drugs in aqueous solution which can be atomized into a finely dispersed mist (aerosol).

INHALER. Any device for administering substances in gaseous, vapour, or aerosol form by *inhalation.

INHERITANCE is the process of genetic transmission to offspring from parents. See GENETICS.

INHIBITION. The act of influencing in a negative direction, of diminishing, restraining, or extinguishing altogether an event, action, or process, as for example in relation to neuronal activity.

INJECTIONS, whereby a substance is introduced into part of the body under pressure, usually with a *syringe, can be made into almost any tissue or organ; thus they can be intradermal, subcutaneous, intramuscular, intravenous, intra-arterial, intraperitoneal, intrapleural, intra-articular, intrathecal, etc. the site varying with the purpose and nature of the injection. Injections are distinguished from *infusions by the fact that the latter are introduced under pressure of gravity alone.

INJURY. Harm, hurt, damage or impairment; trauma.

INNER EAR comprises the *cochlea, vestibule, and *semicircular canals, enclosed within the *temporal bone of the skull. The inner ear subserves the functions of hearing and balance. See OTORHINOLARYNG-OLOGY.

INOCULATION is the introduction into a living organism or culture medium of foreign material, particularly of a disease agent, *vaccine, *serum, or *microorganisms.

INQUEST. A judicial inquiry (in the medical context) into the cause of death, usually by a *coroner.

INSANITY is a social and legal term for madness, lunacy, or unsoundness of mind. The original complete form was 'insanity of mind', sanity being an archaic word for health. Definition of insanity usually turns on a person's lack of responsibility for his actions. The term has no precise medical connotation.

INSECTS AS VECTORS OF DISEASE. The class Insecta (six-legged arthropods with head, thorax, and abdomen, and usually but not invariably winged) contains more than a million species, but most of those of importance as disease vectors in man belong to three orders. These are: the Hemiptera (see BUG and LOUSE), the Diptera (see FLIES and MOSQUITOES), and the Siphonaptera (see FLEAS). Two other orders, the Hymenoptera (bees, wasps, ants) and the Coleoptera (beetles) have some medical significance for other reasons. Ticks, mites, spiders, and scorpions are not insects but *arachnids (eight walking legs). See also ARTHROPODS.

INSEMINATION is the introduction of semen into the female genital tract by natural or artificial means. See ARTIFICIAL INSEMINATION.

INSOMNIA is persistent inability to sleep. See SLEEP.

INSTINCT is, biologically, an innate, inherited, species-typical pattern of behaviour that is independent of reason, experience, and learning and which normally results in achievement of adaptive ends. True instinctive behaviour is impulsive. Colloquially the meaning is wider, and approximates to that of 'intuition', as in for example 'my instinct told me' and 'I instinctively felt'.

INSTITUTE OF MEDICAL LABORATORY SCIENCES, THE (more recently THE INSTITUTE OF BIOMEDICAL SCIENCE), was founded in the UK in 1975. Before that there were bodies concerned with maintaining standards in these sciences from 1912. In that year came the Pathological and Bacteriological Laboratory Assistants' Association, and by 1942 it had developed into the Institute of Medical Laboratory Technology. The increasing importance of laboratory sciences in medical practice, and their relative autonomy from the medical profession led to the formation of the IMLS. Following this the designation of non-medically qualified staff (formerly known as technicians) in the *National Health Service laboratories was changed to that of Medical Laboratory Scientific Officer (MLSO). The profession of medical laboratory science was then established. Its autonomy had been developing since the *Professions Supplementary to Medicine Act of 1960, which by 1963 empowered a Council to register those with sufficient qualifications in a variety of professions, including that of medical laboratory technology. Now the Fellowship of the Institute (FIMLS) gives an applicant admission to the state register. Such registration is required for employment as an MLSO in the NHS. The parallels with other professions are close and comparable organizations exist in many other countries (see, for example, PROFESSIONS ALLIED TO MEDICINE (USA)). The IMLS is essentially an educational body concerned with the maintenance of standards in the profession. It prescribes entry requirements, approves training experience in laboratories and courses in institutions, and sets examinations leading to fellowship and a diploma in medical laboratory management.

INSTITUTE OF NAVAL MEDICINE (INM) of the Royal Navy was founded in 1912 at Greenwich near London, was later moved to Clevedon in Somerset, and is now close to the main naval base at Portsmouth in Hampshire. It is concerned with the health and environment of all naval and Royal Marine personnel and to a lesser extent of naval dockyard workers, who are civilians. The INM pursues its aims through training and research. The environment of sailors in naval ships becomes more complex in submarines, with nuclear power, cramped living quarters, fire hazards, immersion, and extremes of heat and cold (see ENVIRONMENT AND MEDICINE I). It is the duty of the medical service and the INM to react to the problems posed by new technology, to foresee their potential effects, and counteract any potentially deleterious ones. See also DEFENCE MEDICAL SERVICES UK.

INSULA. A triangular area of *cerebral cortex lying in the lateral cerebral sulcus (fissure of Sylvius).

INSULIN, the major *hormone regulating *carbohydrate *metabolism, is secreted by the beta-cells of the pancreatic *islets of Langerhans, whence it was first isolated by *Banting and *Best in 1921. It is a *protein of low molecular weight, consisting of 51 *amino acids in two polypeptide chains. The principal action of insulin is to allow the tissue uptake, utilization, and storage of *glucose, with secondary actions on *fat and protein metabolism. Insulin deficiency leads to *diabetes mellitus.

Until recently all insulin for therapeutic purposes had been obtained by extraction from animal pancreatic glands. It is now possible to produce human insulin on a commercial scale by the techniques of *genetic engineering. The structure of insulin was elucidated by Frederick *Sanger of the Medical Research Council Laboratories in Cambridge, for which, in 1958, he received the first of his Nobel prizes in chemistry.

INSURANCE. See HEALTH-CARE SYSTEMS AND THEIR FINANCING; INSURANCE, LIFE AND OTHER FORMS, MEDICAL ASPECTS.

INSURANCE, LIFE AND OTHER FORMS, MEDICAL ASPECTS. From its earliest days in the latter half of the 18th century, life assurance has had a close association with medicine. Then, doctors were not directly involved in assessing the eligibility of lives to be assured, since this was generally done by the directors of the company who interviewed the applicant and judged his health from his appearance and health history. Although a doctor's advice was sometimes sought, it was not until the early 19th century that a formal medical examination was introduced by the Pennsylvania Company for the Insurance of Lives. A few years later a reference from the family doctor became an added requirement, and the evolution of life and health insurance medicine had begun.

The underwriting process
Proposals for life (or health) insurance have to undergo an underwriting process with the joint aims of identifying risks that are unacceptable and of ensuring that those risks which are acceptable are charged an appropriate premium for the cover. Among a group of applicants for insurance there will be average risks plus a smaller proportion of above- and below-average ones. It is the task of the underwriter, with the assistance of a consulting medical officer, to categorize the applications into risk groups and to calculate terms for abnormal risks. The applications for life assurance accepted on normal terms comprise three subgroups: truly average risks, i.e. those with an average life expectancy; a better-than-average group, presenting risk factors portending exceptional longevity; and a group of slightly under-average lives, whose adverse mortality experience will be balanced by the better mortality of the above-average lives. Of those remaining, applicants presenting a significant extra risk are charged special terms, whereas the small percentage of unacceptable

lives are invited to resubmit a proposal at a later date or are declined outright.

The evolution of life assurance medicine
At the beginning of life assurance the underwriting or 'selection' process was crude and not scientifically based. 'Substandard' lives (those presenting an increased risk) were likely to be declined, although some with minor health impairments were taken on at terms reflecting a cautious underwriting approach. Protein or glucose in the *urine, a personal or family history of *tuberculosis, or a history of *gout or *syphilis were judged to shorten life, and were sufficient reason to reject an applicant. Underweight was viewed with suspicion, and rotundity thought to indicate a strong, healthy constitution.

The first large mortality study, the *Specialized mortality investigation*, published in the USA in 1903, was the first step to better understanding of the influence of various medical conditions on mortality. Inspired by the findings of this study, Dr Oscar H. Rogers and Arthur Hunter of the New York Life Insurance Company developed a system of risk assessment in which debit and credit features were ascribed numerical values expressed as a percentage of normal *mortality for the age of the applicant. Thus was born the numerical system of rating which still forms the foundation of life assurance underwriting today. Since the *Specialized mortality investigation* many other insured-life studies have been carried out, almost all based on North American data; the sheer size of the life insurance market there means that data can be collected in sufficient volumes to derive meaningful results. No longer, however, are insurers able to rely totally on their own past experience for their rating basis. The spectrum of medical disorders is too wide and the rapid pace of developments in modern medicine means that underwriters cannot wait for long-term retrospective studies; they need to respond quickly to the changing prognosis in many medical conditions. Thus they have turned also to published reports of series of patients in clinical settings.

Better understanding of the effects of disease on mortality has led to a great widening of the bounds of insurability in terms of variety of impairments and severity of risk. The process began in the early part of the century. By the 1940s it was realized that *diabetes, the treatment of which had been revolutionized by the introduction of *insulin, was an insurable risk, provided the condition was well-controlled and complication-free. At around the same time, insurers became bolder in their willingness to take on lives with high blood pressure or a history of *coronary heart disease. That boldness continued, embracing such conditions as *cancer treated with apparent success, *stroke, chronic *kidney and *liver disorders, and progressive neurological diseases such as *multiple sclerosis. Nowadays the availability of life insurance is such that few medical conditions warrant outright declinature, although rapidly progressive illnesses, malignancies in their terminal phase, and other cases where average life expectancy is short or uncertain clearly have to be rejected.

Life assurance underwriting has had to change not only in the light of medical advances but also in pace with improvements in public health. No longer is there the emphasis on infectious diseases, and tuberculosis in particular. Although risk pricing is still based largely on the same risk factors, the underwriter is now concerned more with the long-term threats of circulatory disease and cancer, and increasingly with the various causes of death associated with *smoking, *alcohol, *drugs, and other facets of modern life style.

Most life insurance proposal forms ask for details of height and weight, personal medical history, family history (a significant predictor of longevity), and smoking and drinking habits. A comparatively recent innovation is a question concerning *AIDS and *HIV. For about two-thirds of applications, the information given in the proposal is sufficient for the company to offer insurance cover. For the remainder, where the applicant falls into an older age-group, the sum assured is substantial, or there is an actual or suspected health problem, further information is obtained in the form of a report from the regular family doctor and/or a medical examination. The examination covers build, blood pressure, pulse rate, and chemical analysis of the urine for glucose and protein, together with clinical examination of the circulatory, respiratory, digestive, nervous, and genito-urinary systems. Where necessary, the basic tools of the proposal form, *general practitioner's report and medical examination may be supplemented by *electro-cardiograms, *X-rays, microscopic urine analyses, a test for HIV antibodies, or various other tests and reports.

Health insurance

It is not only life assurance that has a strong reliance on medicine. Health insurance in various forms may be attached as additional cover to a life insurance policy or stand in its own right.

Permanent health insurance is a type of disability cover which replaces income lost as a result of the insured's inability to carry out his normal occupation. A regular income is paid until the insured returns to work, dies, or reaches normal retirement age, which-ever occurs soonest. The assessment of risks for per-manent health insurance involves considerations often quite different from those for life assurance. Very often medical conditions have serious implications for disabil-ity yet are associated with little or no extra mortality; examples are *osteoarthritis, lesions of the interver-tebral *discs, and psychoneurotic conditions.

Various occupational features influence the disability risk, such as the presence of health or accident hazards or stress, the occupation's position in the spectrum from sedentary to heavy manual, whether a high standard of overall fitness is required (such as for an airline pilot or professional sportsman), whether exceptional dexterity or excellent vision or hearing are needed, and not least the degree of job satisfaction—which in turn affects propensity to claim and motivation to return to work. Against this background the risk posed by a medical condition needs to be assessed. Its impact may be greatly different depending on whether the insured is, say, an architect, professional footballer, diver, pub-lican, or factory worker. Under-average applicants may be rejected, charged an extra premium, or have their cover restricted in some way, perhaps by means of an exclusion clause.

Permanent health insurance claims require detailed assessment to ensure that the claim is eligible within the terms of the policy and that disability is genuine. Claims in payment need to be monitored to ensure that disability is not unnecessarily prolonged. If need be, the insurer may take steps to help the insured back to work, perhaps part-time at first progressing to full-time. Most companies make use of 'counsellors'—nurses who are trained to advise claimants on their rights to state benefits and to help get the insured back to work as soon as possible, perhaps by identifying an opportunity for alternative or further treatment, or by a programme of *rehabilitation. Regrettably, given that fraudulent claims are not uncommon, part of their role is to check that the claim is indeed genuine.

A recent health insurance innovation is 'dread dis-ease' or 'critical illness' cover, in which a cash lump sum is paid to the insured if he or she is diagnosed as having one of a specified list of 'dread' diseases. Typically the list of insured conditions includes myocardial infarction (*coronary thrombosis), coronary artery bypass sur-gery, stroke, and cancer, but most policies also cover various other serious and disabling conditions. The rationale of the cover is that the policy proceeds can be used to replace lost income, pay for private medi-cal treatment, or help with the costs of coping with severe disability. Because dread disease cover pays on *diagnosis* (without the need to prove disability), it has presented a fresh challenge to underwriters who have to judge whether medical history, current health status, lifestyle, and occupation are likely to predispose to one of the medical conditions covered.

Another relatively new form of health cover is long-term care insurance which is designed to help pay the costs of long-term elderly care. Since this is a new con-cept, policies, premium rates, underwriting and claim handling practice have been devised from scratch, and since applicants are likely to be in older age groups, 55 upwards, and claimants will be mainly in their mid-70s or beyond, long-term care presents underwriters, claims assessors, and medical advisers with yet more new challenges.

The other important form of health insurance is private medical insurance which covers the cost of acute care in private medical facilities. In point of fact, little underwriting is done in respect of private medical insurance, the great majority of applications being accepted without thorough selection but with exclusion of pre-existing medical conditions which may later give rise to the need for in-patient treatment.

Towards the future
Of late the association between medicine and life and health insurance has altered significantly with the advent of new medical conditions (such as AIDS) and changes in the public's attitude towards and perceptions of medical issues.

Potentially, AIDS can have a significant financial impact on life and health insurers, who have had to modify their underwriting practice with new questions on application forms, HIV tests, and special questionnaires and ratings for high-risk individuals. In devising their new approach, insurers have worked closely with the medical profession, seeking expert opinion and collecting statistics from a variety of sources.

There has also been public concern over insurers' reaction to AIDS, and no doubt other issues involving medical *ethics will arise in the future needing effective, yet sensitive handling. The consulting medical officer is no longer merely an adviser on underwriting and claim matters and an occasional examiner of new applicants; this post now has a wider role in shaping the insurer's approach to medical issues which impinge to any extent on life and health insurance, be they as a result of medical advances, changes in the pattern and incidence of disease, new legislation, or consumer influence.

R. D. C. BRACKENRIDGE
PETER MAYNARD

Further reading
Brackenridge, R. D. C. and Elder, W. J. (ed.) (1992). *Medical selection of life risks* (3rd edn). Macmillan, London.
Lew, E. A. and Gajewski, J. (ed.) (1990). *Medical risks: trends in mortality by age and time elapsed*. Praeger, New York.
Singer, R. B. and Levinson, L. (ed.) (1976). *Medical risks: patterns of mortality and survival*. Lexington Books, Mass.
Society of Actuaries/Association of Life Insurance Medical Directors of America (1980). *Blood Pressure Study 1979*. SA/ALIMDA, New York.
Society of Actuaries/Association of Life Insurance Medical Directors of America (1980). *Build Study 1979*. SA/ALIMDA, New York.

INTEGUMENT. *Skin.

INTELLECT. The mind, in reference to its cognitive and rational powers, and particularly to the higher thought processes.

INTELLIGENCE. Intellectual capacity, skill, or ability; the ability to comprehend relationships, understand, and reason. In its lowest form, intelligence is said to be present when an animal is aware, however dimly, of the relevance of its behaviour to an objective. Animal psychologists assess intelligence by the capacity to meet new situations with new adaptive responses and the ability to perform tasks which involve comprehension of relationships, the level of intelligence being proportional to the complexity, or abstractness, or both, of the relationships. Human intelligence is expressed quantitatively by the *intelligence quotient.

INTENSIVE CARE
Introduction
Intensive care, also known as intensive therapy, is the name given to that branch of medicine concerned with the treatment of patients who need, and can benefit from, more specialized attention than is available in the standard medical, surgical, or paediatric ward. These include patients who have undergone major surgery or have sustained bodily injuries (major *trauma) such as those following road-traffic or other accidents. Other patients who may be admitted to the intensive care unit (ICU) are those with life-threatening disease or disturbance of a major bodily system, such as the respiratory system, the heart and circulation, the kidneys, the liver, or the nervous system, or those suffering from accidental or deliberate self-poisoning.

The postoperative recovery room is an important subdivision of intensive care, which is intended for the observation of patients who have undergone surgical procedures under general *anaesthesia. They stay in the recovery room until they have regained consciousness and control of their protective reflexes and are no longer at risk from the effects of anaesthesia or surgery.

The intensive care unit has evolved in response to a number of demands. Medical and surgical treatment are now offered to patients who only a few years ago would have been considered to be beyond the reach of medical aid. This has been made possible by an increased understanding of the *pathophysiology of life-threatening conditions and the means of combating them. These developments have created a need for therapeutic and monitoring techniques which can be used only by specially skilled and experienced staff.

All of the patients admitted to the ICU have one feature in common, which is that their presenting condition is considered to be potentially reversible, provided that life can be sustained until the natural process of healing can take place or the toxic agent which is responsible for the illness can be eliminated.

ICU treatment methods
The treatment that patients receive in the intensive care unit is based upon standard medical and surgical methods, but includes the extensive use of equipment for monitoring (measuring and recording) and therapy (treatment). Continuous recording of the heart activity (*electrocardiography, ECG), respiratory function testing, and the recording of urine output are routinely practised. Other techniques may include intravenous, intra-arterial, intracardiac, and intrapulmonary flow and pressure measurements.

The commonest therapeutic device used is the lung *ventilator, since controlled ventilation (mechanically applied artificial ventilation) is important in the treatment of many life-threatening conditions. Interference with respiratory function caused by diseases, by drugs, surgical operations, or other traumatic processes is very common; patients suffering from major cardio-circulatory disturbances such as haemorrhagic, cardiogenic, or septicaemic *shock may also benefit from controlled ventilation.

Many intensive care units are equipped for other forms of sophisticated technical treatment. These include haemo- and peritoneal *dialysis, which may be used to treat patients who are in renal failure, or to hasten the elimination of poisons taken deliberately or accidentally. Haemofiltration and *plasmapheresis may also be employed.

The ICU creates the need for support services, which include the round-the-clock provision of laboratory and radiological investigations. Most patients in the ICU require several laboratory investigations daily, frequently at very short notice. The most essential biochemical investigations can be performed in the ICU itself; these include blood gas analysis, blood sugar (glucose), and the measurement of sodium, potassium, and other *ions in plasma and urine.

Infections are encountered frequently in the ICU and *cross-infection is a constant, although usually preventable, hazard; support of the *microbiology laboratory is essential. A portable radiographic apparatus and film-processing facilities are usually provided, and image intensification is an invaluable aid to the placing of intravascular catheters.

ICU staffing structure
The most important feature of the ICU is the number, skill, and motivation of its *nursing and medical staff. Each ICU patient requires individual nursing care throughout every 24-hour period. This requirement can be met by the allocation of six trained nurses per bed, to provide cover for day and night duty, which means that the ICU with eight beds requires an establishment of 48 trained nurses, together with domestic, administrative, and technical support.

The medical staffing structure must take account of two aspects: the provision of continuous skilled medical care for the patients, and of training experience for junior doctors. Medical and nursing students must spend an appreciable period in the ICU, and all doctors who intend to specialize in acute medicine, surgery, or anaesthesia should be enabled to spend part of their rotational training in the unit.

In most Western countries, including the UK, the responsibility for the clinical and administrative supervision of ICUs is taken by a fully trained (*consultant in the UK) *anaesthetist. The UK postgraduate examination in anaesthesia (the FRCA) contains sections devoted to instrumentation, clinical measurement, and other aspects of intensive care. Most ICU anaesthetists have gained additional postgraduate experience in cardiovascular, respiratory, and renal medicine, and many are in possession of the MRCP diploma in addition to the FRCA.

In some parts of the USA, Australasia, and Europe, a separate specialty known as 'intensivism' or 'reanimation' has evolved. In the UK there is now a recognized higher professional training programme for doctors who wish to specialize in intensive care, as part of another specialty, usually, although not always, anaesthesia.

ICU design requirements
In the UK it is usually recommended that every general hospital which has more than 400 beds should have one ICU bed for every 100 acute beds, and units of from four to eight beds are the rule. In parts of the USA and Europe, much larger units or several separate units are seen.

It is recommended that each ICU bed area should be not less than approximately 18.5 m^2 (200 sq. ft), which is more than twice the standard ward allocation. In many units, each patient has a separate room. In addition, some special facilities should be provided: these include barrier nursing cubicles to reduce the risk of cross-infection from patients who represent a special hazard, such as those suffering from infective *hepatitis, or grossly infected *burns. Other patients, such as the immunosuppressed (for example, patients suffering from *AIDS or receiving *chemotherapy) who are in danger of cross-infection, may be barrier nursed for their own protection. Air conditioning or efficient plenum ventilation are essential throughout the unit.

The facilities needed at each bed position include piped gases (oxygen, compressed air, etc.) and piped suction; many electrical outlets are needed and *computers are being used increasingly for data storage.

A very large storage area is required, and dirty and clean utility rooms for the cleaning and restocking of equipment are essential. Most ICUs have a small laboratory, office accommodation, and an overnight-stay room for the resident. A staff rest room and a seminar room for teaching purposes are also required. A visitors' room and an interview room must be provided. Finally, the whole department must be designed so that it and its contents can be cleaned easily.

Cost of intensive care
Intensive care is very expensive in staff, space, equipment, and services. The daily cost is of the order of four times that of an equivalent period in an acute medical or surgical ward. This is largely attributable to the salaries of the additional personnel, but also includes the cost of the building, its facilities, and services. A sophisticated ventilator costs approximately £15 000 (US $22 000), and routine monitoring equipment may cost up to £10 000 (US $15 000) per bed.

Drugs and intravenous fluids, including blood products and parenteral feeding materials, also contribute significantly to the cost. Expenditure of this magnitude can be justified only in societies where the general level of medical services is high.

It is now apparent that even the most advanced countries cannot afford the luxury of providing every possible facility in every hospital. The logical development will probably be towards the provision of regional ICUs or of units which serve groups of hospitals. Even very sick patients can be transported safely by properly equipped *ambulance, by sea, or by air, provided that they are fully assessed and their projected needs anticipated before they begin their journey, and are accompanied by a competent medical attendant, usually an anaesthetist.

Potential hazards for the patient

These include those of physical and emotional stress and the risk of overtreatment. The ICU can appear to be a strange and, at worst, hostile environment, although the staff always try to minimize this impression. More obviously, treatment may be physically dangerous; powerful drugs may have powerful side-effects; the use of equipment for life support carries with it a potential for disaster. These complications are uncommon, but the staff must be trained to be aware of their possible occurrence, and of methods to combat them.

The risks of overtreatment

In the ICU, overtreatment means the continued application of supportive measures when all direct and indirect evidence indicates that the patient is going to die, and that this event can be only briefly postponed, at some cost to the patient, his relatives, and the exchequer. With modern techniques and drugs, it is possible to sustain the external manifestations of life (heart beat, peripheral circulation, urine output, respiratory gas exchange) for long periods. Furthermore, it is always much easier to start treatment than to stop it.

These were difficult problems in the early days of the ICU, but enough experience has accumulated to make admission criteria more reliable and to enable medical attendants to recognize when no further benefit can be gained by persisting with treatment.

Most patients who are admitted to the ICU either respond to treatment within a relatively short time or deteriorate rapidly, and their prognosis can be clearly determined. A small number who have multiple systems failure (failure of two or more systems such as the cardiocirculatory system and the respiratory system) may require prolonged treatment and the outcome is uncertain. However, one of the principles of intensive care is that treatment must cause the patient as little distress as possible; this objective is gained by the judicious use of sedative and analgesic drugs.

Staff problems

It has been suggested that the nursing staff of the ICU are at risk of emotional stress because of the close contact they have with their patients and the unavoidably high mortality rate (15–20 per cent) of patients in the unit. However, provided that the staff who work in the ICU are self-selected and properly trained, they soon realize that only by their skills and care can the mortality rate be kept as low as it is. The morale of the unit is sustained by good leadership, organization, in-service training, and a friendly atmosphere.

Lessons from intensive care

Intensive care units are a relatively recent development, but some conclusions can be drawn from the experience now available. In the first place, in the ICU it is possible to maintain life in patients with reversible conditions which would otherwise have been fatal. Example of these include multiple injury, *polyneuritis, accidental or deliberate self-*poisoning, respiratory failure, and *tetanus. There is also evidence that admission to the ICU can shorten the duration of hospital stay and reduce the morbidity and complication rate of many non-fatal conditions, particularly major surgical procedures.

At the other end of the spectrum, it is also possible to distinguish those patients who cannot be helped and, accordingly, to avoid prolonging suffering for the patient and family. By concentrating skills and patients in one area of the hospital, the complications of treatment and their prevention are clearly noticed, as are some of the less obvious problems created by intensive care.

J. C. STODDART

Further reading
Berk, J. L. and Salpiner, J. E. (ed.) (1990). *Handbook of critical care* (3rd edn). Little, Brown and Company, Boston.
Stoddart, J. C. (1975). *Intensive therapy*. Blackwell, Oxford.

INTERFERON. A class of proteins possessing antiviral and antitumour activity produced by *lymphocytes, *fibroblasts, and other tissues. They are released by cells invaded by *virus and are able to inhibit virus multiplication in non-infected cells. Although interferon was discovered by Isaacs and Lindemann in 1957, only recently have sufficiently large quantities become available for intensive study and clinical trial. Interferon preparations have been shown to have some clinical effect as antiviral agents, for example in the common cold and in some *herpes infections, and may ultimately find an established place in treatment. Recent evidence also suggests a role in treating *multiple sclerosis. The preparations so far available have produced side-effects, such as fever, lassitude, and prostration, not dissimilar from those accompanying acute virus infection itself. Interferon is also proving effective in the treatment of various forms of malignant disease, especially hairy-cell *leukaemia; the antitumour effect results from enhancement of cell-mediated immune processes, notably by stimulating the activity of 'killer' lymphocytes.

INTERMITTENT CLAUDICATION is the classic symptom of obstructive arterial disease of the legs. Although claudication literally means limping, intermittent claudication describes a typical cramp-like pain in the calf muscles which seizes the patient after he has walked a certain distance; for any particular patient the distance is often remarkably constant. He is obliged to halt, and resting promptly relieves the pain. The similarity to the pain of *angina pectoris is obvious, and the mechanism—muscle *ischaemia—is the same; an older term for the condition is angina cruris. Most patients with the symptom are suffering from *atherosclerotic disease of the aorto-iliac and femoral arteries; occasionally they suffer from other pathological processes such as *thromboangiitis obliterans. Tobacco-smoking is an important aetiological factor. Like angina pectoris, intermittent claudication rarely results from severe *anaemia without arterial obstruction.

INTERN is the US designation for a medical graduate fulfilling an initial resident appointment in a hospital prior to being licensed to practise medicine independently. The UK equivalent is the house physician or house surgeon (see HOUSE OFFICER) in a pre-registration appointment.

INTERNAL MEDICINE IN THE UK. The phrase 'internal medicine' has never enjoyed widespread usage in the UK; neither is there an alternative descriptive term readily available. In a tradition sanctified by usage, reference is sometimes made to the component parts rather than the overall category. Thus, doctors may be trained in 'general medicine', or one of its subspecialties such as *cardiology, *neurology, *gastroenterology, *paediatrics, or *dermatology. The paradoxical inclusion of the last subspecialty perhaps explains the failure of the term 'internal medicine' to gain widespread acceptance as an adequate categorical description. Like many British institutions, internal medicine has substantially changed its character over the centuries. Lines of demarcation which were originally clear have been lost with the evolution of medical practice: attempts to redraw them inevitably seem arbitrary. Even when such fine distinctions have been made, there are important differences in the range of activities embraced by the term, directly attributable to the features of medical practice in different countries.

The difference in implication of words is evident in the role of the physician. In the UK the practitioner of internal medicine is a physician, i.e. a hospital-based doctor who has undergone an extensive educational programme. Thus, a *general practitioner would not be described as a physician. Elsewhere (e.g. the USA) the word has a much broader meaning. The present discipline of internal medicine therefore reflects the changing status and role of the physician. The initial remit with the founding of the Royal College of Physicians in 1518 emphasized one feature of the physician's work which

has been a source of pride and contention to the present day—the wide understanding of disease by men 'liberally educated', which would animate them in pursuing their enquiries into the nature of diseases and methods of cure for the benefit of mankind (John Freind, quoted by Webster 1977). The distinction between the holistic approach of the physician and that of more narrowly based practitioners of certain technical skills, such as the surgeon or the obstetrician, has been eroded in two ways. One of these, the growth of specialization, has been universally experienced. The other, the development of *general practice (family medicine) is unique to the UK. Both have had a profound effect upon the boundaries of internal medicine.

The explosive growth of physiological and biochemical knowledge which began in the 19th century led physicians to develop special interests. At an institutional level this was recognized by the creation of special hospitals such as the National Heart Hospital (1857), and the National Hospital for Nervous Diseases (1860), when London was the unchallenged centre for medical excellence and a London teaching hospital physician's post was the ultimate ambition of the newly qualified doctor. The status of such posts was nevertheless closely bound up with their general non-specialist nature. This was not simply a historical relic, although tradition undoubtedly played a role. A wide knowledge of disease in all its manifestations, an active interest in science, and final responsibility for overall patient management all contributed to the esteem in which the physician was held. Thus, *neurologists responsible for beds at the National Hospital for Nervous Diseases, or *cardiologists with sessions at the National Heart Hospital would also hold sessions as general physicians at undergraduate teaching hospitals. As long as the growth of science did not have too great an impact upon medical practice this arrangement continued. In the past few decades, however, technology has forced ever greater specialization upon the hospital physician. The pre-eminent status of the generalist has therefore been progressively eroded—not without expressions of dismay and grief in the conservative climate of British medicine. The expression of pride with which such a dominant 19th century figure as Gull could take the 'general view' is still heard in British hospitals, although with decreasing frequency. The *raison d'être* for general medicine has subtly changed, and now it largely exists as the receiving house for acute emergencies which do not obviously require care by one of the subspecialties such as the *nephrologist or the paediatrician. Common conditions which present as emergencies, such as *stroke, drug overdoses, or chest infections, are also commonly cared for by the general physician rather than the relevant specialist, largely for the pragmatic reason that there are insufficient specialist staff or beds to cope with these diseases. All this is a far cry from the dominant status in the British hospital hierarchy held by general physicians until recent years.

I have referred to the general physician as though he/she enjoyed a distinct identity. This is no longer the case. Over the past decade or two it has been reluctantly recognized that general (internal) medical practice has to be associated with practice in one (and sometimes two) subspecialties. Thus the general physician with a special interest in cardiology, thoracic medicine, or gastroenterology has been created. Initially the physician was left to develop special interests reflecting his own predilections and local needs. Now consultant posts advertised in the UK invariably specify a special interest, although general medicine may also be included. Some specialties, such as paediatrics, dermatology, and neurology, no longer have any general medical component in their work. Others, such as cardiology, have had a slightly uneasy relationship at one stage, eliminating general medicine from some *consultant training programmes, but more recently reversing these guidelines. Meanwhile, the training handbook of the Joint Committee on Higher Medical Training (JCHMT) in 1980 listed 17 specialties of adult medicine; in 1982, 24; in 1989 no fewer than 29 disciplines, such as *palliative medicine and *intensive care, were recognized.

The other major influence upon the practice of general medicine and its subspecialties has been the development of general practice. Patients cannot directly seek a medical opinion from a hospital-based specialist in the UK. They have first to be referred by a general practitioner. Direct access to a specialist only occurs when a patient is admitted to hospital as an acute emergency. By reducing inappropriate referrals this arrangement has contributed to the relative cost-efficiency of the British *National Health Service so that a comparatively small proportion of the gross national product has been spent upon maintaining, in most cases, a reasonable standard of medical care. This is reflected in the relative paucity of specialists in most fields of internal medicine for a population the size of that of the UK. It should be emphasized, however, that this is not the sole explanation of the small number of medical specialists. There is also a genuine shortfall in most disciplines when measured against need, as assessed by morbidity and mortality. This deficiency in consultant staffing levels historically showed an impressive consistency with other measures of medical deprivation, in the form of a geographical concentration of staff and resources in London and the south compared with other parts of the country. This has been partly corrected over the past two decades although the imbalance of hospital-based medical staff in central London teaching hospitals in relation to the patient population they serve is presenting increasing problems with the working of the internal market following the Health Service Reforms.

The development of *geriatrics as a subspecialty has also had a major impact upon the practice of internal medicine. The diversion of many younger patients into specialty care left the general physician with a high population of elderly patients to manage. These patients frequently presented serious problems in rehabilitation and social care. The growth in numbers of the very old in both the British and other Western populations has compounded this problem. The specialty of geriatrics was developed as a subspecialty of medicine in response to this need. The relationship between the general physician, most of whose beds are occupied by the elderly, and the geriatrician, whose expertise and training were directed at this group, inevitably proved fraught in many hospitals. The obvious decline in the status of general medicine (as opposed to its subspecialties) aggravated these problems. Was the brief of the geriatrician to treat all patients (including the acutely ill) above a certain age, or did his expertise lie specifically in the disabilities and problems of old age? On the one hand, the fact that geriatricians have been trained in general medicine, and, on the other, the policy of segregating geriatric beds in separate wards (or indeed separate hospitals) with lower levels of nursing and medical staffing, created at the best tension and at the worst a two-tier system in which a development intended to help the elderly provided them with inferior care. This problem is slowly being resolved. A new generation of physicians more intensively involved in their specialty work sees no threat in highly qualified geriatricians treating the acutely ill elderly patient. The *Royal Colleges of Physicians have recommended the integration of geriatric and general medicine, which is somewhat slowly taking place. In many hospitals geriatricians and their colleagues with an additional specialty interest share in the care of emergency admissions. It is a logical development which should have happened more rapidly and earlier. The same could be said of correction of the geographical inequalities of hospital staffing in the UK. In this, as in so many other fields of British medicine, questions of status and intensive, almost reflex, conservatism have retarded the rate of change.

The training of the specialist in general and internal medicine and its subspecialties is now regulated by the JCHMT and its subcommittees. Three years are spent in general professional training and a further 4 years in higher specialist training (which includes 1 or 2 years in general medicine where appropriate to the specialty). These are minimal periods. Often the specialist will spend several years longer and include a period of 2 years or so pursuing a research project in order to obtain an MD degree (a higher, and not a primary, medical qualification in the UK). Unlike some other disciplines, the physicians have been against an examination at the end of this lengthy period of training. There are two persuasive reasons for this. First, it is difficult to envisage realistic career options for those who failed such an examination after a prolonged period of specialty training. Any examination, it is felt, would lack teeth. Secondly, the existence of a major examination in other specialties has tended to dominate the interest of the candidate and has prevented more valuable educational activities, such as the pursuit of a significant research project.

One unsatisfactory feature of training of the 'junior doctor' (who may be in his late 30s) is the relative short-term nature of the posts in which he undergoes training. After his or her *preregistration year as a *house officer, the doctor who wishes to pursue a career as a physician will need to obtain at least three, and perhaps several more, posts against intense competition in some cases as he or she moves from being a *senior house officer to being a *registrar and then a *senior registrar. He or she may have to abandon a career intention if no appropriate post becomes available at the right time, or alternatively may have to spend a considerable period without secure employment waiting for the right job to appear. This leaves junior staff in a vulnerable and uncertain position. The Royal College of Physicians of London is currently introducing a training programme in which registrar and senior registrar posts are integrated. This should alleviate a significant deterrent to pursuing a career in hospital medicine. Here again, however, the wheels of progress have moved extremely slowly. Despite these difficulties, internal medicine and its specialties continue to attract some of the most talented newly qualified doctors. Although the need for change has not always been recognized rapidly and the response to such a need has usually been grudging, the ability to recruit such staff is a powerful testimony to the worthwhile nature of the work.

J. D. SWALES

Further reading
Clark, G. (1964). *History of the Royal College of Physicians of London*, Vol. 1. Clarendon Press, Oxford.
Joint Committee on Higher Medical Training (1989). *Training Handbook 1988/1989*. Royal College of Physicians, London.

INTERNAL MEDICINE IN THE USA
History
The discipline of internal medicine in America is historically linked to the separation of medicine and surgery in the UK and in Germany in the late 19th century. Its early history was characterized by contradictions and ambiguities, questioning whether it should be a generalist specialty or a *consultant specialty. This ambiguity has continued into the late 20th century and is in contrast to the clarity of internal medicine's image in the UK, where the distinction between the family physician generalist and the hospital-based internist consultant has been evident at least since 1914. The *Royal Colleges of Physicians have played, and continue to play, a dominant role in most aspects of internal medicine in the UK but their counterpart organization, the American College of Physicians, has not had a comparably dominant role in the USA. Instead, internal medicine in the USA has been most heavily influenced by the leadership of academic medicine, typically leaders of the

full-time faculties of schools of medicine in research universities.

Full-time academic medicine had become well established in the USA by 1920. Major reforms in medical education began following a report by Abraham *Flexner in 1910. Significant among Flexner's suggested reforms was the need to strengthen the contribution of science to the education of physicians. The resultant linkage of science to medical education occurred at a time when the leadership for internal medicine came from within the academic community. The conjunction of these two historical settings fostered an intimate association between the biomedical sciences and the discipline of internal medicine, an association which persists today.

The major historical influences on the organization of internal medicine in the USA have included the First World War, during which the distinction between an internist and a *general practitioner was defined; the establishment of the Association of American Physicians in 1885; the establishment of the American College of Physicians in 1915; the establishment of the American Board of Internal Medicine in 1936; and, most importantly, the decision by the US government following the Second World War to allow the *National Institutes of Health (NIH) to fund biomedical research in the American universities.

Forces leading to fragmentation
The profound influence of the scientific advances resulting from the large-scale NIH investment in American schools of medicine cannot be overstated. Biomedical sciences grew in breadth and depth, and new disciplines emerged from the old. Scientists soon found it necessary to restrict their research to special areas, and this, in turn, fostered the trend toward specialization in science. With internal medicine so heavily dependent upon science, it followed that the discipline moved in parallel to these trends and that the concept of internal medicine as a 'generalist' field became seriously eroded. Three subspecialty boards were established in 1941. Between 1970 and 1971 the American Board of Internal Medicine increased the number of subspecialty boards to nine thereby rapidly accelerating the trend toward subspecialization in internal medicine.

Another force added to the fragmentation of internal medicine into subspecialty units. This was the advent of new technologies, technologies which have allowed internists to perform procedures heretofore considered to be in the domain of the surgeons. These technologies include as examples the fibre-optic *endoscope and *bronchoscope, and *cardiac catheterization. Furthermore, internists found the compensation for the performance of procedures to be more lucrative than the compensation for the provision of consultative services. The development of certain subspecialties was fostered by these financial incentives, but not all benefited. Thus, some of medicine's subspecialties became financially better off, while others lagged. This situation created further trends toward fragmentation based upon economic reward.

As a result of these and other incentives, most trainees in internal medicine have entered subspecialty training. The declining interest in generalism was to have an effect upon the adequacy of numbers of physicians in the USA who practise as generalists.

Declining interest

As stated above, most individuals who choose to train in internal medicine complete 3 years of general training and then elect to pursue additional training in a subspecialty. Approximately two-thirds of all trainees select this course. The number of American medical school graduates selecting internal medicine as a career has declined between 1986 and 1993. This downward trend is reflective of a broader decrease in American medical students' interest in careers in the principal generalist disciplines (*family medicine, internal medicine, and *paediatrics). The recognition of a decreasing interest of medical students in generalist careers at a time when the nation perceives a need for more *primary-care doctors has aroused a sense of concern among many US health policy and government leaders, whose concerns focus particularly on the balance between the number of generalists and the number of subspecialists in internal medicine. Therefore, the leadership of internal medicine is faced with a two-part problem, too many subspecialists among practising internists, and too few American students interested in studying the discipline at all.

Causes of the problem

Most likely, the underlying cause of the trend away from generalism and towards specialization is the higher prestige and reward accorded to the specialists. Interestingly, this differs from a now historical era of medicine when the opposite was true. The enhanced prestige has been accompanied by a differential payment for services rendered, particularly for specialists who perform surgical procedures. Also, in a nation without controls on its resident training positions and even without a national manpower policy, the number of training positions in US specialties has grown in relationship to the need for hospital manpower to care for the patients of the trainers. This open system of training has not, therefore, constrained the young physicians in training from abandoning the generalist fields.

The development of new technologies has also influenced the attractiveness of many specialties to medical students. New imaging technologies have made *radiology attractive to students, who are understandably excited by the diagnostic and therapeutic potential of this evolving field. The availability of new prosthetic devices has enabled *orthopaedics to contribute substantially to the restoration of function in previously seemingly hopeless situations. These two examples serve to indicate the sort of competition faced by internal medicine as it competes with these and other specialties for new entrants to the field.

Most internists are educated in acute-care hospitals at a time when most of the comprehensive care is provided in a physician's office. This discordance between the site of training and the site of comprehensive care distorts the resident's training experience. Residents see primarily the sickest of patients and experience only a brief episode in the total course of a patient's illness. Medical students state that their clerkship experiences in internal medicine are unattractive because they tend to see very few dramatic medical successes and rarely experience the interpersonal relationships characteristic of a previous era.

Movement toward reform

In 1992 the Association of Professors of Medicine studied the curriculum used to train internists and concluded that there was a need for innovation and change. The professors believe that the prestige of the general internist must be enhanced and they have agreed to exert all appropriate means to increase the proportion of internal medicine trainees who become generalists to 50 per cent of all trainees. This influential group of leaders must confront deeply entrenched subspecialty division leaders, many of whom provide the income for the departments over which the professors preside. Yet, the overwhelming concern for the future of the discipline has lent strength to their efforts.

More broadly, many health-policy leaders, either as individuals or as members of public and private commissions or committees, have advocated urgently needed efforts to restore a better balance between the number of generalists and of specialists. In 1992, the Commission on Graduate Medical Education (COGME) and The Physician Payment Review Commission (PPRC), each a Federal Governmental body, have articulated strong positions on this subject. In the same year, the *American Medical Association, the American College of Physicians, the American Academy of Family Practice, and the Association of American Medical Colleges, each a private-sector organization, have made similar statements. These initiatives have established a political environment within which a broad national policy on generalism could be established. Each of these organizations understands that internal medicine is an essential contributor to the solution of the imbalance problem. Thus, the leadership by the professors of medicine and of others from within the discipline is being prodded by the force of public bodies from the outside.

Difficult choices

Heading into the 21st century, internal medicine in America is once again confronted with the choice of whether it is a generalist discipline encompassing all of the traditional medical subspecialties or whether it is a consultant discipline, in which case it defers to the discipline of family medicine for the provision of general care. American internal medicine would aspire to be both, retaining its subspecialties within the family while contending that it provides general care preferable to that provided by family physicians.

At its founding, the American Board of Internal Medicine intended to certify an élite few internists, to set them above all of the others. Over the history of the American Board it has, instead, conferred its certification upon most internists and added certifications to recognize all of the subspecialists who could pass its examinations. This course of events has diminished the distinction between general internal medicine and family medicine to a significant degree, while enhancing the image of the individual subspecialties.

Internal medicine in the USA, as in the UK, takes great pride in the scholarly and intellectual quality of its practitioners. Despite the growth of other medical specialties and the trend toward subspecialization within the discipline itself, it continues to be apparent to most observers of medicine that internal medicine is the discipline which bonds together all of the physician community, regardless of specialty, by its traditions of scholarship and the intellectual application of its knowledge and skills to medical practice. This co-ordinating function is so valued by the public at large and within the profession that it is hard to imagine that it will, through student disinterest, atrophy further. So much now rests upon the energy and wisdom of the present leaders.

American internal medicine continues to be guided by the professors of medicine. Others serve contributory roles, but it is the academic leaders who possess the solutions to the problems described above. The next few years could well be a watershed in the future of this historic and important discipline.

EDWARD J. STEMMLER

Further reading

Howell, J. D. (1989) The invention and development of American internal medicine. *Journal of General Internal Medicine*, **4**, 127–33.

Inui, T. S. and Nolan, J. P. (ed.) (1992). Internal medicine curriculum reform. *Annals of Internal Medicine*, **116**, 1041–115.

Stevens, R. (1971). Trends in medical specialization in the United States. *Inquiry*, **8**, 9–19.

Stevens, R. (1986). Issues for American Internal medicine through the last century. *Annals of Internal Medicine*, **105**, 592–602.

INTERNATIONAL CLASSIFICATION OF DISEASE.

An internationally agreed system and nomenclature of disease classification for which the *World Health Organization (WHO) is responsible. The tenth revision of the *International Classification of Disease* (ICD) was published by WHO in 1992, together with an *ICD Manual* reviewing the history and principles of disease classification. See also CLASSIFICATION.

INTERNATIONAL MEDICAL ASSOCIATIONS AND ORGANIZATIONS.

Medicine is a social science, and politics are nothing else than medicine on a large scale (Rudolf Virchow, *Die medizinische Reform*, 1848).

Introduction

Doctors trained in Western medicine practise it in a mutually recognizable manner in every sizeable community on the face of the earth. Most of them acknowledge a common debt to the early teachings of *Hippocrates in the island of Cos; to the great early medical schools of *Padua, *Bologna, Leiden, Edinburgh, Paris, and Vienna; and to those individuals who created the major disciplines of medical science: men such as *Vesalius, *Malpighi, and *Morgagni of Italy, *Harvey, *Sydenham, John *Hunter, *Jenner, and *Lister of Britain, *Boerhaave of the Netherlands, *Bichat, Claude *Bernard, and *Pasteur of France, *Rokitansky of Austria, and *Virchow and *Koch of Germany. Doctors acknowledge this international inheritance, but their immediate concern is with each individual patient; only slowly over the centuries have they opened their minds to the health needs of communities and whole nations. Few, even today, comprehend the terrible burden of avoidable disease which affects a large proportion of the people of the world. Fewer still would be likely to subscribe to Virchow's proposition, at the start of this entry. Only too often medicine and politics appear to be fundamentally opposed to one another.

Not compassion for the suffering multitudes, but fear of infection from abroad, has been the main spur to international co-operation in matters of health. Great epidemics often spread from other countries. *Plague which, for example, was largely responsible for the destruction of Greek civilization, which killed one-third of the population of the continent of Europe and of Britain in the *Black Death of the 14th century, and caused nearly 100 000 deaths in London in 1665, was seen to spread periodically and disastrously through Syria, Egypt, and Libya. The waves of Asiatic *cholera, such as that which killed a million Russians in a mid-19th century outbreak, had their origins in Bengal and passed by land to Central Asia and Russia, and by sea to Egypt and the Mediterranean. *Syphilis was first known in France as the Spanish or Neapolitan disease; in England as the French disease. The fearful pandemic of *influenza in 1918-19 was seen by the French as originating in Spain, by the Spaniards as originating in France, by the Americans as from Eastern Europe, and by Europeans as introduced by the American troops arriving in France; it rapidly invaded virtually all countries and is thought to have killed at least 15 million people.

In the 6th century, the Roman Emperor Justinian ordered that travellers coming from areas where epidemics were raging should be isolated in camps until 'purified', at which time each person allowed to leave the camp was issued with a certificate of health. Later, great cruelty often accompanied the enforcement of '*cordons sanitaires*'; anyone escaping from an infected area would be brutally killed. In England, in 1625, when the Court moved to Windsor to avoid the plague, a gallows was erected to hang any person who arrived from London. For many centuries there was great fear of the pestilences spread by annual pilgrimages from many countries to Mecca. Rhodes, in 1304, Ragusa in 1377, and particularly Venice from 1400, instituted *quarantine for ships carrying infected persons, a measure soon taken up in Genoa, Marseilles, London, and elsewhere, which led to many deliberate abuses of the commercial freedom of rival states. It was from fear of epidemics, and exasperation over the iniquities of bureaucracy in regard to quarantine, that medical men were at last allowed by governments to introduce measures of international co-operation in health, in the service of a common humanity.

International medical co-operation

Around 1820–30 the French government began to send doctors to Turkey and the Levant to see what might be done to check the advance of epidemics. In 1831 the very first measure of international co-operation in health led to the establishment in Egypt of the Conseil Sanitaire Maritime et Quarantenaire, a multinational bureau which existed until 1938; its original objective was to prevent cholera among Meccan pilgrims from crossing the Mediterranean. In 1834 a Frenchman, de Ségur Dupeyron, prepared a report recommending that the preventive regulations of different countries be brought into agreed order, and from that time the French government pressed for international discussions on problems of mutual health interest. They were successful, and in 1851 the First International Sanitary Conference was held in Paris, attended by the representatives of 11 nations. Each national delegation included one politician and one doctor; they were given independent votes, so that sometimes a delegation effectively disfranchised itself. A second such conference was attended only by politicians, in the belief that the remaining business was concerned only with the signing of agreements. A total of 14 similar conferences was held up to 1938. They achieved little, but fully established the principle that health measures were a proper subject for discussion between nations. The USA, which organized the Fifth Conference in Washington in an attempt to control the dissemination of *yellow fever, first joined in European discussions at the Ninth Conference in 1894 in Paris. America took an important step in 1902 in helping to establish what became the Pan-American Sanitary Bureau (PASB), consisting of all American nations, for the purposes of 'prevention, control and eradication of diseases' in North, Central, and South America. The Bureau remained in service until 1947 when (as PAHO) it became a regional office of the *World Health Organization (WHO).

As a result of the Eleventh International Sanitary Conference in Paris in 1907 the attending national delegations founded the office International d'Hygiène Publique (OIHP). The nine nations which co-operated in its creation were soon joined by more than 50 others. In addition to collaborating in the control of epidemics, they extended international co-operation to include the standardization of sera, vaccines, and antitoxins, the treatment and control of *leprosy, *tuberculosis, *brucellosis, *typhoid, and *venereal diseases, and the purification of water supplies. OIHP moved into 'temporary offices' in the Boulevard S. Germain in 1907 and was still there when absorbed into WHO 40 years later.

At the end of the First World War, the president of OIHP, Santaliquido of Italy, called for health education 'to repair the conscience of mankind'. Influenza had claimed many millions of dead world-wide; starvation caused human meat to be on sale in markets of the newly created Soviet Union, where the ravages of *typhus were so great that Lenin commented 'either socialism will defeat the louse or the louse will defeat socialism'. The Treaty of Versailles (Article XXIII) included the establishment of a Health Organization of the League of Nations. OIHP was expected to form the nucleus, but the refusal of the USA to join the League of Nations, and America's important continued participation in OIHP, resulted in the parallel existence of both bodies until after the Second World War. Individual doctors did their best to co-ordinate the work of OIHP and the League's Health Organization, and there was no conflict of interests, but their combined efforts fell far short of what might have been achieved by one world-wide organization for health.

Nevertheless, the Health Organization of the League was one of the few positive successes of the period between the two World Wars. It has been said that its total budget over 20 years was no more than the cost of one battleship of the period, but even with such unimaginative and disproportionately tiny funds, it achieved a measure of control over major epidemics—not merely their exclusion from Europe—set standards of nutrition for normal physical and mental development, emphasized the importance for health of adequate housing and clean water supplies, improved the understanding and control of *malaria, leprosy, blindness, and many of the multitudinous infestations, and put in train the world unification of national *pharmacopoeias.

Still, governments remained blind to the opportunities for uncontroversial beneficial actions to relieve many of the miseries of mankind. At the end of the Second World War, when the charter of the United Nations Organization was being drafted, all reference to co-operation in health was omitted until, in July 1946, a few individuals pressed for a World Health Conference out of which the World Health Organization (WHO) was created. There was opposition even to this evident and essential step. The chief of the Pan-American Health Bureau campaigned against WHO as

Principal organs of the United Nations

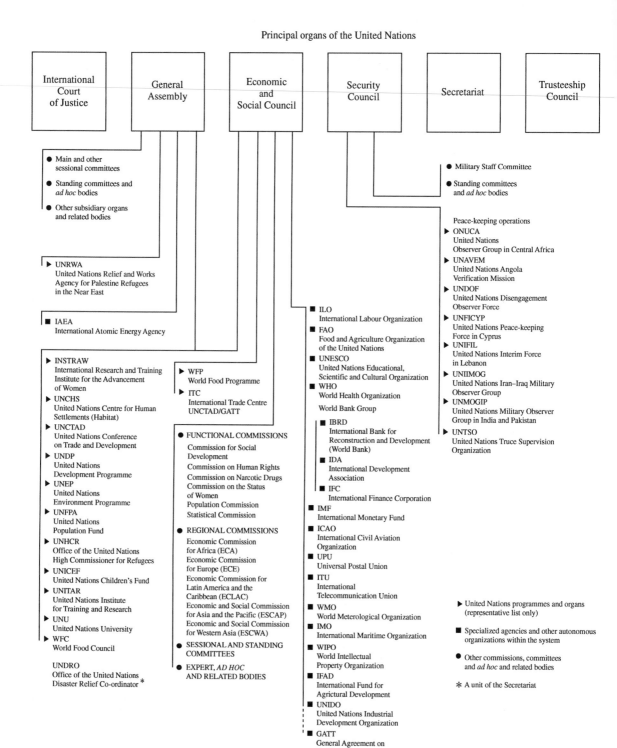

Fig. 1 The United Nations system.

'devised by stargazers and political and social uplifters' and 'advanced internationalists'. The USA feared that WHO would become involved in health insurance and 'socialized medicine' and delayed their entry into WHO for 2 years. Later, the Soviet Union and other Eastern bloc countries withdrew for political reasons for 7 years, and the People's Republic of China (about one-quarter of the world's population) was excluded from effective membership until 1972. Such shortsighted nationalistic politicking was all the more reprehensible because of the example of the United Nations Relief and Rehabilitation Association (UNRRA), which after the war had demonstrated dramatically the feasibility of eradicating malaria from islands such as Sardinia and Mauritius.

The United Nations family

Figure 1 shows the large and disparate range of organizations that currently (1993) make up the United Nations family. WHO is one of a number of special agencies (also including ILO, FAO, and UNESCO) that operate with a degree of distance from the UN General Assembly and its Director General. Typically each such agency has its own membership and governance, which approves its programme of work, sets its budget, and appoints its Chief Officer. While UNO's Economic and Social Council reviews their work, they are not directly accountable to the UN as are, for example, UNDP and UNICEF.

At present, WHO has rather more than 180 member states and an operating budget (1992–1993) of some US$735 million. (The UN budget for the same year was some US$2389 million (£1 = US$1.50), or roughly three times the WHO figure.) Through its six regional committees and regional offices, WHO works with and through the governments of its member states. This is both a weakness and a strength. By comparison with UNICEF, for example, WHO is relatively weak at the project level. Most of its effort goes into assistance to governments, at their request, or to consultations between representatives of governments, facilitated by WHO. Great care is taken at all levels over the production of reports, whether on technical matters or on broader aspects of health policy.

WHO's work on specific diseases has always been strong, illustrated for example by the eradication of smallpox in around 1980, and by the continuing drive against onchocerciasis (river blindness) and poliomyelitis. Nevertheless, the organization recognized long ago that so-called vertical programmes, to tackle specific diseases or conditions, have to be complemented by the integration of these programmes into health systems, and by intersectoral collaboration. Initiatives like women's education and reform, or income generation, can make all the difference to a community's health, but they encompass much more than the health system, traditionally defined. From this awareness sprang the Health for All strategy, formulated by WHO and UNICEF at Alma-Ata in 1978 and formally adopted by the World Health Assembly in 1981. The emphasis of

the strategy is on *primary health care, which includes principles of self-determination, equity and intersectoral collaboration, as well as using simple remedies of proven effectiveness in an integrated health referral system.

It is less clear today where WHO is going next than where it is coming from. These are tough times for international agencies, including WHO, which has been in a zero budget growth situation for some time. Much good work continues, and the health for all strategy has not lost its relevance, but organizations cannot stand still. It needs (as the current Director General, Dr Nakajima, has put it) a paradigm shift to a coherent new vision. Meanwhile, of course, since health is just as surely intersectoral at the international as at the national and local levels, collaboration between WHO and other international agencies is essential. This is obvious in the case of, for example, UNICEF's work on behalf of mothers and children, or the UN Population Fund and Environment Programme, or work for refugees. Less obviously, there has been close co-operation with ILO because of its interest in occupational health and in health insurance; with the Food and Agriculture Organization on nutrition; and with INSTRAW on the advancement of women. Most encouraging currently is the World Bank's growing interest, shared increasingly by other development banks and reflected in the admirable 1993 World Bank report on the health sector, *Investing in health*. It is essential internationally and within countries that health care should not be seen simply as an expensive luxury or a drag on the economy. Investment in health, on the primary health-care model, can make sound economic sense, as judged by the most hard-headed criteria, particularly in some of the poorest countries. In more prosperous countries, health care is too big and complex an economic sector to be safely ignored—as the USA is now recognizing. Moreover, measures of prosperity or economic benefit that ignore health effects are fundamentally flawed. That this should be recognized by the World Bank is a profoundly important advance.

Figure 2, taken from the World Bank report, shows the Bank's estimates of international assistance to the health sector in developing countries, totalling US$4794 million. Of this total, roughly one-third ($1580 million) flows through agencies of the UN. A similar share comes from bilateral agencies, such as USAID, Britain's Overseas Development Agency (ODA), Canada's CIDA, and the comparable donor arms of other national governments in the relatively affluent countries. These agencies constitute an important source of aid, but they often seem as much concerned with the development of national interests as with helping others, and the competition between them can be intense.

The third source of international assistance for health, responsible for roughly one-quarter of the total, is through NGOs and charitable foundations. Table 1 lists some of them, but there are literally hundreds, so that any small selection runs the risk of idiosyncrasy. WHO

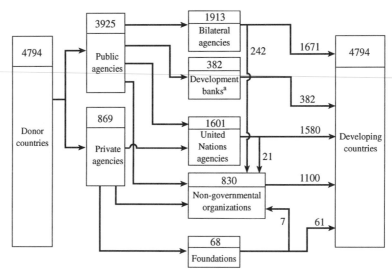

Fig. 2 Disbursements of external assistance for the health sector, 1990 (millions of dollars). [a]Includes US$84 (£56) million in non-concessional loans. (From World Bank 1993, with permission.)

publishes a directory of NGOs with which it is officially related, approaching 200 in the 1990 edition. Pride of place should go to the *Red Cross, established under the First Geneva Convention of 1864 by Henri *Dunant and five other Swiss citizens, inspired by the horrors of the battle of Solferino in 1859, to ensure that the victims of war and other catastrophes would in future be treated 'irrespective of nationality'.

During the First World War, the Red Cross won the enthusiastic goodwill and financial support of countless people, especially in the USA. Its chairman in the USA, Henry Pomeroy Davison, thought that such support would continue in peacetime and he founded the League of Red Cross Societies in 1919 'to anticipate, diminish and relieve the misery produced by disease and calamity' and 'to devise a world health programme'. The League continues to do useful work, but with a fraction of the funds it could valuably deploy.

Private international organizations and foundations
The oldest surviving private medical organization in the world is the Order of *St John of Jerusalem, which was founded in the 11th century and soon had members in many countries. None of the NGOs and foundations listed in Table 1 is anything like so old: a few stem from the 19th century, but nearly all are 20th century creations. Their aims, styles of operation, and levels of funding are widely diverse. What they (and several hundred other organizations) share is that they are active and, in various ways, influential in the field of international health. Many of them are network organizations, e.g. the International Council of Nurses, the International Hospital Federation,

the World Federation of Public Health Associations, and many others, including international organizations for most medical specialties and health-care professions. These associations typically are not well-known to the general public, and are not wealthy; nevertheless, they provide important contacts among countries in their respective fields. International Physicians for the Prevention of Nuclear War may seem a controversial and idiosyncratic example (in Table 1) of this kind, but it earns its place as a winner in its time (1985) of the *Nobel Prize for peace. Arguably the Commonwealth Medical Association, which (as its name implies) is a network organization around the British Commonwealth, is not fully international. From a UK viewpoint, however, it has considerable importance, and its international influence is substantial enough to be recognized by WHO. The Organization for Economic Co-operation and Development (OECD), on the other hand, is primarily a network organization for economic co-operation among the world's wealthier countries. Its interests in social development are subsidiary, but it has produced important and influential comparative statistics for its member countries, and has analysed them thoughtfully. It is currently the best international source for information of this kind.

The international humanitarian relief organizations, which are well-known to the general public, at least in the countries of their foundation, are in a different category. Oxfam and Save the Children are the best-known British examples. Médicins Sans Frontières is primarily a French-speaking organization of physicians and other health professionals committed to relief work,

Table 1 A small selection of NGOs and foundations active internationally in health

Christian Medical Commission
Commonwealth Medical Association
International Council of Nurses
International Hospital Federation
International Physicians for the Prevention of Nuclear War
International Planned Parenthood Federation
League of Red Cross and Red Crescent Societies
Médecins Sans Frontières
Medicus Mundi Internationalis
Metropolis
Organization for Economic Co-operation and Development (OECD)
Oxfam
Save the Children Fund
World Federation of Public Health Associations
Foundations
    Aga Khan
    Carnegie
    Edna McConnell Clark
    Ford
    Hewlett
    Kellogg
    MacArthur
    Andrew Mellon
    Pew Charitable Trusts
    Rockefeller
    Wellcome

even in conditions of great difficulty and some personal danger.

Religious organizations have also been important international actors in health care. The Christian Medical Commission, essentially Protestant, is a major provider of hospital and other medical services, especially in Africa. Medicus Mundi Internationalis is by origin a Roman Catholic example, with branches and affiliated organizations primarily in countries where Roman Catholicism is strong. However, its activities, through its members, go much wider, with 600 developmental projects in East Asia, Africa, and Latin America. The focus is on primary health care and community self-reliance. Nor is this type of international activity confined to Christian organizations. The Aga Khan Foundation, for example, is important in the Moslem world and in any country where there is an Ismaili community.

That takes us into the world of foundations. Some of these, especially the American foundations, are very wealthy indeed, including examples given in Table 1. Typically, these have other objects besides health, and their international coverage is not necessarily comprehensive. Kellogg, for example, includes agriculture and education in its objects, besides health, and is strongest in North and South America, with a considerable interest also in southern Africa. Several of these foundations are concerned with matters that impinge on health, particularly, rather than with health care, education and citizenship. The Rockefeller Foundation has many interests apart from health, where its prime focus is on the poorer countries. Along with a number of other foundations it was recently involved in the International Commission on Health Research for Development, chaired by Dr John Evans, who also chairs the Foundation. Its report, *Health research*, concludes with an agenda for action in terms of international co-operation (among other things).

From a UK standpoint, European organizations are an increasingly important, if (in the world context) somewhat parochial, international forum. The Council of Europe, based in Strasbourg, now has over 30 members, covering a significant number of central, as well as Western, European states. The Council was established in May 1949. It has a Public Health Committee, and organizes regular meetings of Ministers of Health. The Council produces the *European Pharmacopoeia*, and an organ transplant register and bank of rare blood groups. Within Europe, it is the leading international organization on matters of medical *ethics. Initially the European Economic Community (the EEC, now the EU) had no mandate in health. While its membership is much smaller than the Council of Europe, it has for its members (including the UK) much greater international authority. After all, UK laws are, at least in defined fields, subject to Brussels in a way that they certainly are not to the Council of Europe, or even the United Nations. Even though health was outside the competence of the Community initially, under the Treaty of Rome, the activities of its staff (the Commission) nevertheless had substantial implications for health. For example, regulations about the free movement of manpower included physicians and nurses, with mutual recognition of qualifications, at least in theory. Equally, the rulings of the Directorates General of the Commission that dealt with the environment, or with social entitlements, or with the free movement of goods such as pharmaceuticals, all had major implications for health. What the Commission has lacked is any authoritative focus for all its work on health, and any acknowledged authority in this field. The Maastricht Treaty, ratified in 1993, changes this, at least in so far as it prescribes a function for the Community (now the Union) in the field of *public health. Quite what this will mean remains to be worked out, but it will apparently include international activities in relation to 'killer' diseases such as *cancer and *AIDS (perhaps better defined in French as '*les grands fléaux*'). Hopefully, the emphasis will be on European collaboration for *health*, rather than on *health-care provision* or *health financing*, because it is highly doubtful whether standardization of health systems within Europe would be of any real advantage to anyone, whereas intersectoral collaboration to promote health might well be beneficial, if only because no EU country is doing enough of it. More narrowly, there is obviously a strong case for explicit EU collaboration on health problems that move freely across national boundaries, such as AIDS.

Turning back to the broader international scene, it is virtually impossible to do justice to the enormous range and variety of international activities, which increases year by year. Each edition of the *Yearbook of international organizations*—the latest is the 29th edition for 1992–93—illustrates their growing number and complexity. No doubt this trend will continue, as the world becomes more obviously interdependent, and communications become faster and more direct. It is imperative, for reasons of self-interest as well as duty, that the wealthier nations should help the poorer, in order to protect health and life itself. Intense human suffering begets instability. Moreover, in a world where distances stand for little, major epidemics are no respecters of frontiers.

There is also a vast amount to be learned, both by individual health professionals and by whole systems, from international comparisons. The issues of health and health care are so complex, intractable, and subject to change that no nation appears to have found permanent answers to them. That makes it all the more important that we should learn from one another.

Summary

Clinical medicine has always concentrated first and foremost on the individual. Equally important, however, is the health of communities. International contacts are useful for the first, and essential for the second. As the barriers of geographical distance lessen and the world becomes ever more crowded and environmentally more fragile, international contacts in medicine are quite simply indispensable.

G. WOLSTENHOLME
Revised and updated by R. J. MAXWELL

Further reading
Commission on Health Research for Development (Evans, J., Chairman) (1990). *Health research essential link to equity in development*. OUP, New York.
Howard-Jones, N. (1975). *The scientific background of the International Sanitary Conferences 1851–1938*. WHO, Geneva.
Howard-Jones, N. (1978). *International public health between the wars – the organizational problems*. WHO, Geneva.
OECD (1993). *Health system: facts and trends*. OECD, Paris.
Union of International Associations (1993). *Year book of International Organizations 1992/1993*. K. G. Saur, Munich.
United Nations Organization (1992). *United Nations Handbook*. New York.
WHO (1990). *Directory of nongovernmental organizations in official relations with the World Health Organization*. WHO, Geneva.
World Bank (1993). *World development report 1993*: *Investing in health*. OUP, New York.

INTERNIST. A specialist in *internal medicine and its branches, that is the clinical disciplines not requiring recourse to surgical interference. Use of the term is confined to areas of US influence; the equivalent British designation is 'physician'.

INTERSEX is a general term embracing any condition in which a patient manifests some characteristics of the opposite sex, or has mixed sexual characteristics. It has been defined as a state in which any of four criteria fail to agree: viz. chromosomal sex (i.e. *genotype); *gonadal sex; sex of the external *genitalia; and psychological sex (i.e. gender identity). It therefore covers such widely disparate conditions as *hermaphroditism, *homosexuality, transvestism and *gynaecomastia.

INTERVERTEBRAL DISC. See DISC.

INTERVIEW. See COMMUNICATION BETWEEN DOCTORS AND PATIENTS.

INTESTINE. That part of the alimentary tract extending between the pyloric opening of the *stomach and the *anus: it comprises in descending order the small intestine (*duodenum, *jejunum, *ileum) and the large intestine (*caecum, *colon, *rectum, anal canal).

INTIMA. The inner lining of blood vessels in vertebrates, made up of a layer of flattened *endothelial cells surrounded by longitudinal elastic fibres and connective tissue. The full official anatomical name is *tunica intima vasorum*.

INTOXICATION. The state of being poisoned; particularly, the state of being under the influence of *alcohol or other euphoriant substance.

INTRAUTERINE DEVICE (IUD). A contraceptive device, usually in the form of a coil, loop, or spiral made of plastic or metal, designed to be retained in the *uterus. See CONTRACEPTION.

INTRAVENOUS INJECTION. An *injection administered through a hollow needle inserted into the lumen of a *vein.

INTRINSIC FACTOR. A *glycoprotein secreted by the parietal cells of the gastric mucosa as part of the *gastric juice; intrinsic factor is essential for the absorption of *cyanocobalamin (vitamin B_{12}), and its absence leads to *pernicious anaemia.

INTROVERT. One whose thoughts and interests appear to be directed inwards rather than expressed by means of outward action, and who therefore seems internally preoccupied, withdrawn, reserved, or even isolated. The term was used by *Jung, who considered that individuals could be broadly categorized as either introverts or *extraverts. See PSYCHOLOGY.

INTUBATION is the introduction and maintenance of a tube within part of the body, particularly an *endotracheal tube to maintain an *airway for artificial ventilation, administration of general *anaesthesia, etc.

INTUMESCENCE is the process of swelling or the state of being swollen.

INTUSSUSCEPTION is the prolapse or invagination of part of the *intestine into an adjoining segment, a cause of intestinal obstruction, particularly during the first year of life.

INUNCTION is anointing or smearing with *ointment.

INVALID. An individual temporarily or permanently disabled by illness.

INVALIDISM is the state of being a recognized or confirmed *invalid; a state of chronic ill-health.

INVOLUTION is regression or retrograde change in a tissue, organ, or whole organism, either a return to normal size, as in the case of the female reproductive tract following childbirth, or a general degeneration such as that which may accompany senescence.

IODINE. The element iodine (symbol I, atomic number 53, relative atomic mass 126.904) is an essential component of the human diet, being required for the synthesis of the thyroid hormones *thyroxine and *triiodothyronine. The normal daily requirement is about 1 μg/kg of body weight, which in most parts of the world is amply met by ordinary food and water intake; where it is not, iodization of domestic salt is usual and highly desirable, preventing endemic *goitre (thyroid enlargement) which results from dietary iodine deficiency. Iodine in the form of potassium iodide tablets or Lugol's solution (5 per cent iodine in 10 per cent potassium iodide solution) was once used in the preoperative treatment of *thyrotoxicosis so as to reduce thyroid gland vascularity. A radioactive *isotope, ^{131}I, which has a half-life of 8.6 days, is widely used in the diagnosis of thyroid gland conditions, and in the treatment of thyrotoxicosis and thyroid *carcinoma. Topical solutions of iodine have been used for many years as skin *antiseptic agents.

IODOFORM, or tri-iodomethane (CHI_3), was formerly used in topical preparations as a wound dressing by virtue of its weakly disinfectant action. It is toxic when ingested, and local application occasionally results in hypersensitivity reactions.

ION. An electrically charged atom or group of atoms. A positively charged ion, having fewer electrons than required for electrical neutrality, is known as a *cation; a negatively charged one, having more, as an *anion. Thus a *proton is a hydrogen ion, that is a hydrogen atom without its circumnuclear electron, and an *alpha particle is a helium ion. See also ELECTROLYTE.

ION-EXCHANGE is the interchange of *ions of similar charge between an insoluble solid and a solution brought into contact with it. The solid is often a resin or polymer, suitable for the particular exchange desired (ion-exchange resin).

IONIZATION is the formation of *ions, as by *electrolytes in solution. Gaseous ionization is produced by electric sparks, charged particles, *X-rays, *gamma rays, *ultraviolet radiation, etc.

IONIZING RADIATION is *radiation capable of causing *ionization directly or indirectly. Ionizing radiation may be electromagnetic (*X-rays and *gamma rays) or particulate (*electrons, *protons, *neutrons, *alpha-particles, and some other atomic particles). See also RADIATION, IONIZING.

IONOTHERAPY is treatment by the introduction of *ions of various soluble substances into body tissues using an electric current, a process also known as iontophoresis or cataphoresis.

IPECACUANHA is a vegetable preparation; its main active alkaloid is *emetine; it is made from the dried root of the South American plants *Cephaelis ipecacuanha* and *C. acuminata*. In small doses ipecacuanha is thought to be an *expectorant, and it is therefore a constituent of several cough medicines, although its value is dubious. Larger doses are *emetic, and were once used in cases of acute poisoning in order to induce vomiting.

IPSILATERAL. On the same side (cf. *contralateral).

IQ is the commonly used abbreviation of *intelligence quotient.

IRIDECTOMY is surgical removal of part of the *iris.

IRIDOCYCLITIS is inflammation of the anterior part of the uvea, i.e. of the uvea and the ciliary body. See OPHTHALMOLOGY.

IRIDOPLEGIA is paralysis of the muscle of the *iris, so that the *pupil can neither dilate nor contract.

IRIS. The pigmented diaphragm supported by muscle (both circular and radial fibres) which surrounds the *pupil. The iris lies behind the *cornea, and contracts and relaxes to make the pupil constrict and dilate, respectively, thus varying the amount of light admitted to the internal eye. See OPHTHALMOLOGY.

IRITIS is inflammation of the *iris.

IRON. The metallic element iron (symbol Fe, atomic number 26, relative atomic mass 55.847) plays a central role in human metabolism. It is essential to the oxygen-carrying function of *haemoglobin and is a component of various respiratory enzyme systems. Constant dietary replenishment of the body's stores is necessary to prevent depletion, which leads to iron-deficiency *anaemia; more is needed when additional requirements are imposed by growth, menstruation, pregnancy, and bleeding. On the assumption that about 10 per cent of iron in food is absorbed, the upper limits of dietary iron requirements are:

> adults 10 mg/day
> menstruating women 20 mg/day
> pregnant women 50 mg/day
> adolescents 20 mg/day
> infants 1.5 mg/day/kg of body weight

Although there is some degree of physiological regulation of iron absorption according to the state of the iron stores, its scope is limited. In rare cases, usually genetically determined, too much iron is absorbed; this leads to *haemochromatosis or iron-storage disease, colloquially termed 'bronzed diabetes'. A similar condition (*haemosiderosis) can follow multiple blood transfusions.

IRON LUNG is a colloquial term for an early design of *respirator, the Drinker type, in which artificial ventilation is maintained by applying cyclical pressure variation to the interior of a rigid metal cylinder, within which the patient's body, excluding only the head, is enclosed.

IRRADIATION is exposure to *radiation of any kind; in practice it means exposure to *ionizing radiations such as beams of photons, electrons, or neutrons. Artificial radioisotopes are made by irradiating stable isotopes with neutrons. In small doses irradiation may be used to sterilize food, using the sensitivity of biological cells to ionizing radiation.

IRRIGATION is the washing out of a wound, body cavity, or hollow *viscus with a stream of water, saline, or other liquid.

IRRITABILITY. The ability to respond to stimuli, possessed by excitable tissue like nerve and muscle; or an abnormally heightened responsiveness to stimuli on the part of such tissues.

IRRITANT. An agent which gives rise to irritation, particularly chemical irritation of the skin or mucous membranes.

ISAAC JUDAEUS (Isaac Israeli bin Solomon) (*fl.* AD 900). Jewish physician. He was a neoplatonist who wrote notable books on fevers, on the urine, and on dietetics.

ISCHAEMIA (ISCHEMIA) is insufficient blood supply to an area of tissue or an organ, due to obstruction or functional constriction of one or more blood vessels, or as part of a more general circulatory failure. For example, ischaemia of muscle is responsible for the symptoms of *angina pectoris and *intermittent claudication. When sufficiently severe or prolonged, ischaemia progresses to *infarction.

ISHIHARA'S CHARTS are a series of coloured plates made up of spots of various sizes and different colours. They contain patterns, some of which cannot be perceived by individuals with particular defects of colour vision. They are used for the diagnosis of *colour blindness.

ISLETS OF LANGERHANS are clusters of cells scattered throughout the *pancreas. Several types of cell are distinguished in the clusters, of which the most abundant are the beta cells, which secrete *insulin. Others are the alpha cells, which secrete the hyperglycaemic factor *glucagon, and the delta cells, which secrete *somatostatin.

ISOLATION is the separation of the microenvironment of a patient from the general microenvironment of the hospital, either to prevent the escape of microorganisms from the patient ('barrier nursing') or to prevent them from reaching him ('reverse barrier nursing'). The former is required with patients suffering, or suspected to be suffering, from serious communicable disease, the latter when patients are immunocompromised to the extent that normally trivial commensal organisms might cause disastrous *nosocomial (hospital-acquired) infection. Techniques differ in the two cases, but both require impeccable discipline on the part of attendants and visitors.

ISOLATION HOSPITALS were hospitals for the diagnosis, care, and management of communicable diseases into which patients suffering or suspected to be suffering from such diseases were once segregated. Their function has been largely subsumed by isolation units in general hospitals.

ISONIAZID is an important antituberculous chemotherapeutic agent, usually administered by mouth and in combination with other antituberculous drugs.

ISOTOPE. An *atom of the same *element (i.e. having the same atomic number) but differing in mass number from other isotopes of that element. The difference relates to a different number of *neutrons in the nucleus. Isotopes are identical in all chemical properties and in all physical properties except those dependent on atomic mass. Almost all elements occur in nature as mixtures of several isotopes.

ITCH. The cutaneous sensation that provokes an urge to scratch. See PRURITUS.

J

JACKSON, CHEVALIER (1865–1958). American laryngologist. He developed technical procedures for peroral *endoscopy and surgery of the *larynx. He also developed instruments and techniques for endoscopy of the *bronchi and the *oesophagus, especially to remove foreign bodies. See also OTORHINOLARYNGOLOGY.

JACKSON, JOHN HUGHLINGS (1835–1911). British neurologist. He was one of the great pioneer neurologists; he wrote on *speech defects, focal epilepsy ('*Jacksonian epilepsy'), *uncinate epilepsy, and the concept of 'levels' in the nervous system.

JACKSONIAN EPILEPSY is a form of localized *epilepsy, usually caused by a focal lesion in the contralateral motor cortex of the brain. The attack begins as a clonic or repetitive contraction of a group of muscles in the periphery of the body, often the big toe, thumb and index finger, or the angle of the mouth, and then 'marches' up the limb as abnormal excitation spreads through the cortex. The attack may be confined to one limb, may spread to involve the whole ipsilateral side of the body, may sometimes spread to the contralateral side or may terminate in a generalized epileptic fit or *grand mal. Focal motor seizures of this type may be followed by weakness or paralysis of the affected muscles persisting for several hours, known as Todd's palsy or paralysis. The condition was described by John Hughlings *Jackson.

JACOBI, ABRAHAM (1830–1919). German/American paediatrician. He wrote many treatises and books on diseases of children.

JACTITATION. A twitching or convulsive movement of muscles or limbs; alternatively restless tossing about of the whole body.

JAMES, WILLIAM (1842–1910). American psychologist, and brother of Henry James the novelist. He started to study medicine at Harvard, but broke off to explore the Amazon with Louis Agassiz; subsequently he went to Europe to study with *Helmholtz, *Virchow, and *Bernard. He took his MD from Harvard in 1869

but never practised. Indeed his studies seem to have induced a neurosis and he remained at home for some time as a semi-invalid. After teaching physiology at Harvard, he moved on to what was then physiological psychology. By 1890 he published *The principles of psychology*, which helped establish the subject as a science. He then entered a religious phase, applying psychology to religious experience, and these studies with his later works in philosophy started furious arguments. In philosophy he was a pragmatist, judging ideas by their consequences.

JAMESON, SIR LEANDER STARR, BT (1853–1917). British physician and statesman. In 1878 Jameson went out to Kimberley to practise, and there became a close friend of Cecil Rhodes. In 1889 he was sent to win the concession of Mashonaland from Lobengula the chief of the Matabele, and succeeded by curing his *gout. He became administrator of what became Southern Rhodesia (now Zimbabwe). In 1895 he carried out his ill-conceived raid across the Transvaal border ('the Jameson raid'), was defeated, and taken prisoner. He was in Ladysmith during the siege in 1899. Later he entered the South African parliament and in 1904 became prime minister of Cape Colony.

JANET, PIERRE MARIE FELIX (1859–1947). French neurologist and psychiatrist. A pupil of *Charcot, he developed the concepts of psychological *automatism (1889) and *psychasthenia (1903). He held strong views on *hysteria and insisted that sexual inadequacy was a symptom of *neurosis and not the cause.

JARGON APHASIA is a variety of fluent *aphasia in which well-articulated speech is produced but without informational content; it is also known as gibberish aphasia. See LANGUAGE, COGNITION, AND HIGHER CEREBRAL FUNCTION.

JAUNDICE is a yellow discoloration of the *skin and *mucous membranes due to excess of *bilirubin in the blood, also known as icterus. When the cause is obstruction to the flow of bile in the biliary tract (obstructive jaundice), the bilirubin reabsorbed into the blood is of the soluble conjugated form and is therefore excreted by the kidneys, resulting in dark urine (bilirubinuria). At the same time, the stools are pale due to lack of bile pigment in the *faeces. Neither pale stools nor dark urine occur in the other main variety of jaundice, in which the hyperbilirubinaemia is due to excessive destruction of *erythrocytes (haemolytic or acholuric jaundice).

JEFFERSON, SIR GEOFFREY (1886–1961). British neurosurgeon. He occupied the first chair of neurosurgery in the UK, at Manchester, founded in 1939 and was an outstanding clinician and teacher.

JEHOVAH'S WITNESSES are members of a fundamentalist religious sect, the Watchtower Bible and Tract Society, founded about 1879. Jehovah's Witnesses refuse to accept *blood transfusion for themselves or for their children, a difficulty which may in some surgical situations be overcome by using the patient's own blood (removed before operation) or synthetic *blood substitutes.

JEJUNITIS is inflammation of the *jejunum.

JEJUNUM. The second part of the small *intestine, extending from the *duodenum to the *ileum.

JEKYLL, DR, is the antihero of Robert Louis Stevenson's *The strange case of Dr. Jekyll and Mr. Hyde* (1866). Dr Jekyll is a philanthropic and well-liked physician who develops an interest in the dualism of personality. Experimenting with drugs, he succeeds in separating the good and evil sides of his own nature, the latter being intermittently personified as Mr Hyde. The book recounts how Mr Hyde gradually gains the upper hand, culminating in the doctor's self-destruction.

JENNER, EDWARD (1749–1823). British physician and the discoverer of *vaccination. He practised all his life in Berkeley, Gloucestershire. On 14 May 1796 Jenner inoculated James Phipps with material obtained from a *cow-pox vesicle on the hand of Sarah Nelmes; on 1 July, he inoculated him with *smallpox, to which he proved immune (see IMMUNOLOGY). In 1798 he published *An enquiry into the cause and effects of the variolae vaccinae, a disease discovered in some of the western counties of England, particularly Gloucestershire, and known by the name of the cow-pox.* In recognition of his discovery of vaccination he was awarded £10 000 by Parliament in 1802. See also JESTY, BENJAMIN.

JENNER, SIR WILLIAM, Bt (1815–98). British physician. His careful observations on prolonged fevers, along with those of *Gerhard, established the differences between *typhoid fever and *typhus.

JERK. A sudden and brief contraction of a group of muscles of *reflex or involuntary origin.

JESTY, BENJAMIN (1737–1816). Jesty was a farmer of Yetminster and Worth Matravers in Dorset, England. In 1774 he vaccinated his wife and two young children with *cow-pox material, taken from a sore on the udder. He had noted that milkmaids infected with cow-pox rarely contracted *smallpox. This disease was raging in his vicinity at the time, but none of his family contracted it after the *vaccination. He was probably the first formal vaccinator, for Edward *Jenner did not vaccinate until 22 years later. Reviled at first by the local populace, Jesty was ultimately hailed by the Vaccine Pock Institute of London and given two golden lancets. He had used a stocking needle for his wife and children. The Institute was a rival of Jenner's, who vehemently maintained that he was the discoverer of vaccination and successfully claimed money for it from the government. Jesty's experiment was a bold one, even though the immunity of milkmaids was well-known country lore.

JESUIT'S BARK, also known as Peruvian bark and *cinchona bark, is the source of *quinine and other quinoline *alkaloids.

JEX-BLAKE, SOPHIA LOUISA (1840–1912). British physician and pioneer of the right of women to practise medicine. She studied medicine under Elizabeth *Blackwell in New York and in 1869 was accepted for training by Edinburgh University at her second request, but later the Appeal Court decided that the university had acted *ultra vires* in so doing. In 1874 she founded the *London School of Medicine for Women and in 1877 clinical studies were permitted at the London (later *Royal) Free Hospital. In 1876 an enabling act allowed all bodies to examine women in medicine. In 1877 she was permitted to practise; by this time she was an MD Berne. In 1878 she settled in Edinburgh and founded the Women's Hospital and School of Medicine, which survived until the university admitted women in 1894. See also WOMEN IN MEDICINE.

JOGGER'S NIPPLE is irritation of the nipple due to the mechanical friction of clothing during jogging, which is a form of physical exercise achieved by slow running with an up-and-down bouncing movement.

JOHNS HOPKINS HOSPITAL, THE, in Baltimore, Maryland, USA, with its University School of Medicine and University School of Hygiene and Public Health, began under the will of Johns Hopkins, a wealthy businessman, who, when he died in 1873, left $7 million to establish a university and a hospital. The will required careful consideration and expert advice for the site and the building, the provision of physicians and surgeons of the highest character and greatest skill, and a school for nurses. Most far-sighted was his wish that ultimately the hospital would form a part of the medical school of the university. The hospital, opened in 1889, attracted a galaxy of talent, including William *Welch, William *Osler, William S. *Halsted, and Howard A. *Kelly. At first they taught graduate students, and an undergraduate school began in 1893, 4 years after the nursing school. These men and their distinguished pupils inaugurated and carried into practice the idea of the university hospital and medical school with full-time staff who were required to integrate service to patients with research and education. When Abraham *Flexner produced his report of 1910 Johns Hopkins was the model of what was best for the future of medical education. The hospital has expanded its activities into all branches of medicine. Discoveries and advances have included the first use of *rubber gloves in surgery, fundamental work on *rickets, the discovery of epinephrine (*adrenaline) and *heparin as well as many other important developments, but especially well-known is the 'blue-baby' operation developed by Helen Taussig and Alfred *Blalock.

JOINT. Any articulation between two *bones.

JONES, SIR ROBERT, Bt (1857–1933). British orthopaedic surgeon. With Dame Agnes *Hunt he founded the orthopaedic hospital for children at Oswestry in 1900. Robert Jones was one of the great pioneers of *orthopaedic surgery and of the treatment of injuries; he was also an inspiring teacher and many of the distinguished orthopaedic surgeons of the mid 20th century were his pupils.

JOSLIN, ELLIOTT PROCTOR (1869–1962). American physician. Joslin devoted his attention almost exclusively to *diabetes mellitus, working at the New England Deaconess Hospital, Boston. In 1916 he published the first edition of his well-known book *The treatment of diabetes mellitus*, based on his personal observations of more than 1000 patients. Before the discovery of *insulin his treatment was mainly diet and maintenance of low normal body weight. After the discovery of insulin in 1922 he and his colleagues made many important contributions to its clinical use, in particular advocating strict control of the blood sugar. Joslin organized classes for his patients, to instruct them about their disease, the use of insulin, testing for sugar in the urine, etc.

JOURNALS. See MEDICAL JOURNALS.

JUGULAR VEINS are those responsible for drainage of the head and neck. The internal jugular receives most of the blood from the brain, travelling from the skull deep to the sternomastoid muscle to join the subclavian vein. The external jugular is more superficial, draining the scalp and face.

JUNG, CARL GUSTAV (1875–1961). Swiss psychiatrist. Jung had a religious background, with a grandfather, a father, and eight uncles, all pastors of the Basel Reformed Church. He read widely, studied medicine, and later turned away from formal religion, partly by way of spiritualism. Following correspondence with *Freud, a relationship began which lasted for 7 years, before dissolving in acrimony. In 1914 Jung severed his connection with *psychoanalysis, and formed his own school of analytical *psychology. This placed less emphasis on sexual drives starting in infancy, and more on a theory of symbolic *archetypes and the collective unconscious.

K

KAHN TEST. One of a number of serological tests for *syphilis which depend on the fact that in this condition (and in some others) *antibody appears in the patient's *serum directed against a normal component of many tissues called cardiolipin (diphosphatidyl glycerol); when allowed to interact with a suspension of this phospholipid, visible flocculation occurs followed by fixation of *complement. Anticardiolipin antibodies were discovered in 1907 by *Wasserman using a liver extract as *antigen, and the test that bears his name depends on complement fixation. The Kahn test uses overnight incubation. Like the *Wasserman reaction (WR), the Kahn test has been replaced by a simpler, more reproducible, and cheaper slide flocculation version known as the Venereal Disease Reference Laboratories (VDRL) test. Why patients with syphilis should develop antibodies against a normal tissue constituent is not known.

All these serological tests for syphilis can produce false-positive results. More specific are treponemal tests, of which there are now several; these reveal antibody directed against the responsible organism, *Treponema pallidum*.

KALA-AZAR (Hindi for 'black fever') is a serious chronic infection with the protozoan parasite *Leishmania donovani*. Without treatment it carries a mortality rate which may be as high as 90 per cent. It is usually a zoonosis, i.e. a disease of animals which can be transmitted to man. The animals are mostly wild and domestic canines and rodents, and transmission occurs via biting *sandflies of various *Phlebotomus* species. The disease is prevalent in the Mediterranean littoral, East and West Africa, Asia Minor, southern Arabia, India, China, and South America. Also known as visceral *leishmaniasis, kala-azar is predominantly an infection of the reticuloendothelial system; the cardinal features are fever, wasting, anaemia, and enlargement of lymph nodes, liver, and spleen, the spleen in particular often reaching a great size. Hyperpigmentation of the skin of the hands, feet, face, and abdomen is common, accounting for the name 'kala-azar'. Death is usually the result of intercurrent infection, but when diagnosis is made early and treatment (antimony preparations are the first choice but other compounds are

effective in resistant cases) is quickly introduced, almost all patients recover.

KAMIKAZE is used of the Japanese pilots (or their planes, loaded with explosives) who made suicide attacks on enemy targets by crashing into them. The word is used biomedically in a transferred sense, for example 'kamikaze cell'.

KAOLIN is a natural form of hydrated aluminium silicate, $Al_2Si_2O_5(OH)_4$, also known as china clay. Its medical applications are as an ingredient of numerous antidiarrhoeal mixtures and, as a *poultice, in the local application of heat.

KAPOSI, MORIZ KOHN (1837–1902). Hungarian dermatologist. He described many skin diseases including *rhinoscleroma (with Hebra, 1870), multiple haemorrhagic sarcoma (*Kaposi's sarcoma, 1872), and *xeroderma pigmentosum (1882).

KAPOSI'S SARCOMA is a malignant multifocal metastasizing *reticulosis involving particularly the skin and often beginning as reddish soft swellings on the hands or feet. There is a strong association between Kaposi's sarcoma and the *acquired immune deficiency syndrome (AIDS), especially in homosexual men; about 47 per cent of male homosexuals with AIDS develop the condition, as compared with 8 per cent of all AIDS cases.

KAWASAKI DISEASE (OR SYNDROME). A severe illness of unknown cause, usually affecting young children and causing fever, *stomatitis, cervical *lymphadenitis, joint pains, diarrhoea, and a widespread rash. Antibiotics may be of benefit.

KAY-SHUTTLEWORTH, SIR JAMES PHILLIPS, BT (1804–77). British physician and pioneer of public health. He practised in Manchester, where, as medical officer to the Ancoats and Ardwick Dispensary, he witnessed the horrors of the *cholera epidemic of 1832. As a result he published *The moral and physical condition of the working classes employed in the cotton manufacture in Manchester* (1832).

KEATS, JOHN (1795–1821). British physician and poet. He was apprenticed to a surgeon at Edmonton in 1810 and later studied at *Guy's and *St Thomas's Hospitals. He ceased to practise in 1817. He died in Rome in 1821 of pulmonary *tuberculosis, as had his mother and his brother. His chief works were *Poems* (1817); 'Endymion' (1818); 'Ode to a Nightingale' (1819); and 'Hyperion' (1820).

KEITH, SIR ARTHUR (1866–1955). British anatomist. In 1907 he described the *sinoatrial node in the heart with Flack (Keith–Flack node).

KELLY, HOWARD ATWOOD (1858–1943). American gynaecological surgeon. He wrote extensively on diseases of the female genital tract; he also developed methods of inspecting the lining of the *bladder, and of catheterizing the *ureters under direct visualization. He was among the first to employ *radium locally in treating *cancer.

KELOID. Overgrowth of *collagen tissue during the formation of a scar, resulting in the scar being thickened, elevated, and unsightly.

KENDALL, EDWARD CALVIN (1886–1972). American biochemist. He was the first to isolate *thyroxine in crystalline form. He then studied the steroidal compounds in the *adrenal cortex, sharing an interest in this subject with T.*Reichstein of Switzerland. In the mid-1940s he isolated enough *cortisone (then called Compound E) for clinical trial, and gave it to *Hench, who tested it on some patients with *rheumatoid arthritis. The immediate anti-inflammatory effects were spectacular. In 1950 Kendall, Hench, and Reichstein shared the *Nobel prize for this work.

KERATIN is a tough, insoluble but unusually flexible, sulphur-containing protein which is the principal constituent of the outer layer of the *skin (epidermis), the nails, the hair, and the organic matrix of tooth enamel.

KERATITIS is inflammation of the *cornea, the commonest causes being trauma and infectious agents. Keratitis may also be due to nutritional deficiency, sensitivity reactions, neurological conditions causing corneal anaesthesia, abnormal exposure, and lacrimal disorders. Acute keratitis can make the normally transparent cornea hazy with consequent blurring of vision; if resolution occurs with scarring, permanent opacity may result. This can be a danger with any form of keratitis, including *herpes infections. Diffuse interstitial keratitis was a cardinal feature of congenital syphilis (see HUTCHINSON'S TRIAD).

KERATOMALACIA is dryness, softening, and necrosis of the *cornea occurring in severe *vitamin A deficiency.

KERATOSIS is any abnormality of *keratin.

KERNICTERUS describes a condition which may occur in *haemolytic disease of the newborn, when the concentration of unconjugated *bilirubin reaches such high levels that it crosses the blood–brain barrier and causes *brain damage. The parts chiefly affected are the basal nuclei, globus pallidus, putamen, caudate nucleus, and the cerebellar and bulbar nuclei, hence the term 'kernicterus' which is German for 'nuclear jaundice'. Permanent cerebral impairment results and deafness is common.

KETOACIDOSIS. See KETOSIS.

KETONE. Any of a series of organic compounds having the general formula RR' C:O where R and R' are univalent hydrocarbon radicals. An example is *acetone, or dimethyl ketone, which has the formula $(CH_3)_2CO$.

KETOSIS is accumulation in the body of ketone bodies (ketoacids), i.e. *acetone, acetoacetic acid, and beta-hydroxybutyric acid, intermediate products in the breakdown of stored fat. Their concentration in the blood rises, and metabolic *acidosis results. Ketone bodies can then be detected in the urine and (as a characteristic odour) on the breath. The commonest causes are *starvation and uncontrolled *diabetes mellitus (see DIABETIC COMA).

KEYHOLE SURGERY. The journalistic term 'keyhole surgery' has recently come to be applied to what the clinician would now understand as 'minimally invasive' surgery.

A new and general concept of 'minimal invasiveness' in surgery was first proposed by Wickham in 1986 because of the radical changes that had occurred in the treatment of *kidney stones between 1979 and 1983. During this time the major and traumatic operation of open surgical stone removal was at first replaced by the telescopic extraction of stones through tiny 1 cm tracks made from the body surface into the kidney, and secondly by the advent of extracorporeal shockwave lithotripsy. By this latter method stones within the kidney were fragmented by the application of a focused shockwave from outside the body. This shockwave was passed from the generator, either electrical or acoustic, through the soft tissues of the body to impinge on the target stone and produce fragmentation. Particles of stone then passed through the natural urinary passages to the exterior. With the latest machines of this type, called *lithotriptors, no anaesthetic is needed, the patient's body is not invaded, and the whole procedure has become a walk in/walk out event like going to the dentist, but is fully effective in treating the patient's stone disease.

From this sequence of events it became very apparent that a dramatic change had taken place in the therapy of renal stone. Major *trauma had been avoided but the

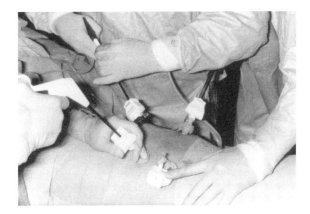

Fig. 1 Keyhole surgery in action through multiple small punctures in the abdominal wall.

same therapeutic effect had been produced. The results of stone treatment by open surgery, telescopic surgery, or lithotripsy were compared in 1986, demonstrating an enormous diminution in mortality and complications if these new procedures were used. The conditions that the patients were suffering from were the same, but the reduction in trauma was achieved purely because the surgery of open access had been replaced by 'minimal access' procedures or 'keyhole surgery'.

On reviewing practices in other specialties at that time it was apparent that similar changes were taking place. For example *gynaecologists were just beginning to control uterine bleeding by coagulation of the uterine lining rather than by removing the whole *uterus. *Orthopaedic surgeons were using a telescopic technique to remove knee cartilages without the need for open operation. Medical *gastroenterologists were removing *gallstones from the *bile ducts with flexible telescopes and retrieval baskets passed through the stomach and *duodenum into the bile duct.

By 1987 it seemed possible to predict the way in which interventional therapy was destined to develop in the next decade (Wickham 1987) and now (1993) many common interventional procedures have already been converted into 'minimally invasive' or 'keyhole' techniques because the resultant reduction in morbidity has become very obvious.

Although a simple telescope had first been used to inspect the abdominal contents in 1901, it was the work of Palmer in France and Semm in Germany in the 1960s and 1970s that initiated the use of ancillary instruments passed through small secondary tubes inserted into the abdominal wall to carry out operative procedures on the female reproductive organs. Why this technique was not seized upon by general surgeons at this time is a mystery. As far as the upper abdomen was concerned, it was left to the medical gastroenterologists and *radiologists in the 1970s to remove gallstones from the bile duct

telescopically by way of the normal gastrointestinal passages. This was followed by direct puncture of the gall bladder with endoscopic stone removal in 1986. Only in 1987, when the removal of the whole gall bladder was carried out by Mauret in France, was the full potential of this technique appreciated. The method was rapidly taken up by general surgeons and the term 'keyhole surgery' coined (Fig. 1), although this was purely one operation out of many that had been developing in other specialties over the preceding 10–15 years. The surgeon now had no need to grope inside the abdomen with his hands, but could observe and carry out his operation remotely by watching a television monitor (Fig. 2).

Telescopic gall-bladder removal is quite a simple operation and is but a further example of the much greater general concept of minimal invasiveness that is now permeating all areas of interventional therapy. Although a considerable part of minimally invasive therapy can be classified as keyhole surgery, i.e. done with a telescope passed into the abdominal cavity, it should be appreciated that many more sophisticated operative techniques have been pioneered in other specialties with the same aim of reducing open surgical trauma, and have been in use for many years. The very delicate operations carried out in the middle ear for many years by ear, nose, and throat surgeons using operating microscopes are a case in point, as is the endoscopic removal of the *prostate which dates back as far as 1927.

Future development
In intestinal surgery for tumours it is now possible to remove the whole of the *oesophagus by endoscope. Segments of bowel may be removed telescopically and joined up again entirely within the abdominal cavity.

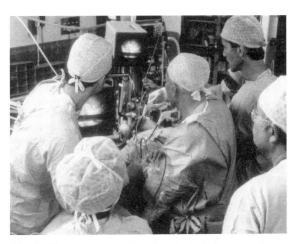

Fig. 2 The surgeon performing 'keyhole' surgery to remove a kidney. Note that everyone is looking at the monitors and not their hands.

Rectal tumours may be removed telescopically through the anus, thus in many cases averting the need for *colostomy or other types of bowel diversion. Diseases of the biliary tract are now almost completely accessible to the endoscopist or interventional radiologist.

In the chest, the lungs, or portions of them, may be removed telescopically, and various forms of heart surgery can be carried out through *catheters introduced into peripheral vessels by the radiologist. Through these catheters balloon dilatation or laser disobliteration of the *coronary arteries can be performed without the gross invasion of the chest cavity as is now required for bypass surgery, which will surely be replaced in the foreseeable future. A blockage in a peripheral artery of the body will be treated by the introduction of telescopes and laser removal of the obstructing tissue without the need for open surgery. Interventional radiologists will also dilate obstructed arteries by balloons and then insert hollow metallic splints to maintain the newly dilated artery in an open position to allow blood flow to resume.

In gynaecology, ablation of the lining of the uterus by *diathermy or *laser coagulation is rapidly removing the need for *hysterectomy which, if required, may be carried out telescopically through the abdominal cavity and the mobilized organ removed by way of the vagina.

In orthopaedics, telescopic examination of the knee and removal of a damaged cartilage are now the norm, but similar techniques are being extended to other joints in the body and it is quite probable that the extensive open operations for the replacement of the hip joint will gradually be replaced by the endoscopic refashioning and relining of joint surfaces with artificial materials or even cartilage grafts.

Ear, nose, and throat, and eye doctors are increasingly using the operating microscope and telescope for their work. Open traumatic procedures for removing the *larynx and large portions of the face for treatment of cancer are rapidly being superseded by internal endoscopic examination and laser dissection or coagulation.

*Neurosurgeons can now remove prolapsed intervertebral *discs using mini-telescopes and micro-techniques on a day-case basis and, ultimately, intracranial brain surgery will be increasingly managed by the endoscope and robot. This catalogue of changes is almost endless and serves to highlight the general concept of minimal invasiveness coupled with instrumental technical advances.

Secondary effects of these techniques upon the health-care process

First, the rapidity of recovery and passage of patients through the treatment sequence is soon going to render the large, hotel type of hospital obsolete. As much as 70 or 80 per cent of this form of intervention can be carried out on a day-case basis in smaller, stand-alone units with good transport access. The emphasis on in-patient nursing care will be less, and will become much more community based, day-case surgery becoming the norm, with the patients being visited postoperatively in their homes. Patients will further benefit as they will be able to decide more easily the timing of their therapy and, with a very short convalescent period, they will be able to return to normal activity much more rapidly.

The type of doctor will also change. Patients may find that their treatment is carried out by a radiologist or even a *technician rather than by the conventional open operative surgeon. Surgeons will need to be trained and retrained as primary microendoscopists or bioengineers rather than as anatomical carpenters as at present.

The specialty boundaries may become quite obscured. For example, skilled endoscopists may well be able to remove a knee cartilage or a kidney stone just as competently as they remove a rectal tumour or a uterus. A new breed of organ-related diagnostic physicians will emerge, while the active interventional therapy may be carried out by a non-organ-orientated endoscopist. Pre-and postoperative care will be supervised by anaesthetists and *intensive care physicians, and not by surgeons.

Health-care funding will need to undergo an appreciable shift from the support of hospital hotel services to the purchase and maintenance of high-technology equipment, such as lasers, robots, videos, and camera systems, coupled with complicated *X-ray machines. The *health economists will need to become accustomed to this necessary relocation of equity from one area to another, and also to promote actively the introduction of significant new technologies more rapidly into the system.

Conclusion

It is now obvious that a complete revolution in interventional medical therapy has occurred in the past decade fuelled by the desire of the doctor to obtain a satisfactory cure without a mutilating operative procedure, and actively aided by the spectacular developments in instrumental technology. There can be little doubt that what makes patients ill during an open operative intervention is the damage caused by the surgeon in achieving his target object. By reducing this surgical trauma, *morbidity and *mortality are vastly reduced. In as far as many procedures are now carried out through small apertures by telescope, they may be categorized as 'keyhole surgery'. Nevertheless this appellation should not be allowed to trivialize and obscure the vast change in attitudes to interventional therapy that may well be as significant as the introduction of the first general anaesthetic in 1846.

J. E. A. WICKHAM

References

Wickham, J. E. A. (1986). Editorial. *British Medical Bulletin*, **42**, 221–2.

Wickham, J. E. A. (1987). The new surgery. *British Medical Journal*, **295**, 1581–2.

KEYNES, SIR GEOFFREY LANGTON (1887–1982). Bibliophile and surgeon. A pioneer at St Bartholomew's Hospital, London, in the 1930s of conservative surgery for *breast cancer ('lumpectomy' instead of radical mastectomy), Keynes also spearheaded the removal of the *thymus gland for *myasthenia gravis. He wrote a major biography of William *Harvey and was also an authority on Sir Thomas *Browne.

KIDNEY. The two kidneys are the principal organs of excretion of water-soluble waste products and regulation of water, sodium, potassium, and hydrogen and their associated anions. Each kidney contains about a million functional units, each comprising a *glomerulus and a *renal tubule. Subsidiary functions include control of the rate of red blood cell production by the bone marrow, and control of the arterial blood pressure. See NEPHROLOGY; PHYSIOLOGY; RENAL FUNCTION TESTS.

KIDNEY DISEASE. See NEPHROLOGY.

KIDNEY FAILURE. See RENAL FAILURE.

KIDNEY TRANSPLANT. See TRANSPLANTATION.

KIENBÖCK, ROBERT (1871–1953). Austrian radiologist. In 1910 he described avascular *necrosis of the lunate bone, one of the carpal bones of the wrist. Lack of blood supply causes the bone to appear smaller and denser on the X-ray plate.

KINESIA. Movement; sometimes used for *motion sickness.

KINESIOTHERAPY is treatment with body movements.

KINETICS is the study of the rates at which chemical reactions and biological processes proceed.

KING'S COLLEGE HOSPITAL was opened in 1840 in Portugal St., Covent Garden, moving to Denmark Hill in South-East London in 1913, partly to provide clinical education for students of King's College in the Strand. This had been founded by Royal Charter of George IV, and it taught basic medical sciences from 1831. In 1908 the Medical School became a School of Medicine in the University of London. Among many famous members of staff was Lord *Lister, who was professor of surgery there when he came to London from Scotland.

KING'S EVIL is another name for *scrofula, which in England and France was supposed to be cured by the King's touch. In England, touching for the King's evil continued from the time of Edward the Confessor until the death of Queen Anne in 1714. A special Office for the ceremony was printed in the Prayer Book until 1719. The practice dated back at least to Clovis the Frank in AD 496, and French kings touched regularly until 1775, the practice being temporarily revived by Charles X in 1824. In 1711, at the age of 2 years, Samuel Johnson was touched by Queen Anne.

KININS. A class of vasoactive endogenous polypeptides formed by the action of proteolytic enzymes on plasma protein precursors. Their production contributes to the *vasodilatation associated with *inflammation and the *hypotension that occurs in states of *anaphylaxis. Their normal function is probably the local regulation of blood flow and glandular function.

KIRCHER, ATHANASIUS (1602–80). Polymath Jesuit priest of Fulda, West Germany. He was an early microscopist. He saw small 'worms' in the blood of plague patients, and various *animalcules in putrefying matter. Probably these were not bacteria, but he postulated that disease was caused by them.

KITASATO, SHIBASABURO, BARON (1852–1931). Japanese bacteriologist. He was the first to obtain a pure culture of *Clostridium tetani* and worked on *immunization against *tetanus and *diphtheria (1890). He isolated tetanus *toxin and proved it could be used to immunize against tetanus. He used killed bacterial cultures for *vaccination and isolated *Pasteurella pestis* in the Hong Kong epidemic of *plague independently of *Yersin (1894).

KLEBS, EDWIN (1834–1913). German bacteriologist. He used plate culture before *Koch; he described the organism causing *diphtheria (the diphtheria bacillus was originally named after him and after *Loeffler who did further work on the organism); and transmitted *syphilis to monkeys, an experiment repeated later by *Roux and *Metchnikoff. He established the importance of the intestinal route for the entry of tubercle bacilli, against the opposition of Koch.

KLEBSIELLA is a genus of Gram-negative coliform *bacilli, species of which are found in the intestinal and respiratory tracts of man, and in association with respiratory tract, urinary tract, and wound infections. *Klebsiella pneumonia* is a severe infection with a high mortality, often occurring against a background of pre-existing bronchopulmonary disease or of chronic *alcoholism.

KLEINE–LEVIN SYNDROME is a rare disorder occurring in young men and characterized by periodic somnolence followed by irritability and excessive eating, often with perverted sexual behaviour. Between attacks, which may last days or weeks, the patient appears normal.

KLEPTOMANIA is a morbid, uncontrollable, and irrational impulse to steal. Shop-lifting is the usual manifestation, though the kleptomaniac may also steal from friends' houses, fellow guests in hotels, and elsewhere. The patient is usually a middle-aged middle-class woman with enough money to buy what she wants. Most are suffering from no other discernible psychiatric condition, whether *neurosis or *psychosis; but shop-lifting is said to occur more often in depressed perimenopausal women. The condition tends to persist in the face of embarrassment and disgrace. The criminal prosecution of such offenders is controversial, and has sometimes led to tragedy, for example suicide. The condition in men differs in pattern, being almost entirely confined to the stealing of books. Shop-lifting is the commonest crime committed by men over the age of 60.

KLINEFELTER'S SYNDROME is a condition, also known as 'seminiferous tubule dysgenesis', of impaired *gonadal development in the male, in which the genetic constitution is abnormal in having one or more extra X chromosomes (see GENETICS). The usual karyotype is 47, XXY. The condition is not familial, and an association with maternal age suggests that at least some cases are due to meiotic non-disjunction during gametogenesis. The extra X chromosome results in atrophy and hyalinization of the seminiferous tubules of the *testis but does not affect the *Leydig cells. Klinefelter's syndrome is a common sex anomaly, occurring in about 0.2 per cent of newborn males.

The cardinal features appear at or after puberty. They are: small, firm testes, *azoospermia, *gynaecomastia, and elevated urinary and serum *gonadotrophins. *Secondary sex characteristics may be poorly developed. Intellectual impairment and *psychopathy are common, and seem to vary directly with the number of X chromosomes; they are least when the karyotype is 47 (XXY) but are increasingly severe with 48 (XXXY) and 49 (XXXXY) genotypes. Klinefelter's syndrome may first be detected when the patient and his partner seek advice for infertility.

KLIPPEL–FEIL SYNDROME is a congenital shortening of the neck due to absence and/or fusion of cervical *vertebrae, conferring a characteristic appearance. Associated anomalies, such as *syringomyelia, are frequently present.

KLUMPKE, AUGUSTA. See DEJERINE, AUGUSTA.

KNOCK-KNEE, or genu valgum, is inward displacement of the knee joints so that they are abnormally close together.

KNOX, ROBERT (1791–1862). British anatomist. He was appointed Conservator of the Royal College of Surgeons of Edinburgh Museum in 1825. The following year he took over Barclay's school of anatomy and rapidly became the leading teacher of anatomy in

the city. Soon the *Burke and *Hare *resurrectionist' scandals involved him in such obloquy that his school was ruined. He left for London and became pathologist to the Cancer Hospital in Fulham in 1856.

KOCH, HEINRICH HERMANN ROBERT (1843–1910). German bacteriologist. In Wollstein, a small town in Posen, he established his own laboratory, culturing *Bacillus anthracis*, the organism of *anthrax (1876), studying sporulation, and developing *photomicrography of bacteria. He isolated *Mycobacterium *tuberculosis* in 1882 and in the same year enunciated the four postulates (*Koch's postulates) to be satisfied before accepting an organism as the cause of a specific disease. In 1883 he visited Egypt and India, where he identified the *Vibrio cholerae* as the cause of *cholera and the Koch–Weeks bacillus as responsible for a *conjunctivitis which was common locally. He noted the presence of amoebae in those dying with *dysentery. On a later visit to Africa he showed that *relapsing fever was due to a *spirochaete carried by a tick, *Ornithodorus moubata*. His latter years were occupied by controversies over *tuberculin, which he prepared in 1891. At first he claimed it as a cure for tuberculosis but was later forced to recant. He denied that the bovine *M. tuberculosis* was pathogenic to man. He was awarded the *Nobel prize in 1905.

KOCHER, EMIL THEODOR (1841–1917). Swiss surgeon, best known for his work on the *thyroid. He carried out over 5000 operations for *thyroidectomy and described postoperative *hypothyroidism (cachexia strumipriva) in 1883. He was awarded the *Nobel prize in 1909.

KOCH'S POSTULATES are the four criteria laid down by Robert *Koch as necessary to prove that a disease is caused by a particular micro-organism.

They are: (1) the organism must be observed in all cases of the disease; (2) it must be isolated and grown in pure culture; (3) the culture must be capable of reproducing the disease when inoculated into a suitable experimental animal; and (4) the organism must be recovered from the experimental animal. See INFECTIOUS DISEASES.

KÖLLIKER, RUDOLF ALBERT VON (1817–1905). Swiss anatomist and morphologist. A pioneer histologist and morphologist, he was the first to describe the structure of tissues in terms of cells.

KOROTKOFF, NIKOLAI SERGEIVICH (1874–1920). Russian physician. Korotkoff, a neglected figure in medical history, reported the technique of blood pressure measurement (*Korotkoff sounds) in 1905 in less than a page of the *Reports of the Imperial Military Medical Academy* of St Petersburg. As far as is known, he made no further contribution to cardiovascular research.

KOROTKOFF SOUNDS are the sounds heard on *auscultation over an artery, usually the brachial, when a pneumatic cuff proximal to it has been inflated to above systolic pressure and then slowly deflated while the cuff pressure is read on an attached manometer. No sound is heard while the cuff pressure exceeds systolic arterial pressure; the level at which faint tapping sounds synchronous with the pulse are first heard is the *systolic pressure. As the cuff is further deflated, the sounds grow gradually louder, then abruptly become muffled and soon disappear; the diastolic pressure is read at the point of disappearance.

KORSAKOFF, SERGEI SERGEIVICH (1854–1900). Russian neuropsychiatrist, best known for his description of alcoholic neuropathy with loss of memory for recent events (*Korsakoff's syndrome, 1887).

KORSAKOFF'S SYNDROME is a condition of severe *amnesia allied to a contrasting background mental state of full consciousness and clear perception. The amnesia relates to recent events, going back for perhaps about a year. A characteristic feature is confabulation whereby the patient gives detailed and convincing but totally fictitious accounts of his recent activity. Korsakoff's syndrome (or psychosis), which is often associated with *Wernicke's encephalopathy and due to *thiamine deficiency, is commonly the result of severe chronic *alcoholism; and the eponym is usually reserved for amnesia with this *aetiology. However, similar amnesic syndromes can occur with intoxication with other poisons, such as lead and carbon monoxide, after subarachnoid haemorrhage, and with various causes of severe malnutrition, including *carcinoma of the stomach and *hyperemesis gravidarum.

KOSSEL, KARL LUDWIG MARTIN LEONHARD ALBRECHT (1853–1927). German biochemist, noted for his work on the chemistry of the *nucleoproteins, during the course of which he discovered adenine, thymine, cytosine, and uracil. He was awarded the *Nobel prize in 1910.

KOUWENHOVEN, WILLIAM BENNETT (1886–1975). American electrical engineer. He was interested in electrical phenomena in animal tissues, and in the problem of *electric shock in man. He helped develop the technique of closed chest *resuscitation for shock victims and the technical details of counter-shock treatment (*defibrillation) to terminate fibrillation in the human heart.

KRAEPELIN, EMIL (1856–1926). German psychiatrist. He published a simple classification of insanity and was the first to draw a fundamental distinction between dementia praecox (now known as *schizophrenia) and *manic-depressive psychosis. His work on the psychiatric aspects of criminology was of great value.

KRAFFT-EBING, RICHARD FREIHERR VON (1840–1902). German psychiatrist. An authority on forensic psychiatry, he published a classical work on sexual deviations, *Psychopathia sexualis* (1876).

KRAUSE, WILHELM JOHANN FRIEDRICH (1833–1910). German anatomist. He described certain specialized sensory nerve end organs (*Krause's bulbs, 1860).

KRAUSE'S BULBS are terminal encapsulated nerve endings, also known as *Krause's corpuscles or bulboid corpuscles. They are thought to function as sensory (touch and pressure) *receptors.

KREBS, SIR HANS ADOLF (1900–82). Anglo-German biochemist. After working in Freiburg he came to the UK in 1933, first to Sheffield; he moved to the chair in Oxford in 1954, where he was director of the *Medical Research Council unit for research in cell metabolism. His two most important discoveries were the cyclic formation of *urea (1932) and the citric acid cycle (Krebs cycle, 1937), the chief source of metabolic energy. He was awarded the *Nobel prize for physiology with F.A. Lipman in 1952.

KROGH, SCHACK AUGUST STEENBERG (1874–1949). Danish physiologist. His researches covered a wide field including the chemical regulation of *respiration, the *pH of blood, the *oxygen consumption of tissues, and chemical changes in *muscle. He is best known for his studies on the physiology of the *capillaries for which he was awarded the *Nobel prize in 1920.

KUPFFER CELL. The representative in the *liver of the *reticuloendothelial system. Kupffer cells are large highly phagocytic pyramidal cells in the lining of the liver sinusoids.

KURU is a uniformly fatal (within months rather than years) cerebral degeneration characterized clinically by severe cerebellar *ataxia and *dementia, and pathologically by a diffuse *spongiform encephalopathy. The disease occurred only among a small group of primitive people in central New Guinea, and has now virtually disappeared. It is transmissible to subhuman primates by inoculation of brain material; the agent is a *prion (slow virus) bearing a close resemblance to that which causes *scrapie in sheep and *Creutzfeldt–Jakob disease in man. The disease resulted from human-to-human transmission by the ritual cannibalistic practice of eating the brains of dead relatives. Like the disease itself, this custom is now virtually extinct.

KUSSMAUL, ADOLF (1822–1902). German physician of wide interests, describing *periarteritis nodosa (1866), *progressive bulbar palsy (1873), *pulsus paradoxus (1873), and *diabetic coma with *ketosis and '*air hunger' (Kussmaul breathing, 1874). He introduced *gastric lavage (1867), *paracentesis of the pleura (1868), and *gastroscopy (1869).

KUSSMAUL BREATHING is a striking form of *hyperventilation, known as air-hunger, characteristic of severe metabolic *acidosis.

KUSTNER, HEINZ (1897–1931). German gynaecologist and obstetrician. Küstner made many contributions, but is remembered for his part in the Prausnitz–Küstner reaction. This is an allergic *hypersensitivity response of the skin when the offending substance is injected into the skin of a susceptible subject. Küstner knew that he could not eat cooked fish without experiencing itching, skin weals, coughing, sneezing, and vomiting, the reaction taking about 12 hours to settle down. Prausnitz, in 1921, took some of Küstner's *serum and some fish and injected the mixture into his own skin. The area became hot, red, and swollen, and the existence of cutaneous *anaphylaxis was established. Similar tests by other investigators followed rapidly. Variants are widely used in the study of allergic diseases (see ALLERGY; IMMUNOLOGY).

KWASHIORKOR. The term 'kwashiorkor' was introduced to describe the syndrome associated with severe protein-energy *malnutrition in children by Cicely Williams, a British paediatrician, in 1934 and originated in the country now known as Ghana (the approximate meaning is 'displaced child'; though not particularly helpful, it has become firmly established). The salient features are generalized *oedema, extreme *apathy, dry, brittle, and reddish hair, and a dermatosis resembling that of *pellagra, with dry hyperkeratotic pigmented lesions. Typically, subcutaneous fat is partly preserved, and *hepatomegaly is common; diarrhoea is almost invariable, and *anorexia is usual. Biochemistry is, as might be expected, considerably disordered, but a low serum *albumin is the central and essential abnormality.

KYMOGRAPHY is the recording of pressure (or other physiological variables) by vertical movement of a stylus on paper wrapped round a mechanically rotating drum, the paper having first been blackened with soot by holding it over a smoky flame.

KYPHOSCOLIOSIS is deformity of the thoracic *spine with abnormal convexity in both the posterior and one of the lateral directions.

KYPHOSIS is deformity of the thoracic *spine causing increased posterior convexity.

L

LABIA. Lips. When otherwise unqualified, taken to refer to the lesser and greater pudendal lips of the female external *genitalia.

LABORATORY MEDICINE. See CHEMISTRY, CLINICAL; MICROBIOLOGY; PATHOLOGY.

LABOUR is the process of childbirth, or parturition, by which a mother expels a *fetus from her *uterus through the *birth canal to the outside world, where it becomes an infant. Labour is divided into three stages. The *first* stage begins with the onset of regular uterine contractions and results in gradual dilatation of the orifice of the uterine *cervix; it ends when the cervix is maximally widened and forms a continuous passage (the birth canal) with the vagina. The *second* stage then begins with the descent of the fetus and ends when the fetus, now an infant, has been completely expelled. The *third* stage is occupied by the expulsion of the *placenta and membranes and ends when contraction of the uterus is completed. See OBSTETRICS.

LABYRINTH. The inner ear, comprising the *cochlea, vestibule, and *semicircular canals, and subserving hearing and balance. See OTORHINOLARYNGOLOGY.

LABYRINTHITIS is inflammation of the *labyrinth, or inner ear. Acute labyrinthitis may follow minor respiratory virus infections, causing *vertigo, nausea and vomiting, and *nystagmus.

LACERATION. A wound caused by tearing of tissue (as opposed to cutting).

LACRIMAL GLAND. Tear gland of the eye.

LACRIMATION. Formation and shedding of tears; weeping.

LACTATION is milk secretion and ejection by the breast. During pregnancy the breasts enlarge under the influence of high levels of *oestrogens, *progesterone, *prolactin, and perhaps placental *gonadotrophin (human chorionic gonadotrophin or HCG). Some milk is secreted into the mammary ducts from the fourth month of pregnancy onwards, but a large surge occurs after *parturition; this increase, coincident with evacuation of the uterine contents, is due to the associated drop in circulating oestrogen levels (it also occurs with abortion after the fourth month). Full lactation in women occurs 1–3 days after delivery, and continues under the influence of prolactin secretion. Suckling stimulates expression of milk from the nipple via the 'milk ejection reflex'; stimuli from sensitive touch receptors in and around the nipple cause secretion of *oxytocin from the posterior pituitary and this causes contraction of myoepithelial cells lining the mammary ducts (genital stimulation in lactating women has the same effect, sometimes causing milk to spurt from the breasts). Suckling reflexly maintains prolactin secretion; prolactin, as well as causing milk secretion, also inhibits *ovulation. Cessation of nursing is followed by a return of *menstruation in about 6 weeks.

LACTEALS. See CHYLOUS VESSELS.

LACTIC ACID ($CH_3CH(OH)COOH$) is a colourless crystalline organic acid formed by bacterial fermentation of *lactose.

LACTOBACILLUS is a genus of non-pathogenic lactose-fermenting *bacteria, species of which occur in the normal intestine.

LACTOSE is milk sugar, a hard white crystalline disaccharide ($C_{12}H_{22}O_{11}$), less sweet than sucrose, found in the milk of all mammals. On hydrolysis it yields *glucose and *galactose. It is often used as an *excipient or a *placebo. Some patients have lactose intolerance because of deficiency of the *enzyme lactase; lactose is then an osmotic *laxative.

LAENNEC, THEOPHILE RENE HYACYNTHE (1781–1826). French physician. He devised the *stethoscope and published *De l'auscultation médiate* (1819). In this book he analysed and described the sounds audible in diseases of the lungs and of the heart, firmly establishing the value of *auscultation. His terminology is still in use today. He died from pulmonary *tuberculosis, a disease of which he had made a profound study.

LAEVULOSE is fructose, or fruit sugar, a sweet crystalline soluble hexose monosaccharide ($C_6H_{12}O_6$) found in ripe fruit, nectar of flowers, and honey. It is converted by the liver to *glucose.

LAG is the delay between a stimulus and an observed reaction, or between any other two causally connected events.

LAHEY, FRANK HOWARD (1880–1953). American surgeon. He founded the Lahey Clinic in Boston and wrote extensively on surgical subjects, especially on surgical treatment of *thyroid disease.

LAMARCK, JEAN BAPTISTE PIERRE ANTOINE DE MONET DE (1744–1829). French naturalist. He contributed to botany by compiling his *Flore française*, based on a new method for identifying and classifying plants; he also contributed to chemistry, meteorology, zoology, and geology. He is chiefly notable, however, for his development of an early theory of *evolution, although he never used the actual term. Lamarck's work was largely neglected even in his lifetime, but was revived later in the controversies that followed Darwin's clearer statement of evolutional theory.

LAMINECTOMY is excision of the posterior vertebral arch, undertaken to expose the *spinal cord, or for spinal or nerve root decompression.

LAMSON, HENRY GEORGE (1849–1882). Doctor-murderer. Lamson qualified in Paris, but was a British subject. He was mentally unstable and a *morphine addict. Unsuccessful in practice in England and increasingly impecunious, he made one unsuccessful attempt to murder his crippled brother-in-law with *aconitine in the Isle of Wight, but eventually murdered him at Wimbledon, near London. The brother-in-law, aged 18, was due to inherit money at the age of 21. If he died before that age it was to be divided between his two sisters, one of whom was Kitty John, Lamson's wife. The trial aroused great interest as the vegetable alkaloid used as a poison was newly discovered, but was identified by forensic science.

LANCET. An influential weekly journal covering general medical topics, founded in 1823 and published in London. The *Lancet* publishes original communications, editorial comment, leading articles, scientific reviews, correspondence, medical news, and occasional papers; and it carries classified advertisements for vacancies open to the medical profession. The *Lancet* was founded by the stormy and controversial physician Thomas *Wakley (1795–1862). See also MEDICAL JOURNALS.

LANCISI, GIOVANNI MARIA (1654–1720). Italian physician. He served a succession of popes, and in 1706 was ordered by Clement XI to investigate the cause of the many sudden deaths occurring in Rome. He showed that they were usually due to heart disease and his *De subitaneis mortibus* (1707) and *De motu cordis et aneurysmatibus* (1728) are among the classics of cardiology. The second gives a good description of syphilitic heart disease. In *De noxii paludum effluviis* (1717) he suggested that *malaria was due to *mosquitoes, noted the pigment in the tissues of malarial patients, advised draining swamps, and advocated the use of *cinchona. He presented his large medical library to the hospital of Spirito Santo (1711).

LANDOUZY, LOUIS THEOPHILE JOSEPH (1845–1917). French neurologist. He described *leptospirosis icterohaemorrhagica (1883) and, with *Dejerine, facio-scapulohumeral *muscular dystrophy (1886).

LANDSTEINER, KARL (1868–1943). Austrian/American pathologist. He transmitted *poliomyelitis from human tissue to monkeys, by intracerebral inoculation. He studied human blood groups, demonstrating the ABO system, thus laying the foundation for safe *blood transfusion. For this work he received the *Nobel prize in 1930. He moved to the USA in 1919 as a member of the *Rockefeller Institute, and continued his immunological research. See IMMUNOLOGY.

LANE, SIR WILLIAM ARBUTHNOT, Bt (1856–1943). British surgeon. He was a brilliant surgical technician of great originality. He devised the 'no-touch operative technique' and an operation for *cleft palate which he carried out on 1-day-old babies. He was a firm believer in the doctrine of '*focal sepsis', a passionate advocate of brown bread, and founder of the New Health Society.

LANGENBECK, BERNHARD RUDOLF KONRAD VON (1810–87). German surgeon. In his time the greatest clinical surgeon in Germany, he founded the *Archiv für klinische Chirurgie* (1861) and the German Society of Surgery, both of which exerted great influence. A brilliant and original operator, he has 21 eponymic surgical procedures named after him.

LANGERHANS, PAUL (1847–88). German physician and pathologist. When working in *Virchow's laboratory in 1869 Langerhans described the pancreatic *islets to which his name is now attached. In 1875 he went to live and practise in Madeira because he had contracted pulmonary *tuberculosis.

LANGHANS, THEODOR (1839–1915). Swiss pathologist. He described the characteristic multinucleate *giant cells of tuberculous lesions.

LANGLEY, JOHN NEWPORT (1852–1925). British physiologist. He was the owner and editor of the *Journal of Physiology* from 1894 until 1925. His researches were mainly on the *sympathetic nervous system, and in 1921 he published the monograph *The autonomic nervous system*.

LANGUAGE is the body of words and word combinations comprising human speech. In most right-handed people, language function resides in the left cerebral hemisphere, although developmental capacity for speech also exists on the opposite side. See LANGUAGE, COGNITION, AND HIGHER CEREBRAL FUNCTION.

LANGUAGE, COGNITION, AND HIGHER CEREBRAL FUNCTION. In humans the *cerebral cortex has developed to its greatest extent, and this can be related to the emergence of language and logical and creative thought. These aspects of cerebral cortical function, together with memory and perceptual processing, are broadly considered under the rubric of higher cerebral function. Advances in *neuropsychology, *neuroanatomy, and neuroimaging (see RADIOLOGY), particularly activation studies using *positron emission tomography (PET), have advanced considerably our understanding of higher cerebral functions and their anatomical correlates. From studies of both normal cognition and careful case studies with circumscribed damage to the brain, information-processing models have been developed for specific cerebral functions (Shallice 1988). It is believed that cerebral cortical function is essentially modular, i.e. that particular circuits of the brain undertake a specific information process and the result of this is then combined with the result of another process in a hierarchical manner (Fodor 1983). There is no assumption that a specific function, or module, has a discrete anatomical location; as the cerebral cortex is a complex neuronal network, the processing may be distributed across a wide anatomical area. However, there is quite clear regional specialization, in that damage to particular cortical areas results in predictable cognitive deficits (McCarthy and Warrington 1990). The concept was developed by the now discredited phrenologists, although the main advance was the demonstration by *Broca in 1861 of the importance of the left frontal area for language. The major example of regional localization relates to cerebral asymmetry, with language and motor programming residing predominantly in the left

cerebral hemisphere. This occurs in approximately 99 per cent of right-handed people and in 70 per cent of left-handed people. By contrast, visuospatial processing is found in the right non-dominant hemisphere in right-handed individuals. Since the days of Broca the map of cortical function has been extended considerably by many techniques, such as activation studies using PET and the study of patients with localized lesions. The latter have most commonly been *tumours or *strokes; the size and site of the lesion dictating the characteristic clinical presentation, which ranges from loss of language, or *aphasia, through to very profound behavioural disturbances with frontal lobe damage. The nature of the lesion will often dictate the speed and extent of the deficit: strokes characteristically result in a sudden loss of function with variable poor recovery; by contrast, tumours will often result in a gradual loss of function, because the slow progression gives more time for the surrounding tissue to compensate. The regional specialization of the cerebral cortex can also give characteristic clinical syndromes due to disconnection of one area from the other by damage to the connecting white matter or fibre tracts, so-called disconnection syndromes. The best examples of this occur in patients with damage to the *corpus callosum. For example, a patient may be unable to name objects placed in the left hand since the sensory information relayed to the right hemisphere is disconnected from the language centre in the left hemisphere. By contrast, such a patient would be able to recognize and name objects in the right hand.

Memory
Memory, like language, is so central to our everyday life and survival that we often take it for granted, and yet memory loss, or *amnesia, may have devastating effects. Although the term memory is used in a general sense, there are, in fact, many types of memory, which can be impaired selectively in different diseases and following damage to different parts of the brain. The type of memory that we all immediately recognize, and which is very important personally, is so-called autobiographical or episodic memory, i.e. memory for those events that happen to us on a day-to-day basis. Structures of the temporal lobes of the brain, particularly the hippocampus and amygdala are central to this memory system. If both temporal lobes are damaged, then such patients may have a profound amnesia for everyday events. The famous case of HM, who had both the amygdala and hippocampus removed bilaterally for intractable *epilepsy, is a tragic example of a man who, while remembering factual knowledge and many motor skills, had no recollection of events on a day-to-day basis. Survivors of *herpes simplex *encephalitis, which also damages the temporal lobes, may present with an identical picture. In these cases memory for facts learnt in the distant past, such as memory for words and general knowledge, remain unaffected. Moreover, motor skills or procedural memory may also be spared.

Patients like HM may be able to learn a new skill, such as a new piano piece, and yet have absolutely no recollection of having done so. Another memory system is short-term or working memory, which provides a brief storage of facts for up to 30 seconds. This is the memory system that would be used to remember a telephone number long enough to dial it, but for redialling later this would need to pass into the long-term, or secondary memory store.

Language

Language is defined as a form of *communication that has grammar and semantics, that conveys meaning that can be abstract, referential (refers to actions at other times or locations), and is understood by other listeners. Speech is the oral-auditory expression and reception of language, but other modalities, such as reading–writing, manual sign language, communication by signals or gestures, navy ciphers, or computer communication, can all be considered to be forms of language. The human evolution of language can probably be related to the emergence of Neanderthal man, based on the anatomical features of the skull, which reflect a well-developed parietal fossa, particularly the posterior inferior portion, which is considered to be a specific human feature. Infants acquire language around the time of myelination of the language areas at 12–24 months, although vocalization and babbling are noted at 3–6 months. Comprehension precedes speech and, by the age of 3 years, speech is well developed and requires very well-coordinated and swift movements of the speech motor apparatus at a time when other motor skills are poorly developed. The ease with which children develop language under variable circumstances has led linguists to suggest that there is an innate capacity for grammar and semantics in the human brain, but if appropriate stimulation is not available, as in the cases of 'Kaspar Hauser' and 'Genie', then language fails to develop, even though non-verbal intelligence is preserved. Incomplete language development in Genie, who was kept in isolation until the age of 14 years, suggests that she had passed the critical age of language acquisition before receiving the appropriate stimulation. Some children with otherwise normal motor development and intelligence have a delay in speaking until 4 or 5 years, so it is important to distinguish these children from those in whom impaired hearing delays language acquisition. Reading and writing are acquired later, and some children have a specific difficulty in reading, referred to as developmental or congenital *dyslexia, which has a high familial incidence and is four times more common in boys than in girls. Dyslexia is often seen within the setting of other more common learning disabilities.

Acquired *dysphasia (impairment of language) is seen most commonly after strokes, when there is often partial recovery, or in association with tumours or degenerative diseases. There have been many clinical classifications of dysphasia, but broadly a distinction is made between a non-fluent and fluent dysphasia. In both cases comprehension may be impaired. With posteriorly placed lesions in the temporal lobe, speech may be fluent but meaningless, and accompanied by a severe comprehension deficit, *Wernicke's aphasia. Speech shows frequent semantic paraphrasias, i.e. substituting of an incorrect but semantically related word, for example 'chair' for 'table'. In addition, there may be phonemic paraphrasias, i.e. substitution of similar-sounding words, such as 'fable' instead of 'table'. Non-fluent aphasias have better preserved comprehension, but low-output and phonemic paraphrasias may be present. Broca's original case (1861) of a non-fluent aphasia was associated with a lesion in the left frontal lobe, and in similar cases articulation is often severely impaired. Global aphasia refers to a severe aphasia with both expression and comprehension being lost; only a few stereotyped utterances may be preserved. In contrast to aphasia, patients with *dysarthria have normal comprehension and syntactical and grammatical construction, but the motor control of speech is disrupted such that speech may be slurred, distorted, and difficult to understand. Impairment of writing, dysgraphia, and impairment of reading, dyslexia, are frequently seen in association with dysphasia, but both can occur in isolation. Acquired dyslexias are associated with lesions in the posterior, dominant parietal lobe.

Cortical motor programming is also localized to the dominant hemisphere, although motor control is related to the motor cortex which controls movement of the opposite, or contralateral, limbs. Dyspraxia is impairment of voluntary movements due to a failure of high-level motor programming. *Apraxia means loss of motor skills. By definition these cannot be diagnosed when there is a significant motor deficit due to *paralysis or diseases of the *basal ganglia and *cerebellum causing movement disorders. Patients with dyspraxia may appear confused when asked to perform a particular task and may have great difficulty with such tasks as using a knife and fork properly.

Visuospatial dysfunction and agnosia

Lesions in the non-dominant right hemisphere are associated with a variety of visuospatial and attentional deficits. Patients may, for example, have an impairment of topographical memory and easily get lost, or they may have difficulty with dressing, so-called dressing apraxia. Prosopagnosia, or failure to recognize faces, is also seen with right hemisphere lesions, and, if severe, patients may be unable to recognize family members by sight, but may immediately do so on hearing their voices. Neglect of contralateral space and of the contralateral half of the body can be a striking feature in some patients with right hemisphere lesions. Thus a patient may forget to put his arm into the left sleeve of his jacket and to shave the left half of his face. Frequently there is an associated left hemiparesis (or *hemiplegia) of which the patient may be unaware and, indeed, may claim that the paralysed limb belongs to somebody else. The denial of a left hemiparesis was referred to as anosognosia by Babinski and the term is now applied generally to a denial or lack of awareness of illness. Another striking example of anosognosia is Anton's syndrome, in which patients have cortical blindness due to damage to the occipital cortex and yet they will deny that they cannot see anything.

*Agnosia refers to a failure of recognition and has been studied in most detail in patients with visual agnosia. One hundred years ago Lissauer drew a distinction between apperceptive and associative visual agnosia, a distinction that has stood the test of time. With apperceptive agnosia the patient has difficulty with forming structural visual percepts and, as such, has difficulty in copying, matching, and identifying any object, and will have particular difficulty if the visual image is degraded or presented from an unusual view. Apperceptive agnosias are found in patients with right parietal lesions. Patients with associative agnosia are rare; in this syndrome the visual percept is normal, but they are unable to recognize the object, which is in a sense stripped of its meaning. Copying and matching, however, are normal. Patients with associative agnosia have usually been reported to have bilateral lesions, but it can be found with a left posterior lesion.

Frontal lobe dysfunction and dementia

The frontal lobes of the brain are concerned with selecting appropriate behavioural responses and inhibiting inappropriate responses, and with utilization of strategies for problem-solving. Patients with lesions in this region may perform well on routine neuropsychological tests of memory, language, and perception, but have profound behavioural difficulties and very poor novel problem-solving strategies, such that they can be quite impaired in everyday life. Patients may appear apathetic with very little motivation or, alternatively, may cause considerable social embarrassment with disinhibited behaviour. With severe frontal lobe syndromes, primitive reflexes may emerge, such as grasp responses to anything placed in the hands and sucking responses for any objects placed in or near the mouth.

The above examples of dysphasias, dyspraxias, memory defects, agnosias, and frontal lobe syndromes all refer to relatively circumscribed neuroanatomical or neuropsychological deficits. Patients with multiple domains of cognitive impairment are said to have *dementia. A variety of definitions has been developed for the term dementia; essentially they require that the patient has normal arousal, i.e. is awake and able to attend to tasks in hand, and also has a number of domains of cognitive impairment, one of which must be memory. The commonest cause of dementia is *Alzheimer's disease, in which there is cell loss and disruption of the synaptic network, particularly in the association areas of the cerebral cortex which are involved with language,

perception, and memory. The other major cause of dementia is so-called vascular dementia, due to multiple strokes or ischaemic changes in the cerebral cortex and the underlying white matter. However, any disease causing diffuse disruption of the neural network can result in dementia and so there are a host of different causes. By contrast to dementia, patients with a confusional state have dramatically impaired cognition, which is in part due to the disruption of their arousal and basic attentional mechanisms. Such patients may exhibit drowsiness or may be in an agitated hyper-aroused state; this is classically seen with alcohol withdrawal as in *delirium tremens. Confusional states are commonly seen with infections and with drug intoxication.

MARTIN ROSSOR

References

Fodor, J. (1983). *The modularity of mind.* MIT Press, Cambridge MA.

McCarthy, R. A. and Warrington, E. K. (1990). *Cognitive neuropsychology: a clinical introduction.* Academic Press, London.

Shallice, T. (1988). *From neuropsychology to mental structure.* Cambridge University Press.

LAPAROSCOPY is visual examination of the peritoneal cavity and the abdominal viscera with an *endoscope (laparoscope) inserted through the abdominal wall. The procedure, also called peritoneoscopy, involves puncturing the abdominal wall and the induction of a *pneumoperitoneum; it can be carried out using only sedation and a local anaesthetic. It is of value in diagnosis, particularly of liver conditions, and can guide a biopsy needle with great accuracy. (See also KEYHOLE SURGERY)

LAPAROTOMY is any surgical incision into the abdominal cavity, particularly when the operation is exploratory.

LAPLACE, PIERRE SIMON, MARQUIS DE (1749–1827). French mathematician. He discovered a theorem still of use in mathematics, while for medicine his value lies in his *Théorie analytique des probabilités* of 1812. This greatly helped on its way the investigation of *vital statistics and *epidemiology.

LARREY, DOMINIQUE-JEAN, BARON (1766–1842). French military surgeon. He introduced the 'ambulances volantes' in 1793 and travelled with the army through Germany, Austria, Spain, and Russia. Napoleon regarded him with affection and respect, leaving him 100 000 francs in his will. He was founder of the new military surgery. He made many clinical observations and was the first to amputate through the hip joint.

LARYNGITIS. Inflammation of the *larynx is not uncommon in the familiar acute viral infections of the upper respiratory tract, adding hoarseness or even *aphonia, pain, dryness of the throat, and cough to the symptoms. In infants laryngitis often causes stridor and the harsh resonant barking cough known as *croup. Laryngeal *diphtheria is now rare, as is chronic laryngitis due to *tuberculosis or *syphilis.

LARYNGOLOGIST. A specialist in diseases of the throat and nose. See OTORHINOLARYNGOLOGY.

LARYNGOSCOPE. Any instrument enabling visualization of the *larynx.

LARYNGOSCOPY is inspection of the interior of the *larynx with an illuminated instrument called a laryngoscope; this is known as direct laryngoscopy. In indirect laryngoscopy the larynx is examined with an angled mirror and reflected light.

LARYNX. The voice-box, situated at the upper end of the *trachea where the latter opens into the throat. The larynx is a valve which closes during swallowing and so prevents entry of food and drink into the lungs. In man it has become specialized so as also to serve voice production. See also EPIGLOTTIS; GLOTTIS.

LASER is *l*ight *a*mplification by *s*timulated *e*mission of *radiation. This produces a powerful, highly directional, monochromatic, and coherent beam of light. The various uses of laser beams in medicine include particularly ophthalmic surgery (see OPHTHALMOLOGY).

LASSA FEVER is one of the much-feared viral haemorrhagic fevers, which occurs sporadically in rural areas of West Africa, notably Nigeria, Liberia, and Sierra Leone. It is due to a small *ribonucleic acid (RNA) virus of the arenavirus group; the animal reservoir is a wild rodent, the multimammate rat, *Mastomys natalensis*, and human infection is thought to occur by contact with infected rat excreta. The clinical manifestations are those of an acute severe illness, with fever, prostration, shock, sometimes *pharyngitis, *proteinuria, *oedema of the face and neck, and haemorrhagic phenomena. The mortality rate in observed cases is high, between 20 and 50 per cent; but subclinical infection with recovery may be commoner than is supposed among inhabitants of endemic areas.

Strict isolation and the administration of convalescent plasma are the main principles of management, together with general supportive care as necessary with any severe illness. In fact, the person-to-person contact risk is probably very small; infection is most likely to spread to those handling specimens of blood, urine, and vomit, as has occurred in some *nosocomial outbreaks. With such specimens the strictest security must be observed.

Work with Lassa fever virus should be undertaken only by the laboratories at the Center for Disease Control, Atlanta, Georgia, USA, or the Microbiological Research Establishment, Porton Down, Wiltshire, UK.

LASSITUDE is a feeling of weakness or exhaustion which can be quite overwhelming. The word derives from the Latin for 'weary'.

LATAH is the Malay name under which a form of religious hysteria (hysterical automatic obedience, often associated with the copying of actions) is known in Java. It may also be characterized by a rapid ejaculation of inarticulate sounds, and a succession of involuntary movements, with temporary loss of consciousness. The condition is said to be prevalent among Malay women and other peoples of South-East Asia.

LATHYRISM is spastic *paraplegia caused by eating peas of the genus *Lathyrus*, notably *Lathyrus sativa*. It has been reported from many parts of the world, including Africa, Iran, India, and some Mediterranean countries. The incidence is said to be higher in times of drought and famine, when consumption of the peas is greater, and when the crop has been subjected to long storage. The toxic substance responsible is thought to be beta-aminoproprionitrile. The condition is progressive, and accompanied by muscle pain, *paraesthesiae, and urinary incontinence.

LATRODECTUS is a genus of venomous spiders which includes *Latrodectus mactans*, the *black widow spider.

LAUBRY, CHARLES (1872–1941). Parisian cardiologist. With others he established the technique of injection of *radiopaque substances into the heart and great vessels for studying their anatomy, paving the way for modern methods of cardiological investigation in the living. In 1939 he published *Radiologie clinique du coeur et des gros vaisseaux*.

LAUDANUM was a famous remedy of *Paracelsus, of which *opium was thought to have been the active ingredient; later the term was used for opiate mixtures; it is now applied to *tincture of opium (containing 1 per cent *morphine).

LAUGHING GAS is nitrous oxide, a widely employed general anaesthetic agent. See ANAESTHESIA.

LAUGHTER is the physical expression (unarticulated sounds, facial contortions, and heaving body movements) characteristic of amusement and mirth, evoked by events, situations, appearances, thoughts, etc. of a ludicrous or incongruous nature or by bodily stimuli such as tickling. Laughter can be pathological as when it is a paradoxical response to situations where grief would be expected.

LAVAGE. Synonymous with *irrigation.

LAVERAN, CHARLES LOUIS ALPHONSE (1845–1922). French physician. Posted to Algeria in 1878, he undertook research on *malaria and in Constantine on 6 November 1880 found the parasite responsible. From 1884 to 1894 he was professor of military hygiene at Val de Grâce, but left the army in 1896 to work at the *Pasteur Institute. He was awarded the *Nobel prize in 1907 for his work on *protozoa.

LAVOISIER, ANTOINE LAURENT (1743–94). French chemist. His researches were important and wide-ranging. In 1775 after a meeting with *Priestley he realized the significance of Priestley's 'dephlogisticated air' which he renamed 'oxygine' in 1787. He showed that the amount of *oxygen absorbed by the body was increased by eating, by physical work, and at low temperatures. He was guillotined in May 1794.

LAW AND MEDICINE (MEDICAL JURISPRUDENCE) IN THE UK. The law regulates, and even limits, many aspects of *medical practice and conduct, and may be called in to evaluate the medical services provided to an individual or class of persons. The fundamental principles of English law stem from Judaeo-Christian concepts of morality as propounded and applied by judges over the centuries—common law—subject to statutes passed by Parliament and, more recently, also EC directives.

Investigations by a *coroner into the causes of an unexpected or unnatural death may include cases where death followed from medical treatment or, indeed, the lack of it. The coroner's *inquest, as its name suggests, takes the form of an inquiry and is not intended to be adversarial in character, although, in practice, the hearing may provide something of a preliminary battleground. The aim and ambit of an inquest are only to establish the cause of death and not to attribute blame or *negligence. However, the proceedings can provide a useful preliminary hearing for the family who believe that negligence was to blame for the death of a relative, similarly, for those representing the doctors or medical carers whose clinical management of the patient was reviewed, giving an indication as to whether a civil claim for negligence could be brought successfully. Very rarely, the evidence may suggest that a party who had responsibility for the medical care was reckless beyond the point of mere inadequacy, and the coroner may halt the inquest and refer the matter to the Crown Prosecution Service for investigation rather than leave the jury to enter a verdict.

Regulation and limits imposed on medical treatment
For instance, the law defines in what circumstances *abortions may be performed and limits other aspects of treatment related to fertility or, indeed, *infertility

(Offences Against the Person Act 1861, as amended by the Abortion Act 1967 and the Human Fertilization and Embryology Act 1990, the Surrogacy Arrangements Act 1985 and the Infant Life Preservation Act 1929). There are also clear legal requirements (and also guidelines) which must be satisfied in cases where mentally ill patients are detained and treated compulsorily against their wishes and/or without their consent (Mental Health Act 1983).

Where disputes arise as to whether medical treatment in particular circumstances (such as an abortion on a mentally handicapped woman who cannot give valid consent) is lawful, a declaration that the treatment is not unlawful may be sought from the High Court and in such circumstances a declaration must be sought where the handicapped woman is under 18 (*F.* v. *West Berkshire Health Authority and Another* [1989] 2 All ER 545; see also *In re B (Wardship) (sterilization)* [1988] 1 AC 199, [1987] 2 All ER 206). Similarly, the approval of the High Court was sought by the doctors and parents of Tony Bland to discontinue medical treatment, which included intravenous feeding and hydration as well as the administration of *antibiotics and other medical measures. Tony Bland had lain in a *persistent vegetative state since April 1989 when he suffered devastating crush injuries at the Hillsborough Stadium disaster (Brahams 1992*a*, 1993; *Airedale NHS Trust* v. *Bland* [1993] 2 WLR 316). In the leading case of *Gillick* the courts were invited to consider whether, and in what circumstances, doctors and others providing *family planning services could do so for children aged under 16, even in cases where they knew that the child's parents objected (Brahams 1985; *Gillick* v.*West Norfolk and Wisbech Area Health Authority and Another* [1986] AC 112, [1985] 3 All ER 402). Where the child has sufficient maturity and understanding, she or he may validly consent to medical treatment, including that associated with family planning, as if of full age. In all these cases the issues were of such public importance and interest that they were taken to and decided upon by the House of Lords.

Actions for compensation
Civil proceedings in the medico-legal sphere are normally brought in the hope of obtaining compensation for injuries suffered in consequence of allegedly negligent medical treatment or, indeed, the failure to provide treatment at all where it was needed. The plaintiff and his family (and it may be the patient's estate if he is dead) may concomitantly hope they will also learn precisely how the injury occurred and hope that by airing this, others may be spared a similar misfortune. All too often, proceedings are commenced following a failure by the defendants to provide a full and adequate explanation of what happened, with, where appropriate, an apology.

Generally, proceedings will be brought in negligence but occasionally there may also arise a claim in battery and trespass to the person—namely that the treatment was given without the patient's consent to it or expressly against his or her stated wishes. If treatment was provided 'privately', then the patient may also sue for breach of contract (it is implicit that contractual obligations will be performed with reasonable skill and care) and there may be precise requirements to visits or the provision of services by a particular doctor which have been breached. If the doctor is unwise enough to 'guarantee' the outcome of any procedure, and this does not materialize, then damages would follow irrespective of whether he was, in fact, negligent. Lawyers recognize that medical procedures may fail, and therefore, guarantees of perfection are never implied into agreements to perform medical procedures, see *Eyre* v. *Measday* [1986] 1 All ER 488. In *Thake and Another* v. *Maurice (1986)* ([1986] QB 644, [1986] 1 All ER 479) the plaintiff succeeded on other grounds.

Criminal recklessness

Occasionally, medical treatment may be judged so grossly negligent as to be criminally reckless. If the patient dies, the doctor may be charged with manslaughter. Recently, there have been several such convictions in the criminal court (Brahams 1990, 1992*b*), two separate cases where death was caused by recklessly negligent provision of *anaesthesia and another death involving two doctors who prescribed gross and inappropriate quantities of psychotropic and hypnotic drugs to a remand prisoner who had recently been weaned off *heroin. These prosecutions may mark something of a growing trend, and in principle there seems no reason to prosecute only in cases where the patient has died rather than having been very seriously injured. In the earlier case of *R.* v. *Bateman* (1925) 94 LJKB 791, the Court of Appeal quashed a conviction of manslaughter, holding that the substandard medical care given by a *general practitioner to a woman in childbirth and afterwards was not so criminally reckless as to justify a conviction of manslaughter.

Negligence

Most treatment in the UK is provided under the *National Health Service (NHS). Under the NHS there will be no contract between the patient and the providers of medical services as compared with the contractual relationship which is created by the provision of medical (and e.g. hospital) services to patients for fees in the private sector. For a claim in negligence to be successful, the plaintiff must prove to the civil standard, namely on the balance of probabilities, that:

(1) the defendant (*doctor, *nurse, *dentist, *chemist, or other health-care provider, etc.) owed him a duty of care;

(2) the treatment/services provided fell below the standard of skill and care reasonably to be expected; and

(3) the patient suffered significant injury, loss, and damage in consequence of the negligent medical care or services provided (or as a result of the lack of provision where this should have been given).

Civil trials for medical negligence or breach of contract are now heard before a judge sitting alone.

Duty of care

In general, the Law does not require doctors to act as good samaritans. Legally they are not under an obligation to volunteer and offer professional help simply because they happen to be present as casual bystanders or passing by when somebody falls ill or suffers an accident. However, *medical ethics does require that they offer help when they are able and, indeed, it could prove embarrassing to a doctor if he were found to have been at the scene of an accident and to have left anonymously before skilled help had arrived (or perhaps was on the point of arrival). That said, many doctors are now worried that, if their intervention proved unhelpful or unsuccessful, they risk being sued for damages. Many who work full-time for the NHS and do not carry private cover would be uninsured when acting outside their employment. There does, however, seem to be a strong case for their employers to extend crown indemnity cover to situations such as these or, alternatively, for all doctors to carry compulsory minimum insurance to cover such eventualities, even after they retire, for minimum premiums.

The fear of a law suit is probably greater than the reality (I know of no reported cases brought against good samaritan doctors in Britain). However, the fear of a negligence claim is none the less understandable in the light of many doctors' privately acknowledged poor expertise in accident and emergency situations and the rise in numbers of claims brought against doctors and hospitals.

In contrast, the law imposes a duty of care on a doctor or other health-care professional where the person requiring attention is already a patient or has presented at the casualty department of a hospital or some other appropriate hospital department or health-care centre. In *Barnett* v. *Chelsea and Kensington Management Committee* (1969) ([1969] 1 QB 428, [1968] 1 All ER 1068) three night watchmen presented themselves at about 8.00 a.m. on 1 January 1966 at a hospital casualty department. They saw the nurse on duty; from their demeanour and the description of symptoms (which included vomiting) provided by one of the men it was clear they were all three feeling ill. The nurse telephoned the casualty officer who told them to go home to bed and call their own doctors. One of them died a few hours later. Death was subsequently found to be due to arsenical poisoning but the evidence showed there was no reasonable prospect of an antidote being given before the death. Thus, although there was a finding by the judge that the defendant health authority, by providing and running the casualty department to which the deceased had presented himself with a complaint of illness or injury, owed him a duty to exercise the skill and care to be expected of a nurse and a casualty officer, and the defendants, through their casualty officer, were negligent and in breach of their duty to examine the deceased and admit him to hospital and treat him, there had been no injury caused by the negligence and breach of duty of care owed because the plaintiff (the deceased's widow) was not able to prove on the balance of probabilities that the death was caused by the negligence.

Once the legal duty of care is in place, the doctor is bound to act with due skill, care, and competence, and must comply with that accepted as proper by a responsible body of medical opinion.

The standard of skill and care: the reasonable doctor test

The standard of care the law expects from any professional, including a doctor or a dentist, will be higher than that expected from the reasonable man or woman in the street. This is because professionals, by definition, hold themselves out as possessing superior skill and knowledge and expect to be retained on that basis. Their competence will be judged by reference to the standards found acceptable by a responsible body of medical opinion (including a minority opinion). In Law, the term 'negligence' does not automatically imply 'neglect' (although this may be a factor), but means simply that the services provided by the professional concerned fell below an acceptable standard of professional conduct judged by his peers. Although there are earlier authorities of historical interest, the cornerstone of all medical negligence claims is the test laid down by McNair J. to the jury in *Bolam* v. *Friern Hospital Management Committee* (1957) ([1957]) 1 WLR 582, [1957] 2 All ER 118) and slightly differently stated 2 years earlier by the Lord President Clyde in the Scottish case of *Hunter* v. *Hanley* (1955) [1955] SLT 213, [1955] SC 200).

In *Hunter* v. *Hanley* the Plaintiff was being treated by Dr Hanley with a course of 12 injections of procaine penicillin in the buttocks with a size 16 needle. In November 1951, during the twelfth injection, the needle broke and remained embedded in her body. She sued in negligence. The trial judge directed the jury that to succeed they had to make a finding of 'gross negligence'. On appeal, this direction was held to be inaccurate and a new trial was ordered. Lord President (Clyde) said:

In the realm of diagnosis and treatment there is ample scope for genuine difference of opinion and one man clearly is not negligent merely because his conclusion differs from that of other professional men, nor because he has displayed less skill and knowledge than others would have shown. The true test in establishing negligence in diagnosis or treatment on the part of the doctor is whether he has been proved to be guilty of such failure as no doctor of ordinary skill would be guilty if acting with ordinary care.

This test was considered by J. McNair in the English case of *Bolam* (which arose from injuries caused by

*electroconvulsion therapy (ECT) given to the plaintiff) who claimed that the administration of the treatment was negligent by reason of the failure to use relaxant drugs or some form of manual control and in failing to warn him of the risk involved before the treatment was given. In the summing-up, the jury were directed:

1. A doctor is not negligent if he is acting in accordance with a practice accepted as proper by a responsible body of medical men skilled in that particular art, merely because there is a body of such opinion that take a contrary view.
2. That the jury might well think that when a doctor was dealing with a mentally sick man and had a strong belief that his only hope of cure was submission to electroconvulsive shock therapy, the doctor could not be criticized if, believing the dangers involved to be minimal, he did not stress them to the patient.
3. In order to recover damages for failure to give warning the plaintiff must prove not only that the failure to give warning was negligent but also that if he had been warned he would not have consented to the treatment.

The jury found for the defendants.

In *Wilsher* v. *Essex Area Health Authority* [1987] QB 730 the Court of Appeal held that the standard of care to be expected had to be judged objectively (the findings on causation by the trial judge were rejected by the House of Lords and retrial suggested but the case was settled). Where the care is provided by a specialized unit, it must be of an appropriate standard to be expected from that unit and not what might reasonably have been expected (subjectively) from, for example, a new junior doctor on the staff who personally had little experience and knowledge. Since the bulk of NHS hospital care is provided by doctors in training, it is imperative that such staff should be properly supervised and must consult senior colleagues when the need arises. Unfortunately, all too often it may be the very ignorance of the junior doctor or nurse which fails to alert him or her to the need for intervention by senior staff. This begs the question of when a junior doctor will be found negligent for failing to recognize the extent of his ignorance and calling for assistance, and how far such decisions should be left to him but anticipated by appropriate review and supervision. *Wilsher* suggests that the *health authority may be directly liable if its organization (and services) are at fault and cause injury, and certainly it is routine for plaintiffs' lawyers to plead that the health authority negligently failed to provide appropriately qualified staff and medical care of a satisfactory standard, and this would seem a powerful submission. However, the only reported decision directly in support of this proposition seems to be *Bull and Wakeham* v. *Devon Health Authority* (Court of Appeal 1989) which related in part to the unsatisfactory organization of the services provided and the siting of those services in relation to one another (*Lancet* 1989).

The House of Lords decision in *Maynard* v. *West Midlands Regional Health Authority* [1984] 1 WLR 634 makes it clear that judges must not merely pay lip service to the test in *Bolam* (and *Hunter* v. *Hanley*), and cannot exercise a preference in favour of one of two or more practices thought proper by a 'responsible' body of medical opinion and in this way find the practice supported by the other view, negligent.

The *Bolam* test applies across the whole spectrum of medical and clinical care and management and does not distinguish between counselling, therapeutic, and non-therapeutic treatment. However, the courts have offered some tempering of *Bolam* in principle at least, with regard to the issue of consent and the minimum amount of information which must be volunteered to a patient who does not ask questions or probe.

Consent

It seems from the House of Lords decision in *Sidaway* v. *Board of Governors of Bethlem Royal Hospital and the Maudsley Hospital and others* [1985] AC 871 that in the case of a lucid patient, before consent can be regarded as 'informed' it must require that sufficient information be given in each case for the patient to make a reasonably informed decision. In that case, the plaintiff, Mrs Sidaway, suffered with persistent pain in her arms and her right shoulder. The source of her pain was diagnosed as pressure on the fourth cervical nerve root. A laminectomy of the fourth cervical vertebra and facetectomy or foraminectomy of the disc space between the fourth and fifth cervical vertebrae was performed. The surgeon freed the fourth cervical nerve root by removing the facets from the fourth vertebra and used a dental drill to free the nerve within the foramen. The plaintiff's spinal cord was damaged and she suffered severe disability in consequence.

She sued the hospital and the surgeon's estate in negligence, originally also claiming battery due to lack of informed consent. The operation was found to have been competently performed; her claim was based on the failure to warn her of the risk of damage to the *spinal cord and subsequent *paralysis. Evidence at trial was that the combined risk was between 1 and 2 per cent and that the risk of damage to the spinal cord alone—the more serious risk—was less than 1 per cent. The trial judge found as a fact that the surgeon had mentioned the possibility of disturbing the nerve root but not of spinal cord damage, and that this was not negligent because there was a responsible body of medical opinion in 1974 that supported this practice. He also found that had Mrs Sidaway been warned of the danger of cord damage she would have refused the operation.

The claim in battery was rejected. It was further argued for Mrs Sidaway that *Bolam* was not the correct test in relation to claims based on a failure to warn and that the disclosure of risks should not have been judged on this basis but by the American 'prudent patient' test, namely the amount of information which objectively would be required by a 'prudent patient' in Mrs Sidaway's position. This submission was rejected roundly at each stage of the litigation and *Bolam* adopted, although in the House of Lords, Lord Scarman said he would have accepted it (but would still not have found for the plaintiff on the facts). However, in the Court of Appeal there were murmurings that doctors could not be allowed to play God, and in the House of Lords, notwithstanding the approval of *Bolam* (and also *Chatterton* v. *Gerson and Another* [1981] 1 QB 432) it was made clear that some risks were so large and so serious that they should be disclosed, e.g. a 4 per cent risk of death and a 10 per cent risk of a stroke—facts taken from actual cases decided across the Atlantic. If these serious risks were not disclosed, then the doctor would have to justify his decision to withhold this information. Furthermore, (per curiam) where a plaintiff asked questions, the doctor was under a duty to answer them truthfully and as fully as the questioner requires—although in practice this will not necessarily require minutely detailed answers but will usually be satisfied by a broad-brush approach, that need not take in for example, research data in the files, see *Blyth* v. *Bloomsbury Health Authority* (1987) PMILL vol. 3 No. 2.

English law proceeds on the basis that a lucid adult is entitled to retain control over what happens to his or her body and that medical treatment which is given without consent is a trespass to the person and a battery. This may also give rise to criminal proceedings where appropriate. However, where the patient consents to undergo medical treatment of the general kind given but later complains that the consent was based on inadequate information (usually warnings of risks of failure), the patient cannot then claim that her consent was vitiated from the start, but must sue in negligence However, compare *Cull* v. *Butler* [1932] 1 BMJ 1195, where specific refusal to undergo a *hysterectomy was ignored (in error), and *Hamilton* v. *Birmingham Regional Hospital Board* (1969) 2 BMJ 456 and *Devi* v. *West Midlands Regional Health Authority* 9 December 1981 CA) where *sterilization was performed without consent. In all these three cases the treatment amounted to a battery and trespass to the person. See also *Allan* v. *Mount Sinai Hospital et al.* (1980) 109 DLR (3d) 634, where an anaesthetic was given without consent and was held to be a battery and trespass to the person and the defendants were held responsible for all the consequences which flowed therefrom, even if not foreseeable.

In an emergency, consent can be deemed if the treatment is required and should not be delayed until consciousness is recovered (as in *Marshall* v. *Curry* [1933] 3 DLR 260) but not merely where it is regarded as convenient and expedient. However, deemed consent is not possible in the face of previously expressed refusals, e.g. by a Jehovah's witness. This is well illustrated by the Canadian case of *Malette* v. *Shulman et al.* (1988) 47 DLR (4th) 18 and see also [1991] 2 Med LR 162, where a casualty surgeon who provided a *blood transfusion to a patient at risk of death following a traffic accident but in knowing disregard of a card refusing acceptance of blood transfusions was successfully sued in trespass.

In the UK the position is similar, although the decision must be proved genuine and not a result of undue influence by a relative, see *Re T* [1992] 3 WLR 782 and notwithstanding the idiosyncratic decision of *In re S* ([1992] 3 WLR 806) (a court decision purporting to declare as not unlawful an operation to perform a *Caesarean section against the wishes of the mother (and her husband) to save the life of the mother and baby (the latter did not survive in any event)) (see also Brahams 1992c). It is notable that in the *Bland* case (*Airedale NHS Trust v. Bland* [1993] 2 WLR 316-400 HL (E), CA and Fam D, Brahams 1992a, 1993) the House of Lords [1993] (and also the Court of Appeal [1992] (Brahams 1993)) emphasized the right to self-determination and the right of a lucid individual to have his or her views respected with regard to acceptance or refusal of medical treatment even if he or she is no longer lucid and mentally capable by the time the issue of whether or not medical treatment should be given has to be decided.

However, though a patient may lawfully refuse treatment and feeding, which may lead to his death, a doctor may not in England and Wales aid or abet a *suicide, albeit that suicide is no longer a crime in itself in England (see the Suicide Act 1961). A doctor may lawfully provide treatment, including drugs, for the relief of *pain which incidentally also have the effect of shortening life, but may not give drugs with the purpose only of ending life, and in this way also the pain and suffering (*R.* v. *Cox* (1992); *R.* v. *Arthur* (1981); Devlin 1985). In *Bland* it was held that medical treatment included drugs and therapy and also nasogastric feeding and other extraordinary measures aimed at hydrating and feeding artificially, and that where a patient gained no therapeutic benefit from continuance of therapy it was lawful to discontinue it, even if the patient was in no condition to refuse or consent.

Children
Under s.8 of the Family Law Reform Act 1969, a child aged 16 and above may consent to medical and dental treatment as if of full age. *Gillick* (*Gillick* v. *West Norfolk and Wisbech Area Health Authority and Another* [1986] AC 112, [1985] 3 AII ER 402) makes it clear that a child below the age of 16 may, where appropriate, also provide a valid consent. Up to the age of 18, the child can be made a ward of court and the court can then override the child and/or its parents in what it perceives as the child's best interests *In re R.* (*A Minor*) (*Wardship: consent to Treatment*) [1991] 3 WLR 592, CA. Lord Donaldson also said (*obiter*), in the case of *R.* that parents could give a valid consent

to treatment in the face of the child's refusal. Recently the courts have reviewed how far the child has the right to refuse treatment thought to be in his interests, and when this would and should be overriden. In *R.* the patient was a psychiatrically disturbed girl of 15 in the care of the local authority who did not wish to ingest antipsychotic drugs. She was overriden, and in any event not found to be *Gillick* competent as her mental condition rendered her without insight and judgment. *In re W. (A Minor) (Medical Treatment) (The Times*, 24 July 1992) the Court of Appeal overrode the refusal of a girl aged 16 to consent on her behalf to necessary treatment for *anorexia nervosa. In that case the judge had found the girl *Gillick* competent but said the court should and would override her refusal in her interests. In the Court of Appeal, Lord Donaldson said the court's inherent powers under *parens patriae* jurisdiction were limitless and extended beyond those of a natural parent. In this case the court disagreed with the trial judge and doubted the girl's competence to give a valid and informed refusal because the nature of her disease would impair her judgement in that it created a compulsion to refuse treatment or accept treatment perceived unlikely to be effective. The Court did not order doctors to treat, but rather authorized them to do so according to their clinical judgement. This was also the approach in the case of *Re J. (A Minor) (Medical Treatment) (The Times*, 12 June 1992) in the case where discontinuance of treatment would allow a very seriously handicapped baby to die (for a useful discussion on the concept of freedom of choice in this context see Lewis 1992).

Although, normally, parents can be expected to consent to medical examination and treatment in the best interests of their children, where a doctor considers that consent is refused against the child's interests, e.g. on religious grounds or to conceal some criminal or other undesirable conduct on the part of the parents or a member of the family, this refusal may have to be overriden if this is an emergency which cannot wait for a court order. However, in such circumstances, a second opinion should be sought and all discussions and relevant history noted and every effort made to persuade the parents to co-operate.

DIANA BRAHAMS

References
Brahams, D. (1985). Contraceptive advice for underage girls. *Lancet*, **ii**, 959.

Brahams, D. (1990). *R.* v. *Adomako* and *R.* v. *Sargent*. Two anaesthetists convicted of manslaughter. *Lancet*, **336**, 340.

Brahams, D. (1992a). Of life and death. *Law Society's Gazette*, 16 December, 3.

Brahams, D. (1992b). *R.* v. *Soha and Salim*. Death of a remand prisoner. *Lancet*, **340**, 1462.

Brahams, D. (1992c). Compulsory intervention during pregnancy. *Lancet*, **240**, 1029.

Brahams, D. (1993). Persistent vegetative state. *Lancet*, **340**, 1534.

Devlin, P. (1985). *Easing the passing*. Bodley Head, London.
Lancet (1989). *Lancet*, **i**, 738.
Lewis, C. (1992). M. H. and D. J. Brahams, *Law Society's Gazette*, 16 December, 27.
R. v. Arthur (1981). *Law Society's Gazette*, 25 November.
R. v. Cox (1992). *Lancet*, 26 September; *Medico-Legal Journal*, **60**, (4), 227; Brahams, D. *Law Society's Gazette*, 30 September, 2.

Further reading
Brahams, D. (ed.) (1989). *Medicine and law*. Royal College of Physicians, London.
Jones, M. (1991). *Medical negligence*. Sweet and Maxwell, London.
Law Commission (1993). *Mentally incapacitated adults and decision making*. Consultation Paper 129. HMSO, London.
Lewis, C. (1992). *Medical negligence*. Tolley, Croydon.
Mason J. K., and McCall Smith, N. (1991). *Law and medical ethics*, (3rd edn). Butterworths, Oxford.
Nelson-Jones and Burton (1991). *Medical negligence case law*. Fourmat Publishing.

LAW AND MEDICINE (MEDICAL JURISPRUDENCE) IN THE USA
Introduction
The practice of medicine in the USA is affected by both federal and state law. On many issues there are variations between the states with regard to specific legal principles, or their application in particular situations, which make it difficult to generalize.

Medical licensure
Licensing legislation for *physicians exists in every state, and for other health professions, such as *nursing, *psychology, *dentistry, and *optometry, in all, or many, states. Licensure for health professionals began in the 19th century and was held valid by the US Supreme Court as a legitimate exercise of the state's police power because its objective is to protect the public from harm likely to follow the ministrations of unqualified and incompetent practitioners.

Licensing boards have increasingly been concerned with matters of professional competence, stimulated by malpractice in rendering health services, and physical and/or mental impairment of licensees. Licensing boards no longer are exclusively composed of members of the licensed profession; usually they also include public or consumer members.

*Malpractice
Malpractice is negligence of a professional. Increased malpractice litigation against physicians and other health practitioners, together with increases in the amounts of verdicts (settlements in the UK) and recognition of new liability theories and additional elements of compensable harm, have resulted in much higher premiums for liability insurance. Unlike Canada and the UK, in the USA an injured person ordinarily has the right to a trial before a jury in a personal injury suit.

For imposition of liability for malpractice, the physician must have failed to meet the standard of care applicable in malpractice litigation; to wit, that degree of care, skill, and judgement generally exercised by competent and skilful practitioners of the defendant's profession, and for harm to be suffered as a result. The standard is frequently stated without reference to the level of practice within the locality, thus acknowledging national standards for professional performance.

Advances in medical knowledge and technology, by maintaining life in circumstances when it previously could not be done, have had profound effects on the amount of damages in malpractice litigation. For example, the cost of rearing a defective child where *amniocentesis was not recommended by the physician to a pregnant woman in the latter part of her childbearing years (thus denying the opportunity to consider whether to undergo an *abortion if the *fetus was defective), has been recognized as compensable harm.

Hospital liability for medical malpractice
Liability is imposed on hospitals for harm resulting from malpractice in the performance of medical services on two bases. The doctrine of *respondeat superior* is applied when the physician is deemed a servant of the hospital because of an employment relationship, or where the trier of fact finds that the physician, although an independent contractor, is the ostensible agent of the hospital because the patient has not selected the physician who has rendered the service and the physician appears to be an employee of the hospital. Liability on a corporate negligence theory is imposed where a patient was injured as the result of malpractice by an independent contractor physician appointed to the hospital's medical staff when the hospital knew, or should have known, that the physician, based on review of prior medical performance or information from other sources, was unqualified or incompetent.

Consent
In traditional consent litigation, the source of law is intentional tort (battery) and the question is whether the patient, or someone legally authorized on his behalf, authorized the procedure performed. However, the greater part of consent litigation deals with informed consent; the issue being whether necessary information was provided when obtaining consent prior to the procedure being performed. Failure to secure informed consent because of inadequate disclosure is viewed as a type of malpractice—an unintentional tort. The test for determining the adequacy of the disclosure in most states is the reasonable patient standard:

. . . the patient's right of self-decision shapes the boundaries of the duty to reveal. That right can be effectively exercised only if the patient possesses enough information to enable an intelligent choice. The scope of the physician's communications to the patient, then, must be measured by the patient's need, and that need is the information material to the decision (*Canterbury* v. *Spence* 1972).

Disclosure elements

The generally recognized necessary elements of disclosure relative to a proposed diagnostic or therapeutic procedure are:

(1) the nature of the patient's condition;
(2) a description of the proposed procedure in language understandable to the patient;
(3) the consequences of the proposed procedure;
(4) the risks associated with the proposed procedure;
(5) feasible alternatives to the proposed procedure; and
(6) the prognosis if the proposed procedure is not performed.

The burden is upon the patient to establish that relevant information was not provided and that, if it had been provided, a reasonable person in the position of the patient, taking that information into consideration, might well not have consented. In informed consent litigation the physician can be held liable for the harm suffered by the patient, even when the procedure was competently performed, because the theory of this litigation is that the patient was denied the opportunity to make an informed decision.

Concern with consent litigation has stimulated use of consent forms, which serve both as a vehicle to provide information to the patient and to document the authorization given. While their use is rarely mandated by law, hospitals generally require their use.

Whose consent is necessary? The consent of a competent adult patient for treatment is effective. For a minor, the general rule is that the consent of a parent or guardian is necessary. However, by virtue of legislation and court decisions, in many situations the consent of a mature minor, alone, can be effective. Where the patient is an adult, incompetent as a matter of law, or incapable of giving an informed consent, consent from a guardian or close relative is ordinarily required or accepted.

Refusal of treatment

An adult patient's refusal of treatment ordinarily will be respected by courts when their intervention is sought by a hospital or physician, unless the patient is deemed to lack the ability to comprehend the ramifications of the refusal, or interests of third parties would be affected. Thus, a court would not countermand an adult patient's refusal of medically necessary blood transfusions on religious grounds unless, for example, the patient were a pregnant woman and the refusal placed a substantially developed fetus in jeopardy. Parental refusal of necessary treatment for a child is subject to court review under state legislation which permits a court to authorize necessary treatment upon finding that, without such treatment, the child is subject to a substantial risk of permanent impairment or death.

Termination or withholding treatment

Increasingly, issues have arisen in the context of not instituting, and terminating, medical measures which are directed toward prolonging the dying process, rather than recovery or improvement in the patient's health. Nearly all states have legislation that recognizes the right of a person under specified circumstances, and by following procedures in such laws, to direct in writing that certain measures should not be employed. Federal legislation requires hospitals and other health-care providers to determine at admission whether the patient has executed an advance directive. In the absence of a patient's advance directive, when the intervention of courts has been sought by another on behalf of a patient, such as a close relative, to have extraordinary medical measures terminated or not instituted, the right has been recognized.

Determination of death and facilitating organ donation

State laws require that ordinarily a physician certify a person's death, which, in addition to irreversible cessation of cardiac and respiratory function, includes *brain death—the irreversible cessation of all brain function, including brainstem activity. Organ *transplantation technology created increased interest in the criteria for determining death because once death is pronounced, with consent as required by state laws that permit donation of bodies or body parts, organs can be removed for transplantation purposes without exposure to criminal or civil liability risks. Federal law requires that requests for donation authorization be made by hospitals in the case of patients who are potential organ donors.

Hospital practice privileges

To practise effectively, most physicians need access to the facilities and services provided by the modern hospital. The hospital governing board has the ultimate governance responsibility according to state law and government agency regulations. In deciding which physicians to appoint to the hospital medical staff, and the extent of the clinical privileges granted them, after recommendation by the organized medical staff, the governing board exercises its discretion.

Legislation, court decisions, state agency regulations, and standards of the Joint Commission on Accreditation of Healthcare Organizations have all served to impose a responsibility on hospitals to evaluate regularly the quality of professional services, including those rendered by physicians, in the interests of protection of patients and avoidance of liability. Evaluation activity— *peer review—has led to the termination of medical staff appointments or restriction of privileges, often followed by litigation by aggrieved physicians who generally seek injunctive relief and money damages, claiming that there has been arbitrary or capricious action. Some litigation by physicians denied practice privileges is founded on claims of anticompetitive conduct violative of the federal antitrust laws. Federal legislation provides qualified immunity to the hospital and participants in the institution's peer review process if they have acted 'in the reasonable belief that the action was in the furtherance of quality health care'.

Reports, testimony, and maintaining patient *confidentiality

Physicians and other health professionals are obliged by ethical principles to maintain the confidentiality of information secured from patients in the course of providing health services. To a substantial degree, practitioner confidentiality obligations are recognized and reinforced by legislation and court decisions, although statutory provisions and court decisions have defined many situations in which disclosure of confidential information is accepted and, in some instances, mandated by law.

Reports

State legislation imposes duties upon physicians and, in some instances, other health professionals and health institutions, to report to governmental agencies cases of specified *communicable diseases, such as *AIDS and *tuberculosis, and incidents of suspected child abuse (*battered babies), and gunshot wounds. Penalties may be imposed upon a person or institution subject to a reporting duty who wilfully refuses to report. Reporting laws ordinarily contain provisions protecting any person making a report pursuant to such laws, absent malice, or from liability to a person the report concerns.

Testimonial privileges

All states have established by statute a privilege that allows a patient to prevent testimony by a physician disclosing information regarding the patient's condition and treatment acquired in the therapeutic relationship. Some testimonial privilege legislation applies to other health practitioners, including dentists, nurses, and psychologists. The contents and scope of such privilege statutes vary considerably from state to state.

Out-of-court disclosure

Disclosure of confidential medical information without the patient's consent may subject the practitioner to liability. If the information disclosed is untrue and injurious to reputation, a basis for liability for defamation is present. Of more significance is the liability risk for unauthorized disclosure of accurate medical information, when its disclosure causes embarrassment to, or offends the sensibility of, the patient, and lacks legal justification. Certain medical information, particularly that dealing with mental illness and treatment, and alcohol and drug abuse, is subject to very stringent federal and state disclosure requirements.

Unauthorized disclosure of medical information is permitted in some situations, such as when a privilege can be asserted because the practitioner making the disclosure has a duty, or legitimate interest, to disclose to a recipient, who has a corresponding interest or duty in the information provided. Courts have recognized a duty on a physician to warn a third person when a patient discloses plans to injure or kill such a person and it is reasonable to believe the patient has both the intent and ability to do so.

Major regulatory programmes

In addition to the statutory and decisional law mentioned previously that affects the practice of medicine directly, a number of encompassing regulatory programmes also have an impact upon the practice of medicine and the provision of health services generally in the USA.

Drugs and devices

Several major items of federal legislation affect the availability and utilization of drugs and various devices (e.g. *pacemakers) used in patient care. For a new drug to enter the channels of interstate commerce it must receive approval of the *Food and Drug Administration. The approval process is to determine whether a new drug is safe and effective before it can be marketed, and it requires testing, including clinical trials. The federal drug legislation also deals with labelling, adulteration, misbranding, and other practices, in order to protect the quality of drugs. The federal programme for devices also requires in some circumstances that clinical testing occur before certain devices can be marketed in interstate commerce. All states have adopted laws regulating drugs; however, the primary regulatory mechanism for new drug products is federal.

Certificate of need

Many states have laws which place restrictions upon hospitals and other health organizations constructing new facilities, acquiring equipment, and instituting new health services. These laws require that a certificate of need be obtained from a state agency if proposed expenditures exceed specified thresholds for capital expenditures or operating expenses of new services. Curtailment of the hospital's freedom to determine the equipment it will acquire and the services to be rendered at its facilities may adversely affect the ability of members of the hospital medical staff to provide particular services to their patients.

Medicare and Medicaid

*Medicare is the federal programme providing health benefits to the elderly. Under Medicare, payments are made to hospitals and other institutional providers for services rendered to the programme beneficiaries, and there is a supplementary programme for paying physicians, other practitioners, and certain other providers for their services. Although Medicare is a financing programme, various restrictions and control measures with regard to the extent of services for which payment is made, and limits upon the amount of payment, have considerable impact on providers. Medicare provides for utilization review, and penalties can be imposed upon institutions and individual practitioners whose conduct in the programme falls within proscriptions of fraud and abuse.

*Medicaid is a state-operated programme in every state, jointly funded by federal and state governments, and subject to extensive federal regulations. The programme is to facilitate through payment mechanisms the provision of health services to those who lack the financial resources to pay for their health services. The scope of the services provided under Medicaid varies to some extent from state to state, and payment levels under Medicaid are lower than the payments medical and other practitioners usually receive for the same services to other patients.

Other

State hospital and *nursing home licensing legislation and regulations, laws and regulations dealing with voluntary and involuntary commitment of the mentally ill, *alcohol and drug abuse control legislation, and a variety of other laws and regulations all impinge upon the practice of medicine. State laws on these subjects vary considerably and the health industry, previously relatively free from government regulation, today is subject to a vast body of regulatory law affecting both institutions and individual health professionals.

N. HERSHEY

References
Canterbury v. *Spence* (1972). 4th Cir. 464, Federal Reporter, 2nd series, 772, 786.

Further reading
Christoffel, T. (1982). *Health and the law*. Free Press, New York and London.
Derbyshire, R. (1969). *Medical licensure and discipline in the United States*. Johns Hopkins Press, Baltimore and London.
Health Law Center (1992). Consent to medical and surgical procedures. In *Hospital Law Manual*, Vol. 2. Aspen Publishers, Rockville, Maryland.
Health Law Center (1992). Medical records. In *Hospital Law Manual*, Vol. 2A. Aspen Publishers, Rockville, Maryland.
Health Law Center (1992). Medical staff. In *Hospital Law Manual*, Vol. 2A. Aspen Publishers, Rockville, Maryland.
Health Law Center (1992). Principles of hospital liability. In *Hospital Law Manual*, Vol. 2B. Aspen Publisher, Rockville, Maryland.
Hershey, N. (1982). *Hospital–physician relationships*. Aspen Publishers, Rockville, Maryland.
Rosoff, A. (1981). *Informed consent*. Aspen Publishers, Rockville, Maryland.

LAXATIVES are agents which promote evacuation of the bowel, also known as aperients, purgatives, or cathartics. They are best classified into: bulk-forming agents (such as unprocessed wheat bran, ispaghula husk, methylcellulose, sterculia); stimulant laxatives (such as bisacodyl, bethanecol chloride, cascara, castor oil, danthron, distigmine bromide, fig, neostigmine, pyridostigmine, senna, sodium picosulphate); faecal softeners (such as dioctyl sodium sulpho-succinate, liquid paraffin); osmotic laxatives (such as lactulose, magnesium salts); rectally administered laxatives (such as bisacodyl suppositories, enemas containing sodium and phosphate, arachis oil, or other substances); and various other laxatives, most of which should be avoided (including preparations containing phenolphthalein, frangula, rhubarb, aloes, colocynth, and jalop). There are innumerable commercial preparations of all the agents mentioned and of mixtures of them, identified by many trade names. In practice, simple constipation is best countered by dietary adjustment: in adults and children by increasing dietary *fibre, in infants by increasing the sugar content of feeds.

LAXITY. Looseness; lack of tension.

LAZARETTES. 'Lazarette' and 'lazaret' are variants of 'lazaretto', meaning lazar house, that is a house or hospital for the reception of poor and diseased persons. 'Lazaretto' has also been used to describe a place of quarantine. The derivation is from Lazarus (Luke 16), the beggar full of sores who was laid at the rich man's gate but who achieved ultimate salvation in Abraham's bosom.

LEAD. Soft bluish-white metallic element (symbol Pb, atomic number 82, relative atomic mass 207.19). Lead has no physiological role, and its salts are toxic (see LEAD POISONING). In industry and commerce lead compounds are used in paint manufacture, in alloys, in lead batteries, in plumbing, and in petrol (antiknock) additives.

LEAD POISONING. Lead is a cumulative poison; chronic lead intoxication, because of its widespread industrial use, was once a common occupational hazard. The cardinal manifestations are *anaemia, abdominal pain (*Devonshire colic), peripheral *neuropathy, renal damage, and cerebral disturbances (saturnine *encephalopathy). The effects of lesser body burdens of lead common to those who dwell in urban environments are not so well established; but public anxiety has led to movements in many countries towards reducing or abolishing altogether the use of lead additives in petrol. See also ENVIRONMENT AND MEDICINE I; OCCUPATIONAL MEDICINE.

LEBER, THEODOR VON (1840–1917). German ophthalmologist. He described degenerative disorders of the retina and delineated their relationships, and made major contributions to understanding of other retinal diseases. He also described a variety of hereditary *optic atrophy to which his name is now attached.

LEECH BOOKS were commonplace books of folk medicine from the Dark Ages of Europe containing accounts of magical and herbal remedies, doubtless repeatedly transcribed. According to Cartwright (*A social history of medicine*, 1977), however, even the Anglo-Saxon leech books contained discernible fragments of *Hippocratic teaching, showing that 'the heritage of Greek medicine was not entirely lost during this period'.

LEECHES. Although leeches (see HIRUDO MEDICIN-ALIS) are pests in heavily infested areas, where they may cause *anaemia due to blood loss, they are not known to be vectors of infectious disease.

LEEUWENHOEK, ANTHONY VAN (1632–1723). Dutch microscopist. Leeuwenhoek was a shopkeeper in Delft. He acquired great expertise in grinding lenses with which he made simple *microscopes capable of a magnification of 200–300. With these he carried out many meticulous studies. He was the first to describe *spermatozoa, *bacteria, striated *muscle, and *capillaries. He is best known for his description of human red blood cells in 1674.

LEFT-HANDEDNESS, or sinistrality, is preferential use of the left hand, often, but not invariably, relating to dominance of the right cerebral hemisphere. See LANGUAGE, COGNITION, AND HIGHER CEREBRAL FUNCTION.

LEGALLOIS, JULIEN JEAN CESAR (1770–1814). French physiologist. He was an early experimental physiologist and showed that respiration was controlled from the *medulla oblongata (1812). He was much impressed by the importance of maintaining an adequate arterial blood supply to the tissues and this led him vigorously to oppose bleeding as a form of treatment.

LEGGE, SIR THOMAS MORISON (1863–1932). First medical inspector of factories in the UK. His work covered a wide range of industrial diseases, with the main emphasis being on the prevention of *lead poisoning.

LEGIONNAIRE'S DISEASE is an epidemic form of *pneumonia caused by *Legionella* bacilli, notably *L. pneumophilia*. Person-to-person spread does not occur, and infection is by droplet inhalation from air-conditioning plants and similar installations. Other modes have not been certainly established, but epidemiological evidence suggests that air-borne dust from excavation sites may be a possibility. *Nosocomial infections have occurred. The disease, which has an untreated mortality rate of about 20 per cent, is characterized by fever, abdominal pain, headache, and pneumonia; in severe cases there is renal, hepatic, and neurological involvement. Legionnaires' disease is so named because of the outbreak that occurred in the summer of 1976 at an American Legion convention in Philadelphia. Many subsequent outbreaks have been recorded.

LEIDY, JOSEPH II (1866–1932). American physician and foremost anatomist. He is credited by some with the discovery of *Trichinella spiralis* in human muscle. He suggested that an illness resembling *pernicious anaemia can be caused by infestation with certain *parasites.

LEISHMAN, SIR WILLIAM BOOG (1865–1926). British bacteriologist and army medical officer. He devised the familiar modification of *Romanowsky's stain (Leishman's stain); he described the causal organism of *kala-azar (*Leishmania donovani*); and elucidated the life cycle of the cause of endemic *relapsing fever (*Borellia duttoni*).

LEISHMAN–DONOVAN BODIES are the intracellular non-flagellate forms (also called amastigotes) of the protozoan parasite *Leishmania donovani*, the causal agent of *kala azar.

LEISHMANIASIS is infection with a *protozoan parasite belonging to the genus *Leishmania*. It occurs in various cutaneous forms, and in the visceral form known as *kala-azar. See also LEISHMAN–DONOVAN BODIES.

LEISHMAN'S STAIN is a microscopic stain consisting of eosin and methylene blue, used particularly for staining blood films.

LENS. The essential element of the dioptric (refracting) system of the eye. Most refraction takes place as light passes through the *cornea but this is a fixed element. The variable-focus lens, the convexity of which alters in response to ciliary muscular tension during the process of accommodation, provides the adjustment necessary to bring the image into sharp focus on the *retina. The lens is a transparent biconvex structure situated between the vitreous body and the anterior chamber of the eye. It consists mainly of elongated, inert cells (lens fibres), which contain large amounts of special lens proteins, the crystallins. Opacity of the lens is termed *cataract, and causes dimness of vision leading to blindness as it progresses. Surgical removal of the lens restores useful vision, only the ability to focus being lost. See OPHTHALMOLOGY.

LEONARDO DA VINCI (1452–1519). Italian artist and anatomist. Leonardo's distinction as an anatomist has only recently been appreciated with the study of his anatomical notebooks now in the Royal Library at Windsor Castle. The anatomical drawings date from 1487, but from 1506 he dissected as an anatomist. See ART AND MEDICINE.

LEONICENUS (Nicolo da Longino) (1428–1524). Italian physician. He was a leading Greek scholar and was largely responsible for the revival of Greek medicine in its pristine form by translation from the original in place of the garbled Arabic versions. He had considerable influence on Montanus and *Linacre. He was criticized for correcting the botanical errors in Pliny's *Natural history*. His *Libellus de epidemia quam vulgo morbus gallicum vocant* (1497) has an excellent account of *syphilis.

LEONTIASIS is the involvement of the face in lepromatous *leprosy, conferring a lion-like appearance.

LEPROSY, or Hansen's disease, is a chronic communicable granulomatous disorder affecting mainly the skin and the peripheral nerves. It is caused by *Mycobacterium leprae*, an acid-fast bacillus, morphologically indistinguishable from the tubercle bacillus. Once common in Europe, it is now largely confined to tropical and subtropical areas; only small geographical foci now exist elsewhere, for example in the USA. The precise mode of transmission remains uncertain, but is from person to person, and close and prolonged contact is thought to be necessary; nasal secretions, in which bacilli can be abundant, are probably involved, but the portal of entry is not known. The situation is complicated by wide variation in individual susceptibility due to immunological factors, and a clinical incubation period which may be as long as 20 years or more. Probably most infections take place in childhood or early adult life. Variation in immune response also accounts for the varied clinical picture, ranging from a florid low-resistance form in which skin lesions are obvious (lepromatous leprosy) to a low-grade high-resistance condition affecting mainly peripheral nerves (tuberculoid leprosy). Although there are about 15 000 000 patients in the world, relatively simple and cheap treatment (with dapsone) arrests the disease and renders it non-infective. There seems no reason why leprosy should not eventually be eradicated completely.

LEPTOSPIROSIS is a zoonotic infection due to a spiral bacterium *Leptospira interrogans*, which commonly infects rats and many other wild and domestic animals, including dogs. Infection in man is usually due to contact of skin or mucous membranes with water contaminated by the urine of infected animals. Many serotypes of *L. interrogans* exist, associated with human infections of varying severity (e.g. *L. icterohaemorrhagica* is usually transmitted to man from rats, dogs, and cats and causes a severe infection long known as Weil's disease; *L. canicola*, from dogs, causes the milder canicola fever; and there are many other clinical variants). The syndromes comprise combinations of lymphocytic *meningitis, *hepatitis, and *nephritis. They range from a mild pyrexial illness to a fulminating fatal infection with *jaundice, *uraemia, haemorrhagic manifestations, and cerebral disturbances.

LEPTOSPIROSIS ICTEROHAEMORRHAGICA. Leptospiral jaundice or *Weil's disease. See LEPTO-SPIROSIS.

LERICHE, RENE HENRI MARIE (1879–1953). French surgeon. He was one of the leading military surgeons in the First World War, and a pioneer of *vascular surgery. He introduced periarterial *sympathectomy and described the clinical picture associated with incomplete obstruction of the bifurcation of the aorta (*Leriche syndrome, 1940).

LERICHE SYNDROME. Fatiguability and pain on exercise in the hips and legs, together with male impotence: this symptom complex is associated with gradual occlusion of the terminal *aorta. There are signs of impaired arterial circulation to the legs.

LESBIANISM is *homosexuality between women, also known as sapphism. Both names derive from Sappho, a Greek lyric poetess who lived in Lesbos during the 7th century BC, and her followers. Its practice has never been a statutory crime in the UK, unlike active male homosexuality.

LETHARGY. Torpor; drowsiness; lack of interest or energy.

LETTSOM, JOHN COAKLEY (1744–1815). British physician. A protégé of John *Fothergill, he founded the General Dispensary in Aldersgate in 1770 and the Medical Society of London in 1773.

LEUCOCYTES are white blood cells or corpuscles. Leucocytes are broadly divided into *granulocytes, *lymphocytes, and *monocytes. See also HAEMATOLOGY.

LEUCOCYTOSIS is an increase in the number of circulating white blood cells (leucocytes).

LEUCODERMA is patchy whiteness of the *skin due to localized loss of *melanin pigmentation.

LEUCODYSTROPHY is a term identifying a group of genetically determined disorders of *myelination within the *central nervous system, leading to generalized disintegration of white matter. They are characterized by severe progressive neurological and mental disturbances.

LEUCOENCEPHALOPATHY is any condition associated with pathological changes in the white matter of the *brain, including those classified as *leucodystrophy.

LEUCOPENIA is an abnormally low concentration of circulating *leucocytes.

LEUCOPLAKIA. Thickened whitish patches on the mucous membrane of the mouth, which cannot be removed by scraping. It may be associated with heavy smoking or other causes of local irritation, and in some patients heralds the development of a *malignant growth. A similar condition can occur in the mucosa of the genital tract in both male and female.

LEUCOTOMY is surgical incision into the white matter of both frontal lobes of the *brain, in order to separate their connections with the *thalamus. The operation was introduced in 1935 by the *Nobel prize-winning Portuguese neurosurgeon *Moniz, and was used thereafter to treat severe, intractable, and progressive psychiatric disorders, particularly severe agitated *depression, chronic *schizophrenia, and intractable obsessional *neurosis. The operation was sometimes dangerous, and often caused undesirable cerebral, personality, and mental side-effects; and its benefits were uncertain. Despite modifications of the procedure, it has now been made largely obsolescent by the advent of effective *psychotropic drugs and even restricted psychosurgical procedures are only now used as a last resort. See also NEUROSURGERY.

LEUKAEMIA (LEUKEMIA) is any malignant disorder characterized by the uncontrolled proliferation of white blood cells or their precursors. Leukaemia is classified according to which type of *leucocyte predominates, for example granulocytic (or myeloid) leukaemia, lymphatic leukaemia, etc.

LEUKOTRIENES are a group of endogenously produced substances related to the *prostaglandins, derived from arachidonic acid in *leucocytes. They are mediators of inflammatory reactions. Leukotrienes A and B are aggregations of neutrophils; C, D, and E are involved in *anaphylaxis.

LEVODOPA or L-dopa is the laevorotatory isomer of the amino acid dopa (3,4-dihydroxyphenylalanine), the precursor of the *neurotransmitter *dopamine. It is the treatment of choice for patients with idiopathic *parkinsonism. It is less effective in postencephalitic parkinsonism and is contraindicated when parkinsonism is drug-induced. It acts mainly by replenishing depleted striatal dopamine, relieving *bradykinesia and *rigidity more rapidly than *tremor. It is now usually given together with an extra-cerebral dopa-decarboxylase inhibitor (carbidopa or benserazide), which minimizes the peripheral side-effects of the drug such as vomiting and cardiovascular effects and allows more of the drug to enter the brain. Other side-effects are involuntary movements and psychiatric complications. About one-third of patients with idiopathic parkinsonism respond dramatically, another third moderately well, and the remainder poorly. Maximum benefit may take some time to become apparent, and there may be some loss of benefit after prolonged treatment.

LEWIS, SIR AUBREY JULIAN (1900–75). British psychiatrist. Founder of the Institute of Psychiatry at the *Bethlem Royal and Maudsley Hospitals, his work as honorary director of the *Medical Research Council Social Psychiatry Unit greatly influenced the development of psychiatry in the UK, and he was recognized as the leading British psychiatrist of his time.

LEWIS, SIR THOMAS (1881–1945). British physician. He was one of the first and most ardent 'clinical scientists'. Noted for his work on cardiac irregularities, he was an early *electrocardiographer, and elucidated *atrial fibrillation. In 1908 Lewis founded the journal *Heart*, which in 1944 became *Clinical Science*.

LEWY BODIES are eosinophilic bodies found in the pigmented neurones of the substantia nigra in patients with Parkinson's disease. When more widely distributed throughout the brain, they may be associated with dementia.

LEYDIG CELLS are the interstitial cells of the male *gonads (testes), which secrete *androgens.

LHERMITTE, JEAN (1877–1959). French neuro-psychiatrist. During the First World War he studied injuries of the *spinal cord, and later made many contributions to neuropsychiatry.

LIBAVIUS, ANDREAS (Libau) (*c*.1560–1616). German physician and chemist. He was one of the founders of the *iatrochemical school. He was an accomplished chemist and his book *Alchemia* (1597) was the most important work on the subject in the 17th century.

LIBIDO is now generally used in medicine to denote sexual drive, energy, or desire, rather than the wider meaning attached to the word in Freudian psychology of psychic energy in general.

LIBMAN, EMANUEL (1872–1946). American physician. He was one of the first American physicians to make use of *blood culture, and wrote extensively about *infective endocarditis, as well as lateral *sinus thrombosis (of otogenous origin)—a disease of utmost gravity in the pre-antibiotic era. With colleagues in pathology he described non-bacterial, or verrucous, endocarditis—a disorder still referred to by the eponym Libman–Sachs disease.

LICENCES FOR ANIMAL EXPERIMENTATION. The *Cruelty to Animals Act 1876 regulated animal experimentation in the UK until superseded by the *Animal Procedures Act. In order to perform experiments on living vertebrates the research worker must be registered and in possession of a licence. In the USA, licensees must comply with the regulations of the Animal Welfare Act (1966) and the National Institutes of Health Policy Issuance 4206. In both countries, licensees must submit an annual report to the appropriate authority and all available evidence suggests that the vast majority of research workers carry out such experiments in a responsible and humane manner. See also EXPERIMENTAL METHOD.

LICHEN. A skin eruption characterized by small firm *papules. Lichen planus, an inflammatory skin disease, is an example: here the papules occur in circumscribed patches; they itch and have a typical blue-violet sheen.

LICHTHEIM, LUDWIG (1845–1928). German neurologist. He attempted an analysis of *aphasia (1885) and described *subacute combined degeneration of the cord (Lichtheim's disease).

LID LAG is a physical sign characteristic of the ophthalmopathy associated with *Graves disease. When the patient is asked to look downwards, the upper eyelids fail to keep pace with the downwards movements of the eyeballs, exposing an area of white sclera. It is also known as von *Graefe's sign.

LIEBIG, JUSTUS VON, BARON (1803–73). German chemist. He was one of the early biochemists and founder of agricultural chemistry. He discovered *chloroform and *chloral (1831), hippuric acid (1829), and *tyrosine (1829). He showed that carbohydrates and fats were oxidized in the tissues. He was unwilling to accept the role of bacteria in putrefaction and is now generally remembered for his meat extract.

LIE DETECTOR. See POLYGRAPH.

LIENORENAL. Connecting the spleen and the kidney, applied particularly to a fold of peritoneum (*ligament) joining the spleen and left kidney.

LIFE is the sum of the distinguishing properties of animate whole organisms such as plants and animals, and their component cells, tissues, organs, and parts. Chief among these are adaptation, growth, and reproductive capacity.

LIFE ASSURANCE is defined as 'An insurance on a person's life; a life insurance policy' (Ogilvie (1882) in the *Oxford English Dictionary)*. In other words the term 'assurance' is restricted to the meaning 'life insurance', while 'insurance' itself when otherwise unqualified means insurance against some event (e.g. loss of property, injury, accident, etc.) other than loss of life. This is the modern though not the historical usage. The *OED* explains the situation thus: '*Assurance* would probably have dropped out of use (as it had almost done in U.S.) but that Babbage in 1826 proposed to restrict *insurance* to risks to property, and *assurance* to life insurance.' The point that Babbage had made (in *Assurance of lives* (1826)) was that life is an all-or-none event, which 'must happen or fail', whereas other, uncertain events 'may partly happen or partly fail'.

LIFE TABLES are statistical tables 'exhibiting statistics as to the probability of life at different ages' (Webster (1864) in the *Oxford English Dictionary*).

LIGAMENT. Any binding or connecting anatomical structure, usually a band of fibrous tissue between bones in the region of a joint.

LIGAND. In pharmacology, ligands are specific chemicals which attach to recognition sites on cell receptor molecules. See PHARMACOLOGY.

LIGATION is the application of a *ligature, that is the tying or binding of a structure.

LIGATURE is any material (catgut, wire, silk, etc.) used to bind, bandage, or tie a structure.

LIGHTENING is the lessening of abdominal distension noted by pregnant women a few weeks before the onset of *labour, associated with subsidence of the gravid *uterus into the *pelvis.

LIMBIC SYSTEM. An imprecisely defined collection of brain structures chiefly concerned with emotional, behavioural, autonomic, and olfactory functions.

LIME JUICE is noteworthy as a dietary supplement empirically used to prevent *scurvy in seamen many years before the existence of *vitamins was postulated and the importance of *ascorbic acid was established as an essential component of the human diet.

LINACRE, THOMAS (?1460–1524). British physician and scholar. With the royal licence he founded the Royal College of Physicians (RCP) on 23 September 1518 and became its first president.

LINCOMYCIN is an *antibiotic introduced in 1963 possessing particular activity against Gram-positive cocci and many anaerobic organisms (See ANTI-INFECTIVE DRUGS). Its use is limited by poor absorbability and by a serious side-effect known as pseudomembranous colitis due to a *toxin elaborated by a lincomycin resistant *clostridium (*Clostridium difficile*).

LINCTUS. A medicine made by mixing a drug with syrup, honey, or other sweet *excipient.

LIND, JAMES (1716–94). British naval surgeon. Although he showed that lemon juice prevented *scurvy in *A treatise on the scurvy* published in 1754, its use was not enforced in the navy until 1795.

LINEAR ACCELERATOR is an apparatus used in *radiotherapy which accelerates *ions to high energies by means of a row of *electrodes having a common axis.

LINGUISTICS is the science of languages. Purists maintain a distinction between 'linguistics' and 'philology', the latter meaning the science of a particular language, or of language-as-communication. But the two words are often used synonymously.

LINIMENT is a liquid preparation for external application to the unbroken skin, which may contain substances with *analgesic, soothing, or *rubefacient properties.

LINKAGE is the association of non-allelic genes with loci on the same chromosome. See GENETICS.

LINNE, CARL VON (Linnaeus) (1707–78). Swedish physician and botanist. He was a taxonomist and systematist who introduced the binomial nomenclature into science, with one name for the genus and one for the species. This he applied to plants in his *Systema naturae* (1735), classifying them by the characteristics of their sexual organs. He extended his scheme to medicine in *Genera morborum* (1763). He devised the term *Homo sapiens*. He was a firm believer in the fixity of species.

LIPIDOSIS is any disorder of *metabolism characterized by the abnormal accumulation of a *lipid in particular tissues, for example *Tay–Sachs disease.

LIPIDS are a group of organic substances, also known as fats, which are esters of *fatty acids and are characteristically insoluble in water but soluble in many organic solvents (such as alcohol, ether, benzene, chloroform, etc.). They are readily stored in the body, where they provide an important reserve store of energy. They are important components of cell structure (especially cell membranes), and serve many other biological functions.

LIPODYSTROPHY is a term embracing various disorders of fat metabolism, the best known of which (progressive lipodystrophy) causes a striking redistribution of subcutaneous fat from the upper half of the body to the lower.

LIPOMA. A benign new growth arising from *adipose tissue.

LIPOPROTEINS are soluble complexes of *lipid and *protein, which, since lipids are themselves insoluble in water, serve as the main lipid transport mechanism in plasma. Lipoproteins vary in composition and hence in physical characteristics; they contain varying proportions of triglyceride, cholesterol, cholesteryl ester, and phospholipid together with one or more of eight major apoproteins. They are usually classified into high density or alpha-lipoproteins (HDL); low density or beta-lipoproteins (LDL); and very low density or pre-beta-lipoproteins (VLDL).

LIQUOR is a term applied to various body fluids but especially to liquor amnii or *amniotic fluid.

LIQUORICE is a preparation of the dried rhizome and roots of leguminous plants belonging to the genus *Glycyrrhiza*. It has been used as a remedy for various ailments at least since the first century, and an active principle, glycyrrhizin, has anti-inflammatory and aldosterone-like properties. Carbenoxolone, a synthetic derivative of glycyrrhizin, is effective in promoting the healing of *peptic ulcer.

LISTER, SIR JOSEPH, Bt, 1st Baron Lister of Lyme Regis (1827–1912). British surgeon and originator of antiseptic surgery. As his surgical practice grew he became more and more concerned by the frequency of suppuration and wound infection in his often insanitary wards. He had reached the conclusion that the cause must lie in the atmosphere when in 1865 Anderson, the professor of chemistry, drew his attention to the work of *Pasteur. He realized at once that the cause of surgical suppuration must be the 'vibrios', as Pasteur called them, which were suspended in the air, and, after careful consideration, he concluded that they could best be destroyed by chemical means. In March 1865 he operated for the first time using *carbolic acid as an *antiseptic. No suppuration followed and thus his argument was vindicated, although a struggle was needed to win complete acceptance.

Later he devised several operative procedures as well as introducing wound drainage and the use of absorbable sutures. In his honour the British Institute of Preventive Medicine was named the Lister Institute.

LISTER, JOSEPH JACKSON (1786–1869). British microscopist and wine merchant. Lister devised the achromatic lens which created the modern *microscope and was responsible for some valuable studies of the mammalian red blood cell. He was the father of Lord *Lister.

LISTERIA INFECTION. See INFECTIOUS DISEASE.

LISTON, ROBERT (1794–1847). British surgeon. Liston was an operator of superlative dexterity, but an indifferent speaker and wrote little. He was the first British surgeon to operate on a patient under *ether anaesthesia. His *splint (the 'long Liston') is still occasionally used today.

LITHIUM is a metallic element (symbol Li, atomic number 3, atomic weight 6.939), one of the alkali metals. It is silvery white and has a melting point of 179 °C; it is the lightest solid known. Chemically it resembles sodium, but is less active. Lithium carbonate is used in the treatment of acute mania, and in the prophylaxis of *manic-depressive illness. Lithium salts have a very narrow therapeutic:toxic ratio and should be used only when facilities for monitoring plasma concentrations are available. Toxic side-effects include *tremor, *ataxia, *dysarthria, *fits, and renal impairment.

LITHOTOMY is the incision of an organ, usually the *urinary bladder, for removal of stone. Before the advent of antiseptic and aseptic techniques made abdominal surgery safe, a perineal approach was necessary; hence the well-known '*lithotomy position'. The operation is honoured with a specific interdiction in the *Hippocratic Oath, which requires that physicians shall 'give way to specialists in this work'.

LITHOTOMY POSITION. This position was formerly employed for the extraction of stones from the *urinary bladder. The patient lies on his or her back with the hips and knees flexed and the thighs abducted and externally rotated.

LITHOTRIPTOR. An instrument designed to break up stones in the kidney, bladder or gall bladder, using electric shock-waves, thus avoiding, in many cases, a surgical operation.

LITTER. A stretcher.

LITTLE, CLARENCE COOK (1888–1971). American biologist. Little's lifelong interest was in mammalian *genetics and *cancer. In 1929 he founded a small research laboratory at Bar Harbor, Maine. There he carried on with experiments in tumour transplantation, and recognized the importance of genetic factors, and of the need to develop inbred strains of mice for such research. The Bar Harbor laboratories eventually supplied inbred strains to workers in many parts of the world.

LITTLE, WILLIAM JOHN (1810–94). British physician. After qualification Little studied in Germany where his *talipes equinovarus was cured by *Stromeyer's subcutaneous *tenotomy. He became interested in the treatment of deformity and on his return to London founded what is now the *Royal National Orthopaedic Hospital (1839). He described congenital *spastic diplegia (Little's disease, 1861).

LITTLE'S DISEASE. See SPASTIC DIPLEGIA.

LIVEDO. Reddish mottling of the skin.

LIVER. The large dark-red glandular organ occupying the upper right-hand portion of the abdominal cavity. Developmentally, the liver belongs to the *gastrointestinal tract, and its primary functions are those of *digestion and *excretion. It has, however, many other important physiological roles, particularly in *protein and *carbohydrate metabolism. It is essential to life. See also GASTROENTEROLOGY.

LIVER FAILURE. The healthy human liver has considerable reserve capacity and remarkable powers of regeneration after injury. Pathological injury must therefore be severe and must damage all hepatic tissue in order for liver failure to occur. When it does so, it is usually a complication of viral *hepatitis (particularly types B and C), but may also occur as a terminal event in alcoholic or non-alcoholic *cirrhosis; it may also result from the ingestion of profoundly hepatotoxic substances, such as *carbon tetrachloride, or occasionally from drug overdosage, particularly with *paracetamol (acetaminophen). The major manifestation of acute liver failure is hepatic encephalopathy or coma. This causes several personality, mental and neurological disturbances, including the important physical sign known as 'liver flap', a coarse bilateral flapping or 'wingbeating' tremor which becomes obvious when the arms are outstretched and the fingers extended and separated. See also ACUTE YELLOW ATROPHY.

LIVER FUNCTION TESTS. A series of laboratory tests usually performed when liver disease is known or suspected, most of which consist of biochemical measurements made on *serum or *plasma. They include measurements of *bilirubin, *alkaline phosphatase, *albumin, *globulin, *prothrombin, various liver *enzymes, *lipids, *lipoproteins, and *mitochondrial antibodies.

LIVER TRANSPLANT. Surgical *transplantation of the liver, now possible in many centres throughout the world, will probably continue into the foreseeable future, since it is unlikely that the multiple and complex functions of the liver can, with present technology, be taken over by totally artificial systems. No other treatment has been found effective for incipient liver failure. Human *allotransplants have proved increasingly successful, but transplantation of baboon liver into human subjects has proved, to date, of temporary benefit only. Nevertheless, and despite a growing number of successes, the difficulties and dangers of liver transplantation are formidable. See TRANSPLANTATION.

LIVINGSTON, SIR PHILIP (1893–1982). Canadian ophthalmologist and aviation medicine pioneer. He became Director-General of RAF Medical Services in the Second World War. His contribution to the testing of *night vision in night fighters and bombers was critical. On his 'retirement' from active duty he returned to his birthplace on Vancouver Island to practise ophthalmology. He also took up writing, and his autobiographical volume *Fringe of the clouds* is English prose at its best.

LIVINGSTONE, DAVID (1813–73). British physician, missionary, and explorer. From the age of 10 years Livingstone supported himself by working in a cotton factory and eventually paid his way through medical school. In 1840 he travelled to South Africa for the London Missionary Society and thereafter undertook many journeys into the interior, especially in what were then called Bechuanaland and Nyasaland. Later he became obsessed with a desire to find the source of the Nile; after one journey in 1871 he had been almost given up for lost when he was found by the American journalist, H.M. Stanley.

LOBE is an anatomical term indicating a major subdivision of an organ or structure, usually having a clear anatomical boundary.

LOBSTEIN, JOHANN GEORG CHRISTIAN FREDRICK MARTIN (1777–1835). German surgeon. He suggested the term '*pathogenesis' and described *osteogenesis imperfecta (fragilitas ossium or Lobstein's syndrome, 1833).

LOCAL ANAESTHESIA (ANESTHESIA) also known as regional or conduction anaesthesia, was discovered some 38 years after general anaesthesia had come into clinical use. It was well known that *cocaine on the tongue produced numbness, as the shrub *Ethythroxylum coca* had for centuries been cultivated by Peruvian Indians high in the Andes and its prepared leaves chewed for their stimulant effect on the brain. In 1884 Carl Koller was working with Sigmund *Freud in Vienna, using cocaine as a treatment for morphine addiction. By animal experiments he showed that the local loss of sensation induced by cocaine could be of value in eye surgery. These findings were announced at an ophthalmological meeting in Heidelberg and by 1885 more than 1000 surgical operations had been performed using topical cocaine. In 1905 the cocaine analogue *procaine, free from the toxic and addictive side-effects of cocaine, was introduced and became the most widely used local anaesthetic for over half a century. Another compound, lignocaine, discovered by Lofgren of Sweden in 1943, is now most often used, but there are others. Local anaesthetics act by blocking conduction in sensory nerves. The block may be of nerve endings (simple infiltration anaesthesia), of whole nerves (regional block), or of spinal segments (extradural and spinal anaesthesia). See also ANAESTHESIA.

LOCAL AUTHORITY SOCIAL SERVICES ACT 1970. This Act, arising out of the reorganization of the UK *National Health Service, required local authorities (metropolitan districts and non-metropolitan countries) to be responsible for those personal social services not directly administered by the NHS, though under the general guidance of the Secretary of State and in liaison with health service agencies. The personal social services include: child care (many aspects); residential services for the elderly and disabled; domiciliary services (e.g. home helps, meals, laundry facilities); care of the handicapped; training (e.g. of social workers, nursery

nurses); voluntary services support and liaison; building and design programmes; urban programmes; care of the homeless; the prevention of illness; the publishing of information about welfare services; and others.

LOCAL GOVERNMENT ACT 1929. This enactment, prepared by the then Minister of Health Neville Chamberlain, finally ended the *poor law system in Britain.

LOCAL GOVERNMENT BOARD. The UK Local Government Board was established in 1871 following the recommendations of Gladstone's Royal Commission of 1869 and combined the oversight of the *poor law system and of *public health. It proved ineffective and was replaced by the *Ministry of Health in 1919.

LOCALIZATION is the assignment or restriction of a disease process to a particular site (organ, tissue, part, area, etc.).

LOCKE, JOHN (1632–1704). British physician and philosopher. He was the 'founder of the analytical philosophy of mind'. His most celebrated work was *An essay concerning human understanding* (1690).

LOCKJAW. See TETANUS.

LOCOMOTOR ATAXIA. Synonym for *tabes dorsalis.

LOCUM TENENS. A medical practitioner undertaking another's professional duties during the latter's absence.

LOEB, LEO (1869–1959). American pathologist. He contributed many studies on tissue growth, and tumour growth, and carried out some artificial cultures of animal cells. He demonstrated an influence of hormones on some kinds of cancer in animals.

LOEB, ROBERT FREDERICK (1895–1973). American physician. He was first to recognize that salt depletion is a central feature of *Addison's disease.

LOEFFLER, FRIEDRICH AUGUST JOHANNES (1852–1915). German bacteriologist. He discovered the cause of *glanders (*Loefflerella mallei*) in 1882 and two years later isolated the *diphtheria bacillus (*Corynebacterium diphtheriae*; *Klebs–Loeffler bacillus) in pure culture. He identified the cause of swine *erysipelas (*Erysipelothrix rhusiopathiae*) and proved that footand-mouth disease was due to a filterable *virus. He attempted to control a plague of field mice in Greece by infecting them with *Salmonella typhimurium*.

LOEWI, OTTO (1873–1961). German pharmacologist. His major discovery concerned the appearance of a chemical substance in the perfusate of a frog's heart following stimulation of its nerve supply that was able to inhibit the action of a second heart receiving the perfused fluid (1921–26); this was later identified as *acetylcholine, which had been isolated by Sir Henry *Dale in 1914. Dale and Loewi were jointly awarded the 1936 *Nobel prize for this work.

LONDON HOSPITAL, THE (NOW ROYAL), was founded in 1740 in the East End of the metropolis. A group of philanthropists met in a tavern in Cheapside and started the hospital with 30 beds. In 1744 it was decided to move the hospital to the fields of White-chapel in a new building. By 1758 it was open with about 300 beds, and the hospital remains on that site. By the beginning of the 19th century The London was England's largest voluntary hospital, with over 900 beds in 1939. Like many other major London hospitals The London has become the centre of a group of hospitals, covering the whole range of medicine and medical education. The associated private medical school which started in 1785 became the London Hospital Medical College in 1876 and was absorbed into the University of London in 1948.

There have been many illustrious members of staff, including James *Mackenzie (cardiology), John *Little (Little's disease), Jonathan *Hutchinson (syphilis, teeth), Morell *Mackenzie (ENT surgery), Hughlings *Jackson (neurology), Robert *Hutchinson (paediatrics), Tudor Edwards (thoracic surgery), and Hugh *Cairns (neurosurgery). For the layman the outstanding tale of the London Hospital will always be the story of the *Elephant Man, a patient deformed by *neurofibromatosis and looked after carefully by Sir Frederick *Treves, the famous surgeon.

LONDON SCHOOL OF HYGIENE AND TROPICAL MEDICINE is a postgraduate school of the University of London. It arose out of the *Athlone Report* of 1921 and the amalgamation of the School of Hygiene, founded in 1925 by the *Rockefeller Foundation, and the London School of Tropical Medicine, which had been part of the university since 1905. The combined school was granted a Royal Charter in 1924. Its headquarters are in Bloomsbury in the heart of London, and it also has the Hospital for Tropical Diseases for its clinical work and investigation. Its work is organized in three divisions: (1) medical statistics and epidemiology; (2) communicable and tropical diseases; and (3) community health.

LONDON SCHOOL OF MEDICINE FOR WOMEN (THE 'ROYAL FREE') arose from the efforts of renowned women who struggled to enter medicine against much opposition—mainly Elizabeth Garrett *Anderson and Sophia *Jex-Blake (see also WOMEN IN MEDICINE). A medical school for women had been started in London in 1874, in the hope that one of the licensing bodies would allow women to sit their examinations. Clinical instruction could not, however,

be given until the Royal Free Hospital agreed, in 1877, to have female students work there. The new institution was called the London (Royal Free Hospital) School of Medicine for Women. It was recognized as a medical school in the University of London Act of 1900. From that time on it has flourished. In 1945 The Royal Charter of 1938 was revised to allow for the admission of men, just as all the other schools changed so that they could admit women. In 1974 the hospital and clinical school moved from their more central site to Hampstead in the suburbs.

LONG, CRAWFORD WILLIAMSON (1815–78). American surgeon and anaesthetist. He discovered the *anaesthetic properties of sulphuric *ether in the early 1840s. He may have been the first to use ether as a general anaesthetic agent, but his report attracted little attention, and the discovery is usually credited to the Boston dentist, W. T. G. *Morton. See ANAESTHESIA.

LONGEVITY. Long life; the condition of being long-lived; it is strongly influenced by *genetic factors.

LONGITUDINAL STUDY. A study in which the same individuals or group of individuals are examined on a number of occasions over a long period of time. See EPIDEMIOLOGY.

LONG-SIGHTEDNESS. See HYPERMETROPIA.

LORDOSIS is exaggerated curvature of the *spine, resulting in abnormal concavity of the lumbar region when viewed from the back.

LOTION. An aqueous solution or suspension for external application to the skin. Lotions cool by evaporation and require frequent re-application.

LOUIS, PIERRE CHARLES ALEXANDRE (1787–1872). French physician. He introduced the 'numerical method' into clinical medicine, thus founding medical *statistics. He analysed large series of cases of pulmonary *tuberculosis (1825) and of *typhoid fever (1829), giving the second the name 'typhoid'.

LOUPING ILL is *encephalomyelitis of sheep and cattle occurring in parts of the British Isles, caused by a tick-borne virus of the flavivirus group. Human infection has occurred sporadically and rarely, and only through occupation.

LOURDES is a place of pilgrimage in France, attracting 3 million visitors each year. In a grotto near the town the young child *Bernadette saw a vision of the Virgin, who spoke to her. Four years later, in 1862, the Pope accepted that the experience was authentic. The girl was canonized in 1933. Many of the sick and ill who visit the Shrine of Our Lady at Lourdes claim cure and relief.

LOUSE. A parasitic insect belonging to the order Anoplura. See BODY LOUSE; CRAB LOUSE; *PEDICULUS CAPITIS*.

LOWER, RICHARD (1631–91). British physician. In 1665 he was the first to undertake direct blood transfusion between two dogs and in 1667, to give the first transfusion of sheep's blood to man in England. He published *Tractatus de corde* (1669).

LOWER MOTOR NEURONES are those *neurones which originate in the anterior horn cells of the *spinal cord and provide the motor nerve supply to skeletal muscles. See NEUROMUSCULAR DISEASE.

LSD. See LYSERGIDE.

LUDWIG, CARL FRIEDRICH WILHELM (1816–95). German physiologist. One of the creators of modern physiology and a teacher of immense influence, he sought to explain all vital processes in physicochemical terms. His own researches were concerned with the circulation and secretion. A man of great ingenuity, he invented the *kymograph (1849), the mercurial blood pump (1859), and the strain gauge (1867), and devised a method of maintaining the circulation in isolated organs (1865).

LUDWIG INSTITUTE. The Ludwig Institute for Cancer Research was established in 1971 as a charitable international medical research organization devoted exclusively to the investigation of *cancer for the benefit of the public. It is not a foundation and does not award grants. The Institute's income is derived from an endowment consisting of assets contributed by Daniel K. Ludwig. The Institute operates through a number of established branches. At present there are eight of these: two in Switzerland, two in the UK, two in Australia, one in Belgium, one in Canada. Additional branches are planned. The branches, the total research costs of which are met by the Institute, work in conjunction with existing hospitals that are themselves organized and operated exclusively for charitable purposes, and are situated in a well-established research environment.

LUES VENEREA. Synonym for *syphilis.

LUGOL, JEAN GUILLAUME AUGUSTE (1786–1851). French physician. Lugol described a solution containing 1 per cent iodine in 2 per cent aqueous potassium iodide (Lugol's solution, 1829) which he recommended for treating *scrofula. Later it was used in *thyroid disorders.

LULLY, RAYMOND (1235–1315). Majorcan *alchemist. He sought the *philosopher's stone which would change base metals into gold, then thought to be a sovereign remedy against most ills. He invented a logic machine which when fed premises spewed out the appropriate conclusions.

LUMBAGO is a pain or ache in the lumbar region (the small of the back). When associated with *sciatica, lumbago is often due to a lesion of an intervertebral *disc. See also BACKACHE; PROLAPSED INTERVERTEBRAL DISC.

LUMBAR PUNCTURE is the insertion of a suitable needle through one of the intervertebral spaces, usually that between the fourth and fifth lumbar vertebrae, into the lumbar *subarachnoid space. The procedure provides a specimen of *cerebrospinal fluid for diagnostic examination, and allows the intrathecal injection of drugs, anaesthetic agents, or contrast medium.

LUNACY is an obsolete term for mental disorder of such a degree as to render the patient incompetent, and to bring him under the guardianship of the state. 'Moral lunacy' is an old psychiatric term equivalent to *psychopathic personality.

LUNACY COMMISSION. In the USA, a committee, usually of qualified psychiatrists, appointed by judicial order to determine the mental state of an individual whose case a court has under consideration. The Lunacy Commission in the UK was a body created by the Lunacy Act of 1845 which was repealed by the *Mental Health Act 1959.

LUNG. See CHEST MEDICINE.

LUNG FUNCTION TESTS. See CHEST MEDICINE; CLINICAL INVESTIGATION.

LUPUS, when unqualified, is an imprecise term suggesting proliferation of facial skin giving a wolf-like appearance. It usually refers to *lupus erythematosus or *lupus vulgaris.

LUPUS ERYTHEMATOSUS is a chronic inflammatory disease of the skin characteristically occurring in a 'butterfly' distribution over the bridge of the nose and the cheeks, marked by red *macules and scale formation with later scarring. See also SYSTEMIC LUPUS ERYTHEMATOSUS.

LUPUS VULGARIS is *tuberculosis of the skin, particularly of the nose and face, characterized by a gradually spreading patch of reddish-brown nodules which on pressure under glass, resemble 'apple jelly'; involution and scarring, and sometimes ulceration, occur in the centre. Tubercle bacilli can be found in the lesions. It is now rare, but responds well to tuberculostatic drugs such as isoniazid.

LUSCHKA, HUBERT VON (1820–75). German anatomist. He investigated the physiology of voice and speech and his name is attached to many anatomical structures; the most familiar is the foramen of Luschka in the lateral recess of the fourth cerebral ventricle.

LUTEINIZING HORMONE (LH) is one of two gonadotrophic *hormones secreted by the anterior *pituitary gland. In both sexes it stimulates secretion of sex hormones by the *gonads; in women it acts with *follicle-stimulating hormone (FSH) to cause *ovulation and is concerned in the subsequent formation of the *corpus luteum. In virtue of its action in men, it is sometimes also known as interstitial cell stimulating hormone (ICSH).

LYDGATE, DR. Dr Tertius Lydgate is a character in *Middlemarch* (1871–72) by George Eliot (Mary Ann Evans), a work which was saluted by Virginia Woolf as 'one of the few English novels written for adult people'. In it George Eliot delineates the detail of life in an English provincial town. Her analysis of the developing medical profession has been praised. Lydgate (allegedly modelled on Sir Clifford *Allbutt) represented a new type of doctor emerging from the surgeon apothecary (one who held diplomas from both the College of Surgeons and the Society of Apothecaries), the forerunner of the enlightened general practitioner of today. See also DOCTORS IN LITERATURE.

LYME DISEASE. See RHEUMATOLOGY.

LYMPH is the fluid drained by lymph vessels from tissue spaces. It is colourless, but sometimes opalescent because of fat particles as in the vessels draining the intestinal villi; the water content is ultimately derived from blood by filtration through capillary walls. Lymph contains a small amount of protein, and a varying number of cells, chiefly *lymphocytes. Because lymphatic *capillaries are much more permeable than blood vessels, the lymph removes large molecules and particles, such as invading bacteria, from tissue spaces.

LYMPHADENITIS is inflammation of *lymph nodes, usually characterized by swelling and tenderness. It is often localized to regional nodes, that is to nodes on lymphatic vessels draining an infected region of tissue or an organ, and is part of the defensive and localizing reaction to infection. Lymphadenitis may also be generalized, as in the virus infection of *infectious mononucleosis (glandular fever). Lymph node enlargement due to pathological processes other than inflammation, such as the *lymphomas or as a result of metastatic spread of *carcinoma, is more correctly called 'lymphadenosis' or 'lymphadenopathy'.

LYMPHADENOMA. Synonym for *Hodgkin's disease.

LYMPHATIC GLANDS. Synonymous with *lymph nodes.

LYMPHATICS. *Lymph vessels.

LYMPH NODES are small (1–25 mm in diameter), bean-shaped organs situated along the main lymphatic vessels, consisting of lymphoid tissue arranged in an outer cortical and an inner medullary area. Several small lymph vessels enter the periphery and a single larger vessel leaves the concavity of the node. Their functions include the filtering off of particulate matter, such as bacteria, from lymph; the addition of *lymphocytes, of which they are the main source, to the peripheral blood; and *antibody production. Lymph nodes occur in mammals and birds but not in other vertebrates. They are part of the *reticuloendothelial and lymphatic systems.

LYMPHOCYTE. A variety of mononuclear non-granulocytic *leucocyte, normally making up about one-quarter of the circulating white blood cell population. Lymphocytes are a major component of the *immune system, and are classified according to origin and function into two major subgroups, designated B (for bursa or bone-marrow dependent) and T (for thymus dependent). B lymphocytes secrete *antibody, while T lymphocytes have several other immunological functions and are further subdivided into cytotoxic (killer), suppressor, helper, and delayed hypersensitivity groups. See IMMUNOLOGY.

LYMPHOGRANULOMA VENEREUM is a venereally acquired infection occurring chiefly in tropical and subtropical countries, due to strains of an organism (*Chlamydia trachomatis*) closely related to those responsible for *trachoma and *non-specific urethritis. Regional *lymphadenopathy a few weeks after infection is the usual first manifestation (a transient primary lesion is noticed in only a few cases), which may be inguinal, perirectal, or pelvic in distribution. Important complications are *fistula formation, lymphatic obstruction with genital *elephantiasis, and rectal stricture. Its many synonyms include: lymphogranuloma inguinale; poradenitis nostras; tropical bubo; and 'fifth venereal disease'. See SEXUALLY TRANSMITTED DISEASE.

LYMPHOMA is a term now applied to any malignant *neoplasm originating from one of the cellular components of the *immune system, including for example *Burkitt's lymphoma, *Hodgkin's disease, and various forms of lymphosarcoma.

LYMPHOSARCOMA. See LYMPHOMA.

LYON HYPOTHESIS. The hypothesis that in female mammalian cells one of the two X *chromosomes is inactive, inactivation occurring at an early stage of development of the embryo and affecting either the paternally derived or the maternal chromosome on a random basis. See also GENETICS; NUCLEAR SEXING.

LYOPHILIZATION is freeze-drying, a method of preservation of biological material by successively freezing and drying in a vacuum.

LYSERGIDE. Lysergic acid diethylamide, or LSD. This hallucinogenic drug is one of the most potent biochemical substances known. Under its influence, subjects experience a '*psychosis in miniature'. Its effects can be dangerous and include panic states, aggression, suicide, and recurrent, sometimes irreversible, psychosis. Tolerance develops with repeated use, and psychological dependence can be extreme; some degree of cross-tolerance occurs with *mescaline and psilocybin. Claims, not fully substantiated, have been made of its value in psychiatric practice. It is said to release repressions, and to be a useful adjunct in treating *alcoholism. Pharmacologically, LSD is a *serotonin antagonist. It is chemically similar to *tryptamine.

LYSIS is the dissolution or decomposition of cells or subcellular structures. See also CRISIS.

LYSOL is a disinfectant mixture of a solution of soft soap (a mixture of the potassium salts of stearic, oleic, and palmitic acids) with the cresols (the three isomers of hydroxytoluene).

LYSOSOME. Small free subcellular vesicle containing digestive *enzymes. See CELL AND CELL BIOLOGY.

LYSOZYME is an *enzyme that destroys or weakens the cell wall of many *bacteria, leading to their rupture and death, and hence functioning as an antibacterial agent; it acts by hydrolysing the complex polymers of amino acids and amino sugars present in cell walls. Lysozyme, also known as muramidase, is found in many mammalian body fluids, including tears and saliva. It is also present in bird egg white. It provides some protection against bacterial invasion.

MACACA. A genus of Old World catarrhine monkeys containing species valued as laboratory animals.

McARDLE'S DISEASE. A rare variety of glycogen storage disease, a group of *inborn errors of metabolism characterized by the accumulation of *glycogen in the tissues. In McArdle's disease, the basic defect is a deficiency of the enzyme phosphorylase in muscle fibres. The manifestations are muscle pain and stiffness increasing during exertion, often with some persistent weakness and wasting. *Myoglobin may appear in the urine.

McBURNEY, CHARLES (1845–1913). American surgeon. His name is associated with acute *appendicitis. *McBurney's point is an area where tenderness is often most marked. He developed the McBurney incision, for removal of the appendix, whereby the abdominal wall is opened by splitting the muscular layers, without cutting across muscle fibres.

McBURNEY'S POINT is the usual point of maximum abdominal tenderness in acute *appendicitis, situated between 35 and 50 mm from the right anterior superior iliac spine on a line between the spine and the umbilicus.

MacCALLUM, WILLIAM GEORGE (1874–1944). American pathologist. MacCallum made several important observations, including: endothelial lining of *lymphatic vessels, the relation between *parathyroid glands and blood *calcium concentration, and studies of the cardiac lesions resulting from *rheumatic fever. He wrote a textbook of pathology that was widely used for many years.

McCARRISON, SIR ROBERT (1878–1960). British physician and nutritionist, who made important studies on endemic *goitre, *beriberi, and many other nutritional problems in India.

McCOY, GEORGE WALTER (1876–1952). American epidemiologist and public health administrator. During work on plague, with W. C. Chapin, he discovered the causative organism of tularaemia, *Pasteurella tularense*, (named for the California county of Tulare, in which it was encountered).

McCRAE, JOHN (1872–1918). Canadian physician and poet. In 1916 at a field dressing station he wrote the poem 'In Flanders Fields'. He died of pneumonia in Boulogne in 1918, and his verses were published posthumously.

McDOWELL, EPHRAIM (1771–1839). American surgeon. He was a pioneer of elective abdominal surgery, without benefit of *anaesthesia or knowledge of measures to prevent *sepsis.

MACEWEN, SIR WILLIAM (1848–1924). British surgeon. Macewen was a pupil of Lord *Lister. He studied the pathology of bone and in 1877 devised the operation of *osteotomy. In 1878 he excised a *cerebral tumour, in 1879 he operated for *subdural haemorrhage, in 1893 he successfully drained a *cerebral abscess and in 1895 he removed a lung for pulmonary tuberculosis.

McGILL UNIVERSITY is in Montreal, Canada. Four Edinburgh-trained physicians, working at the Montreal General Hospital, started lectures on medicine in 1822. In 1829 the Institution which they founded was accepted as the faculty of medicine by the University which grew out of the original McGill College. William *Osler qualified there in 1872 and taught in the faculty from 1874 to 1884. Other hospitals and institutions have been affiliated over the years, one of the more famous being that founded in 1934 by Wilder *Penfield in neurology.

McGRIGOR, SIR JAMES, BT (1771–1858). British army surgeon. During his long military career he served in Flanders, West Indies, India, Ceylon, and Egypt as well as throughout the Peninsular War. He reorganized and greatly improved the army medical services.

McINDOE, SIR ARCHIBALD HECTOR (1900–60). Anglo-New Zealand plastic surgeon. In 1940 he established a centre for plastic surgery at East Grinstead which became world-famous for its care of Royal Air Force personnel.

MACKENZIE, SIR JAMES (1853–1925). British physician. He analysed cardiac irregularities by means of the '*polygraph' which he devised. In 1902 he published *The study of the pulse* and in 1908 *Diseases of the heart.*

MACKENZIE, SIR MORELL (1837–92). British laryngologist. He developed an interest in diseases of the throat and in 1876 founded the Throat Hospital in Golden Square. He became expert in the use of the newly devised *laryngoscope and acquired a large practice in laryngology. In 1887 he was called to Berlin to see Emperor Frederick III. On the basis of a negative biopsy report by *Virchow he declared that the emperor did not have laryngeal *cancer. This view was opposed by the German surgeons and heated arguments ensued. Events proved Mackenzie wrong and he defended himself in undignified pamphlets which earned the censure of the Royal College of Surgeons. See also OTORHINOLARYNGOLOGY.

McKENZIE, ROBERT TAIT (1867–1938). Canadian physician and sculptor. His sculptures of athletes brought him a decoration by the King of Sweden at the Olympic Games of 1912. In the First World War he was a pioneer in *rehabilitation medicine.

MacMICHAEL, WILLIAM (1783–1839). British physician. He was the author of the celebrated *The gold headed cane* (1827), in which the cane recalls the famous physicians who owned it.

McNAGHTEN (McNAUGHTON) RULES were introduced in the UK by the House of Lords in 1843 to clarify the law relating to criminal responsibility and mental state. They state that to establish a defence of *insanity it must be proved that at the time of committing the crime the accused party was labouring under such a defect of reason, from disease of the mind, as not to know the nature and quality of the act he was doing; or if he did know it, he did not know that what he was doing was wrong. These rules were formulated in the light of the case of Daniel McNaghten (also spelt McNaughton), who in the same year had shot and killed Sir Robert Peel's private secretary in mistake for Peel himself. McNaghten was suffering from *delusions of persecution by the Tories, and in consequence was found not guilty and sent to *Bethlem hospital.

MACROGLIA. See NEUROGLIA.

MACROGLOBULIN is globulin of high molecular weight (900 000 to a million), equivalent to IgM. An increased concentration of macroglobulin occurs in certain lymphoproliferative disorders.

MACROPHAGE. A large mononuclear *phagocytic cell occurring in connective tissues and in the walls of blood vessels; it is the essential unit of the *reticuloendothelial system. Macrophages are often mobile, moving by membrane-like pseudopodia; they engulf and remove damaged cells and foreign matter. They develop in the tissues from *monocytes formed in the marrow. The resting tissue forms are usually termed *histiocytes, while in the liver they are called *Kupffer cells.

MACULA. Any spot or discoloured area; more particularly, a small yellowish area subserving visual activity and distinguishable on examining the retina, lateral to and below the optic disc (macula retinae).

MAGENDIE, FRANCOIS (1783–1855). French physiologist. Magendie distrusted all theory and sought to establish facts by experiment and observation. He was a keen and sometimes brutal *vivisectionist; sceptical and contemptuous, he opposed *vitalism and the use of *ether as an anaesthetic, and denied the importance of contagion. He confirmed *Bell's observations on the anterior spinal nerve roots being motor and the posterior sensory (Bell–Magendie law, 1822), and described *decerebrate rigidity (1823) and the secretion of *cerebrospinal fluid. He was a pioneer of toxicology and experimental pharmacology.

MAGGOTS are fly larvae. Infestation of living tissues by maggots is termed myiasis. Many species of fly can cause human myiasis, although in no instance is man either the specific or the only animal host. Open sores and purulent discharges which attract flies are particularly likely to become sites of infestation, usually in the destitute. Several varieties of cutaneous myiasis are described (e.g. creeping, furuncular). Other sites are the nasopharynx, the gastrointestinal and genitourinary tracts, and the eye. The maggots can sometimes cause serious tissue destruction.

MAGIC. Magical thinking or 'magical omnipotence' is recognized by psychiatrists as a normal phase in the mental development of infants and very young children. In older age-groups such archaic, primitive, prelogical thought processes can be a symptom of *schizophrenia and some types of *neurosis.

MAGNESIUM is a white metallic element (symbol Mg, atomic number 12, relative atomic mass 24.312) essential to all life as a constituent of *chlorophyll. It is also an essential component of the human diet (recommended adult intake about 350 mg/day), being required as a *coenzyme in energy metabolism and as an *ion in body fluids (serum level about 2 mEq/l) necessary for the normal function of nerve and muscle cells. Hypomagnesaemia results in a syndrome of nervous irritability like that of hypocalcaemic *tetany. The average Western diet supplies adequate amounts of magnesium, which is present in many foods; cereals, whelks, and coffee powder are among the richest sources.

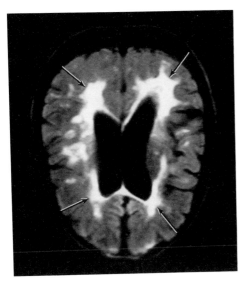

Fig. 1 Transverse image of the brain in multiple sclerosis. The abnormal areas around the ventricles in the white matter appear bright (arrows).

MAGNETIC RESONANCE IMAGING

MAGNETIC RESONANCE IMAGING (MRI) has progressed very rapidly over the past 10 years and is now the imaging technique of choice for *diagnosis of a wide variety of neurological, orthopaedic, oncological, and paediatric problems. Over 6000 systems have now been installed world-wide and an estimated 8–10 million examinations are performed every year. The technique is particularly useful in detecting abnormalities in the soft tissues of the body, and is believed to be without biological hazard. The main barrier to wider use is the high cost of MRI systems.

Mechanism
MRI exploits the fact that the nuclei of the hydrogen atoms in the body behave like tiny spinning magnets and align with the field when the body is placed within a large magnet. When the magnetism of the nuclei is disturbed by a short pulsed magnetic field it returns to equilibrium or 'relaxes' in an exponential fashion. As it does so it induces a small voltage in a receiver coil placed next to the body. The rate of return of the magnetization to equilibrium or relaxation is affected by the local chemical and physical environment of the nuclei. Additional magnetic fields are needed to locate the signal from the nuclei in space, in order to produce an image. Computers are required to reconstruct the images, which are presented on visual display units or radiographic film.

Many disease processes such as *infarction, infection, and *neoplasia prolong the relaxation time of tissues. This is the principal source of tissue contrast on MR images. The MR images are also sensitive to flow effects and molecular diffusion, and can be used to provide specific information on particular concentrations of chemical species within the body.

Whereas most tissues of the body are diamagnetic, and so slightly decrease the magnetic field in which they are placed, this phenomenon does not significantly affect the image. On the other hand, a few substances, such as blood breakdown products containing iron, are paramagnetic and therefore produce relatively large changes in images. Other paramagnetic substances, such as gadolinium diethylenetriamine pentacetic acid (Gd–DTPA), for example, may also be administered as contrast agents to produce similar effects (also see RADIOLOGY).

It is also possible to study nuclei other than hydrogen and obtain information about the concentration of specific metabolites such as *ATP and phosphocreatine.

Applications
In the nervous system, increased relaxation times are seen in infarction, *demyelinating disease, (Fig. 1), infection, *oedema, and *tumours. As a result, the images are very sensitive to the presence of abnormal tissue and the high spatial resolution provides precise location within the brain or spinal cord. Images may be created in any plane; the midline or sagittal plane is particularly well suited to disease in the *spinal cord (Fig. 2).

While calcified tissue usually gives no signal on MR images, soft tissues often give a high signal, and *bone marrow, *ligaments, *cartilage, and muscle are well visualized. This is of importance in assessing injuries to large joints such as the knee and shoulder. As with the nervous tissue, the main change is in the relaxation

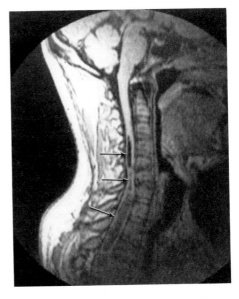

Fig. 2 Spinal cord in syringomyelia. The midline image of the spinal cord shows fluid-containing regions (arrows).

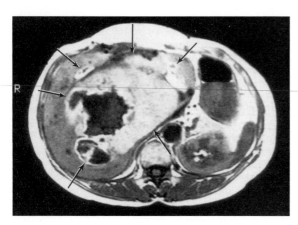

Fig. 3 Transverse image of the upper abdomen in hepatoma (tumour) of the liver. The mass is highlighted (arrows). Note the dark, irregular areas in the mass necrotic (dead) tissue.

times. The images have high sensitivity to the presence of disease, but often more than one disease process can produce the same appearance.

Most tumours show an increase in relaxation time, and can be seen with high contrast (Fig. 3). This can be further increased by the use of injected contrast agents such as Gd-DTPA, which are paramagnetic and increase the speed of the relaxation process. The heart can readily be imaged, and by either synchronizing the imaging process to the heart cycle, or by using very rapid imaging techniques, clear images of the heart can be produced and moving images of cardiac motion can readily be obtained.

The lack of hazard of MRI is of particular importance in *paediatric studies, but care is necessary to exclude ferromagnetic objects from the magnetic field used for imaging, since they may be strongly attracted by the field and behave like missiles.

Future developments
Smaller and more open magnets have been produced recently and these may result in a reduction in the cost of systems. There has also been a strong move towards the use of three-dimensional imaging, which is an efficient method of operation and permits image reconstruction in any plane. It can be combined with display systems to provide image-guided surgery. The versatility of these techniques means that it is possible to obtain *angiograms showing details of blood-vessel anatomy without the injection of any agent. The velocity of flow can be measured with MRI and maps of Brownian motion of water can be produced. Functional studies where changes in brain signal are produced by physiological stimuli can be demonstrated.

It is expected that MRI will continue to expand rapidly. Techniques previously used only in *nuclear medicine and interventional *radiology are now being developed for MRI applications, and a wider range of more specialized systems is now under construction.

R. E. STEINER
G. M. BYDDER

References
Atlas, S. W. (ed.) (1991). *Magnetic resonance imaging of the brain and spine.* Raven Press, New York.
Higgins, C. B., Hricak, H., and Helms, C. (1992). *Magnetic resonance imaging of the body.* Raven Press, New York.
Stark, D. D. and Bradley, W. G., Jr (ed.) (1992). *Magnetic resonance imaging*, (2nd edn), 2 vols. Mosby Year Book, St Louis.

MAGNETISM is the branch of physics concerned with magnets and magnetic fields. See also MAGNETIC RESONANCE IMAGING.

MAGNUS, RUDOLF (1873–1927). German physiologist. Sherrington interested him in the study of reflex maintenance of posture. His fundamental researches were recorded in *Die Körperstellung* (1924).

MAHOMED, FREDERICK HENRY HORATIO AKBAR (1849–84). English physician. He modified the *sphygmograph to enable arterial blood pressure to be measured. This allowed him to explain the association, noted by Richard *Bright, between contracted kidneys and enlargement of the heart—the connecting link being raised blood pressure, or in the language of the day, 'morbid arterial tension'.

MAIMONIDES, RABBI MOSES BEN MAIMON (Abu Imram Musa ibn Maimum; 'Rambam') (?1135–1204). Hispano-Jewish physician and philosopher. Maimonides was born in Cordoba, where he was a pupil of Averroes, moving later to Fez and in 1166 to Egypt. He is buried at Tiberias, where his tomb is still a place of pilgrimage. He codified Talmudic law and wrote on philosophy and theology. His medical writings showed independent and original thought. He was critical of *Galen and published a valuable commentary on the aphorisms of *Hippocrates.

MAINTENANCE THERAPY is the prescription of a drug or drugs on a long-term basis in doses sufficient to sustain a therapeutic effect.

MAJOR HISTOCOMPATIBILITY COMPLEX (MHC). See HLA; IMMUNOLOGY.

MAL. Pain, sickness, disease, etc. (French, e.g. *mal de mer, mal de tête, mal des dents*). *Petit mal and *grand mal are examples of established anglophone usage avoiding the word '*epilepsy'.

MALABSORPTION covers a wide variety of conditions in which there is failure of adequate intestinal absorption of one or more groups of nutrients, with consequent loss of them in the faeces and the development of nutritional deficiency syndromes. *Steatorrhoea is usually present. *Coeliac disease, *sprue, pancreatic insufficiency, lymphatic obstruction, and surgical resection of intestine are examples; but malabsorption has many causes. See GASTROENTEROLOGY.

MALADY. Disease, illness.

MALAISE. Any feeling of being unwell.

MALARIA arises from infection with one or more of four species of protozoal organisms belonging to the genus *Plasmodium* (*P. falciparum, P. vivax, P. malariae, P. ovale*), transmitted by female anopheline *mosquitoes of several different species. Malaria, which is endemic in parts of Africa, Asia, and South and Central America, causes a huge mortality and morbidity; and, world-wide, must be ranked among the outstanding problems of modern medicine. See TROPICAL MEDICINE.

MALE CLIMACTERIC. The waning of sexual activity and interest in the ageing male is normally gradual and progressive, without evidence of any abrupt somatic change analogous to the female *menopause to justify use of the term 'climacteric'.

MALFORMATION. Any abnormality of structure due to faulty development.

MALIGNANT DISEASE is any cancerous disease involving an uncontrolled growth of cells exhibiting *anaplasia, invasiveness, and remote spread (metastasis) (see ONCOLOGY). The term 'malignant' is also applied to non-cancerous conditions having a rapidly progressive and virulent character (e.g. malignant *hypertension, *malignant hyperpyrexia, malignant tertian *malaria).

MALIGNANT HYPERPYREXIA is a rare, genetically determined, complication of general *anaesthesia. See HYPERPYREXIA.

MALINGERING is conscious simulation of mental or physical illness in order to gain some end.

MALL, FRANKLIN PAINE (1862–1917). American anatomist. He made lasting contributions to knowledge of human *embryology, including a method for estimating the age of a human embryo.

MALLOCH, THOMAS ARCHIBALD (1887–1953). American librarian. An arts graduate who later chose to study medicine. Upon graduation in medicine from McGill in 1913 'Young Archie' as *Osler called him, joined the army and served in France. He spent his leaves with the Oslers at Oxford, and used every opportunity to work in the Bodleian Library on his first book *Finch and Baines, a seventeenth century friendship* (1917). Post-war Malloch laboured at Oxford on the great *Bibliotheca Osleriana* with Dr W. W. *Francis and Reginald Hill. Malloch's biographical interests are reflected in his writings on Robin Adair, William *Harvey, and John *Caius, and also in *Short years*, his biography of John Bruce MacCallum, Osler's brilliant pupil who died of *tuberculosis at the age of thirty.

MALLORY, FRANK BURR (1862–1941). American pathologist. He was a master of histological techniques, and among other things, devised the Mallory stain for *collagen. He recognized the importance of phagocytic activity by blood *monocytes, and also played a part in establishing the role of *Haemophilus pertussis* in the aetiology of *whooping cough.

MALNUTRITION is any disorder of *nutrition, applied especially to conditions associated with inadequate intake or defective utilization of food.

MALPIGHI, MARCELLO (1628–94). Italian physician. Malpighi was one of the first microscopists and the founder of histology. In *De pulmonibus observationes anatomicae* (1661) he described the vesicular structure and the capillaries of the lungs. He noted that the blood was composed of a 'host of red atoms' (1661). He described the glomerular tufts of the kidneys (1666) and the Malpighian bodies of the spleen (1666). In *De viscerum structura* (1666) he records probable examples of *Hodgkin's disease. In *De formatio pulli in ova* (1673) he established his place in *embryology.

MALPRACTICE. See PROFESSIONAL MALPRACTICE.

MALTA FEVER. One synonym for *brucellosis.

MALTOSE is a compound *sugar (disaccharide), a molecule of which is made up of two *glucose molecules. It is formed by the action of *amylase on *starch.

MAMMARY GLAND. The specialized milk-producing gland, representing a modified sweat gland, situated on the ventral surface of female members of the class Mammalia, of which it is a defining characteristic. In women, two such glands, together with connective and adipose tissue, form the breasts. Each consists of about 20 lobes, with separate lactiferous ducts opening on to the nipple. See also INFANT FEEDING; LACTATION.

MAMMILLARY BODIES. A pair of small spherical structures forming part of the *hypothalamus.

MAMMOGRAPHY is *radiographic visualization of the *breasts.

MANDIBLE. The bone of the lower jaw.

MANDRAGORA, or mandrake, is a poisonous solanaceous (of the potato family) plant containing several *atropine-like alkaloids (full name *Mandragora officinarum*).

MANDRAKE. See MANDRAGORA.

MANGANESE is a reddish-white brittle metallic element (symbol Mn, atomic number 25, relative atomic mass 54.938). As manganese is required in trace amounts as a *coenzyme in human *metabolism, it is an essential dietary component, although deficiency states have not been demonstrated in man. Excessive intake, which occurs in manganese miners inhaling dust, causes neurotoxicity, the most prominent features being *parkinsonism and mental disturbance ('manganese madness').

MANIA is a mental disturbance characterized by mood elation (euphoria); increased psychomotor activity; increased speed of ideas and thought ('flight of ideas') and rapidity of speech. As in other *psychoses the patient has little or no insight. Moderate elevation of mood and activity is sometimes termed 'hypomania'.

MANIA A POTU is a rare but real syndrome in which the ingestion of *alcohol (sometimes in relatively modest quantity) precipitates an episode of extreme and irrational violence.

MANIC-DEPRESSIVE PSYCHOSIS is a form of mental illness in which periods of *mania (elation and increased psychomotor activity) alternate with periods of *depression (lowering of mood and decreased psychomotor activity); it is also known as 'bipolar affective psychosis'. The term 'manic-depressive' psychosis was introduced in 1896 by *Kraepelin to distinguish this illness from psychoses in which profound mental deterioration occurs (e.g. *schizophrenia).

MANIPULATION. See CHIROPRACTIC; OSTEOPATHY.

MAN-MIDWIFE. Hitherto, an obstetrician or *accoucheur, that is a medical practitioner of *midwifery. The term assumed a wider meaning following the admission (in 1983) of male members of the nursing profession to the practice of midwifery in the UK.

MANNINGHAM, SIR RICHARD (1690–1759). British man-midwife. In 1739 he established the first wards for parturient women in the UK in the parochial infirmary of St James, Westminster.

MANOMETER. Any instrument for measuring liquid or gaseous pressure.

MANOMETRY is the measurement of pressure of liquids or gases: for example, *sphygmomanometry is measurement of blood pressure; the pressure of cerebrospinal fluid is also often measured.

MANSON, SIR PATRICK (1844–1922). British physician and parasitologist. He has been called 'the father of tropical medicine'. He showed the *mosquito to be the vector of *filariasis and suggested its role in *malaria.

MANTOUX, CHARLES (1877–1947). French physician. He devised the intradermal *tuberculin test (1908).

MANTOUX TEST. A form of *tuberculin test.

MAOI. See MONOAMINE-OXIDASE INHIBITORS.

MARASMUS is the term applied to a syndrome of protein–energy malnutrition in children; its essential features are cessation of growth and emaciation without major metabolic disturbances and with retention of both appetite and mental alertness.

MARBURG DISEASE and *Ebola disease are collectively known as African haemorrhagic fever. The two conditions are clinically the same, but the *viruses, although morphologically identical, are immunologically distinct. The first case was reported from Marburg, Germany, in 1967 after contact had occurred between the patient and green monkeys imported from Uganda. Subsequent transmission has been person-to-person. With the best available management, the mortality rate of Marburg disease has been about 30 per cent.

MARFAN, BERNARD JEAN ANTOININ (1858–1942). French paediatrician. He described a disorder marked by bilateral dislocation of the ocular lenses, congenital heart disease, *arachnodactyly, and a tall thin habitus (Marfan's syndrome, 1896).

MARFAN'S SYNDROME. See ARACHNODACTYLY.

MARIE, PIERRE (1853–1940). French neurologist. A brilliant clinician, he described *acromegaly (and linked it with *pituitary tumour) (1886–91), peroneal muscular atrophy (Charcot–Marie–Tooth *disease, 1886), hypertrophic *pulmonary osteo-arthropathy (1890), cerebellar *ataxia (1893), and *cleidocranial dysostosis (1897).

MARIJUANA is a preparation of *cannabis.

MARINE, DAVID (1880–1978). American physician. Following the finding of Baumann, that the thyroid gland contains *iodine, he worked out methods for quantitative analysis of thyroid tissue for iodine content, and found that a low iodine content is associated with *hyperplasia of the glandular elements. This was of primary importance in suggesting that endemic goitre is a deficiency disease. In 1916–17 he was able to demonstrate the prevention of goitre in Ohio schoolchildren by administering iodine; this led directly to the widespread custom of using iodized table salt.

MARTINDALE, WILLIAM (1840–1902). London pharmacist. Martindale was president of the *Pharmaceutical Society of Great Britain in 1899–1900, and compiled and edited the first edition of the *Extra Pharmacopoeia*, published in 1883. Martindale's name has been perpetuated by its attachment to successive editions of this work, which has continued to provide a valuable reference source of information about the properties, actions, and uses of drugs and medicines to medical practitioners and pharmacists alike. Martindale himself had been responsible for producing 10 editions by the time of his death in 1902, after which his medically qualified son, William Harrison Martindale, continued the family association until his own death in 1933. Subsequent editions have been produced by the Pharmaceutical Society of Great Britain. See also PHARMACY AND PHARMACISTS.

MARTYRS, TO MEDICINE. Few medical thinkers and scientists have gone to their deaths on account of their beliefs, although there have been some. For example, *Servetus, a Spaniard who had studied medicine in France, was condemned to death by the Protestant leader John Calvin for proposing (correctly as it turned out) the theory of the lesser or pulmonary circulation of blood, contradicting the teaching of *Galen; he was burned alive in Geneva on 27 October 1553.

MASCULINIZATION is the development of male *secondary sex characteristics, whether normally in the male at *puberty or abnormally in the female; it is synonymous with *virilization.

MASKS are used in medicine, usually either to prevent exchange of air-borne micro-organisms between the wearer's upper respiratory tract and the surrounding air, or for the administration of inhalational anaesthetics or other gaseous mixtures.

MASOCHISM is the achieving of sexual satisfaction from submitting to pain, humiliation, and punishment. The term is derived from the Austrian novelist Leopold von Sacher Masoch (1836–95), whose characters obtained sexual pleasure from cruel treatment.

MASS is the characteristic which confers inertia on a material body. Gravitational mass (equal to inertial mass), determined by Newton's law of gravitation, is that which is actually used in measuring mass and in defining the kilogram, the unit of mass. Scientifically, *weight is the product of a body's mass and the acceleration of free fall (g), but is often used synonymously with mass.

MASSACHUSETTS GENERAL HOSPITAL was founded in Boston, USA, in 1811, although building was delayed by war, so that it was opened to patients in 1821, and became the first teaching hospital of the *Harvard Medical School. The first building was named after its architect Charles Bullfinch. The aims were, and are, to care for the sick; to teach those responsible for that care; to conduct research into the causes, control, and cure of disease. It was there in 1846 that William T.G. *Morton, a dentist, first administered *ether to a patient operated on by John Collins *Warren, so ushering in a new era in surgery (see ANAESTHESIA). The achievement is commemorated in the Ether Dome. *Fitz (1886) identified *appendicitis as an entity, which led to surgery for its cure in an operation which by now has saved millions of lives. In 1905 a Social Service Department was first started; in 1962 there was the first replantation of a severed arm; in 1964 came the first practical method of freezing blood; in 1974 the introduction of *photochemotherapy; and in 1981 the development of artificial skin for grafting. The hospital now has a local, national, and international practice.

MASSAGE is a form of physical treatment, usually manual, by stroking, kneading, pummelling, thumping, pressing, or applying friction to various parts of the body surface. Massage is one technique of *physiotherapy.

MASSEUR (MASSEUSE). Male (female) operator trained in the application of *massage. A masseur may or may not be qualified in *physiotherapy.

MASS SPECTROMETRY. An analytical method which uses the fact that the deflection of any individual *ion in a magnetic field depends on the ratio of the mass of the ion to its electric charge. The material to be analysed is first ionized in a vacuum and the ions are formed into a beam. With suitably disposed magnetic and electrical fields, the beam is then separated into different types of ion according to the mass/charge ratio. Usually the mass spectrum is obtained by deflecting the ions on to a thin slit and measuring the ion current electrically, the magnetic field being varied so as to detect different types of ion.

MAST CELL. A large tissue cell with basophilic granules which on being damaged, or in the presence of *antibody, releases vasoactive amines (*histamine and *serotonin) and *heparin; it plays a part in the inflammatory response.

MASTECTOMY is surgical removal of the breast.

MASTITIS is inflammation of the *mammary gland (breast).

MASTOIDECTOMY is surgical excision of the mastoid portion of the *temporal bone.

MASTOIDITIS is inflammation of the air cells and cavity in the mastoid portion of the *temporal bone.

MASTURBATION is the production of *orgasm by genital stimulation by means other than sexual intercourse. This definition is not restricted to self–stimulation, although this is usually implied.

MATAS, RUDOLPH (1860–1957). American surgeon, chiefly famed for skill in surgery of blood vessels. He devised a method for treating *aneurysms, by stitching the openings of vessels of supply from within the aneurysmal sac, and was credited with the first successful surgical cure of an aortic aneurysm.

MATERIA MEDICA are the substances used in medicine, that is drugs and medicines; it is also the branch of science that deals with the properties and application of these.

MATERNAL DEPRIVATION refers to the deprivation of an infant or child of the stimulation, held to be important to mental and emotional development, normally provided by mother–child interaction.

MATERNAL MORTALITY. The maternal mortality rate is defined as the number of women who die in *pregnancy, *childbirth, or the postnatal period (conventionally defined as the 6 weeks following delivery), per 1000, or more usually today, per 100 000 births. In the past, some countries included deaths from any cause, such as *tuberculosis or heart disease, as well as causes directly related to pregnancy in these calculations. Other countries, including England and Wales, included only deaths directly related to pregnancy (direct maternal deaths); deaths from other causes, known as 'indirect' or 'associated' maternal deaths, were recorded separately. From the early 19th century until the mid-1930s, the maternal mortality rate remained obstinately high, at around 500 per 100 000 births. Unexpectedly, there was no decline in deaths in the early 20th century such as occurred with infant mortality. Since the mid-1930s, however, the maternal mortality rate in all Western countries has fallen steeply, and has stayed at virtually the same annual rate for over 50 years. The many factors responsible for the decline included the *sulphonamides (1937), *ergometrine and *blood transfusion during the Second World War, *penicillin (1945), the virtual abolition of deaths from septic *abortion after 1945, a raised standard of maternal health during and after the war, and much improved systems of maternal care in the community and in hospitals. In Britain, there are now fewer than 10 maternal deaths per 100 000 births. In many parts of the developing world, however, the maternal mortality rate is now as high, or higher, than it was in Europe in the 19th century. It is not often appreciated that at least half a million women still die each year from pregnancy-related causes, because 99 per cent of these deaths occur in developing countries. There is no other public health statistic in which the disparity between developed and developing countries is so wide.

IRVINE LOUDON

MATERNITY SERVICES provided in the UK under the *National Health Service consist of arrangements for regular antenatal and postnatal examinations and treatment, and for delivery. Antenatal care is provided either by the mother's family practitioner or at a hospital out-patient clinic, usually at the mother's choice. Similarly, confinement may take place at home, with the assistance of a midwife and practitioner, or in hospital. In practice, well over 90 per cent of births now take place in hospital, the mother remaining as an in-patient for between 1 and 8 days.

MATRON. See NURSING IN THE UK.

MAUDSLEY HOSPITAL. See BETHLEM ROYAL HOSPITAL.

MAUGHAM, WILLIAM SOMERSET (1874–1965). British physician and writer. He never practised medicine, publishing his first novel *Liza of Lambeth* the year he qualified as a doctor. His most celebrated work was *Of human bondage* (1915), which was said to have sold 10 million copies. In addition to novels and short stories he wrote many successful plays.

MAVOR, OSBORNE HENRY (1888–1951). British physician and playwright. After being professor of medicine at Anderson College, Glasgow, for a short time, he devoted his time to writing plays under the pseudonym of James Bridie. Of his more than 40 plays the best known are *Tobias and the Angel (1930)*, *The Anatomist (1931)*, and *Daphne Laureola* (1949).

MAXILLA. The bone of the upper jaw, which also forms part of the eye socket, the palate, and the nose.

MAXILLARY SINUS. One of the two *paranasal sinuses situated in the body of either *maxilla and communicating with the nasal cavity.

MAXILLOFACIAL SURGERY is the branch of surgery dealing with conditions affecting the face and jaw regions, including *trauma. See PLASTIC AND MAXILLOFACIAL SURGERY.

MAYERNE, SIR THEODORE TURQUET DE (1573–1655). Franco-British physician. He was a meticulous and astute clinical observer who introduced several new remedies including *calomel and 'black wash' (Lotio hydrarg. nig. BP 1949).

MAYO, WILLIAM WORRALL (1819–1911). American surgeon. He was the founder of the *Mayo Clinic in Rochester, Minnesota, where he was later joined by his two sons, WILLIAM JAMES (1861–1939) and CHARLES HORACE (1865–1939). The sons established the Mayo Foundation for Medical Education and Research, affiliated with the University of Minnesota. Charles Horace Mayo was specially skilled in surgery of the *thyroid gland, while William James Mayo had a special interest in surgery of the stomach.

MAYO CLINIC, in Rochester, Minnesota, USA, is one of the great medical institutions of the world. It began with William Worrall *Mayo, who migrated to the USA from Manchester, England. His surgeon sons worked in St Mary's Hospital and in practice, and such was their fame that patients were sent to them from far afield; the use of the term 'Mayo Clinic' crept into general use about 1900. In 1914 the brothers and their associates moved into a purpose-built five-storey building to continue their form of group practice. This was revolutionary because all fees were pooled and the doctors were paid a salary, since they believed that they should not vastly enrich themselves but receive only just and fair compensation for their work. To this end the Mayo Foundation was ultimately started with a large gift from the brothers. This still receives all the income, and administers the Clinic, paying the doctors a salary. The philanthropy does not stop there since the Mayo Graduate School of Medicine was founded in 1915 and the Mayo Medical School (for undergraduates) in 1972, and there is also a Mayo School of Health-Related Sciences. The Clinic is associated with two private hospitals—St Mary's and the Rochester Methodist—which are staffed entirely by Mayo Clinic doctors. There is now a vast range of buildings and services, donated and supported by many benefactors, devoted to the enterprise. The Mayo brothers were legendary in their contributions to surgery, and Edward C. *Kendall and Philip S. *Hench of the Clinic received the *Nobel prize for medicine for their work in isolating *cortisone and using it in the treatment of *arthritis, so opening a new era in endocrinology.

MAYOW, JOHN (1640–79). British physiologist and chemist. He proved that 'nitro-aerial spirit' was removed from air in combustion and in respiration. He published his findings in *Tractatus quinque medico-physici* (1674).

MEAKINS, JONATHAN CAMPBELL (1882–1959). Canadian clinical researcher and medical educator. Wartime service led him to work on 'soldier's heart' and on the treatment of gas warfare injuries to the lungs. He served as dean of medicine at McGill, as director general of medical services for Canada's army, and wrote a textbook, *The practice of medicine*, which went through six editions.

MEALS ON WHEELS provide and transport meals to the elderly and disabled at home through local authority or voluntary agencies.

MEASLES is an acute infectious virus disease conferring lifelong immunity to further attacks. Until the introduction in 1964 of active *immunization, measles (or *morbilli*) in Western urban communities was predominantly a disease of childhood, apart from the first 6 months of infancy, usually protected by persistent maternal immunity; in populations without immunity, all ages are infected. Where most children have been immunized, the incidence has shifted towards the un-immunized young adult population. Measles is a classic *exanthem, i.e. an eruptive fever. Apart from the rash and high temperature, the clinical features are headache, photophobia, catarrhal inflammation of the respiratory tract, and conjunctivitis. The rash usually begins in the mouth, with small white spots (Koplik's spots), and spreads to the face, neck, trunk, and limbs. It is macular and papular in succession, and is followed by desquamation; it is occasionally haemorrhagic. The incubation period is variable but averages about 10–12 days to the onset of symptoms; the disease itself lasts a little longer. Complications are mostly due to secondary bacterial infection (particularly *pneumonia and *otitis media) but *encephalomyelitis occurs in about 0.1 per cent of cases and carries a mortality of 10 per cent. Otherwise, measles is a self-limiting condition from which uneventful recovery is the usual outcome, except in the developing world where it still has a high mortality rate. Rarely, persistence of the measles virus in the body gives rise to *subacute sclerosing panencephalitis many years later.

MEASUREMENT IN MEDICINE is a name sometimes given to medical school or hospital departments specializing in the technology of measurement of physiological or clinical phenomena and the central maintenance of a bank of apparatus for the purpose.

MECONIUM is the green faecal material passed by the newborn infant.

MEDAWAR, SIR PETER (1915–87). British zoologist and immunologist. His work on the rejection of skin grafts in animals laid the foundations of modern cellular immunology, and his subsequent studies of *HLA antigens, along with work on T lymphocytes, led to his being awarded the *Nobel prize for physiology or medicine in 1960. From 1962 he directed the National Institute of Medical Research until severely crippled by illness in 1969, despite which he continued to contribute effectively to immunology and philosophy.

MEDIAN NERVE. An important nerve of the forearm and hand, derived from the *brachial plexus. It supplies most of the muscles of the front of the forearm (flexor) and some small muscles of the thumb; and is responsible for sensation over the skin of the radial (or thumb) side of the hand. The nerve may be injured at various points, but the commonest *lesion is compression as it passes with the flexor tendons through the narrow tunnel at the wrist into the hand—the carpal tunnel syndrome. This causes pain and *paraesthesiae in the hand, and sometimes weakness and wasting of the thumb muscles. It is particularly apt to affect middle-aged women.

MEDIASTINUM. The space between the right and left lungs, and the various structures and tissues which occupy it (including the heart, its great vessels, the trachea, and the thymus gland).

MEDICAID. See GOVERNMENT AND MEDICINE IN THE USA.

MEDICAL ACTS. From the early 16th century, onwards, a series of Medical Acts has been passed by Parliament in the UK to regulate the profession and practice of medicine. The first such statute was the Act of 1511, which provided that none should practise 'physic or surgery' (except graduates of Oxford and Cambridge) unless licensed by the Bishop of his diocese. Candidates for a licence were required to be examined by a special panel convened by the Bishop. Further Acts were passed in 1542, 1858, 1886, 1947, 1950, 1956, 1969, 1978, and 1983. The 1978 Act reconstituted the *General Medical Council and added important provisions to the law concerning standards of professional conduct, registration of doctors whose fitness is impaired, control of medical education, qualifying examinations, overseas doctors, and experience required for full *registration. The 1983 Act consolidated that of 1978 with continuing provisions of those that had gone before.

MEDICAL ADMINISTRATORS. Those engaged in the administration of health and hospital services, whether in the public or the private sector; they may or may not be medically qualified.

MEDICAL ADVISERS. The term has several possible meanings, but applies particularly to that group of doctors employed full- or part-time in the *pharmaceutical industry.

MEDICAL AIDES are paramedical personnel trained to undertake particular aspects of medical work.

MEDICAL ARTISTS. See ART AND MEDICINE; ILLUSTRATION AND PHOTOGRAPHY IN MEDICINE.

MEDICAL ASSOCIATIONS. See MEDICAL COLLEGES, ETC. OF THE UK; MEDICAL COLLEGES, ETC. IN NORTH AMERICA.

MEDICAL AUDIT is the monitoring of outcome in medical practice so as to measure medical competence, efficiency of procedures, etc. See MEDICAL (CLINICAL) AUDIT.

MEDICAL BENEFACTORS. See FOUNDATIONS, AND CHARITIES, ETC.: IN CANADA; IN THE UK; IN THE USA.

MEDICAL BENEVOLENT SOCIETIES are *benevolent societies with one or more specifically medical terms of reference.

MEDICAL BOOKS AND LIBRARIES. Medical writings in various forms have existed from the earliest times. The invention (*c.* 1450) of printing from movable types was the most important factor in the development of books and libraries. Scientific and medical printed books were soon available, at first simply reproductions of the works of ancient writers but soon as an essential factor in the dissemination of developing knowledge. Some books had a profound effect on the medical world.

The *De humani corporis fabrica* of Andreas *Vesalius (1543) marks the beginning of modern anatomy. The French military surgeon Ambroise *Paré wrote several books that added to the knowledge of surgery. They were later (1575) collected and published as his *Oeuvres*.

An outstanding work in the 17th century was William *Harvey's *Exercitatio de motu cordis et sanguinis in animalibus* (1628), in which the circulation of the blood was conclusively demonstrated for the first time. Thomas *Sydenham (1624–89), the 'English Hippocrates', was an outstanding physician who classified diseases, studied patients at the bedside, and made valuable contributions to the literature. A good edition of his collected works appeared in 1848–50.

The development of the microscope in the 17th century led to advances in several fields. In this respect the work of Anthony van *Leeuwenhoek of Delft (1632–1723) and of the Italian Marcello *Malpighi (1628–94) was of particular importance. Giovanni Battista *Morgagni, the founder of pathological anatomy, wrote *De sedibus et causis morborum*, 1761, one of the most important publications in the history of medicine. Herman *Boerhaave of Delft (1668–1738) was an outstanding clinical teacher and a prolific writer.

The works of William *Smellie (1697–1763) and William *Hunter (1718–83) greatly accelerated progress in obstetrics. Hunter's finest work was his *Anatomia uteri humani gravida tabulis illustrata*. The text for this magnificent atlas was published posthumously in 1794. Hunter was also at one time the owner of the Great Windmill Street School of Anatomy, where his brother John (1728–93) taught anatomy and became a great surgeon. He placed surgery on a scientific basis.

After experimenting with a cow-pox vaccine, Edward *Jenner, a country practitioner, introduced *vaccination against *smallpox. This disease had previously been treated by the rather dangerous method of direct inoculation of material from patients suffering from smallpox.

His *An inquiry into the causes and effects of the variolae vaccina*, 1798, heralded one of the greatest triumphs in the history of medicine. Through the efforts of the *World Health Organization (WHO), the global elimination of smallpox was achieved in 1980.

The introduction of surgical *anaesthesia by the Americans C. W. *Long (1842) and W. T. G. *Morton (1846) was another great achievement. It gave the surgeon time—time to examine and operate inside the body and time to employ Lister's 'antiseptic principle' (*Lancet* 1867) for the prevention of wound infection.

Mention has been made of only a handful of the thousands of important publications that have reduced suffering and advanced medicine. References to important texts in medicine and related subjects are recorded in *Morton's medical bibliography* (Norman 1991), an annotated check-list of nearly 9000 such publications.

Throughout Europe, and later in the New World, gatherings of learned men led to the establishment of societies where they met for discussions, conducted experiments, and published their findings. These societies usually developed libraries. The *Royal College of Physicians of London, founded in 1518, has a fine historical and biographical collection. Disputes concerning the Medical Society of London (founded 1773) led to the establishment in 1805 of the (Royal) Medical and Chirurgical Society, one of whose objects was the formation of a good library. The society amalgamated with 14 specialist medical societies in 1907 to form the present *Royal Society of Medicine, which has the largest medical library in the UK.

In 1895 Sir Henry *Wellcome, the pharmaceutical chemist and medical philanthropist, began collecting books, leading eventually to the development of the Wellcome Historical Medical Library in London, now one of the largest and richest collections of medical and scientific historical literature in the world. The United States has rich collections of material in the history of medicine at the National Library of Medicine; the Francis A. Countway Library, formed in 1965 by the fusion of Boston Medical Library (1807) and Harvard Medical School Library (1783); and also at the New York Academy of Medicine Library.

Thornton's medical books, libraries and collectors (Besson 1990) is the standard work on the production, distribution, and storage of medical literature from the earliest times, and aims to record the chief writings of prominent medical authors and to chart the development of medical literature and libraries.

A guide to current material is *Information sources in the medical sciences* (Morton and Godbolt 1992), which provides information on books, journals, abstracts, online and CD-ROM services, audio-visual sources, and historical works available in all branches of medicine and related subjects. It is an evaluative guide rather than a directory of sources, and has 24 chapters contributed by 27 experts in various fields.

Medical librarianship (Carmel, in preparation) is a collective work by and for professional librarians practising in the medical and health-care fields and its American counterpart is the *Handbook of medical library practice* (Darling 1982–88).

The National Library of Medicine

The world's most important medical library, founded in 1836, is the US National Library of Medicine (NLM), Bethesda. The visionary John Shaw *Billings took charge of its 1365 books in 1864, and his monumental achievements include conception and publication of both the *Index-Catalogue of the Library of the Surgeon General's Office* (1880) and, commencing in 1879, *Index Medicus*. The latter is a monthly classified record of the current medical literature.

NLM collects exhaustively in all major areas of the health sciences and its collections now total about 4 million volumes. The progress of medical science worldwide has been facilitated by NLM, and medical libraries rely heavily upon its wide range of bibliographical tools and services.

The *Medical subject headings* (MeSH) thesaurus, on which the indexing of medical literature is based, is unparalleled in its depth and thoroughness. NLM's Unified Medical Language System (UMLS) project focuses on creating new data structures and computer-based tools to facilitate end-user access to computerized information. The number of medical libraries in the UK using the NLM classification almost doubled between 1982 and 1992, reflecting an increasing uniformity and standardization.

NLM has always been at the forefront of implementing new techniques to cope with the exponential increase in medical literature, and its mechanization programme, which commenced in 1960, led to the development of its automated medical literature analysis and retrieval system in 1963 (MEDLARS), and the further development of technology in the 1970s made online searching possible through MEDLINE (MEDLARS onLINE). GRATEFUL MED from NLM is software which enables doctors and health professionals to have low-cost access to MEDLINE direct from their PC.

The UK lacks the focus for health information planning which the USA has in NLM, although the British Library Research and Development Department to some extent defines and addresses the problems of health-related information. However, there is a strong network of medical libraries varying greatly in type and size, with the larger ones being found in the university and private sectors. Libraries of national importance are those of the Royal Society of Medicine, Department of Health and Social Security, with its database DHSS-DATA, the King's Fund Centre, London, and the British Medical Association.

A recent survey identified 686 biomedical libraries and showed that only 158 (23 per cent) had two or more professionally qualified staff. Seventy-five per cent had online search facilities or access to a computer, and 23 per cent had a CD-ROM installation. In the changing educational environment for health-care, strong collections are now being developed increasingly by the new universities (formerly polytechnics), and the large number of small libraries in NHS postgraduate medical centres are normally co-ordinated within regional schemes to raise standards.

The international nature of medical science is recognized by the work of the World Health Organization and its associated library; by the setting up in 1989 of SatelLife (an initiative of International Physicians for the Prevention of Nuclear War) which is an international non-profit organization, which uses micro-satellite technology to provide health information and communication to the developing world, where access to information is so limited and the need so desperate; and finally by the recognition of a European perspective, when in 1984 the European Association of Health Information and Libraries was formally constituted.

Developments affecting medical libraries and their users in recent years have been characterized by:

(1) the accelerating pace of technological change;
(2) new formats of information;
(3) increasing demands by users;
(4) increasing numbers of users;
(5) funding issues;
(6) rationalization and mergers;
(7) structural change occasioned by shifts in government policy; and
(8) the sheer pressure of continuing proliferation of the literature.

These changes are having profound influences on the way libraries operate and the nature of their services.

The technology revolution has seen the widespread introduction of the PC microcomputer in libraries, offices, and homes. This crucial development and the many changes afforded by the confluence of computing and telecommunications technologies, which offer new and powerful ways of finding and managing information, have brought many benefits to library users. The pace of change is rapid and is set to remain so. The advent of the CD-ROM (compact disc read-only-memory) laserdisc technology, the development of interactive video-disc technology, the emergence of many new products including software for personal database management, advances in electronic telecommunications systems, and the appearance of distributed knowledge networks are all part of a new framework for the way information is organized. This developing infrastructure offers users the potential to access a vast array of knowledge from desks or research offices as well as from the library.

The US INTERNET, established in 1983, is a network of computer networks which has grown from 100 (1985) to 2000 (1991), and to 9722 separately run networks (April 1993). It includes the British academic network JANET and represents over 5 million 'connected' individuals.

Some facilities available to UK JANET users are still experimental but very exciting. The Bath ISI Data Service (BIDS) was the first of a series of data deals, bringing *Science Citation Index*, the citation database, and *Current Contents*, the searchable titles to leading scientific and biomedical journals which will shortly include abstracts, direct to the academic community. EMBASE, which overlaps with MEDLINE, also covers European literature not available on MEDLINE, and has recently been mounted over JANET.

Strategic vision for US medical libraries has focused on developing a knowledge management environment to advance science and health by bringing together people, technologies, and processes in useful ways.

The best example of this is IAIMS—the Integrated Academic Information Management System, the pivotal concept of which is transparent integration of access for the individual user to a wide variety of related information required to study and practise health-care and research. Prominent US libraries developing IAIMS programmes are Columbia, Georgetown, and Johns Hopkins universities.

Currently in the UK, all aspects of *medical education are being re-evaluated in the light of the need to exploit the benefits of developing information technology. Furthermore, the whole concept of the work and practice of the traditional medical library has broadened in recent years, as an integrated multidisciplinary approach to library provision is clearly the most cost-effective use of expensive resources such as accommodation, staffing, and IT; services are ideally provided to all groups involved in the delivery of health care from one base. All health-care workers now require the skills and knowledge to use and manage computerized information in their working environment. The availability of so many computerized hospital information management systems means it is now essential for everyone involved in patient-care management to be familiar with computers and able to use available information technologies to empower their roles as health professionals.

In facing these challenges, access to technology in medical libraries must be provided because it is now fundamental to:

(1) the practice of health care in all its aspects;
(2) medical education, undergraduate, postgraduate, and continuing; and
(3) medical research and its application.

The changing educational environment, with its increasing emphasis on self-directed and student-centred learning and the need to demonstrate continuing professional development, is affecting all groups within the health-care professions. There is a realization that the pace of change is so intense that an environment of lifelong learning is being forged, with librarians playing a major role as trainers and catalysts for the development of information awareness at all levels.

Users are finding traditional methods of accessing and

managing biomedical literature inadequate, as paper-based methods are not sufficient to keep up with rapid advances in medical knowledge, and are eager to learn how to exploit available resources, including particularly the CD-ROM which has effectively democratized access to powerful information retrieval tools.

However, changes will be evolutionary and, despite media hype, libraries as physical facilities will continue to exist for the foreseeable future. Less will be bought but users will enjoy much greater access to information. Libraries will continue to offer a range of traditional services, such as interlibrary loans, photocopying, and reference services, together with new products and services.

Users may expect to find much more information in a variety of non-print formats, such as video and compact disc. CD-ROM, the new technology of the 1980s, is now standard in many libraries, and large databases such as MEDLINE and the Cumulated Index of Nursing and Allied Health Literature (CINAHL) are increasingly available for users to search themselves. Multimedia, whereby a user can listen to audio, view still images, see motion video, read text, and scan graphics, is entering the main stream of IT and will be the technology of the 1990s. It will be available in packages for computer-assisted learning (CAL).

The phrase 'the virtual library' has been used to describe a vision of the library in the 21st century. A. J. Harley, Head of Computing and Data Communications for the British Library's Lending Division, defined the virtual library in 1980 by drawing on a computing analogy. Like a 'virtual machine' the virtual library gives its users the 'illusion' of access to resources far greater than those actually present. In the 'ultimate virtual library' the user has 'access to universal knowledge without delay, at his desk'. More recently Naomi Broering of Georgetown University has defined 'a virtual medical library system' as one which will have direct access to many different medical print and non-print formats, bibliographic indexes and abstracts, CD-ROM systems, document delivery full text, electronic journals, medical images, plus e-mail for communications with colleagues. The library environments of the future are under development now and will have the ability to guide users to information sources and to integrate patient care and research systems through powerful and sophisticated computer networks.

As local, national, and international networking infrastructures develop, users may look forward to operating from personal workstations where they can access information and download, manipulate, and transfer it, as well as being able to communicate with colleagues world-wide.

Today is a time of extraordinary upheaval and re-evaluation of traditional roles. New knowledge is being ever more rapidly created and disseminated in non-traditional ways. The shape of the post-Gutenberg era may be decades in the making. Medical libraries must stay abreast of these changes and encourage and expand new applications in ways that facilitate and enhance medical research and practice. Above all, we must embrace wisely those technologies which are adding value to the medical literature and medical media, and remember that at the end of all our work is a patient.

SHANE GODBOLT
LESLIE MORTON

References
Besson, A. (ed.) (1990). *Thornton's medical books, libraries and collectors*, (3rd edn). Gower, Aldershot.
Carmel, M. (ed.) *Medical librarianship*, (2nd edn). Library Association, London, in preparation.
Darling, L. *et al.* (ed.) (1982–88). *Handbook of medical library practice*, (4th edn), 3 vols. Medical Library Association, Chicago.
Morton, L. T. and Godbolt, S. (1992). *Information sources in the medical sciences*, (4th edn). Bowker-Saur, London.
Norman, J. M. (1991). *Morton's medical bibliography. An annotated check-list of texts illustrating the history of medicine*, (5th edn). Scolar Press, Aldershot.

MEDICAL (CLINICAL) AUDIT Ever since men and women first sought help from their relatives and friends for the management of disease, they may be presumed to have been interested in the quality of the help that they have received. When a woman in a primitive society consulted a 'wise woman' about childbirth, for example, she would have some idea of the relative reputation of one wise woman compared with another. As the formalization of health care proceeded, no doubt it became necessary for primitive societies to lay down some boundaries within which their healers could operate, providing also some sanctions if the healers failed to heal. Subsequently *Hippocrates laid down an ethical framework within which we still practise today. Hippocrates also wrote extensively about the outcomes of various diseases, indicating prognostic factors which would influence those outcomes.

Coming closer to the present time, a Royal Charter established the *Royal College of Physicians in 1518. The Statutes of the College have a surprisingly modern ring—one of its purposes is to 'safeguard the health and security of the people'. A system of sanctions was set up so that the Censors of the College could inform the local magistrates of poor-quality practice by quacks. The Censors of the College also had the right to enter the shops of the *apothecaries to inspect their 'drugs and stuffs'.

Throughout the 16th to the early 19th century, *medical practitioners must have practised in relative isolation. Not only was transport between cities poor until the advent of better roads and railways, but there was little interchange of ideas except at the highest reaches of the profession, when learned physicians made surprisingly long journeys and long stays at centres of excellence in London, Edinburgh, The Netherlands,

Paris, and northern Italy. The quality of practice was assessed solely by the local community.

It is, of course, artificial to pick out isolated landmarks in what is a continuous process of evolution in assessing the quality of health-care interventions, but a major landmark must have been the work of Florence *Nightingale. Not only did her work in the Crimea and in London revolutionize the practice of nursing, but she also took an interest in the outcomes of hospital care. It is noteworthy that the *National Health Service in the UK, until very recently, lumped together 'discharges and deaths' as an index of hospital activity. Florence Nightingale kept three categories firmly separate—died, discharged relieved, and discharged unrelieved. Subsequently, Codman, a Massachusetts surgeon, firmly believed that every surgeon should record the outcomes of his operations, and that different outcomes of different surgeons should be compared (Codman 1914). These sensible but revolutionary suggestions did not have a favourable influence upon his surgical career in New England.

An important conceptual advance was the work of Donabedian, who, since the middle 1960s, has written extensively about measuring the quality of medical care (Donabedian 1966). He suggested that quality should be considered under three headings—the structure within which the care was provided, the process of care, and the outcome of care. By structure, he meant not only the physical plant (buildings, X-ray machines, and so on), but also the availability of trained personnel. The process of care is what doctors and nurses actually do with their patients—operations, prescribing the right drugs, and other interventions. The outcomes of care include not only the extent to which disease is eradicated

or relieved, but also a restoration or enhancement of functional status even if the underlying disease cannot be eradicated or relieved. Satisfaction of patients with their care is also recognized as an increasingly important dimension of outcome.

This model, illustrated in Fig. 1, was elaborated further by Maxwell (1984), who pointed out some other dimensions of quality, including financial and geographical access, and that care must be effective, equitable, co-ordinated, and acceptable to those who receive it.

Most audit now takes place within this framework. Medical audit has been defined as 'The systematic, critical analysis of the quality of medical care, including the procedures used for diagnosis and treatment, the use of resources, and the resulting outcome and quality of life for the patient.' (Department of Health 1989).

In practice, in the UK at least, the prefix 'medical' to the word audit has been thought to be too restrictive. Many health-care interventions are the result of team work. It would, for example, be pointless to audit the management of patients with *stroke without considering the contribution of nurses in the acute stage to avoiding pressure sores, and maintaining *nutrition and managing continence, and the role of *physiotherapists and *occupational therapists in helping reduce handicaps consequent upon the disabilities and biological impairments. For this reason, the term 'clinical audit' is increasingly preferred in the UK.

Certain background threads make up the current skein of clinical audit (Kerrison *et al.* 1993). First and foremost is the professional desire to achieve the highest possible professional standards of work. All who work in busy hospitals or in primary care would acknowledge

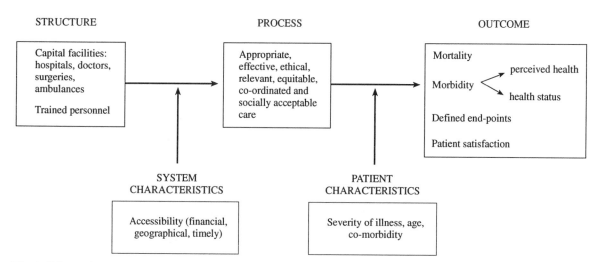

Fig. 1 Schematic representation of some dimensions that should be considered when measuring the quality of care (reprinted from Hopkins 1990, with permission).

that the very pressures of day-to-day work sometimes lead to corners being cut, inadequate information being given to patients, and visits not made. Health professionals need support so that they can stand back from their day-to-day busy activities for a few hours each month in order to inspect the quality of the work that they are doing. To say that one is too 'busy' to evaluate the quality of one's own work is an unprofessional statement. Health professionals must accept that evaluation of their work will sometimes displace an operating session or an out-patient clinic.

The next thread in the skein is related to the control of costs and the allocation of resources. The explosion of health-care costs, particularly in the USA, where health care now consumes nearly 14 per cent of the gross domestic product, has led to complex systems of 'managed health care'. For example, many third-party insurers in the USA now require certain criteria to be fulfilled before they will agree to reimburse the patient for a procedure. There is as yet little evidence that such review criteria significantly influence medical practice. Another intervention in the US is the development of peer-review organizations, which by statute have to review a small proportion of all *Medicare medical records against certain 'quality screens'. These reviews are expensive to undertake, irritate the doctors, and have not been shown to be reliable detectors of overall quality. Costs, or value for money, also underly the government's interest in clinical audit in the UK. The health-service reforms enacted in the NHS and Community Care Act (1990) mean that purchasers (capitation-funded district health authorities and fundholding *general practitioners) can buy health-care interventions from a variety of sources. There is a risk that the providers of health care may provide services that are targeted to low cost rather than reasonable quality. An effective system of clinical audit is therefore a necessary safeguard for the population.

The interest in conserving resources has led to a renewed interest in defining effective health-care interventions. There is little evidence of effectiveness for many of the things which doctors and other health-care professionals do. For example, the evidence that *speech therapy influences the recovery of language after stroke is virtually non-existent. If ineffective treatments were stopped, then more resources would be available for treatments of proven effectiveness. A whole new industry has grown up, on both sides of the Atlantic, of critical appraisal of various health-care interventions. Although praiseworthy, such initiatives will be valueless without taking into account the social culture within which health professionals operate. If a patient takes it into his or her head that he or she needs a *scan for the elucidation of his or her headaches, then it is very difficult in any advanced society to tell him or her that this is not possible, even though all the research evidence shows that, unless certain clinical criteria are fulfilled, scans have very low sensitivity and specificity.

After a critical appraisal of the literature and a definition of the effective health-care interventions, then it is possible to write guidelines for good practice. Audit of the case record will then show whether such guidelines have been followed. There are, however, a number of difficulties about this approach. The cost of record review has already been mentioned. Guidelines are commonly written for 'clean' single disorders, such as *myocardial infarction. However, particularly as the population ages, co-existing disorders (co-morbidities) are very common, and co-morbidities may influence the chosen intervention. Many health professionals are concerned that guidelines give too simplistic an approach to medical practice, and will not encourage individually tailored patient care. There is also a lurking concern that deviation from guidelines may lay the health professional open to subsequent litigation if things do not go well. However, the biggest stumbling block against the more widespread introduction of such audit systems is the difficulty of capturing the information in a way that can be handled by computers. Although it is superficially attractive to suggest that patient characteristics, processes of care, and outcomes of care can be coded, and differences between provider units in their outcomes can then be analysed, there is continuing concern that such an initiative would fail to recognize the individuality of patients' illness and of the biology of their diseases, their concerns, and their preferred outcomes.

Finally, it should be said that deficiencies in patient care are seldom due to consistently poor practice by a single individual. Far more often it is the systems of care that are poor. For example, to fail to act upon a positive laboratory result is clearly poor care. However, the failure may not be due to clinician inactivity, but simply because the hospital information system is incapable of delivering that result in a timely manner. Doctors, nurses, and other health professionals must therefore work alongside managers in improving the systems for delivering health care. At this stage an enormous expansion in health-services research and in the methodology of clinical audit, are needed so that the advances provided by scientific medicine can be translated more effectively into everyday practice.

ANTHONY HOPKINS

References

Codman, E. A. (1914). The product of a hospital. *Surgery, Gynaecology and Obstetrics*, **18**, 491–6.

Department of Health (1989). *Working for patients*. Working Paper No. 6. HMSO, London.

Hopkins, A. (1990). *Measuring the quality of medical care*. RCP Publications, London.

Kerrison, S. Packwood, T., and Buxton, M. (1993). *Medical audit: taking stock*. Health Economics Research Group, Brunel University and King's Fund Centre, London.

Maxwell, R. J. (1984). Quality assessment in health. *British Medical Journal*, **288**, 1470–2.

Donabedian, A. (1966). Evaluating the quality of medical care. *Millbank Memorial Fund Quarterly*, **441** (Suppl.), 166–206.

MEDICAL COLLEGES, FACULTIES, SOCIETIES, AND INSTITUTES OF THE UK. In the Middle Ages, those practising medicine fell into four classes—physicians, surgeons, apothecaries, and quacks. The physicians were learned men with university degrees, well read in the Latin language and literature, and not infrequently in holy orders. The surgeons, often also barbers, practised only the most primitive forms of surgery. The apothecaries' function was to prepare, sell, and administer the drugs prescribed by the physicians, but they naturally acquired some medical knowledge, and began to practise independently. The quacks had no qualifications of any kind. They frequented markets and fairs to offer nostrums, cupping, bleeding, treatment for worms, and pulling teeth.

The physicians naturally considered themselves far superior to the other groups in training, knowledge, and social status. Their patients were mostly drawn from the uppermost social class and its retainers. The great majority of the people were treated either with folk medicine at home or by the lower groups.

In 1511 an Act of Parliament was passed which limited medical practice to those who had undergone strict examination. In the City of London and for 7 miles around, the examination was to be conducted by the Bishop of London or the Dean of St Paul's, with the assistance of four physicians or surgeons. For the rest of England the examination was to be by the bishop of each diocese in a similar manner. The reason why the Church was involved in what might seem a purely medical matter was that the clergy were literate and the organization of the Church throughout the country constituted in effect a civil service.

The Royal College of Physicians was given its royal charter by King Henry VIII in 1518. In the centuries since then many other colleges and faculties have been founded, especially in the past 50 years. All the colleges, which are independent and not under state control, have in common the same aims—to maintain and improve medical knowledge, professional practice, and ethical standards. This they do by education, examinations, research, and example.

As well as the colleges, there are faculties and institutes. The faculties are organizations of workers in the smaller or newer specialties, rather like embryo colleges. In fact, the Faculty of Radiology, founded in 1939, developed into the Royal College of Radiologists in 1975. There are Faculties of Public Health Medicine founded in 1972, with about 2000 fellows and members, and Occupational Medicine founded in 1978, with about 1600 members, linked to the Royal College of Physicians of London.

The institutes are London postgraduate and research organizations which come under the British Postgraduate Medical Federation, in all the main branches of medicine and surgery—cardiology, thoracic (chest) medicine, child health, cancer research, dermatology, dental surgery, laryngology and otology, neurology, obstetrics and gynaecology, ophthalmology, orthopaedics, psychiatry, urology, and accident surgery—based on the appropriate hospitals. There is also an Institute of Basic Medical Sciences—anatomy, pathology, physiology, pharmacology, biochemistry—at the Royal College of Surgeons of England.

Medical societies

There are at least 300 medical societies in the UK. The largest proportion is devoted to the study and furtherance of the numerous specialties in the medical field. The next largest group includes those associated with towns and cities, such as London, Birmingham, Liverpool, Manchester, Bristol, Newcastle upon Tyne, and Edinburgh, and also smaller towns or cities such as Reading, Chester, Bath, York, and Oxford. Then there are those associated with hospitals, and finally a miscellaneous group, concerned, for example, with medical administration, education, medical and scientific films, and cremation.

Some of the oldest societies are listed below with their date of foundation.

The Royal Medical Society of Edinburgh, 1737
Guy's Hospital Physical Society, 1771
The Medical Society of London, 1773
Middlesex Hospital Medical Society, 1774
Edinburgh Harveian Society, 1789
Aberdeen Medico-Chirurgical Society, 1786
Abernethian Society (St Bartholomew's Hospital), 1795
The Royal Medico-Chirurgical Society of Glasgow, 1814
The Hunterian Society, 1819
The Harveian Society of London, 1831
The British Medical Association, 1832
York Medical Society, 1832
Listerian Society (King's College Hospital), 1833
Manchester Medical Society, 1834
The Liverpool Medical Institute, 1837

The Apothecaries' Hall of Dublin

The *Barber-Surgeons Company contained a number of *apothecaries, who were incorporated as a guild by a charter of George II. In 1792 an Act of Parliament constituted the members into the Corporation of Apothecaries' Hall of Dublin. As well as teaching pharmacy, the Hall was also an examining body, and could confer a Licence (LAH Dublin). This was a registrable qualification until 1972, when the examination standard was deemed by the *General Medical Council to be inadequate, and it became no longer registrable. The Hall has premises in Merrion Square, Dublin.

The British Medical Association (BMA)

The Association was founded at Worcester in 1832 by Charles *Hastings. He summoned a meeting of some 50 local doctors, which led to the formation of the Provincial Medical and Surgical Association. The word 'provincial' was stressed because it was felt that doctors in the provinces were neglected, and indeed scorned, by the medical establishment in London. The aims of the Association were 'to promote the medical and allied sciences, and to maintain the honour and interests of the medical profession'. In 1836 a similar and rival organization was formed in London with the name 'The British Medical Association', but in 1855 the provincial association swallowed up the London association and took its name.

Today the Association is best known to the public and to many doctors for its political and organizational activities, and its work to obtain better pay and conditions of service for the medical profession. It has many other activities—scientific, in public health, for medical charities, in insurance, and publishing the *British Medical Journal*, founded in 1840, and other specialist journals. (See MEDICAL JOURNALS.)

The association has fought many battles. In 1867 it ran a campaign against baby-farming, which led to the passage of the Infant Life Protection Act of 1872. In 1909 it published *Secret remedies, what they cost and what they contain*, and in 1912 *More secret remedies*. Both books incurred the wrath not only of the manufacturers, who were in a very lucrative business, but also of the newspapers, which received large advertisement revenue from the trade, and even the Inland Revenue, which received substantial sums from the Stamp Duty on Patent Medicines. Nevertheless, the books did a valuable public service. Many of the secret remedies, although expensive and useless, were at least harmless. Others were undoubtedly harmful—concealed abortion-inducing substances, tonic wines which made unsuspecting invalids consume large amounts of alcohol, children's teething syrups that contained *morphia, and corrosive liquids for application to cancerous growths.

The Association was deeply involved in the discussions and controversies that preceded the *National Health Insurance Act of 1911 and the *National Health Service Act of 1946. Today there are about 84 000 members, that is approximately 72 per cent of practising doctors.

Under the Trade Union and Labour Relations Act, 1974, the Association is listed as a Trade Union, but still remains a Company limited by guarantee, and is not affiliated to the Trades Union Congress. It has premises in Tavistock Square, London, and a library of 80 000 volumes.

The Royal College of Ophthalmologists

The Royal College of Ophthalmologists was formerly a faculty of the Royal College of Surgeons. Founded in 1948 it now has 2700 fellows and members. Its premises are at Cornwall Terrace, London.

The Faculty of Pharmaceutical Medicine

The Faculty of Pharmaceutical Medicine was founded in 1989. Fellows, members, and associates number 680. Quarters are in St Andrew's Place, London.

The Faculty of Public Health Medicine

The Faculty of Public Health Medicine (formerly Community medicine) is concerned with broad questions of health and disease affecting populations, as opposed to the treatment of individual patients. It includes epidemiology, administration, and the study of geographical and occupational problems in the community.

The Society of *Medical Officers of Health and the Society of Community Medicine, with the encouragement of the Royal Colleges of Physicians, united in 1972 to form the Faculty of Community Medicine. The members (MFCM) are admitted after examination, and the fellows (FFCM) are elected from the members, totalling about 2000 altogether. The Faculty has premises in St Andrew's Place, London.

The Medical Society of London

The Society was founded by Dr John Coakely *Lettsom in 1773. The library contains some 30 000 items (see MEDICAL BOOKS AND LIBRARIES). The Society has had four homes, the present one in Chandos Street, London, dating from 1873.

The Royal College of Anaesthetists

The Royal College of Anaesthetists was formerly a faculty of the Royal College of Surgeons. Founded in 1948 it now has 5500 fellows and members. Its premises are in Russell Square, London.

The Royal College of General Practitioners

Proposals for some academic body for general practitioners were first made in 1840, but proved to be abortive. In about 1950 the project was raised again from several quarters. General practice was no longer regarded as the work that doctors did if they did not succeed in becoming consultants or specialists: many of the best students chose general practice as a career. It had become more efficient, much more complex, and in fact a specialty in its own right, yet the 20 000 general practitioners had nothing to bring them together or to organize their work. Despite some opposition from the Royal Colleges of Physicians, Surgeons and Obstetricians the College was incorporated in 1961 and received a royal charter in 1972.

The College has had very beneficial effects on the status, postgraduate training, and morale of general practitioners. It has organized co-operative research projects of value, for example a large and important study of prescription of oral contraception in general practice. The Fellows (FRCGP), members (MRCGP), and associates now number about 17 000. The College has premises in Princes Gate, London.

The Royal College of Midwives

In the 19th century only about 30 per cent of births were conducted by medical men. The great majority of women were attended by *midwives, with very varied standards of training, and in some cases no training at all. Organizations concerned with midwifery came into being only about a century ago. The first Midwives Act concerned with control and training was passed in 1902, another in 1912. In 1941 a College of Midwives was created which, in 1947, became a Royal College.

The Royal College of Nursing

The Royal College of Nursing was founded in 1916 and received a royal charter in 1963. The registered nurses, midwives, and health visitors in the UK together total over 1 000 000. Nurses actually in practice number about 400 000, of whom 298 000 belong to the Royal College of Nursing.

The College's main activities are in education and training, maintaining uniformity of the curriculum, and speaking for the nursing profession. The College has premises in Henrietta Street, London. See also NURSING IN THE UK.

The Royal College of Obstetricians and Gynaecologists

In 1928 application was made to the Board of Trade for a licence to found a British College of Obstetrics and Gynaecology. The Colleges of Physicians and Surgeons strongly opposed the proposal. Their objections arose partly from a long-standing prejudice against specialization, and partly because it was felt that every new college would diminish the status, authority, and dignity of the existing colleges. After much negotiation and argument, the College of Obstetricians was founded in 1929. Opposition and some bad feeling continued until 1937, when the College became the Royal College of Obstetricians and Gynaecologists. Since then the colleges have been in harmony.

There are two grades in the College—members (MRCOG), who have passed an advanced examination in the two subjects, and fellows (FRCOG), who are elected from the members. There is a also a diploma for general practitioners who wish to specialize in obstetrics (DRCOG). The fellows and members number about 8000, of whom 4000 are resident overseas.

The College has a modern building in Sussex Place on the west side of Regent's Park, London.

The Royal College of Pathologists

Pathology is the study of the causes, mechanisms, and processes of disease, that is the laboratory side of medicine. It includes morbid anatomy, histology, haematology, immunology, bacteriology, virology, and clinical biochemistry, all rapidly becoming separate subjects in their own right.

The College of Pathologists was founded as a limited liability company in 1962 and 2 years later received a charter and its present name. There are 9500 associates, who have passed a preliminary examination, members (MRCPath), who have either passed a final examination or submitted original work, and fellows (FRCPath), who are elected after 12 years as members. The fellows and members number about 5400, of whom 1000 reside outside the UK. The College has premises in Carlton House Terrace, London.

The Royal College of Physicians of Edinburgh

The first charter was given in 1681, although attempts to found a college had been going on for the previous 60 years. The charter included provisions for professional examinations, powers to fine unlicensed practitioners, and powers to inspect the drugs in apothecaries' shop. The original fellows numbered 21; today there are over 4000.

At various times the College has founded a library, a natural history museum, a materia medica museum, a dispensary for the sick poor, and a laboratory (which continued until 1950). There are three grades in the College. First, the licentiates, who with the licentiates of the Royal College of Surgeons of Edinburgh and the Royal College of Physicians and Surgeons of Glasgow hold a primary qualification ('the Scottish Triple') (but see Royal College of Physicians of London 'Conjoint'). Secondly, the members, who have passed a more advanced examination in one of several of the main branches of medicine, now held jointly with the London and Glasgow Colleges, so what used to be the MRCP (Ed.) is now the MRCP (UK). Thirdly, the fellows (FRCP (Ed.)) who are selected from the members. The College has had four homes, the present one in Queen Street, Edinburgh, dating from 1846.

The Royal College of Physicians and Surgeons of Glasgow

This College, which fulfils similar functions to those of the Colleges of Physicians and of Surgeons in London, Edinburgh, and Dublin, was founded in 1599. It was originally called the Royal Faculty of Physicians and Surgeons of Glasgow, but the name Faculty came to have a different meaning, so the organization took its present name in 1962. The medical side, like that of the other Colleges of Physicians, has three grades, Licentiates (LRCP (Glasg.)), members (what was the MRCP (Glasg.) is now the MRCP (UK)), and fellows. The surgical side resembles that of the other surgical colleges except that the fellowship examination can be taken in one of several branches of the art—surgery, obstetrics and gynaecology, ophthalmology, otolaryngology, or dental surgery. Fellows and members number about 7800. The College has premises in St Vincent Street, Glasgow.

The Royal College of Physicians of Ireland

The College had its beginnings as a Fraternity of Physicians founded in 1654. In 1667 it received a charter from Charles II and became the College of Physicians in Ireland. In 1890 the name was changed again to the Royal College of Physicians of Ireland.

The functions of the College are similar to those of the London College. They included, from 1692, the right to give a licence to practise in Dublin and for 7 miles around, and the power to fine unlicensed practitioners £5 a month.

There are three grades in the College. The licentiates, with those of the Royal College of Surgeons in Ireland, hold a primary qualification—(LRCPI, LRCSI) (RCPT) ('the Irish Conjoint'). The membership (MRCPI) is achieved by examination. The fellows (FRCPI), numbering about 150, are selected from the members. There are also various specialist diplomas.

The Irish College was the first to admit women, in 1877, as compared with the London College in 1909 and the Edinburgh College in 1925. The College has a building dating from 1864, in Kildare Street, Dublin.

The Royal College of Physicians of London

The Royal College of Physicians of London, the oldest of the Colleges, was founded in 1518 nominally by Henry VIII, but in fact by Thomas *Linacre, an Oxford physician, humanist, and cleric. Originally called the College or Commonalty of the Faculty of Medicine of London, the College acquired its present name in 1682. The charter gave as the objects of the College 'to resist the endeavours of wicked men and especially to repress the audacity of those who profess medicine rather because of their own avarice than in any assurance of a good conscience, whence arise very many ills for the rude and credulous populace'.

Linacre, as the first president, was given powers to fine and imprison those who practised without adequate qualifications. The four censors were empowered to visit apothecaries' shops, inspect the drugs and destroy any not up to standard; these visitations continued until 1858. There were also eight elects, very senior fellows appointed for life, whose chief function was to elect the president, always from among their own number. After 300 years this was realized to be a gerontocracy of the worst kind, and the office of elect was abolished in 1860. Today the president is elected by the general body of the fellows.

In its early days the chief activity of the College was the suppression of unqualified practice, notably by apothecaries. Surgeons were not checked unless they prescribed drugs or attempted to treat internal diseases. The College's efforts became less and less successful because some of the apothecaries were respected practitioners with influential patients and friends, and their status was greatly improved by the foundation of the Society of Apothecaries in 1617. The turning point came in 1704 when the conviction of an apothecary for illegal practice was reversed on appeal to the House of Lords. No more prosecutions were attempted after 1735.

The College did, of course, have other activities. An important contribution was the institution in 1541 of an elaborate system of examinations, with prescribed texts and oral tests. This was 250 years before the older universities replaced their formal medieval disputations by the modern type of examination.

The College has always taken a great interest in public health and preventive medicine; its first report in 1627 was on health hazards in industry; in 1725 it published a report on the evils of gin drinking. More recently it has been active in many fields, especially the dangers of smoking, on which its first report in 1962 was highly influential. Over 60 publications are now in print on such subjects as medical ethics, audit of medical services, dangers of sunlight, sexual abuse of children, fraud and misconduct in medical research, obesity, and care of the disabled.

There are now three grades in the College. The licentiates, along with the membership of the Royal College of Surgeons, hold a primary qualification (MRCS, LRCP, often known as 'the Conjoint'). The 'Conjoint' examination was changed in 1993. The non-university licensing bodies—the Society of Apothecaries and the Royal Colleges of Physicians and Surgeons of Edinburgh, Glasgow, London, and England—have joined in creating a new licensing examination to be held twice a year rotating through the centres in London and Scotland. The resulting qualifications will be (a) LMSSA Lond; (b) LRCP Edin; LRCS Edin; LRCPS Glas; (c) LRCS Eng; LRCP Lond. They will be awarded separately according to where the candidate sits and passes the examination. The 'Conjoint' (MRCS Eng; LRCP Lond) has ceased to exist as a separate examination. The members have passed an examination in more advanced medicine, now held jointly with the Edinburgh and Glasgow Colleges. The fellows (FRCP) are elected from the members. The College also gives, with the College of Surgeons, a number of diplomas in special subjects. There is also a Faculty of Occupational Medicine.

The College started with six fellows; during the 17th and 18th century they numbered 40–60, and in 1828 reached 100. Today there are about 6300 fellows. About 19 600 doctors hold the MRCP (UK). The College has had five homes, the present one, dating from 1964, is in St Andrews Place in the south-east corner of Regent's Park, London. In its long history the College has acquired some 200 portraits and a library of 50 000 volumes, now mainly devoted to medical history and biography.

The Royal College of Psychiatrists

The College is directly descended from the Association of Medical Officers of Asylums and Hospitals for the Insane, which was founded in Gloucester in 1841. There was then virtually no psychiatry outside the custodial care of patients in mental hospitals. In 1865 the Association changed its name to The Medico-Psychological Association, and as the specialty of psychiatry expanded in extent and importance the Association received a charter of incorporation in 1926 as the Royal Medico-Psychological Association. Finally in 1971 a supplemental charter made it a Royal College.

There are three grades in the College: inceptors, who are psychiatrists in training, members (MRCPsych), who have passed an examination, and fellows (FRC Psych), who are elected from the members, the whole numbering over 7000. The College has premises in Belgrave Square, London, with a library of 10 000 volumes.

The Royal College of Radiologists
*X-rays were discovered by Conrad *Roentgen in November 1895. The news spread with remarkable rapidity: an account appeared in a Vienna newspaper on 5 January, in a London newspaper on 6 January, and the first medical X-ray in the UK was taken on the following day. The medical profession at once realized that they had a remarkable new diagnostic tool. In 1897 the Roentgen Society was founded. In 1917 it united with other societies concerned with the study of X-rays, to become the British Institute of Radiology, which received a Royal Charter in 1958. The Institute is concerned with all aspects of X-rays, and its members include radiologists, radiographers, technicians, and manufacturers. Meanwhile, in 1934, the British Association of Radiologists had been formed and in the following year the Society of Radiotherapists, both concerned with the medical aspects of radiology. The two societies united in 1939 to become the Faculty of Radiology of the Royal College of Physicians, which prospered and in 1953 received a charter. Finally in 1975 it received another charter and its present title.

The College has two main divisions—diagnostic *radiology and *radiotherapy. The fellows (FRCR) and members (MRCR) number about 4200. The premises are in Portland Place, London.

The Royal College of Surgeons of Edinburgh
The distant origins of the College lie in the Craft of Barbers and Surgeons founded in 1505. The two occupations remained together for over 200 years, but in 1722 they separated in an amicable divorce. In 1778 the surgeons obtained a Royal Charter as the Royal College of Surgeons of the City of Edinburgh. As the title suggests, the College was connected with the Town Council, rather as a craft guild. In 1851 another charter made the College independent and gave it its present name.

Its licence, with that of the Edinburgh College of Physicians and that of the Glasgow College, formed a primary qualification (LRCP (Ed.), LRCS (Ed.), LRCPS (Glasg.), the 'Scottish Triple', (but see Royal College of Physicians of London 'Conjoint'). Its fellows (FRCS (Ed.)) take an advanced examination. The College has 9300 fellows; it has premises in Nicolson Street, Edinburgh.

The Royal College of Surgeons of England
In London a craft guild of barbers was founded in 1387. Some of its members also practised primitive forms of surgery. The *Barber–Surgeons Company was founded in 1540, and the two occupations remained linked, somewhat uneasily, for 200 years. As the surgeons' art developed, the association with the barbers became increasingly distasteful, and in 1745 the connection was severed by the foundation of the Company of Surgeons. The Barbers' Company still exists as a City Livery Company, but has long ceased to carry out its original functions. In 1800 the Company of Surgeons became the College of Surgeons of London, and in 1843 took its present name as the Royal College of Surgeons of England.

The College has two grades, members who, with the licence of the Royal College of Physicians, hold a primary qualification (MRCS, LRCP) and the fellows (FRCS) who have passed an advanced examination in basic sciences and clinical surgery. The situation is likely to change in the near future. The College is proposing that those who pass an examination 2–4 years after qualification, as is the case at present with the FRCS, shall become members (MRCS) and obtain their Fellowship (FRCS) only after several more years of surgical training in a specialty. At present the FRCS signifies readiness to undertake higher surgical training, in future it will signify its completion. If these proposals are adopted the primary qualification will become LRCS, LRCP.

The College is governed by the president and council, the latter elected by the fellows, of whom there are about 10 000. The library contains some 160 000 volumes.

The original building in Lincoln's Inn Fields, London, dates from 1836. Adjacent to it are extensive modern buildings housing the Institute of Basic Medical Sciences, a residential college, and the laboratories of the *Imperial Cancer Research Fund, which were founded jointly by the Colleges of Physicians and Surgeons in 1902. There are also laboratories at Mill Hill and at Downe, in Kent.

The Royal College of Surgeons in Ireland
As in other parts of the British Isles, surgeons started modestly as an offshoot of barbers, and a Fraternity or Guild of Barbers existed in Ireland in the 15th century. In 1577 Queen Elizabeth I granted them a charter in which was mention of 'the Art of Chirurgery'. In 1780 a number of surgeons constituted themselves the Dublin Society of Surgeons. In 1784 the union between the barbers and surgeons, by then tenuous, was finally broken by the foundation of the Royal College of Surgeons in Ireland by a charter of George III.

The College, with the Royal College of Physicians of Ireland, gives a primary qualification—LRCSI, LRCPI (the 'Irish Conjoint'). There is a higher examination for the fellowship (FRCSI). There are about 4000 fellows.

The College has a building of 1812, with extensive modern additions, in St Stephen's Green, Dublin.

The Royal Society of Medicine

The Society has a complicated parentage. In 1805 there was a secession from the Medical Society of London to form the Medico-Chirurgical Society of London. Despite the split, both organizations prospered. In 1907 the society amalgamated with various specialist societies to form the Royal Society of Medicine. This is reflected in the 37 specialist sections of the Society today. The Society has the largest private medical library in Europe.

The Society now has about 12 000 fellows and about 6000 members in other categories. There are 37 sections which cover nearly all branches of medicine.

The library contains 450 000 books and 9000 periodicals. The Society's present home in Wimpole Street, London, dates from 1912, and has recently been greatly extended.

The Society of Apothecaries

In the 16th and 17th century the physician would sit in a coffee house while the apothecary brought him an account of the patient's symptoms. There was then no physical examination beyond feeling the pulse. The physician prescribed the appropriate remedies, which the apothecary dispensed and administered to the patient. The apothecaries acquired considerable medical knowledge, and it was natural that patients should go direct to the apothecary rather than to the physician.

In 1617 the apothecaries received a charter from James I which founded the Society of Apothecaries and thus greatly raised their status. In 1815 an Act conferred on them the right to give, after due examination, a qualification to practise—licentiate of the Society of Apothecaries (LSA), changed in 1907 to licentiate in medicine and surgery of the Society of Apothecaries (LMSSA). The Society also gives diplomas in industrial health, in venereology, in medical jurisprudence, and in medical history. As well as being a medical corporation, the Society is a City Livery Company, with a hall dating from 1668 in Blackfriars Lane, London.

Undergraduate teaching hospitals and medical schools

In the past there was a clear distinction between 'teaching' and 'non-teaching' hospitals. This is no longer the case. Most undergraduate medical students use more than one hospital. In the following list the principal, or oldest, teaching hospitals in each medical school are listed. Some previously separate medical schools have now been fused and they are listed together below.

London
St Bartholomew's
Charing Cross and Westminster

Guy's and St Thomas's
King's College
Middlesex and University College
Royal Free
Royal London
St George's
St Mary's

Further changes in the organization of London undergraduate medical schools and hospitals are likely following reforms in the National Health Service and the review of London hospitals by the Tomlinson Committee. Charing Cross Hospital may close; St Bartholomew's may change its character from a general hospital, which it has been for 870 years, to a specialist centre. The future of Guy's Hospital is also under debate. At the time of going to press these matters are under review by the government.

Non-London teaching hospitals

Birmingham: Queen Elizabeth Hospital
Bristol: Bristol Royal Infirmary
Cambridge: Addenbrooke's Hospital
Leeds: General Infirmary and St James Hospital
Leicester: Leicester Royal Infirmary
Liverpool: Liverpool Royal Infirmary
Manchester: Manchester Royal Infirmary; Hope Hospital; University Hospital of South Manchester
Newcastle upon Tyne: Royal Victoria Infirmary; Freeman Hospital; General Hospital
Nottingham: Queen's Medical Centre
Oxford: John Radcliffe Hospital; Radcliffe Infirmary
Sheffield: Royal Hallamshire Hospital
Southampton: Southampton General Hospital
Wales: University Hospital of Wales

Scotland
Aberdeen: Aberdeen Royal Infirmary
Dundee: Ninewells Hospital
Edinburgh: Royal Infirmary; Western Infirmary
Glasgow: Royal Infirmary

Northern Ireland
Belfast: Royal Victoria Hospital

Postgraduate teaching hospitals and medical schools
London School of Hygiene and Tropical Medicine
Royal Postgraduate Medical School, London

Designated teaching hospitals (postgraduate)
London
Bethlem Royal and Maudsley Hospital (psychiatry)
Brompton and National Heart (lungs and heart)
Hammersmith Hospital (Royal Postgraduate Medical School)

Hospital for Sick Children, Great Ormond Street
Queen Elizabeth Hospital for Children
London Chest Hospital
Moorfields Eye Hospital
National Hospitals for Neurology and Neurosurgery
Queen Charlotte's Hospital (obstetrics)
Chelsea Hospital for Women
Royal Marsden Hospital (cancer)

British Postgraduate Medical Federation (University of London) Institutes

Cancer Research
Child Health
Dental Surgery
Dermatology
Laryngology and Otology
Neurology
Obstetrics and Gynaecology
Ophthalmology
Orthopaedics
Psychiatry
Urology and Nephrology

Postgraduate medical centres

Regional postgraduate medical centres are found in all NHS regions in England, Wales, Scotland, and Northern Ireland. Each regional centre has a full-time dean, each centre has a part time clinical tutor and specialty tutors.

NHS trusts

Under the reforms of the National Health Service many hospitals and groups of hospitals have been converted into self-governing trusts. In 1992 there were 124 such trusts, together with 18 community health-care and eight ambulance trusts.

A. M. COOKE
D. A. PYKE

MEDICAL COLLEGES, FACULTIES, MAJOR HOSPITALS, SOCIETIES, AND INSTITUTIONS IN NORTH AMERICA. Medical institutions in North America reflect both the social history and intellectual history of the medical profession in the USA and Canada. The similarities and differences of the two countries are mirrored in their institutions and since, in many cases, Canadian organizations were patterned on, or at least strongly shaped, by either US or British models, this discussion will consider Canadian institutions primarily in contrast to those that developed in the US or Great Britain.

While at present the national medical institutions are the most influential and important in both countries, physicians first organized on a local or state and provincial level. Local medical institutions were founded, have served, and continue to serve various purposes—social,

political, and intellectual. The earliest evidence of a medical society in what would become the USA was an organization of practitioners in colonial Boston in 1736, which planned to publish some form of medical literature. There is evidence of similar local groups in New York, Philadelphia, and Charleston, as well as a provincial society founded in New Brunswick, New Jersey. This New Jersey Medical Society was founded primarily to regulate the practice of medicine, and achieved prerevolutionary success when the first colonial regulatory act was passed in 1772.

Similarly, medical schools and *hospitals in colonial North America developed following British models. The earliest hospital founded exclusively as such was the Pennsylvania Hospital, chartered in 1751. Like the voluntary hospitals in mid-18th century English cities, the Pennsylvania Hospital was funded by subscription and cared for the 'worthy' or working poor. Infirmaries evolved in the almshouses to provide places of medical care for paupers. These infirmaries became the city hospitals of the colonial cities—Philadelphia General Hospital and Bellevue Hospital in New York City. There was an asylum in Williamsburg, Virginia, as a place of custodial care of those judged to be insane. Medical schools on the British model were also established in the colonial period. The first was the Medical Department of the College of Philadelphia (later University of Pennsylvania) established by William Shippen and John Morgan in 1765, followed by the Medical Department of King's College (later Columbia University) in New York City in 1767.

The Revolutionary War disrupted most institutions and organizations in the colonies and new beginnings had to be made after the conflict ended. In 1781 the legislature of Massachusetts chartered the Massachusetts Medical Society at the request of 14 Boston physicians who were members of the recently founded (1780) Boston Medical Society. The local society existed for fellowship and mutual enlightenment, but the new state society would issue letters of certification to those individuals who passed a competency examination. The society's qualification had no legal status, uncertified practitioners were still allowed to practise, but it was hoped that the moral force of the society would improve the standards of practice and reduce the practice of irregular practitioners. In 1803 the state society was given the authority to establish subordinate societies, and 18 district societies were organized by 1841. Between 1818 and 1835 the Massachusetts legislature, against the wishes of most members of the society, restricted the right to sue for fees to those certified by the society or those who had graduated from the Harvard Medical School.

*Harvard received endowments for medical instruction from the estate of Ezekiel Hersey in 1770, but made no appointments. The efforts of John Warren to teach anatomy and surgery during the Revolution inspired the Harvard trustees to appoint him as the Hersey professor. Warren was joined by Benjamin Waterhouse and Aaron Dexter to create the Harvard Medical School in 1782. The Harvard School existed amicably with the medical society. As the new nation developed, further medical schools were established, political tension in New York and Philadelphia resulted in rival schools being chartered and competition for students waxed and waned with changing circumstances.

In sharp contrast to the Massachusetts experience, most state societies became embroiled in attempts to restrict the practice of medicine; an idea which usually lacked social and political support. The early New York experience was typical and important well beyond the borders of New York. In 1806 a state society was established with responsibility for regulation. County societies were responsible for examining candidates for admission to the profession, with the state society serving as an appellate body. Because of their licensing authority, county societies, particularly in New York City, became involved in medical school rivalries and suffered from frequent internal battles over control of teaching authority and the profits from medical education. Furthermore, the restrictive legislation became the target of sectarian organizations challenging the regular medical profession in Jacksonian America, and the Medical Society of the Start of New York became synonymous with monopolistic medicine. In 1844 the medical regulatory acts were repealed and the medical societies retreated to become organizations for professional fellowship and educational exchange, but their prestige had suffered extensive damage.

In the face of irregular challenges and the repeal of licensure laws, physicians in many areas formed voluntary associations for fellowship and educational purposes, which served to set apart regular from sectarian practitioners. In New York City the New York Academy of Medicine was founded in 1846 at the urging of several of the leading practitioners. Its by-laws denied fellowship to all irregular practitioners and it could, and did, exercise the moral force in New York City that the Massachusetts Medical Society had never lost in Boston. Voluntary institutions, like the New York Academy, could also influence the *ethics of their membership by internal police powers; for example, the New York Academy denied fellowship to vendors of secret or patent remedies. Initially, such organizations were broadly inclusive, but as they developed they could afford to become selective, and memberships became important social and professional marks of distinction.

There were also local organizations which were never involved in regulatory questions; the oldest of these was the College of Physicians of Philadelphia, founded in 1786. Established along European lines, the College of Physicians had a limited number of fellows and an unlimited number of members. In keeping with its intellectual purposes, the college established a library which

is today one of the nations's great medical bibliographic resources.

In Boston, physicians organized the Boston Society for Medical Improvement in 1803; it was a smaller, less formal group, which met in the homes of members to discuss the medical literature. In 1805 they founded the Boston Medical Library, which they maintained until 1826. Like their Philadelphia counterparts, the Boston physicians recognized the need to provide materials for continuing medical education and worked to ensure access to the latest medical literature. The collections were housed in the Boston Athenaeum from 1826 until 1875, when a second Boston Medical Library was founded by the next generation of physicians, and, like its Philadelphia counterparts, it continues to play a vital role as a regional medical library, particularly since its union in 1965 with the Harvard Medical Library to form the Francis A. Countway Library of Medicine.

In the middle years of the 19th century yet a third type of local medical institution came into existence in urban centres—the research society. Groups of better-trained scientific-minded physicians, many of whom had studied in Paris, organized local societies to which they could report and discuss their clinical and pathological observations and studies. The most dynamic of such groups were the Philadelphia Pathological Society, founded in 1838, the New York Pathological Society, founded in 1844, and the Boston Society for Medical Observation, founded in 1835.

In Canada there were similar provincial or local organizations, but licensure was originally kept separate from societal membership. A medical board was established in Upper Canada (Ontario) from 1881, which was responsible for the examination and certification of practitioners and was an agency of the colonial government. In 1833, a Medico-Chirurgical Society was founded in York (Toronto) which provided a forum for fellowship and professional exchanges. Between 1839 and 1841, when it was disallowed, there was a College of Physicians and Surgeons which examined candidates in the place of the Medical Board and which served as a major professional body. The Provincial Act which had created the college was determined by the Colonial Office, at the request of the Royal College of Surgeons, London, to be too broad and imprecise, thus infringing the rights of the royal college. When the college was disallowed the Medical Board was recreated and the library which the college had begun was given into the custody of the Medico-Chirurgical Society.

Practitioners in various locations realized that real improvement in the social and professional status of the medical profession could best be achieved through collective action on a national scale. It was with such intent that regular correspondence was begun between the medical boards of Upper and Lower Canada in the 1840s; from that correspondence there developed a regulatory co-operative, intended to ensure safe general practice in Canada. In the USA, where regulation and governmental sanction had virtually disappeared, the organizational attempts were all voluntary and positive results developed very slowly.

After the 1844 repeal of the New York Medical Act a young reformer, Nathan Smith Davis, urged the Medical Society of the State of New York to call a convention in New York City. There were 119 delegates from 16 states at the meeting, on 5 May 1846. The group, primarily interested in the reform of medical education, adjourned to permit committee investigation of the various problems and then reassembled in Philadelphia in 1847. They constituted themselves the *American Medical Association (AMA), and through the middle of the 19th century were the collective voice for increased professional awareness and reform in American medicine.

Medical education in 1847 was still based on the 18th century apprenticeship model, in which the preliminary education and qualifications of future practitioners were the responsibility of the individual's preceptor. The schools asked only for a certificate of apprenticeship and the AMA could only encourage both preceptors and schools to strive for higher standards.

The need for reform in medical education was the result of the haphazard development of medical schools in the 19th century. Groups of preceptors obtained charters for proprietary schools and taught each other's apprentices. Schools often developed in small towns which could not support anatomical instruction or organized clinical teaching. Competition among these medical schools and the lack of societal control of *medical practice made educational reform virtually impossible before the Civil War.

In other areas of professional reform, the AMA had more, but still limited success. The organization of the national body lent strength to the formation of local and state societies in areas where none had existed before. In the late 1840s and 1850s, state societies were organized in Alabama, Georgia, Illinois, Indiana, Kentucky, Louisiana, Maine, Michigan, Mississippi, Missouri, North Carolina, Ohio, Pennsylvania, South Carolina, and Virginia; as well as many county medical societies in almost every state.

After the Civil War enforcement of the Code of Ethics on constituent societies was the means by which the profession most effectively opposed irregular and sectarian medical practices—*homoeopathy, *osteopathy, *chiropractic, etc. Even strong state societies, such as the Massachusetts Medical Society, were forced to conform to an increasingly rigid interpretation of the association's code of ethics.

One final area of the association's early reform effort needs to be mentioned—the general efforts to raise the scientific standards of American medicine—but the actual results are extremely difficult to evaluate. The AMA appointed standing committees on the major subdivisions of medicine—medical science, practical medicine (*internal medicine), *surgery, *obstetrics—

the reports of which, as published in the annual transactions, were important reviews of current work in their respective areas of specialization. In 1883 the AMA established the weekly *Journal of the American Medical Association (JAMA)* which increased the association's moral force and scientific prestige among American and foreign physicians.

By the end of the 19th century it had become apparent that the AMA was in serious need of structural and procedural reform. While ostensibly a national organization, it was initially an eastern organization, and by the end of the century an eastern/midwestern organization. Despite some success, the association had not achieved its reform purposes in the first 50 years of its existence and many of its leaders recognized that to succeed it needed a broader professional base and a streamlined organizational structure.

During the latter half of the 19th century other medical institutions, particularly medical schools, proliferated. As the population spread west and south from New England and the Middle Atlantic States, medical schools and other institutions followed. In Chicago, Rush Medical School was founded in 1837 and in the south there were several antebellum foundations, which survived into the present century: the Medical College of South Carolina (1824), Medical College of Georgia (1828–33), and Tulane University School of Medicine (1834) were all important teaching centres. The Morrill Act (1867) creating land-grant state colleges and universities strengthened the schools affiliated with state institutions and resulted in the creation of many of the schools of the Midwest, i. e. Iowa (1869), Minnesota (1888). Similarly, as population density increased, charitable hospitals were established in urban areas. Some were works of civic pride, such as *Massachusetts General Hospital in Boston (1821); others the work of religious groups, such as St Mary's in Rochester, Minnesota, (1887) or the Presbyterian Hospital in New York City (1872). One of the most significant foundations was the *Johns Hopkins Hospital (1889) which, in combination with the Medical School of Johns Hopkins, would inspire change in American medical education. Hospitals of all types grew, especially at the end of the 19th and beginning of the 20th century as antiseptic and aseptic surgery began to revolutionize surgical therapy.

In 1900 the AMA followed the lead of the *British Medical Association and undertook a major reorganization. Under the new plan the AMA became a federation of state medical societies, with membership almost exclusively through membership in a constituent state society. The reorganization of the state societies, based upon constituent local societies, followed, and while executives were elected under the new organizational plan, a compensated secretariat was provided for as well. The membership increased; by 1920 over half on the profession was enrolled in the AMA.

The growing strength of the AMA was one of the most important factors in the achievement of reform in *medical education. Standards were established and medical schools evaluated in the light of those standards. Over the course of the first quarter of the 20th century, the standards were steadily raised and the AMA co-operated with Abraham *Flexner of the Carnegie Foundation in the preparation of his famous 1910 *Report on medical education in the United States and Canada.*

Improvements in medical education continued to concern the AMA throughout the 20th century and, with the increased importance of graduate medical education, the AMA played an active role in the development of standards; but its classic reform problem had been addressed and attention was increasingly focused on other issues. The two issues that most occupied the AMA in the 20th century were: first, the protection of the public in medical matters, particularly its campaign against nostrums and quacks; and, secondly, the questions surrounding compensation for professional services, especially public and private insurance plans and salaried practice.

The newly reorganized AMA was one of the most vocal champions of pure food and drug legislation, and played an important role in the passage of the 1906 Food and Drug Act. Yet, despite its importance as a pioneering piece of legislation, the 1906 Act was in many ways deficient and the AMA continued an active campaign, directed simultaneously at the profession and the general public, against false and misleading claims of patent medicine manufacturers.

The antinostrum crusade took several forms. In the public arena the AMA took full advantage of the 'muckraking' report, *The great American fraud,* by Samuel Adams. Originally appearing serially in *Colliers* magazine from 1905 through 1906, Adams' investigative report was a stirring denunciation of patent medicines and quackery, which the AMA reprinted for public distribution in the years before the First World War. The AMA lobbied against medical patents and adopted a policy of encouraging prescriptions by generic rather than proprietary name—a policy which has been repeatedly debated throughout the 20th century.

The AMA's professional campaign was also multifaceted, including among other things the 1906 establishment of a drug testing laboratory where new and old patent medicines were examined by AMA scientists. Even more effective were the policies adopted by AMA publications, which required drug manufacturers to establish the validity of their advertising claims and the safety of the preparation they advertised. Finally, and perhaps most importantly, the AMA issued an annual volume, *New and non-official remedies,* which provided practitioners with information on drugs. It quickly became the physician's single most important source of drug information and, as such, was a significant listing for every drug manufacturer.

The AMA received high praise for its efforts in the antinostrum campaign and this goodwill was transferred into social prestige and political power. The

AMA's other major thrust of the 20th century—interest in patterns of practice and compensation for professional services—was not as well received by the opinion moulders of American society. Prior to the First World War the membership of the AMA was divided on *national health insurance issues, and as late as 1918 the *JAMA* was editorially favourable toward some form of social insurance programme. However, opposition within the association and anti-German sentiment in the war, (social insurance was first legislated in Bismark's Germany) turned the AMA clearly against federal insurance programmes.

From the 1920s the AMA opposed most challenges to the solo, fee-for-service practitioner, including group practice, contract practice, and both public and private insurance. Medical practice continued to change, the hospital and specialization emerged as the dominant force in medicine, and group practice became more acceptable. The depression of the 1930s made both contract practice and *health insurance important financial options. Private health insurance, such as Blue Cross, was considered less objectionable than state or federally controlled insurance. In recent years the desirability of comprehensive federal health insurance has begun to be re-evaluated by politicians, and the association has shown greater flexibility in considering various alternatives and approaches to compensation, reflecting the changes that society and medical care have undergone and are undergoing.

A comparable organization in Canada was organized on the AMA pattern, although the first unsuccessful attempt antedated the AMA. As early as 1844 William Masden tried to organize the Canadian profession, but it was only after he returned from an AMA meeting in 1867 that he was able to generate sufficient enthusiasm among his peers for an organization. The key factor was probably that a Canadian medical association met a need for professional co-ordination in the newly independent dominion that had not existed to the same degree in the various colonies. One of the principal activities of the Canadian Medical Association (CMA) was the effort to achieve uniformity of registration among the various provinces of Canada, an objective it achieved with the passage of the Canada Medical Act of 1912. Like its American counterpart, the CMA has a long history of concern with quackery and other aspects of public protection in medical matters. It has had a vital interest in public health and has served as the profession's arbitrator in matters of ethics and professional conduct. In these matters it clearly followed the lead of the AMA, and its first code of ethics was modelled on that of the American group.

One final aspect of medical institutions in North America commands attention—the specialty organizations, which are frequently international in scope. Apart from physicians interested in pathological research, the only special interest group within medicine prior to the

Civil War was *psychiatry, and in 1844 the Association of Medical Superintendents of American Institutions for the Insane was organized in Philadelphia. This group has led a continuous existence through several name changes and is today the American Psychiatric Association. The emergence of medical specialization was a slow process—the result of scientific and technical innovation and concomitant social changes. In 1864, one of the earliest specialist societies, The American Ophthalmological Society, was founded. As other specialties developed and achieved a critical mass of specialist practitioners, other specialist societies were organized: the American Otological Society (1868), American Neurological Association (1875), American Dermatological Association (1876), American Gynecological Society (1876), American Pediatric Society (1888), etc.

These groups met annually to exchange specialized knowledge and techniques and to discuss common problems. Frequently they published proceedings or transactions to facilitate further professional exchanges. All were small, usually confined to less than 50 practitioners from the several large cities that existed in late 19th-century America; because of the small size of the emerging speciality the early societies were *de facto* inclusive. Often they met initially in conjunction with the AMA.

In 1880 an exclusive society based on peer-recognized merit in the specialty was organized when Samuel D. Gross invited other leaders of American surgery to meet with him at the AMA meeting, for the purpose of organizing the American Surgical Association (ASA). The membership of the ASA was limited and members were elected by their fellow surgeons. Under the early leadership of Dr Gross the association provided an important forum for scientific discussion.

In 1886, a similar, self-selected group of physicians met as the Association of American Physicians (AAP). At the first meetings the latest studies on the germ theory were presented by American leaders in medical research: George Sternberg, William Councilman, and William *Osler among others. Like the ASA in surgery, the AAP provided an annual forum for presentation and discussion of the latest medical science and its annual transactions made the presentations and discussions available to a wide audience of American practitioners. Such highly selective organizations met important needs but more inclusive groups were also needed, giving rise to the American College of Surgeons (1913) and the American College of Physicians (1915); groups that played a more active role in the social and clinical affairs of the emerging specialties of general surgery and general internal medicine than the highly selective, scientifically oriented groups had done. By the late 20th century these inclusive specialty societies became the chief voice for practitioners.

The progress of medical science also led to the emergence of groups interested in experimental medicine or basic research. The first such group was the American Physiological Society (APS), organized in 1887. The group reflected the emergence of full-time basic science teacher/researchers in American medicine. Out of the APS have come other basic science organizations: the American Society of Biological Chemists (1906) and the Society for Pharmacology and Experimental Therapeutics (1913). Other groups, organized independently of physiology, have used the APS as a clear organizational model, e.g. the Society of American Bacteriologists (1900) and the American Society for Experimental Pathology (1913). Also important in the 20th century was the expansion of *clinical investigation, which gave rise to other exclusive research societies. In 1903, the Society of Clinical Surgery was organized by young, academically oriented surgeons who needed an institution for professional exchange but who were not sufficiently senior to be elected to the American Surgical Association. The Interurban Clinical Club (1905) and the American Society for Clinical Investigation (1908) met similar needs for internists. As the specialty grew, new societies were needed; the next generation formed the Halsted Society (1924) and the American Federation for Clinical Research (1940).

The final specialist institution to emerge was an organization for regulation of the specialty—the specialty board. The first of the boards was the American Board of Ophthalmology, organized in 1916 by the co-operation of the American Ophthalmological Society, the Section of Ophthalmology of the AMA, and the American Academy of Ophthalmology and Otolaryngology. The board was 'to arrange, control and supervise examinations to test preparations for opthalmic practice' and established a pattern of effective specialty certification which virtually every specialty has followed in turn. In Canada, on the other hand, the British model of specialization has played a greater role, and in 1929 the *Royal College of Physicians and Surgeons of Canada was founded to oversee the peer review and certification process.

Medical institutions continue to evolve, emerge, and disappear as the nature of medicine and society undergoes change. The societies discussed above co-operate and compete in a variety of ever-changing ways to shape medical science, education, and practice in late 20th-century America.

DALE C. SMITH

References

Burrow, J. (1963). *AMA: Voice of American medicine.* Johns Hopkins University Press, Baltimore.

Kett, J. (1968). *The formation of the American medical profession: The role of institutions 1780–1860.* Yale University Press, New Haven.

MacDermitt, H. E. (1967). *One hundred years of medicine in Canada 1867–1967.* McClelland and Stewart, Toronto.

Stevens, R. (1971). *American medicine and the public interest.* Yale University Press, New Haven.

MEDICAL CORRESPONDENTS. Contributors to lay newspapers and journals, reporting medical events and advances with professional comment, interpretation, and analysis.

MEDICAL CULTS AND QUACKERY. Just as heretics are unthinkable without the enforcement of religious orthodoxy by the churches, so quacks are essentially products of the development of medical orthodoxy seeking to define and enforce a single proper mode of medical practice: without regulars, no irregulars. In former centuries, at least, it makes more sense to distinguish orthodox medicine from quackery on the grounds of legal and professional exclusion, than in terms of the scientific standing or the success rate of treatments given. It would be historically misleading to imply that official medicine has always been competent whereas fringe medicine has been ineffectual or fraudulent. Unlike, perhaps, the regular profession, fringe medicine has always had notorious black sheep, from the huckstering mountebanks satirized by Ben Jonson and Molière to the 'toadstool millionaires' and 'medical messiahs' who swindled the public in modern America. Yet the regular profession has often appeared mercenary and domineering, and, until the 19th century, it could not reliably counter life-threatening diseases. It is little surprise that irregular healers retained their attractions.

In pre-modern times, the similarities between regular and fringe medicine were no less apparent than the differences. Both evolved a certain showmanship. Orthodox healers of former centuries cultivated a gentlemanly bedside manner, the use of Latin as mumbo-jumbo, the ancestor-worship of *Hippocrates and *Galen, and grave rituals like urine-gazing—all these created the aura of the medicine man *within* the profession, by way of parallel to the quack's alligator, black cats, snakes, or canting neologisms. In centuries in which there was little efficacious *materia medica*, psychological soothing and the placebo effect formed a major component of successful therapy amongst regulars and irregulars alike.

The boundaries between fringe and core medicine have been fluid and shifting. Certain fringe practitioners have sought to ingratiate themselves with the establishment, or at least to bask in its prestige, and many have called themselves Professor or Doctor, without proper justification. Orthodox medicine, for its part, has sometimes seen fit to assimilate fringe practices rather than lose patients *en masse* to marginal medicine. To some degree this happened in the Victorian age with *mesmerism; it may be occurring today with *acupuncture. In short, the historical distinction between medical quackery and orthodoxy has been more sccial than scientific.

From medieval times, all major European nations developed systems of medical licensing, policed by the upper echelons of the medical profession and ultimately sanctioned by kings and governments. Guilds and corporations regulated entry into the profession, and medical oligarchies emerged, exercising a near monopoly of access to promotion, power, and favour, and aiming for a closed shop, to maintain professional standards and protect the public. Numbers were kept small, and fees correspondingly high. This strategy was certainly effective in stigmatizing and marginalizing other healers. But it rarely proved effective as a way of *suppressing* the unorthodox. For, until recently, there never were enough privileged practitioners to meet the overall demand for medical services, especially in rural areas and small towns. With regulars too distant or too expensive, common people had to resort to self-medication and to quacks.

Moreover, in centuries when disease was king and death omnipresent, not only the poor patronized irregular healers. In the case of severe disease, it made sense for all manner of sufferers to shop around. When Prime Minister Sir Robert Walpole found no relief in orthodox medicine for his stomach ailments and kidney stones, he had resort to the quack Joshua Ward's much-touted pills. The physician Sir Hans *Sloane, who rose to become President of the Royal Society and chief endower of the British Museum, had a niece with a spinal deformity. When orthodox treatment failed, he called in the Epsom bone-setter and manipulator, Sally Mapp, who is said to have worked a cure.

Irregular healers have appealed in many ways. Sometimes their cures have appeared extremely modern. Others have been less disgusting and severe than orthodox medicine's heavy artillery of purges, bleedings, and vomits. Certain fringe practitioners, like some evangelical preachers, achieved fashionability. Wealthy invalids with time on their hands would want to sample novel treatments. In the 19th century, Viktor Preissnitz's health-farm hydrotherapy became chic amongst the European élite. In 1 year his patients supposedly included one royal highness, one duke, one duchess, 22 princes and princesses, 149 counts and countesses, 88 barons and baronesses, 14 generals, 53 staff officers, 196 captains and subalterns, 104 high and low civil servants, 65 divines, 46 artists, and 87 physicians. Hypochondriacs might be flattered by the assiduity and attention they received from a polished fringe doctor. Such unorthodox practitioners as Franz Anton *Mesmer (the late-18th century inventor of hypnotism) and his contemporary James *Graham (pioneer of sex therapy) were skilful showmen and actors. Advocate of vegetarianism, mud-bathing, and sexual rejuvenation, Graham combined a marvellous theatrical touch with a sure grasp of audience psychology. Graham presented himself as a high priest at what he called his Temple of Health at the Adelphi, just off the Strand, with a young female priestess who assisted, half-naked, 'at the display of the Celestial Meteors, and of that sacred Vital Fire over which she watches, and whose application in the cure of diseases, she daily has the honour of directing'.

Fringe healers like Mesmer and Graham astutely

addressed themselves to those problems that were the particular ills of high society: ennui, *anxiety, *hysteria, sexual incompatibility, depression, and nervous disorders. By being forced on to the margins, fringe practitioners were almost forced to exploit the opportunities and techniques of the market-place in the era of expanding capitalism. The medical profession ensured the prosperity of those they proscribed.

Unlike licensed medical men, the irregular's fame came entirely from his standing with the public, not his peers. He had to sell his wares in the market. The arts of publicity were crucial. Some, such as the Prussian influenza-curer, Gustavus Katterfelto in the 1780s, exploited penumbra of magic, wonder, and wizardry: black cloaks, snakes, black cats, fuming potions, and electrical sparks. Mountebanks traditionally toured accompanied by monkeys and zanies. Some sought status in the public eye by making the most of being—or pleading to be—foreign and exotic. Thus 'Chevalier' Taylor, the 18th century eye specialist, lectured in pidgin Latin which he confidently, but inaccurately, described as 'the true Ciceronian'. Others sought credit by dropping the names of the powerful and famous. Bottles of 'Daffy's Elixir' had a label stating that 'The Elixir was much recommend to the public by Dr King, Physician to King Charles II, and the late learned and ingenious Dr *Radcliffe'. James Ward, the marketer of the famous 'Pill and Drop', won fame and public confidence after putting George II's dislocated thumb back in place. He also received the testimonies of celebrated men, including the novelist, Henry Fielding.

Quacks traditionally did their business through personal sales. Most were itinerant. The travelling salesman had the aura of mystery. He was elusive to the authorities. Having exhausted one market, he could move on. Increasingly, however, fringe healers settled down, relying upon the publicity apparatus of commercial capitalism, notably the newspapers. 'The Widow READ, removed from the Upper End of Highstreet to the *New Printing-Office* near the Market, continues to make and sell her well-known ointment for the ITCH', announced a Philadelphia newspaper in 1731. Newspaper advertising multiplied the potential market for quack preparations several thousandfold at a stroke. Their nostrums were often sold retail by newspaper publishers and offices.

Soon, some were trying Blitzkrieg advertising. James Eno was the first to use whole-page advertisements in the press for his fruit-salts. 'Professor' Thomas Holloway, who marketed cure-all pills in Victorian England, was spending £20 000 a year on advertising by the mid-19th century. He was the first worldwide advertiser. His name appeared on hoardings in London; it was to be found in newspapers of China, India, and Peru; it even appeared on the Great Pyramid in Egypt. Advertisements were usually festooned with testimonials and other forms of puffery. Quacks pioneered sales gimmicks, including

fancy packaging, appealing brand names, and special offers.

Traditional quackery possessed many apparent advantages. It might appear cheaper than regular medicine. It could be more anonymous, important in the case of embarrassing complaints. Sometimes it appealed to nature. It claimed to conquer otherwise incurable diseases such as *cancer and *tuberculosis. Not least, in an age in which women were excluded from regular practice, the presence of many women quacks in big cities doubtless appealed to female sufferers too embarrassed to take their gynaecological problems to gentlemen surgeons.

Moreover, quacks exploited a psychological appeal, playing upon human unhappiness and unfulfilled expectations, the susceptibilities of the short, the fat, the inarticulate, the impotent, the ageing, the unsuccessful, the shy, the spotty. Sometimes they have played upon fear and shame. Illness, pain, and debility are the wages of evil or ignorance, they claim. Such guilt-inducing ploys have obviously been particularly effective in the case of patients suffering from *venereal diseases, from *alcoholism, obesity, and psychological disorders.

In its individualist and itinerant form, quackery had peaked by 1800. Increasingly, the thirst for non-regular medicine has been satisfied since then by the rise of medical cults, espousing a philosophy of alternative healing, typically linked to specific religious and personal faiths, above all anti-professional, radical modes of self-help. With its appeal to natural and simple cures, *homoeopathy, developed by Samuel *Hahnemann in late 18th century Germany, was one of the first to enjoy a vogue. Hahnemann put forward the principle of treating like with like (for instance, fever-inducing drugs should be used in fever cases), and also believed in the efficacy of very small doses of exceptionally pure drugs, partly because, in his view, orthodox medicine habitually overdosed.

Water cures grew popular. Water has had an enormous cachet as a cure on the medical fringes, regarded as an agent of cleanliness and purification, the matrix of life, and the symbol of baptism and rebirth. It has been deployed in fringe therapies in innumerable ways: pure fresh water has been drunk to cleanse the system, cold water baths have been used in *hydrotherapy; sea water has been taken internally and externally; and, most commonly, healing mineral springs have been promoted. Within temperance and teetotal movements, water became medicinal.

The appeal of the fringe cults has been not just to relieve physical pain, but to make born a new person—even to put the world to rights. Their leaders have been moral, social, and political reformers, wanting to cure ills on the widest possible scale. Pain and suffering have been seen as the consequences of the radical misorganization of society and false values. Society needed to be cured along with the individual. Lydia Pinkham in 19th century America offers a typical instance. Brought up in a Quaker household, at an early age Lydia Pinkham embraced most liberal and humanitarian causes, including abolitionism and temperance. She dabbled with spiritualism and *phrenology, currency reform, and vegetarianism. She launched her own fringe medicine, the Vegetable Compound, quite expressly as part of her own feminist platform. She believed that male doctors were insensitive to female complaints. 'Only a woman understands a woman's ills', she contended. Testimonials from women using the compound confirmed the popularity of a medicine attached to a cause.

Reacting against the early 19th century vogue amongst regulars for 'heroic physic', various health-reform causes sprang up, especially in North America, championed not by physicians but by lay people, disaffected equally with official creeds and regular medicine, and seeking to replace both with a unified, holistic philosophy of spiritual and bodily health, carved out of their own personal experience.

Amongst such sects as the Grahamites and the Thomsonians—both advocates of *herbalism—certain convictions have been widely shared. These sects have argued that civilized man has brought disease upon himself by the 'fall' manifest in modern life-styles: urbanism, greed, speed, excessive meat-eating, and abuse of fermented liquor. By way of remedy, they advocated—on medical, moral, and religious grounds—a return to 'natural' ways of living—vegetarianism, sexual restraint, temperance (both general and specific), the abandonment of stimulants such as tea, coffee, and tobacco. They generally urged an end of artificial and synthetic drugs, trusting to God-given, natural herbal remedies. Homoeopaths insisted upon ultra-pure medicaments, taken in minute quantities; Thomsonians and Coffinites restricted themselves to a few herbal preparations. Influenced by Swedenborgianism, some groups went a stage further, discarding medicines altogether, and trusting to the healing powers of nature, aided by the healing powers of water, prayer, self-control, and spiritual illumination.

The *Christian Science movement exemplifies many of these features. Rejecting the strict Congregationalism of her parents, Mary Baker *Eddy (1821–1910) spent much of her youth sick with non-specific nervous disorders. Regular physicians did her no good. Relieved by homoeopathy, she then undertook a self-healing process, the success of which, in 1866, led her to outline her own system, the creed of which declared that 'there is but one creation, and it is wholly spiritual'. Matter therefore was an illusion; hence there could be no such reality as somatic disease. As explained in her best-selling textbook, *Science and health* (1875), true 'mind healing' would dispel the illusions of sickness and pain. Proclaiming itself the new scientific medicine of the new age, Christian Science owed its high rate of conversions to the 'patient: heal thyself' confidence it inspired.

Especially in 19th century North America, medical cults and fringe religion were typically interlinked. From their early days, both the Mormons and the Seventh Day Adventists voiced their antipathy to regular medicine, Joseph Smith (1805–44) recognizing only roots and herbs, and the Mormons, once in Utah, passing laws restricting the dispensing of most orthodox remedies ('deadly poisons'). Mormons, in particular, championed the constitutional right to resist compulsory smallpox *vaccination. The Adventists, led by Ellen White (1826–1915), proclaimed a 'gospel of health', which particularly valued hydropathic cures. Their Health Reform Institute at Battle Creek, Michigan, was headed by John Harvey Kellogg (1852–1943), brother of the cereal manufacturer.

Why, finally, has the medical fringe enjoyed such a huge and lasting appeal? By being forced out of the élite world of medicine, fringe medicine was actually dumped in the most fertile seedbed of all: the capitalist market-place in the age of rampant capitalism (an arena which orthodox medicine, with its ethical and professional goals, chose to deny to itself). Moreover, fringe medicine often moved into an area of human experience and need largely abandoned by orthodox medicine and orthodox religion alike. Orthodox medicine increasingly treated just the body, in ways unintelligible to the patient. Orthodox religion made promises for an immaterial soul in the hereafter. By contrast, marginal medicine actually appealed to a sense of the whole person—the unity of mental and physical experience—and sometimes also to two other unities: the oneness of the person with the world, and the co-operation of patient and doctor. Quacks often spoke in languages that people understood.

ROY PORTER

Further reading
Cooter, R. (ed.) (1988). *Studies in the history of alternative medicine*. Macmillan, London.
Coward, R. (1989). *The whole truth: the myth of alternative health*. Faber & Faber, London.
Inglis, B. (1979). *Natural medicine*. Collins, London.
Jameson, E. (1961). *The natural history of quackery*. Michael Joseph, London.
Porter, R. (1989). *Health for sale: quackery in England 1650–1850*. Manchester University Press, Manchester.
Young, J. H. (1967). *The medical messiahs: a social history of health quackery in twentieth-century America*. Princeton University Press, Princeton, NJ.

MEDICAL CURRICULUM. See MEDICAL EDUCATION, UNDERGRADUATE.

MEDICAL DEFENCE UNION. The oldest of the three UK medical protection societies. See LAW AND MEDICINE IN THE UK.

MEDICAL DEGREES. See MEDICAL EDUCATION: UNDERGRADUATE; POSTGRADUATE AND CONTINUING.

MEDICAL DINING CLUBS are small, often informal, societies of doctors, which may or may not have a defined scientific purpose.

MEDICAL EDUCATION, POSTGRADUATE AND CONTINUING

The role and responsibilities of the General Medical Council

The UK Medical Act of 1978 gave the Education Committee of the *General Medical Council (GMC) statutory responsibility for co-ordinating all stages of medical education and for promoting high standards of such education. The Education Committee is required by the Medical Act to determine acceptable patterns of experience for general clinical training (the preregistration year), and to issue its determinations as recommendations, to which the examining bodies (the universities and the non-university licensing bodies) must have regard. Recommendations on general clinical training were published in 1987 and in 1992. At intervals of about every 10 years the Education Committee also issues recommendations on basic medical education and, in 1987, it issued recommendations on the training of specialists. In postgraduate education, the Committee stands in a similar relationship to the *royal colleges, faculties and higher training committees as it does to the universities and other licensing bodies in respect of basic medical education.

The stages of medical education—concepts and terminology

Pre-registration training

The pre-registration year (general clinical training) follows immediately after qualification in the UK and completes basic medical education. In this year the doctor's undergraduate education is consolidated and extended during supervised experience as a *house officer in at least two branches of *medical practice, working under provisional registration with the GMC. The year must include a minimum of 4 months' experience in medicine and 4 months in surgery; the remaining 4 months may be spent in any other clinical specialty, including *general practice, approved by the graduate's university. It is, however, usual for the year to be divided equally, with 6 months in each of medicine and surgery. A combination of general and specialty experience (e.g. general medicine and *geriatrics; general surgery and *orthopaedics) is acceptable.

Statutory responsibility for this year rests with the university examining body associated with each health region or area. The postgraduate dean exercises this responsibility on behalf of the university. The most recent *Recommendations on general clinical training* (February 1992) placed particular emphasis on educational supervision, the process and content of training, and on educational standards, opportunities, and objectives. Following satisfactory completion of the pre-registration year, the doctor is eligible to obtain full registration with the GMC.

Postgraduate training

Postgraduate training begins following the pre-registration year. It comprises *general professional training* and *higher specialty training*. In general practice it takes the form of *vocational training*; there is as yet no higher specialty training in primary health care.

(a) General professional training. The meaning of 'general' in this context is not always clear. In most hospital specialties, and particularly perhaps in internal medicine and surgery, it is appropriate to seek 'general' experience before further, more specialized, training. In this sense the term 'basic specialist training' (the 'common trunk' concept promoted by the Advisory Committee on Medical Training (ACMT) of the European Community) is a more accurate description of this phase of postgraduate training. However, 'general professional training' as described in the report of the Royal Commission on Medical Education in 1968 (*The Todd Report*) envisaged a period during which young doctors could obtain a broad range of clinical or laboratory experience in several different specialties before committing themselves to a lifetime in one. There are many advantages to this broader view of general professional training, which remains under discussion.

General professional training (GPT) is undertaken mainly—in some specialties exclusively—in the *senior house officer (SHO) grade. Experience in the *registrar grade increasingly takes the form of higher specialty training. GPT lasts typically for 2 or 3 years, although this period may be extended by 1 or more years because of various circumstances. The governance of GPT rests with the UK royal colleges, and faculties, which are responsible for determining the postgraduate training requirements in their own specialties. In addition to completing the minimum periods of time that must be spent in training posts approved by the appropriate colleges, higher qualifications may also be obtained before entry to higher training. The examinations for these may be of the 'entry' type, such as the MRCP(UK) (Member of the Royal Colleges of Physicians of the United Kingdom), or the 'exit' variety, such as MRCPath (Member of the Royal College of Pathologists). 'Entry' diplomas allow a trainee to enter higher specialty training whereas 'exit' qualifications mark the completion of higher training. In the latter case the acquisition of the first part of the diploma examination allows entry to higher specialty training, and the final part of the examination, leading to the award of the diploma, is completed towards or at the end of it. The UK Royal Colleges of Surgeons now have both an entry and an exit examination; the former, in general surgery, allows entry to higher training in the registrar grade, whereas the latter, in the trainee's surgical specialty, completes postgraduate training.

The colleges are independent bodies, entirely separate from the universities, the *National Health Service (NHS), and governmental control. The colleges lay down the requirements for their examinations, and exercise their governance over GPT by visiting and inspecting posts in the NHS in order to determine their suitability for training. Thus there exists an important means of regulating and of monitoring the quality of training. This gives powerful influence to the colleges, and to those responsible for providing training at the local level, in relation to the NHS authorities which are responsible for providing the necessary resources. The threat of withdrawal of approval for training is serious; it means, in effect, loss of the post.

(b) Vocational training for general practice is in many senses the equivalent of GPT in the hospital service. In the UK it lasts for 3 years overall; 2 years of varied experience in relevant hospital appointments and 1 year as a trainee in general practice, working in a supernumerary capacity under the supervision of a trainer appointed by the regional committee responsible for general practice training.

The hospital component is normally made up of four six-month SHO appointments in specialties appropriate to general practice, and including at least two to be chosen from general medicine, geriatrics, *paediatrics, *obstetrics or obstetrics and gynaecology or *gynaecology, general surgery or accident and emergency, and *psychiatry. These constitute 'prescribed experience'. The usual (although not the invariable) pattern of vocational training is for it to begin with a six-month period in an approved general practice, followed by 2 years in hospital posts, and concluded by a further 6 months attachment as a trainee in general practice. Doctors selected for vocational training schemes may begin their three-year programmes immediately after the pre-registration year. Some doctors, however, prefer to construct their own schemes by seeking a variety of SHO posts, while others may opt to enter vocational training having advanced a considerable distance in hospital training; sometimes, in fact, having completed a substantial proportion or even all of higher specialty training. Doctors who decide to enter general practice after considering or embarking upon other careers may ask for some or all of their hospital experience to be recognized, as 'equivalent experience' if necessary, towards the required training for general practice. The requirement for 1 year as a trainee in general practice is, however, mandatory.

The governance of vocational training for general practice rests ultimately with the Joint Committee for Postgraduate Training in General Practice (JCPTGP), although regional committees and local vocational training schemes have substantial responsibilities. These include the appointment of trainers and trainees, the explicit definition of local criteria for the approval of practices (based on those issued by the JCPTGP),

and the power to visit practices. The SHO posts, which comprise the hospital component of vocational training, must also be approved for training; those specifically designated for vocational training are visited regularly by teams which include representatives from the 'parent' college and a local GP nominated by the Regional or Associate Advisers for General Practice.

Training includes a programme of more formal education based on day, or half-day, release (the content and delivery of these programmes being the responsibility of course organizers) and the progressive assessment of trainees is conducted throughout. At present this assessment is formative, using a variety of methods, although it is likely that summative assessments will be introduced in the future.

The end of vocational training is marked by the issue of a Certificate of Satisfactory Completion. This indicates not only that the requirement as to duration of training has been met but also that performance has been satisfactory. Increasingly the latter criterion is based on formative progressive assessment during the training period. Unlike all other specialties, no formal examination is taken at the end of training; it is possible to become a principal in general practice immediately on completion of vocational training. The Certificate of Satisfactory Completion is, however, regarded as the minimum achievement required by statute; acquisition of the MRCGP (Member of the Royal College of General Practitioners) diploma is regarded as the criterion standard.

(c) Higher specialty training (HST) begins in the hospital specialties when GPT has been completed and the trainee has been appointed to a post approved for HST by the appropriate body. These posts are usually in the senior registrar (substantive or honorary) grade but, increasingly, registrar posts are being approved for higher training. This is now invariably the case in surgery and its specialties. Higher specialty training lasts for 3-6 years, depending on the specialty. At senior registrar level the linking of posts into rotational training programmes is the general rule, and these usually provide experience in both 'teaching' and 'non-teaching' hospitals.

In the case of obstetrics and gynaecology the regulation and governance of higher training are the responsibility of the Higher Training Committee of the Royal College of Obstetricians and Gynaecologists. In other specialties governance rests with the appropriate Joint Committee on Higher Training, which may represent more than one royal college and which also includes representation from other bodies such as professional associations. Each joint committee is supported by a number of Specialist Advisory Committees (SACs), representative of individual specialties, and it is these who, under the aegis of the joint committees, determine the detailed content and duration of training programmes. These details are published at regular intervals by the joint committees.

As with GPT, visits of inspection to training posts, programmes, and rotations take place regularly, at approximately five-yearly intervals. Posts are normally approved, if satisfactory, for 5 years, although the SAC may recommend a shorter period if the visitors have reservations. This allows time for recommendations made by the visitors to be implemented. If the SAC is not satisfied about the quality of training, the joint committee may withdraw recognition.

(d) 'Completion' of training. Over 50 specialties are recognized within the NHS. Although policies differ from specialty to specialty, there is a general tendency for individual royal colleges and joint committees to certify 'completion of training' at the end of the senior registrar period. This '*accreditation' is quite distinct from specialist registration as it is understood in other countries: it denotes that a full sequence of general professional and higher specialist training has been completed, which will normally take a minimum of 6–7 years. In the hospital service only the *consultant has independent responsibility for the care of patients. Legally the only requirement for appointment as a consultant is that the individual should hold full registration with the GMC. However, although accreditation is not mandatory for appointment as a consultant, the advisory appointment committee always pays great heed to the candidates' training and experience. The role of the college assessor on these committees is to advise whether the candidates' training is sufficient to allow their appointment. Accreditation would normally confirm that this was the case.

On 1 January 1991 the GMC introduced a procedure for registration of the completion of specialist training. This is an indicative register, and the designation includes the letter 'T' followed by a further indicator to denote the specialty concerned (e.g. T(GP) indicates completion of vocational training for general practice; T(M) indicates completion of specialist training in medicine). The indicators denote that the doctor has completed the training required for independent medical practice in his or her specialty, whether in hospital medicine, public health medicine, or general practice.

However, during the summer of 1992 the European Commission expressed its concern that the system in place in the UK for the mutual recognition of specialist medical qualifications between the UK and the other member states might not fully comply with the 1975 Medical Directives. While it is not necessarily contrary to Community law to distinguish between those who have completed specialist training and those who are still in training (the GMC's 'T' indicator) there would be an infringement if the UK were not to recognize other member states' certificates as being evidence of completion of specialist training. The directives do not permit a member state to create a higher specialist

training category such as accreditation to which those who have trained in other member states do not have access until they meet UK standards.

In September 1992 the Chief Medical Officer for England established a Working Group to consider the present UK arrangements for postgraduate medical education and career progression in the NHS, taking into account European Community law, and to consider scope for further harmonization of specialist qualifications in Europe. The Working Group was to advise UK Health Ministers within 6 months on any action which needed to be taken. There is no doubt that this heralds major changes in the structure of specialist medical training in the UK, but whatever changes are recommended, the fundamental goal is to preserve, and indeed increase, the high quality of postgraduate training in the UK. Standards will not be compromised.

(e) Training in public health medicine. Until 1974, public health medicine in the UK was practised in local authorities by the department of the *medical officer of health. From 1974 this medical specialty, renamed *community medicine, was transferred into the NHS and certain local authority powers were lost. In 1990, the new name of *public health medicine was adopted, but practised still from within the NHS.

Postgraduate training programmes are organized by regional health authorities and regulated by the Faculty of Public Health Medicine. Doctors are generally expected to have completed at least 2 years' postregistration training in a clinical specialty before starting specialist training in public health medicine. The training programme lasts for 5 years and the first 2 include an academic course leading to Part I of the Membership of the Faculty of Public Health Medicine. During the following 3 years of higher specialist training, posts may be held in academic or service departments, or both. The completion of training, after acquisition of Part II of the membership examination, is marked by accreditation.

(f) University posts. A feature of the British system is the close relationship and extensive interchange between NHS and university appointments. In the clinical departments of the medical schools, appointments are available at junior lecturer and lecturer level which combine teaching and research responsibilities with clinical training. Such posts carry honorary NHS status at an appropriate level, and all such posts, like their NHS equivalents, are approved for training by the appropriate regulating body. It is therefore possible for doctors who have trained in a university post to return to the NHS by being appointed to posts at various levels, including that of consultant. Conversely, many applicants for university posts—including the most senior—come from the NHS. It is also possible to obtain full-time research posts, usually (but certainly not exclusively) held within the universities, and funded

by bodies such as the Medical Research Council or one of the medical research charities, or from some other source, including regional (NHS) research funding. This research will usually lead to the acquisition of a higher university degree such as MD or PhD. Many of these posts are approved for training on an *ad personam* basis. In other cases, experience in full-time research posts is taken into account by the regulating body when the requirements for accreditation are being considered.

Continuing medical education

Once training has been completed, whether in general practice, the hospital service, or in public health medicine, what follows is referred to as continuing medical education (CME). At the moment, although one of the phases of medical education for which the Education Committee of the GMC is responsible, there is no mandatory requirement for independent practitioners in the UK to pursue CME; this is entirely the responsibility of the individual. This is not the case in North America, where relicensure based usually on CME activities is the rule; increasingly, the same principle applies in Australia.

In the UK there has always been an implicit recognition of the fact that the true purpose of CME is ultimately to improve the quality of patient care, through keeping up to date, having the opportunity to compare practice with that of others, and hence to maintain and increase professional standards. Effective CME should properly be based on the principles of adult learning theory, in that it is self-directed, experiential and performance-centred, competency based, and derived from specific learning needs identified by the learner.

CME is also inextricably linked to the process of medical *audit (quality assurance), which is now routine practice in the UK, both in general practice and in the hospital and public health services. CME and medical audit are different but linked aspects of the same process: the setting, evaluation, and improvement of standards. The educational corollaries of the audit process are now universally recognized.

In general practice, the Postgraduate Education Allowance (PGEA) was introduced in 1989. This forms part of the 'target net income' of the practice. In order to qualify for the allowance (which currently stands at £2025 (US$3038)/annum/doctor), general practitioners must participate in an average of 5 days of accredited training per year over a period of 5 years. Courses of CME which count towards the PGEA are approved in England by the regional adviser for general practice; in Scotland this role rests with the postgraduate dean, and in Wales the responsibility is shared between the postgraduate dean and his associate advisor for general practice. There is a considerable financial incentive for general practitioners to achieve the requirements for the PGEA but, although participation levels are high, there is little evidence that the process is truly educational in the terms that were defined earlier for CME.

In the UK, the medical profession is self-regulating, and with this precious principle come both responsibility and accountability. In hospital practice, therefore, personal esteem and peer pressure are powerful incentives for participation in CME. As mentioned earlier, relicensure and recertification are not at present features of the British system. However, a number of royal colleges are pressing for the introduction of mandatory CME linked to recertification, and it seems inevitable that, within a few years, recertification, probably based mainly on participation in CME and related activities, will become the rule. To rely on participation levels and outputs will not, however, be sufficient; attitudes, commitment, and outcomes will be all-important. Nor are the sanctions and rewards ('sticks and carrots') clearly defined. There is, however, a universal move amongst the UK royal colleges to face these important issues head-on.

Mechanisms exist for dealing with doctors whose conduct or standards of professional behaviour, or whose health, give serious cause for concern. In addition, the GMC plans to introduce performance procedures in order to bring the doctor whose general pattern of professional performance raises serious misgivings within the council's jurisdiction. The proposal has been agreed in principle; the details of the procedures are currently under consideration.

The educational process

The educational process takes various forms. First, and most important, is clinical or laboratory apprenticeship, which enables appropriate experience to be obtained. Secondments to provide more specialized experience can be arranged. Secondly, many kinds of day-release and part-time courses are arranged, and library and other educational resources are freely available. Thirdly, many activities take place in hospitals or in general practice which combine teaching with the monitoring of standards. These take the form of case conferences, departmental and interdepartmental meetings, 'grand rounds', journal clubs, and medical audit activities. Fourthly, trainees can participate in nationally or regionally organized conferences and meetings, 'teach-ins', and advanced, 'state of the art' courses. Thus the four strands of service-based learning are evident— experiential learning, resource-based learning, formal teaching, and block learning, the last based usually on study leave. It is certain that this pattern of postgraduate teaching will develop further in the future, as structured training programmes are introduced progressively.

Research is an essential part of training in the NHS and is undertaken either on a full-time or a part-time basis, during tenure of a post in one of the training grades. Periods of elective study either elsewhere in the UK or abroad are also encouraged.

Wide provision is made for the training of doctors who, because of domestic commitments, disability, or other well-founded reasons, are unable to work full-time. This part-time or flexible training is undertaken in supernumerary appointments at SHO, registrar, or senior registrar level. The training programmes are individually planned and are subject to approval by the appropriate regulatory body for examination and accreditation purposes.

The educational context

In the UK, postgraduate training takes place almost exclusively within the NHS. This provides employment for doctors who obtain relevant experience while progressing through the training grades referred to earlier. The principal impediment to improvement in hospital training programmes in all specialties has always been, and remains, the conflict between the service demands placed on trainees and their learning needs. Although changes are essential, these will require careful and sensitive management to avoid losing the great strength of UK training—experiential learning or 'learning by doing'. It is likely that the development of structured training programmes, currently under urgent consideration in the UK, will largely correct the present imbalance between service demands and training needs.

In June 1991 the Department of Health, in agreement with the profession, launched a 'new deal' for junior doctors' hours of work which will reduce, often dramatically, the hours worked each week. Most junior doctors in the UK work an on-call system whereby they are on duty each working day and accept overnight and weekend on-call responsibilities in rotation. A small number of doctors working in specialties where clinical activity is constant, such as accident and emergency, follow a full shift system while others work 'partial shifts' which concentrate most of the junior doctors at the busiest times and ensure adequate time for rest. Since 1 April 1993 no doctors undertaking on-call rotas have been contracted to work for more than 83 hours a week, and this figure must fall to 72 hours by the end of 1994. The maximum contracted hours per week are lower for doctors working full or partial shifts.

With the introduction in the UK of the National Health Service Reforms in 1991 there was considerable anxiety that the introduction of self-governing trusts, working within the NHS as providers of health care, but managed autonomously and free to employ staff on their own terms and conditions of service, would lead to trusts opting out of their responsibilities for training. This was despite many assurances and safeguards emphasized by government. These include a responsibility for trusts to play their part in training the staff they employ, the requirement to use the recognized training grades, and to conform both to national quotas for these grades (see later) and to national agreements on junior doctors' hours of work. Trust hospitals must not cut back on postgraduate training in order to achieve cost reductions, and the Secretary of State for Health has reserve powers to ensure that trusts participate as appropriate in the training of medical and dental staff. Although SHOs are employed at unit (trust or directly (district) managed) level, the employment contracts of registrars and senior registrars are held at regional level, and all staff in the training grades remain subject to nationally agreed terms and conditions of service.

The pessimism and anxiety expressed at the outset have, in fact, largely been without substance. The majority of NHS trusts have, so far, appeared to accept both the importance of postgraduate training and their responsibilities for providing it. Those responsible for the regulation and delivery of postgraduate medical education have, in any case, considerable powers. The process of inspection of posts approved for GPT and HST has already been described; a post which falls short of the requirements set by the relevant regulatory body runs the risk of losing training recognition, and posts which lack this recognition cannot be advertised or filled on a substantive basis. Much more recently, regional postgraduate deans have obtained even greater powers. With effect from 1 April 1993 50 per cent of basic salary costs and 100 per cent of non-recurrent costs of all posts in the training grades, including preregistration posts, reverted from units to region, where they form a postgraduate training budget over which the postgraduate dean exercises overall control. The consequence of these new arrangements is that provider units are reimbursed the training element of salaries of those in the training grades (the proportions referred to above), under a training contract between regions and units, from a budget managed at regional level. These training contracts specify the quality of training that units are expected to provide, including the provision of educational resources, adequate study-leave provision, and protected time for private study and formal education. This procedure allows postgraduate deans to ensure that training standards are maintained and that training is properly evaluated.

Overseas doctors

For immigration purposes, doctors who are EC nationals are classified as 'career' in that they are able to pursue a career in the UK, provided that they hold appropriate registration with the GMC. Overseas nationals from non-EC countries who are entitled to settled status in the UK, and those admitted as doctors to the UK up to 1 April 1985, are similarly classified as 'career'. Other overseas doctors are categorized as 'visitors' and are allowed, with valid GMC registration, to work in the UK in educationally approved training posts in the hospital service for up to 4 years, without the need to obtain a work permit ('permit-free entry'). An increasing number of these doctors come to the UK on a 'sponsorship' basis to obtain training. This does not necessarily imply financial support, but rather that training needs are planned in advance, by arrangement between educational sponsors at home and abroad. Many royal colleges and other organizations such as the British Council also have sponsorship schemes for overseas doctors. Far too often in the past, overseas doctors have arrived in the UK without a prearranged post, without any planned programme of training, and, often, without any clear career plans in mind. This has often led to disappointment and frustration, as these doctors all too commonly occupy those posts that are least satisfactory from the training point of view. It is hoped that the increasing use of organized sponsorship arrangements will do much to avoid these problems.

Manpower planning
Quotas and ceilings
All the training grades in the NHS are subject to restrictions as to the numbers working in each grade. At preregistration and SHO level these are defined as regional ceilings which cannot be exceeded in total number, although relocation of posts among units, districts, and specialties is entirely possible. At registrar level the manpower controls are enforced in England and Wales (the arrangements in Scotland and Northern Ireland are somewhat different) by the imposition of specialty quotas for each region which indicate the maximum number of 'career' registrars that can be employed in each specialty or specialty group. These quotas are set by the Joint Planning Advisory Committee (JPAC) on the basis of advice received from the colleges. Registrars can be employed in excess of these quotas up to the 'baseline' figure agreed between the health region and the Department of Health, but these registrars must be visitors. The principle is that if a specialty includes both career and visiting registrars within a region, a rotational scheme of training should be established wherever possible, so that both career and visiting doctors can receive equality of training. Posts must not be assigned permanently either to career or to visiting registrars; all posts must provide training for both categories and can be filled at any one time either by career or by visiting doctors. Quotas for honorary registrars, both academic and research, are to be issued in the future.

Similarly, quotas are set for all specialties at senior registrar level. These, too, are determined by the JPAC on college advice and, over the past 6 years, there has been considerable redistribution of senior registrars among the health regions. At senior registrar level the specialty quotas include both NHS *and* academic (honorary) posts; there are separate quotas for research which are non-specialty specific. Part-time career registrars and senior registrars in England and Wales are also subject to quotas, defined by specialty or specialty group; both the part-time career registrar quotas and those for part-time senior registrars are issued by JPAC and are held centrally. All quotas, whether for part-time or full-time trainees, or for registrars or senior registrars, are reviewed regularly by the JPAC.

These quota arrangements are linked to an on-going programme of consultant expansion; the aim is that this should proceed at a rate of at least 2 per cent per year. These policies have two principal aims: the first is that consultants should accept a greater direct involvement in patient care and in the direct supervision and training of their junior staff; the second is that, by carefully planning the numbers of doctors in training grades and taking account of career prospects, the length of time spent in training should be reduced and promotion to the consultant grade should become more rapid. The 'support' grades (non-consultant career grades) include the staff grade, associate specialists, and clinical assistants.

The co-ordination and management of postgraduate medical education
Over the past 5 years there have been major developments in the co-ordination of postgraduate medical education (PGME). The responsibilities of the Education Committee of the GMC have already been described, and the other bodies involved in the postgraduate network are the royal colleges and faculties, the universities, the UK Health Departments and the NHS. Thus postgraduate and continuing education are the joint responsibility of the GMC and colleges, which set down minimum training criteria and maintain standards in their own specialties; the NHS and the universities, which jointly provide employment, teaching, and training; the medical profession itself, which is responsible for looking to the quality of its own work; and the Health Departments, which must achieve the necessary manpower integration between the needs of training and those of providing a service. It is evident that the postgraduate network is extremely complex. Furthermore, although the same broad principles apply, the detailed arrangements for the co-ordination and management of PGME are different in Scotland, Wales, and Northern Ireland as compared with England. For these reasons only a general description will be given, based on the English model.

Local arrangements
Each health region in England has a regional postgraduate education committee, which brings together the interests of the royal colleges, through their regional advisers, the NHS, the local medical school, public health medicine, trainees, and the medical profession in general. These committees have a number of subcommittees concerned with the individual specialties, including general practice, which assume general responsibility for working towards the best utilization of the training potential of the specialties throughout the region. The constitution of these subcommittees reflects that of the regional committee, bringing together both college and university interests, as well as those of the health authorities and of trainees. The main tasks of the specialty subcommittees are to arrange and monitor rotational training programmes, organize appropriate courses, assess the progress of trainees, and to provide advice, guidance, and counselling on careers.

In each university with a medical school there is a postgraduate dean or director who functions as the chief executive officer, and often the chairman, of the regional postgraduate committee. Postgraduate deans act as the directors (in some cases holding this formal title) of their postgraduate institutes or departments. Postgraduate deans now hold joint appointments with their university and their regional health authority, and are responsible, in consultation with college and general practice regional advisers, for devising and managing the postgraduate and continuing medical education programmes in their regions. They are the designated budget holders for the postgraduate training budget and use their budgeted money to fund the PGME infrastructure and educational programmes. The postgraduate deans are, *ex officio*, members of their regional manpower committees, thus providing links between medical manpower and its planning and training. Most postgraduate deans now have one or more associate deans, usually with specific responsibilities for a defined aspect of training, such as the preregistration year.

The universities also appoint clinical tutors, on the recommendation of the postgraduate dean. Clinical tutors are based at unit level and are responsible for the running of postgraduate centres; they represent the university and the dean in their unit and have administrative responsibility for the educational budgets devolved to them by their deans. They act as the chief executive officers of their local postgraduate medical education committee.

Central arrangements

The Standing Committee on Postgraduate Medical Education (SCOPME) was set up in August 1988 to replace the Council for Postgraduate Medical Education in England and Wales. Scotland, Wales, and Northern Ireland retain their own Councils for PGME. SCOPME is responsible for advising the Secretary of State on the delivery of postgraduate medical and dental education, taking into account both the standards promulgated by professional bodies and the potential difficulties of reconciling service and training needs. Its members are appointed by the Secretary of State for Health, and the Committee reports regularly, both to the Secretary of State and to the profession.

The roles of the royal colleges, colleges, and faculties have already been referred to: it is they who set down minimum training criteria and maintain standards in their own specialties. Each college appoints regional advisers and college tutors; the former act at regional and the latter at unit or district level, working in close liaison with postgraduate deans and clinical tutors.

The Committee of Postgraduate Medical Deans in England (COPMED) and the Committee of Regional Advisers in General Practice in England (CRAGPIE) are 'free-standing' committees which have informal links with SCOPME on the one hand, and more formal links with the Department of Health on the other. These committees provide a great deal of 'peer support' and peer review.

The Conference of Postgraduate Deans and Directors of Postgraduate Medical Education of Universities of the United Kingdom brings together all of the deans in England, Wales, Scotland, and Northern Ireland, with observers from other bodies, including the UK Health Departments. A similar Conference of Regional Advisers in General Practice also exists. The National Association of Clinical Tutors (NACT) represents these important individuals, and the National Association of Postgraduate Medical Centre Administrators includes those essential staff who administer and manage the postgraduate centres.

Although cross-representation is the rule, the existence of so many different bodies concerned with postgraduate medical education clearly argues the need for rationalization and for a single representative body. It is likely that this will develop in the future.

Postgraduate medical education in Europe

Such education and training exist in all member states, although there is considerable disparity from country to country in relation to the organization of training, its regulation, its duration, and its content. The royal colleges and faculties are unique to the UK and the Republic of Ireland; no similar system operates elsewhere in the EC.

The Medical Directives

These were adopted in 1975 (75/362/EEC and 75/363/EEC). The first of these concerns the mutual recognition of diplomas, certificates, and other evidence of formal qualifications in medicine, and includes measures to facilitate the effective exercise of the right of establishment and freedom to provide services. The second directive specifically addresses the matter of harmonization of standards, both at undergraduate level and at the level of specialist training. The key introductory paragraph here recognizes that medical practice is, in the main, specialized (at that stage general practice was not regarded as a specialty) and it therefore begins by also recognizing the need for co-ordination of the requirements for postgraduate training in specialized medicine. Articles 4 and 5 of the second directive address the important questions of *minimum* length of specialized postgraduate training courses, both for such specialist practice occurring in all member states and for such practice recognized only within some of the states. Most countries exceed these minimum requirements for the duration of training in the specialties listed; this is particularly the case in the UK and Ireland, where there is a general feeling that in some specialties the duration of training required could, with advantage, be shortened.

The Advisory Committee on Medical Training (ACMT)

The Advisory Committee on Medical Training (ACMT) was set up in 1975, following the adoption of the Medical Directives, to advise the European Commission on matters relating to training. The remit of the ACMT, which first met in 1976, is 'to help to ensure a comparably demanding standard of training in the Community, with regard both to basic training and further training'. The Committee has produced a number of important reports, opinions, and recommendations. Three of particular relevance include:

(1) the establishment of competent bodies to set and enforce standards (in the UK this is the GMC);
(2) the establishment, where possible, of a 'common trunk' of training; and
(3) inspection of training posts/centres.

Although the ACMT has recommended longer periods of training than are set out in the Medical Directives, any modifications to training duration are a matter for the competent bodies.

The European Union of Medical Specialists (UEMS)

The European Union of Medical Specialists (UEMS) is a non-governmental body which represents specialists, the term 'specialist' not being defined in any detail. Its member organizations are the national professional associations representing specialists. There are currently 28 'monospecialist sections', which study issues relating to training and practice in specialties which are recognized in at least two-thirds of EC member states. These sections report to the Management Council of UEMS.

Common trunk training

The concept of common trunk training was explained earlier. Although encouraged by the ACMT, there are still considerable disparities, both among specialties and among member states of the EC. In France, for instance, there is no common trunk training in internal medicine, thus leading to early specialization, whereas such training is the normal practice in surgery. In most states, however, and in most specialties, the common trunk exists; it lasts for 1 to 3 years and is followed by a variable period of specialty training. In those countries which have shorter overall periods of training it is usually the early, general element that is restricted. If the duration of training is curtailed in the UK, it is likely that this will mainly affect general professional training, thus leading to the need for more carefully structured and less pragmatic training during this phase of PGME.

Several monospecialist sections of UEMS have outlined structured training programmes; all include a period of general training of 2–3 years' duration, followed by specialist training for 3–4 years. Subspecialty training may extend this, but not invariably so. Most member states of the EC have some type of summative assessment at the end of training, and nearly all have a system of licensure or certification.

Postgraduate medical education in North America

In order to practise medicine, a doctor in North America needs to graduate from an accredited medical school and must obtain a licence to practise. The licence itself is unrestricted, i.e. a doctor may practise in any field and may use the title of specialist merely upon holding a valid licence. However, the desire to establish one's credentials as a specialist who has met some well-defined standard prompted doctors interested in specific areas of medicine to develop a voluntary certification process.

Postgraduate education in the USA is overseen by residency review committees and councils of the American Medical Association (AMA); in Canada it is one of the responsibilities of two organizations; the Royal College of Physicians and Surgeons of Canada (RCPSC) and the Canadian College of Family Practice (CCFP). Individual states or provinces have the legal authority to license physicians, and usually co-ordinate their activities through voluntary membership of a national association such as the Federation of State Medical Boards in the USA and the Federation of Provincial Medical Licensing Associations in Canada. The requirements for licensure typically include:

(1) graduation from an accredited US or Canadian medical school (or a special certification process for graduates of medical schools in other countries);
(2) some amount of supervised postgraduate education in an approved internship or residency programme, sometimes as short as 1 year; and
(3) passing a national examination.

After a phase-in programme which began in 1991, there will only be one national examination programme in the USA (the United States Medical Licensing Examination); in Canada most provinces require doctors to pass the Medical Council of Canada licensure examination.

Specialization

As doctors in North America began voluntarily to limit their practice to a specific specialty, they began to form specialty societies and boards, and to develop formal training programmes for these areas. Soon thereafter, the accreditation of these programmes and the establishment of agencies to oversee formal assessment procedures were introduced in order to ensure the quality of the graduates in the programmes. In the USA there are over 20 specialty boards that certify physicians in various specialties and subspecialties; they co-ordinate their activities through the American Board of Medical Specialties (ABMS). In Canada both the licensure and specialty certification functions are regulated by the RCPSC and the CCFP. This process has been successful in establishing standards for the practice of medicine in North America.

Training is undertaken in the intern and resident grades. This training is more learner-centred and structured than in the UK, thus minimizing the conflict between service provision and training needs. These programmes are, in consequence, shorter than those followed in the UK. Places on training programmes are normally allocated by the National Intern and Resident Matching Scheme, which has operated successfully in the USA for nearly 40 years. A similar matching scheme operates in Canada, and these schemes greatly reduce the anguish, uncertainty, and insecurity often experienced by postgraduate trainees in the UK.

JOHN ANDERSON

Further reading

Commission of the European Communities: The Advisory Committee on Medical Training (1987). *Medical training in the European Community*. Springer-Verlag, Berlin.

Committee of Enquiry into the Regulation of the Medical Profession (1975). *The Merrison Report*. Cmnd. 6018. London.

Department of Health and Social Security (1985). *Joint planning of training grade numbers*. London.

General Medical Council (1992). *Proposals for new performance procedures–a consultation paper*. London.

General Medical Council: Education Committee (1980). *Recommendations on basic medical education*. London.

General Medical Council: Education Committee (1987, 1992). *Recommendations on general clinical training*. London.

General Medical Council Education Committee (1987). *Recommendations on the training of specialists*. London.

NHS Management Executive (1991). *Junior doctors—the new deal*. London.

NHS Management Executive (1991). *Women doctors and their careers–Report of the Joint Working Party*. London.

NHS Management Executive (1991). *Working for patients—postgraduate and continuing medical and dental education*. London.

Joint Planning Advisory Committee (1986, 1987, 1988, 1989, 1990–91). *Reports*. London.

Royal Commission on Medical Education (1965–68). *The Todd Report*. Cmnd.3569. London.

Standing Committee on Postgraduate Medical Education (1990, 1991, 1992). *Reports on the work of the standing Committee on Postgraduate Medical Education*. London.

The 'Tripartite Group' (UK Health Departments, the Joint Consultants Committee, and Chairmen of Regional Health Authorities) (1987). *Hospital medical staffing—achieving a balance: plan for action*. London.

MEDICAL EDUCATION, UNDERGRADUATE
Introduction

Medical education is a tangled web of tensions: academic, professional, political, and personal. Approaches to their solution continue to reflect the diversity of national tradition, attitude, and need.

Professional tensions arise because medicine is a disparate profession. Physicians, surgeons, and general practitioners have their different tasks and different origins; until the 19th century they had distinct pathways of training. Now they start together as medical students and diverge soon after they graduate. In the past they each guarded their professional interests jealously and awarded their own licences to practise; *physicians through powerful royal colleges in London (1518), Ireland (1654), and Edinburgh (1681); *surgeons initially through *Barber-Surgeon Guilds, then through *Royal Colleges of Edinburgh (1778), Ireland (1784), and London—later England (1800); *apothecaries (the forerunners of general practitioners) through their

guild, later, in London, the Worshipful Society of Apothecaries.

On the continent of Europe and in Scotland, medical education has long been university-based. In the remainder of Britain and in Ireland private medical schools associated with teaching hospitals (often with shared staff) and later, especially in London, in hospital medical schools, developed in the 18th and 19th centuries. Private medical schools predominated in the USA until after the First World War when, following stringent criticism of their standard by Abraham *Flexner, university medical schools and their owned, or closely affiliated, hospitals replaced them.

Tension between professional domination of hospital-based education and a more strongly scientific, academic approach continued in Britain until relatively recently, nowhere more strongly than in London, where the principal of London University recorded a conversation in 1944 with

a leading surgeon who pointed out that the London teaching hospitals had clinical facilities which were known all over the world and the Royal Colleges conducted examinations which led to diplomas which were registrable qualifications. Where, I was asked very pointedly, did the University impinge on medical education at all?

The royal colleges regarded the assessment of expertise sufficient for safe practice as their purview. Instinctively, they felt that excessive emphasis on scientific theory would divert interest from practical skills. Further, university matriculation restricted entry to the profession by requiring a higher academic entrance standard than medical schools demanded of their non-university diploma students. In the event, some matriculated students went on to fail their preclinical university examinations in basic medical science and could only then qualify in Britain either by obtaining the conjoint diploma of the Royal Colleges of Physicians of London and Surgeons of England, or the Scottish Triple diploma, offered jointly by the Scottish Royal Colleges, or by becoming a licentiate of the Society of Apothecaries. Having failed the university's halfway hurdle, the route to licensure by graduating in medicine was no longer open to them. A shorter, and thus less expensive, course was an additional attraction of the non-university road into medicine, at least until state grants for student fees and maintenance were introduced after the Second World War.

While much technical progress and the setting of high standards of practice in the past owed little to the universities and much to professional ingenuity, commitment, and ethic, there are increasingly persuasive reasons for learning medicine in the atmosphere of a university rather than of a purely professional school. Medicine, in the words of Professor Owen Chadwick,

needs people who are capable and critical; and it's far more important to the nation that they should be capable and critical than that they should study one particular set of subjects.

With rapid scientific progress in medicine, tension between the academic and professional ethos in undergraduate medical education is not now a burning issue. But a conflict has arisen between developing the intellect with the capability of applying knowledge and skills flexibly in practical settings on the one hand, and the insistent information overload on the other, resulting from the strong, if outdated, tradition that newly qualified doctors should know something about everything. The original reason for a heavily factually based course of education and training was the expectation (indeed the *requirement* in Britain from the Medical Act of 1886 to the regulations of the *General Medical Council (GMC) issued in 1957) that qualification must guarantee the possession of the knowledge and skill requisite for the efficient practice of medicine, surgery, and midwifery, since most doctors immediately entered general practice on graduation so as to earn a living. Since 1953, when doctors on qualifying in the UK were first required on qualifying to complete a preregistration hospital year before entering independent practice, the emphasis has moved more towards education, with less comprehensive instruction. Nevertheless, the demand for greater detailed knowledge has flourished as enthusiastic and burgeoning subspecialties each demand a place in the curriculum. This dilemma was summed up by Sherman Mellinkoff, former Dean of Medicine at the University of California, Los Angeles:

The goal is to produce the physician we should like to see if we were sick. The direction is increasingly toward the creation of an efficient, specialised staff member for a procedure-oriented care facility. The goal and direction have by no means separated, but they are drifting apart.

While the profession is carefully addressing, in partnership with the universities, how best to instil general excellence into students entering a rapidly specializing world, the political paymasters (through the *Department of Health and local health service managers in the UK) and various articulate community organizations are striving to influence what medical students should learn. John Carswell summed up this conflict between universities and government thus:

The state and the universities are like a discontented couple who cannot live without each other: he rich, busy, self-important, preoccupied with office; she proud, independent and in her own opinion beautiful. The state-husband will always complain about her extravagance and inconsistency and the university-wife will endlessly criticise his stinginess, jealousy and philistinism.

The biggest single philosophical advance in undergraduate medical education recently in the UK has been to view as a single entity the process of basic medical education from entry to full registration with the GMC (1 year after graduation), involving the acquisition of clinical knowledge, skills, and attitudes, and their underlying basis in biological, physical, behavioural, and social science. Attention is also being given to ensuring that the final preregistration year of general clinical training ensures a smooth transition from basic medical education to general professional training, and from there to specialist training. These phases of *postgraduate medical education are the financial responsibility of the Departments of Health, operational responsibility being handled jointly between the royal colleges and a regional postgraduate dean appointed by the regional health authority and the university in partnership.

The objective of basic medical education is to produce a broadly educated, critical doctor who, on qualification, can reason, act and recommend safely, sensibly, and sympathetically in the best interests of a patient and of the population at large, offering wise and sensitive advice when, as may happen, the interests of individuals and society appear to conflict. He or she must have the motivation and ability to continue to learn, to manage his or her own professional activities, and to work well as one of a team with others. Such a doctor will also question policies and traditions and will strive to improve standards of care and quality of practice.

With such qualities assured, the new doctor is ready to train for very many specialties in hospital or the community. Some countries, such as China, separate career pathways and training programmes much earlier, even after the first 2 or 3 years of the undergraduate course, with separate streams for *public health, for *paediatrics, and for other specialties. Europe and North America are unlikely to follow this approach, although after graduation their specialty pathways diverge more rapidly and radically than in Britain. Britain still aspires to the totipotential medical graduate, flexible, imaginative, capable of training for any specialty.

Learning medicine involves many personal tensions and can be bewildering, busy, and even at times, frustrating. The initial years in basic science sometimes seem irrelevant to the essentially clinical goal of most students. This is changing: world-wide moves are being made to make the early years more clearly relevant, more inspiring, and better integrated into the essential core of knowledge a doctor needs, without sacrificing scientific credibility. Medicine is a hard taskmaster: fulfilling, adequately (in some countries very well) paid, more secure than many other professions, but both physically and mentally demanding. Medical education must also prepare the doctor for, and help him or her to handle, these personal demands.

Objectives of basic medical education and training
On graduation (which in Europe is also qualification, conferring a legal right to practise under supervision), the new doctor is expected to possess a substantial core of knowledge, to have acquired many practical skills, and to have laid the foundation of appropriately critical, yet sensitive, attitudes to practice, to the advancement of knowledge and his or her own personal development.

Licensure is separate from graduation in the USA

and Canada, but takes place at about the same time. In Canada, graduates take a separate qualifying examination of the Medical Council of Canada which, with the medical degree and a completed year as *intern (*house officer), enables the doctor to become a licentiate of the Council. Each provincial licensing authority reserves to itself the ultimate decision regarding a licence to practise medicine in that province, as do individual states in the USA. Medical graduates in the USA take either the diploma of the National Board of Medical Examiners, or the diploma of the Federation Licensing Exam. They also have to complete an intern year before licensing.

While much of the knowledge and most of the skills might be acquired satisfactorily in a purely professional educational environment, instilling questioning and innovative attitudes is peculiarly a university task. In the words of the UK Committee of Vice Chancellors and Principals:

The most important task of medical education is to give students the aptitude and the motivation for a lifetime of continuing self-education that will fit them for the practice of medicine well into the next century. They must be taught and learn in a context in which they see new knowledge being acquired, assessed and integrated into clinical practice. Research-based education is characteristic of the universities. Clinical academic staff are and must be involved in teaching, research and patient care.

The university setting of undergraduate medical education should also encourage students to reflect on human needs more extensive than those of their immediate patients or local population. They should be trained to examine the world-wide interface between the profession, preservation of health, and prevention and treatment of disease. That this opportunity for reflection is not yet fully harnessed is a reason for using opportunities better. Reflection is the springboard for responsible, educated leadership and action, as the *Times Higher Educational Supplement* put it:

Surely this is an age in which we desperately need more intelligent and trained men and women who can, with courage and some degree of excellent education in the sciences and humanities, confront chaos and assert against the brutalities and miseries of our world some confidence in humanness: in creativity, in the powers of mind and sensibility, in the capacity of human beings to create meanings and values, and to take their fate on themselves. And is university not the place where young men and women are trained in this confrontation with life as teachers, doctors, engineers, lawyers . . .

Superficially, the knowledge required of a doctor seems daunting. In fact, only a fraction of what might be required needs to be on immediate recall, either when serving as a pre-registration house officer or, later, in a chosen specialty—by which time some things will have changed substantially, and more will change over a professional lifetime. None the less, practically all medical curricula are heavily overloaded with information, whether predominantly based on theory, as in Italy

(Table 1), or, as in the UK, emphasizing practical clinical skills (Table 2). The pressure of information still reflects the perceived wish to create a fully trained medical practitioner on qualification. Medical schools have been slow to accept, and qualifying examinations to recognize, that qualification is only the prelude to a period of postgraduate education and not an immediate passport to independent practice. The opportunity to increase education and diminish information and instruction has not yet been fully exploited.

The GMC's last published *Recommendations on basic medical training* (1980) defined the extent of knowledge and skills required to obtain a primary qualification to practise medicine in the UK:

Basic medical education must provide the student with a thorough knowledge of human biology in the broadest sense. He or she should be introduced to the concept of illness and its range and consequences in order to acquire a knowledge and understanding of disease. By the time of qualification, the graduate should have sufficient knowledge of the structure and functions of the human body in health and disease, of normal and abnormal human behaviour, and of the techniques of diagnosis and treatment, to enable him or her to assume the responsibilities of a preregistration house officer and to be prepared for vocational training for a specialty (including general practice), followed by continuing education throughout a professional career. The graduate's knowledge should thus include the basic principles underlying the subjects taught but need not include those detailed aspects which are more appropriate to specialised vocational training.

In order to achieve this object, the GMC has stated that it is necessary for a student to acquire knowledge and understanding of:

(1) the sciences upon which medicine depends and the scientific and experimental method;
(2) the structure, function, and normal growth and development of the human body and the workings of the mind and their interaction, the factors which may disturb these, and the disorders of structure and function which may result;
(3) the aetiology, natural history, and prognosis of the common mental and physical ailments; students must have experience of emergencies and a good knowledge of the commoner disabling diseases, and of ageing processes;
(4) normal pregnancy and childbirth, the commoner obstetric emergencies, the principles of antenatal and postnatal care, and medical aspects of family planning and psychosexual counselling;
(5) the principles of prevention and of therapy, including health education, the amelioration of suffering and disability, rehabilitation, the maintenance of health in old age, and the care of the dying;
(6) human relationships, both personal and communal, and the interaction between man and his physical, biological, and social environment;
(7) the organization and provision of health care in the community and in hospital, the identification of the

Table 1 Medical curriculum in Italy

Year		Semester	
	Preclinical		
1	Medical mathematics; statistics	I	
	Medical physics and chemistry	II	Tests
	Medical biology and genetics		
	Histology; embryology I		
			Examinations
2	Biochemistry I	III	
	Anatomy I		
	Biochemistry II		Tests
	Anatomy II	IV	
	Physiology I		
			Examinations
3	Biophysics; biomedical technology	V	
	Physiology II		
	Microbiology I; immunology		
	General pathology I		Tests
	Microbiology II	VI	
	General pathology II		
	General and practical pathophysiology		
	Introduction to experimental research		
			Examinations
	Clinical		
4	Methodology; clinical laboratory science; pharmacology	VII	
	Infectious diseases		
	Pathological anatomy I		Tests
	Cardiology; angiology; pneumology	VIII	
	Gastroenterology; nephrology; urology		
	Endocrinology; metabolic disorders		
			Examinations
5	Pathological anatomy II	IX	
	General internal medicine		
	Haematology; clinical oncology		
	Clinical rheumatology; immunology		
	Clinical radiology; radiotherapy		
	General surgery		
	Neurology; psychiatry; clinical psychology		Tests
	Dermatology; venereology	X	
	Ophthalmology; ENT; odontology		
	Medical therapy; orthopaedics		
	Geriatrics; health care		
			Examinations

Table 1 (*cont.*)

Year		Semester
6	Internal medicine; paediatrics	XI
	Special surgery	
	Gynaecology; obstetrics	
	Internal medicine	Tests
	Forensic medicine; toxicology	XII
	Hygiene; social and professional medicine	
	Trauma; first aid	
	Special surgery	
	Final examination	Medical degree

Postgraduate mandatory training: an additional 6 months of practical training in general medicine (Tirocinio), followed by:

Examination for professional qualification   'Esame di stato'

need for it, and the economic, ethical, and practical constraints within which it operates; and

(8) the ethical standards and legal responsibilities of the medical profession.

To develop the professional skills necessary:

(1) to elicit, record, and interpret the relevant medical history, symptoms, and physical signs, and to identify the problems and how these may be managed;

(2) to carry out simple practical clinical procedures;

(3) to deal with common medical emergencies;

(4) to communicate effectively and sensitively with patients and their relatives;

(5) to communicate clinical information accurately and concisely, both by word of mouth and in writing, to medical colleagues and to other professionals involved in the care of the patient; and

(6) to use laboratory and other diagnostic and therapeutic services effectively and economically, and in the best interests of patients.

To develop appropriate attitudes to the practice of medicine, which include:

(1) recognition that a blend of scientific and humanitarian approaches is needed in medicine;

(2) a capacity for self-education, so that knowledge and skills may continue to be developed and extended throughout professional life, recognizing an obligation to contribute if possible to the progress of medicine and to new knowledge;

(3) the ability to assess the reliability of evidence and the relevance of scientific knowledge, to reach conclusions by logical deduction or by experiment, and to evaluate critically methods and standards of medical practice;

(4) a continuing concern for the interests and dignity of patients;

(5) an ability to appreciate the limitations of personal knowledge, combined with a willingness, when necessary, to seek further help; and

(6) the achievement of good working relationships with members of the other health-care professions.

Of the many and various practical skills needed by a new doctor, the ability to communicate easily, effectively, and with empathy towards both patients and colleagues is cardinal. Acquisition of a wide range of practical techniques is highly desirable but few are essential, provided house officers are conscientiously supervised by more senior members of the team. The GMC (1992) has described the objectives of education and training in the preregistration year (Table 3), supposedly the final year of basic medical education, but currently considered by house officers themselves more as servitude.

Only when deans, with the support of the GMC, have the courage to use the undergraduate curriculum primarily as a moulding, integrating, and challenging process of learning will the knowledge needed be selectively acquired and effectively assimilated. Likewise, skills are best understood and practised when the context and value of their use are experienced in real situations, especially when the student plays a responsible part in their performance.

Educational approaches

Most medical students learn today much as they learned yesterday. Tomorrow is likely to be different.

The current conventional approach is world-wide, well-tried, solid, and uninspiring, but remarkably cost-effective in terms of resources, which are both limited and diminishing. The curriculum traditionally falls into two main sections—preclinical and clinical. The preclinical course, normally of about 2 years' duration, is concerned with the biological, behavioural, and social

Table 2 The conventional pattern of basic medical education and training as followed in some UK medical schools

	Year	Exams
Preclinical		
Anatomy and cell biology	1	
Biochemistry and molecular genetics		
Physiology and biophysics		Sessional
Biometry and medical statistics		
Psychology; sociology		
		MB Pt 1
Body systems	2	
Pharmacology		Sessional
General pathology		
		MB Pt 2 & 3
Clinical		
Introductory medicine and surgery including communication skills, ethics	3	Course exams
Paediatrics		
Obstetrics and gynaecology		
Psychiatry and neurology		
General practice; public health; accident and emergency	4	
Pathology (histopath.; microbiol.; haematol.; immunol.)		MB Pt 4
General medicine	5	
General surgery		
Elective		
Surgical specialties (ENT*; eyes; orthopaedics)		
Medical specialties (Dermatology; STD**)		
Anaesthetics		MB Pt 5–8
Clinical pharmacology and therapeutics		
General medicine	5	
General surgery		
		Medical degree
		Provisional registration with GMC
Preregistration year	6	
Working as qualified doctor under supervision; 6 months surgery and 6 months medicine, or 4 months surgery, 4 months medicine, and 4 months general practice		
		Full registration with GMC

* Otorhinolaryngology
**Sexually transmitted disease

Table 3 Objectives of the preregistration house officer year

To understand the nature and implications of, and to make an appropriate initial decision about, each problem presented to him or her as a doctor

To plan and carry out, under appropriate supervision, the investigation, treatment, or management of, and rehabilitation after, acute and chronic illness, and to participate in programmes for promotion of good health

To apply knowledge of science and of logical method to the assessment of clinical problems, and to continue to develop the ability to assess the reliability of evidence

To develop knowledge and understanding of disease processes

To maintain attitudes appropriate to the practice of medicine, which include respect for the dignity of the patient and concern for the relatives, awareness of the legal and ethical aspects of medical practice, together with appreciation of the importance and implications of professional confidentiality

To be aware of the limitations of his or her own knowledge and skills and to be ready to seek help

To continue to develop the capacities for self-education and self-audit

To learn effective and economic use of laboratory and other diagnostic and therapeutic services

To learn safe practice in relation to radiation protection, blood products, body fluids, and tissues in the ward and laboratory, and to have regard at all times to the safety of patients and health-care workers

To gain experience in teaching others, effective teamwork, the management and administrative aspects of medical practice, and the work of those bodies which plan, advise, and assist with the organization and provision of health care in the community and in hospital

---

sciences underpinning medicine, in particular, anatomy and cell biology, physiology and biophysics, pharmacology and toxicology, biochemistry and molecular genetics, biometry and statistics, psychology, and sociology. It is preceded in continental Europe and Scotland, where school education is less specialized than in the rest of the UK, by an initial year of chemistry, physics, maths, and biology. Teaching is largely by lectures, seminars, practicals, and demonstrations (often case-demonstrations of a patient to illustrate failure of a normal body mechanism). While too much emphasis is still placed on didactic teaching and too little on learning through self-directed study, the situation has improved since the *Lancet* reported in 1834:

In several of the large recognised schools [of medicine in London] the students are required to pay for, if not to attend, lectures, the delivery of which occupies from ten to twelve hours of cathedral gabble, scarcely relieved by one interruption, save the momentary silence which is occasioned by the change of one gabbler for another . . . thus the student is to be bored from one end of the week to the other with trashy talk which can never reach the understanding or the memory, except through the operation of the sight or the medium of touch.

By tradition, and for organizational reasons, not least that the two sections of the course are mounted on different sites in many universities, the preclinical and clinical periods are distinct. Written, oral, and practical examinations in the basic medical sciences must be passed before commencing the clinical course. Requirements are rigorous, and in the event of first time failure, only one further attempt is normally permitted, 3 months later. The perpetual student is a person of the past. Up to half the students take an additional year of scientific study in depth, either between the preclinical and clinical courses or during the clinical course; this 'intercalated' year leads to a BA, B.Sc., or B.med. Sci. degree.

Separation of the scientific basis of medicine from its clinical application encourages students to regard biomedical science and clinical medicine as distinct entities to be undertaken one after the other, rather than, as is educationally more effective, being integrated to inform each other. The clinical course itself lasts 2 years in North America, between 2 and 3 in the UK, and normally 4 on the continent of Europe.

It is tempting to think that having learned the scientific background, clinical medicine is straightforward. Far from it: clinical medicine is as much art as science, and it can no more be learned purely from books than driving a car can be learned from reading a driving manual and a copy of the *Highway Code*. Trousseau, the distinguished 19th century French physician, who introduced the concept and practice of clinical diagnosis by systematic physical examination, advised students to:

Take care not to fancy that you are physicians as soon as you have mastered the scientific facts; they only afford to your understandings an opportunity of bringing forth fruit, and of elevating you to a high position as a man of art.

The tradition of acquisition of hands-on clinical skills as a cardinal requirement in undergraduate clinical medical education is strongest in the UK, North America, and Australasia. These skills are not taught by lectures but through a carefully supervised clinical apprenticeship, a time-consuming, personal process for which students are divided up into small groups alongside working teams of doctors, normally after a short introductory clinical course outlining and giving initial instruction in the skills to be acquired, especially *communication skills. The introductory course is preceded in many medical schools by a *nursing week during which medical students are attached to wards under the direction of the ward sister (charge nurse) and are assigned the hours and duties of a junior nurse in order to gain insight into ward life and wider everyday aspects of patient care—the aspects which often concern patients most.

Much of the clinical course is occupied by 2 or 3 month attachments of small groups of students to medical teams (or 'firms' in the British system) in a succession of major hospital specialties: general medicine, general surgery, obstetrics and gynaecology, paediatrics, and psychiatry. The purpose of each attachment is to develop skill in clinical diagnosis and care by listening to and talking to patients and by examining them, using similar techniques in all the specialties but adapted to different body systems, age-groups, and attitudes. In doing so, students learn from their teachers how to make decisions in clinical diagnosis, investigation, and total treatment and management, not only of the patient but also of concerned families, friends, and employers ('holistic medicine').

Students are allocated their 'own' patients on the ward. They are expected to listen to their story, to question them, to examine them, and to reach their own judgment on the most likely diagnosis and the alternatives. They should discover what investigations have been ordered and why, and join discussions on the final diagnosis and treatment. Their own notes should record all this and the day-by-day progress of the patient, just as if they were the house officer in charge.

Clearly, this is a patchy way of building up a portfolio of carefully supervised experience, but it is widened by seeing other students' patients on ward rounds and at special case presentations. Reading around each condition seen is very much the student's own responsibility; those with initiative, enquiring minds, and the ability to make short notes about each condition as they come across it are the ones who really learn and who shine in their final assessments or examinations, and thereafter. Students also learn practical techniques such as taking blood and setting up intravenous infusions. Not only do they also see patients at leisure in the wards but they also learn by being attached, one at a time, to the team when on night and weekend emergency admitting duty, in out-patient clinics, and in the operating theatre. In the out-patient clinic they have the opportunity to clerk new patients and to make their diagnosis first before going over each case with a teacher; they also have the opportunity to see a range of conditions in patients who are attending the clinic for follow-up.

In obstetrics, students develop a feel for continuity of care in pregnancy from the antenatal clinic, through delivery to the postnatal clinic; they experience a dimension of health care in which disease plays only a small part. In paediatrics, they begin to acquire the art of dealing with children and with parents; while in *psychiatry, a whole range of different attitudes and skills have to be developed. These five core specialties between them cover a spectrum of all ages and conditions, sufficient for learning all the general lessons of communication, assessment, decision-making, and care which they will need as doctors. While this may be the core of their clinical education, it is by no means all.

Shorter periods are spent in several other disciplines including public health; the purpose is to explore different interfaces in health care, to broaden understanding of ill-health in relation to the patient's environment, to balance individual health against the health of populations, and to provide an opportunity of extending background knowledge of areas about which students learn little in hospital. A month in an accident and emergency department is also popular, especially because students are given responsibility for practical tasks such as suturing and dressing wounds, and, often for the first time, feel useful and valued. Very different, but extremely informative, is the time spent in *general (family) practice, usually partly in an inner-city practice and partly in the country: this offers a different spectrum and context of ill-health, a different approach and priorities, a feeling of continuity and involvement with the community.

*Pathology (histopathology, haematology, microbiology, clinical chemistry, and immunology) is a recurring theme throughout the clinical course. It is often examined separately by written and practical examinations, usually some months before the final clinical examinations, which are currently clustered at the end of the course in most schools, although there are moves to separate them, not least to reduce the stress of such a concentrated test of a massive burden of knowledge and practical skills. The final clinical examinations usually consist of written papers (multiple choice and essay), clinicals, and orals; low marks in either written papers or orals can be compensated, but passing the clinicals is usually essential for qualification.

While some students suffer the preclinical years and enjoy the clinical, it is probably true to say, in the UK at least, that they are often neither stretched intellectually nor inspired. They become competent doctors, but only a few become really innovative. Many seem worn down by the sheer burden of information: they seem to end up less questioning and imaginative than they started; not bored but blunted.

The preclinical course has already improved greatly, partly by introducing many clinical demonstrations to illustrate the consequences of failure of normal physiological or pharmacological mechanisms, or to explore the anatomical disturbances of developmental abnormality or disease, and partly by breaking down the boundaries between departments by teaching integrated body systems instead of complementary topics in isolation. Credit for first integrating the basic medical science disciplines around teaching by organ-systems rests with

Case Western Reserve University in Cleveland, Ohio, in 1950. While each science discipline still claims some teaching time, most preclinical courses now integrate horizontally the teaching of basic medical sciences.

A second and more profound revolution has been to centre the course on illustrative clinical problems, chosen specifically because they are common and multidisciplinary or, alternatively, rare but especially instructive. These are studied from every scientific, clinical, and social dimension, building up systematically over a period of time a sufficient body of basic knowledge of the processes of normality and disease. The cardinal aspects of such a course are the requirement for self-learning and the vertical integration of the basic medical sciences with clinical science, diagnosis, and management. McMaster University School of Medicine at Hamilton, Ontario, was the pioneer in this field, its ideas being further developed at the new Medical School of the University of Newcastle, New South Wales (NSW), in the 1970s. Although the emphasis on self-directed learning and seminar work, rather than traditional lecture-room teaching and practicals, seems highly desirable, there are disadvantages, such as the insecurity felt by students who for some considerable time have a very fragmentary knowledge base. Demands on academic staff for individual supervision and seminar teaching in small groups are also greater than with a conventional curriculum. In 1985 Harvard Medical School launched an innovative alternative undergraduate course along these lines, which was so well received that it replaced the traditional course entirely 3 years later. Most of the innovation is in the early years of the course, the clinical apprenticeship dimension of the later part maintaining its traditional place and importance. The University of Limburg in Maastricht in The Netherlands has also introduced a radically 'problem-based' curriculum. It has also pioneered the teaching of practical skills without intruding on patients in a 'skills laboratory'.

A third, more gradual, revolution has been proceeding at the same time. The Newcastle, NSW, curriculum encouraged substantial participation by general practitioners in the formal course itself and in the purely clinical component. In similar vein, the Harvard curriculum offers a course (half a day per week) on the relationship between patient and doctor, covering cultural, social, economic, and psychological issues around a series of clinical seminars in which patients discuss the impact of illness on their lives and what they expect from their doctors. Hospital out-patient and general practitioner clinics are increasingly being used to enable students to learn clinical medicine in a community context. This development also reflects the diminishing role of hospital admission in patient care and therefore the diminishing opportunity for in-patient clinical teaching. Clearly, there are cost implications, and also increased difficulty in defining the objectives and assessing the effectiveness of such disseminated education and training. Carried further still, some medical schools in relatively less developed countries are moving medical education even more substantially out into the community. While it is important that doctors should be educated to meet the health needs of their country, it is very necessary to be clear about the need for innovative university-educated doctors who will lead and constantly re-educate themselves in a changing world, on the one hand, and the limited role of semi-barefoot doctors trained only to do one particular task at one snapshot in history, on the other.

Mindful of many of these trends, and after consultation with UK medical schools and faculties, the GMC in 1991 recommended in a discussion document (not for the first time, but more firmly) a substantial reduction in the information load of the undergraduate medical curriculum, together with a core course of essential knowledge (occupying about two-thirds of the time) and a range of options for study in depth according to individual appetite and enthusiasm. Learning through critical curiosity is to be central, developed through a substantial component of problem-based learning in the early years and searching analysis in depth and breadth of a succession of clinical case seminars later. The GMC also recommended a wider approach to the understanding of health and disease, including both prevention and management, in relation to social context. It also wished the curriculum to promote deeper knowledge and understanding of scientific method, the ability to evaluate evidence, and the assessment of research method. It is likely that in response to this recommendation (which may ultimately have the legal force of a direction) UK medical schools will substantially change the early years of the curriculum and will introduce more choice throughout the whole of a curriculum planned as a continuum.

Students learn most quickly and effectively when given responsibility. This they can do to a limited extent when acting for a short time as a 'student-assistant', deputizing for a preregistration house officer. But the knowledge and technical skills acquired during the undergraduate course become imprinted and improved during the preregistration house officer year. Experience alone is not, however, always educational; 'experience', said Professor A. C. Dornhorst 'receives more respect than its inevitability deserves'. To benefit fully from experience one must be helped to learn from it. Certainly, the undergraduate medical course needs to be complemented firmly and effectively by a closely supervised year of practical experience as a house officer before full registration as a medical practitioner. This year, properly 'formed', might well be termed 'the finishing school', envisaged by Dr Richard Davies, Fellow of Queens' College, Cambridge, in 1759, about 200 years before the preregistration year became mandatory:

. . . attendance at some public hospital . . . ought to be the finishing school of the clinical physician [for] men should not be sent raw into the world to form their own experience at the hazard of men's lives . . . neither a previous education alone, nor practice alone, can complete the physician, because men may grow old in practice without the capacity to *form* experience, which, in the philosophic sense, is the knowledge of truths established by repeated experiments.

The preregistration year is an essential complement to the undergraduate course. Currently all is not well. It seems that supervision is often inadequate; newly qualified doctors may be required to assume more responsibility than is either appropriate or perhaps safe. Practical techniques, first learned as a student, are not sufficiently checked and improved. Progress may be insufficiently assessed and discussed, and career advice is either not sought or not effectively provided. Even if supervision is adequate, working hours are too long and too intense for optimum educational benefit; tired doctors learn little—and they make mistakes. The average working week for junior hospital doctors in 1992 in Britain was 85 hours; the government is committed to substantial reduction over the next 4 years, but it is not yet clear that this can be done without interfering with educational time or impoverishing educational experience. A major current problem is that much of the working week is taken up with non-educational, repetitive routine duties, more appropriately performed either by non-medical staff or by medical staff other than young trainees at the most formative moment in their professional lives. Finally, although much of the learning is 'by doing', there is also a need for some component of formal education, either to fill gaps in undergraduate education or to prepare for professional responsibilities and dilemmas which can best be fully appreciated for the first time at this stage. The profession and government are acutely aware of the need to improve the preregistration house officer year radically, but the practical problems are formidable.

The undergraduate medical curriculum is superficially similar throughout the European Community but, in practice, doctors reach the stage approximating to the preregistration year with substantially different levels of clinical training and experience, despite having experienced a similar duration of education. While UK graduates are deliberately equipped for the clinical responsibility expected of them as preregistration house officers, graduates in several other countries would not, at that stage, with their more theoretical education, have reached an equivalent point of practical expertise. Each EC member state is obliged to recognize each other's 'diplomas, certificates and other evidence of formal qualifications', but as there may be insufficient local graduates to fill the additional preregistration posts which may be needed in the UK to reduce working hours, and as most EC member states still produce more doctors than they can employ, a real problem of equivalence may lie ahead. Critical scrutiny should be made of the point in the European medical educational processes at which to accept true equivalence. Not to do so is to put political expediency before the safety of patients and to give substance to the comment of that committed European, Sir Rolf Dahrendorf, in regard to 'a move to harmonise medical training with identical numbers of preclinical and clinical hours throughout the community' that 'the underlying approach was as characteristic of European bureaucracy as it was contrary to the best interests of Europe.'

Where do students learn?

There are 28 medical schools in the UK (Table 4) of which one (St Andrews University) only takes preclinical students, most of them going to Manchester for their clinical studies. The curriculum of all these schools is accredited by the GMC. The USA has 127 medical schools and Canada 16. Their educational programmes are accredited by the joint Liaison Committee on Medical Education, sponsored by the Association of American Medical Colleges and the American Medical Association.

Table 4 Annual entry of home students to basic medical science courses in UK medical schools in 1991

Medical school	Annual entry
University of Birmingham	153
University of Bristol	144
University of Cambridge	218
University of Leeds	153
University of Leicester	117
University of Liverpool	147
University of London	
Charing Cross and Westminster	151
King's	103
Royal Free	97
St Bartholomew's	102
St George's	159
St Mary's (Imperial College)	96
The Royal London	73
United Schools of Guy's and St Thomas's	190
University College and Middlesex	194
University of Manchester	175
University of Newcastle upon Tyne	126
University of Nottingham	133
University of Oxford	96
University of Sheffield	128
University of Southampton	124
Queen's University, Belfast	139
University of Aberdeen	155
University of Dundee	101
University of Edinburgh	186
University of Glasgow	223
University of St Andrews	80
University of Wales	136

The number of overseas students permitted at medical schools in the UK is approximately 5 per cent of total intake.

A vigorous debate continues concerning the amount of the undergraduate curriculum which should be based in the medical school, in affiliated district hospitals, or in the community. Views also differ about how much clinical education should be lecture/seminar based and how much should take place in the hospital wards or out-patient clinic—or in general practice.

Traditionally much medical education has been based on the main university hospital. However, for several reasons the work of university hospitals in which undergraduate teaching has been based is reducing: inner-city populations are falling; in Britain, patients who would have come from further afield are being discouraged by the constraints of the National Health Service (NHS) internal market; and high hospital costs are forcing more work into a day-care setting or into the community. Meanwhile the practice of the main university hospitals is becoming increasingly specialized, which may be good for research (although much research is, in fact, into common conditions) and for postgraduate specialty education and training, but not so good for undergraduates who mainly need bread-and-butter medicine and surgery. Complicated problems are, however, by no means inappropriate to the intellectual development of students. In *The Oxford companion to medicine* (1986) Sir John Ellis noted that the main university hospital, or 'university medical centre', sets the standard, by innovation sets the pace, and provides a rare concentration of expertise backed by university departments of every kind. He observed that 'the complex and unusual clinical problem [is] as necessary to education as the simple and common problem is to training.'

Students enjoy spending time at affiliated district hospitals, and their staff, many of whom are excellent and committed teachers, welcome them. Yet the pressure of work is such that teaching time is limited and, experience alone is not sufficient education. A balance must be struck between the two types of teaching opportunity: 'The process of undergraduate medical education requires thought and analysis', said Professor A. C. Dornhorst, 'if we are to concentrate on principles with less detail we cannot afford to subcontract to the same extent'. Most clinical academic staff and their research are concentrated on the facilities and interactive academic environment of the medical school, but it is by no means certain that the university staff could cope with more students when they are already extremely hard-pressed with research and their own service to patients, besides the current level of teaching.

Within the hospital an increasing amount of practice is in clinic and day-care facilities. These resources could be better used for teaching. Special teaching out-patient clinics could be structured to call up successive groups of patients with similar diseases to provide a systematic core of clinical education. Comparatively little service work would be done in these clinics, and out-patient clinic costs would necessarily increase.

Meanwhile, vociferous sections of both profession and public call for more teaching of basic clinical skills to be undertaken in a community setting, especially in general practice. Many general practitioners would be good teachers, and although abnormal clinical signs might be fewer, they would have much to contribute to communication skills and overall assessment of illness. Groups of students would need to be small because of the nature of the consultative relationship. Many practitioners would need to be recruited, and their time is expensive. Ideally, such teaching should be within easy reach of the medical school, yet in most inner cities general practice is least well developed in these areas.

An elective period of between 8 and 12 weeks is a maturing experience for most students; most go abroad. This is quite different from the practice of some continental universities of sending students abroad for up to 1 year to seek unstructured clinical experience without any guarantee of the quality of supervision. A hospital may provide excellent service but may be quite unsuitable for reasons of time, interest, or the extent of the student's previous clinical education, to provide part of the core course. The British elective system (reciprocated with many other countries) is designed normally to give wider perspectives in a short time, rather than to provide specific education in any branch of medicine: it offers an opportunity often to discover the irrelevance of much Western medicine to the health needs of developing countries.

Both undergraduate and postgraduate medical education involve a partnership between different types of hospital and community health care resources in a geographically compact area. Universities are recognizing increasingly their responsibility to help those who teach in this network develop their educational skills, and to set clear educational objectives and means of assessing their achievement.

Selection of students

In most countries medical students are selected on their academic rank-order in school-leaving exams or, in the USA, predominantly on college grades. Singapore limits the number of academic high-fliers entering medicine, taking the view that a substantial proportion of the best brains should, in the national interest, enter more productive scientific disciplines than medicine. The Netherlands experimented with selection by lottery. A limit on the number of medical graduates, and thus on intake to medical school, is imposed in most countries, but some still permit entry as of right to any university course, reducing the number by competitive examination at the end of the first or second year.

High academic grades are required for entry to medicine in Britain, too, but other achievements and qualities are also taken into account. Two-thirds of UK medical schools interview applicants and all schools have available a confidential reference on applicants from head teacher or deputy, whether interviewed or not. Universities in Britain are free to use their own judgment in selecting students for admission. Most British medical schools feel they have a public responsibility to interview and so to gauge as best they can the relative merits and potential of the applicants who are strongest on paper. The task is not to judge absolute suitability or unsuitability but to select in open competition those who on all available evidence would seem to have most to offer to patients, to the advance of medicine, and to the community in which they will live and learn for the next 5–6 years.

The one indisputable merit of interview is that it offers an applicant an opportunity to speak for him or herself and to ask questions, formally at interview and informally outside. It also ensures that all potential entrants visit the school, and meet both students and staff before deciding their own preference. For the medical school, it is useful to be able to probe aspects of the application, such as unexplained gaps, and the extent to which declared interests are real and achievements personal; attitudes and awareness of health and human issues can be explored, together with the degree to which the applicant has researched, considered, and personally made a career choice without undue pressure from others. The ability to pass examinations is important, but both the university course and a medical career require more, in particular, 'an intellect capable of developing good judgment, the ability to see the patient as a whole, the ability to see all aspects of a problem in the right perspective and the ability to weigh up evidence' (Dr John Todd).

A good (but not necessarily outstanding) academic record is needed to secure an interview. At interview wider attributes and personal qualities count most, such as excellence in any hobby, sport, or public service (on the basis that to achieve excellence in anything requires application as well as ability); evidence of perseverance, commitment, and resourcefulness; curiosity, initiative, and enthusiasm; the ability to reason and discuss; and evidence of consideration for others. Most of those offered a place after interview might well have received an offer on their record alone. However, a few individuals with modest academic records demonstrate outstanding personality and commitment at interview and win a place, subject to achieving satisfactory academic grades. A few people, clever on paper, seem so lacking in humanity, sparkle, or motivation, or are so arrogant, that they lose a place through interview which they might otherwise have had.

PETER RICHARDS

Further reading
Black, D. A. K. (1987). *Invitation to medicine*. Basil Blackwell, Oxford.
General Medical Council (1980) Recommendations on basic medical education. *Medical Education*, May.

General Medical Council (1991). *Consultation paper on basic medical education*. London.
General Medical Council (1992) *Recommendations on general clinical training*. London.
Richards, P. (1990). *Living medicine*. Cambridge University Press, Cambridge.
Richards, P. (1992). *Learning medicine 1993*. British Medical Association, London.

MEDICAL EDUCATION OF THE PUBLIC. See HEALTH EDUCATION COUNCIL; MEDICINE AND THE MEDIA.

MEDICAL EVIDENCE. The testimony of medical witnesses often plays an important part in judicial proceedings, both criminal and civil, the doctor appearing either as an expert or a material witness. Although it cannot be regarded as a special class of evidence, it is nevertheless often crucial to the case, for example in assisting a court to determine the nature, extent, and probable outcome of personal injury and hence the amount of any award of damages. Witnesses must endeavour to keep in mind the need to be audible, comprehensible in lay terms, competent, informed, unbiased, honest, and consistent; and that their function is to assist the court to reach a just decision. See LAW AND MEDICINE IN THE UK; LAW AND MEDICINE IN THE USA.

MEDICAL FACULTIES IN UNIVERSITIES. See MEDICAL EDUCATION, UNDERGRADUATE.

MEDICAL FEES. See MEDICAL PRACTICE.

MEDICAL FOUNDATIONS. See FOUNDATIONS AND CHARITIES, IN CANADA, IN THE UK; IN THE USA, ETC.

MEDICAL GODS. Chief among the medical gods of the heroic Greeks was *Aesculapius, god of medicine, formally deified in Athens in 420 BC. Aesculapius, who had been instructed in the healing art by Chiron, a centaur, was the son of *Apollo and Koronis, born according to tradition in the mountains above *Epidaurus. Machaon and Podalirius were his sons, who accompanied Agamemnon on the expedition to Troy. Homer speaks of Machaeon as 'a doctor worth many men at cutting out arrows and laying on gentle drugs', while Podalirius 'had cunning to find out things impossible and to cure that which healed not'. Of the six daughters of Aesculapius, Hygieia, goddess of health, is best known; others were Panacea (the restorer) and Meditrina (the preserver of health). Epigone, wife of Aesculapius, was the 'soothing one'.

MEDICAL GUILDS. Like other trade guilds, these social and professional associations first came into prominence in England in the 14th century and formed the basis of medical organization until the establishment of the *Royal College of Physicians and the United Company of *Barber-Surgeons two centuries later. However, organized guilds of physicians, known as Asclepiads, had existed far earlier in ancient Greece. The most famous flourished on the island of *Cos about 420 BC; the Coan guild, which produced the *Hippocratic Oath, was a closed group of physicians with excellent teaching, training, library, data recording, diagnostic, and treatment facilities.

MEDICAL HISTORY. See HISTORY OF MEDICINE.

MEDICAL JOURNALS. Even if medical research produces apparently important results, the process is incomplete unless these are communicated. Such communication takes several forms: conversation at lunchtime or conferences among colleagues; formal presentation at a workshop or large conference; or publication in a journal. Nevertheless, the aim of communication is not only to present the research findings but also to submit these to informed scrutiny and criticism, which will determine whether they are ultimately incorporated into the body of knowledge (such as important review articles or textbooks) or rejected as unsound.

Hence, despite all the modern developments in communication, publication still has everything in its favour. Articles published in journals can disseminate research findings widely and cheaply, can give them in considerable detail (enabling readers to recalculate the results and to compare them with their own), and can record them in permanent form. Admittedly, there are some disadvantages in publishing articles in journals (delay, for example) but, bearing in mind that the system has continued virtually unchanged for the past 350 years, the scientific community must regard these snags as only minor.

Beginnings
Scientific journals were not introduced straightaway with the introduction of printing in 1454: there was a gap of some 200 years before they began to be published, and of another 20 years before journals that were strictly medical appeared. Before that, scientists had disseminated their work either by having it copied and circulating the manuscript, or, later, by publishing it as a book—as a separate treatise (*tractatus*) or an essay (*exercitatio*)—or by corresponding with one another (although Europe had no postal system at all before 1516). Nevertheless, there were drawbacks to these methods: they were restrictive, or even secretive, confining the new information to a few members of an 'in' peer group; they were slow to disseminate knowledge, or often too expensive or too time-consuming for some authors; and some countries lagged behind others in their ability to offer publication at all. For this reason,

in 1628 William *Harvey had to publish *De motu cordis* in Frankfurt in Latin, as no suitable form of publication was available to him in the UK.

The scientific and medical periodical was a development of the newspaper or newsletter by an individual, a scientific society, academy, or college (the last three were developments of the medieval guilds).

The first independent scientific journal, the *Journal des Sçavans*, was published in France on 5 January 1665, although this was largely the effort of one man, Jean-Paul de la Roque. The same year in Britain, however, a group of scientists in the Royal Society also began publication of its *Philosophical Transactions*; both journals have continued to appear.

First medical journal
For over 100 years most medical men published their work in scientific rather than specifically medical journals, probably because of the great prestige associated with the former and their sponsoring societies. Some medical journals were published—the first two being the *Acta* of the Royal Medical and Philosophical Society of Copenhagen, edited by Thomas *Bartholin, the anatomist, which appeared in 1671, and the second, *Nouvelles Découvertes sur Toutes les Parties de la Médecine*, edited by Nicolas de Blegny, which was published intermittently between 1679 and 1681. Nevertheless, most were short-lived news-sheets of low scientific status, whose titles and places of publication were frequently changed.

The 19th century saw a big expansion in the number of journals published, their origin reflecting the leadership taken by Germany in medical activity: thus, of the total of 436 periodicals published, no fewer than 246 were German, compared with 50 French, 26 British, 22 Dutch, 21 Danish, 19 Austro-Hungarian, and 18 Swiss, the remainder being divided among the other countries (including the first American medical journal, the *Medical Repository*, published in 1797).

Publications of the 18th and early 19th centuries
Such figures, however, might give a spurious importance to the German periodicals, which were often only local news-sheets or aimed as much at the public as at doctors, and many medical men still preferred to publish serious work in prestigious general scientific journals or in pamphlets. As in the 17th century most publications still ceased to appear after a few years. Even as recently as the last quarter of the 19th century, a count showed that, of the 1147 medical journals ever begun, only 250 were still being published (and no fewer than 339 of the 386 journals published in Germany and Austria had ceased to appear).

Nevertheless, the latter part of the 18th century saw two important developments: the beginning of the rise of English as the international language of science (a dominant position it has unquestionably occupied since the First World War), and the formation of a society which was subsequently to publish the first strictly medical journal that still appears today. This, *Transactions of the Medical Society of London*, began publication in 1810.

Establishment of the general journal

The later 19th century saw two important and permanent developments, as well as one which was evanescent: these were, respectively, the establishment of the general medical journal, the beginnings of the specialist journal, and the fleeting appearance of the 'one-man' journal. The general journal may be defined as a publication aimed at all doctors; the specialist journal as one dealing with only a single specialty (such as mental illness or heart disease); and the 'one-man' journal as one written and conducted by a single person (such as Sir Jonathan *Hutchinson's *Archives of Surgery*, 1889–1900).

In the 19th century two editors, both British, bestrode this world like Colossi: Thomas *Wakley, the founder of the *Lancet*, at the beginning of the century, and Ernest *Hart, the editor of the *British Medical Journal*, at its end. Without these last two, the history, standards, and style of medical periodicals might have been very different.

Thomas Wakley's journal, symbolically named the *Lancet*, was first published on Sunday 5 October 1823, with three main aims: to print the lectures given by the teachers of the London medical schools; to publish medical and surgical case reports; and to furnish non-medical comment. His right to print these lectures was challenged by John *Abernethy, the senior surgeon at *St Bartholomew's Hospital. Wakley won this lawsuit, which was to be the first of 10 that he fought, and he also waged campaigns in the *Lancet* against: the medical Establishment (particularly the two royal colleges in London and the worshipful Society of Apothecaries); against privilege, nepotism, and malpractice; and against social evils, such as the adulteration of food, dangers on the railway, and the health hazards of tobacco.

These, together with the publicity aroused by his lawsuits, ensured the *Lancet's* rapid success. By the end of its second year of publication the journal had a circulation of 4000, and Wakley was enabled to carry his battles even further by his election as a Member of Parliament in 1838.

By the time Wakley died, in 1862, he had laid secure foundations for the general medical journal, which aimed at informing, instructing, commenting, and amusing—a mixture of original papers about medical research with up-to-date comment and current news. Such a pattern was to be followed by general journals all over the world, and indeed Wakley would have little difficulty in finding his way around those published today.

The other main general medical journal in the UK, the *British Medical Journal (BMJ)*, was developed from a modest quarterly, the *Midland Medical and Surgical Reporter*, which was first published in 1828. Its anonymous editor was (Sir) Charles *Hastings, a Worcester physician and an almost exact contemporary of Wakley. Four years later, Hastings founded the Provincial Medical and Surgical Association, which subsequently, in 1855, was to be called the British Medical Association (BMA); in 1857 its journal—which had started weekly publication on 9 October 1840—was renamed the *British Medical Journal*.

In 1866 this acquired a brilliant editor in Ernest Hart, a London surgeon who had also worked part-time at the *Lancet*. Hart was to be editor for 30 years and under his leadership the journal was to achieve not only national importance but also international fame. Even if Hart's prose style was less colourful than Wakley's (although his English was crisp and economical), his journal also achieved notable reforms. Like Wakley, Hart campaigned tirelessly against such medico-social evils as baby farming (concealed infanticide), and the lack of health care for paupers; for registration of midwives; and for medical services for the armed forces. He achieved most of his aims, but was equally concerned in the journal to record and comment on medical affairs, in the remotest town in Ireland as well as in the large cities of Europe, India, and the USA. Hart was also called in by the *American Medical Association at the end of the 19th century to advise on how to improve its journal. Today, editors still quote his reply: 'More articles and a bigger wastepaper basket'.

Other major countries also established national general medical journals during this time. In order of their appearance (and under today's title) these were as follows: *New England Journal of Medicine* (1812); *Gazette des Hôpitaux* (1828); *Wiener Medizinische Wochenschrift (1854); Medical Journal of Australia* (1856); *Nederlandsche Tidschrift von Geneesheitskunde* (1856); *Indian Medical Gazette* (1866); *Norwegian Medical Journal* (1881); *New Zealand Medical Journal* (1884); and *South African Medical Journal* (1903).

Rise of the specialist journals

As with the general medical journals, many specialist journals that were launched during the 19th century failed to survive, but some were successful and are still published. By the First World War almost every specialty that was clearly defined already had a journal of its own, usually in both the UK and the USA, and as new specialties came into being, so journals were started to serve them.

During the 1930s and after the Second World War the pace of subdividing medicine into specialties continued to increase, and this was reflected in both the number and character of the specialist journals. In 1900, for example, roughly 1000 biomedical journals had been launched; in 1950, 4000; and in 1970, 14 000; today the total is well over 20 000. Apart from the USA and the UK, other countries also began to publish specialist journals, notably in Scandinavia.

The character of some of the new specialist journals also changed; they became 'superspecialist', or even 'super-superspecialist'. Examples were a specialist journal called *Biochemistry*: a superspecialist version of this might be the *Journal of Carbohydrate Biochemistry*, and the super-superspecialist version the *Journal of Invertebrate Carbohydrate Biochemistry*.

Such journals are all largely devoted to publishing the results of original research. But over the past century several new types of journal have been introduced: the abstract journal (containing summaries of articles usually in one discipline published in a variety of different journals); the didactic or review journal, which aims at updating or instructing doctors, sometimes specifically for higher examinations; and the medical newspaper, which, besides reporting current events, may also contain instructional material or articles written in a radical journalistic style reminiscent of that of Thomas Wakley. Many of these new journals (colloquially known as 'throw-aways') are published by commercial firms primarily for profit.

Crisis in communication

At least 50 years ago it became apparent that the number of scientific journals was increasing both regularly and rapidly—by 6–7 per cent a year, thus doubling in 10–15 years and rising tenfold every 35–50 years. In 1939 the British scientist J. D. Bernal suggested that 'drastic action should be taken to restrict this information explosion', an idea that was repeated by Sir Theodore Fox, a distinguished editor of the *Lancet*. Both Bernal and Fox argued that journals should be classified into archival or recorder publications, and newspaper or current awareness journals. Bernal even suggested that the former could be replaced by a system of distributing abstracts of articles sent to a central source, with interested readers obtaining copies of the full paper on request; some journals have experimented with this idea.

Despite these suggestions the proliferation of journals has continued. Nevertheless, a reverse argument has also been put forward: that the growth of journals is a sign of health rather than disease in the scientific community. Professor Derek de Solla Price, of Yale University, showed that scholars have read and written at much the same rate over the past 3 centuries and for much the same reasons (communication and assessment of results and the prestige of the individual or the research group). New journals are often started because the disciplines of many readers cross fixed boundaries—that they are not, say, pure cardiologists but chemical pathologists or immunologists with an interest in cardiology. The titles and popularity of several recent journals (such as *Prostaglandins*, *Placenta*, or *Hypertension*) illustrate the need for such cross-disciplinary journals.

History has shown, moreover, that, faced with information overload, scientists have always managed to cope. Initially, for example, encyclopaedias were started in order to synthesize all the diverse information available in books and journals; when there were too many encyclopaedias for the individual to cope with, abstracting journals in individual subjects were introduced; and when there were too many of these, the computer databases were devised.

Another traditional factor in this process has been whether the message of the article becomes incorporated into knowledge bases: is it mentioned in the conversation or correspondence of top scientists (the 'invisible colleges') and does it appear as a reference in important review articles and textbook citations? One measure, the Science Citation Index, provides an objective guide to the impact of any article. This is a computer-based study of how many times an article is quoted in subsequent papers. Citation analysis has been developed in the USA by the journal *Current Contents* (a regular publication which lists the articles appearing in a large number of journals).

Together with other techniques, citation analysis has proved an important tool in research into the quality of published work. For bio-medicine, analysis has shown that some quarter to a half of all published articles are never cited even once in the reference lists of subsequent articles; and only 10–15 per cent of articles are considered really important by consensus groups of experts. A future possibility for solving information overload, then, might be to apply some sort of quality control by using citation analysis, indicating in lists of references supplied to scientists how many times individual articles have been quoted. Libraries can also apply similar analysis to determine what journals they should subscribe to.

Weighing in the balance

Today most journals are published by medical associations, specialist societies, commercial publishers, or two of these in collaboration. These appoint an editor and an editorial board, who are usually responsible for editorial policy, and deal with the production, dispatch, and promotion of the journal.

With any journal publishing original work, one of the editor's principal responsibilities is to assess the suitability of articles submitted for publication. Because of the number of these articles, and because when any discipline evolves it becomes increasingly complex and specialist, most editors have to ask experts for their advice—a process known as refereeing, assessment, or peer review.

The questions to be answered by the referee today usually relate to the newness, trueness, and importance of the article. Is the article original—for the world, the continent, or the country—and if not, does its importance overcome this consideration? Is it scientifically correct: are the methods used appropriate and reproducible; did the work conform to internationally accepted ethical codes; is any statistical analysis appropriate; and are the deductions made justifiable from the observations reported? Finally, what is the quality of the writing, will publication add appreciably to knowledge, is the article appropriate to this particular journal, and what is the assessor's own recommendation?

Some journals routinely use two, or occasionally more, outside assessors for refereeing; others use one, with the editor or one of the editorial board also reading the article with these criteria in mind. In some cases a statistician will also be asked to comment on the statistical aspects of the paper. Furnished with all these opinions, the editor alone may take the final decision or may also discuss the article with his editorial board. Five main outcomes are possible: to reject outright with no suggestions about publication in another type of journal (a recommendation usually implying that the article is too poor to be salvaged); to reject with a suggestion that the article would be more appropriately published elsewhere (with or without a detailed report on the article's merits and deficiencies); to offer to see a version revised in accordance with suggestions made by the editor and his team without any commitment to publish; to offer to publish provided that the author(s) will make certain changes to the article; to offer publication unconditionally.

The rejection rate varies according to the type of journal. The major general journals (the *Lancet*, the *New England Journal of Medicine*, the *BMJ*, and the *Journal of the American Medical Association*) offer high and broadly based circulations and rapid publication (within 3–4 months); their rejection rate approaches 85 per cent. The specialty journals have much smaller circulations, usually restricted to those working in the disciplines, and their delay from acceptance of the final manuscript to publication is between 9 and 18 months; their rejection rates vary from 30 to 70 per cent.

Most scientists believe that refereeing is vitally important in ensuring that journals continue to publish work of the highest quality. Given that publication of wrong information can raise false hopes (among the public as well as doctors, for journalists may highlight a research report as 'New hope for cancer sufferers'), the assessor has a great responsibility as a 'gatekeeper'. Even if a journal has a correspondence column in which letters can be published pointing out the errors in an article, harm may have been done already and readers may not see even a prominently printed correction; other scientists may waste much time and money in repeating the work and showing that it is wrong. Despite this, an assessor's work is largely anonymous, unpaid, and unacknowledged, and done largely out of a sense of responsibility to the medicoscientific community; the community and the editors owe them a great debt.

The electronic future
The price of medical journals, like that of almost everything else, has risen enormously, as has their number; thus few monthly journals now cost under $200 (£139) a year and some may charge as much as $1000 (£666) (1992 prices). With a limited budget, libraries have had difficulty in providing a full range of journals, as well as of textbooks and monographs, and in some instances (in the Third World, for example) comprehensive library services have already ceased to exist. Hence for some time both editors and publishers have been concerned to find a way of cutting costs while maintaining high standards.

The first solution adopted was the abstract (or secondary) journal, which printed summaries of articles, taken either from the original paper itself or contributed by experts. This technique has recently been given added impetus by the production of two abstract journals with invited comments by experts—*Journal Watch* and *Journal Club*. Nevertheless, apart from the overheads of the editorial office, the heavy costs of printing, paper, distribution, and storage have remained, and it was natural to turn to the electronic media to try to save money. Computers had already been used to supply the contents of the *Index Medicus* (a monthly volume listing the contents of over 3000 important medical journals) 'on line'. This means that a list of articles on a topic could be obtained via the ordinary telephone service, first displayed on a videoscreen and then printed out, if needed. The next step was to put abstracts into the same system, and probably a third of subscribers to some abstracting services are now on line for this (or receiving tapes for playing in their own computer) rather than receiving the printed version of the journal.

Not unnaturally, people have asked whether entire journals could not be treated in this way. Many editorial offices now use computers for choosing suitable referees and for routine clerical work, such as keeping track of articles submitted or accepted for publication, and would have little difficulty in preparing a journal for transmission either on line or on tape. In 1984 four major journals—the *Annals of Internal Medicine*, *British Medical Journal*, *Lancet*, and *New England Journal of Medicine*—were made available 'on line', although without their illustrations, which had to be supplied separately.

Since then many others have been added. A more radical development, however, and one that has been much discussed, is the true electronic journal. Two journals, started in the UK in the 1980s, pioneered this development, but they also appeared in hard-copy form and did not survive. The *Online Journal of Clinical Trials*, however, has concentrated on publishing an important but small segment of current research. Started in 1992, it will consider rather longer articles than most printed journals; it can receive, peer review, and negotiate on them using online facilities; and once an accepted article has been modified to the editor's satisfaction it can be published without any delay. Sponsored by the American Association for the Advancement of Science, and edited by the distinguished veteran, Dr Edward J. Huth, this journal's progress will be followed with great interest by those of us who believe that part of the future must lie in this direction (particularly given its capacity to contain a sizeable amount of data). However, even this journal has come to an arrangement with the *Lancet* to allow the latter to consider possible parallel publication of independently peer-reviewed shorter versions of some articles. Possibly a need for many authors to achieve a high level of visibility in the conventional medium does not augur well for any rapid development of this idea.

It would be foolish to pretend that journals and editors do not face considerable problems. The economic threats of ever-increasing costs, and the recent inability of some libraries to continue to afford to subscribe even to all major journals, are continually in the background. A second problem is posed by the decline in reprint sales, which is partly because the squeeze on departmental budgets means that less money is available to purchase reprints, and partly because readers may photocopy the article from the journal. Most established mainstream journals do not rely substantially on the sale of reprints for their healthy financial state, but the smaller-circulation journals may rely on this for their survival. More serious, however, is the wholesale photocopying of an entire journal instead of subscribing to it. Photocopying of a single article for individual use is allowed by many countries, but wholesale copying is now widespread in those countries not participating in international copyright agreements, is growing in the rest of the world, and obviously poses a serious threat to all journals. Its solution will depend on an internationally agreed system of regulating photocopying, on establishing a system for royalty payments, and, equally, on being able to police any system that is introduced.

Editors face several problems scientifically, as well. There are often doubts about the effectiveness and fairness of peer review, together with a recent upsurge in the number of known cases of research *fraud— forgery, piracy, and plagiarism of scientific articles. As well as the economic competition of the 'throw-away' journals, there is a possibility that commercial interests may use the new technology to produce for sale online information that is neither validated nor accurate. Even so, to be aware of new threats to standards and to anticipate them has always been part of the task of the editor and his advisers; one recent development has been the formation of editors' associations in Europe, the USA, Australia/New Zealand, the Middle East, and the Far East, where these problems can be discussed.

The first and second international conference on peer review, held in Chicago in 1990 and 1993, respectively, presented much international and original research into this problem, which has aroused a lot of attention.

The dissemination of scientific information has had a vital role in research for a long time. Whatever the challenges, it is in the interests of the entire community that it should continue as rapidly and efficiently as possible.

S. P. LOCK

MEDICAL JURISPRUDENCE. See LAW AND MEDICINE IN THE UK; LAW AND MEDICINE IN THE USA.

MEDICAL OFFICERS OF HEALTH (MOHs) appointed by local authorities and responsible for local matters relating to the public health, were a mid-19th century creation in the UK, largely in response to the great *cholera epidemics which led to the *Public Health Act of 1848. The first MOH had been appointed by Liverpool the previous year, under the Liverpool Sanitary Act of 1846; and a further 35 such posts were created during the next 10 years, the short life of the *General Board of Health. A subsequent Public Health Act, that of 1872, divided the country into a number of districts and required each to appoint its own MOH. The office survived the introduction of the *National Health Service (NHS) in 1948, which left such matters as domiciliary maternity, nursing, and health visiting services, together with child welfare, family planning, vaccination, school health, health education, screening, and other preventive medicine programmes still in the hands of the local authorities. In 1974, however, with the reorganization of the NHS into an integrated and unified structure, these responsibilities passed to health authorities and left only basic sanitation (drainage, sewage, refuse disposal, etc.) to local councils. The MOH thereupon ceased to exist. His place has effectively been taken by a new type of specialist working within the NHS. See PUBLIC HEALTH IN THE UK.

MEDICAL PAMPHLETEERING. During the centuries after the invention of printing, pamphleteering became a popular means of disseminating information and opinions, a pamphlet being a privately printed short booklet either unbound or bound loosely in paper covers. The views thus promulgated were mostly religious or political, usually controversial, but some of medical interest. Among the latter were, for example, Thomas *Percival's exposition of medical etiquette ('Medical Ethics', 1847), John *Snow's account of the true mechanism of cholera transmission ('On the Mode of Communication of Cholera', 1849) and the contemporaneous pamphlet 'concocted on sanitary subjects' by which Sir Edwin *Chadwick was said to have established himself in a position of absolute power on the *General Board of Health. The importance of pamphleteering declined towards the end of the 19th century with the growth of newspapers, magazines, and journals. See also MEDICAL JOURNALS.

MEDICAL PEERS. In 1993, 19 persons were distinguished by dual membership of the medical profession and of the British House of Lords, 15 of whom had had life peerages conferred upon them, the remaining four having inherited their titles.

MEDICAL PHOTOGRAPHY. See ILLUSTRATION AND PHOTOGRAPHY.

MEDICAL PRACTICE. Medicine is a cultural phenomenon, and in each country medical practice has its distinctive characteristics. Cross-national differences may be partly explained by the role of government, the formal organization of health-care systems, or the political ideologies attributed to them. Medical practice rests firmly, however, on the historical traditions of the medical profession and the development of medical education in each country; on the comparative evolution of medical institutions (notably *hospitals) and other health professions (notably *nursing); on definitions of medical care developed by the general public and by the medical profession over many years. It is also influenced by less tangible questions—of social attitudes, ideology, expectations—that make it possible to speak of a national culture or national style.

Patterns of medical practice in two countries, the UK and the USA, are often usefully compared, and their development reflects the influence of contrasting ideologies as well as different structures and methods of financing. The ownership and management of hospitals, for example, are important to medical practice, because of the crucial position of the hospital as the location of advanced medical technology and because of the authority suggested in patterns of ownership. The predominant mode of practice in the USA is private practice: the doctor, working out of his or her own office, also holds a staff appointment at one or more private hospitals, to which he or she may admit patients and care for them while they are there. The predominant mode of practice in the UK is the doctor working for a government health service, with hospital appointments strictly limited and controlled by the National Health Service (NHS).

Medical practice in the UK

Structure and authority are, however, only part of the picture. Tradition adds other notable distinctions. The British medical profession—but not the American—is divided by function into two distinct professional streams: *general, or family, practitioners (GPs), who provide *primary care, and hospital-based *consultants or specialists. GPs work out of offices (known as 'surgeries') or health centres in the community, usually in group practices of three or more doctors, and provide primary access to health services and the most important source of care for the general population. Each member of the population selects and registers with a GP who is technically an independent contractor with the NHS. There are, on average 1860 registered patients per doctor. Family practices may include additional NHS professional staff, notably *district nurses and *health visitors (nurses with special training in health education and preventive care who work primarily with families, young children, and the elderly), but most care is given by (or under the direction of) GPs. When necessary, the physician can access a specialist diagnostic department or refer the patient to a consultant for advice or hospital admission. Consultants or specialists are employed by the NHS on a salary scale which is generally uniform across specialties, and they are based in hospitals with their supporting staff and facilities.

Thus the primary care and the hospital functions are separated, functionally and physically. GPs have a monopoly of patients, while consultants monopolize hospital treatment, apart from a few places where GPs have small numbers of beds. By custom, British patients do not generally have direct access to specialists; a major exception is hospital emergency care. Instead, there is a formal system of 'referral' between GPs and specialists, with the GP acting as gatekeeper and general provider and manager of services, while the specialist has the secondary role of expert. Relatively few physicians are attached to the staff of any given hospital, compared with the USA. The referral system between GPs and consultants is a delicate professional power relationship, built into the profession's traditions, ethics, and expectations. The specialist accepts responsibility for the care of the patient for any necessary hospital treatment, referring the patient back to the GP on the completion of treatment.

The division in British medicine has at least four other important ramifications. First, government policy for many years has been to encourage and stimulate primary care, including the abolition of the wide income gap between GPs and specialists which existed into the mid-1960s. GPs outnumber hospital consultants in proportions of 3:2. To think of medical practice in the UK is therefore still largely to think of care being given in a primary-care setting, with the hospital remaining as a back-up system involving only 10 per cent of patients consulting GPs. The acknowledged role and relative number of GPs give them a legitimate prestige and a power base that does not exist for family practitioners in the USA. Secondly, by its very existence, the primary-care system shapes and defines what doctors do, and how they see the practice of medicine. The patients registered with a group of GPs—perhaps 8000 individuals in a four-person partnership—make up the 'practice', a definable community of care. General practices are not geographically defined, that is there are no rigidly defined boundaries or catchment areas within which patients must sign up with particular physicians; technically each GP or practice group competes with all the rest. An individual is free to choose a practice or practitioner; and the practitioner is free to refuse or accept him. Nevertheless, the responsibility of the general practice group for treating a specified community of patients, sick or well, makes the practice an important concept for British medicine.

Some GPs have accepted additional financial responsibility on behalf of their patients for a range of specialist services. Under the fund-holding scheme introduced with the reforms of the NHS and Community Care Act 1990, volunteer GPs receive a budget from NHS funds with which they negotiate for and buy hospital and consultant services according to their perception of priorities. The practice provides a base for assessing health and disease in the population, which is not available to specialists, who do not see a cross-section of the population but only patients pre-selected by specific conditions. GPs, in contrast, deal with the whole range of problems defined by patients as health or disease.

General practice, with medical records covering the individual health histories of the practice population, also gives doctors the opportunity to undertake community-based research through epidemiological studies. The GP is responsible for the continuing care of individuals and families, the availability of home visiting, and the encouragement of team work in general practice, including district nurses and health visitors (visiting nurses) in the team. The conscious linking of medical and social services through much of the history of the NHS since 1948, and a tradition of work in *public health and public welfare by GPs which goes back to the 19th century, give British medicine a much more distinctive 'social' cast than the more technologically focused medical profession in the USA.

Thirdly, the continuation and support of general medical practice have maintained an intellectual interest in primary care within the culture of the medical profession—an interest which has only recently (and partly) been revived in American medicine, following the acceptance of a specialty of family practice in 1969 and the development of designated family-practice residency positions. Fourthly, the divided structure has established a set of relationships between consultants and hospitals which are quite different from the relationships developed by American specialists. British consultants may work full-time or part-time for the NHS, but all of this work is hospital-based. The consultant is assigned a set number of hospital beds in a given location. These beds become 'his' or 'her' beds, with the consultant or his designates having the sole privilege of admitting patients to them. The British consultant, working with his 'firm' or team of house staff, not only has a more central role in the hospital than the average American specialist but a considerable degree of professional autonomy: a specified territory, a specified staff, and a continuing relationship with the nursing personnel of the one or two wards which contain his beds. Consultants control their own waiting lists. Following the 1990 NHS reforms, opportunities for medical management, including budget-holding for clinical departments, have increased. Medical *audit of the kind familiar in the USA has been comprehensively introduced, but the clinical autonomy of each individual consultant has been retained.

A further observation on the relationship between consultants and hospitals relates to out-patient work. Consultants and their staff see patients in the in-patient wards and in the hospital out-patient department, to which patients are referred by their GPs. Out-patient departments thus act primarily as specialist consultation clinics, not (as in the USA) as sources of both primary and specialist care. British hospitals see relatively fewer out-patients and emergency patients than their US counterparts, but the differential nature of these visits must be stressed. Many large inner-city US hospitals provide a vast amount of primary care to the relatively poor, who would expect to be treated by GPs in the UK.

British doctors can become GP principals after 4 years' post-qualification training in hospitals and primary care, while consultants are appointed by competitive search after at least 8 post-qualification years, frequently longer, in training whose standards are closely controlled by the appropriate royal college. A consultant is regarded as an expert, as reliable, and as competent. There is current concern that too much hospital work is being done by junior hospital doctors (house staff or residents) who are technically in training. Although consultant numbers (19 720 in 1990) have been increasing at a rate of over 2 per cent per annum, the junior workforce has been increasing also. By the 1980s manpower controls were made more stringent in an effort to redress the balance between training posts and career opportunities, and to provide services to patients based firmly on consultant skills and experience. The junior doctors themselves are now more prominent, better organized, and more politically important than they were 20 years ago, a reflection in large part of the expansion of hospital care in British medicine, if not to the extent of the expansion in the USA.

The broader question of the appropriate balance between primary and hospital care has tended to be obscured by the increasing activity and intensity of care in the hospital due to scientific advances and the modernization of services. Hospital lengths of stay have shortened, and *day surgery has been widely introduced during an era when much emphasis has been laid on efficiency, productivity, and value for money. Attention has recently turned towards prevention and primary and community care, partly in the pursuit of a long-term national strategy for health, and partly in a conscious effort to exchange the dominance of hospital-based care for local personalized care wherever appropriate. The importance of public health preventive measures was recognized following an enquiry into the future development of the Public Health function in 1988 and government commitment to priority health goals was published in 1992.

The 1990 NHS and Community Care Act gave new powers and responsibilities to GPs and to local government with effect from 1993 for residential care in the community. Many of these services were formerly within the province of NHS hospitals. There will be considerable effects upon the distribution of doctors and upon the prospects and nature of medical practice. Public health and general practice will be strengthened and are unlikely to be overwhelmed by hospital speciali-zation. A system of manpower control has achieved a fairly even geographical distribution of GPs during the history of the NHS, city-centre practice being the least popular and therefore least well staffed. Hospital spe-cialties have been separately planned, and there remain relatively wide variations in the distribution of hospital medical staff by region, in part the heritage of the dif-ferential distribution of hospitals when the NHS came into being in 1948. Moreover, as might be expected, some specialties are far more popular than others. At one end of the scale, general surgery and obstetrics and gynaecology are highly competitive. At the other are specialties, for example in psychiatry, where posts are unfilled. An impending shortage of UK-trained doctors has been predicted. The number of places in medical schools is centrally controlled and a modest increase to an annual intake of 4470 has been proposed, which includes 340 places for overseas students. Fifty per cent of the UK intake are women. Trends in recent years have lessened the dependence of the NHS on overseas doctors, and equal opportunities for men and women have improved. Women continue, however, to be under-represented in popular specialties.

The great majority of doctors in most countries are male (the former USSR is a notable exception). Almost all nurses and most technical occupations, from physi-cal therapists (*physiotherapists) to laboratory *techni-cians, are predominantly female. Over the past 15 years nurses have become more organized and more assertive in both the UK and the USA; the old image of the nurse as the doctor's handmaiden is rapidly passing away. At the same time, the greater infusion of women into medi-cine is changing the predominantly male image of the physician.

British health care has been subject to considerable criticism in recent years. There is continuing questioning of the relatively low cost of the NHS and the finan-cial stringencies imposed on the service in the 1970s and 1980s. Waiting lists, especially for 'cold' surgery, are still too long, and many regard the numbers of consultants in all specialties to be inadequate. Private hospitals, providing rapid (non-emergency) treatment, have increased greatly in number, and about 15 per cent of the population is now insured for private medical care through either individual or group (employment-based) schemes. Cutbacks in services appear likely in the com-ing decades. Despite rising budgets and the increasing costs of high technology care, the UK spends less than 6 per cent of its gross national product on health services, compared with 14 per cent in the USA. Criticisms of the NHS's social effects are also widespread. The Royal Commission on the National Health Service (1979) noted *inter alia* that, while there is general satisfaction with the health service among patients and workers in the system, social and geographical inequalities in the provision of resources continue to exist. A 1980 report, *Inequalities in health*, found relatively equitable

distribution of health services, but marked differences in health by social class. Such studies led to increas-ing interest in health outcomes and their relationship to medical practice and other influences, especially poverty. The national strategy for health (as opposed to health care) partly addresses these problems. The effects of very radical shifts in resources as a result of the NHS reforms and the introduction of a 'managed mar-ket' cannot yet be foreseen. The philosophy of medical practice in the UK remains that of a low-cost system funded by general taxation, with strong egalitarian aims and comprehensive coverage of the population, which has free access to services. The USA, in contrast, has a relatively high-cost system dedicated to the promotion of scientific excellence with a willingness to provide more services to those who can afford to pay and to leave sections of the population without right of access to care, although this philosophy is now being seriously questioned.

Medical practice in the USA

American patterns of practice reflect a profession strati-fied into specialties. Fully trained doctors work as spe-cialists either in private practice or (about one-third) as hospital staff. A fifth of trained doctors classify themselves as family or primary-care physicians (GPs), but compete with specialists for patients. Practice is typically from doctors' offices in buildings in city or suburban centres close to hospitals, where most have appointments or privileges which allow them to admit and bill patients. The initial offer of medical services is for a fee. Relatively high incomes are earned by US doctors in general, and high technology in hospital care enjoys a high standing. General and preventive medicine have a relatively low status.

While the British system of specialty labelling depends on the existence of specified hospital consultant posi-tions, American physicians may declare their expertise in any specialty they think fit. However, the formal structure of specialties is governed by 22 specialty cer-tifying boards, with functions comparable to the royal medical colleges in the UK. Each offers specialist exami-nations and certificates and participates in a system of approval of hospital training positions. Together, the specialty boards, each an independent professional organization, dominate the structure of medical practice by defining which fields are, and are not, to be recog-nized as having full specialist status.

Such decisions mutually reinforce the controlling structures in American medicine, including the depart-mental structure of medical schools and the establish-ment of specialist departments and training programmes in hospitals. Areas without a specialty board, such as *geriatrics, have a less-than-full acceptance.

While the structure of the NHS in the UK strength-ened the pre-existing position of the GP, the availability of private *health insurance schemes in the USA has bolstered fee-for-service practice. Insurance for medical care, like the provision of services, is fragmented among different agencies, and coverage is only partial.

The structure of private practice has strengthened the traditional American expectation that any physician is free to open up or join a practice anywhere in the USA. Fee-for-service practice and private health insurance schemes, by paying for medical care on the basis of services actually given, have encouraged doctors to develop their own specialist interests to the extent they can market these services to patients. Present patterns of specialist distribution show the relative enthusiasm for *surgery in American medical practice. Over one-quarter of American doctors practise in surgical or related fields, including *obstetrics and gynaecology and *anaesthesia. If British medical practice is typified by the general medical practice consultation, the epitome of American medical practice is the surgical operation. As Bunker has pointed out, in the USA there are relatively twice as many surgeons, and twice as much surgery is done as in the UK.

The American patient seeks not one doctor but an array of specialists, depending on individual perceptions and needs. From the patient's point of view, she/he is a shopper in a market for medical services and may seek, in a year, the independent services of several specialists. *Paediatrics provides general medical care to children and this specialty, together with internal medicine and sometimes with obstetrics and gynaecology, are generally referred to in American debates as primary-care fields. Yet there remains no primary-care *system* or *functions* such as exists in the UK. Recent efforts to encourage 'managed care' through insurance arrangements have attempted to limit patient access to specialists by requiring approval of the patient's primary doctor, in order to make services more cost-efficient. Nevertheless, in most cases the American system puts the onus for choosing the right specialist on the individual patient: the British system puts it on the GP.

American medical specialists practise in remarkable isolation. Typically, once patients consult a physician, they attend him for the duration of the diagnosis and treatment, whether on an out-patient or in-patient basis. When treatment is complete (or before), as determined either by the physician or the patient, the latter is free to select the same, or another, source of care for the next perceived medical incident.

Outside the private medical practice of individual specialists or single specialist groups, two major organizational structures exist in the USA to co-ordinate specialist care in an institutional setting: the hospital out-patient department and/or emergency room and the Health Maintenance Organization (HMO). Since American patients may see specialists in their private offices, the hospital out-patient department, as observed, has a different function in American medicine from that in the UK, where the out-patient department is largely a specialist referral centre. The American out-patient department also acts as a primary

source of care for walk-in patients who prefer to use the hospital rather than seek private specialists. Historically the American out-patient department has served the poor and underprivileged, while private specialists have served the relatively affluent, and this pattern still obtains to some extent.

HMOs, in contrast, represent efforts to provide co-ordinated services for middle-class Americans, at least those able to afford insurance. The HMO is a privately organized health service or network, providing care to subscribers who pay a monthly fee to the HMO, in return for which they become entitled to specified medical care benefits. The organization offers an array of specialists, either working together as a group (as in a private *polyclinic) or affiliated only in the sense that their names appear on a common, approved list. The individual patient, instead of seeking care through a general medical care practitioner (the British model) or through a mix of specialists co-ordinated by himself (the standard American model) thus enrols for care in an organization. Some HMOs own and operate their own hospitals; others admit patients to independent local hospitals under the care of HMO physicians. The current debate about 'managed competition' in the USA as a vehicle for system reform, assumes that the great majority of the population would subscribe to an organized group such as an HMO and that each group would compete with other groups for patients.

Meanwhile, the American system of medical practice remains a pluralistic system of specialists in private practice, each of whom holds one or more hospital appointments (and may belong to several practice networks for purposes of health insurance) and of hospital out-patient departments, which provide substantial services to the poor and under-privileged, particularly in the cities, also of experiments in organized multispecialist systems represented in HMOs and similar ventures.

The private character of American medicine can also be seen in its major institutions. The largest type of US hospital is the not-for-profit acute general hospital, typically run by an independent corporation of local citizens and providing services to a relatively small district or community; these hospitals, which include a small number run by religious organizations, form together with the other type—the company-managed, profit-making, investor-owned hospitals—a powerful group in the structure of American medicine. Both see themselves as part of a generic private sector. An important movement towards mergers, consolidation, and shared services among hospitals in the same area, or through wider geographical chains has, in recent years, led to a position where many American hospitals are now engaged in some form of interinstitutional co-operation. Such moves are particularly important for medical practice at the local level, for co-operation among institutions implies co-operation among medical staffs and, in some cases, consolidation, merger, or closing of hospital departments. With these moves, as well as with other co-operative developments (such as HMOs), or potentially threatening developments (such as the constant threat of cutbacks in *Medicare and *Medicaid) American physicians—with their long tradition of apathy or resistance to organizational changes—are now acutely aware of broader organizational issues in medicine. All of the major professional groups have developed, or are developing, proposals for systematic change.

American hospitals contain, on average, far more concrete symbols of technology than their British counterparts and employ far more personnel. The character of hospitals as high-technology centres pervades the ideology of American medicine.

Fee-for-service practice and private hospitals reinforce the idea that doctors have something useful to sell: a combination of time and technology. The intrinsically business-orientated structure of medical practice is engrained deep in the social system. It is this combination of technology and business that makes practice reform so difficult to achieve in the USA. Attempts to control costs are readily equated with reduction in technology, or 'quality'. In medicine as in other spheres, 'more' is seen as 'better'. Debates about excessive use of technology in the last months of life, prolonging the inevitable process of death, provide one exception to this view, albeit still controversial. There is less concern about the millions of Americans without health insurance than about restricting technology to any group of patients. In parallel, proposals for national change are couched in business-sounding rhetoric, including managed care and managed competition. President Bill Clinton's emphasis on 'fairness' (1993) has added an important new dimension to the constant health-reform debates; it is too early to assess how these will work out.

Both the American and the British practice systems have their advantages and disadvantages. Where the American system works well, with patients referring themselves appropriately to specialists, the patient may receive continuing, high-quality care for a given condition both inside and outside the hospital. On the other hand, the American system imposes major responsibility on the patient to choose the appropriate specialist for a given condition. Little is known as to how well American patients make these decisions, nor what are the ultimate effects. Nor, for that matter, do we have comparable information on general practitioner and specialist care in the UK. However, a striking element of comparison is the relative role of the hospital in the two systems. Whereas the British hospital can be seen as at the fringe of medical practice, the American hospital is central to the practice of medicine, reinforcing the underlying technological character of American medicine, while at the same time underlining the fact that there are few alternative foci for medical practice organization.

While the American hospital remains a logical centre for the organization of health services, and while competition for funds may move some hospitals into new areas, countervailing economic forces may cause contraction in hospital services as a whole, in favour of expanded private practice systems. Academic health centres (university hospitals) have been particularly hard hit by cutbacks in Medicaid payments, and American doctors are well aware of the exigencies of the medical market-place.

American medical practice is beset by uncertainty and with concern about the increasing costs of medical care. A possible surplus of physicians creates anxiety among medical students who end their medical education carrying a potentially massive load of debt. Established practitioners fear increasing competition due to rapid expansion in medical schools (spurred by federal funding) and liberal immigration policies for foreign physicians. Medical incomes have been declining in real terms since the 1970s, although they remain among the highest incomes in the USA (and significantly higher than doctors' incomes in the UK). Doctors, together with hospitals, have also been subjected to considerable criticism since the late 1960s as being at least partly responsible for the rapidly escalating costs of medical services. Lacking an organized health-care system, or for that matter a national health policy, there is no other easy target for patients and politicians to blame.

More generally, the technological, specialized character of American medicine has limited the ability of American doctors to capture public interest in behavioural and social aspects of medicine, for which a growing demand exists. Major industrial firms have developed their own weight control, *smoking reduction, exercise, and *alcohol programmes. Psychologists have moved rapidly into counselling and behaviour modification. Indeed, much of the work now being done in behavioural medicine is being defined as 'education' rather than as 'medicine'. Similarly, programmes for the elderly in areas not regarded as typically 'medical'— such as *day-care centres, clubs, or health information programmes—are unlikely to develop under the aegis of the medical profession. While geriatrics remains a relatively unpopular specialty in the UK, it is doubtful whether physicians in the USA will be a major force for providing health services to the elderly at all. At a time when hospitals and physicians are being criticized for rising costs, American medical practice may not be able to readjust its role towards a more comprehensive view of health as well as sickness. Some of the questions addressed to medical practice are similar in both countries: the appropriate future role of primary care, the relative cost of hospitals, how best to define and organize regional specialty services, or the appropriate geographical distribution of practitioners. Yet review of medical practice in these two countries reminds us forcibly of the tradition of medical practice peculiar to a specific culture.

In both countries the doctor's role is being challenged

on several fronts simultaneously. As other professional groups have become organized and unionized, whether they are laundry workers, nurses, or doctors themselves, the medical profession finds itself as one occupation among many; the traditional dominance of physicians has thus been lessened. Medical audit systems assume that there are standard (ideal) patterns of care and methods of practice regulation. The importance of organizational issues, including the management of capital, cost control, and equitable distribution of health services, has brought politics and economics firmly into the practice picture. Health administrators and politicians have become important decision-makers, yet they must depend, in turn, upon the views of many different occupational, political, and consumers groups. Medical practice, broadly defined, has become a complex web of negotiations among different groups, each perhaps with different ideas of what a health service should be. Thus paradoxically, over the past century the doctor's role in society has become both more and less powerful: more powerful in terms of what she or he can do to affect the health of the individual; less powerful in decision-making within the health-care system.

Future patterns of medical practice will depend on specific compromises reached among the positions of conflicting groups, on prevailing traditions and professional structures in different societies, and on the scope and style of government involvement and intervention. Despite the common problems posed by specialized medicine in different cultures, medical practice will continue to display subtle national differences.

ROSEMARY A. STEVENS
E. ROSEMARY RUE

Further reading
Marsh, G., Wallace, R. B., and Whewell, J. (1976). Anglo-American contrasts in general practice. *British Medical Journal*, **i**, 1321–5.
Public health in England. The report of the Committee of Inquiry into the future development of the public health function ('Acheson' Report) (1988). Cmd 289. HMSO, London.
Stevens, R. (1971). *American medicine and the public interest.* Yale University Press, New Haven.
Townsend, P. and Davidson, N. (eds) (1988). *Inequalities in health: The Black Report* (1982). Penguin, Harmondsworth.
Working for patients. (1989). Government White Paper on the Health Service. Cmd 555. HMSO, London.

MEDICAL PROTECTION SOCIETY. One of the three UK medical protection societies. See LAW AND MEDICINE IN THE UK.

MEDICAL PUBLISHERS. See MEDICAL BOOKS AND LIBRARIES; MEDICAL JOURNALS.

MEDICAL QUALIFICATIONS. See MEDICAL EDUCATION: POSTGRADUATE AND CONTINUING, UNDERGRADUATE.

MEDICAL RECORDS. A medical record is an account, written, dictated, or fed into a computer by a doctor, of the previous medical history of a patient, his or her present illness, and the findings on physical examination (including the results of any tests that have been carried out), together with details of treatment and notes on progress and further developments. It may include entries by other doctors and other health professionals. Nursing records are often included. Since the *National Health Service Act 1946, medical records in the UK (apart from those relating to private practice) have been the legal property, not of the doctor concerned, but of the Secretary of State for Health and Social Security or the Secretary of State for Scotland, custody being delegated through the various health authorities to their appropriate officers. Computerized records now fall within the terms of reference of the Data Protection Act but under the terms of the Access to Health Records Act 1992 patients are entitled to scrutinize manual records relating to them.

MEDICAL REGISTER. In the UK the Medical Register is maintained by the *General Medical Council, and lists all persons legally qualified to practise medicine and hence to fill public office, to use dangerous drugs, to sign death certificates, and to perform certain other duties. See REGISTRATION.

MEDICAL RESEARCH COUNCIL, THE, (MRC) is the principal agency in the UK through which government funds are provided for the support of medical research. It is a quasi-autonomous body responsible, like the other research councils, to the Office of Science and Technology (not the Department of Health), whose ministers appoint the Council's members. A majority of these are doctors and scientists eminent in their respective disciplines but there is a significant leavening of lay members and government representatives. The full-time chief executive, the Secretary, has always been a medical scientist. The MRC gives grants to support work in universities, hospitals, and other institutions throughout the UK and in some other, mostly developing, countries. It also maintains a cadre of full-time permanent research scientists in wholly maintained institutions in the UK and abroad. A national fund for medical research originated with the National Health Insurance Act of 1911. A predecessor body, the Medical Research Committee, was created in 1913. The Medical Research Council itself came into being and was granted a Royal Charter on 1 April 1920. See also FOUNDATIONS, ETC. IN THE UK.

MEDICAL SAINTS. Early Christians invoked medical saints in much the same way as the Greeks and Romans had invoked their gods, healing having been a specific function of the Church since the power to cure was conferred on the 12 disciples (Luke 9:1); and the tradition persisted until modern times. Even at the beginning of the 19th century, for example, Scottish patients with mental disturbances were treated by immersion in the waters of St Fillan's pool, St Fillan being one of the heavenly psychiatrists (another was St Dymphna, who specialized in mental subnormality). The list of saints associated with particular conditions is long: it includes St Margaret of Antioch and St Dorothy, called on during *labour; St Petronilla looked after fevers (as did the mythical St Febronia, descended from the Roman goddess Febris); St Roche and St Sebastian dealt with the prophylaxis and cure of plague; others were St Vitus (nervous diseases), St Lawrence (burns and scalds), St Erasmus (abdominal complaints), St Clare (ophthalmic diseases), St Apollonia (toothache), and St Antony (scurvy). No fewer than four were assigned to *chorea— St Guy, St John, St Anthony, and St Vitus—and two to *erysipelas—St Francis and St Anthony.

MEDICAL SCEPTICS. Playwrights and film makers, philosophers, and social scientists have all delighted in taking a sceptical view both of medicine and of the doctors who practise it. From Molière (*Le médecin malgré lui*) to Alan Bennett (*The madness of George III*), they have poured scorn on the theories and practice of medicine. Satirists have always excelled in poking fun at those who have power over us in society, or at those whom we fear. Doctors amply fulfil both these criteria.

Medicine's critics pose an array of challenging questions. Who determines the aims of modern medicine and what are they? What is the evidence for the success of medical intervention? How does this compare with the improvements in health consequent not on medical discovery, but on social and economic advance? What harm is done by medical care and by the medical profession? Is the cost of health care commensurate with the benefits? Has biotechnology damaged our perception of the human state and redefined what we mean by life and death in mechanistic terms? Are we in danger of dehumanizing the very processes of care? As the power and effectiveness of medical interventions have increased, so medicine itself has come increasingly under sceptical scrutiny. Some have gone so far as to suggest that doctors have created a society of dependent patients, fearful of future disease, ill with the anxiety of it, and prepared to trade autonomous life choices, for the slavery of medical prescriptions.

Such critique has been levelled at medicine by thinkers both within and without the medical profession.

In his Rock Carling Lecture *The role of medicine*, Professor Tom McKeown (1976) advanced the argument that since Descartes medical science has been unhelpfully preoccupied by the image of the patient as a body-machine. Current medical theory postulates that this machine is inherently faulty and requires internal intervention. McKeown argued that this mechanistic approach neglects the powerful determinants of health and illness which are not amenable to medical interventions. He identified four determinants of health

(genetic diseases; conditions associated with the genetically programmed wearing out of organs at the end of life; diseases in which the environmental influences are prenatal; and those in which the environmental influences are postnatal). The ability of modern medicine to intervene is limited largely to the last of the four categories, and McKeown suggested that even here it is easy to overestimate the effects of medical interventions. Although most of the major infections (*pneumonia, *scarlet fever, *measles, and so on) have declined dramatically during the 20th century, the decline was already well established before the introduction of immunizations and *antibiotics. At the time of *streptomycin introduction in 1947 the major decline in the incidence of *tuberculosis in the UK had already taken place.

Professor Archie Cochrane, in his Rock Carling Lecture (*Effectiveness and efficiency*) (1972), made a plea for greater scientific scepticism in the evaluation of health care. With hindsight, it is relatively easy to look with horror on the excesses of unscientific medical care. The bleeding, cupping, and purging of earlier centuries were treatments based on imaginative theory, unsupported by evidence. The death of Charles II at the hands of his doctors is said to have been infinitely more cruel that that of his father at the hands of an executioner.

In the 1930s *tonsillectomies and *circumcisions were carried out with no doubt the best of intentions, but on the basis of faulty clinical reasoning and no evidence of benefit. From the 1970s onward there has been a dramatic increase in interventive *obstetrics, and in particular of *Caesarean sections, with little proven effect on infant or maternal *morbidity and *mortality. McCormick and Skrabanek (1990) have challenged the evidence that *screening for breast and cervical cancers, now public policy in the UK, does more good than harm. Cochrane's argument was that in the absence of a rigorous method of evaluation, both doctors and the public are easily seduced into enthusiasm for health-care policies and therapeutic interventions, which are based only on hope and belief.

Zola (1972) and others have criticized the medical profession for having 'medicalized society'. In the 19th century the relationship between social conditions and disease was increasingly understood and acknowledged. *Public-health doctors became social reformers, and *Virchow, a pathologist and public-health reformer, wrote 'Medicine is a social science, and politics nothing but medicine on a grand scale'. In the 20th century, new insights into the causes of chronic disease focused on the habits of human behaviour—concerning diet, exercise, cigarette smoking, sexual intercourse, and so on. These human behaviours have been labelled 'risk factors' by doctors, who in the pursuit of disease prevention prescribe how we should live our lives. Summing up the evidence on so-called 'risk factors' in the development of coronary-artery disease, a physician (Myers 1968) has composed the following profile of a low-risk individual:

. . . an effeminate municipal worker or embalmer completely lacking in physical or mental alertness and without drive, ambition, or competitive spirit; who has never attempted to meet a deadline of any kind; a man with poor appetite, subsisting on fruits and vegetables laced with corn and whale oil, detesting tobacco, spurning ownership of radio, television, or motorcar, with full head of hair but scrawny and unathletic appearance, yet constantly straining his puny muscles by exercise. Low in income, *blood pressure, blood sugar, *uric acid and *cholesterol, he has been taking nicotinic acid, pyridoxine and long term anti-coagulant therapy ever since his prophylactic castration.

The critique of medicine in general has found a particular focus in the field of mental health. Psychiatrists, such as David Cooper (1967), Thomas Szasz (1961), and R. D. Laing (1960), challenged the very concepts and practices of contemporary *psychiatry. It is argued that the attempt to conceptualize a schizophrenic experience as a disease, using physical disease as the model, is not only misleading and fruitless, but also repressive. The control of feelings and behaviour by drugs has been compared with the use of physical constraints in the past. Foucault (1967) argued that the introduction of the madhouse into European society was part of a movement to shut away the social and political deviants in an age when social conformity was deemed an economic necessity. He described this as 'the great containment' and traced a direct line of development from leper colony, or lazar house, to madhouse, workhouse, and hospital (Foucault 1973). During the bleakest years of the USSR, political dissidents were treated as psychiatric patients, their protest hidden in psychiatric institutions and muted by the administration of the major *tranquillizers.

Perhaps the most trenchant scepticism about the benefits of medicine in the medical profession was voiced by the moral philosopher Ivan Illich (1976). He made much use of the term 'iatrogenic'—a word derived from Greek roots, and meaning 'caused by doctors'. He listed three levels of iatrogenic damage.

First, he described clinical iatrogenesis, by which he meant the physical damage caused by the remedies that doctors employ. Illich was referring to the fact that many of the drugs that doctors use have unwanted effects which cause inevitable damage. In addition, drugs may be prescribed inappropriately, or the patient may mistakenly take an overdose, so that iatrogenic disease becomes a growing epidemic alongside the very advances of medical treatment and burgeoning of new health-care institutions.

Secondly, Illich listed social iatrogenesis. This is what Zola and others have described as the medicalization of life, the creation of dependency on medical institutions, and so on. Illich's third category was cultural iatrogenesis. This he described as the expropriation of health:

When dependence on the professional management of pain, sickness and death grows beyond a certain point, the healing power in sickness, patience in suffering and fortitude in the face of death must decline. These three regressions are

symptoms of third-level iatrogenesis: their combined outcome is Medical Nemesis.

Despite the exaggerations of many of the attacks on medicine and the medical profession, despite the obscure language of some of the philosophers, and the barbed tongue of the playwrights, the medical sceptics are the allies of good-quality medical care, not its enemies.

The keystone of modern experimental research in medicine, as in all sciences, is the mounting of a challenging critique by the scientist himself, on his own working methods, data, and conclusions. Scepticism is therefore an integral component of scientific thought. It is essential to the biomedical advances of the 20th century, and in the future it will ensure the limitation of medicine's potential harm, and the maximizing of medicine's potential good.

MARSHALL MARINKER

References
Cochrane, A. L. (1972). *Effectiveness and efficiency*. The Nuffield Provincial Hospitals Trust, London.
Cooper, D. (1967). *Psychiatry and anti-psychiatry*. Tavistock Publications, London.
Foucault, M. (1967). *Madness and civilisation*. Tavistock Publications, London.
Foucault, M. (1973). *The birth of the clinic*. Tavistock Publications, London.
Illich, I. (1976). *Medical nemesis*. Marion Boyars, London.
Laing, R. D. (1960). *The divided self*. Tavistock Publications, London.
McCormic, J. and Skrabanek, P. (1990). *Follies and fallacies in medicine*. Tarragon Press.
McKeown, T. (1976). *The role of medicine*. The Nuffield Provincial Hospitals Trust, London.
Myers, G. S. (1968). In *Life, death and the doctor*, (ed. Lasagnal), pp. 215–16. Alfred Knopf.
Szasz, T. (1961). *The myth of mental illness*. Harper and Row.
Zola, I. K. (1972). Medicine as an institution and social control. *Sociological Review*, **20**, 487–504.

MEDICAL SOCIETIES. Local provincial medical societies were active in England in the latter part of the 18th century, and increased during the first part of the 19th. Most were at first mainly concerned with the lending of books and journals but later developed into societies for both scientific discussion and mutual protection. One such was the Worcester Medical and Surgical Society, founded by Charles *Hastings in 1816, which became the Provincial Medical and Surgical Association in 1832 and the British Medical Association in 1855. See also MEDICAL COLLEGES, ETC: OF THE UK; OF THE USA.

MEDICARE. See GOVERNMENT AND MEDICINE IN THE USA; MEDICAL PRACTICE.

MEDICINE AND STAMP COLLECTING. In May 1990, the 150th anniversary of the world's first adhesive postage stamp—the famous Penny Black of Great Britain—was celebrated. This initial stamp featured the head of Queen Victoria, as it was considered that a bust design would be the most difficult one to forge. Over the years since then, almost every country world-wide has developed a postal system and issued its own distinctive postage stamps to pay for its use. Because Great Britain pioneered the use of stamps, it is the only country in the world where the Universal Postal Union does not insist that the country's name appears on their stamps—only the monarch's head is necessary.

For the first 50 years or so after the Penny Black was issued, it was possible to collect an example of almost every stamp issued throughout the world. By the turn of the century, sheer issuance volume dictated that many collectors started limiting their field of interest. In the early days, this limitation was frequently geographical—Europe, the Americas, one country and its colonies, were all examples that were frequently chosen. Gradually, however, postal administrations realized that stamps could have a secondary use as an effective public information, publicity, and advisory medium; alternatively they could be used for propaganda.

The diversity, artistry, and attractiveness of the designs—particularly of stamps on the hundreds of thousands of items of mail crossing international borders—stimulated the interest of recipients into saving them and trying to acquire similar ones. Almost any theme imaginable has, at one time or another, been depicted on stamps, and many doctors, not surprisingly, stick to stamps which have a medical theme. Much fun can be

had in the detective work involved in tracking down an elusive reference or stamp issue. The American Topical Association—among others—has published handbooks dealing with various aspects of medical philately. Several journals are published, the monthly *Scalpel and Tongs* in America, or the quarterly *Medi-Theme* in the UK.

The Medical Philately Study Group, which publishes *Medi-Theme*, was founded in 1982. It has a world-wide membership. It maintains contact with similar groups, such as *Scalpel and Tongs* in America, Philatelia Medica in Germany, Groupe Santé in France, and Esculapio Filatelici in Italy. Illustrations of some stamps with a medical theme are reproduced in Fig. 1.

Until the beginning of this century, many postal administrators considered that letters could spread disease. To disinfect the mail, various methods were used. These included, amongst others, first slitting the surface of the letters or punching holes in them with a 'rastel', then fumigating by superheated steam, sprinkling with vinegar, chloride of lime or other chemicals, or toasting them over heat. They could also first be handled with tongs. The Disinfected Mail Study Circle (founded in 1974) publishes a quarterly journal *Pratique*.

JAMES DUNLOP

MEDICINE AND THE MEDIA. In 1907 William *Osler warned medical students of the dangers of interacting with the media. 'In the life of every successful physician,' he said, 'there comes the temptation to toy with the Delilah of the Press—daily and otherwise. There are times when she may be courted with

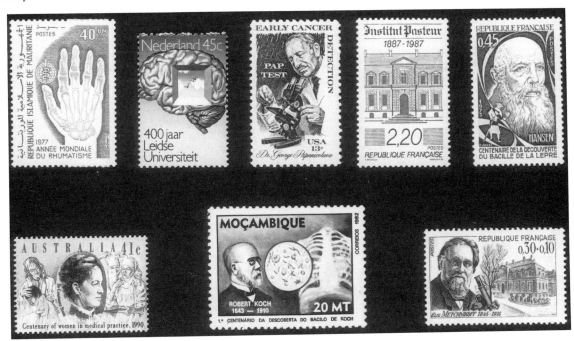

Fig. 1 Stamps with a medical theme.

satisfaction but beware: sooner or later she is sure to play the harlot and has left many a man shorn of his strength, viz the confidence of his professional brethren.' When *Your life in their hands*, a television programme that filmed surgical cases, began in Britain in 1958 many doctors, including the editor of the *British Medical Journal* (*BMJ*), condemned it for spreading anxiety and *hypochondriasis.

Yet by the 1970s Charles Fletcher, one of Britain's most distinguished physicians and the first presenter of *Your life in their hands*, was advising that 'Every doctor should now be willing to collaborate with the media today in public education about what medicine has to offer in prevention and cause of disease.' By the 1980s *Jimmy's*, a series of transmissions from St James's Hospital, Leeds, was one of the most popular programmes on British television; a week of special broadcasts from Hammersmith Hospital in the 1990s was watched by half of the population; and a medical programme that advertised for a medically qualified presenter received dozens of applications.

Coverage of health matters in the media has grown dramatically in the past 50 years. Nowadays most newspapers have at least one health correspondent; in addition, each week they devote one or more pages specifically to health matters. The broadcast media devote just as much space to health, and a survey by NBC in 1983 found that 81 per cent of the general population wanted more news about health and medicine—compared with 31 per cent wanting more politics and 29 per cent more business coverage. Hospitals and surgeries are also regularly the setting of soap operas and dramas.

The news media range over the whole field of health, but there is a bias towards the new and the dramatic. Thus new and risky surgical operations—particularly, in the past 20 years, *transplants—receive a great deal of coverage, while the more mundane, for instance, *mental illness and the problems of *ageing, receive much less attention. 'Lifestyle' issues, such as smoking, drinking, diet, and exercise, are widely covered on both news and feature pages. Many of the news stories are derived from *medical journals, particularly the weekly general medical journals, but an increasing number of organizations—professional associations, *research institutions, and *pharmaceutical companies—are keen to use the media to promote particular issues and to raise their own profile.

What is the effect of this increasing media coverage of health matters? The usual answer is that people are better informed about health, more able to take charge of their own health, and more likely to be discerning and critical consumers of health-care services. This may be true, but scientifically sound studies of the effects of increased health coverage in the media are scarce. Indeed, some of the few who have written extensively on this topic have argued that the mass of material may actually reduce understanding of health issues— partly because of the way material is selected and partly because of the inevitable tension between the scientific complexities that underlie medical stories and the need for short, clear, and exciting stories.

Certainly, the result of using the mass media for *health education has been disappointing. Thus, for instance, doctors thought that once the evidence was gathered on the harmful effects of smoking some powerful messages through the media would solve the problem. But this was not the case, and research has shown that simply transmitting messages through the media— either through advertising or editorial coverage—is not enough on its own to change behaviour. Rather, media coverage 'sets the agenda' and supports efforts made by other means, through community health workers, for instance.

Although it is hard to be sure about the overall effects of health coverage in the media, there have been some examples of the media having had important effects on particular issues. A television programme first suggested that children around nuclear installations may be at increased risk of *leukaemia and some solid *cancers. Doctors and others might have complained that the programme was sensational and scary, but its central proposition turned out to be true even if the risks proved much less than was originally suggested. Unfortunately, television programmes are not good at conveying the size of a risk, and pictures of young children dying of cancer inevitably have an impact that dull statistics cannot match.

The media have also played a vital role in highlighting the brutal regimes of some of Britain's special hospitals, but some programmes have been less successful. Thus uproar was caused by a television programme that argued that clinical methods for diagnosing *brainstem death were inadequate. The number of organs available for transplantation fell, but British neurologists insisted that the programme had given a wholly false impression of how brainstem death was diagnosed. The criteria for diagnosing brainstem death were subsequently revised, and the programme makers might argue that the programme was thus justified. And it was another television programme, about a small boy who urgently needed a liver transplant, that increased the supply of organs for transplantation.

Another issue that angered many British doctors was the widespread media coverage of brain damage supposedly caused to children by *whooping cough *vaccine. Eventually, a court decided that the evidence for the vaccine causing brain damage was virtually nonexistent, but by this time the number of children being vaccinated had fallen dramatically, resulting in another epidemic. In all of these cases, the media would argue that they were simply reflecting debates going on among doctors, and that they have a public duty to do so—even if public anxiety is created.

One particular conflict between doctors and journalists has been over the publication in the mass media of studies reported in medical journals. The editors of journals make journalists wait until the studies are published in their journals—arguing that the peer-review process will then make it more likely that the study is sound, and that if doctors have the full scientific paper, they will be better able to make up their own minds on the studies than if they simply read a few paragraphs in a newspaper or see a brief comment on television. Journalists argue that studies of importance to the public should be reported immediately and should not have to wait for the peer-review process. Some journals have refused to publish papers if the findings have been leaked to the press, but a system has now been devised by the International Committee of Medical Journal Editors for allowing publicity before publication in restricted circumstances.

Ironically, one of the few circumstances where a scientifically sound study has shown a positive effect of publicity has to do with the widespread reporting of such stories from medical journals. Researchers showed that studies selected from the *New England Journal of Medicine* for reporting in the *New York Times* were more likely to be cited in scientific journals than articles not selected. And it wasn't that the journalists were simply selecting the most important studies, because those selected but not reported—at a time when the *New York Times* was on strike—were not better cited.

The relationship between the media and doctors is likely to remain fraught—and perhaps it should be so—but we are unlikely to return to the days of Osler and see doctors ignoring the media. Extensive coverage of health matters will certainly continue.

RICHARD SMITH

Further reading
Karpf, A. (1988). *Doctoring the media: the reporting of health and medicine*. Routledge, London.
Klaidman, S. (1991). *Health in the headlines: the stories behind the stories*. Oxford University Press, New York.

MEDICINE IN AFRICA. Medical education and care in Africa vary from one country to another. In East Africa they have long been under the influence of the Nile civilization and its tradition of medicine. In West Africa medicine was more primitive and traditional. In the 17th century, health officers arrived with colonists (Portuguese, French, British, or German) and with military units. Some *missionary organizations sent nurses and some doctors, who treated infections and parasitic diseases. However, *malnutrition, *schistosomiasis, *malaria, *onchocerciasis, infantile *diarrhoea, *trypanosomiasis, *treponematosis, *leprosy, *tuberculosis, and, more recently, *AIDS, remain major problems in central West and East Africa.

North Africa was served by several famous medical doctors and scientists during the Middle Ages. Arabic medicine (in Spain, Morocco, Tunisia, and Egypt) was of a high standard (a medical golden age). Hospitals were built and organized in a comparatively modern manner and were managed by doctors who examined the patients regularly and presented their findings to the students (doctors in training). This Hippocratic tradition spread to the medical schools of southern Europe. Progressively, thereafter, the situation in North Africa deteriorated.

The situation in southern Africa was influenced by the methods and principles of the different colonial powers. In South Africa, and in adjacent states, once colonies but now independent, two types of health-care services developed alongside traditional medicine: free governmental medical care was provided for the indigenous population, but this was all too often rudimentary, while modern, well-developed, private medical care was offered to the settlers (and the more affluent of the indigenous population) (the first heart transplant in the world was done by Barnaard in South Africa in 1970).

After the Second World War, with the flowering of political independence, modern medicine spread, leading to the creation of several faculties of medicine in most African countries. The training programmes were usually based on the Western model. In most cases, depending upon the political and social situation in the country concerned, health-care provision was organized as a social service rather than depending upon a private system. However, the budget of such public systems still provides only 50 per cent of total expenditure on health, so that services are largely concentrated in cities, and provision in rural areas is often inadequate, sometimes non-existent.

The percentages of world population in the developed and developing countries are 33.4 and 66.6 per cent, respectively; while the comparable percentages of trained medical manpower (doctors) are 74.4 and 25.6 per cent. As a result, most African countries have a large number of inhabitants per medical doctor (range: 1 for 14 000–50 000, varying between individual countries). In some countries there is one hospital per 200 000–1 200 000 inhabitants, and one primary medical-care centre per 6500–150 000 inhabitants. In addition, medical manpower is concentrated largely in the hospitals, in contrast to the primary health-care centres. This produces an unbalanced health system.

The consequence of increasing health-care costs in developing countries, and the reduction of the funds coming from international organizations (UNICEF, WHO, PNUD, FAO) and other programmes (EC, USA, Russia, France, Switzerland, Germany, UK, China) has been a progressive reduction in public health-care provision. Primary health care and a general immunization and vaccination policy have been the principal goals of African health policy (aiming at a welfare state). However, most health departments in Africa are now unable to pay for an adequate primary health-care system. Hospital budgets are insufficient and equipment inadequate. In many countries only the more affluent and privileged have access to private medicine of an adequate standard.

Free, government-provided, medical services reach only 40 per cent of the population of Tunisia, for example. A higher rate is achieved in some other countries, but in none is coverage complete. The general organization of Tunisian health-care services is, however, relatively simple. Vaccination campaigns are organized regularly. Primary health-care centres, where accessible, are open to anyone who needs medical assistance. Routine blood tests and chest X-rays are free. If more sophisticated investigations are required, the medical staff in the primary-care centre can arrange transfer of the patient to a regional and/or national hospital or institute. The services delivered in such referral centres depend on the availability of funds for the purchase of equipment, medical and nursing supplies, and drugs. Theoretically, all patients in Tunisia have free access to government hospitals or institutes, including those who have public (40 per cent) or private (10 per cent) insurance. Several private clinics exist which are well-equipped (X-ray, CT scan, angiography, sonography, and Doppler scanning) and are authorized to deliver medical and surgical services on repayment for all groups of patients. Many patients, however, prefer the public hospitals if they need complicated surgery, or when they have severe medical conditions, but use the facilities of private clinics to reduce waiting time when requiring simple elective surgery or treatment for other non-urgent conditions.

Some countries have many different types of hospital: army hospitals, police hospitals, engineers' hospitals, etc., each with part-state and part-private sections. Thus in Egypt, for example, the organization of medical practice is mixed private and public in both primary care and in hospital. In Algeria, Morocco, Tunisia, and in most of the predominantly Black countries the two sectors are completely distinct. Doctors working in the governmental system are unable to work in private practice, while those in private practice have no access to governmental services.

In conclusion, medical and health care is difficult and variable from one country to another in Africa, depending on the political system of the countries concerned and their economic prosperity.

M. BEN HAMIDA

MEDICINE IN AUSTRALIA. Australia enjoys a very high standard of health care. Infant mortality rates average 7.1 per 1000 live births. Standardized annual death rates are 662 per 100 000 population. Life expectancy at birth is 74.3 years for males and 80.3 years for females. Health care expenditure is 8 per cent of gross domestic product (compared with 6.0 per cent for the UK and 14.0 per cent for the USA). The doctor–population ratio, at 1:440, is the second highest in the world, after Belgium.

Australia is a net exporter of health and medical services. This applies both to Australian-trained doctors (as well as other health professionals) who practise in many parts of the world; and also to *medical education in both undergraduate and postgraduate fields, where doctors from other countries are trained in Australian medical schools. In addition, there is significant treatment, on a fee-for-service basis, of foreign patients.

Constitutionally, Australia is a commonwealth; it is a federation of seven states and one territory. Most matters relating to medicine and health are state-controlled. Historically, there have been state differences in the delivery of medical and hospital services since 1946, when (with a federal government funding supplement) Queensland introduced a completely free, hospital-based medical service.

In 1975, the commonwealth government instituted a national health scheme (Medibank), funded by a 1 per cent health levy on income tax assessments. This continues (since 1 February 1984 as Medicare) and provides a basic refund (as a percentage of the scheduled fee set by Government) to health practitioners, including doctors and allied health workers such as physiotherapists. Medicare does not include dental expenses.

Clinical medicine in Australia hinges on the pivot of the local *general medical practitioner (GP), over 90 per cent of whom are trained in Australia. There is a common standard of clinical medical care throughout the nation. Some 6.5 per cent of all consultations with general medical practitioners ('doctors of first contact') result in a referral to a specialist; and 2 per cent of such initial GP consultations involve secondary referral to other health professionals, such as *speech therapists, *physiotherapists, or *occupational therapists.

General and medical demography
The Australian population consists of 16.85 million people, of whom 77.6 per cent are Australian-born (Tables 1 and 2). Immigration has been a dramatic feature of the Australian demographic profile since the end of the Second World War.

Table 1 Some medico-demographic features of the Australian population

Total population	16.85 million
Aboriginal Australians and Torres Strait Islanders	238 600 (1.4% of total population)
Number of doctors	38 400
Doctor : population ratio	1:440
Percentage of population outside capital cities	43
Percentage of doctors in rural areas	23
Percentage of population having private health insurance	45

Table 2 Birthplace, by country, of the Australian population. The contemporary Australian population is more than 95 per cent Caucasian. One in every eight Australians is not Australian-born. Data derived from the 1986 *Australian Commonwealth Governments Census of Population and Housing*

Birthplace	Percentage
Australia	77.6
UK and Ireland	7.2
Asia	3.0
New Zealand and Oceania	1.7
Italy	1.6
Europe (unspecified)	1.4
Yugoslavia	1.0
Greece	0.9

There are 238 700 Australians of Aboriginal and Torres Strait Islander descent, or 1.4 per cent of the general population, currently living in Australia (1990 census figures). This group lives primarily in rural or outback communities. Infant mortality rates are higher (up to 25 per 1000 live births) and life expectancy at birth (e.g. 45 for Aboriginal males) is less for Aboriginal Australians than for those of European origin.

There are currently 38 000 doctors in Australia. Twenty-three per cent of these live outside capital or major provincial cities. Forty-three per cent of the general population live outside capital cities.

Health responsibilities
Three groups provide and control health care in Australia—the federal government, the state government, and the private sector. The federal government controls the datum of fees charged by doctors through its scheduled fees list. This is a guide only, as fees are at the discretion of individual medical practitioners. Reimbursement through the federal government's Medicare health scheme, is, however, linked to this list of scheduled fees. The federal government also controls the entry of foreign doctors into Australia; and the health standards of immigrants and health aspects of customs and quarantine. The latter is of major importance as Australia, an island continent, is free from *rabies, *cholera, and many of the tropical and subtropical viral encephalitides, and also from many of the great medical and veterinary scourges such as foot-and-mouth disease, swine fever, Newcastle disease, and anthrax. The last case of indigenous malaria occurred in 1962. All incoming air-flights to Australia are fumigated with insecticide.

The federal government provides complete health coverage for members of the armed services, and complete health care (including hospital in-patient care) to veterans of the armed services of Australia, through the health division within the Department of Veterans'

Affairs. Through the armed services, health and medical care are also provided to some overseas countries. The federal government also provides health care through aid organizations, such as the Australian Development and Assistance Bureau. This aid is targeted particularly to countries in the Indo-Asian-Pacific region. The federal government funds, and by its funding processes controls, undergraduate medical education in Australia.

State governments provide a range of health services, including the provision of government (public) hospitals, throughout the nation. These provide full in-patient and out-patient services, in a hierarchical system of referral and sophistication, with all capital cities having at least two tertiary referral hospitals. Such hospitals also provide the infrastructure for the training of medical students; and provide the infrastructure and control the training and placement of new and graduate doctors in the state (public) hospitals. Medical boards exist in all states and are arms of the state government. They set and control standards of professional competence and practice, establish registers of doctors legally entitled to practise, and supervise professional ethical and disciplinary issues. The legal implications of medical practice are controlled by medical tribunals in each state capital city, these having the status of a court-of-law. State governments also have responsibility for providing integrated medical services, such as psychiatric services, school health services, Aboriginal health services, preventive medicine, and *forensic medicine. The current trend is towards 'regionalization' throughout the various State Health Departments in Australia, with the establishment of autonomous regions (based on primary populations ranging from 100 000 to 500 000 persons). In this system of regionalization, each region (state-funded) is responsible for all aspects of preventive and clinical care, with the exception of teritary referral institutions such as high-dependency neo-natal units, spinal units, burns centres, and specialized surgical units such as those providing *cardiothoracic surgery and *neurosurgery.

There are more than 1000 local governments in Australia, and these retain responsibility for local preventive health issues relating to water supply, sewerage, food safety, and local environmental safety.

The private sector of health and medicine is very important in the Australian context. Although both major parties in the Australian political scene champion the concept of socialized medicine, the ethos at the patient level is of privately sought individual medical care. The place of the local general practitioner remains pre-eminent in the Australian health-care system, against this background. Many non-governmental institutions have evolved to provide health care for geographically or socially disadvantaged groups.

One of the most important of these non-governmental medical institutions is the Royal Flying Doctor Service (RFDS) of Australia, which was established in 1928 in Cloncurry, in Queensland. The RFDS

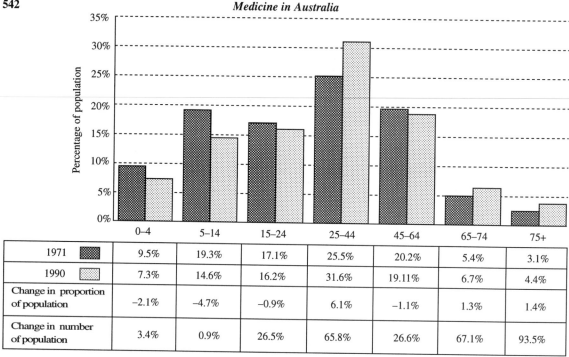

	0–4	5–14	15–24	25–44	45–64	65–74	75+
1971	9.5%	19.3%	17.1%	25.5%	20.2%	5.4%	3.1%
1990	7.3%	14.6%	16.2%	31.6%	19.11%	6.7%	4.4%
Change in proportion of population	–2.1%	–4.7%	–0.9%	6.1%	–1.1%	1.3%	1.4%
Change in number of population	3.4%	0.9%	26.5%	65.8%	26.6%	67.1%	93.5%

Age group (years)

Fig. 1 Age profile of the Australian population, with secular trends (from Birdges–Webb *et al.* 1992).

operates with up to 45 per cent federal government funding, up to 45 per cent state government funding, with the balance (in practice, between 10 and 20 per cent) raised by voluntary contributions from the Australian public. The RFDS operates from 13 bases throughout the nation. Current statistics include:

Number of Royal Flying Doctors	24
Number of nurses	48
Aircraft	37
Pilots	63
Annual patient contacts	153 000

The RFDS provides telephone medical consultations to the outback; conducts routine clinics, including *immunizations, child health clinics, *family planning consultations, and preventive medicine; medical consultations and treatment of all types; and emergency transport and treatment of the sick and injured.

Historically, much private health care was provided by various 'lodge' systems in Australia, and these have evolved to private health-insurance companies. Hundreds of disease-specific voluntary patient advocacy and support groups exist in the country. Private philanthropic funding is very important for both health care and research. The annual budget of Rotary International (Australia) now exceeds 10 million Australian dollars, specifically targeted to medical research. Similarly, Lions International (Australia) funds medical

research and patient-care facilities, targeted particularly to disease-specific areas such as eye diseases and the preservation of vision; and research into, and help with, the clinical management of patients with chronic renal disease.

Payment for health care in Australia

Total health expenditure in Australia is 25 billion Australian dollars ($25 000 000 000) (US$18.75 billion, £12.5 billion). Two-thirds of this expenditure is on patients over 60 years of age; and an estimated one-half of the total health-care expenditure occurs during the last year of life, on average during the eighth decade.

The overall cost of health care is shared almost equally between the three contributors to medicine:

Federal government	35.9%
State government	33.5%
Private sector	30.6%

The federal government contributes to health-care costs through taxation; and, from taxation and levy revenue, maintains a form of national health service (Medicare, see above). The cost of drugs is covered, in part, to 'public' patients attending general hospitals and to certain other disadvantaged members of society, under another federal government scheme called the Pharmaceuticals Benefits Scheme. This currently contributes 1600 million Australian dollars to subsidies for prescribed pharmaceutical products in Australia.

The federal government controls part-reimbursement of medical costs—consultations, allied health costs, pathology services, and surgery—through a list of scheduled fees. The principles of the Medicare scheme consist of:

1. Reimbursement to patients of 85 per cent of the scheduled fee—the patients paying their private medical practitioner in the first instance, and reclaiming costs from the government; or sending their accounts to the Government Medicare Office who will give to the patient a cheque for 85 per cent of the scheduled fee, which the patient then passes on (with the balance from his or her own purse) to the doctor concerned.
2. Doctors are encouraged not to bill patients directly, but to 'bulk bill' directly to the government. This fundamental core of socialized medicine has generally been resisted by the medical profession. Exceptions occur in the case of impecunious or other selected groups of patients; and in a number of instances where entrepreneurial medical services have been set up to take advantage of the system where no 'bad debts' occur. There has been considerable debate in this context about the risks of overservicing in such a 'bulk bill' socialized system of medicine.
3. Patients are treated free of charge in public hospitals. This point has been the subject of considerable state-to-state variation. In some states (e.g. Queensland) public hospital patients are treated free of charge without any means test, but with no Medicare documentation changing hands. In other states (e.g. New South Wales) patients are subject to a means test before treatment is offered free in public hospitals, and the federal government is billed through the Medicare system.
4. Private medical and hospital insurance is not tax-deductible. This is a point of major philosophical difference between the two major political parties in Australia. The medical profession generally strongly supports private health and medical insurance, and government measures to promote this.
5. The Medicare scheme is funded by a 1.25 per cent levy surcharge on taxable income. When introduced, the Medicare tax levy was 1 per cent on taxable income for tax payers in Australia. With the increasing sophistication of medicine and increasing costs of delivering the technology and hardware from new medical research, it is anticipated that this Medicare levy will rise inexorably.

The political philosophy of the federal government in office in Australia in the past 15 years has been socialized medicine, but with freedom of choice for patients for the selection of both doctor of first contact and

Table 3 National health-care costs in Australia, as a percentage of the total budget (from the *National Health Strategy* 1992)

Hospital costs	44
Medical costs	18
Pharmaceuticals	9
Administration	9
Nursing home	8
Dental hospital and services	5
Community health	4
Other professional services	3

for specialist referrals. A Medicare card is issued to everyone aged 16 years or older. A uniform system of scheduled fees operates in all states. Some 3.8 million Australians (of the total 16.8 million in the general population) hold pensioner cards or sickness benefit and health care cards. These provide special benefits for pharmaceutical costs; and many doctors voluntarily charge such patients the scheduled fee only.

With the inevitability of increasing costs in medicine, the principle of universal socialized medicine has had to be progressively modified. The Medicare rebate for pathology services has been lowered; private hospital bed subsidies have been abolished; and a patient contribution of $2.50 (US$1.88, £1.25) per item has been introduced for pensioners in the Pharmaceutical Benefits Scheme.

Tension has existed for the past 2 decades between the Australian Medical Association (comprising some 70 per cent of the practising medical profession in Australia) and the federal government-in-office, concerning the broad philosophies of socialized medicine, which the Australian Medical Association does not, in principle, espouse. Hospitals constitute the biggest call on the Australian health-care budget. The costs of health care are shown in Table 3.

Diseases and ill-health

The leading causes of death in Australia are summarized in Table 4. The principal international index of a nation's health, the infant mortality rate, is currently 7.1 deaths per 1000 live births, and has fallen to this level from a level of 10.5 deaths per 1000 live births, over the past decade. Infant mortality rates measure the combined effect of antenatal care of pregnant women, perinatal care of mother and infant, the incidence of congenital abnormalities, and the sudden infant death syndrome. In Australia, deaths from congenital abnormalities are 1.9 per 1000 live births, and those from the sudden infant death syndrome are 1.6 per 1000 live births. Among the young (up to age 25) violent trauma remains the major cause of death. Comparative studies of the cause of death in all age-groups are shown in Table 5.

Medical education

There are 11 undergraduate medical schools in Australia. These range in size from those with an intake of 60 students per year (e.g. Flinders University in Adelaide and the University of Tasmania in Hobart) to 240 (e.g. the University of Sydney). The criteria for selection to medical schools vary but in all such schools most students are selected by the criterion of academic achievement at the competitive matriculation examinations. All schools have subquotas for 'mature age' students, and for 'disadvantaged and refugee' students. The ethnic mix of students entering medical school does not reflect that of the general population. Sixty-five per cent of medical students at the University of Sydney are of Asian ethnic origin, whereas the figure is less than 15 per cent at the University of Tasmania.

The medical course in all Australian universities lasts 6 years, but educational philosophies differ from university to university. Some (e.g. Flinders in Adelaide and the University of Newcastle in New South Wales) adopt a 'problem-oriented' approach from the first year. Others (e.g. the universities of Melbourne and Queensland) adopt a more 'pyramidal' approach, with students learning the basic physical sciences, then the basic biological sciences, then the applied clinical sciences, and finally clinical medicine. Currently, there is a net intake of some 200 medical graduates from overseas into Australia, the equivalent of approximately the annual output of one average medical school. There is also a move towards the establishment of medical education as a postgraduate degree in Australia. Three medical schools (Sydney, Queensland, and Flinders) intend to make medicine a postgraduate degree. It is anticipated that this will be implemented in 1997 and will generally

follow the North American system (as opposed to that of Britain and Europe). Entry to these new courses will follow the acquisition of a basic BA or B.Sc., with selection by an aptitude test and personal interview. The proposed 'postgraduate' medical courses in Australia will be of 4 years' duration.

Postgraduate medical education in Australia is comprehensive and vigorous, and a full and complete postgraduate education to full registration as a specialist is available for all specialties. Such training is provided under the auspices of the various royal colleges, e.g. the Royal Australasian College of Surgeons, the Royal Australasian College of Physicians, the Australian College of Paediatrics, and many other similar professional bodies. Training in general practice is conducted by the Royal Australian College of General Practitioners and also by the (federally funded) Family Medicine Programme, a major postgraduate education scheme introduced in 1972.

Future special targeted groups for health in Australia include federal-funded programmes targeted to 'at risk' groups of special need. These include the National Aboriginal Health Strategy, the National Women's Health Programme, and the National Campaign against Drug Abuse. This last is currently funded with 33.4 million Australian dollars (US$26 million, £17 million) of federal money, annually.

The National Better Health Programme aims to achieve a better standard of health for all Australians, with an emphasis on lower socio-economic groups, and with a strong preventive medicine ethos. This programme concentrates on five priority areas—controlling high blood pressure; improving nutrition; the prevention and early detection of malignant diseases; geriatric health; and the prevention of accident injury and trauma. In recent years, this programme has had

Table 4 The eight leading causes of death in Australia (from the Australian Bureau of Statistics *Causes of death, Australia 1991*)

Cause	Standardized death rate (per 100 000 general population)	Percentage of total deaths
Malignant neoplasms	174	26.3
Ischaemic heart disease	167	25.5
Cerebrovascular disease	65	10.0
Chronic obstructive airways disease	33	5.0
All accidents and violent deaths	27	4.0
Specific motor-vehicle accidents	13	1.9
Suicides	13	2.0
Diabetes mellitus	13	1.9

Table 5 Relative percentages of the major causes of deaths, by selected age-groups, in Australia (modified from the Australian Bureau of Statistics *Causes of death, Australia 1991*)

	Age groups (years)			
	1–14	15–24	25–44	75 and over
Malignant neoplasms	14	7	24	19
Ischaemic heart disease	0	1	7	29
Cerebrovascular disease	0	1	3	14
Obstructive airways disease	2	2	1	5
Accident and trauma	42	46	20	2
All other causes	42	43	45	31
Total	100	100	100	100

annual funding of 39 million Australian dollars (US$29 million, £19.5 million), from both commonwealth and state sources.

J. PEARN

Further reading

Bridges-Webb, C., Britt, H., Miles, D. A., Neary, S., Charles, J., and Traynor, V. (1992). Morbidity and treatment in general practice in Australia 1990–1991. *Medical Journal of Australia (suppl).*, **157**, S1–S56.

Castles, I. (1992). *Causes of death. Australia 1991*. Canberra, Australian Bureau of Statistics, Catalogue No. 3303.0. Summary of findings: 1–3.

Committee of Inquiry into Medical Education and Medical Workforce Australian (Commonwealth Govt of Australia) (*The Doherty Committee*). (1988). Australian Medical Education and Workforce into the 21st Century. (*The Doherty Report*). Australian Government Publishing Service, Canberra.

Gillespie, J. A. (1991). *The price of health. Australian Government and Medical Politics 1910–1960*. Studies in Australian History Series. Cambridge University Press, Sydney.

Health Care Evaluation Branch (Department of Health, Housing, Local Government and Community Service, Commonwealth Government of Australia) (1992). *The Australian health scheme: an overview*. Dept Health, Housing, Local Government and Community Services, Canberra.

Herron, J. (1991). Current problems in health care—government criteria in resource allocation today and in the future. **31**, 351–4.

Patrick, R. (1987). *A history of health and medicine in Queensland 1824–1960, Australian and New Zealand Journal of Obstetrics and Gynaecology* p. 454. University of Queensland Press, Brisbane.

Royal Flying Doctor Service of Australia (Australia Council) (1992). *Annual report 1992*. RFDS National Office, Sydney.

Sax, S. (1990) *Health care choices and the public purse*. Allen and Unwin, Sydney.

Scotton, R. B. (1974). *Medical care in Australia*. Sun Books Melbourne (with the Applied Economic and Social Research Institute, University of Melbourne).

MEDICINE IN FRANCE
History

The formal teaching and practice of medicine in France effectively began in the city of *Montpellier, an old town in the south of France, the first city where medicine was officially developed and recognized. St Bernard reported that, from 1153, people went to Montpellier for health care. In 1220, 30 years before the university began, the first great school of medicine was founded there, with a chancellor at its head. The school of medicine was the first in Europe and students came from many countries. The most famous physicians and surgeons were de Villeneuve and Mendeville (who was Philippe le Bel's physician and wrote a treatise on surgery), and Guy de Chauliac who wrote a treatise entitled '*Grande chirurgie*'. Mendeville and Guy de Chauliac had different approaches; the former recommended suture of wounds, whereas the latter thought that wound suppuration was preferable. A second school of medicine was created in Paris in 1270.

In the succeeding centuries many famous Frenchmen illumined the history of medicine, notably Ambroise *Paré, the great surgeon who achieved much outstanding work, author of the famous sentence 'I looked after him, God cured him'; Jean *Fernel (1497–1558), who studied and taught physiology; la Mettrie and his work '*L'homme machine*'.

During the French Revolution, schools of medicine were closed and medical journals forbidden. As with all other professions, the art of healing could be practised by anyone. Medicine was in a parlous state. But, after Robespierre's fall, a physician named Foucroy protested and obtained permission from the Convention for the re-opening of three faculties (Paris, Montpellier, and Strasbourg), with the creation of chairs and professors paid by the state. The 'medicine of observation' developed, with the increasing practice of dissection. The state ordered the nomination of professors of clinics in hospitals. Childbirth became a medical discipline, and Baudelocque was given a departmental chairmanship in Paris. He created the Port-Royal maternity hospital, which is still well known. Teaching was given in French in place of Latin, and the Church no longer had authority over faculties and hospitals.

Notable figures in this intermediary period were *Pinel, head of the first French psychiatric school, who delivered mental patients from chains, and *Bichat, who identified the various tissues of the human body. Corvisart, Napoleon's physician, used percussion in thoracic disease. *Laënnec perfected *auscultation, studied *tuberculosis, and died after contracting the disease. He was a monarchist and a religious man; hence he was severely criticized by *Broussais, a republican and an atheist of violent character. Bouillaud demonstrated the relationship between rheumatism and cardiac inflammation.

At the beginning of the 19th century several French physicians enhanced the reputation of French medicine, and surgeons such as *Larrey, Desault, and *Dupuytren created a brilliant surgical school.

Due to *Magendie and, above all, Claude *Bernard (1813–78) an experimental revolution followed, with the study of many aspects of human physiology, including the recognition of the endocrine glands and the concept of function of the different organs. Bernard's *Introduction à la médecine expérimentale* (1865) became the standard reference work on physiology.

At the same time, the occurrence of great *epidemic diseases, mainly *smallpox, *cholera, *tuberculosis, and *typhoid fever, gave rise to increasing concern for *public health. Hygiene chairs were founded in every faculty. The French Academy of Medicine was founded in 1820 by Louis XVIII, with representatives of all human health disciplines: physicians, surgeons, pharmacologists, veterinarians, physicists, and chemists. Thus, in the 19th century, with so many scientists, clinicians, or researchers, France had achieved a prominent role in European medicine.

Soon afterwards research in laboratory medicine began to develop. *Pasteur (1822–95) defied the concept of spontaneous generation, very popular at this time, identified the cholera germ, and, most important of all, carried out the first vaccination against rabies. He received many distinctions and honours and became famous throughout the world as a benefactor of mankind. In 1888, the Institut Pasteur was built with public grants and research activity has continued there ever since.

Research in chemistry promoted major therapeutic developments. Pelletier and Caventou identified emetine and quinine, digitalin was discovered by Nativelle, and Pravaz perfected the use of syringes. Major advances were also made in human physiology. Marey studied human gait; Chauveau, cardiac contraction; Poiseuille and Potain, blood pressure. Because of the work of Pean, visceral surgery became a routine procedure.

Clinics continued to develop rapidly through the teaching of highly qualified clinicians such as *Dieulafoy. *Duchenne was interested in paralysis, and described a disease later called Duchenne's disease (*muscular dystrophy). *Charcot had enormous prestige and founded a great neurological school to study several diseases later named after him. Together with *Dejerine, Pierre *Marie, and *Babinski, Charcot ranks among the great pioneers of neurology in France. *Broca was also prominent in studying aphasia. *Esquirol was one of the first psychiatrists. In yet another field, Orfila created a reliable school of legal medicine, the only one in Europe. *Venereal diseases were observed by Ricord and Fournier among others.

At about this time, some physicians also became interested in preventive medicine, and Dunant created the private organization called 'la Croix Rouge' (the *Red Cross). In 1896, Imbert in Montpellier and Beclère in Paris were the first to use X-rays in clinical practice, and Beclère organized training in *radiology in Paris. Later, Pierre and Marie *Curie discovered radium.

Meanwhile, the Institut Pasteur had become a great centre for biological research. In 1921, the introduction of a vaccine against tuberculosis (*BCG) by *Calmette and *Guérin was a major development. A student of Pasteur, *Metchnikoff, inaugurated the first steps in immunology, and was soon followed by Fernand Widal and Charles *Richet. D'Arsonval contributed new knowledge in *medical physics, Nicolle and Deve made important contributions to parasitology.

In 1902, in France, several new laws introduced an important new system of *public health, *hygiene, compulsory protective inoculations, social security, and the foundation of an international office of public health.

Recent developments in medical education, care, and organization

During the second part of the 20th century, many advances have been made in medical knowledge and techniques which cannot be adequately summarized here. To mention only a few, they include a vaccine against *poliomyelitis (Lépine 1954), the discovery of the *HLA system (Dausset 1958), the relationship between *Down's syndrome and *chromosome 21 (Turpin and Lejeune 1959), advances in the clinical treatment of mental diseases (Delay and Deniker 1952), new developments in nephrology (Hamburger), and the introduction of organ transplantation.

In 1958, at Robert Debré's instigation, the practice of public medicine in university hospitals was, for the first time, controlled by law. According to law, physicians must comply with three tasks, namely, patient care, medical education, and research. Great hospitals became centres of training and research. Two systems of medicine, public and private, became more or less smoothly complementary.

In 1968, following major student unrest, the official university organization was modified; chairs were changed into flexible professorships and hospital physicians into hospital practitioners. For the first time, faculties became teaching and research units (Unités d'enseignement et de recherche, UER) and later units of training and research (Unités de formation et de Recherche, UFR). The medical curriculum was extensively modified. The former system (*externat* and *internat des hôpitaux*—externship and internship) was replaced by a system which is supposed to be more democratic, with no '*externat*' examination, but an '*internat*' examination with a limited number of places in specialized medicine and an 'internship' in general medicine for all students.

The present medical system is very complex. There are private hospitals or clinics and public hospitals, called university hospitals in towns where a university is situated and regional hospitals in other towns. There is also an intermediate system in private, non-profit hospitals. The practice of private medicine requires the degree of doctor in medicine. In public medicine, postgraduate students are appointed assistant residents, university lecturers, '*chefs de cliniques*' (assistant professors for 2 years, renewable), hospital practitioners (either full-time or part-time), and professors of the university at three levels (first class, second class, exceptional, and with other levels in each class).

Hospital health care is run by an administration called '*l'assistance publique*' (public health care) with a general manager appointed who cannot be a medical practitioner. The UER manager elected as dean of the school of medicine is responsible for university medical teaching and postgraduate education. The medical council of the hospital plays an advisory role alongside the manager of '*l'assistance publique*'.

Graduate and postgraduate examinations are organized in the UFR under the control of professors. The '*concours d'internat*' varies according to modalities which are increasingly modified towards a regional organization. University hospital practitioners, or professors, are nominated by the CNU (National Council of the Universities), which includes elected and appointed members organized in sections and subsections.

The National Institute for Medical Research (INSERM), runs several laboratories partly related to, and situated in, the university hospital system; the managers of units are sometimes independent. In the same way, a number of research laboratories of the National Centre for Scientific Research, CNRS, are staffed by university hospital practitioners.

The 'order of physicians' (ordre des médecins—the regulatory authority) is divided into a national order and regional orders, and deals mainly with the legal and ethical aspects of the medical profession.

Training sessions are organized by regional associations, providing postgraduate medical training to give practitioners up-to-date information on medical knowledge and new techniques. The practice of private medicine is not age limited, whereas in hospitals, the age limit is 65 years.

French medicine is presently among the best in the world in many fields. Research activity is well developed in several centres concerned with major current medical problems. The health and social security system ensures social protection. The state is responsible for legislation and bears overall responsibility for health care. This responsibility is divided between two ministries: the Ministry of Health and the Ministry of Education, which is responsible for the university-level education of health professionals. Recently, a ministry of high-level education and research has been created, which carries the responsibility of defining the priorities in various fields of research, of following major advances, and of adapting and modernizing medical education.

GEORGES SERRATRICE

MEDICINE IN GERMANY, AUSTRIA, AND SWITZERLAND
The countries
The present Federal Republic of Germany (FRG) was forged in 1990 through the union of the old FRG, or West Germany (which comprised 62.7 million inhabitants and 11 states, or *Länder*, including West Berlin), and the German Democratic Republic (GDR), or East Germany (which had been a centralized state of 16.4 million inhabitants and which now consists of five additional federal *Länder*). The diametrically opposed forms of political organization in East and West Germany after 1945 gave rise to two completely different health-care systems. Since 1990 all legal and administrative precepts of the old FRG have also applied to the five new *Länder* created on the territory of the former GDR, but a number of important dissimilarities still exist and must be kept in mind in the following account.

The Republic of Austria with its current borders has existed as a federal state essentially since 1918, when the Hapsburg monarchy collapsed after the First World War. The country consists of nine *Länder* (provinces, or states) and a population of 7.8 million (1991). Switzerland, largely unchanged since the 16th century, has been a federal state since 1848, is composed of 26 cantons, and has a population of 6.8 million (1990). Additional general demographic data are given in Table 1.

In the 9th and 10th centuries, what eventually came to be known as the Holy Roman Empire of the German Nation emerged from the partitioning and gradual dissolution of the Carolingian empire after Charlemagne's reign. As Christianization in Europe proceeded, the empire extended further and further eastward, chiefly along the Baltic coast, throughout the 12th century. In the 14th century, its dominions stretched nearly to present-day St Petersburg, encompassing what is now Germany, Austria, Switzerland, the Czech Republic, eastern France, the Low Countries, and parts of northern and central Italy.

In 1291, three of Switzerland's original cantons formed a league that became the nucleus of the Swiss Confederation. It grew in the wake of the Reformation and was virtually independent of the empire from 1499 on. Exacerbated by the wars of the Reformation in the 17th century, devolution of the Holy Roman Empire continued until approximately 300 principalities, dioceses, and free imperial cities existed within its borders. Austria remained the single major power and ruled vast territories of southern Europe for hundreds of years. Besides Austria, Saxony and Bavaria were the

Table 1 Life expectancy in Germany, Austria, and Switzerland

Country	Life expectancy at birth (in years)				Population (%) 1990	
	1950–54		1989		0–14 Years	>65 Years
	Male	Female	Male	Female		
Germany						
FRG	65.3	69.4	72.6	79.2	15.1	15.4
GDR	66.2	70.8	70.1	76.4	19.7	13.1
Austria	63.6	68.6	72.1	78.9	17.4	15.0
Switzerland	67.7	71.7	74.1	81.3	16.4	15.0

only German-speaking regions of relative note in terms of wealth and population. Not until the rise of Prussia in the course of the 18th century did the Hapsburg monarchy of Austria have to contend with a military and political rival as well. After liberation from Napoleonic supremacy in 1814, Prussia gradually grew to become the predominant and, in the 1860s, the prevailing political force in the unification of Germany.

Wars fought under this Prussian leadership shifted Germany's political boundaries repeatedly. They expanded northward towards Denmark in 1864 and westwards towards France in 1870–71, culminating in the German Empire, often called the Second Reich (empire) to indicate its descent from the Holy Roman Empire of medieval times. In the First World War this Reich, too, spread eastwards—into Polish, Czech, Slovak, and Russian regions.

The end of the First World War saw the disintegration of the multi-ethnic Hapsburg empire. It was carved into several independent states, Austria itself becoming a republic with borders much as they are today. The defeated German Empire also vanished and was superseded by a republic in 1918 and, in 1933, by a third empire—the Third Reich.

In the reorganization of Europe after the allied victory over Germany in the Second World War, considerable areas of the Third Reich in the east were ceded to, and subsequently integrated into, the Soviet Union and Poland. These regions, which no longer have German-speaking population groups, became indisputable parts of those two countries upon the signing of the peace treaties formally ending the Second World War. The two German states established in 1949, the FRG and the GDR, each existed as a part of its respective postwar power bloc, the capitalist West and the socialist East. The border between the blocs separated West and East Germany and, for a time, divided the world in half.

A brief history of medicine

Medical activity goes back as far as our first human ancestors, a fact deduced from the 100 000-year-old bones of *Homo sapiens neanderthalensis*, some of whose remains have been discovered in Germany. Humans wounded or crippled when young were able to survive for up to 60 years of age, although they undoubtedly required intensive care and help both during their affliction and long thereafter.

The earliest documents from German-speaking areas show that Benedictine canon of the 6th century required all monasteries to have rooms especially set aside as an infirmary. Ground plans of the monastery at St Gallen, dated to the 9th century, designated such sick rooms, along with a separate kitchen, separate bath, a herb garden, physician's quarters, and a building for bloodletting.

In the 12th century, after the monasteries had been the main centres of medical activity for centuries, intense discussion of clerical medical activity was prompted at several councils, because of the mortal danger posed by operations performed by physicians. From 1215 on, clerics were prohibited from performing surgery and were denied even the right to receive medical training. For centuries thereafter, theoretical medical studies at the university were strictly disassociated from the various surgical techniques, which were not practised by physicians. Simultaneously, the functions relating to the further development of medicine passed from the clergy to the temporal schools of classical medicine in the universities being founded at that time.

One cannot overestimate the impact of serious *epidemics, above all, the *plagues. The first great wave of plague reached Germania in the 6th century AD. The second plague epidemic in central Europe, which raged between 1347 and 1532, coincided with a 30 per cent mortality rate in the population as a whole. As in Nuremberg and Strasbourg in 1349, it led, among other things, to fanatical pogroms directed primarily against the adherents of the Israelite faith, who were held responsible for the calamity. Other *infectious diseases, particularly *leprosy, led to the banishment of many people. In the 14th century, there were centres in Constance and Cologne to which people diagnosed (in effect, condemned) as having leprosy were obliged to travel in order to be committed to special *hospitals for life. Hospitals were established and run throughout the German-speaking realm as far as Ebling on the Baltic Sea (in today's Poland), mostly by the knightly orders that originated during the Crusades.

The first German universities—Prague (1348), Vienna (1365), and Heidelberg (1386)—offered formal medical studies lasting 4–5 years, though the courses consisted solely of theoretical lectures. In the hospitals, however, physicians had no significance whatsoever for centuries to come. Not until the 16th century do records indicate the presence of permanently employed hospital physicians. Before that time, few towns had their doctors look after hospital patients as well, and even then just occasionally.

In the field of medicine, the renaissance of the sciences in the 16th century is inseparably linked with the name of Andreas *Vesalius (1514–64), who came from a family originally from Wesel on the Lower Rhine. He travelled throughout Europe during his years of study and, at 30 years of age, continued to do so as personal physician to Charles V and, later, to Philip II. He can be regarded as the father of modern anatomy and, hence, of knowledge about the morphology and structure of the human body.

One of Vesalius's key contemporaries in medical thought was a man from the Swiss town of Einsiedeln, Theophrast von Hohenheim (1493–1541), known as *Paracelsus. Paracelsus became an outspoken critic of the traditional concept that the maintenance of health depended upon the harmony of the four bodily *humours—blood, phlegm, choler (yellow bile), and melancholy (black bile). At one point he served as town physician in Basel, and was active for some time in various cities in southern Germany, Switzerland, and Austria between Nuremberg and Vienna. Challenging long-unquestioned notions about the origins of diseases, he advocated the *experimenta ac ratio*—personal experience and one's own thinking.

The medical breakthroughs crucial to the further development of the field in the German-speaking world came from Vienna in the latter half of the 18th century. They included the regular observation of patients, the continual examination and pathological–morphological tracking of the clinical course of diseases, and discriminating diagnostic methods using technical aids. Yet another contribution by Viennese medicine came from the obstetrician Ignaz *Semmelweiss (1818–65). As the first person to realize that dreaded childbed fever (sepsis) coincided with infections conveyed by a physician's hands, he developed the basic principles of *asepsis.

One of the pre-eminent bases for *homoeopathy, a widely practised tenet of medicine in Germany, is vitalism's concept of health and disease, which constituted the climax of 18th century experiments in theoretical medicine. It was substantiated by the Thuringian Christoph Hufeland (1762–1836), a personal physician at the royal court in Berlin in the early 19th century and chief physician of the Collegium Medico-chirurgicum, which predated Berlin's university.

The century of the Enlightenment, the era of enlightened absolutism, also marked the birth of the modern hospital. The advent of this new philosophy, in which medicine was deemed a servant of the state, can be seen as the occasion for the building of the first state hospitals, such as the *Charité in Berlin in 1727. The new state health institutions also assisted the universities in teaching. In addition, medicine promoted the health of people working in the burgeoning manufacturing sector. The fundamental elements of health care and social welfare were laid down as 'medical policy' by the Viennese physician Johann Peter Frank (1745–1821).

The principles of physiology as an empirical science are associated with Johannes *Müller (1801–58) and his school of thought in Berlin. Berlin was also home to Rudolf *Virchow (1821–1902), who pioneered the modern concept of pathological processes—by emphasizing that diseases arose not in organs or tissues in general but in their individual cells—and tirelessly campaigned for socially responsible health policy derived from medical knowledge. Another figure from the international heyday of medicine in Berlin was Robert *Koch (1843–1910), who discovered many pathogens of prevalent diseases and did more than anyone to establish the science of *bacteriology.

In the early 1880s, protracted disputes with a strong labour movement led the chancellor of the German Reich, Otto von Bismarck, to initiate uniform social legislation aimed at providing workers with extensive accident protection, health care, old-age insurance, and disability benefits. In the health policy of many countries today, it still serves as a model of comprehensive social welfare.

The organization of health care
General
The health-care systems of the FRG, Austria, and Switzerland have many features in common. Unlike their counterparts in eastern Europe and many countries of western Europe, they are not state-run. Instead, they are based on statutory social insurance, meaning that the government itself has little political authority and responsibility for shaping it directly. By virtue of the federal system, a number of those competencies lie with the states and cantons and with local authorities. The independence of the lower administrative echelons is greatest in Switzerland and least in Austria.

The most sweeping statutory and state-monitored social insurance is in Austria, where it embraces 99.8 per cent of the population. The system is both compulsory and comprehensive, guaranteeing broad coverage in case of illness. The system has 19 sickness funds, which are regionally and directly responsible above all for a few large hospitals and a small number of professional units, and which are run by the beneficiaries themselves. In Germany 90 per cent of the population has statutory health insurance, which is carried by 1164 health sickness funds (1990). The majority of the remaining population is also covered against costs and risks to income in case of illness. In Switzerland it is true that merely 30 per cent of the population, including the sizeable group composed of all foreign workers who have temporary residence permits, are compulsory members of one of the some 375 recognized sickness funds created for this purpose, but 95–98 per cent of the Swiss are protected by some sort of health insurance. Unlike their counterparts in Austria and Germany, however, Swiss patients must carry a substantial share of the costs directly: 10 per cent of all out-patient medical charges and costs of medication as well as other fees, and all benefits in kind for accidents and dental treatment. The expenses of hospital services in particular must be met by optional supplementary insurance.

For lack of space, this article will focus mainly on the health-care system in Germany. However, apart from the characteristics already mentioned, the situation in the other two countries does differ in important respects. In Austria, for example, in-patient and out-patient health care are not strictly differentiated, as is the case in Germany. On the whole, the medical associations in Austria have less influence on the structure of health care than they do in Germany, so most hospitals are able to give professional medical

Table 2 Development of the relationship between generalists and specialists within the group of private physicians, and total of all physicians in the Federal Republic of Germany before 3 October 1990

	1960	1970	1980	1990
Private physicians				
General practitioners	27 592	25 539	26 853	31 837
Specialists	15 026	20 763	32 924	43 414
Total	42 618	46 302	59 777	75 251
All physicians	74 486	92 773	139 452	195 254

treatment to out-patients. Similarly, most Swiss hospitals can help treat out-patients. One peculiarity is that medication can be dispensed by the practising physicians themselves, the number of whom is growing. In 1981 one-third of Switzerland's private physicians accounted for approximately 20 per cent of the sales of medicaments in the country. The strong position of the chemical and pharmaceutical industry is considered responsible for this.

The health-care system in detail

In Germany, government facilities represent only a tiny share of the health-care institutions, which are customarily set up and run by private or independent non-profit (charitable) organizations. All out-patient care is handled exclusively by private physicians. Table 2 summarizes the ratio of private physicians to specialists.

It is clear from this table that the *specialists outnumber the *general practitioners, and that this disproportion has swelled with the vast increase in the total number of doctors, and the static population growth. Because all patients have free direct access to all private physicians, much family-doctor care is undertaken also by specialists, notably internists, *paediatricians, *gynaecologists, and to some extent, by *orthopaedic surgeons, dermatologists, and *psychiatrists. Private physicians own their own practices, including all the equipment, and are the employers of the personnel working for them. All private physicians caring for patients covered by statutory sickness funds are part of the Association of Sickness Fund Physicians, an organization administered by the physicians themselves. The Association of Sickness Fund Physicians monitors the bills written by the physicians and pays the individual physicians for their services, using a schedule of fees to distribute the total lump sum allocated to it by the sickness funds. This system of payment, which is based essentially on compensation for individual services rendered, has been heavily criticized in recent years because it has been shown to inflate the volume of medical services in relation to the number of licensed physicians. At the end of 1992, physicians were practically unrestricted in setting themselves up in private practice.

The hospitals solely responsible for in-patient care are organized by three main groups of institutions: public (cities and local communities), independent non-profit (such as Church-affiliated organizations and the German Red Cross), and private. For historical reasons, the share of hospital beds represented by each of these three groups varies in the *Länder* of the FRG. Whereas public institutions account for the biggest share in the *Länder* of northern Germany and those of eastern Germany (i.e. the GDR until 3 October 1990), independent, non-profit institutions constitute the largest share in western and southern Germany (see Table 3).

Except for the 35 university hospitals, hospitals give out-patient treatment in emergencies only. Under certain circumstances, psychiatric care and out-patient operations are possible (for cost reasons). In recent decades the number of hospital beds has steadily declined, for medical innovations have provided ways to treat many diseases satisfactorily on an out-patient footing. Table 4 presents some of the data on hospital services.

The hospitals are financed through the 'dual system'. Construction and capital costs for major equipment are

Table 3 Number of hospitals and hospital beds in Germany before 3 October 1990

	Former FRG	Former GDR	Total
Public			
Hospitals	897	339	1 236
Beds	282 076	143 996	426 072
Charitable			
Hospitals	978	75	1 053
Beds	216 286	10 921	227 207
Private			
Hospitals	1 006	2	1 008
Beds	107 437	260	107 697
Grand total			
Hospitals	3 092	418	3 510
Beds	660 735	156 957	817 692

Table 4 Hospital services in Germany before 3 October 1990

Service	No. in the FRG	No. in the GDR	Total
Beds			
1970	683 254	190 025	873 279
1990	660 735	156 957	817 692
In-patients treated			
1970	8 871 018	2 312 772	11 183 790
1990	13 194 122	2 444 415	15 638 537
Patient days			
1970	220 826 000	56 316 000	274 725 000
1990	208 576 000	42 579 000	251 950 000
In-patients treated per 1000 inhabitants			
1970	154.0	–	–
1989	213.3	–	–
Hospital beds per 10 000 inhabitants			
1970	112.0	–	–
1990	106.9	–	–
Average length of stay (in days)			
1970	24.9	23.3	24.6
1990	15.8	17.8	16.1
Average utilization of beds (%)			
1970	88.5	81.2	86.9
1990	86.5	73.7	84.2

covered by the government, provided that the hospitals are included in the hospital supply plan administered by the health minister of the *Land* in question. In each *Land* this schedule is reviewed and readopted every few years. It contains the state's input on the need for beds in the individual specialties as projected on the basis of demographic development, primarily age cohorts, and the other health-care institutions involved. A hospital's running costs (e.g. salaries and non-durable medical supplies) are met by the hospital allowance to be paid by the sickness funds. This allowance is a lump sum paid per bed per day of hospital confinement, and is normally the same for all departments of the hospital. It is negotiated between the representatives of the hospital associations and the statutory sickness funds. The hospital must document its ordinary business expenses so that the sickness funds can approve the allowance for the following calendar year.

The *public health service is left basically with supervisory and preventive functions. One of its supervisory responsibilities is to monitor all health institutions for compliance with hygiene regulations, building codes, and other provisions. The public health service is also concerned with monitoring infectious diseases and, increasingly, with gathering data for the health-assessment reporting being developed in the *Länder*. A great defect of the manner in which data are presently gathered is that no relationship can be established between, for instance, mortality and living conditions.

One of the central prevention-oriented responsibilities of the public health service is to give check-ups to pre-school and school-aged children, as well as to support and promote health awareness.

Health-care funds are raised by legally established provident institutions, namely, those dealing with statutory health insurance, statutory accident insurance, statutory retirement insurance, and statutory unemployment insurance. In essence, these institutions arose from the disputes between the state and the labour movement during the industrialization of Germany in the latter half of the 19th century. Since its advent in the 1880s, the social safety net has been extended to nearly all occupational groups. By the 1960s practically 98 per cent of the population had total coverage. Either for reasons of occupational status or because of income that falls below an income-adjusted threshold set annually by the government, 90 per cent of the population is covered by statutory health insurance. All unemployed family members are insured as well. An additional 9 per cent of the population is either entitled to total state health coverage as civil servants or is voluntarily insured by statutory or private health insurance. Health-insurance benefits cover:

(1) all treatment by physicians and dentists;
(2) drugs, with a mandatory additional payment of up to approximately 10 per cent;
(3) dentures, up to approximately 50 per cent of the cost;

Table 5 Development of expenditures on health benefits in the Federal Republic of Germany before 3 October 1990

Year	Total health benefits (in million DM)	Percentage of GNP	Compulsory sickness funds (in million DM)
1970	70 596	6.4	24 712
1980	195 661	9.2	88 427
1989	276 807	9.2	127 579

* DM = £2.40

(4) medication and adjuvants, between 90 and 100 per cent of the cost (e.g. *physiotherapy, spectacles, and artificial limbs);

(5) hospitalization, up to 100 per cent (with a comparatively small mandatory additional payment of no more than DM 121 per year); and

(6) sickness benefits up to approximately 80 per cent of the patient's income (in cases of protracted illness, disbursement begins on the day that the patient's salary is no longer paid by the employer—for most employees, after 6 weeks).

Total expenditure on health benefits has soared in recent decades, but their percentage of West Germany's gross national product has remained about the same (see Table 5).

The current discussion of health policy revolves mainly around four problems:

1. The volume of out-patient services is steadily increasing because the number of physicians has continued to grow whereas the population at large has not.

2. The inordinately high percentage of specialists among the physicians is leading to an excessive number of unnecessary and expensive diagnostic and therapeutic measures.

3. Physicians are prescribing too many drugs whose effectiveness has not been proven, whose effects are even classified as rather detrimental, or whose use by the patient is altogether negligible.

4. The health-insurance system is burdened by the growing share of old people who can no longer look after themselves adequately. They do not actually need long-term medical treatment but are hospitalized anyway for lack of other facilities (such as affordable accommodation designed to permit care for elderly occupants). This issue is to be solved by the introduction of insurance, conceived specifically to provide for such care.

UDO SCHAGEN

Further reading

Abholz, H. -H. *et al.* (ed.). *Jahrbücher für kritische Medizin.* [*Yearbooks for critical medicine*], 2 vols per year, 1970–93. Argument, Hamburg.

Federal Minister for Labor and Social Affairs (ed.) (1991). *Übersicht über die soziale Sicherheit* [*Survey of the social safety net*]. Bundesminister für Arbeit und Sozialordnung, Bonn.

Schneider, M. *et al.* (1992). *Gesundheitssysteme im internationalen Vergleich* [*An international comparison of health systems*]. BASYS, Augsburg.

MEDICINE IN GREECE
The Pre-Hippocratic (or Homeric) period

Ancient Greek medicine derived knowledge from many older sources. Greeks, because of their geographical location, were exposed to the influence of Egyptian, Babylonian, Mesopotamian, Phoenician, and Minoan (Cretian) civilizations. They also learned from ancient Jewish medicine.

Pre-Hippocratic medicine was connected with Greek mythology and the temples of *Aesculapius, the god of medicine. Aesculapius was the patriarch of a large family, who had health and medical functions: his wife, Epione, soothed pain; his daughter, Panacea, had a cure for everything; Hygeia, another daughter, whose domain was public health and the prevention of disease, fed the temple serpents; Telesphorus cared for convalescents; Podalirius was an army surgeon and psychiatrist; and, lastly, Machaon was the surgeon of whom Homer wrote in a famous line of the *Iliad* (II. XI: 514): 'A doctor is a man worth many others'.

The Hippocratic period

The mythological period of Greek medicine was followed by a long, sacerdotal period with priest–physicians. Aesculapius left numerous successors, the Asclepiades, who continued his work. Their activities were mainly psychotherapeutic and were practised in health centres situated near the sea, or near springs in several regions by the Mediterranean Sea.

Along with sacerdotal medicine, a kind of secular medicine also developed, and under the influence of naturalist philosophers—often named 'physiologists'—medicine progressively lost its religious character. Consequently, the Aesculapian medicine of the Ionian school in Asia Minor, the Pythagorean school of Croton in Magna Graecia (now southern Italy), the Empiricism of the school of Cnidos were the precursors of the Hippocratic period.

Hippocratic medicine was founded in the 5th century BC on the basis of Greek physical philosophy. The most important difference between Pre-Hippocratic and Hippocratic physicians was that the former were solely respected craftsmen, the latter both craftsmen and philosopher–physicians.

*Hippocrates the Coan (Fig. 1) (born around 460 BC), was the founder of scientific medicine which flourished in Pericles' 'golden age' of Greece. This was a true medical philosophy, different from religion, metaphysics, and pure philosophy. Hippocrates declared that 'the philosopher–physician is equal to the gods' (ἰηρός γάρ φιλόζοφος ἰζόδεος); nature was 'the teacher of all teachers' and 'the physician of our diseases', and he viewed the doctor as 'Nature's helper'. He observed diseases with the eye of a naturalist and established rules by which the physician would know what to expect and what to do at the right time.

His monumental work *Corpus Hippocraticus*, consisting of about 60 treatises (although evidently the work of many medical writers, Hippocrates must have been the author of those valued most highly), offered for the first time a combination of medicine, science, and human art, also relating professional medicine to medical ethics. Evidence was also provided on the growth of scientific enquiry in early Greek thought.

*The Hippocratic Oath, although just one page long, is a monumental code of medical ethics, which established the pattern of deontology (ethics) of the medical profession throughout the ages.

Hippocrates based his medical doctrine on three principles: the patient is a psychosomatic entity, disease is governed by rules, and the physician is nature's helper and a servant of the medical art.

The following Hippocratic messages are most important and valuable even to current medicine: 'The physician must investigate the entire patient and his environment'; 'The physician must assist nature which is the physician of the diseases'; 'For where there is love of man there is also love for the medical art'; 'The physician must benefit and not harm the patients'; 'The physician must co-operate with the patient, with the patient's attendants and external circumstances'; 'Nothing happens without a natural cause'; and 'Medicine is the most noble of all arts'.

Twenty-five centuries later, his teachings are still of great importance, not only in medicine but also in specific aspects referring to the ecology of the environment and atmospheric pollution. Also, his teaching that 'What drugs will not cure, the knife will; what the knife will not cure, the cautery will; what the cautery will not cure must be considered incurable' had a prophetic value for modern surgery in the treatment of coronary artery and other diseases. Furthermore, the recent tendency towards predictive medicine is well illustrated in his work 'on predictions' and the example of a patient who was about to die and for whom the physician made the predictive diagnosis: 'This man is not going to die, but is going to become blind'.

His first aphorism contains the essence of Hippocratic philosophy: 'Life is short; and the art long; and the

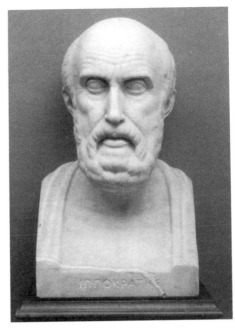

Fig. 1 Hippocrates (by permission of the International Hippocratic Foundation of Cos).

right time an instant; and treatment precarious; and the judgement difficult. It is necessary for the physician not only to provide the needed treatment but to provide for the patient himself and for those beside him and to provide for his outside affairs'.

Hellenistic (Alexandrine) period

After Hippocrates' death, his doctrine continued to flourish and also to influence philosophical thinking, as evidenced by the most reliable authorities such as Plato (427–347 BC), *Aristotle (384–322 BC), and his pupil Theophrastus (372–287 BC). Aristotle, the philosopher, was the son of a physician to the King of Macedonia, a pupil of Plato, and a tutor of Alexander the Great in Macedonia. Aristotle's main psychosocial doctrines were influenced by Plato, who is regarded as 'the follower of Hippocrates' and who was, in turn, influenced by Socrates (470–399 BC), a contemporary of Hippocrates. According to *Galen, Aristotle's teleological treatment of the parts of the organism was derived basically from Hippocrates. Aristotle contributed greatly to the development of *embryology, and believed that the spirit (or pneuma), which is part of the soul, does not depend on any organ. On the other hand, his treatise *History of animals* reveals his great knowledge and talent in animal anatomy, which justly gave him the title 'Father of Zoology'. With the 'Father of the Science of Botany', Theophrastus, the purely biological school of Aristotle may have come to an end

Alexander the Great, Macedonian King and conqueror (356–323 BC), a pupil of Aristotle, was among his most famous disciples. The Alexandrian school replaced the schools of Cnidos and Cos, for two principal reasons: first, Alexandria, with its famous library and its invaluable museum, served as the meeting place of the most eminent scholars of the world, thus becoming a new Athens; secondly, the dissection of human bodies was legalized—old 'taboos' collapsed and Alexandria became the capital of anatomy and physiology.

*Herophilus and *Erasistratus (3rd–4th centuries BC) were among the most celebrated physicians of the Alexandrian school. Herophilus, influenced by the school of Cos, was more of an anatomist than a physiologist, while Erasistratus, influenced by the school of Cnidos, was more of a physiologist. Their medical knowledge was not only because of their access to the library of Alexandria, but also because of many years practising the dissection of human bodies. Although rivals, their remarks and discoveries complemented each other. Both of them, spirited with the ambition that Greek science should embrace the world in its entirety and in unity, tried and successfully imposed their principles on medicine by teaching that 'the only fruitful medical method of thinking is that which views man in his entirety'.

The high standards and value of medicine in the Hellenistic period are shown by the fact that *anatomy and *physiology did not make any significant progress in the 400 years separating Herophilus and Erasistratus from Galen (2nd century AD).

Greco-Roman (Galenic) period

The Greco-Roman period of medicine is marked by Galen (Clarissimus Galenus) who was born (around AD 129) in Pergamos of Asia Minor and became famous as a physician in Rome in the Emperor's court. His Latin name, Galenus, comes from the Greek *'galenios'* which means serene or calm. The so-called 'prince of physicians' was also a prolific writer. He said that 'true medicine is the friend of moderation and the discipline of truth'. He was interested in, and made significant contributions to, many medical disciplines, such as anatomy and physiology (which were inseparable for him), *pathology, and therapeutics. Galen admired and carefully studied Hippocrates: 'Hippocrates showed the road, but as he was the first who discovered it, he could not go as far as he had wished.' Galen's physiology was greatly influenced by the fashionable Hippocratic theory of the four humours. The work of Hippocrates was more synthetic, whereas that of Galen was more analytical. A fundamental difference was that illness was located in an organ or a system for Galen, while illness was something of a general affliction according to Hippocrates.

Galen's ideas dominated medical thought far into the 16th century and can be considered as precursors of modern experimental medicine.

Byzantine period

Many historians report that after Galen, medicine experienced a period of decadence and made no progress in the years of the Byzantine Empire.

It is often stated that medicine in this period ceased to be scientific, experimental, or philosophical, and instead became dogmatic under the influence of Christianity, and that there were no famous physicians.

This is not correct, as is illustrated by Oribasius, a native of Galen's birthplace, who studied medicine in Alexandria, discovered many new diagnostic and therapeutic medical and surgical methods, was an enemy of empirical medicine, and established himself as an eminent physician of this period.

Byzantine medicine, dominated by the spirit of 'love for one's neighbour', was profoundly humanitarian but also Galenic and Hippocratic in character. It preserved the tradition of Hellenic medicine and passed it on into western Europe. It supported social welfare and the development of hospital medicine. New cures were discovered. Christianity appreciated the importance of human life and started a new period of hope and giving, as summarized by the word 'caritas' (charity).

Neo-Hellenic period

Modern Greece was officially recognized as a sovereign and independent country in 1830, 9 years after the revolution leading to liberation from 400 years of Turkish rule.

Physicians initially were heterogeneous, insufficient and unequally distributed. They were: physicians who had practised medicine during the Turkish occupation; foreign physicians, postgraduates mainly of European medical schools, who came to Greece to help with the revolution and stayed after the liberation; Greek national physicians from Europe who returned to Greece; Bavarian physicians and pharmacists serving in the Greek royal court of the Bavarian king; and, finally, empirical physicians who were licensed by the government to practise medicine.

During the Turkish occupation, many talented young Greeks studied medicine in renowned French and Italian universities, with financial support of Greek communities abroad and philhellenes (friends of Greece). Alexandros Mavrokordatos (17th century), Emmanouil Timonis, and Iakovos Pilarinos (who in the 18th century described a method for the prevention of smallpox) were among the most famous of them.

The first medical school (1837) and the Athens Medical Society (1835) were fundamental in the development of medicine in Greece. Many of the new Greek medical graduates continued their studies either in France and Germany (19th century) or in Britain and the USA (20th century). George *Papanicolaou (Pap test) of Cornell University, is one of many examples.

There are today seven medical schools in Greece, which produce more physicians than are needed. This is in addition to those who study medicine abroad either for a better education or because of failing local entry exams. This has now created a crisis, with 35 000 medical specialists or non-specialists (only 450 have the specialty of a general physician) for a population of 10 000 000 people. Specialists with unequal degrees of medical skill and experience are unequally distributed, with half of them practising in the capital, Athens. Despite some recent improvements, medical care outside the big cities is often appalling. Most Greeks seek medical advice and treatment in the big cities, mainly Athens and Thessaloniki. The crisis of confidence between people and physicians is reflected by the large number of patients who travel abroad, hoping for better management and even cure. This happens despite the availability of some excellent modern and well-equipped hospitals with highly qualified physicians in Greece. Nearly all Greeks have medical insurance, which is usually job-related; there are over 10 major organizations, such as IKA (Organization for social security), OGA (Organization for Agricultural Insurance), and other similar bodies for civil servants, bankers, etc. Private medicine is flourishing and practised by nearly all. Recent legislation does not allow physicians employed in state hospitals to practise privately; those in academic medical positions do. In 1983 a National Health System (NHS) was introduced by the Socialist Government. Most private non-profit making hospitals were nationalized. New private profit-making hospitals were outlawed and the existing ones were not allowed to expand or to change their services. Private bed numbers fell from 42 per cent of the total in 1980 to 30 per cent in 1990 but privately owned high technology diagnostic medical centres flourished. Also, the terms of medical employment have changed. The lack of organization of medical care and the influence of factors other than qualifications and efficiency in the appointment of senior medical, academic and administrative staff have a negative influence upon practice and especially upon academic medicine, despite the evident high potential for improvement and devoted physicians. As a compensation, a great number of Greek physicians distinguish themselves abroad in keeping with their tradition, as exemplified by Galen who was born in Pergamos, studied medicine in Alexandria, and became famous in Rome.

S. G. MARKETOS
C. P. PANAYIOTOPOULOS

MEDICINE IN ITALY
History
Choler, *melancholia, and *phlegm are words still in use today. Pythagoras introduced them in the 6th century BC, while teaching at his famous medical school in Crotone, at that time Magna Graecia, on the humours that influence human behaviour. Among the followers of Pythagoras, Empedocles from Agrigento, an anatomist, embryologist, and physician, was possibly the most illustrious, his reputation still living well into the Middle Ages.

Besides its impact on the Magna Graecia medical culture, Greek influence was also predominant in Roman medicine, as *Celsus points out in his *De re medica* (*c.* AD 30), an historical appraisal and a *summa* of the medical and surgical knowledge of his time, highly considered as a textbook right up to Renaissance times. *Galen, who worked in Rome in the 2nd century AD, was of Greek origin. Very few men have influenced the progress of medical sciences as Galen did.

It is hard to separate history from legend in assessing the evidence of medical achievements in the Dark Ages.

Perhaps the most important factor was the spread of Christianity, which emphasized giving help and relief to sufferers as one of the works of mercy. Benedictine monks were particularly active in this field: hospices and hospitals were built along the main routes of the early Middle Ages, to assist travellers and pilgrims. Some still exist, while traces of others can still be found in place names today.

The Crusades prompted the institution of the Knights Hospitalers' Orders, devoted to the assistance of merchants, soldiers, and pilgrims. The Order of the Knights of Jerusalem, then of the Knights of Malta, founded by Amalfi merchants, is still operative today.

Greek and Arabian medical traditions merged in the first medical school in Italy, established in Salerno, around the turn of the 10th century AD, initially supported by the Benedictines of Monte Cassino. It was the first and only European institution where a degree in medicine could be obtained, and it attracted medical scholars from the whole of Europe. Graduates of the school worked in Italy, France, Germany, and England. In England, the court physician at the time of Edward the Confessor was a Salerno graduate.

From Salerno stemmed the medical school at the University of Bologna, founded in the 12th century. Bologna was possibly the first university fitting the modern idea of such an institution. A century later, professors and students overflowed from Bologna to Padua. Bologna and Padua became the most important centres of medical studies in Italy. For several centuries, the use of Latin as the language of science fostered a great mobility of teachers and students among the universities of Europe, such as Paris and Montpellier in France, Cambridge and Oxford in England, a distinguished example being William *Harvey.

Later, universities were founded in Naples (1225), Siena (1241), Perugia (1266) (where, for the first time the denomination *Universitas studii* was used), Florence (1320), Pisa (1338), and Pavia (1361).

Several Renaissance painters and sculptors were keen students of anatomy. Among them, *Leonardo da Vinci has a place of outstanding importance for his drawings and descriptions. The career of Leonardo marked a turning point in medical research and started the quest for instruments of investigation. Galileo *Galilei built a thermometer and a microscope. Marcello *Malpighi, professor at Bologna and correspondent of the *Royal Society, published a treatise on macroscopic and microscopic pulmonary anatomy in 1661.

Rather than '*Anatomicorum princeps*'—as he has been considered by some—Bologna professor Giovanni Battista *Morgagni was a pathologist, a pathophysiologist, and a clinician. His *De sedibus et causis morborum per anatomen indagatis* represents a landmark of medical knowledge. His interests encompassed all fields of medicine, and several diseases still bear his name. The spread of medical knowledge later gave rise to medical schools of distinction and renown all over the world, in France, England, Spain, Germany, and America.

It is not possible to report in this brief outline all the achievements of Italian medicine in modern times. Nevertheless, not to mention the name of Camillo *Golgi would be a serious omission. A histologist who worked at Pavia, his name is linked to the study of the nervous system and of subcellular organelles. Working in Rome with Giovanni Battista Grassi and Ettore Marchiafava, Golgi also made a contribution to studies on *malaria, then a major health problem in Italy.

The organization of health care

In 1978, Law No. 833/78 replaced the previous system of health insurance with the Sistema Sanitario Nazionale (SSN for short) (national health system), which provides health assistance for every citizen. The organization of the system depends on the state and, at peripheral levels, on the regional and local councils and Unita Sanitarie Locali (USL) (Local Health Units).

According to a 1991 survey (ISIS 1991), the USLs directly manage 972 hospitals throughout the national territory. Twenty-six scientific institutes devoted to health care and 40 hospitals run by religious orders or religious organizations are also included in the SSN. In addition, the SSN has made reciprocal agreements with 643 privately owned clinics. University hospitals take part in the SSN in two ways: eight university hospitals are managed directly by the universities (for instance at Naples) and are bound to the SSN by special agreements; all other university hospitals are managed by the local USLs, on the basis of agreements between the universities and the regions. There are 440 181 beds available under the SSN, only

16.5 per cent of them being privately owned (October 1991).

Employees and nurses of the SSN are hired according to their qualifications, on the basis of regular civil service collective contracts. Each USL decides which positions within its organization are to be occupied by full- or part-time physicians.

National collective agreements determine the optimum physician:potential patients ratio and, consequently, the number of part-time physicians that can be hired by each USL for general practice and paediatrics, their terms of employment, the limitations on private practice, and the conditions governing the work of specialists. Citizens are free to choose their doctor, within the limit of the established number of patients per physician. Upon doctors' requests, the USL authorizes hospital admissions as well as access to laboratory and instrumental investigations. In most of these latter cases, a percentage contribution (colloquially named 'ticket') must be paid by the patients for these services and for prescriptions. Exceptions can be granted on the basis of income and, for certain income brackets, also in the case of diseases requiring continuous treatment. As a result, about one in four of the Italian population is exempted.

Private practice is open to all physicians who do not belong to the SSN. Special regulations allow private practice 'within the walls' to full-time SSN personnel.

SSN funding (Fondo Sanitario Nazionale—National Health Fund) is made up by contributions paid by employers and workers and social contributions and subsidies from the state. Some USLs also derive income from different sources.

Table 1 compares health expenses in Italy, the EEC, and USA. Data refer to 1987 (ISIS 1991).

Medical education

All medical schools in Italy are controlled by the state and confer a legally recognized degree. The control of the state is exercised by the Ministry of University and Technological Research, which approves the statutes of each university, publishes details of, and controls, the competitive examinations for academic posts, and ratifies the nominations made by the faculties.

Table 2 shows the distribution of the universities having a medical school. In some instances, courses are also

Table 1 Health expenses in Italy, EEC, and USA in 1987

	% of GIP*	Million L/inhabitant**	% State participation
Italy	7.24	1.09	79.15
EEC	7.45	1.01	78.09
USA	11.18	2.66	41.43

* Gross internal product.
** The average is estimated for the purchasing power. One pound sterling (US$1.50) is roughly equivalent to 2200 L.

Table 2 Distribution of medical schools in Italy

Region	Main campus	Branch
Piedmont	Turin	Novara
Lombardy	Brescia	
	Milan	
	Pavia	Varese
Veneto	Padua	
	Verona	
Friuli Venezia	Trieste	
Giulia	Udine	
Emilia Romagna	Bologna	
	Ferrara	
	Modena	
	Parma	
Liguria	Genoa	
Tuscany	Florence	
	Pisa	
	Siena	
Marche	Ancona	
Umbria	Perugia	
Lazio	Rome 'La Sapienza'	
	Rome 'Tor Vergata'	
	Rome 'Sacro Cuore'	
Abruzzo	Chieti	
	L'Aquila	
Campania	Naples	Naples II
Puglia	Bari	
Calabria	Reggio	Catanzaro
Sardinia	Cagliari	
	Sassari	
Sicily	Catania	
	Messina	
	Palermo	

held in branches, located in neighbouring cities. The data refer to 1990. The curricula of degree courses in medicine and surgery were profoundly modified in 1986, in view (among other things) of the requirements of the European Community. The courses are spread over 6 years, the total number of teaching hours being 5500. Basic subjects are taught in the first 3 years and clinical, preventive, and social medicine in the last 3 years. Each year, faculties establish the maximum number of places for new students who are admitted to the first year after a placement test. The degree is conferred after all curricular requirements have been completed and a thesis has been discussed. Graduates work for 6 months in university clinics or in selected SSN hospitals before taking their board examination.

Postgraduate specialization schools are established in every faculty. The establishment of the schools and their statutes are submitted for approval by the Ministry.

Graduates may apply for doctoral courses (Dottorato di Ricerca). Two or more universities agree to operate doctorate courses in various fields of research. Students follow their research programmes, attending the laboratories of the participating universities. At the end of the course, a national committee, appointed for each doctorate, evaluates the work carried out, on the basis of both the published papers and of the doctorate thesis. The doctorate is intended as a title to obtain an academic position.

Most universities have undergraduate courses aimed at training personnel to work in the SSN or as technicians in university departments. It is beyond the scope of this article to give a full account of these schools (see Bompiani *et al.* 1992).

ALESSANDRO POLLERI
MARIA VITTORIA GIANELLI

References
Bompiani, A., Carinci, P., and Ghetti, V. (ed.) (1992). *Diplomi universitari e scuole dirette a fini speciali della Facoltà di Medicina*. Francoangeli, Milan.
ISIS (1991). *Mensile di Sanita Pubblica*, 10–11, 15–48.
Istituzione del servizio sanitario nazionale, Law No. 833 (1978). *Gazzetta Ufficiale*, 360.
Modificazioni all'ordinamento didattico universitario relativamente al corso di laurea in medicina e chirurgia, Decree No. 95 (1986). *Gazzetta Ufficiale*, 83.

MEDICINE IN JAPAN

Ageing of the Japanese population—present and future

Until the end of the Second World War in 1945, Japan was considered to be one of the most civilized nations in the Orient, as there was much interest and concern about public health in the private and public sectors alike. However, the reality was somewhat different. Tuberculosis and other acute infectious diseases ranked high among the causes of death, and the infant mortality rate was also high. The average life expectancy in 1935 was less than 50 years (46.92 for males and 49.6 for females).

After the Second World War there were several fortunate influences brought to bear on health care in Japan, including financial and administrative assistance from the USA, and dramatic advances in the chemotherapy of infectious disease. In addition, birth control guidance, improvement of environmental hygiene, mass examination for tuberculosis control, and increased opportunities for regular health check-ups for the early detection of adult chronic diseases such as hypertension, malignancy, cardiac disease, and diabetes became possible. Also, through increased health education and public awareness about the prevention of chronic disease, the lifespan of the Japanese began to extend steadily after a decade after the end of the Second World War. This upward trend continued, and in 1991 the average life expectancy of the Japanese had reached 76.11 years for males (compared with 72.0 for the Caucasian male population of the USA) and 82.11 years for females (78.8 for American Caucasian females). Thus, Japan ranked first in the world in terms of longevity of its population. The consequence of this achievement, however, was a rapidly ageing population structure. Some of the reasons underlying this notable change were:

(1) a drastic decrease in deaths from tuberculosis and other infectious diseases;
(2) a marked decline in the infant mortality rate; and
(3) the homogeneity, lack of poverty, and lack of disadvantaged groups in Japanese society.

The high infant mortality rate in the past was partly due to the fecundity of Japanese women, and partly to common infant deaths resulting from infectious diseases and malnutrition. In infants less than 12 months old, the mortality in 1925 was 150 per 1000 live births. In 1940 it had fallen to 90/1000. The decline was very rapid after the Second World War; in 1960 it was 30.7/1000, and in 1985 5.3/1000. Such a rapid decline was not seen elsewhere in the world, and today Japan ranks among the nations with the lowest infant mortality rate.

The adult mortality rate in the population was 14.6 in 1947, 2 years after the Second World War, but had fallen to 6.7 in 1991 (compared with 8.8 in the USA in 1988). This notable decline in mortality, together with the rapid decline in infant mortality mentioned above, reflects the striking improvements achieved in general health conditions in Japan during these periods.

Changes in the causes of death in the Japanese

Tuberculosis, pneumonia, and other infectious diseases were the principal causes of death of the Japanese until around 1950. However, deaths due to cerebrovascular disease (CVA) increased rapidly, and in 1951 this became the commonest cause of death, while cancer ranked second, and third was cardiovascular diseases. In 1981 cancer ranked top, followed by CVA and cardiac disease. Since 1981 deaths from malignancy have increased steadily, cardiac diseases are now ranked second, while CVA is third.

What reasons underlay the rapid decrease of CVA deaths in the 1970s, which had long been the principal cause of death in Japan? First, the dietary habits of the Japanese, with a high salt intake (average 15 g/day) have changed, and the intake gradually decreased to 12 g/day through extensive health education. Secondly, regular health examinations, focusing on blood pressure measurement, which became widely available to the general public from 1955, allowed the early detection and treatment of hypertension, thus reducing CVA deaths. The resultant decrease in deaths from hypertensive cerebral haemorrhage in the middle-aged population helped to extend the average life expectancy of the Japanese. Cardiac disease is now the second most important cause of death in Japan, but compared to the high incidence in Europe and the USA, it is still relatively low.

As for malignant disease, stomach cancer ranks highest, followed by lung cancer, but as gastrointestinal X-rays and gastroendoscopy screening have become readily accessible to the general public, more and more early cases are discovered and successful surgery can be performed. Also, the decrease in salt intake, as well as westernization of dietary habits, are assumed to be contributory factors tending towards a gradual decrease in cases of stomach cancer; but colon cancer cases are steadily increasing.

Medical problems in Japan

Japanese medical care costs much less than in the USA and other Western countries. Japan had a per capita annual health-care expenditure in 1989 of US$1035 (£1 = US$1.50) compared with the American figure of US $2350. Surgical operation rates and their costs in Japan are about one-quarter of those in the USA. This is because of the control of the Ministry of Health and Welfare over medical fees and all other charges in Japanese medicine. However, annual medical expenditure has gradually increased up to US$1729 billion (¥ 21 790 billion) in 1992, and the costs of medical care of the elderly over the age of 65 reached 29.4 per cent of the total annual medical expenditure in Japan. (US$1=¥ 126.)

The number of hospital beds in Japan is the highest of any country in the world. The average length of hospital stay in Japan was as long as 22.8 days in 1992, and cost per in-patient per day was US$114 (¥ 14 400), bearing in mind the longer hospital stay when compared with the USA; the cost of one out-patient attendance was US$46 (¥ 5900).

Japanese patients stay in hospitals for an unusually long time when compelled to be admitted because of illness; however, this may be offset against their total vacation time. The Japanese are seen much more often by doctors in primary care or hospital out-patients than in other Western countries. They each visit their doctors 12.9 times yearly. There are about 210 000 doctors serving a population of 123 million in Japan, while there are only about 800 000 nurses, including both registered and 'practical' nurses. They are compelled to work hard and to carry a heavy physical load due to a chronic shortage of hospital nurses. As, in consequence, graduate nurses do not stay long in their posts, many big hospitals have had to close some wards.

As there is a universal health insurance system controlled by the Japanese Government anyone can be seen in the out-patient departments of most hospitals or dispensaries at any time. However, they often have to wait 2 or 3 hours for 3 minutes' consultation with doctors as there are so many out-patients. The income of doctors i.e. the fees payable for out-patient consultations is calculated according to the number of consultations and not by the length of time required for each consultation.

The Japanese health-care insurance system is very much welcomed by the elderly as virtually all of their medical costs are covered by the government.

Some personal thoughts on improvement of care of the elderly in Japan

Today Japan faces a growing problem of how to provide medical and welfare care for an ageing population. The administrative measures needed to cope with this situation are lagging behind need. Although the proportion of people over 65 in the whole of Japan is still just 13 per cent (1992), in some remote rural areas, where there is a population drift to the cities, villages may have more than 20 per cent.

As the elderly population increases, so do the costs of medical care. The Ministry of Health and Welfare is now studying how best to curtail this increase. The entire population is at present covered by one or other of the health insurance organizations, and medical costs are paid to the hospitals and physicians on a fee for item of service basis. This method is under review by a joint commission comprising representatives from health insurance organizations, hospital authorities, the Japan Medical Association, and learned societies.

The current proportion of the Japanese gross national product spent on medical care is 8.0 per cent (1990), but it is becoming increasingly difficult even to maintain this level. A rise is considered to be inevitable by most doctors. The Japanese government, however, proposes that it will be able to keep such expenditure below 7 per cent. Amendment of the Health and Medical Services Law for the Aged and an increase in the number of intermediate nursing homes are some of the principal measures proposed in order to curtail any future rise in medical expenditure.

It is also considered possible to improve welfare and medical care by some redistribution of medical expenditure. Japan has twice as many hospital beds per unit population as the USA, and too many elderly people are long-stay residents in hospital. It is intended to reduce hospital admissions and to shorten lengths of stay by options such as the provision of intermediate nursing homes and improved community care with visiting nurses. The government will be asked to provide adequate financial assistance to the private sector, which will build and run the intermediate nursing homes. The qualified registered nurses who gave up work after marriage will be encouraged to offer home-care nursing, assisted by trained helpers, publicly subsidized; voluntary workers will also be encouraged to help.

The social security budget in Japan is comparatively much smaller than that of many Western nations; if increases in medical expenditure can be rationally and effectively curtailed, it should be possible to increase the budget for social security benefits, including community care.

Another essential will be improved housing conditions. In an urban environment, high-rise apartments should be planned in order to secure extra living space. More elderly people live with their children in Japan when compared with most Western nations. If this is to be maintained, larger family homes will be needed in addition to trained helpers subsidized by public funds, to assist the daughters or daughters-in-law who care for the elderly. Housewives and elderly people who are healthy enough to work could be recruited for this purpose.

As the age of retirement in Japan has been increased from 55 to 60 in recent years and may soon rise to 65, it will be increasingly important to create a social structure offering opportunities for work, social activities, and learning for the elderly. The new intermediate nursing homes should be provided in urban environments whenever possible, so that the elderly in these homes can be in touch with their younger relatives, and arrangements should be made for elderly people of experience and ability to assist in youth educational programmes. These social activities will give the elderly people a chance to find a meaning in life and at the same time help them to stay mentally young.

Public awareness about the causation of disease and about appropriate programmes for early detection of diseases is now improving in Japan as the general public now attach great importance to better health. Circumstances are now right to provide programmes of health education and health promotion.

As 96.2 per cent of Japanese junior high school graduates now enrol in institutions of higher education, there are now many people who understand the value of efforts for protecting and preserving health and for aiming at a longer and better life. Much more emphasis on practical methods of improving physical and mental health are still needed. For such a campaign to be successful it will be necessary to recruit and train volunteer health leaders from the general public.

Medical education in Japan

Contemporary Japanese medical education is based on Western medicine; yet, until 120 years ago, medicine in Japan was predominantly of Chinese origin. Chinese medicine was brought to Japan in AD 554, but medicine did not develop extensively before 1550.

From 1641 on, with the arrival of Dutch physicians, Dutch medicine was introduced and spread in Japan, centring on Kyushu Island in the south. This, in turn, led to the founding of private medical schools. In 1849, smallpox vaccine was imported into Japan, and was eventually used throughout the country.

In 1870, shortly after the ascension of Emperor Meiji, the Japanese government decreed the adoption of German medicine. The first medical school specializing in German medicine was founded in 1877 in Tokyo (the predecessor of the Faculty of Medicine, Tokyo Imperial University), with professors of medicine recruited from Germany. Subsequently, national medical schools were built in cities such as Kyoto, Sendai, Sapporo, and Fukuoka.

By 1939, there were 13 medical schools in Japan. However, during the Second World War the number of medical schools was increased to 34, in order to train military doctors. The newly founded schools were called 'medical technical schools'; their curriculum was compressed and shortened by 2 years.

As the war progressed, the number of Japanese medical schools further increased to 51. After the war, the system was changed under the guidance of the Allied Occupation Forces. Under the new system, a student enters medical school after graduation from high school, takes 2 years of a pre-medical course, and then proceeds to the four-year medical school curriculum. Under this system, medical education takes a total of 6 years.

While prewar Japan adopted predominantly the German style of medical education, during the postwar era this was rapidly replaced by the English-American style.

Before the Second World War a licence to practise medicine was conferred automatically on all graduating students of medical schools. A change took place after the war, so that only those who completed a year of rotating internship after graduation became qualified to take the medical licensing board examination and to obtain a licence to practise.

In 1963, the internship programme was abolished as the result of opposition by the interns, who were receiving a year of training without pay. Since then, the students take the national medical licensing board examination immediately after graduation. Those who qualify receive a stipend while training in university hospitals or other public or private teaching hospitals.

As Fig. 1 shows, the number of medical schools in Japan increased rapidly after 1940, totalling 46 in 1969. But a shortage of doctors became apparent in rural areas, so government policy was implemented to allocate at least one medical school for each prefecture. Between 1970 and 1979, the number of medical schools was increased to 80, including 50 national or prefectural medical schools, and 30 private ones; this system continues today.

The enrolment of students increased proportionally, reaching 8360 in 1981. The government considered this to be a surplus, and the schools were advised to cut back on admissions, resulting in a decrease in the number of medical students to 7845 in 1992. The teacher–student ratio in medical schools is 1 to 3.3.

It is estimated that in 1990 there were 210 000 physicians in Japan. As the total population of Japan is 123 million, there are 58.6 doctors per 10 000 population, fewer than in Great Britain and the USA.

Characteristics of Japanese medical education and clinical medicine

Prewar Japanese medical schools tended to value basic medical science. This was a characteristic of German medical education, resulting to some extent in a lack of bedside training.

During the postwar era, a large number of medical personnel came to Japan from the USA for the purpose of advising Japanese schools on their development. Medical textbooks and journals published in the UK and

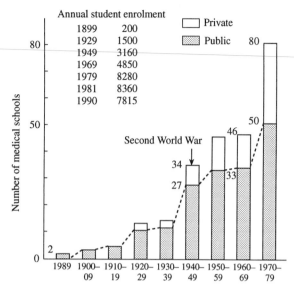

Annual student enrolment	
1899	200
1929	1500
1949	3160
1969	4850
1979	8280
1981	8360
1990	7815

Fig. 1 Private and public medical schools in Japan, and annual student enrolment.

the USA were imported. Exposure to such literature on the part of Japanese physicians and medical students during the postwar era seems to have increased their regard for clinical medicine.

However, it is my opinion that in Japan, dedication to the teaching of clinical medicine on the part of the staff is still lacking, particularly when compared with the situation in the UK and the USA. Furthermore, Japan is 30 years behind the USA in the institution of specialist training programmes. This is attributed to the attitude of the medical school professors, who over-encourage young students to pursue basic medical research rather than to acquire clinical skills from an early stage in their training.

Most drugs prescribed in Japan are pharmaceutical products of western origin. But Chinese herbal medicine, as well as moxibustion and *acupuncture, have been covered by health insurance for the past 10 years. Thus the application of both Western and Oriental-style medical treatment is gradually gaining ground in present-day Japan.

SHIGEAKI HINOHARA

MEDICINE IN NEW ZEALAND. Professional issues of medicine and health feature greatly not only in contemporary New Zealand life and society, but also in its history. New Zealand has led the world in the area of many health issues; and for a country relatively small in size and population, its spearhead influence on the standards of world health has been very significant.

Health and medical standards are amongst the highest in the world. Life expectancy at birth is 75 years of age, and the infant mortality rate is currently 8.1 per 1000 live births. This latter is the lowest infant mortality rate, in a multiracial society, in the world. These salutary indices are due to a combination of a temperate climate, low population density, an historical commitment to health as a major focus of societal goals, a classless society, and a high standard of living. The average hourly earning rate in New Zealand is 14.8 dollars per hour.

New Zealand has been a world leader in racial tolerance, universal adult suffrage, and in social welfare issues such as old age pensions, child welfare, and accident compensation issues.

New Zealand was the first country in the world, in 1893, to introduce voting for women in national elections. In 1899, the ex-goldminer and Prime Minister, Richard John Seddon, introduced old age pensions, another world first. The initial formulation of the structure of the atom—a nucleus with orbiting electrons— was formulated by Lord Rutherford, a physicist from Christchurch in New Zealand's South Island. On this discovery alone, undertaken collaboratively with the Dane, Niels Bohr, depends much of modern medical technology and hardware. The establishment of the Royal New Zealand Society for the Health of Women and Children (the Plunket Society) in 1907, and the training of Karitane Nurses which followed, was another world first. This latter provided every family in the nation with a standardized universal system of free neonatal and infant care, based on home visiting by trained nursing staff. In 1972, the New Zealand Parliament passed the Accident Compensation Act, then unique in the world, which provided compensation for all injury without the need for recourse to legislation. In the 1980s the country made a courageous attempt to become nuclear-free, and history may judge that pioneering stance as another great health milestone in the history of humankind. New Zealand has been rightly called the 'social health laboratory of the world'. Sir Edmund Hillary, the first conqueror of Mount Everest (in 1953) went on to provide extensive health services for Nepal. Sir Arthur *McIndoe contributed new techniques to plastic and reconstructive surgery; and Sir William Liley has contributed enormously to neonatal medicine.

Legislation and health

Modern New Zealand was established in 1840, when a group of Maori Chiefs signed the Treaty of Waitangi with the British Crown. The New Zealand Land Wars (1860–81) were followed by decades of *rapprochement*. In spite of legislative and some public conflict, the Race Relations Act of 1961 affirmed total and absolute equality for all races in the nation.

Matters of health are involved at three levels—the National Department of Health, area health boards, and health departments in territory councils. The National Department of Health administers relevant health legislation, funds health and medical programmes, and ensures the provision of essential services.

The nation is divided into 14 area health boards, which are funded by federal money from the Department of Health's budget. These area health boards are responsible for providing a full range of hospital, community, public health, and preventive medicine services. In addition to providing treatment, they are responsible for health promotion and health education—themes that are very strong in the societal mix of New Zealand, when seen in a world perspective. There are 74 city or district territory councils, each with its own local health department. These latter administer, *inter alia*, local food safety, refuse control, water supply quality, and sewerage.

The pivot of New Zealand's medical care is the local *general medical practitioner. Very importantly, dental care is provided free to dependent children under 18 years of age throughout the country. Eight per cent of the cost of all pharmaceuticals is met through public funding. A number of private hospital systems are also subsidized from the public purse. Forty-five per cent of the population has private health insurance, but this meets only 3.5 per cent of the total cost of the national health and medical care expenditure.

New Zealand has a history of vigorous voluntary and self-help organizations in health. Such institutions as the Royal Plunket Society, the New Zealand Family Planning Association, the New Zealand AIDS Foundation, Children's Health Camps, *Red Cross, and the Order of *St John play major roles in pre-hospital care, medical education, preventive medicine, and counselling and support services. The nation has been at the world forefront of the more general issues of equality of women in the health and medical services, the welfare of children in society, and preventive health issues such as fluoridation of water supplies. New Zealand was one of the first countries in the world formally to enshrine a Commission for Children in the national legislature. Funding for health services is largely provided from income tax. Essentially, 80 per cent of New Zealanders are of European descent, with 10 per cent of the population identifying as Maori. English is universally spoken, but Maori is also an official language, now taught in all New Zealand schools. The current ethnic mix is shown in Table 1.

The 1991 Census revealed that 85 per cent of the population live in urban areas, with 68 per cent living in main urban areas, such as major cities and large provincial towns. Of the New Zealand population of 3.37 million, some 885 000 live in Auckland. In Wellington, the nation's capital, live 326 000.

The New Zealand birthrate is 17.62 per 1000 population. The total fertility rate is 2.61, being the average number of births a woman would have if exposed to the current fertility rate. The ex-nuptial birthrate is

Table 1 The ethnic composition of New Zealand (compiled from data in *The New Zealand Year Book 1993*)

		Percentage
European		78.8
Maori		9.6
Pacific Islanders (Samoans, Tongans, Cook Islanders, and Niveans)		3.7
Chinese		1.0
Indian		0.8
Fijian		0.1
Other		6.0
Total population	3 373 929	100

52.05 per 1000 non-married women in the 15–49 year age-group.

The total population life expectancy at birth is 72.4 years for males and 78.3 years for females. The average age at death is 69.7 years. There is some racial inequality in these health statistics. The life expectancy for Maori males is 67.4 years and for Maori females 72.4 years. Currently, the average age of new mothers at the birth of their first child is 28.0 years. The infant mortality rate is 8.1 per 1000 live births.

Diseases and morbidity

The leading four causes of death in New Zealand are ischaemic heart disease, malignant *neoplasms, *respiratory diseases, and *cerebrovascular disease. New Zealand has always had a high rate of *coronary heart disease, believed to be associated with a relatively high *per capita* intake of saturated animal fats. Current death rates, by disease, are shown in Table 2.

With general improvement in health and public education about smoking and diet, death rates from heart

Table 2 Rank order of the leading causes of death in New Zealand (compiled from the New Zealand's Government's *National health statistics*, 1990 data)

	Death rate per 100 000 general population
Ischaemic heart disease	201.3
Malignant neoplasms	199.1
Respiratory diseases	77.2
Cerebrovascular diseases	76.9
Other forms of heart disease	32.4
Motor vehicle accidents	22.5
All other accidents and trauma	17.9
Diabetes mellitus	13.3

disease have fallen from a crude death rate of 300 per 1000 population in 1960, to the current level of 201 per 1000.

The overall infant death rate of 8.1 per 1000 live births, includes a perinatal death rate of 2.8 per 1000, and a sudden infant death syndrome rate of 2.7 per 1000. Maternal death rates are 15 per 100 000 live births.

Because of the leading role that New Zealand has taken in accident compensation and prevention, considerable statistical detail is available from the New Zealand Accident Compensation Corporation. The current road toll in New Zealand is 650 killed annually, with 16 700 injured. Road deaths contribute 2.0 per cent of all deaths in the general population (New Zealand Police data). *Suicide rates in New Zealand are 12.2 per 100 000 general population.

Children's hospital rates vary according to race, with the admission rates for Maori children approximately double those of non-Maori children. Annual hospital discharge rates for children, per 100 000 age-specific child population, are: under 1 year, 526.0; 1–4 years, 155; 5–9 years, 69; and 10–14 years, 50.

Doctors and *medical education

There are 10 330 doctors in New Zealand, and 7170 hold Annual Practising Certificates. Practice in medicine is governed by the Medical Practitioners Act of 1968. Of the medical practitioners who are currently registered to practise medicine, 26 per cent are women. Of all the doctors in New Zealand, 34 per cent are in active full-time general medical practice and of these 24 per cent are women. Health care provided by the local general medical practitioners is partly funded from the public purse, as are referrals to specialists. Eighty per cent of the cost of all drugs is met from public funding.

Doctors and matters dealing with medicine come under the jurisdiction of the Medical Council of New Zealand. Similarly, there is a *Nursing Council of New Zealand, and currently 44 800 nurses own Annual Practising Certificates. The New Zealand *Physiotherapy Board examines, registers, and regulates the conduct of physiotherapists, of whom there are 5 130 in New Zealand.

New Zealand has seven universities, including two (Otago and Auckland) with medical schools. The University of Otago Medical School was established in Dunedin in 1887, and has major teaching campuses in the cities of Dunedin, Christchurch, and Wellington. The University of Auckland Medical School is in Auckland itself. The medical course is a standard six-year course, with a further registration year, after which time doctors are registered by the Medical Council of New Zealand. There is a system of conditional registration, allowing certain doctors to practise in an approved hospital only. The Medical Council of New Zealand has disciplinary powers and functions as a court or tribunal, with subsequent right of appeal to the High Court of New Zealand.

There is a net export of New Zealand medical graduates to overseas. There is also a system of vigorous postgraduate education, conducted both locally by local medical societies and by various professional colleges.

Health care

There are two principal levels of health-care payment in New Zealand—government-funded and service from the private sector. Government-funded health-care systems are means tested. Those people who have a demonstrably low income or who are on social welfare benefits are issued with the Community Services Card. Those who possess this card are eligible for free hospital services and receive a subsidy of NZ$12 per visit to their local general medical practitioner. For prescription charges, card holders are charged a maximum of NZ$5 per item, with no family or individual having to pay for more than 15 prescriptions in 1 year. (NZ$2.55=£1/US$1.50.) For those who do not hold Community Services Cards, there are significant rebate services for all medical charges, for specialist and allied health professional charges, and for hospital admission. Subsidies (for the general population who do not hold the Community Services Card) are calculated on a *per family* rather than an individual rate. The general medical services subsidy of NZ $15 is payable for children's visits to the doctor. The treatment of accidents remains largely free.

J. PEARN

Further reading

Department of Social Welfare (NZ) (1992). *The Community Services Card* [brochure], March. Department of Social Welfare, Wellington.

Department of Statistics (NZ) (1993). *The New Zealand Official Yearbook 1993*. [Te Pukapuka Houanga Whaimana o Aotearoa], (96th ed) 139–180. Dept of Statistics, Auckland (NZ).

Ministry of External Relations and Trade (HM New Zealand Government) (1991). About New Zealand. Ministry of External Relations Wellington (NZ). [Available at New Zealand Consulates and Government Offices in all countries.]

New Zealand Health Information Service (NZHIS) (1993). Annual Reports entitled:
Hospital and selected morbidity data
Mental health data
Cancer data
Mortality and demographic data
Fetal and infant death data; also
Health points (since August 1992)—two-page fact sheets. Department of Health, Wellington (NZ).

Pearn, J. H. (1992). Courage and curiosity: Surgeon-explorers in Australia and New Zealand. Part 1. Discovery and bridgehead. *Australian and New Zealand Journal of Surgery*, **62**, 219–234. Part II. The science of the outback. *Australian and New Zealand Journal of Surgery*, **62**, 304–10.

MEDICINE IN POLAND
The history of medicine in Poland

In 1364 King Kazimierz the Great created in Cracow the first university with a medical faculty, now known as Jagellonian University. Even earlier, 'Nicolai from Poland' published a medical treatise, containing a polemical critique of Hippocrates in verse. During the Renaissance, numerous medical books were published: J. Strus, *Sphymicae artis*, in Basel, 1555; S. Petrycy described venereal diseases in 1591; in 1613 the first handbook of hygiene was published; and J. Uwiecki published *De morbo irae et curatione eiusdem*, a psychiatric handbook, in 1597. The University of Lvov was created in 1661. In 1750–53 in Leszno *Primitiae Physico-Medicae*, the first Polish medical journal, was published.

During the time of unrest in Poland (17th and 18th centuries) little was done in medicine, but in 1775 under 'The Hospital Constitution', the first official statutes of a health service were established, by Parliamentary Act.

At the end of the 18th century Poland lost its independence, and was subordinate to the authority of neighbouring states during the entire 19th century. This greatly influenced the development of science in the country. However, even during that period some important discoveries were reported by Poles. In 1875 W. Mayzel published the first report on mitotic division of animal cells. In 1881 L. Rydygier adopted stomach resection for the treatment of peptic ulcer. In 1895 N. Cybulski and W. Szymonowicz participated in the discovery of *adrenaline in the adrenal gland. In 1897 E. Biernacki elaborated his clinical *erythrocyte sedimentation test. In 1911 K. Funk was the first researcher to use the term 'vitamin'. Medical faculties were created in Warsaw in 1798 and in Wilno in 1803.

After Poland again became an independent state in 1918, five medical faculties were organized (Warsaw, Cracow, Lvov, Wilno, and Poznań). Three pharmaceutical and two dental schools were also created. Between 1920 and 1939 a health-care system was established, based on individual and collective insurance. A network of private and social health-care units was organized. Scientific research was also developing. In 1920 R. Weigl elaborated a very effective vaccine against *typhus. In 1925 L. Hirszfeld and H. Zborowski published their hypothesis on immunological conflict between mother and child.

The period of the Second World War was a very tragic one for Polish medicine. During it Poland lost approximately 20 per cent of its population, 40 per cent of its doctors, 30 per cent of its pharmacists, and 20 per cent of its nurses. Teaching of medicine and medical research nevertheless continued under these extremely difficult conditions though universities were closed and research was banned by the Germans. Clandestine medical faculties continued, almost secretly, to graduate new doctors (Warsaw and Cracow); a Polish Medical Faculty of émigrés was created in Edinburgh. In the ghettos of

Warsaw fundamental studies were carried out on the influence of hunger on the body.

In 1950 the medical and pharmaceutical schools were separated from their parent universities as medical academies subordinated to the Ministry of Health and Welfare. In 1958 the Polish Academy of Sciences founded a separate Division of Medical Sciences.

Health care in Poland today

The development of health care in Poland has been determined by the provision in the constitution that entitles every working citizen to free medical care, and by the economic situation of the country. Financing of the system comes from the state budget, and varies from 5 to 7 per cent of the total budget (GNP). For that purpose, the employers (until recently mainly state enterprises), pay an insurance premium of some 4.3 per cent of the total wage bill.

Organization of health services, sharing of resources, and their utilization are supervised by the Minister of Health and Social Welfare, who also exercises control over medical schools of the universities, the research institutes, and the directors of regional administration offices who deal with management of the territorial organization of health services. Separate organizations provide health care in the Ministry of National Defence, the Ministry of the Interior, and in the Polish State Railways, according to long-lasting tradition.

The organization of health care has depended, in recent years, on the establishment of integrated health-care complexes, one for every 200 000–500 000 of the population. These organizations provide access to primary medical care and to secondary care in internal medicine, *paediatrics, *surgery, and *gynaecology and *obstetrics at a basic level (some 6600 out-patient clinics in 670 hospitals). In dentistry the basic care units provide some 270 000 consultations and therapeutic procedures per year. Emergency medical aid is provided by 59 ambulance-service stations with 4877 ambulance cars, and 79 aeroplanes and helicopters. Some 420 000 consultations and therapeutic procedures and 37 000 patient journeys are provided in a year.

In the individual provinces, there are hospitals with more specialized out-patient clinics (*cardiology, *oncology, *ophthalmology, *laryngology, *dermatology, *neurology, etc.), each providing medical care to between 1 and 4 million of the population. Departments of medical schools, research institutes, and the Polish Academy of Sciences (approximately 40 units in all) offer specialized treatment, exercise specialist supervision, provide consultations, and prepare expert opinions at the request of state authorities.

Industrial health care provides some 29 000 consultations and prophylactic procedures per year. The health-care system also provides some 3500 *pharmacies, employing 8300 pharmacists. In some regions, mainly in big cities, alongside the state health service, so-called medical co-operatives operate, providing over 450 000

consultations and therapeutic procedures in return for payment.

Blood collection, partial processing, and distribution are dealt with by 24 blood-donation stations and 479 blood-collection units. A total of 531 000 litres of blood are collected each year.

*Public health services (prevention of infectious diseases, including vaccination, health education, inspection of water supply and food production, and evaluation of the country's epidemiological condition) are the responsibility of the Chief Public Health Medical Officer. These services have 385 laboratories spread across the country.

The Ministry also supervises rehabilitation and sanatorium care (some 100 sanatoria in health resorts, which admit some 670 000 patients per year).

Some 12 000 doctors, pharmacists, and other specialists are involved in teaching medicine and pharmacy (in 12 medical schools or academies with some 35 000 students). In addition to standard undergraduate courses, there is also a well-developed system of postgraduate training and continuing education for physicians in several dozen specialties and subspecialties. For many years, postgraduate medical training centres have organized training courses, specialist examinations, and have evaluated the need for such education.

The health services in Poland thus employ a total of some 79 000 physicians (i.e. in a ratio of 19.5:10 000 population), 19 000 dentists (4.6:10 000), 16 000 pharmacists, and 194 000 nurses.

In 1989 the medical societies were re-established in Poland, providing self-government of the medical profession, including responsibility for supervising undergraduate and postgraduate training courses, exercising inspection of professional liability of the physician, and taking care of their professional interests. New legislation concerning medical professional activity and the organization of health care has been proposed. Self-government of pharmacists and nurses has also been established.

Recently the health-care system has been undergoing substantial transformation as a result of the changed political system. The state health service units have been undergoing restructuring and some have been replaced by private institutions (in 1992, approximately 1000 new units were created). In general, the state system of health care is being partially replaced or supplemented by a system based on individual obligatory and/or voluntary insurance contracts. In the near future, the services rendered by private institutions as well as by the state system will be covered by insurance companies.

The health condition of the population in Poland may be illustrated by the following indices (according to Zea books: *Health protection* 1990; *Chief Census Bureau* 1991). The standardized total death rate in Poland is 1145.2/100 000 population, with death from circulatory failure accounting for 605.2, neoplasms for 209.5, and injuries and poisoning 72.9; the neonatal mortality rate amounts to 1614 per 100 000 live births. The incidences of certain infectious and other diseases (number of cases per 100 000 population) are as follows: tuberculosis, 46.9; viral hepatitis, 57.6; venereal diseases, 26.9; measles, 2.7; rubella, 41.0; salmonelloses, 99.2; and mental diseases, 375.3 (of these, the incidence of alcohol psychosis is 21.5).

Scientific activity in medicine is carried out in three sectors which have different tasks. In the 12 medical schools the academic units are usually also research laboratories, and participation in research projects is a basic duty of the teachers. Hence, the faculties of medicine employ most medical research workers. The research projects carried on in these schools are extensive and cover all branches of clinical and theoretical medicine. The second sector engaged in medical research includes the independent institutes supervised by the Minister of Health and Social Welfare. The research projects carried out at the 14 institutes, which employ 1000 researchers, aim, above all, at solving the key problems of health protection in Poland. The institutes also provide expert opinions to the Minister of Health, e.g. the State Institute of Hygiene serves the Chief Public Health Medical Officer and the Institute of Cardiology or the Institute of Oncology, apart from carrying on teaching and specialized out-patient clinics, conduct epidemiological studies. The third medical research sector comprises the institutes of the Polish Academy of Sciences (PAS). Five PAS institutes, employing some 600 researchers, deal mainly with basic biomedical research, concentrating, for example, on mechanisms regulating homeostasis, on neurobiology, on immunology. One PAS institute deals with experimental and clinical pharmacology; some others combine research with clinical topics (e.g. the Neurosurgical Clinic in Warsaw, the Genetic Clinic in Poznań). Moreover, the PAS has organized a network of scientific committees and boards in which some 1500 scientists participate. Forty medical periodicals are published (some 100 000 scientific and research papers per year). Both research and publishing activity in Poland have had a long tradition, dating back to the 13th century.

On behalf of the Government of the Republic, scientific research in Poland is supervised by the Committee for Scientific Research, a body partly elected and partly appointed, which deals mainly with apportionment of state resources for research. The above-mentioned sectors of medical research receive their resources from the Committee.

This extensive system is, on the one hand, underfinanced and has recently suffered reductions; nevertheless it has enjoyed many successes. Special mention should be made of spheres in which equal-terms co-operation has been established with other countries. These include: research in neuroregulation of biological processes, nervous system ischaemia, transplantation immunology, autoaggressive diseases, epidemiology of cardiovascular diseases, epidemiology of neoplasms, genetically determined muscle diseases, studies on arterial hypertension, and banking of tissue and organs for transplantation.

MIROSLAW MOSSAKOWSKI
JANUSZ KOMENDER

MEDICINE IN SCANDINAVIA. Scandinavia comprises Denmark (population, 5.1 million), Finland (5 million), Iceland (255 000), Norway (4.2 million), and Sweden (8.5 million). Sweden has the oldest and Iceland the youngest population. The life expectancy has grown in all five countries and is now 73 years for males and 79.3 years for females born in 1990. The 0–14-year-olds' share of the total population has decreased significantly since 1970, whereas the proportions of 65–79-year-olds and 80-year-olds and more are increasing. This trend will continue at least until 2025.

The political structure and the strong ties existing between the Nordic countries have influenced the development of medicine in Scandinavia. Denmark and Norway formed a political union between 1380 and 1814, with Copenhagen as the political and medical centre. Finland was part of Sweden from 1154 until 1809, when it became an autonomous grand duchy subordinated to Russia. Norway and Sweden were forced into a political union in 1814. Norway again became an independent nation in 1905, Finland in 1917. Iceland was first an independent nation, then became part of Norway, following it into the Danish–Norwegian kingdom, persisting as a part of Denmark until 1944, when the country again became independent.

History of medicine

Trepanned skulls from prehistoric times have been found in Denmark, Norway, and Sweden. In 1939, a neolithic skull was found during excavations near Kirkenes in Finmark, Norway. Similar operations were performed all over Europe, using the same and similar techniques, apparently with some knowledge of *anatomy. Accordingly, an exchange of professional knowledge must have taken place in prehistoric times.

The earliest sources of information about the history of medicine in Scandinavia are based upon the Edda, a collection of old verses and sagas (850–1050), the sagas (1050–1350), and written laws (1050–1350). The most famous doctor in the saga period was Hrafn Sveinbjornsson in Iceland, who was killed in 1213. He had travelled extensively in Europe and is known to have removed concretions from the urethra and performed venesection and cauterization.

In northern Europe, medicine grew up mainly in religious institutions such as monasteries and abbeys. Scandinavia became Christian around AD 1000 and medical institutions were therefore slow to develop. Several monasteries were built in Scandinavia during the 12th and 13th centuries. Archaeological excavations at Vadstena in Sweden and Øm and Æbeltoft in Denmark

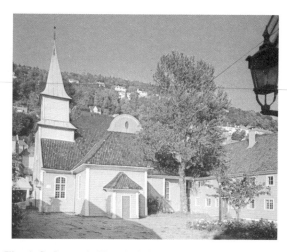

Fig. 1 St Jørgen's Hospital, Bergen, Norway (now a medical museum).

have reported that care and treatment of patients were part of their activities. Although the Church opposed the practice of medicine by monks, especially surgery, several skeletons found at the Cistercian abbey at Øm indicate that surgical treatment had been given. Surgical instruments were found both in Öm and at Æbeltoft, in Vreta and Gudhem in Sweden, and at Varna in Norway. The oldest monastery in Norway to offer medical treatment was the Augustine abbey at Halsnoy, an island south of Bergen. It was founded in 1164 and closed at the Reformation.

Leprosy was widespread in Scandinavia during the 13th century. Patients were excluded from social life by law, but were taken care of at St George's institutions. Denmark had 35 institutions dedicated to St Jørgen (St George). They were all closed with the Reformation. The first leprosy hospital in Bergen was established in 1266, but St Jørgen's hospital was first mentioned as a leprosarium in 1411. It remained a hospital for leprosy until the disease was eradicated from Norway, and is today a medical museum (Fig. 1).

The order of St Anthony was known for the care and treatment of diseased people, especially those suffering from ergotism (*ignis sacer*) and others who were crippled by disease or injury. Nonneseter abbey in Bergen and Maarkor in Denmark belonged to this order.

With the Reformation in 1536, all monasteries were closed. The first hospitals to be built in Scandinavia after the Reformation were established for academic purposes. Uppsala in Sweden had the first, Nosocomium academicum. It was built in 1717. It was followed by the Serafimerlasarettet (Seraphim Lazaret) in Stockholm in 1752. Serafimerlasarettet had eight beds but could take 15 patients, two in each of seven of the beds. In 1765, the number of beds was increased to 40.

The Royal Fredrik Hospital in Copenhagen was opened in 1757 and had 158 beds. It was not built for academic purposes but nevertheless became an important centre for the training of surgeons. The General Hospital in Copenhagen was opened in 1769 with 300 beds, mainly for poor people. Untrained washerwomen were first to be involved in nursing hospitalized patients. Nursing was slow to develop. The organization of deaconesses was founded in Germany in 1836 and had branches in Stockholm (1851), Copenhagen (1863), and Oslo (1868).

The University of Uppsala was founded in 1477 but had no chair in medicine until the 17th century. Therefore, Sweden did not train academically qualified physicians in the 16th century. The University of Copenhagen was founded in 1479 during the reign of Christian I. It had four faculties, one of them medicine. However, no physicians graduated before the Reformation in 1536. The university was reopened by King Christian III in 1537. It soon had a dominating position in Scandinavia, with anatomists such as Nicolaus Stenonius and Thomas *Bartholin. They, and several of their colleagues, had been students at various universities in Europe, such as Rostock, Paris, Leiden, and Montpellier, and they integrated Copenhagen in the common European medico-cultural tradition. Oluf Rudbeck in Uppsala was an equally prominent figure in Swedish medicine. He built the first anatomical theatre in Uppsala in 1662 and he is also remembered as the first to describe the *lymphatic vessels.

The University of Åbo (Turku), Finland, was opened in 1640 and Lund, Sweden in 1666. However, Lund remained, for a long period of time, mainly a theological school.

As in most European countries, surgery was from the beginning performed by a heterogeneous group of academically unqualified men. In Scandinavia, the surgeons organized guilds of surgery just before, or during, the 16th century—in Stockholm, 1496; Copenhagen, 1506; and Bergen, 1597. A three-year apprenticeship followed by 4 years abroad were required in order to qualify as a surgeon. Surgeons were allowed to treat cutaneous lesions, perform venesection and cupping, and to remove stones from the bladder and urethra. They were not permitted to treat internal diseases. On the other hand, surgery could be performed only by those trained in the discipline.

Surgeons were not admitted to the universities. The training of surgeons was reformed during the 18th century. A separate Academy of Surgery, independent of the university, was opened in Copenhagen, and a Director General appointed (Fig. 2). The Faculty of Medicine protested vehemently. However, in 1785, the first professor at the Academy of Surgery was accepted as equal to the professor of medicine. The Academy of Surgery was closed in 1842 and all medical training transferred to the Faculty of Medicine. In Sweden, surgery was accepted by the Medical Collegium in 1797. The Karolinska Medico-surgical Institute in Stockholm was founded in 1810 and was co-ordinated with the Faculty of Medicine in 1874.

The 18th century was important for the development of medicine in Scandinavia. Maternity clinics were built in Copenhagen in 1750 and in Stockholm in 1775. The first such clinics were established to provide homes for unmarried pregnant poor women and to prevent the killing of newborn babies, which was not uncommon. The first Medical Acts of Denmark (and with it, Norway) were written in 1674, declaring that only those who had graduated at, and defended a doctoral thesis at, the University of Copenhagen were allowed to practise as physicians. This was changed in 1788, when physicians became civil servants and did not need a doctor's degree. The first hospital in Norway was the Rikshospitalet (National Hospital) in Oslo. It was opened in 1826 as a university hospital for the first Norwegian university, which opened in 1813.

Towards the end of the 19th and the early 20th centuries social security and medical treatment became part of the official health policy of the Scandinavian countries. Many of the first hospitals were private, owned by religious organizations, but the state, and then also the counties, expanded the hospital system and took over the private hospitals. Contacts between the Scandinavian countries have been very close in medicine. As a result, the hospital systems in the Scandinavian countries have developed in parallel. This has led to a similar, often identical, structure.

In 1989, Denmark had 487 beds in general hospitals per 100 000 population; Finland, 519; Iceland, 475; Norway, 397; and Sweden, 452. *Psychiatry was slower to develop. Legislation for psychiatric patients came in Finland in 1841, in Denmark in 1852, and in Norway and Sweden in 1854. In 1989, the number of beds in psychiatric hospitals per 100 000 inhabitants was 102 for Denmark, 258 for Finland, 180 for Iceland, 88 for Norway, and 216 for Sweden.

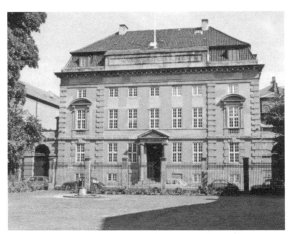

Fig. 2 The Royal Surgical Academy, Copenhagen, Denmark.

Organization of health services in the Nordic countries

Some features of the health services in Scandinavia are common to all countries. Services are given according to law and most are financed by the government. Treatment of disease is either financed by the government or through compulsory health insurance schemes. The health and social security systems are similar in terms of benefits, services, and their availability. Health services are based upon a combination of municipal primary health systems, county-based hospital services in both general secondary care and psychiatry, while advanced medicine (tertiary care) is associated with the regional hospitals, which are also university hospitals and research centres.

In all Scandinavian countries, an amount is charged for treatment and purchase of medicine. Wages or a cash allowance are given during sickness to employees. All five countries have well-developed hospital services with advanced specialist treatment. Specialist treatment outside hospitals is also offered.

*Primary health care is a public matter in all Scandinavian countries. In Finland, Iceland, Norway, and Sweden the major part of the treatment takes place at publicly run health centres, while in Denmark it is provided by *general practitioners and practising specialists.

In all five countries there are programmes of prevention for mothers and infants, school health care, and dental care for children and young people. Similarly, in all countries there are preventive *occupational health services and general measures of environmental protection. Social security has had an increasing share of the gross domestic product (Table 1).

Denmark

There are three political and administrative levels of the health service. The state is responsible for legislation and bears overall responsibility for health care and supervision. The responsibility of the state is divided among several ministries. The Ministry of Health has the responsibility for hospital care, *public health care, training of *nurses, *postgraduate medical education, and the part of the national health insurance which finances the general practitioners, *dentists, etc. The Ministry of Social Affairs holds the responsibility for nursing homes and housing for old people, the Ministry of Labour for the occupational health services, the Ministry of Education for the university education of

Table 1 Social security as percentage of the gross domestic product in the Scandinavian countries, 1987

Denmark	Finland	Iceland	Norway	Sweden	Mean
27.4	25.7	16.9	26.2	34.7	26.2

Source: Ministry of Social Affairs and Health (1992). Social security in Finland 1989 and 1990, Publication No. 7, p. 138.

health professionals and the Ministry of Environment for environmental hygiene.

The counties are responsible for most health-care services. According to the Hospital Act, all general and psychiatric hospitals are run by the counties. An exception to this is the State Hospital of Copenhagen (Rigshospitalet) which is run by the state in close collaboration with the counties. This hospital is under the Ministry of Health. Highly specialized hospital functions are centralized to five major hospitals in the country. Hospital treatment is free of charge.

Private, non-profit hospitals have so far been run as a part of the public hospital service, according to an agreement with the counties. At the end of the 1980s, however, a private profit hospital was set up, and more were planned. Treatment in private hospitals is paid for by the patients themselves, without public subsidies.

National health insurance is financed by taxes. It ensures that patients who do not need hospital treatment get a number of services, either free of charge or with a reduced fee. Furthermore, the cost of many medicines is partly covered.

The municipalities are responsible for the primary and public health-care systems, home nursing, *paediatrics, child dental care, and school health care. Most nursing homes and other local services for the elderly are also under the responsibility of the municipalities. Drugs are sold by public, controlled pharmacies.

Finland

The health services come under the Ministry of Social Affairs and Health, which has under it the National Agency for Welfare and Health. The Ministry of Education is responsible for the university education of health personnel and the National Board of Education, under the Ministry of Education, for postgraduate medical education. The Ministry of Environment is responsible for environmental hygiene.

For regional administration, the country is divided into 12 provinces, each with its own Department of Social Affairs and Health. These departments administer state appropriations and form an administrative intermediate authority in the field of public health care, as well as approving regional plans. The specialized central hospitals are run by a federation of municipalities. Each hospital handles the most common clinical specialties. There are five university hospitals, in Helsinki, Turku, Oulu, Kuopio, and Tampere.

The municipalities are responsible for organizing health and social services and for general public health (environmental health). The municipalities have established health centres that operate either independently or in collaboration with adjoining municipalities.

The primary health-care system is based upon health centres. It includes the primary health-care services, such as maternal and child services, school and student health services, care of those engaged in active employment, health care of the elderly, health information, other preventive measures (*vaccination, *screening, etc.), primary medical and nursing services and medical rehabilitation, dental care, and *ambulance services. The major part of dental care for adults is performed by private practitioners.

Iceland

The Icelandic Ministry of Health and Social Insurance has the responsibility for health care. The field of responsibility of the Ministry includes all general matters of health, primary medical care, preventive measures, the appointment of physicians, the Directorate General of Health, the Medico-Legal Council, hospitals and sanatoria, nursing homes and homes for old people, dental treatment, sales and control of drugs, insurances, and the State Assurance Institute (Riksforsikringsanstalten).

With the exception of a few private institutions, the hospitals are run by the state. The two main hospitals are the State Hospital and the Municipal Hospital in Reykjavik.

In 1990, the operation of independent health centres was entirely subordinated to government administration. Since 1991, the state has taken over other health centres, as well as the municipal hospitals. Today the state is responsible for almost all health services and is covering all expenses in connection with their daily operation, while the municipalities are still paying 15 per cent of all expenditure for investment and maintenance. However, the actual administration of health services has been decentralized to a great extent to special boards in the districts.

Primary health care is divided into eight regions, which are later to be divided into 31 areas with a total of 83 health centres. Of these, nine will be in Reykjavik. Dental treatment is usually given by dentists in private practice in their own clinics.

The Ministry of Education is responsible for health education. Postgraduate medical education takes place mainly abroad.

Norway

Political responsibility for the national health services in Norway rests with the Social and the Health Departments. They bear the main responsibility for matters concerning economy, planning, and other issues of political importance concerning health. The Directorate of Health is in charge of the overall professional supervision of the health service in Norway. Each county has a state-employed County Medical Officer, with responsibility for supervision of health status and health services in the county. The County Medical Officer is also an advisor to local and central health authorities.

The health system is regionalized. There are five health regions in Norway, each with its regional hospital, which is also a university hospital. All regional hospitals are owned by the respective counties, except for the State Hospital in Oslo (Rikshospitalet) which is the regional hospital for health region I, but is owned by the state in close collaboration with the county. The state also runs a few specialized hospitals. The regional hospitals are dependent upon substantial block grants from the state, which cover up to 50 per cent of the running costs.

The counties are responsible for the operation of specialist and dental treatment. They are authorized to plan and run health institutions, specialist health services, medical laboratories, ambulance services, and to provide advice and guidance to the local health services in fields such as paediatrics, geriatrics, etc. The county authorities also have a duty to ensure that dental health services are available to all living in the county. Dental services are performed either by the counties' own employees or private dentists who work according to an agreement with the county.

The municipalities are responsible for primary health care: health promotion and the prevention of disease or infirmity through environmental health care, family health services, school health services and health information, diagnosis and treatment of sickness, injury, and infirmity, medical rehabilitation, nursing, and care. The local health authorities may organize these services by employing their own personnel or by making an agreement with self-employed personnel. The responsibility for the prevention of disease and for treatment of patients rests with the local authorities, but the patients are referred for specialist treatment in hospitals or university clinics whenever needed. Pharmacies are mainly private but subjected to strict public control.

Sweden

Here also, the state bears the political responsibility for the hospital and health services. The National Board of Health and Welfare is the central supervisory authority for the health and hospital services. The central supervisory authorities within environmental and health protection are, in addition to the National Board of Health and Welfare, the National Environmental Protection Board, the National Board of Occupational Safety and Health, the National Food Administration, the National Institute of Radiation Protection, the Chemical Inspectorate, and the National Drug Inspectorate. The corresponding regional responsibility lies with the provincial authorities.

The health and hospital services under the county councils are divided into the regional hospital service, the provincial hospital service, and the primary health service. The county councils and the independent municipalities bear the final responsibility for the health and hospital services.

There are six regional hospitals, each associated with a university. However, the universities are run by the state, while the university hospitals are regional. These hospitals provide advanced and specialized diagnostics and treatment, as well as general central hospital functions.

The provincial hospitals comprise both more specialized hospitals covering all the province and hospitals covering only part of the province. Medical treatment is provided within most specialties, both for in-patients and at the out-patient clinics. Psychiatric treatment, which is often divided into sectors, belongs under the provincial hospital service.

Private health and sickness care exists on a limited scale. There are a few places at private nursing homes. About 15 per cent of all medical consultations take place with private practitioners. In addition, there are physiotherapists in private practice. Within dental care, half of the dentists are private practitioners.

JOHAN AARLI

References

Gotfredsen, E. (1964). *Medicinens historie*. Arnold Busck, Copenhagen.

Ministry of Social Affairs and Health (1992). *Social security in Finland 1989 and 1990*, Publication No. 7, Helsinki.

Nordic Medico-Statistical Committee (NOMESKO) (1992). *Health Statistics in the Nordic Countries 1990*, p. 84.

MEDICINE IN SOUTH-EAST ASIA. Geographically, South-East Asia comprises the Indochina Penisula and the islands and peninsulas to the south-east of the Asian continent. The region extends over 2000 miles (3200 km) from north to south and 3500 miles (5600 km) from east to west, and encompasses the mainland nations of Thailand, Myanmar (Burma), Vietnam, Laos, Cambodia, (West) Malaysia, and the island nations of the Philippines, (East) Malaysia, Singapore, Indonesia, Brunei, Borneo (Indonesia), Timor, and a number of smaller islands. Most of South-East Asia has a stable, homogeneous tropical climate with the region's average monthly temperature of around 27 °C. It is also ethnically very diverse and the populations speak many diverse languages, belonging to five main language groups, namely Sino-Tibetan, Mon-Khmer, Thai, Vietnamese, and Austronesian (Malay–Polynesian). The total population of the region in 1992 was approximately 400 million, with Indonesia the most populated at 187.4 million, followed by Vietnam (71.3 million), Thailand (58.3 million), Myanmar (42.9 million), Malaysia (18.7 million), Cambodia (8.7 million), Laos (4.3 million), Singapore (3.1 million), and Brunei (0.3 million). The statistics given in Table 1 show the comparative status of various South-East Asian countries.

The development of medical education

In the early stages, medical education and health services in South-East Asian countries followed the trends of the former Western colonial powers. Their influence in these two areas can still be traced up to the present day. Western medicine came to South-East Asia along with the arrival of European merchants seeking to explore and dominate the region, particularly in the 16th century. Thus merchants of British, Spanish, and Dutch origin were the main groups travelling back and

Table 1 Some statistical information about the countries of South-East Asia

	Population growth (annual) (%)	Population/doctor	Infant mortality /1000 live births	Literacy (%)
Brunei	2.8	1 323	8	85.1
Cambodia	2.2	27 000	116	48.0
Indonesia	1.8	7 238	65	85.5
Laos	2.9	6 495	97	83.9
Malaysia	2.6	2 656	3	78.5
Myanmar	2.1	3 350	65	81.0
Philippines	2.3	1 016	40	93.5
Singapore	1.1	753	6	90.7
Thailand	1.4	4 631	24	93.0

forth between Europe and the islands and peninsulas of the region. Conflicts of interest eventually brought to the region the naval fleets of those European powers, resulting in colonization of most South-East Asian nations. It was not until the latter half of the 19th century that the first medical school was founded in South-East Asia. After several epidemics, a school of medicine was established in Batavia by the Dutch in 1851. However, lessons of modern Western medicine may have been taught earlier in Bangkok by Dr D. B. Bradley (1804–73), a well-known MD of New York University, who first arrived in Bangkok in 1835 and spent most of his life there. He was the owner of the first printing press in Thailand and published a number of treatises on medicine in the Thai language. The Dutch school in Batavia was attached to the military hospital and Dutch military physicians were the teachers. The purpose of the school was to train native practitioners, mainly in order to formalize widespread smallpox vaccination. At first the course lasted for 2 years, leading to the title of Doktor Djawa or Javanese physician; these doctors were trained to diagnose common diseases, to perform minor surgery, and to treat some illnesses. By 1875 the course was extended to 6 years with Dutch as the main language of instruction. In 1902 the school, having been reorganized with more buildings added, was renamed School tot Opleiding van Inlandsche Artsen (School for the Training of Native Physicians) and the course was extended to 9 years after elementary school; a three-year preparatory course equivalent to junior high school was compulsory before students were allowed to enter the six-year medical school course. In 1913 the Dutch colonial government established a second medical school in Surabaya, East Java, named Nederlandsch–Indische Artsen School (Netherlands–Indies School of Physicians.) Both schools later became faculties of medicine in the Universiteit van Indonesie which was also established by the Dutch. The medical school in Surabaya later became a Faculty of Medicine of the University of Airlangga. In 1948 the Republic of Indonesia opened a new faculty of medicine in

Jogjakarta in the newly established Universitas Gadjah Mada with Bahasa Indonesia (Indonesian language) as the language of instruction. All other medical schools came into being after Indonesia officially gained its independence in 1949; by the end of the 1990s there were altogether 24 medical schools in Indonesia, 14 belonging to the government and 10 private, altogether producing approximately 1100 doctors each year.

The oldest private medical school in the region was established in November 1871 at the University of Santo Tomas in Manila, the Philippines, under the auspices of the Roman Catholic Church. In June 1907, a second medical school sponsored and controlled by the government of the Philippines was opened in accordance with Act No. 1515 of the 'Philippine Commission'. The College, then under the University of the Philippines, was renamed the College of Medicine and Surgery in 1910; since March 1923 it has been officially known as the College of Medicine of the University of the Philippines. These two medical schools were the main producers of doctors for the country for several decades. The past quarter of a century has seen some 25 privately owned medical schools opened to local as well as to a large number of foreign students who have sought to enter the medical profession and then to return to practise in their homelands. Of the total of 26 medical schools in existence in the Philippines in 1992, only the College of Medicine of the University of the Philippines was controlled by the government; all of the schools together produced more than 4000 new doctors each year.

The development of medical education in Thailand, the only country in South-East Asia which avoided Western colonization, took a different course. The oldest medical school, originally known as Pattayakorn Medical School and shortly thereafter renamed the Royal Medical School, was established in the capital city of Bangkok by the royal decree of King Chulalongkorn the Great of Thailand in 1890 at Siriraj Hospital. This hospital had been founded by the same king 2 years earlier upon the tragic death, at a very young age, from diarrhoea, of his beloved son, Prince Siriraj. The most prominent turning point in medicine in Thailand was due to the achievements of Prince Mahidol of Songkla, who initiated and, together with Prince Jainad, carried out successful negotiations with the Rockefeller Foundation. That foundation, for a 12-year period, from 1923 to 1935, helped the Royal Medical School at Siriraj Hospital in Bangkok to upgrade its standards to those of American medical education at that time. At one time labelled as 'the poorest I have ever seen' by Dr Victor Heiser, a Rockefeller Foundation representative visiting the region, the Royal Medical School was greatly modernized and improved. It became a Faculty of Medicine of Chulalongkorn University, which was founded in 1916 by King Rama VI in commemoration of his father. In 1943, by an Act of Parliament, the Faculty of Medicine and Siriraj Hospital were transferred to the newly established University of Medical Sciences which eventually set up two more medical schools, one based at the Thai Red Cross Chulalongkorn Hospital in Bangkok and the other at the northern city of Chiang Mai. The past few decades have seen six more medical schools established, two in the provincial cities of Songkhla in the south and Khon Kaen in the north-east, the others being in Bangkok, one of which belongs to the army. Recently a private medical school belonging to Rangsit University was opened but has yet to receive approval by the Thai Medical Council. From the eight government medical schools in existence in 1992, the number of doctors produced was approximately 900. All graduates of government medical schools are automatically given a licence to practise by the Thai Medical Council.

Medical education in Malaysia and Singapore developed similarly as the two countries together formed a federation in the British Empire until independence in 1957. Western medicine was introduced to Singapore by Thomas Prendergast, a subassistant surgeon who accompanied Sir Stamford Raffles when he landed in Singapore in 1819. From 1870, suitably qualified young men were sent annually by the government to the Madras Medical College in India to train as assistant surgeons. In 1905, the Straits and Federated Malay States Government Medical School was founded in Singapore. After the school received a large donation in 1912 from the King Edward VII Memorial Fund, the name of the school was changed to King Edward VII Medical School in 1913, and to the King Edward VII College of Medicine in 1921. In 1949, the College of Medicine amalgamated with the Raffles College to become the University of Malaya, and became its Faculty of Medicine. In 1959, the University of Malaya established two largely autonomous divisions, one in Kuala Lumpur, the other remaining in Singapore. Before Singapore became an independent republic in 1965, the school became in 1962, the Faculty of Medicine of the University of Singapore, which again, in August 1980, through the merger with Nanyang University became the National University of Singapore. The University of Malaya in

Kuala Lumpur soon founded a new medical school in 1972. The past two decades have seen two more medical schools established in Malaysia under the National University of Malaysia, Universiti Kabangsaan, in Kuala Lumpur, and the Universiti Sains Malaysia, originally in Penang Island but later moved to Kota Baru in Kalantan State in the north-east of West Malaysia.

In Myanmar (Burma) the first medical school was established in the capital city of Rangoon at the turn of the century when the country was still a British colony. Like Singapore and Malaysia, early doctors who came to Myanmar were from Britain and were followed by those qualified from various medical schools in India; during the colonial period this reflected the policy of the British government. The development of medical education in Myanmar has been hampered considerably by several incidents when, due to political unrest, universities were closed, sometimes for prolonged periods. There are at present only three medical schools in Myanmar, two in Rangoon and one in Mandalay, qualifying about 550 doctors a year.

The programmes of training

The curricula of medical schools in South-East Asia were influenced by the various stages of development and prevailing trends in each individual country. The systems of education in these schools varied considerably and still reflect the influence of the countries of colonial domination which, in most cases, were British, American, or Dutch. In the Philippines, the required admission standard into the University of Santo Tomas School of Medicine in 1871 was an AB degree, which at that time was considered as equivalent to a full high school course as given in the USA. The curriculum in medicine consisted of a one-year 'ampliacion' or premedical course followed by a five-year course in Medicine leading to a diploma of 'Licencado en Medicina', which is equivalent to a Bachelor of Medicine. An extra year was needed to obtain the doctorate (MD) degree. Some time after the American occupation of the country, the curriculum of the Santo Tomas University Medical School was revamped, so that all graduates in medicine were awarded the diploma of MD. A number of American-based foundations, particularly the Rockefeller Foundation, enabled the College of Medicine of the University of the Philippines to upgrade its manpower and facilities until, at one time, the college was said to be the best medical school in the region. The current medical curriculum leading to the Doctor of Medicine degree of all the medical schools in the Philippines is similar to that in the USA, namely that a B.Sc. degree is a prerequisite for admission; there follows a four-year curriculum, consisting of a two-year preclinical period and two-year clinical period, followed by 1 year of internship. An examination is required for a licence to practise in the Philippines. A large number of native MD graduates have emigrated to practise medicine outside the Philippines, mainly the

USA. The administration of medical schools and the curriculum in the Philippines is guided and controlled by two important bodies, namely the Board of Education and the Association of Philippine Medical Colleges.

The medical curriculum in the Indonesian medical schools is, in general, based upon the European model, being divided into premedical, preclinical, and clinical phases. The minimum required period to complete the medical course is 6–7 years which also includes internships in teaching hospitals. While medical education is the responsibility of the Ministry of Education and Culture, most teaching hospitals are managed by the Ministry of Health or by the Provincial government. The responsibility of generating, implementing, and co-ordinating policy in relation to the training of doctors and dentists lies with the Consortium of Medical Sciences, a government agency under the aegis of the Ministry of Education and Culture.

In Thailand the medical curriculum of the Royal Medical School in Bangkok, when it first opened in 1890, began differently as the school had to induct students not familiar with modern Western medicine into a three-year course combining components of Western and traditional medicine. It was only after the subsequent developments funded by the Rockefeller Foundation that the medical profession became attractive to students as the medical curriculum was then similar to American medical education, namely a four-year course consisting of 2 years' preclinical and 2 years' clinical training. However, a Bachelor degree was not required for admission into the medical school, only 2 years in a medical science course before entering medical school, and there was no internship period. The First National Conference on Medical Education held in 1956 recommended several amendments in the medical curriculum and, through a total of five national conferences held to date, a number of substantial changes have been introduced into all medical schools. They have included the introduction of internship in 1961, compulsory government service for all graduates in 1968, and the realignment of the entire medical curriculum of all medical schools into a six-year course consisting of one-year premedical training, a two-year preclinical, and a three-year clinical course incorporating the internship period, as introduced in 1980. Recently, some medical schools in Thailand have opted for a problem-based curriculum. The reintroduction of The Thai Medical Council Act 1968 has imposed several regulations and professional standards to which all medical schools must comply. The university administration system in Thailand is under the responsibility of a separate Ministry of University Affairs headed by a cabinet minister. A Consortium of Medical Schools was set up recently to co-ordinate educational and administrative matters relevant to medical schools.

Malaysia, Singapore, and Myanmar share a similar pattern of undergraduate medical education, reflecting the system of medical education in Britain. The entry requirements into the medical schools include the local Higher School Certificate or the British General Certificate of Education Advanced Level or equivalent examinations. The medical curriculum leading to an MB,BS (or MD) degree generally takes 5 years, consisting of a two-year preclinical and three-year clinical period. To obtain a licence to practise, graduates must complete 1 year of internship (housemanship) in a recognized hospital. In Singapore, English is the language of instruction whereas the Malaysian language is used in medical schools in Malaysia. There has also been a trend to adopt the problem-based curriculum, particularly into the newer medical schools in Malaysia. The medical degree of the medical schools in Singapore is at present recognized by the General Medical Council of Great Britain as a primary qualification for the purpose of full registration, enabling its medical graduates to be eligible for registration in the UK and some other Commonwealth countries.

Postgraduate education

The systems of postgraduate medical education in South-East Asian countries differ greatly. The only common features are trends towards medical specialization and those 'academic' qualifications leading to higher degrees, namely the M.Sc. or Ph.D., or diplomas in subjects related to medical, clinical, preclinical, and allied fields. The higher and postgraduate degrees and diplomas are generally under the responsibility of the individual university or institution concerned. Examples of such academic qualifications are master and doctorate degrees of public health, higher degrees and diplomas of tropical medicine and hygiene, or nutrition at present being offered by a number of universities and institutions in the region.

In South-East Asia, 'professional' medical education, where a period of clinical training is obligatory, is generally under the responsibility of the respective Medical Councils or other similar professional bodies. In Indonesia, the Consortium of Medical Sciences is responsible for the residency training programme in some 20 specialties. On the other hand, the Philippine Medical Association, through its affiliate societies, as well as the Board of Education, is responsible for the training of medical specialists. In Malaysia and Singapore, the university still remains the sole source of training with the granting of the Mastership diploma in various clinical specialties. The Thai Medical Council, an autonomous body, is responsible for the residency training programme in some 30 specialties and subspecialties in the country. A formal specialist training programme does not exist in Myanmar and the Indochinese countries.

The period of training leading to specialist qualifications varies greatly in countries of South-East Asia. In Thailand, the Thai Medical Council sets a flat three-year formal training programme in all major specialties. However, doctors who have practised in their own specialty for a period of 5 years and have passed the required examinations are granted equivalent specialist diplomas. Holders of the Thai Medical Council specialist diplomas are entitled to admission as fellows of relevant royal colleges or colleges. In Indonesia and the Philippines, a period of training ranging from 3 to 4 years, depending on specialty, is required. The period of training required for the fulfilment of the Mastership qualification in Malaysia and Singapore is 2 years. However, doctors who have spent time in general practice are also eligible to take the Mastership examination.

One notable trend in medicine in South-East Asian countries during the past decades has been in the area of regional co-operation; this has been achieved through the many regional professional bodies, such as the Medical Association of South-East Asian Nations, through which a large number of academic and social activities are jointly carried out on a regular basis. Such activities have strengthened the development of various aspects of medicine in South-East Asia.

ADULTA VIRIYAVEJAKUL

MEDICINE IN SPANISH-SPEAKING COUNTRIES

During the government of Emperor Octavius Augustus and following the defeat of the resisting Cantabrians and Asturians, its original inhabitants, the Iberian peninsula finally became part of the political, cultural, and economical structure of the Roman Empire in 19 BC.

Subsequently, the humoral-based *Hellenic medicine practised by the Roman conquerors co-existed with the old, traditional pre-Roman therapies related to the worship of water and mountains, which prevailed in the less civilized and romanized areas of the country. In the larger urban zones the colonizers built ambitious public works to improve hygiene and sanitary conditions; such were the aqueducts of Segovia and Mérida, and the dam of Proserpina which supplied water to Mérida. In addition, public baths were built in other towns and many hot-water sources were exploited for potential therapies, demonstrated by the abundant votive stars found around these sources of water. Additionally, many surgical instruments, similar to those found in distant provinces of the Roman Empire, have also been found. These findings demonstrate the extent of diffusion and acceptance of the Hellenistic-Roman type of medicine in the Iberian peninsula. Nevertheless, the distance of these provinces from Rome delayed the programme of romanization and, consequently, the practice of medicine was not as contemporary as that practised in other territories of the empire, such as southern France.

After the fall of the Roman Empire, settlement of the Visigoths (originating in Germania) in Hispania (5th century AD) was followed by a period of cultural stagnation similar to that which occurred throughout the entire Christian world. During this period the most important Spanish contribution to medical knowledge was the concept that Saint Isidore of Seville (560–636) included in his *Etimologies*, a primitive medical encyclopaedia

which was soon widely referred to throughout Europe. While the book lacked originality, it was a useful synthesis, and Saint Isidore presented the ideas of some of the later Roman authors (e.g. Cecilio Aureliano, Sorano) in a very comprehensive manner.

In the year AD 711 many inhabitants from North Africa, having been converted to the Islamic faith, invaded the Iberian peninsula. The so-called Arabic domination of Spain lasted over 700 years and so intensively influenced the language and life-style that its effects may still be easily identified today.

The geographical location of Spain allowed intellectual and cultural exchange with other European countries; this was very fruitful for the development of science and medicine. Arabic medicine, which resulted from the assimilation of Hellenic medicine by the oriental cities of Resaina, Nissibis, and Gondishâpur, was soon accepted. Several clinicians (Averroes, Avenzoar) and surgeons (Abulcassis) wrote books which were widely read during the Middle Ages and the Renaissance. Hispano-arabic physicians, especially Averroes, in accordance with the Islamic ideal of the *hakim* (a physician simultaneously interested in all aspects of knowledge and enquiry, including theology), contributed greatly to the development of philosophical thought.

Military campaigns directed towards the expulsion of Muslims from the peninsula which, especially during the 11th century, constituted the *Reconquista*, provided a decisive impetus to the diffusion of classical medicine as reinterpreted by Arab physicians, throughout those countries remaining under Latin influence.

In different Spanish centres (Tarazona, Barcelona, Tarragona, Ripoll), but very specifically in the city of Toledo, work on translating Greek philosophy (Aristotle and Plato) and science into Latin from Arabic texts soon emerged, thereby prompting a wide diffusion of classical culture. Translation of the *Koran* was also regarded as fundamental in efforts to refute the Islamic faith and convert the Muslims to Christianity. Simultaneously, versions of medical texts (*Galen, Ionnitius, and *Avicenna, and a number of Hippocratic texts) decisively contributed to the incorporation of classical medicine into western European countries. For several centuries, translations written in Toledo, later corrected by commentators during the Renaissance, became the textbooks used to train successive generations of European physicians.

The subdivision of the Iberian peninsula into independent kingdoms allowed individual contacts between scholars from the eastern regions of Spain with those in the rest of Europe; such was the case with Arnau de Villanova (1235–1312), considered one of the most illustrious representatives of medieval scholastic medicine.

The many Jewish settlements in the Iberian peninsula determined the character of Spanish medicine from the Middle Ages onwards, due to the outstanding 'art of healing' of the Jewish physicians. The presence of Jewish physicians was habitual in Spanish society.

Some openly expressed their traditional religious beliefs (*Maimonides), yet others converted to Christianity, either sincerely or under pressure. Some of these physicians endured great conflicts under the Inquisition and its religious intolerance.

The first universities created in Spain (13th–14th century), emulating those already existing in Europe, contributed to the institutionalization of medicine as a discipline of academic standing. At the University of Salamanca, the Chair of Physic (medicine) was soon recognized, although it was never accorded the distinction of other disciplines such as law and theology. Despite these advances, it should be pointed out that the Islamic tradition (characterized by a more faithful adherence to the Arabic medical textbooks and Arabian Galenisms) prevailed for several centuries.

However, as a consequence of the development of medical humanism after the 15th century, revisions of the original Greek and Latin texts became the norm; although later than in Italy, some Spanish universities (Valencia, Alcalá, and, to a lesser extent, Salamanca) joined in the movement of correcting the original Greek texts by producing rigorous critical editions.

The 16th century undoubtedly represented the most brilliant period of Spanish medicine, paralleling the political hegemony and intervention in Europe which existed from the reigns of the Catholic kings (1476–1516) to that of Charles I (1517–55). The decisive factor leading to this scientific development was the movement of many Spanish physicians throughout Europe (P. Pintor, J. Almenar, G. Torella, L. Alderete, A. Laguna). Although Latin continued to be the scientific language *par excellence* until the 18th century, the peninsular languages (Castillian, Catalonian, and Portuguese), in differing degrees, although still lacking precision and maturity, gradually became the vehicle of scientific communication.

Until the 18th century, the *Protomedicato* served as the supreme political-administrative institution, exercising all medical and *public health responsibilities. During this period the political establishment completely controlled the training of professionals (*protomedicos* examined all university graduates before authorizing their professional activity) as well as various aspects of sanitary activity (inspections carried out by the *protomedicos* and their delegates).

Dating from the reign of Phillip II (1556–98), a gradual process of isolationism contributed to the progressive marginalization of Spanish medicine and its exclusion from the innovative methodology which nourished medicine and science in the 17th century. Faithful to the so-called 'authorities', a highly systematized practice of medicine was imposed, impermeable to all innovation; capacity for dialectic argument was given precedence over observation and experimentation. This process was challenged by minority groups (*novatores*) in the later decades of the 17th century, but with little effect until more enlightened rulers came into power after 1750. The hiring of foreigners to fill offices and various occupations, including medicine, promoted this change. Moreover, the need for a more professional army motivated the state's interest in the training of surgeons; as a result, colleges of surgery were founded (Cadiz, 1748; Barcelona, 1760) and introduced new teaching methods. These new institutions were able to introduce learning techniques traditionally avoided in the universities.

Political confrontations in the 19th century between the partisans of an absolute monarchy and those who backed a mere liberal constitution had undesirable consequences upon medicine and public health. Successive purges and exiles generated such insecurity that any climate conducive to reflection and study was unthinkable; universities suffered a major loss of independence and teaching facilities. Many properties belonging to the Catholic Church were also confiscated (*desamortización*), and the institutions established under its auspices were transferred to civil authorities. This instability meant that European science reached Spanish culture only after considerable delay. Only after the restoration of the Bourbon lineage in 1874 did progress become possible.

Until 1936, the year in which the Spanish Civil War began, there were uninterrupted attempts to further Spanish participation in, and knowledge of, European medicine and science. In the area of basic science, the outstanding histologist, S. Ramón y *Cajal (1854–1934), founded a brilliant school of research and was the main instigator, as President of the Board of Advanced Studies, of programmes of research abroad for young scientists. The lack of a complex public health infrastructure allowed a much more restricted international reputation for the work of other able professionals: G. Marañón, T. Ortega, G. Pittaluga, and A. Márquez. The Spanish Civil War resulted in the nearly total dismantling of weak existing structures. Emigration of intellectuals was widespread from schools of medicine (especially among the basic disciplines) and also among professionals in many clinical specialties. The years immediately following the war were marked by international isolation and recurrent economic crises. Economic development only began in the 1960s. Various campaigns of preventive medicine were implemented (eradication of *malaria in 1964, systematic *vaccination of the infant population). A public assistance (national insurance) system was put into effect which covered the entire population, and new hospitals and centres for primary care were created. The incorporation of new generations of professionals, trained, for the most part, in other European or American centres, and the ever-increasing dedication of public funds to health (the Health Ministry was created in 1977), has characterized medicine in Spain during the past 2 decades.

Medical care and training in present-day Spain

At the present time, there are 26 public medical schools in Spain and a private one in Pamplona, created by the

Opus Dei in 1954. In order to enter one of the medical schools, after finishing the baccalaureat, the students have to pass a national examination in science and the humanities, and are accepted or rejected according to their scores. Once accepted they have to complete a six-year academic programme to obtain their licence in medicine. The first 2 years are dedicated to basic disciplines (anatomy, physiology, biochemistry, genetics, etc.) and the following 4 years, in addition to theoretical lectures, involve the students in clinical activities within the hospitals associated with each medical school.

On completion of medical studies an official licence to practise medicine and surgery is granted. However, most students receiving this licence, in order to obtain specialty training, apply to a national postgraduate specialty programme known as MIR (Médicos Internos y Residents). This postgraduate programme, lasting 3–6 years, takes place in hospitals accredited by the national committee for each specialty. Every year some 20 000 young physicians apply to enter these programmes, which have a training capacity for 4000 doctors. Once specialty training is completed, physicians have the alternative of occupying hospital positions, starting their own private practice, working for private insurance companies, or joining local governmental medical facilities.

Medical care in Spain is offered both in publicly and privately administered institutions. Public health care is delivered through the National Institute of Health, within the Ministry of Health. A network of publicly owned health facilities encompasses the entire territory of Spain and is administered both at a federal and regional level. All Spanish citizens are covered by this system and contributions are made through the workplace by the employer and by the employee as part of a national Social Security programme. All medical specialties are covered, with the exception of dentistry and optical services. Patient care starts with primary medical care, but can also provide major hospitalization. Eighty to ninety per cent of medication is also provided.

A private patient-care system exists in parallel with the National Health Care system. It takes the form of a fee for item of service system, provided by insurance companies or private physicians.

South America

Since the discovery of America in 1492, the development of the continent has been indivisibly linked to the history of Spain. Apart from the prolonged political dominance over much of the newly discovered continent, a lasting bond was created by the use of a common language. One of the more significant and lasting examples of this symbiosis was the creation of various universities (Santo Domingo, Mexico, and Lima). These basically reproduced the Hispanic model of the University of Salamanca, which, in turn, imitated the medieval model of Bologna, wherein jurisprudence studies were given priority over those of medicine. For this reason, only some of the universities (Mexico, Lima, Guatemala, and Quito) offered studies in medicine, while others were quite late in offering these studies in their curricula (Havana, Caracas). European humoral medicine of Hippocratic–Galenic origin was first introduced by the doctors who arrived on the new continent (Álvarez Chaca arrived in Columbus' second trip, 1493) and subsequently by the universities created in the New World. Numerous European diseases reached the new continent and decimated local populations, isolated since their crossing of the Bering Straits (*measles, *leprosy, *smallpox, *influenza), while others were brought back to Europe with increased virulence (*syphilis). The Africans shipped to America for slave labour carried their own diseases (*yellow fever), as well as contributing to the ethnic mix. The great interest with which European doctors studied American therapeutic products was rapidly reported and widely distributed in various publications by the Sevillian doctor N. Monardes (1493–1588).

During the 18th century, the most ambitious campaign undertaken by the Spanish Crown in the colonies was the expedition of vaccination (1803) directed by Dr F. Balmis; lymph vaccine was transported first to America and then to Asia (the Philippine Islands, then under Spanish control) to try to combat smallpox, which had previously been introduced there by the colonists.

Medical education in Mexico

Two stages may be identified: the colonial and the republican. In 1533 the first university in the American continent was founded in 'Nueva Espana' (now Mexico), entitled the Royal and Pontifical University. In this university a medical school was inaugurated in 1519 and the opening lecture was given by Professor Juan de la Fuente, who received a salary of 150 gold pesos annually as chairman of the 'Catedra Prima'. In 1598 Dr Juan Plasencia established the second chair, entitled 'Visperas'.

In 1768, under the responsibility of two surgeons, Antonio Vezquez de Leon and Domingo Rusi, the Royal College of Surgery was founded, following the pattern of the same institutions in Barcelona and Cadiz. The 'Real Hospital de los Naturales' was used for patient care, and the first chair (Clinical Surgery, Operations and Legal Medicine) was inaugurated in 1770.

The Medical School and the College of Surgery functioned independently. In the medical schools a six-year programme of training was required but only 4 years in the College of Surgery. In 1833 the two institutions merged and a unified degree of Medical Doctor and Surgeon was granted. While this process evolved in Mexico City, in 1792 a medical school was established in Guadalajara under the auspices of the Royal Literary University.

The Republic of Mexico became an independent free and confederate state in 1824, 3 years after Mexico became independent from Spain. The first elected authorities created a new medical school in Oaxaca in 1827, followed by others in Nuevo Leon (1828), Morella (1829), Yucatan (1833), and San Luis de Potosi (1877).

This course of events developed in a similar manner in other Latin American countries as they each gained their independence from Spain.

Medical education in Venezuela

Venezuela was discovered by Columbus during his third voyage in 1498. There are records indicating that until 1763 medical practice was carried out by individuals acting empirically and independently. The following merit mention: surgeon Alonso and the pharmacist Bernal were the first Europeans to practise medicine in Venezuela; Don Diego Montes 'The Venerable' (1531) treated poisoned arrow wounds by using *cauterization; in 1696 surgeon Guerra Martînos performed the first *autopsy in Venezuela on a person who had died of *yellow fever ('black vomiting'); Albertus Millier, a physician from Vienna, signed a death certificate on a patient believed to be the first documented case of tuberculosis in Venezuela; the first *craniotomy was performed in Caracas by Pedro Roberto Diget on 5 April, 1736; in 1908 Dr Balmis began a programme of smallpox vaccination.

In 1763 the first organized teaching of medicine at university level was developed by Dr Lorenzo Campins y Ballester, who established a 'licence' in the so-called 'Protomedicato de Medicina' following Spanish and European models. In 1827, after Venezuela became an independent nation, Dr Vargas, Rector of the Central University of Venezuela, created a faculty of medicine, where modern teaching techniques were used. Many other medical schools and hospitals were also founded in other cities. At the end of the 19th century the influence of French medicine was clearly gaining ground, and hospitals began to be considered as health and rehabilitation centres and not mere asylums. All these institutions were financially supported by the government. In 1922, there were 482 physicians, increasing to 1452 in 1947, and to 14 771 in 1978 for a population of 8 million.

Several other important events also deserve mention. In 1904 the National Academy of Medicine was founded, and in 1930 the Ministry of Health was created, followed by a compulsory public Health Insurance programme. In 1954 the Institute of Neurology and Cerebral Research was inaugurated.

More recently, the influence of the North American method of teaching and practising medicine has been clearly apparent. Many private hospitals have been developed to compensate for the administrative difficulties of the public institutions.

Conclusion

The process of emancipation and independence of the colonies from Spain in 1821 promoted a nationalist tide which also sought to develop science and health. The political convulsions suffered by most of these countries, however, proved a decisive factor in the relegation of social as well as scientific development. The first medical schools in Spanish-speaking American countries imitated European, principally French, models. However, influence of the USA in the 20th century has resulted in the current general acceptance of that model. Numerous medical doctors, researchers, and teaching professionals, exiled after the Spanish Civil War and the Second World War, relocated in various Latin American countries, which profited greatly from their expertise. In recent decades, political instability and economic crises have forced many young Latin American doctors to emigrate to the USA where working conditions and research possibilities are more attractive.

Acknowledgement

The authors are grateful to Professor Ricardo Rangel for the note on Mexico and to Professor Pedro Ponce for that on Venezuela.

ALBERTO PORTERA-SÁNCHEZ
ANTONIO CARRERAS PANCHÓN

MEDICINE IN THE ARAB WORLD. The contribution of Arabic medicine to the evolution of medical knowledge is immense. Arab conquests in the 7th century came at a time when the Graeco-Roman civilization was plunging deep into decline and chaos. Europe was entering the Dark Ages and it needed a saviour to preserve the classic civilizations of Greece and Rome which were quickly disappearing. The Arabs, with their new religion, conquered most of the known world within a few decades. Their empire extended from the Ganges across Asia, North Africa, and south-western Europe. They spread their faith into China and as far west as the Pyrenees. During the 8 centuries of their empire, medicine flourished, among other scientific and literary endeavours. The new rulers of the empire quickly took to the civilizations they conquered. Graeco-Roman, Alexandrian, Byzantine, Persian, Indian, and other cultures were assimilated and cultivated. This was helped by the relative freedom under which Muslims as well as non-Muslim scholars could work. Islam accepted Christianity and Judaism as fellow religions worshipping the same god, and followers of these monolithic faiths could practise their religion in the Muslim state. Islam encouraged scientific and medical endeavours with clear messages in the *Holy Koran* 'and if any one saved a life, it would be as if he saved the life of all people' (section 5, Surat Al-Maida, verse 32). Medicine was practised by physicians who were outside the immediate control of the mosque, in contrast to the view of the Christian Church which prevailed in Europe for several centuries, where medicine was in the hands of the priests who looked at the human body as a sin, disease as a curse, and suffering a virtue. It is amazing that within a century the Arab nomad conquerers were transformed into benevolent rulers who nurtured and protected the arts and sciences. The libraries, institutions, and universities created in major cities were remarkable.

The initial advances in medicine were quickly established. These involved primarily the translation of Graeco-Roman works into Arabic. *Hippocrates and *Galen were thus faithfully translated and preserved. The translations were, by and large, performed by *Nestorian Christians and Jews. Nestorians were the followers of a Syrian monk, Nestour, who became patriarch of Constantinople in AD 428. He was excommunicated in AD 431 for heresy, his followers were persecuted and fled to Mesopotamia and Persia. They were educated in Greek culture and spoke Syriac, which is a close cousin of Arabic and Hebrew, all being derived from Aramaic. They were the link between the fast-disappearing Greek culture and the newly rising Arab Muslim civilization.

Sedillot (*Histoire des Arabes, Paris, 1854*) said:

What especially characterised the Baghdad school at its beginning was the truly scientific spirit which presided over all. To go from the known to the unknown, then from effects to causes and only to admit as true what had been demonstrated by experimental work, such were the principles taught by the masters. During the ninth century the Arabs were in possession of this fruitful method which a long time afterward was to be in the hands of modern investigators, the instrument of their finest discoveries.

Hunayn Ibn Is 'haq (Johanitius AD 809–873) is considered by many to be the initiator of the renaissance in the East. He was a Christian born in Al-Hira (southwestern Iraq). The quality and the breadth of his work make him the principal figure among many scholars who were the custodians of the Graeco-Roman culture and its translation into Arabic. His books on medicine alone numbered 84; they included many translations of Galen, Hippocrates, and Plato. He also produced original contributions such as *Masail fi al-Tibb* (*Questions in medicine*) and *Al-Asher Maqalat fi al-Ayn* (*Ten dissertations on the eye*). It is said that he was paid by the weight of his writings in gold; hence he used coarse paper and wrote in large letters.

The practice of medicine during the early part of Islam was influenced by the sayings (Hadith) of the Prophet Mohammed (AD 570–632). These have the power of law to Muslims:

Science is the remedy for the infirmities of ignorance, a comforting beacon in the height of injustice. The study of the sciences has the value of a fast; the teaching of them has the value of prayer; in a noble heart they inspire the highest feelings and they correct and humanise the perverted.

His sayings on medicine were collected in *Al-Tib al-Nabawi* (*Medicine of the prophet*). The practice of medicine evolved quickly. It began early in the 8th century by the establishment of the first hospital in Damascus by the Caliph Al-Walid I in AD 707. The golden age of the Arab civilization was undoubtedly during the reign of Haroon Al-Rashid in Baghdad, AD 787–810. Baghdad was the centre of culture and

science. During that time the Persian element was added by the Barmakids who were the wazirs (ministers) of the caliphs. The famous Persian School of Medicine in Jundisapur was gradually transferred to Baghdad. The first of the most famous medical family to come to Baghdad from Jundisapur was Jerjis Ibn Bakhtyishu. The Bakhtyishu dynasty spanned 250 years; Nestorian Christians, they were the most famous and powerful physicians. The grandson Gibrail Ibn Bakhtyishu was the chief physician to the Caliph Haroon Al-Rashid. His annual income was recorded at 4.9 million Dirhams (silver coin). He became the caliph's principal physician after curing his favourite wife from an hysterical paralysis.

Medical education and practice were initiated in hospitals, which were built, endowed, and administered by the state. There was regular inspection and certification. Adhudi, Al-Rashid, Al-Muqtadiri in Baghdad, Al-Mansuri, Al-Nasiri, Al-Qashashin in Cairo, Al-Nuri in Damascus were but a few. In the city of Baghdad, on the orders of the caliph, a census of all practising physicians was made in AD 949. This followed a reported medical mistake leading to a patient's death. There were 860 physicians, excluding those directly working for the government service. They were recertified and licensed. It is of interest to note that physicians were licensed to practise their specialty only after an examination. The Arabs were the first to recognize surgery and its practice as part of medicine, which was not the case in Europe with its barber-surgeons even many centuries later.

The practice in hospitals was the backbone of medical learning. Each of the famous doctors was chief physician at a hospital. Al-Razi (Rhazes), Ibn Sina (Avicenna), and Ibn Nafis were notable in the East; Al-Zahrawi (Abulcassis), and Ibn Zuhr (Avezoar) in the West. Several books on hospital organization and management were written, but unfortunately few survived. Al-Razi's book on *Sifat Al-Bimaristan* (*Characteristics of the hospital*) is an excellent example. The word *Bimaristan*, or *Maristan* in Persian, means home for the sick. Al-Razi was chosen to head the old Hospital in Baghdad after a careful selection among 100 applicants. The best description of hospitals across the empire is found in the writings of the most famous Arab traveller, Ibn Jubayer, who was born in Valencia and died in Alexandria (AD 1145–1217).

It is very difficult to choose the most representative works to cover the many centuries of the Arab Renaissance. Most of the books and manuscripts have been lost. This was mainly due to the massive destruction by the Moguls in the East when Holagu (AD 1258) plundered and burned Baghdad, and later to the fanatical destruction of the Moorish culture by the later conquerors in south-west Europe. Andalusia was reported to have had 70 libraries. One of those, the library of Caliph Al-Hakem II in Cordova, had 500 000 books and manuscripts, most of which have disappeared. Another difficulty encountered in trying to form a clear picture of the state of medicine is that many books and manuscripts were rewritten several times over the years, and later Latin translations were inaccurate and at times misleading. It is difficult to find identical copies of the same work.

It must be remembered that many physicians, translators, and scientists were not ethnic Arabs, or in many cases Muslims, but Nestorians, Christians, Jews, Persians, and of other races. The freedom to pursue their endeavours was only possible through the relative tolerance of Islam. With this in mind it is difficult to choose those individuals who contributed most to the progress of medicine during the Arab civilization. This choice is helped by the excellent biographical texts, exemplified by the work of Ibn Usaibiah (1203–70), *Oyun Al-Anba'a fi Tabaqat Al-Atibba'a (Fontes relationum de classibus medicorum; Original news on the classes of doctors)* in which he gave biographies of over 400 physicians. Amongst other biographers who included many physicians in their works is Ibn Khallikan (1211–82) in his book *Wafiyat Al-Ayan (Deaths of notables)*, which listed the biographies of 870 distinguished people.

Perhaps four major texts dominated the period and were the principal medium of transmitting Graeco-Roman, Byzantine, Persian, and Indian medical knowledge into Latin. They added an Arabic dimension on clinical observation as well as original surgical, medical, anatomical, therapeutic, and prognostic contributions.

The first was *Al-Hawi (Liber continens)* by Abu Baker Mohammed Ibn Zakariya Al-Razi (Rhazes, AD 865–925), who was born, as his name implies, in Al-Razy in Persia. He quoted at length from Greek, Persian, and Indian sources. In addition to his encyclopaedic work, he produced more specialized succinct monographs such as his masterpiece *Al-Judari wa-Al-Hasbba (Smallpox and measles)*. This is probably the most concise treatise of Arabic medicine and its last Latin edition was printed in 1866. His clinical abilities were best exemplified in his book *Burr al-Sa'ah (Cures in an hour)* in which he described all conditions which a physician can cure in an hour. His other major text, *Al 'Mansuri (Liber al-Mansorum)*, although smaller than *Liber Continens*, probably had more influence on European medicine, especially the School of *Salerno. Al-Razi held the view that fever was not a disease but showed that the body was working to bring about a solution to the disease (*Liber continens*, Book XXIII, 347). He was the first to describe the *recurrent laryngeal nerve and thought it originated near the *trachea.

The second major text was *Kamil al-Sinaah al-Tibbiya*, also known as *Al-Kitab Al-Maliki (The complete medical profession; or Liber regius)*. It was written by Ali Ibn Abbass Al-Majusi (died AD 994, Haly Abbas) who was a Persian Magian (Zoroastrian). His detailed descriptions of urinary catheterization, tuberculous lymph node excision, and breast cancer removal are a joy to read. The best translation into Latin was

by Stephen of Antioch. Other translators were not so scrupulous and some claimed the work for themselves.

The third, and probably best-known, text is *Al-Qanoon fi al-Tibb (The canon of medicine)* by Abu Ali Al-Hussain Ibn Abdulla Ibn Sina (Avicenna, AD 980–1037). Born in Balkh near Bokharra, he practised all over Persia, and wrote in Arabic not only on medicine but on philosophy, logic, astronomy, music, and mathematics. Perhaps the best Western Renaissance equivalent figure was *Leonardo da Vinci. His intellect and early scientific achievements are legendary. Avicenna's eccentricities made him move to many countries and cities. It has to be mentioned that his works were kept and conserved only through the dedicated work of his companion and biographer Abu Ubayid Al-Juzjani who first met him in AD 1002.

The Canon of medicine was the principal medical text in the Arab world and Europe for around 8 centuries. The brilliance shown in classification, presentation, argument, and subtleties deeply impressed medical scholars. *Osler stated that 'The Canon was the Medical Bible for a longer period than any other book'. His original descriptions included: *anthrax, *meningitis and its differentiation from meningism, central and peripheral facial weakness, the six motor muscles of the eye globe, pleurisy, pneumonia, and intercostal neuralgia. Ibn Sina's description of various causes of *jaundice as due to blood corruption (haemolytic), toxic, and retention of bile covered nearly all known causes of the condition. Other interesting works included a delightful book *Urjuza fi al-Tibb (Poems in medicine)* where he covered current medical knowledge in 1314 verses of poetry. Other works include *Al-Adwiah al-Qalbia (De viribus cordis; Cardiac drugs)*.

The fourth major work was *Al-Taysir fi al-Mudawat wa-al-Tadbir (Facilitation, treatment and organization; Facilitatio)* written by Abu Marwan Ibn Malik Abu al-Ala Ibn Zuhr (Avezoar, AD 1094–1162), who was born in Seville and was a member of a distinguished family of physicians. This book was complemented by his contemporary and countryman Ibn Rushd's (Averroes, 1126–98) book, *Al-Kulliyat fi al-Tibb (Generalities in medicine)* which was published in the same era. Ibn Zuhr was the first to describe *pericarditis, including pericardial effusion.

Surgery owes much to Abul-Qasim Khalef Ibn Abbass Al-Zahrawi (Abulcassis) who was born in a suburb of Cordova and died in AD 1013. His writings and books are voluminous and highly technical. *Al-Tasrif Lemen Ajeza un Al-Taleaf (Practical guide for those who cannot be authors)* was translated into Latin by Gerard of Cremona and influenced medical teaching in medical schools such as those of Salerno and *Montpellier. One of his important dictums stated 'If anatomical knowledge is ignored mistakes will be made and the patient will be killed'. His detailed descriptions of surgical procedures and their contraindications are precise and clear. Although his anatomy and basic surgery were based on Galen and Paul of Aegia, he went much further in describing exact operative detail and illustrations of surgical instruments. He wrote on surgical treatment of liver abscess, *goitre, *Pott's disease, *hydrocephalus, and tracheostomy, as well as on obstetrics and on performing craniotomy when the fetal head was too large.

Other names that should be mentioned include Ibn Nafis, the celebrated physician of the 13th century, who was the dean of the Mansoori Hospital in Cairo and was the first to describe the pulmonary circulation and clearly showed that blood is aerated in the lungs. He disagreed with Avicenna on the blood supply of the heart muscle and suggested the existence of the coronary circulation. Rabbi Musa ibn Maymoon (*Maimonides 1135–1204) was a Jewish physician born in Cordova who became a physician to Salah al-Din Al-Ayoobi (Saladin) in Egypt. His claim to fame, in addition to his distinguished medical works such as *Fusool Musa* (*Moses' aphorisms*), was his philosophical book on religion, *Dalalat al-Haireen* (*Guides to the perplexed*). His works showed evidence of independent original thought and were translated into Latin, Hebrew, French, and German.

*Pharmacy as we know it today was started as a separate discipline by the Arabs. The use of chemicals, including sugars and alcohol, to make potions was introduced. The discipline was separated from medicine for the first time and placed under state control and licensing. Ibn-Albitaar (born in Malaga and died in Damascus, AD 1197–1248), a worthy successor of Dioscorides, was the Inspector of Pharmacists in Cairo; he travelled far and wide in search of new plants and remedies. His book, *Al-Jamie le Mufradat Al-Adwia wa Al-Agthia* (*The corpus of simples*), included over 1400 different drugs. This work was translated into French by Leclerc (Paris 1877). Many drugs and medicines were later imported into Europe. This commerce was very large and formed one of the chief sources of income for the Italian maritime republics during the Renaissance.

The Arabic era eventually came to an end and its cultural heritage was transferred to Europe. This happened over centuries, in both the East and the West, but mostly in south-west Europe. Gerbert of Aurillac (AD 930–1003), who later became Pope Sylvester II (AD 999), travelled to Toledo and brought back Arabic knowledge to medieval Europe. The Crusaders did not really contribute to translation, most of which was carried out in Spain. The School of Translators in Toledo under Archbishop Raymond and Gerard of Cremona (AD 1114–87) was the main venue for transmitting Arabic and Greek writings to Latin. Le Clerc (1876) said, 'The Arabs thus repaid unto the Christians of the Western world the services formerly rendered to them by the Christians in the East'.

There were major differences between the Eastern Arabic Renaissance, which began in the 8th century, and the Western Latin Renaissance 6 centuries later. In the Eastern Renaissance Greek texts were highly valued

and sought after and Caliphs searched high and low for Greek masterpieces. In the Western Renaissance Arab texts were treated with suspicion and were much less regarded. The schools of translators in the East were organized and well financed, mainly in Baghdad, while in the West they were more individual in different monasteries and universities. Moreover, Arabic was a live and vibrant language which lent itself to development, while Latin, into which the works of Western Renaissance were translated, was a dead language only used in the Church and in science.

After the demise of the Arab empire in the East, followed by the decline of the Moorish rule in Andalusia, Arab medicine as well as science and literature virtually went into hibernation. During the following 8 centuries of Ottoman rule, there was little scientific advancement within the Arab world; on the contrary the previous achievements declined and practically disappeared.

It was only late in the 19th century that Western medicine started to filter back to the Middle East and North Africa. Currently there are two basic schools of medicine in the Arab world. By and large, following colonial influence in the late 19th century, there is an English-speaking school in the East (Egypt, Iraq, Saudi Arabia, etc.) and a French-speaking influence in the West (Morocco, Tunisia, Algeria, etc.). Medical education is taught in English or in French with one or two exceptions, where it is taught in Arabic.

Health care is generally provided by the state, with varying degrees of efficiency. The health-care systems reflect the prosperity of various Arab countries and their population demography. In the North African countries, where most of the Arab population resides, state medicine is mainly preventative and is directed towards primary care. The more expensive curative medicine is mainly provided by the private sector and is out of the reach of many citizens. In the East, oil wealth improved the standards of living and medical care is provided free at the point of delivery to all citizens. The Arab world, especially in the east, still imports medical technology and personnel from many parts of the world. However, many Arab physicians today receive undergraduate medical training locally, and postgraduate medical education is gradually becoming available in many Arab countries. An attempt to co-ordinate organized postgraduate training across the Arab world is underway under the auspices of the Arab Board of Postgraduate Medical Education. It is clear that the wheel of history has turned full circle and the Arabs are again receiving medical knowledge from outside Arabia as they did 12 centuries earlier. The main difference now is in the international revolution of communication and contact, which surely makes future Arabic contributions to the advancement of medicine a part of the global effort.

Thus it can be said that Arabic scholars kept the torch of science aglow during the Dark Ages. They saved knowledge which otherwise would have been irretrievably lost, and gave it back after many improvements. Their contributions to the evolution of medical knowledge are unparalleled.

RA'AD A. SHAKIR

Further reading
Castiglioni, A. (1947). *A history of medicine*, (2nd edn). Knopf, New York.
Cumston, C.E. (1927). *An introduction to the history of medicine*. Knopf, New York.
Elgood, C. (1951). *A medical history of Persia and the Eastern Caliphate*. Cambridge University Press, Cambridge.
Hitti, P.K. (1991). *History of the Arabs*, (10th edn). Macmillan, London.
Khairallah, A.A. (1946). *Outline of Arabic contributions to medicine and the allied sciences*. Beirut.
Leclerc, L. (1876) *Histoire de la médecine arabe*. Leroux, Paris.

MEDICINE IN THE EC (EU). The European Community (EC) (more recently called the European Union (EU), though many still prefer the familiar EEC or EC), created as an economic and political response to the devastation of the Second World War, has a growing influence in the 1990s. Health is not exempt from this process of change. This article describes the health systems of the Community and the EC's role in health affairs, and considers likely developments and problems in response to changes taking place within the Community as a whole.

The history and institutions of the Community
The Treaty of Rome in 1957 bound six countries in a Common Market, whose economic success encouraged six more (including the UK) to join between 1973 and 1985. The free market for labour and services in Europe has continued to grow as more countries have become 'associated' with the Community, and the controversy surrounding the expansion of the EC's political and social dimensions has not inhibited new applications for membership, several of which have recently been successful at the time of writing.

The EC's executive arm is the European Commission. This relatively small but powerful Brussels-based bureaucracy polices the implementation of Community law throughout the EC, issues directives to member states, and drafts laws for the Council of Ministers and the European parliament to consider. The Council is the forum in which government ministers of the 12 member countries take decisions on the Commission's proposals, while the elected members of the parliament have growing power to amend legislation and to regulate expenditure by the Commission.

The current and future powers of the EC in health affairs
So wide is the EC's influence that it is perhaps surprising how little formal power it has in the field of health. The Rome Treaty left health care under national control, and even now none of the Commission's 23 Directorates-General (DGs) has overall responsibility for health issues, which are camouflaged within the activities of DGs covering areas such as education, consumer protection, social affairs, research, and freedom of movement. Since the agreement on a 'Single European Act' in 1987, the pace of integration has quickened and the Commission has had more to say on matters affecting health. The Maastricht Treaty would accelerate this process; clause 129 gives the EC the legal basis for the first time to introduce legislation on 'public health'. The clause is couched in general terms, and the Commission is unlikely to set up a new DG or appoint a health Commissioner, but, none the less, there are implications for professional and consumer groups who want to influence European health systems through the EC institutions.

The organization of health care in the Community
Doctors throughout the EC may have a common intellectual heritage and shared values, but national health-care systems remain diverse. Some are variants on the UK model of a monolithic *national health service, but most are social security systems in which a patient consults a doctor in 'free practice', recouping the fees from compulsory *health insurance funds. Some systems are in rapid evolution, even turmoil, and everywhere governments are trying to contain spiralling health-care costs, to introduce market forces into health care, and to bring health professionals under greater control of lay managers.

How doctors are represented in the Community
Through the Standing Committee of Doctors of the European Community—also known as the Comité Permanent (CP)—the 12 national doctors' associations try to speak to the EC institutions with a single authoritative voice. The variety of health systems can make this difficult to achieve. Other bodies represent particular groups of doctors: UEMS (specialists), UEMO (general practitioners), PWG (junior hospital doctors), and so on, each with its own structure and agenda, but all channelling their views to the EC institutions through the CP. They work best as think tanks and ginger groups. For example, the PWG has strongly influenced the profession's views on medical manpower planning and on quality in *postgraduate medical education, and it was under prolonged UEMO-led pressure that the Commission issued a Directive in 1986 (EEC 1986) which required doctors to have specific training before entering general practice in any EC country—an important measure for raising standards in primary care.

Medical education and manpower in the EC
All EC countries except Luxembourg have medical schools, but there are great national differences in how these select, train, and assess medical students. Postgraduate specialist training varies even more. These

differences have undoubtedly slowed the harmonization of *medical education in the Community.

The number of doctors in the 12 existing EC countries has trebled since the 1950s to almost a million, but the resources needed to make use of their skills have not kept pace. Concern is growing about medical unemployment and underemployment, not only for the human and economic waste of keeping doctors idle, but also because a doctor cannot maintain high standards over a professional lifetime in the face of a dwindling case load. The UK has avoided serious difficulties by matching medical school intake with predicted future demand for doctors, but few other EC countries have tried to do this. Some cannot constitutionally limit access to higher education purely on planning grounds, but also the very concept of manpower planning is alien to insurance-based, private practice systems in which market forces prevail. The ratio of doctors to population shows a three-fold variation over the EC, with the most congested medical labour markets in countries with few controls over the supply of doctors.

Not surprisingly, perhaps, there is currently a complete absence of medical manpower planning at Community level. Ironically, the present glut of doctors may be followed early next century by a shortage, as those in the 'bulge' retire. Better planning at national and Community level is urgently needed to ensure that there then will be enough doctors to meet health needs.

Freedom of movement and harmonization of standards
The completion of the 'single market' in 1992 marked the achievement of a central aim of the Community—the abolition of national barriers to the movement of labour. In fact, doctors who are both nationals of an EC country and have obtained a primary medical qualification in an EC country have been free to practise throughout the Community under Directives issued in 1975 (EEC 1975). It is striking how few have done so; for example, some 1000 EC doctors (mostly from Germany, The Netherlands, Ireland, Greece, and Spain) work in the UK—1 per cent of the medical workforce. Nearly all are in junior hospital training posts, and most (but not all) will return to their own countries. The outflow of UK doctors to other EC countries has been negligible, and migration elsewhere in the EC is also low. Practical matters such as language, local ties, and pressure from the crowded medical labour market still decide where doctors live and work.

Not only doctors (and other health professionals) have the right to migrate. Some health managers are marketing their services internationally, and a growing number of patients are now being treated in a country other than their own.

If professionals have the right to move freely within the Community, the public has a right to expect similarly high standards of education and training, no matter where in the EC their doctor has qualified. Recognizing this, the Commission set up the Advisory Committee on

Medical Training (ACMT) 'to help ensure a comparably demanding standard of training in [all member states of] the community'. Unfortunately, medical training differs enormously in detail throughout the Community, so that the criteria allowing countries to recognize each other's basic and specialist medical qualifications under the 1975 directives were necessarily couched in vague terms and based on the duration, rather than the quality, of training. Training time correlates poorly with educational quality, and pressure is growing for another look at this issue.

For various reasons, the ACMT's own recommendations on specialist training (Advisory Committee on Medical Training 1978,1983,1986) have been implemented only patchily; real harmonization remains elusive. A recent initiative from the UEMS has set up, through its 'monospecialist sections', a network of European Boards to assess and certify doctors completing specialist training, and (a new concept in most EC countries) to visit and inspect the quality of training given by hospitals and institutions. Public and professional interest alike demand that the emphasis must now be not only on harmonizing but on raising standards of education and practice in the Community.

Medical ethics—consensus and differences
The Treaty of Rome was silent on medical *ethics, and the Commission has therefore had little to say on the subject. Doctors have been keener to explore the ethical implications of medical developments, but at least as many problems as solutions have emerged. Legal, religious, and historical obstacles have made it impossible to secure consensus on *abortion, *in vitro fertilization (IVF), and *euthanasia, and even in less contentious areas such as patient *confidentiality and organ donation only limited progress has been made towards a common European stance. These and other relevant issues are regularly considered by the Conférence des Ordres, a body representing the European medical regulatory authorities.

Doctors continually face new ethical challenges. Issues arising from the changing relationship between doctor and patient, and from the relative scarcity of health resources will severely test the profession's ability to reach a common European view—and one which can be accepted by the public and politicians.

Public health and the EC—a brave new world?
The EC's role in co-ordinating efforts against *public health scourges is in its infancy. The Community's greatest chance of success will be against the most obvious challenges. Professionals easily see the value of co-ordinating efforts against *AIDS and *cancer, and the *Chernobyl disaster helped politicians to realize that threats to the public health do not respect national boundaries, and that action against them must have an international dimension. Action plans like 'Europe against Cancer' and the campaign against

AIDS have shown the potential for the EC institutions to co-operate with individual countries and the *World Health Organization to achieve defined public health goals, and the research budget needed to support this work has doubled in the past 5 years.

On a smaller scale, regulations under the umbrella of 'consumer protection' have let the EC influence health indirectly in areas as diverse as health and safety at work, food additives, drug safety, and the quality of drinking water. Here the Commission's role evokes a mixed response, with vocal groups in most countries ready to denounce such regulations as bureaucratic interference in the rights of individual countries and their citizens, even as antidemocratic.

At a time when the Community is changing more rapidly and in more fundamental ways than ever before, these views perhaps reflect uncertainty about how far and how fast moves towards greater European integration should go. This question goes far beyond the arena of health, but how it is answered may have consequences for how we deliver and receive health care in the future.

DOUGLAS GENTLEMAN

References

Advisory Committee on Medical Training (1978). *Report and recommendations on the general problems of specialist training.* Commission of the European Communities, Brussels.

Advisory Committee on Medical Training (1983). *Second report and recommendations on the training of specialists.* Commission of the European Communities, Brussels.

Advisory Committee on Medical Training (1986). *Third report and recommendations on the conditions for specialist training.* Commission of the European Communities, Brussels.

EEC (1975). Council Directives of 16.6.75. 75/362/EEC and 75/363/EEC. *Official Journal of the European Communities,* **L167,** 1–16.

EEC (1986). Council Directive of 15.9.86 on specific training in general medical practice. 86/457/EEC. *Official Journal of the European Communities,* **L267,** 26–8.

MEDICINE IN THE FORMER SOVIET UNION
For many decades, official propaganda depicted the development of medical science and health care as highly successful achievements which demonstrated that the Soviet state had a paramount concern for the well-being of its citizens. Only with the advent of *glasnost* during the latter 1980s did highly placed individuals admit that in these areas the USSR lagged behind leading industrial countries, and that, due to neglect and misguided strategies, there was now a public health crisis of major proportions.

The many and serious defects identified at this time can be linked, directly or indirectly, to a single underlying cause. This is the earlier extirpation of 'civil society', with its opportunities for independent pressure groups to influence policy, achieved as the leadership of the one-party state turned to repression and terror in order to gain its objectives.

To a major extent, traditional medical ethics were suspended as the masters of the Soviet state abolished 'bourgeois' practices and obliged doctors to act as agents of social control. That role was especially evident in connection with the certification of short-term illness amongst the working population.

In medicine, as in other sectors of the economy, the former intelligentsia ceded position to Soviet-trained 'specialists' whose loyalty to the behests of the state took precedence over professional commitment. As the largely agricultural country was urbanized and industrialized at break-neck speed under Stalin's tyranny, a vast increase in the number of medical graduates occurred, with the emphasis on quantity rather than quality. A concomitant feature of this expansion was the mobilization of women, which reduced and then reversed the earlier preponderance of men in the ranks of this occupational group.

By the start of the Second World War, *morbidity and *mortality data showed a marked improvement over the appalling figures of some 20 years earlier. This alteration was doubtless influenced, in part, by the greater availability of health care. However, a highly selective emphasis could be seen in the concentration of resources in urban areas, with health care at the workplace very much to the fore, and neglect of the rural population. For vast numbers of peasants, the health service comprised no more than the local *midwife or *feldsher who, as in Tsarist days, was their doctor-surrogate.

At that time—and during subsequent decades—the health service had a low priority rating in respect of public expenditure. This also holds true for medical and pharmaceutical research, although development in those fields was retarded at least as much, if not more, by another negative influence. That was the intellectual and physical isolation from the West which Stalin imposed on scientists as one aspect of his intention to create 'socialism in one country'. Such a culture made it possible for T. D. Lysenko to elaborate a distinctive Soviet 'science' of plant-breeding, the practical applications of which were implemented by the authorities—with predictably disappointing results. As for medical specialties, research work in *psychiatry probably suffered most due to the obligation to accommodate particular restrictions and perversions which Marxist–Leninist doctrine entailed.

The death of Stalin in 1953 was not followed by fundamental changes in this sector; the 'administrative-command' system continued to promote an essentially quantitative approach to the planning and delivery of health care. Over the 40 years between 1950 and 1990, as can be seen from Table 1, enormous increases were recorded in the leading 'production' indicators. The supply of hospital beds nearly quadrupled, while the number of doctors (including dentists) rose by well over four times, as did the number of 'middle-grade medical personnel'.

Table 1 Basic indicators of Soviet health service development 1950–90 (in thousands)

End of year	1950	1960	1970	1980	1985	1990
Doctors	236.9	385.4	577.3			
Dentists:						
higher grade[†]	10.4	16.2	39.6	997	1170	1279*
lower grade[‡]	17.7	30.1	51.5			
Pharmacists						
higher grade[†]	12.2	26.5	47.7	75.2	91.0	118.0
lower grade[‡]	44.9	74.3	120.1	164.7	180.3	200.0
Middle grade						
medical personnel§	719	1388	2123	2814	3159	3420
Hospitals	18.3	26.7	26.2	23.1	23.3	24.1
Hospital beds	1011	1739	2663	3324	3608	3832
Units providing out-patient care by doctors and dentists	36.2	39.3	37.4	36.1	39.1	
Attendance per shift	–	–	–	4333	4874	5585

* Includes 41 000 lower-grade dentists.
† With higher education.   ‡ With specialized secondary education.
§ This category consists mainly of feldshers, feldsher-midwives, midwives, environmental health officers, nurses, medical laboratory technicians, radiographers, and dental technicians.
Sources: *Narodnoe khozyaistvo SSSR* for various years.

To set these figures in perspective, it is essential to relate them to a population base. The quotient of doctors to population reached 44.2 per 10 000 persons by 1990, among the highest in any country. However, cross-national comparisons need to take into account various peculiarities of medical practice in the USSR, such as the fact that Soviet doctors undertook a range of duties from which their Western counterparts were partly or wholly exempt.

By 1990, the quotient of hospital beds to population had also reached a very high level, at 132.6 per 10 000 persons. Over the decades, the increased supply of beds, predictably enough, gave rise to a substantial growth in the annual number of persons admitted to hospital as in-patients. By the mid-1980s this figure had reached the equivalent of about one-quarter of the total population.

The heavy reliance on hospitalization also reflected a negative factor, namely the absence of a single type of doctor of first contact who could provide continuity of care and be responsible for deciding whether the patient's condition called for referral to a hospital-based specialist. Here it should be noted that, as part of the strategy of training large numbers of doctors to work essentially as technicians, the regime had abolished the traditional single-door entry to medical practice and had split up training as between separate, if overlapping, courses. Thus at the end of the Soviet period almost all medical students undertook their training in one of the following broad areas: therapeutics, paediatrics, dental surgery, and hygiene, sanitation, and epidemiology.

From Table 2, a most important qualification emerges

about the provision of Soviet health care, namely the vast extent of spatial variation in the supply of leading 'inputs'. While overall responsibility rested with the USSR Health Ministry, the 15 republics which composed the Union had substantial freedom of manoeuvre regarding the development of this service as one sector of their economies. So even at the end of Soviet rule a massive gap could be found between the best and the least well-supplied republics, and that was despite the issue by the central ministry (in 1979) of planning guidelines which would have much reduced the variation. In 1990 the actual range for the supply of doctors was 32. 1, as against 10.9 in the plan—which amply demonstrated the ineffectiveness of the attempt to introduce 'territorial justice' in this sector.

In the early post-war period the introduction of *sulphonamide preparations and *antibiotics probably made an important contribution to the improvement in the summary measure of public health, average expectation of life. However, the Soviet Union never came near to catching up with the West with regard to pharmaceutical research. Up to the end of Soviet rule, modern *drugs for the advanced treatment of illness were frequently unobtainable due to systemic failures of production and distribution. The same explanation applies in respect of the chronic shortages of medical equipment and instruments, including even the most basic.

In their economic development strategy, the masters of the Soviet state gave totally excessive emphasis to investment in the military–industrial complex at the expense of measures which could prevent or mitigate the onset of illness, and save lives. One particularly telling consequence of this imbalance was that in the USSR termination of pregnancy rather than *contraception constituted the main form of family limitation. (Data for the Russian Federation show that legally induced abortions exceeded live and stillbirths by a ratio of two to one in 1990.)

After the Second World War the average expectation of life improved up until the mid-1960s, but the picture thereafter gave the lie to propaganda about the Soviet state as a uniquely effective guarantor of its citizens' well-being. By 1979–80 life expectancy for Soviet men stood at 62.2 years, in contrast to an average of 70.7 years for the USA, France, Great Britain, Japan, and West Germany—all major industrial countries. At that time Soviet women had a life expectancy of 72.5 years, as against the average of 77.7 for the five comparator nations.

A very similar picture emerges from the time-series for the infant mortality rate (IMR), which provides a litmus test for the general level of a country's socio-economic development, as well as for the standards of its maternity and child health services. In 1990 the USSR reported an IMR as high as 22 deaths of infants under 1 year per 1000 live births, and that was calculated on the basis of a less rigorous methodology than is used elsewhere. Even so, the rate was some 2.2–5 times higher than in the five nations named above. In Central Asia the reported levels far exceeded those in

Latvia, Belorussia, and Estonia. Indeed, official statisticians calculated that if the levels in the latter republics obtained throughout the USSR, the average expectation of life would improve by a whole year.

Pre-revolutionary Russia had some of the worst morbidity rates in Europe, and the record shows that the Soviet Union ended its existence in the same mode. For example, the incidence of *tuberculosis, although declining, remained relatively high (the death rate from this disease was 2–10 times higher than in the five comparator nations named above). In 1990 outbreaks of *diphtheria and even of *cholera occurred in European Russia, with subsequent deaths. Towards the less serious end of the spectrum, in 1988 there were 1.8 million reported cases of severe intestinal infections, the result mainly of low standards of hygiene in population centres, at reservoirs, and in the food-processing industry. The increased prevalence of serum *hepatitis in the same year was said to be due mainly to the absence of disposable syringes, and of other disposable items and sterile equipment.

Following the coming to power of Mikhail Gorbachev in 1985, senior medical officials recognized the need for massive 'top-down' reform of Soviet medicine. In 1986 the then USSR Health Minister, S. P. Burenkov, declared that 'For society today what is important is not how many there are of us [doctors] but how we work and the quality of the medical care which we provide'. His successor, Yevgeni Chazov, earned an honourable place

Table 2 Planned and actual ratios for key health service indicators, by Union Republic in 1990 (per 10 000 population)

Planned	Hospital beds		Doctors*		Middle-grade medical personnel	
	Actual	Planned	Actual	Planned	Actual	Planned
Russian Federation	138.6	137.5	42.2	46.9	144.0	122.6
Ukraine	135.7	135.5	40.0	44.0	131.5	117.5
Belorussia	136.8	132.3	38.6	40.5	129.5	115.6
Uzbekistan	134.0	123.7	35.1	35.8	124.1	110.7
Kazahkstan	137.2	136.2	37.3	41.2	133.9	123.9
Georgia	129.0	110.7	38.8	59.2	121.9	118.3
Azerbiadzhan	128.2	102.2	35.6	39.3	116.5	98.9
Lithuania	141.1	124.4	40.9	46.1	136.2	127.4
Moldavia	135.0	131.4	35.5	40.0	128.2	118.6
Latvia	142.6	148.1	43.7	49.6	142.0	117.4
Kirgizia	131.2	119.8	34.8	36.7	122.9	104.9
Tadzhikistan	135.7	105.8	32.8	27.1	114.2	80.3
Armenia	128.7	89.8	38.5	42.8	117.9	103.0
Turkmenia	133.7	113.3	34.5	35.7	125.0	105.0
Estonia	141.0	121.0	42.5	45.7	140.3	96.2
USSR	136.8	132.6	39.8	44.2	136.0	118.3

* Includes two grades of dentist.
Sources: *Narodnoe khozyaistvo SSSR v 1990 g.* and *Osnovnie Ustanovki k sostavleniyu pyatiletnevo plana razvitiya zdravookhraneniya i meditsinskoi nauki na 1981–1985 gg.*

in the historical record for his unstinting efforts to raise the levels of public spending on the health sector and to achieve radical improvements in public health through a wide range of new policies which were unveiled in 1987. Amongst the changes envisaged were: the requirement of higher standards in medical schools; the introduction of family doctoring; and improvement in the training of health service managers.

Chazov also recognized the need for a massive shake-up in the field of medical research. In his judgement, only some 50–60 institutes were producing work of high quality, while 100 were engaged on routine practical questions and a further 80–100 could simply be closed down without any loss.

At this point it is appropriate to caution against a grandly dismissive attitude towards the fundamental and applied research carried out by Soviet medical scientists. While propagandists certainly made exaggerated or untenable claims about achievements in this field (as in others), it will not do to ignore the genuine success stories. Here a few examples must stand for all. In 1982 a Soviet team was able to surprise American experts by demonstrating the first ultrasonic heart examinations to be carried out in space. Even in the unsettled early days of Bolshevik rule, A. L. Myasnikov pursued his investigations into the role of cholesterol in the aetiology of atherosclerosis, publishing his results in 1923. The research of A. F. Samoilov, undertaken in the 1920s, has a seminal value today for the guidance it affords in resolving questions of electrocardiographic diagnosis and in discovering new antiarrhythmic agents.

It is also to Chazov's credit that he attempted to modernize ossified organizational and operational practice by facilitating the creation of large-scale experiments in new forms of health-care finance and delivery. (Among the key ideas tried out was that of the 'internal market'.) However, his successor, I. N. Denisov, went a stage further by elaborating a Union-wide scheme for what was termed 'insurance medicine'. In essence this entailed substantially supplementing the government's budget allocations with item-for-service payments from the compulsory insurance of employed persons.

It can be shown that the scheme received support from numbers of rank-and-file doctors who, in the 'new times', were now free to organize themselves on an independent basis and give public expression to their collective views. The All-Union Association of Soviet Doctors, which came into existence in April 1990, had amongst its stated aims professional self-improvement, self-defence functions, and 'active participation in the development of the science and practice of medicine with the objective of protecting the population's health'.

In 1991 the nationality-based republics of the former military superpower became independent sovereign states, and hence were free individually to perpetuate or renounce any aspect of their Soviet past. At the time of writing, the Russian Federation intends to introduce a scheme of 'insurance medicine', a key feature of which would be the patient's right of free choice of medical practitioner and free choice among the appropriate health-care institutions. Many of those, it can be added, appear liable to privatization and commercialization as part of the government's overall economic strategy.

At present, the power of Russia's central government has been so weakened that the Russian Federation may even fragment as the Soviet Union did. In that case, its larger regions, such as Siberia, and the 'autonomous republics' (homelands of ethnic minorities) will manage health-care provision—like other services—having regard to their own political and economic circumstances. If such a fragmentation does take place, it will surely have the effect of deferring the renaissance of Russian medicine. In the meantime, affluent industrialized countries have a moral obligation to ameliorate, as best they can, the harrowing public health situation which is one consequence of the failure of 'the Soviet experiment'.

MICHAEL RYAN

Further reading
Feshbach, M. and Friendly, A. (1993). *Ecocide in the USSR*. Basic Books, New York.
Golyakovsky, V. (1984). *Russian doctor*. Hale, London.
Knaus, W. A. (1981). *Inside Soviet medicine: an American doctor's first-hand account*. Everest House, New York.
Ryan, M. (1989). *Doctors and the state in the Soviet Union*. Macmillan, London.
Ryan, M. (1993). *Social trends in contemporary Russia; a statistical source-book*. Macmillan, London.

MEDICINE IN THE INDIAN SUBCONTINENT

India is a unique country where various stages of evolution of medical treatment modalities still coexist. It is like a museum of medicine. Empirical, magical, priestly, religious, and scientific medicine are practised simultaneously in different parts of the country. Ayurvedic medicine and homoeopathy are given almost the same importance, as is modern allopathy, by the government of India. There are also many experts in the Unani system of medicine.

The ancient Indian physicians used medicine derived from vegetable products, animal products (such as flesh, fat, bone marrow, horns, hoofs, hair, skin, and urine), and earthly products (such as gold, silver, copper, lead, iron, and arsenic). Some practise these ways of treatment even today. Yogic and tantric medicine are still in vogue.

Ayurveda—the art of healing

The origin of the art of healing in India is steeped in obscurity. 'Ayurveda' means 'knowledge of life'. The Vedas are believed to contain knowledge of divine origin, pertaining to all aspects of human life, which was passed on by the gods to certain sages, who became teachers and passed on the knowledge to their disciples. Ayurveda is attributed to Lord Brahma (considered as creator of the universe in Hindu mythology) and can be traced back about 8000 years. It deals with the diagnosis and treatment of various diseases.

The ayurvedic system of medicine is widely practised in South-East Asia. According to Ayurveda, there are two schools for healing, i.e. the school of physicians (*Atreya sampradaya*) and the school of surgeons (*Dhanvantari sampradaya*). The specialists mentioned include those from *internal medicine (*Kayachikitsa*), *paediatrics (*balachikitsa*), psychological medicine or *psychiatry (*grabhchikitsa*), *otorhinolaryngology and *ophthalmology, *surgery (*shalyatantra*) *toxicology, *geriatrics (*jarachikitsa*), and the sciences of eugenics and aphrodisiacs (*vorishyachikitsa*). The pathogenesis of all diseases is explained on the basis of three basic constituents of the physiological system—motion (*vatta*), energy (*pitta*), and inertia (*kapha*).

It is claimed that, during the days of Gautama Buddha, there were two great centres of learning for medicine in India, namely Taxila in the west, with Atreya as professor of medicine, and Banaras or Kashi in the east, with Susruta as the teacher of surgery. Atreya, the most prominent amongst the teachers of Ayurveda, is often regarded as the father of Indian medicine.

The main source of our knowledge of ancient Indian medicine is from original contributions of Charaka and Susruta. *Charaka Samhita* is a comprehensive and monumental work on the Indian system of medicine, and represents a collective view of the writings of various workers from the 120th century BC to the 15th century AD. Susruta was a great surgeon, teacher, and an admirable author. Although Susruta's concepts of anatomy and physiology were primitive by modern standards, he was able to give excellent descriptions of a variety of surgical techniques. He performed surgery on the nose, ear, eyes, ligated blood vessels, set fractured bones, applied forceps in labour, and performed caesarean sections.

Susruta Samhita is the only excellent work available on the subject of ancient Indian surgery (*Shalya-Tantra*). It was translated into Arabic before the end of the 8th century AD, and was called '*Kitab-i-Susrud*'. It deals elaborately with fetal development, human anatomy, and the functions of the body. It gives detailed descriptions of various diseases of men, women, and children. Charka's *Materia Medica* consists mainly of vegetable products, although animal and earthly materials have also been mentioned. Commentary on '*Charka Samhita*' by Chakrapanditta, written in 1066 AD, is still considered to be the best document on ancient Indian medicine. Ayurveda describes two types of examination: examination of the patient (*rogi pariksha*) and examination of disease (*rog priksha*). It is undertaken to determine the state of various vital functions of the body, and the diagnosis of various diseases. Examination of the eyes, body structure, urine, and faeces has also been mentioned.

Patients were usually treated at their place of residence in Vedic and post-Vedic times. Hospitals for the care of sick people came into existence for the first time in India during the reign of King Ashoka in 274–236 BC. In Ayurvedic literature there is no mention of nurses or female attendants, although male attendants were mentioned. Specialization is not a new concept introduced by the present generation, as is commonly believed. Consultant physicians or specialists existed in the old Indian medicine system as well. Physicians and surgeons trained by the medical and surgical schools of Taxila and Banaras practised side by side with the priestly physicians. They described the diagnosis of *ascites by percussion and treatment by *paracentesis. The relationship between an enlarged spleen and liver and ascites was well recognized during Susruta's time. There was also mention of treatment of *bladder stones through an incision on one side of the perineum, intestinal perforation, *plastic surgery of the nose and ears, reduction of *fractures, and *obstetrical surgery for extrauterine pregnancy. The menace of unqualified practitioners of medicine, i.e. quacks, which even now is rampant in the Indian subcontinent, was described even in post-Vedic times. They were responsible for bringing the entire medical profession of the time into disrepute.

Various treatments practised by Ayurveda specialists included the administration of 'digestives', the creation of thirst, hunger, emesis, purgation, *enemas, and blood-letting. Great stress was given to the regulation of diet. The medicines were prepared by practitioners of Ayurveda in their homes. Large-scale production of ayurvedic drugs is now undertaken in modern factories. There are around 4500 pharmacies in South-East Asia. Some such factories in India are under government control. The cost of drugs and the fees of physicians are much less in ayurvedic than in conventional medical practice.

Unani system of medicine

The system of Greek medicine which developed during the Arab civilization is called Unani medicine. The European historians call it Arab medicine. This system is most prevalent in Pakistan, although many practitioners can be found in India as well. The Arab physicians followed the humoral theory of Greek medicine to explain health and disease. The human body is supposed to be composed of four elements (*arkan*), named *mitti* (earth), *pani* (water), *hawa* (air), and *aag* (fire). Temperature (*mizaj*) occupies a very important place in the Unani system. The basic philosophy is that the body functions properly only when there is a balance between physical and spiritual functions.

The medicines used in the Unani system are mainly of herbal origin, but animal, mineral, and marine drugs are also used ('marine drugs' are those prepared from marine plants or animals). These drugs do not have a rapid action.

Medical education and practice

Ancient India

Admission to medical schools in ancient India was very difficult. Students were required not only to select the textbook (*sastra*) but also the teacher. There were strict criteria for this selection. The 'pupil–teacher relationship' of ancient times was highly individual, prolonged, and close. The ideas were individually transferred from teacher to pupil. The entire personality, knowledge, behaviour, and character were literally passed on to the disciple 'for better or for worse'. This system was later changed to the monastic or institutional system of teaching, after the establishment of ancient Indian universities at Taxila (for medicine) and Banaras (for surgery). Small groups of pupils were usually selected with care and trained. The present-day system of teaching medicine is an extension of the old monastic system. According to *World Health Organization (WHO) data, there are 108 undergraduate teaching institutions in the traditional system of medicine in India, awarding degrees after 4.5 years of training in Ayurveda/Unani Siddha. There are two postgraduate institutes awarding postgraduate degrees. The Ayurveda University at Jamnagar in the state of Gujarat, is the only one of its type in the world. Currently there are more than 460 000 practitioners of traditional medicine in India, but only 271 000 are registered under State Boards. The majority of these are ayurvedic practitioners. There are around 150 000 homoeopathic practitioners in India.

The government of India has listed traditional remedies for purposes of providing primary health care. There are separate directorates for the traditional system of medicine in all states of India. There are 215 hospitals and 14 000 dispensaries in the country providing traditional medical care.

Modern allopathic medicine

The allopathic system of medicine has evolved in more technologically advanced nations and societies. It is difficult to pin-point the exact time when allopathy, or so-called Western medicine, separated from traditional medicine, from which it evolved thousands of years ago. It is only in the past 100 years or so that the allopathic system has gradually overshadowed all other systems of medicine, owing to adoption of modern scientific methods. Growth has been rapid in the past 50 years.

Western medicine was introduced into India by European medical men in the 17th century. Gabriel Boughton, a surgeon of the English ship *Hopewell*, was probably the first to treat the badly burned daughter of Emperor Shah Jahan in AD 1636. He, in turn, obtained permission for his company to trade in Bengal and the foundation of the East India Company was laid. Nicolos Manucci was the physician to Shah Alam, the eldest son of Aurangzeb, from 1678 to 1682. Nawab Haider Ali and Tipu Sultan in southern India also had several European medical men in their service. John Martin Honigberger served the Sikh Darbar of Maharaja Ranjit Singh in the Punjab from 1839 to 1849. These physicians and surgeons received consultation fees in kind or cash right from the beginning.

There are now approximately 150 allopathic medical schools in India, recognized by the Indian Medical Council, the supreme All-India body which is the watchdog of the standard of allopathic medical education and service in India. Approximately 14 000 medical students graduate every year in allopathic medicine from recognized medical schools.

Medical services in India

The delivery of medical services in India is today imparted according to the following stages:

Stage I. Primary medical care in vast rural India is provided through the Primary Health Centres (PHC), which are all located in the villages. Each PHC looks after 3–5 rural dispensaries. Trained medical graduates man these centres and dispensaries.

Stage II. These are country and district hospitals where medical services are provided by specialists in medicine, *surgery, *obstetrics and gynaecology, *ophthalmology, *otorhinolaryngology, and *dentistry; a substantial investigative infrastructure and facilities for in-patient care are available.

Stage III. Medical services of a much higher standard are provided in larger (500–1000 bed) hospitals attached to the medical schools. Medical services of a superspecialist (*tertiary care) nature are offered at these institutions.

Stage IV. There are a few medical institutions of national importance (centres of excellence) where medical services of the highest order, including neurosurgery, cardiac bypass, and organ transplant surgery are offered to referred patients. These institutions train specialists and superspecialists. There are about half a dozen institutions of this type in this vast country of almost 880 million people.

The government of India also recognizes ayurvedic and homoeopathic medicine, and appoints trained graduates in these systems, along with allopathic graduates, to the primary health centres, country, and district hospitals.

The British type of national health service does not exist in India despite the fact that before independence India was governed from Britain. However, medical services in government hospitals (central or state government) in India are provided free of charge, except for nominal charges for rich and upper middle-class patients (who are in the minority). There are a few hospitals in the private sector which impose substantial charges and cater only for the upper strata of society.

J. S. CHOPRA
S. PRABHAKAR

Further reading

Bannerman, R. H., Burton, J., and Wen-Chieh, C. (1983). *Traditional medicine and health care coverage*. World Health Organization, Geneva.

Filliozat, J. (1964). *The classical doctrine of Indian medicine*. M. Manoharlal, New Delhi.

Vakil, R. J. (1966). *Our glorious heritage*. Times of India Press, Bombay.

MEDICINE MEN. Medicine man is a synonym for *witch doctor, that is a person in primitive societies who combines the functions and powers of physician, magician, and priest.

MEDICINES ACT 1968. This major piece of UK legislation made new provision with respect to medicinal products and related matters, and established the *Medicines Commission. The Act was in eight parts, the various matters covered being as follows: constitution, terms of reference, functions, and committees of the new Commission (part 1); licences and certificates relating to medicinal products, including clinical trials and medicinal tests on animals (part 2); further provision relating to sale, supply, importation, and other dealings in medicinal products (part 3); pharmacies, including their registration, disqualification, and use of titles (part 4); containers, packages, and identification of medical products (part 5); promotion of sales of medicinal products (part 6); the *British Pharmacopoeia* and other publications (part 7); and other miscellaneous provisions (part 8). See also PHARMACOLOGY; PHARMACY AND PHARMACISTS.

MEDICINES COMMISSION. The Commission was established by the UK *Medicines Act 1968; it was to consist of not less than eight members appointed after consultation with appropriate organizations to provide expertise and experience in the following areas: the practice of medicine (other than veterinary medicine); the practice of veterinary medicine; the practice of pharmacy; chemistry other than pharmaceutical chemistry; and the pharmaceutical industry. The administration, terms of reference, and duties of the Commission were defined in the Act.

MEDICO-LEGAL MATTERS. See FORENSIC MEDICINE; LAW AND MEDICINE IN THE UK; LAW AND MEDICINE IN THE USA.

MEDITATION is exercise of the mind in deep reflection or contemplation; in transcendental meditation, a state of mental peace is induced by repetition of a mantra (a Sanskrit syllable or word).

MEDIUM. A nutritive substance on or in which microorganisms, cells, or tissues may be cultured.

MEDLARS is an acronym for Medical Literature Analysis and Retrieval System, a computer system enabling the biomedical literature to be searched, analysed, and extracted according to the specifications of the user. Medlars is based on the US National Library of Medicine in Washington, DC, but can be interrogated by users in other countries via linkage with appropriate terminals.

MEDULLA OBLONGATA. The lowermost part of the *brain, connecting the *spinal cord with the *pons. As well as ascending and descending nerve tracts, it contains the vital nerve centres controlling blood pressure, respiration, and cardiac action.

MEDULLOBLASTOMA. A malignant *tumour of the *cerebellum occurring particularly in children. Like other brain tumours arising in the posterior cranial fossa, it tends to obstruct the circulation of the *cerebrospinal fluid and to cause early signs of increased intracranial pressure.

MEGACOLON. Abnormally large and dilated *colon, a condition which may be either congenital or acquired. The former, also known as Hirschsprung's disease, is due to absence of the normal nerve plexus in a portion of the terminal bowel; this results in a contracted segment of varying length extending proximally from the *anus with massive dilatation of the colon behind it. Acquired megacolon can result from severe chronic *constipation of whatever cause.

MEGALOBLASTIC ANAEMIA is any of a group of *anaemias in which megaloblasts (large nucleated immature precursors of abnormal red blood cells) are present in the bone marrow. Most such anaemias are due to deficiency either of *cyanocobalamin (vitamin B_{12}), as in *pernicious anaemia, or of *folic acid, as in megaloblastic anaemia of pregnancy. See also HAEMATOLOGY.

MEGAPHAGIA. Grossly increased consumption of food, sometimes but not necessarily associated with increased hunger. See BULIMIA.

MEIOSIS is *cell division in which the chromosome complement of the two daughter cells is half that of the parent. It occurs in sexual reproduction, subsequent union of two *gametes restoring a full complement in the *zygote.

MELAENA (MELENA) is the passage of black or very dark *stools, usually owing to the presence of altered blood arising from *haemorrhage in the upper gastrointestinal tract or to taking *iron compounds.

MELANCHOLIA is a state of mental dejection, misery, or *depression.

MELANIN is the dark brown pigment responsible for the colour of skin, eyes, hair, nipples, and other structures. It is synthesized in several steps from the *amino acid *tyrosine in cells called melanocytes; its formation is stimulated by *melanocyte-stimulating hormone (MSH) and is promoted by sunlight, which causes tanning.

MELANOCYTE-STIMULATING HORMONE (MSH) is a *peptide hormone secreted by the anterior *pituitary gland which controls the activity of the *melanin-producing cells of the skin and other tissues.

MELANOMA. A tumour of *melanin-containing cells.

MELLANBY, SIR EDWARD (1884–1955). British medical scientist and administrator. He showed that *rickets was due to deficiency of *vitamin D. He proved to be a forceful and stimulating secretary of the *Medical Research Council and during his tenure of the post initiated the *National Institute for Medical Research.

MEMBRANE. Any thin sheet-like layer of tissue lining or enclosing an anatomical structure, or a layer of material acting as a partition or boundary.

MEMORY. The process of remembering is a complex mental function that includes at least the following steps: recognition, registration, short-term retention, long-term retention, retrieval, and activation (or expression). Defects in memory called amnesias and dysmnesias are characteristic of many organic brain disorders. Even very small lesions in particular areas of the *temporal lobes can cause dysmnesic syndromes without disturbing other mental functions.

MENARCHE is the first appearance of *menstruation.

MENDEL, JOHANN GREGOR (1822–84). Austrian geneticist. Mendel was raised in very poor circumstances; in 1843 he entered the monastery at Brno. For some 10 years he experimented, crossing plants, cultivating them, and testing at least 28 000. The paper in which he formulated what is now known as Mendel's law—*Versuche über Pflanzen-Hybriden* (1866)—was ignored until 1900 when discovered separately by de Vries, Correns, and Tschermak. Mendel ranks as the founder of *genetics.

MENIERE'S DISEASE. A condition due to excessive fluid (hydrops) in the *labyrinth of the inner ear. It causes variable hearing loss and *tinnitus, and disabling paroxysms of *vertigo. Ménière's disease affects mainly older adults.

MENINGES. The three membranes enveloping the *brain and *spinal cord, known (from within outward) as the pia mater, the arachnoid mater, and dura mater, respectively. The arachnoid is connected to the pia by

a cobweb-like network of fine threads (hence 'arachnoid'); the intervening subarachnoid space is filled with *cerebrospinal fluid.

MENINGIOMA. A tumour arising from the meninges of the *brain or *spinal cord, usually benign and slow-growing but disturbing function because of its space-occupying effect.

MENINGITIS is inflammation of the *meninges, clinically manifest by severe headache, *photophobia, and neck stiffness, sometimes with head retraction.

Meningitis can be caused by infection with many micro-organisms including viruses, bacteria, protozoa, and fungi. The clinical picture varies with the nature and severity of the infection. Meningeal involvement may be merely an incident in a generalized infective illness; or it may be the dominant or presenting feature, particularly when the causative organism is the *meningococcus (*Neisseria meningitidis*), which has a specific affinity for the meninges, or with a number of virus infections. The illness may be mild and self-limiting in viral meningitis (also known as aseptic or benign lymphocytic meningitis) provided the substance of the brain does not also become inflamed (encephalitis). On the other hand, bacterial meningitis can be a severe and dangerous disease with a high mortality and sometimes with a legacy of permanent neurological disability.

MENINGOCELE is herniation of the spinal *meninges through a congenital defect in the posterior wall of the spinal canal. See SPINA BIFIDA.

MENINGOCOCCAL MENINGITIS is *meningitis due to the *meningococcus (*Neisseria meningitidis*), also called epidemic cerebrospinal meningitis or cerebrospinal fever. One of the commonest forms of pyogenic meningitis, it occurs in both sporadic and epidemic outbreaks, predominantly in children and young adults. It was formerly an extremely dangerous disease, but the outlook was dramatically improved first by *sulphonamides and later by *antibiotics, the mortality rate coming down from about 75 per cent (often with severe neurological damage in the survivors) to the present figure, which is about 5 per cent or less. A vaccine against some types is being introduced.

MENINGOCOCCUS, or *Neisseria meningitidis*, is the agent of *meningococcal meningitis; it may also cause *septicaemia without meningitis, *pneumonia, and other infections. It is a *Gram-negative *diplococcus, often seen intracellularly in stained smears.

MENINGOMYELOCELE is herniation of the spinal *meninges and the *spinal cord through a congenital defect in the posterior wall of the spinal canal. See SPINA BIFIDA.

MENISCUS. One of two crescent-shaped cartilaginous structures found in the knee joint attached to either side of the upper (articular) surface of the tibia.

MENOPAUSE. The female *climacteric, when physiological cessation of *menstruation and *ovulation occurs, usually though not invariably in the second half of the fifth decade.

MENORRHAGIA is excessive or prolonged loss of blood with *menstruation.

MENSTRUATION is the periodic physiological discharge of blood and mucous membrane from the *uterus, recurring at approximately four-week intervals throughout the reproductive period of women, that is from the *menarche at *puberty to the *menopause, or about 30 years. The sudden destruction of the uterine mucosa represents the end of the luteal phase of the cycle which follows *ovulation and during which the uterus is in a state of readiness for possible implantation of a fertilized ovum. The menstrual cycle, which is under hormonal control, is a variant of the *oestrous cycle which occurs in sexually mature females of many other mammals; it is confined to catarrhine primates (Old World monkeys, anthropoid apes, and humans).

MENTAL DEFICIENCY is a term formerly used to denote deficiency of intellectual function, but now it has been largely superseded in the UK by 'mental handicap' or 'people with learning difficulties'. Another alternative is 'mental retardation' which is also used in the USA and in many other countries.

MENTAL DEFICIENCY ACTS 1913–1938 provided legislation in the UK regarding mental disorder before they were repealed by the *NHS Act 1946 and the *Mental Health Acts of 1959, 1960, and 1975, which superseded them.

MENTAL DISEASE is any disorder of the mind, congenital or acquired.

MENTAL HEALTH ACT 1959. This major piece of UK legislation repealed the Lunacy and Mental Treatment Acts 1890 to 1930 and the *Mental Deficiency Acts 1913–1938, making fresh provision for the treatment and care of mentally disordered persons and management of their affairs. Mental disorder was defined and classified to include mental illness, arrested or incomplete mental development (excluding severe subnormality), and *psychopathic disorder, when these were of a nature or degree to require, or be susceptible to, medical treatment or other special care or training. Among the provisions of the Act were the dissolution of the former *Board of Control and the setting up of Mental Health Tribunals for each hospital region of England and Wales.

MENTAL HEALTH ACT 1983. An enactment, most of the provisions of which came into force on 30 September 1983, which consolidated the UK law relating to mentally disordered persons and in particular the greater part of the *Mental Health Act 1959 and of the *Mental Health (Amendment) Act 1982.

MENTAL HEALTH (AMENDMENT) ACT 1982. This Act implemented proposals set out in a UK government White Paper *Review of the Mental Health Act 1959* (Cmnd. 7320) published in September 1978. It amended the *Mental Health Act 1959 and made substantive new provisions in a number of respects, as follows: to empower courts to remand accused persons to hospital for a report on their mental condition, or for medical treatment; to enable courts to send a convicted person to hospital temporarily in order to decide whether it is appropriate to make a hospital order in respect of him; to make further provision in respect of the removal of patients to and from the UK; to amend and extend the powers of Mental Health Review Tribunals; to specify certain forms of medical treatment for which consent must be given; to impose a duty upon district health authorities to provide after-care services; to impose a duty upon the Secretary of State to draw up a code of practice; to provide for the Secretary of State to establish the Mental Health Act Commission; and to amend the law relating to electoral registration and voting in the case of voluntary mental patients.

MENTAL NURSING. See NURSING IN THE UK; NURSING IN THE USA.

MENTAL RETARDATION is a term used for mental subnormality or handicap (i.e. a deficiency of intellectual function).

MENTAL SUBNORMALITY is the term which the *Mental Health Act 1959 used instead of 'mental deficiency'. It was defined as a state of incomplete or arrested development of mind.

MEPACRINE is a synthetic antimalarial drug introduced and used for many years as an alternative to *quinine but now superseded. It also has *anthelminthic properties and has a limited role in the treatment of *Taenia* and *Giardia* infestations.

MERALGIA PARAESTHETICA (PARESTHETICA) is numbness, tingling, and burning discomfort over the surface of the outer aspect of the thigh on one or both sides. It is due to entrapment and compression of the lateral femoral cutaneous nerve and occurs most often in obese patients, especially those who wear tight corsets or belts, but also in rowers.

MERCAPTOPURINE is an *antineoplastic and *immunosuppressive agent that acts by interfering with *deoxyribonucleic acid (DNA) synthesis. Its main use is as a remission-maintenance drug in acute *leukaemias.

MERCURY is a liquid metallic element (atomic number 80, relative atomic mass 200.58; symbol Hg), commonly known as quicksilver. Mercury compounds found widespread application in medicine in the past, but because of their toxicity are now no longer used. Mercury poisoning is a hazard of certain occupations. The manifestations of poisoning include *tremor ('hatter's shakes'), psychic disturbances known as *erethism ('mad as a hatter'), *ataxia due to cerebellar degeneration and other effects on the central nervous system, inflammation of the gums, discoloration of the lens of the eye, kidney disorders, and skin sensitization.

MERRISON REPORT may refer to either of two reports, both of UK Royal Commissions, of which Sir Alec Merrison was the chairman. One (1975) concerned the regulation of the medical profession in the UK, and resulted in reorganization of the *General Medical Council. The other (1979) was an inquiry into the operation of the *National Health Service. See GOVERNMENT AND MEDICINE IN THE UK.

MESCAL BUTTONS are the flowering heads of the peyote cactus *Lophophora williamsii*, the source of the alkaloid *mescaline.

MESCALINE is a toxic and hallucinogenic *alkaloid derived from the cactus *Lophophora williamsii*. Intoxication with mescaline induces *hallucinations, particularly of music and colour.

MESENCHYME is embryonic connective tissue of the *mesoderm, consisting of irregularly branching cells in a jelly-like matrix. It gives rise to connective tissue, blood vessels, cartilage, bone, etc.

MESENTERY. The double layer of *peritoneum attaching the *intestine and other abdominal organs to the posterior abdominal wall; it contains the blood vessels and nerves supplying these viscera.

MESMER, FRANZ ANTON (1734–1815). Swiss physician. He was inspired by *Mead's book on the influence of the planets on the body. He used magnets to draw out the 'animal gravitation' which he later called '*animal magnetism'. This view was satirized in Mozart's opera 'Cosi fan tutte'. Finally his hands took the place of the magnet and with them he claimed to infuse 'mesmeric fluid' (the origin of the term 'mesmerism'). Expelled from Vienna in 1778 he established a clinic in Paris which attracted a large following, including Marie Antoinette. The Revolution and the disapproval of orthodox practitioners forced him to leave France for Switzerland.

MESMERISM is a synonym for *hypnosis.

MESODERM. The middle of the three germinal layers of the embryo, in between the *ectoderm and the *endoderm. From it are derived muscle, cartilage, bone, blood, blood vessels, kidney, gonads, peritoneum, pleura, pericardium, connective tissue, and other structures.

MESOMORPH is one of the three constitutional types in W. H. Sheldon's (1940) classification (the others being *ectomorph and *endomorph). There is a supposed predominance of those tissues derived from *mesoderm (particularly muscle, cartilage, and bone) resulting in a powerful and compact body build.

MESOTHELIOMA. A highly malignant *tumour arising from mesothelium (the epithelium of the serous membranes, i.e. *pleura, *peritoneum, *pericardium) which, in pleural mesothelioma, is strongly correlated with exposure to asbestos.

MESSENGER. A biological substance or molecule carrying *genetic information, such as 'messenger RNA' (usually abbreviated to mRNA) which carries blueprints for polypeptide synthesis from *chromosomes to *ribosomes. See CELL AND CELL BIOLOGY; RIBONUCLEIC ACID.

METABOLIC RATE. The rate of *energy consumption by the body, usually calculated from the rate of *oxygen uptake.

METABOLISM. The sum of the chemical processes occurring within a living organism.

METAMORPHOSIS is a period of rapid transformation, particularly from larval to adult form (e.g. tadpole to frog).

METAPHASE. The second phase of *mitosis and *meiosis, when the *chromosomes are arranged on the equator of the spindle. See CELL AND CELL BIOLOGY.

METAPLASIA is the transformation of the type of cell in a tissue, particularly to an abnormal form.

METASTASIS is the remote spread of a *tumour or *infection from its primary site; the micro-organisms or malignant cells travel in blood or lymph, setting up distant foci of disease. The capacity to form metastases is a defining characteristic of malignancy in tumours, i.e. cancers.

METATARSUS. That part of the foot which consists collectively of the five long bones (metatarsals) and associated structures, and articulates proximally with the ankle (tarsus) and distally with the toes (phalanges).

METAZOA comprise all multicellular animals (cf. *Protozoa) except the sponges (phylum Porifera), which, because of their totally different organization and separate evolution, are sometimes regarded as a separate division of the animal kingdom known as the Parazoa.

METCHNIKOFF, ELIE (1845–1916). Russian microbiologist. His early work was on the development of invertebrates, but he later became interested in the *mesoderm. He observed *phagocytosis (a word he coined in 1880), noted the *macrophage, and believed that immunity depended solely on cellular mechanisms (see IMMUNOLOGY). His views were expressed in *L'immunité dans les maladies infectieuses* (1901). He was awarded the *Nobel prize in 1908.

METHACHOLINE is a cholinergic drug, i.e. one with effects like those of *acetylcholine.

METHADONE is a synthetic *narcotic *analgesic, similar to *morphine and *heroin in its pharmacological and addictive properties; it is widely used as a substitute for them in treating *addiction.

METHANOL is methyl alcohol, or wood spirit (CH_3OH), obtained by the destructive distillation of wood; it is a clear, colourless, flammable liquid, widely used as an industrial solvent. Although it has pharmacological effects similar to those of ordinary (ethyl) alcohol (*ethanol), it is very toxic, and as little as 15 ml may be fatal. It has a particular affinity for the optic nerve, and can produce temporary or permanent blindness. It may contaminate inefficiently distilled alcoholic beverages (its boiling point is 14 °C lower than that of ethanol), and is widely available as methylated spirits, a mixture of methanol and ethanol.

METHICILLIN is a semisynthetic penicillinase-resistant *penicillin (trade name: Celbenin®), of value in treating infections due to penicillinase-producing *staphylococci. It is not acid-stable and must be given by injection. See also ANTI-INFECTIVE DRUGS.

METHIMAZOLE is a drug which blocks the synthesis of *thyroid hormone by the thyroid gland, hence used in the treatment of *thyrotoxicosis.

METHODISTS. Adherents to a school of medical thought which flourished in the 1st century BC in Rome, at the time of *Aesculapius. Its basis was the simplistic doctrine of *strictum et laxum*, disease being due either to narrowing (*status strictus*) or relaxation (*status laxus*) of the body's internal pores.

METHOTREXATE is one of the *antimetabolite group of drugs, used to treat acute lymphatic *leukaemia (particularly with meningeal infiltration) and various other types of *cancer, and as an *immunosuppresive agent.

METHYL ALCOHOL. See METHANOL.

METHYLATED SPIRIT is an *alcohol mixture used as a liquid fuel, consisting (by volume) of 90 per cent *ethanol, 9.5 per cent *methanol, 0.5 per cent pyridine (to destroy palatability), and small amounts of petroleum and methyl violet dye. Industrial methylated spirit is 5 per cent methanol in ethanol and is free from pyridine.

METRITIS is inflammation of the *uterus.

METRONIDAZOLE is an antimicrobial drug active against anaerobic bacteria and protozoa.

MEYER, ADOLPH (1866–1950). American psychiatrist. He developed a school of psychiatry called psychobiology, stressing the need to consider all facets of a person's experience and physical state in determining the cause of psychological or psychiatric manifestations.

MEYER, KARL FRIEDRICH (1884–1974). American microbiologist and epidemiologist. He was an immensely productive investigator, and even after retirement published more than 200 scientific articles. His work concentrated on infections which can be transmitted from animals to man, including *glanders, *encephalitis, *brucellosis, *coccidiomycosis, *plague, *psittacosis, *rabies, and *anthrax.

MEYER, WILLY (1858–1932). American surgeon. He introduced certain urological technical procedures into American practice, such as catheterization of the male ureter. He devised a new operative procedure for radical resection of the breast. His special interest was thoracic surgery; he helped to devise an improved negative-pressure cabinet.

MEYNERT, THEODOR HERMANN (1833–92). Austrian neuropsychiatrist. He wrote extensively on the anatomy and physiology of the brain (1865–72) and many cerebral structures bear his name. He described *amentia.

MHC. See MAJOR HISTOCOMPATIBILITY COMPLEX.

MIASMA is a supposed harmful gas or effluvium emanating from cesspits, rubbish dumps, decaying matter in the earth, etc., held at one time to be responsible for disease (e.g. *malaria). The idea that all disease could be explained in this way was current in the 18th and early 19th centuries—the theory of miasma, or pythogenic theory.

MICRENCEPHALY (MICROCEPHALY). Smallness of the brain.

MICROBE. Any micro-organism (i.e. *bacterium, *virus, *protozoon, etc.), particularly, in lay usage, one capable of causing disease. See MICROBIOLOGY, MEDICAL.

MICROBIOLOGIST. A doctor or scientist specializing in the study of micro-organisms (*viruses, *bacteria, *fungi, and *protozoa).

MICROBIOLOGY, MEDICAL. Medical microbiology involves the study of *micro-organisms that colonize or infect humans, the mechanisms by which they cause disease, the body's response to infection, and specific antimicrobial prevention and *treatment. These organisms are a minute proportion of those that form a part of the ecosystem of our planet, but they include representatives of *bacteria, *viruses, *fungi, and *protozoa. This article will be restricted to consideration of bacteria and viruses.

The bacteria range in size from about 1/2000 to 1/100 mm. They generally divide by binary fission, and have a simple genetic apparatus and none of the larger cytoplasmic organelles that characterize *cells of plants and animals. Most bacteria synthesize all the components needed for their reproduction and can grow in artificial media outside the body. A few, such as the organisms causing *typhus and *chlamydial genital infections, can grow only in living host cells.

The viruses range in size from about 1/30 000 to 1/3000 mm. They comprise a nucleic acid genome of either *DNA or *RNA (but never both) surrounded by a protein coat. They disassemble when they enter a susceptible animal cell and replicate by subverting the genetic control of the host cell to produce all their own structural components. In some cases, viruses become latent by integrating their DNA or DNA transcripts of their RNA into the host cell *chromosome.

The origin of medical microbiology
Before the latter part of the 19th century, diseases that we now know to be *infectious were frequently attributed to *miasmas, physiological imbalances, genetic inadequacies, evil spirits, or divine interventions. Nevertheless, some students of disease recognized that many were contagious and made recommendations, such as *quarantine, for their control, on the basis that some unseen transmissible agents were involved. Before disease-causing microbes were discovered, it was also recognized that recovery from certain diseases was associated with resistance to acquiring the disease a second time, and deliberate inoculation of material from *smallpox lesions into the skin of healthy individuals (variolation) was practised in many societies. This somewhat hazardous procedure usually resulted in a mild or localized form of the disease with protection against a subsequent severe form. The discovery by Edward *Jenner (1749–1823) that the same effect could be obtained by *vaccination with material from cow-pox lesions of cattle laid a firm base for subsequent attempts to produce artificial active *immunity to infectious diseases, and vaccination on a world-wide basis led to the ultimate conquest of smallpox.

The discovery of micro-organisms
Although scattered reports of observations of microbial life antedated his work, Antony van *Leeuwenhoek (1632–1723) must be considered the father of microbiology. His occupation was in drapery and local government but his avocation was in lens-making, and he contrived a series of single-lensed microscopes that allowed him to see and study the shape, size, and movement of a variety of microscopic 'animalcules' from human body and the environment. These studies were published in a series of reports to the Royal Society. Unfortunately, he maintained close secrecy about the manufacture of his lenses and the illumination system that he used, and few corroborative studies were reported until the compound multilensed microscope was developed a century later.

The influence of Pasteur and Koch
The seminal discoveries in medical microbiology were those of Louis *Pasteur (1822–95) in France and of Robert *Koch (1843–1910) in Germany. Pasteur was trained as a chemist and first worked with microbes in a series of studies that showed that alcoholic fermentation was due to the action of living microscopic yeast cells rather than to purely inanimate chemical processes. This success was followed by a series of elegant experiments which laid to rest the widely held view that micro-organisms (and indeed some insects) arose spontaneously from decaying organic matter.

Pasteur then demonstrated that micro-organisms were responsible for some ailments of great importance to French industry and agriculture, ranging over diseases of wines, silkworms, sheep, and cattle. Early recognition of the significance of these studies to human disease by Joseph *Lister (1827–1912) led him to develop a system of *antiseptic *surgery to prevent the surgical wound infections which were a prevalent and lethal complication of surgery at the time.

Pasteur's crowning achievements were the development and exploitation of techniques to reduce the virulence of infectious organisms without eliminating their capacity to produce immunity to subsequent infection with fully virulent strains. In this way, he developed vaccines for the control of chicken *cholera and *anthrax in sheep, and for preventing *rabies in humans who had been attacked by rabid canines. Much of Pasteur's work involved the growth of bacteria and yeasts in liquid culture, and in the process he developed methods of sterilization and of 'pasteurization' that formed the basis of those in use today.

Robert Koch, a younger contemporary of Pasteur, was trained as a physician, and made some of his key discoveries in an improvised laboratory in the small town of Wollstein as a district health officer. He isolated and characterized the bacilli of anthrax, and *tuberculosis, and demonstrated their causative roles by a series of rigid and imaginative experiments. He was a superb technician and developed new procedures for staining, visualizing, and growing bacteria, and for solidifying liquid culture media with agar. This latter procedure was a critical advance because many specific bacterial infections occur in sites in which other non-pathogenic microbes are also present. By spreading such mixtures on the surface of sterilized agar media and incubating at body temperature, colonies of distinctive shape, size and colour developed from well-separated microbes of the different species. Each such colony comprises billions of progeny of the original organism, is visible to the naked eye, and pure cultures were obtained by transferring a few of the constituents of the colony to another medium. This process, using the type of culture dishes described by Richard *Petri in 1887, remains a central step in the isolation, characterization, and study of pure cultures of bacteria.

The work of Pasteur and Koch was rapidly recognized in their times, and considerable resources in the form of institutes, assistants, and support of students were placed at their disposal. Each of their laboratories trained large numbers of investigators who, in turn, made critical discoveries on the causes, transmission, *epidemiology, and sometimes control of common *infectious diseases. The impact of this work towards the end of the 19th century is hard to overstate. The bacteria causing *diphtheria, *typhoid, cholera, *tetanus, *gonorrhoea, epidemic *meningitis, *dysentery, and *plague, and the *staphylococcus and *pneumococcus, were isolated and characterized, to mention but a few. The disease manifestations of diphtheria and tetanus were shown to be due to specific *toxins made by the causative bacteria, and *antibodies produced in animals against the toxins (*antitoxins) were shown to neutralize their effects, and were introduced into therapy. In 1884, Hans Christian *Gram (1853–1938) developed a staining method in use today which clearly distinguished two classes of bacteria which are now termed Gram-positive and Gram-negative. The period was one of extraordinary scientific ferment. Congresses of microbiology were held, courses taught, journals initiated, and textbooks written, and the aura of mystery and inevitability that had accompanied outbreaks of *epidemic infections was replaced by the knowledge and understanding on which their control could be based.

Bacteriology in the 20th century
The period 1900–44 was one of extension, consolidation, and refinement of the rapid advances made at the end of the previous century. Many more bacterial causes of disease were discovered, including those of *whooping cough, *tularaemia, *syphilis, and *leptospirosis. There were major advances in methods of culturing bacteria. Selective media were developed that allowed preferential growth of organisms such as the typhoid or dysentery bacilli in the presence of the much larger numbers of harmless normal microbial inhabitants of the lower intestine. Methods were developed for easily producing an environment completely free of oxygen to allow the growth on solid media of anaerobic bacteria, such as those causing *gas gangrene, *tetanus, and *botulism, that die in the presence of oxygen.

The period also saw the development of many new methods to help identify bacteria. Procedures for detecting their ability to break down substances such as complex carbohydrates were developed, and sero-identification methods were introduced in which specific antibodies produced in animals were used to determine whether the *antigen(s) that elicited them were present in an organism. Such tests allowed differentiation of species which closely resembled each other in shape, size, and Gram staining (e.g. the colon *bacillus, the typhoid bacillus, and dysentery bacilli), and were critical to advances in bacterial *taxonomy, and to tracing the *epidemiology of infectious diseases. Electron microscopy, with a resolving power of 100 times that of the light microscope, was developed in the 1930s, and opened the way to later studies on bacterial structure.

Since the mid-1940s, there have again been dramatic advances in medical bacteriology, particularly in knowledge of bacterial structure, *genetics and pathogenesis of infection, and in diagnostic procedures.

Bacterial structure
The anatomy and chemical composition of bacteria have been clarified by electron microscopy and the ability to separate and analyse different structural components. They have been shown to have complex outer layers, with characteristic differences between Gram-positive and Gram-negative species. Many bacteria possess rotating flagella that endow them with motility, and many have external surface components that mediate attachment to target host cells or prevent ingestion by *phagocytes. In the cytoplasm are found the bacterial *genome, which is a very large, circular, tightly packed double-stranded DNA molecule, lacking a surrounding membrane, and large numbers of protein-synthesizing *ribosomes that differ in structure from those of plants, animals, and fungi. The cytoplasm also frequently contains small, circular DNA molecules, termed plasmids, which can carry genes encoding properties such as *antibiotic resistance or virulence, which allow the organism to survive and grow under conditions that are otherwise adverse. A prototypic bacterium is illustrated in Fig. 1.

Bacterial genetics
In the late 1940s and 1950s there were strong disagreements as to whether commonly observed bacterial variation in different environments was a result of random *mutation and selection or some form of adaptation that could be inherited. The issue had been partly resolved in 1943 in a series of elegant experiments by

Salvador Luria and Max Delbruck, but the occurrence of random mutations was conclusively proved by Joshua and Esther Lederberg in 1952. It was later shown that the genetic complement of bacteria was much more plastic. Bacterial viruses from one strain could infect another of the same species and in the process carry over a piece of the donor genome which could integrate into that of the recipient and transfer a property (e.g. antibiotic resistance) from the donor. This process was termed transduction. Likewise, building on the work of Frederick Griffith in 1928, it was shown in 1944 by Oswald *Avery, Colin MacLeod, and Maclyn McCarty that DNA extracted from one strain of a bacterial species could enter another and endow it and its progeny with a characteristic of the donor. Thus, DNA was shown to be the genetic material of bacteria. In 1947 Joshua Lederberg and Edward Tatum showed that some bacteria could conjugate and that part of a chromosome copy could be transmitted unidirectionally from one to the other. This was later shown to be determined by an inherited factor in the donor now known to be a plasmid.

Plasmids have been found to play critical roles in infectious diseases and their treatment. In 1959–60 Tsutomu Watanabe and other workers in Japan showed that multiple antibiotic resistance could be transferred within and between species in nature and in the laboratory. This phenomenon is due to transfer of a plasmid carrying *genes encoding the resistances. Bacteria that acquired the resistance plasmid could then, in turn, serve as a source of multiresistance to other bacteria.

Plasmids replicate in the bacterial cell as it divides and are thus part of its genetic make-up. The genes that they carry are generally inessential to the bacterium under optimal conditions for growth, but provide it with protection against some environmental insults (e.g. antibiotics), or facilitate the ability of a potentially disease-causing bacterium to damage its host, for example, by encoding a toxin. It is now known that some important genes are carried on transposons,

which are short segments of plasmid that can excise and integrate into other plasmids or into the organism's nuclear DNA. These jumping genes enormously enhance the genetic capacities of bacteria to survive and thrive under unusual conditions at a rate that could never be achieved by random mutation and selection. They are thus of great significance to the evolution of bacterial infectious diseases and to our ability to treat them.

Virology

The first half of the 20th century brought significant advances in the understanding of viruses and viral disease. Towards the end of the 19th century, it had already been shown that mosaic disease of tobacco plants and foot-and-mouth disease of cattle were caused by agents that could not be seen with the light microscope, could pass through filters that would hold back known bacteria, could not grow in artificial culture, but could be transmitted to the host species from which they were derived. Early in the 20th century the term 'virus' was restricted to infectious agents with these properties, and the first demonstrated mammalian viral diseases were of animals because transmission could be demonstrated experimentally in their non-human hosts. Viruses of bacteria that caused them to break down (bacteriophages) were discovered by Frederick Twort in 1915 and by Felix d'Herelle in 1917. These were much studied later as useful models for other viral infections, and, because of their specificity, as markers in epidemiological studies of bacterial diseases. Bacteriophages can serve as vectors for the transfer of genetic material between bacteria, and some encode toxin production by certain disease-causing bacteria, such as the diphtheria bacillus.

As early as 1913 there had been limited success in growing viruses in slices of living tissue maintained in special culture media, but survival was short, and contamination with bacteria or fungi was an almost inevitable complication. In 1931, Ernest Goodpasture and his colleagues overcame these difficulties by the use of embryonated hen's eggs to grow the virus of fowl pox. This technique was refined by Macfarlane *Burnet, and a range of viruses, including those of *influenza, *herpes simplex, smallpox, and vaccinia, were grown and studied in the various membranes of the developing chick embryo. It was by then recognized that viruses multiplied only within living cells of the host, and could not be grown in artificial culture. The tobacco mosaic virus was the first virus to be seen by electron microscopy, in 1939. Subsequent refinements have demonstrated all known viruses, including some that have not been grown in cell culture.

Viral structure

Viruses vary in size, but have two common structural arrangements as shown in Fig. 2. They contain a nucleic acid core of either DNA or RNA (but never both)

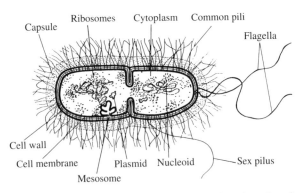

Ribosomes   Cytoplasm   Common pili
Capsule
                                    Flagella

Cell wall

Cell membrane   Plasmid   Nucleoid   Sex pilus
        Mesosome

Fig. 1 The structure of a dividing bacterium (reprinted with permission from Sherris, 1990).

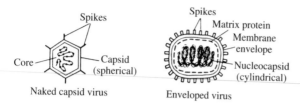

Fig. 2 The structure of two basic types of virus (reprinted with permission from Sherris, 1990).

within a protein coat, of which the subunits are organized in icosahedral or helical symmetry. Some viruses are also surrounded by membranes that they acquire as they emerge from the host cell or its nucleus. As with bacteria, surface structural components of viruses are responsible for specific attachment to the host cells that they will be infecting.

Viral genetics
The genome of viruses is smaller and less complex than that of bacteria, reflecting the smaller size of viruses and the contribution of the host cell to viral replication. Mutations in the viral genome are common, particularly in RNA viruses. Results include the minor year-to-year changes in the influenza virus that partially circumvent immunity from previous infections, the very large numbers of rhinoviruses of the common *cold, variations in the *HIV virus that occur during the course of infection (which complicate the search for effective vaccines), and the development of resistance to antiviral agents.

A more fundamental genetic change can occur when two different viruses infect a cell simultaneously. Their genetic material may then be rearranged to encode a virus with properties different from its progenitors and against which immunity directed towards others recently encountered is ineffective. This is a relatively infrequent event but appears to have been the origin of the disastrous 1918–19 influenza *pandemic and the Asian influenza epidemic of 1957.

Cell-culture techniques
With the advent of potent non-toxic antibiotics, the possibilities of growing human and animal cells in uncontaminated cultures became more practical. In 1949 John Enders, Frederick Robbins, and Thomas Weller first grew the *poliomyelitis virus in cultures of monkey kidney cells, and set the stage for the development of the first poliomyelitis vaccine by Jonas Salk in 1955. There followed extensive experiments to develop different cell lines for viral growth. Some have limited periods of survival on subculture, probably because of genetic programming. Others, derived from malignant tumours, are 'immortalized', and HeLa cells, for example, have been maintained in culture for over 30 years. Cell culture has now been used to grow the great majority of viruses known to produce disease in humans.

Just as some bacteria may require particular culture media for growth, different viruses may grow in cells derived from different sources. Their effect on the cells can vary from destruction, through the development of altered surface properties, to infections that can be demonstrated only by resistance of the cell to infection with another virus. The type of virus responsible for the effects on cell cultures or experimental animals can be determined serologically: for example by neutralizing its effects with specific antisera. In some cases, serological procedures such as immunofluorescence are used to demonstrate viruses within the infected cells. Bulk cell cultures permit the purification of considerable quantities of viral particles by physical separation techniques, and these procedures have been used in detailed structural and chemical studies of viruses and in vaccine production.

Viral replication
Within the past 40 years or so, the mechanisms by which viruses are reproduced have been clarified. Unlike bacteria, which multiply by binary fission, viruses lack the complement of *enzymes and structures needed for reproduction, and replicate by programming the cell they infect to synthesize and reassemble new viruses, often in very large quantities. Viruses are then usually released from the cell, often following its destruction, and can then infect other cells.

With some viruses, infection of host cells can result in a state of latency in which the cell seems unaffected. This can result from integration of viral DNA, or of a DNA transcript of viral RNA, into the host cell genome, by viral DNA adopting a plasmid-like state within the cell, or by viral replication occurring very slowly in concert with cell division.

Latency is involved in the relapsing nature of *cold sores and genital herpes infection, in the reactivation of the *chickenpox virus after many years to produce shingles (*herpes zoster), and in the long period between initial HIV infection and the development of overt disease. Some viruses that integrate into the host cell genome induce changes that lead to certain kinds of tumour. Most examples of these occur in animals, but two unusual types of *leukaemia in humans have been shown to be caused by specific viruses, and other viral infections are less directly associated with the development of malignancy.

The pathogenesis of bacterial and viral diseases
To produce disease in an otherwise healthy person, pathogenic bacteria and viruses must first evade a variety of host defences. For example, the skin can be breached by wounds or insect bites; organisms causing intestinal disease are usually quite resistant to the acids and enzymes of the stomach; and the ciliated cells of the trachea and bronchi that protect the lungs may be damaged or destroyed by an infecting organism. Most pathogenic bacteria and all viruses must then attach

to the surface of specific target cells to initiate infection. This process involves a complementary association between microbial surface structures, such as bacterial pili or viral capsid spikes, and particular molecular configurations of host cell membranes.

The next stage of infection requires multiplication of the infecting organism. Bacteria may multiply on the epithelial surface to which they have attached, within their target cells, or in the underlying tissues. Viruses replicate within their target cells, damage or destroy them, and then spread to attack neighbouring cells. Invasive infections with both bacteria and viruses involve lymphatic or blood stream spread, followed by continued multiplication in more remote susceptible cells or tissues. A variety of tissue and cellular defences must be evaded for multiplication to proceed. For example, some bacteria possess capsules that render them insusceptible to phagocytosis, some produce toxins that kill phagocytes, and some inactivate antibodies that may attack them.

The mere multiplication of an organism does not necessarily produce disease. This can result from the production of one or more specific toxins (e.g. diphtheria or cholera), from direct destruction of target cells by a virus (e.g. influenza), from the damaging effects of the inflammatory responses of the host (e.g. pneumococcal *pneumonia), or from hypersensitive immune reactions to the infecting organism (e.g. tuberculosis and some viral diseases).

Bacteria that can cause disease in healthy individuals are a very small proportion of those inhabiting the body. Their virulence is determined by several genes, some of which may be plasmid-borne. The ability of the host to withstand infection or to control an infectious disease is also complex, and depends on the many components of an intact cellular and humoral immune system. In recent years, an increasing number of severe infections with organisms previously considered of little or no pathogenic potential have been encountered in those whose immune systems are compromised by disease, cancer *chemotherapy, or *immunosuppresive drugs. The most important and accelerating cause of these opportunistic infections is the HIV virus of *AIDS. A large proportion of those who succumb to AIDS die of one or other of a variety of infections due to organisms that rarely, if ever, cause disease in health. Some of these infections are acquired from normal microbial inhabitants of the body, some from the environment, and some are reactivations of latent viruses or bacteria. These patients are also unusually susceptible to old epidemic diseases, such as tuberculosis, because of their deficiencies in cell-mediated immunity.

New developments in the detection and identification of micro-organisms

Laboratory diagnosis is still primarily based on direct microscopic detection, staining reactions, cultural characteristics, biochemical reactions, seroidentification, and serodiagnostic procedures. All but the last of these reflect properties encoded in the organism's genome. Recently, more direct approaches to detecting the make-up of the genome have become available, and these promise to revolutionize the discipline as methods become simpler and costs reduced.

The nucleic acid genomes of bacteria and viruses can be partially purified, digested with endonuclease enzymes that break them at specific sites, and then examined electrophoretically in a gel to determine the mobility of the resulting fragments. This produces a specific 'fingerprint', and a comparison can be made between an unidentified strain and a reference strain to determine whether or not they are identical. More simply, the DNA can be treated to yield fragmented single strands, and then tested to determine whether those from the different organisms can revert to the double-stranded state. The degree of homology achieved correlates with the degree of relationship between the two organisms. These approaches are changing our understanding of the evolution and taxonomy of micro-organisms. A simpler application of these methods can be used to detect and characterize plasmids. Many bacteria contain one or more plasmids of various sizes, and these are represented in the immediate progeny of the organisms. Plasmid DNA can be separated from chromosomal DNA and examined by gel electrophoresis. Migration is directly related to plasmid size and is consistent for the same size of plasmid from different strains. Thus the procedure can be used in current epidemiological studies to trace the source or spread of a given organism, or to trace the source or spread of resistance plasmids between different species of bacteria. Endonuclease treatment of plasmid DNA before electrophoresis increases the assurance that plasmids from different strains are identical in composition as well as size.

Identification of an organism, or even of the presence of specific genes in the genome of an organism, can often be accomplished by the use of a probe. This is a segment of single-stranded DNA or of ribosomal RNA complementary to a specific portion of the genome of the organism to be detected, or to the gene that is being sought. Probes are produced by genetic engineering techniques or synthetically, and are combined with a radioactive or other label that allows their easy detection. When applied to the products of digested DNA or even to disrupted organisms, the presence or absence of DNA complementary to that of the probe can be determined by methods that detect the label.

The most dramatic diagnostic application of molecular techniques has been the development of the polymerase chain reaction (see GENETICS). Starting with as few as one or two organisms, repetitive enzymic amplification steps produce very large numbers of DNA copies of specific parts of a bacterial or viral genome. These copies are then available in sufficient amounts to allow a DNA sequence analysis and lead to an identification that could not otherwise have been made. This technique has been used, for example, to detect minute amounts of HIV virus and *hepatitis C virus in human serum. Even more dramatically, it has allowed identification of non-viable organisms in tissue samples, and detected organisms that have never been isolated and allocated them to known taxonomic groups by determining the base sequences of highly conserved parts of their genomes.

Many other new diagnostic procedures have come into use in recent years, based on serological methods that have allowed the detection of very small amounts of microbial components and of the antibodies that they elicit. Antibodies labelled with fluorescent dyes can allow single organisms to be identified microscopically, and other labelling procedures can detect soluble microbial products or specific antibodies. Combinations of immunological and electrophoretic procedures can speed the detection of microbiological antigens in clinical material, or separate different microbial antigens so that the specificity of antibodies in serum against the different components can be determined. Using these approaches, the diagnosis of the commonest forms of childhood meningitis can be made from the *cerebrospinal fluid within an hour or two, and the serological diagnosis of HIV virus infection confirmed with a high degree of reliability.

The chemotherapeutic revolution

The development of effective antimicrobial agents was probably the most significant development in medicine in the mid-20th century. Most bacterial infections became amenable to treatment, and antiviral agents of increasing effectiveness have become available or are under development. Antimicrobials as a group have allowed the development of organ transplantation and anticancer chemotherapeutic regimens that would otherwise have been impossible because of the disastrous effects of infections in these situations.

Selective toxicity

Chemotherapy of infectious diseases with naturally occurring antibiotics or synthetic antimicrobial compounds (these will be referred to as antimicrobics) depends on greater toxicity for the microbe than for the host. Paul *Ehrlich (1845–1915), first described the principles on which chemotherapy should be based and discovered the first effective (although toxic) antisyphilitic drug, *arsphenamine, in 1909.

All the major classes of antimicrobics since discovered act on certain structural or physiological characteristics of the microbe that are either absent from the host cell, or are represented in the host in a less susceptible form. Most effective antibacterial agents (see ANTI-INFECTIVE DRUGS) exploit the uniqueness of the cell wall, the differences between bacterial and host ribosomes, or differences in the enzymes involved in nucleic acid synthesis, replication, or transcription. Selective

toxicity is rarely absolute because many antimicrobics damage particular host tissues if given in excessive amounts: however, for a broad group of cell-wall active agents, such as penicillin, the difference between effective and toxic levels is very great. Selective toxicity of antiviral compounds has been more difficult to achieve, because the mechanisms of viral replication and assembly utilize the same or similar metabolic processes to those of the cell they infect. Nevertheless, a number of synthetic antiviral compounds are now available. Most act by interfering with invasion of the cell by viruses, with replication of viral nucleic acids, or with viral assembly, but many have some toxicity to host cells (see ANTI-INFECTIVE DRUGS).

*Interferon, discovered in 1957 by Alick Isaacs, is one of a class of naturally occurring antiviral proteins produced by host cells in response to viral infections. It serves as an early host defence against viral infection, and has proved of value therapeutically in some infections due to the herpes group of viruses. It can now be manufactured by genetic engineering techniques, and its more ready availability is permitting wider trials of its role in viral therapy and in the treatment of some cancers.

Antimicrobial resistance

Antimicrobial resistance is a growing problem. When each antimicrobic was first introduced, its activity against particular groups of organism was generally predictable. For example, almost all strains of pathogenic staphylococci were susceptible to penicillin. However, within a few years of the introduction of penicillin most strains of staphylococci were found to be resistant to penicillin and often to other antimicrobics with antistaphylococcal activity. Despite the efforts of the pharmaceutical chemists, micro-organisms have shown sufficient genetic versatility to find mechanisms of resistance to almost all new agents—sometimes rapidly but sometimes only after decades of use. Resistance may result from low-frequency mutations in the bacterial or viral genome, but bacterial resistance is more often plasmid-mediated. Some plasmids may carry genes encoding resistance to as many as 15 antimicrobics. On transfer to another organism, a plasmid and its encoded resistance becomes part of the genetic make-up of the recipient.

Resistance becomes important with antimicrobic treatment of an infection because resistant strains or variants can multiply and cause continuation or relapse of the disease. Plasmid-mediated resistance amplifies the problem and the plasmid can spread to organisms that are normal inhabitants of the body (e.g. the colon bacillus) and thus increase the reservoir of resistance genes. Spread of resistant organisms between individuals in hospitals or community epidemics often occurs, and is facilitated by widespread use of antimicrobics to which the infecting strain is already resistant and which destroy competing normal inhabitants of the body. A similar situation occurs in cattle and poultry receiving antibiotic food supplements, and multiresistant *Salmonella* can be selected and transmitted to humans through contaminated meat or eggs, causing disease, often in epidemic form.

On a community-wide scale, the resistance problem involves failure to prevent spread of infecting organisms, the extensive and often inappropriate use of particular antimicrobics in medicine, and, to some extent, their non-medical use in animal husbandry.

J. C. SHERRIS

Further reading

Dixon, B. (1979). *Magnificent microbes*. Atheneum, New York.

Lechevalier, H. A. and Solotorovsky, M. (1974). *Three centuries of microbiology*. Dover Publications, New York.

McNeill, W. H. (1976). *Plagues and people*. Anchor Press/Doubleday, Garden City, NY.

Rosebury, T. (1969). *Life on man*. Berkley Publishing, New York.

Sherris, J. C. (ed.) (1990). *Medical microbiology. An introduction to infectious diseases*, (2nd edn). Appleton and Lange, Norwalk, CT (previous publisher, Elsevier, New York).

Tortora, G., Funke, B., and Case, C. (1992). *Microbiology*, (4th edn). Benjamin/Cummins, Redwood City, CA.

MICROCOCCUS. A very small *coccus.

MICROGLIA. One of the two components of *neuroglia, the supporting tissue of the central nervous system. Microglia contains cells of mesodermal origin which have a *phagocytic function, similar to *macrophages elsewhere.

MICROMANIPULATOR. An apparatus which attaches to a *microscope and allows manipulation of objects within the field of view.

MICROMELIA is a congenital *deformity characterized by tiny or vestigial limbs.

MICRO-ORGANISM is the general term for any microscopically small organism. Micro-organisms include *viruses, *bacteria (including *rickettsiae), *yeasts, and *protozoa.

MICROSCOPE. The study of structure is essential to the study of biology and medicine. Although the naked eye can discern much detail in tissues, etc., it is only with the use of optical aids, the microscope in its various guises, that we can determine cellular and subcellular structure. In addition to the standard light microscope, which, using transmitted light and a system of lenses, allows magnification of up to 1000, modern electron microscopes, of both the transmission and scanning varieties, provide magnifications of as much as 100 000. For descriptions of other techniques of microscopy including dark ground, fluorescence, polarized light, phase contrast, and interference methods,

see More (1986). Also see ANATOMY; HISTOLOGY; MICROBIOLOGY, MEDICAL; PATHOLOGY.

Reference

More, I. A. R. (1986). Microscope. In *The Oxford companion to medicine* (ed. J. Walton, P. B. Beeson, and R. Bodley Scott). Oxford University Press.

MICROSCOPY is the examination of structure with optical and other types of enlarging instruments which enable visualization of detail indistinguishable by the unaided eye. See MICROSCOPE.

MICROSURGERY is the surgery of minute structures for which the surgeon's vision must be assisted by a *microscope.

MICROTOME. An instrument for cutting thin sections of objects or tissues for microscopic examination.

MICROTUBULE. One of many tubular structures lying within the *cytoplasm of a cell which may be distinguished on electron *microscopy as part of the cell's internal architecture, sometimes referred to as the cytoskeleton. Microtubules, which consist of a protein, tubulin, have a structural function; they are, for example, responsible for the spindle formation in *mitosis and for the organization of cilia and flagella. See CELL AND CELL BIOLOGY.

MICTURITION. Urination; the act of passing *urine.

MIDBRAIN. The mesencephalon, the uppermost part of the *brainstem; it comprises the tectum or roof and the two cerebral peduncles.

MIDDLE EAR. The tympanic cavity, a cavity in the *temporal bone of the skull which separates the *tympanic membrane (eardrum) from the inner ear; the space is bridged by the three auditory *ossicles, which transmit the sound vibrations. The cavity communicates with the mastoid antrum, an air space in the mastoid portion of the temporal bone, and with the *Eustachian tube.

MIDDLESEX HOSPITAL, THE, London, was founded in 1745. It was at first situated in a small street off Tottenham Court Road, serving the slums nearby. The first lying-in beds in a general hospital in the UK were opened there in 1747, and it was then called The Middlesex Hospital for Sick and Lame and Lying-in Married Women. The notable obstetrician William *Hunter worked there. A new hospital was built on the present site, and was opened in 1757. In 1791 Samuel Whitbread, the brewer, gave money to endow a ward for patients suffering from *cancer. They were often excluded from other hospitals as there was no cure and they stayed for a long time as in-patients. The hospital was rebuilt on its present site in 1924. The hospital's medical school began at the foundation and was rebuilt in 1960. In 1982 the hospital combined with University College Hospital nearby to pool their resources for service, teaching, and research. The schools are part of the University of London.

MIDWIFE. A nurse qualified to assist patients during *childbirth and to provide antenatal and postnatal care. See NURSING IN THE UK; OBSTETRICS.

MIDWIFERY. *Obstetrics, the branch of medicine concerned with pregnancy, childbirth, and the puerperium.

MIDWIVES ACT 1951. This UK act consolidated previous Midwives Acts, notably those of 1907, 1915, 1918, 1921, and 1936. The main provisions included: establishment of a Central Midwives' Board; prevention of persons other than a state-certified midwife, currently on the roll of midwives, from attending a woman in childbirth, except in an emergency or under the direct supervision of a doctor; requirement of midwives to summon medical aid if necessary, etc.

MIGRAINE is a common periodic disorder of which the main feature is one-sided *headache (*migraine* is the French equivalent of the Greek *hemicrania*). The headache is severe and often incapacitating; it can last for up to 24 hours or more, and is frequently accompanied by photophobia, nausea, vomiting, and prostration. Classically the patient experiences some warning of an impending attack—this prodrome can take various forms, but most often involves visual or sensory phenomena (loss of part of the field of vision, bright or coloured lights and geometric patterns, the so-called 'fortification spectrum', or tinglings and pins and needles in the lips or hands). In individual patients, certain precipitating factors may be defined; but these seem to have no common denominator. Migraine is unpleasant and often temporarily disabling; it is not, however, life-threatening, and may lessen or disappear with advancing age. The mechanism is unclear, but it is generally agreed to be primarily a vascular phenomenon of constriction and later dilatation affecting the arteries supplying the head. There is a strong familial influence.

MIKULICZ-RADECKI, JOHANN VON (1850–1905). Polish surgeon. One of the leaders in abdominal surgery, he devised the *oesophagoscope and was the first to operate in a mask and cotton gloves. He described the enlargement of lacrimal and salivary glands known as *Mikulicz's syndrome (1892).

MIKULICZ'S SYNDROME is bilateral diffuse swelling of the *salivary and *lacrimal glands from any cause (e.g. *sarcoidosis, *lymphoma, *leukaemia, *collagenosis, *Sjögren's disease).

MILIEU INTERNE (sometimes *milieu intérieure*) means 'internal environment', and was used by the French physiologist Claude *Bernard to denote the physicochemical composition of the body fluids and its physiological constancy. See HOMEOSTASIS.

MILITARY MEDICINE. See ARMED FORCES OF THE USA, MEDICAL SERVICES; DEFENCE MEDICAL SERVICES (UK).

MILK is the maternal mammary gland secretion which is the natural food of young mammals. The precise composition of milk varies according to species; for example, although human milk has approximately the same fat content as cow's milk, it contains twice as much carbohydrate and half as much protein. See also INFANT FEEDING; LACTATION.

MILK OF MAGNESIA is a white suspension of magnesium hydroxide in water, used as an *antacid and *laxative.

MILLER, HENRY GEORGE (1913–76). British neurologist. He was a man of great personal charm and legendary mordant wit. Although speaking was his true element, he also wrote with elegance, on both neurological topics and more general matters; among his books were *Early diagnosis* (1960), *Modern medical treatment* (1962), *Diseases of the nervous system* (with W. B. Matthews, 1972), and *Medicine and society* (1973). Many of his other contributions to medical literature were on *multiple sclerosis and accident neurosis. After his death in 1976, tributes written by friends and colleagues were published by the *British Medical Journal* under the title *Remembering Henry*.

MILLIN, TERENCE JOHN (1903–80). Irish surgeon. He introduced the then revolutionary retropubic approach to removal of the *prostate gland. This allows access to the organ, which is frequently enlarged in older men, causing obstruction to urinary outflow, by getting into the space behind the pubic bone and in front of the bladder. Before this the gland was reached by incising the bladder wall. The Millin operation was tidier and carried fewer complications. It became standard international surgical practice. He made several other urological advances, including total bladder resection for *cancer.

MINAMATA DISEASE. An outbreak of methyl mercury poisoning in a fishing village in Minimata Bay, Japan, during the 1950s, was associated with severe neurological manifestations. It was due to the discharge of an industrial mercury compound which contaminated the fish. See also POISONING.

MINERAL SPRINGS supply natural water containing

appreciable concentrations of salts and gases dissolved from the rocks and soil through which it has flowed. The discovery of such springs and their supposed medicinal qualities dates from earliest history; *Hippocrates in 400 BC described contemporary watering places in his work *Airs, waters and places*, and *Pliny in AD 77 wrote about the mineral springs of Europe. Many springs discovered by the Romans are still well known, for example, those at Aachen (Aix-la-Chapelle) and Baden-Baden in West Germany, at Spa in Belgium, and at Bath in England. Others whose waters have achieved world renown include Harrogate, Vichy, Dax, Selzer, Bad Pyrmont, Ems, Wiesbaden, Baden (Switzerland), and Carlsbad (Czechoslovakia). In the USA, mineral springs have not been exploited to the same extent. Of about 8800 which exist, only some 400 have been used commercially. A few are well known, such as Saratoga Springs, New York, and White Sulphur Springs, West Virginia.

MINER'S NYSTAGMUS is a form of *nystagmus (a rapid tremor of the eyeballs independent of and not affecting normal ocular movements) which used to be an occupational disease of coal miners. It was due to the poor light in which many miners worked; when lighting conditions improved, the condition disappeared. Miner's nystagmus was a 'prescribed disease' in the UK under the *National Insurance (Industrial Injuries) Act of 1946.

MINISTRY OF HEALTH. Successor of the *Local Government Board and predecessor of the present *Department of Health, the Ministry was established by the Ministry of Health Act of 1919. See also GOVERNMENT AND MEDICINE IN THE UK.

MINOT, GEORGE RICHARDS (1885–1950). American physician. Following G. H. *Whipple's demonstration that liver is beneficial for anaemia of blood loss, in 1926 Minot (with W. P. Murphy) tried a liver diet in patients with *pernicious anaemia. They achieved cures of what had hitherto been a fatal disease. For this work, Minot, Murphy, and Whipple received the *Nobel prize in 1935.

MIOSIS (sometimes spelt 'myosis') is contraction of the *pupil.

MIOTIC. Any agent causing pupillary constriction.

MIRACLES are acts of healing considered to have been brought about by an other than natural agency.

MISCARRIAGE. Spontaneous *abortion.

MISSIONARIES, MEDICAL, MISSION HOSPITALS, AND MISSIONARY SOCIETIES. Western standards of social welfare and medical care embody Christian values. Christ showed compassion for the poor, the disabled, and the outcasts of society; he healed the sick and taught his disciples to do likewise. Early Christians became the first medical missionaries. During an outbreak of bubonic *plague in Alexandria in 256 AD, when most citizens fled the city, only the Christians stayed to care for the victims, and many lost their own lives as a result. By the 4th century they had established community *nosokomeia*, places for care of the sick. The modern hospital developed from medieval monastic institutions. During the Reformation 'the disendowment of hospitals was more injurious to the poor than the disendowment of monasteries' (Trevelyan 1946). When Christian missionaries went to what is now termed the 'Third World', they found appalling medical need; by the beginning of the 20th century most missionary societies had medical departments.

Before the 19th century, Western medicine had little to offer. But the advent of scientific medicine coincided with the Industrial Revolution, expanding trade, geographical exploration, and increased world awareness by the West. One of the first missionary doctors was Dr John Thomas, who accompanied the Baptist William Carey to India in 1792. The Edinburgh Medical Missionary Society, founded in 1841, was the first such medical society in Britain. The Church Missionary Society, established in 1799, let nearly a century pass before developing a medical outreach, which subsequently became very extensive.

Some individuals of true greatness devoted their lives to service abroad and became an inspiration to others. David *Livingstone (1813–73) is often remembered as an explorer of Central Africa and the Zambezi. Initially based at mission stations, his early journeys were undertaken to discover locations where further healthy bases might be established, many missionaries having died from *malaria. He is also remembered as a pioneer in the fight against slavery, for his epic endurance to the end, then for the story of how devoted Africans carried his embalmed body 1500 miles through unfriendly territory to the coast: his final resting place is in Westminster Abbey.

Albert *Schweitzer was a doctor of philosophy and of theology, a famous organist and authority on Bach when, at the age of 30 years he decided to become a medical student and to devote the rest of his life to service in Africa. He reached Gabon in 1913, built a hospital at the remote location of Lambaréné, described in his book *On the edge of the primeval forest*, and died there in 1965, aged nearly 90. A truly Olympian character, awarded the *Nobel Peace Prize, his personal philosophy was contained in three simple words, 'reverence for life'.

Sir Wilfred *Grenfell (1865–1940) was a pioneer physician to the fishing villages of Newfoundland's Labrador coast. Known as 'Grenfell of Labrador', his missionary work there attracted hundreds of Canadian, American, and British doctors, nurses, and medical students.

Mission hospitals played a significant role in medical education. Of necessity many nursing schools were established. Dr Peter Parker founded the Ophthalmic Hospital in Canton in 1834; of him it was said 'he opened the gates of China with a lancet, when European cannon could not heave a single bar'. Medical schools developed in China at Canton (1866), Tientsin (1881), Mukden (1884), and Soochow (1894); the first Chinese to graduate (1892) (in Hong Kong) was *Sun Yat Sen, who became the founder of the Chinese Republic. The Peking Union Medical College (1906) established very high standards. Women of India had often been denied medical attention because of *purdah*. Recognizing their plight, women missionaries founded two medical schools for the training of female doctors, at Ludhiana (1894) by Dame Edith Brown and at Vellore (1918) by an American doctor, Ida Scudder. The Vellore hospital became the Christian Medical College of South India, of international repute.

Most mission hospitals remained small in size and located in rural areas. The influence of medical missionaries is often remarkable and out of all proportion to their numerical strength. By Western standards the staffing ratio of doctors is very low in relation to clinical demand. The better the hospital, the greater is the demand, patients often travelling great distances. A major problem of developing countries is that although the central government provides hospitals in the capital and main provincial towns, rural areas are poorly served. The further from the main towns, the more pressing are the medical needs, and it is here that most medical mission hospitals are sited. Many have outlying dispensaries and maternity centres or mobile clinics; roads are often poor, transport is scarce and expensive, so basic medical help needs to be reasonably close to hand.

The extent and nature of medical problems (and inherent personal dangers) facing missionary doctors and nursing sisters have often been daunting, particularly in the early days when understanding of tropical diseases and their treatment was relatively poor. Since 1967 a *WHO campaign has eliminated *smallpox world-wide; advances in therapy have greatly reduced the incidence of conditions such as *sleeping sickness and *yaws; diseases such as *leprosy, *schistosomiasis, *filariasis, *amoebic and bacillary *dysentery can be cured. *Tuberculosis, now rare in Western society, is still rampant in many areas of the world. *AIDS threatens devastation in developing societies.

*Leprosy is a particular disease in which medical missions have played an important and often pioneering role. This was so even before specific treatment was available, and isolation in leper colonies was usual: the name of Father Damien is remembered in this context. In India the Mission to Lepers, established in 1873, became The Leprosy Mission in 1966; many pioneers in the treatment of leprosy during that period were missionaries. Of recent years Paul Brand in Vellore has been a leading figure in reconstructive surgery, physiotherapy, and rehabilitation of deformed victims of leprosy. Mother Teresa's name is associated with leprosy, with rescue of abandoned babies, and those dying in destitution on the streets of Calcutta. The Salvation Army's world-wide care for the poor and deprived is well known.

Another area of great concern has been child welfare. The synergy of poverty, *malnutrition, and endemic disease leads to very high mortality for the 'under-fives' (Wilkinson 1969). Experience with static and mobile child welfare clinics has shown that much of this is preventable. Professor David Morley's *Paediatric priorities in the developing world* has been influential in governmental organization of health planning.

Where medical cover is limited, conditions requiring surgery often present at an advanced stage; for example, *hernias, uterine *fibroids, and *thyroid tumours may be massive. *Cataract is common in tropical countries; Sir Henry Holland performed 60 000 cataract operations in India. The Commonwealth Society for the Blind provides clinics in some mission hospitals. In the pioneer days it was often the dramatic successes of surgery that made Western medicine, and particularly preventive measures, acceptable to other cultures.

Despite the pressure of heavy workloads, there have been outstanding contributions to research. Sir Patrick Manson, to many 'the father of tropical medicine', went to China in 1865, aged 21 years, to help an overworked missionary, studied filariasis and discovered that a mosquito carries the causative parasite. In the early 1920s Sir Clement Chesterman was a pioneer in the use of *tryparsamide for the cure of sleeping sickness in the Congo. In 1958 Denis Burkitt in Uganda described the malignant tumour which now bears his name (*Burkitt's lymphoma). There have been many other contributions to medical literature (see Davey *et al*. 1985).

Medical needs of developing countries have always been great, but of recent years there has been tragic exacerbation by the twin horrors of drought and civil war. These have led to catastrophic levels of malnutrition and suffering which can only be met through massive international assistance by the *Red Cross, United Nations (International) Children's (Emergency) Fund (Unicef), the American government, antifamine agencies such as *Oxfam, the French and German equivalents, and emergency organizations such as Médicins sans Frontières. Amongst mission hospitals there is greater co-ordination of resources, such as the bulk purchase of drugs by interdenominational Joint Mission Hospital Equipment Boards, aid in staffing by Voluntary Service Overseas (VSO), financial assistance by Christian Aid, other charities, and the UK Ministry of Overseas Development.

The pioneering days of medical missionaries may have passed, but their work goes on, with increased emphasis on preventive medicine. In many hospitals the need for expatriate assistance has lessened as skilled indigenous medical staff have become available. Teaching hospitals are now usually managed by central government. Some hospitals in Nigeria are jointly run by Church and state. The Christian College at Vellore, with over 1000 beds and 350 doctors, is still supported by the Church of South India. There is a general devolution of responsibility from Western missionary societies to overseas churches. But in poorer developing countries the medical needs of rural areas are still very great.

Early in the 20th century, mission hospitals were in the vanguard of recognizing, meeting, and raising awareness of medical problems in developing countries. Increased media coverage has very literally 'brought this home' to everyone; meeting those needs has become a shared responsibility for all of us.

J. L. WILKINSON

References

Davey, F., Browne, S. G., and Thompson, W. A. R. (1985). *Heralds of health*. Christian Medical Fellowship, London.
Feschotte, J. (1955). *Albert Schweitzer*. Black, London.
Macnair, J. I. (1954). *Livingstone's travels*. Dent, London.
Morley, D. (1973). *Paediatric priorities in the developing world*. Butterworth, London.
Trevelyan, G. M. (1946). *English social history*, (2nd edn). Longmans, Green & Co., London.
Wilkinson, J. L. (1969). Children in hospital in Sierra Leone: a survey of 10 000 admissions. *Transactions of the Royal Society of Tropical Medicine and Hygiene*, **63**, 263–9.

MISUSE OF DRUGS ACT 1971. See DRUG REGULATION.

MITCHELL, SILAS WEIR (1829–1914). American neurologist. Mitchell carried out detailed studies of nerve injury at a special hospital in Philadelphia during the American Civil War. Later he became interested in functional *neuroses in women, and advocated treatment by prolonged bed rest. He described *erythromelalgia and various peripheral *neuropathic syndromes. He also wrote several popular novels and books of poetry.

MITE. See *ACARUS*.

MITHRIDATICUM was a universal *antidote and prophylactic against poisoning; it was a medieval concoction of 72 ingredients. The name (alternatively mithridate, mithridatium, mithridaticon, etc.) derives from Mithridates VI, King of Pontus and Bythinia (120–63 BC) who was said to have rendered himself proof against poisoning by repeatedly taking small doses of antidotes.

MITOCHONDRIA are spherical, rod- or thread-shaped organelles found in the cytoplasm of all living cells except bacteria and algae. Mitochondria are the main sites of generation of energy from oxidative metabolism of foodstuffs. As well as the many enzymes needed for this function they contain *ribonucleic acid and

*deoxyribonucleic acid and can replicate proteins. Mitochondria (singular: mitochondrion) have a distinctive structure on *electron microscopy. See CELL AND CELL BIOLOGY.

MITOSIS is *cell division (strictly, cell nucleus division) in which the nucleus divides into two identical daughter nuclei, each with the same number of *chromosomes as the parent and having identical characteristics. It is the normal method of tissue growth.

MITRAL STENOSIS is narrowing of the orifice of the mitral valve, obstructing the diastolic flow of blood from the left atrium into the left ventricle (see VALVES, CARDIAC). In consequence, the cardiac output is restricted and the pressure behind the obstruction rises, causing pulmonary venous congestion. Prominent among the symptoms are fatigue, *haemoptysis, and *dyspnoea (including sometimes the paroxysmal nocturnal dyspnoea known as cardiac *asthma). The outlook for patients with mitral stenosis, which is almost always a delayed result of *rheumatic fever in earlier life, has been dramatically improved by the advent of surgical techniques for relieving the obstruction.

MITTELSCHMERZ is an abdominal pain experienced by some women midway through the menstrual cycle, caused by the process of *ovulation. See also SAFE PERIOD.

MIXTURES are liquid medicinal preparations containing two or more ingredients.

MÖBIUS, PAUL JULIUS (1853-1907). German neurologist. He described *ophthalmoplegic migraine, the Leyden–Möbius type of *muscular dystrophy (1879), weakness of convergence in *thyrotoxicosis (Möbius's sign, 1886), and also congenital absence or *aplasia of facial, bulbar, and other muscles (Möbius syndrome).

MOIR, DAVID MACBETH (1798-1851). British physician and writer. He is mainly remembered for his literary pieces, contributed in large numbers to *Blackwood's Magazine* and many other periodicals, often with the signature of Δ (Delta). He also published verse and a novel *Mansie Wauch*.

MOLAR. A solution containing 1 *mole of solute per litre. See also TEETH.

MOLE. That amount of a substance which has a mass in grams equal to its relative molecular mass (molecular weight).

MOLECULAR BIOLOGY is the study of the chemical structures and processes underlying biological events, in particular the formation, organization, and activity of the macromolecules essential to life such as *nucleic acids and *proteins; and the detailed structure and function of *chromosomes and subcellular *organelles.

MOLECULAR BIOLOGY IN MEDICINE
Introduction
While it is always difficult to know just when a scientific movement starts, the origin of the molecular biological revolution is usually attributed to the observation by Griffith in 1928 that it is possible to 'transform' a 'rough' strain of a *bacterium—the *pneumococcus— (which lacks a capsule and is not harmful to mice) into a 'smooth' strain (which has a capsule and kills mice) by injecting living rough organisms with dead smooth organisms into a mouse. This phenomenon is an example of what is now called genetic engineering, and it is worth pointing out, to those who are worried that genetic engineering is new and man-invented, that bacteria have long used this 'technique'.

A group at the Rockefeller Institute for Medical Research led by Oswald Avery, another bacteriologist, repeated these experiments and showed that similar transformation would occur in the test-tube and that detergent extracts of the smooth organisms were effective. They went on to demonstrate—to their own great surprise and to the even greater surprise of the scientific community—that the active principle in the extracts of the smooth bacteria was *DNA, a material which had previously been believed to have only a structural function. This single experiment convinced most of the scientific community that DNA was the material of which *genes were composed and gave rise to an intense interest in the chemistry and structure of this class of nucleic acid. This led to the elucidation in 1953 of the 'double-helix' structure by Watson and Crick, based on the crystallographic studies of Rosalind Franklin and Maurice Wilkins. Because this structure carried with it the mechanism by which DNA could replicate and maintain its specific sequence, it had an enormous influence and rapidly led to deciphering of the genetic code and of the mechanism of *protein *synthesis. This revolution of the 1950s and 1960s was an analytical revolution which enabled scientists for the first time to analyse the structure of genes. It led eventually to the development of practical mechanisms for sequencing DNA by Gilbert and by Sanger, and in this way opened the way to what is now called the Human Genome Project, whereby it is intended that eventually the whole human genome will be sequenced.

However, it was not this revolution which allowed manipulation of genes. A second revolution occurred in the 1970s. It arose from the discovery of plasmids— spontaneously occurring pieces of bacterial DNA, which transmit, among other things, *antibiotic resistance from one organism to another; the discovery of 'restriction' *enzymes, which bacteria use in order to destroy DNA foreign to them, cutting the DNA at specific sequences which they do not have in their own DNA; and the discovery of the enzyme 'reverse transcriptase'. This enzyme is capable of transcribing *RNA into DNA, which is the opposite direction to the usual sequence in protein synthesis and is a trick used by a family of viruses, including the *virus causing *AIDS. The discovery of plasmids, of restriction endonucleases, and of reverse transcriptase together made it possible to manipulate genes at will, and the consequences of this 'genetic engineering' have been even greater than that of the analytical revolution, and have given rise to the biotechnology industry.

The discovery some 10 years ago of the polymerase chain reaction, which allows genes to be amplified without having to clone them in bacteria, is a further striking advance in our ability to analyse and manipulate genes, and the technology that has become available in these ways has had truly remarkable effects on the practice of biology and medicine. David Weatherall has written elsewhere in this volume about the new *genetics and I will here consider applications in other fields that have arisen from the new technology and are changing the practice of medicine.

The production on a pharmaceutical scale of natural products that normally occur in minute amounts
There are a large number of potent biological molecules made by both plants and animals which were discovered by virtue of their biological activity but which occur *in vivo* at such low concentrations that purification by conventional techniques was extremely difficult and production in pharmaceutical amounts either impossible or extraordinarily expensive. Two important and overlapping groups of such molecules are *hormones and cytokines.

Although some major protein hormones had been purified before the advent of biotechnology and one, insulin, was in common use as a drug, many others were first made in substantial amounts by biotechnology. One good example is erythropoietin, a hormone, made in the kidney, which enhances blood production. Its deficiency in chronic renal disease gives rise to an *anaemia which was once difficult to treat. Erythropoietin made by biotechnology has had great success as a drug in correcting this anaemia. Similarly, growth hormone used for treating dwarfism in children can be made by genetic engineering. This is both potentially cheaper than extracting it from large numbers of human *pituitary glands and, furthermore, is free of the danger of having the hormone contaminated with the agent that causes *Creutzfeldt–Jakob disease—the human equivalent of 'mad cow' disease—which, tragically, contaminated several batches of human growth hormone extracted from pituitary glands.

Cytokines are also intercellular messengers but, unlike hormones, they are not secreted into the general circulation but act locally in their own micro-environment. For this reason they tend to be produced in even smaller amounts than hormones, and until the advent of molecular biology most of them were unknown. It is a remarkable triumph of the new technology that many such novel biological compounds have been produced whose existence had often not previously been suspected. Such compounds include: (at a minimum) three *interferons (INF), originally described as antiviral agents but which have major actions on cell function; 12 interleukins (IL); various colony-stimulating factors (CSF); the two species of tumour necrosis factor (TNF) and three members of the 'tumour growth factor β' family. Together these are responsible for many aspects of cell differentiation and activation.

The initial attempt to use cytokines as pharmacological agents was disappointing. It turned out that they were quite capable of producing severe toxic reactions. For example, one of the early discoveries that came from the purification of an interferon was that the symptoms associated with viral infections are not due to the virus itself but to the high concentration of interferon produced. While it may be reassuring to patients with viral infections to know that they feel ill because their host response to the virus is vigorous, it does limit the use of larger doses of these materials for therapeutic purposes. Furthermore, it turns out that at high doses the biological activities of cytokines are multiple and overlap, and it is difficult to find compounds that have a single effect. Nevertheless, increasing experience has produced, and will continue to produce, therapeutic uses for both the cytokines and, perhaps particularly for inhibitors of their action (Haworth *et al.* 1993). Interleukin-2 has found a use in *tumour therapy, as has tumour necrosis factor. However, perhaps more striking is the use of *antibodies to tumour necrosis factor in the treatment of septic shock in experimental animals, and there is preliminary evidence of its efficacy in human *rheumatoid arthritis. A few examples of the pharmaceutical uses of the common cytokines are shown in Table 1. However, many of the more recently described factors are too new to have been properly evaluated for therapeutic use, and the evaluation of potent agents is a time-consuming step-by-step procedure. The optimal way of using even those agents currently used is still being studied.

Novel ways of making antibodies

A quite separate revolution in the 1970s arose from the original work by Kohler and Milstein which led to the development of *monoclonal antibodies—individual antibodies which can be produced in substantial amounts. The original techniques were cell biological and the antibodies were made from mouse tumour cells after fusion with individual antibody-forming cells. Although the technique enables a tremendous spectrum of antibodies to be made, it has a disadvantage in that it is restricted to antibodies that mice can make; this excludes some antibodies which may be wanted in man, for example antibodies to the rhesus blood groups.

Secondly, the antibodies made are murine and these are recognized antigenically as foreign by humans, so that their use as therapeutic agents in man is limited. Molecular biological techniques have largely overcome these problems and it is now possible to make chimeric antibodies of which the great majority of the molecule is human and only small regions in the 'business end' come from the mouse. Such chimeric antibodies are proving extremely useful for therapy and are likely to become increasingly widely used in a number of diseases. However, even more substantial innovations are at hand. Winter and his colleagues (Winter and Milstein 1991) have devised methods of making antibodies that circumvent immunization altogether. This is done by constructing enormous phage libraries displaying random associations of amino acids within the binding regions of antibodies displayed on *bacteriophage. It is possible to select with antigens those *immunoglobulins that react specifically and at high affinity with the *antigens involved. Having selected the binding-site fragment, this can then be engineered into antibody molecules containing regions with effector properties of one's choice. Eventually, these techniques for obtaining antibodies will be more powerful, quicker, and cheaper than current techniques and will allow us to foresee the generation of virtually unlimited arrays of antibody molecules directed against any chosen antigenic pattern. Since antibodies can inactivate biological molecules, and antibodies to hormone and cytokine receptors can frequently act as 'agonists' (drugs that produce the same effects as biologically active molecules), the therapeutic implications of this are immense and a whole branch of the biotechnology industry devoted to the use of antibodies is rapidly growing up.

New vaccines

So far the greatest contribution made by medical intervention to human health has been the introduction of active immunization against *infectious disease. Starting with *smallpox vaccination in the 18th century, many

Table 1 Examples of therapeutic uses of cytokines

IFN-α	To convert hepatitis B antigen-positive carriers
	Hairy-cell leukaemia
IFN-β	Multiple sclerosis
IFN-γ	Chronic granulomatous disease
IL-2	Cancer therapy—generation of lymphokine-activated killer (LAK) cells
TNF-α	Cancer therapy
	Infections with *Pneumocystis* and *Toxoplasma* (mice)
CSFs	Marrow stimulation after chemotherapy

There are also uses for antibodies to cytokines and for cytokine inhibitors, e.g. anti-TNF-α for rheumatoid arthritis (in humans) and septic shock (in mice).

major lethal diseases have been eliminated by vaccination. These include smallpox, *yellow fever, *polio, *diphtheria, and more recently *measles and *hepatitis B and A. Where these diseases persist it is because vaccination is not effectively used for a variety of social and environmental reasons. Traditionally, vaccines have either been living attenuated organisms (smallpox, yellow fever, polio, and measles), inactivated organisms (polio), or (more or less) purified proteins, such as the toxins of diphtheria and *tetanus suitably modified, or the hepatitis B surface antigen. There are, however, many infectious diseases which have not so far yielded to vaccination. These include some viral infections, the most notable perhaps being the new retroviral infection with *HIV that gives rise to AIDS, and many diseases due to parasites, both protozoal and metazoal, which are of enormous importance, particularly in the Third World. These include *malaria, *leishmania, and *schistosomiasis. It seems likely that novel approaches to vaccination are required to produce effective vaccines, and molecular biology has allowed a number of highly ingenious approaches.

In the first place, the attenuation of organisms to make them incapable of producing disease, while still giving rise to immunity, can now be approached in much more scientific ways by the deletion or modification of particular genes. It is also possible to incorporate important antigenic portions of one parasite into another organism, which can then be used to introduce it into its host. There has been widespread experimentation with the *vaccinia virus (used for immunizing against smallpox) aimed at introducing into it antigens which can immunize against other diseases and removing from it those genes which, in a small number of cases, give rise to complications such as *encephalomyelitis. While no such vaccines are yet in use in man, there is a successfully engineered vaccinia vaccine incorporating portions of the *rabies virus which is used in the form of infected bait to control rabies in the wild population of animals in continental Europe, and which is proving highly successful.

It is also possible to make, by the techniques of molecular biology, isolated proteins which can be used as immunogens to protect against disease. This has proved highly successful with hepatitis B, and the widespread immunization of populations against hepatitis B is also certain to be the first successful intervention in preventing human cancer. The primary hepatoma, which is common in the Far East and in Africa, depends for its development on the liver cells having been infected with hepatitis B virus. If hepatitis B can be eliminated from the population, most hepatomas would not occur.

Two problems with much of the new technology are: first, that it is extremely expensive and therefore will be difficult to apply to the Third World; and secondly that it requires cold storage of the vaccines for their delivery. Currently an extremely ingenious technology is being explored which overcomes these difficulties. This is to incorporate the DNA coding for immunizing antigens in plasmids which normally grow only in bacteria, and to inject these into animal muscle. Muscle is made up of interconnecting cells, so that injections into muscle always end up with the material being inside the cell; in these circumstances it can be shown that plasmids are able to express the proteins they code for at least for some time and thereby make, within the immunized host, the antigens to which an immune response is desired. Plasmids, being pieces of bacterial DNA, are cheaply and rapidly grown in bacteria, and being solely DNA they do not require refrigeration. If this technology can be made to work and demonstrated to be safe, it may represent a major advance in introducing vaccines on a massive scale without enormous economic cost.

DNA fingerprinting

The work of Alec Jeffreys (1991) created an entirely novel way of uniquely identifying human beings. This is the technique known as DNA fingerprinting, which relies on the fact that we all contain within our genomes multiple, and highly variable, repeats of small sequences of DNA whose real function *in vivo* is unknown and which are relatively unstable, so that an individual's pattern of these constitutes a 'finger print'. Professor Jeffreys has developed a number of ingenious techniques by which such fingerprints may be created and in so doing has produced a true revolution in *forensic medicine. It is now possible positively to match human tissue (and this includes *semen) with a particular individual where DNA is available; to do rigorous tests for genetic relationships, such as paternity; and potentially to identify an individual from a single cell, be it a hair, a drop of saliva, or a piece of dandruff. These techniques have already proved very valuable in investigations of crime; but they have many other potential uses for the identification of individuals or the establishment of relationships between them.

Genetic manipulation of cells and animals—gene therapy

The new techniques of gene manipulation make it possible to alter the genetic composition of a living cell with capacity for growth, and therefore to introduce genes that will function into the tissues of living animals and humans. This carries with it the promise of being able to treat single-gene genetic disease. Indeed, the first experiments involving testing an immune disease deficiency due to the deficiency of a particular enzyme (adenine deaminase) and the treatment of *cystic fibrosis by introducing into lung cells the normal form of the gene that is deficient in this disease, are already being undertaken. Although there are formidable practical difficulties in targeting genes in humans, the prospect of being able to treat serious, life-endangering diseases such as *muscular dystrophy and the *haemoglobino-pathies is now very apparent, and one can be optimistic that some forms of this therapy will become available within the next decade. Although some disquiet about genetic manipulation of somatic cells has been expressed from time to time, there is a wide consensus, not only among the medical profession, but among the whole community interested in bioethics, that somatic cell therapy of serious disease carries no significant ethical problems. There is similar agreement that trying to modify the *germline* of humans, i.e. to create by genetic manipulation individuals with 'desirable' traits is, for the foreseeable future, not permissible. On the other hand, genetic manipulation of the germline in both plants and animals is being widely undertaken for a variety of purposes, many of which are agricultural and not directly relevant to this discussion.

There is, however, growing interest in the prospect of preparing genetically modified farm animals, particularly pigs, whose organs can be used for transplantation into man. The reasons why pig kidneys and pig hearts cannot be transplanted into humans are now moderately well understood and it is at least potentially feasible that a relatively modest number of genetic manipulations will make such organs suitable for *transplantation into man. Primarily these are likely to concern the introduction of the human pattern of complement control proteins into the pig, and the modification of certain carbohydrate-modifying enzymes to produce a human pattern of heterophile (carbohydrate) antigens. There is compelling evidence that the supply of human organs is inadequate and will become more inadequate for the treatment of human renal and heart disease (not to mention transplantation of some other organs such as pancreas and pancreatic islets) where there is a growing demand for such treatments. If this form of treatment can indeed be made to work, it is likely to prove of great benefit in this very successful branch of human surgical intervention.

Tumour suppressor genes

A major field of investigation that has arisen from the study of molecular biology is the discovery and analysis of genes that play a role in both the induction and the prevention of *cancer: oncogenes and tumour suppressor genes. Oncogenes were first recognized in viruses that can give rise to tumours in animals, where it became apparent that these viruses contained in their own genome homologues of host cellular genes which in their own host presumably have functions other than giving rise to cancer. A systematic analysis of the phenomena has shown, perhaps disappointingly, that there is a very substantial number of such genes and, inasmuch as their natural function is known, they are all concerned with various aspects of the regulation and control of the growth of normal cells. A number of them are enzymes that phosphorylate a particular amino acid, tyrosine, in other proteins. This is a common and

important mechanism of controlling the activation status of proteins. From work of this kind, a great deal has been learnt about the control of cell activation and also a great deal about genetic predisposition to individual tumours.

It has further become clear that there is a related class of genes whose products serve to hinder tumour induction and whose malfunction predisposes to tumour formation. The nuclear protein, p53, is a particularly striking example of a tumour suppressor, and abnormal forms are common in many forms of human cancer (Lane 1992). It seems likely that knowledge gained in this way will, in the foreseeable future, certainly allow us to detect people who are at particular risk of developing particular tumours and who may therefore require a particular form of medical surveillance and also possibly even intervention in the formation of individual tumours.

PETER J. LACHMANN

References

Haworth C., Maini, R. N., and Feldmann, M. (1994). Prospects for cytokines in human immunotherapy. *The cytokine handbook*, (ed. A. W. Thompson). Academic Press, London.

Jeffreys, A. J. (1991). In *DNA fingerprinting; approaches and application*, (ed. T. Burke., G. Dolf, and A. Jeffreys) Birkhauser, Basel.

Lane, D. P. (1992). p53, guardian of the genome. *Nature*, **358**, 15–16.

Winter, G. and Milstein, C. (1991). Man made antibodies. *Nature*, **349**, 293–9.

MOLECULE. The smallest portion of a substance which can exist without losing its chemical identity.

MOLLUSCUM CONTAGIOSUM is a skin eruption caused by a virus and seen most commonly in children. It is characterized by the appearance of persistent rounded umbilicated *papules from which cheesy material can be expressed.

MONAKOW, CONSTANTIN VON (1853–1930). Russian neurologist. Much of his research was on the localization of function in the *cerebrum and later on the *extrapyramidal motor system (1924). He discovered the cuneate nucleus (von Monakow's nucleus) and the rubrospinal tract (von Monakow's bundle, 1909).

MONDEVILLE, HENRI DE (*c.* 1260–1329). French surgeon. He was a practical common-sense surgeon who tried to avoid *suppuration of wounds, advocating meticulous cleanliness. His *Cyrurgia* deals with anatomy, surgical pathology, wounds, and injuries. It circulated in manuscript but was not printed until 1892. He was a founder of the surgical fraternity of the Collège de S. Côme and of great influence in his time.

MONGOLISM is an outmoded synonym for *Down's syndrome.

MONILIASIS. See CANDIDA.

MONITORS are pieces of apparatus designed for continuous measurement or display of particular indices of physiological function, such as heart rate, arterial blood pressure, arterial oxygen tension, electrocardiogram, etc.; they are used for constant surveillance of patients under *intensive care, general *anaesthesia, etc.

MONOAMINE OXIDASE (MAO) is an *enzyme which catalyses the breakdown of monoamines, such as *adrenaline, *noradrenaline, *serotonin, *dopamine, and *tyramine. *Antidepressant drugs belonging to the *MAOI group inhibit the action of monoamine oxidase.

MONOAMINE-OXIDASE INHIBITORS (MAOIs) such as phenelzine, iproniazid, tranylcypromine, etc. are *antidepressants.

MONOCLONAL ANTIBODIES are completely homogeneous *antibodies, that is with specificity for a single *antigen. The production of monoclonal antibody has been made possible by the discovery (1975) of the 'hybridoma' technique, in which a B-*lymphocyte sensitized to a particular antigen is 'immortalized' by fusion with a *myeloma cell (from a cultured cell line), establishing a *clone of cells able to produce large quantities of an antibody of single specificity. Monoclonal antibodies are of great therapeutic and diagnostic potential. See IMMUNOLOGY; MOLECULAR BIOLOGY AND MEDICINE.

MONOCYTE. A mononuclear phagocytic *leucocyte, the largest nucleated cell of the blood. Monocytes are formed in the marrow and migrate to the tissues, where they become *macrophages.

MONONUCLEOSIS is an increase in the number of *monocytes in the blood. See INFECTIOUS MONONUCLEOSIS.

MONOPLEGIA is *paralysis of one limb.

MONRO, ALEXANDER 'PRIMUS' (1697–1767). British anatomist and surgeon. Monro studied under *Boerhaave at Leiden and became professor of anatomy and surgery to the Surgeons' Company of Edinburgh in 1719 and the first professor of anatomy to the university the next year. He was the founder of a dynasty of anatomists who occupied the chair for 126 years with great distinction.

MONRO, ALEXANDER 'SECUNDUS' (1733–1817). British anatomist and physician. The son of *Monro 'primus' with whom he worked as joint professor of anatomy from 1755 to 1767, thereafter occupying the chair alone until joined by his son in 1800. He studied in London under William *Hunter as well as in Paris, Leiden, and Berlin. He described the communication between the two lateral *ventricles of the brain known now as 'the *foramen of Monro' (1783).

MONRO, ALEXANDER 'TERTIUS' (1773–1859). British anatomist. He became his father's assistant in 1798, conjoint professor of anatomy in 1800, and sole professor of anatomy in the University of Edinburgh from 1817 to 1846. He was less gifted, less successful, and less popular than his forebears.

MONSTER. An obsolete term for an infant born with severe developmental abnormalities.

MONTESSORI, MARIA (1870–1952). Italian educationalist. She was the originator of the well-known system of teaching which bears her name, and was the first woman in Italy to graduate in medicine, which she did from the University of Rome in 1894. Her methods were originally devised for educating backward children and proved so successful that she developed them for application to normal children of lower age-groups.

MONTPELLIER, in the south of France, is famed in medicine for carrying the torch of learning, especially during the difficult years of the 13th and 14th centuries, leading up to the Renaissance. Its medical school probably began in the 12th century and may have been inspired by *Salerno. Geographically the university was well placed between Italy and Spain, where much of the Arabic tradition in medicine remained. Many famous doctors studied there. John of *Gaddesden, who became professor at Oxford in the 14th century, was one. So was Guy de *Chauliac, who became physician and chaplain to Pope Clement VI at Avignon, and made contributions to surgery, inventing a rope suspended over the bed of a patient by which he could lift himself up. Other students and visitors were Andrew *Boorde, who became physician to Henry VIII, and wrote *The breviarie of health*; *Paracelsus; Sir Thomas *Browne; Sir Theobald Turquet de *Mayerne, physician to James I; Thomas *Sydenham; and Desgenettes, later physician to Napoleon. The medical school still exists and flourishes.

MONTREAL GENERAL HOSPITAL, THE, was founded in 1819 and is Canada's oldest teaching hospital. Students were admitted in 1821 when four professors were imported from the University of Edinburgh. The school became part of *McGill University in 1829, and remains so. There are now schools in all other health-care disciplines. Patients come from the province of Quebec, eastern Canada, and the north-eastern USA. There is a large research programme carried out in purpose-built accommodation, as well as extensive teaching facilities. There are 785 beds for all specialties except paediatrics. Sir William *Osler was pathologist and physician on the staff from 1874 to 1884. Carcinoembryonic antigen was discovered there by P. Gold and S. O. Freedman.

MOOD is the state of *emotion or affect of an individual.

MOORE, FRANCIS (1647–?1717). British physician and astrologer. Moore practised in Lambeth as a physician, astrologer, and schoolmaster. He published *Almanac kalendarium ecclesiasticum* (1699) and *Vox stellarum* (1700) which still appears as **Old Moore's almanac*.

MOORE, JOHN (1729–1802). British surgeon. He wrote travel volumes which were well received. He was a friend of Smollett, whose biography he wrote, and he met and corresponded with Samuel Johnson, Lord Byron, and other 18th century literary and other personages. He wrote novels as well, which enjoyed praise in his time.

MORAN, LORD. See WILSON, CHARLES McMORAN.

MORBID ANATOMIST. A pathologist, that is an expert in the anatomy of diseased tissues.

MORBID ANATOMY is that part of pathology which deals with the anatomy of diseased tissues.

MORBIDITY has been defined by the World Health Organization (WHO) as 'any departure, subjective or objective, from a state of physiological well-being'. In this sense it is synonymous with 'sickness', 'illness', 'disease', etc.

MORBUS. Disease.

MORGAGNI, GIOVANNI BATTISTA (1682–1771). Italian physician and pathologist. His book *De sedibus et causis morborum per anatomen indagatis* (1761) records the *post-mortem findings in some 700 cases and attempted, for the first time, to correlate the anatomical lesions with the symptoms experienced. Morgagni was the first to describe cerebral *gumma, cardiac valvular lesions, syphilitic *aneurysms, *acute yellow atrophy of the liver, and *tuberculosis of the kidney. He has been described as 'the father of morbid anatomy'.

MORGAN, THOMAS HUNT (1866–1945). American geneticist. He became a leader in the modern era of genetics research, chiefly as a result of work with *Drosophila*, in which he was able to identify the roles of certain *genes. For this work he received the *Nobel prize in 1933.

MORIBUND. About to die.

MORNING SICKNESS is nausea, particularly in the mornings and sometimes with vomiting, experienced by some healthy women during early pregnancy.

MORON is an obsolete term for a mentally subnormal patient with a mental age of between 7 and 9 and an *IQ between 50 and 69.

MORPHIA. See MORPHINE.

MORPHINE is a powerful *narcotic, *analgesic, and highly addictive drug occurring naturally as an *opium alkaloid. Because of its unrivalled capacity to relieve *pain, it is an invaluable drug despite its drawbacks; apart from *addiction, these include respiratory depression and constipation.

MORPHOEA (MORPHEA) is localized *scleroderma, characterized by circumscribed patches of skin *fibrosis.

MORPHOLOGY is the science of shape, form, structure, and homologies.

MORRIS, SIR WILLIAM RICHARD, Bt (1st Viscount Nuffield) (1877–1963). Morris started his own bicycle repair business in Oxford at the age of 16, and 30 years later his factories were producing 50 000 Morris motor cars a year. In his lifetime he gave away £30 million, including £2 million to found a clinical medical school at Oxford in 1936, and £250 000 to the Royal College of Surgeons in 1948.

MORTALITY. 'The ratio of the total number of deaths in a year in a given population, from a particular cause, group of causes, or all causes, to the total population' (World Health Organization 1971). The 'crude mortality rate' is the number of deaths per thousand total population during a given year. The 'age-specific mortality rate' is the number of deaths which occur in a year to a thousand persons of a particular age or age-group (see also EPIDEMIOLOGY).

MORTON, WILLIAM THOMAS GREEN (1819–68). American dentist and anaesthetist. He discovered the anaesthetic properties of *ether, and used it in dental extractions. In 1846 he administered ether to a patient at the *Massachusetts General Hospital, while the surgeon John Collins *Warren removed a vascular tumour from the patient's neck. There were many observers present and this episode, together with Morton's later teaching, did much to convince surgeons of the value and uses of general *anaesthesia.

MORTUARY is a building or set of rooms for the temporary reception of dead bodies.

MOSAICISM is a genetic abnormality in which an individual possesses two or more cell lines which are genotypically distinct, but are derived from a single zygote. See GENETICS.

MOSQUITO. A family (the Culicidae) of delicate two-winged flies or gnats with aquatic larvae, some species of which bite and suck the blood of mammals, including man. It contains a number of genera of medical importance. Chief among these are: *Anopheles*, many species of which are vectors of *malaria and some of *filariasis; *Aëdes*, species of which transmit *viral diseases such as *yellow fever, *dengue, several varieties of *arbovirus *encephalitis and *encephalomyelitis as well as filariasis; and *Culex*, species of which transmit viral diseases and filariasis. The nuisance value of biting mosquitoes can also be considerable.

MOTION SICKNESS is the familiar syndrome experienced by susceptible individuals when travelling by motor vehicle, train, aeroplane, or ship, or in other ways subjected to unusual motion and disorientating stimuli. Although the mechanism of motion sickness is not precisely understood, abnormal stimulation of the vestibular balancing system (see LABYRINTH) plays an important part. Symptoms are various and unpleasant; they usually include malaise, sweating, salivation, nausea, and vomiting. See also ENVIRONMENT AND DISEASE I.

MOTOR NEURONE DISEASE is a progressive degenerative disorder of the central nervous system involving both upper and lower motor neurones. The conditions known as amyotrophic lateral sclerosis, progressive muscular atrophy, and progressive bulbar palsy are clinical varieties of motor neurone disease (though in the USA the first of these terms is often used instead of motor neurone disease to designate the whole spectrum). See NEUROMUSCULAR DISEASE.

MOUNTAIN SICKNESS. See AEROSPACE MEDICINE; ALTITUDE SICKNESS; ENVIRONMENT AND DISEASE I.

MOURNING is the outward expression of *grief, modified by custom, culture, or religion.

MOYNIHAN, SIR BERKELEY GEORGE ANDREW, Bt (1st Baron Moynihan of Leeds) (1865–1936). British surgeon. He founded the Association of Surgeons of Great Britain and the *Journal of Surgery*. He introduced *rubber gloves to British surgeons.

MRI. *Magnetic resonance imaging.

MSH. See MELANOCYTE-STIMULATING HORMONE.

MUCOCELE. A *cyst or dilated cavity distended with clear mucoid fluid.

MUCOSA. Mucous membrane. See MUCUS.

MUCOUS MEMBRANE. Any of the epithelial linings of the body containing *mucus-secreting glands.

MUCUS is a slimy solution of mucins, a group of glycoproteins (also called mucopolysaccharides), secreted by unicellular glands known as goblet cells found in vertebrate epithelial linings or mucous membranes.

MULLER, HERMAN JOSEPH (1890–1967). American geneticist. The early part of his scientific career was spent at Texas University, where he carried out fundamental studies on *genes, gene mutations, genetic linkage, and genetic recombination (see GENETICS). His work on the production of gene mutations in *Drosophila* by *X-rays was later to bring him the *Nobel prize for medicine (1946). In 1933, at the age of 43, he left the USA for Moscow, becoming senior geneticist at the Institute of Genetics of the Academy of Sciences of the USSR. Four years later he went to the Institute of Animal Genetics in Edinburgh, where he was lecturer and research associate from 1937–40, before returning to the USA, to Amherst College. In 1945 he became professor of zoology at Indiana University. His later years were marked by involvement in controversial issues: he proposed the establishment of a sperm bank to perpetuate the genetic characteristics of outstanding men, and was an early opponent of the use of nuclear weapons.

MÜLLER, JOHANNES PETER (1801–58). German physiologist. Müller was one of the great teachers of physiology who believed that philosophical speculation had no place in science and that the foundation of the science was observation and experiment. His *Handbuch der Physiologie des Menschen* (2 vols, 1833–40) was a landmark in physiology. He confirmed the *Bell–Magendie law; studied *colour vision (1826) and *phonation (1835); and enunciated the law of specific nerve energies (1840), which states that, however stimulated, a nerve will give rise only to its specific single sensation.

MULTIPLE BIRTH. The birth of two or more offspring from a single *pregnancy. The incidence of multiple birth (normally about 1 in 80 for twins, 1 in 80×80 for triplets, 1 in $80 \times 80 \times 80$ for quadruplets) is increased after taking drugs which stimulate *ovulation. See FERTILITY DRUG.

MULTIPLE INJURIES. See CRUSH SYNDROME; SURGERY OF TRAUMA.

MULTIPLE MYELOMA. See MYELOMA.

MULTIPLE SCLEROSIS is a common chronic neurological disorder, often remittent but usually ultimately progressive, affecting scattered areas of white matter throughout the brain, spinal cord, and optic nerves. The primary lesion is loss of *myelin, with inability of the affected fibres to conduct impulses, followed by sclerosis or scarring. The onset is usually in early adult life and the disease thereafter runs a variable course, often remittent at first but usually with gradually increasing disability; the average duration is 35 years. The essential feature of the signs and symptoms is their multiple nature, indicating involvement of widely separated regions of the nervous system (the condition was formerly termed 'disseminated sclerosis'); the functions most consistently impaired are those relating to the pyramidal motor tracts, the cerebellum, and the optic pathways, leading to weakness or paralysis of the limbs, incoordination, and visual defects. The cause of multiple sclerosis is unknown. Current evidence seems to indicate a combination of immunogenetic and infective influences.

MUMMIES are bodies (of human beings or animals) which have been preserved by *embalming according to the Ancient Egyptian or some similar method before burial; sometimes also used to mean bodies which have been desiccated by exposure to sun or air, or those which have been preserved by embedment in ice.

MUMPS, also known as epidemic parotitis, is an acute infectious disease, mainly of childhood, affecting predominantly the salivary glands. The causative virus is one of the *Paramyxovirus* genus; spread is from person to person by droplets, and there is no animal reservoir. The clinical manifestations are those of a mild virus infection together with pain and swelling of the salivary glands, especially the parotids. The condition is usually self-limiting, and the prognosis excellent. Occasionally complications ensue; these include *orchitis (in post-pubertal males), *pancreatitis, *thyroiditis, *meningitis, and *encephalitis. An attack of mumps usually confers life-long immunity.

MÜNCHAUSEN, HIERONYMUS KARL FRIED-RICH FRIEHERR VON (1720–97). German swashbuckler. Münchausen was renowned for his mendacious fables of his prowess as a soldier and sportsman. They became legendary when published in London in 1785 by Rudolf Erich Raspe (1737–94). Patients who tell fantastic and patently untrue tales of their illnesses have been said to suffer from *Münchausen's syndrome.

MÜNCHAUSEN'S SYNDROME is a condition in which patients repeatedly present themselves to hospitals, often seeking admission and operation for an acute abdominal emergency or sometimes manifesting apparently disabling neurological symptoms. Their symptoms may be so convincing that *laparotomy or some other invasive procedure is undertaken, when no organic disorder is found. Such patients wander from

hospital to hospital, until they find one at which they are not known and recognized. The abdomen may bear several surgical scars. Münchausen's syndrome is probably to be regarded as a bizarre form of *malingering, though it is sometimes associated with *addiction to powerful analgesics. Most such individuals are suffering from *psychopathic personality or personality defect.

MUNDINUS (Mondino de Luzzi; also Liucci or Liuzzi) (*c.* 1270–1326). Italian anatomist. He taught anatomy at Bologna. He was the first to introduce the systematic teaching of the subject into the medical curriculum and carried out dissections himself. *Anatomia Mundini* (1316) remained the dissector's handbook for 200 years and passed through 39 editions although it contained many errors and followed *Galen slavishly.

MUNTHE, AXEL MARTIN FREDRIK (1857–1949). Swedish doctor and psychiatrist. He is remembered especially for his book of reminiscences called *The story of San Michele* (1929), the place being the name of his villa on the isle of Capri. The book is sensitive and delicate, with a charming and charmed view of life and death as a doctor sees it.

MURMUR. A noise additional to the normal heart sounds heard on *auscultation over the heart or vessels and recurring with each cardiac cycle. The presence of a heart murmur does not necessarily indicate heart disease.

MURPHY, JOHN BENJAMIN (1857–1916). American surgeon. He is chiefly remembered for his contributions to surgery of the biliary and gastrointestinal tracts. 'Murphy's sign', of *gall-bladder inflammation, is pain on inspiration when an examiner is exerting manual pressure below the right rib margin. He devised a clamp which was helpful in suturing the severed ends of the intestine.

MUSCA is a genus of two-winged flies, including the common housefly (*M. domestica*). See FLIES; MAGGOTS.

MUSCARINE is a toxic *alkaloid which occurs in the attractive but poisonous fairy-tale toadstool fly agaric (*Amanita muscaria*). The pharmacological effects of muscarine mimic those of *acetylcholine released at postganglionic *parasympathetic nerve endings, the *receptors related to which are therefore termed 'muscarinic' (to distinguish them from the acetylcholine receptors in autonomic ganglia and at neuromuscular junctions, which are 'nicotinic')

MUSCLE is the main contractile tissue of the body, consisting of elongated muscle fibres which on stimulation become shorter and thicker. It is of three types: voluntary or striated muscle, largely under conscious control;

cardiac muscle, which is responsible for the autonomous rhythmic contraction of the heart; and involuntary or smooth muscle, which confers contractility on the walls of blood vessels and hollow organs such as the alimentary tract and the urinary bladder, and which is under the control of the *autonomic nervous system. See also NEUROMUSCULAR DISEASE.

MUSCLE SPINDLE. A specialized neuroreceptor of skeletal *muscle responsible for monitoring muscle length. The spindles are intramuscular sense organs consisting of special, short, slender muscle fibres and specialized sensory nerve endings enclosed in a cellular and connective tissue capsule.

MUSCULAR DYSTROPHY is the name covering a group of primary degenerative *myopathies, all of which are genetically determined. See NEUROMUSCULAR DISEASE.

MUSEUMS, MEDICAL. To most people, a museum is just a place one visits to see objects on display, but it is actually much more than a simple exhibition. The objects have been acquired carefully, to a definite plan. They have had to be entered in a register or *computer, and looked after (guarded against decay, theft, fire, flood, and the like; and kept so they can be found when needed). Some of them are displayed and written about, but facts about all must be discovered. In a medical museum, the objects are themselves 'medical' or have medical connections of some kind. There are really two main kinds of such museums: those dealing especially with objects from the history of the subject, and those specializing in normal or pathological specimens.

Before the 19th century most museums were really only displays of curiosities, all mixed up to titillate the curious. One of the first true medical museums to be organized to a proper theme was that of John and William *Hunter, developed to provide systematic instruction in *anatomy, for medical students in London. This collection became the core of the museum of the *Royal College of Surgeons of England, and much of it survives there to this day. Many medical schools and colleges throughout the world, but especially in Europe, also have such museums. A few museums combine specimens with historical material; the *Royal College of Surgeons of Edinburgh is one well-known example.

Keeping museums going is a very expensive process nowadays. If specimens are included, they have to be made and maintained by specialist *technicians, and the work is very time-consuming and highly skilled. Qualified staff have to explain the specimens, either in person or by means of labels and longer texts and diagrams. Work with microscopes and other special apparatus is required, and a great deal is always going on behind the scenes, not least because of the need to keep up to date.

If museums have historical material, it has to be looked after just as carefully, because much of it may be irreplaceable, and much of it is almost certainly delicate. Virtually all known materials have been used to make medical equipment, and some on display or in store might be 400 years old; some may even be thousands of years old, if the museum includes objects from ancient Egypt, for example. Specialist technicians must look after the fabric of the objects, and others must guard them—some are worth many thousands of pounds. Above all, the curators must be knowledgeable about them, and able to tell others what is known.

There are museums dealing with the *history of medicine in its widest sense all over the world; 'medicine' includes many separate subjects, such as *surgery, *pharmacy, *midwifery, and *nursing, as well as subdivisions of each. There are preserved pharmacies everywhere, and a host of smaller museums dealing with some aspects of medical history, or preserving famous buildings once used as medical schools or other medical or fringe medical establishments. They are found, for example, in such widely scattered places as Lhasa, Melbourne, Delhi, Beijing, Padua, Cleveland (Ohio), Pavia, Washington (DC), Lyon, Göteborg, Budapest, Barcelona, and Utrecht. Larger ones, with displays derived from a number of different sources, are at Vienna, Paris, Leiden, Zurich, and Ingolstadt. The largest in the world is in London—the Wellcome Museum of the History of Medicine, at the Science Museum.

The Wellcome Museum owes its existence to Sir Henry *Wellcome, who was the wealthy owner of a pharmaceutical company, and who had a passion for collecting, and the means to satisfy it. The medical core of his objects was transferred to the Science Museum in 1977—more than 150 000 objects covering all countries, historical periods, and specialisms. The museum caters for young general visitors, and for specialist adults equally. Most need to visit only the large public galleries, with over 5000 objects on display. Each item is carefully labelled (few things are as mystifying as an unlabelled pile of surgical instruments on a glass shelf), with plenty of illustrations showing them in use and providing background information also. Many are shown in their context, in full-scale reconstructions, or in models.

When the museum was first opened, in London in 1913, very little of the wall was left uncovered, and cases were crammed full of poorly labelled objects. This might have been what was wanted at the time, for those visiting such museums were a highly selected group. Nowadays the visitors are of all kinds from all over the world, and careful selection of objects and full explanations guard against the too-rapid onset of 'museum fatigue'.

Some visitors need behind-the-scenes access. This might include discussions with specialist curators, visits to the very large stores to look in detail at objects in some numbers, liaison with historians, talks with designers, and a myriad of other individual arrangements. In this way, the Wellcome Museum is just like any other specialist medical museum, but on a rather larger scale!

Why all this effort? In the case of museums full of anatomical and pathological specimens, much of the work is concerned with teaching. Undergraduates have to be able to recognize parts of the body and their relationships to others, for obvious reasons. To see a good preparation is most revealing, and even inspiring. Those more senior may be working for an advanced qualification, and must have so much more knowledge. Pathological specimens have a special importance nowadays, for so many diseases widespread only a few years ago are now very uncommon, and the preservation of reference specimens is clearly important, as they can be so much more revealing than a picture. If specimens were made by famous workers, that also is important, as their technique might be as interesting as the organ itself.

In the case of the historical object, perhaps each could be considered as a 'crystal of history'. If an object made or used by a famous doctor is handled, it may give a clue to technique which no amount of book reading could offer. Merely to see such an object provides many visitors with a sense of history and even of awe. In the Wellcome Museum, for example, is the microscope used by *Pasteur, the antiseptic spray used by *Lister, the first-aid kit which *Livingstone took across Africa with him, the first brain-*scanner, an iron artificial limb from the 16th century—to name only a very few, all compelling attention and stimulating imagination. For the specialist, to use historical equipment is to understand better what was done with it, and what were its limitations.

Nowadays we are all very much better off, medically speaking, than were our ancestors of the 19th century, and so much better off than those of 3 centuries ago that we cannot really envisage how truly awful life could be then, and how short and troubled existence commonly was. To visit museums of medical history brings it home, showing how some of the progress has been achieved.

B. BRACEGIRDLE

Further reading
Bazin, G. (1978). *The museum age*. Desoer S. A., Brussels.
Science Museum (1982). *The Wellcome Museum of the History of Medicine*. Science Museum, London.

MUSHROOMS AS CAUSE OF POISONING. See POISONOUS FUNGI.

MUSIC AND MEDICINE. The practice of medicine and music have often gone hand in hand. Many doctors have also been musicians. The first five professors of music at Oxford were all physicians, and over the years the roll of medico-musical practitioners includes, among others, Thomas *Campion, Oliver *Goldsmith, Robert *Boyle, *Auenbrugger (libretti), *Bartholin (a study on the Grecian double flute), von *Helmholtz, *Billroth, *Borodin, Albert *Schweitzer, William Wallace, Sir Francis *Champneys, Alan Tyson, T. J. Walsh, Jules Stern, Van Osdol, Harold Sternlicht, and Peter Ichentahl. Doctors' orchestras have been founded in Vienna, New York, and London. There are numerous flourishing, and highly competent, hospital choirs.

To balance this practitioner roll, there is an equally impressive history of medico-musical traditions: the lore on proportions and balance, for example, as developed by the Pythagoreans; the different types of *shaman and their drums; the role of mantric sound-syllables and rhythms for inducing healing through altered states of consciousness. In many cultures, medicine and music are combined in ceremony (the priest doctors of ancient Egypt or the medicine men of the American Indians) or in the aegis of one particular god in a pantheon: Apollo in Greece; Saraswati in southern India.

What are some of the issues at the back of this medico-musical association?

An underlying principle of medicine concerns the relation between normal and abnormal. Doctors' knowledge of the normal arises from a study of the *anatomy, *physiology, and *psychology of the human body and mind (the psyche-soma). This knowledge provides an essential base for understanding what can go wrong in the psyche-soma. Equally, their study of what goes wrong, the abnormal, often provides doctors with unexpected insights into the normal.

When applied to music, this relationship in medicine between the normal and abnormal works in a variety of ways. The core of music has to do with sounds, which we perceive primarily through our ears and our faculty of hearing. Our understanding of the anatomy and physiology of hearing, and of those occasions when hearing is disturbed (as in the medical specialty of *audiology) can contribute directly to this core of music.

The fact, for example, that we have two ears which combine to provide us with a single hearing field (our binaural hearing) has important consequences for the localization of sounds in space, a problem which has inspired many musicians including Gabrieli, Berlioz, and Stockhausen. The simultaneous presentation of more than one melody has, in counterpoint, proved a bedrock for Western European music. The exercise of separating these two streams of sound and feeding one into the left ear and the other into the right (so-called dichotic listening) has offered one approach to exploring how the different sides of our *brain may function.

From medicine we learn that a complex faculty such as hearing is intricately connected with many other systems in the psyche-soma: neurological connections in the brain; systems which underlie our capacity to move, dance, and sing; or systems whereby we experience and express emotions or understand and articulate *speech. Just as the material of music draws deeply on expansions such as silence, noise, repetition (rhythm), contrast (variation), so our medical understanding of what we are about when we are making or listening to music draws on these many fields which abut on and expand that of 'pure' hearing.

One example of this inter-connectedness may be seen in the phenomenon of synaesthesia, that capacity to combine sensory modalities, to hear sounds in colour or as tactile textures. The phenomenon has intrigued musicians from the early Renaissance days of word-painting to Scriabin and Messiaen. It plays an important role in song-writing, where the aim is clearly to bridge the two languages of words and music. Studies on synaesthesia illuminate our understanding of our earliest steps in symbolizing and in integrating our verbal self with those other selves (like the musical one) which pre-date our use of words.

Other approaches to the connection between the *language of music and words have been pursued by *laryngologists and *neurologists. The first are engaged, with singers, on such issues as *phonation, the neuro-muscular basis of vocal mechanics, the adaptation of the voice to the ever-expanding demands put on it; and with *paediatricians and child *psychiatrists, on the analysis and synthesis of voice sounds, the formation of everyone's idiosyncratic cry, which, in certain instances, can assist in the *diagnosis of a particular disease.

Neurologists have explored certain abnormalities of musical experience (the '*amusias') along lines similar to those undertaken into the abnormalities of speech (the '*aphasias'). The distinctions they outline point to the various, often clearly defined, problematic areas: vocal amusia, the loss of the ability to sing; instrumental musical or receptive amnesia, the loss of the ability to play an instrument, to recognize a familiar tune, or to discriminate melodic patterns; musical *alexia and musical *agraphia, the loss of the ability to read or write down a series of notes; basic disorders of rhythm entailing a failure to reproduce rhythmic patterns or to distinguish between them; tone-deafness, which may have a *genetic origin.

Besides the amusias, another abnormality which may throw light on the neural basis of music is those rare types of *epilepsy which are triggered off by music ('musicogenic epilepsy'), which may be accompanied by auditory *hallucinations (and hence lie on the boundary of physiology and psychology), and which are associated with disturbances in brain rhythms in either temporal lobe.

Further insights into this neural basis for our musical experiences and for the way our hearing and listening link with other systems are coming from increasingly detailed studies on how the normal and abnormal brain function. These studies entail observing the blood flow (and hence the activity) of different sites in the brain when different mental activities are undertaken, such as listening to pitches of individual notes, to sequential patterns of notes, to a piece of music, or such as listening to music in our head as when we are composing music. An overriding impression from any of these studies is the wide ramifications of networks involved and the speed at which they operate.

Music is inseparable from dance, and though we may take it in through our ears, we respond to it through our whole body. This embodied response is reflected not only in these wide-ranging networks of neurological studies but also in the many body-parts which are employed in playing different instruments, and so in the many occupational hazards to which musicians are prone, and for which they may consult their medical practitioners. Indeed, the list of these hazards comes to read like a medical textbook and a course in how to avoid them (including techniques for correct posture and relaxation) has now become part of a musician's training.

The musician's use of the doctor's skills is complemented by the doctor's use of the musician's art. Music has been used as a general environmental sedative, especially in centres for disturbed children and adults; in *intensive care as a means of reaching a *comatose patient; in the *obstetric wards through simulated heart-beat sounds or other 'lullabies' for babies before and after delivery; and in *anaesthesia to counter pre-operative tension especially during an operation under local anaesthesia such as a *cataract.

For the blind, musical scales have been used in electronic travel aids to display distances between objects; for the mentally handicapped, music has proved valuable in operant *conditioning and learning programmes. It may, especially as rhythm, enter the treatment of *stuttering or, as melodic intonation, that of aphasia. Associated with play, music may provide a channel of access to autistic or withdrawn children.

Along with the other arts therapies, music can serve as a means of creating a shared 'potential space' in which patients can feel safe enough to explore their identities. In this space, through music, the therapist seeks to mirror or resonate aspects of the situation which, until then, were hidden for both therapist and patient alike.

Through music, then, it is claimed that, from our earliest years, we can expand our embodied self; can enhance our capacity to feel; and can develop our acquisition of social and intellectual skills. The task of consolidating such claims by logical and statistical techniques which would satisfy a traditional scientist is formidable. So far the verification of propositions about the efficacy of music as a therapeutic tool rests largely on ostensive definition and empirical results: 'We've tried this here and it works'.

R. N. T. HIGGINS

Further reading
Clynes, M. (ed.) (1983). *Music, mind, and brain*. Plenum Press, New York.

Critchley, M. and Henson, R. A. (1977). *Music and the brain*. William Heinemann, London.

Handel, S. (1991). *Listening: an introduction to the perception of auditory events*. MIT Press, Cambridge, MA.

Sloboda, J. A. (1985). *The musical mind: the cognitive psychology of music*. Oxford University Press, Oxford.

Sloboda, J. A. (ed.) (1988). *Generative processes in music: the psychology of performance, improvisation, and composition*. Clarendon Press, Oxford.

MUSTARD, WILLIAM T. (1914–88). Canadian surgeon. A pioneer in the surgery of congenital heart disease, he developed the 'Mustard operation' for transposition of the great vessels.

MUSTARD GAS is the vapour from a poisonous blistering liquid, dichlorodiethyl sulphide $(CH_2Cl.CH_2)_2S$. Occupational exposure is carcinogenic.

MUTAGEN. Any agent that increases the frequency of genetic *mutations: the agent may be chemical (e.g. *mustard gas) or physical (e.g. *ionizing radiation). See also AMES TEST.

MUTATION. An abrupt change in *chromosomal *DNA. A mutation restricted to a single *gene will, by altering its DNA sequence, produce a corresponding alteration in the amino acid sequence of the protein coded for by that gene. Most mutations are of this single-gene type, but grosser structural alterations in chromosomes (e.g. inversion, translocation) may also occur. The significant mutations are those which occur in the *gametes or their precursor cells, since these will be inherited. In nature, mutations are rare, random events which provide the basis for evolution by *natural selection. Environmental *mutagens can greatly increase the frequency of mutations. See also GENETICS.

MUTISM is dumbness, the state of being unable to or of refusing to speak.

MYALGIA is *muscle pain.

MYASTHENIA GRAVIS is an *autoimmune disorder characterized by muscular weakness and fatiguability. See NEUROMUSCULAR DISEASE.

MYCOBACTERIUM is a genus of *Gram-positive *acid-fast *bacilli which includes the causative organisms of *tuberculosis (*M. tuberculosis hominis* and *M.t. bovis*) and *leprosy (*M. leprae*).

MYCOLOGY is the study of fungi.

MYCOPLASMA is a genus of micro-organisms, the smallest free-living organisms known. They are distinguished from *viruses in being able to grow in artificial media, i.e. outside cells, and from *bacteria (with which they are nevertheless usually classified) in having no cell wall. Many are animal parasites or saprophytes. One species, *Mycoplasma pneumoniae*, is an important cause of respiratory infection in man; another, *Mycoplasma hominis*, is thought to be a possible cause of some cases of *non-specific urethritis.

MYCOSIS is any disease caused by a *fungus.

MYCOSIS FUNGOIDES. A malignant T-cell *lymphoma affecting primarily the skin, although lymph nodes and some viscera may also be involved.

MYCOTOXIN. Any toxic substance produced by a *fungus; the *aflatoxins and the *ergot alkaloids are examples. See also POISONOUS FUNGI.

MYDRIASIS is dilatation of the *pupil.

MYDRIATIC. An agent which dilates the *pupil.

MYELIN is the fatty substance, consisting of various *lipids in combination with *protein, which forms the sheath enveloping all larger *axons of *nerve cells in the nervous system of vertebrates. By isolating the axons from the body fluids, it enables them to conduct impulses more rapidly than smaller non-myelinated fibres. In demyelinating diseases such as *multiple sclerosis there is patchy loss of myelin with consequent impairment of neural function.

MYELINATION is the development of *myelin sheaths.

MYELITIS means inflammation either of the spinal cord or of the bone marrow, according to context.

MYELOGRAPHY is *radiographic visualization of the *spinal cord after injection of a *contrast medium into the *subarachnoid space.

MYELOMA. Any *tumour arising from *bone marrow. Multiple myeloma is a malignant neoplasm of *plasma cells (active antibody-secreting B *lymphocytes) usually occurring at several bony sites, causing bone destruction and abnormal secretion of immune *globulins.

MYENTERIC PLEXUS. See AUERBACH.

MYIASIS is the infestation of living tissues by fly larvae. See MAGGOTS.

MYOCARDIAL INFARCTION.
See CORONARY THROMBOSIS.

MYOCARDITIS is inflammation of heart muscle.

MYOCARDIUM is the muscular tissue of the heart.

MYOCLONUS. Sudden involuntary contractions of groups of *muscles causing jerking movements.

MYOFIBRIL is one of the fine threads, about one micrometre thick, a number of which together make up a striated *muscle fibre.

MYOGLOBIN is the oxygen-carrying pigment of *muscle.

MYOKYMIA is the spontaneous contraction of small bundles of muscle fibres (*fasciculation), particularly in the lower eyelid and calf muscles. It is a benign condition, often accompanied by *hyperhidrosis. Other rare forms of myokymia also occur, one in association with *myotonia, another, facial myokymia, giving a rippling or undulating movement of the facial muscles.

MYOMA. A tumour arising from *muscle tissue.

MYOPATHY. Any disease of muscle. In practice, the term is restricted to muscle disorders other than those secondary to disordered function of the central or peripheral nervous system. See NEUROMUSCULAR DISEASE.

MYOPIA is near-sightedness, in which the refractive power of the eye relative to its length is too great and distant objects come to a focus in front of the retina. It is corrected by concave (negative) spectacle lenses. See OPHTHALMOLOGY.

MYOSIN is a major protein component of the *myofibrils of *muscle. Together with another protein, actin, it provides the muscular contractile mechanism, the myosin molecules sliding along actin filament to produce shortening of muscle fibres (the sliding filament hypothesis). See NEUROMUSCULAR DISEASE.

MYOSITIS is inflammation of *muscle. See DERMATO-MYOSITIS; NEUROMUSCULAR DISEASE.

MYOTONIA is a form of delayed relaxation of voluntary muscle. See NEUROMUSCULAR DISEASE.

MYOTONIA CONGENITA is a congenital form of *myotonia, usually inherited as an autosomal *dominant condition (Thomsen's disease), although a *recessive variety also occurs. See NEUROMUSCULAR DISEASE.

MYOTOXIC describes an agent toxic to muscle tissue.

MYXOEDEMA (MYXEDEMA) is adult hypothyroidism, which results from deficient or absent function of the *thyroid gland. The cardinal features are: weakness and lethargy; mental dullness and memory loss; weight gain; dry, coarse, and puffy skin; cold intolerance; hoarseness of the voice; and severe constipation. The diagnosis is confirmed by finding a low level of *thyroxine in the circulation; treatment is by replacement therapy with that hormone.

MYXOMA. A *tumour of primitive *connective tissue cells.

MYXOMATOSIS is an infectious viral disease of rabbits, originally described in Brazil but now widespread (and artificially introduced into several countries in order to control the rabbit population). It causes fever, swelling of mucous membranes, and skin tumours resembling *myxomas; it has a high mortality rate. It is not pathogenic to man.

MYXOVIRUS is one of a large group of *ribonucleic acid (RNA) *viruses which includes those of *influenza and *mumps and some of those associated with the common *cold.

NAEGELI, OTTO (1871–1938). Swiss haematologist. His book *Lehrbuch der Blutkrankheiten und Blutdiagnostik* (1931) was the bible of *haematology for many years. He described myelomonocytic *leukaemia and a cell called the micromyeloblast.

NAEVUS (NEVUS). Birthmark; any congenital mark or discoloration on the skin or mucous membrane of the mouth.

NAILS, like hair, are composed of *keratin and their normal growth is sensitive to the general state of *nutrition; transverse furrows often follow acute severe illnesses, after growth is resumed. In iron-deficiency anaemia they become characteristically soft and concave (koilonychia). Nail changes occur in many cutaneous disorders, particularly *psoriasis and fungus infections such as *ringworm.

NALIDIXIC ACID is an oral antibacterial drug of value in urinary tract infections. See ANTI-INFECTIVE DRUGS.

NARCISSISM, or excessive self-love, is held by some psychoanalysts to be regression to or persistence of a normal early phase of *psychosexual development. In Greek mythology Narcissus was a youth who fell in love with his own image reflected in a fountain and pined away until transformed into the flower of the same name.

NARCOANALYSIS is *psychoanalysis assisted by the administration of a drug (usually a short-acting *barbiturate like thiopentone sodium) which causes mental disinhibition and so facilitates expression of thoughts, ideas, and memories.

NARCOLEPSY. Periodic attacks of an uncontrollable urge to sleep during normal waking hours. It is often associated with *cataplexy. See also SLEEP.

NARCOSIS is stupor or insensibility produced by drugs which depress the central nervous system.

NARCOTIC. Any drug which produces *narcosis. The term is often used synonymously with 'narcotic analgesic' to mean a drug like *morphine, used primarily to relieve pain. As morphine and related compounds are strongly addictive, 'narcotic' is sometimes loosely used for any drug of *addiction.

NASOPHARYNX. The part of the *pharynx lying above the soft palate and behind the nose.

NATIONAL ACADEMY OF SCIENCES (NAS). A private organization of scientists and engineers in the USA dedicated to the advancement of science and its use for the general welfare. The Academy, with its headquarters in Washington, DC, has an official advisory role to the US government on matters concerned with science and technology; it was given its charter by Congress in 1863. Membership is conferred on the basis of major contributions to scientific research or development, and is by election only; members at present number about 1250. The NAS brings together scientists and engineers to exchange information and to further research by means of institutes, boards, committees, subcommittees, panels, and *ad hoc* groups. It is organized into scientific sections; these include sections of mathematics, astronomy, physics, engineering, geology, chemistry, botany, geophysics, biochemistry, neurobiology, population biology, evolution, medical genetics, anthropology, psychology, social and political studies, and economic sciences. The Institute of Medicine was organized under the NAS charter in 1970. It studies public health policy, with special emphasis on the provision of adequate health services for all sectors of society. It has about 300 members.

NATIONAL BLOOD TRANSFUSION SERVICE. In England and Wales, the National Blood Transfusion Service (NBTS) operates in conjunction with the Department of Health and 15 regional blood transfusion centres to provide a service for the collection (from voluntary unpaid donors), storage, and distribution of blood and blood products. There is a separate Scottish National Blood Transfusion Service with five regional blood transfusion centres and a headquarters laboratory.

NATIONAL BOARD OF HEALTH (USA). See HEALTH, NATIONAL BOARD OF (USA).

NATIONAL FORMULARY, BRITISH. See PHARMACY AND PHARMACISTS (UK).

NATIONAL FORMULARY (USA). The *United States Pharmacopoeia* has been published since 1820, and has gone through many editions. Its purpose has been to describe drugs regarded as appropriate and essential by the medical profession. Presently it is revised at five-year intervals, but supplements are issued when appropriate. In 1888 the first *National Formulary* of unofficial preparations was published by the American Pharmaceutical Association. For some time the *Pharmacopoeia* was looked upon as limited to the 'best' drugs, whereas the *Formulary* included some 'second best' agents, approved by some, but not all, of the profession. Gradually a tendency developed for the *National Formulary* to emphasize the standards for inactive ingredients (excipients) used in making drug dosage forms. In 1975 the US Pharmacopoeial Convention, Inc., took over publication of both reference works, and in 1980 they were published together in a single volume. This presented standards of strength, quality, and purity for about 2800 drugs. There is a Committee on Revision, which distributes proposed revisions for both publications, and invites comments before issuing supplements or new editions.

NATIONAL HEALTH INSURANCE ACT 1911. Lloyd George's famous enactment represented a landmark in developing state provision for health in the UK. Because of fierce opposition from the medical 'establishment', including the *British Medical Association, the Act did not come into force on the appointed day (12 July 1912) but was delayed until late 1913. By this time there were 15 000 000 insured persons, and the government had recruited 10 000 general practitioners willing to participate. Under the Act, insured workers (wage earners with an income of less than £160 per annum, excluding civil servants and teachers) but not their families, were entitled to free advice and treatment from 'panel doctors' and to sickness benefit paid through approved societies such as trade unions, workmen's clubs, etc. Hospital treatment for the seriously ill or injured was not included. Panel doctors were paid an annual capitation fee of 7s. 6d. per patient. Another pioneering feature of the Act was the provision of a subsidy for medical research of 1d. per patient per annum; from this modest beginning, the *Medical Research Council eventually emerged.

NATIONAL HEALTH SERVICE ACT 1946. The National Health Service (NHS), which came into being in the UK on 5 July 1948, was established under this Act. It followed, and was largely based on, the *Beveridge Report* of 1942 and a subsequent government White Paper of 1944. It became:

the duty of the Minister of Health to promote the establishment in England and Wales of a comprehensive health service designed to secure improvement in the physical and mental health of the people and the prevention, diagnosis and treatment of illness and for that purpose to provide or secure the effective provision of a service in accordance with the provisions of the Act. Service so provided shall be free of charge, except where any provision of the Act expressly provides for the making and recovery of charges.

The NHS comprised: central administration; hospital and specialist services; the health services of local health authorities; general medical, dental, and pharmaceutical services; and mental health services. The administrative bodies for hospitals were Regional Hospital Boards, with Boards of Governors and Hospital Management Committees; those for general practice, Executive Councils; while the Local Health Authorities administered personal health services.

The provisions of the 1946 Act were later much altered under amending Acts of 1973, 1977, and 1991, but the basic principles underlying the provision of a National Health Service remain. See also GOVERNMENT AND MEDICINE IN THE UK; HEALTH-CARE SYSTEMS AND THEIR FINANCING.

NATIONAL HOSPITALS FOR NERVOUS DISEASES, THE, arose from the amalgamation of several hospitals. The National Hospital for the Paralysed and Epileptic was founded in 1860 and had eight beds in Queen Square in London. The London Infirmary for Epilepsy and Paralysis was founded in 1866 in Marylebone, moving to Maida Vale in 1903. These two hospitals founded neurology and neurosurgery as independent specialties in the UK. In 1948, with the advent of the *National Health Service, they were amalgamated under one Board of Governors, becoming then the National Hospitals for Nervous Diseases. Their research and postgraduate medical educational activities were brought together in 1951 under the Institute of Neurology, as part of the British Postgraduate Medical Federation, a school of the University of London. Recently, the name of the hospital in Queen Square has been changed to the National Hospital for Neurology and Neurosurgery.

Among the great names in neurology who worked in these hospitals were John Hughlings *Jackson, David *Ferrier, Henry *Head, Charles Edouard *Brown-Séquard, James Collier, S. A. Kinnier *Wilson, and Gordon *Holmes, while in the early years of neurosurgery Victor *Horsley was pre-eminent.

NATIONAL INSTITUTE FOR MEDICAL RESEARCH. The National Institute for Medical Research (NIMR), Mill Hill, London, is the UK *Medical Research Council's major institute for research in the basic laboratory sciences subserving medicine. The concept of such an institute dates from the beginning of the Council itself, immediately prior to and following the First World War. The first of the Institute's two sites, at Hampstead, was occupied in 1920; in 1949, it moved to larger purpose-built accommodation in Mill Hill, six miles further north of central London. Many noted biomedical scientists worked at the NIMR. The first three directors, spanning the period from 1928 to 1971, were Sir Henry *Dale, Sir Charles Harington, and Sir Peter *Medawar. Among the many topics upon which major research achievements were initiated or developed were: the methonium compounds, which provided the first effective treatment of *hypertension; the isolation of *ergometrine; many physical methods including *ultramicroscopy and gas *chromatography; *protein synthesis; *vitamin D; virology, particularly with respect to *influenza and transmissible tumours; *immunology and the discovery of *interferon; *insulin and *carbohydrate metabolism; sex *hormones and reproductive physiology; environmental physiology; and methods for biological standards and control. See also RESEARCH INSTITUTES.

NATIONAL INSTITUTES OF HEALTH (NIH) arose out of a small bacteriological laboratory at the Marine Hospital, Staten Island, New York, established by the US government. It was for research into *cholera and other *infectious diseases. For its first 25 years it concentrated on these, but in 1891 it moved to Washington, DC, as the Hygienic Laboratory. It gradually expanded its interests into *public health under the auspices of the US Public Health Service. In 1930 the name was changed by enactment to National Institute of Health, with the wide remit of 'ascertaining the cause, prevention and cure of disease'. Later the NIH moved to Bethesda, Maryland, where it now employs a staff of over 12 000, some in the Clinical Centre. As funding for research has become increasingly a government concern its administration was handed over to the NIH, which supports research in universities, hospitals, and medical centres of all kinds. With the addition of the National Heart Institute, the National Cancer Institute, and some others the enterprise became the National Institutes of Health. See also RESEARCH INSTITUTES.

NATIONAL INSURANCE ACT 1946. This was an enactment arising out of the *Beveridge Report*, which formed the legislative basis of the British version of the 'welfare state' that has existed since 1948. The Act, largely replaced by the National Insurance Act 1965, established an extended system of national insurance providing pecuniary payments by way of unemployment benefit, sickness benefit, maternity benefit, retirement pension, widows' benefit, guardian's allowance, and death grant; it also provided for making payments towards the cost of a *national health service. Earlier legislation regarding unemployment insurance, national health insurance, widows', orphans', and old age pensions was repealed by the Act.

NATIONAL INSURANCE INDUSTRIAL INJURIES ACTS. These UK Acts, beginning with that of 1946, replaced the Workmen's Compensation Acts 1925–45, repealing most of their provisions, and established a system of compulsory insurance against personal injury caused by accidents arising out of and in the course of an insured person's employment and against prescribed diseases and injuries due to the nature of a person's employment. Compensation was in the form of insurance benefits administered by the state. The Acts were in turn superseded by the Social Security Acts of 1975 and 1978.

NATIONAL MEDICAL ASSOCIATIONS. See MEDICAL COLLEGES, ETC. OF THE UK; MEDICAL COLLEGES ETC. IN THE USA.

NATURAL CHILDBIRTH, also known as the Grantly Dick Read method, was first advocated by Read in 1933. The principle is the avoidance of pain and muscular tension by relaxation methods that allow birth to proceed naturally and render *analgesic drugs unnecessary. Some advocates also feel that the mother should be allowed to choose her own posture during labour.

NATURAL SELECTION is the process by which life forms best adapted to their environment survive and reproduce in the greatest numbers, propagating their *genetic characteristics. Genetic *mutations producing new characteristics favourable to survival and reproduction are propagated, those unfavourable are not. Charles *Darwin in 1859 proposed natural selection as the principal mechanism of evolutionary change and hence as the origin of species.

NATUROPATHY is a system which eschews the use of medicinal drugs and the consumption of other than 'natural' foods.

NAUSEA is an unpleasant sensation of being about to vomit, sometimes culminating in the act of vomiting. The original meaning was seasickness.

NECROBIOSIS is the formation of circumscribed degenerative lesions of skin *collagen, seen particularly in diabetic patients.

NECROLOGY. A death roll, an obituary notice, or a history of the dead.

NECROPHILIA is a pathological liking for dead bodies, or a sexual perversion involving intercourse with corpses.

NECROPSY. Synonym for *autopsy.

NECROSIS. Death of tissue.

NECROSIS, AVASCULAR. *Necrosis due to failure of blood supply.

NEEDLE. Any slender sharp metal instrument for puncturing or suturing; or when hollow, for injecting or aspirating.

NEGATIVISM is pathological resistance to suggestion; in pronounced cases the patient does the opposite of what he is asked to do. The same term is sometimes used to denote an abnormal state in which a patient consistently does what he ought not to do (with food, faeces, etc.).

NEGLIGENCE is an act or state of being neglectful, of duty, dress, cleanliness, etc. See also PROFESSIONAL NEGLIGENCE; LAW AND MEDICINE IN THE UK; LAW AND MEDICINE IN THE USA.

NEGRI, ADELCHI (1876–1912). Italian pathologist. While assistant to *Golgi, Negri discovered the *rabies corpuscles (Negri bodies) in the pyramidal cells of *Ammon's horn in the brains of animals dying of rabies. They are recognized as pathognomonic of this disease. Negri died of pulmonary *tuberculosis aged 35.

NEISSER, ALBERT LUDWIG SIEGMUND (1855–1916). German dermatologist and bacteriologist. Neisser discovered the bacterial cause of *gonorrhoea, since named *Neisseria gonorrhoeae*, in 1879 when pelvic infections and vaginal discharges were not understood. He also investigated *syphilis and worked with *Ehrlich on the use of arsenicals; he advocated the therapeutic value of mercurials, to prevent the worst manifestations of *neurosyphilis. In 1880 he identified *Mycobacterium leprae* which Hansen had seen in 1873 but had not thought to be the cause of leprosy. He was associated with von *Wassermann in devising his serological test for syphilis.

NEISSERIA is a genus of aerobic Gram-negative *diplococci which includes the important pathogens of *gonorrhoea (*Neisseria gonorrhoeae*) and *meningococcal meningitis (*N. meningitidis*).

NELATON, AUGUSTE (1807–73). French surgeon. He introduced the rubber *catheter (1860) and was one of the first to use electrocautery. He popularized *ovariotomy in France and invented a bullet-seeking probe which was first used on Garibaldi at Aspromonte in 1862. A line joining the anterior superior iliac spine and the ischial tuberosity is still commonly called Nelaton's line.

NEMATODE. Any member of the large phylum Nematoda, which consists of roundworms, threadworms, and eelworms, many, but not all, being endoparasitic in plants and animals. Those of medical importance include *Ascaris, *Strongyloides, *Ancylostoma, *Toxocara, *Trichinella (the agent of *trichiniasis), the several species causing *filariasis, and some others.

NEOMYCIN. A member of the *aminoglycoside group of antibiotics which is considered too toxic to be administered parenterally. Its use is therefore confined to topical application in infections of the skin and mucous membranes, and to sterilization of the intestine before bowel surgery or in hepatic failure. See also ANTI-INFECTIVE DRUGS.

NEONATE. An infant in the first 4 weeks of life.

NEOPLASM. Any tumour or new growth, whether or not malignant. See ONCOLOGY.

NEOSTIGMINE is a synthetic quaternary ammonium compound with cholinergic effects, used in treating *myasthenia gravis and other conditions. It is an *anticholinesterase, i.e. it inhibits the enzyme which destroys *acetylcholine.

NEPHELOMETRY is the optical measurement of turbidity in suspensions by means of light scattering.

NEPHRECTOMY is surgical removal of a kidney.

NEPHRITIS is any inflammation of kidney tissue. When otherwise unqualified, it usually means one of that group of disorders collectively known as glomerulonephritis. See NEPHROLOGY.

NEPHROGRAPHY is the radiographic visualization of the kidneys, on plain X-ray films or with the assistance of *pyelography, *arteriography, or *computed transaxial tomography.

NEPHROLITHIASIS. The presence of *calculi within the kidney and upper urinary tract.

NEPHROLOGIST. A specialist in kidney diseases.

NEPHROLOGY is the study of the *kidneys, their structure and function in health and disease from fetal development to the *atrophy of old age. The word is used in this full sense in the title of societies and publications, e.g. the members of the International Society of Nephrology include *physicians, *surgeons, *pathologists, anatomists, physiologists, biochemists, immunologists, geneticists, and epidemiologists, united in their interest in the kidneys. 'Nephrology' is also used in a restricted sense to denote the subspecialty of medicine practised by renal physicians. Surgeons who operate on the kidneys and urinary tract are called *urologists.

The recent history of nephrology

In *The Oxford companion to medicine* (1986), Sir Douglas Black gave an elegant account of the dawn of nephrology and its rapid advance in the 19th and early 20th centuries. There were some outstanding leaps forward, such as the description of the glomeruli by Marcello *Malpighi in 1661, but many bright flashes of inspiration left little permanent illumination until the work of Richard Bright in the 19th century (Berry and Mackenzie 1992) and his contemporaries, pupils, and successors (Cameron 1988). Despite many important advances in the century after Bright, our understanding of kidney disease was still rudimentary at the start of the Second World War. No effective treatment existed for any form of renal disease until the introduction of *sulphonamides for urinary *infection in 1936. Since then there have been major advances in the understanding and management of many aspects of renal disease.

Acute renal failure

In 1941, during the London Blitz, Bywaters and Beale described acute renal failure due to crush injury. In subsequent studies Bywaters discovered the mechanism of acute renal failure in this condition, caused by massive destruction of muscle, now called rhabdomyolysis. Rational conservative treatment by diet and fluid balance was developed in The Netherlands and by Graham Bull and his team at Hammersmith Hospital in the early post-war years. *Haemodialysis was first used as a temporary replacement of renal function in 1943 and became available as a routine treatment from the mid-1950s, followed by peritoneal dialysis (1960s) and haemofiltration (1980s).

Chronic renal failure

Renal *transplantation was first used successfully in identical twins in Boston in 1951 and became an effective treatment between unrelated individuals from the mid-1960s (Morris 1988). From 1960 haemodialysis was used for chronic renal failure and replaced the excretory function of the kidneys sufficiently to allow survival for decades. Peritoneal dialysis was developed at about the same time but became a serious alternative to haemodialysis only after the introduction of continuous ambulatory peritoneal dialysis in the late 1970s. The development of drugs to control *hypertension had a major impact on the morbidity and the rate of progression of chronic renal failure from the 1950s. The role of low protein dieting in slowing the progression of chronic renal disease was subjected to many controlled trials in the 1980s and early 1990s, showing probable benefit (El Nahas *et al.* 1993).

Renal *pathology

Renal *biopsy (taking a small sample of kidney tissue by a needle for histological study) was introduced by Iversen and Brun in Denmark in the 1950s. This made possible the study of renal disease at all stages of the illness and greatly expanded knowledge of the natural history of renal diseases and their response to treatment.

Glomerulonephritis (nephritis)

This term describes the diseases, formerly lumped together as Bright's disease, in which the glomeruli

are affected by inflammation and scarring. With the aid of renal biopsy they have been sorted into many distinct types, which respond in different ways to treatment with drugs.

One form of nephritis has been prevented, at least in developed countries. The advent, in 1944, of *penicillin, which is effective against streptococcal infection, greatly reduced the incidence of post-streptococcal nephritis, making it a rare disease. Another form of nephritis responded consistently to treatment; in minimal change disease, in which the slight abnormalities in the glomeruli are seen only by electron microscopy, response to *corticosteroids is rapid and complete, though periodic relapse is common. This was a disabling and often fatal illness, affecting mainly young children, until the introduction of corticosteroids in 1950. Massive loss of proteins in the urine caused *oedema (due to loss of *albumin), susceptibility to infection (due to loss of *immunoglobulins), clotting (due to loss of inhibitors of clotting), and other complications. Similar symptoms occur in any disease causing heavy proteinuria and are known collectively as the *nephrotic syndrome.

A major step forward was the demonstration by Keith Peters and his colleagues at Hammersmith in 1975 that two of the most aggressive forms of glomerulonephritis, *Goodpasture's syndrome and systemic *vasculitis, could be reversed by a cocktail of immunosuppressive drugs and plasma exchange. Immunosuppression has also brought steady improvement in the treatment of glomerulonephritis complicating generalized diseases such as systemic *lupus erythematosus and Wegener's granulomatosis. However, for most of the common, slowly progressive, forms of glomerulonephritis the benefits are uncertain and side-effects prohibitive. Much has been learned about the immunological mechanisms that cause these diseases, but safe treatments to reverse these processes have yet to be devised.

Urinary infection (*cystitis)

This commonest of all diseases of the urinary tract responds rapidly to many of the antibacterial drugs that have followed sulphonamides into clinical practice. However, antibacterials are a mixed blessing; while curing the existing infection they predispose to subsequent infections by altering the bacterial population of the bowel. Advances have included the development of drugs such as trimethoprim and the quinolones which reduce the bowel population of invasive organisms, and the recognition that 3 days of treatment cure cystitis just as effectively as longer courses.

An uncommon effect of urinary infection is scarring of the kidneys (chronic *pyelonephritis) sometimes leading to kidney failure. Work in the 1950s and 1960s, particularly at University College London, showed that this process usually started in infancy. It results from delayed development of a valve at the lower end of the ureter, where it enters the *bladder. This causes reflux of urine from the bladder up to the kidneys during urination; if the urine is infected, *abscesses form in the kidneys and lead to scarring. Operations to restore valvular function have a high success rate, but controlled trials have so far shown only minor effects on the natural history of the illness.

Drug-induced damage to the kidneys

Most drugs, or their metabolites, are excreted through the kidneys, and some are concentrated during this process. Some very valuable *antibiotics, anticancer drugs, and immunosuppressants damage the kidneys if used at high dose or for prolonged periods; regular measurements of their blood concentrations are needed to prevent this side-effect.

In 1953 Spühler and Zollinger in Switzerland noticed a high incidence of fatal kidney scarring in people who consumed large quantities of headache powders and similar pain-killers, a practice common among watch-makers. Epidemics of this disease—analgesic nephro-pathy (Stewart 1993)—were described from many coun-tries, particularly Australia, Scandinavia, Belgium, and Germany. In the worst-affected areas it became the commonest cause of renal failure. Fiscal control of the sale of analgesic mixtures and the withdrawal of phenacetin, the principal component believed to be the cause, has been followed by the gradual decline of this disease, which is now rare in the UK and most other countries.

Genetic diseases of the kidney

Genetic diseases of the kidney are the leading cause of renal failure in childhood, but much the commonest is polycystic kidney disease, which presents in adult life; it accounts for about 8 per cent of cases of renal failure in the UK. Over 100 dominant or recessive diseases and chromosome disorders affecting the kidney are listed in standard textbooks (Cameron *et al.* 1992). The *gene affected in polycystic disease has been located on *chromosome 16, and those for several rarer diseases have been cloned. So far no major changes in treatment have resulted, but *genetic counselling and *prenatal diagnosis are rapidly improving.

Endocrine functions of the kidney

The existence of *renin has been known for almost a century, but its chemical nature, the site of its secretion in specialized cells of the afferent arteriole, and its function have been worked out over the past 50 years. It cleaves angiotensinogen to produce angiotensin-1, which is further split to angiotensin-2 by angiotensin converting enzyme (ACE). Renin is secreted in excess when the renal arteries are narrowed and in some types of chronic renal disease, raising *blood pressure. The development of ACE inhibitors which interrupt this pathway has been an important advance in treating high blood pressure.

The role of the kidney in stimulating the formation of red blood cells was proposed in 1906, but the isolation of *erythropoietin, the determination of its chemical structure and its site of secretion in peritubular cells, the cloning of its gene and its production in cultures of mon-key kidney cells into which the human gene had been implanted are triumphs of the past 20 years. Erythro-poietin is expensive, about £3000 (US$4500) per annum per patient, but is now given to those with *anaemia due to renal failure with a striking improvement in quality of life.

*Bone disease and hypertrophy of the *parathyroid glands are manifestations of renal failure that have been studied since the 1930s. The great steps forward were: the discovery by Fraser and Kodichek in 1970 that the kidney was the organ that converted vitamin D to its active form, calcitriol; and the synthesis and marketing of calcitriol by Roche. Reduced formation of calcitriol in chronic renal failure releases the parathyroid glands from control by this hormone and their overactivity softens the bones. Administration of calcitriol or its precursor, alfacalcidol, in renal failure prevents or heals this variety of bone disease.

The work of the renal physician

Cystitis is usually treated by general practitioners. The other conditions listed above are referred to renal phy-sicians for diagnosis and treatment. Most of their work-load consists of the treatment of acute and chronic renal failure. Acute renal failure is often a complication of life-threatening diseases such as infections, major sur-gery, accidental *trauma, and accidents of childbirth and abortion; the last is now rare in the UK. The incidence of renal failure rises steeply with age, as does its mortality, which remains high (about 40 per cent) because of the severity of the primary disease.

Chronic renal failure has over 100 causes, in addi-tion to the genetic diseases. The common ones are glomerulonephritis, *diabetes, hypertension, chronic pyelonephritis, polycystic disease, urinary obstruction, and 'cause unknown'. The incidence rises steeply with age, and is about three times higher in immigrants from countries in Africa, the Caribbean, and the Indian sub-continent than in Caucasians in the UK. The preferred treatment of irreversible chronic renal failure is renal transplantation, but it is limited by the supply of donor kidneys, so in many countries few patients over 60 receive a transplant. While awaiting a transplant, or indefinitely in those who do not receive one, renal excre-tory function is replaced by 'renal dialysis', while the endocrine functions are replaced as described above.

Renal dialysis

The title is a condensed sentence; it means 'purification of the blood in renal failure by dialysis or/and filtration'. It is achieved by one of three methods described below.

Haemodialysis

Blood is taken from a suitable vessel and pumped over a semipermeable *membrane which allows the passage

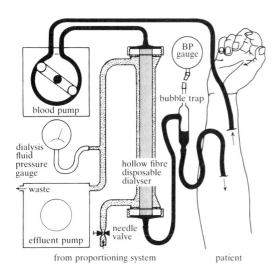

Fig. 1 A modern haemodialysis circuit (simplified). Blood is taken from the arterial tube and pumped through the hollow-fibre disposable dialyser before returning through an air trap to the patient. Dialysis fluid flows in the opposite direction from a proportionating system, which produces it from water and concentrate.

of the small molecules which accumulate in renal failure but retains the larger proteins and blood cells. As it passes down the tube it is 'washed' by a stream of fluid on the outer side of the membrane that carries away the waste products. This dialysis fluid contains solutes such as sodium and dextrose in the same concentrations as normal blood so that they are not lost from the body. Some substances such as *amino acids and *vitamins are omitted from the fluid to save cost; they are lost during dialysis but are replaced by eating a good diet or taking supplements.

The early history of haemodialysis and peritoneal dialysis has been described by Drukker (1988). The first successful human dialysis was made possible by the pioneer work of Willem Kolff, who calculated the area of cellulose membrane needed for human dialysis in Groningen in 1938. He then faced the problem of supporting 30 metres of sausage skin without creating a large and unstable extracorporeal blood volume. Undeterred by many failures, he perfected his design during the Second World War and used it in 1943.

Figure 1 shows a modern successor to Kolff's machine. His 30 metres of sausage skin are replaced by an artificial kidney in which the blood passes through a bundle of hollow fibres in a tube about 25 cm long and 3 cm wide. The ancillary equipment (not all shown in Fig. 1) includes: a roller blood pump which propels the blood through the artificial kidney at 200–400 ml/min; a sensor on the arterial line which detects negative pressure and

sounds an alarm; a pressure gauge on the return line which detects obstruction to flow; an ultrasonic monitor to detect air or froth in the bubble trap and prevent air embolism; sensors which monitor the temperature and ionic concentration of the dialysis fluid; a proportioning pump which makes dialysis fluid from purified water and concentrate; and a dialysis fluid pressure gauge. The transmembrane pressure—which determines how much water is removed by filtration—is derived from the two pressure gauges, monitored continuously, and adjusted electronically.

A water purification system turns tap-water into ultra-pure water by successive filtering, softening, reverse osmosis, and deionization. Failure to take these precautions in the early years of dialysis led to epidemics of aluminium poisoning (causing anaemia, bone pain, fractures, and fatal *dementia—so-called dialysis *encephalopathy); *haemolytic anaemia from zinc or copper from pipes and storage tanks or chloramines from water disinfection; pyrogen reactions from bacterial growth; and other syndromes caused by contaminants in tap-water.

Kolff's original artificial kidney saved the lives of many patients with acute renal failure, but he and others were defeated in their attempts to treat the commoner condition of chronic renal failure because they ran out of blood access sites. This problem was solved in 1960 by Scribner and Quinton in Seattle who devised the shunt shown in Fig. 2. It was the mainstay of regular haemodialysis for the next 6 years but was plagued by recurrent clotting and was replaced by the Cimino–Brescia fistula (Fig. 3). For short-term access in acute renal failure a silastic tube is inserted through the subclavian or jugular vein into the superior vena cava.

Patients in chronic renal failure require dialysis for about 4 hours three times a week, and must restrict their intake of water, salt, potassium, and phosphate between dialyses. The widely used cellulose membranes do not allow the passage of larger weight substances, which therefore accumulate to high levels. One of these, β2-microglobulin, is deposited in fibrillar form around bones and joints, causing bone pain, fractures, and

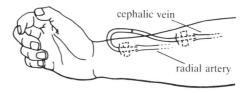

Fig. 2 The original Quinton–Scribner shunt for haemodialysis. Silastic tubes with stabilizing wings and teflon tips have been inserted into the radial artery and cephalic vein and connected end-to-end. They are disconnected and attached to the machine during the procedure.

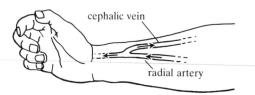

Fig. 3 Cimino–Brescia fistula. Arterial blood flows through the surgically created fistula into the cephalic vein, into which needles are inserted.

nerve compression after about 5 years of dialysis. The use of more expensive, high-permeability membranes retards the development of this 'dialysis amyloid' at the cost of more complicated monitoring.

Haemofiltration

With a high-permeability membrane it is possible to operate a circuit like that in Fig. 1 but with no dialysis fluid. Ultrafiltrate is squeezed out of the blood by high transmembrane pressure, measured, and discarded. It is replaced by an electrolyte solution infused into the arterial, or return, line. Haemofiltration is more expensive than haemodialysis, but it removes larger molecular weight substances better than diffusion, and is used preferentially in some rich countries. In the UK it is used almost exclusively to treat acute renal failure, because the system can run slowly throughout the illness. This allows high-volume intravenous feeding in patients unable to eat and drink.

Peritoneal dialysis

The *peritoneum is a natural membrane though which solute exchange can take place between blood in capillaries under the peritoneum and fluid introduced into the peritoneal cavity. However, the high urea content of the blood in renal failure creates an osmotic pull so that some fluid is transferred into the patient. To prevent this, and to extract water from the patient, an osmotic agent is added to the fluid. This is usually dextrose, which is cheap and effective but has the following disadvantages:

(1) a lot of dextrose is absorbed, blunting appetite and causing obesity; and

(2) if the peritoneum is damaged by infection, dextrose is absorbed more rapidly and loses its osmotic effect.

Alternatives which have recently reached the market are amino acids and Icodextrin®, a glucose polymer of higher molecular weight than dextrose.

For the treatment of acute renal failure, peritoneal dialysis is used with hourly exchanges of about 2 litres of fluid, which is efficient but expensive and limits mobility. Figure 4 shows the system used for continuous ambulatory peritoneal dialysis (CAPD) which is the method

used to treat chronic renal failure. Two litres of fluid are infused into the peritoneal cavity, left for about 5 hours (8 hours overnight), then drained out, measured, and discarded. Between exchanges the patient leads a normal life. The main complication of CAPD is peritonitis. The silastic catheter, which remains in the abdomen, is readily colonized by bacteria from the skin, which escape the body's defences by forming a protective layer of slime. The introduction of the disconnect system shown in Fig. 4 has greatly reduced, but not eliminated, this problem.

DAVID KERR

References

Berry, D. and Mackenzie, C. (1992). *Eponymists in medicine: Richard Bright 1789–1858. Physician in an age of revolution and reform.* Royal Society of Medicine Services, London.

Cameron, J. S. (1988). The nephrotic syndrome. A historical

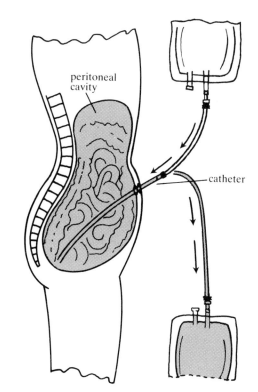

Fig. 4 The principle of CAPD. Two bags, the upper one containing 2 litres of fluid, joined by a Y-shaped tube, are attached to the indwelling silastic catheter. The peritoneal contents are drained into the lower bag (upper tube clamped). About 50 ml of fluid from the upper bag are flushed through the Y connector (the indwelling catheter is clamped). The rest of the 2 litres are run into the peritoneal cavity (the lower tube is clamped). The bags and Y connecter are disconnected and the catheter capped and protected.

review. In *The nephrotic syndrome* (ed. J. S. Cameron and R. J. Glassock), pp. 3–56. Marcel Dekker, New York.

Cameron, J. H. (ed.) (1993). *Analgesic and NSAID-induced kidney disease.* Oxford Monographs in Clinical Nephrology 2. Oxford University Press, Oxford.

Drukker, W. (1988). Haemodialysis: a historical review; and Peritoneal dialysis: a historical review. In *Replacement of renal function by dialysis*, (ed. J. F. Maher), (3rd edn.) pp. 20–80; 475–515. Martinus Nijhoff, The Hague.

El Nahas, A. M., Mallick, N. P., and Anderson, S. (ed.) (1993). *Progression in chronic renal failure.* Oxford Monographs in Clinical Nephrology 1. Oxford University Press, Oxford.

Morris, P. J. (ed.) (1988). *Kidney transplantation. Principles and practice*, (3rd edn.). W. B. Saunders, Philadelphia.

Stewart, J. S., Davison, A. M., Grunfeld, J.-P., Kerr, D. N. S., and Ritz, E. (ed.) (1992). *Oxford textbook of clinical nephrology.* Oxford University Press, Oxford.

Walton, J., Beeson, P. B., and Bodley Scott, R. (eds) (1986). *The Oxford companion to medicine.* Oxford University Press, Oxford.

NEPHRON. See RENAL TUBULE.

NEPHROSIS is, strictly, any disease of the kidney; it is commonly used synonymously with *nephrotic syndrome.

NEPHROTIC SYNDROME is a syndrome of *oedema, *albuminuria, and hypoalbuminaemia due to increased permeability of the renal glomerular basement membrane to *protein. See NEPHROLOGY.

NEPHROTOXIC describes an agent that is poisonous to kidney tissue.

NERVE CELL. See NEURONE.

NERVE FIBRES are the individual components of nerves; each fibre consists of a fine thread-like process (an *axon or a *dendrite) of a nerve cell (*neurone) surrounded, in the case of larger fibres, by a sheath of *myelin. Each axon or motor (efferent) fibre conducts impulses away from its cell body, and does so independently of other fibres in the nerve. Dendrites (sensory or afferent fibres) conduct towards their cell body. The myelin sheath, when present, provides high-resistance insulation from tissue fluids and enables greater conduction speeds.

NERVE GAS. One of a group of volatile liquids which are severely toxic by virtue of their anticholinesterase action; they inhibit the enzyme *cholinesterase which normally inactivates the neurotransmitter substance *acetylcholine. Hence acetylcholine accumulates in excess, and causes cholinergic paralysis.

NERVES are bundles of sensory and/or motor nerve fibres with connective tissue and blood vessels, each nerve running in a common sheath of connective tissue.

Within a nerve each nerve fibre conducts impulses independently of its fellows.

NERVOUS BREAKDOWN is an imprecise term denoting any acute and incapacitating emotional or mental disturbance.

NERVOUSNESS is a state of undue excitability, irritability, or restlessness.

NERVOUS SYSTEM. The *central nervous system (*brain and *spinal cord) and the peripheral *nerves considered together, including the *autonomic nervous system.

NERVOUS SYSTEM, CENTRAL. See CENTRAL NERVOUS SYSTEM.

NERVOUS SYSTEM, PERIPHERAL. The neural elements of the body (see NEURONE) and their supporting tissues considered collectively, excluding those contained in the *brain and *spinal cord and also excluding the *autonomic nervous system.

NESTORIAN MEDICINE. The Nestorian Christians were followers of Nestorius, Patriarch of Constantinople, who in AD 431 was denounced by the Council of Ephesus for his heresy (that Christ had two distinct natures, divine and human). The doctrine, however, continued to flourish in Syria and the East, and the Nestorians, debarred from eminence in Church and State, turned to medicine. The medical school and hospitals at Edessa (Urfa, the 'Athens of Syria') were taken over, and a school was established which for a time rivalled that of Alexandria. Despite the success of Nestorian practitioners, they were expelled from the empire in 489 by Emperor Zaro at the instigation of the orthodox Bishop Cyril. The Nestorians then moved to Persia, where they established further medical schools, the most famous being that at Jundishapur. Here the most liberal-minded Christians came together with advocates of Greek free thought and the ancient knowledge of the East—Hindu physicians were to be found among the professors. For 2 centuries the Nestorians translated Greek medical texts into Arabic, thus contributing to the flowering of Arabian medicine in the 7th century and long afterwards.

NETTLE RASH is the familiar rash which occurs when *histamine is released on pricking the skin by the hairs of the nettle, indistinguishable from that of *urticaria. See ALLERGY.

NEURALGIA is any pain originating in a nerve (all pain is, of course, conducted by nerves).

NEURAL TUBE DEFECT is a congenital anomaly resulting from defective development of part of the posterior wall of the spinal canal or the vault of the skull. See ANENCEPHALY; SPINA BIFIDA.

NEURASTHENIA is a term, now obsolete, introduced by G. M. Beard in 1867 to describe a condition he thought was due to exhaustion of nerve cells; its major manifestations were fatiguability and weakness combined with other ill-defined symptoms.

NEURECTOMY is the surgical excision of part of a *nerve.

NEURILEMMA. A thin outer *membrane which encloses the *axon, and the *myelin sheath when present, of individual peripheral nerve fibres. It is also called the sheath of *Schwann.

NEURINOMA. A *tumour arising from the outer sheath of a peripheral *nerve fibre (the sheath of *Schwann or neurilemma), also known as a neurilemmoma, schwannoma, or neurofibroma.

NEURITIS is inflammation of a nerve or nerves. The term is sometimes loosely used to embrace other non-inflammatory lesions of the peripheral nervous system which would more properly be termed '*neuropathy.'

NEUROANATOMY is the anatomy of the *nervous system.

NEUROBLASTOMA. A highly malignant *tumour, occurring most often in children under 4 years of age, most often in the *adrenal medulla, or sympathetic chain, less often in the brain.

NEUROCHEMISTRY is the chemical physiology of nervous tissue.

NEURODERMATITIS is any skin disorder due to, or aggravated by, mental or emotional factors; the term is sometimes used more specifically to denote *atopic *eczema (atopic dermatitis).

NEUROENDOCRINOLOGY is the study of the interactions between the *nervous system and the *endocrine organs, of which the most important is that between the *pituitary gland and the *hypothalamic region of the brain.

NEUROEPIDEMIOLOGY is the *epidemiology of diseases of the nervous system.

NEUROFIBROMA. A tumour arising from the *Schwann cells of peripheral or cranial nerves.

NEUROFIBROMATOSIS is a genetically determined disorder, inherited as an autosomal *dominant characteristic, of which the major manifestations are multiple benign tumours attached to peripheral or cranial nerves

(neurofibromas) and pigmented skin patches ('café au lait' spots). Neurofibromatosis is also known as von *Recklinghausen's disease. Two types exist (type I and II) which are clinically and genetically distinct.

NEUROGENETIC is a synonym for (the preferable) 'neurogenic', meaning either originating in the nervous system or giving rise to nervous tissue.

NEUROGLIA is the supporting tissue of the *central nervous system, analogous to *connective tissue elsewhere. Two components are recognized: macroglia, of ectodermal origin like other neural tissue, the cells of which (astrocytes and oligodendrocytes) are concerned with *myelin formation and various metabolic functions; and microglia, containing mesodermal cells similar to *macrophages.

NEUROLEPTIC. One of the group of drugs used to modify the manifestations of *psychoses, known alternatively as 'major tranquillizers' or 'antipsychotics'. See TRANQUILLIZERS.

NEUROLOGIST. A physician specializing in diseases of the nervous system.

NEUROLOGY
Introduction
Neurologists diagnose and treat diseases affecting the *brain, *spinal cord, peripheral *nerves, and *muscles. Disordered thought processes or emotions are treated by psychiatrists, although the two specialties overlap, particularly in relation to dementia or psychosomatic symptoms. Modern neurologists interact closely with related specialists: with *neurosurgeons in treating *tumours and *subarachnoid haemorrhage; with neuroradiologists, who image structural disease of the brain and spinal cord; and with *neurophysiologists, who investigate blackouts using *electroencephalography and diseases of nerve and muscle using nerve conduction studies and *electromyography. Diagnosis in neurology is founded on clinical principles, attending closely to the patient's history and to careful physical examination. The advent of non-invasive investigations, such as *computerized tomography (CT) and *magnetic resonance imaging (MRI) scanning of the brain and spine, means that most neurological diagnoses can be made on an out-patient basis. Fortunately, most patients with neurological symptoms do not have disabling or fatal illness. Bodily symptoms are commonly encountered which result from stress and other mild psychological disorders. Neurology presents doctors with richly varied challenges: refined clinical skills are essential, effective treatments are increasingly available, ingenious medical engineering can minimize disability, everyday practice confronts complex ethical issues, and neurobiological research promises to revolutionize our understanding of neurological diseases.

Historical aspects

The diagnostic foundations of modern clinical neurology arose in mid-19th century Berlin and London. Treatises attempted to classify neurological diseases in terms of their symptoms and physical signs, and to correlate these with the *pathology of the autopsied brain. For instance, Reynolds realized that brain tumours could both diminish normal brain function, by causing *paralysis, and increase brain activity by inducing epileptic *convulsions. *Brown-Séquard realized that distinctive combinations of muscle weakness and loss of sensation resulted from different patterns of damage to pathways of the spinal cord. *Erb, Westphal, and *Gowers realized that absent tendon reflex jerks signified disease of the nerve roots or peripheral nerves, whereas unusually brisk *reflexes reflected spinal cord damage. In 1896 *Babinski realized that if the great toe extended as a result of stroking the sole of the foot, it was a clear sign of damage to the spinal cord or brain; his sign has been revered by neurologists ever since. The *ophthalmoscope came into use in the second half of the 19th century; swelling of the optic nerve head was recognized to reflect raised pressure within the skull due to brain tumours, chronic *meningitis, or *hydrocephalus. In 1888, Gowers published his famous 'Manual' of diseases of the nervous system; his compilation laid the basis of present-day diagnostic neurological practice. He summarized the principal signs and psychological deficits resulting from damage to different parts of the brain. This was crucial for guiding neurosurgical operations in the decades before *radiologists developed X-rays for locating brain tumours. During the latter half of the 20th century, radiologists have developed *angiography to visualize the blood vessels of the brain, and *CT and *MRI to visualize tumours and other structural abnormalities of the brain and spinal cord.

Blackouts and epilepsy

Attacks of unconsciousness present a common diagnostic problem for neurologists. Common causes include *epilepsy, irregular heart rhythms, and simple *faints. Epilepsy results from storms of uncoordinated electrical discharges in the brain. Sudden loss of consciousness results from epileptic discharges throughout the whole brain. This involves either momentary 'absence' or 'petit mal' attacks, in which the patient becomes blank and inaccessible for a few seconds, or 'grand mal seizures' with falling and violent limb shaking, often associated with tongue-biting and urinary incontinence. In contrast, focal epileptic discharges produce diverse symptoms, depending upon where they arise in the brain. These range from repetitive limb twitchings, to episodes of automatic behaviour or stereotyped *hallucinations. Seizure discharges can be detected by electroencephalography (EEG). The diagnosis of epilepsy generally depends upon a characteristic description of attacks provided by the patient or a witness. The cause of epilepsy is usually unidentifiable and is only occasionally genetic, but sometimes it results from structural brain disease, such as *trauma or tumours detectable by brain scans. Modern antiepileptic drugs, principally phenytoin, carbamazepine, and sodium valproate, either abolish or diminish seizures in most patients. A few patients are unresponsive to drug therapy and may be considered for neurosurgical treatment, particularly if their attacks arise within the temporal *lobes of the brain.

Modern treatment of epilepsy usually permits patients to follow a normal life-style, thankfully abolishing the old stigma that epilepsy represents a form of insanity. In most countries, patients with epilepsy are barred from driving until free of seizures for 2 years, and for many this constitutes the main disability caused by their epilepsy.

*Headache and *migraine

Headache and facial pain are two of the commonest symptoms encountered in everyday neurological practice. Most headaches do not signal medically serious disease, although they may cause considerable distress and disability. The commonest headaches are migraine and muscle tension headache.

Simple migraine

Simple migraine causes discrete bouts of intense throbbing headache, each lasting between 3 hours and 3 days. These are generally associated with nausea or vomiting and dislike of loud noises or bright lights. The headache is often one-sided, at least at the onset. In *classical migraine* such headaches are preceded by a prodromal visual disturbance lasting 15 to 30 minutes, manifesting as holes in the visual field, tunnel vision, brightly coloured spots (photopsia), or zig-zag lines (fortification spectra). Occasionally the prodrome involves temporary speech loss, pins and needles, or limb weakness. Migraine tends to run in families. Attacks may be associated with the menstrual periods, or are occasionally precipitated by cheese, chocolate, or wine. Drugs to treat individual attacks include simple painkillers, ergotamine, and sumatriptan. Patients disabled by frequent severe attacks should eliminate identified precipitating factors and may prevent attacks by taking daily prophylactic medications such as propranolol or pizotifen.

Tension headache

Tension headache consists of a tight band or pressure sensation encircling the head; brief bouts of this will be familiar to most people. When chronic, it is present in varying severity on most days, and tends to worsen throughout the day. The cause of tension headache is not clear, but sustained contraction of scalp muscles is often blamed. It may occur in depressive illness or anxiety states, but is usually encountered in hard-working yet otherwise well-balanced individuals.

Treatment may include advice about reducing stress, undertaking regular physical exercise or relaxation, and low-dosage antidepressant drugs such as amitriptyline.

Only occasionally does headache signify serious disease requiring investigation with brain scans or *lumbar puncture. Headache of abrupt onset, often during physical exertion, occurs in *subarachnoid haemorrhage. Gradually worsening daily headache, worse on awakening, occurs when raised pressure within the skull results from brain tumours, abscesses, hydrocephalus, or benign intracranial hypertension. Meningitis causes headache associated with neck stiffness and dislike of bright lights. In elderly patients, giant-cell *arteritis may cause severe scalp tenderness, and prompt steroid treatment is essential to forestall blindness due to involvement of the arteries to the eye.

*Strokes

Strokes are sudden neurological disturbances due to diseased brain blood vessels. Those resulting from blocked brain arteries are termed 'ischaemic strokes'. If brain arteries burst, blood clots form either within the brain, an 'intracerebral *haematoma', or within the meningeal membranes surrounding the brain a 'subarachnoid haemorrhage'. The ischaemic and haemorrhagic forms are clearly distinguishable by brain scans. Stroke is a common cause of severe disability and death, particularly in the elderly. For reasons not wholly clear, stroke is gradually becoming less common in Western countries.

Ischaemic strokes

Ischaemic strokes cause loss of neurological function in the part of the brain deprived of its blood supply. Commonly there is weakness of one side of the body (*hemiplegia) or difficulty with speech (*aphasia) when a middle cerebral artery is blocked, or loss of half of the field of vision (*hemianopia) if a posterior cerebral artery is blocked. Small blood clots, called emboli, are the usual cause of blocked brain arteries. Emboli usually come from a diseased heart, or from narrowed *carotid arteries in the neck. Once an embolus has lodged in a small artery, the surrounding area of brain dies, permanently losing its function. No treatment is known to prevent brain death once an embolus has firmly lodged. Fortunately, emboli sometimes break up and pass onward, restoring blood flow. If this occurs within the first few hours, complete recovery of neurological function quickly follows. If complete recovery occurs within 24 hours, such attacks are termed 'transient cerebral ischaemic attacks' (TIA). TIAs do signal an increased risk of permanent stroke in the future. Prompt assessment is required to identify any reversible risk factors. If the emboli arise from a severely narrowed internal carotid artery, surgical reboring (carotid *end-arterectomy) can reduce the risk of further TIAs or

future stroke. Patients can reduce their risk of further strokes by taking daily low-dose *aspirin which beneficially affects blood coagulation.

Subarachnoid haemorrhage

Subarachnoid haemorrhage is the commonest form of haemorrhagic stroke and occurs when weakened arteries rupture into the meningeal coverings around the brain. It causes an abrupt severe headache, and sometimes instantaneous death. Brain scans may visualize the haemorrhage, and lumbar puncture detects blood in the spinal fluid. The source of the bleeding is pin-pointed by angiographic X-rays of brain blood vessels. Most usually it arises from a distended weakened artery wall, termed an *aneurysm. This can be repaired or occluded neurosurgically to prevent recurrence. Less frequently the haemorrhage comes from a longstanding tangle of blood vessels called an arteriovenous malformation or *angioma. Some patients have a normal angiogram; often they are smokers or oral contraceptive consumers, and they have a better long-term outlook. Subarachnoid haemorrhage is a serious condition and permanent brain damage may occur eventually even in those who survive the initial haemorrhage intact. Continued presence of blood in the meningeal coverings of the brain can induce spasm of other brain arteries many days later, resulting in secondary ischaemic strokes.

Multiple sclerosis

Multiple sclerosis is due to episodes of damage to patches of myelin in the white matter pathways of the brain or spinal cord. This demyelination blocks the transmission of nervous messages in the affected pathway. The underlying cause of multiple sclerosis is not known, but the leading contenders are an autoimmune attack by the body upon its own myelin or the effects of a viral infection or a combination of the two. It is commonest in temperate countries. Multiple sclerosis usually causes a succession of attacks affecting different sites in the nervous system. Particularly vulnerable are the *optic nerves, with loss of vision; the spinal cord, causing limb weakness and impaired urinary control; and the brainstem, causing loss of balance and co-ordination. Partial recovery occurs after each attack, and this may be speeded by short courses of treatment with *steroids. A diagnosis of multiple sclerosis is based upon a history of relapsing and remitting symptoms affecting at least two separate areas of the brain or spinal cord. Investigations may support this clinical diagnosis; delayed visual *evoked responses may reveal slowed transmission along optic nerves affected by a previous silent attack. MRI shows widespread plaques of *demyelination.

The clinical course and severity of multiple sclerosis are quite unpredictable for any individual patient. At the mildest extreme, a patient may experience only two episodes of demyelination. At the other extreme, severe disability can result from progressive accumulation of widespread plaques of demyelination. Such patients often become wheelchair bound, and clumsiness may limit the use of their hands. Most patients with multiple sclerosis fall between these two extremes. These range from those who have a few attacks during their lifetime but no significant residual disability, to those in whom numerous attacks have caused a degree of permanent disability but who remain reasonably independent. No treatment is known to prevent further attacks of multiple sclerosis or to enhance the degree of eventual recovery from each attack. There is no clear evidence that dietary manipulations are effective, although supplementation of polyunsaturated fatty acids has been popular with some. For those who are cruelly disabled by multiple sclerosis, often as young adults, skilled *rehabilitation can minimize the degree of disability. It is possible that β-*interferon, though prohibitively expensive, may be shown to modify the course of the disease.

Neurodegenerative diseases
Certain disabling neurological diseases result from progressive death of specific groups of nerve cells in the brain or spinal cord. These neurodegenerative diseases are particularly common in the elderly. They include the memory loss of *Alzheimer's disease, the movement disorder of *Parkinson's disease, and the muscle weakness of *motor neurone disease. They usually occur spontaneously and inherited forms account for less than 10 per cent.

Alzheimer's disease
Alzheimer's disease is the commonest cause of *dementia. Memory is lost along with other cognitive abilities such as calculation, reasoning, or insight. Ultimately the personality disintegrates. *Neurones are lost from the cerebral cortex and some subcortical structures, and microscopy reveals characteristic 'neurofibrillary tangles'. Although Alzheimer's disease itself is not treatable or preventable, brain scans may reveal alternative causes for dementia, such as multiple small strokes, or hydrocephalus which may improve after neurosurgical shunting to drain the distended cerebral ventricles.

Parkinson's disease
Parkinson's disease involves a 'pill-rolling' *tremor of the hands, 'lead-pipe' rigidity of the limbs, and slowed movements causing reduced facial expression and blinking, small handwriting, poor manipulation, and a slow, shuffling gait. It results from loss of the neurones in the substantia nigra of the brainstem which normally secrete *dopamine as their *neurotransmitter. Microscopy of surviving neurones shows characteristic *Lewy body inclusions. Parkinsonian symptoms improve substantially with *levodopa medication which supplements the deficient dopamine. Later in the disease, levodopa becomes less effective, and patients' responses may fluctuate dramatically. Similar parkinsonian syndromes

can be a side-effect of major tranquillizing drugs used in *psychiatry, which block dopamine's actions.

Motor neurone disease (amyotrophic lateral sclerosis)
In this disease the muscles atrophy and weaken. This follows death of the motor neurones directly supplying the muscles and of the upper motor neurones in the brain which control those lower motor neurones. The disease starts either in a limb with weakness, or in the bulbar (throat) muscles with difficulty in speech production, eating, swallowing, or breathing. It does not affect skin sensation, the control of urination, or sexual function. Mental faculties are preserved, highlighting the distress of patients who are fully conscious of becoming prisoners in bodies they can no longer move. No cure is known for motor neurone disease, and no way is known of arresting the inevitable deterioration.

Infections
Meningitis
Meningitis is an infection of the meningeal membranes covering the brain. It may be caused by *bacteria, *viruses, or *fungi. The range of infections has widened now that many patients have impaired immune defences due to drugs taken after organ *transplantation or to *AIDS. Bacterial meningitis is a serious disease causing permanent brain damage or death unless diagnosed promptly and treated with antibiotics. Initial symptoms of headache, fever, neck rigidity, and intolerance of light may progress to coma within hours. Diagnosis is by lumbar puncture, yielding cerebrospinal fluid containing copious inflammatory cells and bacteria; *Haemophilus*, *Neisseria*, *Pneumococcus*, and *Tuberculosis* species are the commonest causes.

Encephalitis
Encephalitis is an inflammation within the brain, either due to invasion by viruses (such as *herpes simplex) or as a remote effect of viral infections elsewhere in the body (such as *measles). Headache, fever, and seizures develop, often with speech difficulties, confusion, or *coma. Often the exact *virus responsible for acute encephalitis is not identifiable. The antiviral drug *acyclovir treats the herpes simplex form; most patients with encephalitis receive this nowadays pending accurate virological diagnosis. Without treatment, encephalitis may cause death, or leave residual memory disturbances, epilepsy, or parkinsonism. Fortunately, many patients now recover from encephalitis.

The brain can be affected by some slowly progressive infections. *Creutzfeldt–Jakob disease is due to a subviral particle called a prion, and causes dementia accompanied by sudden 'myoclonic' limb jerkings. *Subacute sclerosing panencephalitis is due to latent measles virus infection of the brain, also causing myoclonic jerking and intellectual decline; it is extremely rare in children previously immunized against measles. *HIV infection can cause a slowly progressive dementia. Slowly progressive leg weakness (tropical spastic paraplegia) results from infection with another retrovirus, HTLV-1.

MICHAEL DONAGHY

Further reading
Matthews, W. B. (1978). *Multiple sclerosis – the facts*. Oxford University Press, Oxford.
Sacks, O. (1990). *Awakenings*. Harper, New York.
Spillane, J. D. (1981). *The doctrine of the nerves*. Oxford University Press, Oxford.
Walton, J. N. (ed.) (1993). *Brain's diseases of the nervous system*, (10th edn). Oxford University Press.

NEUROMA. A *tumour arising from nervous tissue, usually from elements of the *neuroglia.

NEUROMUSCULAR DISEASE
Introduction
There are three forms of muscle in the human body. The heart is composed of cardiac muscle; there is smooth, unstriated, or involuntary muscle in the wall of the stomach and intestine. But much of our weight is made up by voluntary or skeletal muscle under the control of the will; there are hundreds of individual muscles which control movements of the eyes, face, mouth and throat, trunk, and limbs. Voluntary movement is initiated in the motor cortex of the *brain, from which impulses travel down through the *brainstem and *spinal cord in upper motor *neurones of the pyramidal (corticospinal) tract; these impulses excite activity in the anterior horn cells of the spinal cord grey matter, from which arise the motor roots and *nerves which form the final common path of motor activity. One such cell and its nerve fibre, or *axon, is called a lower motor neurone. The motor nerve fibres are each covered with a sheath of *myelin, regularly interrupted at nodes of Ranvier; this sheath is formed and enveloped by Schwann cells. Impulses travelling down a lower motor neurone reach the neuromuscular junction or motor end-plate (where a nerve fibre joins a muscle). Release of *acetylcholine at this junction, if adequate in amount, initiates an action potential, which leads on to contraction of muscle fibres and hence to movement. A motor unit of voluntary activity consists of one anterior horn cell, its axon, and the group of muscle fibres which it innervates. Under normal conditions muscle fibres cannot contract singly. Firing of one anterior horn cell causes contraction of all of the muscle fibres of the unit, producing an action potential which can be recorded electrically. Each muscle fibre is made up of many *myofibrils as well as *nuclei, specialized *cytoplasm called sarcoplasm, and other *organelles, including *mitochondria. The myofibrils contain thick filaments of a *protein called myosin and thin filaments of actin: these filaments interdigitate, sliding upon one another so that the myofibril and hence the muscle fibre shortens when it contracts. Myosin filaments are attached to prominent Z bands regularly throughout each muscle fibre, producing a striated appearance. Each fibre is covered by a *membrane called sarcolemma, which has an outer basement membrane and an inner plasma membrane.

The neuromuscular diseases involve the motor unit (Fig. 1). The pathological process may involve the anterior horn cells, the motor roots or nerves, the neuromuscular junctions, or the muscles themselves. Viruses, such as that of *poliomyelitis, may attack the anterior horn cells (or the motor nuclei of the cranial nerves which are functionally similar). The degenerative diseases affecting these cells are called motor neurone diseases or spinal muscular atrophies; those affecting peripheral nerves are *neuropathies; and those primarily involving muscle, *myopathies.

Disease or death of anterior horn cells or division of their axons causes denervation (loss of nerve supply) of a muscle. It can then no longer contract: it

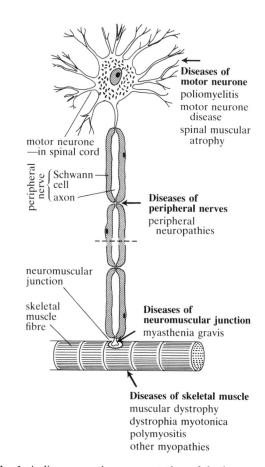

Diseases of motor neurone
poliomyelitis
motor neurone disease
spinal muscular atrophy

motor neurone —in spinal cord

peripheral nerve { Schwann cell / axon

Diseases of peripheral nerves
peripheral neuropathies

neuromuscular junction

skeletal muscle fibre

Diseases of neuromuscular junction
myasthenia gravis

Diseases of skeletal muscle
muscular dystrophy
dystrophia myotonica
polymyositis
other myopathies

Fig. 1 A diagrammatic representation of the lower motor neurone, neuromuscular junction, and voluntary muscle, and some of the commoner diseases which affect this neuromuscular system.

is paralysed and wastes progressively. Total denervation gives *paralysis, partial denervation weakness; the wasting is denervation *atrophy. Myasthenia gravis, in which transmission from nerve to muscle is impaired, gives weakness without wasting but is characterized by fatiguability (weakness increasing progressively following repeated contraction). Primary myopathies, such as the *muscular dystrophies, cause both weakness and wasting.

Diagnostic methods

Diagnosis depends first upon analysis of the clinical and family history and upon physical examination to detect wasting and/or weakness of individual muscles. Methods exist for assessing the strength of most muscles and for eliciting tendon *reflexes (tendon jerks), as well as for measuring the perception of different types of *sensation. Clinical diagnosis depends upon recognizing different patterns of involvement of nerves and muscles.

Several hundred neuromuscular diseases are now recognized and many biochemical or other tests may be needed in addition to clinical examination for diagnosis. The three principal diagnostic investigations are: first, estimation of blood levels of *enzymes such as creatine kinase. In many myopathies, and some motor neurone disorders, creatine kinase is greatly increased in the blood.

Secondly, electrophysiological methods are invaluable. Measurement of the rate of *conduction of the nerve impulse in peripheral nerves is helpful, especially in neuropathy. In those which affect predominantly the myelin sheath (demyelinating neuropathies) the rate of conduction is slowed. *Electromyography is also invaluable; it involves inserting a needle electrode into a muscle and amplifying the electrical activity recorded at rest and during contraction, with visualization on a cathode ray *oscilloscope.

Thirdly, perhaps of greatest diagnostic value is muscle *biopsy. This involves removing, either by needle or surgically, a muscle sample which can then be studied biochemically and microscopically. In most neuromuscular diseases abnormalities are found in sections appropriately stained and examined under the light microscope. Within the past 25 years, histochemistry (a method of staining muscle fibres to demonstrate their enzymatic content) and electron microscopy have added new dimensions to biopsy diagnosis, as has immunochemistry. Histochemistry has shown that human muscle consists of two major fibre types which are randomly distributed in a chequerboard pattern: type I fibres depend upon *aerobic metabolism and have a high concentration of oxidative enzymes, while type II fibres have a high concentration of *glycogen and depend upon *anaerobic metabolism. These are differentially affected in various diseases. Electron microscopy has demonstrated many hitherto unsuspected morphological abnormalities in skeletal muscle, especially in some congenital, non-progressive myopathies which can cause the so-called *floppy infant syndrome (see below). Immunochemical staining for dystrophin (see below) is probably now essential in identifying Duchenne and Becker dystrophy.

Motor neurone disease

This condition, also called motor system disease, is a progressive degenerative disorder of unknown cause, usually developing in middle or late life; it involves both the upper and lower motor neurones. The lower motor neurone lesions give weakness and wasting of muscles in the head, neck, and limbs, while involvement of upper motor neurones causes *spasticity or increased tone (resistance to stretch) in the limbs. When the condition begins with weakness, wasting, and *fasciculation of limb muscles, it is often called progressive muscular atrophy; when it begins with spasticity in the extremities, and weakness and wasting appear late, it is called amyotrophic lateral sclerosis; when it first affects muscles of speech and swallowing, spreading to the limbs later, it is called progressive bulbar palsy. The term 'amyotrophic lateral sclerosis' is used in the USA to identify all forms of the disease, while 'motor neurone disease' is preferred in the UK. Although its effects may be modified by appropriate drugs and appliances, no curative treatment is known; the disease is remorselessly progressive and is often fatal within 2–5 years or rarely 10 or more years after the onset; patients usually die from *respiratory infection. The condition is usually sporadic but occasionally affects more than one member of a family.

Spinal muscular atrophy

Several varieties of spinal muscular atrophy occur in infancy, childhood, and adult life, which affect selectively the anterior horn cells of the spinal cord but not the upper motor neurones; very occasionally, motor nuclei of cranial nerves are also affected, giving difficulty with speech and swallowing, less often impaired ocular movement or facial weakness. Most types of muscular atrophy are genetically determined and of autosomal *recessive inheritance due to a *gene located on *chromosome 5; dominant inheritance is uncommon; very rarely the condition is *X-linked. Werdnig–Hoffmann disease (the severe infantile form) begins before birth or just afterwards, causing diffuse muscular weakness, hypotonia, progressive paralysis, respiratory insufficiency, and usually death before the end of the first year of life. Milder varieties, causing localized, restricted, or more diffuse weakness of limb and trunk muscles, may begin in later infancy, childhood, adolescence, or adult life.

The neuropathies

In the spinal canal, the posterior roots carry sensory information into the spinal cord, the anterior roots motor impulses which leave it. They combine into spinal nerves at each segment of the spinal column and leave by intervertebral foramina where they may be compressed by *prolapsed intervertebral discs, giving upper limb pain when this occurs in the neck or *sciatica when it occurs in the lumbar *spine. Spinal nerves in the cervical (neck) and lumbar regions come together to form the brachial and lumbo-sacral plexuses; those in the dorsal region form intercostal nerves (which lie between the ribs). From the plexuses, peripheral nerves arise, most containing both motor fibres concerned with initiating and controlling movement, and sensory fibres centrally conveying feeling from the joints, muscles, skin, and other structures.

The term 'neuropathy' embraces all pathological processes involving peripheral nerves. In traumatic neuropathies, peripheral nerves are damaged by physical injury; in the compression neuropathies, peripheral nerves are compressed due to disease in a joint or in other organs. The ulnar nerve, which passes behind the inner side of the elbow (the 'funny bone') can be irritated at this point, giving tingling and pins and needles in the little and ring fingers, and sometimes wasting of small hand muscles. Compression of the median nerve in the *carpal tunnel at the wrist, due to swelling of flexor tendon sheaths resulting from overuse, can give pins and needles which often waken the patient from sleep and which involve particularly the thumb, index, middle, and ring fingers.

When arteries carrying blood to peripheral nerves (the vasa nervorum) are affected by disease, the function of several such nerves may become defective through *ischaemia (mononeuritis multiplex). This can occur in *diabetes mellitus but more often in inflammatory arterial disease, such as *polyarteritis nodosa or other forms of *arteritis, or in infections like *leprosy.

There are many inflammatory and metabolic disorders involving peripheral nerves more diffusely, called 'the polyneuropathies'. Sometimes the myelin sheaths of the nerves are most affected (the demyelinating polyneuropathies): in other cases, the axons are primarily involved (the axonal neuropathies). A common acute or subacute demyelinating neuropathy is the so-called *Guillain–Barré syndrome in which, in severe cases, there is also progressive weakness with tingling and pins and needles in the extremities, developing rapidly over a few days, sometimes leading to paralysis of all four limbs and even of the respiratory muscles, requiring assisted respiration. Usually motor weakness is more severe than sensory impairment. Usually, if serious complications such as respiratory weakness can be prevented or controlled, recovery is ultimately complete. *Steroid drugs are of no value but plasma exchange (*plasmapheresis) may help.

The potential causes of polyneuropathy are legion. Deficiency of *vitamin B_1, either nutritional or due to chronic *alcoholism or to heavy metal poisons (lead, arsenic, gold, etc.), competitive *inhibitors of the vitamin, can cause a severe axonal neuropathy which is often sensory at the outset but later involves motor

nerves. *Uraemia also causes an axonal neuropathy, while the neuropathy which often complicates type 1 diabetes mellitus involves both myelin and axons. Drugs can also cause polyneuropathy. One such is *isoniazid, but there are many others. Vitamin B_{12} deficiency in *pernicious anaemia also produces a sensory polyneuropathy as one manifestation.

There are also many forms of genetically determined polyneuropathy, some predominantly motor and some sensorimotor (including Charcot–Marie–Tooth disease, a benign condition in which muscular weakness and wasting are limited to muscles below the knees and those of the hands). Various forms of *hereditary sensory neuropathy have also been described. Similar changes sometimes occur in the neuropathy of *leprosy. Polyneuropathy is also a common, non-metastatic complication of *malignant disease.

The muscular dystrophies

The muscular dystrophies are a group of primary, degenerative myopathies, all genetically determined. Rare forms are limited to the external ocular muscles (ocular myopathy and the even rarer oculopharyngeal variety). Rarely, too, dystrophy affects predominantly the distal limb muscles (distal myopathy). The commonest varieties are the so-called Duchenne and Becker *X-linked varieties, the autosomal *recessive limb-girdle type, and the autosomal *dominant facioscapulohumeral form.

The Duchenne type, being X-linked, affects virtually only boys. Some do not walk until 18–20 months of age. By about the age of 3 years all affected boys have difficulty in walking, with frequent falling, clumsy running, difficulty in climbing stairs, and in rising from the floor. Enlargement of calf muscles is common, but there is selective wasting and weakness in upper and lower limb muscles in a consistent pattern. Most patients are confined to a wheelchair by the age of 10 and few survive beyond the age of 20–25. Although the longevity and quality of life in such patients have been improved by modern *rehabilitation, no effective treatment is known, but gene therapy may soon become possible. Death is either due to respiratory infection or to the involvement of heart muscle.

Isolation and characterization of the Duchenne gene in 1987 by Kunkel and his colleagues at Boston Children's Hospital, USA, soon led to the discovery that a protein, later called *dystrophin, an important structural component of the sarcolemmal plasma *membrane, was totally absent in boys with Duchenne dystrophy and greatly reduced in those with the Becker type and in many female carriers of the Duchenne gene, some of whom showed variable degrees of muscular weakness (manifesting carriers). An immunochemical method of staining using monoclonal *antibodies raised against dystrophin has added precision to diagnosis by muscle biopsy. Isolation of the gene has also made possible the accurate identification of female carriers (especially among the sisters of dystrophic boys), half of whose sons would be expected to develop the disease, while half of their daughters would also be carriers. Antenatal diagnosis in pregnant carriers is now possible using *chorionic cell biopsy which is feasible earlier in pregnancy than *amniocentesis, thus making possible selective *abortion only of affected males. *In vitro fertilization of ova from carriers, followed by embryo biopsy, is also making it possible for such women to have unaffected sons and non-carrier daughters. Experiments in gene replacement in mice and dogs with an X-linked dystrophy due to dystrophin deficiency suggest that *gene therapy in human subjects may not be far away.

The Becker variety is also X-linked but is much more benign and of later onset.

The limb-girdle variety begins either with selective involvement of shoulder girdle muscles (the scapulo-humeral form) or in the pelvic girdle muscles (the pelvifemoral form), spreading to the other group later. It, too, is much more benign than the Duchenne type, often leading to a wheelchair existence in middle life, and death before the normal age. By contrast, the facioscapulohumeral variety, of dominant inheritance and due to a gene on chromosome 4, is severe in some individuals but mild in others, who may even go through life without recognizing that they have the disease in a restricted form.

Myotonic disorders

Myotonia is a form of delayed muscular relaxation; after the patient is asked to relax, there is an after-contraction which can be recorded electrically. A patient being asked to open a hand after gripping an object is unable to do so quickly and the fingers uncoil slowly. A tap on the tongue or on a limb muscle produces a dimple which slowly disappears. Sometimes myotonia is generalized from birth and no other disability develops. In this condition (myotonia congenita) the prognosis is excellent, but the myotonia, worse in cold weather, restricts movement. In some families, myotonia congenita is dominantly inherited (Thomsen's disease). There is also a recessively inherited variety which develops later in childhood and is also benign. Myotonia can be relieved by drugs such as *quinine, procainamide, or *phenytoin, but the response is variable.

In dystrophia myotonica (myotonia atrophica, Steinert's disease), myotonia is often limited to the hands, and may indeed be clinically unobtrusive or detectable only by electromyography. Facial weakness, *cataracts, weakness of sternomastoid muscles, and distal wasting and weakness of limb muscles develop usually in adolescence or early adult life. This condition is progressive, disabling, and uninfluenced by treatment; most patients die before the normal age. Infants of mothers with myotonic dystrophy may be very 'floppy' or hypotonic at birth, and often show marked developmental delay before developing the typical manifestations of myotonic dystrophy in adolescence. Recent identification

of the gene for this disease on chromosome 19 suggests that gene therapy may ultimately be possible.

Inflammatory myopathy

While viral diseases of muscle, such as *Bornholm disease (an acute *myositis with fever, causing difficulty in breathing and pain in the chest wall and *diaphragm for a few days, and which is due to the *Coxsackie A3 virus) occur, and while *influenzal myositis (in Western countries) or pyogenic myositis due to *Staphylococcus aureus (in tropical countries) are other recognized forms of inflammatory myopathy, the commonest inflammatory myopathy in Western countries is polymyositis. This is an *autoimmune disease in which *lymphocytes in the blood become sensitized against muscle and invade and damage it—there is often, but not always, muscle pain and tenderness with diffuse, non-selective weakness of proximal limb muscles. Sometimes there is difficulty in swallowing and inflammation of the skin, when the condition is called *dermatomyositis. This condition can occur at any age, but in middle or late life it often complicates malignant disease in the lung or elsewhere. Treatment with drugs such as *prednisone and *immunosuppressive agents like *azathioprine is usually successful, except in patients with associated malignant disease which determines the *prognosis.

Infestation with *Trichinella spiralis* (trichinosis or *trichiniasis), due to eating contaminated pork, can mimic polymyositis. *Polymyalgia rheumatica, a disease of the elderly, gives diffuse muscle pain which restricts movement but produces no weakness; the erythrocyte sedimentation rate is greatly raised, and the response to steroids is immediate.

Myasthenia gravis

Myasthenia gravis is another autoimmune disease; circulating *antibodies form against the acetylcholine *receptor on the surface of muscle fibres with which acetylcholine (released at the end-plate) combines. This antibody coats the receptors so that acetylcholine cannot have its full effect; the muscles become weak and fatiguable; repeated contraction causes increasing weakness. Typically the condition, commoner in females and beginning at any age, affects external ocular muscles, with drooping of the eyelids towards the end of the day, with or without double vision (diplopia). Often there is difficulty in speaking, swallowing, and chewing (chewing difficulty increasing during a meal is almost diagnostic). Variable weakness of limb muscles without wasting is also common, always accentuated by exercise.

The diagnosis of myasthenia gravis is confirmed by estimating circulating antibodies in the blood and clinically by injecting intravenously edrophonium chloride (Tensilon®); this reverses the weakness, if only for a few seconds or minutes. This drug inhibits cholinesterase, the enzyme which breaks down acetylcholine. Sustained benefit can be produced by longer-acting drugs such as pyridostigmine. In the long term, it is more effective to remove surgically the *thymus gland which produces the white blood cells or T *lymphocytes, which, by interacting with B lymphocytes, help to produce the antibodies. Steroid drugs and immunosuppressants are also helpful. In an acute emergency, *plasmapheresis can be of temporary benefit.

The floppy infant syndrome

There are many benign congenital myopathies of variable severity and rate of progression associated with specific structural abnormalities in muscle fibres; myotubular or centronuclear myopathy, central core disease, and nemaline myopathy, are three examples.

Metabolic and endocrine myopathies

Weakness of proximal limb muscles is often seen in patients with *thyrotoxicosis, but improves as this is treated. By contrast, diminished thyroid activity (*myxoedema) can cause slowness of muscular contraction and relaxation, with muscular enlargement (Hoffman's syndrome). Increasingly severe muscular pain during exercise, eventually preventing movement, is seen in *McArdle's disease due to deficiency of the enzyme phosphorylase; *glycogen accumulates in the muscle and cannot be broken down. Other enzymatic defects affecting muscle glycogen breakdown have similar effects.

Other metabolic disorders of muscle include the familial periodic paralyses of dominant inheritance, in which episodes of diffuse muscular weakness are precipitated by exertion or by a heavy *carbohydrate meal. In some, the attacks are accompanied by a rise in serum *potassium (the hyperkalaemic type), in others by a fall (the hypokalaemic type). In each type, attacks can be prevented by treatment with drugs which promote potassium excretion, such as *acetazolamide.

Several muscle disorders are associated with abnormalities of *fat metabolism. An inherited deficiency of carnitine (essential for *fatty acid metabolism) causes excess storage of neutral fat in skeletal muscle, causing muscle weakness. Sometimes this is improved by oral carnitine.

Several metabolic myopathies may mimic clinically limb-girdle or facioscapulohumeral dystrophy in which abnormal mitochondria can be identified by biochemical and morphological studies. The mitochondria may be increased or abnormal in size and shape, often containing large crystalline inclusions. Many different systemic and intramuscular biochemical abnormalities have been identified in such cases. Deficiencies of several enzymes of the cytochrome electron transport chain have now been recognized in patients with mitochondrial myopathy, and knowledge is extending rapidly. Effective treatment may well be introduced for some such conditions within the next few years.

JOHN WALTON

References

Dyck, P. J., Thomas, P. K., Griffin, J. W., Low, P., and Poduslo, J. F. (ed.) (1992). *Peripheral neuropathy*, (3rd edn). W. B. Saunders, Philadelphia.

Harper, P. S. (1989). *Myotonic dystrophy*, (2nd edn). W. B. Saunders, Philadelphia.

Mastaglia, F. L. and Walton, J. N. (ed.) (1992). *Skeletal muscle pathology*, (2nd edn). Churchill Livingstone, Edinburgh.

Walton, J. N., Karpati, G., and Hilton-Jones, D. (ed.) (1994). *Disorders of voluntary muscle*, (6th edn). Churchill Livingstone, Edinburgh.

NEURONE (NEURON). A *nerve cell, comprising a cell body with several short processes (dendrites) and one long one (the axon) which together with its sheath forms a *nerve fibre. Neurones generate, receive, and transmit nervous impulses.

NEUROPATHOLOGY is the study of the structure and morphology of diseases of the nervous system.

NEUROPATHY is any pathological condition affecting the peripheral nervous system, motor, sensory, or autonomic. Common causes include *diabetes mellitus, *alcoholism, *malnutrition, *genetic abnormality, *carcinomatosis, and mechanical pressure on nerves; but there are many others. See NEUROMUSCULAR DISEASE.

NEUROPHARMACOLOGY is the study of the action of drugs on the *nervous system.

NEUROPHYSIOLOGY. The physiology of the nervous system. Clinical neurophysiology embraces techniques such as *electroencephalography, *electromyography, and related disciplines.

NEUROPSYCHIATRY is that branch of medicine the practitioners of which are skilled in the disciplines both of *neurology and *psychiatry.

NEUROPSYCHOLOGY is the study of the psychological effects of organic brain disease.

NEURORADIOLOGY is the *radiology of the *nervous system.

NEUROSIS is one of a group of psychological disorders, also known as 'psychoneuroses', distinguished from the *psychoses by retention of insight, contact with the environment, and sense of reality. The neuroses may be regarded as a quantitative exaggeration of normal reactions to events and situations (such as anxiety, sadness, and fear) not qualitatively different from them. See PSYCHIATRY.

NEUROSCIENCE
Introduction

In 1971, attendance at the annual meeting of the American Society for Neuroscience was approximately 1500, whereas in 1990 it was over 12 000; clearly, neuroscience can be considered among the fastest growing areas of science. Unlike other branches of science, which differ from each other in the way they describe the physical world, neuroscience is defined solely by its object of study: the central and peripheral nervous systems. Many of the more basic branches of science, from *molecular biology, chemistry, and physics right through to *psychology, *psychiatry, and information technology, are brought together to attempt to elucidate the central question of how the brain works. We can tackle this problem by exploring events either at the level of single cells, i.e. from the 'bottom up', or at the level of functioning systems, i.e. from the 'top down'.

The 'bottom up' approach: single cells
The human brain consists of some 200 billion *neurones, which are outnumbered 10:1 by 'glial' cells (from the Greek for 'glue'). These non-neuronal cells make up half the bulk of the central nervous system and play a range of critical roles in ensuring that the environment of the neurone remains benign. The critical difference between neurones and *glia (neuroglia) is that neurones have the ability to communicate with each other over long distances.

The well-established view of neuronal communication is that it comprises an alternating sequence of electrical and chemical events. An electrical impulse (an '*action potential') in the first neurone causes release of a chemical *neurotransmitter, which crosses a narrow gap (at a *synapse) to the second neurone, where it then causes a transient change in the electrical properties. Twenty years ago the popular view was that, in this way, cells either inhibited or excited each other in a digital on/off fashion. However, if this was the case, it was puzzling why transmitter molecules were used at all. Since these substances require large amounts of energy for their manufacture and disposal, a reasonable alternative might simply have been for electrical current to spread passively from one neurone to another: this scenario of 'electrical transmission' does occur to a certain extent in the central nervous system. However, chemical transmission is by far the most prevalent.

Much research in neuroscience is now focused on understanding the full significance of chemical transmission. A key clue is provided by the diversity seen from one neuronal population to another, which would be completely unnecessary for the simple one-to-one relaying of signals. This diversity is expressed in at least three ways: in basic cell shape (morphology), in the chemical neurotransmitters and their *receptors, and in the electrical conductances of the *cell membranes of neurones.

Morphological diversity
Almost all vertebrate neurones are polarized and have the same basic design, comprising an input region (dendrites), a central processing area (cell body or soma), and an output region (axon). However, this basic design is expressed in a variety of shapes, and such morphological diversity reflects a high degree of functional specialization. Synaptic boutons (swellings that derive from close contacts) along the axon serve as the point of communication between one neurone and another neurone, or between a neurone and an effector tissue, such as *muscle or *gland. Most neurones have a single axon, although it frequently branches many times so that many other neurones can receive synaptic input from a single neurone. A typical neurone in the *cerebral cortex may give rise to more than 1000 such boutons, and these will form synaptic contacts with several hundred other nerve cells, illustrating divergence. Since any particular neurone will only form a limited number of synaptic contacts (around 10) with another individual neurone, while the recipient neurone has several thousand such contacts along its dendrites and on its cell body, it is clear that convergence is also an important principle in neural networks. i.e. each neurone receives input from several hundred other neurones. As we have understood more about the neural networks in the nervous system, it has been found that the connections between neurones are far from random: divergence and convergence combine with the high specificity of neural connections to provide sets of organizing principles for the different parts of the central nervous system. For example, it seems as if there is a basic circuit for the cerebral cortex and another basic circuit for a subcortical group of brain structures, the *basal ganglia.

Morphological diversity is most apparent in the pattern formed by the axons of neurones. In this respect, there are two major classes of neurone: first, those with very long axons (up to several centimetres) that pass from one region of the central nervous system to another, or pass from the central nervous system to peripheral tissues (projection neurones); secondly, those whose axons remain within the region wherein the cell body lies (local-circuit neurones or interneurones). The shape of the axonal arborization of the local-circuit neurones reflects their role. For example, in the cerebral cortex some axons innervate mainly the cell body and proximal dendrites of other neurones, giving a basket-like appearance (the basket cells of Ramon y *Cajal), while the terminal branches of another type of local-circuit neurone hang in rows, giving the appearance of a chandelier (Fig. 1). These chandelier cells have been found to have the most specific targets of any neurone yet studied in the brain: they form synaptic contacts exclusively with the initial segments of the axons of other neurones in the cortex. The initial segment of the axon is the part that connects the axon to the cell body and has a very high density of ion channels; these ion channels open when the cell body is electrically depolarized above a particular threshold, and their opening generates the action potential that then propagates along the axon towards the boutons. The

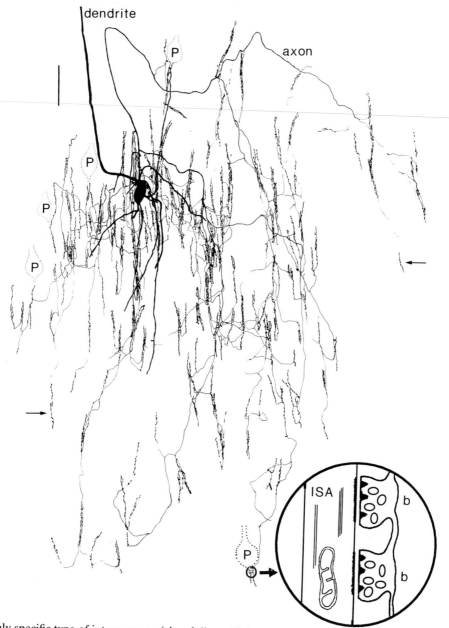

Fig. 1 A highly specific type of interneurone (chandelier cell) in the hippocampus of the monkey. The neurone was impregnated by the Golgi procedure and was first drawn through the light microscope and then examined in the electron microscope. The cell body (soma) of the neurone is shown by the black oval structure on the upper left. Several dendrites (thicker lines) and a single axon leave the soma. The axon of the chandelier cell branches many times to give a dense network of fine collateral branches, of which more than 200 were observed in this case. Each collateral branch of the axon gives rise to specialized segments (two of which are indicated by arrows) that are approximately vertical and contain several swellings (varicosities). Examination of these varicosities in the electron microscope showed that they were boutons (b) containing elliptical-shaped synaptic vesicles, and that each bouton formed a synaptic contact with the initial segment of the axon (ISA) of another type of neurone, a pyramidal neurone (see inset). Some cell bodies of the pyramidal neurones are shown in outline (dotted, P). The initial segment of the axon is where the action potential is generated. Since each chandelier cell innervates several hundred pyramidal cells, it is ideally suited to influence the firing of a whole population of pyramidal neurones. The scale bar on the upper left indicates 50 μm. The inset is a drawing from the electron microscope, with a magnification of 15 000. (Courtesy of P. Somogyi (1983). *Brain Research*, **259**, 137–42).

highly specific innervation of this part of the neurone by the chandelier cell suggests that its function is to regulate the initiation of action potentials. Since each chandelier cell innervates the initial axonal segments of many other neurones (divergence), the chandelier cells might be involved in synchronizing the firing of whole groups of neurones. The transmitter used by the chandelier cell is *GABA (gamma-aminobutyrate), which is the most widespread inhibitory transmitter in the central nervous system. The transmitter used by the neurones that are innervated by chandelier cells (pyramidal neurones) is *glutamate, the most widespread excitatory transmitter in the central nervous system.

Chemical diversity

There are approximately 50 putative transmitters in the brain, the principal classes of which are *amino acids, *amines, *peptides, and *purines. Larger molecules, *proteins, can also play a part in influencing the excitability of the neurone, and even very small molecules, such as nitric oxide, play a role in communication between neurones. The transmitters (such as glutamate and GABA) that excite or inhibit other neurones, although widespread, are in a minority. Almost all the other transmitter substances in neurones play a different role: they act to modulate the responses of neurones to these excitatory or inhibitory transmitters. The actions of chemical transmitters are mediated through chemically sensitive sites (receptors) at synapses on the target cell. For each transmitter substance there are several different types of receptor, activation of each of which has a different effect. There are two main classes of receptor, those that control the opening of ion channels (see below) and so influence the electrical properties of the membrane directly, and those that cause changes in the activities of *enzymes within the cell which, in turn, may lead to changes in the properties of ion channels or to other longer-term effects within the cell. The diversity of transmitter receptors greatly enlarges the scope of the modulatory actions of chemical transmitters; it also makes it possible for *pharmacologists to design drugs that are very specific in their effects.

Chemical diversity is often associated with morphological diversity: thus, different transmitters and different receptors are found in neurones with different shapes and different patterns of axonal arborization. Neurones may thus not only have a morphological 'signature' but also a chemical signature. It has also been found that the same neurone may contain two (or even more) transmitters, one of which may be an inhibitory or excitatory transmitter while the other(s) may play a modulatory role.

Diversity of ion channels

The excitability of neurones is ultimately dependent on a wide range of electrical conductances, in the form of ion channels in the membrane, in addition to those responsible for the classical action potential. While the action potential itself is 'all-or-nothing', i.e. digital, these additional conductances are, broadly speaking, 'analogue' and are carried mainly either by *potassium or *calcium ions passing through their respective channels. Different types of potassium and calcium channels can be regulated either directly by the voltage across the nerve cell's membrane, or indirectly by specific transmitters.

Potassium conductances tend to maintain the neuronal *status quo*, calcium conductances to innovate. The efflux of potassium ions from the cell acts to stabilize the cell by hyperpolarization and/or by making the cell more leaky so that electrical signals have less impact. Conversely, the entry of calcium ions into the cell triggers off a host of reactions both at the level of the membrane and also within the interior of the cell, thus leading to a range of changes in the actions of enzymes or in the manufacture of proteins, which in turn can cause long-term changes in both neuronal structure and function.

Although all neurones generate action potentials, different neuronal subtypes each have a different constellation of these analogue conductances. Hence, it is possible that each neuronal type has its own electrophysiological signature that determines the degree and manner to which it will be able to respond to incoming signals. In certain neurones, an interplay of calcium and potassium conductances can cause the cell to be 'autorhythmic', i.e. to oscillate in its excitability independent of any inputs.

Another important aspect of these analogue conductances is their location. For example, we now know that the dendrites are not just passive cables which transmit incoming signals up to the region of the cell body. Rather, specific conductances are generated in this region, remote from the cell body. The function of these conductances is not yet fully known. However, it is now established that they can play a valuable part in the local integration and filtering of signals, before they are transmitted to the cell body. Furthermore, dendrites can also play a double role in that they can serve not only as a postsynaptic target but also a presynaptic element, by releasing substances in a non-classical fashion.

The dendritic release of substances is different from that at the classical synapse in that it can affect large groups of neurones simultaneously, without producing any conspicuous change in their rate of firing. Rather, the action of dendritically released substances appears to be to bias or 'modulate' the cell to any subsequent inputs. In this way neuronal communication can be described not only in terms of space, how cells form contacts with each other, but also in terms of the passage of time, depending upon the rate of diffusion of substances released from dendrites.

A recent advance at the cellular level in neuroscience has been to build a 'silicon neurone' which has the great advantage over more conventional (digital) computer models of the brain in that it can generate analogue conductances comparable to the ones described above.

On the other hand, replication of the chemical phenomena that occur within and between neurones has as yet defied synthetic reproduction. The electrical events, as in the real brain, can only ever provide a footprint of the chemical phenomena.

We are now beginning to understand the interplay of electrical and chemical events at the cellular level. A good example of a recent advance is the phenomenon of 'long-term-potentiation', where prior stimulation of a neurone, either in the living animal or in isolated brain tissue, causes it to be more sensitive to subsequent stimulation for several hours afterwards. This potentiation of the response is caused by the entry of calcium ions through a special channel (coupled to a particular type of glutamate receptor) which is only activated following the priming of the initial stimulation. The adaptation of neurones seen in long-term-potentiation is likely to play an important part in some forms of memory.

In summary, although the cellular approach gives us insights into the mechanisms by which neurones interact over space and time, we now need to know how these mechanisms are translated into 'phenomenology', recognizable 'functions' in the outside world.

The 'top down' approach: integrated systems

The brain can be divided up anatomically into conspicuous gross regions that are readily visible to the naked eye. However, how this anatomical compartmentalization relates to functions remains a mystery. For example, we know that *Parkinson's disease is associated with loss of cells in a specific region (the *substantia nigra) and that *Huntington's *chorea is due to cell loss in yet another (the striatum). However, we do not yet know precisely how either of these regions actually contributes to the generation of movement.

There are three main techniques used to elucidate the 'function' of a brain region. Electrical stimulation is of limited use since it frequently results in no behaviour whatsoever, or entails the use of electrical current spread vastly exceeding what would occur normally. The second approach is to study the effect of lesions, either experimentally induced or as the result of various types of pathological change. This process, however, has been likened to taking the valves from a wireless that then started to howl, and saying that the function of the valve was to inhibit howling. Finally, it is possible to record the electrical activity of single cells in an identified brain region and to correlate the activity with any ongoing movement. The problem with this third approach is that we have no idea how representative a single neurone is out of a population of millions. It is unlikely, given the considerations in the preceding section, that all cells will function identically. Rather, it is likely that each cell plays a different part in a unified team. Until we can identify the team, any information detected from single cell activity should be interpreted with caution.

An alternative approach has been to adopt the opposite strategy. Instead of finding the function of any one brain region, we can start with a known function and find out where in the brain it is mediated. One of the most successful illustrations of this approach has been with the 'function' of vision. Interestingly enough, however, there is no one single area of the brain devoted to vision, but at least 30 different areas that process, partly in a parallel (or simultaneous) way, partly in a serial (or sequential) way, different aspects of incoming signals, such as their colour, their shape, or their movement. Similarly, for the 'function' of movement, we know that one brain region (*cerebellum) is important for the type of movements that require ongoing sensory feedback, such as tracking type movements. On the other hand, another region (basal ganglia) is vital for the generation of 'spontaneous' movements that are not locked in to any sensory cues. Still another brain region (*motor cortex) controls the actual co-ordination of muscles. A third example of distributed, parallel processing is in memory, where different brain regions have been shown to be associated with memories for, again, different aspects of an object.

Just as 'normal' functions can be 'assigned' to several different brain regions, so can certain abnormal functions, in particular those affecting higher functions of the human brain. *Schizophrenia, for example, involves structural abnormalities in the temporal lobe that influence the functioning of a neural network involving the basal ganglia and the prefrontal cortex. *Alzheimer's disease also involves structural changes in the temporal lobe, but, in addition, there is a loss of specific neurones that project from certain subcortical regions to the cortex. Hence there would appear to be no one single area underscoring either schizophrenia or *dementia.

Although there is overwhelming evidence that certain brain functions and dysfunctions are distributed throughout the brain, we are left with the problem that our final awareness is of a complete, unified world. The critical problem, then, at this level of neuroscience is to explore how the fragmented, parallel components are resynthesized.

Future prospects

We have seen that a major problem at the cellular level is to understand how neuronal mechanisms, i.e. physical events, are transformed into functions. In a similar fashion, although at a more macro level, the main problem with the systems approach is to see how the participation of identified physical brain regions is co-ordinated to produce conscious awareness. In both cases the answer lies in trying to see individual components, be they individual cells or individual brain regions, as part of a larger whole rather than as isolated entities in their own right.

Progress in this direction is well illustrated, for example, by recent experiments on regions of the brain associated with vision. Neurones in different regions can form into groups whose activity is synchronized so that they oscillate at the same frequency in response to certain visual stimuli. An important aspect of these observations is that the groups formed are transient, depending on the prevailing conditions. Hence the same neurone could participate in different groups, thus affording the brain an enormous economy in how neurones are used. Transient neuronal groupings have also been demonstrated optically, by means of fluorescent dyes. Hence it could be the case that these large and transient aggregates form the functional unit where parallel signals are resynthesized and where a unified consciousness emerges. At this point, however, neuroscience gives way to philosophy, at least for the moment.

S. A. GREENFIELD
A. D. SMITH

Further reading

Levitan, I. B. and Kaczmarik, L. K. (1991). *The neuron: cell and molecular biology*. Oxford University Press, Oxford.

Scientific American (1993). Mind and brain. Readings from *Scientific American*. W. H. Freeman, New York.

Zeki, S. (1992). *A vision of the brain*. Blackwell Scientific Publications, Oxford.

NEUROSURGERY, CURRENT PRACTICE

History

Neurosurgery is a young field of medicine, less than a century old. The pioneering efforts of several general surgeons to operate upon the brain were possible because of the development of *anaesthesia in 1846 and the introduction of Listerian aseptic surgery. The enormous gains in understanding of clinical *neurophysiology and neurological localization in the brain came just before and were equally important to the development of surgery on the brain. Sir William *MacEwen was the first to describe successful removal of intracranial *tumours. His success with treatment of brain and spinal *abscesses remains remarkable. *Godlee is generally credited with having been first to operate upon an intrinsic brain tumour. Sir Victor *Horsley was the first surgeon to devote a substantial part of his practice to neurological diseases. Horsley developed the concept of stereotactic localization of subcortical structures. He was successful in the treatment of intracranial granulomas and the first to operate to cure *epilepsy. Horsley pioneered neurosurgical approaches to the posterior fossa and was the first to localize and remove a *spinal cord tumour. He established neurosurgery as a surgical discipline, but it remained for Harvey *Cushing to make it a specialty.

In 1901, Harvey Cushing returned to *Johns Hopkins after a year of research with Kocher. Against the advice of his chief, William *Halsted, he elected to limit his practice to neurological diseases. During the succeeding 12 years in Baltimore, he applied the meticulous anatomical surgical techniques of Halsted to the

nervous system and reduced the enormous morbidity and mortality of neurosurgical procedures of that time to levels which rivalled those possible today. Cushing's influence extended further than neurosurgery, for he introduced the *sphygmomanometer for the measurement of *blood pressure and added blood pressure recording to the pulse and respiration anaesthesia records he had already devised for the operating room. He introduced the use of *X-rays for localization into surgical practice, and the use of physiological saline in surgery. His greatest contribution was the discovery of the hormonal nature of the *pituitary gland and the definition of the diseases of the pituitary. These great accomplishments are all well known. It is less appreciated that Cushing with his mentors, Halsted and *Osler, founded the Hunterian Surgical Laboratory at Johns Hopkins and originated the concept of the trained clinician/scientist in academic medicine.

In 1912, Cushing went to Boston to the Peter Bent Brigham Hospital, where he continued his innovations. The use of suction in surgery and the application of electrocautery for *haemostasis both came from his operating room. Cushing and his colleagues published extensively on the pituitary and its disorders. His book, *The pituitary body* (1912), founded the field of surgical *endocrinology. His surgical experience led to a classification of *gliomas, a detailed description of acoustic *neuromas, and a clarification of *meningiomas. Through his efforts a school of surgery developed which soon became world-wide. Cushing drew students from many countries and they in turn spread Cushing's concepts that neurological patients required dedicated surgeons and special departments for their care.

The early field of neurosurgery

These first neurosurgeons were only able to treat a limited number of neurological diseases. Operations for trigeminal neuralgia (*tic douloureux) were common and were extensively detailed in the literature. Cushing's interest in the pituitary led many of his followers to concentrate upon these relatively rare tumours. Some meningiomas located in favourable areas could be totally removed and others were at least partially removable. Gliomas were usually treated by lobectomy if possible, by internal decompression, or by simple cranial decompression when a deep-seated tumour could not be found. Acoustic tumours were operated upon by an intracapsular route. Neurosurgeons treated *trauma, and *haematomas were successfully removed.

During these early days most neurosurgery was palliative. Pituitary tumours were sometimes cured, but recurrence was more probable. Only the most favourable meningiomas could be removed totally. Acoustic tumours and gliomas were virtually never palliated for more than a short time. Trauma producing simple extradural or subdural haematoma could be treated effectively, but all other forms of severe cerebral *trauma were almost invariably fatal.

The change from palliation to cure

Walter *Dandy, a pupil of Cushing and his successor at Johns Hopkins, was responsible for the philosophical change that moved neurosurgery from a palliative field to its modern concepts of accurate localization and surgery for cure. In 1918, Dandy introduced the new technique of *ventriculography which, for the first time, allowed the accurate preoperative localization of intracranial masses. To his belief that preoperative localization was mandatory for successful surgery, Dandy added the concept that the goal of every operation should be cure of the offending lesion. He was successful in total removal of acoustic tumours. He was the first to operate upon arteriovenous malformations and the first to clip an intracranial *aneurysm. Through his operations for *tinnitus and *vertigo, Dandy established the concept of functional neurosurgery. In addition to these remarkable surgical feats, Dandy performed an equally remarkable laboratory investigation which established the causes of *hydrocephalus and is fundamental to our understanding of the circulation of the *cerebrospinal fluid.

Imaging the nervous system

Prior to Walter Dandy's time, all cerebral localization was carried out by assessing the neurological history and determining the attendant signs. This was a fallible technique in the best of hands, and many of Cushing's operations were simple decompressions when the tumour could not be found. Abnormalities seen on plain radiographs of the skull followed. Dandy's ventriculography allowed accurate localization of intracranial lesions and remained a standard technique until the 1970s. In 1931, Egas *Moniz and Almeida *Lima introduced cerebral *angiography, which demonstrated all kinds of vascular lesions and, after refinement, assessment of the cerebral circulation. *Myelography with positive contrast agents was introduced by Siccard and Forrestière. This technique allowed localization of spinal lesions.

The first functional technique for cerebral localization was *radioactive brain scanning. The accumulation of a radioactive material following intravenous injection could be imaged to provide additional information about intrinsic abnormalities which might be difficult to demonstrate because of a paucity of anatomical distortion.

Early angiographic studies were limited by the contrast agents available and the need for direct vascular puncture. Development of safe contrast agents was paralleled by the use of intravascular *catheters. Simple catheter techniques were soon replaced by flexible catheters which could be manipulated into individual brain vessels from a distant source, such as the femoral artery in the groin. Angiography became safe, much less painful, and highly specific. These dramatic advances prepared the way for the endovascular therapeutics of today.

Similar advances occurred in myelography. The first agents were unsatisfactory, but the introduction of

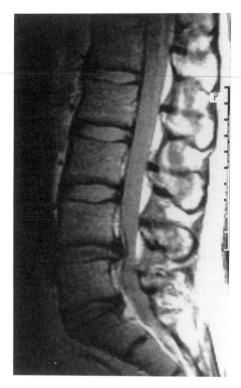

Fig. 1 MRI representation of the spine, demonstrating a substantial disc protrusion at the L4–5 level. MRI demonstrates the outline of bones and all soft tissues with virtual anatomical accuracy.

iodized oil (pantopaque) made myelography practical and safe. However, these oils had the disadvantage of being poorly absorbed by the body. They now have been replaced by water-soluble agents which are readily excreted. Each new agent has fewer problems than the last it replaced, and myelography has become less and less complicated.

Until the early 1970s air studies, angiography, and myelography were the standard diagnostic techniques upon which neurological localization and neurosurgery depended. In the early 1970s *computerized axial tomography (CAT) was introduced and a revolution in imaging began. The CAT *scan utilizes a computer to capture and display the large amount of information generated by X-rays passing through the body which cannot be displayed on conventional film. The capture of these images and the techniques for their display were the work of Hounsfield, although advances have occurred widely in the imaging industry since his original monumental contribution. The CAT scan (now more often called simply *CT) revolutionized intracranial and spinal imaging. Bony structures are seen with remarkable clarity. The brain and spinal cord are visualized well. Many substances, such as cerebrospinal fluid or blood, are easily differentiated. For the first time the intracranial tumour and all of its effects upon the brain could be seen. Spinal cord tumours were seen less well, but the combination of CT imaging with water-soluble myelography provided superb visualization of intraspinal structures. The accuracy of CT scanning was remarkable. For the first time the brain and spinal cord could be seen with a test that was generally safe and painless. The impact upon the field of neurosurgery was enormous. For the first time neurosurgeons could accurately assess the results of trauma, the location of tumours and their effects upon the rest of the brain, the presence of blood and the location of haematomas, the degree of hydrocephalus, and the source of spinal fluid obstructions, congenital abnormalities of the brain, and, of equal importance, the postoperative status of the brain of patients who were not doing well after surgery. The accuracy of CT scanning changed the focus of *neurology and neurosurgery from diagnosis to treatment.

The addition of *magnetic resonance imaging (MRI) was equally revolutionary. CT scanning was so accurate that most were surprised when MRI added increased anatomical clarity to the imaging process. Not only were intracranial abnormalities seen with detail unimagined before, but the normal structures of the brain were visualized with great accuracy. Functional abnormalities, such as the plaques of *multiple sclerosis, or small lesions, such as those of subclinical strokes, leave changes which can be seen. Furthermore, exposure to *radiation is avoided by the use of magnetic fields. The current techniques of magnetic resonance imaging provide the anatomical standard by which all other localizing studies are judged (see Figs 1–3). The neurosurgeon can now rely upon precise diagnosis and accurate localization so that the surgical incisions can be minimized, important surrounding structures identified

in advance, and a rapid postoperative assessment of patients with problems is available.

In the late 1980s the concept of three-dimensional reconstruction of both CT and MRI images was developed. The computer programmes to carry out these reconstructions now allow anatomically accurate reconstruction of images of the head, skull, brain, and its appendages with virtual anatomical accuracy.

Neurosurgery as a mature specialty
During the period from the end of the Second World War until the mid-1970s, neurosurgery matured as a field, and remarkable advances in the treatment of neurosurgical diseases were made throughout the world. The techniques were largely those of Harvey Cushing and Walter Dandy modified by outstanding surgeons in many countries. Surgery for trigeminal neuralgia, operations upon pituitary tumours, removal of intracranial and spinal tumours, and the treatment of trauma were all important aspects of neurosurgery. Trauma, in particular, was studied extensively during and after the Second World War and in the lesser wars that followed. However, a number of new areas were added or developed from earlier beginnings.

Operations on the herniated spinal disc
In 1934, Mixter and Barr described operations for the removal of the ruptured intervertebral *disc which

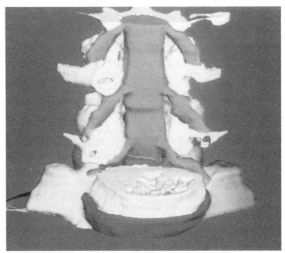

Fig. 3 This representation of a myelogram is a three-dimensional reconstruction. The bones of the spine are white and the dural sac and exiting nerve roots are shown as grey, branching tubes. The apparent removal of bone has been carried out electronically by subtracting information from the routine CT scan and producing this 'electronic laminectomy' to allow the nervous structures to be examined.

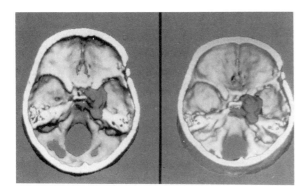

Fig. 2 This three-dimensional representation of the base of the skull has been generated from routine CT scans. The calvarium has been electronically removed to show the skull base. The dark tumour seen on the right side of the base was a meningioma.

had herniated into the spinal canal. The recognition of the herniated disc as a frequent cause of disabling *lumbago and *sciatica received immediate surgical attention throughout the world. The herniated lumbar, and subsequently the cervical, disc became a principal focus for neurosurgeons, particularly in North America. Surgery for these disc protrusions remains an important part of neurosurgical practice today.

*Psychosurgery

Egas Moniz and Almeida Lima introduced frontal *leucotomy for the treatment of psychiatric disease in 1935. Surgery on the frontal and temporal lobes and the thalamus was explored broadly in the 1940s and 1950s. While the techniques were of great value for many patients, psychosurgery has virtually disappeared, for reasons which are at once pharmacological, social, and political.

*Stereotaxis

Stereotactic localization of subcortical structures had been in laboratory use since the time of Horsley and Clarke. Through the 1940s and 1950s, a number of surgeons developed instruments that allowed the destruction of deep brain targets for the treatment of tremors and other forms of abnormal movement, and for pain and epilepsy. The techniques were most widely employed for the tremor of parkinsonism, and thousands of patients world-wide were treated. The development of effective medication virtually eliminated stereotaxis by the mid-1970s. It is now undergoing a modest rebirth.

Epilepsy

Convulsive seizures are among the oldest afflictions of recorded history and certainly one of the most dramatic. Epilepsy was a major study of early neurologists and Horsley attempted to treat epilepsy in the earliest days of neurosurgery. However, it remained for Wilder *Penfield and many colleagues at the Montreal Neurological Institute to make the study and treatment of epilepsy a serious surgical venture. Penfield made great contributions to this field by establishing the first extensive cerebral localizing maps for man, categorizing the epilepsies, and providing relief for many afflicted patients. The rise in epilepsy surgery was paralleled by the development of more effective anticonvulsant drugs and the need for epilepsy surgery diminished somewhat. Nevertheless, the techniques of temporal lobectomy, hemispherectomy, and removal of isolated abnormal areas of cortex for the control of epilepsy all became standard neurosurgical procedures.

Pain

Treatment of trigeminal neuralgia was one of the first operations to interest neurosurgeons. Foerster described the effects of dividing spinal nerves for the relief of pain. Spiller suggested division of the anterolateral quadrant of the spinal cord (the lateral spinothalamic tract) on the basis of observations made in a patient with bilateral spinal tuberculomas. Neurosurgeons prided themselves upon their skill in doing this operation (cordotomy) for the relief of pain, usually the pain of *cancer. Many elaborate anatomical schemes to assure division of appropriate fibres were published. The operation was very successful and a great help to cancer sufferers. Mullan suggested performing the operation percutaneously by means of a needle inserted into the spinothalamic tract. This operation became so popular that it supplanted the open operation. More recently, the development of long-acting narcotics for the relief of cancer pain has reduced the need for cordotomy.

Neurosurgical interest in trigeminal neuralgia continues. Sweet popularized the technique of percutaneous radiofrequency destruction of the fifth cranial nerve. Rather than the open operations utilized by earlier surgeons, Sweet devised a technique of insertion of a fine needle carrying a radiofrequency current behind the Gasserian ganglion through a foramen at the base of the skull. The technique has been modified by utilization of the injection of noxious agents, and in one form or another the percutaneous procedure has virtually eliminated trigeminal surgery.

An alternative has been the development of microvascular decompression by Janetta. It is theorized that trigeminal neuralgia often results because abnormal blood vessels compress or irritate the trigeminal nerve in the posterior fossa. Janetta has devised ways of moving these nerves using microsurgical techniques through a limited exposure. While the pathogenesis of the condition is still debated, there is little doubt that the operation is successful and does not carry the risk of facial sensory loss which may attend the other techniques.

Neurosurgeons have also pioneered the use of pain-relieving procedures which attempt to alter nervous system function by electrical stimulation. A variety of devices to be placed around peripheral nerves, over the spinal cord, or within the brain, are available and have been in use for more than 20 years. They remain helpful in a limited number of patients, but are the province of a small number of experts.

Diversion of the cerebrospinal fluid

Hydrocephalus was understood after the pioneering work of Dandy, and many neurosurgeons attempted to relieve the problem. Cushing and Dandy used open craniotomy to puncture the lamina terminalis, thus opening the ventricles into the subarachnoid space. A variety of techniques to divert the spinal fluid into some other body cavity were proposed, but none were effective until the development of valved systems that allowed the controlled delivery of excess spinal fluid into the vascular system or abdomen. There are now several of these shunts available. All share the basic concept of a valve that regulates pressure or flow, thus controlling the flow of fluid from the ventricle into a body cavity where it can be absorbed. Because of the reduced number of complications, the *peritoneum is now the most common site of diversion. Hydrocephalus has been changed from a uniformly fatal or disabling disease into one in which a child may be restored to relatively normal function.

Congenital anomalies
The successful treatment of other forms of congenital anomaly of the nervous system has been equally dramatic. Myelomeningocele was at one time almost always fatal because of infection. While nervous system function cannot be restored, it is possible to prevent complications, treat the other anomalies, and allow these children to live a worthwhile life by repair of the spinal defect. Craniosynostosis, the premature closure of skull sutures which produces marked skull deformities, can be repaired as well. Surgery for these skull abnormalities has now been developed to the point that even the most complicated, involving skull and face, can be repaired with reasonable results. These children, who previously would have been relegated to the life of a freak, are made to look very acceptable.

Ischaemic disease of the brain
Surgery in the neck on the blood vessels supplying the brain has been in common use for over 40 years. Operations on the vertebral system are usually limited to unusual abnormalities and are the province of a small number of highly specialized vascular surgeons. By contrast, stenotic disease at the carotid bifurcation has been treated by general surgeons, vascular surgeons, and neurosurgeons throughout this period of time. Carotid *endarterectomy was extremely popular and was one of the most common operations. The concept was the prevention of stroke, not the improvement of neurological function. In the recent past, extensive studies have demonstrated the validity of endarterectomy for patients with more than 70 per cent narrowing of the carotid artery. Additional studies are under way to investigate the question of whether restoration of blood flow will be beneficial in patients with less than 70 per cent *stenosis who have had ischaemic symptoms, and in the asymptomatic patient who has stenosis.

Aneurysms and arteriovenous malformations
Walter Dandy first demonstrated the feasibility of surgery to occlude cerebral aneurysms and remove arteriovenous malformations. The focus of neurosurgery in the 1950s and 1960s was largely upon these two abnormalities, and many of the most famous surgeons of the time were vascular surgeons.

The early operations were often complicated and mortality was high. Ligation of carotid and vertebral arteries in the neck was employed as an alternative to try to reduce the pressure within the aneurysm and thus reduce the risk of haemorrhage. Other surgeons attempted to wrap the intracranial aneurysms after exposure because of the lack of adequate metal clips for their occlusion. McKenzie, Olivecrona, and Norlèn all introduced new clips which improved the surgeon's chance for aneurysmal obliteration. Scoville developed the concept of the spring-loaded clip, and now many other prominent surgeons have produced individual clips and entire systems of clips for use in aneurysm surgery. Improvement in anaesthetic techniques, use of *hypothermia, the new clips, and the reduced risk of angiography all allowed successful treatment of aneurysms and arteriovenous malformations during this period.

Magnification, microscopic anatomy, and the development of modern neurosurgery
By the early 1960s, several neurosurgeons had suggested that magnification with an operating microscope would be advantageous in many neurosurgical procedures. Yasargil, after a year of study in Vermont with Donaghy, returned to Zurich where he began to apply microsurgical techniques in all kinds of neurosurgical operations. Microscopes had to be modified for neurosurgery, the instruments devised and developed, and the anatomy understood in an entirely different way. His results in aneurysm and acoustic surgery demonstrated such an advantage over existing surgical techniques that microsurgery soon became the standard and formed the basis for the enormous improvement in treatment of neurosurgical diseases which has occurred in the past 20 years.

Aneurysms and arteriovenous malformations
During the early history of aneurysm surgery it was not clear that operation resulted in an advantage over the natural history of the disease. The long-lasting study of *subarachnoid haemorrhage, aneurysms, and their therapy, sponsored by the National Institutes of Health, demonstrated the advantage of surgery if done with a small resultant morbidity and mortality. The microsurgical techniques and the surgical skills pioneered by Yasargil produced a morbidity and mortality of less than 10 per cent and allowed most competent neurosurgeons to carry out these operations, which had been the province of only a few master surgeons before. Many of the famous neurosurgeons of the past 20 years have been aneurysm surgeons, as this field became the glamour subspecialty of neurosurgery. Entire systems of instrumentation, including greatly improved aneurysm clips were developed, anaesthetic techniques were improved, and the postoperative management of complications has made the same dramatic strides as has surgery.

The principal cause of mortality in those patients who survive the first subarachnoid haemorrhage is from rebleeding. Study of the natural history, coupled with improvements in management techniques, have allowed aneurysms to be treated on an urgent basis, thus eliminating the rebleeding risk. The second major problem is vasospasm, which produces ischaemic stroke. Allen introduced calcium-channel-blocking agents for the prevention of these ischaemic effects, providing the first reasonable treatment for this dreaded complication. It is now understood that maintenance of blood volume and blood pressure is also important for the maintenance of blood flow, and vasospasm, which produced serious consequences in at least 20 per cent of post-surgical aneurysm patients, is now a much less frequent cause of concern.

The same microsurgical techniques that allowed the precise identification and obliteration of aneurysms, have been helpful for the treatment of arteriovenous malformations. Individual blood vessels can be identified and controlled, and the treatment of these vascular anomalies in the brain is now feasible. Some surgery had been done earlier, but the published series did not clearly improve upon the natural history of the disease in most instances.

Tumours of the cerebellopontine angle
Tumours of the acoustic nerve have been a neurosurgical challenge since the days of Harvey Cushing, who treated them with subtotal removal, but preserved and improved cranial nerve function. Walter Dandy demonstrated that total removal and cure was possible, but at the expense of facial paralysis. This remained the standard until the microsurgical era, when total removal became routine, and the surgeon was able to focus upon preservation of cranial nerves. Modern microsurgeons save the facial nerve routinely, cure is expected, mortality has almost disappeared, and currently the surgical challenge is to preserve or restore hearing which is still lost in most patients.

Tumours of the skull base
The broad variety of tumours that occur at the base of the skull were treated ineffectually until the recent past. Many of these are benign, but eventually cause death of the patient by inexorable progression of loss of cranial nerve and, finally, brainstem function. Neurosurgeons and *otorhinolaryngologists have combined to develop a variety of new surgical techniques which are quite different from traditional neurosurgical operations. Some require operating through the mouth, dividing both the upper and lower jaw, operating through the face or sinuses, or surgical exposures around the eye, and are combined with extensive dissections in the neck. These radical operations now allow successful surgery on tumours that were considered inoperable a decade ago. There is still debate about how radical this surgery should be for the benign meningiomas which are slow growing. Nevertheless, it is obvious that many patients for whom no satisfactory therapy was available only a short time ago, can benefit from this surgery by cure or long-term palliation. This field is the most technically challenging left in surgery and the major surgical advances of the near future are likely to be here.

Intramedullary spinal cord tumours
Enhanced MRI has revolutionized the surgeon's ability to diagnose and understand tumours occurring within the spinal cord. The nature of the tumour can be guessed with accuracy and its extent measured with certainty. Microsurgical techniques, coupled with spinal cord monitoring, allow delicate dissection of tumour with continuous assessment of spinal cord function. The favourable tumours that are encapsulated can usually be removed with only a limited risk of paralysis. Gliomas which infiltrate the cord are generally not curable, but palliation with preservation of function is possible. Successful surgery for these tumours is a product of developments in the past 10–15 years.

Brain and spinal cord trauma
One of the areas of greatest advance in neurosurgical practice has been in the field of trauma to the nervous system. These advances have not come from technical surgical achievements, but are based upon clinical research, which has greatly increased our understanding of the pathophysiology of injury to the nervous system.

The pathological consequences of injury to the spinal cord have been studied in great detail and are now well understood, although as yet nothing can be done to restore function in most cases. Collins and his associates have demonstrated a beneficial effect of steroids administered in very high doses immediately after the injury. This is the first demonstration that any treatment is of benefit in severe spinal cord injury.

Even more progress has been made in the area of brain injury. While it is also true that a seriously damaged brain will not recover and regeneration is not possible, the secondary effects of brain injury are now much better understood and can be treated. This is because some neurosurgeons have led the way by studying and understanding the complex relationships between increased pressure within the skull secondary to injury, its effects upon blood flow, and its mechanical effects upon the brain. These studies have led to techniques for ameliorating the damaging effects of all these factors upon potentially recoverable brain cells. The declining spiral that these patients typically present can be controlled and reversed. Hence there has been a dramatic improvement in the mortality and morbidity of serious head injury.

The management of gliomas and chemotherapy
Much effort has been expended in the management of gliomas, but these intrinsic brain tumours remain an unresolved problem. The immediate effects of tumour growth can be palliated by surgery. There is some evidence that radiation therapy is beneficial for slow-growing gliomas, and it is certainly beneficial in the

short term in more malignant tumors. Many chemotherapeutic agents have been tried, but to date, the only tumours commonly cured by chemotherapy are medulloblastomas in children. Such treatment continues to be under intense study. Nevertheless, the malignant gliomas remain among the most devastating of all known neoplasms.

What is new in the field of neurosurgery?
Endovascular therapy
The techniques of catheter manipulation within arteries supplying the nervous system has greatly improved the treatment of many kinds of vascular abnormality and some tumours. Spinal cord arteriovenous malformations can often be treated by obliteration of nutrient vessels, rather than by open surgery. A combination of surgery and endovascular obliteration is sometimes required, but reduction of blood flow generally makes surgery much safer. Equal success has occurred in the treatment of cerebral arteriovenous malformations. It is now common for these blood vessel abnormalities to be treated by a combination of endovascular obliteration produced by the injection of sclerosing agents, with techniques to occlude feeding vessels. Sometimes the malformations can be successfully treated by these methods alone. In other patients, total removal may be required, but the surgery is made much safer by gradual occlusion of the feeding vessels of the malformation. Focused radiation techniques for small areas of residual malformation can then be added. Such combined methods have greatly reduced mortality and morbidity for patients harbouring these lesions.

There have also been attempts to treat aneurysms by inducing intravascular thrombosis, rather than by direct surgery. Success here is much less obvious. Some aneurysms have been occluded by one or more balloons expanded within the lumen of the abnormality, or by balloon occlusion of feeding vessels when feasible. The injection of thrombogenic materials into saccular aneurysms has also been employed. At present none of these techniques is as effective as direct surgery for most aneurysms, but these methods of treating aneurysms without craniotomy are still being explored.

Stereotaxy and stereotactic radiosurgery
There has been a modest rebirth of stereotactic techniques for the treatment of movement disorders and pain. Increased understanding of the pathways important in the generation of movement disorders has led to more defined target points for destructive lesions used to treat these abnormalities of movement, such as tremor in parkinsonism. Implantation of stimulating devices in the thalamus or periaqueductal grey matter of the brainstem has also been employed for the treatment of otherwise intractable pain.

Stereotactic *biopsy of tumours is now feasible. Visualization on CT or MRI with control of stereotactic sampling by these images, has made the technique

much more accurate and much safer than the free-hand needle biopsy techniques employed in the past. This allows tumours to be identified with safety and avoids craniotomy in some patients when other techniques, such as radiation therapy, are to be used.

Stereotactic craniotomy is also being developed. Tumours are localized by a stereotactic technique and approached through very limited exposures. This limited exposure provides an added margin of safety for the patient, but it is uncertain whether the biological behaviour of tumours so treated has been changed.

Epilepsy and the study of brain function
There has also been a resurgence of interest in epilepsy surgery. Modern techniques of monitoring electrical activity of the brain have been developed. Grids of electrodes are inserted surgically over the brain surface. Patients can then be monitored for as long as several weeks. This has replaced the technique of such monitoring in the operating room which allowed examination of patients under highly artificial circumstances for only short periods of time. More data have been obtained from centres employing these techniques in a few years than were developed in the great studies of Wilder Penfield over his entire career. New insights into the localization of language and memory function are accumulating rapidly.

Spinal reconstruction
For many years spinal surgery consisted of the excision of herniated discs, the treatment of trauma, the removal of tumours, and correction of a few congenital or acquired spinal anomalies. In the past 5 years, new methods of reconstruction of the spine have been developed. There are now many metal systems of screws, plates, rods, wires, nuts, and bolts which allow the spinal surgeon to fix the unstable spine in order to correct anatomical abnormalities. Because of improved methods of fixation, decompressive techniques have grown more radical. There has been a broad emphasis in neurosurgery and in *orthopaedics upon appropriate spinal reconstruction following surgery for trauma and tumours. There has also been a dramatic increase in the ability to deal with the consequences of degenerative spinal disease. The long-term efficacy of many of these reconstructive systems remains to be proved, but increased interest in spinal reconstruction has brought great hope for the future treatment of chronic spinal pain.

Monitoring techniques
One major advance of the past 10 years has been the development of electrical techniques that allow continuous assessment of spinal cord posterior column function, spinal cord motor function, of the visual and auditory systems, of brainstem function, and of the integrity of peripheral and cranial nerves. Surgeons are now able to carry out operations on the spinal cord with

increased safety because the transmission of electrical signals can be recorded continuously. Nerve roots can be manipulated with greater safety while recording electrical activity in the roots at risk. Surgeons operate upon acoustic tumours while regularly assessing seventh nerve function and auditory potentials. Peripheral nerve function can be evaluated after they have been exposed. These techniques are being continuously refined to increase intraoperative safety further.

Three-dimensional imaging of the nervous system

The three-dimensional techniques now available in CT scanning have improved dramatically the imaging of the nervous system and its surrounding bony structures. Three-dimensional imaging in the brain is now accurate enough to be called 'frameless stereotaxis'. The accuracy is so great that the surgeon can have an exact understanding of the location of tumours. Furthermore, this system can be used in the operating room to demonstrate exactly where a tumour is located, thus guiding the surgical exposure. Three-dimensional imaging has also proved invaluable for such long-standing spinal problems as assessment of the continuity of fusion, bone, or the size of a neural foramen.

What are the developing areas of greatest interest?

It seems likely that the genetic basis of some brain tumours will soon be elucidated. Surgical cure of gliomas is unlikely, so the development of gene therapy may be promising. Some work has been done upon the genetics of the nervous system tumours which complicate *neurofibromatosis. Spinal reconstruction is likely to develop explosively. Techniques that attempt to restore function after spinal injury may emerge. The development of new materials, either biodegradable or absorbed into normal structures, will be crucial. Understanding the causes of spinal pain is a major challenge. The development of robotic control in the operating room is another area of great potential. Frameless stereotaxis and the accurate localization of tumours by computers using three-dimensional images is already a reality. Stereotactic radiosurgery will probably be revolutionized in the near future by the development of greater accuracy in the focusing system. Functional imaging is likely to be the next step in diagnostic radiology. The brain can now be portrayed with great anatomical accuracy by CT and MR scanning. The next step will be to demonstrate the metabolic state of the brain and to define both acute and chronic biochemical aberrations.

Conclusion

Neurosurgery is barely 100 years old and has been a mature specialty for less than 50 years. Modern neurosurgery began with the advent of magnification techniques and is less than 30 years old. The first 30 years of the specialty were devoted to diagnosis, understanding the diseases to be treated, and palliative surgery. Walter

Dandy introduced the concept of imaging the nervous system and curative surgery which dominated the field until the 1960s. The addition of magnification methods to the neurosurgical armamentarium brought emphasized maintenance on the integrity of the small discrete areas of the nervous system and has reduced mortality and morbidity of neurosurgical procedures to levels that seemed unattainable only a few years ago. The new imaging techniques have revolutionized diagnosis, so that most patients are seen in the early stages of their disease when satisfactory treatment is much more likely. Thus the field of neurosurgery has changed with each generation. The surgeons trained by Harvey Cushing found their methods out-moded by Walter Dandy's new concepts. Emphasis on the meticulous neurological examination by Cushing was replaced by the need for a detailed knowledge of anatomy, as demonstrated by ventriculography and angiography. Much of the neurosurgeon's time was spent in performing these diagnostic studies. CT and MRI rendered these tests obsolete and have made diagnosis much more simple. The emphasis now can be upon forms of treatment and expected outcomes, rather than diagnosis.

More recent developments in the field have changed the role of the neurosurgeon yet again. Endovascular techniques and stereotaxis require new skills and less direct surgery. Spinal reconstruction is a new and exciting field. Functional imaging provides a new level of understanding of the pathophysiological effects of neurosurgical diseases and the consequences of their treatment.

Neurosurgery has changed from a field characterized by uncertain diagnosis and treatment, with very high mortality and morbidity, to one of precise diagnosis and localization with mortality and complication rates which are lower than those of many much simpler specialties. Magnification, understanding the microscopic anatomy, development of new micro-instruments, and an emphasis upon delicate surgical techniques have led to the development of a field of surgery technically unmatched in history. Neurosurgery has redefined itself every 25–30 years. The era of magnification is now nearly 30 years old. The new field of neurosurgery, which is likely to replace it, will emphasize minimally invasive techniques to preserve, restore, and improve lost or impaired neurological function.

DON M. LONG

Further reading

Fox, W. L. (1984). *Dandy of Johns Hopkins*. Williams and Wilkins, Baltimore.

Fulton, J. F. (1946). *Harvey Cushing. A biography*. C. C. Thomas, Springfield, IL.

Long, D. M. (1991). Historical vignette, the Johns Hopkins Hospital. *Journal of Neurosurgery*, **75** (1), 160–1.

Walker, A. E. (1967). *A history of neurological surgery*. Hafner, New York.

Wilkins, R. H. and Rengachery, S. S. (1985). *Neurosurgery*. McGraw-Hill, New York.

NEUROSYPHILIS is *syphilis affecting the central nervous system, the chief clinical varieties being *meningovascular syphilis, *tabes dorsalis, and *general paralysis of the insane, although the distinctions are not always clear-cut. The latter two are manifestations of late (quaternary) syphilis.

NEUROTOXIC describes any agent which is toxic to nervous tissue.

NEUROTOXIN. Any substance which is poisonous or destructive to nervous tissue.

NEUROTRANSMITTERS are chemical substances released in minute amount at the endings of *nerve fibres in response to arrival of a nerve impulse; in the case of a *synapse, the neurotransmitter diffuses across the synaptic cleft to bind with *receptors on the postsynaptic cell membrane and initiate excitation of the postsynaptic cell. At other types of nerve ending, it similarly causes excitation of the adjacent effector organ. A number of substances able to act as neurotransmitters have been identified, the best known of which are *adrenaline, *noradrenaline, *acetylcholine, and *dopamine.

NEUTROPHILS are *granulocytes (polymorphonuclear leucocytes) with fine neutral-staining granules. See HAEMATOLOGY.

NEW ENGLAND JOURNAL OF MEDICINE. See MEDICAL JOURNALS.

NEWTON, SIR ISAAC (1642–1727). British scientist. He was one of the great scientists of all time, epitomizing the revolutionizing of thought in the 17th century. Newton's contributions were to optics, mechanics, astronomy, and mathematics. He analysed light into its component colours and believed that it consisted of particles emanating from its source. He invented calculus before Leibniz, who discovered it independently. He is especially remembered for his enunciation of the laws of motion and the law of gravity. These explained much of the behaviour of the material world, and occurrences in orbits of astronomical bodies. His most famous work is that called *Philosophiae naturalis principia mathematica* (Mathematical principles of natural philosophy) published in 1687.

NIACIN is one of the vitamins of the B group (vitamin B$_3$), deficiency of which results in *pellagra. It is a mixture of nicotinic acid and nicotinamide, into which nicotinic acid is converted in the body. Nicotinamide is required for the synthesis of an important *coenzyme, nicotinamide adenine dinucleotide (NAD), which plays a vital role in energy formation and storage. Niacin is widely available in the diet and is not destroyed by cooking or standing; deficiency is rarely encountered in the West except in chronic *alcoholism and intestinal *malabsorption. Elsewhere it tends to be associated with a maize-dependent diet.

NICOLAS, JOSEPH GUILLAUME MARIE (1868–1960). French dermatologist. With *Favre, Nicolas described a sexually transmitted disease in which the lymph nodes in the groin enlarge and subsequently break down to discharge via multiple sinuses on the skin. Originally named after these two men, it is now called *lymphogranuloma venereum.

NICOTINAMIDE. See NIACIN.

NICOTINE is a natural alkaloid, first isolated from the leaves of the *tobacco plant (*Nicotiana tabacum*) in 1828. It has complex pharmacological actions, the major component of which is transient stimulation followed by more persistent depression of all autonomic ganglia. It has no therapeutic application. Its medical importance lies in its toxicity and in its presence in tobacco. That nicotine makes a major contribution to the addictive properties of tobacco (including *snuff as well as that smoked in cigarettes, cigars, and pipes) is now well established. It is less clear to what extent it is an aetiological agent in the serious diseases associated with tobacco smoking, such as lung *cancer, other cancers, chronic pulmonary disease, *coronary heart disease, peripheral vascular disease, and deleterious effects on fetal growth. The other toxic components of tobacco smoke, particularly tar and *carbon monoxide, are the major factors in these conditions. Hence the widespread, and not entirely unsuccessful, use of nicotine-containing chewing gum and skin patches as substitutes for cigarette-smoking, which is the most dangerous form of tobacco use.

NICOTINIC ACID. See NIACIN.

NIGHT BLINDNESS, also known as nyctalopia, is a manifestation of *vitamin A deficiency. Vitamin A, or retinol, is essential for the proper functioning of the retinal receptors known as *rods, which subserve vision in dim light (see OPHTHALMOLOGY).

NIGHTINGALE, FLORENCE (1820–1910). British pioneer of nursing. After some years of doubt she became convinced that her vocation was to nurse. Family resistance was overcome with difficulty. In 1853, after a visit to the Institute of Protestant Deaconesses at Kaiserswerth, she was appointed Superintendent of the Hospital for Invalid Gentlewomen in Harley Street, London. Her success there inspired Sidney Herbert, the Secretary at War, to ask her to organize the nursing services in the army hospitals in the Crimea, where the appalling conditions had recently been revealed in articles in *The Times*. She established herself and her 38 nurses at *Scutari, where 5000 sick and wounded came under her care. In February 1855 the death rate of soldiers admitted to the hospital was 42 per cent; by June of that year it had fallen to 2 per cent. Miss Nightingale became a legendary figure, and on her return to England a fund, totalling £50 000, was raised which she used to establish, in 1860, an institute for the training of nurses at *St Thomas's Hospital, London.

Thereafter she took no part in public life, seldom leaving her sickroom, from which, nevertheless, there issued a stream of reports and recommendations dealing with sanitary reform in army and civilian life. See also NURSING IN THE UK.

NIGHT TERRORS, also known as *pavor nocturnus*, are a sleep disturbance of young children characterized by a state of terror suddenly interrupting normal sleep and accompanied by screaming, shouting, or groaning. The episode is usually followed by a return to sleep without a period of wakefulness. The child subsequently has complete amnesia for the event; this distinguishes *pavor nocturnus* from the more familiar nightmare. See also SLEEP.

NIGHT VISION. See OPHTHALMOLOGY.

NITROFURANTOIN is an antibacterial drug effective against many organisms causing urinary tract infection. See ANTI-INFECTIVE AGENTS.

NITROGEN is the invisible and almost inert gaseous element (relative atomic mass 14.0067, atomic number 7, symbol N) which comprises about 80 per cent of atmospheric air. As an essential constituent of *nucleic acids and *proteins, nitrogen is vital to all living organisms. It is of particular medical importance in the pathogenesis of *decompression sickness.

NITROGEN MUSTARD. See ALKYLATING AGENTS.

NITROUS OXIDE, laughing gas, or nitrogen monoxide (N_2O), was suggested as an anaesthetic agent by Sir Humphry *Davy in 1800 and successfully used in 1844 by Horace *Wells, a dentist of Hartford, Connecticut. It is still a valuable inhalational general analgesic and anaesthetic. See ANAESTHESIA.

NITS are the ova or eggs of lice, particularly of the head louse, *Pediculus capitis*. Nits are easily recognized as small rounded bodies firmly adherent to the hair shafts.

NOBEL PRIZES FOR PHYSIOLOGY OR MEDICINE. See Table 1.

Table 1 Nobel prizes for physiology and medicine, 1901–93

1901	Emil von Behring (Germany)	Diphtheria antiserum
1902	Ronald Ross (UK)	Mosquito and malaria
1903	Niels Ryberg Finsen (Finland)	Ultraviolet light in lupus vulgaris
1904	Ivan Petrovich Pavlov (Russia)	Conditioned reflex
1905	Robert Koch (Germany)	Tuberculosis
1906	Camillo Golgi (Italy) and Santiago Ramon y Cajal (Spain)	Structure of nervous tissue
1907	Charles Louis Alphonse Laveran (France)	Malarial parasite
1908	Paul Ehrlich (Germany)	Immunity
	Elie Metchnikoff (France)	Phagocytosis
1909	Theodor Kocher (Switzerland)	Thyroid disease
1910	Albrecht Kossel (Germany)	Bases of nucleic acid
1911	Allvar Gullstrand (Sweden)	Physical properties of lens
1912	Alexis Carrel (USA)	Vascular suture
1913	Charles Richet (France)	Anaphylaxis
1914	Robert Bárány (Austria)	Vestibular apparatus
1915	No award	
1916	No award	
1917	No award	
1918	No award	
1919	Jules Bordet (Belgium)	Lysis by complement
1920	August Krogh (Denmark)	Contractility of capillaries
1921	No award	
1922	Archibald Vivian Hill (UK)	Production of heat in muscles
	Otto Meyerhof (Germany)	Lactic acid metabolism
1923	Frederick Grant Banting and John James Richard Macleod (Canada)	Insulin
1924	Willem Einthoven (Netherlands)	Electrocardiography

Table 1 (*cont.*)

1925	No award	
1926	Johannes Fibiger (Denmark)	Discovery of the *Spiroptera* carcinoma
1927	Julius Wagner-Jauregg (Austria)	Malaria treatment of dementia paralytica
1928	Charles Nicolle (France)	Transmission of typhus fever by the louse
1929	Christiaan Eijkman (Netherlands)	Discovery of the antineuritic vitamin
	Frederick Gowland Hopkins (UK)	Discovery of growth-stimulating vitamins
1930	Karl Landsteiner (Austria)	Human blood groups
1931	Otto Warburg (Germany)	Intracellular respiration
1932	Charles Sherrington and	Function of neurones
	Edgar Douglas Adrian (UK)	
1933	Thomas Hunt Morgan (USA)	Function of chromosomes
1934	George Hoyt Whipple, George Richards	Liver treatment of pernicious anaemia
	Minot, and William Parry Murphy	
	(USA)	
1935	Hans Spemann (Germany)	Embryonic development
1936	Henry Dale (UK) and	Chemical transmission of nerve impulses
	Otto Loewi (Austria)	
1937	Albert Szent-Györgyi (Hungary)	Studies on vitamin C
1938	Corneille Heymans (Belgium)	Respiratory reflexes
1939	Gerhard Domagk (Germany)	Antibacterial action of sulphonamide
1940	No award	
1941	No award	
1942	No award	
1943	Henrik Dam (Denmark)	Discovery of vitamin K
	Edward A. Doisy (USA)	Chemical structure of vitamin K
1944	Joseph Erlanger and Herbert Spencer	Studies of single nerve fibres
	Gasser (USA)	
1945	Alexander Fleming, Ernst Boris Chain,	Antibacterial action of penicillin
	and Howard Walter Florey (UK)	
1946	Hermann Joseph Muller (USA)	X-ray induced mutations
1947	Bernardo Alberto Houssay (Argentina)	Role of anterior pituitary in carbohydrate metabolism
	Carl F. Cori and Gerty T. Cori	Carbohydrate metabolism
	(USA)	
1948	Paul Müller (Switzerland)	DDT as an arthropod poison
1949	Walter Rudolf Hess (Switzerland)	Hypothalamus and autonomic function
	Antonio Egas Moniz (Portugal)	Prefrontal lobotomy
1950	Edward Calvin Kendall, Philip Showalter	Adrenal hormones
	Hench (USA), and Tadeus Reichstein	
	(Switzerland)	
1951	Max Theiler (USA)	Yellow fever vaccine
1952	Selman Abraham Waksman (USA)	Discovery of streptomycin for tuberculosis
1953	Hans Adolf Krebs (UK)	Citric acid cycle
	Fritz Albert Lipmann (USA)	Coenzyme A in intermediary metabolism
1954	John F. Enders, Frederick C. Robbins,	Poliovirus in tissue culture
	and Thomas H. Weller (USA)	
1955	Hugo Theorell (Sweden)	Oxidizing enzymes
1956	André Fédéric Cournand, Dickinson	Cardiac catheterization
	Woodruff Richards (USA),	
	and Werner Forssmann (Germany)	
1957	Daniel Bovet (Italy)	Synthetic vasoactive drugs
1958	George Wells Beadle and	One gene–one enzyme concept
	Edward Lawrie Tatum (USA)	
	Joshua Lederberg (USA)	Bacterial genetics

Table 1 (*cont.*)

Year	Laureate(s)	Contribution
1959	Severo Ochoa and Arthur Kornberg (USA)	Biological synthesis of the nucleic acids
1960	Frank Macfarlane Burnet (Australia) and Peter Brian Medawar (UK)	Acquired immunological tolerance
1961	Georg von Békésy (USA)	Physiology of the cochlea
1962	Francis Harry Compton Crick, Maurice Hugh Frederick Wilkins, and James Dewey Watson (UK)	Molecular structure of DNA
1963	John Carew Eccles (Australia), Alan Lloyd Hodgkin, and Andrew Fielding Huxley (UK)	Ionic mechanisms affecting nerve cell membrane
1964	Konrad E. Bloch (USA) and Feodor Lynen (Germany)	Metabolism of cholesterol and fatty acids
1965	Francois Jacob, André Lwoff, and Jacques Monod (France)	Genetic control of synthesis of viruses and enzymes
1966	Francis Peyton Rous (USA)	Cancer-producing virus
	Charles B. Huggins (USA)	Hormonal treatment of cancer
1967	Ragnar Granit (Sweden), H. Keffer Hartline, and George Wald (USA)	Chemical and physiological processes in the eye
1968	Robert W. Holley, H. Gobind Khorana, and Marshall W. Nirenberg (USA)	How genes control cell function
1969	Max Delbrück, Alfred Hershey, and Salvador Luria (USA)	Use of phage in studies of inheritance
1970	Julius Axelrod (USA), Bernard Katz (UK), and Ulf von Euler (Sweden)	Chemical mediators of nerve transmission
1971	Earl W. Sutherland, Jr (USA)	Mechanism of hormone action: cyclic AMP
1972	Gerald M. Edelman (USA) and Rodney R. Porter (UK)	Structure of immunoglobulins
1973	Nikolas Tinbergen (UK), Konrad Z. Lorenz, and Karl von Frisch (Germany)	Studies of animal behaviour, instinct
1974	Christian de Duve (Belgium), Albert Claude, and George E. Palade (USA)	Cell biology
1975	David Baltimore, Renato Dulbecco, and Howard M. Temin (USA)	Interaction of tumour viruses and nucleic acids in cells
1976	Baruch S. Blumberg (USA)	Discovery of hepatitis B virus
	D. Carlton Gajdusek (USA)	Slow-acting viruses
1977	Rosalyn Yalow (USA)	Radioimmunoassay
	Roger Guillemin and Andrew Schally (USA)	Isolation of hypophyseal peptides
1978	Werner Arber (Switzerland), Hamilton Smith, and Daniel Nathans (USA)	Restriction endonucleases
1979	Allan MacLeod Cormack (USA) and Godfrey Newbold Hounsfield (UK)	Computer-assisted tomography
1980	George Snell, Baruj Benacerraf (USA), and Jean Dausset (France)	Immunogenetics: the histocompatibility complex
1981	Roger Sperry (USA)	Cerebral hemispheric function
	David Hubel and Torsten Wiesel (USA)	Mechanisms of vision
1982	Sune Bergström, Bengt Samuelsson (Sweden), and John Vane (UK)	Prostaglandins and biologically related substances
1983	Barbara McClintock (USA)	Mobile genetic elements
1984	Niels Jerne (Switzerland)	Concept of the 'network theory' of the immune system
	Cesar Milstein and Georges Koehler (UK)	Production of monoclonal antibodies

Table 1 (*cont.*)

1985	Michael Stuart Brown and Joseph Leonard Goldstein (USA)	Cholesterol metabolism
1986	Stanley Cohen (USA) and Rita Levi-Montalcini (Italy)	Mechanisms regulating cell growth
1987	Susumu Tonegawa (Japan)	Genetics of antibody diversity
1988	Sir James Black (UK)	Design of new therapeutic compounds
	Gertrude Belle and George Herbert (USA)	Design of new drug treatments
1989	John Michael Bishop and Harold Eliot Varmus (USA)	Derivation of oncogenes
1990	Joseph E. Murray and Thomas Edward Donnall (USA)	Organ transplantation
1991	E. Neher and B. Sakmann (Germany)	Ion detection in cell membranes
1992	Edwin Krebs and Edmond Fisher (USA)	Protein enzymes
1993	Richard Roberts and Philip Sharp (USA)	Genes, DNA, and introns

Note: The nation listed refers to the site of the prize-winning work, not the birthplace of the scientist.

NOCARDIOSIS is a subacute or chronic suppurative infection of the lungs which may spread to the central nervous system or other body sites, more likely to occur, and taking a severer course, in immunocompromised patients. It is due to an aerobic, Gram-positive, filamentous bacterium, *Nocardia asteroides*, commonly present in soil.

NODE. Any small mass of differentiated tissue.

NODULE. A small palpable mass.

NO-FAULT COMPENSATION. As the name suggests, no-fault compensation is the label given to a variety of alternatives to traditional litigation which grant compensation to personal injury victims without the requirement that such victims prove their injuries were caused by the fault of someone else. No-fault compensation schemes have grown up as a consequence of the criticism that the elusive search for fault wastes resources and leaves a high proportion of accident victims uncompensated.

No-fault schemes first appeared in workers' compensation plans of the turn of the century, and have since spread to almost every field of endeavour in which human activity has been shown to cause personal injuries. The actual workings of such plans vary widely, depending on the heads of compensation offered (medical expenses, loss of earnings, etc.), the prerequisites to a successful claim (automobile accidents, adverse effects of drugs, etc.), the degree of seriousness of injuries covered (many North American automobile plans leave the most serious injuries to the traditional tort system), and whether the plan is compulsory for all potential victims. A crucial distinguishing factor, and the focal point of the controversy regarding no-fault compensation, is the extent to which a no-fault plan takes away the right to sue.

New Zealand's comprehensive no-fault system
Worthy of closer scrutiny as representative of many common features of no-fault plans is the accident compensation system which came into force in New Zealand in 1974. This legislated scheme purports to provide compensation for all personal injuries caused by accident occurring in New Zealand or suffered by New Zealand residents travelling overseas. The level of compensation is not high, being reduced from that offered by the scheme prior to its 1992 revision, and in no way matching that of a common law award of damages. Compensation will be given (but only to prescribed maximum levels) for medical treatment and *rehabilitation costs occasioned by an accident. The corporation that administers the scheme is likewise authorized to pay for vocational retraining programmes for injured workers and additional matters, such as home help and child care expenses, etc.

The largest source of compensation under the New Zealand scheme is that of loss of earnings. A successful claimant will receive 80 per cent of earnings lost as a result of his or her injuries, such compensation continuing to the age of qualification for national superannuation. Needless to say, various limitations on the entitlement exist. As always, there is a prescribed maximum amount payable. At six-monthly intervals there will be a medical assessment of the degree of the claimant's capacity for work. If that capacity is 85 per cent or more, earnings-related compensation shall cease, regardless of the lack of any opportunities for employment. In the case of a fatal accident where loss-of-earnings compensation would have been payable to the victim had he or she survived, a percentage of such compensation will be payable to the victim's surviving spouse and dependants for limited periods of time. Additional benefits payable in the event of a death arising from a personal injury are a funeral grant of NZ$1900 and sums of NZ$4000 to a surviving spouse and NZ$2000 to each surviving child. (NZ$2.55 = £1/US$1.50)

Although the scheme formerly provided for lump-sum payments of up to NZ$27 000 for 'non-economic' losses such as pain and suffering, this head of compensation has now been abolished. In its place is a periodic payment known as an 'independence allowance', which is available to all claimants who have suffered a degree of disability of 10 per cent or more. The amount payable is small, being a percentage of the maximum of NZ$40 per week (for 100 per cent disability) depending on the actual degree of disability.

The no-fault debate

Two substantial criticisms of New Zealand's scheme can be made, which likewise exist to challenge many of the less comprehensive versions of no-fault compensation plans in place in other jurisdictions. The first is the legislated exclusion of claims for personal injury 'caused wholly or substantially by gradual process, *disease* or infection' except in the case where such injury has arisen in the course of employment, a 'medical misadventure', or is 'a consequence of personal injury or treatment for personal injury'. This exclusion of disease claims from New Zealand's scheme is indefensible on any ground other than that of the scheme's limited resources—why should the *cancer sufferer be forced to accept (if eligible) the meagre assistance of a social welfare benefit, while the drunken daredevil injured by his or her foolishness receives the greater compensation offered by the no-fault scheme? The unfairness of the disease exclusion exerted an obvious influence on court rulings as to the scope of the scheme prior to its 1992 reworking, resulting in some surprising rulings in favour of claimants who sought cover for 'personal injuries by accident' which the lay person might suspect were no more than the effect of disease. Thus compensation was granted to a woman with a history of back trouble who suffered pain upon bending down to pick up milk bottles; to a child who suffered an apnoeic attack (cessation of breathing) due to unknown causes; to the woman who did not give her informed consent to a novel form of treatment for cancer; and to the woman who suffered a 'nervous breakdown' in the middle of a gruelling management course.

The 1992 legislation has attempted to exclude such veiled disease claims by introducing more restrictive definitions of 'accident' ('. . . the application of force or resistance external to the human body . . .'), 'medical misadventure' (in addition to medical negligence, a medical mishap will be covered only if its consequence is both severe and rare, occurring in 1 per cent or less of cases of similar treatment), and 'personal injury' (which, as to mental injuries, includes only those suffered as a consequence of actual physical injuries to the claimant). In all probability, however, the unfairness of the disease exclusion will continue to be one of several factors blurring the dividing line between cover under the scheme and the lack thereof.

The second major criticism of the New Zealand scheme focuses on the legislated bar to litigation for damages (other than for punitive damages) 'arising directly or indirectly out of personal injury' covered by the scheme. Serious questions have been raised about the desirability of a system of no-fault compensation such as that in place in New Zealand, where the victim of rape, gross medical *negligence, or automobile collisions involving alcohol cannot sue for full compensation. Such results appears particularly incongruous in a legal system which unhesitatingly accepts the propriety of the civil lawsuit for property damage (such as damage to *the automobiles* involved in a collision) and a host of other interests protected by the law.

Despite 20 years of operation of the New Zealand scheme and its intense study by other jurisdictions, it remains unique as to its scope of operation and extent of the bar on litigation. Although the 1974 Report of the Australian National Committee of Inquiry, chaired by Mr Justice Woodhouse (who likewise chaired the 1967 New Zealand Royal Commission which preceded the New Zealand scheme), recommended a full no-fault system for Australia, including compensation for disease, its recommendations were not acted upon. The exhaustive inquiry into compensation for personal injury conducted by the English Royal Commission chaired by Lord Pearson rejected the New Zealand approach in its 1978 Report. Despite the fact that the *British Medical Association and the UK *Royal colleges support the introduction of a no-fault scheme, this proposal is, to date, opposed by the UK government, if only on the grounds of cost.

Mention must be made, however, of the most positive aspect of the New Zealand scheme. This is its relatively low cost, which is not merely a function of the modest benefits payable. By largely doing away with the need to determine fault, administration costs are low—amounting to 6 per cent of expenditure in 1991. This is a substantially lower percentage than that found in compensation systems requiring proof of fault.

Sweden's no-fault insurance regime

In contrast to New Zealand's extreme form of no-fault compensation, Sweden employs a multilayered system of accident *insurance to achieve many of the same goals. At the primary level is a universal social insurance providing generous cover for losses caused by disease, accident, or death. Because it compensates without reference to fault, there is no incentive to sue for many minor personal injuries. This universal social insurance is supplemented by four further insurance schemes which aim to compensate personal injury victims at a level comparable to that achieved through a tort action, without the necessity of proving fault. The cover provided by these supplemental schemes is aimed at work-related injuries and disease, traffic accidents, medical and dental treatment injuries, and injuries caused by any manufactured drug. Although only traffic accident insurance is compulsory, the influence of the other schemes is wide as most individuals claim under the schemes which are negotiated on their behalf through collective agreements (work injuries), their county council (medical injuries), or the agreement reached between the drug manufacturers and a consortium of insurance companies (pharmaceutical injuries).

Tort law survives in Sweden to compensate the accident victim who can prove fault in the few areas falling outside the focus of the no-fault insurance schemes. There are differing rules governing the right to sue of a participant in each of the four voluntary schemes. Thus the worker covered by a scheme forming part of a collective agreement will be precluded from suing his or her employer, but the victim of a medical injury does not forgo the chance to sue, although such suits are now rare, given the liberal amounts awarded under the scheme.

Although the Swedish version of no-fault compensation may be criticized for favouring some particular sorts of injuries, thereby raising the predictable problems of demarcation of cover, it may appear to some a more palatable form of no-fault compensation than that in place in New Zealand. Its administrative costs are comparably low. The no-fault systems of both countries aim to achieve the laudable goal of an equitable system of loss-spreading whereby society undertakes to compensate its members for *all* those personal injuries which are an inevitable part of daily life in our modern world.

R. MAHONEY

References
ACC v. *Mitchell* [1992] 2 NZLR 43.
ACC v. *E* [1992] 2 NZLR 426.
Brahams, M. (1988). The Swedish 'no fault' compensation system for medical injuries'. *New Law Journal*, **138**, 31.
Donselaar v. *Donselaar* [1982] 1 NZLR 97.
Green v. *Matheson* [1989] 3 NZLR 564.
Hellner, J. (1986). Accident compensation: the Swedish alternative. *American Journal of Comparative Law*, **34**, 613–35.
Oldertz, C. (1986). Security insurance, patient insurance, and pharmaceutical insurance in Sweden. *American Journal of Comparative Law*, **34**, 636–56.
Sugarman, S. D. (1989). *Doing away with personal injury law*. Quorum Books, New York.
Wallbutton v. *ACC* [1983] New Zealand Accident Compensation Reports 629.

NOGUCHI, HIDEYO (1876–1928). American bacteriologist and immunologist, born in Japan. Noguchi joined Simon *Flexner at the University of Pennsylvania, then moved with him in 1904 to the newly opened *Rockefeller Institute in New York. He was affiliated with that institution until his death in 1928, which resulted from *yellow fever in West Africa while he was carrying out experiments regarding the aetiology of that disease. He and Flexner confirmed that *Treponema pallidum* is the cause of *syphilis, and Noguchi later demonstrated the organism in brain tissue from a patient with *dementia paralytica. In Peru he discovered that a species of *Bartonella* is the cause of *Oroya fever. He also recovered *Leptospira icterohaemorrhagica* from cases

diagnosed clinically as yellow fever, and thought this to be the cause of the disease.

NOISE is defined, medically speaking, as sound of intensity sufficient to disturb and/or discomfort the listener. Excessive noise can cause transient or permanent deafness. For example, young people habitually exposed in discotheques, etc. to amplified sound of 85–100 *decibels (dB) for long periods suffer impairment of hearing acuity (a whisper is up to 30 dB, a normal voice 30–50 dB, a shout about 100 dB). Any noise of 80 dB or more is likely to produce deafness if exposure is prolonged indefinitely. Limits can be set for maximum permissible noise emission in a stated period (e.g. 90 dB in a shift of 8 hours in a working environment). Residents in the vicinity of a motorway should not be exposed to more than 70 dB. In the UK control of noise emission is provided for under Part III of the Control of Pollution Act 1974, which replaced the Noise Abatement Act 1960. Noise control is largely the responsibility of local authorities, the Department of the Environment being the relevant department of central government. Also see ENVIRONMENT AND MEDICINE I.

NOMA is an infective gangrenous ulceration of the mouth, occurring chiefly in children with severe malnutrition.

NOMENCLATURE OF DISEASE. See CLASSIFICATION.

NON-ACCIDENTAL INJURY. See FORENSIC MEDICINE; SURGERY OF TRAUMA.

NON-SPECIFIC URETHRITIS is now a common sexually transmitted disease, often abbreviated to NSU (or NGU, for non-gonococcal urethritis). Almost half the cases are caused by the agent of *trachoma (*Chlamydia trachomatis*), a small proportion by that of *trichomoniasis, and the remainder probably by an organism known as *Ureaplasma urealyticum*, which is often non-pathogenic. See also SEXUALLY TRANSMITTED DISEASE.

NOORDEN, CARL HARKO VON (1858–1944). German physician. He devised a dietary regimen for the treatment of *diabetes mellitus which was widely used.

NORADRENALINE (NOREPINEPHRINE), one of the *catecholamines, is the major *neurotransmitter of the *sympathetic nervous system; it is released at the terminals of the postganglionic fibres, and by the adrenal medulla. Its effects are mainly alpha-adrenergic (see ADRENERGIC BLOCKADE), and it is a powerful elevator of arterial pressure. It is known in the USA as norepinephrine. See also ADRENAL GLAND; ADRENALINE.

NOREPINEPHRINE. See NORADRENALINE.

NORTRYPTILINE is a tricyclic *antidepressant drug.

NOSOCOMIAL INFECTION is an infection acquired in hospital (for which 'nosocome' is an obsolete term).

NOSOLOGY is the nomenclature and *classification of diseases.

NOSTRADAMUS, MICHAEL (Notrèdame, Michel de) (1503–66). French physician and astrologer. He studied medicine at *Montpellier and remained in the town during an epidemic of *plague; this won him enough popular approval to force an unwilling faculty to accept him. After marrying a rich wife in 1547, he turned from orthodox medicine to astrology and casting of horoscopes.

NOSTRUM. A quack remedy (literally 'our own').

NOTHNAGEL, HERMANN KARL WILHELM (1841–1905). German physician. He is remembered for his description of unilateral *oculomotor paralysis associated with ipsilateral cerebellar *ataxia in lesions of the superior cerebellar peduncle of the brain (Nothnagel's syndrome).

NOTIFIABLE DISEASE. See NOTIFICATION OF DISEASE.

NOTIFICATION OF BIRTHS AND DEATHS. See OFFICE OF POPULATION, CENSUSES, AND SURVEYS; REGISTRAR GENERAL; REGISTRARS OF BIRTHS AND DEATHS; REGISTRATION ACT 1836.

NOTIFICATION OF DISEASE. Most countries require notification of certain *communicable diseases to local or central government health authorities. Six such conditions are internationally notifiable to the *World Health Organization: these are *plague, *yellow fever, *smallpox, *cholera, louse-born *relapsing fever, and louse-borne *typhus. A further 20 or so are notifiable in the UK, and about twice that number in the USA. In the UK certain occupational diseases and all cases of *cancer are also notified and registered. Some countries make provision for any condition to be temporarily or regionally notifiable.

NOVOCAINE is a proprietary name for the local anaesthetic agent *procaine.

NOVY, FREDERICK GEORGE (1864–1957). American microbiologist. In 1892 he was appointed professor of bacteriology in Michigan, one of the first Americans to hold such a title. He studied anaerobic bacteria, and described a *Clostridium, later called *Clostridium novyi*. Later he developed culture media for *protozoans, *trypanosomes, and *leishmanii. He also discovered the causative agent of American *relapsing fever.

NOXA. Any agent harmful to the body (plural noxae).

NSAID is the acronym for *n*on-steroidal *anti-inflammatory *d*rug. NSAIDs, most of which are also analgesic, are used in the treatment of musculoskeletal disorders; *acetylsalicylic acid (aspirin) is the prototype. Many compounds are now available. See PHARMACOLOGY.

NUCLEAR MAGNETIC RESONANCE. See MAGNETIC RESONANCE IMAGING (MRI).

NUCLEAR MEDICINE is a medical specialty that uses radioactive materials in *diagnosis, *prognosis, and treatment. Nuclear medicine studies are often presented in the form of pictures, called nuclear images. These are based on the use of the 'tracer principle', invented in 1913 by the Hungarian, Georg de *Hevesy, for which he was awarded the *Nobel prize in 1943. Using the 'tracer principle', Hevesy discovered that living organisms, including the human body, are characterized by a continual turnover of the chemical molecules that make up the body. In a healthy person, there is a delicate balance between the rate of formation and rate of breakdown of the body's chemical constituents. This is called the 'dynamic state of body constituents', the examination of which is the basis for the practice of nuclear medicine.

Since the treatment of many diseases is chemical or pharmacological, it becomes more and more appropriate that chemistry should be widely used in diagnosis and in the planning and monitoring of treatment. The ability to measure *in vivo* chemistry provides a new approach to the design and development of *drugs. It is now possible to determine the relationship between a specific molecular structure and the pharmacological effects of the drug. Radiotracer techniques can be used to classify patients in terms of biochemical abnormalities, and to plan and monitor the effects of treatment.

Radiopharmaceuticals

In nuclear medicine studies, one traces the amount, distribution, and physiological reactions of radioactive substances within the body. With the technology of nuclear medicine it is possible to examine many chemical reactions occurring within the cells of the body. Radioactive tracers, such as glucose, fatty acids, *amino acids, *peptides, and *nucleic acids make it possible to examine the growth and development of the organs of the body, their regeneration and repair when injured, and the response to drugs.

Radioactive *isotopes* are atoms of a given chemical type that emit gamma, beta, or alpha *radiation in the process of *radioactive decay*. Radium and uranium are naturally occurring radioactive atoms; iodine-131, carbon-11, and technetium-99m are examples of man-made radioactive atoms. Radioactive atoms or molecules emit electromagnetic radiation, similar to *X-rays, called photons, or radioactive particles, called alpha or beta particles. Different chemical forms of the same atom are called *isotopes*. A specific radioactive atom is called a *radionuclide*. Radioactive isotopes of practically every element became available at the end of the Second World War, as a result of the wartime invention of the nuclear reactor. Another source of radioactive tracers is the cyclotron, which can be turned on and off in a manner similar to an X-ray machine, whenever the radioactivity is to be produced. Radioactive atoms decay by changing energy states; the rate of change is described by the *half-life* of the radionuclide. In the process of radioactive decay, a *parent radionuclide* decays to a *daughter*. Specific parent/daughter systems include the widely used technetium-99m daughter that is obtained from the parent molybdenum-99. In modern medical practice, about 75–85 per cent of the examination of patients with radioactive tracers involve the use of this radionuclide.

A few radioactive isotopes are used in patient studies in the elemental form. The most important examples are isotopes of iodine for diagnosis and treatment of *thyroid disease. Most studies require that a specific compound be labelled with a radioactive isotope. The compound is selected on the basis of its known physiological or pharmaceutical action or its predicted biological distribution. It is possible to label such small quantities of drugs or other useful compounds with large amounts of radioactivity that injection of the radiopharmaceutical produces no physiological response in the patient. The drug 'traces' the function or biochemical process of interest, but does not interfere with it.

Radiopharmaceuticals can be used safely in medical diagnosis because they disappear rapidly from the body by the process of radioactive decay. Many radiopharmaceuticals also have short biological half-lives, which means they are metabolized and excreted from the body quickly. The combination of the physical and the biological half-life determines the effective half-life of a radiopharmaceutical and the radiation burden to the patient. This is expressed in terms of rads, rems, grays, or sieverts.

Positron-emitting radionuclides, such as carbon-11 (half-life, 20 minutes); flourine-18 (half-life, 110 minutes); and oxygen-15 (half-life, 2 minutes), are produced by a particle accelerator, usually a cyclotron. The radionuclide is then incorporated rapidly into molecules, such as glucose, oxygen, amino acids; neurotransmitter precursors, such as L-Dopa; or drugs, such as *N*-methyl-spiperone, which bind to dopamine receptors. After injection of the patient, a positron emission tomographic (PET) scanner is used to create serial images that portray the distribution of the radioactive tracers at various times after injection, during which time the radioactive molecules take part in biochemical processes in the brain (Fig. 1). Quantitative data are derived from computer analysis of the emitted radioactivity, and converted into 'functional' or 'biochemical' images of the human brain in action. Such images make it possible to relate behaviour to brain chemistry, and brain chemistry to behaviour.

PET studies fall into three categories: regional blood flow, substrate metabolism, and chemical information transfer. In the latter category, PET is beginning to play a major role in establishing the biological correlates of neurological and psychiatric disorders, and may help to monitor the effects on brain chemistry of drugs in the treatment of *depression, *Parkinson's disease, *epilepsy, *Alzheimer's disease, and *substance abuse. PET studies of the heart are making it possible to distinguish dead, non-viable tissue from regions of the *myocardium which would benefit from surgery to restore blood flow to these cells. Metabolic studies in patients with *cancer help establish the spread of disease or the effectiveness of treatment.

Radiopharmaceuticals designed to bind to specific receptors on cancer cells, such as somatostatin receptors in neuroendocrine *tumours, are being used to target specific features of *tumour cells, leading to effective means of treatment. PET can often detect chemical abnormalities before anatomical changes have occurred. The diagnosis of the presence and extent of disease can be made earlier, at a time when treatment is most likely to be effective.

Instrumentation

SPECT (single photon emission computed tomography) and PET instruments are similar to computed tomography (CT) scanners or *magnetic resonance imaging (MRI) devices, but measure photons coming from radioactive decay of a radioactive tracer administered to the patient, rather than X-rays going through the patient

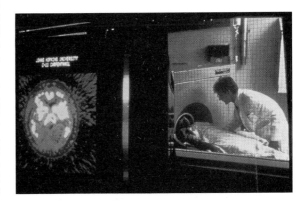

Fig. 1 A positron emission tomography (PET) study performed after injecting the patient with carbon-11 labelled carfentanil shows the distribution of mu opiate receptors (yellow colour) in the brain.

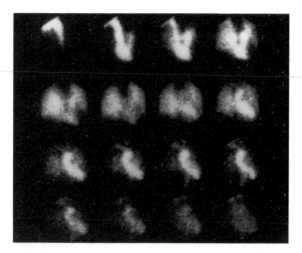

Fig. 2 Serial one-second images were obtained after a bolus injection of technetium-99m-labelled red blood cells. The passage of blood through the chambers of the heart can be followed, and the size and function of the chambers assessed. Further computer processing produces numerical data which permit objective evaluation of the patient's cardiac function.

(CT) or radiowaves coming from the patient (MRI). In some cases the imaging detector rotates around the patient. At other times large radiation detectors are kept stationary. Computers are used to portray the chemical reactions going on within organs being examined.

Patient studies

To perform a nuclear medicine study the patient is injected with a radiopharmaceutical, which is selected to examine a specific biochemical or physiological process. As the radiopharmaceutical reacts in the chemical process under investigation, the radioactive atom emits gamma rays or positrons that are measured with radiation detection instruments. Computers then convert the measurements into 'functional' or 'biochemical' pictures of processes going on within the patient's body.

Among the most common diseases encountered by nuclear physicians are: thyroid disease, cancer, and coronary artery disease (Fig. 2). The general approach of nuclear medicine is to define normal regional function or *biochemistry in normal persons, detect deviations from the normal, and characterize diseases in terms of how the findings differ from normal, using established statistical criteria. This 'physiological' approach is in contrast to the 'ontological' approach, which views disease, such as cancer, as something foreign that has invaded the body.

For example, hyperthyroidism is an increased rate of incorporation of iodine into the thyroid, where it is converted to abnormally increased amounts of the thyroid

hormone, thyroxine. In hypothyroidism, this reaction is abnormally low, and the patient has a deficiency of thyroxine.

Other imaging techniques, such as CT and MRI, define disease on the basis of abnormal structure. The anatomical detail obtained from these techniques provides structural detail often surpassing that seen by surgeons at the operating table.

Nuclear medicine techniques can be used to assess the effectiveness of surgery, *radiotherapy, and *chemotherapy, and can document the extent of disease, and progression or regression in response to different forms of treatment (Fig. 3). Such data permit modifications of the treatment plan sooner than can be determined by the clinical response of the patients or changes in the size of the abnormalities. Thus, treatment need no longer be based solely on clinical response, gross morphology of the lesions, and histopathological examination of

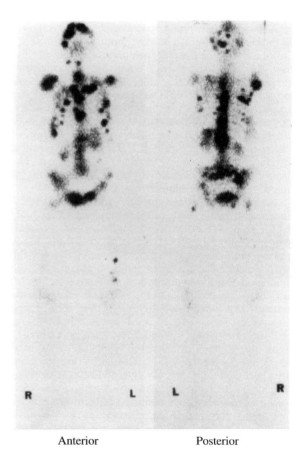

Anterior   Posterior

Fig. 3 A bone scan obtained in a patient with breast cancer reveals widespread metastatic disease, with increased metabolism in the ribs, skull, and other bones.

biopsies. Biochemical characterization of abnormalities, such as cancer, is becoming a new method for classifying patients and their diseases, and for planning and monitoring their treatment.

HENRY N. WAGNER, Jr.

JULIA W. BUCHANAN

References

Phelps, M. E., Mazziotta, J. C., and Schelbert, H. R. (1986). *Positron emission tomography and autoradiography: application in the brain and heart*. Raven Press, New York.

Wagner, H. N. Jr (1989). Nuclear medicine. *Journal of the American Medical Association*, **261**, (19), 2860–2.

Wagner, H. N. Jr (1990). Merrill Sosman Lecture. Drugs, behaviour and brain chemistry. *American Journal of Roentgenology*, **155**, 925–31.

Wagner, H. N. Jr and Conti, P. S. (1991). Advances in medical imaging for cancer diagnosis and treatment. *Cancer*, **67**, 1121–8.

Wagner, H. N. Jr, Buchanan, J. W., and Espinola-Vassallo, D. (1986). *Diagnostic nuclear medicine: patient studies*. Year Book Medical Publishers, Chicago.

NUCLEAR SEXING. Determination of genetic sex by examining the nuclei of somatic cells, usually in a stained smear from the buccal mucosa. In normal females many nuclei show a small stainable body (Barr body) lying in close relationship to the nuclear membrane. This is a condensed mass of chromatin representing one of the two X *chromosomes in an inactive form. In males, who have only one X chromosome, Barr bodies are absent and the smear is said to be 'chromatin negative'. See also GENETICS.

NUCLEIC ACIDS are naturally occurring compounds present in the *chromosomes or *ribosomes of most cells and responsible either for storing genetic information or translating it into the structure of proteins. See DEOXYRIBONUCLEIC ACID (DNA); RIBONUCLEIC ACID (RNA).

NUCLEOLUS. A small dense body distinguishable within the nucleus of most cells, concerned with the synthesis of ribosomal ribonucleic acid.

NUCLEOPROTEINS are compounds consisting of a *nucleic acid in combination with a *protein.

NUCLEUS. The cell nucleus is a membrane-bounded body found within the *cytoplasm of most biological cells, of both plants and animals (termed *eukaryotic* on that account). It contains the *chromosomes. In the non-dividing cell, the nucleus is spherical or ovoid by light microscopy and usually appears homogeneous except for one or more denser bodies termed nucleoli and granules of heterochromatin; when fixed it contains a darkly staining basophilic network. At the onset of mitosis or meiosis, the chromosomes separate and become visible. See CELL AND CELL BIOLOGY.

NUFFIELD, LORD. See MORRIS, WILLIAM.

NUFFIELD PROVINCIAL HOSPITALS TRUST. Founded by Lord Nuffield in 1940, the Trust's original purposes were defined as 'the co-ordination on a regional basis of hospital, medical, and associated health services throughout the provinces; the making of financial provision for the creation, carrying on, or extension of such hospital, medical, and associated health services as are necessary for such co-ordination; and the promotion of improved organization and efficient development of hospital, medical, and associated health services throughout the provinces' (provinces being taken to mean outside the Metropolitan Police District of London). Since the foundation of the *National Health Service in 1948 led to the effective regionalization of the health services in the UK, the main purpose of the Trust has been to assist the development and improvement of hospital and other health services generally and the encouragement of health services research, interpreted in the widest sense. The making of grants has been a major function, usually, although not invariably, to university departments. More recently, the adoption of an 'institute' role in relation to policy exploration has resulted in a programme of seminars, lectures, and conferences and in a series of Trust publications. The Trust has also established working groups in topics within its main interests.

NURSE-PRACTITIONER. A qualified nurse whose role in the provision of primary health care has been enlarged beyond that traditionally assigned to the nursing profession, embracing functions normally carried out by medical practitioners, for example the making of diagnoses and the prescribing of medicaments. See NURSING IN NORTH AMERICA.

NURSES ACTS 1943–1969. Following the original UK Nurses Registration Act of 1919, a series of Nurses Acts were passed in 1943, 1949, 1957, 1961, 1964, and 1969. Their provisions included the enrolment of assistant nurses, reconstitution of the General Nursing Council, reorganization of the Register of Nurses to include male nurses, financial support for training and the inspecting of training schools, evaluation of nurses trained outside the UK, and abolition of the annual retention fee.

NURSES AGENCY ACT 1957. This UK Act introduced regulation of agencies for the supply of nurses. Persons carrying on such an agency must be licensed annually by the appropriate local authority. The licensing authority may inspect records and premises of agencies. Selection of nurses to be provided for each particular case must be made by or under the supervision of a registered nurse or general medical practitioner, and prescribed records must be kept. Any person supplied with a nurse must be advised in writing as to his or her qualifications. The Act prescribed penalties for contraventions of its provisions.

NURSING HOME ACT 1975. This UK Act consolidated previous legislation concerning nursing homes contained in the *Public Health Act 1936 and the *Mental Health Act 1959. A nursing home is defined as any premises used or intended to be used for the reception and provision of nursing for persons suffering from any sickness, injury, or infirmity but excluding NHS hospitals. Maternity homes are included, and mental nursing homes are also defined. Powers of registration, control, and inspection of nursing homes had already been conferred on the Secretary of State for Health and Social Services under the *National Health Service (Reorganization) Act 1973.

NURSING HOMES. Small private hospitals.

NURSING IN THE ARMED SERVICES. See ARMED FORCES OF THE USA: MEDICAL SERVICES; DEFENCE MEDICAL SERVICES (UK).

NURSING IN NORTH AMERICA
Introduction
This is an introduction to North American nursing in relation to the types of educational preparation required (differentiating the types of individuals who are called nurses and their educational preparation) to practise as a registered nurse, as well as the types of advanced education available to registered nurses. In addition to basic and advanced education, nursing specialization is discussed.

The USA and Canada are similar, but also different. Registered nurses in the USA have little difficulty practising their profession, or achieving advanced education, in Canada. The reverse is equally true. Registered nurses move across the national border with ease and frequency. Yet, the historical development of nursing has differed and the means of advancing the profession have had different emphasis. For a full description of these differences, as well as the historical development of nursing in North America, see Schlotfeldt (1986).

Educational preparation of the registered nurse
In North America there are five different routes to becoming licensed as a registered nurse. Graduates of all five programmes are eligible to sit for the national licensing examinations. The traditional route, now becoming more rare, is the 2–3 year hospital training school programme. This programme was developed from the Florence *Nightingale model and was the primary method of achieving nursing education until the 1970s, when baccalaureate education began to be seen as the preferred route. Hospital students are taught by faculty members employed by the hospital, and learn their skills in the hospital. The training programmes prepare general duty nurses able to staff the hospital in all areas: *paediatrics, *maternity, *surgery, *medicine, *orthopaedics, and so on.

The second route, which became popular in the 1970s, is the two-year community college programme. These programmes are more prevalent in the western US where there are more community colleges providing the first 2 years of university education than in any other region. University and college education are similar concepts in North America. Both offer post-secondary education programmes. The two-year college offers either the first 2 years of university education in a community college, or two-year technical programmes such as engineering, draughtsmanship, and nursing. Small, privately endowed 4-year baccalaureate programmes are frequently called colleges, although some are entitled 'universities'. 'University' is frequently reserved for large state or provincially funded schools that offer graduate degrees, specifically the Ph.D. Students receive the Associate of Arts (or Associate of Science) degree common to community colleges. Community colleges have a planned curriculum, including introductory courses in *anatomy and *physiology, *sociology, English, chemistry, and biology. Community colleges usually develop contract systems with nearby hospitals for student clinical experience. University faculty members are present in the setting where the student obtains the clinical experience. Faculty members are present to answer questions, observe performance, and provide consultation. Some universities also contract for *preceptors* in the clinical setting to assist in the teaching of students. A preceptor is an employee of the hospital or agency in which the student is placed for clinical experience. The preceptor provides the clinical supervision that would otherwise be provided by the faculty person. Preceptors are carefully selected by the faculty for their clinical skills and educational background before being appointed to the position. Preceptorship is becoming more common as a teaching aid in clinical placements.

The third route, preferred today, is the baccalaureate programme, in which students are treated as any other university student receiving a bachelor's degree in the sciences. Nursing is considered to be an applied science and is granted the degree, Bachelor of Science in Nursing. These programmes of study, like their science counterparts, usually take 4 years to complete, although some take 5 years. Students will take their basic physical and social sciences with other university students and take their nursing subjects from the nursing faculty. If the university has an affiliated hospital, many students will do their general nursing in that institution. Many schools, however, do not have hospitals, so university schools will contract with community hospitals and agencies to provide clinical experience. Students are then rotated through various hospital departments and out-patient or community clinics and agencies during the school year, in conjunction with their course work. All students will be exposed to nursing of children, the childbearing family, chronic and acute illnesses in adults, women's health, mental health (psychiatric nursing), and community health nursing. The emphasis, in the university setting, is on health promotion and disease prevention. Acute care, nursing interventions, nursing theory, and *rehabilitation or home and chronic care are also part of the curriculum.

The prerequisites to entry into these three programmes or routes to achieving licensure are:(1) a high school education, or the equivalent; (2) good marks; and (3) prerequisite course work.

The fourth route is specifically designed for those individuals already possessing a bachelor's degree. There are a few generic master's programmes in nursing (i.e. McGill University, Yale University) where the individual can take a 2–3 year course, receive a master's degree (M.N. or M.Sc.—Applied) in nursing and sit for the licensing examination. Generic nursing programme refers to the basic nursing education leading to licensure as a registered nurse. The standard required courses and clinical experience mandated by the state board of nursing and the national accreditation board comprise the *generic curriculum*. Usually, the applicant with a bachelor's degree in another field will apply to either an Associate of Arts degree programme or to a baccalaureate degree programme for their nursing education, as these schools are easier to access.

The last route for obtaining a basic nursing education, is to apply to one of three schools in the USA (Case Western Reserve University in Cleveland, Ohio; Rush Presbyterian Hospital in Chicago, Illinois; and the University of Colorado in Denver) which offer the Doctorate of Nursing (DN or ND) degree. These programmes range from 3 to 6 years in length. They prepare the individual to sit for the licensing examination and require a bachelor's degree (in any field) as a prerequisite for admission.

Baccalaureate education is the preferred route for obtaining the education and practice necessary to practise nursing, and both Canada and the USA have set the year 2000 as the deadline to achieve this goal. Baccalaureate education, unlike the hospital training programmes and the community college programmes, includes preparation for community health nursing in its curriculum, introduces students to nursing research, and expects the baccalaureate graduate to use research findings as the basis for practice.

Pre-baccalaureate education (hospital training programmes, 2-year community college programmes), as a result, are either being phased out or are evolving in creative ways, to provide a route of entry into the baccalaureate programme. Many hospitals and community colleges are collaborating with baccalaureate schools of nursing to provide the first 2 years of the baccalaureate programme, while the university provides the last 2 years. In this way the various curricula become standardized, textbooks and lectures become equivalent. Students may choose not to continue toward a baccalaureate programme or may take extra course work and sit for their examinations. In many schools of nursing offering the baccalaureate degree, places are reserved for the registered nurse from a community college or hospital school who wishes to continue his or her education in nursing. They are called post-basic students (Canada) or RN Completion (US) students. In this way, North American schools are attempting to assist registered nurses to meet the bachelor's degree requirement by the year 2000.

The licensed vocational nurse (LVN), practical nurse (LPN), and nursing assistant (NA)

To assist the registered nurse, a series of assistant positions were created. The licensed vocational nurse (LVN) or licensed practical nurse (LPN) in the USA, and the nursing assistant (NA) in Canada, have all received 1 year of coursework and experience in general nursing. They are all qualified to be employed in hospitals and *nursing homes, to give general nursing care, medical treatment, and to dispense medications. In many in-patient facilities, they staff the institution under the direction of one registered nurse who serves as the director of nursing. They are trained in special training programmes and are licensed by examination.

In the USA, the Veterans Administration Psychiatric Hospitals had educational programmes for nursing assistants that combined a teaching programme with clinical experience. These programmes were 2 years in length and prepared the candidate to assist the registered nurse in the in-patient care and treatment of the psychiatric veteran.

Nurse's aides are another category of nursing assistant. Aides are trained by the employing institution for direct patient care and maintenance of the patient's environment. These training programmes rarely last more than 6 months, some are as short as 2 weeks. The aides may give bed-baths, feed and dress patients, take temperatures and *blood pressures, or they may be limited to transporting patients and changing water. Each institution determines the degree of responsibility of the nurse's aide. In some nursing homes, all patient care is given by nurse's aides under the supervision of the LVN. Many aides, through years of experience in the same institution, become knowledgeable about patient care, and are very proud of their profession. Others simply seek this field of employment during their school years as temporary employment.

Licensure

In North America, RN is reserved for the basic license to practise general nursing in a particular state or province. The license is conferred upon a qualified applicant upon completion of a required (and/or accredited) course of studies and satisfactory performance in the licensure examination. Annual fees are paid to maintain licensure. In the USA evidence of continuing education in nursing is part of the maintenance of current licensure.

Basic licensure does not cover advanced practice or clinical specialization. Specializations such as *mid-wifery or *nurse practitioner roles require an additional programme of required coursework and clinical experience, and a further examination before certification.

Advanced education

Because basic or generic nursing students are being prepared at the bachelor's, master's, and doctoral levels, there must be qualified faculty members prepared to teach them. Teachers in faculties of nursing are being required to obtain graduate education in nursing (preferably both the master's and doctoral degrees) with at least one graduate degree in nursing. Baccalaureate students expect their teachers to be better educated than they are, and they expect them to be better educated in nursing. There are some differences in Canada and the USA in the style and content of the master's and doctoral degrees in nursing, but the two countries also have much in common.

Entry into a master's programme in nursing requires a bachelor's degree in nursing, or its equivalent (equivalence is established by the admissions committee in each school). The degree is course-based, and may or may not require a research project, culminating in a master's thesis. In many American schools, the applicant identifies a clinical area in which she or he wishes to become a specialist. The programme of study (coursework and clinical experience) is already prescribed. The student passes the requisite number of courses for the degree, which varies from 1 to 2 years in length. Schools may or may not require a final comprehensive examination or a research project. In contrast, Canadian schools emphasize the research component of the degree, with either a research project or a master's thesis requisite to the degree. Although there are required courses in nursing theory and research methods, there are fewer required courses than in the American schools. Students may choose among a variety of course options to fulfil a content requirement, while many American schools will specify which course will meet the requirement. Length of the programme varies in the Canadian schools depending upon the research topic chosen for study. A comprehensive examination may or may not be required, but the student is expected to defend a thesis.

Some schools of nursing in North America also provide advanced preparation for those wishing to pursue a career in nursing education or administration. These specialties are frequently part of the master's degree in nursing, and usually require additional coursework and supervised experience. If no specialization is available within a nursing programme, administrators and educators will seek advanced preparation from schools of education.

Entry into a nursing doctoral programme in the USA and Canada is based upon successful completion of a master's degree (preferably in nursing). In the USA, individual universities will determine which degree the faculty can confer: the Ph.D. in nursing, the DNSc. or DNS (Doctor of nursing science), or the DSN (doctor of science in nursing). The requirements for these degrees are similar. All require a doctoral dissertation.

Doctoral programmes in nursing vary between the two countries. In Canada, where the first Ph.D. in nursing programme was started at the University of Alberta in 1992, the emphasis is again upon the research undertaken by the candidate, rather than required coursework. Entrance into one of the five Canadian Ph.D. programmes is based upon an earned master's degree in nursing, or its equivalent. There are very few required courses, compared with their American counterparts, and coursework is determined by the candidate in consultation with the faculty supervisor. In the USA, there are more than 40 doctoral programmes in nursing. Coursework is required at the doctoral level and is based upon coursework completed at the master's level. Students are not usually admitted post-baccalaureate to a doctoral programme. The supervisory committee and the dissertation chair may be determined after the first year of coursework.

Clinical specialization in nursing

In both Canada and the USA, clinical specialization is available to any registered nurse. The types of specialties are predetermined by educational preparation. Thus, all specializations are available to the baccalaureate-prepared nurse while only some are available to the diploma or hospital-trained nurse. Some specializations are achieved through experience, others are available only through advanced education.

Generalist

All graduates of all generic nursing programmes are considered to be generalists. They have been educated to work in almost any in-patient setting. New graduates are expected to learn the particular skills requisite to the new posting, as is any new employee. In fact, most hospitals have an orientation programme for new employees and/or new graduates. Although the educational institution has introduced the new graduate to the concepts and skills necessary for a new practitioner, there is no claim that the new graduate is skilled in every possible clinical area or in every possible clinical procedure or treatment. No generic programme claims to meet the needs of all possible employing institutions. Instead, the programmes claim to have prepared the new practitioner to be able to find the help needed if he or she does not know how to do a particular assignment. Most educational institutions cannot afford to prepare a practitioner who is capable of being a skilled practitioner in all areas. To prepare a generalist at the entry level who is skilled in most areas of practice, would require the same length of programme as is currently the base for the nursing doctorate.

Specialist

(a) Clinical specialist. There are several avenues to becoming a *clinical* specialist. Clinical specialization may be gained through years of clinical experience in an area and/or through educational programmes at the post-basic or graduate level. In the USA, specialization is most frequently seen as part of graduate education in nursing, which includes supervised clinical experience in the area. In some cases, later certification of this specialization may be obtained through advanced supervised practice over time (sometimes 2 years) followed by an examination. The areas in which graduate students may specialize are wide, including midwifery, maternity nursing, mental health nursing, *intensive care nursing, *community health nursing, *gerontology nursing, *cancer nursing, and so on. Within each of these areas there are further areas of specialization.

In Canada, the same specialties are found; however, there is also a *psychiatric nursing clinical specialty at the primary basic education level. Clinical specialization is offered at both the graduate level and the post-basic level. Certificate programmes include such areas as perinatal intensive care nursing and midwifery. There are a few training schools for psychiatric nursing still in existence in which students specialize in this field throughout their training and receive a minimum of general nursing preparation. These nurses sit for a different examination and receive a different licence. They are paid on a different pay scale and have a different professional union. They receive a diploma or certificate but do not receive a university degree of any kind. At the time of writing, an effort is being made to bring these psychiatric nurses into mainstream nursing by providing them with an educational experience at the university similar to that of the post-basic nurse. These psychiatric nurses may then sit for the national licensing examination to become registered nurses. The training programmes for registered psychiatric nurses in psychiatric institutions are expected to die out or to shift their focus to the training of psychiatric aides or nursing assistants.

A second area of clinical specialization, in Canada, that does not require advanced education, is the outpost nurse. These nurses live and work in the Yukon and the Northwest Territories, providing primary care to populations having no physicians within hundreds of miles. In emergencies, patients are flown south to the nearest medical centre for care. Otherwise, nurses provide all health-care services. There are advanced training programmes for nurses (2 years) in this field (at Dalhousie University) based upon 2 years' experience in the north.

The third method of achieving clinical specialization is through clinical experience in an area. Nurses become knowledgeable about a clinical specialty from working with clients and physicians, but are never directly rewarded for this knowledge and are never certified for this specialty.

(b) Nurse practitioner. The title, nurse practitioner, in the USA is reserved for a special form of clinical specialization. (Nurse practitioners are not physician's assistants, although many have confused the two groups. Physician's assistants are trained by physicians in schools of medicine to meet their special needs. This is not true of nurse practitioners.) The programmes for nurse practitioners are usually reserved for post-basic students or graduate students. The emphasis is upon skill development in primary health care as well as in physical assessment and intervention into minor medical problems. Nurse practitioners are well qualified to work independently in outpost nursing or in remote rural areas. Final examinations and certification are required for qualification. Medical group practice offices in the USA will have nurse practitioners and physicians working together, each having his or her own clients. Nurse practitioners are capable of seeing and examining most patients, referring patients they cannot handle to the physician.

Accreditation of schools of nursing

All schools of nursing in the USA must receive national evaluation every 7 years. Accreditation is serious in that students who graduate from an non-accredited school may be denied admission to advanced education. New schools of nursing or new programmes must be evaluated at or before the third year of the programme. Deans of schools of nursing meet regularly (in state, regional, and national fora) to discuss changes in regulations and changes in education. In addition to the national accreditation process, state boards of nursing regularly review the schools of nursing in their states to determine whether the schools are following the changes in the requirements for licensure. These reviews are more frequent than the national reviews. Finally, universities regularly review the programmes and curricula of their various schools, faculties, and departments. Schools of nursing are not exempted from this review process.

All three reviews require a statement of the goals and objectives of the school, a discussion with faculty members and students, including: (1) demographic data and scholarship; (2) explanations of any changes since the previous review; and (3) a discussion of the courses and clinical placements. Course outlines, for every course taught in the school of nursing (clinical and academic), are prepared according to a standard format. Student evaluations of each course are made available to the review team. When the review team arrives at the school for the on-site visit, students, faculty, and administration in every programme are interviewed. The review team will give a final oral report to the school before departure, as well as their recommendation regarding accreditation. The school can provide additional documentation to the review committee as needed.

The difference between Canada and the USA is that schools of nursing in Canada are evaluated for national accreditation voluntarily. The onus of lack of accreditation is the same in both countries.

Summary and conclusions

There are five distinct routes to preparation of the registered nurse in North America, one of which, the ND, or Doctor of Nursing, is available only in the USA. Registered nurses in either country may practise nursing in the other country or be admitted to advanced education programmes. National reciprocity is based upon the similarity of the educational programmes leading to licensure. Both countries offer course-based master's and doctoral programmes based upon the baccalaureate degree in nursing. These advanced degrees in nursing focus upon nursing specialties, advanced practice, theory, and research. The intent of all levels of nursing education is to improve nursing practice.

PAMELA J. BRINK

References
Kerr, J. R. and MacPhail, J. (1991). *Canadian nursing: issues and perspectives*. C. V. Mosby, Ottawa.
Schlotfeldt, R. M. (1986). Nursing in the USA and Canada. In *The Oxford companion to medicine*, (ed. J. Walton, P. B. Beeson, and R. Bodley Scott), pp. 893–902. Oxford University Press, Oxford.

NURSING IN THE UK. The emergence of nursing as a role for a trained skilled person occurred during the second half of the 19th century, as the result of an outburst of scientific and medical discoveries, and of the social pressures resulting from the Industrial Revolution and its related events.

Throughout the centuries, the women in a household cared for the sick of their family, just as they fed and clothed them in health. The care of the indigent and homeless sick devolved mostly on religious communities until the Reformation. The nursing historian finds much of interest in these times, but this account will be confined to the 19th and 20th centuries.

Florence *Nightingale wrote in 1892:

There comes a crisis in the lives of all social movements. This has come in the case of nursing in about thirty years. For nursing was born but about thirty years ago. Before it did not exist, though sickness is as old as the world.

She was alluding to the establishment of the first nurse-training school at *St Thomas's Hospital in 1860. She recognized that there was a body of nursing knowledge, manual skills, and ethical principles that could be taught; she had the influence, following her work in the Crimean War, to persuade people to believe her. Moreover, she showed in her *Notes on nursing*

that nursing knowledge could be objectively defined and based on scientific rules.

At one time, men could be divided into landed gentry, merchants and shopkeepers, and 'others'. The Industrial Revolution saw the rise of a prosperous middle class of manufacturers who began to seek professional advancement for their children. Medicine attracted many applicants, all able to pay for hospital experience, and doctors soon needed to divide beds among themselves for teaching purposes. In the first half of the 19th century, hospitals in London and the big provincial cities had so many medical students that there was no need of nurses, except as unskilled attendants. One effect of this surge of medical training was that acute medicine and surgery provided all the 'interesting' cases and 'good teaching material', and the chronic sick, the enfeebled aged, and the psychiatrically ill were not wanted in the voluntary hospitals. This had far-reaching effects, felt even today in the *National Health Service, and in the lack of esteem felt for some specialties like *geriatric care, in which the need is very great.

There were two important facts that made nursing women's work. First, nursing was always seen as part of domestic household work; secondly, as Josephine Butler noticed in 1866 (*Education and employment of women*, London, 1866, p.3), then there were 2.5 million women, mostly spinsters and widows, seeking means of support through work.

Working-class women might hope to find employment in factories where, although badly paid and overworked, they met outside their homes, and learned the facts of industrial life. Middle-class women could be governesses, often working only for their keep, or clerks working a 60-hour week for 12 shillings. A few tried to gain registration as doctors, and many began to realize that without a vote women had no political power. When, during the Crimean War (1854–56), Florence Nightingale showed that there was work that intelligent women could do in hospital, so enthusiastic was the response that by the 1890s more women wanted to nurse than could be trained.

Miss Nightingale wrote to Benjamin Jowett in 1889, 'When very many years ago I planned a future, my one idea was not organising a hospital but organising a religion'. Thus for nearly three-quarters of a century nursing in the UK was fashioned by a great pioneer and by the social trends of Victorian England. Nurses were to be women, and dedicated to their work; they were thus doubly vulnerable to economic exploitation, and remained so until the middle of the 20th century.

Our feelings and ideas about pre-Nightingale nursing derive from two sources. One is fiction; how powerful is the image of Sairey *Gamp, and of the women whom Scrooge saw quarrelling over his clothes after his 'death'. The other is fact. *St Bartholomew's Hospital, London, has continuous records from 1549; from the accounts of the governors' meetings one can picture the work of the sisters (charge-nurses) who lived in a room off their wards, gave simple care, fetched the patient's food from the buttery, washed their ward linen, and spent their 'spare' time in spinning. Much unpretentious care was given, often with heroism in times of plague and pestilence.

Miss Nightingale's new recruits were, not unnaturally, rather disdainful and disapproving about those whom they were replacing. Their predecessors might have been forgiven for some of the ways in which they maintained fortitude in days before *anaesthetics and *antiseptics. A sister wrote in 1902 about what she saw on entering the first school at St Bartholomew's Hospital in 1877.

Drunkenness was very common among the staff nurses, who were chiefly of the charwoman type, frequently of bad character, with little or no education, and few of them with even an elementary knowledge of nursing . . . One woman I remember who came some little time after I did, and under whom I worked, had been a lady's maid, and had never done a day's nursing. She was, however, of a decidedly superior class to any of the others . . . Nursing, as you understand it now, was utterly unknown. Patients were not nursed, they were attended to, more or less . . . The work was very hard—lockers, locker boards and tables of course to scrub every day. No, we did not as a rule scrub the floors, though I have scrubbed the front ward of Matthew on a special occasion before 6 a.m. . . . The patients had their beds made once a day, the bad ones had their sheets drawn at night . . . then you thought nothing of having fourteen or fifteen poultices to change. All wounds of course suppurated, and required poulticing two or three times a day . . . the thermometers in use then were very much longer than those in use now, and had to be read while in position, as they ran down at once when removed from the mouth or armpit. They cost 12/6d each. The sisters and nurses never used a thermometer, the dressers and clerks took the temperatures when required.

This was the nursing scene in 1877. Infection, both medical and surgical, was rife. The nurse worked long hours at hard work with little reward. Light was, however, breaking on the hospital scene. Anaesthesia had arrived to relieve the lot of the patients and of surgeons; the nature of infections such as *typhoid and *cholera began to be understood. Doctors were now able to cure. The nurse stopped scrubbing the floor, and began her role by taking over duties delegated from the doctor, so becoming the servant of the doctor rather than of the patient. This relationship was facilitated by the fact that doctors were men and nurses women, each readily accepting the Victorian mode of dependency.

State registration
Nursing in the 1880s and 1890s involved physical and mental stress. *Streptococcal infections were dangerous, so *scarlet fever, *nephritis, and *rheumatic fever afflicted them. Septic fingers were painful and disabling, *diphtheria and *tuberculosis could still be fatal. Chronic foot pain was a common cause of drop-out until working hours became reasonable a century later.

Yet these women found time not only to upgrade hospital care, but to dream of professionalism. They thought and talked about the content of nursing, how long training should be, how to establish higher education (was it possible that there might one day be university degrees in nursing?). Above all, they thought about statutory training and state registration.

Miss Nightingale had little use for registration until, late in her life, she recognized it as inevitable. She still thought of nursing as a kind of religious life for spinsters: when they married, they left nursing. Mrs Bedford Fenwick, the great proponent of registration and professionalism, throughout a long life wrote, spoke, and worked unceasingly, seeking support, helping to promote bills, and finally living to see state registration attained in 1919. She was the first nurse on the register of the *General Nursing Council (GNC).

Overseas nursing
By the close of the 19th century British nurses were being appointed to work for the government in the (then) British colonies. Before state registration in 1919 these nurses had no agreed corpus of nursing knowledge to teach, and some simply imparted what they had learnt at home. It was possible to hear African students describing how to give a bed-bath, beginning 'First close the nearby windows', as if they were in Liverpool or Glasgow.

The overseas nurses had to adapt not only to climatic extremes and diseases they had never known before, but to different social systems. It seemed unnatural to some cultures to cherish the diseased and sickly, and the physical care involved in nursing was a task for menials, not for the educated. Women in many societies could not nurse men, so male students had to be recruited. Mission hospitals and mission nurses contributed along with colleagues in the Overseas Nursing Association to the growth of indigenous nursing patterns. Hong Kong was the first colony to obtain reciprocal registration with the GNC in 1935. Great advances were made between the First and Second World Wars. Many people came to train in the UK, and returned to train others.

At the turn of the century British nurses taught and trained their colleagues overseas. Eighty years later nurses of the Third World may have things to teach us. Developing countries may believe that prestigious hospital buildings for the sick are an out-of-place export from older societies, and that resources can be more profitably used on *immunization, *health education, *dietetics, and *antenatal and *midwifery services. In such cultures nurses have a key role, and British nurses may yet learn from them how nursing skills are best deployed.

The turn of the century
By the end of the 19th century the new nurse of Florence Nightingale's ideals had displaced the pre-Crimean one as the model (Fig. 1). Hospitals and their matrons

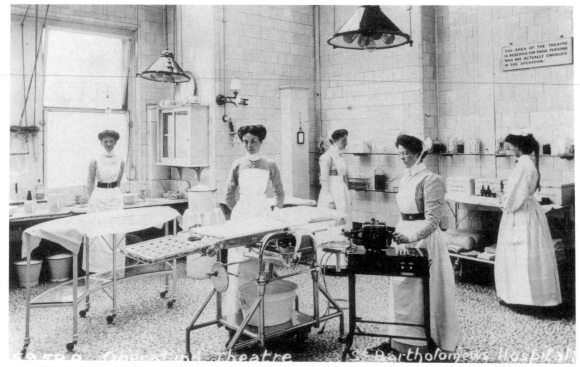

Fig. 1 The coming of anaesthetics and asepsis began the emergence of a technical role for the nurse, as shown in this photograph of an operating theatre at St Bartholomew's Hospital. (Reproduced by permission of the Medical Illustration Department, St Bartholomew's Hospital, London.)

(nurses in charge of hospitals) were much concerned with the length of nurses' training and had a vested interest in making it lengthy, as the pay of the probationer was minute, and if she formed a major part of the work force, this helped impecunious hospitals. The period of training successively rose from 1 to 2 and then to 3 years. This was the limit of acceptability, except in the fashionable teaching hospitals, which were able to require a fourth year as a staff nurse.

Many organizations were formed to further the aim of state registration, but nurses were also concerned with other activities including the struggle for votes for women in the UK, and formulation of their own role and the best means of educating them for it. Mrs Bedford Fenwick was an international as well as a national protagonist of registration, and keenly interested in education. In the *Nursing Record*, which she edited and mostly wrote for nearly half a century, she gave book prizes for published 'case studies' as a means of encouraging nurses to observe their patients and their illnesses, and to record the results of care. She said at the International Council of Nurses in 1907:

To enumerate our most pressing needs; we require preliminary education before entering hospital wards; we need postgraduate education to keep us in the running; we need special instruction as teachers to fit us for the responsible positions of

sisters and superintendents; we need a state-constituted board to examine and maintain discipline in our ranks, and we must have legal status to protect our legal rights and to ensure us ample professional autonomy.

All her aims have now been realized, but the first decade of the 20th century, was a time of increasing anxiety as the shadow of approaching war inhibited action in many spheres. Many accounts appeared of what was happening to bedside nurses in the closed world of hospital wards and nurses' homes. The work still retained the dual aspect of domestic work and personal care (Fig. 2). The following account was written by a woman who began to train in 1916, and who later headed Lady Minto's Indian Nursing Service. She says of her probationer days:

Life was hard. Cleaning and washing patients, making beds, giving bedpans, and then cleaning again . . . lockers, brasses, mackintoshes, spittoons. Very seldom were we probationers allowed contact with anything interesting or instructive. Many fell by the way, as often as not because of the ward sisters' stinging sarcasm. Medical students suffered in the same way, but they were in the wards each day for a short time only.

With our long hours on duty, one particular patient depended so much on the personal touch of the individual nurse. We really did see them through their illness, which I think made our job so absorbingly interesting. We were at

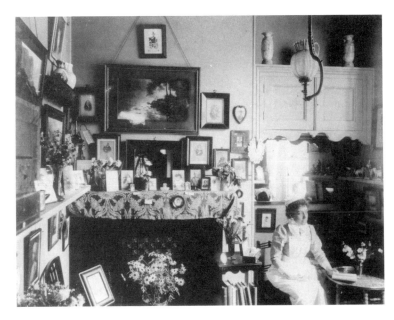

Fig. 2 Nursing as a vocation. The sister in the early 20th century divided her life between the patients in her ward and her sitting room which led off it. (Reproduced by permission of the Medical Illustration Department, St Bartholomew's Hospital, London.)

their bedside each day for ten to thirteen hours . . . and for twelve hours on night duty . . . we became part and parcel of their sufferings.

Treatments included saline infusions, bread, linseed and kaolin poultices, and mustard plasters. I have seen cupping done to relieve congestion and have myself applied leeches.

Lest indeed it should be thought that skilled sustained personal attention was unlikely to be curative, she also related how in 1923 in India she was sent to nurse an engineer's wife with blackwater fever at a small coalfield in the hills. She went up to the bungalow in a coalbucket, together with the coffin which it was thought her patient would need very soon. A week later the nurse triumphantly sent the coffin down again empty.

In the wards probationers (student nurses) worked under continual blame and criticism. It was as if training had to be made as rigorous as possible, so that only the strongest survived. It is sometimes said that this was the result of rule by elderly spinsters, but this is a simplistic view. Medical students were managed in much the same way by the consultants: ward rounds were often painful occasions, when learners were held up to ridicule in front of their patients.

This relationship with seniors had to be borne in surroundings of pain and death, so what induced young women to support it? The challenge to endure is always powerful, and patients were always appreciative. Juniors had great camaraderie among themselves, and this

was especially evident among those who joined on the same day. Nurses of a 'set' often remained friends for life, and enjoyed recounting stories of the hardships they had endured. They called each other by their surnames, as girls then did at university, in imitation of men.

The First World War and after

The effect of the First World War on nursing was tremendous. Nurses were needed in unprecedented numbers, and the Voluntary Aid Detachment (VAD) founded by the British *Red Cross met part of the demand. Male nurses from mental hospitals left to join the services, as did many from general hospitals. There were 2 million casualties on the Western Front alone, mostly adult men, so that there were many spinsters and widows who would have to earn a living after the war.

During the war women proved themselves in many fields. The vote could no longer be withheld, and the nurses' demand for state registration had to be granted.

The College of Nursing was founded in 1916 to further nursing interests, and now survives as the Royal College of Nursing (RCN), the main professional body concerned with educational policy, ethical standards, and conditions of service. In 1920 a General Nursing Council was established to supervise instruction and examinations, and to compile a register of trained nurses.

Nurses in the thirties were aware of social trends envisaging a welfare state with more state control of individuals, but were busy with their own internal problems of registration, curriculum development, and education. Those who worked in larger general and teaching hospitals remember this as a time of stability in a world that was about to explode. Hours were still long and pay low, but the nursing role was well established: it was to give comfort; the patient always came first. Nurses did not run unless there was a fire or *haemorrhage. Such axioms were not thought of as clichés, but as truths to be followed.

'Good nursing' might still save lives for which no medical cure existed. *Diabetes was treated by *insulin, but lobar *pneumonia patients still suffered a long dangerous illness culminating in a crisis, through which nurses hoped to bring them. Healthy young men who had a *hernia operation stayed in bed until the stitches were removed. A drug called *prontosil had been discovered which could cure infections. *Blood transfusion was becoming common, so surgical *shock was retreating. Lung surgery was becoming safer, and heart surgery was on the horizon.

One of the most disturbing things nurses then had to learn was that comfortable bed-rest might be lethal, and that nursing care which encouraged immobility was a disservice. Venous *thrombosis and pulmonary *embolism, and many other less dangerous but uncomfortable conditions, were attributed to bed-rest. Early mobility for patients made nurses question their clinical practices in many fields.

The Second World War and after

Recruitment remained difficult all through the war, and civilian hospitals had a particularly hard time. In 1944 it was decided to direct nurses to priority areas, but the opening of the Second Front changed the picture, and in 1945 came peace.

During the war women won advancement in many fields, while sharing the hardships of the battlefield and the prisoner-of-war camps. Many new forms of work were opened up to women, and in the years of full employment they had no difficulty in finding skilled jobs. Nursing had lost its old appeal as the major field of work open to women. It was now seen as an area of low pay with hard work in Victorian premises, and many women were no longer eager to tolerate such conditions.

In an endeavour to fill vacancies, more auxiliaries and students were recruited, so that the ratio of untrained and trained staff altered for the worse. The age of entry was lowered in the hope that there were many young people who went elsewhere because they were too young to nurse. Headmistresses now saw nursing as an occupation for the undereducated and were unwilling to help intelligent candidates to nurse.

The inauguration of the NHS in 1946 should have been a time of hope. A free health service was to be one basis of the new caring society, but nurses and doctors were depressed and anxious. Assistant nurses were now a statutory grade, working for enrolment with the GNC. One-year 'crash' courses for people with wartime nursing experience abounded. 'Cadet' schemes for children leaving school were legion, in the hope that bridging the gap between school and hospital would keep up numbers. All these increased the imbalance between untrained and trained staff. Those who qualified and remained in nursing were promoted early and without training to posts of responsibility. In some areas the number of patients awaiting admission was high and the staff meagre.

A change came, too, in the traditional role of the nurse. *Antibiotics and *renal dialysis and other technical procedures were entering common use. Cure became commoner, and the quality of nursing care of less obvious importance to the outcome of an illness, if not to the well-being of the patient during it.

Suggestions and proposals for the ailments of the nursing profession were not lacking. Doctors, the general press, political parties, trade unions, nursing journals, the RCN, and the GNC all took part. Many thought that more money for staff would solve all problems, others that harsh prevailing attitudes must be cured. Some wanted the training lengthened, some shortened. All wanted the syllabus reorganized, but not all in the same direction. Everyone agreed that many students were unequal academically to the demands of the syllabus; their eventual failure was traumatic and discouraged recruitment, but if they were not recruited, there was no one to do the work. Matrons went on recruiting missions to Africa, the West Indies, and Asia seeking potential students, pupils, and auxiliaries, and tutors found that they must teach English as well as nursing. Overseas men and women who became state registered acquired a qualification recognized at home, but others did not, which caused ill feeling. Patients and some nurses did not understand each other's cultural back-ground or language.

One estimate suggests that in the 1960s 35 per cent of the nursing force came from overseas. Wastage in 1961 was 39 per cent overall, and many registered nurses went to the USA, Canada, and Australia, where conditions were better and salaries higher. This further increased the imbalance between trained staff and learners.

In 1962 the GNC reintroduced the educational entrance test, which prevented the recruitment of inadequate people who could be used for their services for a year or two and then discarded. Nurses began to express their need for an education affording proper professional status, and appropriate financial reward.

Changes in the population were also to have a profound effect on the task of the nurse, but this was not yet mirrored in the syllabus. The birth rate had fallen, people lived longer, and old people had problems finding a place in the small houses in which their children lived. About a third of all hospital admissions were for mental disease or handicap, but these facts were not reflected as yet in the nurse-training syllabus, which was still based on the 'acute hospital'.

Psychiatric nurses

The plight of the mentally ill has varied across the centuries, but has always been sad. When England consisted predominantly of small rural communities, some eccentricity of behaviour or lack of intelligence was generally tolerated. With the coming of the Industrial Revolution and the growth of cities, the insane were confined in institutions. Since derangement of behaviour was a common sign of insanity, the uninformed often felt that this could be altered if the patient so wished, and if he did not he was either perverse or possessed. Fear led to brutality, and those who tended the insane were custodians rather than nurses.

The hospitals were built very much to a pattern, standing in large grounds with a water tower as a conspicuous feature. Doctors and nurses were isolated from the rest of medicine, and male and female nurses married and lived in tied cottages around the grounds. The inmates, often confined for quite trivial reasons, were there for long periods, even for life. The philosophy was to provide a safe, quiet life for the inmates. As a medical specialty, psychiatry was not held in great esteem and those who practised it often showed little interest in nursing.

Outbursts of rage and violence were handled by isolating the patient in a padded cell. These were still in use even in the 1940s, and there were some doctors and nurses who defended their use, believing that segregating the violent prevented the spread of excitement to other patients, and allowed a sobering-up period.

As the mid-century approached, the wind of change blew through psychiatric hospitals, and cure of several forms of mental disease became possible. *Syphilis, which had caused *general paralysis of the insane, could be cured by *penicillin. Many new drugs were introduced for the control of *depression, *anxiety, *schizophrenia, and violent behaviour (see PSYCHIATRY).

The later years of the 20th century have been marked by a revolution in the care of the mentally ill and handicapped. It is now evident that many such individuals are capable of leading full lives in the community with professional help and supervision, and with the tolerance of the general public. This has resulted in the dispersal of patients from the large hospitals on the margins of towns, where they were formerly segregated. It may be too early as yet to assess fully the outcome of this radical policy. Undoubtedly, total success cannot be expected; some fail to gain acceptance outside hospital, and many add to the numbers of homeless sleeping rough. We know that adequately funded and staffed community services are needed; so also is the goodwill of ordinary people, who, when asked 'Am I my brother's keeper?', are prepared to answer 'Yes'.

Men as nurses

When Florence Nightingale led her regiment of women into hospitals, these were staffed only by attendants. Women were in desperate need of work so as to earn a living, just as medical advances increased the scope of work available; they were not willing to surrender such work to men without a struggle, and they conducted for many years a determined campaign against them. In this they were assisted by several circumstances. First, nursing was so poorly paid that men who could gain a better reward did so. Secondly, nursing had the image of being a female occupation.

There is, of course, no reason why men should not display devotion and tenderness. If we think of paediatric nursing, people are fathers as well as mothers. Once one accepts that at bedside level men and women can contribute equally, doubts about the role of men in nursing disappear. Obviously they can also be managers, administrators, and professors.

In 1947 the Queen's Institute first accepted men as students for district nursing, and from 1961 they were able to train as health visitors. In 1960 the Royal College of Nursing amended its charter enabling it to accept male nurses as members.

The last bastion of female exclusiveness to fall was midwifery, and a few men have qualified. While it does not at the moment seem likely that they will ever be very numerous, no one finds it odd that men should become *obstetricians, and it is natural that some men should want to be midwives.

In 1980 men formed about one-sixth of the nursing force. One important social fact influencing their distribution is that men do not have their service interrupted when children arrive, and those who seek promotion tend to have a more straightforward path than married women. There are, therefore, many men seeking promotion away from bedside nursing. Hence for social reasons, men are more numerous in administrative grades than at student level.

The part played by men in securing more realistic salary scales should also be recorded. They have always formed an important element in mental nursing, where union organization was strongest. They spoke with a united voice, represented themselves as heads of families, and rejected the popular view that as nurses worked for love they did not need financial reward.

Role of the nurse

Medical and scientific advances in the second half of the 20th century have given the nurse marvellous opportunities in care, but have also presented her with acute practical and ethical problems of which her predecessors could not have dreamed. The student nurse must today have experience not only in her training hospital, but also in elements of psychiatric nursing, midwifery, community service, and the care of the old. When she is registered she can take certificates in a variety of specialties, and can consider whether she works not just in hospitals, but with the armed services, in occupational health, with a primary-care team, the prisoner service, overseas nursing, or in the community. If she chooses the last, she can be a *health visitor, a *district nurse, a midwife, or work in a *family planning clinic.

The work of the district (community) nurse has changed in content and method. People live longer, to suffer more *degenerative diseases; in many areas there are large immigrant populations with pressing problems, especially among women. Some diseases disappear, some make sporadic reappearances; some problems, like baby-battering, come increasingly to attention. Nurses increasingly work as a part of a team with general practitioners and health visitors. The ability to consult with fellow professionals is a stimulus to maintain standards and increase knowledge.

The hospital nurse is in charge of her environment, and the patient comes as a client. The district nurse is in a different position: she can enter a patient's home only by invitation, and if her services and attitudes are not acceptable she can be refused admission. She has, however, unrivalled opportunities to give total care. She sees the patient's life-style, his social problems, and those of his family and relatives. A great deal of the nursing in the UK is done by relatives in the home, many of whom need the support of the nurse over technical procedures, and advice and teaching on how to cope with problems.

Reorganization

The hospital ward is the centre in which nurses learn most of their art and science, and is where the general public most often meets them. The ward sister was traditionally the linchpin in this important setting, and up to the Second World War stayed in her post for years, often living in a bed-sitting-room attached to the ward, and devoting her life to it. Consultants depended on her clinical judgement; she was the stable element on the ward team, often at great personal sacrifice. She had no nursing superior but Matron.

The Salmon Report, published in 1966, dealt with the structure of the hospital nursing service from ward sister upwards, and proposed how administration and management were to be structured. Sisters were now to be nursing officers of both sexes, nursing officers managed a group of wards, senior nursing officers co-ordinated their work and were responsible to a principal nursing officer. After a brief pilot trial, in 1967 the Salmon structure was implemented.

The results were painful in many ways. People who liked bedside nursing saw that pay and pension prospects demanded that they move up the promotion ladder. Matrons disappeared: unit officers took on management positions without formal training. Senior nurses had to reapply for their own re-named positions, and sometimes found themselves rejected after years of performing their duties apparently to everyone's satisfaction. In 1979 came a major health service reorganization which produced nursing posts at District, Area, and

Regional levels. There were more vacancies than there were adequately prepared nurses to fill them; the same applied to the medical and financial officers who made up the management teams.

The 1970s were a time of crumbling attitudes and beliefs, and awakening of economic awareness. Hospitals were previously built in the belief that there would always be a supply of low-paid workers to move goods by hand, and of student nurses to do most of the nursing. Now everyone was working shorter hours, earning bonuses and overtime pay, and union activity in hospitals was increasing. Although one may regret the loss of some earlier attitudes, the 'good old days' were not always good for nurses. They no longer fill matron's inkwells, or put buttons on consultants' white coats. They have many problems still to solve: one is how to press for salary rises when they cannot bring themselves to take industrial action. Another is how to maintain morale in the face of recurrent reorganization.

The bedside nurse today

While morale is not high among senior nurses, it is possible to perceive at the basic clinical level an air of hope and of independent self-awareness among professional nurses that is quite new. During the last 35 years nurses have seen an immense change in all aspects of medical and surgical care, and very important questions were posed as techniques such as renal dialysis, positive pressure ventilation, and cardiac monitoring became available. The nurse had to ask herself whether her task was to tend mechanical appliances or to give traditional nursing care to a patient while a technician looked after the machines.

Cardiac resuscitation in its early stages caused much anxiety and heart-searching for nurses, and also for medical staff. If ineffective, nurses felt defeated: if successful, they sometimes found they had restored a life of handicap. Once the technique was routine, patients approaching their end might have their life prolonged for a few days at the expense of destroying the peace and quiet that everyone deserves. Similar fears and queries arose when donor kidneys first came into demand for kidney transplants.

With experience, along with good communication with doctors, improving methods and understanding, such problems are resolved and previous anxieties are allayed; nevertheless, new ones constantly arise. Thus appropriate care for the handicapped newborn causes much discussion.

Nurses cannot surrender their consciences to medical instructions, and are morally and legally responsible for their own actions and decisions. Perhaps it is this approach to professional maturity that has made nurses question their real function, and to find an answer in the rather pedantically named Nursing Process.

Once nurses were asked in state examinations, 'What are the signs, symptoms, and treatment of (e.g.) diabetes mellitus?' Today this would seem strange: diseases occur only when they are manifested in people, and it is people, not diseases, for whom nurses care. When someone comes into hospital, nurses assess from a written nursing history the problems that the nurse can possibly solve; set a series of goals they may hope to reach; use, in attaining these goals, the very best nursing care they can give; review these goals and their methods of reaching them; and afterwards assess how successful they were in attaining them.

It is not only in general hospitals that this ambition to formulate and give the best and most personal care is pursued. In psychiatric and mental deficiency hospitals, and in the community, the same kind of movement is going on to increase the quality of care and hence the level of professional satisfaction. Perhaps we can hope that the winds of administrative change will blow less frequently for a few years, and that the grades that at present are going through a difficult and discouraging stage will find more satisfaction.

Professional preparation

The formulation of examinations that determined suitability for state registration were formerly prescribed by the GNC, but are now the responsibility of its successor organization, the United Kingdom Central Council (UKCC) for nursing, midwifery, and health visiting, a statutory body concerned not only with education but also, like the *General Medical Council, with conduct and discipline. Once practical tests of nursing skill were conducted in the classrooms of schools of nursing, where nurses were asked to lay trays and trolleys showing their knowledge of procedures. Since the syllabus was updated only at intervals, nurses might find their professional competence being tested by questions on obsolete methods.

As nurses gained insight into the uniqueness of their possible role, they refined the methods of evaluating professional competence. On-going assessment of practical skills in giving and planning individual care, knowledge of responsibilities for drug therapy, ability to plan for a group of patients, and for the nurses who give that care, has taken the place of classroom tests. This assessment takes place in the wards and among patients for whom the candidate is working.

As academic entry standards for nurses have risen, so it seemed increasingly inappropriate that intelligent women should have to choose between an academic education and work which they had a deep desire to undertake. Courses shared between a university and a school of nursing, which would lead to a degree and to state registration as a nurse were approved increasingly. The number of applicants for these courses was an indication of the desire for advanced education by nurses, and demand for places has continued. Apart from the number of courses based in schools of nursing, there are professors of nursing in several universities in England, Scotland, and Wales.

There are also now opportunities to take a master's degree or a doctorate (e.g. Ph.D.) in many universities. Some of these are taught degrees that offer clinical nursing as a specialty. When nursing degrees were established, some objected that graduate nurses would speedily desert clinical nursing for administration. This has not proved to be the case: many people who want to gain degrees as well as nursing qualifications have clinical nursing in hospital or the community as their primary interest and when the Open University was established, many nurses, some of whom were very senior, enrolled for part-time degrees, and had a high level of success, in spite of the length of study involved. Now, under 'Project 2000', proposed by the UKCC and approved in principle by government, all nurses in training will in future become students rather than workers, and it seems likely that nursing will soon become an all-graduate profession.

Looking to the future

Looking at nurses around the world, one sees that their work, reward, and status are influenced by many factors: by the structure of society; by views on women's work and position; by the gross national product; by the resources available for the health services; by whether the country is northern or southern, industrial or agricultural; by life expectancy; and by the nature of the health problems to be attacked. Developed countries that have conquered the major infections are struggling with illness caused by the environment and the machines they have created, and by problems such as smoking, alcohol, and drug abuse. All countries are concerned about providing medical care by the state for those unable to pay for it themselves, and about the relationship between state care and private medicine; none are sure how hospitals should be planned, or what is the best size.

How is the trained nurse seen today by the public and by her peers? In the 19th century the qualified nurse's tradition had three historical strands—domestic, military, and religious. Today the domestic element has largely disappeared; caps and aprons are rarely seen. 'Officer' as a title with its connotations of rank, is used only by the armed forces. The religious component is largely confined to *hospice care, where it still makes an important but ecumenical contribution.

Hospital schools of nursing have joined to form colleges, most affiliated to, or part of, a university or college of further education. Most student nurses still pursue the traditional three-year syllabus, but there are many university courses leading to a degree. Under Project 2000, programmes are offered by approved colleges under which students take a three-year course, of which the first year is common ground, while the next 2 years are devoted to general, psychiatric, and mental handicap experience.

Provision of hygienic care, and those tasks which were the sole work of the nurse up to the 19th century have been largely delegated to health-care assistants.

The trained nurse sees herself as ascertaining needs, planning their fulfilment, teaching, superintending, and assuring quality of care.

Many highly skilled practical tasks are still performed by the trained nurse. Most of us have seen her/him at work, caring for someone who has had a heart operation or has sustained injuries requiring intensive care on a life-support system. We all recognize the special skills required of nurses in such settings.

Those of us attending hospital find that the word 'patient', with its connotation of suffering, is tending to give place to 'client'. We are likely to be greeted by a nurse who gives us her name and tells us that she will be the one in charge of us, to whom we should refer any problems. She will, with her team, plan our nursing care, work with our doctor, give us advice on health, and arrange necessary care after our discharge. Many of us are also likely to meet the practice nurse, a colleague of our *general practitioner. She may run clinics of her own on immunization, diagnostic tests, child care, and minor dressings.

Nursing is influenced by social changes (e.g. the increasing age of the population, the arrival of *AIDS), by medical advances (e.g. the range of organ transplants and joint replacements), by political decisions (e.g. the creation of Hospital Trusts), as well as by the views of individual nurses about their respective roles. Prophecy is rash, but it seems likely that the next 50 years will see increased professionalism, with emphasis on planning, management, and health-care teaching. It would perhaps be unwise, however, to preclude the possibility that the electronic technician and engineer may take over some high-tech tasks, just as surgeons envisage the employment of robotics in some routine parts of operations. Perhaps then the nurse will once again be increasingly concerned with personal care, like her medieval predecessor.

WINIFRED HECTOR

Further reading
Abel-Smith, B. (1960). *A history of the nursing profession* Heinemann, London.

Baly, M. E. (1980). *Nursing and social change*, (2nd edn). Heinemann, London.

Baly, M. E., Robottom, B., and Clark, J., (1981). *District nursing* (2nd edn). Heinemann, London.

Henderson, V. (1966). *The nature of nursing*. National League for Nursing Press, New York.

NUTRITION of either plants or animals consists of taking in, absorbing, and utilizing food substances. The science of nutrition involves the knowledge and understanding of these processes. To use this knowledge appropriately requires additional information about the composition of food stuffs and an appreciation of the interaction of cultural, religious, socio-economic, political, and environmental influences that determine the food intake of an individual.

The science of nutrition

Like other biological disciplines, the science of nutrition is founded upon the base of pre-existing observations and knowledge of related fields, including chemistry, botany, *physiology, *anatomy, medicine, agriculture, and health sciences, indeed, virtually the whole of biology. Nutrition is not, as is so commonly mis-stated, a new science, inasmuch as many of the basic concepts were recognized centuries ago. The breadth and diversity of roles whereby processes of nutrition influence health have been more generally defined and have become of great public interest within the 20th century. The general public's interest in, and concern for, health and for the control of chronic diseases (e.g. *cardiovascular diseases, *cancer, and emotional and mental conditions, etc.), combined with the awareness of the news media, have aroused expectations (sometimes unjustifiably) of unprecedented benefits arising from food and dietary manipulation. Accordingly, there is a growing appreciation of the need to incorporate sound nutrition science education into the curriculum at both pre-university and university, as well as professional, levels of instruction.

Essential nutrients and deficiency diseases

Curative and, at a later date, preventive roles of certain foodstuffs in relation to a specific disease or syndrome have been recognized (e.g. fresh vegetables and citrus fruits in scurvy, preparations of iron for *chlorosis (iron-deficiency anaemia) and of *iodine and iodine-containing foods for *goitre). Investigations of these and other similar relationships in man and animals led to recognition of a category of 'essential nutrients', the absence of which from the diet would result in a particular disease syndrome. Observations of such relationships stimulated subsequent studies in experimental animals of the effects of deliberate removal of a dietary constituent, and the seeking of an analogous syndrome in man. Continuing critical scientific research expands and refines knowledge of the essential nutrients, and quantifies dietary requirements. Some substances have, mistakenly, been deemed essential nutrients, but later findings have negated such conclusions. Conversely, elements remain that require critical assessment as to their essential role, if any. Animal species differ appreciably in their need for a particular dietary compound or substance, just as they display marked differences in reaction to individual *drugs. Hence, a disease syndrome produced by deprivation of a nutrient in one species may not be manifest in another species.

Specific disease syndromes caused by deficiencies of essential nutrients were gradually identified during the final decades of the 19th century and, primarily, during the 20th century. Experimental studies in laboratory animals have provided the necessary evidence for elucidation of the nature of the essential nutrients and their metabolic roles. Table 1 summarizes the most widely

Table 1 Characteristic features of well-recognized vitamin or mineral deficiency diseases

Deficiency disease	Nutrient deficient	Clinical characteristics
Scurvy	Vitamin C (ascorbic acid)	Perifollicular petechiae; swollen, red gums that bleed easily; lassitude, general weakness; haemorrhage in the joints; loosening of the teeth; plasma vitamin C virtually undetectable
Beriberi	Vitamin B_1 (thiamine)	Peripheral neuritis; loss of deep tendon reflexes (especially lower extremities); oedema; cardiac enlargement (right-sided); tachycardia; increased pulse pressure; low erythrocyte transketolase activity; low urinary thiamine
Wernicke–Korsakoff syndrome	Vitamin B_1	History of alcoholism; disorientation, confusion; ataxia, severe loss of memory; confabulation; abnormally low erythrocyte transketolase
Ariboflavinosis	Riboflavin	Lesions at corners of mouth (angular stomatitis or cheilosis); photophobia with pericorneal injection; seborrhoeic dermatitis; glossitis; increased *in vitro* stimulation of erythrocyte glutathione reductase activity by flavin adenine dinucleotide
Pellagra	Niacin (nicotinic acid, nicotinamide) (or the precursor amino acid, tryptophan)	Symmetrical dermatitis of exposed surfaces of hands, arms, lower extremities, face, and neck; diarrhoea; glossitis, anxiety, hallucinations, dementia; low urinary *N*-methyl-nicotinamide
Tropical sprue Macrocytic anaemia of infants Pernicious anaemia of pregnancy	Folic acid	Steatorrhoea (sprue); glossitis; macrocytic anaemia; weakness; weight-loss, debility; low levels of folate in blood serum and erythrocytes
Anaemia of vegetarians	Vitamin B_{12}	History of strict vegetarianism; weakness; macrocytic anaemia; glossitis; megaloblastic changes in bone marrow; low levels of serum vitamin B_{12}
Pernicious anaemia	Conditioned deficiency of vitamin B_{12}	Macrocytic anaemia; megaloblastic marrow; glossitis; peripheral neuritis; evidence of spinal cord degeneration; atrophy of gastric mucosa; gastric achlorhydria; lack of gastric 'intrinsic' factor and decreased absorption of labelled vitamin B_{12}; low levels of serum vitamin B_{12}
Convulsive seizures in infants	Vitamin B_6 (pyridoxine, pyridoxal, pyridoxamine)	Convulsive seizures in infants: convulsions in deprived adults; neuropathy of lower extremities in older subjects under treatment with isoniazid; cheilosis and seborrhoeic dermatitis; low levels of pyridoxal phosphate in plasma or whole blood
Xerophthalmia	Vitamin A (retinol; precursor, carotene)	Night blindness; corneal dryness, dullness, corneal ulceration, degeneration, perforation; conjunctival Bitot spots; blindness; low serum vitamin A levels; defective dark adaptation

Table 1. (*cont.*)

Deficiency disease	Nutrient deficient	Clinical characteristics
Rickets and osteomalacia	Vitamin D (various forms; exposure to ultraviolet irradiation, sunlight)	Defective calcification of bones: enlarged epiphyses with uncalcified cartilage; enlargement (beading) of costochondral junction of ribs: bowing of legs in young children; in adults bone deformations due to softening and stress; pseudo-fractures; characteristic changes in bones on radiography; elevated alkaline phosphatase activity and low concentration of 25-OH-D in plasma
Hypoprothrombinaemia (haemorrhagic disease of the newborn; hypoprothrom-binaemia associated with biliary obstruction or malabsorption)	Vitamin K	Haemorrhagic tendency, bleeding: low level of prothrombin in plasma; prolonged blood clotting time; in adults associated with defective gastrointestinal absorption (biliary obstruction, sprue, other cause of steatorrhoea, or liver disease) or with anticoagulant therapy
Microcytic hypochromic anaemia	Iron	Lassitude, weakness, pallor, other general symptoms of anaemia; history of diet deficient in iron in infants and children; in adults usually associated with chronic blood loss; low blood haemoglobin: red blood cells pale, small, low in haemoglobin; low level of iron in serum, increased levels of iron-binding protein, transferrin
Dwarfism, sexual infantilism of adolescence	Zinc	Growth failure; delayed sexual maturation of adolescents; impairment of wound healing; low levels of zinc in plasma and in red blood cells.
Acrodermatitis enteropathica	Genetically conditioned zinc deficiency	In weanling infants; severe rash around body orifices; diarrhoea; failure to thrive; skin infections; death; responds to zinc or zinc picolinate
Endemic goitre	Iodine	Enlargement and hypertrophy of the thyroid gland; usual onset girls 12–18 years, boys 9–13 years of age; endemic in iodine-deficient geographic areas; persists throughout life; secondary thyrotoxicosis may develop as may carcinoma; low urinary excretion of iodine; increased uptake of labelled iodine by thyroid
Cretinism	Iodine	In endemic goitre areas; iodine-deficient mothers may produce offspring who are mentally retarded, becoming dwarfed, with empty, expressionless faces, saddle noses, with widely set eyes, drooling, open mouth, with or without thyroid enlargement

occurring, well-established syndromes of malnutrition due to deficiency of a vitamin or mineral.

The table includes examples attributable to simple dietary lack, as well as others that are 'conditioned' in that they result from some abnormality that decreases the absorption of the nutrient, increases its loss from the body, or otherwise interferes metabolically with it fulfilling its physiological role. As an example, *vitamin B_{12} deficiency results in macrocytic *anaemia and in neurological changes. It may be due to simple dietary deficiency as a result of prolonged adherence to a strictly vegetarian regimen, because vegetables are not a source of this essential nutrient. This deficiency may also occur after surgical removal of a patient's stomach, because the stomach is the source of a factor necessary for absorption of the vitamin, and following its removal there is impairment of vitamin B_{12} absorption. It may also occur in individuals having an intact stomach but *atrophy of the gastric mucosa, with resulting decreased secretion of the intrinsic factor necessary for absorption of the vitamin. These latter two mechanisms are examples of 'conditioned deficiencies' that occur despite adequate intake of the vitamin in the foods consumed.

Concept of 'safe and adequate intake'

The biological effect of an ingested substance, even of essential nutrients, is determined by the quantity ingested. Excessive quantities of any food constituent can be harmful; in some instances the harmful effects of excess first attracted the nutritionist's attention, the physiological essentiality only later being recognized. Two examples are:

(1) the early recognition of mottled enamel of the teeth and the syndrome of *fluorosis due to excessive intake of fluoride, and subsequent recognition of the essentiality of adequate fluoride for minimizing dental decay and preserving normal tooth and bone structure; and
(2) the earlier delineation of selenosis among grazing animals in areas of high soil content of selenium, and later the demonstration in both experimental animals and man of a requirement for small trace quantities of this element.

Recognition of the sometimes narrow range between the minute intake that fulfils the requirement and the excessive intake of the nutrient that is toxic has led to incorporation into statements of dietary standards of 'estimated safe and adequate daily dietary intakes'.

The principle behind 'a safe and adequate intake' concept is important, not only in relation to trace minerals and some vitamins but also for other nutrients that sometimes are misadvisedly advocated as beneficial in mega-doses. Protection of the consumer against harmful effects of overdosage lies behind governmental regulations that control enrichment levels of foodstuffs, the limiting of foods that may be enriched, the permitted claims pertaining to high-dosage supplements, as well as the controlled use of nutrients in some non-food items.

The concept of safe and adequate levels of intake is applicable not only to the micronutrients but also to the more commonly regarded macronutrients. These include the consumption of energy-providing foodstuffs ('total calories', whether provided by *carbohydrates, including sugar (4 calories/g), fats (9 calories/g), protein (4.0 calories/g), or alcohol (7.0 calories/g). Physiologically, energy supplied in excess of the individual's requirement as determined by age, activity, gender,

and other factors, is stored as body fat, and persistent intake of excess results in obesity. Variation in the caloric needs to meet daily expenditures are such that setting of a maximum quantitative intake limit is impracticable. The appropriate guide for the individuals is, then, personal awareness and judgement of body change as sensed by self-inspection, alterations in weight, or awareness of the fit of usual clothes.

Dietary standards

Tables of dietary standards have long been devised, and today are commonly set forth as quantitative guides for the intake of nutrients by persons according to categories of age, gender, physiological state, and activities that may influence needs. The purposes and use of dietary standards vary, and have evolved, from perhaps the simplest purpose 'to prevent dietary disease', to feed categories of individuals (e.g. armies, naval personnel, nations), to maintain health and working capacity in adverse economic circumstances, to provide for planning agricultural production to meet national food needs, to maintain optimal health status for a measurable maximum number of individuals, to serve as guides for the planning of specific-use diets, and to design educational or regulatory devices such as labelling. It is evident that the form and content of such standards as the recommended dietary allowances (RDA) of the Food and Nutrition Board, National Academy of Sciences, or standards of international agencies such as *WHO, or those of individual nations, may differ, depending upon the intended purpose and use as well as the evidence considered in arriving at the approximations.

Tables 2 and 3 are cited as examples of the recent most inclusive and quantitatively generous allowances. These are designed 'for the maintenance of good nutrition of practically all healthy people in the United States' and are not to be interpreted as *requirements* necessary to prevent deficiency states.

Scientific evidence considered in developing the various statements of national, international, and specific-purpose nutritional standards includes data from and knowledge of:

(1) the nutrient content of foods;
(2) essential nutrients, precursors, metabolism, and interconversion and stability;
(3) food and nutrient intakes of populations;
(4) clinical and laboratory assessments;
(5) clinical and metabolic knowledge of relevant levels of nutriture;
(6) experimental studies of deficiency syndromes;
(7) therapeutic response to differing levels of intake;
(8) existing data concerning relevant studies of nutrient balance, half-life, turnover, and storage of nutrients;
(9) general public health statistics pertaining to populations and experimental subjects; and

Table 2 Food and Nutrition Board, National Academy of Sciences – National Research Council recommended dietary allowances,* (revised 1989)

Category or condition	Age (years)	Weight† (kg)	(lb)	Height† (cm)	(in)	Protein (g)	Fat-soluble vitamins Vitamin A (µg)	Vitamin D (µg)	Vitamin E (mg)	Vitamin K (µg)	Water-soluble vitamins Vitamin C (mg)	Thiamin (mg)	Riboflavin (mg)
Infants	0.0–0.4	6	13	60	24	13	375	7.5	3	5	30	0.3	0.4
	0.5–1.0	9	20	71	28	14	375	10	4	10	35	0.4	0.5
Children	1–3	13	29	90	35	16	400	10	6	15	40	0.7	0.8
	4–6	20	44	112	44	24	500	10	7	20	45	0.9	1.1
	7–10	28	62	132	52	28	700	10	7	30	45	1.0	1.2
Males	11–14	45	99	157	62	45	1000	10	10	45	50	1.3	1.5
	15–18	66	145	176	69	59	1000	10	10	65	60	1.5	1.8
	19–24	72	160	177	70	58	1000	10	10	70	60	1.5	1.7
	25–50	79	174	176	70	63	1000	5	10	80	60	1.5	1.7
	51+	77	170	173	68	63	1000	5	10	80	60	1.2	1.4
Females	11–14	46	101	157	62	46	800	10	8	45	50	1.1	1.3
	15–18	55	120	163	64	44	800	10	8	55	60	1.1	1.3
	19–24	58	128	164	65	46	800	10	8	60	60	1.1	1.3
	25–50	63	138	163	64	50	800	5	8	65	60	1.1	1.3
	51+	65	143	160	63	50	800	5	8	65	60	1.0	1.2
Pregnant						60	800	10	10	65	70	1.5	1.6
Lactating	1st 6 months					65	1300	10	12	65	95	1.6	1.8
	2nd 6 months					62	1200	10	11	65	90	1.6	1.7

Table 2 (*cont.*)

Category or condition	Age (years)	Water-soluble vitamins				Minerals						
		Niacin (mg)	Vitamin B_6 (mg)	Folate (µg)	Vitamin B_{12} (µg)	Calcium (mg)	Phosphorus (mg)	Magnesium (mg)	Iron (mg)	Zinc (mg)	Iodine (µg)	Selenium (µg)
Infants	0.0–0.4	5	0.3	25	0.3	400	300	40	6	5	40	10
	0.5–1.0	6	0.6	35	0.5	600	500	60	10	5	50	15
Children	1–3	9	1.0	50	0.7	800	800	80	10	10	70	20
	4–6	12	1.1	75	1.0	800	800	120	10	10	90	20
	7–10	13	1.4	100	1.4	800	800	170	10	10	120	30
Males	11–14	17	1.7	150	2.0	1200	1200	270	12	15	150	40
	15–18	20	2.0	200	2.0	1200	1200	400	12	15	150	50
	19–24	19	2.0	200	2.0	1200	1200	350	10	15	150	70
	25–50	19	2.0	200	2.0	800	800	350	10	15	150	70
	51+	15	2.0	200	2.0	800	800	350	10	15	150	70
Females	11–14	15	1.4	150	2.0	1200	1200	280	15	12	150	45
	15–18	15	1.5	180	2.0	1200	1200	300	15	12	150	50
	19–24	15	1.6	180	2.0	1200	1200	280	15	12	150	55
	25–50	15	1.6	180	2.0	800	800	280	15	12	150	55
	51+	13	1.6	180	2.0	800	800	280	10	12	150	55
Pregnant		17	2.2	400	2.2	1200	1200	320	30	15	175	65
Lactating	1st 6 months	20	2.1	280	2.6	1200	1200	355	15	19	200	75
	2nd 6 months	20	2.1	260	2.6	1200	1200	340	15	16	200	75

* The allowances, expressed as average daily intakes over time, are intended to provide for individual variations among most normal persons as they live in the USA under usual environmental stresses. Diets should be based on a variety of common foods in order to provide other nutrients for which human requirements have been less well defined.

† Weights and heights of reference adults are actual medians for the US population of the designated age. The use of these figures does not imply that the height-to-weight ratios are ideal.

Table 3 Estimated safe and adequate daily dietary intakes of selected vitamins and minerals*

Category	Age (years)	Vitamins		Trace elements†					
		Biotin (μg)	Pantothenic acid(mg)	Copper (mg)	Manganese (mg)	Fluoride (mg)	Chromium (μg)	Molybdenum (μg)
Infants	0–0.4	10	2	0.4–0.6	0.3–0.6	0.1–0.5	10–40	15–30
	0.5–1	15	3	0.6–0.7	0.6–1.0	0.2–1.0	20–60	20–40
Children and	1–3	20	3	0.7–1.0	1.0–1.5	0.5–1.5	20–80	25–50
adolescents	4–6	25	3–4	1.0–1.5	1.5–2.0	1.0–2.5	30–120	30–75
	7–10	30	4–5	1.0–2.0	2.0–3.0	1.5–2.5	50–200	50–150
	11+	30–100	4–7	1.5–2.5	2.0–5.0	1.5–2.5	50–200	75–250
Adults		30–100	4–7	1.5–3.0	2.0–5.0	1.5–4.0	50–200	75–250

* Because there is less information on which to base allowances, these figures are not given in the main table of RDA and are provided here in the form of ranges of recommended intakes.
† Since the toxic levels for many trace elements may be only several times usual intakes, the upper levels for the trace elements given in this table should not be habitually exceeded.

(10) comparative demographic information.

Considered scientific judgement of such composite information permits consolidation of valid standards of defined needs of nutrients.

Non-essential but beneficial dietary considerations
Astute observers detected long ago a relationship between food habits and health. *Hippocrates (460–370 BC) observed, 'Growing bodies have the most innate heat, they therefore require the most food, for otherwise their bodies are wasted. In old persons the heat is feeble, and therefore they require little fuel, as it were, to the flame, for it would be extinguished by much.' The modern tools of *epidemiology and experimental science are identifying associations between quality of health and foods consumed that do not reflect the recognized essential nutrients in the diet. These associations exist for elevated serum *cholesterol levels and a high intake of dietary fats, especially the saturated *fatty acids; conversely, high intakes of the polyunsaturated fatty acids (chemically referred to as *n*-3 and *n*-6 fatty acids) in fish by the indigenous Esquimo population of Greenland, or the experimental dosing of European or American subjects with supplements rich in these fatty acids, result in lowering of serum levels of low-density lipoproteins (LDL). This is a phenomenon regarded as beneficially reflecting a lowered risk of cardiovascular disease. Similarly, much epidemiological and other evidence now indicates convincingly that moderate intake of alcoholic beverages is associated with a desirable increase in the high-density fraction (HDL) of cholesterol in the serum. Experimental laboratory investigations have demonstrated an anticancer property that may be associated with a variety of foods and beverages, including members of the brassica family (broccoli), and other common foods or beverages (e.g. coffee). Some of these compounds have been identified chemically, others are under intensive evaluation (e.g. carotenoids). The ultimate significance of such biologically active substances in foods remains to be ascertained through future research. Proper understanding of these must include assessment of both potential beneficial and toxicological properties for experimental animals and man.

The growing complexity of knowledge of essential nutrients, of dietary risk and beneficial factors, and of the pathogenesis of chronic diseases reinforces the wisdom of the advice of the Roman writer, *Celsus (25 BC–AD 50), concerning eating patterns that:

A man in health, who is both vigorous and his own master, should be under no obligatory rules . . . His kind of life should afford him variety. It is well to avoid no kind of food in common use; to attend at times a banquet, at times to hold aloof; to eat more than sufficient at one time, at another no more . . .

W. J. DARBY

Further reading
Cronin, F. J. Francis, J., and Shaw, A. M. (1988). Summary of dietary recommendations for healthy Americans. *Nutrition Today*, **23**, 26–34.
Beaton, G. H. (1991). Human nutrient requirement estimates. *Food, Nutrition and Agriculture*, **1**, 3–15.
Brown, M. L. (ed.) (1990). *Present knowledge in nutrition*, (6th edn), p. 632. International Life Sciences–Nutrition Foundation, Washington, DC.
Food and Nutrition Board, National Research Council (1989). *Recommended dietary allowances*, (10th edn), pp. 284. National Academy Press, Washington, DC.
Gurr, M. I., (ed.) (1988–91). *Nutrition Research Reviews*, Vols 1–4. Cambridge University Press, Cambridge.
Weisell, R. C. (1991). Trace elements in human nutrition. *Food, Nutrition and Agriculture*, **1**, 25–9.

NUTTALL, GEORGE HENRY FALKINER (1862–1937). Anglo-American bacteriologist. He carried out important researches on *immunology, *parasitology, and *insects as vectors of disease. He founded the *Journal of Hygiene* in 1901 and *Parasitology* in 1908.

NYCTALOPIA is a synonym for *night blindness.

NYMPHOMANIA is intense sexual excitement in a woman, indiscriminately directed at any man (or, in 'inverted nymphomania', at any woman) and unrelieved by *orgasm. Nymphomania is a rare episodic state which may have an organic basis (e.g. drug *psychosis, *encephalitis, neurological temporal lobe lesions) and is to be distinguished from female hypersexuality, which is simply one end of a normal distribution curve.

NYSTAGMUS is a rapid *tremor of the eyeballs independent of normal ocular movements. Nystagmus is classified according to its direction (horizontal, vertical, rotatory), character (e.g. oscillatory, phasic), and any precipitating factors.

NYSTATIN is an *antibiotic agent obtained from the mould *Streptomyces noursei*. It is active against a number of *yeasts and *fungi but is used mainly against *Candida* infections, by topical application to the skin and mucous membranes. It is ineffective by mouth and is too toxic for parenteral use. see ANTI-INFECTIVE DRUGS.

OBESITY is excess body fat. The weight/height^2 index (body mass index or BMI) is a better indication of obesity than body weight alone in adult men and women (but not children). It is usually arbitrarily defined as existing when body weight exceeds 120 per cent of ideal weight; expressed as BMI in kg/m^2 of body surface, this value is 27 for men and 25 for women. Alternatively reference can be made to the widely available Metropolitan Life Insurance Company Tables, which provide guidelines for acceptable weight ranges at different heights. Whatever definition is used, obesity is very prevalent among Western populations, particularly in the middle-aged. It is an important health hazard and carries an increased risk of premature death. It has been estimated that life expectation diminishes by about 2 per cent for each kg of body weight above normal. Among the major associations of obesity are *coronary heart disease, *hypertension, *diabetes mellitus, *osteoarthrosis of weight-bearing joints, several forms of *cancer (colon, rectum, and prostate in men; breast, uterus, and cervix in women; and some less common cancers), and *gall-bladder disease. Liability to *varicose veins, menstrual abnormalities, and respiratory disorders is also increased, and surgical operations carry a greater than normal risk.

OBJECTIVE. In an optical system such as a *microscope, the objective is the lens or complex of lenses that is nearest the object being examined.

OBSCENITY is that which is filthy, disgusting, or offensive to the senses or sensibilities. It is notoriously difficult to define except in a specific cultural context. According to current English law, material 'shall be deemed to be obscene if its effect . . . is, if taken as a whole, such as to tend to deprave and corrupt persons who are likely . . . to read, see or hear the matter contained or embodied in it'.

OBSESSION. A pathologically persistent or recurrent idea, which may be emotionally generated and which sometimes leads to irrational action.

OBSTETRIC FORCEPS. Any of a variety of instruments designed to assist in the extraction of the fetal head during childbirth. See OBSTETRICS AND GYNAECOLOGY.

OBSTETRICIAN. A medical practitioner specializing in the medical care of pregnancy and childbirth. See OBSTETRICS AND GYNAECOLOGY.

OBSTETRICS AND GYNAECOLOGY. Despite its double name, obstetrics and gynaecology is a single specialty and most of its practitioners are both obstetricians and gynaecologists. Obstetrics deals with pregnancy and childbirth, the word probably deriving from the Latin *obstare*, to 'stand before': the midwife (*obstetrix*) 'stood before' the woman to receive the baby. Gynaecology (from the Greek *gyne*, 'woman') deals mainly with reproductive disorders of non-pregnant women, but also includes problems in early pregnancy.

OBSTETRICS
History
In early times women in labour were attended by relatives or uneducated midwives. (The word 'midwife' derives from the Anglo-Saxon *mid*, 'with' and *wif*, 'woman'). Some Greek and Roman physicians taught midwifery, but doctors, being male, were excluded from attending childbirth until the 16th century. The first book on midwifery was printed in 1513 in Germany. Ambroise *Paré (1510–90), a French military surgeon, founded a school for midwives in Paris. In 1572 a French Huguenot family, the *Chamberlens, fled to England with the forerunners of modern obstetric *forceps, which were their family secret.

Accoucheurs (male midwives) became fashionable in France in the 17th century. A surgeon attended a mistress of Louis XIV in 1663 and an accoucheur, Mauriceau, published a treatise on midwifery in 1668.

In England in the 18th century the secret of the obstetric forceps became public although their use remained controversial. The first British school of midwifery was founded in 1725 in London and the first chair of midwifery in Edinburgh in 1726. Queen Charlotte's Hospital, Britain's first maternity hospital, was founded in 1739. In that year William *Smellie, a Scottish doctor, set up a school of midwifery in London, and in 1752

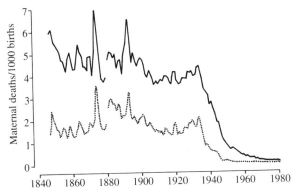

Fig. 1 Maternal mortality rates in England and Wales, 1847–1984. The rate from all causes is shown by the bold line, and the death rate from puerperal sepsis by the dotted line. In spite of social and medical advances, both rates hardly changed between 1847 and 1937. (Redrawn from *Report on confidential enquiries into maternal deaths in England and Wales 1982–84*, p. 141. HMSO, London.)

he published his *Treatise on the theory and practice of midwifery*. Smellie (1697–1763), 'the master of British midwifery', was a man of humanity and common sense but was violently opposed by some local midwives. One of his pupils, William *Hunter, a fellow-Scot and older brother of the famous surgeon John, became very popular and by the latter part of the 18th century *accoucheurs* were fashionable in England.

In the 19th century labour was still dangerous. Among the poor, rickets caused pelvic deformities. In maternity hospitals many women died of puerperal fever, whose contagious nature was recognized by Alexander Gordon of Aberdeen in 1795 and Oliver Wendell *Holmes in the USA in 1843. In 1861 *Semmelweiss in Vienna reduced deaths from puerperal fever by reducing cross-infection with methods such as hand-washing.

Midwifery became a compulsory subject for medical students in 1833 in Scotland and 1866 in England. In 1847 James Young *Simpson, professor of midwifery in Edinburgh, used *chloroform to relieve labour pain. He met strong opposition from doctors and clergy until Queen Victoria requested it at the birth of her seventh child.

Obstetrics was limited to childbirth itself until the 20th century, when antenatal care was introduced. In 1901 R. W. Ballantyne set aside a bed for antenatal patients in *Edinburgh Royal Infirmary. Antenatal clinics were opened in Boston, Sydney, and Edinburgh in 1911, 1912, and 1915, respectively. Obstetrics remained a branch of surgery until 1929, when the *Royal College of Obstetricians and Gynaecologists was founded.

The history of obstetrics is closely linked with that of midwifery. Midwives were mostly illiterate 'Sarah Gamps' until the 19th century, when several European countries introduced regulations for their training and control. Attempts to do the same in Britain failed, but in 1872 the Obstetrical Society of London began issuing certificates of competence to midwives. The Midwives Institute was set up in 1881. At last, in 1902, the Midwives Act made state registration compulsory and set up a Central Midwives Board to regulate midwifery. The Midwives Institute became the College of Midwives in 1941, the prefix 'Royal' being added in 1947.

Maternal mortality

Throughout history childbirth has been dangerous for women, but after 1930 there was a remarkable improvement in Britain. The *maternal mortality rate (MMR)—the number of women dying per 100 000 deliveries—in Britain until 1935 was around 500 but nowadays it is only 8 (Fig. 1). The MMR remains high in many developing countries, and in parts of Africa it is still around 500. The reasons for the fall in Britain are numerous. The health of the population has improved but the fall is probably due more to specific measures. For example, infection can now be treated with *antibiotics, and bleeding by *blood transfusion. Legalization of *abortion in 1967 eliminated criminal abortion as a cause of maternal death.

Since 1952 a national Confidential Enquiry into Maternal Deaths has examined each death and issued regular reports with recommendations for improvements. Haemorrhage and infection are now relatively rare causes: in recent years the commonest causes have been venous *thrombosis, raised *blood pressure, and deaths associated with *anaesthesia.

Perinatal mortality

Childbirth is 100 times more dangerous for the baby than the mother. The perinatal mortality rate (PMR) is the number of stillbirths and deaths in the first week of life per 1000 deliveries. In 1935 the PMR in England and Wales was 70, and in 1990 it was 8.3. The three main causes of perinatal mortality—low birth weight, lack of oxygen *in utero*, and congenital abnormalities—are discussed below.

Obstetric techniques

Obstetric forceps were first used on living babies by the Chamberlens. They were modified during the 18th and 19th centuries but the forceps in use today are similar to those designed by Simpson 150 years ago. Most forceps require the baby's head to be facing towards the mother's back but in 1916 Kjelland, a Norwegian obstetrician, designed forceps for use when the baby's head is facing to the side or to the front.

The vacuum extractor (or ventouse), invented by Malmstrom of Sweden in the 1950s, has a suction cup which is applied to the baby's head. After recent improvements, studies have shown that it causes less trauma to the mother than forceps delivery, although the baby may suffer mild ill-effects from bruising of the scalp.

Caesarean section got its name from the Lex Caesarea, a law dating from the 7th century BC that if a pregnant woman died, the baby should be removed and buried separately. The first well-attested case in Europe was that of Jacob Nufer, a Swiss sow-gelder, who successfully operated on his own wife in 1500. The procedure was not done with any regularity until the 1880s, at which time 'classical' caesarean section involved a lengthwise incision in the *uterus. This does not heal well and may rupture in subsequent labour. In 1906 the modern 'lower segment' operation was introduced, in which the incision is in the fibrous lower part of the uterus.

Current practice
Antenatal care

The emphasis in modern obstetrics is on preventing problems. The purposes of antenatal care are to treat symptoms during pregnancy, to screen for maternal and fetal complications, and to help prepare a couple for childbirth and childrearing.

At a prepregnancy clinic checks are made on a woman's health, obstetric history, and immune status (e.g. to *rubella). Women with a history of genetic disease can receive counselling and, if necessary, diagnostic tests. Those with pre-existing disease such as diabetes may need alteration of their treatment.

The pattern of antenatal clinic visits varies between countries but in Britain a woman usually attends first around the 12th week of pregnancy, monthly until the 28th week, fortnightly until the 36th week, and weekly thereafter. The midwife, general practitioner, and hospital clinic share the care, depending on local arrangements and individual risk factors. The trend nowadays, for low-risk women, is towards fewer visits and less hospital care.

Investigations at booking (the first visit) include tests for *anaemia, *syphilis, rubella, and blood grouping. If a woman's blood group is *Rhesus negative and her baby is Rhesus positive, she could develop *antibodies against the baby's red blood cells, leading to fetal anaemia which may be lethal. Such 'Rhesus isoimmunization' has been almost eliminated by a national prevention programme: Rhesus-negative women are injected with a small amount of antibody to destroy fetal cells in the mother's blood before they stimulate an immune reaction.

(a) **Prenatal diagnosis.** Around 2 per cent of babies have major congenital abnormalities, such as *Down's syndrome or *spina bifida. The risk of some of these can be reduced, e.g. women planning a pregnancy are now advised to take supplements of folic acid to prevent spina bifida, but for the remainder all we can do is make the diagnosis as early as possible, when the woman can be offered the option of terminating the pregnancy.

In chromosomal abnormalities, the baby's cells contain abnormal genetic material due to failure of the *chromosomes to distribute themselves correctly at conception. Most cause *miscarriage but a few are compatible with life, e.g. Down's syndrome, in which there is an extra chromosome 21. Chromosome abnormalities can be diagnosed in various ways. Pre-implantation diagnosis can be performed after *in vitro* fertilization (IVF): in the laboratory one cell is removed from a very early embryo; the chromosomes are examined and if they are normal the embryo can be placed in the womb. Chorion villus sampling (CVS) can be done from the eighth week of pregnancy: a sample of placental tissue is removed via a needle inserted through either the vagina or the abdominal wall. Chromosomes from these rapidly dividing cells can be examined directly by microscopy. Amniocentesis involves removing some amniotic fluid via a needle through the abdominal wall. Cells shed from the fetus can be cultured and examined, which takes longer than direct examination after CVS. Amniocentesis, formerly restricted to the 15th week of pregnancy or later, can now be done as early as the 10th week.

Anatomical abnormalities can occur in fetuses with normal or abnormal chromosomes. The commonest types are abnormalities of the nervous system (e.g. spina bifida) or the heart: others include cleft palate or club foot. They are present from the early weeks of embryonic life but become detectable only when the structures are large enough to be seen on ultrasound scans.

(b) **Obstetric *ultrasound.** During the Second World War echoes from high-frequency sound waves were used to detect submarines. In the 1950s in Glasgow Professor Ian Donald modified the technique to make measurements on the fetus in the amniotic fluid. In the early days a single beam of ultrasound produced blips on an oscilloscope screen, but today's machines give detailed moving images, allowing diagnosis of anatomical abnormalities and accurate assessment of fetal growth and of the position of the placenta. Ultrasound has transformed obstetrics and is now widely used in gynaecology and other specialties.

(c) **Complications of pregnancy.** At each antenatal visit the size of the uterus is assessed. A large uterus may mean multiple pregnancy, excess amniotic fluid, or a large baby, and a small uterus may mean the baby is failing to grow. This can be checked by ultrasound. Checks are also made on the woman's blood pressure and urine for signs of pre-eclampsia—a condition in which the blood pressure rises and protein appears in the urine and which, untreated, can progress to eclampsia (convulsions). In the later weeks checks are made for breech presentation, which is present at the end of 4 per cent of pregnancies.

Care in labour

About 600 000 babies are born in Britain every year, most of them in hospital. The move towards 100 per cent hospital deliveries accelerated in the 1960s as doctors and women perceived hospital as safer for the baby. There is now concern that home delivery should remain as an option for women who want it, although hospitals are becoming less institutional to strike a better balance between safety and a relaxed environment.

(a) Normal labour. Labour has three stages, the first lasting from the onset until the uterine cervix is fully open. During the second stage (which ends at delivery of the baby), the woman feels the urge to push. The third stage is from delivery of the baby to delivery of the *placenta. In Britain women in labour are cared for mainly by midwives, who as independent practitioners are not required to seek medical help unless they feel this is necessary.

Pain relief in labour. There is much variation in the amount of pain experienced during labour and much debate about the best form of pain relief. Methods include psychoprophylaxis, painkilling drugs such as pethidine, inhaled gases, and *epidural analgesia. General anaesthesia is nowadays rarely used for instrumental delivery and many caesarean sections are carried out using epidural block. General and epidural anaesthesia are administered by specially trained anaesthetists.

For epidural analgesia a fine *catheter is inserted between the vertebrae and a painkilling drug is infiltrated around the roots of the nerves leading from the uterus. This can give complete freedom from pain but may interfere with the second stage of labour by abolishing the urge to push, and therefore this increases the chance of an instrumental delivery.

Fetal monitoring. The simplest way to monitor the baby's condition during labour is by the midwife listening to its heartbeat through a stethoscope. Electronic monitoring of the fetal heart rate became widespread in the 1970s. During labour uterine contractions can reduce blood flow to the placenta, interfering with the baby's oxygen supply and altering its heart rate, but abnormalities may have no sinister cause and an electronic monitor (cardiotocograph, CTG) can cause unnecessary concern. CTG abnormalities can be checked by taking a sample of fetal blood for measurement of oxygen levels but this facility is not available in all hospitals.

Active management of labour also became widespread in the 1970s and 1980s. Often a woman's first labour is slow because the uterus does not contract strongly, although subsequent labours are usually much more efficient. 'Active management' of a first labour involves early diagnosis of slow progress and the use of oxytocin, a natural *hormone, to strengthen the contractions. It reduces the need for instrumental delivery or caesarean section, but oxytocin has to be given by intravenous drip and some women see active management as excessive medical intervention.

(b) Complications of labour. Some complications such as malpresentation (e.g. breech presentation) may be anticipated in the antenatal clinic, but some are unpredictable. For example, rarely the umbilical cord may drop into the vagina when the waters break, or more commonly heavy bleeding may occur immediately after delivery (postpartum haemorrhage). The most common indications for intervention nowadays are fetal distress or failure to progress.

Fetal distress means the baby shows signs of lack of oxygen, such as a slow heartbeat or the passage of meconium (bowel contents) *in utero*. These signs can occur, however, when the baby's oxygen levels are normal. Failure to progress in labour means the cervix fails to dilate beyond a certain point, due either to poor contractions or to the baby being too big for vaginal delivery. 'Slow progress', however, can be a subjective diagnosis. Thus both these indications may be arbitrary.

If delivery is necessary in the first stage of labour, caesarean section is required. In the second stage vaginal delivery may be assisted by forceps or vacuum extraction, but caesarean section may be preferred to a potentially difficult instrumental delivery. Rates of caesarean section have risen steadily in many developed countries. In Britain in the 1950s 5 per cent of babies were born by caesarean section but by 1990–91 the rate had risen to 13 per cent. In the USA the rate has risen to 25 per cent. The rise has been blamed on overenthusiastic obstetricians, but recent research shows that women are unwilling to accept even a low risk to their baby, and many prefer caesarean section when a mild complication is detected.

The puerperium

This refers to the time from delivery until the woman's genital tract returns to normal, usually around 6 weeks later. In the early days after delivery emotional lability is usual but true puerperal *psychosis is uncommon. Infection of the womb, the cause of the once-dreaded puerperal fever, is now infrequent and can be treated with antibiotics. In Britain fewer than 50 per cent of women breast-feed, although hospitals are now having some success in increasing this figure.

Future trends

There is a stark contrast between the obstetric needs of countries like Britain and those of developing countries, where the MMR is high and many women suffer complications such as vesicovaginal *fistula (bladder damage during labour). The *World Health Organization estimates that world-wide half a million women die every year as a result of pregnancy, one a minute, and wants to halve this total by the year 2000. This will mean improving maternity services, raising the status of women in some cultures, and providing easy access to cheap contraception.

In Britain, by contrast, the trend is towards reducing medical intervention without compromising safety. Research studies to distinguish useful from unnecessary intervention involve large numbers of women and sophisticated statistical analysis, and several studies may have to be combined to obtain clear answers. Obstetric and midwifery practice is increasingly being guided by such research. At the same time, women have high expectations and any adverse outcome of pregnancy may lead to litigation. Huge awards have been made to 'brain-damaged' babies, but it is now recognized that only a small proportion of cases of *cerebral palsy are due to obstetric causes.

GYNAECOLOGY
History
Gynaecology developed during the 19th century as a specialized branch of surgery. Around 1800 the vaginal speculum was first used to inspect the walls of the vagina. Dilatation of the cervix was carried out in 1832 in Edinburgh. In the 1840s James Marion *Sims of Alabama developed an operation for vesicovaginal fistula. Sims was one of the founders of the Women's Hospital in New York, the world's first hospital devoted to gynaecology. By 1888 an operation had been devised for the repair of uterine prolapse, a condition in which the womb protrudes through the vagina because of weakness of its supporting ligaments.

Abdominal gynaecological surgery developed at the same time. In 1809 Ephraim *McDowell of Kentucky carried out the first successful operation for removal of a large ovarian *cyst. The mortality of such operations remained high, however, until late in the 19th century. Lawson *Tait of Birmingham, England, carried out *hysterectomy for uterine *fibroids in 1874 and the first successful operation for *ectopic pregnancy in 1883. By the end of the century surgical gynaecology was established and early in the 20th century large operations were being performed, such as radical hysterectomy for cancer of the cervix, pioneered by *Wertheim of Vienna. Medical gynaecology developed after the discovery of the sex hormones in the 1920s, leading to innovations such as the *contraceptive pill in the 1950s.

Current practice
Gynaecology now encompasses surgical operations, hormonal and other medical treatments, and broader issues—*family planning, health *screening, and treatment at the *menopause—which demand an understanding of the aspirations of women in modern society.

The menstrual cycle
The human menstrual cycle has considerable potential for going wrong, and even when normal can cause

women discomfort and inconvenience. At *puberty the *hypothalamus (an area at the base of the brain) produces a hormone to activate the *pituitary, a gland under the brain which stimulates the ovaries to secrete oestrogen, a female sex hormone which thickens the endometrium (the lining of the womb). The average age at menarche (the first menses) is now 13, having been higher earlier this century. Regular ovulation begins about 15 and the ovaries fail at an average age of 51.

Menstrual disorders
Menstrual bleeding can be too heavy (menorrhagia), absent (amenorrhoea), infrequent (oligomenorrhoea), or too frequent (polymenorrhoea). The amount of blood lost at menstruation is normally less than 80 ml. In clinical practice the menstrual flow is not measured objectively, the gynaecologist being guided by the history given by the woman.

Medical gynaecology. Most of the hormones controlling the cycle can be given pharmacologically. In cases of amenorrhoea or oligomenorrhoea ovulation can be induced by stimulating the ovaries. The commonest menstrual disorder, menorrhagia, may be treated by suppressing the ovaries with the contraceptive pill. Endometriosis, a painful condition in which endometrium grows outside the uterus, may be treated by suppressing the ovaries or pituitary.

Menopause
The 'menopause' is the last menstrual period, and the 'climacteric' is the phase when the periods become irregular before stopping altogether. Menstruation ceases because the ovaries run out of eggs. Withdrawal of oestrogen causes hot flushes and in the longer term increases the risk of *osteoporosis (loss of bone) and heart disease. These risks can be reduced by giving oestrogen as hormone replacement therapy (HRT). If this treatment were widely adopted, it could substantially alter disease patterns in older women by reducing osteoporosis and heart disease.

Surgical gynaecology
The range of gynaecological operations is wide, although some, such as ventrosuspension (an operation to change the position of the uterus) are now performed much less frequently than in the past.

Hysterectomy is the commonest major operation carried out in Britain and the USA, apart from caesarean section. In Britain 66 000 hysterectomies are performed every year and in the USA 25 per cent of women reach the menopause through hysterectomy. The commonest indication is menstrual disorder, although fibroids (benign tumours of uterine muscle) are often also present.

Pelvic floor repair includes various operations performed for *prolapse of the uterus or vaginal walls. Part of the vagina is removed, the muscles are tightened, and hysterectomy may be performed at the same time.

Dilatation and curettage ('D&C') is less frequently performed now than formerly because of better medical treatment for menstrual disorders. The cervix is stretched with graduated dilators, and a curette, a small spoon-shaped instrument, is used to remove tissue from the uterine cavity.

(a) Minimally invasive surgery. Nowadays an increasing amount of gynaecological surgery is being carried out by 'minimally invasive' techniques.

Laparoscopic surgery. A laparoscope is a kind of telescope which is inserted into the abdomen, usually near the umbilicus. Laparoscopy was popularized in Britain by Patrick Steptoe in the 1960s. Until recently it was mainly used for inspection of the pelvic organs and for sterilization, which involves blocking the Fallopian tubes by electrocoagulation, elastic rings, or metal clips. Recently, larger operations, including hysterectomy, have been carried out either via the laparoscope or with its help. It is still too early to say to what extent such surgery will replace conventional techniques.

Hysteroscopic surgery. Although hysterectomy is commonly performed for menorrhagia, removal of the entire uterus is really unnecessary because only the endometrium bleeds. A hysteroscope is an instrument for looking inside the uterus through the cervix, and it can be used, along with a laser or electrocautery, to remove the endometrium, including the deepest layer, to prevent regrowth. Transcervical resection of the endometrium takes as long as a hysterectomy but, because no abdominal incision is involved, the woman can return home much sooner after operation.

(b) Gynaecological emergencies. The most frequent reasons for emergency gynaecological admission are abdominal pain or vaginal bleeding. In a woman of reproductive age pregnancy testing is usually done. Tests for human chorionic gonadotrophin, a hormone produced only by pregnancy tissue, are now so sensitive that they can detect a pregnancy before a woman misses a period.

About 20 per cent of all pregnancies end in clinically recognizable miscarriage, and unless bleeding stops quickly, curettage is necessary. Ultrasound scanning can differentiate miscarriage from ectopic pregnancy.

After conception, the fertilized egg takes 3–5 days to pass down the Fallopian tube into the uterus. One in 400 pregnancies implants in the tube—an ectopic pregnancy. The tube is too delicate to sustain the pregnancy; as it stretches, pain occurs, and tubal rupture may lead to fatal bleeding. Formerly the treatment was to remove the tube by open operation, and often this is still necessary. It may be possible, however, to remove the tube by laparoscopic surgery or to remove the pregnancy and leave the tube intact, albeit with an increased risk of another ectopic pregnancy.

In the non-pregnant woman, pelvic pain is often attributed to pelvic inflammatory disease, but this is probably over-diagnosed. Ovarian cysts may cause sudden pain due to rupture, twisting, or bleeding. Causes of abnormal bleeding are hormonal imbalance, heavy menstruation, or, less commonly, disease such as uterine or cervical *cancer.

Subspecialties

(a) Reproductive medicine. This subspecialty includes treatment of infertility, disorders of ovarian function, and the menopause.

Infertility. About one in six couples has difficulty in achieving pregnancy. Investigation involves semen analysis and tests of ovulation and the Fallopian tubes. At present little can be done to improve a poor sperm count. Ovulation can be induced with drugs, although careful monitoring is necessary to prevent multiple ovulation. Blocked tubes can be treated surgically, but the Fallopian tubes are small and delicate and if damage is severe the chances of conception are low.

In the 1980s Patrick Steptoe, working in Oldham, and Robert Edwards of Cambridge University developed *in vitro* fertilization (IVF). IVF involves removing an egg (or eggs) from the ovary, fertilization with sperm in the laboratory, and replacement of the fertilized egg in the uterus. The technique was difficult to develop because the egg can be fertilized only at exactly the right moment after the preovulatory surge of hormones. Even in nature, couples trying for pregnancy have no more than a one-in-three chance of conceiving in a single cycle, and it is unlikely that IVF will achieve better than this. Several attempts may be needed, but IVF is expensive and highly stressful for the couple.

(b) Gynaecological *oncology. Oncology is the study of cancer. Gynaecological oncology is concerned with prevention, early detection, and treatment of cancer of the reproductive organs. (In Britain breast cancer is dealt with by general surgeons, not gynaecologists.)

Cancer of the cervix is usually caused by the human papilloma *virus, transmitted by sexual intercourse. Most cases occur after a premalignant phase lasting about 10 years, which can be detected by scraping cells from the cervix and examining them under a microscope. This is the basis of cervical screening. Formerly, cervical smears were taken when a woman happened to consult a doctor, but nowadays, with systematic screening, GPs call all their women patients for smears every 3–5 years.

If a smear is abnormal, the cervix is examined at a hospital clinic through a *colposcope, a low-power binocular microscope which allows biopsies to be taken from abnormal areas. Without this it would be necessary to take a cone *biopsy, which removes the entire circumference of the cervix in order to be sure of including any

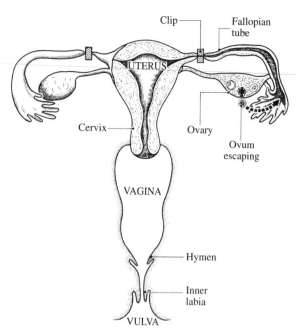

Fig. 2 Diagram of the female genital tract. In the operation of sterilization, the Fallopian tubes are blocked (e.g. by clips, as shown) to prevent the sperm from fertilizing the egg (ovum).

abnormal area. If a colposcopic biopsy is abnormal, a larger area is removed by laser or *diathermy.

Cervical cancer is treated by *radiotherapy, although for early disease radical surgery is an alternative.

Cancer of the endometrium (or body of the uterus) may be due to prolonged stimulation by natural oestrogen, from ovarian cysts or ovarian dysfunction. HRT with unopposed oestrogen is also a risk factor, but nowadays if a woman has a uterus her HRT will include progestogen, a hormone similar to progesterone, which is produced after ovulation. Cancer of the endometrium usually reveals itself early by bleeding. Treatment is by hysterectomy, often combined with radiotherapy.

Cancer of the ovary usually does not become apparent until an advanced stage, when it presents as abdominal swelling. Treatment is by surgery and *chemotherapy. Attempts at early detection involve blood tests for biochemical markers released by the cancer, and ultrasound scanning of women with raised levels. So far such screening is still experimental.

Rarer gynaecological cancers include choriocarcinoma, a tumour of pregnancy tissue, which is lethal if untreated but responds well to chemotherapy. Vulval cancer usually affects older women, and treatment is wide excision of the vulval skin. Vaginal cancer is extremely rare, but cases have been reported in women whose mothers were treated for threatened miscarriage with DES (diethylstilboestrol), an artificial oestrogen.

(c) Urogynaecology. Urinary incontinence is a common problem in women, as the muscles of the pelvic floor can be weakened by childbirth or lack of hormones after the menopause. Urodynamic investigation (measurement of bladder pressure) can distinguish different types of *incontinence. Urge incontinence (oversensitivity of the bladder) is treated by drugs and bladder retraining. Stress incontinence (weakness of bladder supports) is usually treated by an operation to strengthen the bladder neck.

(d) Fertility control. In view of the world's problems with overpopulation, fertility control is a most important part of modern gynaecology.

Contraception is best provided by general practitioners, family planning doctors, or, indeed, over the counter, but gynaecologists have a role in training—particularly in the insertion of intrauterine contraceptive devices. The Royal College of Obstetricians and Gynaecologists has a Faculty of Family Planning founded in 1993.

Sterilization is popular in Britain. Every year about 90 000 female sterilizations are performed and a similar number of *vasectomies. About 50 per cent of couples over 40 have opted for sterilization. Female sterilization is carried out by laparoscopy under general anaesthesia, often as a day-case procedure (Fig. 2). Long-term aftereffects are rare and the failure rate is less than 0.5 per cent.

Termination of pregnancy is a more accurate term than 'abortion', which, strictly speaking, means miscarriage. In Britain the Abortion Act of 1967 allows abortion if two doctors agree that continuing with the pregnancy would be harmful to the health of the woman or her existing children. In Britain about one in three women will have an abortion at some time in her life, usually before the age of 25: about 170 000 abortions are carried out every year and the abortion rate is 13/1000 women aged 15–45. In the US the rate is 24/1000, and in Russia, 124/1000.

Up to 12 weeks of pregnancy abortion is carried out by suction, often as a day-case procedure. After 12 weeks, drugs (prostaglandins) are used to induce abortion. Before the 9th week, medical termination can be carried out using mifepristone ('RU486'), a progesterone antagonist, followed by prostaglandin. Medical abortion is available only in hospitals and clinics licensed under the Abortion Act.

(e) *Sexual medicine. In spite of today's open attitude to sex, many couples still have difficulties. Common problems in gynaecological practice include vaginismus (involuntary tightening of the vaginal muscles making penetration difficult or impossible) and lack of libido. A history of sexual or physical abuse in childhood may present in later life as sexual difficulty or pelvic pain, and such patients are best referred to a psychiatrist.

For simple vaginismus, teaching a woman to use vaginal dilators may be effective.

Future trends
The demand for surgical treatment of menstrual disorders seems likely to continue, although minimally invasive surgery will increase. There will be a continuing demand for assisted conception, but male infertility remains a challenge. The most urgent need is to provide realistic sex education for young people to help them avoid unwanted pregnancy and sexually transmitted disease, but this requires action from society at large.

J. DRIFE

Further reading
Chamberlain, G. (1992). *ABC of antenatal care*. British Medical Journal, London.
Department of Health (1991). *Report on confidential enquiries into maternal deaths in the United Kingdon 1985–87*. HMSO, London.
Enkin, M., Keirse, M., and Chalmers, I. (1989). *A guide to effective care in pregnancy and childbirth*. Oxford University Press, Oxford.
Symonds, E. M. (1992). *Essential obstetrics and gynaecology*, (2nd edn). Churchill Livingstone, Edinburgh.

OBSTRUCTIVE JAUNDICE is *jaundice due to obstruction to the flow of *bile, for example, obstruction of the biliary tract by *gallstones, *carcinoma of the head of the *pancreas, or many other possible causes operating within or outside the liver. As the *bilirubin reabsorbed into the blood is of the soluble conjugated form, it is excreted by the kidney causing dark urine. However, the stools are pale due to lack of bile pigment in the faeces.

OCCIPITAL LOBE. The hindmost part of each *cerebral hemisphere, the cortex of which contains the primary receptive area for the sense of vision.

OCCIPUT. The posterior projection of the head.

OCCLUSION is the closure, obstruction, or blocking off of an opening, passage, or cavity.

OCCULTISM is the doctrine and practice of the ancient and medieval reputed sciences involving secret and mysterious agencies, or their modern equivalents, such as magic, alchemy, astrology, theosophy, etc.

OCCUPATIONAL CRAMP has long been believed to be a form of occupational *neurosis in which muscular spasm occurs in groups of muscles involved in a particular occupational task when an attempt is made to undertake that task, although the same muscles function normally under other circumstances. Writer's cramp is the best known example but many other forms occur in musicians, typists, etc. Many authorities believe that these conditions are forms of focal *dystonia and not of emotional origin. (Stoker's cramp is due to salt depletion and does not come under this heading.)

OCCUPATIONAL DISEASES OF FARM WORKERS. Agricultural workers, by virtue of their occupation, are exposed to many more infective and parasitic agents than the general population. They may thus be at greater risk of contracting such conditions as *brucellosis, *glanders, *erysipeloid, *ringworm, *orf, *cow-pox, *tetanus, *hydatid disease, etc. An allergen associated with mouldy hay accounts for *farmer's lung'. See also OCCUPATIONAL MEDICINE.

OCCUPATIONAL MEDICINE
From industrial disease to occupational health
Occupational medicine is that branch of medicine concerned with the effects of work on health, and the effects of health on the ability to work. It is essentially a discipline in *preventive medicine. The evolution of the concept of occupational health, initially from observations on industrial disease, can be traced from antiquity.

Historical development
Occupation has always exerted a profound influence on the pattern of life and death. *Hippocrates in 'Airs, waters and places' made observations on the effects of environment on health and the quality of life, but did not focus specifically on the occupational environment. However in 370 BC he described severe *colic in a worker who extracted metals, and may have been the first to recognize *lead as the cause of this symptom.

Cinnabar, the red sulphide of mercury, had been mined in Almaden, Spain, since Phoenician times and was used by the Romans as a durable pigment, together with red lead and other metallic compounds, to decorate buildings. Pliny, in the 1st century AD, described *mercury poisoning as a disease of slaves, for the mines of Almaden, contaminated with mercury vapour, were too unhealthy for Roman citizens to work in. He also described workers with lead oxides (used as pigments) tying up their faces in loose bags to avoid inhaling the poisonous dust.

The Middle Ages saw the development of metalliferous mining in central Europe. In *De re metallica*, published in 1556 and translated into English by a past president of the USA and his wife (Hoover and Hoover 1912), Agricola gave a detailed description of the mining, smelting, and refining of gold and silver. Agricola described the methods employed for ventilation, and illustrated primitive methods of personal protection in a series of wood-cuts. He described mining accidents and major disasters in mines, later to become all too familiar. He described also the harmful effects of dry dust inhalation, giving rise to difficulty in breathing and destruction of the lungs. A little later, *Paracelsus, a Swiss physician, wrote on the occupational diseases of mine-workers, smelter-workers, and metallurgists, giving a detailed description of mercurialism.

However, Bernardino *Ramazzini is generally acknowledged as the father of occupational medicine. Ramazzini practised as professor of medicine in the University of Modena, and later held the chair of medicine in Padua. His *De morbis artificum diatriba*, published in 1700, added one important question, 'What is your occupation?', to Hippocratic history-taking (Farrington 1941). He described in his treatise 54 different occupations associated with particular diseases, and included a description of the ill-effects on surgeons of rubbing into the skin mercurial ointments in the treatment of *syphilis, of the diseases of the mirror-makers of Venice, and a chapter on the diseases of learned men.

The insanitary and polluted condition of the new towns, and the working conditions in mines and factories, which followed the Industrial Revolution, pioneered in Britain, were aptly described by Charles Dickens. At that time, epidemics of *cholera, *tuberculosis, and *typhus, known as factory fever, were common. The pioneer of industrial medicine in the UK was Charles Turner *Thackrah, who published in 1831 *The effects of the principal arts, trades and professions and of civic states and habits of living, on health and longevity, with suggestions for removal of many of the agents which produce disease and shorten the duration of life.* Thackrah was a contemporary of *Addison, *Bright, and the poet Keats at Guys Hospital in London, and later was the founder of the Leeds School of Medicine. He wrote on the dust diseases of the lungs of miners and the grinders of metals using sandstone wheels, the forkgrinders of Sheffield dying before the age of 40. In his observations on the association of silica-dust inhalation with tuberculosis, giving rise to rapidly lethal silicotuberculosis, Thackrah antedated the current concern in developing countries where occupational exposures interact with endemic disease and *malnutrition to give rise to more severe disease.

Reform of the squalid conditions in the working environment was initiated, not by knowledge of industrial disease, but by public awareness of the outrageous exploitation of child labour in mines, factories, and mills. The humanitarian efforts of Robert Owen, Lord Shaftesbury, and others led to the first effective Factory Act of 1833, which set the minimum age of employment at 9 years, prohibited night work below 18 years, and restricted work to 12 hours a day. The Act established a Factory Inspectorate, and the Factory Act of 1844 led to the appointment of certifying surgeons.

The scandal of the climbing boys who swept the chimneys, immortalized in English literature, was finally brought to an end in 1875 when Lord Shaftesbury introduced a bill requiring chimney sweeps to hold a work licence. One hundred years previously, Percivall *Pott, by means of pertinent epidemiological observations, linked scrotal *cancer to ingrained soot in the skin, and provided the first evidence of an environmental cause for cancer. His work was followed by that of Butlin, who in 1892 showed that pitch, tar, and mineral oil also caused skin cancer, opening the road to work on experimental *carcinogenesis.

At the turn of the 20th century industrial disease and,

in particular, lead poisoning were rife in the UK, claiming many lives every year. Thomas *Legge, appointed first medical inspector of factories in 1898, introduced the notification system for certain industrial diseases, enabling attention to be drawn to the work site for control measures to be instituted. As a result, lead poisoning, responsible for nearly 4000 notified cases with over 100 deaths annually in the early 1900s steadily declined in frequency despite greatly increasing use of lead.

While the classic industrial diseases have declined in incidence in the UK and other industrialized countries during the 20th century, they have not been eradicated. In developing countries undergoing rapid industrialization, gross occupational disease may be seen on a scale not seen in the UK since the industrial revolution. With the decline in frank industrial disease in the UK, the increased surveillance of exposed workers has shown an increasing prevalence of subclinical effects, manifested by biochemical or other measurable changes, the health significance of which is not always apparent. New industrial diseases have also developed, related to modern technology, unknown even a century ago.

*X-rays were discovered in 1895 and *radium isolated in 1898 but the physicists working with newly discovered ionizing radiation knew nothing of its biological effects. The first case of skin cancer resulting from X-irradiation was reported in 1902, and by 1922 over 100 radiologists were estimated to have died from their occupational exposures. Pierre *Curie experienced radium dermatitis and both Marie Curie and her daughter died of *leukaemia. In a New Jersey factory between 1916 and 1923, girls pointed their brushes, dipped in radioactive paint, between their lips, in the production of luminous dials, resulting in death from *aplastic anaemia and bone *sarcoma some years later. More recently, *radiation sickness and deaths have occurred following exposure in nuclear energy establishments. An increased risk of developing leukaemia has been observed in the children of parents employed in the nuclear industry, but whether a causal relationship exists has yet to be determined (Roman *et al.* 1993).

Musculoskeletal disorders (repetitive strain injury) in workers, attributed to cumulative trauma, have been increasing markedly in relation to a changing work environment characterized by a requirement to perform more repetitive tasks at a faster pace (Millender *et al.* 1992).

While asbestos has been processed since ancient times, its increasing usage in modern technology since the late 19th century has given rise to heavy dust inhalation, with the progressive recognition of *asbestosis, its association with bronchial carcinoma, and, as late as 1960, its causal relationship with malignant *mesothelioma. As mesothelioma may develop 40 or more years after initial exposure to asbestos, the mortality from this condition, currently rising, is expected to continue to rise at least until the end of the century.

Technological development makes it likely that new occupational diseases will develop in the future; an effective monitoring system for new chemicals and processes, and constant vigilance by clinicians, hygienists, and epidemiologists, are required to prevent or to minimize such diseases.

The role of international agencies

A joint International Labour Organization, *World Health Organization committee (ILO/WHO, 1950) defined occupational health as:

The promotion and maintenance of the highest degree of physical, mental and social well-being of workers in all occupations; the prevention among workers of departures from health caused by their working conditions; the protection of workers in their employment from risks resulting from factors adverse to health; the placing and maintenance of the worker in an occupational environment adapted to his physiological equipment and, to summarise, the adaptation of work to man and of each man to his job.

This definition advances the concept of occupational health beyond the prevention of occupational disease, and introduces the promotion of positive health and the concept of fitting the job to the worker. WHO has had, since its inception, a major role in the field of occupational health. A global medium-term programme for workers' health covering the period 1984–89 aimed at the development of occupational health programmes as an integral part of health service infrastructure. Emphasis has been placed on 'work-related diseases' rather than purely occupational diseases, to include psychosocial hazards, reproductive hazards, and the application of ergonomics to health promotion. WHO produces, among other publications in this field, a series of monographs on environmental health criteria through its International Programme for Chemical Safety (IPCS) and a series on the evaluation of carcinogenic risk of chemicals and processes through the International Agency for Research on Cancer (IARC, WHO).

The International Labour Organization (ILO), also based in Geneva, is best known to occupational physicians through its occupational safety and health series of publications, and, in particular, through the ILO international classification of radiographs of the pneumoconioses, whose standard films have been widely used in epidemiological studies.

The interaction between industrial activity and the environment, between occupational health and environmental health, can be well illustrated by reference to the activities of the International Register of Potentially Toxic Chemicals of the United Nations Environment Programme (IRPTC, UNEP). A list of environmentally dangerous chemicals and processes of global significance, distributed to world governments, includes lead, mercury and cadmium, carbon dioxide, oxides of nitrogen, sulphur dioxide and its derivatives; and what has been termed the injudicious use of pesticides, which still give rise to poisoning on a large scale in many parts of the world.

The Council of the European Community issued, in 1980, a directive on the protection of workers from risks related to exposure to chemical, physical, and biological agents at work. A series of individual directives followed, aimed at establishing limit values for occupational exposure to a number of chemical agents, e.g. lead and asbestos, and for the appropriate health surveillance of workers. Occupational health guidelines for chemical risk have been defined under the EEC's (now EU's) Environmental Chemical Data and Information Network (ECDIN). These guidelines advise on pre-employment and periodic medical examination and biological monitoring procedures, giving action levels where these are available (Commission of the European Community 1983).

Occupational health is co-ordinated through the Health and Safety Directorate, Directorate-General V of the Commission of the European Communities centred in Luxembourg, although research in this field is the priority of Directorate General XII in Brussels.

Occupational health in the UK

At the present time, some 155 000 people in Britain are in receipt of industrial injuries benefit, and about 200 000 are involved in industrial accidents sufficiently severe for them to be reported to the Health and Safety Executive. While back pain and psychiatric disorders are the most common, *dermatitis accounts for about 60 000 cases per year, cancers contributed to by occupational exposures about 5000, and occupational *asthma about 1500 cases per year (Seaton 1993).

Occupational medicine was originally excluded from the National Health Service (NHS), and again excluded after its reorganization in 1982. The larger, privately controlled industries and those publicly controlled, such as the National Coal Board and British Rail, developed their own non-statutory occupational health services. In several areas, health services for groups of smaller industries were organized on a co-operative basis. However, many of the smaller plants, where the worst working conditions could be found, had, and still have, minimal cover by *general practitioners with part-time appointments in industry, and some have no cover at all.

While physicians with full-time appointments in occupational health services will have received appropriate training, some doctors with part-time appointments have had no such occupational health training. Occupational medicine is now an accredited specialty in the UK and other countries of the European Community. The Faculty of Occupational Medicine at the *Royal College of Physicians, London, is responsible for academic standards. The faculty awards an associateship (AFOM) and a membership (MFOM) by examination and a fellowship (FFOM) by election. Candidates for the AFOM are required to have completed 2 years in approved full-time posts or part-time pro rata to be eligible. The *Royal College of Nursing awards the Occupational Health Nursing Certificate (OHNC) to nurses who have completed 2 years post-registration experience in nursing followed by a full- or part-time course. Training for a career in occupational hygiene is provided at both undergraduate and postgraduate level by a number of universities, and a professional qualification is awarded by the British Occupational Hygiene Society and the Institute of Occupational Hygienists.

During the first half of this century, successive legislation on matters related to health and safety built a cumbersome legal edifice which had many inadequacies and omissions. The report of the Committee of Enquiry on Safety and Health at Work was followed by a new, broadly based enabling Act, the Health and Safety at Work etc. Act of 1974, aimed at covering all persons at work. The Act encompassed for the first time people working in hospitals and schools and included the control of processes which may affect the health and safety of the general public, such as emissions into the atmosphere, the discharge of toxic substances into waterways and on land, and the transport and storage of potentially dangerous materials. The Health and Safety at Work etc. Act set up the Health and Safety Commission, answerable to the Secretary of State of the Department of Employment. The Commission is a tripartite body representing trade unions, employers, and local authorities. The operational arm, the Health and Safety Executive (HSE), is responsible for implementing the advisory functions of the Commission and for enforcing the statutory provisions. The Employment Medical Advisory Service (EMAS), which superseded the old medical inspectorate of factories and which had been set up by a separate act the preceding year, forms the medical arm of the HSE. EMAS is responsible for advising the HSE, doctors, employers, workers, and unions on health matters related to employment.

An important and innovative feature of the Health and Safety at Work etc. Act is the placing of the onus of responsibility on the employer to ensure, as far as is reasonably practicable, the health, safety, and welfare of his employees, and also of persons not in his employ with access to his premises. The employee has a duty to take reasonable care and to co-operate with others to ensure that the required measures are complied with. Furthermore, the Act is also designed to protect the general public from risks to health or safety resulting from the activities of persons at work.

A series of regulations and approved codes of practice have followed the Health and Safety at Work etc. Act. In 1988 the Control of Substances Hazardous to Health (COSHH) Regulations introduced a requirement for employers and the self-employed to assess the risks arising from exposure to substances hazardous to health. An approved code of practice followed to provide practical guidance with regard to control of exposure to suspected specified carcinogens.

A framework directive, agreed by the European Council of Ministers in 1989, has been followed by a series of six 'daughter' directives as part of the European Commission's programme of action on health and safety. The resultant new regulations, which came into force in the UK in January 1993, introduce new approaches, clarify, and make more explicit current health and safety law, but do not replace, for example, the COSHH regulations. In brief, the Management of Health and Safety at Work Regulations, 1992, require a risk assessment to be performed, and where five or more employees are involved, for this to be recorded. Health and Safety arrangement and health surveillance must also be defined, and appropriate information must be given to employees. Other regulations operative from January 1993 are the Workplace (Health Safety and Welfare) Regulations, 1992; the Manual Handling Operations Regulations, 1992; the Personal Protective Equipment at Work Regulations, 1992; the Provision and Use of Work Equipment Regulations, 1992; and the Health and Safety (Display Screen Equipment) Regulations, 1992. There has been, in the past, no specific legislation with regard to display screen equipment, which definition extends beyond the typical office visual display unit, to include, for example, a microfiche viewer. There are currently more than 8.5 million display screens in use in the UK. Adverse health effects have centred on upper limb disorders, visual discomfort, and stress-related symptoms. The regulations require consideration of work-station design, the working environment, relevant human factors, and an appropriate safety audit. Adverse health effects related to work with display screen equipment may be considered an example of a new industrial disease related to modern technology, but then, as Ramazzini observed in the early 18th century, 'where clerks incessantly drive the pen over paper, intense fatigue of the arm develops because of continuous strain upon the muscles and tendons, which eventually may lead to failure of power in the hand'.

G. KAZANTZIS

References

Commission of the European Community (1983). *Occupational health guidelines for chemical risk*. Luxemburg.

Farrington, B. (1941). The hand in healing. A study in Greek medicine from Hippocrates to Ramazzini. *Proceedings of the Royal Institution of Great Britain*, **32**, 60–91.

Hoover, H. C. and Hoover, L. H. (ed.) (1912). *Georgius Agricola: De re metallica* (translated from the first Latin edition of 1556). The Mining Magazine, London.

Millender, L. H., Louis, D. S., and Simmons, B. P. (ed.) (1992). *Occupational disorders of the upper extremity*. Churchill Livingstone, London.

Roman, E. *et al*. (1993). Case-control study of leukaemia and non-Hodgkin's lymphoma among children aged 0–4 years living in West Berkshire and North Hampshire health districts. *British Medical Journal*, **306**, 615–21.

Seaton, A. (1993). Occupational medicine – let's keep our white coats and stethoscopes. *Occupational Medicine*, **43**, 63–4.

OCCUPATIONAL NURSING. See OCCUPATIONAL MEDICINE.

OCCUPATIONAL PHYSICIAN. A physician specializing in the health of the working population and in diseases associated with occupational environments. See OCCUPATIONAL MEDICINE.

OCCUPATIONAL THERAPISTS. Occupational therapy is defined by the American Occupational Therapy Association as a method of treatment for the sick or injured by means of purposeful occupation. The goals are to arouse interest, courage, and confidence; to exercise mind and body in healthy activity; to overcome disability; and to re-establish capacity for industrial and social usefulness. Occupational therapists have traditionally taught handicrafts, but the scope has been widened to include physical exercises, games, music, and household and industrial skills. They also advise upon adaptations to the home and workplace and the provision of aids to disabled or handicapped people.

OCULAR. Pertaining to the eye.

OCULIST. A specialist in diseases of the eye; an ophthalmologist. See OPHTHALMOLOGY.

OCULOMOTOR PARALYSIS. The oculomotor (or third cranial) nerve supplies all the extrinsic muscles of the eye, that is those responsible for eye movements, with the exception of the superior oblique muscle (supplied by the trochlear or fourth cranial nerve) and the lateral rectus (supplied by the abducens or sixth cranial nerve). When a lesion affects the oculomotor nerve alone, the paralysed eye is deviated laterally and downwards and there is loss of upward, downward, and medial movement; in addition, there is complete *ptosis with *mydriasis and loss of *pupil reactivity.

OD is a hypothetical force (also called the odylic force) postulated by von Reichenbach (1788–1869), said to permeate all nature and to be manifest in individuals of sensitive temperament; it was invoked to explain the phenomena of *mesmerism and animal magnetism.

ODONTOLOGY is the scientific study of the teeth.

ODOURS. Awareness of odours is often useful in medicine, as in daily life. Characteristic smells on the breath occur after the use of tobacco, alcohol, and cannabis, the stale odour of acetaldehyde being a delayed sign of alcohol indulgence. Volatile drugs, such as paraldehyde and various anaesthetic agents, are usually obvious; the sweetish smell of acetone may indicate ketosis due to diabetes or starvation; lead poisoning is said to confer a metallic odour on the breath (*halitus saturninus*), and poisoning with arsenic, selenium, phosphorus, and tellurium can be suggested by a smell akin to that of garlic; *foetor hepaticus* is a musty smell characteristic of severe liver disease with encephalopathy, thought to be due to the presence of mercaptans in the expired air; foul-smelling breath (*foetor oris* or halitosis) can occur in apparently healthy individuals but also results from sepsis of teeth, gums, sinuses, and respiratory tract.

OEDEMA (EDEMA) is excess fluid in the tissue spaces. A sufficient accumulation in the subcutaneous tissues causes visible swelling. The fact that this is due to excess extracellular fluid and not to any other cause is confirmed by the characteristic sign of 'pitting on pressure'; firm pressure with a finger or thumb maintained for at least five seconds causes a depression in the swollen area which takes some minutes to disappear after pressure is removed. Oedema may be localized, due to local vascular causes such as venous or lymphatic obstruction, or generalized, implying overall body retention of fluid and electrolytes. The latter occurs, for example, in some heart and kidney disorders, although there are many other causes. The distribution of oedema fluid is influenced by hydrostatic factors. It thus accumulates in the relatively lax tissues under the skin, and especially in dependent parts (feet, ankles, and lower legs in the ambulant patient; over the sacral and pelvic regions in those confined to bed).

OEDIPUS COMPLEX is the term for the complex of a child's emotions associated with a subconscious desire for the parent of the opposite sex, which, if not resolved, may, according to Freudian theory, lead to feelings of guilt and difficulty in forming normal sexual relationships.

OESOPHAGOSCOPY (ESOPHAGOSCOPY) is *endoscopy of the oesophagus.

OESOPHAGUS (ESOPHAGUS). The gullet, that part of the alimentary tract which connects the *pharynx with the *stomach; it consists of a musculomembranous tube running downwards through the *mediastinum and passing through the *diaphragm.

OESTROGEN (ESTROGEN). Any substance, natural or synthetic, which produces changes in the female sexual organs similar to those produced by oestradiol, the natural *hormone of the vertebrate *ovary. The main actions of oestrogens are: development of female *secondary sexual characteristics; stimulation of vaginal cornification, myometrial hypertrophy, and endometrial hyperplasia (which may be followed by withdrawal bleeding); and inhibition of *follicle-stimulating hormone secretion by the anterior *pituitary gland, suppressing ovulation. Oestrogens are also produced by the *placenta, and in small amounts by the *adrenal cortex and *testis. Indications for their therapeutic use include; oral *contraception; *menopausal symptoms and *osteoporosis; certain cases of breast and prostate *cancer; certain cases of *dysmenorrhoea and *menorrhagia; and inhibition of *lactation. Many doctors now advise their use as hormonal replacement therapy (HRI) in post-menopausal women.

OESTRUS (ESTRUS). The brief period (usually 1 or 2 days) during which female non-human mammals evidence sexual desire and are receptive to copulation. Oestrus, which coincides with *ovulation, is part of a physiological cycle characteristic of sexually mature female mammals (the oestrous cycle), of which *menstruation may be regarded as a variant.

OFFICE OF POPULATION, CENSUSES AND SURVEYS (OPCS). This UK government department, which incorporates the General Register Office, is responsible for the regulation of civil marriages, the registration of births, marriages, and deaths in England and Wales, and control of the registration services; the analysis of vital medical and demographic statistics and publication of reports thereon; the periodic census of the population; research into the attitude and circumstances of the general public or of particular groups of individuals. The director of the OPCS is also *Registrar-General for England and Wales.

OIL. Any greasy liquid which is insoluble in water and soluble in *alcohol and *ether. Mineral oils are mixtures of various *hydrocarbons, while animal and vegetable oils are simple *lipids, mixtures of fatty acid glycerides distinguished from fats only by their liquidity.

OINTMENT. Any greasy water-insoluble preparation, usually containing medicinal substances. The commonest base is a mixture of liquid, soft, and hard paraffins.

OLDBERG, ERIC (1901–86). American neurosurgeon. Harvey *Cushing's last chief resident at the Peter Bent Brigham Hospital, 1929–30. Professor and Chairman, Department of Neurology and Neurosurgery, University of Illinois College of Medicine. He trained more than 80 neurosurgeons, many of whom pursued careers in academic neurosurgery.

OLD MOORE'S ALMANAC was the best known early English almanac published by the Stationers' Company. Francis *Moore was a physician, astrologer, and schoolmaster who published it, containing weather predictions, in order to promote the sale of his pills. The first number was completed in July 1700 and contained predictions for 1701. The front cover of the edition for 1791, in the possession of W. Foulsham & Co. Ltd, carries a twopenny duty stamp and reads:

Vox Stellarum: or, a Loyal Almanack for the Year of Human Redemption M, DCC, XCI. Being the Third after Bissextile or Leap-Year. In which are contained All things fitting for such a Work; as, a Table of Terms and their Returns; The Full, Changes, and Quarters of the Moon; The Rising, Southing,

and Setting of the Seven Stars, and other Fixed Stars of Note; the Moon's Age, and a Tide Table fitted to the same; The Rising and Setting of the Sun; the Rising, Southing and Setting of the Moon; Mutual Aspects, Monthly Observations; and many other Things, useful and profitable.

There are a number of current versions, containing many predictions besides the weather.

OLD VIENNA SCHOOL. The 'old Vienna school' of medicine was established about the middle of the 18th century by two able physicians, van *Swieten and de Haen, both of whom had been trained in Holland. Hospitals and clinics were established, and the *Allgemeines Krankenhaus, Vienna's famous general hospital, was founded in 1784. This hospital alone was dealing with 14 000 patients a year by the end of the century, when Johan Peter *Frank was the director. Joseph Leopold *Auenbrugger was a young physician there when he described his invention of *percussion for elucidating obscure diseases of the chest. During the first quarter of the 19th century, while clinical medicine was reaching new heights in London and Paris, the Vienna school lapsed into a period of relative inactivity, until reinvigorated by the work of *Rokitansky and *Skoda.

OLFACTION is the sense of smell.

OLFACTOMETER. An instrument for measuring the acuity of *olfaction.

OLIGODENDROGLIA is one of the component elements of *neuroglia, the supporting tissue of the nervous system; its cells (oligodendrocytes) are responsible for the formation of *myelin in the white matter of the brain and spinal cord.

OLIGOPHRENIA. Mental subnormality or handicap—an obsolete term.

OLIGURIA is the passage of abnormally small quantities of *urine.

OMBUDSMAN. The appointment in the UK of an ombudsman, more formally known as the Health Service Commissioner, was provided for under the *National Health Service (Reorganization) Act 1973. His function is to investigate complaints arising primarily from administrative failure or error, and not those involving clinical matters or family practitioners, for which an established system for dealing with complaints already existed. The responsibilities of the Commissioner, whose security of tenure can be disturbed only by Parliament, extends to Wales and Scotland, with offices and representation in those countries. Of cases investigated and reported on, most have involved waiting-list errors, inadequate records, and inadequate information given to patients' parents or relatives. Many have resulted from faults which were easily remediable.

OMENTUM. A loose fold of *peritoneum, associated with a variable amount of *adipose tissue, which hangs down from the *stomach and *colon within the abdominal cavity.

ONANISM is the extravaginal depositing of semen (see Genesis 38:9), as in *masturbation or *coitus interruptus.

ONCHOCERCIASIS is infestation with the adult worms and microfilariae of the *nematode parasite *Onchocerca volvulus*. It is endemic in tropical communities living within a few kilometres of fast-flowing water, the breeding environment required by the blackfly (*Simulium damnosum*), which is the vector of the disease. The most important complication of onchocerciasis is loss of vision due to microfilarial invasion of the eye ('river blindness').

ONCOGENES are viral *genes, that is segments of *deoxyribonucleic acid (DNA), thought to be capable of inducing malignant transformation in cells.

ONCOLOGIST. A physician, surgeon, or radiotherapist who specializes in the diagnosis and treatment of cancer. See ONCOLOGY; RADIOTHERAPY.

ONCOLOGY: CANCER, NEOPLASTIC DISEASE, MALIGNANT DISEASE
Introduction
Oncology is a word derived from the Greek, *onchos*, a lump, or *tumour. Oncology is the study of *cancer. Cancer is a proliferation of cells which grow in an uncontrolled manner, invading local tissues and spreading widely through the blood or *lymphatics to produce secondary deposits, or metastases, in distant parts of the body. The *cells composing the tumour grow better than normal cells, and have either partially or completely escaped the complex mechanisms of restraint that control growth in normal cells.

History
While cancer was known to ancient civilizations, and descriptions occur in medieval manuscripts, the disease as it would be defined today was established as an entity by the great German *pathologists of the 19th century. They described the cellular nature of cancer, and classified cancers including *leukaemia, a cancer of the blood in which *white blood cells become malignant, and *lymphomas, which are cancers of the lymph nodes.

At the beginning of the 20th century, most major forms of cancer had been described, and attention focused on finding the cause and introducing treatment. In 1775, Percivall Pott had described the association of soot with cancer in chimney sweeps, and *environmental hazards soon became recognized, such as shale oil (associated with skin cancer), radioactive ores (causing *lung cancer in miners), beta-naphthylamine (used in the rubber industry, and causing *bladder cancer in workers), and cigarettes (linked to lung cancer, as described by Doll and Bradford Hill). Research on the causes of cancer began with the testing of various chemicals. Benzpyrene was shown by Kennaway to be the constituent of coal tar which produced experimental skin cancer in animals. It was found that not only chemicals could cause cancers, but also *viruses. Early experimental sarcomas produced by the Rous sarcoma virus were followed by the identification of many others in the laboratory. Later, the realization that a particular form of lymphoma described by Burkitt was caused by the Epstein–Barr virus in man, showed that the study of oncogenic viruses was no longer of academic interest only. Recently, human T-cell leukaemia has been found to be due to the virus HTLV-1, which is acquired in southern Japan and the West Indies. Neither chemicals, *radiation, nor viruses account for the majority of cancers in adults, however, and the search for environmental hazards continues.

In children, some forms of cancer can be shown to be inherited. A rare eye tumour, retinoblastoma, is inherited on *Mendelian lines as a dominant characteristic, i.e. in a family where one parent carries the abnormal *gene, half the children will have the tumour. The specific abnormality on *chromosome 13 in these patients has been defined and shown to be a specific loss in the *DNA content of the nucleus. Other such losses, or deletions, have been identified in families where the unfortunate members suffer a wide variety of different malignancies. The common feature of these inherited cancers is a deletion of a part of the *genome, or total DNA content, which is responsible for suppressing the development of cancer.

Techniques in *molecular biology now enable the most intimate structures of the cancer cell to be explored. Two mechanisms seem likely to be involved at the molecular level in the cancer cell. In the first, parts of the genome involved in cell growth become activated, and these so-called 'proto-oncogenes' produce cell constituents which give the malignant cell a growth advantage over the normal cell. In the second mechanism, described above, parts of the genome which are concerned with regulating growth (so-called 'suppressor' genes) are lost, and the cell escapes from their restraining influence. These mechanisms are now ripe for exploitation as a means of curing cancer.

Different types of cancer
Normal tissues can be divided into those that make up the body structure (bone, muscle, fibrous tissue, fat, etc.) and those that cover or line the airways, the intestinal tract, the urinary tract, with a thin sheet of *epithelium. When structural tissues become malignant, they are called *sarcomas—thus, bone sarcomas (osteosarcomas) and fat sarcomas (liposarcomas)—whereas epithelial cancers are called *carcinomas—thus, lung carcinoma, arising from the epithelium lining the main

airways or bronchi; breast carcinoma, arising from the ductal tissue in the breast; carcinoma of the *stomach and *colon, arising from the respective epithelial linings of these organs.

Sarcomas are more commonly seen in children, and spread via the bloodstream, whereas carcinomas are more commonly seen in adults, and usually (but not always) spread via the lymphatics. In general, the sarcomas are less well differentiated, i.e. it is harder to see from which tissue they are derived, but on the other hand (especially in children) they respond better to treatment with *chemotherapy (anticancer drugs). In adults, carcinomas respond less well to chemotherapy, and some show resistance to these agents from the start, while others develop resistance very quickly.

Management of cancer
Diagnosis
The proper management of cancer depends on an accurate diagnosis, which should never be made without looking at the tumour cells under the microscope. Many techniques are now refining the process so that the study of markers on the surface of the cell, demonstration of the presence of chemicals within the cell (*cytochemistry), changes in the number or configuration of the chromosomes in the *nucleus (*cytogenetics), or demonstration of deletions or *translocations in chromosomes by molecular biology are all of increasing importance.

Staging
In order to compare results, generally agreed staging systems are essential. In their simplest form, staging schemes define tumours as either confined to the tissue of origin, or having spread to local tissues and organs (hence regional spread), and finally as having metastasized. In the case of so-called 'solid' tumours, which arise from one primary site and spread locally and then to other parts of the body, staging is very important. It will influence the type of treatment recommended, and will usually be a very important factor in determining survival or prognosis. Clinical oncology employs staging as a shorthand to compare treatment programmes. No ideal treatment exists for any form of cancer at the moment, and every advance in therapy has to come from so-called 'trials' of treatment. Refinements of staging are produced for every cancer, and international staging systems such as the TNM (tumour, nodes, metastases) staging classification, and the Ann Arbor (named after a place) for *Hodgkin's disease, have been widely accepted.

Definition of response
Just as staging is a shorthand enabling patients to be compared, so response to treatment has its own notation. A 'complete response' indicates that all clinical symptoms, the examination of the patient, and the relevant investigations, show no evidence of the cancer. A 'partial response' is when the disease has decreased by

more than half its original extent, while stable disease, and no response are self-explanatory. The efficacy of a programme is usually measured in response rate, which is the total of complete response and partial response results. In general, the possibility of curing a particular cancer only arises when the number of patients obtaining a complete response on a treatment programme is high, and even then complete response may not be translated into a high proportion of cures, because of the relative inadequacy of present methods of detecting residual cancer. Where a marker is produced, such as the substances beta-human chorionic gonadotrophin and *alphafetoprotein, in patients with testicular cancer for example, disappearance of these substances correlates well with the eventual cure of the patient.

Performance status
Performance status defines the state of a patient's health. It may be a good indicator of a patient's ability to stand modern intensive therapy and to benefit from it in terms of survival. The concept of performance status was first introduced by Karnofsky (Table 1). Patients at the top of the table usually respond well to therapy, while those in the middle do not. Patients in the lower part of the table may not be helped by therapy, and may be better managed by supportive care.

Table 1 Karnofsky performance status

100	Normal, no complaints
90	Able to carry out normal activity; minor symptoms of disease
80	Normal activity with effort; some symptoms of disease
70	Cares for self; unable to carry on normal activity or work
60	Requires occasional assistance, but is able to care for most of own needs
50	Requires considerable assistance and frequent medical care
40	Disabled; requires special aid
30	Severely disabled; hospitalization probably needed
20	Very sick; needs in-patient hospitalization
10	Moribund; fatal processes progressing rapidly

Specific treatment
The history of the development of cancer therapy is a story of the use of increasingly sophisticated surgical techniques for the removal of cancer, more powerful and controlled radiation beams of different types for its localized destruction, the development of naturally produced and synthetic chemotherapeutic agents which inhibit and then kill malignant cells, and the introduction of naturally occurring constituents which control cells,

the so-called '*cytokines', of which *interferon is an example.

Although these modalities will be dealt with under separate headings, programmes involving two or more treatment methods together are now becoming common.

(a) Surgery. Until the beginning of the 20th century, surgery was the only effective means of treating cancer. It will remain important as the main means whereby *biopsy (removal of a small sample of tumour) can be effected for diagnostic purposes. When technically possible, surgery can be used to remove the whole of a tumour if it is confined to the primary site. Chemotherapy is used, particularly in early stage childhood tumours, to reduce the size of a tumour so that it can be removed with the least possible damage to surrounding tissues. There is now a trend for surgery to be more limited; for example, where appropriate, the tumour alone is removed from a breast, rather than removing the whole breast, or a long bone in the limbs, affected by tumour, is removed and replaced by a prosthesis, rather than performing an *amputation.

(b) Radiotherapy. The discoveries of *X-rays by *Roentgen (1895) and of *radioactivity by the *Curies in 1899 were followed, in a very short space of time, by their application to medicine. Radiotherapy was available as a treatment for tumours in the first decade of the 20th century. Tumours may respond to electromagnetic radiation (X-rays) or to particles (electrons or beta-rays, protons, neutrons, and alpha particles). Radiation may be delivered by injected *isotopes (e.g. radioiodine), by machines producing high-energy X-rays, by radiation sources such as radioactive cobalt, and by *cyclotrons producing particles such as protons or neutrons. With the exception of isotopes, both tumour and normal tissues in the radiation field will be affected, and in order to reduce the damage to normal tissues within the field of therapy, the dose is fractionated, i.e. a patient will be treated once or twice a day over a period of time. Normal tissues, which recover more rapidly than tumour tissues, are thus less likely to be seriously damaged. Radiotherapy is primarily indicated for small, localized tumours, and is the treatment of choice for retinoblastoma (small tumours in the retina), or laryngeal carcinoma (small tumours in the larynx), which are cured in more than 90 per cent of cases.

(c) Chemotherapy. The fact that mustard gas could shrink lymphoid tissues was already known before derivatives were produced during the Second World War. Nitrogen mustard was found to be effective in the treatment of disseminated lymphoma. Before 1946 disseminated malignancy was incurable, but the use of nitrogen mustard made it possible to affect the course of cancers such as Hodgkin's disease and leukaemia, which have already disseminated when the patient is first seen. In 1948 a report came from the USA of a drug very similar to folic acid, called aminopterin, showing that it could produce a complete response or remission in children with acute lymphoblastic leukaemia. Within 2 years the first of two major families of anticancer drugs, the alkylating agents and the antimetabolites, were in use. *Choriocarcinoma, a rare cancer of women, was shown to be curable using methotrexate, an antimetabolite, and disseminated Hodgkin's disease was found to be curable when combinations of anticancer drugs, including nitrogen mustard, vincristine (a plant product), procarbazine, and prednisolone, were used in short courses. The principles of multidrug therapy were successfully applied to lymphomas and leukaemias, and then to testicular cancer, the commonest malignancy of young men, where high cure rates were obtained even with disseminated disease.

(d) Adjuvant therapy. The possibility that even when cancer is detected early, spread may occur in the form of small foci of tumour, so-called 'micrometastases', which are undetectable by current methods, suggested that treatment with chemotherapy at this stage would be highly successful in improving the cure rate. This hypothesis was confirmed in a study of children with *Wilms' tumour (a sarcoma of the kidney) treated at Boston Children's Hospital. Following removal of the kidney tumour, adjuvant chemotherapy was given, and it proved possible to increase the cure rate for Wilms' tumour from 40 to over 80 per cent.

This principle has been applied to adult solid tumours, notably breast cancer. While individual trials have not shown the dramatic improvement seen in children's tumours, nevertheless, overviews of large numbers of trials have shown a 10 per cent saving of lives at 10 years in those women given some form of adjuvant chemotherapy.

(d) Drug resistance. The generally disappointing results in common tumours such as lung cancer, gastrointestinal cancer, renal cancer, and *melanoma have intensified the search for the reason why these cancers either fail to respond to powerful anticancer drugs or, having once responded, become resistant. The ability of the cell to pump out toxic materials has been shown to be due to a number of mechanisms, but in particular to *glycoprotein, a chemical pump in the membrane of the cell. Tumour cells can increase the production of these cell-membrane pumps, and thus become immune to the effect of chemotherapy. Drugs such as verapamil and cyclosporin A are being investigated for their ability to inhibit the activity of the glycoprotein pumps. Drug resistance has become an important area of cancer research.

(e) Hormones. The beneficial effects of *oestrogens on advanced prostatic cancer were first shown in 1941. Hormone-dependent cancers such as *prostate cancer, breast cancer, and endometrial cancer, have been controlled successfully, often for worthwhile periods of time, by hormonal manipulation, but unfortunately they are not cured by these agents. Since the treatments are well tolerated, they may be the first choice; for example, in elderly postmenopausal women *tamoxifen, a synthetic oestrogen, is a highly satisfactory treatment, producing a high rate of response with long-term control.

(f) Cytokines. It is becoming apparent that the growth of cells is controlled by a network of complex substances produced in the microenvironment by a variety of different cells, of which lymphocytes form an important group. These 'interleukins' can be shown to affect tumours, and a large number have now been described. Interleukin-2 has been introduced recently into clinical practice. Cytokines such as interferons have also been used and are curative in some rare forms of leukaemia, such as hairy-cell leukaemia, and will control chronic myeloid leukaemia for some time.

(g) Monoclonal antibodies and immune modulation. Other approaches to the cure of malignancy, such as *antibodies targeted against tumours, and stimulation of the host's own immunological responses, have been disappointing so far in the clinic, although they have given a great deal of insight into tumour behaviour.

Shimkin (1986) concluded that the control of many forms of cancer would be achieved by clinical and scientific research by the end of the 20th century, and I see no reason to disagree.

                                           J. S. MALPAS

Further reading
Franks, L. M. and Teich, N. (ed.) (1986). *Introduction to the cellular and molecular biology of cancer.* Oxford University Press, Oxford.
Shimkin, M. B. (1986). Oncology (neoplastic diseases). In *The Oxford companion to medicine,* (ed. J. Walton, P. Beeson, and R. Bodley Scott). Oxford University Press, Oxford.
Williams, C. J. (ed.) (1992). *Introducing new treatments for cancer: practical, ethical and legal problems.* Wiley, Chichester.

ONYCHIA is infection of the matrix of a finger- or toe-nail.

OOCYTE. Ovarian cell, precursor of the *ovum.

OOPHORECTOMY is the surgical removal of one or both *ovaries.

OPENING SNAP. A discrete short high-frequency sound heard on cardiac *auscultation following shortly after the second heart sound, associated with mitral valve opening at the beginning of *diastole. An audible opening snap at or near the apex of the heart is a characteristic sign of *mitral stenosis.

OPERATING THEATRE. A room designed and equipped for the purpose of carrying out surgical operations, usually with anterooms for anaesthetic induction, recovery, surgical and nursing staff, etc.

OPERATING THEATRE ATTENDANTS. Ancillary staff attached to operating theatres; theatre orderlies.

OPERATION. Any surgical procedure.

OPHTHALMIA. Any severe inflammatory condition of the eye. Ophthalmia neonatorum refers to acute purulent conjunctivitis developing in infants within a few days of birth as a result of direct infection from the mother's birth canal, due for example to *gonorrhoea.

OPHTHALMOLOGIST. A medically qualified specialist in diseases of the eye; an oculist. See OPHTHAL-MOLOGY.

OPHTHALMOLOGY. Vision is the most important of the traditional five senses in the human, and eyesight is responsible for almost 50 per cent of the total sensory input from the external world to the internal world of the conscious human being. As a result, loss of vision or the prospect of loss of vision can cause great anxiety and can greatly exacerbate mental stress or mental illness. As early as 1550 BC, the Egyptians had outlined in the Ebers Papyrus a list of recognized eye diseases, and Alexander in 327 BC, during his campaign along the Indus River, commented on the knowledge of eye disease amongst Indian physicians. The Chinese were also aware of ocular disease and had described *cataract even before the Indian physicians. Hippocrates described the *anatomy of the eyeball and the *optic nerve, and for a period of some 2000 years his teachings held sway. In 1847 Charles Babbage, an Englishman, suggested that it would be possible to view the back of the eye through the pupil, using a perforated mirror; this was elaborated on by von *Helmholtz in 1851, triggering a massive increase in the knowledge of ocular disease.

Anatomy and physiology of the visual system
The eye has the very important function of converting the images of the external world into electrical signals. The electrical impulses from the eye are transmitted up the optic nerve to a junction with the optic nerve from the other eye, where at least 50 per cent of the nerve fibres cross to relay to the opposite side of the brain. This crossing is called the optic chiasm. The nerves then travel as a bundle of fibres, called the optic tract, until they come to a relay station called the lateral geniculate ganglion, where a rearrangement of the fibres takes place. The messages are then transmitted through another fan-shaped bundle of nerve fibres, called the optic radiation, to the occipital lobe of the brain, where more processing is carried out by the visual cortex. At this level, vision consists of very crude images of light and dark, and for vision to occur as we know it,

the messages have to be passed on to a number of other areas in the brain. These include an area in the temporal lobe of the brain where visual memory is situated, and the parietal lobe of the brain where vision is related to other forms of sensory input and where our ability to recognize symbols needed for reading and writing are situated. There are also connections to the anterior part of the brain, the frontal lobe, where conscious imagery is processed further.

Anatomy and physiology of the eye

The eyeball (Fig. 1) consists of three separate concentric layers, modified anteriorly to form the transparent cornea which allows the passage of light. The outermost layer, the sclera, is a tough, fibrous, protective envelope consisting of collagen and referred to in lay terms as 'the white of the eye'. The innermost layer, the *retina, is designed to be light sensitive and has the ability to convert these light signals to electrical coded signals for transmission to the higher visual centres. The intervening layer, the choroid, is very vascular. In its anterior part it forms the ciliary body and part of the iris. The bulk of the space in the eyeball is occupied by a transparent gel, the vitreous humour, while in the anterior part of the eyeball there is a cavity between the *cornea and the *lens, the anterior chamber, filled with clear circulating fluid—aqueous humour.

For light to reach the retina it must pass through four transparent media; in order:

1. The cornea, which is the transparent part of the sclera at the front of the eye and which is responsible for 75 per cent of the refracting (focusing) power of the eye.
2. Aqueous humour, a clear fluid which nourishes the avascular cornea and lens, and creates a pressure within the eye to keep the eye in shape. Aqueous humour is produced by modified muscle called the ciliary body and passes through the pupil, draining through the angle between the cornea and the iris into the canal of Schlemm.
3. The lens, a pea-sized structure made of proteins inside a capsule, which is responsible for 25 per cent of the focusing power of the eye. The lens can alter its shape in order to focus on the retina, and as it becomes stiff with age the ability to focus lessens (presbyopia).
4. The vitreous humour, a clear gel in which opacities can develop in older age or in short-sight (myopia), when the opacities are called vitreous floaters.

The iris is a circular muscle with a hole in the centre, the *pupil, which regulates the amount of light entering the eye and also helps in focusing on near objects by contracting its size. The retina is a complex, three-layered structure lining the inside of the eyeball. The deepest layer contains the rods and the cones, which are responsible for picking up light signals from the external world. Rods are responsible for night vision and cannot perceive colour, whereas cones are responsible for day vision and can perceive colour. In the centre of the retina there is a modified anatomical area called the *macula, which is responsible for the greatest clarity of vision. This area has no retinal blood vessels and relies on its nourishment by diffusion from the choroid, whose main functions are:

(1) to act as a source of nutrients for the overlying retina;
(2) as a heat exchanger to dissipate the heat released by the absorption of light.

The other two layers in the retina, the bipolar cell layer and the ganglion cell layer, modify the signal from the rods and cones and send the message along the optic nerve to the visual cortex.

Refractive errors

Approximately one-third of the population do not see clearly because of refractive errors, resulting either from differences in the size of the eyeball in relation to the focusing power of the eye, or changes in the curvature of the cornea or lens. Under normal circumstances the cornea and the lens focus the object of regard clearly on the macular area. If this does not happen, a blurred image results. There are three main types of refractive error—myopia, hypermetropia, and astigmatism.

Myopia

Myopia (short-sight) is often a hereditary condition which results in the eyeball being too large for the refracting power of the eye, such that images are focused in front of the retina and not on it. The eye can be made emmetropic (normally refracting) by using a spectacle lens which diverges light rays in the first instance, to cause the point of focus to be further back and on the retina. The same effect can be produced by contact lenses which change the curvature of the cornea, or by refractive surgery where the curvature of the cornea is altered by surgical means or by a laser. The large eyeball of myopia is more likely to be the seat of retinal detachment, macular haemorrhage, or chronic

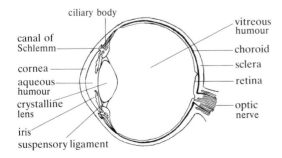

Fig. 1 Vertical section through the eyeball.

open-angle *glaucoma, as well as vitreous degeneration with vitreous floaters.

Hypermetropia

Hypermetropia (long-sight) occurs when the eyeball is too small in relation to the refracting components of the eye, such that the point of focus is behind the retina. Hypermetropia can be neutralized by the use of lenses which converge rays of light to a greater degree than the cornea and lens of the eye concerned, such that the point of focus is brought to bear on the surface of the retina. Contact lenses can be used for this, and corneal surgery to a lesser degree at the present time. The ability of aqueous humour to drain out of the eye in a small hypermetropic eye can be impaired and can lead to acute narrow-angle glaucoma in a very small number of hypermetropic individuals.

Astigmatism

Astigmatism occurs when the curvature of the cornea is different in one direction than in another. This leads to differential refraction and a blurred image, and can be offset by the provision of cylindrical lenses in glasses to correct the defective meridian of corneal curvature. Astigmatism can be combined with myopia and hypermetropia and can be corrected by spectacle lenses, contact lenses, or, more unpredictably, corneal surgery.

Visual failure

Visual failure in the developed world occurs more commonly in the elderly and is in many cases age-related, whereas visual failure in the developing world occurs in the younger age-groups, often related to infection and malnourishment. The three main causes of visual failure in the elderly in the developed world are cataract, senile macular degeneration, and chronic open-angle glaucoma.

Cataract

As stated above, the lens in the eye, approximately the size of a pea, is totally transparent and made up of proteins. As age progresses, the proteins break down and opacities begin to develop in the lens, sometimes in the centre, the nucleus, and sometimes in the lens material surrounding the nucleus, the cortex. As the opacities increase, the ability of light to pass through the lens decreases and slow visual failure occurs. Present techniques of cataract surgery involve the removal of the lens through a small incision in the cornea, but leaving the posterior capsule of the lens—the envelope which surrounds the lens matter—intact. A plastic lens is inserted into the space to compensate for the lens that has been removed. The power of the lens to be inserted has to be accurately determined and this is usually done by the use of ultrasound. If it is not possible to insert an intraocular lens for technical reasons, the loss of the natural lens can be compensated for by a contact lens or by spectacle lenses, these last being somewhat unsatisfactory because of magnification of the image and problems of distortion. Occasionally, the posterior capsule of the implanted lens thickens again and a hole has to be made in the capsule to allow good vision to return; this is usually done using a laser on an out-patient basis. Cataracts can also occur as a result of injury to the eye and can occur at birth as a result of maternal infections in pregnancy, e.g. german measles, or as a hereditary trait in certain families.

Senile macular degeneration

The macula depends solely on diffusion from the choroid for its nutrient supply, and if this diffusion is impaired, degeneration can result with resultant impaired central vision. Macular degeneration is age-related and comes on insidiously, often making itself manifest by distortion of central vision which progresses to a blank spot in the centre of vision. The patient is unable to read, but yet can see around and about and can navigate fairly easily. In one type of macular degeneration, small new blood vessels grow, and occasionally this is amenable to treatment using a laser, but the vast majority of cases are untreatable. In myopia, macular degeneration occurs as a result of macular haemorrhage more frequently than in the non-myopic population. Some patients benefit from the use of magnifying aids for reading and there are new closed-circuit television aids for reading, which are also of help.

Chronic open-angle glaucoma

In some individuals the drainage of aqueous humour becomes defective and the intraocular pressure slowly rises to somewhere in the region of 30–40 mm of mercury. This pressure, if continued for a number of years, causes the blood vessels supplying the optic nerve, as the optic nerve enters the eyeball, to be squeezed, and the optic nerve suffers as a result. This optic nerve damage manifests itself as field defects, i.e. deficiencies in the field of vision which relate to nerve fibre damage. One per cent of the population over the age of 40 develop open-angle glaucoma in the fullness of time, and the incidence rises with age. The treatment can be medical or surgical. Medical treatment consists of drops, which improve the efficacy of the drainage mechanism in the eye, and surgery takes the form of an artificial drainage system created by a carefully sculpted gap in the sclera, called a fistula.

Acute visual failure

Acute visual failure can arise as a result of markedly increased intraocular pressure over a short period of time, acute narrow-angle glaucoma; as the result of a sudden shut-down of circulation within the eye; or acute inflammation of the optic nerve.

Acute narrow-angle glaucoma

Acute narrow-angle glaucoma occurs in small eyes (hypermetropic) and is the result of an abnormality in the basic architecture of the drainage mechanism whereby this mechanism shuts off suddenly and the intraocular pressure rises to somewhere in the region of 50–60 mm of mercury. This causes acute pain and a diminution of vision due to the cornea becoming cloudy as a result of water being forced into it and making it less dehydrated. The treatment is medical in the first instance, to reduce the formation of aqueous humour and to try to improve the outflow so that the pressure becomes normal at which time the pain decreases and vision improves. However, the condition is likely to occur again if surgical intervention is not undertaken, and modern techniques involve the use of a laser to create a small hole in the peripheral iris which allows free drainage of aqueous humour from behind the iris to in front.

Retinal vascular occlusions

Retinal vascular occlusions cause sudden visual failure. The commonest is a central retinal vein occlusion, which may be related to high blood pressure, arteriosclerosis, raised intraocular pressure that makes the circulation sluggish, or any condition which thickens the blood, such as an increase in protein or blood cells within the bloodstream. When a central vein obstructs there is marked congestion of the blood vessels as they leave the eye and loss of vision results, which is usually permanent. Much less common is obstruction of the central retinal artery, which causes sudden visual loss as a result of it being occluded as it enters the eye, more commonly as a result of emboli—small particles of blood clot or degenerate arterial wall which are carried into the small blood vessels, resulting in blockages.

Inflammation of the optic nerve

The commonest inflammation of the optic nerve, resulting in visual failure, is optic neuritis which, in turn, is most commonly related to *multiple sclerosis. In this condition, the inflammation occurring in the optic nerve results in the loss of special sheaths around the nerve fibres that allow them to conduct impulses at a rapid rate. The condition is usually unilateral, the patient is in a younger age-group, and he or she complains of loss of central vision with occasionally slight pain in the eye on movement, as a result of inflammation of the coverings of the optic nerve being stretched because of swelling. Vision usually recovers in 6–8 weeks in the majority of cases, but inflammation may recur over a number of years.

Retinal detachment

In a previous section, mention was made of a higher incidence of retinal detachment in short-sighted individuals. Retinal detachment is the result of a retinal hole caused by degeneration of the vitreous humour and pulling on the peripheral retina. Fluid from the vitreous humour leaks through the hole into the deeper layers of the retina and strips the retina off the underlying deeper layers like wallpaper off a wall. The patient is aware of an area of poor vision which slowly gets larger and, if the hole is not sealed, total visual loss can occur. The aim of treatment is to seal the hole to stop further leakage of fluid into the retina, using extreme cold (cryotherapy) or laser treatment.

Squint (strabismus)

In the human, both eyes look ahead and the field of vision of one eye coincides to a marked degree with that of the other, overlapping by some 85 per cent. This allows stereoscopic vision to take place and is usually the rule in hunting animals that need precise depth perception to catch their prey. The ability to move the eyes together depends on complex centres in the mid-brain relaying messages from the eyes to the muscles that move the eyes. If this process is disrupted in any way, the eyes do not move together and a squint will result, so that the eyes are not directed at the same point. A squint may be due to:

(1) a paralysis of one of the muscles responsible for moving the eye (paralytic squint);
(2) a poor retinal image in one or both eyes, so that the images cannot be superimposed properly, due to, for example, refractive error or cataract; or
(3) where there is a disturbed relationship between accommodation, i.e. the ability to focus and the ability of our eyes to converge, such as happens when reading (concomitant strabismus).

This last type of squint is commoner in children. In an eye which squints, the brain is faced with a double image and in children under the age of 7 the brain is able to blot out the image from the squinting eye. If the squint is not detected, the vision in the squinting eye becomes poorer and poorer until it is amblyopic—a lazy eye. After the age of 7 the prospects of restoring vision to an amblyopic eye are very poor indeed. The aim of treatment is to make the child use the lazy eye by patching the good eye under close supervision until the vision is as good as it was prior to the squint. If a squint is still present at that stage, surgery may be necessary.

Systemic diseases

Many systemic diseases have effects on the eyes; diabetes is one of the commonest.

Diabetes

There are two main types of *diabetes, namely insulin-dependent and non-insulin-dependent. Both types can have ocular effects. Cataract is more common in both types than in the general population. Small retinal blood vessels are susceptible to damage in long-standing diabetes. There are two forms of retinopathy, namely non-proliferative, which is by far the commoner, and proliferative. In non-proliferative retinopathy, the small blood vessels leak and cause fluid and fat to accumulate in the retina, disturbing vision; whereas in proliferative retinopathy, because small blood vessels become occluded and low oxygen levels result, the growth of new blood vessels is stimulated. These blood vessels are much less robust than normal and can cause haemorrhages, which in turn cause a great deal of internal damage both to the retina and to the eye as a whole. As a consequence, patients with diabetes are now regularly screened for ocular complications, and if diabetic retinopathy is diagnosed, many such patients receive laser treatment on an out-patient basis. The aim of the treatment is to obliterate the new blood vessels and to destroy areas of the retina where low oxygen levels are occurring; this is successful provided the condition is diagnosed early enough.

World-wide problems of visual failure

The problems outlined above relate in the main to the developed world. The developing world faces many problems of visual failure. Cataract is widespread and surgery is often not available, so many millions of cataract sufferers do not have vision restored because of lack of resources. *Trachoma, a *chlamydial infection, affects 500 million people in the world, 2 million of whom are classified as blind. This disease, which is spread by flies, is much accentuated by poor socio-economic circumstances. In undernourished populations, *vitamin A deficiency is widespread, leading to opacification of the cornea as a result of drying of the eyes secondary to the vitamin deficiency. A small vitamin supplement added to the daily diet obviates this visual failure and, if instituted world-wide, would prevent blindness in 250 000 children annually. River-blindness (*onchocerciasis) is a parasitic infection, spread by flies, which occurs in central tropical Africa and in central America. The parasite causes inflammation within the eyes and in their blood vessels. *Leprosy, which is curable, accounts for approximately 500 000 cases of blindness in the world each year. It is a chronic bacterial infection, leading to invasion of nerves by the bacteria. This leads to problems in closing the eyes, so that the cornea becomes dry and opaque, while in other cases inflammation in the eye leads to blindness.

A. L. CROMBIE

OPHTHALMOPLEGIA is paralysis of one or more of the muscles of the eye.

OPHTHALMOPLEGIC MIGRAINE is a variety of severe *migraine, in which *oculomotor paralysis develops during the attack. It is postulated that the oculomotor nerve is compressed by swelling of, or around, the internal *carotid artery.

OPHTHALMOSCOPE. An instrument which enables inspection of the interior of the eye.

OPIATE is an imprecise term often employed to mean any drug or mixture of drugs which is either *hypnotic or *addictive, whether or not derived from or related to the *opium alkaloids.

OPIE, EUGENE LINDSAY (1873–1971). American pathologist. He made important contributions to knowledge in several fields, including *tuberculosis, *pancreatic dysfunction, and the processes of pyogenic and granulomatous inflammation.

OPISTHOTONOS is spasm of extensor muscles along the length of the body, which then rests on the *occiput and heels with the back arched. It typically occurs in *tetanus and *strychnine poisoning.

OPIUM is an extract of the capsules of the opium poppy (*Papaver somniferum*). It is the source of the narcotic, analgesic, and addictive opium alkaloids, such as *morphine, *codeine, *papaverine, *apomorphine, and about 15 others.

OPPENHEIM, HERMANN (1858–1919). German neurologist. He described *amyotonia congenita (Oppenheim's disease, 1900), and an alternative method of evoking the plantar reflex (Oppenheim's reflex, 1902).

OPPORTUNISTIC INFECTION describes infection by micro-organisms whose normally low pathogenicity is enhanced by depression of the host's humoral or cellular immune defences, such as occurs in immune deficiency syndromes and following the administration of immunosuppressive drugs. The systemic *mycoses, such as *aspergillosis and systemic *candidiasis, *toxoplasmosis, *cytomegalovirus infection, and *pneumocystis pneumonia are examples. See IMMUNOLOGY.

OPSONIZATION is the process whereby bacteria or other particles are coated with an *antibody protein or a component of the *complement system (opsonins) and thus rendered susceptible to *phagocytosis by polymorphonuclear *leucocytes or *macrophages.

OPTIC ATROPHY. Primary optic atrophy is the abnormal ophthalmoscopic appearance of the *optic disc resulting from degeneration, demyelination, or compression of fibres of the optic nerve. The disc shows a white pallor with sharply demarcated edges and reduced vascularity; the lamina cribrosa and physiological cup are prominent. Particularly when *multiple sclerosis is the cause, the pallor may be more obvious in the temporal halves of each disc. It is usually possible to distinguish this appearance from that of secondary optic atrophy, which is a sequel of long-standing *papilloedema. In this case the pallor is more grey, and the lamina cribrosa and disc margins are poorly demarcated.

OPTIC CHIASM is the X-shaped formation presented by the two *optic nerves at the point of crossing (decussation) of the fibres from the inner halves of the retinae.

OPTIC DISC. The head (or commencement) of the *optic nerve in the centre of the *retina, as seen on ophthalmoscopic examination of the optic fundus with the instrument directed a little inwards from the axis of the eye. It is a well-demarcated, round or slightly oval, pale area with the blood vessels of the retina radiating outwards from its centre. Inspection of the optic disc is an essential part of routine physical examination. Abnormalities of diagnostic significance include *optic atrophy and *papilloedema. See also OPHTHALMOLOGY.

OPTIC FUNDUS. The interior aspect of the back (fundus) of the eye, as seen magnified some 20 times on ophthalmoscopic examination. The *optic disc, the *macula, and the retinal blood vessels radiating outwards from the centre of the disc are the most obvious features, displayed against the red background of the choroid (the vascular coat of the eye) seen through the transparent *retina. See also OPHTHALMOLOGY.

OPTICIAN. One who supplies spectacles. In the UK, an ophthalmic optician tests sight, prescribes glasses, and supplies them. In some countries such an individual is called an optometrist. A dispensing optician does not test sight, but supplies glasses on the prescription of others. See GENERAL OPHTHALMIC SERVICES.

OPTIC NERVE. The second cranial nerve, consisting of *nerve fibres conveying impulses from the light-sensitive *receptors (rods and cones) of the *retina. The optic nerve runs backwards from the eye to meet its fellow from the opposite side at the *optic chiasm, a point of *decussation; here the fibres from the inner half of each retina cross over to join the uncrossed fibres of the outer halves, forming right and left optic tracts. Thus, while each optic nerve consists of fibres from the eye on the same side, the right optic tract carries fibres from the right halves of both eyes (representing the left visual field), and vice versa. See also OPHTHALMOLOGY.

OPTICS is the study of light.

OPTOMETRY. Testing vision, especially in order to detect refractive errors, and the correction of such errors by the provision of appropriate spectacles or lenses.

ORAL PHASE is a psychoanalytical term for the earliest stage of psychosexual development, occupying approximately the first year of life, during which pleasure is obtained by oral activities. It is succeeded by the anal phase.

ORBIT. The bony cavity occupied by the eyeball and its appendages, formed by the apposition of eight of the skull bones.

ORCHIDECTOMY is excision of one or both *testes.

ORCHITIS is inflammation of the *testes.

OREGON HEALTH CARE. See ETHICAL ISSUES IN MODERN HEALTH CARE.

ORF is a contagious pustular dermatitis of sheep, a virus infection to which goats are also susceptible. The lesions occur on hairless areas, particularly around the mouth and hooves. It can be transmitted to man, when it usually causes a single *maculopapule on the hand or arm; this becomes vesicular (forms a blister) and harmlessly resolves.

ORGAN. Any multicellular part of an animal or plant which forms a separate structural and functional unit, for example liver, kidney, lung, etc.

ORGANELLE. A persistent structure with specialized function forming part of a cell, for example a mitochondrion, liposome, ribosome, centriole, flagellum, etc. (see CELL AND CELL BIOLOGY). An organelle in a cell is analogous to an organ in a whole organism.

ORGANISM. Any living animal, plant, fungus, bacterium, or virus.

ORGANIZER. Any part of an *embryo which performs an induction on another part, that is which influences its differentiation.

ORGANOTHERAPY is the treatment of disease by administration of extracts of animal organs, usually *endocrine glands, now replaced by the use of pure *hormones.

ORGASM is the culmination or climax of sexual intercourse, arousing an intensely pleasurable sensation in both sexes, and accompanied in the male by ejaculation of *semen.

ORIBASIUS, (?325–?403). Byzantine physician. He did much to establish the authority of *Galen and his book *Synagogae medicae* was widely used in the Latin West and by the Arabs.

ORIENTAL SORE. One of the several names for cutaneous *leishmaniasis.

ORIGIN OF SPECIES, THE, is the classic work of Charles *Darwin, published in 1859, in which he proposed *natural selection as the main mechanism of evolution. The full title was *On the origin of species* *by means of natural selection, or the preservation of favoured races in the struggle for life.*

ORNITHOSIS. See PSITTACOSIS.

OROYA FEVER is a bacterial infection characterized by fever and *haemolytic anaemia, confined to certain parts of South America. The causative organism is a small Gram-negative bacillus *Bartonella bacilliformis*, transmitted by species of biting *sandfly, particularly *Phlebotomus verrucarum*.

ORTHODIAGRAM. An undistorted *X-ray silhouette made by tracing the outline of an organ or structure on a fluoroscopic screen.

ORTHODONTICS is the branch of *dentistry concerned with the correction of irregularities of the teeth and jaws.

ORTHOPAEDICS (ORTHOPEDICS). Orthopaedics is concerned with injuries and disorders of the musculoskeletal or locomotor system. This not only includes bones and joints, classically in the management of *fractures and *arthritis, but also those structures which involve stability and movement of the human frame, i.e. the ligaments, muscles, tendons, and nerves. The blood vessels and skin, which are necessary for the nutrition and protection of the musculoskeletal system, are secondarily involved in surgical procedures.

Orthopaedic surgery involves operations not only on the limbs but also on the spine, pelvis, shoulder girdle, and, in trauma work, the head. The spine can be approached surgically from the back directly, and from the front through the chest and abdomen. Therefore the orthopaedic surgeon may be called upon to explore almost any part of the human body.

The word 'orthopaedics' is derived from the Greek words *orthos*, meaning straight or free from deformity, and *paideia*, meaning the rearing of children. It was first used by Nicholas André, who was professor of medicine in the University of Paris in 1741, when describing the art of correcting and preventing deformities in children (André 1741) and was particularly related to spinal deformity or *scoliosis.

Definition
Orthopaedics is the specialty concerned with the development of the form and function of the human frame and its investigation, preservation, and restoration by medical, surgical, and physical means.

There are two main components of the specialty: elective orthopaedics and traumatology. The former is mainly concerned with diseases and disorders of the musculoskeletal system, for example, arthritis, bone infection and *osteoporosis, whereas the latter is concerned with injuries, be they of single bones or of the whole body.

History of orthopaedics
Orthopaedic conditions have been known from very early times. Primitive man obviously suffered from fractures but the first reports of injuries are found in the Edwin Smith papyrus, thought to have been written by *Imhotep in approximately 2000 BC (Breasted 1922). The account involves 48 cases of injuries and treatment amongst labourers on the great pyramids in Egypt and included head and spine injuries, fractures of the limbs, and flesh wounds.

The work of the Hippocratic school (460 BC to 370 BC) is well known, and includes volumes on joints, fractures, levers as well as the management of spinal deformity, particularly that resulting from *tuberculosis. There are illustrations of treatment of spinal deformities on a scamnum with the use of windlass traction to the hips and shoulders combined with forceful direct *manipulation of the spinal deformity.

From this time physicians avoided the treatment of fractures and this fell into the hands of bone-setters. In addition, other non-qualified groups such as the truss-makers and the instrument-makers who generally made devices for correcting deformities such as splints, braces, and artificial limbs, were also involved in the management of factures and deformities. It appears that bone-setting is is old as man himself and the modern equivalent of the bone-setters are the *osteopaths and *chiropractors who developed in England during the 18th and 19th centuries. They concerned themselves with the treatment of orthopaedic conditions and not with the setting of fractures. None of these groups, however, cut or operated on their patients. An important dynasty began with Evan Thomas (d. 1814) of Anglesey in Wales. His great grandson was Hugh Owen *Thomas (1834–91) of Liverpool who was a medical graduate and the first real exponent of orthopaedics in Great Britain. However, his contribution was mainly in the area of splints and many ingenious devices for correcting deformities. In particular he decried manipulation and advocated 'prolonged, enforced, and interrupted' rest of the affected part. Whilst he was acceptable to the medical profession, he was a difficult man personally who was frequently at odds with the Establishment. It therefore fell to his nephew, Sir Robert *Jones, who was a man of charm and tact, as well as great ability, to develop many of Hugh Owen Thomas' ideas and to establish a medical and operative basis for modern orthopaedics. He founded the Liverpool School of Orthopaedics following his outstanding success as Director of the Medical Services in the First World War (Watson 1934).

Friction between the medical profession and bone-setters and barbers continued throughout the mediaeval period and culminated in England in the separation of the Barbers from the Surgeons in 1745. The *Apothecaries Act of 1815 ordered that surgeons should have the same courses of higher study as physicians, prompted by the success of Napoleon's army doctors who had dual training. In 1858, with the advent of the Medical Register, surgeons and physicians were forbidden to collaborate with unqualified practitioners. This caused the bone-setters and other non-qualified practitioners to become ostracized although the physicians had maintained very little interest in treating deformities and fractures. This situation changed owing to the activities of William *Little (1810–94), the founder of the London School of Orthopaedics, who had a club foot secondary to poliomyelitis (Bentley 1991). He could not get surgical treatment for this in England and therefore visited Stromeyer of Hanover in 1836, where his foot deformity was corrected by open operative division of the Achilles tendon. Little then introduced open operative orthopaedic surgery to Britain in the following year.

The teaching of the bone-setters and manipulators was that every joint that was 'put out' had to be 'put in' by jerky passive manipulation. This could be well illustrated by a torn *cartilage in a locked knee, when a click would accompany the reduction of the cartilage into the correct place. The displacements of the joints, however, have never been demonstrated, and the snap or crack associated with rapid manipulation of joints is a normal phenomenon but has been interpreted as in some way beneficial to the patient.

Until the 20th century surgeons were largely concerned with the surgery of battle. There was no special segregation of surgeons into orthopaedic surgeons. Thus some of the early contributions on fractures were by surgeons who were extremely general in their practice, such as Percivall *Pott (1714–88), who was renowned for his description of fractures and *dislocations of the distal tibia, William Hay (1736–1819), who first used the term 'internal derangement of the knee', and Sir Astley *Cooper (1768–1841), who described disarticulation of the hip and the pathogenesis of non-union of femoral neck fractures, which are still a great cause of disability in contemporary practice. Sir Benjamin *Brodie (1786–1862), who was incidentally a friend of the Thomas family, wrote on diseases and infections of the joints and is best remembered for his description of chronic bone infection.

The foundation of orthopaedics in Britain
Orthopaedics began in different parts of the country simultaneously. William Little was the founder of the London School of Orthopaedics and was originally a physician at the London Hospital. He established open surgery in Britain for club foot and founded the first orthopaedic infirmary in London in 1838. Subsequently this became the Orthopaedic Institute in 1840, and was renamed the Royal Orthopaedic Hospital in 1845. In 1851 the City Orthopaedic Hospital was founded because of the demand for treatment, and the National Orthopaedic Hospital was also founded around that time. In 1905 the Royal and National Hospitals fused to become the Royal National Orthopaedic Hospital,

which exists to this day as the major orthopaedic institution in London and the south of England. This was joined by the City Orthopaedic Hospital in 1907 and a new purpose-built hospital was opened by King Edward VII in 1909.

The British Orthopaedic Association
An association of orthopaedic surgeons, the British Orthopaedic Society, was formed in 1898, but this was disbanded owing to lack of support in 1909. Orthopaedics came of age in Britain only following the First World War. This was due to the stimulus of Robert Jones, who was appointed Director of Medical Services in the First World War on the basis of his extensive experience of treating injuries during the building of the Manchester ship canal between 1892 and 1898. He was a nephew of Hugh Owen *Thomas and was sent by his parents to Liverpool at the age of 17 to read medicine and to live with his uncle. He subsequently entered practice with his uncle in Nelson Street and proved not only to be a superb surgeon, but also a man with great administrative gifts. He founded the first purpose-built orthopaedic hospital for children at Heswell in 1900, and subsequently the world-famous orthopaedic hospital at Oswestry in collaboration with Dame Agnes Hunt, who was a formidable and gifted organizer and had, until that time, run her own nursing home for cripples at Baschurch.

Robert Jones's success in the First World War was his ability to organize the care of the wounded and, in particular, to develop the use of the Thomas splint designed by his uncle, which, when placed on the limb of an injured soldier, would prevent movement and reduce infection. Soldiers were removed from the front-line to base hospitals without any treatment to the wound to begin with, and the incidence of gas *gangrene, and therefore amputation of the leg, was reduced from 80 to 20 per cent.

Following the war Jones, with the help of G. R. Girdlestone of Oxford, who had originally been a general practitioner in Oswestry, where he met Jones, established a national plan of orthopaedic hospitals and departments for the treatment and *rehabilitation of war casualties, and later for children and others with conditions such as *poliomyelitis, chronic infection, and tuberculosis. The major specialist units were established at Oswestry, the Royal National Orthopaedic Hospital in London, and Oxford. By the end of the war there were nine military hospitals with 30 000 beds; subsequently, these were taken over as the major orthopaedic units throughout the country.

Following the success of orthopaedic surgery during the First World War, Robert Jones and colleagues set up the British Orthopaedic Association in 1918. This was a key development in the quality of care, training, and research in orthopaedics in the UK. Screening of infants for the prevention of congenital dislocation of the hip introduced by van Rosen in Malmo also made a great impact on the practice of orthopaedic surgery.

However, the conditions listed above are still rampant in the developing world. Aggressive early operative treatment of the tuberculous spine pioneered by Hodgson in Hong Kong has improved the outlook enormously for those fortunate enough to have access to the facilities. Screening for patients with scoliosis to check for progression has not been so successful. The surgical treatment of spinal deformity, pioneered in the USA by Harrington and others, has provided spectacular results for a condition formerly considered untreatable. Anterior spinal devices, such as that developed originally by Dwyer in Australia, and modified since, have also made spinal deformity treatable in almost every case, although the cause often remains unknown.

As trauma care has moved largely to the care of the aged and to the young involved in road-traffic and other accidents, the challenge for orthopaedics has been in managing *osteoarthritis of major joints, which has led to dramatic developments in the past 30 years.

Total hip replacement (THR)

The concept of hip replacement has been around for many years; Robert Jones attempted the replacement of the surface of the joint with gold foil. In the 1920s and 1930s Smith-Petersen of Boston developed a cup which was placed between the surfaces of the hip joint, originally using such materials as ivory, glass, and bakelite, and finally vitallium alloy. However, this provided only a lining between the femoral head and the socket of the joint, and often resulted in *necrosis of the femoral head and rapid wear of the socket, with recurrence of pain. In 1946 the Judet brothers of Paris introduced a femoral head replacement made of polymethylmethacrylate, the same material as that used for bone cement. This gave excellent results but failed after a few years with serious inflammation and destruction of the surviving bone.

It became apparent that both sides of the hip joint would have to be replaced, and Philip Wiles (1890–1967) of the Middlesex Hospital performed six metal replacements in the 1930s, using a *prosthesis which was fixed to bone with screws. Although his results were reasonably successful, the prosthesis always became loose in the bone, producing pain, and his work was interrupted by the Second World War. A prototype total hip replacement, made entirely of metal and fixed with bone cement, was devised and implanted by McKee of Norwich in 1940. The major step forward came in the 1950s when Sir John Charnley (1911–92) combined metal femoral components with a plastic socket to produce a 'low friction' prosthesis compared with those of metal-on-metal (Charnley 1961). His first experiments, using Teflon® sockets were a disaster, with rapid destruction of the material and the surrounding bone. He then tried HDP (high-density polyethylene) as a socket material and fixed the components with bone cement (polymethylmethacrylate), which had already been used by dentists to fix teeth. The experience with Teflon® made Charnley cautious, but gradually the metal-on-plastic hip emerged as being superior to the metal-on-metal, since the lower friction produces less stress on the cement–bone interface and therefore has less tendency to loosen. However, evidence is increasing of failure of the prosthesis over the long term owing to wear of the polyethylene and the inflammatory and irritant effects of the particles on the surrounding bone, leading to loosening of the prosthesis and damage of the bone.

Hence new materials will be required to improve hip replacement and some preliminary work on ceramics as a bearing material, in various parts of the world but especially in Europe, have indicated a lower wear rate.

The initial concept of changing a total hip replacement for a new one after 10 years, which was predicted by Charnley, has not become a reality. When cemented prostheses become loose there is usually great difficulty in replacement because the bone has been damaged by the loose fragments of HDP and cement, and also it is difficult to remove all the cement. Although new ultrasound systems are available to remove cement, they are not generally available, and in any event the bone quality is poor at the end of the second operation. This has led to a great interest in non-cemented, close-fitting prostheses, but experience over 10 years suggests that these suffer, first, from the early problem of persistent pain in the thigh, so that the patient never walks as freely as one with a cemented hip, and, secondly, from the problem of loss of bone, especially in the femur, because of stress shielding, which occurs with a stiff metal prosthesis in the pliant bone of the femur. Thus bone wastage and eventual collapse occur. These problems have not been solved; despite this, a patient with a cemented THR can, if early complications are avoided, expect a 95 per cent chance of 10 years of trouble-free performance from the total hip replacement.

Other joints, such as the knee, the elbow, the shoulder, the small joints of the hand, the wrist, and the ankle, can be replaced, but only the knee joint replacement produces a success rate comparable with that of the hip.

Contemporary trauma

A major persistent problem in trauma is the treatment of complications of increasing age, especially of osteoporosis in women. Roughly 30 per cent of orthopaedic beds in the UK are occupied by patients with fractures of the neck of the femur, and other fractures such as spinal, wrist, and shoulder fractures occur increasingly commonly in the older age-groups. Whether the advent of *hormone replacement therapy (HRT) will affect this in future is uncertain, but the fundamental biological problem, rather than technical expertise, is the probable limiting factor in trauma of the aged.

In the meantime, major advances in the management of fractures have occurred, with the development of precision methods of rigid fixation of fractures by plates and screws from the AO School in Switzerland. Also, intramedullary nailing, developed initially in Germany, and external fixators attached to the bones by pins placed into the bone have been developed, making great contributions in trauma management. Fractures are now treated much earlier by operation, resulting in a lower complication rate and quicker rehabilitation, allowing an early return to employment. Also, there is increasing evidence that early internal fixation of fractures in multiple injuries increases the chances of survival.

Minimally-invasive surgery and *arthroscopy

A current major vogue is to perform operations through smaller and smaller incisions (*key-hole surgery), based on the concept of less damage to the skin and surrounding tissues and rapid recovery because pain is much less. The development, particularly of the arthroscope, which is a telescope adapted for use inside joints, has been dramatic in the management of knee disorders. A major factor was the invention of glass cold light sources by Hopkins; previous instruments had depended on electric circuits which were difficult to sterilize and to maintain. Thus, since the early 1970s, pioneered by Jackson in Canada, (Jackson and Abe 1972), the diagnosis and management of 80 per cent of knee disorders can be performed without open operation.

The use of the arthroscope and miniature cameras and visual display units enables the surgeon to operate by looking at a television screen rather than down the telescope. This also allows onlookers, including the operating assistants, to see the operation, and is invaluable for teaching. The television image can also be transmitted by close-circuit television or other types of linkage.

Academic orthopaedics
Teaching and training
The importance of study of the musculoskeletal system has not been appreciated fully in the undergraduate curricula of most universities in the USA and some in the UK. Orthopaedics is still considered to be a specialty of general surgery in these universities, where teaching is still dominated by traditional medical and surgical disciplines and lags behind the current developments in clinical and educational practice.

Postgraduate teaching
For postgraduates, orthopaedics in the USA and the UK has been a leading specialty in developing high-quality teaching and training. This was especially possible in the UK, because in NHS hospitals large numbers of in-patients and out-patients were treated in units with few doctors. This led to a high concentration of clinical cases, which enabled a graduated, supervised training in principles of trauma and orthopaedics. In the 1960s Sir Frank Holdsworth in Sheffield devised the then revolutionary scheme of rotation of surgeons in training

at intervals of 6 or 12 months between different surgical units, to maximize their surgical exposure in the shortest possible time (Holdsworth 1967). This scheme is now an integral part of all surgical rotations in the UK and in many other countries, resulting in a greatly increased quality of training.

In the late 1970s the first national examination in orthopaedics—the FRCSOrth.—was established at the Royal College of Surgeons of Edinburgh. This eventually became the intercollegiate examination of the four Royal Colleges of Edinburgh, London, Glasgow, and Dublin and has, since 1990, been a requirement for all young orthopaedic surgeons in training in the UK.

Research in orthopaedics
Most research in orthopaedics has been clinically orientated. The presence of an NHS system in the UK made clinical studies relatively easy, and the willing involvement of successive generations of patients has facilitated this process. The prospective controlled randomized *clinical trial arose in Britain because of the ready access to large numbers of patients treated in NHS hospitals, and is now the basis of all prospective clinical studies in medicine. In orthopaedics, as early as 1922, Robert Jones realized the importance of the academic aspects of orthopaedics by founding the Board of Orthopaedic Studies in Liverpool University and the M. Ch. Orth. (mastership in orthopaedics) degree of Liverpool University. The first Chair of Orthopaedic Surgery was set up in Oxford in 1939, founded by Lord Nuffield, who was a personal friend of G. R. Girdlestone, who in turn a personal friend of Robert Jones. The Liverpool chair was founded 1 year later and others have been established slowly, so that now 18 exist in the UK. Only one other department (University College, London) runs a higher degree course (M.Sc. in orthopaedics).

The British Orthopaedic Research Society was formed in the 1960s by a group of 22 surgeons, and has developed into an active, multidisciplinary society for all those having an interest in orthopaedic research, be they surgeons, physicians, engineers, or biologists, holding regular meetings twice a year.

Orthopaedics world-wide
Throughout the past 30 years, orthopaedics has developed world-wide, particularly in America, which now has the largest academy in the world, with over 20 000 members and an Orthopaedic Research Society of commensurate size. The development of orthopaedics is in an early stage in developing countries. Nevertheless, there is great international collaboration among the orthopaedic associations and among individuals sponsored by governments and by their specialist orthopaedic associations, so that schemes for training of overseas doctors exist in the Royal College of Surgeons of London and in the American Academy of Orthopaedic Surgery.

The British Orthopaedic Association has over 1000

fellows and 2000 other members in the UK and abroad. Although a professional organization and a charity, it has increasingly involved itself in all aspects of the development of orthopaedics, including especially teaching and education, research, fund-raising for research through its biannual Great Hip Walk, and political matters which affect all orthopaedic surgeons and their patients. It has also developed into nine specialist societies, which reflect increasing superspecialization into groups concerned chiefly with hip surgery, knee surgery, spinal surgery, foot surgery, children's surgery, and hand surgery, since increasingly orthopaedic surgeons develop a special interest in addition to their general orthopaedic responsibilities.

Manpower and services

A major contemporary difficulty for orthopaedics in the UK is a shortage of manpower; there being only one orthopaedic consultant per 66 000 of population compared with an average of one per 30 000 in Europe and one per 10 000 in the USA. This situation has arisen because of the policies of successive governments and has resulted in an average of waiting times for major elective orthopaedic procedures, such as total hip replacement, of 6–12 months throughout the UK. The situation will be gradually improved by the planned shortening of postgraduate training, in line with Europe, to 6–7 years, provided the will is present to create the finance and infrastructure required. Certainly, the increasing specialization necessary for maintaining up-to-date expertise and satisfying increasing patient demand for orthopaedic services requires consideration. A recent extensive review of trauma services in the UK revealed a serious lack of expert medical personnel, equipment, and poor overall planning, resulting in over 100 000 cases of 'preventable' disability per annum (McKibbin 1992). This requires a response from health-care planners.

The future

The exciting and explosive developments in orthopaedics and trauma surgery, especially in the past 20 years, have greatly increased the capacity of orthopaedic surgeons and their associated health-care professionals (*nurses, *physiotherapists, and health-care planners) to prevent and treat promptly an array of previously serious and untreatable injuries and disorders of the musculoskeletal system. Health-care planners need to devise ways of providing the best treatment for the greatest number of patients, but at the same time preserving excellence of standards of teaching, education, research, and development as a vital part of future planning. The problem of providing adequate services in developing countries remains and, as in other aspects of human activity, represents a challenge for the 21st century (Bentley 1994).

GEORGE BENTLEY
SIMON DONELL

References

André, N. (1741). *L'Orthopédie, ou l'art de prévenir et de corriger dans les enfants, les difformités du corps.* A. Millar (1753), London.

Bentley, G. (1991). William John Little. In *Dictionary of national biography*. Oxford University Press, Oxford.

Bentley, G. (1994). *The British Orthopaedic Association, Europe and the 21st century.* Presidential Address, BOA Annual Scientific Meeting, Wembley. 11 September 1992. *Journal of Bone and Joint Surgery, Orthopaedic Proceedings*, Suppl. 1, **76B**, 59–60.

Breasted, J. H. (1992). The Edwin Smith papyrus. *New York Historical Society Quarterly Bulletin*, **6**, 5.

Charnley, J. (1961), Arthroplasty of the hip – a new operation. *Journal of Bone and Joint Surgery*,.

Holdsworth, F. W. (1967). The training of the orthopaedic surgeon. *Journal of Bone and Joint Surgery*, **49B**, 188.

Jackson, R. W. and Abe, I. (1972). The role of arthroscopy in the management of disorders of the knee. *Journal of Bone and Joint Surgery*, **54B**, (2), 310–22.

McKibbin, B. (ed.) (1992). *The management of skeletal trauma in the United Kingdom.* British Orthopaedic Association Report.

Watson, F. (1934). *The life of Robert Jones.* William Wood, Baltimore.

ORTHOPAEDIC (ORTHOPEDIC) SURGEON. One who specializes in the surgery of the skeletal system, its articulations, and its associated structures. See ORTHOPAEDICS.

ORTHOPNOEA (ORTHOPNEA) is the inability to breathe easily except when sitting upright.

ORTHOPTICS is the remedial training of the eye muscles. See also OPHTHALMOLOGY.

ORTOLFF OF BAVARIA (*fl.* 15th century). A successful writer of medical books living in Würzburg, Ortolff is best known for his *Artzneibuch* (1477) a popular textbook of medicine. In *c.* 1500 he published *Frauenbüchlein oder wie sich die schwangern Frauen halten sollen*, a guide for pregnant women.

OSCILLOGRAPH. Any instrument for recording electrical variations (oscillations).

OSCILLOSCOPE. A cathode ray tube which displays electrical variations.

OSLER, SIR WILLIAM Bt (1849–1919). Anglo-Canadian physician. Osler began his medical training at Toronto, moving to Montreal, where he graduated MD McGill in 1872. After touring the European medical centres for 2 years he returned to Canada as professor of the Institutes of Medicine in *McGill University, becoming physician to the *Montreal General Hospital in 1878. His reputation grew so rapidly that after 6 years he was invited to the chair of medicine in the University of Pennsylvania and 5 years later to become foundation professor and physician at the *Johns Hopkins University Hospital at Baltimore. During his 15 years in this post he influenced medical teaching throughout the USA, combining the bedside methods of the English school with the laboratory associations of the German. Here too he wrote his work *The principles and practice of medicine* (1892) which was the model for all later textbooks.

In 1904 he moved to the Regius chair of medicine at Oxford, where his antiquarian and literary tastes had leisure in which to develop. His success in the UK was no less than in the USA. He expanded the preclinical departments at Oxford and helped to overcome the University's traditional suspicions of 'the sciences'. He was largely responsible for founding the Association of Physicians of Great Britain and Ireland and the *Quarterly Journal of Medicine*. He was among the first to study the *platelets (1874), to describe *hereditary haemorrhagic telangiectasia (Osler–Rendu–Weber disease, 1901), *polycythaemia vera (Vaquez–Osler's disease, 1903), and *infective endocarditis (*Osler's nodes, 1909).

OSLER'S NODES are painful pea-sized nodules in the pads of the fingers and toes which sometimes appear and disappear (after hours or a day or two) in *infective endocarditis, of which diagnosis they are strongly suggestive. *Osler's view that they represent the effects of minute *emboli from the infected heart valves was almost certainly correct.

OSMOLALITY (OSMOLARITY) is the number of osmotically effective (see OSMOSIS) dissolved particles per unit quantity of a solution, expressed either as (milli) osmols per kilogram of solvent (osmolality) or as (milli) osmols per litre of solution (osmolarity). The osmol is the standard unit of osmotic pressure, being equal to the gram molecular weight divided by the number of particles or ions into which a substance dissociates in solution.

OSMOSIS is the flow of water (or other solvent) through a semipermeable membrane, i.e. one which permits passage of the solvent but not of the substance dissolved. When solutions of different strength are separated by such a membrane, solvent flows from the weaker to the stronger until they are of equal molecular concentration. The pressure which must be applied to the stronger solution so as to prevent such flow is termed the osmotic pressure.

OSSICLE. Any small bone, but particularly those of the *middle ear.

OSSIFICATION is the formation of new bone, which normally takes place in pre-existing *cartilage or fibrous tissue.

OSTEITIS is inflammation of bone.

OSTEITIS DEFORMANS is a synonym for *Paget's disease of bone.

OSTEITIS FIBROSA CYSTICA is the name given to the radiological and pathological changes in bone structure characteristic of *hyperparathyroidism, sometimes also known as von *Recklinghausen's disease of bone.

OSTEOARTHRITIS. See OSTEOARTHROSIS.

OSTEOARTHROSIS is a chronic degenerative non-inflammatory condition of joints frequently known also as 'osteoarthritis'. Some degree of osteoarthrosis is almost universal in older age-groups and may be regarded as the inevitable result of wear-and-tear; when severe, it is an important cause of disability. Genetic factors probably influence the rate and degree of degenerative change, as do abnormal stresses on joints, for example the weight-bearing joints in *obesity.

OSTEOCHONDRITIS is literally, inflammation of bone and cartilage; in practice, it is applied to a heterogeneous group of conditions associated with *necrosis of these tissues (also known as osteochondrosis).

OSTEOGENESIS IMPERFECTA is a genetic condition, usually transmitted as an autosomal *dominant trait, in which the bones are abnormally brittle and fragile, and repeated fractures cause skeletal deformities. In one of the two main varieties, known as osteogenesis imperfecta congenita, the fractures begin *in utero* and the baby is born with deformities; in these cases, another characteristic finding is a blue discoloration of the *sclera (white) of the eye. In the other, osteogenesis imperfecta tarda, the appearance of fractures is delayed until the child begins to walk. The condition, the pathophysiology of which is not understood, is also known as fragilitas ossium.

OSTEOLOGY is the study and knowledge of bones.

OSTEOMA. A non-malignant *tumour of bone.

OSTEOMALACIA is softening of bone due to inadequate absorption and utilization of *calcium; the usual cause is deficiency of *vitamin D. Osteomalacia is the adult equivalent of *rickets in childhood.

OSTEOMYELITIS is inflammation of bone and the *marrow, usually due to a pus-forming *staphylococcal or *streptococcal infection. It is now less common and much less dangerous than it was before the advent of *antibiotic therapy.

OSTEOPATHY is a system of therapy founded by an American country practitioner named Andrew Taylor Still (1828–1917) based on the manipulation of skeletal structures. Still's original hypothesis, that all diseases were explicable on the basis of faulty structural relationships and would therefore yield to physical manipulation, has little credence today. However, modern osteopaths justifiably claim considerable success in the treatment of certain painful conditions involving bones and joints. The profession now requires a long prescribed programme of training in the UK, the USA, and many other countries, and is subject to statutory regulation. See COMPLEMENTARY MEDICINE.

OSTEOPETROSIS, also known as Albers–Schönberg or marble bone disease, is a rare, genetically determined disorder of bone function in which there is a failure of normal bone resorption, so that it becomes excessively dense. In the severe or malignant form of the condition, the bone marrow and its blood-forming tissue are obliterated and cranial deformities appear in early childhood. Milder syndromes occur in which the dense bone (which is more brittle than normal) is detected on radiography following a fracture, or in which the presentation is with *osteomyelitis.

OSTEOPOROSIS. In osteoporosis bones become porous, reduced in amount, and fragile. This occurs most often in women after the menopause.

Bone strength relies on mineral (calcium) deposited on *protein (*collagen), analogous to reinforced concrete. A vital difference is that bone is alive, constantly being removed and replaced by specific cells which determine its growth, shape, amount, and repair.

With age, the density (and size) of the skeleton increases to reach its peak at about 30 years, and then slowly declines. The rate of loss is constant in men; in women it temporarily increases in the postmenopausal decade as *oestrogen production virtually ceases.

Osteoporosis is a major cause of *fractures, and women have more fractures than men; peak bone mass is less, bone loss is more, and life span is greater. Fractures of the hip, spine, and forearm are common and related to osteoporosis. A hip (neck of femur) fracture makes it impossible to walk, requires surgery, and increases disability and mortality. The cost of hip fracture is enormous: in America their primary care has been estimated at US $6 ($4) billion per year. Vertebral (spine) fractures are less disabling and occur earlier than hip fractures. Progressive loss of bone leads to vertebral collapse, reduced height, and back pain. Forearm fractures often occur when the arm is extended to prevent a fall.

Apart from osteoporosis, falls are an important cause of fracture, especially in the elderly. Their frequency can be reduced by life-style changes (i.e. reduced *alcohol intake), by treating medical conditions (e.g *anaemia, *hypertension), and by altering the environment (avoid *hypothermia, improve illumination); and their effects by protection (for instance, pads over the upper thighs).

Prevention of osteoporosis begins in childhood and depends on a high peak bone mass and a low rate of loss. Bone mass depends on the optimum interaction between genetic and mechanical factors, modified by *diet and *hormones. It is increased by good *nutrition, sufficient *calcium, and plenty of exercise during growth; and reduced by excessive alcohol, by drugs, immobility, poor nutrition, and oestrogen lack—as in *anorexia nervosa and excessive exercise.

From the age of 30 these risk factors also accelerate bone loss, as do medical conditions such as excessive *corticosteroids, *thyroid overactivity, defective intestinal absorption (*coeliac disease), and early natural or surgical *menopause. Bone is lost when removal exceeds formation and the treatments of osteoporosis attempt to correct this.

Thus weight-bearing exercise stimulates bone-forming cells and reduces bone loss at any age. Likewise, sodium fluoride stimulates bone formation but the new bone is abnormal and the fracture rate is not reduced. In contrast, bone removal (resorption) is slowed by hormone replacement therapy (HRT) in women, by additional calcium, by the hormone calcitonin, and by cyclical use of simple inorganic compounds known as phosphonates.

Since oestrogen deficiency is the likely cause of accelerated bone loss after the menopause it is logical to give oestrogen to prevent it. However, an unwelcome effect of replacement oestrogen is an increase in *cancer of the uterus (endometrial cancer). Clearly this does not occur when the uterus has been removed *(hysterectomy); but if it has not, *progestogen is necessary to abolish the cancer risk, and this often produces regular or irregular bleeding. In addition, more than 10 years of oestrogen replacement may produce a slight increase in breast cancer. The advantages of long-term oestrogen are that it prevents bone loss, reduces femoral neck fracture, and, importantly, reduces death from heart attacks and similar events (cardiovascular mortality) by half. For women who have had a hysterectomy these advantages are considerable; for those who still have a uterus the acceptability of oestrogen plus progestogen remains low and the cardiovascular advantages have yet to be proved. This does not deny the usefulness of short-term HRT for menopausal symptoms.

Many women take little calcium in their diet (with the fashion for weight reduction and high-fibre diets); however, much current evidence suggests that bone loss can be slowed by additional calcium, either in the diet or as tablets.

Calcitonin is a hormone which directly suppresses the bone-resorbing cells and, given by repeated injection, produces a temporary increase in bone density. Unfortunately it is expensive and has troublesome side-effects. Calcitonin nasal sprays, being developed, should be more acceptable.

Where HRT is inappropriate or unacceptable, an increasingly used non-hormonal treatment is the bisphosphonate disodium etidronate Didronel®. Bisphosphonates are simple inorganic compounds which are incorporated into bone and reduce the activity of its cells. Oral Didronel® is given in repeated cycles for 2 weeks out of 15 with additional calcium. There is evidence that the amount of bone in the spine increases, whereas fracture rates decrease.

In practice, the prevention of bone loss—and by implication the reduction of fracture—depends on common-sense advice. It assumes that no obvious medical cause has been missed, and recommends exercise at all ages, sufficient calcium, the avoidance of recognized risk factors (especially smoking); and where appropriate and acceptable, HRT. Many problems remain unsolved, such as bone density screening to detect persons with low bone mass, and the role of long-term HRT in women with intact uteri.

ROGER SMITH

Advice about osteoporosis is provided by the National Osteoporosis Society, PO Box 10, Radstock, Bath BA3 3YB, UK.

Further reading

Lauritzen, J. B., Petersen, M. M., and Lund, B. (1993). Effect of external hip protectors on hip fractures. *Lancet*, **341**, 503–5.

Riggs, B. L. and Melton, L. J. (1993). The prevention and treatment of osteoporosis. *New England Journal of Medicine*, **327**, 620–7.

Smith, R. (1990). *Osteoporosis*. Royal College of Physicians of London, London.

OSTEOTOMY is the surgical cutting of bone.

OTITIS is inflammation of part of the ear, as in otitis externa, otitis media, and otitis interna. See OTORHINOLARYNGOLOGY.

OTOLOGIST. A physician or surgeon specializing in conditions affecting the ear. See OTORHINOLARYNGOLOGY.

OTOLOGY is the branch of medicine dealing with the ear. See OTORHINOLARYNGOLOGY.

OTORHINOLARYNGOLOGIST. A specialist in diseases of the ear, nose, and throat. See OTORHINOLARYNGOLOGY.

OTORHINOLARYNGOLOGY (THE EAR, NOSE AND THROAT; ENT). Given the frequency with which this region of the head and neck is afflicted by common and often serious diseases, it is surprising that the specialty has existed as a recognizable entity for less than 100 years. Indeed, it is only within the past 2 decades that the otorhinolaryngologist has developed into a well-trained clinician able to care for a wide-ranging group of complex illnesses. Even so, the amount of time devoted to the training of medical students in this discipline (and its sister specialty *ophthalmology)

is minimal and to the disadvantage of the *general practitioner.

Aural *surgeons, those concerned primarily with the ear, had been appointed to British hospitals by 1851 but were invariably *physicians, as were those dealing with the *larynx, or voice box. However, the founding of specialist hospitals, Moorfields for diseases of the eye and ear being the first in 1805, did much to provide the foundations for later developments. However, early practitioners faced enormous difficulties in developing a specialty primarily concerned with organs hidden from view and whose function was largely conjectural. To many doctors, as well as the public, ENT surgery meant wholesale removal of the *tonsils and *adenoids, enthusiastic but useless *sinus procedures, and *mastoid operations. The discovery of *antibiotics, confidently predicted to result in the demise of otorhinolaryngology, together with the application of modern technology, have led to meteoric developments in the specialty, which now covers areas far outside the ear, nose, and throat.

Although the singing teacher Manuel Garcia is credited with the use of the first mirror for visualizing the larynx, the invention of electric light in 1879 made examination of these 'secret places' feasible. Utilization of the Zeiss stereoscopic *microscope in 1923 led to modern *microsurgery of the ear, while the development of *anaesthesia and antiseptic techniques led to safe major surgical operations. There can be few specialties which have undergone such dramatic changes within such a short space of time and which now cover such a wide range of conditions. In the larger centres, this has resulted in surgeons confining their interests to a particular field, or even age-group. Aural surgeons deal with the ear whereas audiological physicians deal with non-surgical aspects of hearing and balance. Rhinologists deal with disorders of the nose, including *allergy; the laryngologist specializes in head and neck diseases, including *cancer, and the paediatric otolaryngologist is concerned primarily with the young. All have benefited from the improvements in *biotechnology which have been the hallmark of the latter part of this century.

Otology today

Prior to the discovery of antibiotics, all ear inflammations were viewed as potentially serious because of the risk that the patient might develop *mastoiditis, which in turn could lead to intracranial complications such as *meningitis or a cerebral *abscess. Spread throughout the bloodstream (*septicaemia) could also occur, and was invariably fatal. The introduction of *sulphonamides and then *penicillin markedly reduced these complications, and now all cases of acute infection of the middle ear are treated with antibiotics. Most occur in children, with complete recovery but some develop a sterile effusion behind the *tympanic membrane, leading to deafness. The treatment of this condition, often called 'secretory *otitis media', or 'glue ear', by the insertion of ventilation tubes or 'grommets' is now said to be the commonest operation performed under general anaesthesia throughout the Western world. These tubes act by equalizing air pressure on both sides of the tympanic membrane, allowing resolution and absorption of the exudate. Failure to control this condition leads to hearing loss which may persist if treatment is delayed. Despite the use of a wide range of new and potent antibiotics, chronic infection of the middle ear remains a continued cause of ear discharge. With improvements in community health and standards of living, the number of affected patients is decreasing, except perhaps in the poorer parts of the larger cities. Training in the use of the operating microscope and increased knowledge of the underlying *pathology of middle-ear disease have led to a reduction in the number of patients requiring radical surgery, and the emphasis today is on reconstruction of the middle ear rather than ablation. Magnification with good illumination allows accurate assessment of disease, with preservation of healthy tissue and repair of the tympanic membrane or missing *ossicles (see below).

Sound reaches the inner ear by transmission from the tympanic membrane via three bones, or auditory ossicles. The last of these, the stapes, so-called because of its stirrup shape, fits neatly into the bony capsule surrounding the *cochlea or organ of hearing. Vibrations transmitted to the fluid within the cochlea stimulate the sensitive ends of the auditory nerve and are eventually recognized as sound by the brain. Conductive *deafness is a result of any interference with transmission of sound by the ossicles, and fixity of the stapes due to the formation of new bone, called *otosclerosis, has now become amenable to surgical correction. Previous attempts at removing the stapes failed because of trauma to the sensitive inner ear or through infection. Today, *stapedectomy and replacement by a *prosthesis, which may be made of Teflon®, fat, connective tissue, gelatin sponge, or other materials, offer patients an excellent prospect of long-term improvement of hearing.

In more affluent countries, increasing scientific knowledge has led inevitably to better control of disease and an increase in our life expectancy. This has not, however, been accompanied by a lessening of the degenerative process which is an integral part of human life. Our hearing ability probably starts to decrease early in life, and severe hearing impairment, often accompanied by *tinnitus, is now a important cause of social deprivation in the elderly. In addition, many drugs have proved to be ototoxic, producing permanent deafness, and in recent years much attention has been paid to the development of cochlear implants aimed at bypassing the damaged inner ear. Research has been expensive and dependent upon biomedical engineering expertise. However, as a result of close co-operation between otologists, auditory physiologists, and electronic engineers, practical implants have been developed and increasing clinical experience is producing encouraging results, although a replacement for the highly sophisticated human cochlea can never be anticipated.

Audiological physicians

Not all otologists wish to be surgeons, and the need to make accurate measurements in testing hearing and balance, as well as assessing the need for hearing aids, has led to the emergence of a relatively new specialty. Until 50 years ago hearing was estimated by using the conversational or whispered voice. Tuning forks were used to differentiate between conductive and inner ear deafness, and accurate assessment was unpredictable. The invention of the valve amplifier, now superseded by complex computer-driven audiometers, provided instruments capable of objective measurements, not only of hearing but of signals generated within the cochlea, brainstem, or even the brain.

Dramatic progress has also been made in the design of *hearing aids. At the inception of the *National Health Service (NHS) in 1948, free aids were available but were bulky, unattractive, and unsophisticated in design. Today's aids are worn behind the ear and the response can be varied to suit individual hearing loss, although non-NHS aids are still more sophisticated, and expensive.

About one in 10 000 live births produce children with impaired hearing and, although uncommon, early testing of 'at risk' babies is essential for effective *rehabilitation. Audiological physicians, with their technical expertise, are playing a vital role in accurate assessment of these problems, as well as the more obscure conditions affecting the cochlear and vestibular systems. Unfortunately, they tend to be situated in larger centres because of the cost and sophisticated equipment that is essential for accurate assessment. However, the increase in life expectancy is resulting in larger numbers of politically influential 'senior citizens' who expect relief from the deafness and balance disorders which so commonly occur in the elderly.

The rhinologist

If punishment for real or imagined crimes is to serve as a warning to others, then it must be permanently visible but leave the victim alive, 'a high noticeability but low morbidity'; thus *amputation of the nose has enjoyed popularity in all cultures for at least 1500 years. Indeed, it has been said that the history of nasal amputation is the history of *rhinoplasty, now becoming so popular for cosmetic reasons. Until recent years this might be said to be the one aspect of rhinology to have made steady progress within the last century.

Nasal allergy has proved to be a fruitful field for enthusiastic practitioners from a wide variety of specialties, although differential diagnosis of much nasal pathology has awaited the arrival of the well-trained surgeon knowledgeable in the *anatomy, *physiology, and *pathology of this region.

Today's rhinologist is skilled in the use of fibre-optics

for inspection of the nasal passages and in functional surgery, and is able to measure ciliary mucosal transportation and other physiological characteristics of the nasal *mucosa. An awareness that nasal function and that of its related sinuses is dependent upon preservation of protective tissues, which in the past have been so ruthlessly destroyed, has led to a new cognizance of the need for 'conservation surgery'. This is now possible because of the development of suitable instrumentation and improved illumination, although, since success is frequently measured subjectively, the dangers of excessive enthusiasm are inherent in what is an anatomically complex and potentially dangerous region of the head and neck.

Common nasal pathology, such as benign polyps, was recognized in Ancient Egypt, and they were removed with a knotted cord. However, the function of the nasal sinuses and research into nasal physiology have attracted only slight attention in the past, despite the increasing prevalence of naso-sinus allergy and infection. Differentiation between the seasonal type of allergy and the commoner vasomotor rhinitis is now of importance in view of the plethora of antihistamine drugs available 'over the counter'. Identification of a true allergic response requires both time and experience and most rhinological clinics will be staffed by an *immunologist as well as a surgically trained rhinologist. The art and science of rhinology are undergoing major refreshment at this time, and this is one area within the specialty that can be expected to show significant progress within the next decade.

The laryngologist—head and neck surgeon

In most countries, surgeons receive a broadly based training in ENT, with a few then obtaining special training in one of an increasingly large number of subspecialties, of which laryngology is the most popular. Such individuals are concerned primarily with complex problems within the head and neck, although there are no strict boundaries to their expertise. Within the past 20 years this aspect of the ENT surgeon's work has expanded astonishingly, largely at the expense of the *plastic and general surgeons. All *neoplasms within the head and neck, with the exception of the eye, will be treated, although in most instances this will require a combined approach with a *radiotherapist, medical *oncologist, *neurosurgeon, and other experts. Rarely is the laryngologists' interest restricted to the larynx, and they are more accurately called 'head and neck' surgeons.

As a distinct specialty, laryngology only existed once indirect examination of this organ became possible, by the use of the laryngeal mirror in 1854. Even then only a few exceptional individuals acquired sufficient dexterity to remove the more accessible benign *polyps and other lesions. However, with the development of anaesthesia and illuminated instrumentation, direct visualization became feasible, and endoscopic examination of this region is now a standard procedure. The commonest cancer found within the head and neck is in the larynx, invariably associated with smoking. Originally treated by surgical excision, *radiotherapy is more usually the first line of attack in the UK, with surgery for failures. Even so, modern procedures will frequently allow preservation of some voice. Long-term survival is far better than in lung cancer, the other major smoking-related cancer, but rehabilitation following laryngectomy is restricted by loss of voice. Today, total removal of the larynx is usually accompanied by restoration of the voice using a 'plastic shunt' between the *trachea (windpipe) and *oesophagus (gullet). This technique has been perfected to a stage where most well-motivated patients can expect to achieve a reasonable voice, although *speech therapy, which requires no artificial aids, remains effective in many patients.

Although age-related cure rates have changed little for most cancers within the head and neck, more effective local excision is possible with the development of sophisticated operations involving the skull base or translocation of the stomach into the neck. Even with better local control of the cancer, however, late spread around the body remains a prime cause of failure, for cancer *chemotherapy has proved to be of little help for most head and neck tumours.

Perhaps the greatest progress has been made in the field of rehabilitation, where the patient can now confidently expect to achieve acceptable levels of appearance and function after the most radical of operations. This has been made possible by improvements in prosthetics as well as plastic reconstruction of surgical defects. However, the feasible limits of excision have now been reached, and further progress awaits basic information from the *molecular biologists and possibly a new approach to cancer therapy.

Paediatric otolaryngology

An appreciation that children are not simply young adults has led to some ENT surgeons restricting their practice to a younger age-group and the diseases that are present in childhood. Paediatric otolaryngology began in eastern Europe shortly before the Second World War and, although now recognized as an independent subspecialty, it has been slow to develop in the UK.

Removal of the tonsils and adenoids, once the mainstay of ENT surgery, has shown a welcome decline in popularity, coincidental with an appreciation that recurrent upper respiratory infections may be the means by which the child acquires immunity. The indications for this procedure have never been quantified, despite which it still appears with some regularity on most operating lists.

Possibly the most important role played by the paediatric otolaryngologist is in the care of the very young child with congenital lesions of the ear, nose, and throat, where specialized facilities and expertise have markedly reduced the risks of treatment. The child and its parents have the right to expect to receive the very best advice and treatment available, and the paediatric otolaryngologist based in a paediatric hospital is in a unique position to offer this expertise.

There can be few specialties which have undergone such dramatic developments within the past 2 decades as otorhinolaryngology. From humble beginnings, often confined to relatively untrained practitioners, limited in both diagnostic opportunities and surgical possibilities, it has blossomed to become one of the most progressive of all the surgical specialities. Although such extraordinary progress cannot be expected to continue in otology, with the possible exception of cochlear implants, or head and neck surgery, still awaiting a cure for cancer, rhinology may be the growth area in the next decade. There can be no doubt that the future has much in store for this specialty.

DONALD HARRISON

Further reading
Harrison, D. F. N. (ed.) (1988). *Dilemmas in otorhinolaryngology*. Churchill Livingstone, London.
Hinchcliffe, R. and Harrison, D. F. N. (ed.) (1976). *Scientific foundations of otolaryngology*. Heinemann, London.
Maran, A. G. D. and Lund, V. J. (1990). *Clinical rhinology*. Thieme, New York.
Scott Stevenson, R. and Guthrie, D. (1949). *A history of otolaryngology*. Churchill Livingstone, Edinburgh.

OTOSCLEROSIS. A cause of deafness, in which an abnormality, sometimes genetically determined, of the surrounding bone hinders the movement of the *stapes, one of the tiny *ossicles which transmit sound vibrations from the eardrum to the inner ear. Surgical treatment can be of help. See OTORHINOLARYNGOLOGY.

OTOSCOPE. An instrument for inspecting the external auditory canal and eardrum.

OVARIAN CYST. Benign ovarian cysts may occur at any age, although they are most common between 35 and 55. Often they produce no symptoms, and thus may become very large before the patient notices something amiss. Her increasing girth, often ascribed to obesity, may be commented on by friends. Or she may develop pressure symptoms (e.g. breathlessness, indigestion, piles, swelling of the legs, varicose veins) as a result of the size of the tumour. Backache may occur, but frank pain and menstrual abnormality are uncommon.

OVARIAN FOLLICLES is an alternative term for *Graafian follicles. See also OVULATION.

OVARIECTOMY is the surgical removal of one or both *ovaries (synonymous with oophorectomy).

OVARIOTOMY is a surgical incision into the *ovary, usually to remove an ovarian tumour; the word is sometimes used synonymously with *oophorectomy.

OVARY. The ovary is the female *gonad, a paired organ situated one at each side of the *uterus below the opening of the *Fallopian tube. During the 30 or more years of female reproductive life, from *menarche to *menopause, ovulation, the production of a single ovum, occurs once a month. Like the male gonad, the ovary, in addition to the production of *gametes, has an *endocrine function, secreting the *hormones responsible for female *secondary sexual characteristics.

OVERLAYING is suffocation of an infant by lying on top of it.

OVULATION is extrusion of an oocyte (egg or ovum) from a *Graafian follicle on to the surface of the *ovary, whence it passes via the *Fallopian tube into the *uterus. Ovulation occurs once a month on about the 15th day of the menstrual cycle throughout the female reproductive period (from *menarche to *menopause). It is marked by slight *pyrexia and in some women by *mittelschmerz. Maturation of Graafian follicles is under the control of *follicle-stimulating hormone secreted by the anterior *pituitary gland. See also FERTILITY DRUG.

OVUM. The female reproductive cell or *gamete. During the reproductive period of the human female, a single ovum is released from one or other *ovary at monthly intervals on or about the 15th day of each menstrual cycle.

OWEN, SIR RICHARD (1804–92). British physician and naturalist. He was made superintendent of the natural history department of the British Museum in 1856. Owen was the leading comparative anatomist of his time in Europe.

OXALATE. Any salt of oxalic acid. Excessive secretion in the urine (hyperoxaluria) can result in the formation of calcium oxalate stones in the urinary tract. See UROLOGICAL SURGERY.

OXFAM was started in 1942 as the Oxford Committee for Famine Relief by a few citizens who decided to do something to help hungry children in Greece, then under Nazi occupation. From that time it has come to be a household word, distributing over £20 million each year. Its aims are 'To relieve poverty, distress and suffering in any part of the world . . .' It is essentially a fund-raising and grant-giving body, the money coming from private (often small and multiple) donations and from an immense amount of voluntary work. The employed staff is relatively small. The policy is to assist personal and local endeavours of the poor to help themselves. In several areas of the world there are field directors: they are approached with projects needing support, and also seek them out in order to give assistance to agencies working locally who are most likely to understand the problems. These field directors evaluate the projects and make recommendations to the central committees of Oxfam. Often small grants may help enormously in such matters as sanitation, the building of latrines, irrigation, and buying seed or implements for agriculture.

Although most of its work is of this kind, Oxfam is also one of the first to receive calls for help when disaster strikes as in famine, drought, flood, earthquakes, and wars, with their terrifying human aftermaths. Then food, blankets, tents, medical supplies, engineers, and doctors are often supplied in very short time. There are standby teams of volunteers for this type of relief. Similar organizations, such as Médecine sans Frontières (France), exist in many other countries. See also MISSIONS AND MISSION HOSPITALS.

OXIDATION is the combination of *oxygen with a substance, or the removal of *hydrogen from it. The term is also used more generally to signify any reaction in which an atom loses electrons, for example the change of iron from the ferrous (Fe^{2+}) to the ferric (Fe^{3+}) state.

OXIMETER. A photoelectric instrument for measuring the *oxygen saturation of *haemoglobin. The technique is called oximetry.

OXOSTEROIDS are metabolic products of *hormones, the urinary content of which is derived chiefly from *corticosteroids but partly also from *testosterone; their measurement provides a rough indication of *adrenocortical function.

OXYGEN is a gaseous element (atomic number 8, relative atomic mass 15.9994, symbol O), which is odourless and invisible. Oxygen is the most abundant element in the Earth's crust including the seas and the atmosphere; it constitutes 20 per cent by weight of atmospheric air. It is chemically very active; both combustion and *respiration involve combination with oxygen. All known forms of life (except some bacteria) depend on a supply of oxygen to provide energy by metabolism of *glucose or some other nutrient. In man, oxygen is absorbed into the bloodstream through the lungs and transported in combination with *haemoglobin to the tissues. Pure oxygen is of therapeutic value in many situations.

OXYGEN DISSOCIATION CURVE. The sigmoid curve describing the relationship between the partial pressure of *oxygen and the volume in reversible combination with unit mass of *haemoglobin (or the percentage saturation of haemoglobin with oxygen). The shape and position of the curve are influenced by a number of variables, most notably temperature, pH, and pCO_2.

OXYTOCIN is one of the two hormones secreted by the posterior lobe of the *pituitary gland; it initiates *labour at the end of pregnancy, stimulates uterine contraction, and also plays a part in *lactation.

OXYURIS is the *threadworm or pinworm, *Oxyuris* (or *Enterobius*) *vermicularis*.

OZONE is a form of molecular oxygen with three instead of two atoms (symbol O_3). It is very active chemically and a powerful oxidizing agent, sometimes used as a disinfectant. Ordinary air contains only minute amounts; higher concentrations are irritant to the lungs.

P

PABULUM. Food of any kind.

PACCHIONI, ANTONIO (1665–1726). Italian physicist and anatomist. In 1692 he described the protrusions of *arachnoid membrane now known as *Pacchionian bodies.

PACCHIONIAN BODIES are small granulations associated with the *arachnoid mater of the *meninges, through which the *cerebrospinal fluid is reabsorbed into the venous circulation.

PACEMAKERS. The normal cardiac pacemaker is a collection of cells situated in the wall of the right atrium called the *sinoatrial node; it has a greater inherent rhythmicity than any other part of the *myocardium and it therefore initiates the wave of excitation which produces each contraction of the heart. Artificial pacemakers are electrical devices for providing regular external stimuli in order to maintain an adequate heart rate in patients with *heart block, in whom inherent rhythmicity has partly or completely failed. See also CARDIOLOGY.

PACING is maintaining the heartbeat by repetitive stimulation of the myocardium with a *pacemaker.

PADUA, in northern Italy, had a university founded there in 1222, the second oldest in Italy. It was part of the movement which led to the Renaissance, and had a long tradition in science and medicine. *Galileo was professor of mathematics. Andreas *Vesalius was professor of anatomy and his book *De fabrica* marked the beginning of scientific medicine. Gabriel *Fallopius followed Vesalius in the chair. *Fabricius ab Aquapendente taught William *Harvey when he visited, and perhaps gave the Englishman the idea of the valves in veins. Other famous visitors were Thomas *Vicary, John *Caius, and Sir Thomas *Browne. *Santorio was there and *Fracastoro, and *Morgagni, the founder of pathology, was professor of anatomy in 1721. Bernardino *Ramazzini in 1700 published the first work on *occupational diseases. For two or more centuries work coming from Padua was a key to much of the history of medicine during the Renaissance and after.

PAEDERASTY (PEDERASTY) is anal intercourse between a man (the paederast) and a boy.

PAEDIATRICIAN (PEDIATRICIAN). A physician specializing in children's diseases. See PAEDIATRICS.

PAEDIATRICS (PEDIATRICS)
Paediatrics (pediatrics) and paediatricians (pediatricians)
Paediatrics is that sphere of medical practice which applies to infants and children. Nomenclature varies among different countries and institutions, and among different aspects of medical practice. The term 'child health' is sometimes used interchangeably with 'paediatrics', or sometimes to indicate an approach in which maintenance of health is given somewhat greater emphasis in relation to the treatment of disease.

The term *paediatrician (pediatrician)* is taken to mean a physician who spends the bulk of her or his time working with children. In a number of countries paediatricians play a prominent part in the primary medical care of children, whether prevention or treatment, and this is the predominant situation in North America. In the UK primary care for children is predominantly provided by general practitioners, and this is increasingly also the case for their primary preventive care. Paediatricians in the UK work mainly in hospital in-patient and out-patient practice, although in recent years the number of paediatricians specializing in community paediatrics—community paediatricians—has increased markedly (see below). Paediatricians, especially at university hospitals and to a greater extent in North America, have become specialized by disease group or organ system, as in paediatric oncologist (*cancer and *leukaemia), paediatric *neurologist (brain, nerve, and muscle disorders), and paediatric *gastroenterologist (intestinal disorders). Neonatology is a numerically important branch of paediatrics, specializing in the disorders of the newborn; perinatologists, a rarer group, involve themselves in care both *in utero* and immediately after birth. Child psychiatrists are the equivalent of paediatricians within *psychiatry. Paediatric *surgery, paediatric *anaesthesia, and other paediatric specialties are continuing to evolve, practitioners being sometimes full-time in paediatrics at big centres but in smaller units working only part-time in the child specialty.

There is a widespread belief, supported by some research data, that, for rare or complicated disorders, the chances of successful treatment and of family satisfaction are greater when paediatric expertise in the various specialties is available in 'tertiary referral' centres. These are usually university-associated children's units or hospitals, ideally in close proximity with *obstetric departments (for complex neonatology) and specialized adult facilities, e.g. *neurosurgery and *cardiac surgery, with which their paediatric counterparts can co-operate. The success of such specialized children's centres is contributed to by the availability of paediatrically trained nursing staff and similarly expert personnel in *physiotherapy, *radiography, and *nutrition. The availability of laboratory personnel experienced in the range of disorders and the micro-methods appropriate to paediatric material is also important. For more common conditions, the view is that facilities close to the patient's home are needed to allow the close integration between primary care and hospital services necessary for effective treatment of patients with *asthma, *pneumonia, or *gastroenteritis, who only sometimes need admission to hospital, usually being safely treated at home. Such secondary care, or district units as they are, known in Britain, provide for the substantial majority of hospitalized children and for the medical care of the great majority of newborn babies; only those with severe disease or very low birth weight are referred to the tertiary centre. These units also provide a useful focus for the provision of community paediatric services, although these are sometimes organized from other premises.

Recently, several different professional strands have all contributed to similar child-health goals. In the UK for example, child psychiatry has evolved from the convergence of paediatric aspects of psychiatry with the child guidance movement. Within community paediatrics there has been an analogous convergence between preventive paediatric services, formerly organized by local government, and hospital paediatricians interested in health maintenance and the reduction of the impact of handicap on individual children.

Death and disease in childhood (see Campbell and McIntosh 1992)

The tasks of paediatrics can be put in context by consideration of child death, child disease, and child handicap. The picture is strikingly different in the industrialized world today (where most paediatricians work) compared with that in the past. The change reflects the currently successful abolition of the complex and devastating interaction of *malnutrition, infection, and poverty on children's health and survival seen historically in all countries and continuing over much of the poorer world today. Paradoxically, the fall in child mortality has resulted in a lower proportion of children in the population of the industrialized world; 23 per cent of its population in 1988 was under 14 years of age, compared with, for example, Africa's 47 per cent. These differences are because of a higher birth rate and a lower child survival in the latter. The figures for developed countries a century ago were similar to those in Africa today.

Death

In Britain today 29 per cent of all childhood deaths occur in the first month of life and predominantly follow problems *in utero*, being due to birth before development is complete (premature or pre-term delivery), malformation (congenital abnormality), or poor growth (intrauterine growth retardation). About half the deaths in the remainder of the first year are also from these causes; most of the others are either from unexplained sudden infant death (*cot death) or from respiratory infection, such as pneumonia. In later childhood the picture is quite different. Accidents are overwhelmingly the commonest cause of deaths, accounting for nearly 40 per cent of deaths in children between 10 and 15 years of age, followed by cancer and by the late death of children who have survived through the early years of life but who were malformed at birth or irreversibly damaged by problems following premature delivery.

Disease and handicap

About 30 per cent of children thought by their parents to be ill enough to see a doctor have a cold or sore throat, while about 1 in 10 have earache. Only 1 in 20 attend for a skin disorder or for gastroenteritis, while 1 in 100 are thought to have a urinary infection. Of children ill enough to be admitted to hospital, about one-third have a chest disorder of some kind, and one-tenth are admitted because of injury, intestinal disorder such as *diarrhoea or *appendicitis, or to have their tonsils out.

Amongst children attending school who are examined to review their health, mild disorders are quite common. The great majority have some dental decay, although this is less in areas where fluoride is added to the drinking water. About 12 per cent need spectacles and a further 2 per cent are colour blind. Four per cent of school children are diagnosed as asthmatic (a higher proportion have some degree of asthmatic chestiness), and the same number are so fat as to be classed as obese. One in 10 5-year-olds wets the bed, but this figure drops to 1 in 100 by the time of leaving school. One child in five is identified at some stage in childhood as being sufficiently disturbed as to have a behaviour disorder interfering with their progress or happiness. Just under 1 per cent of children have a severe ongoing handicap. Of these, two-thirds are mentally handicapped, just under half have fits, a quarter are blind or severely deaf, and 1 in 10 have handicapping abnormalities of their bones, including arthritis. Such well-known but relatively rare conditions as *cystic fibrosis, *muscular dystrophy, or *phenylketonuria affect even fewer children.

In terms of quantity, most medical care of children is given outside hospital. The average child in Britain sees a general practitioner four times a year, visits a hospital once every 5 years, and is admitted to hospital only once per childhood. Such hospital stay is likely to last approximately 4 days; it was three times as long in 1955.

History of paediatrics

Because of the extreme dependency of the human offspring, cultural procedures have developed in human societies which help to give parents confidence to face the awesome responsibilities of discharging their obligations to the new baby. The methods have always covered the care of the normal, with extra measures for dealing with signs and symptoms, that is with appearances and behaviour regarded as not normal. Lists of these abnormal happenings date from the earliest human records. Both in the Egyptian *Ebers Papyrus, dating from the first half of the 16th century BC, and in the slightly later Berlin Papyrus on mother and child, there are sections on the diseases of infancy. In Indian and Chinese manuscripts, and to a lesser extent in the Talmud, diseases of children are described and discussed. *Hippocrates in his '*Aphorisms*', notably in the fragment 'On Teething', shares responsibility for the kind of list which persisted with relatively little change, either in its content or in the accompanying recommendations, from classical times down to the middle of the 16th century AD. This constitutes external rather than internal medicine: sores, rashes, lumps, and bumps seen and felt from the outside without the use of artefacts or any exploration within.

Rosen von Rosenstein (1706–73), Professor of Medicine at Uppsala, Sweden, was a founder of modern paediatrics as a medical specialty, writing, in 1765, the textbook entitled (in English translation) *The diseases of children and their remedies*. A private hospital for the treatment of children was opened in Vienna in 1787. Half a century later, public children's hospitals followed in Berlin (1830), St Petersburg (1834), and Vienna (1837), but it was the French who led the way.

After the Revolution, in 1802, the French government founded a hospital for sick children (Hôpital des Enfants Malades) in Paris. The assumption of responsibility by government ensured continuity and sufficient resources to make possible the study of diseases of children. From 1838 to 1843 Barthez and Rilliet published their three-volume work on the diseases of children, which remained the bible for doctors for the next 25 years. It was a time of French pre-eminence in clinical medicine and in physiology.

By contrast, in England such endeavours were left to private charity. In fact a *Foundling Hospital had been opened by Thomas *Coram in London in 1745. Attempts to gather sick children together, so that doctors might learn by experience how to treat them and to compare the success of different treatments, were made

by George *Armstrong in 1769 and by John Bunnell Davis in 1815; both proved abortive. It was not until 1852 that Charles *West opened the Hospital for Sick Children in *Great Ormond Street. In all these plans, the objective was first and foremost to cut down the high infant and child mortality rates by improving the skill and knowledge of the doctors, but this was by no means the sole objective. Mothers were instructed about hygiene and the general care of children and there were opportunities for the training of nurses. However, although the hospitals provided centres in which medical and *nursing skills could be fostered, it was soon evident that their contribution to falling death rates would be small. Indeed, hospital admission could itself engender *epidemics of *infectious diseases, often fatal. The solution was to be sought and found elsewhere in the better ordering of the public health.

Paediatrics and paediatricians had made an earlier and more encouraging start in the USA, where an American Pediatric Society held its first meeting in 1889, the *Archives of Pediatrics* having been founded 5 years earlier. The members of the society, like the contributors to the journal, were physicians with a 'special interest in the study of diseases in children'. Nevertheless, much time and space were devoted to infant feeding. Hygiene, public health, and child labour were, even at that time, recognized as appropriate subjects for discussion, but the doctors' chief concern was disease. The first American children's hospital was opened in Philadelphia in 1855.

In Austria and in Germany the approach was more academic. The problems of infant nutrition and of infant feeding were joined with studies of the diseases of the newborn and of the early childhood years. The lead which these countries took over France, where modern medicine had found its first home, remained with them until the First World War, when it crossed the Atlantic. Abraham *Jacobi, L. Emmett *Holt, Henry Koplik, J. Lewis Smith, William *Osler, not all confining their work to children, had, among others, laid firm foundations upon which the next generation built the science of paediatrics while not neglecting the art. The culmination came when John Howland (1873–1926) established the Harriet Lane department of paediatrics at *Johns Hopkins Hospital in Baltimore in 1912. Notable paediatric contributions in both medicine and surgery are owed to others. In Japan the children's hospital of Tokyo National University celebrated its centenary in 1989.

Over the past century *medical journals have become a key element in the spreading of good practice and in reporting research findings. There are currently some 60 paediatric journals, although most widely important research is reported in only a few if these. Arguably the first of these was the *Jahrbuch für Kinderheilkunde*, first published in Germany in 1868, which subsequently became *Annales Paediatrici* and then evolved into the present-day *Pediatric Research*.

Frederic *Still in London and John Thomson (1856–1926) in Edinburgh were the first two British specialists in diseases of children. The others, who acted as physicians in the children's hospitals, were general physicians (internists) with a special interest in sick children—and particularly in recognizing such modifications of adult illnesses as occurred during childhood, in illnesses which seemed mainly or only to affect children, and in congenital malformations. Still described a children's form of *rheumatoid arthritis in his MD thesis in 1896. *Mental deficiency (handicap) was a special interest, not in its own right but when it formed one of a collection of congenital defects. Only Thomson, in his pamphlet *Opening doors* (1923), aimed to tell parents what they could do to help their disabled child.

The real function of the children's specialists in those early days remained general medicine applied to the special age-group which began at birth, although many years were to pass before the *obstetricians relinquished their nominal responsibility for the newborn. When the special age-group ends is still undecided, the onset of *puberty being one obvious determinant. The development of adolescent medicine as a further specialization has only a limited following.

The introduction of effective *immunization began with diphtheria toxin–antitoxin mixtures. During the 1920s, *clinical trials were made on selected populations. A major preoccupation was the risk of *serum-sickness, a complication of immunization noted by von *Pirquet in Vienna in 1905 and leading him to his conception of *allergy. The general adoption of active immunization took many years. Its introduction found the general public, and even the doctors, somewhat suspicious despite the century-long experience of *smallpox vaccination. Protection against *tetanus and, to a lesser degree, against whooping cough (*pertussis) became available, but it was not until the 1940s that the vaccine being offered in the UK was accepted by the majority as safe and beneficial. As late as 1951, *poliomyelitis epidemics (first noted in 1910) swept the USA and Sweden, inducing the sort of community panic which we associate with the *plagues of the Middle Ages and leaving a trail of death and serious motor handicap. Since the introduction of the *Salk vaccine, first described in 1953, these catastrophes have become part of history.

The problems posed by *tuberculosis were different. *Consumption had been recognized in classical times and tuberculous disease of bone has been diagnosed, with as much certainty as is possible, in the third millennium BC. *Koch identified the tubercle bacillus, publishing his researches in 1882. Infection was spread by coughing and, less commonly, by drinking infected milk, and by the dawn of paediatrics tuberculosis had established itself as a community as well as a family disease. Certainly, among urban populations almost every child, either as a baby or at some time before maturity, would encounter and be challenged by the tubercle bacillus. Some babies succumbed; others overcame the challenge, becoming sensitized, so that their response to further almost inevitable encounters led to an altered reaction; this, through the results of his tuberculin test, confirmed von Pirquet in his belief in his concept of allergy. At first a whole system of special clinics and dispensaries was aimed at treatment of the individual patient. Later, mass *radiography led to early case-finding, better segregation of open cases (patients with bacilli in their *sputum), and a reduction in the sources of infection. Grandfather coughing by the fireside was removed and his opportunities for infecting his grandchildren were lessened. The discovery of an effective *antibiotic (*streptomycin) by *Waksman in 1944 provided a final touch, but the rise in drug-resistant tuberculosis associated with the disease in *HIV immunocompromised individuals may mean that the story of childhood tuberculosis is not finally closed.

Although these astonishing successes neither originated in children's hospitals, nor directly involved paediatrics, they greatly influenced the health of children. At the same time, further researches had put into the doctors' hands other antibiotics, so that the treatment of most non-viral infections could be safely done at home by family doctors or, if in hospital, within a much shorter time and with less resulting debility. These advances, with the reduction in tuberculosis, effective treatment of *meningitis, the virtual disappearance of acute gastroenteritis, *osteomyelitis, and *rheumatic fever with its tendency to cause *valvular disease of the heart, reduced the demand for hospital beds and therefore for the hospital paediatrician of later childhood.

Community paediatrics

This subspecialty has evolved to address medical issues which have historically been dealt with inadequately in Britain both by general practitioners and by hospital-focused paediatricians. These include the surveillance of the child population as a whole for presymptomatic or early signs of disorder, by what has come to be known as *screening, for conditions such as deafness, metabolic disorder, poor growth, and developmental delay. The balance of benefit–cost and inconvenience and timing of this have been the subjects of considerable thought recently (Hall 1991). Health education and disease prevention, including advice on the feeding of babies, immunization, and advice on accident prevention have been other important roles. In more recent years child protection has become an important focus of work, in conjunction with the law courts and other social agencies attempting to ameliorate conditions for children in families where violence or neglectful parenting puts the child's health or development seriously at risk, and has extended into the controversial area of abusive adult–child sexual interactions. The amelioration of the impact on the child and family of severe handicap is another important role, as is the overlapping task of educational medicine, giving medical advice on the diagnosis and management of children who are performing unexpectedly poorly at school. Again, community paediatrics has a joint role with educational psychologists, *social workers, and, of course, parents in this area. Historically community paediatric services were provided as an aspect of local government. Over the past 20 years there has been a gradual but somewhat erratic evolution of services towards surveillance, prevention, and education, predominantly provided by the primary health-care team of general practitioner and specialized nurses and health visitors. Handicap, specialized educational medicine, and child protection are predominantly provided by specialist community paediatricians, often working as part of a team with general paediatricians based on a district paediatric unit. Another development of recent years has been the establishment of specialized paediatric nurses, providing a link between home-based and hospital-based treatments with other specialized nurses such as asthma nurses, diabetes nurses, or cancer nurses.

(the late) A. WHITE FRANKLIN
R. D. H. BOYD

Further reading
Campbell, A. G. M. and McIntosh, N. (ed.) (1992). *Forfar and Arneil's textbook of paediatrics*, Churchill Livingstone, Edinburgh.
Hall, D. M.B. (ed.) (1991). *Health for all children*, (2nd edn). Oxford University Press, Oxford.
Nichols, B. L., Ballabriga A., and Kretchmer, N. (ed.) (1991). *History of paediatrics: 1850–1950*. Nestlé Nutrition workshop Series 22. Raven Press, New York.
Still, G. F. (1931). *The history of paediatrics*. Oxford University Press, London.

PAEDOPHILIA (PEDOPHILIA) is the sexual orientation of adults towards children.

PAGET, SIR JAMES, Bt (1814–99). British surgeon. During his apprenticeship, to a local surgeon, Charles Costerton, he and his brother Charles published *The natural history of Yarmouth* (1834). While still a student, he discovered and described *Trichinella spiralis*. In 1843 he became one of the original fellows of the Royal College of Surgeons and accepted the post of warden of the residential college for students at St Bartholomew's. Paget catalogued the pathological museums at St Bartholomew's Hospital and at the Royal College of Surgeons and in doing so acquired a knowledge of *pathology unrivalled by any other surgeon. His name is still attached to a number of disorders. He was the first to describe *fibrosarcoma of the abdominal wall (*Paget's recurrent fibroid, 1851); a superficial *necrosis of bone (Paget's quiet necrosis, 1870); an eczematoid cancerous lesion of the nipple (*Paget's disease of the nipple, 1874); and osteitis deformans (*Paget's disease of bone, 1876).

PAGET'S DISEASE OF BONE is a not uncommon skeletal disorder, particularly in later life, of unknown cause. There is patchy increase in bone vascularity accompanied by uncoordinated bone resorption (osteolysis) and new bone formation (osteosclerosis). Bone pain, weakness, deformity, and pathological fractures may result; there are typical X-ray changes and a raised serum *alkaline phosphatase level. The condition, also called osteitis deformans, has been shown to respond to treatment with *calcitonin.

PAGET'S DISEASE OF THE NIPPLE is a condition presenting as an apparent superficial inflammation of the nipple region in middle-aged women but due to underlying cancer of the breast, usually an *adenocarcinoma of the ducts.

PAGET'S RECURRENT FIBROID is a *fibrosarcoma recurring in scar tissue following earlier removal.

PAIN
Definition
Pain has been defined by the International Association for the Study of Pain as an unpleasant sensory and emotional experience associated with actual or potential tissue damage or described in terms of tissue damage. Pain is the prerogative of man because he *perceives* pain, whereas animals respond to a noxious (painful) stimulus. Hence animals do not, as far as we are aware, perceive pain and therefore pain in animals is called nociception (the *response* to a noxious stimulus). This basic difference was reinforced by *Pavlov in the early part of the 20th century, when he gave dogs electric shocks before he fed them. Initially this produced a painful response, withdrawal, and vocalization, but after a time the painful response was replaced by a joyful response, salivation. Thus he proved that in dogs the response to a noxious stimulus could be changed from nociception to pleasure. This difference between pain and nociception has important connotations when research in animals is extrapolated to man. Pain and nociception are not the same; they are related in some way but the relationship may not be a direct one.

The basis of research into pain has been the relationship between the stimulus and the perception of pain. However, in only one of the three different types of pain—operative, acute, and chronic—is this relationship direct. This is best explained by the patient's response to *surgery, a noxious stimulus which is followed by pain in almost a graded fashion. As most, if not all, surgery is performed under general *anaesthesia (therefore the patient's response to the noxious stimulus is assessed by the anaesthetist who infers that the patient is or is not feeling pain), then this, as with animals, is nociception (the response to a noxious stimulus). In this situation there is progressive damage and the pain provides some protective function to the organism. The second type of pain is acute, a good example of which is the pain associated with a broken limb, which is made worse by movement but not necessarily relieved by rest. The movement-associated pain is protective in that the *fracture may heal more quickly and effectively if the limb is rested. The stimulus here is related to the response. However, there is another pain associated with the fracture. This is the dull, aching pain which is not associated with any external stimulus but in some way must be related to the trauma itself. It is difficult to see a protective function for this pain, apart from reminding the patient of the injury. Postoperative pain is similar in all respects to this.

The third type is chronic pain, where there is no relationship as yet described between the stimulus and the response. If, for example, we take the pain associated with *arthritis, there is absolutely no correlation between the pain and the degree of arthritis found on *radiographs. Chronic pain does not provide any protective function for man. Indeed, if the analogy is continued with arthritis, rest, which relieves the pain, increases the demonstrable destruction, while exercise, which increases the pain, is associated with less destruction in the long term. Chronic pain appears to have no positive advantages for man; indeed, it appears to be totally nihilistic. Furthermore, there is no evidence that animals suffer chronic nociception (pain); thus it is difficult to establish any logical phylogenetic reason for chronic pain. Phylogenetically, operative pain is a result of civilization. Acute pain provides some advantages for man, whereas chronic pain seems to provide only disadvantages and, as such, chronic pain may be a random error in the system.

Theories
Broadly, there are two basic theories of pain perception:

(1) the specific theories, which state that pain is a specific sensation which has specific *receptors (nociceptors) and is transmitted along specific neural channels to specific areas of the brain.
(2) the pattern theories, which state that pain is perceived as a result of all the information available to the brain at that time—thus most, if not all, receptors can transmit pain—and that there are no specific neural pathways within the central nervous system.

It is obvious that there are many variations on each of these themes, and that there are also theories which encompass elements of both the specific and the pattern theories. The 'gate' theory of pain, proposed by Melzack and Wall in 1965, is a pattern theory which, thus far, has stood the test of time. Basically, it stated that the perception of pain could be modified at the first junction, i.e. the spinal cord. They further proposed that this modification of the pain was a result of all the information available at that time from within and from outside the patient. It was the first theory

which included chronic pain as part of its basis and interestingly, it was the first theory to be proposed by a psychologist (Melzack) and an anatomist/physiologist (Wall), thus highlighting the importance of the two elements of pain—physical and emotional. This theory has been shown to be correct in that both pain and nociception can be modified at the first junction, the dorsal horn of the *spinal cord. The two major criticisms of the theory are that it is too simple, and that the inhibition shown in the diagram is presynaptic. The first of these criticisms is valid and the second is debatable. Be that as it may, the 'gate' theory focused attention on the dorsal horn of the spinal cord, with the resulting development of spinal *analgesia.

Figure 1 shows the areas of the nervous system where pain can be interrupted, with the two fundamental elements being the *axons (nerve fibres) and the *synapses (junctions). Until the 'gate' theory, most of the research involved modification of the axons, where local anaesthetics work, but since 1965 most of the

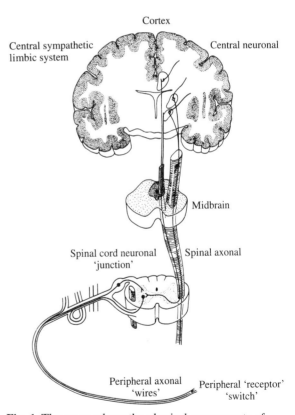

Cortex

Central sympathetic limbic system

Central neuronal

Midbrain

Spinal cord neuronal 'junction'

Spinal axonal

Peripheral axonal 'wires'

Peripheral 'receptor' 'switch'

Fig. 1 The areas where the physical components of pain may be interrupted: at the receptors (switch), axons (wires), or neuronal synapses (junctions). The emotional components of a patient's pain may be modified in the brain, but the precise area or areas involved remain to be defined.

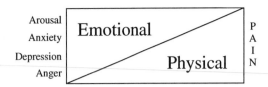

Fig. 2 The two components of pain, physical and emotional (the patient's response to the pain).

research has revolved around modifications at the junctions (synapses).

Therapy

The two components of pain, physical and emotional, are always present, but both components do not always need treatment. Pure physical pain probably does not exist (Fig. 2) because there is always an emotional component (albeit very small). By the same token, pure psychogenic pain probably does not exist, because there is always a physical component. This latter observation is reinforced by the fact that most, if not all, of the behavioural modification programmes designed to teach patients to cope with their pain have a physiotherapeutic basis. There are four basic mood dimensions—arousal (how alert or drowsy is the patient), anxiety (how relaxed or tense is the patient), depression (how happy or unhappy is the patient), and aggression (how angry or comfortable the patient feels towards his fellow man). All these mood factors have an unpleasant extreme which is therefore painful and so will need treatment. These unpleasant mood factors are always part of pain but do not always need treatment. They form the emotional response to the physical stimulus. The decision as to whether this emotional response requires treatment needs to be assessed in each patient.

The physical component always requires treatment because all patients believe that there is a physical basis for their pain and they are correct. However, the physical component may not be the major element. The art in treatment of patients with pain rests in identifying which is the more important element, and then in designing the treatment programme to deal mainly with that element, while also treating the other components. There are four basic strategies for dealing with the physical component of a patient's pain:

(1) physical, for example electrical stimulation;
(2) pharmacological;
(3) injections;
(4) surgery.

There are three basic strategies for dealing with the emotional component of a patient's pain:

(1) reassurance;
(2) pharmacological;
(3) professional counselling.

Operative pain

In this situation, where the stimulus is directly related to the response, patients most commonly require general or local anaesthesia in order to provide analgesia. However, simple operations have been performed using electrical stimulation to provide the analgesia. *Acupuncture has also been used to provide analgesia for operations. Although it is not effective in all patients, it has been reported that the use of a strong magnetic field can provide anaesthesia for some patients. Electrical stimulation, acupuncture, and magnetic fields are in some way related to physical therapy, general anaesthesia is based on the use of drugs, and local anaesthesia generally requires injections. On the emotional side, in some circumstances it is possible for some patients to use self-hypnosis to control their pain during surgery; however, antidepressant and anticonvulsant drugs are unable to provide anaesthesia for surgery. In susceptible patients it is possible to perform operations under hypnosis, the most sophisticated form of counselling.

General anaesthesia is believed to have its effects on the synapses whereas local anaesthesia affects the axons. Under general anaesthesia the patient's response to pain is assessed and so, strictly speaking, it is nociception; the anaesthetist infers from the physiological responses that the patient is or is not feeling pain and takes the appropriate action. The physiological mechanisms underlying general anaesthesia have not been defined. It is at least one stage further on than *sleep and we do not yet fully understand the physiological mechanisms of sleep. It is most likely that general anaesthetics have their effect throughout the central nervous system, presumably via a non-specific (global) effect on synaptic transmission. Electrical stimulation presumably has its effect via the axons, while magnetic fields are believed to have their effect via the central nervous system, and are somewhat analogous to general anaesthetics. It is believed that acupuncture has its analgesic effect via a similar mechanism to that underlying hypnosis. The mechanisms by which self-hypnosis and hypnosis provide analgesia are not understood, but are believed to lie at a cortical level.

Acute pain

The most common acute pain is that following surgery (postoperative pain) and so this model will be used to illustrate our understanding of the physiology of acute pain and its relief. The natural history for most acute pain is for it to resolve with time as part of the natural healing process. There is no evidence that the treatment of the pain *per se* has any effect on its duration. Thus the treatment of acute pain is the treatment of the symptom while the body's 'healing' processes resolve the underlying cause of the pain, in this situation the surgery. Usually there are two different types of post-operative pain; the first is the dull ache which is present all the time and the second is the pain that is related to movement.

With the dull ache there is no obvious relationship between the stimulus and the response; it is presumably related to the local trauma of the operation, whereas the second pain has an obvious stimulus. There is a wealth of medical evidence to support the importance of early mobilization following surgery and so there is a need to control this pain to enable the patients to move. Fortunately, the natural history of the duration of this movement pain is generally shorter than that of the dull, aching pain. There is a third type of pain which, uncommonly, follows any trauma and that is a neuralgic (neuropathic) pain. It is related to nerve (axon) damage and is generally not relieved by conventional analgesia; hence this pain may persist and become chronic.

Not all patients require or demand postoperative analgesia: approximately 25 per cent of patients do not require postoperative analgesia irrespective of the operation (stimulus). The explanation for this observation is unknown, but at one end of the spectrum it is that the patients do not have any pain and at the other they do not wish to have any treatment for the pain. Most patients fall in the middle of this spectrum and have varying combinations of both these factors. These patients expect to have pain postoperatively and believe that the pain is a normal consequence of their surgery. They would prefer the pain to any possible complications of the therapy for the pain. In their own words, they would prefer to put up with the pain as they know that it will get better with time.

Movement pain

The physical methods for treating pain, such as acupuncture and electrical stimulation, are not very effective for this type of pain. Nevertheless, they are worth trying in those patients who do not wish to use drugs. Their success rate is low but there is a small group of patients in whom they will be effective. The most common method of dealing with pain is pharmacological, and the most commonly used drugs are the opiates (narcotics). Morphine is the standard for this group of drugs and it is usually given as an injection (these injections may be intermittent or continuous). Intermittent intramuscular injection is the technique commonly used in most hospitals. However, there has been a tendency towards using continuous infusions of morphine or similar drugs, usually intravenously and, most commonly, via patient-controlled analgesia machines. These machines circumvent most of the disadvantages of the intermittent injections and give the individual patient control over his or her pain and pain relief. It is interesting to note that even with these machines most patients do not give themselves complete pain relief; they titrate themselves to an acceptable level of pain, which is different for each individual. No study involving patient-controlled analgesia has ever produced complete pain relief, but these studies have produced patient satisfaction, which is a different issue.

The aim of patient-controlled analgesia is to maintain a steady blood concentration of the opiate, to provide background analgesia and then, when the patient is about to move, or when the pain increases, the patient gives himself or herself a boost of the drug to prevent or control the pain. It is generally very effective, but because there are so many variables (the patient, the operation, the pain, and the drug used to mention but a few), it is not 100 per cent effective in all patients. However, it has been an important advance. Patients receiving patient-controlled analgesia are more satisfied with their pain relief than are those patients who are having conventional, as required, dosing with the same opiates. There are a number of different machines on the market, of varying degrees of sophistication, all of which have advantages and disadvantages. As these machines are mainly managed by the nursing staff, it is imperative that they should be aware of the limitations of the machine that they are using. Thus it is common for a particular hospital or ward to standardize the machines they use in order to limit possible complications. It is common in most large hospitals to have a pain control team to supervise their use. The membership of this team varies, but the basic team consists of a doctor and a nurse. The doctor's role is to control the prescription of the drug or drugs and to liaise with other medical staff, while the nurse ensures that the patients and machines are being monitored effectively and also liaises with the nurses on the wards. It is common practice in most hospitals for the team, or at least a member of the team, to visit or review each patient every day while they are receiving patient-controlled analgesia.

It is possible to use injections of local anaesthetics around the appropriate nerves to provide analgesia for postoperative pain and, with modern technology, a catheter can be placed near the nerve so as to provide continuous nerve blockade. This provides good pain relief but has the disadvantage of causing numbness in the distribution of the nerve; if the nerve has a motor component then weakness or paralysis of the muscles supplied by that nerve ensues. In theory it is possible to block any nerve in the body to provide pain relief, but it is unusual for the pain following surgery to be limited to the distribution of one nerve. Hence the most common nerve-blocking technique used for postoperative pain is epidural catheterization. Spinal nerves pass from the spinal cord via the epidural space to supply various parts of the body and so local anaesthetics can be placed in the epidural space to block the appropriate nerves. Epidural analgesia is most often used for women in childbirth. There have been two major improvements in this technique. The first is the use of epidural opiates in conjunction with the local anaesthetic and the second is the use of constant infusions of local anaesthetic and opiates. In the latter situation patient-controlled analgesia machines can be used to provide the patient with control over his or her pain and pain relief.

This movement-related pain generally resolves within the first 48 hours of surgery, and so the patient is left with the aching type pain, which also resolves with time.

The aching pain

This pain is generally relieved by orally administered drugs. The two major groups used are the minor opiates and the non-steroidal anti-inflammatory drugs. Physical methods such as acupuncture and transcutaneous electrical nerve stimulation are more likely to be effective for this pain.

The neuralgic pain

This pain may be relieved by transcutaneous electrical stimulation or acupuncture. It also generally responds to the unconventional analgesics, the antidepressants and the anticonvulsants. It does resolve with time, but the sooner the patient is given a clear explanation of the cause of the pain and provided with effective therapy, the sooner it will resolve.

There are specific surgical procedures for specific acute pains, for example removal of a lumbar disc protrusion that is pressing on a nerve root and causing pain in the leg (*sciatica). A description of all the operations for different acute pains is beyond the scope of this article. The unpleasant emotional component of acute pain is the patient's anxiety about the connotations of the pain and, as soon as it is possible, he or she should be informed of possible causes and their meaning. The patient may need pharmacological treatment and/or counselling to help them cope with the information, although most often patients respond to reassurance.

Chronic pain

Chronic pain is that pain which has persisted for at least a month despite all conventional treatment and investigation. Chronic pain may be acute pain which persists (that is the pain may persist because the appropriate treatment for the cause of the pain or for the pain itself, has not been prescribed). It may persist because the patient is intolerant of the correct treatment or does not wish to use it. The therapy prescribed for patients with chronic pain is, by and large, symptomatic. The cardinal rule when a patient's pain is being treated symptomatically is 'that pain must not be treated symptomatically if there is a definitive treatment for the cause of the pain'. This is also the cardinal rule of the pain clinic, where the more difficult chronic pain therapeutic problems are referred. Pain clinics may be defined as the workplace of a group of health professionals who treat patients with chronic pain symptomatically. Chronic pain does not appear to provide any benefits to the patient—it is destructive, both physically and emotionally, for most patients. The classic example of this is 'osteoarthritis', where there is very little (if any) relationship between the radiological evidence of destruction and the pain, and, in addition, the less mobility in these joints the greater the destruction in the long term.

Therapy of chronic pain

Transcutaneous electrical stimulation provides adequate analgesia in 30 per cent of the patients in whom it is used; it has only two major side-effects—allergy to the tape or allergy to the jelly—both of which are surmountable. Acupuncture also works consistently for chronic pain. All injections, be they acupuncture, placebo, or active, are capable of producing long-term pain relief. Unfortunately, it is not possible to predict those in whom these techniques are going to be effective. As far as pharmacological therapy is concerned, it is important to exclude the powerful conventional analgesics, because of the risk of addiction, but most patients with chronic pain are insensitive or intolerant to these drugs. There are a number of unconventional analgesics, including the antidepressants and the anticonvulsants. The anti-convulsants have been used effectively to treat trigeminal neuralgia for 30 years because conventional analgesics were shown to be ineffective. There are many other types of pain which respond to these drugs either individually or in combination.

Most often axonal blockade involves the injection of local anaesthetics which will abolish the pain, albeit briefly. Patients may be made numb, yet do not achieve lasting analgesia. In such situations, it is possible to say that the pain is not coming from where the patient is feeling it. Thus, in the first instance, axonal blockade is diagnostic but occasionally it is therapeutic in that the pain does not return when the local anaesthetic wears off. In a number of patients who do not obtain analgesia while numb, it is possible to stop their pain with the injection of drugs, such as morphine or other analgesics, around the spinal cord (neuronal blockade). With modern technology, catheters can be implanted around the spinal cord to provide a continuous infusion for long-term pain relief. The duration of this effect at present is not good enough to recommend its use in most patients with non-malignant pain. Nevertheless, in the future these systems will improve. There is, however, a small but consistent group of patients who only obtain adequate pain relief when they are asleep, and it is not possible to provide this group with adequate analgesia. Neuronal blockade, however, will in all cases of pain stop it for the duration of the blockade. The most complete form of neural blockade is general anaesthesia, but this is inappropriate for patients with chronic pain. Operative procedures for the relief of chronic pain such as division of nerves or sensory pathways in the spinal cord are time-limited in their beneficial effects because the nervous system is designed to overcome destructive procedures. Therefore these procedures should be reserved for patients with limited longevity. Unfortunately, even in these patients the success rate of surgery for chronic pain is not 100 per cent; at best it is 80 to 90 per cent.

A clear explanation of the emotional component of chronic pain is often enough to enable some patients to cope with this aspect. It should be pointed out that it is normal to be chronically anxious, unhappy, and frustrated by the situation. It is also important to tell the patient that these mood factors are unpleasant and, as such, are part and parcel of their pain. The decision in an individual patient as to whether the emotional components need specific treatment should be discussed with him or her. Drug therapy for this emotional component involves the use of antidepressants, which also help the anxiety and the unhappiness. There are at the present time no drugs available to control anger. The only therapy for frustration is professional counselling, which also may help to allay anxiety and unhappiness. Its object is to enable the patient to cope with the pain and the problems it creates. It is not designed to relieve the pain *per se*.

In summary, the treatment of all three types of pain should involve management of both the physical and emotional components. The art lies in identifying which of the two components is the more important (Fig. 2).

The future

It is possible to relieve operative pain in all patients. Adequate pain relief can be provided for most patients with acute pain, remembering that not all patients wish to be totally pain-free. As far as chronic pain is concerned, effective short-term pain relief is achievable for most patients; it is the provision of long term relief that awaits further technological advances. With increasing knowledge the medical profession will improve its ability to treat patients with pain more effectively.

CHRIS GLYNN

Further reading
Wall, P. D. and Melzack, R. (1989). *Textbook of pain*. Churchill Livingstone, Edinburgh.

PALAEOPATHOLOGY (PALEOPATHOLOGY) is, strictly speaking, the study of disease in human (and animal) remains. A less restricted view of palaeopathology, however, is to consider it as that part of medical history which deals specifically with the history of disease and, to this end, to utilize all the relevant information, documentary, pictorial, or pathological.

For many years ancient human remains were treated more as curiosities than as serious objects for study, and it was not until the end of the 19th century and the beginning of the 20th that the subject became established as an academic discipline. This development was stimulated by the discovery of the huge burial grounds in Egypt; examination of many human mummified remains identified lesions characteristic of various disease states; this was work with which the name of Sir Marc Armand Ruffer (1859–1917) is particularly associated. Ruffer is usually credited with coining the term 'palaeopathology' but, in fact, he was anticipated by R.W. Shufeldt, writing in the *Popular Science Monthly*, an American magazine, in 1893.

In the 1930s and 1940s palaeopathology languished somewhat, but was revived in the 1950s in both Europe and North America. In the past 20 years or so, the discipline has become greatly more rigorous, and epidemiological techniques have begun to be employed, so that it is now concentrating more on populations than on individual skeletons with interesting *pathology, which formerly tended to be the case.

A number of problems beset palaeopathologists in their work. The first and most obvious is that they are able to deal only with those diseases which affect the skeleton; this is a substantial minority of all those which are found in the International *Classification of Disease (ICD). Those who examine mummified remains are in a slightly more favourable position for they do have soft tissues to examine, but the numbers of these remains are so few, compared with the numbers of skeletons available for study, that they contribute little to the overall picture, certainly so far as population data are concerned. For this reason, attention has to be given to the relatively small number of conditions that affect the skeleton and, of these, the joint diseases and especially *osteoarthritis, which is always abundant in any group of skeletons, are the most important. Erosive arthropathies do occur, but seldom, and their diagnosis is often problematical. *Rheumatoid arthritis has also been reported by some authors, but the number of cases that are recognizable as conforming to modern clinical criteria is extremely small; claims for high prevalence rates amongst some North American indigenous populations have not been accepted by all authorities, and there have been no convincing cases found in the UK to date.

Injury to the skeleton is also commonly encountered, both accidental and deliberate. Much can be learned about the practice of bone-setting in earlier populations by the state of healing of fractured bones and their alignment, and by whether they have become secondarily infected. It is clear from the extremely good results which appear to have been achieved that many former populations had access to individuals with considerable skill in reducing and setting broken limbs, and presumably not all had formal medical education. Injuries received on the battlefield are also relatively common in some periods, and judicial injury in the form of beheadings and hangings may also be observed.

The second difficulty for palaeopathologists concerns *diagnosis. There is nothing to help them except the morphology of the lesions and, to some extent, *radiography, although this is often not as helpful as might be supposed. Not only does this paucity of information greatly limit the ability to reach a diagnosis in the first place, it also renders difficult any comparison with prevalence rates in contemporary populations in whom diagnosis frequently relies either on the patient's history or the results of biochemical or other tests. Thus, comparing the frequency of osteoarthritis in a skeletal population with that reported from either a hospital or a general practice population is extremely problematical since the groups are similar in almost no respects. Nor is the comparison with data obtained from radiological surveys reliable since it has been shown that the palaeopathologist is able to pick up many more lesions than are visible on *radiography.

Nor is there any relief when comparing data with the results of the early palaeopathologists. Wood Jones, in one of his accounts of the pathology of the skeletons from Nubia, stated that rheumatoid arthritis was the most common disease. It is certain that he was referring to osteoarthritis, not the disease that is nowadays known as rheumatoid arthritis. Differences in diagnostic fashion and in the preferences of particular palaeopathologists make comparison, if not impossible, then certainly imprecise. Because of this, some attempts have been made to introduce operational definitions of disease into palaeopathological practice. A start has been made with the arthropathies, and one is gradually being adopted for osteoarthritis; it is hoped that acceptable criteria for defining some of the *infectious diseases may follow.

Despite the difficulties inherent in the subject, however, palaeopathologists have made important contributions to the understanding of disease in the past and have made significant contributions to the knowledge of pathological processes in bone. The most notable example has been the work of Møller-Christensen, who provided a detailed description of the bone changes in *leprosy based on his study of skeletons from a leper hospital in Denmark.

The most interesting areas for future work in palaeopathology concern the extraction of organic compounds from bone. For example, it is has been possible to recover mitochondrial *DNA, *albumin, IgG, *haemoglobin, osteocalcin, and *myeloma protein from several thousand-year-old human bones, and there seems little doubt that other compounds will also soon be extracted.

H. A. WALDRON

Further reading

Møller-Christensen, V. (1965). New knowledge of leprosy through paleopathology. *International Journal of Leprosy*, **33**, 603–10.

Rogers. J., Waldron, H. A., Dieppe, P., and Watt, I. (1987). Arthropathies in palaeopathology: the basis of classification according to most probable cause. *Journal of Archaeological Science*, **14**, 179–93.

PALATE. The partition separating the oral and nasal cavities; it comprises a bony portion in front (the hard palate) and a fleshy portion behind (the soft palate). The latter is drawn up during swallowing to occlude the back of the nose.

PALLIATIVE THERAPY is treatment undertaken with the objective of relieving symptoms, particularly when these are painful or in some other way distressing,

but in the knowledge that it will not affect the outcome of the disease.

PALMER, WILLIAM (1824–56). British physician and poisoner. He was found guilty on circumstantial evidence of poisoning his wife in 1854, and his brother and his friend James Parsons Cook in 1855. He was believed to have murdered 13 persons in all.

PALPATION is the act of examining by touch.

PALPITATION is subjective awareness of the heartbeat, usually as an unpleasant thumping sensation in the chest or at the root of the neck. It occurs in normal subjects when the force of the beat is abruptly increased, as by emotion or on lying down in bed. *Extrasystoles often cause palpitation, as may other disturbances of cardiac rhythm.

PALSY. Paralysis.

PALUDRINE® is a proprietary name for *proguanil, a drug used in the prevention and treatment of *malaria.

PANCREAS. A large elongated glandular structure situated transversely at the back of the abdominal cavity, behind the stomach. Its function is primarily digestive; its secretion, pancreatic juice, contains several digestive *enzymes and passes into the *duodenum via the pancreatic duct. The pancreas also has an endocrine function, secreting *hormones directly into the bloodstream. These hormones are elaborated by cells scattered throughout the gland, in clusters called the '*islets of Langerhans', and are chiefly concerned with regulating *carbohydrate metabolism; they include *insulin, *glucagon, and *somatostatin.

PANCREATITIS is inflammation of the *pancreas.

PANDEMIC. An epidemic of intercontinental or worldwide proportions. See EPIDEMIOLOGY.

PANEL PRACTICE was a general medical practice which provided advice and treatment to insured wage-earners under the terms of the *National Health Insurance Act 1911, implemented in 1913.

PANNICULITIS is inflammation of the subcutaneous layer of fatty tissue.

PANNUS. A layer of *granulation tissue which develops over the *synovial membrane of joints in *rheumatoid arthritis and which contributes to their immobilization; also, a layer of granulation tissues infiltrating the *cornea in *trachoma and obscuring vision.

PANTOTHENIC ACID is a member of the water-soluble *vitamin B complex, an essential component of the human diet as part of the *coenzyme A molecule. It is, however, so widely available in food that spontaneous deficiency is unknown.

PAPANICOLAOU, GEORGE NICHOLAS (1883–1962). American pathologist. His best-known work was on the exfoliative *cytology of the *vagina and the uterine *cervix. He demonstrated changes in vaginal epithelium at different phases of the menstrual cycle, and developed a cytological test for malignant change in the uterine cervical epithelium. This test has been widely employed for early detection of malignant change, and is often referred to as the 'Pap smear' (see CERVICAL SMEAR).

PAPAVERINE is an *opium alkaloid, but with a pharmacological action quite different from that of *morphine; its major effect is to relax involuntary muscle, and it has been used mainly as an *antispasmodic in ischaemic conditions due to arterial spasm.

PAPILLA. Any small nipple-like protuberance.

PAPILLOEDEMA (PAPILLEDEMA) is oedematous swelling of the *optic disc, due to raised intracranial pressure compressing the *optic nerve; the cause is usually a space-occupying lesion such as a tumour inside the skull, but it may also result from malignant *hypertension or from *thrombosis of the central vein of the *retina.

PAPILLOMA. A small wart-like benign *tumour derived from *epithelium.

PAPOVAVIRUS. A group of small *deoxyribonucleic acid (DNA) *viruses, many of which have the capacity to cause *tumours in animals (e.g. *papilloma, *polyoma, *sarcoma, *warts).

PAPPENHEIM, ARTUR (1870–1916). German haematologist. A leading young haematologist, he founded the journal *Folia haematologica* (1904), and published a superlative *Atlas der menschlichen Blutzellen* (1905–12). He invented the specific stain for *plasma cells (Unna–Pappenheim stain). He died of *typhus contracted on active service.

PAPULE. A pimple; a small circumscribed lump on the skin.

PAPWORTH VILLAGE COLONY. A village settlement for patients with stable *tuberculosis founded in 1916 by Pendrill Charles Varrier-Jones and later moved to Papworth in Cambridgeshire. It comprised residential cottages, workshops, and a sanatorium and hospital; it enabled such patients to live a relatively normal working and family life while remaining under strict medical supervision. It may be regarded as the forerunner of the modern *rehabilitation centre. Papworth Hospital is now a major cardiothoracic centre where, for example, heart and lung *transplantation is performed.

PARA-AMINOSALICYLIC ACID (PAS) is an antibacterial agent formerly used in the treatment of *tuberculosis but now replaced in drug combination regimens by agents that are more effective, less toxic, and easier to take, such as *ethambutol.

PARACELSUS, THEOPHRASTUS PHILIPPUS AUREOLUS BOMBASTUS VON HOHENHEIM (1493–1541). Swiss physician. Paracelsus, always known by this assumed name, began practice in Strasbourg but in 1527 was appointed town physician and professor of medicine in Basle. He so outraged his colleagues by burning the works of *Galen and *Avicenna and by admitting *barber-surgeons to his lectures, which were delivered in the vernacular, that he was forced to flee in 1528. Thereafter he wandered through Central Europe as an itinerant practitioner. Paracelsus has been called the 'Luther of medicine'. Coarse-fibred but violently articulate, he defied the authority of Galen and Avicenna, condemning all medical teaching not based on experience. In so doing he opened the door to the renaissance of medical thought. An able doctor and a competent chemist, he introduced *laudanum, *sulphur, lead, and *mercury into Western therapeutics and popularized tinctures and salts. He associated *cretinism with endemic *goitre and distinguished mental defect from acquired mental illness.

PARACENTESIS is the release of fluid accumulated in a body cavity (e.g. *pleural, *peritoneal) by puncturing and draining through a needle or tube.

PARACETAMOL is one of the two most important non-narcotic *analgesic drugs in current use, the other being *aspirin. Paracetamol, also known under the trade name of Panadol® in the UK and as acetaminophen in the USA, is less irritant to the stomach than aspirin. Unlike aspirin, it has no significant anti-inflammatory action. Its chief disadvantage is the danger of overdosage, which can cause serious liver damage.

PARAESTHESIAE (PARESTHESIAE) are abnormal skin sensations variously described as tingling, prickling, burning, or 'like pins and needles'.

PARAGONIMIASIS is infestation with a hermaphroditic *fluke (trematode worm) of the genus *Paragonimus* (e.g. *P. westermani, P. uterobilateralis*), which inhabits the lungs and occasionally other tissues of various mammals, including man. Lung flukes have a remarkable life cycle, requiring two intermediate hosts, the first being (as with other trematodes like *bilharzia) an appropriate freshwater snail, the second a freshwater crustacean (crayfish or crab). Human infestation is acquired by eating inadequately cooked crabs or crayfish, and must be differentiated from other chronic lung diseases, particularly *tuberculosis.

PARA-INFLUENZA VIRUS is one of a group of viruses, in which four distinct types have been recognized, belonging to the family of *paramyxoviruses. Para-influenza virus is a common cause of respiratory infections, ranging from the common *cold to *pneumonia; type 2 is particularly associated with *croup in children.

PARALDEHYDE is a rapidly acting and powerful *sedative drug, which occurs as a liquid with an unpleasant smell and taste. It is for this reason administered rectally or by parenteral injection. It is particularly useful for controlling acute mental disturbance, and is relatively safe.

PARALYSIS is loss of function in a muscle or group of muscles.

PARALYSIS AGITANS is idiopathic or primary *parkinsonism, also known as Parkinson's desease. It is one of the commonest neurological conditions, particularly in the elderly, among whom its prevalence is about 0.5 per cent. The aetiology is unknown.

PARALYTIC SHELLFISH POISONING. See RED TIDE.

PARAMEDICAL describes non-medical personnel engaged in ancillary or supportive tasks. So-called 'paramedics', who usually have basic nursing qualifications, nowadays undergo further training in *resuscitation and other techniques of emergency care.

PARAMYOCLONUS MULTIPLEX is a form of progressive *myoclonus in which repetitive sudden involuntary contractions of muscle groups occur first in the shoulder girdle and later involve the muscles of the trunk, limbs, face, and neck. It is now more often called hereditary essential myoclonus.

PARAMYXOVIRUS. A group of single-stranded *ribonucleic acid (RNA) viruses which includes the *para-influenza, *mumps, *measles, canine distemper, and *rinderpest viruses.

PARANASAL SINUSES are the cavities, lined with mucous membrane and containing air, which communicate with the nasal cavity; they are the ethmoidal, maxillary, frontal, and sphenoidal sinuses.

PARANOIA in its pure form is a rare variety of *schizophrenia, commonest in men over the age of 30. The patient builds up an increasingly elaborate delusional system, which may have its origin in some genuine grievance but which is beyond all bounds of reality. The delusions of persecution (and of grandeur, often also present) may, however, long remain concealed from others if not openly expressed, since the patient may appear mentally normal in all other respects; even to the extent that homicidal attempts may be the first manifestation. Certain political assassinations have been explained on this basis. Paranoid reactions also occur in *depression, *alcoholism, and *senile dementia.

PARAPARESIS is partial *paralysis of the lower half of the body.

PARAPHIMOSIS. Strangulation of the glans of the *penis by a retracted tight foreskin (*prepuce).

PARAPHRENIA is a form of *schizophrenia occurring in later adult life and more commonly in women, characterized by wildly improbable delusions of persecution (see PARANOIA).

PARAPLEGIA is *paralysis of the lower half of the body.

PARAPSYCHOLOGY is the study of *extrasensory perception and allied phenomena (clairvoyance, telepathy, etc.) which appear to transcend natural laws.

PARAQUAT is a highly toxic bipyridyl contact herbicide used in various proprietary weedkiller preparations (e.g. Gramaxone®, Weedol®). It is very irritant externally and can cause corneal damage if it gets into the eye; ingested, even a small amount is lethal. Liver, kidney, and lung are all severely affected; the liver and kidney may recover, but the damage to the lung is irreversible. The lesson that stands out from a review of paraquat deaths in the UK is that paraquat solutions should never be decanted into soft-drink bottles.

PARASITE. An organism living in or on another and obtaining food from it; a parasite may or may not harm its host, but confers no benefit upon it. Parasites of man include bacteria, viruses, fungi, protozoa, and metazoa (multicellular organisms), notably worms.

PARASYMPATHETIC NERVOUS SYSTEM. Part of the *autonomic nervous system, which regulates the involuntary activity of glands, smooth muscle, and cardiac muscle. The parasympathetic system derives from the cranial and sacral parts of the neuraxis (cf. the *sympathetic system which is associated with the thoracic and lumbar segments). The nerves involved are the third, seventh, ninth, and tenth *cranial nerves (the oculomotor, facial, glossopharyngeal, and vagus nerves, respectively) and the second, third, and fourth sacral nerves. The effects produced by stimulation of parasympathetic fibres include: visual accommodation by constricting the pupil and focusing the lens; salivary secretion; slowing the heart and decreasing its force of contraction; decreasing pulmonary ventilation; increasing digestive activity; emptying the bladder and rectum; and penile erection.

PARATYPHOID FEVERS are a group of enteric fevers allied to *typhoid fever but generally milder. They are due to infection with species of *Salmonella* other than *Salmonella typhi*.

PARATHYROIDS. The *endocrine organs controlling *calcium homeostasis. The parathyroid glands are small yellowish bodies attached to the posterior surface of the *thyroid gland; there are usually four in all, arranged in two pairs, but the number is variable. The glands secrete the hormone parathormone. Its essential function is to counteract any tendency of the blood calcium to fall. It thus promotes the release of calcium from bone, enhances absorption of calcium from the gastrointestinal tract, promotes renal tubular reabsorption of calcium, and increases renal phosphate and bicarbonate excretion.

PARAVACCINIA VIRUSES are the putative agents, non-bacterial and non-vaccinial, of rashes occasionally associated with *vaccination.

PARE, AMBROISE (?1510–90). French surgeon. He acquired a reputation for skill, judgement, and probity in both the court and the army. Probably the greatest surgeon of the 16th century, Paré revolutionized the treatment of wounds, abandoning the use of the cautery for simple dressings. He recommended ligature of the vessels, devised many types of *prosthesis, and advocated *massage. Also see SURGERY

PAREGORIC is a camphorated tincture of *opium, an old remedy for diarrhoea (consisting of powdered opium, anise oil, benzoic acid, camphor, ethanol, and glycerin).

PARENCHYMA is the distinctive tissue characteristic of an organ and responsible for its functioning.

PARESIS. Partial *paralysis.

PARINAUD, HENRI (1844–1905). French ophthalmologist. He described *conjunctivitis due to contact with animals and an *ophthalmoplegia due to paralysis of the external rectus muscle of one eye with spasm of the internal rectus of the other.

PARITY is the condition of having borne children (e.g. nulliparous, multiparous, etc.).

PARK, MUNGO (1771–1806). British physician and explorer. His first exploration of the Niger was from 1794 to 1797, when he returned to England and gained some renown by his book *Travels in the interior districts of Africa* (1799). In 1801 he set up in practice in Peebles, but in 1805 accepted an invitation to organize another expedition to find the source of the Niger. He was killed with all his companions by natives at Boussa.

PARK, WILLIAM HALLOCK (1863–1939). American bacteriologist and public health authority. He was an early worker in the manufacture and use of *diphtheria *antitoxin, and an influential authority in determining policy aimed at control of *tuberculosis, diphtheria, and *poliomyelitis.

PARKINSON, JAMES (?1775–1824). British physician and palaeontologist. Parkinson practised in Hoxton, where he recorded the first recognized case of fatal perforative *appendicitis in 1812, and published in 1817 *An essay on the shaking palsy* (*Parkinson's disease). He was an original observer with radical political views. He collected fossils and wrote a three-volume work *Organic remains of a former world* (1804–11).

PARKINSON, JOHN (1885–1976). English physician. He was a founder of *cardiology in the UK, being physician to the cardiac department at the London Hospital and president of the Cardiac Society.

PARKINSONISM is a characteristic constellation of neurological signs due to disease or degeneration of the *basal ganglia of the brain (often referred to as the 'extrapyramidal' motor system), particularly of that part known as the substantia nigra. The condition is associated with a reduction in the *dopamine content of nigral *neurones and is often alleviated by the administration of the dopamine precursor *levodopa or by one of its analogues. The four major features of the syndrome are: muscular rigidity, bradykinesia (paucity and slowness of voluntary movement), a slow tremor at rest (especially of the arms and hands), and postural deformities. The patient's appearance, with a mask-like face, a short shuffling gait, and a 'pill-rolling' tremor of the hands, is familiar and unmistakable. *Transplantation into the brain of fetal brain tissue is being explored experimentally.

Parkinsonism may be divided into three main groups: the first is idiopathic or primary parkinsonism, also known as Parkinson's disease or *paralysis agitans; in the second group, parkinsonism is the result of a known aetiological agent, such as *encephalitis lethargica (pandemics of which occurred between 1919 and 1926), or intoxication with *manganese, or certain drugs (particularly neuroleptic agents such as *phenothiazines); and the third group comprises a few more widespread degenerations of the central nervous system (including cerebral vascular disease) in which parkinsonism is only one part of the clinical picture, along with, for example, *dementia, cerebellar *ataxia, *opthalmoplegia, etc.

PARKINSONISM–DEMENTIA COMPLEX is a syndrome characterized by three main features: memory impairment, progressing to severe *dementia; urinary *incontinence; and gait abnormalities resembling those of *parkinsonism. Radiologically there is evidence of dilatation of the cerebral ventricles; the condition may result from occult (or normal pressure) *hydrocephalus, and can be ascribed to *cerebrospinal fluid outflow obstruction. The association of dementia with features resembling those of parkinsonism also occurs in patients with widespread degenerative central nervous system changes due, for example, to arteriopathy. A variety of progressive parkinsonism with dementia believed to be due to to an unidentified environmental agent occurs in the Chamorro people of the Pacific Mariana islands.

PARKINSON'S DISEASE is idiopathic or primary *parkinsonism.

PARONYCHIA is pyogenic infection of the nail folds.

PAROSMIA is any disturbance of the sense of smell.

PAROTID. The largest of the three pairs of *salivary glands, situated below and in front of the ears.

PAROTITIS is inflammation of one or both *parotid glands, the commonest cause of which is infection with the *mumps virus.

PAROXYSM. A temporary but violent attack, for example of coughing.

PAROXYSMAL HAEMOGLOBINURIA (HEMO-GLOBINURIA) is the excretion of free *haemoglobin in the urine following episodes of intravascular *haemolysis; haemoglobin is released into the plasma and passes into the glomerular filtrate. In the condition known as paroxysmal nocturnal haemoglobinuria (the Marchiafava–Micheli syndrome), red blood cell destruction occurs usually, though not invariably, at night and is due to the action of activated *complement on an abnormal population of red cells. The cause of this condition is unknown, but evidence of general bone marrow depression is often present. *Phlebothrombosis, especially involving hepatic and mesenteric veins, is a common complication. Among several other varieties of paroxysmal haemoglobinuria are those precipitated by exposure to cold (due to a complement-fixing antibody often associated with a viral or syphilitic infection) and by prolonged or vigorous exercise ('march' haemoglobinuria, due to mechanical damage to red cells).

PAROXYSMAL NOCTURNAL DYSPNOEA (DYS-PNEA) is paroxysmal breathing difficulty due to episodic failure of the left ventricle with consequent pulmonary congestion and oedema, formerly known as *cardiac asthma. The nocturnal incidence of the symptom, related to *orthopnoea, occurs when the patient, having gone to sleep propped up on pillows, slips down into full recumbency during the night. He awakes gasping for breath and usually seeks relief by sitting on the side of the bed; so intense may be the feeling of suffocation that he rushes to open a window and leans out to breathe. The symptom is characteristic of conditions which put a burden on the left ventricle, such as arterial *hypertension and aortic *valve disease.

PARR, THOMAS (?1483–1635). Born at Winnington, Shropshire, he acquired fame as 'Old Parr' and claimed to have 'done penance in a white sheet' for begetting a bastard when he was aged 105. He was taken to London by the Earl of Arundel and presented to the King. He died of the unaccustomed rich diet. William *Harvey carried out a post-mortem examination.

PARRY, CALEB HILLIER (1755–1822). British physician. He was the first to describe *exophthalmic goitre (1786), *facial hemiatrophy (1814), and *megacolon (1825, posthumously).

PARTHENOGENESIS is the development of an unfertilized *ovum into an individual (*parthenos* = virgin). Parthenogenesis occurs normally in some plants and animals, in which conventional sexual reproduction (providing the genetic recombination desirable for evolution) takes place at other times. The phenomenon may be induced artificially in ova which are not normally parthenogenetic, including those of some mammals, by various techniques (cooling, pricking, acid treatment, etc.).

PARTNERSHIPS are a long-established feature of *general medical practice in many countries. They have increased greatly in number in the UK since the inception of the *National Health Service. More than 80 per cent of family doctors now work in partnerships.

PARTURITION is childbirth. See LABOUR.

PARVOVIRUS. A group of very small single-stranded *deoxyribonucleic acid (DNA) *viruses widely distributed in vertebrates.

PAS is an acronym representing both *para-aminosalicylic acid and *periodic acid–Schiff.

PASSAGE (usually with French pronunciation) means the process of passing micro-organisms through a number of successive hosts or cultures, either in order to maintain them or with the objective of modifying their virulence.

PASTE. A semiliquid medicinal preparation intended for external application. Pastes usually contain finely powdered solids such as zinc oxide and starch and are fairly stiff; they are useful for circumscribed lesions such as those which may occur in *psoriasis and chronic *eczema.

PASTEUR, LOUIS (1822–95). French chemist and microbiologist. In 1857 he was made director of scientific studies at the Ecole Normale. He showed that fermentation in wine, beer, and milk was due to micro-organisms (see MICROBIOLOGY) which were not spontaneously generated but normally abounded in the atmosphere (1864). This work inspired *Lister to introduce *antiseptic methods in surgery in 1865. Pasteur was called by the government to investigate the disease of silk worms which was bringing ruin to the French silk industry. By 1868 he showed that there were two distinct microbial diseases, and also how the diseased stock could be detected early and the infection prevented. By this time he had become professor of chemistry at the Sorbonne. In 1865 he sustained a stroke resulting in a left hemiparesis but recovered sufficiently to return to work. His interest in pathology grew and in 1877 he identified the causes of *anthrax and fowl cholera and developed protective *vaccination against them. His celebrated studies in *rabies began in 1882 when he showed that the *virus was present in the nervous tissue of affected animals and that it became attenuated when such tissue was exposed to heat. Injections of the heated material would then protect animals against infection. On 6 July 1885 he successfully applied this preventive method to a 9-year-old boy, Joseph Meister, the first patient to receive it.

PASTEURELLA. A genus of micro-organisms causing disease in domestic animals including birds (canaries, fowl, ducklings, and geese). The causative agent of *plague, *Yersinia pestis*, was formerly known as *Pasteurella pestis*.

PASTEUR INSTITUTE, THE, in Paris, was founded in the lifetime of Louis *Pasteur, and he was its first director. Pasteur attracted many top-class scientists and set up five departments: for microbe research in general; applied to hygiene; for microbial morphology; for microbe technology; and for rabies. Among the first five researchers were *Roux and *Metchnikoff. Other now world-famous names from the Institute were *Yersin, *Bordet, Nicolle, d'Hérelle, *Calmette, *Guérin, *Laveran, Bovet, Jacob, Lwoff, and Monod, eight of whom won *Nobel prizes in physiology or medicine.

Now the Institute is a private state-approved foundation. There are eight departments: bacteriology and mycology; ecology; virology; immunology; molecular biochemistry and genetics; molecular biology; experimental physiopathology; and a clinical department. The hospital facilities were started in 1900. The Institute was instrumental in assisting the Institut du Radium to apply Marie *Curie's discoveries to medicine. There are also Pasteur Institutes in Lille and Lyon, and elsewhere in the world, which, although independent, have associations with the Paris institute. Several are in developing parts of the world, involved especially in public hygiene, sanitation, and control of infection. See also RESEARCH INSTITUTES.

PASTEURIZATION is partial sterilization by heating, particularly of milk, to a temperature and for a period of time which is sufficient to destroy most pathogenic *bacteria (although not their spores). Thirty minutes at 60 °C is usual; 15 seconds at 72 °C is also employed.

PATELLA. The knee cap, the sesamoid bone embedded in the common tendon of the extensor thigh muscles (quadriceps femoris).

PATHOGEN. Any agent of disease, but particularly a disease-producing micro-organism.

PATHOGENESIS. The mode of production or development of a disease; the developing pathological process.

PATHOGNOMY is knowledge of the clinical manifestations of diseases.

PATHOLOGICAL ANATOMY is a synonym for *morbid anatomy.

PATHOLOGIST. A specialist in *pathology.

PATHOLOGY is the study of disease processes and how they affect the cells, tissues, and organs of living things. Diseased cells, tissues, and organs are studied for many reasons, but the principal motive is to discover in what ways they have become abnormal and whether they could be returned to normal, and/or whether the abnormality could have been prevented.

In modern medicine in the UK, pathology has become divided into five fields: chemical pathology (clinical *chemistry), *haematology, *immunology, medical *microbiology, and histopathology, although in many countries 'pathology' is used to mean solely histopathology. Sometimes this area of pathology is qualified as anatomical pathology or tissue pathology, particularly in the USA. Anatomical pathology is one of 26 medical monospecialties recognized by the European Union; the other pathology specialties come under bio-pathologie médicale. Anatomical pathology is practised almost exclusively by medically qualified pathologists (see below).

Morbid anatomy
Used in the sense of anatomical pathology, pathology encompasses the study and dissection of diseased organs

and tissues at the level of the naked eye (macroscopic). This sort of study has fascinated scholars from *Celsus in ancient times, through Michelangelo and *Morgagni (1682–1771), who was the first to correlate symptoms in life with anatomical changes, to the present. It has long been referred to as 'morbid anatomy', that is, *anatomy that has become deranged, distorted, or disturbed over time by one or more of the seven disease categories (see below). Matthew *Baillie published the first comprehensive book on morbid anatomy in 1793 and the first professor of 'pathological anatomy' (Lobstein) was appointed in Strasbourg in 1819, to be followed by Carswell at University College, London in 1829 and Herbert Mayo at King's College in 1830. Today most morbid anatomy departments have changed their names because 'morbid' is regarded as a distressing word, too much associated with death and dissection.

Morbid anatomy is particularly the province of the post-mortem room. The post-mortem examination (synonyms: autopsy, first used 1678; post-mortem (1850); necropsy (1856)) is an important method of establishing what disease processes were present at the time of death, from which, together with microscopical examination of selected tissues and organs (see below) and any other information or evidence that may be collected, the 'cause of death' may be deduced. As we do not know what constitutes 'life' or 'death', what actually causes death in its final moment cannot be known, although cessation of cerebral function, the circulation, and breathing are obviously part of it. Death is thus a cessation of function, while the post-mortem examination deals with structural changes in the organs and tissues, from which the functional changes must be assumed. As every pathologist who conducts post-mortems knows, there are sometimes too many structural changes and sometimes too few to provide a coherent explanation as to why death occurred. In these cases the cause of death must take on the nature of a 'best guess'. Unfortunately, this undermines the general belief, so assiduously cultivated by popular fiction and television characters, that all human mysteries can be unravelled by post-mortem examination.

Since post-mortem examinations began to be performed routinely in some countries, particularly Germany and Austria, at the beginning of the 19th century. (*Rokitansky is said to have performed 30 000 himself in Vienna), correlation of the pathological findings with the clinical signs, symptoms, and test results has contributed a great deal to medical knowledge of individual diseases. From that start, however, the 'post-mortem rate', that is the number of post-mortems as a proportion of deaths, rose to a peak after the Second World War but then declined; now it may be as low as 5 per cent in many hospitals in the Western world. This decline occurred partly because physicians and surgeons believed that the greatly improved methods of investigating patients in life left little that was not known to be discovered after death. That this may not be true emerges from reports from various countries that up to 25 per cent of post-mortems reveal, on the one hand, serious, sometimes treatable, disease that was not suspected in life and, on the other, that confident diagnoses made in life may be wrong.

The UK *National Health Service (NHS) reforms of the late 1980s accepted post-mortem examinations as a form of audit of clinical practice, and it is likely that a certain number of post-mortems will always be required for audit purposes. Post-mortems have always provided the most reliable information on causes of death for the *Office of Population, Censuses and Surveys (OPCS) for England and Wales, which otherwise relies on what is entered on the death certificate. The deaths-by-cause data, published annually by Her Majesty's Stationery Office (HMSO), are very valuable for the epidemiological study of disease and its trends. In recent times confidential enquiries, first into maternal deaths, more recently into perioperative deaths and perinatal deaths, which have greatly contributed to our understanding and prevention of such deaths, have relied heavily on post-mortems not being missed. Such targeting of post-mortems is likely to be more fruitful than the performance of post-mortems on an arbitrary percentage of cases. Furthermore, the individual post-mortem examination is most successful when the clinicians target it at specific questions unanswered in life—serendipitous findings may be illuminating and good for teaching but usually come into the 'so what' category.

In England and Wales, moreover, the fall in post-mortem rates has been smaller than that experienced elsewhere, because the rules of death certification and their interpretation by the local Registrars of Births, Marriages and Deaths require that many hospital cases are reported to the *coroner, who usually orders a post-mortem examination. In 1993, for example, at King's College Hospital in London, the post-mortem rate was 50 per cent (of 1495 cases), of which 33 per cent were coroner's cases and 14 per cent fetal or perinatal cases, but only 7 per cent non-coroner's, adult cases. For non-coroner's cases, the next of kin or a reliable relative must give consent; failure to ask for consent, and refusals, often on religious grounds, are among factors that determine the post-mortem rate.

The deaths considered above are generally due to natural causes, although the picking up of deaths from unnatural causes is part of the function of such post-mortems. Deaths from unnatural causes, including homicide, *poisoning, road accidents, and so on, come into the realm of *forensic pathology (which is part of forensic science) and are also the province of the coroner. He generally employs pathologists who are trained in forensic work, who may be retained by the Home Office, and who are experienced in giving evidence at inquests and in the criminal courts, to perform these post-mortems, usually in close collaboration with the police. In Scotland the Procurator-Fiscal fulfils the role of the coroner, but orders post-mortems on cases of natural death less often.

The coroner system has been widely adopted and adapted throughout the world, particularly where there has been British administration. An alternative system, that of the medical examiner, is seen in some of the states of the USA. In this system, cases are handed to the medical examiner's department which also investigates them and presents the results in court.

Histopathology

Histopathology, the term that is often used to replace morbid anatomy but actually complements it, is the study of diseased cells, tissues, and organs at greater magnification than can be managed by the naked eye, that is, microscopically. Its normal counterpart is *histology, which has the same relationship to histopathology as anatomy to morbid anatomy (see above). Compound microscopy was known from the end of the 15th century. Van *Leeuwenhoek made the first of his *microscopes in 1673, and described red cells (7 micrometres (μm) diameter) in 1674, thus leading eventually to the cellular theory of plant and animal tissues as propounded by *Schwann in 1837 and carried forward in its application to diseased tissues in men by great men such as *Virchow (1858). Microscopists have extended their range from light microscopy (resolution down to 0.5 μm) into electron microscopy, to 'see' on a cathode-ray tube intracellular details down to the level of large molecules (resolution down to 2 nanometres (nm)). An advance of the 1980s was the introduction of the confocal laser scanning microscope, with which thick sections of tissue rendered fluorescent in various ways can be 'optically sectioned', that is, thin sections of tissue within the section can be scanned and visualized electronically. The images of such optical sections can be stored in a computer and superimposed to produce three-dimensional images of the cells and tissues under study.

Although fresh and even living cells and tissues can be observed microscopically, they are virtually translucent and devoid of detail. It is usually more convenient to 'fix' them in a preservative such as 10 per cent formaldehyde solution, cut them into thin slices or sections (usually 5–10 μm thick for light microscopy or 0.1 μm for electron microscopy), stain them to pick out the components of interest, and mount them on glass slides with a glass coverslip to maximize their optical properties. For electron microscopy the sections are mounted on copper grids. From *Virchow's time until recently staining was largely empirical, often with aniline dyes, but first *histochemical and enzyme histochemical techniques and then *monoclonal antibodies capable of labelling specific *antigens (immunohistochemistry) became available for identifying cellular and tissue components. In the 1980s the development of *molecular biology produced the technique of *in-situ* hybridization to identify specific lengths of *DNA and *RNA.

Categories of pathological change

All anatomical pathology is included within seven disease categories: (1) exogenous, (2) congenital, (3) inflammatory, (4) circulatory, (5) metabolic, (6) degenerative, and (7) neoplasia. These categories are not mutually exclusive; for example, the pathology of *cirrhosis of the liver includes aspects of all seven categories. Nevertheless, to be able to categorize a disease pathologically greatly enhances one's ability to think constructively about it and to devise ways of studying, diagnosing, treating, or preventing it.

Exogenous (including iatrogenic) disorders

Pathological effects are frequently the result of injurious influences from outside the body. Physical agents include heat, cold, accidental, deliberate, or occupational injuries from blunt or sharp objects, and various forms of *radiation, such as sunlight and ionizing radiation. Chemical agents include all forms of chemical substances, including poisons and substances that are abused, such as *alcohol and the constituents of glue, or inhaled or ingested at work, such as asbestos fibres or coal dust. *Micro-organisms, including bacteria, viruses, protozoa, and fungi, and the *toxins they produce are important exogenous causes of disease. Finally, an important and easily forgotten type of exogenous damage is that caused to patients by health professionals during surgery or other treatments, or by the prescription of drugs and medicines, either through wrong dosage or as side-effects or adverse reactions to the correct dosage—this form of disease is termed iatrogenic. *Iatrogenic disease may therefore be of physical, chemical, or microbiological origin.

Congenital disease

Congenital disease includes inherited disease, determined by the *genome inherited from the parents, such as *haemophilia; developmental abnormalities and syndromes, such as *congenital heart disease; and sundry abnormalities acquired before birth, such as heart failure due to *rhesus incompatibility, or during birth, such as brain damage due to lack of oxygen. The pathologist must remember that developmental abnormalities are often multiple, and should follow clues such as the presence of an extra digit.

Inflammatory conditions

*Inflammation is the reaction of tissues and organs to various agents, including infecting organisms such as *bacteria, *viruses, *protozoa, and *fungi, and injuries such as wounds or fractures. It may be acute, as in *abscesses or *pneumonia, or chronic and scar forming, as in *tuberculosis or chronic ulceration. Some of the body's reactions to injury are mediated by immune processes designed as defence mechanisms; these may, however, themselves become disturbed and cause inflammation, especially if the immune process wrongly comes to regard body components themselves as inimical. *Rheumatoid arthritis is believed to be an example of such an '*autoimmune' disease.

Circulatory disorders
Diseases of the circulation include bleeding (*haemorrhage), which may result from injury or have a hereditary origin as in haemophilia, and inappropriate clotting (*thrombosis). A thrombus may obstruct the blood supply to an organ, as when it occurs in one of the coronary arteries that supply the heart muscle, with severe or fatal consequences. Alternatively a thrombus, particularly in a leg vein, may break off into the blood stream and circulate until it is caught in a branching or narrowing blood vessel and, again, the blood supply is blocked; circulating material is called an *embolus, which may consist of thrombus or other substances. Pulmonary embolism, i.e. thrombus blocking the main artery to the lungs, is a feared and potentially fatal complication after surgical operations and injuries. After much study by clinicians and pathologists, deep leg-vein thrombosis and consequent pulmonary embolism have been greatly reduced by using rhythmically inflated boots during surgery, and making patients move their legs and walk much earlier than used to be the practice.

Metabolic conditions
Abnormal *metabolism or handling of nutrients and chemical substances by the body, such as *diabetes or *gout, generally have a genetic basis but may be initiated by additional factors, such as viral infections. Some, such as *phenylketonuria, should be screened for in early life. Others, such as *uraemia, are the result of damage to specific organs, in this case the kidneys, but can affect a wide range of organs and tissues.

Degenerative conditions
Degenerative pathology is the result of wear and tear, and therefore occurs in older people. For example, the *cartilage that covers the bone ends in joints is prone to wear out, especially in people who have used their joints a great deal in sports or through being overweight. This leads to *osteoarthritis, which is not the same as *rheumatoid arthritis, an inflammatory autoimmune disease of the joints (see above).

Neoplasia
The mechanisms that control cell division are complicated and are still being worked out (see also ONCOLOGY). It is obvious that very fine control is needed to build a human being from a fertilized egg, and that many things could go wrong. Similarly, after development is complete, cells in the various organs and tissues are constantly dividing to replace worn out and dying cells, particularly in the blood, skin, and intestinal tract. Cells that are lost through injury or disease are replaced by cell division, which then stops. Sometimes cell division occurs inappropriately, so that too many cells are produced; this is called *hyperplasia. Sometimes the cell

division gets completely out of hand and does not stop; this is called neoplasia (new growth). The usual lay term for a *neoplasm is a *tumour, although 'tumour' is also used less precisely to mean a swelling of any sort. If the neoplastic cells infiltrate the surrounding tissues and/or are carried to other parts of the body through the lymphatic, venous, or arterial vessels and continue dividing there (a *metastasis, metastases), this is malignant neoplasia or *cancer. If they merely divide locally without spreading into neighbouring tissues or further afield, this is benign neoplasia. Benign neoplasms may have deleterious and even fatal effects, but technically they are not cancers. It is believed that neoplasia arises as a result of a change, or series of changes, in the *genome of a single cell, the progeny of which then behave in a neoplastic way, which is generally irreversible. Neoplasms, including malignant neoplasms, can be produced experimentally in animals and in cell culture by physical means, ionizing radiations, chemicals, dietary substances, drugs, and viruses, thus tending to confirm with varying degrees of conviction that similar associations in man are causal.

Neoplasms, particularly malignant neoplasms, have many effects on the body, only some of which are understood. Much depends on the doubling time of the tumour cells. As a rule of thumb, death can be expected when the tumour burden (original, primary, tumour plus metastases) reaches 10 kg, but it is often not clear, clinically or at post-mortem, exactly why the patient died when he or she did and not earlier or later.

A vast amount of clinical, experimental, and epidemiological research is devoted to the study of cancer, in order to find ways of preventing, curing, and alleviating or palliating the suffering it causes. For the individual patient and for this research effort it is a *sine qua non* that cells and tissues are examined microscopically to be sure that it really is cancer that is being dealt with and not one of the other forms of tissue pathology described in this section. This form of diagnosis, together with the identification of other features indicating the prognosis of the neoplasm, i.e. how one may expect it to behave, calls for the particular skills and experience of the surgical pathologist, i.e. the anatomical pathologist in his role of examiner of tissues or cells (see below) obtained by the surgeon or other clinician in life for diagnostic purposes. Such a piece of tissue taken for diagnosis is called a *biopsy.

Aetiology and pathogenesis
Pathologists are particularly called upon to explain the causation of diseases. *Aetiology is the term, first used in 1684, to describe the branch of medical science which investigates the causes and origins of diseases. Pathogenesis is the term, first used in 1876, to describe the progression or development of pathological changes once something has gone wrong with the normal structure or function of the cells. It is, therefore, one thing

to try to elucidate the cause of a disease, but quite another to study its progression or natural history, and how the latter may be altered by different factors, including treatment. The useful terms aetiology and pathogenesis should not, therefore, be used loosely or interchangeably.

Relative frequency of pathological categories

In the OPCS's annual report for 1992, there were 558 313 deaths in England and Wales, 16 681 from exogenous causes (injury and poisoning), 1565 from congenital anomalies, 254 683 from circulatory disease, 10 605 from metabolic diseases, and 145 963 from neoplasms. The numbers of deaths from inflammatory diseases and degenerative diseases are not given separately. The death statistics are also broken down further to show the relative frequency in men and women, in age by decade, and in geographical location. Other relevant information, which would be useful but which is not available, is the relative frequency in ethnic groups, and breakdowns by dietary, alcohol, and smoking habits, and by occupation.

Specialization

Until the 1930s many physicians and surgeons not only carried out post-mortems but also many of the simple pathological tests that were then available. General or all-purpose pathologists had, however, been gradually emerging during the early 20th century, alongside pathologists specializing in microbiology and anatomical pathology, particularly in the universities, medical schools, and teaching hospitals. Since 1948 the activities of the anatomical pathologists have traditionally included casework with living and dead patients, usually together with teaching and research, in collaboration with virtually every other medical specialist and general practitioner, since anatomical pathology underlies all their work.

With the enormous expansion of pathological knowledge in this period, however, anatomical pathologists have begun to form subspecialties, that is, after a general postgraduate anatomical pathology training, to concentrate on one specific part of anatomical pathology. Forensic pathology was the first subspecialty, with pathologists such as Sydney Smith and *Spilsbury becoming famous between the wars. Cytopathology is emerging as a separate subspecialty and merits further consideration below. Perinatal and paediatric pathology have become acceptable subspecialties. Otherwise, apart from *neuropathology, which is concerned with the central nervous system, peripheral nerves, and voluntary muscles, and which is well entrenched, only a few enthusiasts have been able to establish a career in the pathology of a single organ or system, usually in specialist hospitals. However, it seems likely, particularly with the present trends in the development of training and examination or accreditation systems in this country and Europe, that anatomical pathologists devoted solely to diagnosis, teaching, and research in skin pathology, gynaecological pathology, bone and joint pathology, gastrointestinal pathology, ophthalmological pathology, cardiovascular pathology, lung pathology, liver pathology, kidney pathology, or, cutting across these lines, tumour pathology and paediatric pathology, will be needed to provide a service of sufficient quality.

Cytopathology

In histopathology the diagnosis calls for the study of both the cells and the extracellular structures in the tissues and their relationships to each other. Cytopathology, on the other hand, is a branch of histopathology that deals with cells obtained in such a way that their normal histological or histopathological relationships are lost. Cytopathological preparations obtained by scraping the cells off the surface of the uterine cervix (neck of the womb) with a spatula, so-called cervical smears, are the best known. Papanicolaou popularized this technique in 1928, and the stain named after him is still widely used. But cells may be obtained if necessary from almost any surface by scraping, brushing, or irrigating, from inside organs and tissues by sucking with a syringe and needle (fine-needle aspiration cytology), and from urine or body fluids, such as *cerebrospinal fluid (by lumbar puncture), followed by centrifugation. However obtained, the cells are smeared on to slides, stained, covered with a coverslip, and studied microscopically.

Cytopathology is used particularly for the initial diagnosis of cancer. The recognition of cells, sometimes just a few cells among many non-malignant cells, as being malignant is, however, subjective and not easy. Most clinicians therefore think it wise, before the patient undergoes irreversible surgery or potentially harmful radiotherapy or chemotherapy, to confirm the diagnosis by taking a piece of tissue by biopsy (see above) for histopathological examination as well.

Cervical screening

In the initial stages of cancer of the cervix the malignant cells are confined to a small area of the surface. At this stage the cancer can be completely eliminated and therefore cured. The authorities in British Columbia were the first to try to perform cervical cytology on all the women in their population at regular intervals and to see if the incidence and mortality of cancer of the cervix fell. By 1964 the incidence had fallen, but to prove a reduction in mortality has always, for various reasons, presented more of a statistical challenge. Cervical cytology screening programmes were subsequently introduced into the UK. In England and Wales, however, the annual mortality from cancer of the cervix has fluctuated around 1900 for the past decade. There has been much argument about the screening programmes, but under the new general practitioner contract bonus payments are made to those screening 50 or 70 per cent (a higher payment) of the women on their patient lists. The work is labour-intensive and subjective, and a proportion of false positive and false negative results is inevitable in spite of quality control and quality assurance procedures. Many women, often those most at risk, are not reached by the screening programmes. From the cytopathologist's point of view, it would be a great advance if the abnormal cells, which are found in only about 7 cases per 1000, could be separated for separate study, or if the slides could be scanned mechanically or by computer. There has been much research on these lines but a sufficiently reliable solution has not yet been found.

Breast screening

Deaths from cancer of the female breast in England and Wales have gradually risen from 12 513 in 1981 to 13 663 in 1992. Many of these cancers can be recognized in X-ray pictures (*mammography) before they can be felt, and, after confirmation of the diagnosis by fine-needle aspiration cytology and/or biopsy, excised. Following the Forrest report in 1988, a national breast screening programme offering mammography to women aged 50–64 was set up in the UK. The effect of this programme on the mortality from this disease in the UK has yet to be seen, although in other countries, particularly Sweden, the mortality has been lowered.

The path to a career in pathology

During their training, medical, dental, and veterinary students attend classes in anatomy, histology, and pathology, in which they have to show competence. After reaching the medical, dental, or veterinary register in Britain, they may choose to specialize in pathology. This is achieved by obtaining a junior post in open competition in a district general or teaching hospital, and then working towards the two-part examinations in pathology organized by the *Royal College of Pathologists, which may be completed after 5 years' approved time in the specialty; the College may also approve time spent in pathology laboratories in other countries. The first part of the examination, which includes all aspects of histopathology, including cytopathology, may be taken after 3 years. After 2 more years the second part may be taken in one of the subspecialties mentioned above, or by the production of a research degree (MD or Ph.D.) relevant to pathology. The diploma of membership of the Royal College of Pathologists (MRCPath) is then awarded, with automatic elevation to the fellowship (FRCPath) after 12 years. In practice, the holder of the MRCPath diploma is an acceptable candidate for a career (consultant) post in district general or teaching hospitals. Under the directives of the European Union, training in any member state is mutually recognized and the pathologist is entitled to practise in any member state after 4 years of approved training.

The *Royal College of Pathologists

The Royal College of Pathologists was founded in 1962 to be responsible for the standards of practice of all the pathology specialties (see above), to monitor postgraduate training programmes, to set the examinations for specialist recognition, and to advise the authorities about matters of concern to pathology and its practice. The College is particularly involved at present, together with many other organizations, with the inspection of pathology laboratories throughout the country, to ensure that minimum standards are met, and, for the same purpose, with the question of continuing medical education.

Conclusion

The medical specialty of anatomical pathology complements anatomy and histology and, encompassing morbid anatomy and histopathology, including cytopathology, underlies the whole practice of medicine. In most countries its training and practice are regulated by the government; in Britain by the Royal College of Pathologists. Its practitioners are to be found in every general hospital, teaching hospital, and medical school world-wide. In addition to their day-to-day casework, pathologists are usually enthusiastic teachers of undergraduates and/or postgraduates, and also do a variable amount of research work, often in collaboration with clinical colleagues. There are several major journals devoted to pathology, and many smaller, more specialized ones. As the subject started to acquire definition in the 19th century and to be particularly associated with post-mortem work, it has acquired an old-fashioned aura, which, in the era of molecular biology, is not justified; furthermore, its old tasks of tissue diagnosis, prognostication, and the elucidation of aetiology and pathogenesis, are no less essential and exciting today.

W. F. WHIMSTER

Further reading

Foster, W. D. (1982). *Pathology as a profession in Great Britain and the early history of the Royal College of Pathologists*. Royal College of Pathologists, London.

Knight, B. (1983). *The coroner's autopsy*. Churchill Livingstone, Edinburgh.

MacSween, R. N. M. and Whaley, K. (eds) (1992). *Muir's textbook of pathology*, (13th edn). Edward Arnold, London.

Wheater, P. R., Burkitt, H. G., and Daniels, V. G. (1987). *Functional histology. A text and colour atlas*, (2nd edn). Churchill Livingstone, Edinburgh.

Wheater, P. R., Burkitt, H. G., Stevens, A., and Lowe, J. S. (1991). *Basic histopathology. A colour atlas and text*, (2nd edn). Churchill Livingstone, Edinburgh.

PATHOLOGY TECHNICIANS. See TECHNICIANS; PATHOLOGY.

PATHOPHYSIOLOGY is the physiology of disordered function.

PATIENTS. Earlier usage of the world 'patient' to mean any suffering or sick person is now obsolete, the term now being restricted to one under the care of a medical attendant.

PATIENTS' ASSOCIATION, THE

was started in 1963 in the UK because of anxieties about patients in the *National Health Service (NHS) possibly being used without their informed consent in medical experiments, and as the results of the *thalidomide tragedy came to light. There has always been concern that the near monopoly of health care of the NHS in the UK could lead to an overemphasis on the welfare of the providers to the relative neglect of those for whom they should care. Patients' rights to care, consideration, courtesy, and good facilities may be swamped by health professionals' interests, and organizations to further these. This can occur through ignorance and insensitivity. The Patients' Association attempts to prevent and remedy these proper causes of complaint. It is a voluntary body which relies on subscriptions from its members and aims to 'represent and further the interest of patients: give help and advice to individuals: acquire and spread information about patients' interests: promote understanding and goodwill between patients and everyone in medical practice and related activities'. It has had success in focusing attention upon the rights and interests of a potentially neglected group. It promotes its aims by using all organs of the *media, advising individuals who feel they have legitimate complaints, and by making suggestions for improvements and innovations to health institutions of all kinds.

PATIENTS, NOTABLE (ILLNESSES OF THE FAMOUS).

A tiny number of individuals have a claim to historical immortality solely because of their medical conditions. The name of James Phipps would be entirely forgotten but for the fact that he was the first individual to be vaccinated against smallpox by Edward *Jenner. Alexis St Martin, a French-Canadian fur trapper, is remembered because a gunshot wound created a gastric fistula that exposed the workings of his stomach and enabled the American doctor, William *Beaumont, to make pioneering observations upon the physiology of digestion.

But if sicknesses have won very few people celebrity, the ailments of the illustrious have been of perennial interest; eminent physicians have written at length about their distinguished patients (Lord *Moran on Winston Churchill being a prime instance), and medical historians, amateur and professional, have published widely on the maladies of the mighty. The reasons for this are many. All the trivia of eminent people attract attention. As we know very well in these days of media voyeurism about *AIDS, the private lives of prominent people become appropriated into the public domain. Along similar lines, it was noted two centuries ago that the sicknesses of the eminent create fashions in complaints. 'Various distempers in certain ages and countries have had the fashion on their side, and have been thought reputable and desirable', observed the notable clinician, William *Heberden:

some maladies have been esteemed honourable, because they have accidentally attacked the great, or because they usually belong to the wealthy, who live in plenty and ease . . . when Louis XIV happened to have a fistula, the French surgeons of that time complained of their being incessantly teased by people, who pretended, whatever their complaints were, that they proceeded from a fistula: and if there had been in France a mineral water reputed capable of giving it them, they would perhaps have flocked thither as eagerly as Englishmen resort to Bath in order to get the gout.

The medical histories of the great also attract attention because they are exceptionally well-documented, affording rare shafts of light into the generally poorly recorded practice of medicine in former centuries. We know, for instance, that only after the death of Queen Victoria did her physician, Sir James Reid, discover that she had a ventral hernia and a prolapsed uterus—clear proof that he had never once given her a full physical examination. This instance may well indicate just how recently physical examinations have become a normal aspect of medical practice—although, equally, it might point to an eccentricity of the queen and the power of the throne to command physicians.

Or take James Boswell. Because he kept such copious diaries we know that Dr Johnson's biographer was a habitual sufferer from venereal infections. Boswell was 'clapped' on no fewer than 19 occasions. What forms of treatment did he undergo? For his youthful bouts of 'Signor Gonorrhea', Boswell religiously went to regular surgeons, such as Andrew Douglas in Pall Mall. Douglas initially treated him with purges, put him on a light diet, and ordered bed rest; many years, many claps, later, having changed his strategies, Douglas was to try injecting fluids into the urethra.

When he was infected in Italy, Boswell went to the very best surgeon—James Murray, personal physician to the Old Pretender—and secured an audience with no less eminent a man than *Morgagni, the father of pathological anatomy. On later occasions, Boswell waited upon regular surgeons, such as Peter Adie in Edinburgh and Daniel Johnstone in Ayr. By 1767, Boswell, still only 25 years of age, had his seventh attack, and paid a visit to the Edinburgh surgeon, Duncan Forbes. On a later occasion he consulted the great Percivall *Pott, perhaps the most illustrious surgeon in Britain. On the point of marriage, he consulted a whole gaggle of doctors to ensure he was infection-free.

But Boswell also, just to make sure, travelled to London to purchase some bottles of Kennedy's Lisbon Diet Drink, a popular nostrum vended by Gilbert Kennedy, graduate of both of Rheims and Oxford. The Diet Drink consisted of sarsaparilla, sassafras, liquorice, and guaiac wood, and cost half a guinea a bottle; Boswell was instructed to drink two bottles a day.

When his regular doctors, such as Sir John Pringle,

tried to dissuade him from taking it, Boswell mounted a defence of Kennedy's mixture. 'It is amazing', he recorded in his journal, 'to see a man of Sir John's character so impregnated with partiality as to refuse its just credit to a medicine which has undoubtedly done wonders'. Boswell noted that Pringle had been equally 'prejudiced' against Keyser's pills, another remedy for venereal disease that he had mooted taking. Boswell wanted to believe that self-interest underlay the doctors' distrust of such proprietary cures. As early as 20 January 1763, when being treated by Douglas, he had reflected his doubts. Douglas was his 'friend'; yet he behaved not as a friend, but in the 'opposite character' of a surgeon, 'Douglas as a surgeon will be as ready to keep me long under his hands, and as desirous to lay hold of my money, as any man.'

Matrimony did not put a conclusion to the clap, and subsequent attacks saw Boswell often consulting Pringle and Douglas, who, despite being orthodox, by now had his own personal injection fluid ('a secret known to only a few'). But by this stage—maybe less sanguine about the doctors, or simply feeling that intimate familiarity had made him an expert—Boswell also took to self-medication, something probably connected with reading in 1786 John *Hunter's *Treatise on the venereal disease*. Boswell modified his views in course of time. As with whores, so with cures, Boswell tried them all. Here, Boswell's eminence, his contacts, and the fact that he was a compulsive recorder of his own experiences, enable us to piece together a scene of the medical jigsaw all too often lost.

Studying the ailments of the great is also fascinating because it provokes speculations as to how far the diseases of the great have changed the course of history. The Ottoman leader, Bajazet, was deterred by an attack of *gout from marching into central Europe; upon this, Edward Gibbon (himself a sufferer) observed in his *Decline and fall of the Roman Empire* that 'an acrimonious humour falling on a single fibre of one man may prevent or suspend the misery of nations'. In 1920, King Alexander of Greece died from the bite of his pet monkey. His death triggered a series of events that led Churchill, obviously recalling Gibbon, to comment that 'a quarter of a million persons died of this monkey bite'. Others would, of course, counter that it is not the accidents of the individual but grand impersonal forces that are the true agents of historical change. Had Lenin not died prematurely in 1924, following three strokes, Stalinist totalitarianism would not have been averted; rather, it would now be known as 'Leninist'.

Not least, the diseases of the famous entice attention because they provoke questions as to how far the personalities and careers of notable people were affected by such ailments and infirmities. It has been suggested, for instance, that on his later voyages James Cook (who successfully ensured adequate vitamin C for his sailors) was suffering from serious dietary deficiencies: worms may have deprived him of *niacin and *thiamin. To these have been attributed an increased tetchiness and failure of judgment that may have precipitated the series of blunders that led to his death at the hands of the Hawaiians in 1779.

Even with extremely conspicuous and often well-documented individuals, it is often hard to formulate a retrospective diagnosis upon their illnesses and cause of death, to say nothing of the possible effect of ailments upon their lives and minds. Despite the spilling of a vast amount of ink, there is absolutely no agreement as to the cause of Mozart's death; kidney disease and heart disease are widely suggested, but some still believe that he was poisoned, perhaps by the rival composer, Salieri. Both Friedrich Nietzsche and Robert Schumann died insane, but autopsies did not clearly establish the causes of their conditions. Although it is widely assumed, there is no convincing proof that Nietzsche's growing paralysis was the long-term aftermath of a syphilitic infection picked up from prostitutes (although Nietzsche himself seems to have given currency to this view).

In many cases, confusion seems to proliferate rather than to become resolved. There is no doubt that Charles *Darwin suffered, in the last 50 years of his life, from seriously debilitating conditions, including headache, vomiting, dyspepsia, nausea, lassitude, palpitations, and other nervous afflictions. Some historians and biographers believe his condition was organic, perhaps the consequence of *Chagas' disease, contracted from a bite from an insect, *Triatoma infestans*, suffered while on the pampas in South America, or perhaps the result of self-dosing with proprietary medicines containing *arsenic. Other psychobiographers suggest that Darwin's malady was essentially psychogenic. Some have argued that the morbidly oversensitive Darwin never successfully mourned the early death of his mother. Others believe that the strain of developing the scandalous theory of evolution by natural selection precipitated nervous collapse. Still others suggest that Darwin's invalidism, whatever its cause, was an instance of 'creative malady', a disorder not too serious to preclude work but sufficient to protect the naturalist from official appointments and other interruptions and calls on his time. Indeed, no small number of eminent people have probably been the beneficiaries of such therapeutic 'creative maladies'—Florence *Nightingale, for instance, who took to her bed soon after her return from the Crimea, and exercised power during the rest of her extremely long life as an invalid whose malady was never satisfactorily diagnosed.

Certain disorders have long been seen as top people's diseases. At least since the Renaissance, gout (as William *Heberden noted) was viewed as a mark of good living and fine pedigree (it was regarded as a hereditary disorder). 'Gout is the distemper of a gentleman', insisted Lord Chesterfield, 'whereas the *rheumatism is the distemper of a hackney coachman'. The great English clinician, Thomas *Sydenham, himself a sufferer, noted of gout, 'what is a consolation to me, and may be so to other *gouty* persons of small fortunes and slender abilities, is that kings, great princes, generals, admirals, philosophers and several other great men have thus lived and died'. In *Bleak House*, Dickens' old county baronet, Sir Leicester Dedlock, reflects that 'all the Dedlocks in the direct male line through a course of time during and beyond which the memory of man goeth not to the contrary, have had the gout'. Gout was widely seen as one of the 'diseases of civilization'—others included *hypochondria, nervous disorders, and *neurasthenia—that supposedly occurred disproportionately in wealthy rather than poor nations, in the upper rather than the lower classes, and especially amongst gentlemen and ladies of talent, sensibility, and imagination.

Associations between eminence and sickness were particularly stimulated by the theory of the 'mad genius'. Originating in Plato's concept of 'divine furor' and the Aristotelian notion of black bile (one of the *humours), the notion became popular in the Renaissance that geniuses were typically afflicted with melancholy. It required a malady of the soul to fire the imagination to that pitch of intensity and unworldliness required to produce great art or poetry, or indeed to be a distinguished religious prophet. In his *Lives of the artists*, Vasari noted the oddities of many of the distinguished painters of the Renaissance. Much was later made of the idiosyncrasies of Sir Isaac *Newton as a typical absent-minded scientist. The 'mad poet' appeared in Georgian England with William Collins, Kit Smart, William Cowper, and William Blake, rather as the 'mad king' appeared with George III in Britain and Christian VII in Denmark. Many early 19th century Romantics positively celebrated the idea that it was the artist's fate to soar spiritually only at the cost of physical decomposition and a premature death. *Tuberculosis and *syphilis became the fashionable disorders of Romantic and Bohemian intellectuals and artists (Keats, Chopin, Schubert, Baudelaire, Flaubert, the Brothers Goncourt, Alphonse Daudet, and so on).

Two new twists were added to these concepts around the turn of the 20th century. On the one hand, 'degenerationist' psychiatrists, notably followers of Cesare Lombroso, began to suspect the sanity of almost anyone eminent in the arts. And, at the same time, *Freud's investigations of the workings of the unconscious claimed to confirm that there was something neurotic about the urge to produce great art, and furthermore cast suspicion upon the very urge to greatness, leadership, and power. Freud's study of Leonardo implied that his artistic creativity arose from sexual confusion, which had its roots in immature homosexual tendencies; and his investigation of Woodrow Wilson seemed to attribute the American President's need to exercise power to unresolved personal and sexual tensions with his father. The one-time colleague of Freud, Alfred *Adler, focused his attentions upon the psychopathology of power, and Wilhelm Reich analysed fascism as a form of megalomania. Over the past 50 years, there has

been a plethora of studies purporting to explain the public careers of politicians, statesmen, generals, artists, and media stars in terms of their supposed unhappy childhoods, sexual inadequacies, neurotic disorders, or physical defects. Eminent people, nevertheless, remain willing to expose themselves in the *psychiatrist's chair, perhaps revealing that the chief disorder of famous people is exhibitionism.

ROY PORTER

Further reading
Clare, A. (1992). *In the psychiatrist's chair*. Heinemann, London.
Colp, R. Jr., (1977). *To be an invalid*. University of Chicago Press, Chicago.
Moran, C. M. W. (1966). *Winston Churchill: the struggle for survival 1940–1965*. Constable, London.
Nisbet, J. F. (1900). *The insanity of genius and the general inequality of human faculty physiologically considered*. Grant Richards, London.
Ober, W. B. (1979). *Boswell's clap and other essays: medical analyses of literary men's afflictions*. Carbondale Southern Illinois University Press, Carbondale, Ill.
Pickering, G. (1974). *Creative malady*. George Allen & Unwin, London.

PATRICIDE is the killing of one's father.

PAUL OF AEGINA (*fl.* AD 640). Greek physician. He compiled the *Epitomae medicinae libri septem*, a medical encyclopaedia, much of which was drawn from Pribasius. It was extensively quoted by the Arabs. His writings support *Galen, but give clear and original descriptions of surgical procedures. His *materia medica* comes from *Dioscorides.

PAUL, JOHN RODMAN (1893–1971). American physician and epidemiologist. He devoted much attention to the *epidemiology of infections within families and school groups. His studies of *streptococcal infections at different age periods did much to clarify the association of beta-haemolytic streptococcal infection with *rheumatic fever. In the course of these studies he and Bunnell discovered heterophile *antibodies in patients with *infectious mononucleosis (for some time called the Paul–Bunnell test). Later he developed the technique of 'serological epidemiology', that is testing sera for specific antibodies in samples obtained from various age and population groups from different parts of the world.

PAUL–BUNNELL TEST. A test for the presence in serum of the sheep erythrocyte *agglutinins (heterophil antibodies) characteristic of *infectious mononucleosis.

PAVLOV, IVAN PETROVICH (1849–1936). Russian physiologist. His early work was on the circulation and control of blood pressure but he soon turned to the physiology of digestion where his skill as an animal operator enabled him to make notable advances. For this work he was awarded the *Nobel prize in 1904. The latter part of his working life was occupied by his researches on *conditioned reflexes, the topic for which he is now particularly remembered.

PEARL, RAYMOND (1879–1940). American biostatistician. He was a pioneer in statistical treatment of biological phenomena, including human fertility, population changes, and mortality.

PEARSON, KARL (1857–1936). British biologist and mathematician. He founded the journal *Biometrika* in 1901 and was an influential teacher of *statistics and biometry.

PECTORILOQUY is the transmission of the spoken voice through the chest wall, which can be assessed by both *palpation and by *auscultation. When even a whisper is clearly articulated and heard through the stethoscope, the sign of 'whispering pectoriloquy' is said to be present; it suggests abnormally increased sound conductivity between bronchi and surface due, for example, to consolidation of the intervening lung *parenchyma (as in lobar *pneumonia).

PEDIATRICS. See PAEDIATRICS.

PEDICULUS CAPITIS, the head louse, is a species closely related to the *body louse but its habitat is restricted to the hair of the head; unlike the body louse, it is not a vector of disease. Infestation with head lice, common under institutional conditions, is of great nuisance value and socially distressing. The active parasites are easily recognized with the naked eye, as are the eggs or nits which adhere firmly to hair shafts.

PEDICULUS CORPORIS. See BODY LOUSE.

PEDICULUS PUBIS. See CRAB LOUSE.

PEDIGREE ANALYSIS is the study of the blood relatives of a patient with a particular disease in order to determine whether it is likely to be of genetic origin and, if so, the likely pattern of inheritance (e.g. autosomal dominant, autosomal recessive, sex-linked recessive, polygenic, etc.). The analysis, to be reliable, requires observation (preferably direct) of sufficient members (preferably all) of several successive generations of the family; and partial as well as complete expressions of the abnormality must be sought. The original patient is known as the index case, the proband, or the propositus. See GENETICS.

PEDODONTIST. A dentist specializing in the dental care of children. See DENTISTRY.

PEDUNCLE. A stalk or stem; any stem-like structure serving as attachment, for example of a tumour.

PEER REVIEW. Assessment of the quality of one's work by colleagues of comparable standing and experience (one's peers).

PELIOSIS RHEUMATICA. Henoch–Schönlein (allergic or vascular) purpura associated with non-migratory polyarthritis, chiefly of the knees and ankles; it is also known as Schönlein's disease or purpura rheumatica.

PELLAGRA is the deficiency syndrome resulting from lack of *niacin in the diet; niacin (or vitamin B_3) is the generic term for nicotinic acid and its physiologically active amide nicotinamide. The cardinal manifestations, often accompanied by those due to deficiency of other dietary components, are thickness, roughening, and pigmentation of exposed skin areas (pellagra = 'rough skin'), inflammation of the tongue, diarrhoea, and mental disturbances leading to *dementia. Pellagra is rarely encountered under conditions of Western civilization except when secondary to *alcoholism, intestinal *malabsorption, or one or two rarer conditions. Elsewhere it is associated particularly with maize-dependent diets. See NUTRITION.

PELVIMETRY is measurement of the dimensions of the *pelvis, of particular importance in *obstetrics.

PELVIS. The lower part of the trunk of the body, i.e. the region bounded by the two hip bones and the sacral and coccygeal portions of the spine.

PEMOLINE is a weak central nervous system *stimulant.

PEMPHIGUS is a descriptive term for skin diseases characterized by prominent blister formation.

PENFIELD, WILDER GRAVES (1891–1976). Canadian neurosurgeon. The first director of the Montreal Neurological Institute. In the course of craniotomies performed under local anaesthesia, for treatment of focal *epilepsy or for removal of *tumours, he was able to derive important new information about areas of cortical function.

PENICILLAMINE is a *chelating agent, used to treat heavy metal poisoning and other conditions (such as *Wilson's disease) where chelation is desired. It has also been used in the treatment of *rheumatoid arthritis. It is an *amino acid obtained from the hydrolysis of *penicillins.

PENICILLIN was the first of the *antibiotics (1941), for which the 1945 *Nobel prize was awarded to *Fleming,

*Florey, and *Chain. The name is now a generic term for a large number of derivatives of 6-amino-penicillanic acid obtained naturally or semisynthetically from the moulds *Penicillium* and *Aspergillus* (the original penicillin G was from *Penicillium notatum*). They exert their antibacterial action by interfering with the synthesis of an essential component of bacterial cell walls known as peptidoglycan; there is no action against cells of host tissues except in a few individuals with a specific *allergy to the penicillin molecule. Collectively, the penicillins have a wide spectrum of activity against micro-organisms: it includes particularly those which are Gram-positive (staphylococci, streptococci, pneumococci) but also some which are Gram-negative (meningococci, gonococci); and some *spirochaetes (including that responsible for *syphilis), some *clostridia, and some *fungi. Antibacterial spectra vary between different penicillins. See also ANTI-INFECTIVE DRUGS.

PENIS. The male external organ of micturition and copulation, developmentally homologous with the female *clitoris. (Phallus is not an exact synonym, being reserved for the erect penis.)

PENNSYLVANIA, THE MEDICAL COLLEGE OF, was founded in 1850 as the Female Medical College of Pennsylvania. Among the Quakers of Philadelphia, women were accepted more as the equals of men than in most other societies. Many male Quaker doctors were more willing to take women as apprentices— the pattern of medical education of the time—than other contemporaries. However, as in Europe, women still found difficulty in obtaining degrees from medical institutions. An Act of incorporation was granted in 1850 by the Legislature with very little opposition. Forty women began medical studies in the first year. The Civil War temporarily closed the College, but then, under a succession of able deans, it flourished. One was Ann Preston who founded The Women's Hospital in 1861, to provide clinical facilities for education because of male opposition to women attending the practice of other hospitals in Philadelphia. By 1867 the name was changed to that of The Women's Medical College of Pennsylvania. In 1969 the name was changed again to that of The Medical College of Pennsylvania. Men were then admitted to its courses, to its staff, and to the offices of dean and president.

PEPSIN is one of the important enzymes of *digestion, secreted by the *stomach and responsible for breaking down *proteins into *polypeptides.

PEPTIC ULCER is ulceration of the stomach, lower oesophagus, or first part of the duodenum, that is those parts of the gastrointestinal tract subjected to the action of the *hydrochloric acid and *pepsin secreted by the stomach. Peptic ulcer is common: between 10 and 20 per cent of the population develop an ulcer at some time in their lives. Duodenal ulcers are commoner than those in the stomach (gastric ulcers), although this ratio varies between different populations. Men are more often affected than women, particularly in the case of duodenal ulcer. Symptoms vary in severity, and tend to be remittent. Chief among them is periodic epigastric pain which at its worst can be disabling. The major complications are haemorrhage, perforation into the peritoneal cavity, and obstruction at the outlet of the stomach (pyloric stenosis). The causation of peptic ulcer is not well understood and is probably complex. Mental and emotional stress is usually held to play a part. It is also known that genetic factors are also important, while recently infection with a micro-organism, *Helicobacter pylori* has also been implicated.

PEPTIDE. A compound of two or more *amino acids linked together by peptide bonds; a peptide bond (−CO. NH−) is formed from the union of the carboxyl group (COOH) of one amino acid with the amino group (NH_2) of another, water (H_2O) being lost in the process. Peptides are classified according to the number of amino acid residues (or cores) they contain, for example dipeptides, octapeptides, polypeptides, etc.

PERCEPTION. Appreciation of a sensory stimulus.

PERCIVAL, THOMAS (1740–1804). British health reformer. He holds an important place in epidemiology for his analysis of *bills of mortality from 1772–76, and for his *Code of medical ethics* published privately in 1794, and later in 1803.

PERCUSSION is a standard method of physical examination whereby the resonance of structures lying beneath the body surface is assessed by striking it to elicit a sound. The usual technique is to lay one hand on the surface with the fingers separated, and to tap the middle phalanx of the middle finger with the tip of the other middle finger.

PERFUSION is the blood flow through an organ, tissue, or part.

PERGAMUM was the capital city of an ancient kingdom in Asia Minor (alternative spelling Pergamon). Pergamum is famous for the school of sculpture which flourished there in the 3rd and 2nd centuries BC; for the early Church which was founded there in the 1st century AD; and for having been the birthplace of *Galen in AD 131.

PERIARTERITIS is inflammation of the outer arterial wall and of the tissues immediately surrounding it.

PERIARTERITIS NODOSA is the term formerly used for *polyarteritis nodosa.

PERIARTHRITIS is inflammation of the tissues immediately surrounding a joint.

PERICARDIAL EFFUSION is the accumulation of fluid within the *pericardium, which may accompany *pericarditis or occur as part of generalized fluid retention. Rapid or large accumulations cause *tamponade.

PERICARDITIS is inflammation of the *pericardium; it may be involved in many pathological processes, infective and otherwise. Pericarditis may be incidental to some other major illness (*coronary thrombosis, *renal failure, *carcinoma, *trauma, etc.) or may present *sui generis*. When the latter is the case, the commonest causes are *rheumatic fever, *virus infection, and *tuberculosis.

PERICARDIUM. The fibroserous membrane enclosing the heart; like the serous membranes of the *pleura and the *peritoneum, it has parietal and visceral layers, which move against each other and which are separated by a potential space.

PERIMETRY is measurement of the field of peripheral vision.

PERINEUM. The surface area of the pelvic outlet, comprising the region between the external *genitalia in front and the *anal orifice behind.

PERIOD. Any interval of time. The more precise physical definition is the constant time interval between recurrences of a periodic (regularly repetitive) function such as, for example, *menstruation.

PERIODIC ACID–SCHIFF REACTION. A histological staining technique for revealing *glycogen, neutral *polysaccharides, and *glycoproteins in tissue sections. The section is treated first with periodic acid and then with Schiff's reagent (a fuchsin stain for detecting *aldehydes).

PERIODIC DISEASE is a syndrome of unknown aetiology characterized by various combinations of fever, joint pain, oedema, vomiting, and abdominal pain. The symptom complex recurs and subsides at regular intervals in individuals, who otherwise appear perfectly healthy.

PERIODIC RESPIRATION is any pattern of breathing in which a period of hyperventilation alternates with one of hypoventilation and/or apnoea. *Cheyne–Stokes respiration is the most familiar type.

PERIODONTICS. See DENTISTRY

PERIODONTIST. See DENTISTRY

PERIODONTITIS is inflammation of the tissues surrounding and supporting the teeth, a major cause of dental trouble and tooth loss. See DENTISTRY.

PERIOSTEUM. The thin sheath of specialized connective tissue carrying blood vessels and nerves which envelops all bones. Its integrity is essential for new bone formation in adult life and therefore for the healing of fractures.

PERIPHERAL VASCULAR RESISTANCE. The overall resistance offered to blood flow in the periphery of the blood vascular system, determined by the state of contraction or relaxation of the *arterioles. The peripheral vascular resistance may be roughly assessed as the ratio of the mean arterial blood pressure to the total peripheral blood flow (normally identical to the *cardiac output). In arterial *hypertension, it follows that if the cardiac output is normal, the total peripheral vascular resistance must be abnormally raised.

PERISTALSIS. The wavelike contractions of involuntary muscle which continually pass along the long axis of tubular organs, notably the *gastrointestinal tract, propelling the contents in a forward direction.

PERITONEAL DIALYSIS. See RENAL DIALYSIS.

PERITONEOSCOPY is synonymous with *laparoscopy.

PERITONEUM. The serous membrane of the abdomen, consisting of a parietal layer lining the abdominal and pelvic walls, continuous with a visceral layer which encloses each abdominal structure. The layers are mobile relative to each other, and a potential space exists between them (the peritoneal cavity).

PERITONITIS. Inflammation of the peritoneum, usually resulting from the rupture of a hollow viscus such as the *appendix.

PERMEABILITY. A structure is said to be permeable to a substance if it allows that substance to pass through it.

PERNICIOUS ANAEMIA (ANEMIA) is *megaloblastic anaemia due to impaired absorption of *cyanocobalamin (vitamin B_{12}), caused in turn by a gastric defect in which there is *achlorhydria (an important diagnostic feature), and the *gastric juice is also deficient in 'intrinsic factor', a protein substance which promotes B_{12} absorption. The aetiology is unknown, but it is probable that *autoimmunity plays a part. The essential features are those of severe and progressive anaemia; the red blood cells are abnormally large (macrocytosis), so that the mean corpuscular volume is raised. Neurological symptoms may develop, due to *neuropathy or to degeneration of the lateral and posterior columns of the spinal cord (subacute combined degeneration of the spinal cord). Pernicious anaemia (or Addisonian anaemia as it is also called, *Addison having described the condition in 1849) was almost invariably fatal until the classic discovery by *Minot and Murphy (1926) of the effect of feeding liver, a landmark which led ultimately to the identification of vitamin B_{12}.

PERSEVERATION is the persistent repetition of words or actions despite the patient's efforts to say or do something else.

PERSISTENT VEGETATIVE STATE. A permanent state of 'mute, mindless wakefulness' in which the brain-stem continues to function but the cerebral cortex is, for practical purposes, totally destroyed, usually as a consequence of severe *head injury, *anoxia, or severe brain disease.

PERSONA is the term used by *Jung to signify the set of attitudes adopted by an individual to fit the role he perceives for himself in society; in other words, the 'persona' is the personality displayed to the world, as opposed to the inner or unconscious personality, which Jung termed the 'anima'.

PERSONALITY is an inclusive term used to indicate the totality of behavioural, attitudinal, intellectual, and emotional characteristics of an individual.

PERSPIRATION. Sweat, *sweating.

PERTUSSIS is a synonym for whooping cough. Pertussis is a highly contagious infection of the respiratory tract with a marked predilection for infants and young children, usually conferring lifelong immunity. It is caused by the bacterium *Bordetella pertussis*, formerly known as *Haemophilus pertussis*. The common name derives from the characteristic inspiratory whoop which follows the prolonged and distressing spasms of coughing. Whooping cough is a dangerous as well as an unpleasant disease; serious complications can occur during the acute illness, which has a significant mortality, and leaves some patients with a lifelong legacy of crippling respiratory disability. Active *immunization effectively reduces both frequency and severity. This should be initiated at the age of about two months.

PERTUSSIS VACCINATION. Active immunization against whooping cough using a killed suspension of *Bordetella pertussis*. See PERTUSSIS.

PERUVIAN BARK is a synonym for cinchona bark (Jesuit's bark, etc.). See QUININE.

PERVERSION. Deviant sexual behaviour, that is other than normal sexual intercourse. Many such deviations

are no longer regarded as either pathological or socially unacceptable and the less pejorative term 'sexual deviance' is often preferred.

PES CAVUS. Increased concavity of the longitudinal arch of the foot.

PESSARY. A vaginal *suppository, or a mechanical device inserted into the *vagina to provide tissue support or to prevent insemination of the *uterus.

PETECHIA. A tiny reddish punctate spot in skin or *mucous membrane due to capillary *haemorrhage.

PETERS, JOHN PUNNETT (1887–1950). American physician. His scientific interests lay in body fluid and in renal disease, leading to the publication of *Body water*; but he had wide interests in the application of chemistry to clinical medicine, expressed most fully in his collaboration with van *Slyke, in *Quantitative clinical chemistry*. The two volumes, *Methods* and *Interpretation* were indispensable handbooks from their first appearance in 1931.

PETHIDINE is a synthetic narcotic analgesic with actions similar to, but somewhat less potent than, those of *morphine; like morphine, it is highly addictive. Its analgesic effect is prompt but short-lived and therefore not suited to the relief of pain due to terminal *malignant disease. It is widely used in *obstetric analgesia, and is the analgesic of choice when intracranial disease is known or suspected. Pethidine is also known as meperidine or Demerol® (in the USA).

PETIT, JEAN LOUIS (1674–1760). French surgeon. In 1731 he founded L'Académie des Chirurgiens. He published *L'art de guérir les maladies des os* (1705). Petit invented the screw-tourniquet, undertook the first *mastoidectomy in 1736, and distinguished *cerebral compression from *concussion. The anatomical area bounded by the iliac crest, the latissimus dorsi muscle, and the external oblique muscles is known as Petit's triangle.

PETIT MAL is a specific form of minor *epilepsy, characterized by temporary lapses of consciousness lasting only a few seconds and beginning and ending abruptly; the patient, usually a child or young adult, may be unaware that anything has happened and carry on with whatever he or she was doing. Attacks may occur only occasionally, or many times a day. Petit mal, also known as 'absence seizure', is associated with a characteristic *electroencephalographic (EEG) pattern.

PETRI DISH. A circular flat-bottomed vertical-sided shallow glass dish with a slightly larger glass cover of similar shape, in which micro-organisms are cultured on a nutrient medium.

PETTENKOFER, MAX JOSEF VON (1818–1901). German physician and hygienist. He founded the Institute of Hygiene in Munich in 1879. Although one of the pioneers of hygiene, he did not accept that some diseases had a bacterial cause, believing them to be of chemical origin. To prove his point he drank a pure culture of *Vibrio cholerae* and suffered no ill-effect. In addition to his contribution to public health, most of his researches were in *metabolism.

PETTY, SIR WILLIAM (1623–87). British physician and political economist. A distinguished administrative and financial reformer, Petty was a pioneer political economist who urged the need for statistical data. He was also an ingenious inventor; he designed a double-keeled vessel and tried to install power in a ship.

PFEIFFER, RICHARD FRIEDRICH JOHANNES (1858–1945). German bacteriologist. In 1892 he described the *influenza bacillus (*Haemophilus influenzae*), now known not to be the cause of influenza, and in 1896 *Micrococcus catarrhalis*. He established the life cycle of *Coccidium oviforme* in rabbits in 1892, and described *bacteriolysis in 1894.

PFLÜGER, EDWARD FRIEDRICH WILHELM (1829–1910). German physiologist. He was especially interested in respiratory gaseous exchange and was responsible for the concept of *respiratory quotient.

pH is a measure of *hydrogen ion concentration expressed as its negative logarithm to the base ten. A solution with a pH of 7 is neutral. Solutions with a pH of less than 7 are acidic and those with a pH of more than 7 are alkaline.

PHACOMATOSIS is a term which embraces a number of genetically determined neurological disorders associated with multiple *hamartomas of the skin and eye. They include *neurofibromatosis and *tuberous sclerosis, and are also known as the neurocutaneous syndromes.

PHAEOCHROMOCYTOMA (PHEOCHROMOCYTOMA). A *chromaffinoma of the *adrenal medulla or *sympathetic ganglia which secretes excessive quantities of *adrenaline and *noradrenaline, causing episodic or persistent *hypertension.

PHAGOCYTE. Any cell able to ingest foreign materials. Many cells have this property to some degree, but the most intensely phagocytic are the *polymorphs, the *monocytes, and the *macrophages (the 'professional' phagocytes).

PHAGOCYTOSIS is the process by which a *phagocyte engulfs into its cytoplasm other cells, bacteria, or other particulate matter by flowing all around the foreign object, forming a vacuole.

PHALLUS. The erect *penis; a word used most often in the context of its ancient symbolism.

PHANTOM LIMB. An illusion of the presence of an amputated limb, which may be associated with pain, aches, or *paraesthesiae referred to the absent part.

PHARMACEUTICAL INDUSTRY. In the 1990s the pharmaceutical industry has three outstanding characteristics: it is highly successful, it is completely international, and it is centrally dependent on its research and innovation. Understandably, these three characteristics are closely interlinked. First, the world-wide growth of the industry since the 1940s has resulted from its major role in the discovery and development of the vast majority of modern medicines in use today. In turn, the cost of the research involved is such that new medicines must be sold in all countries if this initial investment is to be recovered. And the risks of failure in research are such that high returns are necessary to attract this investment in the first place. However, the very success of the industry, and the central role that its discoveries play in the practice of medicine, have given rise to economic and ethical difficulties. The growth of the modern industry, its organization and activities, and the controversial issues which surround it will be discussed briefly in this article.

Present structure
The industry is very varied, with a low concentration in terms of share of the market. The main central core focuses on the development, manufacture, and marketing of new *prescription medicines. There are between 100 and 200 principal international companies making up this sector of the industry, with several hundred more with smaller research facilities or which concentrate on formulating existing medicinal chemicals into new preparations.

In addition, there is an important sector of the industry which produces medicines based on older established active ingredients, and which advertises them under brand names direct to the public (so-called 'over-the-counter' or OTC preparations). Thirdly, there are the manufacturers of so-called 'generic' medicines—preparations sold under their official *pharmacopoeial names. Again, these are based on well-established chemical ingredients, and are made available for prescription in cases where the doctor has not specified a particular manufacturer's brand.

These three main groups of manufacturers—of branded prescription medicines, nationally advertised medicines, and 'generic' preparations—show a considerable degree of overlap, with the same companies often involved in all three types of business. It should also be pointed out that over a period of years the medicines manufactured by the 'generic' companies will originally have been developed as innovations within the research-based sector of the industry. Hence the seminal role of research for the industry as a whole. As far as the research-based innovative core of the pharmaceutical industry is concerned, there is a very striking international geographical pattern. Throughout the latter part of the 20th century, only five countries in the world have dominated the scene. These are the UK, France, West Germany, Switzerland, and the USA.

There is likely to be one major change in this international pattern of the pharmaceutical industry in the 1990s. This is the development of the Japanese industry. There seems little doubt that the Japanese pharmaceutical industry plans to follow the example of its motor car, motor cycle, and electronics industries in penetrating deeply into world markets.

The role of research

Huge sums of money are involved in pharmaceutical research. A recent study indicated that on average in 1987 it cost US$231 (£154) million to develop a single new pharmaceutical chemical compound (Di Masi *et al.* 1991).

With such large sums of money at stake, it is important to understand the process of pharmaceutical innovation in the industry today. There are broadly three approaches, which overlap to some extent. The first is to screen compounds from a wide variety of sources for potential pharmacological activity. For example, a company may take compounds occurring in nature (such as salicylic acid), modify them, and then see what pharmacological actions the new compounds have on animals; or a company manufacturing synthetic agricultural chemicals may randomly test these to see if they have any pharmacological activity. Secondly, and more specially, a company may take a new compound with a known pharmacological action and then modify it chemically to see how its activity is affected. The third broad approach to pharmaceutical innovation appears on theoretical grounds to be the most scientific, although it is not always the most effective in practice. This is the specific synthesis of compounds which are expected from a scientific hypothesis to have a particular pharmacological action.

Once a 'product candidate' has been identified and synthesized as a result of one of these three approaches, there starts the very long and painstaking task of testing the chemical compound for any warning signs of toxicity and for its pharmacological effectiveness, first in human volunteers and then in patients. This whole process is now estimated on average to take about 10 years between the first synthesis (and patenting) of the compound and its eventual marketing in the form of a pharmaceutical preparation. The great majority of hopeful new approaches fail in this latter testing stage, either because the chemical does not live up to its early promise as an effective treatment, or because it proves toxic to some species of animal, or because it causes untoward adverse *side-effects during *clinical trials in man. This is an important aspect of the element of risk which justifies the higher than average returns from the few medicines which do eventually reach the market. There is also, of course, the risk that serious adverse effects may become apparent after the medicine has been put on the market. Apart from the seriousness for the patients and prescribers, this again is a commercial catastrophe for the manufacturer, who will usually have to discontinue sales of the product.

Economic factors

This raises the question of the economic environment which is necessary to support the pharmaceutical industry's investment in research. It is now generally accepted economic theory that any industry which is based on innovation must be protected from the unfettered forces of pure price competition (Schumpeter 1942). The mechanism for providing this protection is through the use of patents and brand names. These give the innovator the exclusive right to sell his innovation for the period of the patent life, and continue to give him some protection from imitators through the use of the brand name after the patent has expired.

In the UK and the rest of Europe, patents give the innovator 20 years of exclusivity to sell the new medicine. In the USA, the period is 17 years. However, as has already been pointed out, about 10 years of this period are taken up with the development and testing of the medicine. Thus in the UK, Japan, and the USA there have been moves to try to get the period of patent protection to run from a later date—for example, when the medicine is first tested in man rather than when it was first synthesized. As a result it is possible to get up to 5 years' extension of patent life under new laws in the USA and in the European Community.

The use of brand names in prescribing has recently been a controversial issue. Clearly, brand names are intended to give the original pharmaceutical manufacturer some extra financial return, beyond that obtainable under patent, so branded prescription medicines are more expensive than the 'generic' alternative produced by other companies once the patent has expired. In addition, brand names guarantee the reliable source of the medicine and ensure that the patient receives exactly the same formulation each time the medicine is dispensed. Medicines dispensed under their generic name may have significant variations in their pharmacological action even when they contain exactly the same amount of active chemical ingredient. These variations arise from differences in the method of formulation of the medicine by different manufacturers, all of which will nevertheless comply with the official standards set out in the pharmacopoeia. The use of the specific manufacturer's brand name in prescribing and dispensing avoids the risk of variation, as the medicine will, in this case, be manufactured in exactly the same way. On the other hand, the prescribing or dispensing of the cheaper unbranded medicines can save either the health service or the patient money. This raises the whole question of the appropriate profitability of pharmaceutical companies and the balance between a natural desire to have a 'cheap drug bill' and the importance of continuing to finance industrial pharmaceutical research.

All countries in Europe have some sort of comprehensive health service, under which medicines are provided free or at a nominal cost. The USA is, to a large extent, an exceptional case, in that the patient still often pays directly the full cost of the medicines prescribed. In the case of non-prescribed, nationally advertised medicines, of course, in all countries the patient pays the full price for the medicine which he or she purchases.

Under the European health services, a variety of measures have been taken to try to reduce the cost of the pharmaceutical service. Perhaps the best balanced and most sophisticated of the arrangements has existed in the UK, where under the Pharmaceutical Price Regulation Scheme each manufacturer negotiates annually with the Department of Health and Social Security over the appropriate level of prices and profit for all its sales to the British *National Health Service (NHS). This scheme is renegotiated at regular intervals to try to ensure that this proper balance is still being achieved.

On the other hand, West Germany, The Netherlands, and Sweden have introduced schemes under which patients are only reimbursed for the price of the cheapest equivalent medicine which is available and must pay the difference if they wish to have the more expensive medicine actually prescribed by the doctor. Countries such as Belgium, France, and Italy also have much stricter controls on the individual prices of prescription medicines. In general, there continues to be a debate on the best method of getting pharmaceuticals as cheaply as possible, without at the same time inhibiting the pharmaceutical industry's ability to invest in continuing and increasingly expensive research. However, there is an unfortunate desire for some countries which do not themselves have a strong research-based industry merely to want to pay the lowest possible prices for their medicines.

Safety of medicines

Apart from economic considerations, an important aspect of the development of the pharmaceutical industry over the past 20 years has been the effort devoted to trying to make medicines as safe as possible. In 1961 the *thalidomide disaster focused world-wide attention on the ability of medicines to do harm as well as good. Since 1961 much stricter government controls have been introduced in all countries to try to prevent any adverse effects occurring with medicines. Nevertheless, the pharmaceutical manufacturers need continually to emphasize that they cannot develop absolutely safe

medicines. Like any form of therapy, medication can involve risks.

Before concluding this article, two special subjects are worth mentioning. The first is the role of the pharmaceutical industry in the Third World, and the second is the prospect of future progress for the industry in its contribution to therapeutics.

The Third World

In the Third World there are overwhelming medical problems. These stem from a shortage of medical personnel and facilities, and from a serious maldistribution of these scarce resources between the privileged urban areas and the neglected rural districts. It has been suggested that the inappropriate marketing of medicines and even of medicinal foods (e.g. infant foodstuffs) by the industry has added to these problems, and pharmaceutical manufacturers are very sensitive to these criticisms. The industry has, therefore, introduced recently a Code of Marketing Practice to apply to Third World countries. This is similar to, but less stringent than, similar codes of practice which have been operated for many years in some developed countries such as the UK. The intention is to ensure that medicines are never advertised for inappropriate indications or without due attention being paid to their possible risks.

More positively, the pharmaceutical industry is trying to step up its research programme into methods of preventing or curing the specifically Third World health problems, and is co-operating with WHO in training pharmaceutical personnel for the less developed countries.

Prospects for the future

To return to the Western world, and looking to the future, there seem to be tremendous prospects for advances over the next 20 years from pharmaceutical industry research. These advances, like progress in the past, will come from an effective collaboration between academic medical scientists and the pharmaceutical industry. The former very often produce the basic knowledge from which pharmaceutical progress can develop. The latter have the resources and the expertise to convert this basic knowledge into new therapeutic substances.

One important area for such co-operation is in relation to *molecular biology and *genetic engineering. The fundamental understanding of the chemistry within the human cell which has emerged in the past 30 years is now reaching a stage where it is starting to lead to treatments for *virus diseases, many more *cancers, and *autoimmune disorders. Another important area is in brain biochemistry, where there are prospects of effective therapy for *schizophrenia, senile *dementia, and the addictive diseases, such as *alcoholism.

Thus, in conclusion, the modern international pharmaceutical industry seems to have a flourishing future ahead of it. There are economic problems which it must overcome, such as some countries' obsessional desire to obtain 'cheap drugs'. But on the whole, the prescription medicine manufacturers have a good relationship with their immediate 'customers', the medical profession. As the predominant source of most of the new medicines in the past 40 years, and as the probable source of all important pharmacological advances in the next 40, the pharmaceutical industry has, on balance, positive, and should continue to make, a very strong, positive, and beneficial contribution to the progress of medicine.

G. TEELING SMITH

References

Di Masi, J. A., Hansen, R. W., Grabowski, H. G., and Lasagna, L. (1991). Cost of innovation in the pharmaceutical industry. *Journal of Health Economics*, **10**, 107–42.

Schumpeter, J. (1942). *Capitalism, socialism and democracy.* Harper and Row, New York.

PHARMACIST. A druggist, pharmaceutical chemist, or (formerly) an *apothecary, that is a person qualified and licensed to make up prescriptions and to dispense medicinal substances. See PHARMACY AND PHARMA-CISTS.

PHARMACOGENETICS is the study of genetically determined variation in individual responses to drugs.

PHARMACOKINETICS. The dynamics of drug distribution in biological systems. See PHARMACOLOGY.

PHARMACOLOGY is the scientific study of the effects of chemical substances on living systems. The chemicals which pharmacologists investigate include normal constituents of the body, compounds derived or extracted from animals and plants, substances synthesized by chemists, or (increasingly) products produced by specially adapted cell systems of bacterial, yeast, or mammalian origin and encompassed by the term biotechnology products. The biological systems studied by pharmacologists range from microbiological organisms, parts of cells, intact cells and organs, to whole animals and populations.

Pharmacology underpins the applied sciences of toxicology, clinical pharmacology, and therapeutics. Toxicology is the study of poisons or potential poisons. Toxicologists are concerned not only with the potential adverse effects of drugs, but also with the possible hazardous properties of household and industrial chemicals, food additives, pesticides, herbicides, environmental pollutants, and cosmetics. Clinical pharmacology is the study of the effects of drugs in man, and is especially involved with those actions which lead to therapeutic benefits or adverse reactions. Clinical pharmacologists have a special interest in evaluating and optimizing the efficacy and safety of drugs during their clinical use. Clinical pharmacologists may also study the consequences of drugs used in populations (pharmacoepidemiology) either in relation to monitoring their safety (pharmacovigilance) or to their cost-effectiveness (pharmacoeconomics). Therapeutics is the branch of medicine concerned with the treatment of disease, and, although intimately involved with pharmacology and clinical pharmacology, it also includes non-pharmacological treatments (e.g. *physiotherapy, *psychotherapy).

Nomenclature and classification

Like other chemicals, drugs have formal scientific names which describe, precisely, their structure. Examples include N-acetyl para-aminophenol and acetylsalicylic acid. These, however, are too cumbersome for routine clinical use and consequently 'trivial' names are assigned to chemicals that are to be used as medicines by the British Pharmacopoeal Commission. Examples of what are properly known as British Approved Names (although sometimes referred to as 'non-proprietary' or 'generic' names) include *paracetamol (for N-acetyl para-aminophenol) or *aspirin (for acetylsalicylic acid). The pharmaceutical company that manufactures and sells a particular drug frequently does so under a 'brand' or 'proprietary' name which is a registered trade mark: Panadol, Panasorb, and Calpol are all brand names of products containing paracetamol.

Drugs can be classified in three ways. The therapeutic class describes the condition, or symptoms, for which the drug is used (e.g. oral *contraceptives, *analgesics, antidiabetic agents, or *anticonvulsants). Some drugs, however, are useful in a range of disorders, or form subcategories within a single therapeutic class. These can be classified on the basis of their pharmacological actions (e.g. *diuretics, *antihistamines, anti-inflammatory drugs). Within therapeutic or pharmacological classes, drugs may be further classified according to their chemical family (e.g. *sulphonylurea* antidiabetic agents, *thiazide* diuretics).

Basis of drug action

There are, broadly, five ways in which chemicals produce pharmacological effects:

(1) physical effects;
(2) chemical neutralization;
(3) binding to specific *receptors;
(4) chemical incorporation;
(5) *enzyme inhibition.

Physical effects

Some commonly used therapeutic agents produce their effects by a purely physical action. Despite the relative simplicity of this mechanism such drugs retain an important place in therapeutics. Thus, substances which physically alter the volume and consistency of *faeces are used to treat disorders of the bowel: blood and blood substitutes replace the circulating blood volume after *haemorrhage or fluid loss; topical emollient creams and ointments may restore some of the physical properties of damaged skin.

Chemical neutralization

Some drugs act by neutralizing substances within the body. The simplest form occurs when alkalis are used to treat symptoms due to excess acid in the stomach. Oral administration of alkaline mixtures containing sodium bicarbonate, magnesium trisilicate, or aluminium hydroxide will neutralize hydrochloric acid in the stomach and relieve the pain of *peptic ulceration or *heartburn.

A more sophisticated form of neutralization occurs with drugs that combine, sometimes very specifically, with (usually noxious) chemicals in the body. The process not only renders the noxious chemical innocuous, but usually converts it into a form that can be more readily removed from the body by renal excretion or hepatic metabolism. Examples include drugs which combine (chelate) with heavy metals and are used to treat lead, mercury, and thallium *poisoning. In the past few years specific *antibodies have been developed to neutralize unwanted substances in the body. Digoxin antibodies have been developed to treat poisoning with this drug, and antibodies to toxic substances released by bacteria are currently under development.

Specific receptors

Most drugs produce their effects by interacting with specific and discrete parts of cells. Receptors are large molecules (usually proteins) that bear recognition sites for specific chemicals known as 'ligands'. The binding of a ligand to its receptor initiates a train of events resulting in a characteristic response, such as muscular contraction or *glandular secretion. Agonists are ligands which mimic the action of a natural hormone or neurotransmitter, and examples include salbutamol (a bronchodilator) or *morphine (an analgesic). By contrast, antagonists are ligands that bind to specific receptors without stimulating the tissue. They produce their effects by displacing naturally occurring agonists and thus preventing their action. The antiulcer drug cimetidine, and the antipsychotic agent haloperidol, are typical antagonists.

Although the existence of specific receptors has been suspected for over a century, it is only relatively recently that they have been isolated and characterized. Several different types of receptor are recognized.

(a) Neurotransmitter receptors. Within both the central and peripheral nervous system communication between nerve cells, and between nerves and their effector organs (e.g. muscle, glands), is achieved by chemical means. When a nerve impulse reaches the end of a nerve fibre, a specific chemical (neurotransmitter) is released which diffuses across the synaptic cleft to an adjacent nerve, muscle, or glandular cell. The neurotransmitter then interacts with, and stimulates, its specific receptor lying within the postsynaptic nerve or muscle cell membrane. Many neurotransmitters are now known, but the most important and ubiquitous include *noradrenaline, *acetylcholine, *dopamine, glutamate, gamma-aminobutyric acid (GABA), 5-hydroxytryptamine (*serotonin), and *enkephalin. These are all agonists and their effects are terminated either by metabolism by specific enzymes situated close to the receptor (e.g. acetylcholinesterase for acetylcholine), or by 're-uptake' into the presynaptic neurone via a specific transport mechanism (e.g. noradrenaline).

One of the most important observations in modern pharmacology is that receptors which are specific to a particular neurotransmitter may also be tissue, or functionally, specific. Thus acetylcholine receptors in the heart differ from those in voluntary muscle, despite being stimulated by the same agonist. Noradrenergic receptors which, on stimulation, produce constriction of blood vessels are known as alpha-noradrenergic receptors; noradrenergic receptors in the heart and lungs are structurally different and are known as beta-noradrenergic receptors. Furthermore, cardiac beta-receptors (known as beta$_1$-receptors) are different from those in the lungs (beta$_2$-receptors). Subclasses of receptors for acetylcholine, dopamine, GABA, and serotonin are also well-characterized.

The characterization of the receptor subclasses has been of great pharmacological (and therapeutic) importance. Agonists and antagonists specific to particular receptor subclasses have been developed, and this has permitted compounds to become available that are targeted to particular organs or functions. This, in turn, has meant that new drugs have emerged with highly specific actions, and which avoid the adverse consequences of wider receptor interactions.

(b) Ionophore receptors. The membranes of many (if not most) cells contain proteins which, on 'activation', allow ions (especially sodium, potassium, calcium, chloride) to pass freely across the membrane and cause some cellular action. Some of these ionophores are activated by specific ligands, such as acetylcholine or GABA, and form part of the receptor complex. Others are not activated by ligands but by other cellular events such as *depolarization. Local *anaesthetic agents (e.g. lignocaine) block sodium channels in nerve fibres and hence prevent the transmission of nerve impulses. A major class of antihypertensive agents (the so-called calcium-channel blockers) prevent the movement of calcium ions into vascular smooth muscle and thus prevent its contraction. Drugs which act on potassium and chloride channels are currently under development and may have important therapeutic properties.

(c) Hormone receptors. Many *hormones, including sex hormones and *insulin, exert their effects by interacting with specific receptors. In many instances, pure preparations of natural hormones are themselves valuable therapeutic agents, and examples include cortisol, thyroxine, and insulin. Some, however, are so rapidly metabolized that they are ineffective unless given by intravenous infusion. Synthetic analogues which retain the chemical configuration required for antagonist activity, but which are resistant to metabolic degradation, have achieved wide use. This particularly applies to the synthetic *oestrogens and *progestogens used in oral contraceptive products.

Synthetic hormone antagonists are also available and have been used, particularly in the treatment of certain hormone-dependent *tumours. The oestrogen antagonist tamoxifen is valuable in the treatment of certain forms of breast *cancer; and the androgen antagonist, cyproterone acetate, is used for prostatic cancer in men.

(d) Transport receptors. The transport of certain substances across cell membranes is mediated by specific 'pumps'. Drugs that inhibit the re-uptake of noradrenaline or serotonin into presynaptic nerve terminals are widely used as *antidepressants.

Chemical incorporation

Some of the most effective anticancer drugs produce their effects by undergoing incorporation into molecules which are critical to cell division. Alkylating agents all possess the property of forming strong (covalent) linkages with the primary genetic material deoxyribonucleic acid (*DNA), producing a major distortion of function in cell division. Antimetabolites are chemical analogues of the purine and pyrimidine bases which are essential components of DNA. They are incorporated into DNA and then miscode genetic information and cause cellular death. Cancer cells are distinguished from normal cells by their uncontrolled division. They are, therefore, preferentially affected by anticancer drugs acting by chemical incorporation. However, other rapidly dividing normal cells in the body may also be influenced, resulting in serious adverse reactions, including loss of hair, sterility, and depression of *bone marrow function.

Enzyme inhibition

The formation and breakdown of most bodily constituents are catalysed by proteins known as *enzymes. An enzyme usually displays a high degree of specificity for a particular reaction, and contains an 'active site' which mediates its catalytic action.

Many important drugs produce their therapeutic effects by inhibiting the action of enzymes. Such drugs bind to an enzyme's active site and prevent the normal substrate gaining access to it. Because of the high specificity of most enzymes, it is frequently possible to achieve comparable specificity of drug action.

Drugs which are enzyme inhibitors produce their effects by one of two mechanisms: they either prevent the metabolism of some active natural substance; or they impede the synthesis of a normal body constituent. Some drugs inhibit the enzymes responsible for the metabolism of neurotransmitters. Monoamine-oxidase inhibitors (used to treat depression) and cholinesterase inhibitors (used to reverse muscle relaxants after general anaesthesia) block, respectively, the metabolism of noradrenaline and acetylcholine. This leads to persistence of these neurotransmitters and hence an increased intensity of their action.

Many drugs inhibit the synthesis of critical physiological substances, and thus produce therapeutic effects. *Penicillins and *cephalosporins inhibit a bacterial enzyme responsible for cell wall synthesis. Ciprofloxacin, and other members of the same class of antibiotics, inhibit the bacterial enzyme which coils DNA. The antiviral agent, *zidovudine (AZT), used to treat *AIDS, inhibits an enzyme responsible for converting the RNA of human immunodeficiency virus into a form that can be inserted into human DNA. The nonsteroidal anti-inflammatory drugs, such as aspirin and ibuprofen, inhibit the formation of some of the mediators of inflammation, fever, and pain (*prostaglandins). The anticancer agent, methotrexate, inhibits the enzyme responsible for the synthesis of DNA precursors. Many other important drugs act by inhibiting enzymes, and this general mechanism is second, in importance, only to interaction with specific receptors.

Drug handling

Drugs may be administered either locally or systemically. Local administration is intended to confine a drug to the diseased organ or tissue; topical skin preparations, nose drops, or vaginal pessaries are typical examples. After so-called 'systemic administration' either orally (by mouth), or parentally (by injection), drugs reach their intended site of action via the bloodstream; they will also, however, inevitably reach other tissues where they may cause unwanted effects. In recent years it has become apparent that the intensity and duration of effect of many drugs depend on their handling within the body, which, in turn, is regulated by the processes of drug absorption, distribution, and elimination.

Absorption

Most drugs are given orally and must pass through the stomach before undergoing absorption in the upper small intestine. Conditions which delay gastric emptying, such as food, fear, pain, nausea, and fever will delay both the absorption and therapeutic effects of a drug. Intestinal absorption of most drugs occurs by simple diffusion across the mucosal lining of the gut. Drugs which, for physicochemical reasons, do not readily diffuse across the mucosa, will be retained in the intestinal tract and excreted in the faeces. Such drugs will not, therefore, reach the circulation, and must be given by injection if a systemic effect is required. On the other hand, non-absorbable antibiotics can be effective in the treatment of intestinal infections.

Drug molecules which cross the lining of the gut must pass through the liver before reaching the systemic circulation. Some drugs are so avidly metabolized within the cells lining the gastrointestinal tract, or by the liver, that only a small fraction of an oral dose is available to exert a systemic effect. With glyceryl trinitrate (see Table 7) this fraction is so minute that no systemic effect is observed; however, sucking a tablet of glyceryl trinitrate under the tongue avoids 'presystemic' destruction because the blood draining the mouth bypasses the liver and flows directly into the main circulation.

Distribution

Once drugs reach the bloodstream they are distributed, to a greater or lesser extent, to various tissues and organs. The degree to which a drug penetrates individual organs and cells is governed by many factors, including the chemical properties of the drug, the structural characteristics of the tissue, and its blood supply. Even within the blood, many drugs are loosely bound to red blood corpuscles or *plasma proteins which can therefore act as a 'reservoir'. Penetration of drugs into the brain is restricted by 'tight junctions' between cells lining the cerebral blood vessels, and only those compounds which are sufficiently soluble to dissolve in the lipid membrane of this so-called 'blood–brain barrier' are capable of producing pharmacological effects within the central nervous system.

The principles governing drug distribution are put to practical use both in selecting drugs for individual patients, and in the development of new drugs. Thus, the selection of an *antibiotic appropriate for treating bacterial *meningitis is determined (at least in part) by its capacity to cross the blood–brain barrier. In the context of new drug development, the relatively recent introduction of two new histamine$_1$-antagonists (terfenadine and astemizole), which do not cross the blood–brain barrier and are thus devoid of the sedating effect of their predecessors, offer substantial hope to sufferers from hay fever.

Elimination

Once drugs have been absorbed into the systemic circulation, various physiological and biochemical processes act to eliminate them from the body.

Drugs are eliminated from the body either by renal excretion or by metabolism.

(a) Renal excretion. Some drugs are excreted in unchanged form by the kidneys. In the presence of renal disease, however, renal drug excretion rates fall and half-lives become longer. Consequently, higher blood levels and more intense pharmacological effects (including adverse reactions) may occur. It is therefore necessary to reduce the dosages of drugs undergoing renal excretion, if toxicity is to be avoided, in patients with disordered kidney function. The immature kidney of the newborn infant, and the 'normal' decline in renal function which occurs with advancing years, also render the very young and the elderly susceptible to drug toxicity if conventional adult dosages (even allowing for difference in body weight) are given. Fortunately, kidney function can be reasonably well predicted from simple blood tests, and drug toxicity due to 'relative overdosage' of renally excreted drugs in the newborn, the elderly, and the patient with kidney disease, is largely avoidable.

(b) Metabolism. Most drugs used in clinical practice undergo metabolism in the liver before their degradation products (metabolites) can be excreted in the urine. Often these metabolites are pharmacologically inactive, and drug metabolism is therefore frequently regarded as a detoxification mechanism. In recent years, however, it has become apparent that some drugs are themselves biologically inactive, and that their pharmacological effects are produced by their metabolites. Furthermore, in an increasing number of instances, drug metabolites have been shown to possess a similar pharmacological profile to that of their parent drug, or even to cause toxic adverse effects.

A wide variety of drug metabolic pathways have developed during evolution—probably as a protection against toxins in food and the environment. The detailed metabolic fate of a particular drug may therefore be extremely complex, and drug metabolites themselves often undergo further biotransformation before they can be excreted by the kidneys. Despite this, it is usually possible to identify a drug's 'major' metabolic pathway and its corresponding metabolite. Clinical pharmacology and therapeutics, however, remain bedevilled by two major problems—differences between individuals in rates of drug metabolism, and differences between species in both rates *and* routes of drug metabolism.

During the past 25 years it has been apparent that, even amongst healthy individuals, there are marked interpersonal variations in the rates at which people metabolize drugs via specific pathways of biotransformation. This is partly due to genetic factors, and partly due to environmental influences which we face in everyday living. Although the relative importance of nature and nurture differs for different metabolic pathways, the therapeutic consequences are similar. Individuals who are 'slow' metabolizers of a particular drug will tend to achieve higher blood drug levels and greater risks of suffering toxicity; 'rapid' metabolizers will have lower blood levels, and greater risks of therapeutic failure.

The genetic control of drug metabolism varies qualitatively for different pathways, and quantitatively for different races. Known environmental factors influencing individual pathways include cigarette *smoking, *alcohol, exposure to certain environmental pollutants (e.g. pesticides), *other* drugs taken at the same time (e.g. oral contraceptives), certain foods (e.g. brassica vegetables), and the relative proportions of dietary protein and carbohydrate. Add to this the obvious effects of liver disease, the less obvious effects of cardiac, respiratory, and renal disease, and changes attributable to gender and age, and it becomes clear that the ability of any one individual to metabolize a particular drug can be difficult to predict, particularly when he or she is ill. Where the margin between therapeutic failure (due to a relative underdosage) and toxicity (due to relative overdosage) is large, such differences may be important only for a few individuals lying at the extremes of rapid and slow metabolism. Where the margin of safety is small, special steps must be taken to ensure therapeutic efficacy or safety.

Scientific basis of therapeutics
Efficacy
Until about 1950, most therapeutic remedies were introduced into clinical practice on the basis of anecdotal evidence. The effects in a few patients would be observed and, if apparent benefit occurred, others with the same disease would then be treated. This approach to the demonstration of efficacy of a new, or established, remedy is now regarded as hopelessly unreliable and has been responsible, over several thousand years, for the adoption of much useless treatment. First, the natural progression of most disease is extraordinarily variable. Even patients with lethal forms of cancer may quite spontaneously have prolonged periods of remission; patients with less life-threatening conditions (including many psychiatric, neurological, rheumatic, dermatological, and cardiac disorders) also have long remissions, or the disease may even show spontaneous arrest; furthermore, many everyday illnesses, such as the common infectious diseases of childhood or musculoskeletal injuries, usually recover without (or despite) medical intervention. Under these circumstances the apparent demonstration of recovery, remission, or reduction of symptoms in a few patients forms no basis for the scientific proof of efficacy. Secondly, the demonstration in the laboratory that a particular drug has pharmacological properties which are likely to be useful in certain diseases, is no reason for assuming therapeutic efficacy, even though it might represent a valid reason for careful clinical studies. Not only may man fail to respond in the same way as laboratory animals, but he may also experience severe adverse effects which outweigh the drug's benefits. Thirdly, drugs are often used in conjunction with other therapeutic manoeuvres, such as bed-rest, nursing care, physiotherapy, or other drugs. Comparisons between patients treated with a new drug, and previous experience (often referred to as 'historical' controls), can readily be confounded by

such changing factors. Furthermore, the psychological effects of using a new drug are so profound, in both patient and doctor, that unintentional bias on the part of both parties may lead to erroneous conclusions. Patients with primarily subjective symptoms such as *anxiety, *depression, *pain, *insomnia, and *nausea often show some improvement even when given tablets or capsules containing no active pharmacological ingredient. This so-called '*placebo' response does not mean that the particular symptoms are nonexistent, or overplayed, but is a demonstration of the power of the optimistic psyche to influence subjective sensations.

The randomized controlled *clinical trial is a technique for examining efficacy which aims to eliminate all these sources of bias. Its evolution over the past 30 years owes much to the late Sir Austin Bradford Hill, and represents one of the most important advances in medical science in the 20th century. Its principles have been used not only to evaluate the efficacy of drugs and other therapeutic manoeuvres (*surgery, physiotherapy) but also in the fields of *public health, education, social sciences, and even the penal system. The technique is as follows: patients with a particular disorder, and who are reasonably homogeneous (i.e. alike in relevant characteristics), are randomly allocated to two (or more) treatment groups. One group receives the particular drug under study, and other groups receive either no drug, a *placebo, or a comparative drug. The outcome in the patients in each group is then compared statistically, and the likelihood of any difference occurring as a result of chance is calculated: if the probability of a difference occurring by chance is less than 1 in 20, then the 'null' hypothesis (i.e. that there is *no* difference between treatments) is usually rejected. If further analysis of the study shows flaws, then this conclusion may be revised: for example, subsequent examination of the patients' records may show that, fortuitously, those with less severe forms of the disease were—despite 'random' allocation—allocated to one treatment group.

Various additional measures are frequently adopted in randomized controlled trials to eliminate confounding factors. Very often, and especially where subjectivity by the patient or investigator might introduce bias, the patient and the doctor are kept ignorant of the treatment group to which the former has been randomly allocated. This so-called 'double-blind' technique can be undertaken by ensuring that the patients in the control group receive a drug, or placebo, that is similar in appearance, smell, and taste to that given to the test group. A further refinement, often adopted in studying the efficacy of a drug which produces symptomatic relief of a chronic disorder (e.g. arthritis or high blood pressure), is the 'crossover trial'. In this technique, the patient is treated with both the test drug and, on a separate occasion, the control drug. Thus, patients act as their own controls, but the method is obviously ethically inapplicable in circumstances where a cure resulting from the use of the drug is highly probable.

Table 1 Some drugs used in the treatment of gastrointestinal disorders

| Therapeutic class | Pharmacological class | Drugs | |
		Generic name	Brand names (UK examples)
Antiulcer agent	Antacid	Aluminium hydroxide	Aludrox®
Antiulcer agent	Antacid	Magnesium trisilicate	
Antiulcer agent	Histamine (H₂) antagonist	Cimetidine	Tagamet®
Antiulcer agent	Histamine (H₂) antagonist	Ranitidine	Zantac®
Antiulcer agent	Mucosal protective	Tripotassium dicitratobismuthate	De-Not®
Antiulcer agent	Mucosal protective	Sucralfate	Antepsin®
Antidiarrhoeal	Opioid	Codeine phosphate	
Antidiarrhoeal	Opioid	Loperamide	Imodium®
Laxative	Bulking agent	Ispaghula husk	Isogel® Metamucil®
Laxative	Stimulant	Senna	Senokot®
Laxative	Osmotic laxative	Lactulose	Duphalac®

Table 2 Some drugs used in the treatment of cardiovascular disorders

| Therapeutic class | Pharmacological/chemical class | Drugs | |
		Generic name	Brand names (UK examples)
Antiarrhythmic	Local anaesthetic	Lignocaine	Xylocard®
Antihypertensive	Angiotensin-converting enzyme inhibitor	Captopril	Capoten®
		Enalapril	Innovace®
Antianginal	Nitrate	Glyceryl trinitrate	Sustac®
Antianginal	Nitrate	Isosorbide dinitrate	Cedocard®
Antianginal	Calcium antagonist	Nifedipine	Adalat®
–	Beta-noradrenoceptor antagonist	Atenolol	Tenormin®
–	Diuretic	Bendrofluazide	Aprinox®
–	Diuretic	Frusemide	Lasix®
–	Cardiac glycoside	Digoxin	Lanoxin®
–	Anticoagulant	Heparin	Hepsal®
		Warfarin	Marevan®

Ideally, a randomized controlled trial should use a placebo as the control treatment. This not only allows a smaller number of patients to be studied (because the difference in response between the groups is likely to be larger) but also allows a more accurate estimate to be made of adverse effects. In circumstances where no effective form of alternative treatment is available, there can be no moral or ethical objection to the use of a placebo, provided that patients have freely given their consent to participate. Where effective alternatives are already available, then the control group is normally treated with a comparative drug. The fact that in one randomized controlled trial the difference between the test group and the control group is 'statistically significant' does not necessarily prove that the new treatment is effective, because, even in the absence of bias, any conclusion is based on an assessment of probabilities. It is customary, therefore, for new drugs to be assessed

Table 3 Some drugs used in the treatment of respiratory disorders

| Therapeutic class | Pharmacological class | Drugs | |
		Generic name	Brand names (UK examples)
Bronchodilator	Beta-adrenoceptor agonist	Salbutamol	Ventolin®
Bronchodilator	Cholinergic antagonist	Ipratoprium bromide	Atrovent®
Bronchodilator	Phosphodiesterase inhibitor	Theophylline	
Bronchodilator	Inhaled corticosteroid	Betamethasone valerate	Bextasol®
Bronchodilator	Mast-cell stabilizer	Sodium cromoglycate	Intal®

by several independent clinical trials. When the aim of a trial is to show that the test drug is as effective as an established remedy, the statistical technique is to calculate the probability of no difference, and this requires much larger numbers of patients within each group. Finally, it is important to appreciate that although a new drug may be '*statistically*' better than placebo, this result may not be *clinically* significant: in the case of a new drug for obesity, an average weight loss of 1 kg (2.2 lb) over 3 months compared with a placebo may be statistically significant, but is of little clinical relevance as the amount of weight loss over so long a period would be regarded as inadequate.

Drugs in common use to treat infections and disorders of the various body systems are listed in Tables 1–8.

Adverse reactions

Unwanted and unintended effects of drugs given as normal therapeutic doses are known as adverse reactions (often inaccurately described as side-effects). All drugs will produce, at least in some individuals, adverse reactions which can be classified into one of two types.

(a) Type A reactions are augmented pharmacological effects which are exaggerated, but otherwise predictable responses. They are usually manifestations of pharmacological effects which are observed when larger than normal doses are given. Examples include low blood pressure (*hypotension) resulting from the use of antihypertensive agents, hangover effects from *hypnotics, or constipation with opioid analgesics. They occur either because of enhanced sensitivity of the particular tissue or organ at which the drug acts, or because the individual displays unusual 'handling' of the drug. Individuals who eliminate the drug slowly will be at particular risk.

Type A reactions are usually common, predictable from the known pharmacology of the drug, reproducible in animals, and rarely dangerous. Although

they usually disappear when the drug is stopped, they are not necessarily an indication to withdraw the drug altogether—merely that the dose should be reduced.

(b) Type B reactions are bizarre responses that are unrelated to the drugs' known pharmacological properties. They are often unpredictable, and can rarely be reproduced in experimental animals. Typical examples include *rashes with antibiotics. They are not apparently dose-dependent, are often serious, and are usually an indication to stop the drug completely.

Common adverse reactions, occurring more often than once in 500 patients, are usually recognized during early clinical trials. Indeed, safety evaluation has now become an important and integral component of clinical trials for efficacy because it is possible in this setting to adopt objective criteria for their detection. Thus, investigators will record the frequency of any adverse clinical events in both the test and control groups: a statistically significant increase in the frequency of particular symptoms or abnormal laboratory tests amongst patients treated with the test drug strongly suggest an adverse reaction. In this manner, it is possible to identify previously unsuspected adverse reactions and to obtain some estimate of their frequency.

Reactions occurring more rarely can be extremely difficult to recognize. For statistical reasons, if a reaction occurs once in 1000 treated patients, 3000 of these treated patients would have to be observed to be 95 per cent certain of seeing the reaction in one. If the potential reaction is indistinguishable from a common naturally occurring disorder, then the number of subjects required could run into tens of thousands. Several techniques have been devised to solve this problem. In the wake of the *thalidomide tragedy, the UK Committee on the Safety of Medicines set up a spontaneous reporting system whereby all doctors are asked to inform the Committee, in strict confidence, about any suspected adverse reaction they encounter. Although

Table 4 Some drugs used in the treatment of central nervous system disorders

Therapeutic class	Pharmacological/ chemical class	Drugs	
		Generic	Brand names (UK examples)
Hypnotic	Benzodiazepine	Temazepam	Eukypnos®
Anxiolytic	Benzodiazepine	Diazepam	Valium®
Anxiolytic	Benzodiazepine	Lorazepam	Ativan®
Antipsychotic	Dopamine antagonist	Haloperidol	Haldol®
Antidepressant	Tricyclic drug	Amitriptyline	Tryptizol®
Antidepressant	Tricyclic drug	Dothiepin	Prothiaden®
Antidepressant	Monoamine-oxidase inhibitor	Phenelzine	Nardil®
Antidepressant	Selective serotonin re-uptake inhibitor	Fluvoxamine	Faverin®
Antiemetic	Cholinergic antagonist	Hyoscine	
Antiemetic	Dopamine antagonist	Metoclopramide	Maxolon®
Analgesic	Prostaglandin synthetase inhibitor	Aspirin	Solprin®
		Ibuprofen	Brufen®
Analgesic	Opioid	Codeine	
Anticonvulsant	Hydantoin	Phenytoin	Epanutin®
Anticonvulsant	Iminostilbene	Carbamazepine	Tegretol®
Anticonvulsant	GABA transaminase inhibitor	Valproate	Epilim®
Antiparkinsonian	Dopamine precursor	Levodopa	Sinemet® Madopar®
Antiparkinsonian	Cholinergic antagonist	Orphenadrine	Artane®

GABA, gamma-aminobutyric acid.

Table 5 Some drugs used in the treatment of infections

Therapeutic class	Pharmacological/ chemical class	Drugs	
		Generic name	Brand name (UK examples)
Antibacterial	Penicillins	Benzylpenicillin	Crystapen®
		Ampicillin	Penbritin®
Antibacterial	Cephalosporins	Cephaloridine	Ceporin®
Antibacterial	Tetracyclines	Oxytetracycline	Imperacin®
Antibacterial	Aminoglycosides	Gentamicin	Genticin®
Antibacterial	Sulphonamides	Sulphamethoxazole	
Antituberculous		Isoniazid	Rimifon®
		Rifampicin	Rifadin®
Antifungal agent	Imidazole	Miconazole	Manistat®
Antiviral agent		Acyclovir	Zovirax®
Antiviral agent	Reverse transcriptase inhibitor	Zidovudine	Retrovir®
Antiprotozoal agent	Antimalarials	Primaquine	
Antiprotozoal agent	Antimalarials	Proguanil	Paludrine®
Antiprotozoal agent	Amoebicides and trichomonacides	Metronidazole	Flagyl®
Antihelminthic	Ascaricides	Piperazine	Antepar®
		Thiabendazole	Mintezol®

Table 6 Some drugs used in the treatment of musculoskeletal disorders

Therapeutic class	Pharmacological/ chemical class	Drugs	
		Generic name	Brand names (UK examples)
Non-steroidal anti-inflammatory	Salicylate	Aspirin	Solprin®
Non-steroidal anti-inflammatory	Propionic acid derivative	Ibuprofen	Brufen®
Non-steroidal anti-inflammatory	Acetic acid derivative	Diclofenac	Voltarol®
Non-steroidal anti-inflammatory	Indolacetic acid derivative	Indomethacin	Indocid®
Non-steroidal anti-inflammatory	Oxicam	Piroxicam	Feldene®
Antirheumatic	Gold salt	Aurothiomalate	Myocrisin®
Antirheumatic	Chelating agent	Penicillamine	Distamine®
Antigout	Xanthine oxidase inhibitor	Allopurinol	Zyloric®

Table 7 Some drugs used in the treatment of malignant disease

Pharmacological/ chemical class	Drugs	
	Generic name	Brand names (UK examples)
Alkylating agent	Cyclophosphamide	Endoxana®
	Melphelan	Alkeran®
Cytotoxic antibiotic	Doxorubicin	Adriamycin®
	Bleomycin	
Antimetabolite	Methotrexate	
	Mercaptopurine	Puri-Nethol®
Vinca alkaloids	Vincristine	Oncovin®

it has generated useful information, this method is uncontrolled and can lead to bias; consequently, other methods are usually needed to confirm or refute an association between drugs and suspected adverse reactions. A method which has proved to be particularly valuable once such a hypothesis has been generated, is the 'case–control' study. In this, the frequency of takers of a drug amongst patients developing a particular condition is compared with the frequency of takers of the same drug in patients who do not suffer from the condition. The technique can be quick and effective, as was the case with the association between blood clotting and the contraceptive pill. The second technique is the cohort study, where a large group of patients starting treatment with a drug are followed for months or years. This approach can not only confirm suspected adverse reactions and recognize previously unsuspected reactions, but can also estimate their incidence. Against

this are the considerable logistic problems that arise in identifying the appropriate patients and arranging for their long-term follow-up.

In the UK, at the same time a new drug is marketed for widespread use, the benefit–risk ratio will have been carefully considered by the Committee on Safety of Medicines and found to be favourable. Where it is found to be unfavourable, the drug is refused a marketing licence. For reasons discussed above, this decision is in many respects a provisional one and, with time, the assessment may change. Thus, rare but important adverse effects may appear when many thousands of patients are treated, as some adverse effects may manifest themselves only after many years of continuous use, or safer drugs may become available. Where the benefit–risk ratio appears to become unfavourable, the Committee on Safety of Medicines may recommend changes in the terms under which the drug

Table 8 Some drugs used in the treatment of endocrine disorders

| Therapeutic class | Pharmacological/ chemical class | Drugs | |
		Generic name	Brand names (UK examples)
Antidiabetic	Insulin	Neutral insulin	Actrapid®
		Insulin zinc suspension	Monotard®
Antidiabetic	Sulphonylurea	Tolbutamide	Rastinon®
		Glibenclamide	Daonil®
Antidiabetic	Biguanides	Metformin	Glucophage®
Antithyroid		Carbimazole	Neo-Mercazole®
Steroids	Glucocorticoids	Prednisolone	Prednesol®
		Cortisone	Cortisyl®
Steroids	Oestrogens	Ethinyloestradiol	
		Mestranol	
Steroids	Progestogens	Norethisterone	
		Medroxyprogesterone	
Steroids	Androgens	Testosterone	
		Methyltestosterone	

can be marketed, or may recommend to the Secretary of State for Health that its licence be revoked or suspended.

M. D. RAWLINS

Further reading
ABPI Data Sheet Compendium (1993–94). Datapharm Publications, London.
British National Formulary (1993). British Medical Association and The Pharmaceutical Society of Great Britain, London.
D'Arcy, P. F. and Griffin, J. P. (ed.) (1986). *Iatrogenic diseases*, (3rd edn). Oxford University Press, Oxford.
Davies, D. M. (ed.) (1991). *Textbook of adverse drug reactions*, (4th edn). Oxford University Press, Oxford.
Dollery, C. T. (1991). *Therapeutic drugs*. Churchill Livingstone, Edinburgh.
Dukes, M. N. G. (ed.) (1988). *Meyler's side effects of drugs*. Excerpta Medica, Amsterdam; Elsevier, New York.
Martindale: the extra pharmacopoeia, (30th edn) (1993). Pharmaceutical Press, London.
Speight, T. M. (1982). *Avery's drug treatment*, (3rd edn). ADIS Press, Auckland; Churchill Livingstone, Edinburgh.

PHARMACOPOEIA. A compilation of recognized drugs, giving data relevant to preparation, recognition, standards of purity, dosage, storage, and labelling. See also *BRITISH PHARMACOPOEIA; NATIONAL FORMULARY (USA); NATIONAL FORMULARY, BRITISH*.

PHARMACOPOEIA COMMISSION. A body set up under the *Medicines Act 1968 charged with the responsibility, under the authority of the Health Ministers, of preparing new editions of and amendments to the *British Pharmacopoeia* (previously the responsibility of the *General Medical Council).

PHARMACY ACTS 1852, 1868, 1954. These UK statutes are analogous to the *Medical Acts. They concern the education, qualification, standards, conduct, and control of the pharmaceutical profession and the powers and duties conferred on the professional body for pharmacy, the *Royal Pharmaceutical Society of Great Britain. See PHARMACY AND PHARMACISTS.

PHARMACY AND PHARMACISTS (IN THE UK). 'What medicine owes to pharmacy it owes chiefly to the Pharmaceutical Society of Great Britain', said the *Lancet* on the occasion of the society's centenary in 1941. A fine tribute indeed to an organization that continues to serve the medical profession well because it does so through its service to the pharmaceutical profession; service which is informed by a conscious need to put the public interest in the forefront when policy decisions are made.

The Royal Pharmaceutical Society of Great Britain
The Royal Pharmaceutical Society of Great Britain, as it is now known, is unique because it combines, largely through the fortuitous mutations of history, functions for the pharmaceutical profession similar to those performed separately for the medical profession by the *British Medical Association (BMA) and the *General Medical Council (GMC), plus a law-enforcement role, but with no direct part in negotiations over remuneration. The society does, of course, represent the views of the profession to government departments and to other professions.

How did the Pharmaceutical Society arise and what are its functions? The answers to these questions may help to demonstrate the multifarious activities of pharmacists, how they are educated and trained to meet their responsibilities, and what those responsibilities are.

The society was founded in 1841 at a time when no pharmaceutical profession as such existed in Britain. The pharmacists' true predecessors were the *apothecaries, who had largely, though by no means entirely, become medical practitioners. The bulk of *drugs were supplied by chemists and druggists, who were thus fulfilling as best they could the role being vacated by the apothecaries. Unfortunately, many of the chemists and druggists were inadequate to the task. Indeed, John Savory (the name is perpetuated in the chain of pharmacies known today as Savory and Moore) was the instigator in 1830 of a proposed petition to the government to introduce a bill to regulate the practice of pharmacy, pointing out 'the prevalence of ignorant and incompetent persons calling themselves chemists and druggists'.

The opportunity for the foundation of the Pharmaceutical Society was provided by proposed legislation that threatened to bring chemists and druggists under the control of apothecaries and to prevent them from counter prescribing—a prohibition that would, in the words of Jacob Bell (chemist and druggist of Oxford Street, London, and the true founder of the society) have deprived the poorer classes of the benefit of medicine altogether.

Although the immediate threat of legislation was lifted through the opposition of chemists and druggists, the latter realized that the problem could reappear. Hence they supported the foundation of a permanent body to represent their interests. The Pharmaceutical Society was thus established on 15 April, 1841, gaining its Royal Charter in 1843.

Jacob Bell recognized that the key to professional status lay in education. For that reason, the new society inaugurated in 1842, at its headquarters in Bloomsbury Square, a school of pharmacy which, since 1949 has been the School of Pharmacy of the University of London. The school's professors have been recognized as teachers of the university since the beginning of the century, and the school has been awarding London University degrees since the 1920s.

With the physical takeover of the school by the university in 1949 and its move to new premises in Brunswick Square in the 1950s, the society's own scientific activities were reorganized in a new department called the Department of Pharmaceutical Sciences.

A main function of the department is the compilation of scientific publications, including the *British national formulary* (published jointly with the *BMA), *Clarke's isolation and identification of drugs*, and *Martindale* (the Extra *Pharmacopoeia) which is claimed to be 'the world's most comprehensive source of drug information in a single volume' (and a massive and massively authoritative volume it is). It is also available 'on-line' and in a CD-ROM version.

The department is also responsible for a medicines testing laboratory and a pharmaceutics laboratory (both housed in the society's Scottish Department headquarters in Edinburgh). The former provides an analytical service principally to the Medicines Control Agency of the Department of Health.

The society's library, founded in 1841, is now part of the Department of Pharmaceutical Sciences and includes an information office.

The department organizes all kinds of scientific meetings, including postgraduate schools. When required, advisory committees or working parties are set up by the department on matters of current concern.

The society also conducts the annual British Pharmaceutical Conference held to discuss scientific and professional matters. Periodicals published by the Society include the weekly *Pharmaceutical Journal*, the monthly *Journal of Pharmacy and Pharmacology*, and the occasional *International Journal of Pharmacy Practice*.

The society is actively engaged in developing the practice of pharmacy in each of its branches (described in detail later) and in promoting continuing education for practising pharmacists. It offers various research scholarships and two practice research awards.

As has been said, the society performs functions analogous to those discharged on behalf of the medical profession by the *GMC. Thus, the society is responsible for maintaining the registers of pharmaceutical chemists and pharmacy premises.

Education

Anyone who has been awarded a degree in pharmacy in the UK which has been approved by the society, and who has completed satisfactorily a year of pre-registration training, can be registered by the society as a pharmaceutical chemist (pharmacist).

In approving pharmacy degrees, the society does not impose a model syllabus but is concerned mainly that, whatever the course, the student must receive a sufficiently broad understanding of the scientific principles and techniques of the pharmaceutical sciences to become, after postgraduate training in practice, a competent pharmacist. The course is expected to provide students with a comprehensive knowledge of, and expertise in, all aspects of the preparation, distribution, and action and uses of drugs and medicines, both human and veterinary.

Each school receives, at intervals of no more than 5 years, a visiting party from the society which examines the facilities and discusses with academic staff and students the agreed programme.

The society describes four main elements to be included in the course and provides a broad indication of the scope of each element, as follows:

1. Chemistry of drugs, of other constituents of medicines, and of biological systems. The sources, structures, and properties of chemical substances

of natural and synthetic origin used in medicine; the relevant molecular structure of, and the molecular interactions of, drugs in biological systems, including the principles of pharmacodynamics, *pharmacokinetics, and drug design (see also PHARMACOLOGY); physicochemical aspects of drugs and of biological systems, including chemical kinetics and thermodynamics; chemical stability; analytical methods; physical and chemical tests and other aspects of specifications for drugs.

2. Medicines design and manufacture; materials, methods, and quality standards. Physical, chemical, and biological properties of materials, formulations, and devices used to deliver biologically active molecules. Biopharmaceutics and pharmacokinetics in relation to drug absorption and disposition, formulation criteria, and dosage regimens. Evaluation and control of physical, chemical, and biological degradation of drugs and medicines; principles of preservation against microbial contamination. Design and standardization of medicines for administration to the body by different routes, and to specific target sites. Technical specifications for pharmaceutical excipients, including water. The influence of pharmaceutical and biochemical engineering processes on product quality, including biological safety, bioavailability, dosage uniformity and stability; principles and evaluation of aseptic procedures and sterilization processes in the preparation of pharmaceutical, surgical, and medical products and devices. Immunological products. Radiopharmaceuticals. Quality assurance of pharmaceutical products and processes; packaging, good manufacturing practice, environmental control, pharmacopoeial and regulatory requirements.

3. Action and uses of drugs, medicines, and other products. Cell biology; human and mammalian *physiology, *biochemistry, *pathology, and *pathophysiology, as a basis for the understanding of disease and of the *pharmacology of drugs. Biological methods of measurement of drug activity; chemical, physical, biochemical, and biological aspects of the actions of drugs and other agents in man, animals, and plants. Immunological aspects of disease and *chemotherapy. The therapeutic uses and adverse reactions of drugs and medicines, their relevance to the treatment of humans and animals. Concepts of clinical pharmacy, including the rational use of drugs in patients. The existence of, and opportunities for, misuse and abuse; drug dependence. Principles of treatment of disease, focusing on the process of problem-solving; *therapeutics associated with clinical *toxicology and *epidemiology.

4. The practice of pharmacy: includes the law, *ethics and practice of pharmacy, and social and behavioural sciences.

The society expects each of the first three elements to be given approximately the same emphasis in the core curriculum and recognizes that part of the final year might be devoted to the study of one principal subject. Also, those components of the undergraduate course which collectively deal with the actions and uses of drugs and medicines are expected to occupy about 35 per cent of the whole course, irrespective of the degree of specialization in the final year.

There are 16 schools of pharmacy in the UK, all in universities. Each has its own entrance requirements, which are usually three 'A' levels, including chemistry plus any two subjects from a biological science, mathematics, and physics. Alternatively, applicants may offer an equivalent combination of two 'A' levels and two 'AS' levels, provided that chemistry and another science are included at 'A' level and that not more than one non-science subject is offered at 'AS' level. Most institutions also accept equivalent Scottish 'Highers'.

The three- or four-year courses lead to a Bachelor of Science (B.Sc.) honours degree in pharmacy or a Bachelor of Pharmacy (B.Pharm.) honours degree, according to the school of pharmacy attended.

Persons registered as pharmacists automatically become members of the Royal Pharmaceutical Society. The number of members at the end of 1992 was approximately 39 000.

The society's Statutory Committee is the equivalent of the GMC's Disciplinary Committee. The Statutory Committee has power over pharmacists and corporate bodies owning pharmacies, and may disqualify both. The society issues a code of ethics which is intended to set the standard of professional conduct, and with which pharmacists are obliged to conform.

Register of pharmacies

The society is required by statute to maintain a register of pharmacies, as has been mentioned. The pharmacies (and the premises of agricultural merchants, saddlers, and feed compounders, for whom the society also maintains registers) are visited regularly by members of a corps of 26 inspectors maintained by the society. The society is responsible for enforcement of certain provisions of the *Medicines Act, particularly those relating to the sale and supply of medicines that can be sold only in pharmacies, and the sale, supply, or administration of prescription-only medicines. There are about 12 000 pharmacies currently on the register of premises, each required to be under the personal control of a pharmacist, and in each of which sales of medicines that can be sold only in pharmacies must be sold by, or under the supervision of, a pharmacist.

By far the largest proportion of pharmacists are engaged in what is called community or retail pharmacy. The number is about 20 000. Hospitals employ about 5000; industry, 1400; and wholesaling and teaching, smaller numbers still. There are large numbers of registered pharmacists who no longer practise; and substantial numbers live overseas.

How pharmacy practice has changed

Pharmacy practice has changed dramatically since the start of the century, when the physician's therapeutic armamentarium was largely galenicals—infusions, tinctures, extracts and powders of crude, mainly vegetable drugs. It has to be remembered, however, that the active ingredients of many vegetable drugs—*morphine from opium and *quinine from cinchona bark, for example— were isolated during the early 19th century. Indeed, it was the development of organic chemistry in the 19th century that led to the pharmaceutical revolution of the 20th century, with its synthetic chemical medicines. The first was *arsphenamine, discovered by Paul *Ehrlich in 1904, and better known as Salvarsan (salvation of humanity against syphilis). In the 1930s came the antibacterial *Prontosil® in Germany and the *sulphonamide M&B 693 in the UK. The development of *penicillin in the 1940s was followed by a plethora of other valuable medicines in what has been called the 'first therapeutic revolution'.

At the same time, the compounding of medicines has moved largely from the pharmacy to the pharmaceutical factory. Even in the 1950s, compounding was being performed in the pharmacy—ointments, plasters, pills, powders in single dose form, capsules, cachets, mixtures, and emulsions.

Now, however, apart from a tiny percentage of prescriptions, if any of those operations are required they are performed in pharmaceutical factories, along with the principal dose form, the tablet. Incidentally, the tablet machine dates from the 19th century. Such manufacturing as continues in hospital pharmacies, apart from specialist items, is now limited to a few centres.

So, in the first half of this century, the pharmacist performed his supply role of compounding and dispensing medicines. One of his main concerns was physical incompatibilities in prescriptions. Today, one of the pharmacist's principal concerns is pharmacological incompatibilities. The therapeutic revolution has compelled the pharmacist to concentrate on clinical aspects of medicines—a necessity that was foreseen by the more perspicacious in the 1930s.

The enormous expansion in the numbers and varieties of potent medicines has made the task of the pharmacist much more difficult. Apart from the danger of confusion between closely similar names, there is the complexity of dosage regimens and the problem of pharmacological incompatibilities and drug interactions. Labelling also may now be much more complex.

Today, the essential knowledge for the pharmacist, as for the prescriber, is pharmacokinetics (what the body does to medicines) and pharmacodynamics (what medicines do to the body) (see PHARMACOLOGY). That is taken care of in the pharmacist's education as has been shown above, with roughly one-third of the pharmacy syllabus, so far as it concerns the pharmaceutical sciences, dealing with clinical aspects of medicines.

A leading British medicinal chemist (Professor Arnold Beckett) has said that the education of the pharmacist should lead to his being an expert in drugs and the expert in medicines. What he meant was that only the pharmacist was the expert on the formulation of medicines. Incorrect formulation or storage could lead to incorrect bioavailability. The educational programme should, therefore, according to Professor Beckett, emphasize the factors and principles of drug formulation and bioavailability. Bioavailability is the release of the products of the metabolized drug to the body tissues. For example, the breakdown of the first antibacterial Prontosil® into sulphanilamide was responsible for its activity.

The historical changes just discussed have affected all branches of pharmacy, including industrial pharmacy which effected them. Yet, the basic responsibilities of the pharmacist in respect of the dispensing of prescribed medicines remain the same. Those responsibilities include, first, quality assurance of the medicines supplied and, secondly, security of the patient, which requires constant vigilance on the part of the pharmacist and a duty to query any prescription with the prescriber if there is any cause for doubt whatever.

Indeed, in a case heard in the High Court in 1982 concerning an overdose of Migril®, the substantial damages awarded against the prescriber were only slightly greater than those against the pharmacist concerned.

While hospital consultant physicians may acquire an expert knowledge of the relatively narrow range of medicines they prescribe, the general medical practitioner is in a rather different situation, faced as he or she is with a wider range of problems. The value of the hospital pharmacist to the hospital doctor is discussed later. In the case of the general medical practitioner, the community pharmacist can, and does, provide welcome prescribing advice. He may do so by studying prescribing habits and highlighting the medicines that are not being used but could, with advantage, be utilized, and, on the other hand, explaining why some medicines should not have been used. Pharmacists can also give advice on the sometimes vexed question of prescribing by generic rather than brand names.

Another important function of the community pharmacist is that of counter prescribing, or as it is now known, 'responding to symptoms', a preferable term because it is perhaps more accurate. The pharmacist can supply symptomatic treatment with advice to consult a doctor if the symptoms persist. On the other hand, should the pharmacist suspect that the symptoms reflect a serious condition, and one where treatment of the symptoms might merely suppress the warning signs, he should not supply a medicine but advise the patient to see a doctor. The pharmacist has been aided in recent years by the transference of certain prescription-only medicines to the pharmacy medicines category, i.e. medicines that may be sold over the counter to the general public by a pharmacist. Pharmacists are also allowed to supply small quantities of prescription-only medicines under certain conditions in an emergency.

Community pharmacists also have a role in providing some health screening tests and in advising the public generally on health matters such as *diet, *family planning, baby care, and oral hygiene. The community pharmacist may also provide an advisory service to nursing homes, etc., concerning the storage and administration of medicines.

Hospital pharmacy

The therapeutic revolution has greatly affected hospital pharmacy. Until the mid-1960s, hospital pharmacists rarely left their departments. It was then realized that if the pharmacist's knowledge was to be utilized more fully and sensibly, it would be necessary that he should be clearly seen as part of the patient-care team, meaning basically that he would be included in the prescriber–nurse–patient situation on the ward. Hence the emergence of the ward pharmacist, who has developed into the clinical pharmacist.

The fundamental task of the clinical pharmacist is to promote safe, effective, and economical medication. That means advising the doctor on prescribing, and nurses, and perhaps patients, on administration. Clinical pharmacists advise on the initiation of therapy, prevent prescription errors, and may deter unnecessary medication. They may also provide a therapeutic drug monitoring service for certain medicines; this is a pharmacokinetic service designed to control dosage where the safety and effectiveness of a particular medicine present special difficulties.

Apart from the clinical activities undertaken by hospital pharmacists, they are also responsible for the purchase of medicines, the supply of medicines to the wards for general use and for individual in-patients, and also the dispensing of medicines for out-patients. Pharmacists are also responsible for the prescription and supply of total parenteral nutrition for individual patients. They also maintain quality assurance facilities and perform a limited amount of manufacture.

Some pharmacists specialize in radiopharmacy—the preparation of radioactive diagnostic and therapeutic agents. Most large hospital pharmacies maintain a drug information service for their own and their hospital colleagues' use. Like community pharmacists, hospital pharmacists are available to nursing homes, etc., in a mainly advisory capacity.

*Pharmaceutical industry

The pharmacist's educational background equips him to engage in almost every department of the pharmaceutical industry. Many are engaged in general management, many in research. Formulation naturally attracts some pharmacists. Others are concerned with process and packaging development, production, quality assurance, marketing, and regulatory affairs (licensing of medicines).

By way of illustration of the contribution of pharmacists to the pharmaceutical industry, it may be mentioned that the top British company, Glaxo, was very much the creation of a pharmacist, the late Sir Harry Jephcott. Moreover, the way to its current success was paved largely by another pharmacist, Sir David Jack, FRS, recently retired research director of the Glaxo Group. He was brought into Allen & Hanburys (A&H) (a subsidiary of Glaxo) by the late C. W. Maplethorpe, also a pharmacist, and then managing director of A&H. Maplethorpe was a former president of the Pharmaceutical Society, the first president of which, in 1841, was William Allen, FRS, who was the Allen of Allen & Hanburys.

ROBERT BLYTH

PHARMACY AND POISONS ACT 1933. This UK Act, together with the subsequent Poisons List Order and Rules 1966–68, established control of the practice of pharmacy and the sale and supply of 'poisons'. Under the Act, a Poisons Board was created with authority to draw up a Poisons List. The List recognizes two classes of substance: those used in medical, dental, and veterinary practice and restricted to sale by registered pharmacists; and those in common domestic use, which may be sold by persons registered by local authorities. Restrictions on sale and supply vary with the nature of the substances, and certain exemptions are made. Subsequent relevant legislation was contained in the Pharmacy and Medicines Act 1941, the *Medicines Act 1968, and the *Poisons Act 1972. See PHARMACY AND PHARMACISTS.

PHARYNGITIS is inflammation of the *pharynx.

PHARYNGOSCOPY is visual examination of the *pharynx.

PHARYNX. The cavity lying behind the nose and mouth and providing the passage of communication from them to the *larynx and the *oesophagus respectively; it is thus a channel both for respiratory gases and for food and drink, common to the respiratory and alimentary tracts. It has a muscular wall lined internally with mucous membrane and is usually divided into three zones: the nasopharynx (above the level of the soft *palate); the oropharynx (between the palate and the upper edge of the *epiglottis); and the hypopharynx (below the upper edge of the epiglottis).

PHASE CONTRAST is a technique of microscopy which allows structural boundaries to be visualized without special staining, based on the use of phase differences of reflected and transmitted light waves passing through and around the objects under study.

PHENACETIN is an aspirin-like *analgesic and *antipyretic drug (*p*-ethoxyacetanilide, also known as acetophenetidin), which, though widely used for many years after its introduction (in 1887), is no longer recommended; taken over long periods, it can cause serious damage to the kidneys (analgesic nephropathy). *Paracetamol is now the preferred alternative to *aspirin.

PHENELZINE is one of the monoamide-oxidase inhibitor group of *antidepressant drugs.

PHENINDIONE is one of the oral *anticoagulants, also known under the proprietary name of Dindevan®. Because of occasional hypersensitivity reactions, the *coumarin group of drugs (e.g. *warfarin sodium) is usually preferred.

PHENOBARBITONE is a long-acting *barbiturate, now rarely used, except in some cases of *epilepsy.

PHENOCOPY. A characteristic, indistinguishable from one which is normally genetically determined, produced by environmental causes.

PHENOL (C_6H_5OH), formerly known as carbolic acid, is a powerful *antiseptic with a characteristic smell. It is poisonous when ingested. See also LISTER.

PHENOLPHTHALEIN. See LAXATIVES.

PHENOME is a term used in classification systems to denote a group of organisms related by *phenotype.

PHENOTHIAZINE is the parent compound of several drugs, of which the prototype is *chlorpromazine, used primarily to treat *psychoses. The phenothiazine derivatives belong to that group of drugs known variously as major *tranquillizers, antipsychotics, or neuroleptics.

PHENOTYPE. The sum of the observed characteristics of an individual, whether of genetic or environmental origin. See GENETICS.

PHENTOLAMINE is an alpha-adrenergic blocking agent; its main use is in the diagnosis and management of *phaeochromocytoma.

PHENYLBUTAZONE is a potent *non-steroidal anti-inflammatory drug (NSAID), once extensively used to treat rheumatic disorders, being particularly effective in *gout and *ankylosing spondylitis. It has, however, various serious side-effects; of the adverse reactions reported, blood *dyscrasias (aplastic anaemia, agranulocytosis, thrombocytopenia) are the most important and have caused some fatalities. In the UK the drug was withdrawn from general use in March 1984. Its use is now restricted to ankylosing spondylitis and its supply limited to hospitals.

PHENYLKETONURIA is a genetically determined inability to metabolize L-phenylalanine, which, unless detected and treated soon after birth, results in mental retardation. See INBORN ERRORS OF METABOLISM.

PHENYTOIN is a drug widely used in the control of *epilepsy, also known under the proprietary names Epanutin® or Dilantin®. It is ineffective in absence seizures (*petit mal).

PHILIP, SIR ROBERT WILLIAM (1857–1939). British physician. He opened the first tuberculosis dispensary in the world in Edinburgh in 1887 and the first in London in Paddington in 1909.

PHILOSOPHER'S STONE. A putative object or mineral substance capable of effecting the transmutation of base metals into gold. It was the ultimate goal of *alchemy and the quest for it was chief among the preoccupations of alchemists ('philosophers'). Some felt that the stone, when found, would also prove to have the power to cure all diseases and to prolong life indefinitely.

PHIMOSIS. A *prepuce, of which the orifice is too small to permit retraction over the glans penis, the usual justification for *circumcision other than that performed on religious or tribal grounds.

PHLEBECTOMY is the surgical excision of part or all of a vein.

PHLEBITIS is inflammation of a vein; it may be due to trauma or infection, or may follow *thrombosis. In either case, since inflammation favours secondary thrombosis, the condition is usually one of 'thrombophlebitis'. The alternative term 'phlebothrombosis' is reserved for cases of venous thrombosis without signs of inflammation.

PHLEBOGRAPHY is the radiographic visualization of veins after filling them with a radiopaque material.

PHLEBOTHROMBOSIS is venous thrombosis without obvious inflammation. See PHLEBITIS.

PHLEBOTOMUS. See SANDFLY.

PHLEBOTOMY is a synonym of *venesection.

PHLEGM was one of the four *humours of early medical science; in modern lay usage, it is equivalent to *sputum.

PHLEGMON. See CELLULITIS.

PHLOGISTON was the supposed principle of combustion, postulated by *Stahl at the beginning of the 18th century to be present in all combustible substances and to be liberated during combustion.

PHLS. See PUBLIC HEALTH LABORATORY SERVICE.

PHOBIA. A pathological fear of a particular class of objects or situations unrelated or disproportionate to any threat it presents. Common phobias are fear of heights, open spaces (agoraphobia), enclosed spaces (claustrophobia), cancer, snakes, syphilis, and very many others. Phobias when disabling may require psychiatric attention.

PHOCOMELIA is a severe congenital anomaly in which the limbs fail to develop, so that the hands and feet may be directly attached to the body. See THALIDOMIDE.

PHONATION is the production of voice sounds.

PHONETICS is the study of voice, vocal sounds, spoken language, and pronunciation.

PHONOCARDIOGRAPHY is the recording of the sounds generated by the action of the heart.

PHOSGENE is carbonyl chloride ($COCl_2$), a colourless poisonous gas with a smell of musty hay. See CHEMICAL WARFARE.

PHOSPHATASE is the term for a large group of *enzymes, widely distributed throughout the body, which split *phosphate from its organic compounds (esters).

PHOSPHATE. Any salt or ester of phosphoric acid (H_3PO_4).

PHOSPHENE is a visual sensation appearing with the eyes shut, not due to the penetration of external light.

PHOSPHORYLATION is the introduction of a phosphate group into an organic molecule.

PHOTOCHEMOTHERAPY is the treatment with drugs which induce sensitivity to light, particularly natural or artificial ultraviolet radiation. For example, members of the psoralen group of drugs are used in combination with long-wave ultraviolet radiation (the combination known for short as PUVA) in the treatment of *psoriasis.

PHOTOMETER. An instrument for measuring luminous intensity, usually by comparing two light sources.

PHOTOMICROGRAPHY is photography with the aid of a *microscope. Photographs so obtained are called photomicrographs.

PHOTOPHOBIA is intolerance of bright light.

PHOTOSENSITIVITY is abnormal sensitivity of the skin to light, particularly sunlight.

PHOTOSYNTHESIS is the process, on which all forms of life (except certain bacteria) depend, by which green plants utilize the energy of sunlight to synthesize carbohydrate from atmospheric carbon dioxide and water. Chemically the reaction is a complex one and not fully understood; the presence of *chlorophyll, however, is essential.

PHRENIC NERVE. A long nerve which arises in the neck from the cervical plexus; it runs downwards to enter the thorax and traverses the length of the *mediastinum to reach the *diaphragm. It carries sensory fibres from the pleura, pericardium, and peritoneum and makes connections with the sympathetic plexuses; but its chief importance is that it provides the motor innervation of the diaphragm, right and left phrenic nerves supplying the respective hemidiaphragms.

PHRENOLOGY is a pseudoscience which purports to relate mental development and mental faculties to the external configuration of the skull.

PHTHISIS is an archaic term for pulmonary *tuberculosis.

PHYCOMYCOSIS is a broad term covering infection with several fungal species; it is almost always 'opportunistic', i.e. it occurs in individuals whose immune defences (see IMMUNOLOGY) have been compromised by pre-existing disease or exposure to immunosuppressive agents.

PHYSIC is an archaic term meaning *internal medicine, that is medicine practised by physicians in the UK and by internists in the USA.

PHYSICAL EXAMINATION is ordinarily taken to mean examination of the patient using the examiner's five senses aided only by the portable tools of his trade such as *stethoscope, tendon hammer, *ophthalmoscope, etc., and excluding special investigative techniques like lumbar puncture, blood biochemistry, radiography, electro-cardiography, etc.

PHYSICIAN. In the UK, one who practises internal medicine or one of its subspecialties, as distinct from surgery and obstetrics; in the USA, any qualified medical practitioner.

PHYSICIANS TO THE SOVEREIGN. See ROYAL MEDICAL HOUSEHOLD.

PHYSICK, PHILIP SYNG (1768–1837). American surgeon, sometimes called the father of American surgery. He was responsible for developing many practical procedures and technical devices useful for the practice of surgery in the pre-anaesthetic era. Among these were methods for dealing with fractures and dislocations, amputations, design of instruments for removal of bladder stone, absorbable suture materials, and curved suturing needles (see also SURGERY).

PHYSICS, MEDICAL (AND SOME CONTRIBUTIONS OF ELECTRONICS AND ENGINEERING TO MEDICINE)
Introduction
Medical physics involves a critical mass of highly qualified, skilled, and caring medical physicists and technologists, from a variety of physical science and engineering disciplines, dedicated to serving patients, their consultants, *general practitioners, and the community.

In case the need for such multidisciplinary expertise is not obvious, it may be helpful to think of the human body in technological terms. The body can be regarded as a machine controlled by the world's most sophisticated microcomputer (the brain), about the size of a large grapefruit and largely self-programmable. The machine is self-propelled in any direction with a forward speed of up to 20 m.p.h. or so. It is largely waterproof, entirely rustproof, and semi-immersible. Control is effected, with automatic feedback, through self-adjusting binoculars and by auditory, olfactory, and tactile signals. The machine is equipped with a pair of sophisticated remote manipulators. It is powered by a wide variety of fuels (ideally unleaded). The machine can self-replicate and, although no guarantee is provided, has an expected lifetime of about 70 years. To a large extent, the machine is self-repairing. However, in the event of a malfunction, diagnosis of the problem (and its rectification) should be achieved ideally without 'lifting the bonnet' and with minimal damage to external bodywork. However, no manuals relating to construction, function, or repair are provided. In these circumstances, there is clearly a need for multidisciplinary collaboration among scientists, technologists, and other health-care professionals.

Hospitals generally comprise many departments spanning the lifetime of our human machines, from *antenatal care through obstetrics and gynaecology to (eventually) geriatrics. In between, there are about 30 departments specializing in diagnosing the problems with components of the human system and in their repair, modification, replacement, or other treatment. Practically all of these departments, as well as the community in general, can (and generally do) benefit from the careful application of science and technology by the medical physics department.

To meet the challenge of this wide-ranging spectrum of demands for support or assistance, medical physics comprises some 20 specialisms or subspecialisms, which are not compartmentalized, generating instead multidisciplinary collaboration and cross-fertilization. As, perhaps, the best way of gaining an understanding of medical physics, we shall briefly 'visit' the more major specialisms, illustrated in Fig. 1 together with some of their contributions.

Medical physics specialisms
Radiotherapy physics
*Radiotherapy physics applies its expertise in measurement to the treatment of *cancer by means of *radiation, ensuring that the dose delivered to a *tumour corresponds accurately with that prescribed by the radiotherapist, and that treatment is planned and treatment aids constructed to minimize adverse effects on healthy tissues nearby. Mould room staff create plastic shells moulded, for example, to the patient's head, which subsequently ensure that the tumour remains exactly in the radiation beam by preventing patient movement during treatment. Operational responsibilities are also undertaken for intracavitary therapy, using radioactive sources rather than external beams, for example in the *cervix or *uterus, as well as for maintenance of the complex therapy machines.

Diagnostic radiology physics
Diagnostic *radiology physics seeks to optimize the images from X-ray exposures while minimizing the radiation doses to patients within programmes of quality assurance.

Radiation protection
Radiation protection is provided to ensure the safe use of all types of radiation. Monitoring of hospital staff and workplaces is undertaken. Advice is provided to health authorities, local authorities, and the public, particularly on major nuclear installations.

Radioisotopes
Radioisotopes are exploited by administering small amounts of radioactively labelled pharmaceuticals, preferentially taken up by specific body organs and tissues (such as the heart, kidneys, lungs, and bone), to image or examine the organs and their dynamic function for diagnosis of a wide range of diseases. Radioisotopes are also administered internally for the treatment of cancer and other diseases. Also see NUCLEAR MEDICINE.

*Ultrasound
Expertise is applied to quality assurance of ultrasonic equipment in hospitals, in undertaking highly specialized examinations, and in developing new equipment and clinical imaging applications.

Bioengineers
Bioengineers provide expertise in mechanical engineering, including supervision of wide-ranging workshop skills. As part of the contributions to *rehabilitation

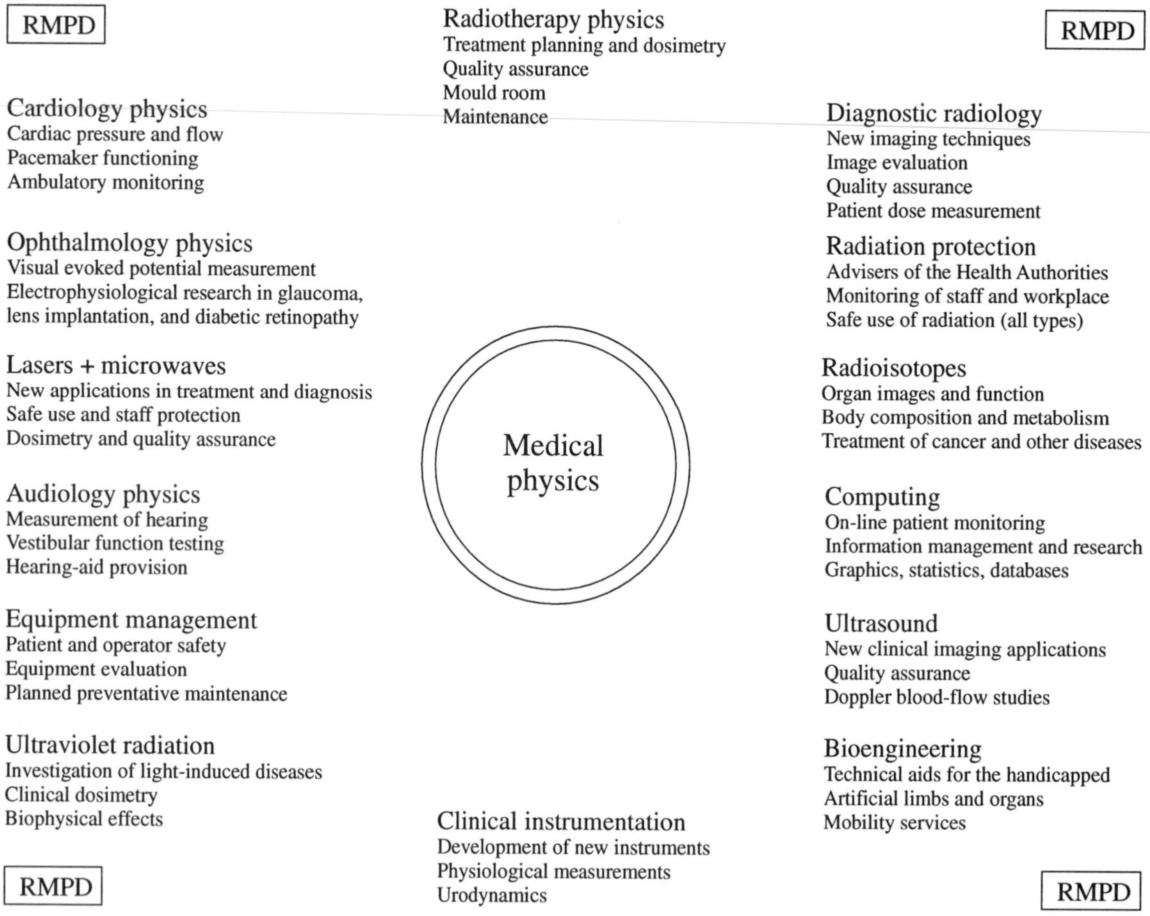

RMPD

Radiotherapy physics
Treatment planning and dosimetry
Quality assurance
Mould room
Maintenance

RMPD

Cardiology physics
Cardiac pressure and flow
Pacemaker functioning
Ambulatory monitoring

Diagnostic radiology
New imaging techniques
Image evaluation
Quality assurance
Patient dose measurement

Ophthalmology physics
Visual evoked potential measurement
Electrophysiological research in glaucoma,
lens implantation, and diabetic retinopathy

Radiation protection
Advisers of the Health Authorities
Monitoring of staff and workplace
Safe use of radiation (all types)

Lasers + microwaves
New applications in treatment and diagnosis
Safe use and staff protection
Dosimetry and quality assurance

Radioisotopes
Organ images and function
Body composition and metabolism
Treatment of cancer and other diseases

Audiology physics
Measurement of hearing
Vestibular function testing
Hearing-aid provision

Medical physics

Computing
On-line patient monitoring
Information management and research
Graphics, statistics, databases

Equipment management
Patient and operator safety
Equipment evaluation
Planned preventative maintenance

Ultrasound
New clinical imaging applications
Quality assurance
Doppler blood-flow studies

Ultraviolet radiation
Investigation of light-induced diseases
Clinical dosimetry
Biophysical effects

Bioengineering
Technical aids for the handicapped
Artificial limbs and organs
Mobility services

Clinical instrumentation
Development of new instruments
Physiological measurements
Urodynamics

RMPD

RMPD

Fig. 1 Components of a regional medical physics department (RMPD).

engineering activities, technical aid services develop individually designed devices as aids for everyday living or mobility for disabled people, or modify suitably commercially available aids for their use. In some centres, responsibility is taken for the provision of powered wheelchairs, the repair of all types of wheelchairs, and advice in quality aspects of artificial limbs.

Cardiology physics
*Cardiology physics provides specialist advice and facilities for clinical measurement and diagnosis in the cardiac investigation laboratories, open-heart theatres, intensive and coronary care units, and for cardiac pacing and 24-hour heart rhythm analysis.

Ophthalmology physics and audiology physics
*Ophthalmology physics and *audiology physics provide and develop state-of-the-art procedures for assessing visual and hearing ability and causes of impairment. Electrophysiological measurements, using electrodes

attached to the head to detect the minute impulses generated by external stimuli (evoked responses), have added greatly to the long-established test procedures.

Laser physics
Laser physics advises on safety and develops new procedures in the diagnostic and surgical use of lasers.

Photobiology
Photobiology is concerned with therapy using ultraviolet radiation in dermatology, especially for psoriasis. Patients with skin diseases caused by exposure to sunlight are investigated. Methods of dosimetry and also of measuring the effectiveness of sunscreens have been developed.

Clinical instrumentation and physiological measurements section
This is involved in the development of new instruments and procedures for physiological measurements, such

as intracranial pressure, blood oxygen concentrations, and blood flow in skin using lasers. The innovative nature of such work often leads to devices potentially capable of commercial exploitation. See also CLINICAL INVESTIGATION.

Computing
Computing is used for processing on-line data from patient monitoring, information management, and research. Advice and assistance are commonly provided to clinical specialties and management.

Equipment management
Equipment management is essential to ensure patient and operator safety, including equipment developed by departments themselves. Evaluation of commercial instruments and planned preventative maintenance are undertaken.

Summary
These specialisms are able to draw collaboratively on the different expertise of one another to provide multidisciplinary solutions to complex clinical problems, or in establishing new services. There is a natural cross-fertilization among the experts of each specialism, often leading to valuable, exciting, and innovative developments or improvements in patient care. Such skills and expertise are rare, diverse, and invaluable. Their integration, as a critical mass within medical physics departments, is essential to the exploitation of modern medicine for the care of patients and people with disabilities in the community.

KEITH BODDY

PHYSIOGNOMY. The face or countenance, particularly viewed as an index to mind or character.

PHYSIOLOGIST. A scientist who studies the functions of living organisms; in the medical context, one concerned with the normal functions of the human body. See PHYSIOLOGY.

PHYSIOLOGY
Introduction
Physiology is the science of functions and related phenomena of living organisms and their parts. This clearly differentiates it from *anatomy, which is the science of form and structure. Although physiology involves both plant and animal studies, this article is concerned only with animal physiology.

From ancient times man has been interested in the workings of the human body and those of other animals. However, physiological studies and understanding have followed the discoveries of physics and chemistry. Indeed, techniques developed by physical scientists have often been used, albeit in modified form, to obtain a better understanding of life processes.

An example is the early development of microscopic lens systems, which ultimately led to magnifications which permitted the enunciation of the *cell doctrine. The realization that complex living organisms consisted of myriads of individual cells led ultimately to Claude *Bernard's insistence on the importance of the 'internal environment', within which the cells live their individual lives.

Physiology once embraced all that was known of the processes of living organisms, but the growth of knowledge has inevitably led to the division of physiology into a number of specialist disciplines. An early specialization was biological chemistry. Now *biochemistry is almost invariably treated as a distinct, related subject. As a consequence, physiology has tended to move more towards biophysical studies.

There follows a brief description of some of the topics in physiology taught to first-year medical students. Although frequently described as human (or medical) physiology, many of the advances in our understanding came about as a result of *animal experiments. The following descriptions relate to healthy normal young adults. No reference is made to specialized fields, such as reproductive, fetal, or developmental physiology.

The concept of an internal environment
Of the 65 kg weight of a typical young adult human, about 40 kg (60 per cent of the total body weight) is water. The water is distributed among three compartments: intracellular water, which accounts for 70 per cent of the total body water; interstitial water, which makes up 24 per cent; and blood plasma, which accounts for the remaining 6 per cent.

Intracellular water is contained within the myriads of individual cells which make up the body, all of which are surrounded by interstitial water. Because of the exchange between the individual cells and the interstitial fluid (the fluid being water together with the substances dissolved in it), an individual cell can sustain its life processes. In turn, the interstitial fluid is in dynamic equilibrium with the water and dissolved small molecules of the blood plasma contained within the capillaries of the circulation.

Although water can move freely between compartments, as determined by osmotic and hydrostatic forces, the variety and concentration of the dissolved substances differ markedly from compartment to compartment. Intracellular fluid has a higher concentration of potassium, magnesium, phosphate, and sulphate *ions than extracellular fluid (the interstitial fluid and the plasma). In contrast, the extracellular fluid contains higher concentrations of sodium and chloride ions than intracellular fluids. Plasma, although having similar concentrations of most solutes to those in interstitial fluid, differs from the latter in containing significantly more dissolved *protein—the plasma proteins. The important role of the plasma proteins in the interchanges between blood and interstitial fluid will be discussed later.

The importance of the exchanges between cells and the interstitial fluid and the exchanges between the interstitial fluid and the circulating plasma cannot be overstated. From the interstitial fluid the cells obtain the materials they need for their continuing well-being, and the cells excrete their waste products into the interstitial fluid. The relative constancy of the interstitial fluid is, in turn, determined by the exchanges between it and the circulating blood. Subsequently the blood has to rid itself of waste products it has received from the interstitial fluid, notably via the lungs and kidneys, and it must replace those materials which have been removed from the plasma to meet the metabolic requirements of the cells. To this end the blood obtains *oxygen from the lungs and other materials either directly from the digestive system or, more commonly, indirectly from intermediate body stores (e.g. *glucose from the liver).

Thus the primary role of each of the circulatory, respiratory, renal, and digestive systems is to contribute towards the maintenance of an internal environment within which the cells of the body can survive and carry out their characteristic activities. The normal regulation of these physiological systems and their response to altered circumstances, for example, sudden exercise or transient dehydration, takes place below the level of consciousness and is determined by alterations in the activity of the *autonomic nervous system (see later) or components of the *endocrine system.

An additional requirement for the internal environment is the maintenance of a constant temperature. The high thermal capacity of water is important in this, but an increase or decrease of body core temperature also changes the activity of the autonomic nervous system aimed at minimizing the deviation from the normal set point of 37 °C.

Blood

In a typical adult weighing 65 kg, the blood volume is approximately 5 litres. Of this half consists of formed elements and half is plasma. The formed elements, all of which are formed in the red *bone marrow, are of three types, the red cells (*erythrocytes), the white cells (*leucocytes), and the *platelets (thrombocytes).

The red cells, which individually have a life span of roughly 120 days, greatly increase the oxygen-carrying capacity of the blood. Plasma, when subjected to the partial pressure of oxygen normally present in the *alveoli of the lungs, can carry about 3 ml of oxygen/l. Blood containing a normal number of red cells ($\approx 5 \times 10^{12}$/l) and a normal *haemoglobin concentration (150 g/l), can carry 200 ml of oxygen/l. Haemoglobin is a globular iron-containing protein which combines reversibly with oxygen. The amount of oxygen combining with haemoglobin depends upon the partial pressure of oxygen to which the protein is subjected. Haemoglobin also plays an important role in buffering the *carbon dioxide entering the blood.

The white cells are of a variety of types (*neutrophils,

*eosinophils, *basophils, *lymphocytes, and *monocytes). In total they normally number between 5 and 10×10^9/l. The white cells play a protective role, and their numbers may be greatly increased by infection.

The platelets are small fragments of cytoplasm derived from large multinucleated cells (the megakaryocytes) which are found exclusively in the red bone marrow. Between 200 and 400×10^9 platelets/l are normally present. They have two important roles in *haemostasis: to seal small breaches which may result from wear and tear in the integrity of the capillary endothelium, and to play a part in the process of blood clotting (coagulation).

Plasma is the watery solution within which the formed elements of the blood are transported round the circulation. It consists of roughly 91 per cent by weight of water, 7–8 per cent of protein, approximately 0.9 per cent NaCl (in ionized form), and, in smaller concentrations, numerous other solutes including ions, glucose, *amino acids, blood fats, *vitamins, and *hormones. The plasma also contains important *buffer systems (notably the bicarbonate and phosphate systems) which minimize the change of hydrogen ion concentration (pH) when stronger acids or alkalis are added to the interstitial fluid (and hence the plasma) as a result of cellular activity.

The cardiovascular system

The cardiovascular system comprises the heart and the blood vessels (arteries, arterioles, capillaries, and veins). Functionally there are two circulations, the pulmonary and the systemic. The pulmonary arteries convey venous blood from the right side of the heart to the lungs, where carbon dioxide is released from the blood into the alveoli. Simultaneously with the unloading of carbon dioxide, the blood (by virtue of its haemoglobin content) takes up oxygen from the alveolar gas mixture. The resulting arterial blood (i.e. blood containing effectively its maximum content of oxygen) is returned via the pulmonary veins to the left side of the heart. The systemic circulation comprises the *aorta, which accepts the arterial blood leaving the left side of the heart; the arteries, into which the aorta divides; the complex arterial tree, which conveys the blood to all parts of the body; the arterioles; the capillary network surrounding the cells; and the veins, which convey the venous blood back to the right side of the heart.

The heart

The two circulatory systems share a common pump, the heart. The heart is in fact a double pump, a right-sided pump providing the pulsatile force which moves the venous blood returning from the systemic circulation through the pulmonary vessels, and a left-sided pump which receives the arterial blood returning from the lungs and propels it round the systemic circulation. The two pumps work in unison so that at each beat the volume of blood ejected from the right side of the heart into the pulmonary circulation accurately matches the volume of blood ejected by the left side of the heart into the systemic circulation.

The heart has four chambers, a right atrium and a right ventricle (the right heart), and a left atrium and a left ventricle (the left heart). The walls of these chambers consist of a muscular *syncytium (the cardiac musculature), but the musculature of the two atria is separated from the muscular syncytium of the ventricles by a connective tissue band which completely encircles the heart.

During a single cardiac cycle there is initially a period when all of the cardiac musculature is relaxed. This is known as *diastole. During this time venous blood is returning to the right auricle from the systemic circulation and passing passively into the right ventricle. Similarly, on the left side of the heart arterial blood is returning from the lungs to the left atrium and passing into the left ventricle.

Atrial contraction (atrial *systole) is initiated by an electrical wave which starts at the sinoatrial node (a region of specialized muscle fibres situated in the right atrium). The wave spreads throughout the atrial syncytium, causing the atrial muscle to contract and complete the filling of both ventricles with blood. Because of the connective tissue ring electrically separating the atria from the ventricles, the electrical wave cannot pass directly from the former to the latter save by a single band of specialized conducting tissue known as the *bundle of His. Towards the end of atrial contraction the electrical wave passes down this bundle and spreads throughout the ventricular muscle. Ventricular contraction ensues and both right and left intraventricular pressures rise as a result. Blood is prevented from returning from the ventricles to the atria by the closure of the atrioventricular valves. When the right intraventricular pressure exceeds the pressure in the pulmonary artery and the left intraventricular pressure exceeds the pressure in the aorta, the pulmonary and aortic valves open and blood is ejected from the ventricles into the respective circulations. At the conclusion of ventricular contraction the ventricular muscle relaxes and the heart returns to the diastolic state. As the intraventricular pressures fall, blood is prevented from returning from the pulmonary artery into the right ventricle or from the aorta into the left ventricle by the closure of the pulmonary valve and the aortic valve.

In a healthy young adult at rest, a complete cardiac cycle occupies about one second or slightly less, producing a heart rate of 60–70/minute. During each ventricular ejection phase about 70 ml of blood (the stroke volume) are ejected into each of the pulmonary and systemic circulations. It is the ejection of blood into the systemic circulation which can be appreciated as the *pulse at the wrist (or in any other artery). Multiplying the heart rate by the stroke volume gives the value of the cardiac output expressed in l/min. With the values quoted above the cardiac output would be 4.2 l/min.

Both the heart rate and the stroke volume (and thereby the cardiac output) can be considerably increased during exercise and the recovery period thereafter.

The systemic circulation

The aorta, which receives the blood pumped out by the left ventricle, contains much elastic tissue in its wall and can therefore accept the stroke output by 'giving' to accommodate the increased volume. Between ventricular contractions the elastic wall exerts pressure on the contained blood, ensuring its onward movement. The arteries, and more especially the much smaller diameter arterioles, present a resistance to this onward flow. The impedance offered by the sum of all the arterioles is known as the total peripheral resistance, and, as a result of it, the pressure in the main arteries falls only gradually from the highest level reached during left ventricular systole to a level at which the fall is interrupted by the following ventricular contraction. The highest and lowest pressures measurable (directly or indirectly) in a major artery during a single cardiac cycle are known as the systolic arterial *blood pressure and the diastolic arterial blood pressure respectively (frequently shortened to systolic and diastolic pressure). Typical values for a healthy young adult would be 120 mm mercury (mmHg) systolic and 80 mmHg diastolic. Such an arterial blood pressure is typically written as 120/80.

Although the blood flow in the major arteries is pulsatile, the repeated divisions of the arterial tree, together with the resistance to flow offered by the arterioles, progressively diminishes both the pulsatile nature of the flow and the pressure exerted by the blood on the wall of the vessels. By the time blood reaches the capillaries its flow is linear and the pressure (at the arterial end of the capillary) is about 32 mmHg.

The exchange at capillary level between the plasma and the interstitial fluid depends upon the interplay of hydrostatic and osmotic pressures. Owing to the plasma proteins, whose molecules are too large to pass through the single-cell endothelial lining of the capillary walls, the blood has a total osmotic pressure which exceeds that of the interstitial fluid (which has a negligible protein content) by some 25 mmHg. At the arterial end of a capillary the hydrostatic force (the capillary blood pressure) is 32 mmHg. Since the hydrostatic pressure exceeds the inward osmotic pull of 25 mmHg there is a net movement of water, together with the smaller molecules dissolved in it (including oxygen), out of the arterial end of each capillary. By the time the blood reaches the venous end of a capillary its hydrostatic pressure has fallen to a value of 18–19 mmHg. The excess osmotic pressure of the plasma over that of the interstitial fluid remains at about 25 mmHg, so there is a net flow of water and dissolved substances, including carbon dioxide and other cellular waste products, from the interstitial space into the blood. This continuous replenishment of the materials needed by cells and the removal of their waste from their environment is central to the internal environment, and the *raison d'être* for the circulatory system.

Finally, the systemic veins return the venous blood (blood from which some of the oxygen content has been removed and to which the waste product carbon dioxide has been added) to the right atrium. The central venous pressure (the pressure in the right atrium during diastole) approximates to zero.

The pulmonary circulation

Compared with the systemic circulation the pulmonary circulation is a low-pressure system. The pulmonary arterial pressure is about 25/10 mmHg compared with a systemic arterial pressure of 120/80. As a result, the mean capillary blood pressure in the pulmonary circuit is only 10 mmHg, and therefore well below the excess osmotic pressure of the plasma throughout the length of the capillary. Hence the alveolar air sacs of the lungs remain 'dry' and the unloading of carbon dioxide from the blood into the alveoli is facilitated, as is the uptake of oxygen by the blood from the lungs.

Finally, the lungs, like all other organs, receive an arterial blood supply from the systemic circulation to serve the metabolic need of their constituent cells.

Circulatory control systems

The arterial blood pressure at any instant is determined by two factors, the value of the total peripheral resistance (the resistance to the forward flow of the blood offered by the arteriolar tree) and the cardiac output. Both factors can undergo change.

The walls of arterioles contain involuntary (smooth) muscle, under the influence of *nerve fibres of the autonomic nervous system (the *vasomotor nerves). Altered discharge along the latter may cause the smooth muscle of the arteriolar walls either to relax (producing vasodilatation) or contract (producing vasoconstriction). Changes in the autonomic nervous system can bring about vasodilatation of the arterioles supplying one organ or region of the body and vasoconstriction elsewhere. By such changes more of the cardiac output may be diverted from one region to another without producing a significant change in the total peripheral resistance.

The heart rate and the force of ventricular contraction are also under the control of the autonomic nervous system. By virtue of altered activity in autonomic nerve fibres terminating around both the sinoatrial node and the ventricular muscle, the heart may be caused to increase in rate from 60 or 70 beats/minute to 180 beats/minute and the stroke output to increase from 70 ml/beat to 140 ml/beat. Acting together, these two changes can increase the cardiac output sixfold, from 4 l/min to 24 l/min.

However, the arterial blood pressure would rise significantly if the cardiac output was increased sixfold without any change in the total peripheral resistance. This is avoided by sensory end-organs (see later), which sense blood pressure, situated in the walls of both central arteries and large veins. The information from these sensory end-organs is conveyed via sensory nerves to the cardiovascular centre in the brainstem. As a result of this, adjustments are made to the patterns of discharge in the autonomic nerve fibres to both the heart and the arterioles, which result in appropriate co-ordinated changes in both cardiac output and total peripheral resistance. Since the heart is constrained to maintain both a near constant arterial pressure and central venous pressure, the average pressures at the arterial and venous ends of the capillaries are kept within the limits that permit effective exchanges between the blood and tissue fluid.

It is self-evident that for these exchanges to be satisfactory the blood reaching the arterial end of the capillaries must be of constant composition. It must contain an adequate quantity of oxygen to satisfy the needs of the cells, together with the necessary fuel (typically glucose) from which the cells can obtain energy by oxidation. There must also be the building blocks (such as *amino acids) which the cells may need to undertake anabolic (protein-building) tasks. The arterial blood must also have been adequately 'cleared' of waste products (such as carbon dioxide, hydrogen ions, etc.) which are present in excess in venous blood. The relative constancy of arterial blood is ensured by the activities of three other physiological systems, the respiratory system, the renal system, and the gastrointestinal system (the last supplemented by the functions of the liver). The tasks undertaken by these systems will now be outlined.

The respiratory system

The respiratory system is responsible for external respiration. This entails the transfer of oxygen from the atmospheric air to the blood and the removal of excess carbon dioxide from the blood to the atmosphere. This exchange is effected by the respiratory cycle of inspiration (during quiet respiration this is brought about by a contraction of the diaphragm), expiration (which, during quiet respiration, is passive and due to diaphragmatic relaxation), followed by a pause.

During inspiration, air is drawn into the lungs via the airways. The inspired air, reaching the smaller bronchioles, exchanges by gaseous diffusion with the air in the terminal air sacs (the alveoli). Because the tidal airflow does not reach the alveoli, the composition of the alveolar air retains an effectively constant composition throughout the respiratory cycle. The mixed venous blood entering the arterial end of the pulmonary capillaries is brought into contact with alveolar air. As a result of partial pressure differences between the blood and alveolar air, carbon dioxide leaves the blood and enters the alveolar air, while oxygen moves in the opposite direction. Subsequently, as a result of gaseous diffusion, the tidal expired air contains more carbon dioxide and less oxygen than the inspired air.

At rest the body requires about 250 ml of oxygen/minute. A similar volume of carbon dioxide is produced, the exact volume depending on the substrate being oxidized. These values may be greatly increased during exercise.

Normally the rate and the depth of respiration are controlled automatically by the partial pressure of carbon dioxide in the arterial blood. This is sensed by the respiratory centre (which, like the cardiovascular centre, is situated in the brainstem). If this partial pressure rises above its normal arterial level of 40 mmHg, the respiratory exertions are increased. However, since the diaphragm is a skeletal muscle, external respiration can, to some extent, be brought under voluntary control. This is necessary in order to phonate and carry on a conversation. Similarly, the breath can, within limits, be held, or voluntary hyperventilation can be undertaken. However, at rest, during moderate exercise, and during sleep, external respiration continues automatically and without conscious intervention.

The renal system
Each normal adult *kidney contains many functionally important units, known as *nephrons. The first part of each nephron consists of a tuft of capillaries (the glomerulus) and here an ultrafiltrate of the plasma is formed. This ultrafiltrate has a composition similar to plasma save that it contains no plasma proteins (the molecules of which are too large to pass through the capillary wall). Once formed, the ultrafiltrate passes along the lumen of a structure known as the loop of Henle. During its passage the ultrafiltrate is subjected to a process of selective reabsorption. Some solutes for which the body has a continuous need (e.g. glucose) are totally reabsorbed. Others which are waste products of metabolism (e.g. urea) are not subjected to any active reabsorption (although some molecules may pass back by passive diffusion) and are consequently excreted. Several important constituents of the ultrafiltrate are reabsorbed depending upon the body's need for them. Examples include sodium and water. Specialized cells of the loop of Henle are 'informed' how much of the material to reabsorb from the glomerular filtrate through the circulating levels of specific hormones (mineralocorticoids produced by the cortex of the *adrenal gland in the case of sodium, and *antidiuretic hormone from the posterior *pituitary gland in the case of water). For example, drinking a large volume of water will reduce the *osmolarity of the blood and interstitial fluid. The reduced osmolarity is detected by osmoreceptors and results in a decreased release of antidiuretic hormone by the pituitary gland. Consequently, the reabsorption of water from the ultrafiltrate formed by the glomeruli will be reduced and the excess water excreted, together with other unwanted materials, in the urine.

The gastrointestinal system and the liver
The gastrointestinal tract converts the food that is eaten into molecules that can be absorbed, either actively or passively, through the walls of the small intestine and passed into the capillaries of the *splanchnic circulation. Thus through multiple digestive enzymes and the mixing achieved by intestinal movements, complex *carbohydrates are converted into monosaccharides, fats into either chylomicrons or to glycerol and fatty acids, and proteins into amino acids. The movements of the *gut, which both mix the food with the digestive enzymes and also move the contents along the length of the bowel (peristaltic waves), are produced by the smooth muscle of the gut wall. This involuntary muscle, like that of the arteriolar wall, is under the control of the autonomic nervous system, and gut movement may be increased or decreased by changes in autonomic activity. The juices containing the digestive enzymes which are secreted into the mouth (saliva), stomach (gastric juice), and intestine (pancreatic juice, bile, and succus entericus) are produced under the control of either the autonomic nervous system or local hormones (e.g. gastrin).

Substances transported across the intestinal wall, which include water, vitamins, trace elements, etc., as well as the three primary foodstuffs, pass to the liver via the portal vein.

The liver is a major metabolic organ and is important in regulating the composition of the blood plasma. The liver is responsible for the synthesis and regulation of the plasma proteins. It also acts as a storage site for several substances, whose concentration is carefully regulated in the plasma (e.g. the blood glucose level, which is set by the hormones glucagon and insulin). The liver is also responsible for the production of *bile and is a major site for detoxification.

The autonomic nervous system
All these physiological systems (the cardiovascular system, the respiratory system, the renal system, and the gastrointestinal system) are together responsible for maintaining an internal environment in which all the cells of the body can function optimally. The regulation of these systems is, with the exception mentioned for respiration, undertaken below the level of consciousness. Even when asleep, adjustments made in the autonomic nervous system or in the production of individual hormones ensure the continued constancy of the environment in which the cells of the body exist.

The output of the autonomic nervous system is determined by sensory inputs received from many sources (pressure *receptors in the walls of central arteries and great veins, stretch receptors in the lungs, etc.) but the autonomic nervous system is entirely motor (efferent) in function.

The autonomic integrating centres (where sensory inputs are received and motor outputs are determined) lie within the central nervous system but are subcortical in location (e.g. the cardiovascular centre referred to earlier is situated in the brainstem). The efferent motor fibres of the autonomic system fall into two groups, the *parasympathetic fibres and the *sympathetic fibres. The former leave the central nervous system either accompanying specific *cranial nerves (third, seventh, ninth, and tenth) or via some sacral spinal motor nerves (second, third, and fourth). Together these two parts are known as the craniosacral parasympathetic outflow. The sympathetic fibres leave the spinal cord with the thoracic motor spinal nerves.

All tissues that receive an autonomic innervation show intrinsic (spontaneous) activity. Such structures which have been mentioned include cardiac and involuntary (smooth) muscle and some secreting cells of the gastrointestinal tract. For example, if all the autonomic nerve fibres innervating the heart are cut, the heart continues to beat, albeit at a fixed rate. For an innervated structure, any increase in the autonomic nervous discharge increases, or decreases, the activity of that tissue. A tissue innervated by the autonomic nervous system receives both a sympathetic and a parasympathetic supply, and the influence of the two innervations is antagonistic. If an increased impulse discharge along the sympathetic innervation increases the inherent activity, increased parasympathetic activity will decrease it. For example, with an initial heart rate of about 100 beats/minute enhanced sympathetic activity in the fibres to the heart will increase the heart rate, and enhanced parasympathetic activity will decrease it. However, the sympathetic innervation does not enhance the activity of all the tissues it innervates: sometimes the parasympathetic innervation is excitatory and the sympathetic inhibitory.

The provision of the ideal internal environment carries substantial 'self-interest' for the systems discussed, since their cells share that environment. However, that environment also encompasses the cells belonging to two further systems which play no major part in its maintenance. Both the systemic nervous system and the skeletal muscular system are pivotal to human life as we know it, and without Claude *Bernard's 'milieu interieur' the nerve cells and skeletal muscle fibres could not survive. These will now be considered briefly.

The systemic nervous system

The systemic nervous system comprises the central nervous system (the *cerebrum, the *brainstem, and the *spinal cord—all protected by bony enclosures) and the *peripheral nervous system. The peripheral nervous system includes all the nerve fibres and *neurones lying outside the central nervous system, with the exception of those belonging to the autonomic nervous system. Functionally the peripheral nerve fibres either convey information towards the central nervous system (sensory nerve fibres) or convey motor impulses (motor fibres) from the central nervous system to skeletal (striated) muscle.

The sensory system

Throughout the body there are scattered many thousands of sensory end-organs. Each is specifically sensitive to one type of environmental change. For example, in the walls of some large arteries there are pressure-sensitive end-organs which measure the pressure the contained blood exerts on the arterial wall. There are sensory end-organs situated in the carotid arteries which measure the oxygen tension of the blood. The nerve impulses discharged from these end-organs enter the central nervous system and connect to higher centres but do not impinge on consciousness. The information conveyed is used to determine motor discharges in the two divisions of the autonomic nervous system.

Other sensory end-organs, such as those in the skin, are sensitive to touch, and rise or fall in temperature and pressure. The nervous discharges from these sensory endings are conveyed via a series of nervous pathways to the sensory cortex of the appropriate cerebral hemisphere. Here, and in the light of experience, the sensations reach consciousness and are interpreted. Similarly, the sensory inputs from the special sense organs (eyes, ears, tongue) have distinct regions of cortical tissue to which their impulses are passed and at which 'interpretation' (again in the light of experience) can take place. How this is achieved is not fully understood. Neither is the mechanism by which past sensory inputs (memories) are stored, although this appears to take place in the cerebrum.

The motor system

Adjacent to the sensory area in each cerebral hemisphere is the motor cortex. Here learned patterns of motor activity (movements) are stored as they are learnt during childhood development. Such learned movements can subsequently be produced at will by causing a discharge of nerve impulses to pass down a pathway to the appropriate level of the spinal cord. Here the descending fibres of the upper motor neurones make contact with the nerve cells of the lower motor neurones which convey the instruction to contract to the appropriate skeletal muscles.

The skeletal musculature

Skeletal muscles account for roughly half the body weight. Unlike cardiac and involuntary muscle (both of which exhibit spontaneous activity), skeletal muscle remains at complete rest until caused to contract by the arrival of one or more impulses along its motor nerve innervation (lower motor neurone). In a muscle capable of discrete movements, a single motor neurone may innervate only a few skeletal muscle fibres, but in a large, powerful muscle, a single motor neurone may innervate several hundred muscle fibres. A single motor neurone and the group of muscle fibres it innervates is known as a motor unit. The strength and duration of a skeletal muscle contraction are determined by the number (and size) of the motor units activated, and the number and frequency of the motor nerve impulses reaching those motor units.

A. J. BULLER

Further readings
Bern, R. M. and Levy, M. N. (1993). *Physiology*, (3rd edn). Mosby Year Book, London.
Fulton, J. F. (1966). *Selected readings in the history of physiology*, (2nd edn). Thomas, Springfield, Illinois.
Hodgkin, A. L., *et al.*, (1977). *The pursuit of nature: informal essays on the history of physiology*. Cambridge University Press, Cambridge.

PHYSIOTHERAPIST. A person trained and qualified in *physiotherapy.

PHYSIOTHERAPY is treatment by physical methods such as exercise, massage, muscular re-education, heat, electrical stimulation, etc. Physiotherapy is one of the recognized *professions supplementary to medicine, and in the UK it is under the control of the Chartered Society of Physiotherapy.

PHYSOSTIGMINE. See ESERINE.

PIA MATER. The innermost of the three *meninges, which envelop the *brain and *spinal cord.

PICA is an appetite perversion characterized by a craving for particular, often bizarre, articles of diet. Children with pica sometimes attempt to eat material or articles that could not be regarded as food. Pica is not uncommon in pregnancy.

PICK, ARNOLD (1851–1924). Czech neuropsychiatrist. He described presenile *dementia with focal cerebral atrophy (Pick's disease, 1892).

PICK, LUDWIG (1868–1935). German pathologist. He described a *sphingomyelin storage disorder (Niemann–Pick disease, 1927).

PICKERING, SIR GEORGE WHITE (1904–80). British physician. His interests were mainly in cardiovascular disease and his book *High blood pressure* (1955) was widely acclaimed. He did much to encourage continuing education in medicine by advocating the building of postgraduate centres.

PICKLES, WILLIAM NORMAN (1885–1969). British general practitioner. The first president of the UK College of General Practitioners (see PRIMARY MEDICAL CARE), Pickles practised for 53 years in the village of Aysgarth, Wensleydale, Yorkshire. His book, *Epidemiology in a country practice*, threw original light on the spread of infection in a rural district. 'Rural districts, where the population is thin and the lines of intercourse few and always easily traced, offer opportunities which are not to be met with in the crowded haunts of large towns.' He knew everyone in Aysgarth and, with his wife, kept meticulous records. There is an admirable quality of simplicity in his research methods and writing. His book survives as a classic.

PICKWICKIAN SYNDROME. The syndrome of *obesity, *cyanosis due to *hypoventilation, and somnolence. Other features are excessive eating, fatiguability, breathlessness, carbon dioxide retention, secondary *polycythaemia, pulmonary hypertension, and eventually *cor pulmonale. The syndrome is named with reference to Mr Wardle's boy Joe, in *The posthumous papers of the Pickwick club* by Charles Dickens, published in 1837.

PIGMENTATION is abnormal coloration of skin or mucous membranes due to the deposition of a pigmented substance. In many cases this is dark brown and due to *melanin (melanoderma), which is responsible for normal skin pigmentation; increased activity of the melanocytes (see SKIN) may be due to local factors such as irritation or may be generalized due to increased secretion of *melanocyte-stimulating hormone (MSH) by the anterior pituitary. Thus patchy or diffuse melanoderma can occur in many conditions, including sunburn, pregnancy, menopause, old age, Addison's disease, multiple neurofibromatosis, pediculosis ('vagabond's disease'), malaria, pellagra, diabetes mellitus, carcinomatosis, and others, as well as in some primary skin diseases. Pigmentation may also be due to iron-containing derivatives of *haemoglobin, such as haemosiderin; this is seen following skin and subcutaneous haemorrhages, and in *haemochromatosis or 'bronzed diabetes'. Other metals which may be deposited in the skin causing pigmentation include silver (argyria), bismuth, and mercury.

PIKE'S PEAK is a mountain in Colorado (4298 m) where much physiological work on the effects of exposure to high altitude was carried out, such as the studies of J. S. *Haldane in 1912 on acclimatization. See ENVIRONMENT AND MEDICINE I.

PILES. See HAEMORRHOIDS.

PILL, THE. When not otherwise qualified, the contraceptive pill. See CONTRACEPTION.

PILLS are small, spherical or ovoid masses, designed to be swallowed, used to administer pharmaceutical agents. The active substance (or substances) is mixed with a vehicle, the excipient, to confer cohesion and firmness. 'Pill' is sometimes loosely used synonymously with *tablet.

PILOCARPINE is an *alkaloid with cholinergic effects, used in *ophthalmology to cause *miosis in the treatment of *glaucoma.

PINCUS, GREGORY (1903–67). American biologist and endocrinologist. His main interest was in the properties of the steroid *hormones, especially in connection with function of the *gonads. He made fundamental contributions to the development of *contraceptive methods, using oral *steroid preparations.

PINEAL. The pineal body, a small structure protruding from the centre of the brain, derived embryologically from the *ependyma of the third ventricle. Although its tissue is rich in various *neurotransmitter substances and it is innervated by postganglionic *sympathetic fibres, its precise function in man is still uncertain. However, it secretes the hormone melatonin and is believed to be concerned with *gonadal function, with *circadian rhythms, and with variations in skin *pigmentation.

PINEALOMA. A rare *tumour, sometimes a true neoplasm of pineal *parenchyma, more often a *teratoma, sometimes with other cellular elements predominant. Precocious puberty is an occasional association.

PINEL, PHILIPPE (1745–1826). French physician. In 1793 he was given charge of the insane at the Hospice de Bicêtre and in 1795 at the *Salpêtrière. At both he instituted a new era in *psychiatry by his strenuous opposition to violent methods of treatment, and by insisting that the chains of all patients be removed. He made an attempt to devise a Linnaean *classification of diseases in his *Nosologie philosophique* (1789).

PINK DISEASE. See ACRODYNIA.

PINK EYE. Acute *conjunctivitis.

PINNA. The external and visible part of the ear.

PINTA is a skin disease of tropical South America, disfiguring but with little effect on general health. It is caused by a *spirochaete (*Treponema carateum*) closely related to those of *syphilis and *yaws.

PINWORM. See THREADWORM.

PIORRY, PIERRE ADOLPHE (1794–1879). French physician. He invented the '*pleximeter' and wrote *Traité sur la percussion médiate* (1828) on its use.

PIPE-SMOKING is a less dangerous method of *smoking tobacco than cigarettes, probably because less inhalation of smoke occurs in lifelong pipe smokers. Another factor may be the lower temperature of combustion in the bowl of a pipe. The mortality rate of pipe smokers is higher than that of non-smokers but the increase is small compared with that for cigarette smokers. However, cigarette smokers who change to pipe-smoking as an alternative to giving up smoking may not improve their health and life prospects much, as an established inhalation habit is usually transferred to other methods of smoking.

PIROGOFF, NIKOLAI IVANOVICH (1810–81). Russian surgeon. One of the most important figures in Russian medicine, he was an educationalist and a supporter of women's role in medicine. A skilled surgeon, he is known for his osteoplastic amputation of the foot (Pirogoff's amputation, 1854) and for his attempt to induce *anaesthesia by administering *ether rectally (1847).

PIRQUET, CLEMENS FREIHERR VON (1874–1929). Austrian paediatrician of Vienna. Pirquet described a test for *tuberculosis in which the surface of the skin is scarified through two drops of old tuberculin, an *antigen. A positive result was when after 24–48 hours the site of the scratches showed a red inflamed papule with a central areola. This test confirmed previous tuberculous infection, but did not show whether the disease was active. Pirquet was a founder of the study of *allergy.

PITCAIRN, DAVID (1749–1809). British physician. He was the first to note that lesions of the heart valves followed *rheumatic fever. His father, Major Pitcairn, was killed at Bunker Hill in 1775 and his brother, Robert, was the first to sight Pitcairn Island on 2 July 1767 which was thus given his name.

PITCH is the quality of a sound determined by the frequency of vibration of its source; a high frequency produces a sound of high pitch.

PITUITA. Secretions of *mucus; *phlegm.

PITUITARY GLAND. The pituitary gland, or hypophysis, is located at the base of the brain, attached by a stalk to the *hypothalamus. It is the most complex *endocrine gland, having several functions including the control of several other glands ('the leader of the endocrine orchestra'). It has two major components, the anterior lobe or adenohypophysis and the posterior lobe or neurohypophysis. The anterior lobe, which is itself regulated by the hypothalamus, secretes several important hormones. These include the following seven: growth hormone (somatotrophin or GH), which is essential for normal growth and also influences carbohydrate metabolism; *prolactin (lactogenic hormone), which regulates the secretion of milk; *adrenocorticotrophic hormone (ACTH), which controls the secretion of hormones from the adrenal cortex; two *gonadotrophic hormones, one of which (*follicle-stimulating hormone or FSH) controls the formation of ova by the ovary in the female and sperms by the testis in the male, and the other (*luteinizing hormone or LH) the secretion of sex hormones by the gonads; *melanocyte-stimulating hormone (MSH), which controls the pigment-producing cells of the skin; and *thyrotrophic hormone (TSH), which stimulates thyroid gland activity.

The neurohypophysis stores and releases two hormones: *oxytocin, which initiates labour at the end of pregnancy, stimulates uterine contraction, and also plays a part in lactation; and *antidiuretic hormone (ADH), which stimulates renal retention of water and has a blood-pressure-raising effect.

PITYRIASIS is any skin disease characterized by the formation and shedding of branny scales.

PLACEBO. A treatment known to be without effect given to a patient either merely to please him or her, or else to serve as a 'control' treatment in comparison with a potentially effective substance or method which is being subjected to *clinical trial. In the latter case, the aim is to eliminate the 'placebo effect'; that is, the improvement which many patients exhibit merely because they are taking or undergoing something which they believe will do them good.

PLACENTA. The placenta unites the mammalian *fetus to the maternal *uterus and serves as its organ of respiration, nutrition, and excretion. The placenta, developed from fetal tissue, is in close contact with the maternal blood circulation so that diffusion of oxygen and nutrients (but not cells or particulate matter) can occur in one direction and of carbon dioxide and urea in the other. It contains a dense network of fetal blood vessels which communicates with the remainder of the fetal circulation through the umbilical arteries and vein. The placenta also acts as a maternal endocrine organ, producing *hormones (*gonadotrophin, *oestrogen, *progesterone) needed to maintain pregnancy. The placenta is extruded shortly after the birth of the infant (the 'afterbirth'); it then weighs about 0.6 kg and is disc-shaped, about 2 cm thick and 16 cm in diameter.

PLACENTA PRAEVIA (PREVIA) is an abnormally situated *placenta, lying across or adjacent to the opening of the *uterus. It is a cause of haemorrhage in late pregnancy or during labour, and may necessitate *caesarean section.

PLAGUE is a severe *bacterial infection due to the organism *Yersinia pestis* (formerly known as *Pasteurella pestis*). It is endemic in parts of South-East Asia and Africa, and occurs sporadically elsewhere. Primarily a disease of wild rodents, transmission to man usually occurs through the bite of a *rat flea, causing the variety known as bubonic plague, in which regional *lymphadenitis (bubo) is prominent. When the condition becomes septicaemic and pneumonic, person-to-person transmission occurs by droplet infection.

Untreated, the mortality rate is high; but it responds well to early *antibiotic therapy. See also BLACK DEATH.

PLANIGRAPHY is the radiographic visualization of structures in a single plane of the body, as in *tomography.

PLANIMETER. A mechanical integrating instrument which measures surface areas by using a movable tracing arm.

PLANTALGIA is pain in the sole of the foot.

PLAQUE, DENTAL. See DENTISTRY.

PLASMA is the liquid which together with the suspended cells comprises blood. *Serum is plasma without *fibrinogen, after the latter has been removed in clotting. See HAEMATOLOGY.

PLASMA CELL. A B-*lymphocyte in its most active antibody-secreting form. See IMMUNOLOGY.

PLASMAPHERESIS is whole-body *plasma exchange, the plasma being replaced with fresh frozen plasma or some other osmotically appropriate fluid.

PLASMID. An extrachromosomal genetic element existing and replicating autonomously in the cytoplasm of a cell. Bacterial plasmids are closed loops of *deoxyribonucleic acid (DNA) consisting of only a few *genes, capable, for example, of conferring antibiotic resistance on the host cell; they are used in *genetic engineering.

PLASMODIUM is the genus of *protozoal parasites which includes the causative organisms of *malaria.

PLASTER is fabric coated with an adhesive substance for application to the skin, for protection and treatment. See also PLASTER OF PARIS.

PLASTER OF PARIS is made from powdered calcium sulphate ($CaSO_4.^{1/2}H_2O$), obtained by heating gypsum, or hydrated calcium sulphate ($CaSO_4.2H_2O$), to 120–30 °C so that it loses three-quarters of its water. On mixing with water, plaster of Paris sets and rapidly hardens. It is particularly useful for making casts and bandages for purposes of immobilization.

PLASTIC AND MAXILLOFACIAL SURGERY. Plastic surgery is a medical specialty with ancient roots. The Egyptian papyri describe physicians who specialized in the treatment of fractures of the facial bones, war injuries, and accidents. Their methods of repair have been studied by students of medicine (Gnudi and Webster 1950).

Plastic surgery is sometimes defined as 'that branch of medicine which seeks to correct congenital or acquired deformities in order to improve function, appearance, or both'. It deals with defects of the body surface and of the underlying bones and muscles. Although it is, in large measure, concerned with deformities involving the face, the head, and the neck region, it also includes the treatment of deformities of the hands and feet, the breast, body contours, and the external genitalia. Deformities inhibit function by making an individual feel that his or her physical image is inadequate. The word, plastic, basically means 'form', and it is the form of the human face and body that primarily concerns the plastic surgeon.

Aristotle, in his treatise *On the parts of animals*, stated, 'Art indeed consists in the conception of the result to be produced before its realization in the material.' That ability is a quality much needed by the plastic surgeon. It is a quality that should distinguish the artist from the technician. In 1798, Desavit first used the term 'plastique' in a medical paper and, in 1838, Zeis published the first *Handbuch der plastischen Chirurgie*. Plastic surgery was entirely reconstructive until the 20th century. In recent decades, the reliability and safety of this branch of surgery have advanced to such a degree that elective cosmetic (aesthetic) surgery is now highly reliable and extremely popular. Such surgery always carries some risk and should not be undertaken unless that patient's sense of deformity is producing significant emotional problems. These problems may lead to inhibitions that significantly affect the patient's behaviour and personal relationships—inhibitions that are often eliminated by appropriate surgery.

During the 8th century AD, Arabian scholars, with the rise of Islam, provided Arabic translations of the work of the famed Indian practitioner, Sushruta. Thus, Europeans and, in particular, Italians, including the Branca family of Sicily and Gaspare *Tagliacozzi of Bologna, became familiar with ancient methods of plastic surgery that had been developed on the subcontinent of India (Gnudi and Webster 1950).

In 1597, Gaspare Tagliacozzi published his treatise entitled *De curtorum chirurgia per insitionem* (Fig. 1). This marvellous work established him as the first modern plastic surgeon. He described the use of flaps of skin and fat taken from the upper arm to reconstruct the nose. He employed a technique of moving these flaps of skin in stages to make the operations more successful. Tagliacozzi, like William *Harvey, another great medical pioneer, was ridiculed and persecuted for his 'heresies'. Following his death, there was a decline in science and medicine throughout all of Europe, including the practice of plastic surgery. This lasted throughout the 17th and 18th centuries. During these dark times, surgeons reported the mythical use of reparative tissue taken from a slave or person other than the patient and used for grafting.

In the 13th century, it was common practice in India to punish convicted criminals by amputation or mutilation of body parts. A frequent punishment for adultery was amputation of the nose. As in modern times, adultery was not limited to the poorer classes and, as a result, demand emerged for physicians with skill in the surgical replacement of the human nose. The cost of surgery was no problem for the prince or maharajah who had lost his nose. This 'demand' produced specialists in what we now call 'plastic surgery'.

Hindu religious law prohibited those belonging to the higher levels of the caste system from touching human blood. It was left to the lowly tile makers (belonging to the seventh caste) to develop the necessary surgical skills for rebuilding the nose. Over a period of many generations, these surgical skills were developed and passed down from father to son, unbeknown to the Western world of medicine.

In 1794, two British physicians, travelling in India, were invited to witness one of these nasal reconstructions, performed in the Indian foothills of Mahvatta. They were astonished when they saw this operation. The patient was held on the ground by four strong men as the surgeon quickly cut free most of the skin from his forehead, leaving it attached only by a small bridge at the medial eyebrow region. The skin was then turned, folded, and roughly shaped into the form of a nose before fastening it to the scarred skin in the central face. Stitches and thorns were used to fasten the new nose into position and the patient's forehead

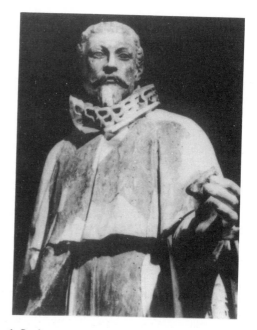

Fig. 1 Sculpture at the University of Bologna, showing Gaspare Tagliacozzi as he holds the model of a human nose and contemplates the problem of its reconstruction. He is known today as the father of modern plastic surgery.

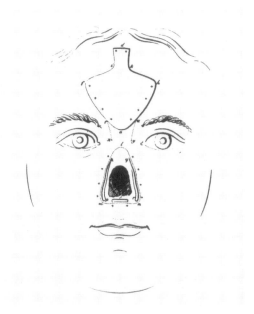

Fig. 2 Illustration from Von Graefe's book, *Rhinoplastik* (1818), shows his diagram on the forehead to outline the shape of the skin needed to rebuild the nose.

was then dressed and allowed to heal over a period of weeks. The pedicle of skin remaining between the eyes was divided 25 days later. When this dramatic operation was reported subsequently by those English physicians in the *Gentleman's Magazine* in London (1794), it was met with disbelief and ridicule. Only after some years was the validity of the report established. To this day, we know this technique of transferring forehead skin to reconstruct the nose as the 'Indian method of rhinoplasty'.

Dr Joseph Carpue, a noted English surgeon, intrigued by this report from India, devoted the next 20 years of his life to confirming the details and methods that were used. Finally, he attempted the operation himself in September in 1814. His patient had been an officer in the Egyptian army who had been treated for syphilis by the use of mercury. This medication had caused the loss of his nose.

In an operation lasting exactly 37 minutes, Dr Carpue cut and elevated skin from the forehead and sewed it into new incisions that he made into that part of the patient's face which surrounded the defect caused by the missing nose. When the dressing was removed 3 days later, the patient exclaimed, 'My God, there is a nose'. This operation and a second one performed by Carpue in 1815 marked the introduction of major reconstructive plastic surgery into Western medicine (Carpue 1816).

During the 19th century, several other European surgeons made great contributions to the specialty of plastic

surgery. These included von Graefe and his publication of *Rhinoplastik* in 1818 in Germany (Figs 2 and 3). His younger contemporary, Dieffenbach (1845), ingeniously extended the principles of nasal reconstruction to other types of defects, especially those involving the face and lips.

In France, Dupuytren (1832) developed new methods for treating burns and for relieving severe contractures of the hands. At the same time, von Langenbeck was making major contributions to the closure of congenital clefts of the palate in children.

On 8 December 1869, Reverdin gave the first demonstration of free skin grafting in the human. Ollier, in 1872, and *Thiersch, in 1874, published extensions on this technique to show that larger grafts and grafts containing dermis (the deepest layer of the skin), as well as epidermis, could also be used. In England, Wolfe (1876) first described the use of the full-thickness skin graft for the treatment of eyelid deformities.

Early plastic surgery in the USA and UK
In the USA, specialization in plastic surgery appears to have developed as a result of the stimulation by William Stewart *Halsted at the Johns Hopkins University School of Medicine. He encouraged one of his younger associates, Dr John Staige Davis, to limit his practice to plastic surgery. Dr Davis published, in 1919, the first textbook in English on plastic surgery, entitled, *Plastic surgery–its principles and practice*.

When the First World War broke out in 1914, Dr

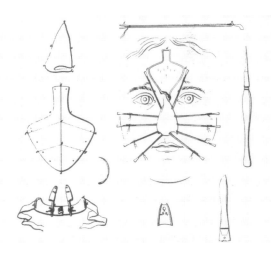

Fig. 3 The forehead flap has been transferred into the nasal defect. Small fish-tailed wooden sticks are used to allow daily tightening and loosening of the stitches. The lower left-hand corner pictures a splint to maintain the nostril air-passages during the healing period. This is a modification of the ancient Indian method of rhinoplasty described in Susruta.

Davis and Dr Morestin of France were the only two recognized specialists in plastic surgery among the allied forces. Trench warfare in France produced a staggering number of maxillofacial wounds, and most military surgeons did not know how to deal with these problems. Morestin, a native of Martinique, conducted an active plastic surgery programme at the military hospital of Val-de-Grace in Paris (Morestin 1915). He died, prematurely, in the great influenza epidemic in 1917, but not before he had interested a British physician, Sir Harold *Gillies, in plastic surgery. Gillies subsequently established a military plastic surgery centre at the Queen Mary Hospital in Sidcup, Kent. At this hospital, many young plastic surgeons, such as Kilner and McIndoe, Ferris Smith from the USA, Waldron and Risdon from Canada, and Pickerill from Australia, learned many of the operative methods and skills of reconstructing patients who had received severe war injuries.

During the First World War, Varstad Kazanjian, a dental surgeon from the Harvard Dental School, was working at Etaples near Boulogne. He applied his knowledge of prosthetic *dentistry to the early treatment of gunshot wounds of the jaws, and perfected new methods of splinting jaw fractures that were associated with massive loss of bone. He developed principles that are still in use 60 years later (Kazanjian and Converse 1974). When the USA entered the First World War in 1917, Surgeon-General *Gorgas organized a section on oral and plastic surgery for the US military forces. Vilray P. Blair, of St Louis, headed that section and chose Robert H. Ivy as his assistant. Five years earlier (1913), Blair had published a classic book entitled *Surgery and diseases of the mouth and jaws*.

In the 1920s and 1930s, John Staige Davis and Vilray Papin Blair, in the USA, and Harold Delf Gillies in England, were the best-known leaders in the developing specialty of plastic surgery. Each made important and original contributions to the application of plastic surgical principles to correct the deformities of civilian life. Gillies (1920) helped to pioneer the development of the tube pedicle flap, while in 1929 Blair and his associate, Barrett Brown, developed the technique of cutting and using large, thin sheets (split thickness) of skin to resurface the open wounds of patients with major burns. In 1939, Earl Padgett and an engineer, George Hood, developed the first mechanical dermatome that could be used for taking large sheets of split-thickness skin grafts. The invention of the dermatome made it possible for surgeons with only modest surgical skill in plastic surgery to harvest skin grafts for covering large skin defects. During the Second World War, this device saved many lives and limbs.

Cosmetic, or aesthetic, plastic surgery began to develop during the period between the World Wars. A German surgeon in Berlin, by the name of Joseph, was developing the modern method of corrective rhinoplasty, permitting the operation to be carried out by means of incisions hidden within the nose (Joseph 1931).

Two surgeons from the USA, Aufricht and Safian, observed and further developed his methods.

In 1937, Vilray Blair and 12 other senior American plastic surgeons established The American Board of Plastic Surgery. At the end of the Second World War there were still only 200 American surgeons who could meet the qualifications for certification by that board.

By 1951, only two plastic surgeons had been appointed as full-time heads of plastic surgery divisions in American medical schools (Robert McCormack at the University of Rochester in New York and Milton Edgerton at The Johns Hopkins University in Baltimore, Maryland). Academic plastic surgery was still in its infancy. Over the ensuing 40 years, 6000 additional American and Canadian plastic surgeons have received plastic surgery board qualified training, and over 100 American medical schools now have appointed full-time specialists in plastic surgery. Several universities have given plastic surgery full departmental status. Hospitals in Canada, England, Scotland, Ireland, France, Italy, and Japan have also established postgraduate training programmes for plastic surgeons.

One of the largest medical centres during the Second World War was The Valley Forge General Hospital at Phoenixville, Pennsylvania. The chief of its plastic surgery section, Dr Barrett Brown, and his associate, Dr Bradford Cannon, trained many young general surgeons in reconstructive surgery. When those medical officers returned to civilian life, they applied these wartime surgical techniques to civilian problems, such as cancer of the head and neck, industrial and automobile injuries, aesthetic and body contour surgery, and even to correction of deformities caused by metabolic and vascular diseases such as *arthritis and *stroke. It is noteworthy that Dr Joseph E. Murray, one of the plastic surgeons trained at Valley Forge during the Second World War, was later awarded the 1990 *Nobel prize in Medicine for his continuing contributions to organ transplantation—the first plastic surgeon so honoured.

During the years just before the Second World War Drs Sterling Bunnell, Alan Kanavel, and Summer L. Koch had pioneered advances in surgery of the hand in the USA. Enormous progress was made during that war in rebuilding the injured hand. For the first time, hand surgery became a major part of the work of plastic surgeons throughout the world. In the 1950s, William Littler inspired many young plastic surgeons to become serious students of surgery of the hand. In the 1960s, Paul Brand, working in Vellore, India, first demonstrated that the hand and facial deformities of *leprosy could be greatly relieved by techniques of plastic surgery. This gave millions of leprosy victims new hope.

Following the Second World War, many new medical centres sprang up in Europe to recognize the specialty of plastic surgery. Burian established a department at Charles University in Prague in 1948. In Vienna, Eiselsberg, Pichler, and Esser developed facilities in the specialty. In Germany, Schuchardt established a plastic clinic in Hamburg to treat soldiers who had been injured on the Russian front. Wassmund, in Berlin, continued the plastic surgery methods originally started by Axhausen.

Several French surgeons had been trained in plastic centres, either in the UK or in the USA immediately following the Second World War. They then established a new French school of plastic surgery under the leadership of Morel-Fatio and Claude Dufourmental. At about this same time, in South America, plastic surgery was being developed and demonstrated by Hector Marino and Malbec. This world-wide activity led to the founding of the first International Association of Plastic Surgeons in 1960. The new and burgeoning specialty of plastic surgery in Japan soon developed too, as a result of the leadership of Sechii Ohmori.

Modern plastic surgery

Today, plastic surgery includes much more than those traditional fields relating to reconstructions of the nose and correction of fractures and deformities of the facial bones and jaw. Plastic surgeons now treat patients needing complex reconstructions of the hand, paraplegics needing repair of pressure sores, or those needing grafting of wounds resulting from frost-bite and major thermal burns. Other plastic surgery patients require the replacement of skin, fat, and muscle, and later bone reconstruction or repair of damaged peripheral nerves. In the 1950s and 1960s, plastic surgeons made substantial contributions to the treatment of patients with head and neck malignancy by developing methods of immediate and sophisticated reconstruction of the face and jaw. These procedures reduced deformity and helped patients regain the ability to talk, swallow, breathe, and control saliva.

The broadening scope of plastic surgery requires long years of diversified training of its practitioners. This need was recognized by the American Board of Plastic Surgery. It has required aspiring plastic surgeons to take a long period of training in general surgery prior to entering additional years of residency in plastic surgery.

Today, plastic surgery plays an academic role in almost every large medical centre throughout the USA. Plastic surgeons are involved in major reconstructive surgery throughout the body, and they are also engaged in basic research, studying wound healing, tissue *transplantation, biology of implantation of synthetic materials, *genetics, human *embryology and development, speech pathology, and, most recently, the new fields of microsurgery and craniofacial surgery. This last subspecialty has, for the first time, made possible the correction of severe deformities seen with many birth defects that require repositioning of parts of the cranium, orbits, and facial bones. Craniofacial surgery became more effective with the establishment of multidisciplinary teams of plastic surgeons, neurosurgeons, and ophthalmological surgeons. Plastic surgeons are now able to translocate and reposition the human eye without loss of vision. These techniques were pioneered by Tessier in France and by Edgerton and Converse in the USA in the late 1960s and early 1970s (Kazanjian and Converse 1968).

Unfortunately, the general public, even to this day, tends to think that plastic surgeons are concerned primarily with aesthetic surgery. Recently liposuction aesthetic surgery has been developed to permit removal of unwanted body fat. Orthognathic surgery now allows repositioning of the jaws and teeth to remodel facial contours. Many advances in cosmetic surgery were introduced by plastic surgeons who first developed those techniques while doing craniofacial reconstructions. The value of broad surgical training for plastic surgeons is evident.

Aesthetic surgery is an important subdivision of plastic surgery. Its primary goal is to improve the emotional health and self-imagery of the patient. When properly selected, these patients show enormous psychological and vocational gains following operation. The lay public has come to appreciate the value of these procedures and, hence, the demand for aesthetic (cosmetic) surgery continues to increase.

Pope Pius XIII stated, on 14 October 1958, 'if we consider physical beauty in its Christian light, and if we respect the condition set by our moral teachings, then aesthetic surgery is not in contradiction to the will of God, in that it restores to perfection that greatest work of creation, Man'.

MILTON T. EDGERTON

References

Blair, V. P. (1913). *Surgery and diseases of the mouth and jaws.* Kimpton, London; Stenhouse, Glasgow.

Carpue, J. C. (1816). *An account of two successful operations for restoring a lost nose from the integuments of the forehead.* Longman, London. Reprint (1990), Classics of Surgery Library, Birmingham Alabama.

Davis, J. S. (1919). *Plastic surgery – its principles and practice.* P. Blakiston's Sons, Philadelphia.

Dupuytren, G. (1832–1834). *Leçons orales de clinique chirurgical faites à l'Hôtel-Dieu de Paris.* Ballière, Paris.

Edgerton, M. T. (1974). The role of plastic surgery in academic medicine. Presidential address. *Journal of Plastic and Reconstructive Surgery,* **54**, 523.

Edgerton, M. T. Udvarhelyi, G. B., and Knox, D. L. (1970). The surgical correction of ocular hypertelorism. *Annals of Surgery,* **172**, 473.

Gentlemen's Magazine (1794). A communication to the editor, Mr Urban, signed B. L. and dated 9 Oct. 1794. London.

Gnudi, M. T. and Webster, J. P. (1950). *The life and times of Gaspare Tagliacozzi.* H. Reichner, New York.

Joseph, J. (1931). Nasenplastik und sonstige Gesichtsplastik nebst einem Anhang über Mammaplastik. *Ein Atlas und Lehrbuch.* Kabitzch, Leipzig.

Kazanjian, V. and Converse, J. (1968). *Plastic surgery.* Saunders, Philadelphia.

Kazanjian, V. H. and Converse, J. M. (1974). *The surgical treatment of facial injuries,* (3rd edn). Williams and Wilkins, Baltimore, Maryland.

Morestin, H. (1915). La reduction graduelle des difformités tégumentaires. Reprinted in *Bulletin Memorial Société Chirurgie*, **41**, 1233.

Ollier, L. (1872). Greffles cutanée ou autoplastique. *Bulletin Academie Médecine*, **1**, 243.

Reverdin, J. L. (1870). Greffes épidermiques; expérience faite dans les service de M. le docteur Guyon. *Bulletin Société Impériale Chirurgie*.

Tagliacozzi, G. (1597), *Du Curtorum chirurgia per Insitioneum*. Venice.

Tessier, P., Giot, G., Rougerie, J., Delbet, J. P., and Pastoriza, J. (1967). Osteotomies cranio-naso-orbital-faciales. *Annales Chirurgie Plastic*, **12**, 103.

Von Graefe, C. F. (1818). *Rhinoplastik; oder, Die Kunst den Verlust der Nase organisch zu ersetzen in ihren früheren Verhäultnissen erforscht und durch neue Verfahrungsweisen zur höulherne Volkommenheit geföurdert*. Realschulbuch-handlung, Berlin.

PLATELETS are the smallest cellular elements of the blood, minute non-nucleated fragments (also called thrombocytes) formed from larger bone-marrow cells (megakaryocytes). Platelets play an important role in blood coagulation and in certain immunological reactions. See HAEMATOLOGY.

PLATT, ROBERT (Baron Platt of Grindleford, life peer, 1967) (1900–78). English physician. As the first full-time professor of medicine in Manchester, he attained a national reputation as an outstanding clinician, and an adviser on medical education and research. He was president of the Royal College of Physicians of London from 1957 to 1962, during which time the College became much more active in postgraduate education, and acquired premises to enable it to fulfil this task—the building designed by Denys Lasdun on the east side of Regent's Park. During his presidency the College set up a committee 'to report on *smoking and *atmospheric pollution in relation to carcinoma of the lung and other illnesses'; the publication of the report on *Smoking and health* in 1962 was a landmark in creating public awareness of the dangers of smoking.

PLEOCYTOSIS is an increase in the number of cells in the *cerebrospinal fluid.

PLEOMORPHISM. Occurrence in a number of different forms.

PLETHORA. Congestion with blood.

PLETHYSMOGRAPHY is the recording of changes in the total volume of an organ or part, often used as a measure of blood flow through it (e.g. finger plethysmography).

PLEURA. The serous membrane lining the interior of the thoracic cavity (parietal layer) and enveloping the lung (visceral or pulmonary layer). The layers are continuous with each other and move against each other as the lung expands and contracts during breathing. They enclose a potential space known as the pleural cavity.

PLEURAL CAVITY. The potential space enclosed by the visceral and parietal layers of the *pleura.

PLEURAL EFFUSION is an accumulation of fluid within the *pleural cavity. See also PLEURISY.

PLEURISY is inflammation of the *pleura. In dry pleurisy, the inflamed surfaces move against each other causing a characteristic sharp pain on breathing, and on *auscultation a pleural friction rub can often be heard. These manifestations disappear when fluid accumulates in the pleural cavity (pleural effusion); the chief signs are then a marked impairment of resonance on *percussion and diminution of breath sounds on *auscultation.

PLEURODYNIA is pleural pain, often used synonymously with *Bornholm disease.

PLEXIMETER. The object which is tapped during examination by *percussion; this is usually the middle phalanx of the examiner's middle finger (the pleximeter finger) but sometimes a small plate pleximeter is substituted.

PLEXUS. Any network of vessels or nerves.

PLINY THE ELDER (Gaius Plinius Secundus) (c. AD 23–79). Roman natural historian. Pliny served in the army and later as a proconsul in Spain and Africa. He wrote an encyclopaedic natural history, *Naturalis historia*, in 37 volumes. Books XX–XXXII deal with medicine. He died from exposure to fumes from the eruption of Vesuvius.

PLOMBAGE is surgical *occlusion with inert material (plombe) of a cavity in the body, for example in bone, or in the thorax round a collapsed lung.

PLUMBISM. *Lead poisoning.

PNEUMA was a supposed all-pervading vital principle central to a Graeco-Roman theory of medicine widely accepted during the 1st centuries BC and AD. Pneuma was carried around the body in the nerves and underwent changes in particular organs; at death it left to rejoin a universal stockpile. The doctrine was promulgated by *Erasistratus and others.

PNEUMATISM was a school of medical practice based on the theory of *pneuma.

PNEUMATURIA is the passage of air or other gas in the urine.

PNEUMOCOCCUS is a Gram-positive diplococcus, the official name of which is now *Streptococcus pneumoniae*. A facultative *anaerobe, it is responsible for most cases of lobar *pneumonia, some other bacterial pneumonias, and some serious infections elsewhere in the body, including meningitis.

PNEUMOCONIOSIS is a lung disease produced by the inhalation and pulmonary deposition of dusts, of occupational or other environmental origin. The extent of interference with lung function depends on the nature and size of the dust particles and the pulmonary reaction to them. Thus some pneumoconioses are relatively innocuous, such as those due to carbon particles (anthracosis) and to iron dust (siderosis). Others, like *silicosis and *asbestosis are much more serious. See OCCUPATIONAL MEDICINE.

PNEUMOCYSTIS is a genus of micro-organisms thought to be *protozoa but of which the life cycle has not been established with certainty. *Pneumocystis carinii* is the causative agent of a life-threatening form of *pneumonia (pneumocystosis) which characteristically occurs as an *opportunistic infection in patients with congenital immunodeficiencies and those under treatment with immunosuppressive agents; it has been reported in as many as half the patients with the *acquired immune deficiency syndrome (AIDS). In healthy subjects, infection is probably asymptomatic.

PNEUMOENCEPHALOGRAPHY is the *radiographic demonstration of *brain structures through visualization of the cerebral ventricles and subarachnoid space after replacement of *cerebrospinal fluid with air or other gas.

PNEUMOMEDIASTINUM is the presence of air in the *mediastinum, usually due to *trauma involving the bronchial tree (also known as mediastinal *emphysema).

PNEUMONECTOMY is surgical removal of a lung.

PNEUMONIA is inflammation of the parenchyma of the lungs, that is the alveoli and interstitial tissue, due to infection with micro-organisms. The term '*pneumonitis' is almost synonymous, but strictly speaking means inflammation of lung tissue from any cause. Almost any micro-organism can cause pneumonia, including many bacteria, viruses, rickettsiae, and fungi.

PNEUMONITIS is inflammation of the parenchyma of the lungs from any cause, including chemical and physical agents. The term *pneumonia is sometimes used synonymously but usually implies inflammation due to infection with micro-organisms unless otherwise specified. An alternative usage restricts the meaning of pneumonitis to mild segmental inflammation.

PNEUMOPERITONEUM is air in the *peritoneal cavity. Artificial pneumoperitoneum is sometimes induced

in order to assist *radiological diagnosis; it was formerly a common procedure in the treatment of pulmonary *tuberculosis, to help in immobilization of the lung.

PNEUMOTHORAX is the presence of air in the *pleural cavity. Normally the subatmospheric pressure in the potential *pleural cavity keeps the parietal and visceral pleural layers in close apposition. If a communication develops between the cavity and the atmosphere, air is sucked in, and the elastic lung collapses; since the respiratory movements of the chest wall can no longer expand it, it ceases to function. If the communication acts as a valve, gas pressure builds up within the cavity, displacing the *mediastinal structures to the opposite side and interfering with circulation (tension pneumothorax). Pneumothorax can result from penetrating chest wounds, from various lung diseases (particularly *emphysema), and in otherwise healthy subjects probably as a result of minor congenital weaknesses in the lung wall which rupture under strain (spontaneous pneumothorax). An artificial pneumothorax can readily be induced by inserting a hollow needle through the chest wall; this was formerly used as a method of resting the lung in the treatment of pulmonary tuberculosis, and sometimes in diagnostic *radiology.

PODAGRA. Synonym for *gout.

PODIATRY is the US term for *chiropody.

POIKILODERMA is any variegated or mottled appearance of the skin.

POISEUILLE, JEAN LEONARD MARIE (1797–1869). French physiologist. He devised a mercury *sphygmomanometer in 1828, and enunciated his law, which stated that the rate of flow of a liquid in a tube is given by the formula: $\pi p r^2 / 8 l \mu$, p is the pressure of the liquid, r the radius of the tube, l its length, and μ the coefficient of the liquid's viscosity.

POISONING

All substances are poisons; there is none which is not a poison. The right dose differentiates a poison and a remedy.
Paracelsus (1493–1541)

Introduction
This important principle was set out almost 500 years ago, but acute poisoning, both from *drugs and other substances, remains a major problem in health care; one of the targets set out in the UK government's White Paper *The health of the nation* is to reduce by 15 per cent the overall *suicide rate, which is due, in large part, to self-poisoning by drugs, chemicals, or motor vehicle exhaust gas (*carbon monoxide).

In adults, most poisons are self-administered, usually

deliberately with suicidal or 'parasuicidal' intent. Accidental exposure, through work or environmental contamination, is uncommon. However, inadvertent acute or chronic exposure does occur, usually through occupational exposure to chemicals, but sometimes when members of the public are exposed to toxic chemicals, for example, garden materials or cleaning agents. Environmental pollution is a rare cause of exposure to toxins, but one that causes great public concern; incidents at Seveso in Italy, involving dioxin, and, more recently, at Bhopal where isocyanate was released, are prominent examples. Poisoning in children is invariably accidental, but occasionally may be a feature of child abuse. The homicidal use of poisons, once very common, is now rare. Table 1 shows the nature of the agents involved in calls to the Newcastle Poisons Centre in 1991.

*Epidemiology

Poisoning is a major component of the workload of accident and emergency departments, and it is a major cause of admission to medical units. In London, it is estimated to account for more than 10 per cent of acute adult medical admissions. Deliberate self-poisoning is the second most common cause of death in young adults.

Hospital admissions for poisoning in the UK rose steadily in the 1960s and 1970s, reaching a peak of 120 640 admissions per annum in 1978. Since then, there has been a modest decline in admission rates. Since some poisoning incidents are handled by *general practitioners (GPs) and are not referred to hospital, and because not all cases seen at accident departments are admitted, the true incidence of ingestion of toxic agents may be 2–3 times the hospital admission rate, i.e. it is estimated that there may be more than 300 000 poisoning incidents per annum in the UK.

Most patients admitted to hospital for self-poisoning are young, particularly in the 15–25 age-group. Women outnumber men in all age-groups, with the exception of young children; there is a particular predominance of women in the 15–45 age-group.

Since the early 1970s, mortality from acute poisoning has been more or less constant at about 4000 deaths per annum, although the pattern of agents causing these deaths has changed markedly; carbon monoxide and *barbiturates are now involved less frequently, while deaths from *analgesic drugs and *antidepressants have increased. Because of the effectiveness of current techniques of *resuscitation, supportive treatment, and, where appropriate, the use of antidotes, *mortality in poisoned patients admitted to hospital is very low, less than 1 per cent. In a study of 737 patients admitted to hospital in Newcastle, only three (0.4 per cent) died. Most deaths from poisoning (about 80 per cent) occur at home.

About 13 000 children are admitted to hospital each year in the UK because of actual or suspected ingestion of a poison, the vast majority being less than 5 years of age, and up to 39 000 poisoning 'incidents' may take place each year, although the majority are poisoning 'scares' involving little risk of harm to the child, rather than true poisoning. Most cases occur in the home, often when the substances involved are not in their usual storage place or container. There has been a gradual, but not dramatic, decline in hospital admission of poisoned children, which may be due, in part, to the increasing use of child-resistant containers for medicines and other household products. Mortality in cases of childhood poisoning is lower than for adult poisoning. Between 1974 and 1980 only 69 children under the age of 5 years died from poisoning by drugs, and 11 after ingesting non-medicinal substances. Carbon monoxide, however, continues to be the major cause of fatal poisoning in children, causing more deaths than those from all other chemicals and drugs combined. Poisoning incidents in children usually involve exploratory behaviour, and ingestion of relatively small quantities of household materials that are often innocuous. In contrast to adults, young children are much more likely to ingest household products such as bleaches, detergents, white spirit, disinfectants, or cosmetics. Nevertheless, serious poisoning involving toxic chemicals or drugs such as iron, analgesics, and antidepressants does still occur. The resulting morbidity, distress to children and their families, and cost to the NHS dictate that health promotion programmes should include awareness and prevention of child poisoning.

Table 2 shows the range of agents that had been taken by 737 poisoned adults admitted to hospital in Newcastle. It can be seen that drugs, particularly analgesics and *benzodiazepine sedatives (such as diazepam or nitrazepam) are frequently involved in adult self-poisoning. Adults frequently take overdoses of medicines that have been prescribed for themselves or their relatives, and patterns of poisoning therefore reflect the therapeutic use of drugs. Thus poisoning by barbiturates, once a major cause of death, is seldom seen now, since these toxic drugs are much less often prescribed than previously. In contrast, poisoning by benzodiazepines is very common, although these drugs are relatively safe and mortality is correspondingly low. There has also been an increase in the incidence of

Table 1 Calls to Newcastle Poisons Centre 1991

Agent	% of calls
Industrial chemicals	11
Pesticides	2
Household agents	21
Cosmetics/personal hygiene products	4
Drugs (including drugs of dependency)	55
Plants/animals	5
Other poisons	2

poisoning by analgesics and antidepressants, reflecting growth in the prescribing of these drugs.

In the UK, alcohol is taken in addition to a drug overdose in about 60 per cent of male and about 40 per cent of female cases; and many poisoning incidents involve more than one drug.

The pattern of poisoning may be very different in other countries; in many developing countries, poisoning by herbicides and pesticides is very much more common than in the UK.

Treatment of poisoning

There are four general principles in treating poisoned patients. These are: first to provide general first aid and to support the patient's respiratory and cardiovascular functions; secondly, to minimize any direct effect of the poison, for example, caustic effects of an alkali on the skin or gastrointestinal tract, or *fits caused by drugs acting on the nervous system; thirdly, to reduce the amount of poison entering the body by reducing its absorption from the gastrointestinal tract; and, fourthly, to reduce the toxic effects of the poison after it has been absorbed, either by the use of an antidote, or by increasing the rate at which the poison is eliminated from the body.

Initial management

In all but the simplest of cases, medical advice is essential. If a significant quantity of a drug has been ingested, then it is likely that some form of hospital admission will be indicated. Most depressive drugs produce their maximum effect within 3 or 4 hours after ingestion, and the patient may be asleep, deeply unconscious, or even dead within this time. However, some poisons, such as

Table 2 Agents taken by 737 poisoned patients admitted to hospital in Newcastle

	Number	Percentages
Alcohol	324	43.9
Antibiotics	40	5.4
Antidepressants	125	17.0
Aspirin	105	14.2
Benzodiazepines	371	50.3
House/garden agents	29	3.9
Neuroleptics	36	4.9
Non-steroidal anti-inflammatory drugs	32	4.3
Paracetamol	241	32.7
Sedatives	38	5.2
Other	184	25.0

Many patients took more than one agent; percentages refer to the number of patients who ingested a particular product as part of an overdose.

*paracetamol, take several hours, or even days, for their effects to become evident. It is therefore important to seek advice in any suspected poisoning, even if the patient appears normal.

Induction of vomiting by first aiders is best avoided. There are some materials, for example, petroleum products, in which inhalation of vomit containing the toxin may be more dangerous than allowing it to remain in the gastrointestinal tract. The use of saline is ineffective, dangerous, and potentially lethal, as large quantities of salt may be absorbed. Copper sulphate is an equally obsolete and dangerous emetic. Similarly, the use of stimulants such as hot coffee is inappropriate; the amounts of *caffeine present have no therapeutic effect and again, should the patient vomit, there is a risk of inhalation of vomitus.

It is important that those looking after a poisoned person are not contaminated by the toxin. In the case of carbon monoxide exposure, immediate steps should be taken to provide adequate ventilation. In the case of exposure to corrosive materials, care should be taken to ensure that the first-aider does not also suffer burns or other skin damage.

Some poisoned patients will present with breathing difficulties or low blood pressure and resuscitation is the immediate priority. Initial management should include a risk assessment, which will involve taking a detailed history of the amount and type of poison, and the route of exposure. It is useful here if any containers and residual contents accompany the patient to hospital. Obtaining a reliable history can be difficult. There is often considerable uncertainty about what, if any, poisons children have ingested; and adults may be very drowsy or uncooperative. Laboratory analysis is of little value as a diagnostic tool, although once the nature of the poison is known, blood concentrations can be a valuable prognostic indicator and aid to monitoring treatment. Changes in the level of consciousness, or other physical signs such as skin colour and heart rate, may be indicators of the severity of poisoning.

Hospital management

Treatment of the poisoned patient in hospital comprises supportive and symptomatic care, together with (where appropriate) measures to prevent or reduce absorption of the toxin, measures to enhance the rate of elimination, laboratory investigations, and the use of antidotes. Seriously poisoned patients require expert supportive care, with particular emphasis on maintenance of an adequate airway and breathing, avoidance of low blood pressure, management of cardiac rhythm disturbances, convulsions, hypothermia, metabolic and fluid balance.

(a) Prevention of absorption of the poison. Three techniques have been traditionally used to minimize absorption of poisons from the gastrointestinal tract: gastric lavage, *emetic drugs, and adsorbent materials such as

Fuller's earth or activated charcoal. Despite their use for many years, there is considerable controversy over the effectiveness of these techniques. In particular, there is increasing recognition that gastric lavage and the use of emetics are of little value in many poisonings, as there is little objective evidence that either technique successfully removes large amounts of drug from the stomach, particularly if there has been any substantial delay in starting treatment.

In gastric lavage (stomach washout) a large-bore tube is introduced into the stomach, and fluid is passed down the tube, which is then lowered to allow the fluid plus stomach contents to run out. The patient needs to be conscious because of the risk of aspiration into the lungs, or, if unconscious, then the lungs need to be protected by passage of a cuffed *endotracheal tube into the airway by an *anaesthetist. Gastric lavage has been very commonly (but often inappropriately) used in acute poisoning. However, there is little evidence of its efficacy, and the procedure is traumatic. Moreover, it is now known that some of the lavage fluid passes from the stomach into the duodenum, sometimes taking tablets with it and thereby contributing to more rapid absorption. Gastric lavage is therefore increasingly used only in selected patients; these include cases where large numbers of tablets have been taken that may adhere in the stomach (e.g. *aspirin), or large overdoses of drugs (such as *morphine and some antidepressants) that may delay gastric emptying.

Ipecacuanha is an emetic drug which stimulates the part of the brain that produces vomiting. It is taken as an oral mixture and produces vomiting after a time delay, usually about 10–20 minutes. It can produce prolonged vomiting which is distressing for the patient and, like lavage, the evidence of its effectiveness in removing poisons is weak. Nevertheless, ipecacuanha is often used in children, where it is still regarded as the method of choice when gastric emptying is indicated. It should not be used when petroleum products or corrosive agents have been taken. In the USA, ipecacuanha is frequently used as a first-aid measure, and many domestic medicine cabinets contain a supply of ipecacuanha syrup. Its use for this purpose is not recommended in the UK, however, because of the risk of prolonged vomiting or other complications, and the need for a degree of training to determine when it may be contraindicated.

Activated charcoal is very finely powdered charcoal that binds many drugs and chemicals, making them unavailable for absorption from the gut. Charcoal is useful in many, although not all, drug poisonings and is increasingly used as a first-aid measure. As with other techniques used to reduce the absorption of poisons, the earlier charcoal is given, the greater its effect. It can be given to children in a fizzy drink to make it more palatable. In contrast to emetics and lavage, charcoal is also effective at absorbing drugs in the duodenum and small intestine; repeated doses can therefore be useful when delayed- or sustained-action tablets have been taken, as

these continue to release drug for several hours after they have left the stomach. Fuller's earth is used as an oral adsorbent in paraquat poisoning.

(b) Enhanced elimination of the poison. Toxins in the blood are normally eliminated from the body either by excretion in the urine, metabolism in the liver, or a combination of both. There are at present no effective techniques for increasing the rate of drug metabolism, but several methods of enhanced elimination are available that mimic or accelerate urinary excretion. These include attempts to increase urinary excretion by increasing the flow rate (forced *diuresis) and also by changing the pH (acidity or alkalinity) of the urine for alkaline or acid drugs, respectively. Once very popular, these techniques are now less widely used, because it is difficult in practice to achieve the required changes in acidity or alkalinity, and the procedures themselves are not without hazard; there is a consequent risk of metabolic disturbances and fluid overload that can, in some circumstances, be more hazardous than the poison being treated.

An alternative approach is haemodialysis, which removes the drug or chemical from the blood using a *dialysis (artificial kidney) machine, or haemoperfusion, in which blood is passed through a plastic column containing granules of activated charcoal. While both of these techniques are safe and effective in the management of some forms of poisoning, for example, with aspirin, *theophylline, and ethylene glycol (antifreeze), they are not universally applicable because the chemical nature and pattern of distribution of many poisons in the body render them inaccessible to removal by these techniques.

The removal from the body of iron and of heavy metals such as mercury and lead can be accelerated by using a sequestering or chelating agent. These are drugs, usually given intravenously, which bind the metal, minimize its toxic effects, and increase its availability for excretion by the kidney. Chelating agents can themselves be toxic, and their use therefore requires a careful assessment of the severity of the poisoning that is being treated. Nevertheless, serious iron or heavy metal poisoning will usually be treated with agents such as desferrioxamine (iron poisoning), dimercaprol (mercury), or sodium calcium edetate (lead).

(c) Laboratory investigations. Analysis of body fluids to detect or measure toxic materials is only indicated if the diagnosis is in doubt (where, in any case, routine laboratory analysis is often unhelpful) or, more commonly, where the poison is known and the symptoms are serious enough to warrant active treatment using specific antidotes, haemodialysis, or haemoperfusion. Laboratory investigation can be time-consuming and expensive, and often yields information of only limited value. In particular, the concept of a 'toxic level' upon which treatment decisions can be based is sometimes misleading; laboratory data should always be viewed in the context of the history, the patient's clinical condition, and conventional biochemical indicators such as blood chemistry and blood oxygen concentration. Nevertheless, interpreted intelligently, blood concentrations can be valuable in the management of several poisons, notably iron, paracetamol, aspirin, digoxin, and theophylline. These investigations are available in most hospital laboratories, and more specialized analyses can be provided at regional or supraregional centres.

(d) Use of antidotes. An antidote can be defined as an agent which neutralizes the effect of a poison. It may produce this effect in a number of ways, but the action is usually specific to a single chemical or group of related chemicals. Although the view is widely held that the use of antidotes is central to poisons treatment, in fact specific antidotes are available for only a relatively small range of poisons (Table 3). The effects of morphine, *pethidine, and related opiate analgesics can be completely and safely reversed using a specific opiate antagonist, naloxone, which acts on opiate receptors in the brain. Naloxone is itself without side-effects, and should be used whenever there is the possibility that opiates have been taken; a positive response to naloxone is diagnostic of opiate overdose.

The potentially lethal liver toxicity of paracetamol in overdose can be prevented in many cases by using a specific antidote. This neutralizes the toxic product (metabolite) of paracetamol formed in the liver, which is responsible for the liver damage that paracetamol produces in overdose (although not in conventional therapeutic doses). Two such antidotes are currently available, acetylcysteine (the preferred treatment) and methionine.

Ethanol (alcohol) is used to counteract the toxic effects of ethylene glycol (antifreeze) or *methanol. These chemicals produce their serious toxicity by being converted to toxic intermediate compounds; ethanol competes for the same metabolic pathways, but produces relatively harmless metabolites. In this way it prevents the toxic metabolites from being formed. Other treatment, such as haemodialysis, can then be used to eliminate the poison. Oxygen (hyperbaric when available) is used to treat carbon monoxide poisoning; it acts by displacing carbon monoxide from binding sites on enzymes where it exerts its toxic effect.

Immunological techniques, where a protein (antiserum) binds and inactivates a specific poison were originally developed for the management of snake envenomation. They have recently been extended to other forms of poisoning, notably with the cardiac drug, digoxin. A preparation of digoxin antibodies is available which binds digoxin, making it inactive, and increases its elimination by the kidney. These techniques are an attractive approach to the treatment of poisoning, but they are only appropriate when the poison is very potent, i.e. relatively small amounts of the toxin are present, which is the case with snake venoms and digoxin.

Prevention of poisoning

Poisoning incidents can be prevented by taking measures to ensure that drugs or other poisons are labelled, stored, and used safely. There is evidence that the increasing use of child-resistant containers has reduced the risk of ingestion of poisons by children.

The pharmaceutical and chemical industries go to great lengths to provide appropriate packaging and labelling for their products, and it is therefore worrying that both drugs and other products are often transferred to other containers within the domestic environment. The practice of storing household or garden products in used drink containers is particularly hazardous, as is the practice of mixing prescribed medicines in the same container; these practices often feature in cases of accidental poisoning.

There has been some interest in attempting to reduce the potential for acute poisoning by the inclusion of antidotes in particularly toxic products. The best examples of this are the herbicide *paraquat, and the analgesic paracetamol. Paraquat is used extensively in horticulture and agriculture, and is particularly toxic. When taken in its liquid concentrated form, it invariably causes fatal lung and kidney damage, and the granular formulations used in domestic gardening are also hazardous. In an attempt to reduce the mortality from paraquat poisoning, paraquat formulations now contain an emetic agent, the aim being to induce vomiting in an individual who has consumed the product. There is, however, no evidence as yet that this measure has altered the mortality from paraquat poisoning.

Following the same principle, the paracetamol antidote methionine has been included in a new paracetamol formulation (Pameton®). Methionine acts by preventing the potentially lethal toxic effects of the paracetamol

Table 3 Some antidotes known to be effective in acute poisoning

Poison	Antidote
Paracetamol	N-acetylcysteine
	Methionine
Opiates	Naloxone
Carbon monoxide	Oxygen
Mercury/arsenic	Dimercaprol
Lead	Sodium calcium edetate
Iron	Desferrioxamine
Digoxin	Digoxin-specific antibody
Organophosphate	Atropine
insecticides	Pralidoxime

overdose on the liver, but has no effect on the normal therapeutic action of the drug. The theory is that individuals who overdose will then consume equivalent amounts of the antidote. However, although this product is now on sale in the UK, it has not been widely adopted either by the general public or by the medical profession, and there is no evidence to date of any impact on the mortality or morbidity from paracetamol poisoning. In any case, such measures are not a substitute for continuing educational and public health programmes on poisoning.

In the months following an acute self-poisoning incident, up to a third of patients may repeat the episode. Effective primary care, psychiatric, or social work follow-up as appropriate is therefore essential to prevent recurrence of self-poisoning. Given adequate aftercare, including effective treatment of any *depression, re-poisoning rates should be less than 10 per cent.

International aspects

Self-induced, industrial, and environmental poisoning is by no means a problem that is restricted to the developed world. Widespread availability of agricultural and industrial chemicals in developing countries carries with it corresponding health risks. The appropriate labelling of products, ensuring that guidelines on safe handling of chemicals are followed, and access to information for health workers, may all present problems in developing countries. These issues have been recognized by the *World Health Organization, the International Labour Organization, and the European Community, and these agencies are working together through the International Programme on Chemical Safety which aims to improve awareness on chemical safety issues, and to develop strategies to disseminate information about poisoning and its management for health staff in developing countries.

Within Europe, the European Commission now requires member states to produce standardized reports on the frequency and nature of poisoning exposures within Europe. In this way it can monitor changing trends in acute and chronic poisoning, and can develop Europe-wide strategies, where appropriate, to deal with the public health issues that may arise.

Poisons centres

Provision of accurate, timely advice is often essential for the effective management of acute poisoning. The constituents of marketed chemical products are often complex, and toxicology is a specialized area of biomedical science; thus most developed countries now have a system of poisons information centres. These can provide data on a 24-hour basis on the ingredients of products, their toxic properties, and appropriate clinical management. Many centres can also advise on, or provide, appropriate laboratory investigations, and can also arrange for referral to specialized treatment units if necessary. In the UK, poisons centres operate

Table 4 United Kingdom National Poisons Information Service (NPIS)

Belfast	Royal Victoria Hospital
Birmingham	Dudley Road Hospital
Cardiff	Llandough Hospital
Edinburgh	Royal Infirmary
Leeds	General Infirmary
London	Guy's Hospital
Newcastle upon Tyne	Royal Victoria Infirmary

as a national network, the National Poisons Information Service (NPIS). Table 4 lists the seven constituent centres of the NPIS. These centres share a common database (Toxbase, developed by the Scottish Poisons Centre in Edinburgh) and they also have access to a recently developed computer system for the identification of solid dosage forms of drugs (tablets and capsules) which is frequently a problem when patients have taken unidentified drugs. Poisons information services within the European countries meet regularly to share experience on poisoning.

J. M. SMITH
D. N. BATEMAN

Further reading

Ferguson, J. A., Sellar, C., and Goldacre, M. J. (1992). Some epidemiological observations on medicinal and non-medicinal poisoning in preschool children. *Journal of Epidemiology and Community Health*, **46**, 207–10.

Hawton, K. and Fagg, J. (1992). Trends in deliberate self-poisoning and self injury in Oxford, 1976–90. *British Medical Journal*, **304**, 1409–11.

Meredith, T. (1991). Epidemiology of poisoning. *Care of the Critically Ill*, **7**, 97–8.

Tibballs, J. (1989). Epidemiology of acute poisoning. *Medicine International*, **61**, 2496–8.

Wynne, H., Bateman, D. N., Hassanyeh, F., Rawlins, M. D., and Woodhouse, K. W. (1987). Age and self-poisoning: The epidemiology in Newcastle upon Tyne in the 1980s. *Human Toxicology*, **6**, 511–15.

POISONOUS FUNGI. The ingestion of poisonous fungi is uncommon, but can be deadly. Most non-edible fungi are either unpleasant or uninteresting but are non-toxic or only mildly so. The highly poisonous species are all gill fungi, the commonest (to which about 90 per cent of deaths are attributable) being *Amanita phalloides* (death cap), of which one cap may be fatal. Other closely related but much rarer species are *Amanita virosa* (destroying angel) and *Amanita verna* (fool's mushroom). *Amanita pantherina* (panther cap) can cause severe *atropine poisoning, but fatalities are rare. The same applies to the attractive-looking fairy-tale mushroom *Amanita muscaria* (fly agaric), which also contains *muscarine. Other species (e.g. *Russula emetica* and some *Gyromitra* spp.) contain thermolabile toxins and are consumed by some after cooking. *Coprinus atramentarius* contains *disulfiram (Antabuse®) and thus causes symptoms of poisoning when ingested with alcohol. Any species of fungus, including the familiar cultivated and wild mushrooms, may be responsible for food *allergy in susceptible individuals.

POISONOUS PLANTS. Poisoning by plants is uncommon, occurring most often in children. Nevertheless, many plants contain poisonous compounds in their roots, leaves, flowers, seeds, or fruit, and may under certain circumstances, for example, when used in 'bush tea' infusions, cause toxic syndromes. These include: the Solanaceae, many of which contain mixtures of alkaloids such as *atropine, *hyoscyamine, *scopolamine, and *nicotine, examples being *Atropa belladonna* (deadly nightshade), *Solanum dulcamara* (woody nightshade or bittersweet), *Hyoscyamus niger* (henbane), *Datura stramonium* (thorn apple), *Nicotiana tabacum* (tobacco), *Capsicum* spp. (e.g. tabasco), *Scopolia* spp; *Cytisus laburnum* (laburnum), which contains the neurotoxic alkaloid cytisine, also found in broom and lupin seeds; *Conium maculatum* (hemlock), which contains conitine, also neurotoxic; *Cicuta virosa* (water hemlock or cowbane), which has caused fatalities by virtue of its highly poisonous cicutoxin; *Oenanthe crocata* (water dropwort), which has a similar toxin; *Aconitum napellus* (monkshood), which contains aconite; *Colchicum* spp. (autumn crocus or meadow saffron), which contains *colchicine; *Digitalis purpurea* (foxglove) and *Nerium oleander* (oleander), which contain *cardiac glycosides; *Cannabis sativa* (hemp, marijuana, etc.), which contains *tetrahydrocannabinol and related compounds; *Senecio longilobus* (ragwort), once used as an emmenogogue, and *Crotalaria* spp., infusions of which cause hepatic veno-occlusive disease; *Bighia sapida* (ackee), the unripe fruit of which contains hypoglycine, the causative toxin of Jamaican vomiting sickness; *Lathyrus* spp. (sweet peas) which cause spastic paraplegia (see LATHYRISM); *Argemone mexicana* (mexican poppy), a contaminant of mustard oil, which contains sanguinarine and interferes with carbohydrate metabolism causing an 'epidemic dropsy' syndrome resembling acute wet *beriberi; and very many others, including the familiar medicinal plants rhubarb, cascara, and senna.

POISONS. See POISONING.

POISONS ACT 1972. This UK Act consolidated the provisions of the *Pharmacy and Poisons Act 1933, in particular those concerning the Poisons Board, Poisons List, and Poisons Rules. Local authorities were required to keep a register of persons entitled to sell non-medicinal poisons, and requirements for such persons were detailed.

POISONS BOARD. A body established under the provisions of the *Pharmacy and Poisons Act 1933.

Section 17 of that Act gave the Board authority to draw up a Poisons List classifying substances according to medicinal and non-medicinal use.

POISSON, SIMEON DENIS (1781–1840). French mathematician. Poisson started medicine but failed to complete his studies. For medicine his important contribution was the Poisson distribution, still much used in *statistics and *epidemiology.

POLARIZATION. For polarization of nerve and muscle cells, see DEPOLARIZATION. Polarization of light signifies the restriction to one plane of the vibrations of light waves.

POLIOMYELITIS is an acute *virus infection, also known as infantile paralysis, with a world-wide distribution confined to primates. Spread is from person to person, the portal of entry being the gastrointestinal tract. In the vast majority of instances, infection produces either no symptoms at all or only those of an influenza-like illness or febrile digestive upset. Some patients, however, manifest signs of *meningitis and a proportion of these develop the motor paralysis which was the much feared complication of the epidemic disease in communities with good sanitation (and hence a low level of naturally acquired immunity) before the advent of active *immunization programmes. The prevention of paralytic poliomyelitis, with its acute dangers and its frequent legacy of crippling disability, is a triumph of public health and community medicine. In countries able to maintain vaccination campaigns, the disease has been virtually eliminated. See EPIDEMIOLOGY; INFECTIOUS DISEASES; MICROBIOLOGY.

POLIOVIRUS, of which there are three serotypes, is a small non-enveloped RNA virus belonging to the *enterovirus genus. It is the causative agent of *poliomyelitis.

POLITZER, ADAM (1835–1920). Hungarian physician and *otologist. He described the cone of light seen in the normal eardrum, and the hearing, on swallowing, of a tuning fork placed centrally on the forehead in only the normal ear. Still in use is his bag used for inflating the middle ear through the *Eustachian tube.

POLITZERIZATION is the inflation of the middle ear using a soft rubber bag (Politzer bag).

POLLEN is formed of the microspores of seed plants (Gymnospermae and Angiospermae) containing male gametophytes, carried by wind or insects to ovules or stigmas for germination. Many pollens are potent allergens. See ALLERGY.

POLLUTION. Man has always tended to defile the natural environment in which he has evolved, and the rapid progress of science and technology during the 20th century has brought new assaults on the human eco-system: examples are radioactive fallout from nuclear weapon testing; river pollution from industrial waste; lead pollution of the atmosphere by the internal com-bustion engine; persistent contamination of the envi-ronment by chlorinated hydrocarbon insecticides such as DDT; noise pollution by jet aircraft; sea and coastal pollution by fuel oil leakage; and many others. Nearly all are of medical importance. See ENVIRONMENT AND MEDICINE I.

POLYA, EUGENE ALEXANDER (1876–1944). Hun-garian surgeon. In addition to valuable experimental work on *pancreatic *necrosis, he devised an operation for *gastrectomy with implantation of the gastric rem-nant end-to-side into the *jejunum (Polya's operation).

POLYANDRY. Multiple husbands. See POLYGAMY.

POLYARTERITIS is multiple inflammation of arteries. Polyarteritis nodosa (also known as periarteritis nodosa and Kussmaul's disease) is an uncommon but serious autoimmune disorder in which focal and inflamma-tory lesions occur in small- and medium-sized arteries throughout the body. It is one of group of collagen or connective tissue diseases. See RHEUMATOLOGY.

POLYARTHRITIS is *arthritis involving a number of joints simultaneously.

POLYARTHROPATHY is any pathological condition affecting more than one joint.

POLYCLINIC. A term generally used to designate a building designed to offer out-patient (as distinct from in-patient) investigation and treatment in a wide variety of medical disciplines.

POLYCYSTIC DISEASE is an inherited condition, in which the kidneys show multiple cyst formation with or without similar changes in the liver. There are two forms, which appear to be distinct entities. Childhood polycystic kidney disease (PKD) is rare, and the pat-tern of inheritance is that of an autosomal *recessive trait. Death occurs in childhood or adolescence, from renal failure in younger children, but in adolescents more often from the liver lesions, which lead to portal hypertension and liver failure. Adult PKD, on the other hand, is fairly common, accounting for about 5 per cent of all patients treated in *renal dialysis and transplan-tation units. It is inherited as an autosomal *dominant trait, and as the condition does not become manifest until well into adult life, after the reproductive period, its transmission is assured. The clinical manifestations include pain and swelling in the loins, *haematuria, urinary infections, renal *calculi, *hypertension, and eventually renal failure. Genetic counselling must be directed at the children of patients, who have a one in two chance of transmitting the genetic defect to their own offspring and of subsequently becoming affected themselves.

POLYCYTHAEMIA (POLYCYTHEMIA) is an in-crease above normal in the total circulating *red blood cell mass. Often the increase is an adaptive reaction to prolonged shortage of oxygen, as for instance in those who live at high altitudes and in heavy smokers; a simi-lar reaction occurs in some forms of chronic heart and lung disease, and in patients with congenitally abnormal types of *haemoglobin. Polycythaemia vera is the name given to a condition in which an increase in red cell mass appears to be primary and purposeless, analogous to the increase in white blood cells that characterizes *leukaemia.

POLYCYTHAEMIA (POLYCYTHEMIA) VERA is primary *polycythaemia, also known as polycythaemia rubra vera, erythraemia, and Vaquez–Osler disease.

POLYDACTYLY is a congenital anomaly associated with extra fingers and/or toes.

POLYGAMY is the practice of having more than one spouse concurrently, subdivided into polyandry (several husbands) and polygyny (several wives). Where poly-gamy is customary it can sometimes be seen to have had some biological, if not ethical, justification.

POLYGENIC describes an inherited characteristic which is controlled by a number of genes, each with a small but additive effect. See GENETICS.

POLYGRAPH. An instrument for simultaneously re-cording several physiological variables, such as arterial pulse and pressure, central venous pulse, respiratory rate, skin conductivity, etc. Polygraphs intended to reveal the physiological concomitants of anxiety are known as lie-detectors.

POLYMERASE. An enzyme which catalyses the con-version of nucleotides to polynucleotides.

POLYMERASE CHAIN REACTION. A technique commonly employed in *molecular genetics through which it is possible to produce copies of DNA sequences rapidly.

POLYMORPH is an abbreviation for polymorpho-nuclear *leucocyte (neutrophil *granulocyte).

POLYMORPHISM is the occurrence within a species of widely different inherited forms, the rarest of them too common to be maintained by recurrent mutation. See GENETICS.

POLYMYALGIA is pain in several muscles simultaneously. Polymyalgia rheumatica is a specific syndrome of later life associated with pain in the muscles of the limb girdles and generalized muscle stiffness after brief periods of immobility.

POLYMYOSITIS. See DERMATOMYOSITIS; NEUROMUSCULAR DISEASE.

POLYNEURITIS is inflammation of many nerves simultaneously. In practice, it is synonymous with polyneuropathy. See NEUROMUSCULAR DISEASE.

POLYNEUROPATHY. See NEUROMUSCULAR DISEASE.

POLYOMA VIRUS is a tumour-producing virus of the *papovavirus group, endemic in mice.

POLYP. A protrusion of *mucous membrane occurring in the nose and elsewhere.

POLYPEPTIDE. A *peptide containing a number of *amino acid residues.

POLYPHARMACY is a deprecatory term for the simultaneous prescription of several medicines.

POLYPOSIS is the occurrence of multiple *polyps, particularly a genetically determined disorder (polyposis coli) in which multiple adenomatous polyps develop in the *colon and become malignant unless removed surgically.

POLYSACCHARIDE. Any of a large class of naturally occurring complex *carbohydrates whose molecules derive from the condensation of four or more simple *sugar molecules (monosaccharides). *Starch, *glycogen, and *cellulose are polysaccharides; so are the components of dietary *fibre.

POLYUNSATURATED FATS are *fats containing *fatty acids in which there is more than one double bond between carbon atoms, at which addition can occur. The best dietary sources of polyunsaturated fatty acids are vegetable oils, such as those derived from sesame, soya, sunflower, and corn (maize). The prevailing view that it is desirable to increase the ratio of polyunsaturated fat to saturated (i.e. no double bonds) fat in the human diet is based on evidence that a high intake of saturated fat is associated with a high plasma *cholesterol level, increased blood coagulation indices, and increased morbidity and mortality from the effects of *atherosclerosis, particularly *coronary heart disease. Polyunsaturated fatty acids lower total plasma cholesterol and reduce blood clotting indices.

POMPHOLYX is a recurrent *eczematous condition characterized by small *vesicles on the palms and soles.

PONS. That part of the brainstem which connects the *midbrain above with the *medulla oblongata below and lies in front of the *cerebellum.

POOR LAW COMMISSION. A body established by the Poor Law Amendment Act 1834. The commission had been proposed by Edwin *Chadwick; it had three members, and Chadwick himself was appointed secretary. It existed until the Poor Law Board was created in 1847. The powers of the latter were in turn transferred to the *Local Government Board in 1871.

POOR LAWS. A series of enactments which spanned more than 500 years and which provided increasingly comprehensive official arrangements for the relief of poverty, the roots of the present-day social security system of the UK. The Poor Law Act 1388 was passed in the wake of the *Black Death (the pandemic of plague of 1346–50) and was essentially a law against vagrancy, designed to restrict the mobility of labour. Among many later pieces of legislation, two landmarks were the Poor Law Act of 1601, the famous '43rd of Elizabeth', and the great Poor Law Amendment Act 1834, which set the framework of social welfare in the UK for the next 100 years. The poor laws effectively came to an end in 1929 when the Local Government Act disbanded the Poor Law Unions and the *Boards of Guardians (which administered the workhouses), establishing Public Assistance Committees instead; local authorities took over the poor law infirmaries as municipal hospitals. See also GOVERNMENT AND MEDICINE IN THE UK.

POPPY. Any plant of the genus *Papaver* (which includes the *opium poppy *P. somniferum*) or of the related genera *Meconopsis* and *Glaucium*.

POPULATION. All the inhabitants of a given country or area considered together, or the number of such inhabitants; more generally, the whole collection of units from which a sample may be drawn. See EPIDEMIOLOGY; STATISTICS.

PORNOGRAPHY was originally the description of the lives and practices of prostitutes. Pornography now has a wider meaning which may be defined as the depicting (verbally or visually) of events calculated to arouse sexual excitement in the reader, listener, or beholder. Pornography flourishes in most modern societies in one form or another, often illegally, but opinion on such matters as its harmfulness or value remains widely polarized.

PORPHYRIA is any condition in which there is excessive production and excretion of porphyrins or their precursors, porphyrins being intermediate compounds formed in the synthesis of the principal (in man) respiratory pigment *haem. The biochemistry of the various types of porphyria is complex; most are *inborn errors of metabolism, and are due to inherited enzyme deficiencies, although some are acquired from the ingestion of toxic substances. They are usually classified into erythropoietic and hepatic types, according to whether the main site of abnormal porphyrin production is the *bone marrow or the *liver. The clinical manifestations of the porphyrias are various and diverse; they include cutaneous *photosensitivity and other skin disorders, attacks of acute abdominal pain, *polyneuropathy, and neuropsychiatric abnormalities. The urine may be reddish orange or brown, or may darken visibly while standing in the light.

PORPHYRINS are a class of naturally occurring pigments derived from pyrrole. They are the basis of respiratory pigments in plants and animals, including *chlorophyll (in which the porphyrin molecule is linked to a magnesium atom) and the *haem of *haemoglobin (where the link is to *iron). See also PORPHYRIA.

PORTAL HYPERTENSION is elevation of pressure in the portal vein, due to obstruction to flow in the small tributaries of the vein within the liver, for example as a result of hepatic *cirrhosis. Among the consequences of portal hypertension are *ascites, *splenomegaly, and varicose dilatation of the venous anastomoses at the junction of the *oesophagus and *stomach, which may lead to severe haemorrhage.

PORTAL VEIN. A short, wide venous channel, formed by the union of veins draining the *stomach, *intestine, and *spleen, that conducts blood (containing the nutrients derived from *digestion) to the *liver.

PORTERS are various hospital ancillary staff who undertake duties as well as gatekeeping, such as the transport of patients between departments.

PORTIER, PAUL-JULES (1866–1962). French immunologist. Portier discovered, together with Charles Robert *Richet, the phenomenon of *anaphylaxis, a term which they introduced to describe hypersensitivity to a foreign substance induced by previous exposure to that substance. The work, which was published in 1902, resulted in Richet being awarded the *Nobel prize in 1913.

PORTWINE STAIN. A bluish-red area on the skin due to a capillary *haemangioma. When on the face, and following the sensory distribution of one division of the *trigeminal nerve, it is diagnostic of the Sturge–Weber syndrome, in which similar vascular anomalies occur in the underlying *meninges and *cerebral cortex and cause generalized or focal *epilepsy, sometimes with

contralateral *hemiplegia, mental retardation, and cerebral *calcification on X-ray.

POSITRON. A positive *electron; an elementary particle with the same mass as an electron and an electric charge of equal magnitude but opposite sign. Some unstable nuclides have a deficit of neutrons, and decay by conversion of *protons to *neutrons and positrons, with emission of the positrons as positive beta-particles. Positrons themselves do not decay, but on passing through matter they collide with negative electrons, as a result of which both particles are annihilated with the production of two photons of electromagnetic radiation in the form of *gamma rays emitted at an angle of 180° to each other. It is these 180° simultaneous gamma rays which are detected in *positron emission tomography (PET), using positron-emitting isotopes of carbon, oxygen, and nitrogen in labelled compounds injected into the patient.

POSITRON EMISSION TOMOGRAPHY (PET SCANNING). A sophisticated and expensive technique of imaging, especially of the brain, which gives evidence relating to regional tissue function and *metabolism. Its prohibitive cost and comparative lack of resolution when compared with *CT and, more especially, *MRI scanning mean that it is largely a research tool rather than a diagnostic method. It is available in relatively few centres across the world, but is yielding valuable new information about biochemical changes in the brain in conditions such as *parkinsonism and *Alzheimer's disease. See also NUCLEAR MEDICINE.

POSTERIOR FOSSA when otherwise unqualified means the posterior cranial fossa, the floor of the posterior subdivision of the cranial cavity (containing the *cerebellum, *pons, and *medulla oblongata).

POSTERIOR ROOT GANGLIA. The *ganglia found on the posterior roots of the *spinal nerves, also known as the spinal ganglia. They contain the cell bodies of the sensory *neurones of the nerves.

POST-MORTEM EXAMINATION is synonymous with *autopsy and necropsy.

POSTURE is the general attitude, position, and deportment of the body, normally maintained by unconscious reflex activity.

POTAIN, PIERRE CARL EDOUARD (1825–1901). French physician. He is remembered now for his apparatus for aspiration of *pleural effusion. He described an 'air *sphygmomanometer' in 1889.

POTASSIUM is a soft, white, very reactive element (symbol K, atomic number 19, relative atomic mass 39.102), a member of the alkali metals. It is the main intracellular *cation of most living tissues; chemically it resembles sodium, which is the main extracellular cation. As with sodium, the movement of potassium ions across cell membranes is fundamental in neuromuscular excitation (see DEPOLARIZATION). Because of its physiological importance, depletion of body potassium (hypokalaemia) is a dangerous disorder of *electrolyte balance which must be corrected by the administration of potassium salts.

POTASSIUM, SERUM. See HYPERKALAEMIA; HYPOKALAEMIA.

POTENCY refers particularly to the strength of medicinal agents, and to the ability to have *orgasm in sexual intercourse (see IMPOTENCE).

POTENTIAL means possible as opposed to actual; it is often an abbreviation of 'potential difference', the electrical equivalent of hydrostatic pressure difference.

POTENTIATION is the promotion of a pharmacological effect by the action of another drug or agent; it is applied similarly to physiological and biochemical effects.

POTOMANIA is a morbid craving for alcoholic drink; it is virtually synonymous with *dipsomania.

POTT, PERCIVALL (1714–88). British surgeon. He forbade the use of the *cautery and is responsible for describing the following eponymic disorders: *Pott's fracture, which he is said to have sustained himself (1750); *Pott's puffy tumour (abscess overlying local osteomyelitis of the skull, 1768); chimney sweep's cancer (epithelioma of the scrotum, 1775); and *Pott's disease (tuberculosis of the spine, 1779).

POTT'S DISEASE is *tuberculosis of the spine; it is rare now in the USA and the UK, but is still important elsewhere in the world. The initial site of infection is usually in the anterior part of a vertebral body, spreading through the intervertebral disc to an adjacent vertebra. The bone may collapse causing anterior angulation and a characteristic hunchback deformity. The '*cold abscess', which may also spread to structures beyond the spine, can compress the spinal cord, causing weakness or paralysis of sphincters or legs ('Pott's paraplegia'). The ultimate response to antituberculous chemotherapy and immobilization is often good, obviating the need for surgical intervention unless paralysis has occurred.

POTT'S FRACTURE is a serious ankle injury in which the foot is forcibly bent outwards with respect to the lower leg. The outer leg bone, the fibula, is fractured above the ankle: on the inner side of the ankle, either the lowest part of the tibia is broken off or else the medial ligament is torn. The ankle is then unsupported and may dislocate.

POTT'S PUFFY TUMOUR (TUMOR) is an extradural *abscess resulting from *osteomyelitis of the skull, causing the syndrome of localized headache, tenderness, and *oedema over the affected area.

POUCH OF DOUGLAS. The fold of *peritoneum which dips down between the *rectum and the *uterus.

POULTICE. A hot dressing for application to the skin either for the purpose of *counter-irritation or in order to increase local blood flow.

POUPART, FRANCOIS (1616–1708). French surgeon and anatomist. He gave his name to the *inguinal ligament (Poupart's ligament).

POWDERS are mixtures of powdered medicinal substances, sometimes with adjuvants such as diluents and dispersing agents. They may be soluble, dispersible, or effervescent, and are normally intended for oral administration. They are usually mixed with water beforehand except in the case of some veterinary powders which are mixed with the animal's feed. The degree of comminution of powders is expressed with a 'sieve number' in millimetres (mm) or micrometres (μm), which is the nominal aperture size of the finest sieve through which the whole of a particular powder will pass.

POWER, SIR D'ARCY (1855–1941). British surgeon and medical historian. He was an editor and biographer of great erudition.

POX is a name used for several diseases characterized by 'pocks' or eruptive *pustules on the skin; the term persists only in compound form, for example *chickenpox, *cow-pox, *smallpox, etc. It was once used as a synonym for *syphilis.

POXVIRUS. A group of related, large deoxyribonucleic acid (DNA) *viruses, which includes the causative agents of *vaccinia, *smallpox, and a number of animal pox infections.

PRACTITIONER (of medicine) is a term denoting a person entitled to practise, although not necessarily engaged in active medical practice. The term is also used in other professions (e.g. *nurse practitioner).

PRAUSNITZ, CARL WILHELM (1861–1933). German hygienist and bacteriologist. He was a pioneer in hygiene and epidemiology, pushing through reforms in food control, sewage, drainage, ventilation, and lighting systems, as well as *infectious disease prevention.

PRAXIS. Practice as distinct from theory; also, a collection of examples for practice. Or, alternatively, skilled voluntary movement, lost in *apraxia.

PRECIPITANT. Any substance or agent responsible for precipitation, whether of a visible deposit in a solution, or of an event such as the sudden onset of a disease.

PRECIPITINS are *antibodies which, when they react with their homologous *antigen, produce a visible aggregate of antigen–antibody complex.

PRECLINICAL EDUCATION. See MEDICAL EDUCATION, UNDERGRADUATE.

PRECOCITY. Premature development.

PREDNISONE is a synthetic glucocorticoid (see CORTICOSTEROIDS). Like cortisone, it is an 11-keto compound and is not itself biologically active, requiring *in vivo* conversion to the 11-betahydroxyl compound prednisolone in order to exert its pharmacological effects.

PREGNANCY is the condition of being with child or young, that is having within the body a fertilized *ovum (zygote), a developing *embryo, or a growing *fetus. See OBSTETRICS AND GYNAECOLOGY.

PREGNANCY TEST. Several tests have been developed to detect pregnancy, most of which use chemical, *bioassay, or (more recently) *radioimmunoassay techniques to estimate *hormone levels in urine or plasma.

PREMATURE BABY. A viable infant born before full term, that is after a gestation period of less than 38 weeks. Prematurity is also defined by reference to birth weight as less than 2.5 kg (5.5 lb).

PREMATURE BEAT. See ECTOPIC BEATS.

PREMENSTRUAL TENSION is a syndrome occurring in the few days before *menstruation and usually ascribed to salt and water retention associated with the hormonal changes at that time; symptoms vary but often include headache, insomnia, fatiguability, and emotional liability.

PREPUCE. The foreskin, the loose fold of skin that covers the glans penis in uncircumcised men.

PRE-REGISTRATION HOSPITAL APPOINTMENTS are resident medical and surgical hospital appointments which must be completed by those newly graduated in medicine in order to obtain admission to the UK Medical Register. See GENERAL MEDICAL COUNCIL; MEDICAL EDUCATION, POSTGRADUATE AND CONTINUING, UNDERGRADUATE.

PRESBYOPIA is the visual impairment resulting from old age. With advancing years, the power of the lens to focus near objects is gradually lost owing to decreasing elasticity, and corrective spectacles are required for close vision (reading, needlework, etc.). See OPHTHALMOLOGY.

PRESCRIPTIONS are written directions for the preparation, supply, and administration of medicines. In the UK, a prescription for a controlled drug may not be dispensed by a pharmacist unless the requirements of Regulation 15 of the Misuse of Drugs Regulations 1973 are met. The prescription must be handwritten in ink, or be otherwise indelible, must give the name and address of the patient, the dose and quantity of the drug to be supplied in both words and figures, and must be signed with the doctor's full signature. Controlled drugs include cocaine, narcotic analgesics, and amphetamine and related compounds; controlled drugs are identified by the letters CD in the *British national formulary*. Many other drugs are 'prescription only' medicines. These include most of the other potent drugs used in medical practice (e.g. antibiotics, hormones, vaccines, hypnotics, etc.). See PHARMACOLOGY; PHARMACY AND PHARMACISTS.

PRESENIUM. The period of life preceding old age.

PRESENTATION, in medicine generally, means the complex of symptoms and signs which first manifests a disease process. In obstetrics, it denotes the part of the fetus presented to the birth canal at the onset of labour (see OBSTETRICS AND GYNAECOLOGY).

PREVALENCE is the number of instances of illness or of persons ill, or of any other event such as accidents, in a specified population, without any distinction between new and old cases. The prevalence may be recorded at a stated moment ('point prevalence') or during a given period of time ('period prevalence'). When the term 'prevalence' is used without qualification, it means 'point prevalence'. When prevalence is expressed as 'prevalence rate', the denominator used is the number of persons in the specified population at the given time; or in the case of period prevalence, the average number of persons during the defined period or the estimated number at the mid-point of that period (Hogarth (1978), *Glossary of health care terminology*, World Health Organization, Copenhagen). See EPIDEMIOLOGY.

PREVENTIVE MEDICINE attempts to control disease by identifying and eliminating causes. Since potentially remediable causes range from such factors as ignorance, poverty, poor sanitation, and maladministration on the one hand, to minute gene aberrations on the other, the scope of preventive medicine is boundless. The catalogue of past success, such as the elimination of *smallpox in 1980, needs no rehearsal. Instead it should be emphasized that present knowledge has by no means been fully exploited. This applies to many promising and intellectually exciting new developments (e.g. the application of molecular biological techniques to *trophoblast biopsy in early pregnancy), but still more to mundane matters of *health education with respect to alcohol and tobacco, legislation further to reduce road-traffic casualties, fluoridation of drinking water, and very many others. See PUBLIC HEALTH MEDICINE.

PRIAPISM is persistent, often painful, penile erection.

PRIAPUS is equivalent to *phallus, from Priapus the Greek and Roman god of procreation.

PRICKLY HEAT is an itchy rash of erythematous papulovesicular type due to obstruction of the ducts of the sweat glands and escape of sweat into the *epidermis. Prickly heat is associated with prolonged excessive heat load.

PRIESTLEY, JOHN GILLIES (1879–1941). English physiologist. He served with distinction during the First World War, towards the end of which he collaborated with J. S. *Haldane in studying the after-effects of gas poisoning. With Haldane he also established the dominant role of *carbon dioxide in determining the depth and frequency of *respiration.

PRIESTLEY, JOSEPH (1733–1804). British scientist and theologian. He was a distinguished chemist, discovering 10 new gases including *carbon monoxide, sulphur dioxide, and *nitrous oxide. He noted that air was 'vitiated' by combustion or respiration, but could be 'restored' by growing green-leaved plants in it. He showed that a 'new gas which was better to breathe than common air' was formed on heating nitre (1771) or mercuric oxide (1774). Unable to cast off the phlogiston theory, he called this gas 'dephlogisticated air'. *Lavoisier, after conversation with Priestley, immediately appreciated its importance and gave it the name of *oxygen.

PRIMAQUINE is a synthetic antimalarial drug, used particularly in the eradication of benign tertian *malaria after primary treatment with *chloroquine.

PRIMARY HEALTH CARE. See PRIMARY MEDICAL CARE.

PRIMARY MEDICAL CARE (GENERAL MEDICAL PRACTICE OR FAMILY MEDICINE). The term 'primary (medical) care' has come into use during the past 25 years on both sides of the Atlantic. It stands for those medical services to which people normally have direct access and is contrasted with 'secondary care' (services normally reached by referral). This distinction is particularly clear in the UK, where primary services are mainly found outside hospitals

and are 'generalist' while secondary services are mainly located inside hospitals and are divided into numerous specialized branches, such as *surgery, *obstetrics, or *gynaecology. The distinction is less clear cut in the USA, where people, when ill, have much more direct access to specialists at present.

Until recently the distinction between primary—generalist services outside hospital and secondary—specialist services inside has been confined within the medical profession—primary services implying those offered by '*general practitioners' (Europe, including the UK) or '*family physicians' (the USA and Canada). The change of emphasis to primary care has come about because of the ever-increasing need for inter-professional collaboration. The primary-care team (for instance, in the UK) includes professionals other than general practitioners—nurses of several sorts, midwives, receptionists, managers, and sometimes social workers. The World Health Organization (WHO) has been an important influence in this change. Recently, by substituting 'primary *health* care' for 'primary *medical* care', the WHO has sought not only to emphasize prevention and health maintenance but to advocate more active involvement of the population and of departments of government, such as education or housing, since they influence health and health care.

Since the general practitioner or family physician is still at the centre of any primary-care team, the essential features of this role must be outlined. It provides 'personal, primary and continuing medical care to individuals, families and a practice population, irrespective of age, sex and illness . . . The general practitioner includes and integrates physical, psychological, and social factors in his/her considerations about health and illness . . . He/she will know how and when to intervene through treatment, prevention, and education to promote the health of patients and their families' (Leeuwenhorst European Study Group 1977).

Primary care and secondary care have features distinct from each other, but they are not alternatives for providing what people in any country need today. Because of the increasing complexity of medical and nursing knowledge and skills, both are essential and each complements the other. Without the generalist, 'access to services becomes more difficult, care becomes fragmented and depersonalised, there is decline of comprehensive management, costs mount without any measurable health benefits.' (J. Fry, writing of Sweden at an earlier time when an almost completely specialized medical service was attempted).

Origins in the UK
The term 'general practitioner' was unknown in the UK before 1800 and came into use increasingly between 1820 and 1830, becoming firmly established by 1840 (Loudon 1986). It provided a title for a role which had been developing throughout the previous century.

Before 1800, the medical profession had been divided

into three groups—physicians, members of a learned profession with a background of university education, who dealt with internal disorders; surgeons, craftsmen whose sphere was external disorders and any condition requiring manual interference; and tradesmen apothecaries, whose legal role was to dispense physicians' prescriptions, but who, 100 years earlier, had won the right to visit, advise, and prescribe, provided that they charged only for medicine prescribed. But by 1800, two of these three groups—surgeons and apothecaries—had merged. Most surgeons treated three or four medical cases for every surgical one. Thus most medical men were already undertaking much of the same kind of practice involving all branches of medicine.

In 1858 a common medical register was established for the first time (see GENERAL MEDICAL COUNCIL). Thereafter there was a common category of 'doctor' but, within that term, social and functional distinctions persisted and developed.

Origins in the United States
In America, in contrast to England or Scotland, there was no similar hierarchy of *physicians, *surgeons, and *apothecaries; attempts to found such hierarchies failed. Medical practice meant general practice. But there was a constant preoccupation about the boundary distinguishing 'regular' from 'irregular' practitioners who, in the 17th century, in the absence of sufficient regulars, had necessarily provided a form of care for a growing population (some of them had been clergymen). Both sorts of practitioner were trained by apprenticeship. Before 1765, when the first medical school was established in Philadelphia, a university education for medicine could be had only in Europe, notably at Edinburgh.

In 1860, American doctors were all typically general practitioners; there were few full-time specialists. Outside the major cities hospitals were few (a total of 178 reported in the USA in 1873). Specialization began to develop from 1870 onwards. By 1909 there were more than 4000 hospitals. The identity of the general practitioner now came into question, especially in cities. Could he survive as the mainstay of practice, when specialists provided skills of higher technical quality? The increasingly clear division of role which gradually emerged in the UK between generalists and specialists, with a well-recognized system of referral between them, did not emerge in the USA.

The rapid development of surgery and *anaesthetics faced general practitioners with a crucial choice. Some persisted in undertaking large surgical operations, thereby incurring criticism from better-trained surgeons for attempting things beyond their competence and training; others turned away from surgery and concentrated on the role of generalist diagnostician, family advisor, and counsellor, acting as a foil to specialists of all kinds. Nevertheless, most hospitals continued to offer access to general practitioners, even for surgical operations.

The founding in 1913 of the *American College of Surgeons was followed in 1915 by the *American College of Physicians. Specialists in internal medicine who made up the membership of the latter college considered themselves not to be general practitioners. They concentrated on the physiological and chemical basis of disease. General practitioners were specifically excluded.

Thus, even before the First World War, the position of the general practitioner was already difficult in cities. Generalists and specialists competed for the same patients, but specialists charged higher fees, even when they were doing the same tasks. The role of general practitioner was contracting, without new skills being acquired to replace those lost to specialists.

Developments since the Second World War in the UK
1948—the start of the National Health Service (NHS)
In jumping to 1948, two influences of great importance must be mentioned—first, the impact of the sciences of physics, chemistry, and biology on medical thinking and practice; secondly, the introduction in 1911 of a *National Insurance system for employed people (not for their families). The first influence threatened, the second helped to preserve the role of the general doctor.

The sciences, steadily contributing to the capacity of medicine to manage more diseases effectively, contributed also to the development of specialization within the medical profession. Specialization was largely confined to doctors working in hospitals, teaching hospitals especially. Distinguished by longer training and by a monopoly of teaching and research, they increasingly acted as consultants, to whom difficult problems and patients requiring either special techniques or admission to hospital were referred by their general practitioners. By 1948 the division of the profession into two tiers, related by the process of referral, was clearly defined. Direct access to specialists now seemed a logical further development, especially as this was happening in some other countries. The survival of the general doctor's role was questioned.

But in the meantime, National Health Insurance had, since 1911, obliged all employed or self-employed wage-earners to pay contributions which entitled them to register with a general practitioner for medical care, free at the time of use. The NHS extended this entitlement to the whole population. Almost all of the population registered with a general practitioner under the NHS and therefore, for the first time, had access to a personal medical adviser without any financial barriers. Linked with the strong tradition of referral and referral back, the position of the general practitioner was in fact preserved. 'The physician and surgeon retained the hospital, while the general practitioner retained the patient' (Stevens 1966).

The state of general practice at the start of the NHS was described by Brotherston (see COMMUNITY MEDICINE IN THE UNITED KINGDOM in *The Oxford companion to medicine* 1986) as 'a cottage industry' with doctors working single-handedly or in small partnerships, isolated from each other and from the development of medicine, unless they held a part-time hospital appointment. Most had chosen this career as a second or third option. Work was divided between insured wage-earners and 'private patients', many of whom could not afford to pay adequate fees.

1948–88—from general medical practice to primary medical care

There have been many changes, with general agreement that most, if not all, have been for the better. The most obvious ones have been:

(1) achieving an even distribution of practices across the country and an increase in the ratio of doctors to patients registered with them;

(2) larger partnerships of doctors and, more importantly, their close association with other professionals (see below);

(3) the development of special postgraduate training, now obligatory, and extensive opportunities for career-long re-education; and

(4) improvement of premises and equipment.

In contrast with almost every other comparable country, the relative importance of primary care within the whole service has slowly increased, the morale of those involved rising in parallel, and recruitment gaining in both numbers and quality.

The system of referral and referral back between generalists working in small units outside hospitals and specialists based in hospitals is recognized as an advantage by both sides. It can provide patients with both a personal doctor and full access to specialist care (on average one in 20 consultations give rise to a referral). Meanwhile the 'gate-keeping' and preventive roles of primary care help to limit the cost of secondary specialist care in hospitals.

During this period, as hospital care has become increasingly specialized, the role of the general practitioner has become increasingly distinct. Proximity to the community served, accessibility and personal availability to a known list of patients are linked with a relatively continuous relationship with individuals and often with whole families. Training for a very broad remit supports the duty to assess whatever problem a patient chooses to present, its nature and urgency, and the doctor's own capacity to cope with it or the need to seek further help. Since one in three patients now brings multiple problems to one consultation, judging their interrelationship and relative importance—co-ordination of care—becomes increasingly necessary. None of these things is so easily provided by any specialist. Taken together, they form the distinctive contribution of the personal doctor and they complement the strengths of specialization.

Among the very broad range of problems dealt with in primary care for people of all ages, including children, two-thirds might be judged to be minor and only one-third major or long-term. But long-term illness, much of it severe, falls increasingly into the field of primary care. Except in remote districts, major and middle-grade surgical operations became the sole province of the specialist surgeon after 1948. The same trend occurred later in *obstetrics, most births now taking place in hospital under specialist and *midwife care. Antenatal and postnatal care are, however, shared with general practitioners, some of whom continue to deal with normal births in hospitals. In contrast, the role of the general practitioner and the primary-care team in internal medicine, especially in diagnosis, has increased with direct access to all the simpler investigative techniques. Changes in public opinion and in medical training have brought more recognition of psychosocial problems, greater understanding, tolerance, better use of the doctor–patient relationship, of simple *psychotherapy, and of drugs which help *depression and *anxiety.

General practitioners looked after an average registered list of 2500 patients in 1950, and 1965 in 1990, by which date they were consulted on average four times a year by each patient. They see 70 per cent of the patients on their list at least once a year. The mean length of consultations has been rising, but is still only 8 minutes, compared with 15 minutes in the USA or 13 minutes in France. But one in every six consultations is conducted in the patient's home and lasts longer. Night visits are done by the doctor or by an appointed deputy. Only about 15 per cent of general practitioners now work without being in partnership with another doctor. The proportion of women doctors had risen to 16 per cent in 1981 and 22 per cent in 1988.

General practitioners, many of whom in 1948 opposed the start of the NHS had, by 1988, become its firm supporters, largely satisfied with their conditions of service. They were appointed by Family Practitioner Committees (FPCs) (part lay, part medical) but they had remained (and still remain) independent contractors, entitled to take on clinical or other work within or outside the NHS. Within it they are accountable for carrying out agreed terms of service. Control was light during the 40 years in question. If they do not meet these terms, a local disciplinary machinery exists. In more serious breaches, the case goes to the *GMC.

Most of the general practitioner's income is in fact derived from the NHS. Whereas in 1948 remuneration was based almost entirely on the number of patients registered with each doctor (capitation—a fixed sum per year per patient), it has since been based in almost equal parts on capitation, an element of salary, and payments for items of service (mostly preventive). The triple method of payment combines the different motivations which belong to each separate method. Total remuneration is lower than that of an American doctor, but this has not been the cause for organized discontent since 1965. Nor can it be said that UK practitioners are poverty-striken, as were many of their predecessors in the 19th century.

The population has valued the NHS highly throughout these years. The relationship between general practitioners and the population at the national level has been the subject of many sociological or 'consumer' surveys. The predominant response has always been one of approval, but with specific and consistent criticisms—for instance, about hurried consultations.

Interprofessional collaboration

Although primary medical care must include the casualty departments of hospitals, since people have direct access to them, they will not be considered here.

The change from single-handed general practice (with the doctor's wife often acting as receptionist) to partnerships of four or more practitioners (group practice) and closer collaboration with *district nurses, practice nurses, *health visitors, midwives, community psychiatric nurses, counsellors, receptionists, and sometimes *social workers, has been a leading feature of frontline medicine in the UK since 1960.

Regrettably it is not possible here to trace the history of these other professional groups, in parallel with what has been written about the history of general practice. Important contributions can be found in Abel-Smith (1960) and Baley (1980).

Group-practice premises and health centres, examples of which can now be found throughout the UK, are now designed to accommodate members of the 'primary-care team.' Their composition and the quality of collaboration within them vary greatly, but the general trend is clear. When care is increasingly transferred from hospitals to homes, places of work, and small community institutions, such teams form an essential resource, whether because of the size of the task or because a wider range of knowledge and skills is needed than can be provided only by doctors.

Teamwork demands organization, training, and regular times for reflection and discussion together. These needs are not yet properly recognized. Moreover, there is potential conflict between care given by a group of professionals and the needs of many patients and clients for a personal, continuing relationship, without which some problems encountered in primary care cannot be resolved or relieved.

Organizing change

The many changes that have come about in general practice and primary care in the UK under the NHS have been first stimulated by organizations other than the government. The *British Medical Association (BMA) negotiated particularly important reforms in 1964. A fundamental and continuing influence has come from the *Royal College of General Practitioners, founded in 1952. It has been the main force in creating a special three-year programme of vocational training—now obligatory for all principals (independent practitioners)

in the NHS—and in offering a postgraduate diploma. It has encouraged and organized a wealth of research in a field where there was previously almost none. It has brought general practice and primary care into all medical schools as a routine element in the undergraduate curriculum. These developments have helped to clarify the role of the general practitioner and to revive the confidence which was waning in the 1950s. Together with improvements in pay, they have been the main cause of a large shift in the career preferences of final-year medical students towards this role in medicine—a shift which has so far been unique among comparable countries.

Developments since 1988

Government intervention, which since 1948 had been limited and mainly beneficial, became intense in the last years of the Thatcher government, which had an unassailable parliamentary majority. A new contract was partly agreed and partly imposed on general practitioners. It strongly reinforced two trends which the medical profession was already pursuing; (1) towards more prevention and health promotion; and (2) towards performance review ('quality assessment and assurance'; 'audit'). It also introduced a major experiment in creating 'budget-holding practices', i.e. larger group practices which were offered an annual budget to cover not only their own running expenses, but to contract with hospitals for certain types of specialist care. This, if widely extended, must further alter the balance between primary and secondary care, but it also requires much greater financial management from a practice, with new staff arrangements. In the meantime the powers of FPCs (now called Family Health Service Authorities) have been considerably increased.

The size of the changes introduced, their nature, and the manner in which they were hurriedly imposed without adequate consultation, have so far had a very negative effect on the workload and morale of general practitioners. Equally radical changes have been made in the management of the whole service and in hospitals. In principle, the aim has been to increase efficiency by introducing more competition through what is described as the internal market. The influence of economists has been paramount in these changes. But it is too early to assess the long-term influence on the effectiveness of the service, on the satisfaction of patients, doctors, and nurses, or on costs.

Developments since the Second World War in the United States

The bias towards specialization had started before the Second World War. Whereas the proportion of self-designated generalists among all physicians in active practice was 90 per cent in 1940 and 46 per cent in 1960, it was 34 per cent in 1986 (some so included were also part-time specialists) (Stevens 1971; Moore 1992).

As the number of general practitioners declined, the mantle of primary care was necessarily assumed by *paediatricians, internists, *psychiatrists, *obstetricians, and other specialists. Patients, seeing that such doctors were plentiful and better trained, bypassed the general practitioner (in 1967, however, 41 per cent of the adult population still reported that they had one).

An organized response to this situation had started in 1945, when a Section of General Practice was at last formed within the *American Medical Association. In 1947 the Academy of General Practice was formed. It moved to establish a recognized special function for the general practitioner, later to be called 'family physician'. A specialty certifying board was established in 1970; it required 3 years of graduate training and a re-test every 6 years. The behaviour of 'consumers' did not immediately fall in with these efforts to strengthen the family physician's position in medical care.

The formation of the Academy of General Practice (later of Family Medicine) caused a reaction in the American Boards of Internal Medicine and Pediatrics (many of whose diplomates were already engaged in primary care) to modify their intrahospital orientation and to provide a rival type of general care. They also modified their requirements, so that 4 years' training in each of the two specialties brought eligibility for joint certification.

Rivalry for the function of medical generalist between family physicians, on the one hand, and internal medicine specialists and paediatricians, on the other, became an obvious feature of American medicine. There has since arisen a new specialty of emergency medicine. The pattern thus remains confused and confusing to the observer.

Primary care in the USA today

Differences from the UK in the distribution of illnesses are slight (Marsh *et al.* 1976), but the American doctor sees a much higher proportion of well people for 'check-ups'. The working day is longer, but fewer patients are seen—the average consultation lasting at least twice as long as in the UK. More physical examinations and tests are done, not least because of greater competition between doctors and a much greater level of litigation against them by patients. House calls make up 0.5 per cent of patient contacts, compared with about 15 per cent in the UK, but primary-care physicians can, and regularly do, provide care to their patients in hospitals. Although nurses work in the consulting suite, it is unusual to find district nurses or *public health nurses attached to a group practice.

The American patient, at least in cities, has a far greater choice of direct access in primary care—between a family physician, an internist, a paediatrician, a gynaecologist, even a surgeon or a psychiatrist. Thus the patient, rather than any doctor, manages access to specialist care. Nevertheless, in many parts of the country choice is limited or non-existent because of maldistribution of doctors, or because of the high cost of care or lack of sickness insurance.

The most important recent change has been the growth of health maintenance organizations (HMOs)— 9.1 million members in 1983 to 35 million in 1990. Most HMOs rely on generalist physicians to provide primary care in their delivery systems. Yet the proportion of American medical graduates choosing any form of primary-care career continues to drop below the level required.

The future

Two important themes can be traced through this account of general and family practice in two countries—the balance between specialist and generalist practice on the one hand, and the balance between organized care and the doctor's independence on the other. Specialists have increasingly dominated the American care system. Trends in the UK continue to increase the relative importance of the generalist. Which emphasis produces the highest overall quality of care is still a matter of belief rather than one of evidence or agreed judgement. High health-care costs are compelling both policy makers and business community in the USA to consider a major redirection in medical manpower policy (Mullan 1992). Meanwhile the WHO, since the Alma Ata Declaration of 1978, has promoted primary care as the central function and main focus of every country's health system.

JOHN HORDER

Acknowledgement
I am very grateful to Dr Gordon Moore (Harvard Medical School) and to those whose help was acknowledged in the edition of 1986.

References
Abel-Smith, B. (1960). *A history of the nursing profession.* Heinemann, London.
Baly, M. E. (1980). *Nursing and social change* (2nd edn). Heinemann, London.
Leeuwenhorst European Study Group, (1977). The work of the general practitioner. Statement by working party of the second European Conference on the teaching of general practice – 1974. *Journal of the Royal College of General Practitioners*, **27**, 117.
Loudon, I. (1986). *Medical care and the general practitioner 1750–1850.* Clarendon Press, Oxford.
Marsh, G. N., Wallace, P. C., and Whewell, J. (1976). Anglo-American contrasts in general practice. *British Medical Journal*, **1**, 1321–5.
Moore, G. T. (1992). The case of the disappearing generalist: does it need to be solved? *The Millbank Quarterly* V. **70**, (2), 362–79.
Mullan, F. (1992). Missing: a national medical manpower policy. *The Millbank Quarterly*, **70**, (2) 381–9.
Stevens, R. (1966). *Medical practice in modern England.* Yale University Press, New Haven.
Stevens, R. (1971). *American medicine and the public interest.* Yale University Press, New Haven.
Stevens, R. (1986). In *The Oxford companion to medicine* (ed. J. Walton, P. B. Beeson, and R Bodley Scott) (medical practice). Oxford University Press, Oxford.

PRIMIDONE is a drug used in the control of some types of *epilepsy, also known under the proprietary name Mysoline®.

PRINCIPAL. A partner or established single-handed practitioner (as distinct from an assistant or trainee) in a *general medical practice in the UK.

PRINCIPLES AND PRACTICE OF MEDICINE is the title of the famous textbook of medicine published in 1891 by Dr (later Sir) William *Osler, the Canadian-born physician, who became professor of medicine successively at the universities of *McGill, Pennsylvania, *Johns Hopkins, and Oxford, where he occupied the regius chair. The last edition to be published during Osler's lifetime was the eighth in 1912; the ninth appeared in 1920 shortly after his death. The book was subsequently revised by McCrae and later by *Christian up until 1939. It was revived again after the Second World War by Harvey and colleagues from Johns Hopkins. The same title was given to a textbook published in 1952 (and later proceeding to many editions) by Sir Stanley Davidson, as a multi-author work originating primarily from the departments of medicine and therapeutics of the University of Edinburgh.

PRINGLE, SIR JOHN, Bt (1707–82). British physician and theologian. In 1742 he was appointed physician to the army commander on the continent. At the battle of Dettingen (1743) in Germany he proposed that military hospitals be sanctuaries, which was accepted by the French commander. This was the forerunner of the idea of the *Red Cross, which was established in 1863. He was present at the battle of Culloden in 1745. In 1752 he published *Observations on the diseases of the army*, which helped improve the environment of serving men and military hospitals and their practice. In a paper read at the Royal Society he used the word 'antiseptic' for the first time.

PRION. A tiny virus-like transmissible agent made up of hydrophobic protein and containing no DNA or RNA. Prions are now believed to cause disorders such as scrapie, kuru, and Creutzfeldt–Jakob disease, once called *slow virus infections.

PRISON MEDICINE. Prisoners have much higher rates of health problems—particularly substance abuse, mental disorders, suicide, and communicable diseases—than people in the community. Yet providing a high-quality health service in prison is difficult because conditions are often exceedingly poor, resources are scarce, the needs of security often conflict with the needs of health, attracting high-quality staff may be difficult, and separation from the health service for the ordinary community may mean that the prison health service sinks to a lower standard. In addition, practising medicine in prison presents many ethical problems.

The few comparisons that have been made between the health of prisoners and people in the community show a higher rate of most problems among prisoners. In particular, *HIV infection is much more common among prisoners, mainly because intravenous drug abuse is common. Responding to HIV may be difficult in prison because security staff and other prisoners may insist, through ignorance and hostility towards those infected, that patients with HIV are isolated. Furthermore, prison authorities are often unwilling to allow condom distribution and needle exchange within prisons for fear of seeming to condone illegal activities.

Abuse of *alcohol and illegal drugs is common among prisoners because addiction often leads people to crime to support their habit, because intoxication may lead to crime, because *substance abuse itself may be a crime, and because drugs are freely available within many prisons. Treating substance abuse in prison is difficult—partly because no drugs (even alcohol) are supposed to be available and partly because abstinence within the highly abnormal environment of prison may not lead to abstinence on release.

Mental health problems are very common among prisoners. Poor mental health, particularly what psychiatrists call personality disorders, may lead to crime, but in many societies prison also serves as a sump for people with chronic mental disorders who have nowhere else to go. Furthermore, the appalling and frightening circumstances of most prisons aggravate and create mental health problems. Treating mental health problems is difficult because facilities are so poor and because—at least in British prisons—psychotic prisoners cannot be treated against their will.

The high prevalence of prisoners with mental health problems has long been recognized but has proved an extremely difficult problem to solve. Prison reformers and doctors lament that mentally ill people should have to be managed in such unsuitable circumstances, but the mental health services in the community are often unable or unwilling to accept mentally disordered offenders.

*Suicide among prisoners is several times higher than in the community, and prison health services have made many attempts to reduce the suicide rate. One strategy is to identify and observe closely prisoners at risk of suicide, but this strategy has not proved particularly successful because those at risk are not easy to identify and, even if identified and observed, a determined prisoner can still kill himself. An alternative strategy has been to try to humanize prisons, making it less likely that prisoners will be driven to suicide. This is a major undertaking, and suicide rates remain high in most prison systems.

Most prisoners are adult men, but adolescents and women may also receive custodial sentences. Most authorities try hard to keep young people out of institutions, recognizing that many become 'schools for criminals' with three-quarters or more of the young people re-offending after release. Women in prison are likely to be treated on a medical rather than punitive model—but often with little success. The same high rates of mental disorder, substance abuse, and HIV infection are seen among women, and there are additional problems of genitourinary infection (many are prostitutes) and of what to do with prisoners who are pregnant or have young children. The trade-off between wanting to keep women with their children and not wanting to expose children to highly unnatural surroundings is difficult.

The Health Service for Prisoners in England and Wales is proud of being the oldest civilian medical service in the country. It has its roots in the tireless work of the prison reformer John Howard at the end of the 18th century. He exposed the appalling condition of the prisons, and even before his famous book *The state of the prisons* had been published in 1777 his work had led to the 1774 Act for Preserving the Health of Prisoners in Gaol and Preventing the Gaol Distemper. This Act and others required all prisons to appoint a surgeon or apothecary. Transportation to New South Wales came to an end in 1840, and the prison system was taken over by the government in 1877. The prison medical service began at this time and looked after prisoners within extremely strict regimens.

The founding of the *National Health Service (NHS) in 1948 presented an opportunity for the Prison Medical Service to be absorbed into the new service, but this did not happen. Since then there has been a continuing debate over whether the health services for prisoners should be provided by the NHS. The Home Office, which looks after the Health Service for Prisoners (as the Prison Medical Service was renamed in 1992), argues that the Home Secretary must be able to run a health service as he, and not the Secretary of State for Health, is ultimately responsible for the health of prisoners. In addition, prison medicine is thought to demand special skills, and there are anxieties that the NHS would not be able to provide as good a service to prisoners as can the Health Service for Prisoners. Those who favour fusing the two services argue that a service separated from the main NHS will inevitably sink to a lower standard, and that doctors employed full-time by the prison service may find themselves putting the interests of prisons before those of prisoners. Although the Home Office has held off from full fusion of the two services, it has reformed the Prison Medical Service into the Health Services for Prisoners, which will pay more attention to health promotion.

Finally, doctors working in prisons face formidable ethical problems. Most prisoners see doctors as members of the prison system and are unbelieving of their assertions that their first priority is to their patients. Problems arise, for instance, when doctors have to declare prisoners fit for punishment or when they are asked to force-feed prisoners on hunger strike. There are also severe problems with confidentiality, and research in prisons may be very difficult because of doubts over the validity of informed consent—might the prisoner be consenting only because he fears reprisals if he does not?

RICHARD SMITH

PRIVATE PRACTICE. See MEDICAL PRACTICE.

PRIVY COUNCIL. Originally the private council of a sovereign with the function of advising on the administration of government. In the UK, the Privy Council is a body of advisers appointed by the sovereign; it includes certain members by usage, such as the princes of the blood, the archbishops, and the chief officers of past and present ministries of state. Its functions are now either purely formal or are carried out by committees; and Privy-Councillorship is mainly a personal dignity conferred in recognition of eminent public service. At present, the Privy Council numbers about 380 members, but is summoned as a body only in order to sign the Proclamation of the accession of a new sovereign or when the sovereign announces an intention to marry. The number normally summoned is four (the Lord President and the ministers chiefly concerned with the particular business), the quorum being three.

Committees of the Council, the most important of which is the Judicial Committee, are responsible *inter alia* for dealing with appeals from the disciplinary bodies concerned with medicine, dentistry, and the professions supplementary to medicine (see GENERAL MEDICAL COUNCIL).

PROBANG. A flexible instrument made of whalebone with a sponge, ball, or button at the end for introduction into the pharynx and oesophagus to apply medication, to extract a foreign body, or to push obstructing material down into the stomach. The probang was invented by the Welsh judge Walter Rumsey (1584–1660), who named it provang but his reasons for doing so are not known.

PROBE. Any surgical instrument used primarily for exploratory purposes; any instrument or method used for exploration (e.g. in biology, genetics, electronics, space research, etc.).

PROBENECID is one of the uricosuric drugs, i.e. substances which, by blocking the renal tubular reabsorption of urate, promote the excretion of *uric acid in the urine. It is of value in treating the hyperuricaemia of *gout. Probenecid also blocks the tubular excretion of certain *antibiotics, notably the *penicillins and *cephalosporins, and may be given in conjunction with these drugs to raise their blood concentration.

PROCAINE is the earliest (1905) and one of the most successful synthetic local anaesthetic agents, widely used for more than 50 years but now superseded by newer drugs. See LOCAL ANAESTHESIA.

PROCARBAZINE is an antineoplastic drug used chiefly to treat *Hodgkin's disease. Because it has an action like that of *disulfiram, alcohol should be avoided during its administration.

PROCESS. A projection, prominence, protuberance, outgrowth, extension, etc. of or from the main body of an anatomical structure.

PROCHASKA, GEORG (1749–1820). Czechoslovakian physician and physiologist. He was one of the first to recognize the integration of function in centres of the brain and showed that movements could be initiated in parts of the brain lower than the *cerebrum.

PROCIDENTIA is a severe degree of *prolapse of the *uterus or *rectum, with most or all of the organ exteriorized.

PROCTITIS is inflammation of the *rectum.

PROCTOLOGIST. A surgeon specializing in anorectal disorders.

PROCTOLOGY. The study of disorders of the anus and rectum.

PROCTOSCOPY is inspection of the *rectum with an illuminated *speculum.

PRODROMES are premonitory symptoms or signs heralding the onset of some disease; the word is often used in the Greek form 'prodromata', and also adjectively as 'prodromal'.

PRODUCT LIABILITY. See PHARMACEUTICAL INDUSTRY.

PROFESSIONAL CONFIDENCE is the principle that information obtained by doctors, and by extension, by their non-medical colleagues, during the course of their professional duties shall not be disclosed to others without the consent of the patient concerned, unless there are overriding moral or legal considerations to the contrary. The author of the *Hippocratic Oath enshrined this principle in the following words: 'All that may come to my knowledge in the exercise of my profession or outside of my profession or in daily commerce with men, which ought not to be spread abroad, I will keep secret and will never reveal.' See also ETHICS AND MEDICINE; GENERAL MEDICAL COUNCIL.

PROFESSIONAL EXAMINATIONS are those which must be passed for professional qualification.

PROFESSIONAL MALPRACTICE (alternatively 'malpraxis') is a term which embraces all forms of medical misconduct including *professional negligence. It is not confined to the latter term, nor does it have a specific English legal connotation. Improper advertising by a medical practitioner, for example, can be described as professional malpractice. It is, however, extensively used in the USA in connection with legal actions involving the unintentional sort of negligence. See LAW AND MEDICINE IN THE UK; LAW AND MEDICINE IN THE USA.

PROFESSIONAL NEGLIGENCE is defined as a failure of the doctor to exercise reasonable skill and care resulting in injury to the patient. Under English law, negligence as so defined constitutes a tort or civil wrong (i.e. not a crime), and a civil action is necessary for the patient to obtain redress. In England, a judge alone determines liability and the amount of damages to be paid, the former requiring a judgement about the standard of care which can be regarded as reasonable under the particular circumstances and the latter an assessment of an adequate level of compensation for whatever injury has been suffered; in other countries, including Ireland and the USA, a jury is also involved. Proof of negligence requires the existence of a professional duty towards the patient, a breach of that duty, and injury to the patient resulting from that breach. Actions must be brought within 3 years of the act complained of, or within 3 years of the plaintiff becoming aware of the harm resulting from it. Some countries, (e.g. Sweden, New Zealand) operate schemes of 'no-fault' compensation for patients suffering the consequences of medical accidents. See LAW AND MEDICINE IN THE UK; LAW AND MEDICINE IN THE USA; NO-FAULT COMPENSATION.

PROFESSIONAL PROTECTION SOCIETIES are organizations which, in return for subscription to membership, provide doctors and dentists in the UK and some other countries (e.g. Australia, Canada, France) with indemnity against the results of legal actions involving professional negligence and some other matters, with medico-legal advice, and with legal representation when necessary. Three such organizations, which are not insurance companies, exist in the UK; they are the Medical Defence Union, the Medical Protection Society, and the Medical and Dental Defence Union of Scotland. Since 1990 doctors in the UK employed in the *National Health Service (NHS) are covered by Crown indemnity but still require cover from these organizations in relation to professional activities outside the NHS. Elsewhere, for example in other European countries and in the USA, professional liability indemnity is provided by commercial insurance companies; this may be much more expensive and is a more restricted service than that provided by the protection societies.

PROFESSIONS ALLIED TO MEDICINE (IN THE UK).

Before 1936 there was no regulation of paramedical occupations in the UK. In 1936 the British Medical Association (BMA) formed the Board of Registration of Medical Auxiliaries and, in 1954, employment in the NHS was limited to those registered with the Board.

Modern health care requires the service of a great many professionals alongside *doctors, *dentists, *nurses, and *midwives. Some of these professionals are regulated by the *Professions Supplementary to Medicines Act (1960). The subjects covered are *chiropody, *dietetics, medical laboratory technology, *occupational therapy, *physiotherapy, *radiography, *remedial gymnastics, and (since 1967) *orthoptics. Each of these professions is regulated by an autonomous board whose functions are to identify and register persons competent in these occupations; to approve qualification and training standards; and to enforce professional discipline. While it is not mandatory for any individual practising in these professions to be registered, the NHS employs only registered practitioners. Such practitioners are required to observe a code of conduct which stipulates that patients may only be treated when referred, that diagnosis and treatment are limited to what the practitioner has been trained to do, and that the practitioner does not represent himself or herself as competent to treat disease.

The Boards' most important functions are to approve training and the qualifying standard. They approve the courses to be followed. For dietitians this is either by a university degree in dietetics or nutrition followed by practical work, or by a postgraduate diploma in dietetics taken after a basic science degree. The adequacy of the training is determined by the Dietitian's Board who also register. Medical Laboratory Scientific Officers are registered with the Medical Laboratory Technicians' Board. Candidates have to have either a Higher National Certificate (or Diploma) in Medical Laboratory Sciences or an appropriate university degree, and must also pass an oral examination based on 1–2 years' training in an approved clinical laboratory. Radiographers register with the Radiographers' Board, the entry qualification being (until 1994) the Diploma of the College of Radiographers or a degree in diagnostic or therapeutic radiography accredited by the Board. For the five other professions, the examining body which grants the qualification is the main or sole professional institution for that specialty. These institutions are the Society of Chiropodists, The British Orthoptic Council jointly with the British Orthoptists Society, the Chartered Society of Physiotherapists (including since 1986 the former Society of Remedial Gymnasts) and the College of Occupational Therapy. In addition to these eight specialties there are many other specialty groups, members of which play important roles in modern medical care. These include:

Art, music, and drama therapists
Clinical psychologists
Clinical scientists (including clinical biochemists, clinical engineers, clinical microbiologists, medical physicists, and scientists in blood transfusion, clinical immunology, haematology, laboratory genetics, and tissue typing)
Dental hygienists, surgery assistants, and technicians
Medical technical officers (including operating department assistants, pathology technicians, perfusionists, and specialized technicians in audiology, cardiology, clinical instrumentation, gastroenterology, neurophysiology, imaging, lasers, nuclear medicine, radiotherapy, rehabilitation engineering, renal dialysis, respiratory physiology, and ultrasound)
Opticians
Pharmacists
Social workers
Speech therapists

All of these professions require specialized training. Examples are as follows:

*Opticians

There are two professional grades. The ophthalmic optician is trained to distinguish between ocular and other causes of visual disability, to test visual acuity, and to prescribe and fit spectacles and contact lenses. An ophthalmic optician can only practise if registered with the General Optical Council. To obtain registration a candidate needs 4 years' training by attending either an approved university course, or a diploma course in accordance with the requirements of the British College of Ophthalmic Opticians. The dispensing optician is not permitted to prescribe or test sight but is trained to fit spectacles, contact lenses, and other ophthalmic appliances. The training period, as stipulated by the College is 2 years.

Pharmacists

To practise as a pharmacist requires regulation by and membership of the *Royal Pharmaceutical Society of Great Britain. This is usually achieved by obtaining a degree in pharmacy or the Society's own diploma, followed by 1 year's practical experience. Pharmacy assistants, who work under the supervision of a pharmacist, carry out dispensing, stocktaking, and similar work. Certificates of proficiency are awarded—after part-time courses taken while employed—by the Society of Apothecaries, the City and Guilds Institute of London, and the Scottish Technical Board.

Clinical psychologists

Many clinical psychologists never work in the NHS. All possess a first university degree in *psychology, together with appropriate postgraduate clinical experience, often involving the acquisition of a Master's degree achieved after additional years of full-time study experience. Since 1987 the British Psychological Society has been empowered, by the Privy Council, to maintain a Register of Chartered Psychologists. The society's Diploma in Clinical Psychology is recognized by the General Whitley Council as a mandatory qualification for trainees to enter qualified clinical psychologist grades in the NHS. The society, in collaboration with the universities, maintains the standard of postgraduate courses.

Speech therapists
The College of Speech and Language Therapists was established in 1948. It is the body responsible for the accreditation of undergraduate and postgraduate courses and examinations leading to the qualification to practise as a speech therapist. It maintains a register of qualified therapists.

Clinical scientists
Many life scientists work in a pathological specialty and develop methods for examining patient specimens in order to diagnose the basis of disease or disorder; physical scientists are mainly concerned with the application of radiation or engineering principles to visualize parts of the body, to measure metabolic processes more directly, or to destroy cancerous tissue. In both groups of scientific disciplines there are many kinds of specialization and specialized application, as the above listing of scientists' titles in the health service shows. Graduates with a suitable first or further degree(s) in science are recruited through a national clearing house into a small number of training posts in accredited hospital departments in one of the listed specialties. Here they undergo an intensive 2–3 year basic training to set them on the road towards the provision of scientific advice, the conduct of research and development related to clinical problems, and the management and delivery of the clinical services based on their discipline. Graduation from basic training, sometimes with an M.Sc. but in every case with assessment of competence on the job by senior members of the profession, leads to appointment to a professional grade where training continues for another 4–6 years. Chartered physicist/chemist/engineer status or membership of the *Royal College of Pathologists is expected before a career post is obtained.

Medical technical officers
Technicians make physical or physiological measurements on patients or instruments in the wide variety of clinical specialties illustrated above, most of which are diagnostic of faults in apparatus or which, alternatively, help doctors to diagnose faults of metabolism, anatomy, or physiology. Technicians work under the direct or indirect supervision of doctors or clinical scientists. They are recruited either from school-leavers with GCSEs or A levels in one or more sciences or from science graduates, and undergo a two year training which supplements their knowledge of anatomy, physiology, and pathology, and enables them to acquire the techniques both of making the measurements and ensuring their accuracy

and reliability. Currently, the exit qualification from the training period is being defined as a National Vocational Qualification (level III) in the specialty; higher qualifications are being developed.

Neither clinical scientists nor medical technical officers need to be registered to work in the health service. Clinical scientists' appointment and promotion is closely controlled by a system of peer review using panels of national assessors, lists of whom are held by the UK departments of health.

M. E. ABRAMS

PROFESSIONS ALLIED TO MEDICINE (IN THE USA). In the USA the allied health professions have developed rapidly, especially in the past 2 decades. This development has been an expression of the rapid expansion of a team approach to health care.

The Committee on Allied Health Education and Accreditation (CAHEA), sponsored by the *American Medical Association (AMA), functions to accredit educational and training programmes in co-operation with various medical specialty societies and allied health professional organizations. These groups, together with the CAHEA, sponsor review committees in each of the fields. Allied health educational programmes are sponsored by many kinds of institutions, ranging from hospitals to colleges and universities, as well as proprietary schools, medical schools, blood banks, government institutions, and others. Altogether, 20 review committees evaluate about 2800 accredited programmes located in more than 1500 sponsoring institutions. The AMA reported (1992) that more than 22 000 physicians and 40 000 allied health professionals teach in these allied health educational programmes. Some 1700 allied health professionals and physicians participate annually as volunteers in the evaluation of some 900 programmes. Educational standards, including the qualifications of programme directors, medical directors, and other programme officials and faculty, are published periodically, along with requirements related to curriculum, resources, financing, and records.

The occupations for which CAHEA currently accredits educational programmes are as follows:

Anesthetist's assistant	Medical technologist
Athletic trainer	Nuclear medicine technologist
Cardiovascular technologist	Occupational therapist
Cytotechnologist	Occupational therapy assistant
Diagnostic medical sonographer	Ophthalmic medical technician/technologist
Electroneurodiagnostic technologist	Perfusionist
Emergency medical technician—paramedic	Physician assistant
Histological technician/technologist	Radiation therapy technologist

Medical assistant	Radiographer
Medical illustrator	Respiratory therapist
Medical laboratory technician (degree)	Respiratory therapy technician
Medical laboratory technician (certificate)	Specialist in blood bank technology
Medical record administrator	Surgeon assistant
Medical record technician	Surgical technologist

In addition to the above activities, CAHEA conducts surveys and studies to identify and address current and projected shortages of allied health personnel, periodically revises its published standards, and conducts site visits as part of the accreditation process.

JEREMIAH A. BARONDESS

Further reading
American Medical Association (1992). *Allied health education directory*. American Medical Association, Chicago.

PROFESSIONS SUPPLEMENTARY TO MEDICINE ACT 1960. This UK Act established a co-ordinating council to supervise a number of registration boards who register members of the supplementary professions and regulate their professional education and conduct. Candidates for appointment by *National Health Service or local authorities who belong to these professions must appear on the appropriate register. Those covered include chiropodists, dietitians, medical laboratory scientific officers, occupational therapists, physiotherapists, radiographers, remedial gymnasts, and orthoptists. See PROFESSIONS ALLIED TO MEDICINE (IN THE UK).

PROFESSORIAL UNITS are hospital units in the various clinical disciplines staffed in whole or in part by doctors, scientists, technicians, and (very occasionally), nurses employed by a university, as well as by staff employed by the hospital, of whom one or more is of professorial rank.

PROGERIA is premature senility. One variety, the Hutchinson–Gilford syndrome, is a rare type of *dwarfism of unknown aetiology with a characteristic appearance of premature old age and of a 'plucked bird'. It develops early, during the third and fourth year of life, and most patients die in childhood or adolescence (the median age at death is 13 years). Degenerative disturbances, particularly *atherosclerosis with cardiovascular and cerebrovascular manifestations, are common. Another, unrelated, condition known as Werner's syndrome, develops in early adult life. This is inherited as an autosomal *recessive trait, but again the fundamental defect is unknown. All the changes of cell senescence occur: there is premature greying, hair loss, hearing loss, teeth loss, *cataracts, *arthritis, *osteoporosis, *diabetes mellitus, and premature *atherosclerosis. Many affected individuals develop malignant tumours, especially *sarcomas. Werner's syndrome is sometimes called 'adult progeria' to distinguish it from the childhood syndrome.

PROGESTERONE is the body's principal progestational *hormone, i.e. the hormone which prepares the *endometrium for implantation of the fertilized *ovum. This preparation occurs during the second half of each menstrual cycle throughout the reproductive period of life, under the influence of progesterone secreted by the *corpus luteum formed in the ovarian follicle after *ovulation; if pregnancy supervenes, the corpus luteum and progesterone secretion persist. Progesterone ($C_{21}H_{30}O_2$) is also produced by the *adrenal cortex and *placenta. Because they inhibit ovulation, progestational substances are widely used in oral *contraceptive formulations.

PROGESTOGENS are natural or synthetic substances with progestational activity.

PROGNATHOUS. Having protruding jaws.

PROGNOSIS is the forecasting, or forecast, of the future course and the outcome of a disease.

PROGRESSIVE BULBAR PALSY. See MOTOR NEURONE DISEASE; NEUROMUSCULAR DISEASE.

PROGRESSIVE MUSCULAR ATROPHY. See MOTOR NEURONE DISEASE; NEUROMUSCULAR DISEASE.

PROGUANIL is an antimalarial drug used in *prophylaxis (daily dosage) and treatment in areas of British influence but rarely in US practice. Proguanil is also known under the proprietary name of Paludrine®.

PROHIBITION is used to mean interdiction by law of the manufacture, importation, or sale of alcoholic drinks for common consumption. In the USA, it was enforced between 1920 and 1933, in accordance with the 18th Amendment to the US Constitution. During this period the manufacture and sale of drinks containing more than 0.5 per cent of ethyl alcohol were illegal. It ended with the 21st Amendment, on 5 December 1933.

PROKARYOTES are cellular organisms without a distinct nucleus or nuclear membrane, whose genetic material is in the form of haploid *deoxyribonucleic acid (DNA) (unpaired chromosomes). Bacteria and blue-green algae are prokaryotes; all other cellular organisms, plant and animal, are *eukaryotes. See CELL AND CELL BIOLOGY.

PROLACTIN is the lactogenic hormone secreted by the anterior lobe of the *pituitary gland, which controls the secretion of milk by the *mammary glands of the postpartum female.

PROLACTINOMA. A *pituitary tumour which secretes *prolactin.

PROLAPSE is a falling or slipping down of an organ; when otherwise unqualified, it usually means prolapse of the *uterus, a not uncommon condition in multiparous women in which the uterine cervix descends to or beyond the vaginal orifice. Rectal prolapse through the anus occurs sometimes in children.

PROLAPSED INTERVERTEBRAL DISC, also known as 'prolapsed nucleus pulposus', 'herniated nucleus pulposus', or 'slipped disc', is a common cause of acute back pain, particularly in the cervical and lumbar regions, and of radicular or nerve root pain, particularly that which is felt along the distribution of the sciatic nerve (sciatica). Each intervertebral disc is a tough flexible pad lying between the bodies of adjacent vertebrae (see SPINE); it consists of a soft centre, the nucleus pulposus, surrounded by a circular ring of fibrous tissue, the annulus fibrosus. The latter is at its weakest posteriorly, and if a particular strain is put on it, for example by bending, it may allow the nuclear pulposus to bulge backwards. Depending on whether this bulge (or hernia) is in the midline or to one or other side of it, it can press on the spinal cord itself or on one or more spinal nerve roots. When in the lumbosacral region, lumbago and/or sciatica can result, together with, in many cases, objective evidence of interference with sensory and motor nerve pathways. A similar situation commonly arises in the cervical spine. Involvement of the relatively more rigid thoracic spine is less common.

PRONTOSIL® was the proprietary name for the prototype *sulphonamide introduced in the early 1930s, no longer in use.

PROPHYLAXIS is the prevention of disease, or the preventive treatment of a recurrent disorder.

PROPRANOLOL is a drug which causes beta-adrenergic blockade (see ADRENERGIC BLOCKADE; BETA-BLOCKERS); it is used in many conditions where this pharmacological effect is desired (e.g. *hypertension, *angina, *arrhythmias, *myocardial infarction, *thyrotoxicosis, psychiatric disorders, etc.).

PROPRIETARY MEDICINES. See DRUGS; PHARMACEUTICAL INDUSTRY.

PROPRIOCEPTION is the reception of sensory information by structures (proprioceptors) within the tissues, especially that relating to the movement and sense of position of parts of the body.

PROPTOSIS is forward displacement of the eyeball.

PROSECTOR. One who dissects a body for anatomical or pathological demonstration.

PROSTACYCLIN. Prostaglandin I_2.

PROSTAGLANDINS are a group of related complex *fatty acids found in most human tissues. They may be regarded as local tissue *hormones, sharing some of the characteristics of hormones and of *neurotransmitters. They are subdivided into six types, labelled A to F, the degree of saturation of the side-chain being in each case designated by the subscript 1, 2, or 3 (e.g. PGE_2, etc.). They have many biological effects, possibly by influencing the activity of the enzyme *adenyl cyclase. These include effects on vascular permeability, blood pressure, acid secretion by the stomach, platelet aggregation, body temperature, the action of certain hormones, and uterine contractility. The action of prostaglandin preparations on the pregnant uterus is employed therapeutically to procure abortion and to induce labour.

PROSTATE. A gland of the male reproductive system of mammals, which contributes its secretion (acid phosphatase, citric acid, and proteolytic enzymes) to *semen. It surrounds the neck of the *bladder and the proximal portion of the *urethra. It comprises both muscle and glandular elements. In man it often becomes enlarged as a result of *hyperplasia in middle and old age, causing symptoms of urinary obstruction which require surgical relief. The prostate may also be the site of bacterial infection (prostatitis) and of *carcinoma.

PROSTATECTOMY is surgical removal of the *prostate gland.

PROSTHESIS. An artificial substitute for a body part.

PROSTRATION is a state of helplessness or total exhaustion.

PROTANOPIA is defective colour vision of the dichromatic type (see COLOUR BLINDNESS) in which red and green sensitivity are lacking.

PROTEIN. Any of a class of very complex nitrogenous organic compounds of high molecular weight (18 000–10 000 000) which are of fundamental importance to all living matter. They consist of hundreds or thousands of *amino acids joined together by *peptide linkage into one or more connected *polypeptide chains which in turn are folded in various ways. The precise sequence of amino acids is identical in each molecule of a given protein. This sequence is determined by the sequence of the nucleotides in the nucleic acid of the *chromosomes of the cells in which the protein is synthesized; three nucleotides code for each amino acid, of which about 20 occur in nature. Most proteins form colloidal solutions in water or dilute salt solutions, except for some with elongated (fibrous) molecules which are insoluble. Proteins are frequently 'conjugated', that is combined with other substances, such as nucleic acids (nucleoprotein), carbohydrates (muco- or glycoproteins), and fats (lipoproteins). Only autotrophic organisms (most chlorophyll-containing plants and a few bacteria) can synthesize amino acids and hence proteins from inorganic constituents; all other organisms are heterotrophic and ultimately depend on the synthetic activities of autotrophic organisms.

PROTEIN–ENERGY MALNUTRITION is a self-explanatory term, often abbreviated to PEM, formerly called protein–calorie malnutrition (PCM). It covers the spectrum of undernutrition, including both the extreme clinical expressions known as *marasmus and *kwashiorkor.

PROTEINURIA. See ALBUMINURIA.

PROTEUS is a genus of Gram-negative bacilli, common in faecal material; most are not highly pathogenic. *Proteus vulgaris* is a fairly frequent cause of *cystitis and is also a secondary invader in some suppurative infections.

PROTHROMBIN is the precursor *enzyme (also known as factor II) of *thrombin. During blood clotting, thrombin catalyses the conversion of soluble *fibrinogen into *fibrin. See HAEMATOLOGY.

PROTON. A stable elementary particle of positive electric charge equal to that of the *electron but of opposite sign. Protons, together with the electrically neutral *neutrons of almost equal mass, make up the nucleus of all atoms; in an electrically neutral atom the number of protons in the nucleus (the atomic number) is equal to the number of planetary electrons. A single proton is a hydrogen *ion, that is, a normal hydrogen atomic nucleus.

PROTOPLASM is the matter of which all biological cells consist; in nucleated cells it is subdivided into that composing the nucleus (nucleoplasm) and that surrounding it (cytoplasm). It is a complex watery *colloid, containing protein, lipids, carbohydrates, nucleic acids, and inorganic salts. It is usually taken to exclude large vacuoles, secretory, and ingested material.

PROTOZOA are unicellular animals, comprising the simplest phylum of the animal world. A few are parasitic in man and therefore of medical importance. They include the causative agents of *malaria, *trypanosomiasis, *leishmaniasis, *amoebiasis, *giardiasis, *toxoplasmosis, and *trichomoniasis. See TROPICAL MEDICINE.

PROTOZOOLOGY is the study of *protozoa, and is a branch of zoology.

PROUT, WILLIAM (1785–1850). British physician and chemist. He was the first 'chemical physiologist'. He showed that the stomach contained free *hydrochloric acid.

PROWAZEK, STANISLAUS JOSEF MATHIAS VON (1875–1915). Bohemian protozoologist. He discovered the cause of *trachoma and fowl pest in 1906. He died of *typhus investigating an outbreak in a Russian prisoner-of-war camp in 1915. Henrique da Rocha-Lima, who also acquired the disease but recovered, discovered the cause and named it *Rickettsia prowazeki* in his honour and in that of H. T. *Ricketts, who also died investigating it.

PRURITUS is itching, which may be generalized or localized to a particular area (e.g. pruritus vulvae, pruritus ani, etc.). It has many causes, including several primary skin diseases and some systemic disorders, such as *diabetes mellitus and *obstructive jaundice.

PSEUDOCHOLINESTERASE is an *enzyme, also known simply as cholinesterase, widely distributed in the body, which inactivates *choline esters. ('True' cholinesterase, which inactivates *acetylcholine, is acetylcholinesterase.) About one person in 300 is deficient in pseudocholinesterase and hence cannot degrade succinylcholine, a muscle relaxant drug often used as an adjuvant in general *anaesthesia.

PSEUDOGOUT is a joint condition of middle and later ages affecting particularly the knees and hips. It tends to be monarticular and may, like gout, occur in acute and painful attacks. Also known as pyrophosphate arthropathy or chondrocalcinosis, it is due to the synovial deposition of crystals of calcium pyrophosphate and other calcium salts.

PSEUDOHERMAPHRODITE. Any case of *intersex other than the rare instances of true *hermaphroditism. Male pseudohermaphrodites are gonadally and genetically male but with female external characteristics; the converse is true of female pseudohermaphrodites.

PSEUDOHYPERTROPHY is a disproportionate enlargement of some groups of muscles which occurs in certain forms of *muscular dystrophy and occasionally in other myopathic and neurological disorders, due to infiltration with other tissue elements. See NEUROMUSCULAR DISEASE.

PSEUDOHYPOPARATHYROIDISM is a rare genetic disorder characterized by abnormal resistance of the tissues to the effects of *parathyroid hormone, simulating *hypoparathyroidism.

PSEUDOMONAS is a genus of aerobic Gram-negative *bacilli widely distributed in the environment, including hospitals. Most do not cause human disease, but one, *Pseudomonas aeruginosa* (formerly known as *P. pyocyanea*), can be the agent of such diverse infections as *endocarditis, *meningitis, *pneumonia, *otitis, wound and burn sepsis, and various types of *nosocomial (i.e. hospital-acquired) infection. The last is particularly liable to occur in ill patients and, because *Pseudomonas* is resistant to many conventional antibiotics, as a 'superinfection' after other organisms have been cleared. *Pseudomonas mallei* is responsible for *glanders.

PSEUDOTUMOUR CEREBRI is a syndrome characterized by manifestations of increased intracranial pressure (headache, vomiting, and *papilloedema) without true localizing signs or any other evidence of a space-occupying lesion such as a cerebral tumour. The syndrome is due to cerebral *oedema and is now more often known as benign intracranial hypertension. Several aetiological factors have been identified, but often the condition resolves without any cause having been established. Treatment with *corticosteroids and/or *diuretics may be needed to reduce the pressure.

PSEUDOXANTHOMA ELASTICUM is a rare *recessively inherited disorder of elastic tissue affecting predominantly the skin, eyes, and vascular system. The name derives from the appearance in early adult life of yellowish *macules and *papules in the skin histologically found to be composed of abnormal *elastic tissue.

PSILOCYBIN is a hallucinogenic agent derived from the mushroom fungus *Psilocybe mexicana*.

PSITTACOSIS is an acute respiratory infection, often with *pneumonia, acquired from birds and due to the organism *Chlamydia psittaci*. The reservoir was originally thought to be exclusively in psittacines (the parrot family) but this is now known not to be so and the more accurate term ornithosis is preferred.

PSORIASIS is a common chronic relapsing skin disease, the cause of which is unknown but which is strongly influenced by *genetic factors. The essential abnormality is an excessively rapid turnover of cells in the epidermal layer of the skin. The rash consists of scattered red papulosquamous patches with silvery scales which do not usually itch and are characteristically concentrated on the extensor surfaces, that is the elbows, knees, and back. The scalp is often affected, the face rarely so. The nails show two typical signs: a deep linear pitting, and separation of the tip from the bed by yellowish keratin. Some patients develop a condition closely resembling *rheumatoid arthritis (psoriatic arthropathy). Psoriasis is common, affecting between 1 and 2 per cent of the population in the USA and Europe. It is very persistent, although temporary remissions are common, both with and without treatment. Other illnesses and stress can precipitate exacerbations.

PSYCHASTHENIA is an imprecise term—'psychic weakness'—introduced by the French psychiatrist Pierre *Janet. As used by him, it embraced all *neuroses characterized by anxiety, phobias, compulsions, and obsessions.

PSYCHE. The mind.

PSYCHEDELIC is a term used of drugs which cause visual *hallucinations, supposedly 'expanding' consciousness and heightening perception. They may also be psychotomimetic, that is produce mental states resembling *psychosis.

PSYCHIATRIST. A medically qualified specialist in mental disorders. See PSYCHIATRY.

PSYCHIATRY is the branch of medicine concerned with mental disorders. In this article, psychiatry is considered from five points of view: the principal psychiatric disorders; the work and training of psychiatrists; the treatments they use; the organization of psychiatric services; and psychiatric research.

Mental disorders

Mental disorders are divided into three groups: severe learning difficulty, personality disorder, and mental illness. The groups are not mutually exclusive; for example, personality disorder and mental illness may occur together.

Severe learning difficulty

Severe learning difficulty (also called mental retardation or mental handicap) is present from the earliest years. It is characterized by abnormally low intelligence and retarded development of other aspects of psychological development evident at or soon after birth. People with severe learning difficulty often have physical handicaps as well, for example problems in walking or controlling the bladder. They also have problems in coping with the demands of everyday life—in milder cases with shopping and travelling, in severe cases even with personal hygiene. In the most severe cases the person may be unable to speak or to control the bladder or bowels. However, most people with severe learning difficulties can live reasonably normal lives provided that they or their families receive some help.

Personality disorders

Personality disorders become apparent from the teenage years. The person is of normal intelligence but his or her behaviour is persistently unusual in some way. Many kinds of personality disorder have been described and two examples will be given. People with antisocial personality disorder (sometimes called psychopathic or sociopathic) are self-centred and heartless, and do not make loving relationships. They are impulsive and do not strive consistently for goals in life. Such people do not feel guilt, and may be callously indifferent to the effects of their actions on others. They make poor parents and may neglect or abuse their children. Another example of a personality disorder is the paranoid type. These people are unduly suspicious and sensitive. They are constantly on the look out for attempts by others to deceive or play tricks on them. They appear secretive, devious, and jealous, and have little capacity for enjoyment.

Mental illnesses
Mental illnesses are disturbances of behaviour appearing after a period of normal development. They may be divided into two groups: psychoses and neuroses, according to two distinguishing features. First, psychoses are generally more severe (they correspond, more or less, to the layman's idea of madness) while neuroses are less severe (corresponding to the layman's idea of nervous problems). Secondly, in *psychosis the person is generally unaware of the extent of his or her illness (he 'loses insight'), while in *neurosis he or she retains this awareness. Each of these two broad classes of mental illness is divided into several further categories, of which some examples will be given.

There are three principal types of psychosis. The first type is called *organic* (this term refers to the presence of a structural abnormality in some organ of the body—in this case in the brain). Organic psychosis is caused by physical disease either affecting the brain directly (e.g. a cerebral *tumour) or indirectly (e.g. toxic substances in the blood resulting from kidney failure). When an organic psychosis develops quickly, the patient is muddled and uncertain of his whereabouts (he is 'delirious'). When an organic psychosis develops slowly there is a gradual decline in all intellectual functions (*dementia), often evident first as poor memory.

In the other types of psychosis, no physical disease can be discovered, so that they are called functional psychoses (the term functional is a term used in medicine to indicate the absence of organic pathology). There are two types of functional psychosis: affective disorders, which are primarily disorders of mood (affect is a technical term for mood), and *schizophrenia. Recently it has become apparent that the distinction between organic and functional psychosis is not absolute. Thus brain imaging and modern techniques of *neuropathology have revealed subtle structural changes in the brain in schizophrenia.

Schizophrenia is a serious mental illness affecting thinking, perception, mood, and initiative. When the illness is acute, the common symptoms include auditory hallucinations (hearing voices) and delusions (false ideas) which are often to do with imagined persecution. In its chronic stage, these symptoms are still present but are often overshadowed by chronic apathy, loss of drive, and social withdrawal.

Affective disorders are of two kinds, *mania and depressive disorder. Some patients experience only the one or the other; some alternate between the two. These alternating disorders are called manic-depressive psychoses. A depressive disorder consists of much more than feelings of sadness. The mood is of profound pessimism often accompanied by thoughts of suicide and severe but inappropriate self-blame. Sleep is disturbed (the patient often wakes very early and cannot go to sleep again), appetite is impaired, and activity is reduced. The picture of mania is the opposite. The mood is usually elated but sometimes irritable, and the person is overactive and inappropriately confident. Some manic patients enter into unsound business schemes, go on spending sprees, or commit other rash and mistaken acts.

Neuroses are subdivided into anxiety disorders, obsessional disorders, and dissociative disorder. Anxiety disorders are dominated by anxious feelings and worrying thoughts, together with the bodily accompaniments of anxiety such as racing heart, dry mouth, and sweating. These sensations are familiar to everyone; the patient with an anxiety disorder experiences more severe and persisting distress in circumstances in which there is no objective reason to be afraid. Obsessional disorders are characterized by repeated intrusive and distressing thoughts, for example blasphemous thoughts and preoccupations with spreading disease by contamination. Such ideas are often accompanied by actions which produce temporary relief from distress: for example, a person with thoughts about contamination may wash his or her hands repeatedly.

In dissociative disorder (also known as conversion disorder, or *hysteria) symptoms characteristic of physical illness occur without any physical cause. For example, patients may be unable to move an arm however hard they try, even though the nerves, muscles, and other structures involved are healthy. Dissociative disorder arises from emotional conflict in the unconscious part of the mind, so that patients are unaware of the emotional causes of their symptoms.

Psychiatrists treat some conditions which do not fall within this scheme of classification. The first is dependence on alcohol or drugs. The second is the disordered pattern of eating found in *anorexia nervosa and *bulimia nervosa. In anorexia nervosa the patient, often a teenage girl, engages in relentless attempts to lose weight through extreme dieting, exercise, and other means. In bulimia nervosa there are episodes of gluttonous eating followed by self-induced vomiting to avoid weight gain. Psychiatrists also give help to people who, although not mentally ill, are passing through a period of intense personal difficulties which have caused emotional distress. Such conditions are referred to as adjustment disorders.

Children suffer mental disorders. In pre-school children these usually involve difficulties with sleeping, eating, and control of aggressive feelings. In older children, most psychiatric disorders fall into two groups. Emotional disorders are characterized mainly by anxiety, unhappiness, and excessive worries. Conduct disorders are characterized by stealing, truancy, and aggressive behaviour.

Mental disorders of these kinds have been found in all countries. Neuroses are more frequent than psychoses, and adjustment disorders are more common still. It has been estimated that about one-sixth of patients attending general practitioners in the UK have some kind of emotional disorder, either on its own or accompanying physical illness.

The view has been expressed that mental disorders do not really exist; they are medical labels attached to unusual behaviour that society cannot tolerate. Three sets of observations indicate that mental disorders are real entities. The first observation will have been made by readers who have met a person suffering from schizophrenia: the severity of the disorder and its sudden appearance in a person who has up to that time lived a socially conforming life are exceedingly difficult to reconcile with the idea that mental illness is merely a label attached to unconforming people. The second observation is that identical forms of mental illness occur at the present time in places with widely different social structures (e.g. rural areas of China and large cities in the USA). The third observation is that the forms of mental illness recorded in the medical writings of previous centuries closely resemble those seen today. There are also observations of a more technical kind, such as the finding of structural changes in the brain of some patients with schizophrenia, which indicate that mental disorders are more than behaviours that society finds inconvenient. Nevertheless, it is true that people can be called mentally ill when they are not. This can happen when a doctor does not examine his patient adequately or fails to use generally agreed criteria for diagnosis. Thus there have been reports of the detention in hospital in some countries of political dissidents who are mentally healthy.

The work of psychiatrists

Psychiatry is a major medical specialty which is divided into subspecialties of general adult psychiatry, child and adolescent psychiatry, psychotherapy, forensic psychiatry, and severe learning difficulties.

Psychiatrists providing general psychiatric services for adult patients work with nurses, occupational therapists, psychologists, and social workers, who together make up a 'mental health team'. In the care of the elderly, the team often includes physiotherapists as well; and in the care of children, teachers. Although most patients are now treated outside hospital, the most severely ill patients still require periods of in-patient care, either in a psychiatric ward of a psychiatric hospital or in a general hospital. Psychiatrists are in charge of these in-patient units but much of their time is spent in treating patients in the community, consulting with general practitioners and with staff looking after patients in hostels or day centres.

Child psychiatrists work mostly with out-patients since few children need to be treated in hospital. They advise parents, schoolteachers, and the staff of children's homes about the care of children with emotional problems, and work alongside *paediatricians in helping handicapped children and those with serious physical illness.

Forensic psychiatrists treat mentally disordered offenders. They see people who are remanded for psychiatric reports by the courts, advise the courts about matters such as the effects of mental disorder on responsibility for illegal actions, and provide treatment especially for the small number of mentally ill or mentally handicapped patients who may be dangerous.

Psychiatrists who treat people with severe learning difficulties are concerned mainly with the treatment of mental disorder and behavioural problems (these occur more frequently in people with severe learning difficulties than in other people.) They help to plan services for people with learning difficulties and for their families, although the provision of many of these services is the responsibility of the educational and social services and of family doctors.

Education and training

All psychiatrists are qualified in medicine and most have undertaken a further period of general medical work before specializing in psychiatry. In the UK, the training of a specialist in psychiatry lasts for at least 6 years. During the first 3 years, the trainee passes through an organized series of posts, chosen to provide wide experience in treating all kinds of psychiatric disorder. At the same time the trainee undertakes a course of academic study leading to an examination. In the UK the final 3 years of training is more specialized, with increasingly greater clinical responsibility and a requirement for some training in research. Similar arrangements exist in other countries, although the details of length of training and timing of professional examinations are not all the same.

At the end of training, most psychiatrists in the UK enter a consultant post in the *National Health Service. In many other countries the fully trained psychiatrist enters private practice, often combining this with a part-time hospital appointment. Consultant psychiatrists keep their knowledge up to date by regular attendance at postgraduate meetings and by reading professional journals.

Some laymen confuse the training of psychiatrists and clinical psychologists. Clinical psychologists are not medically qualified; they begin their training with a three year degree course in *psychology instead of the five year medical course, with its subsequent preregistration year. They then undertake a course in clinical psychology, usually for 2–3 years, instead of the six-year training of psychiatrists. Many also obtain a research degree before entering clinical practice.

Psychiatric treatments

Psychiatric treatments can be divided into three groups: physical, psychological, and social. Sometimes a patient requires only one of these methods; for example, psychotherapy to help with difficulties in personal relationships. In other cases, a combination is needed: for example, drugs to relieve severe depressive symptoms and psychotherapy directed to emotional problems that might lead to further depression. It is a common misconception that there is an inherent conflict between the prescription of drugs and the use of psychotherapy or social measures. On the contrary, a combination is not only compatible in principle but also often necessary in practice.

Physical treatment

This term used to describe the prescription of drugs, the use of electroconvulsive therapy, and the (now very rare) use of neurosurgical operations. In practice nowadays, most physical treatment is with drugs.

Drugs that alter psychiatric symptoms are of four kinds: anxiolytic, which reduce anxiety; antidepressant, which modify depressive disorders; antipsychotic, which relieve symptoms of psychosis; and mood regulators, which prevent relapse in manic-depressive disorders. Each of the main groups of drugs contains many different compounds, most of which differ more in their side-effects than in their therapeutic effects.

Psychotropic drugs provide an effective and safe way of controlling many of the symptoms of illness. Antidepressant drugs have transformed the treatment of depressive disorders. Patients who, in the past, would have remained depressed for months or even years, now usually improve within a few weeks with antidepressant drug treatment. Antipsychotic drugs have also brought about substantial changes in the well-being of schizophrenic patients. Although these drugs do not cure the condition, they calm the patient and reduce the most troublesome symptoms, so that patients can return to life outside hospital, while continuing to take the drugs. However, more than other kinds of psychotropic drugs, antipsychotic drugs have unpleasant side-effects which can cause problems for their long-term use.

Electroconvulsive therapy (ECT) is mainly used in treating the most severe forms of depressive disorder. Antidepressant drugs have replaced ECT for most purposes, being generally as effective. However, their beneficial effects do not appear as quickly as those of ECT which is the best treatment for the most severe and urgent cases. In addition, some patients who fail to respond to antidepressant drugs improve with ECT.

Psychological treatment

Psychological treatment includes counselling, cognitive-behaviour therapy, and dynamic psychotherapy. All three treatments can be given to a single patient or to a group of patients with similar problems, but for simplicity the following account will deal only with individual treatment.

(a) **Counselling.** This is the simplest form of psychological treatment and the one used most often. The essential steps are to relieve distress by allowing patients to talk about their feelings; to help them clarify their ideas and plans, correcting misunderstandings (for example unduly pessimistic views of the outcome of illness), and encouraging self-help. When patients feel overwhelmed by many problems, a 'problem-solving' approach is valuable. In this the problems are defined, possible solutions are considered one by one, a plan of action is worked out with the patient, the plan is acted on, and the results are reviewed. This systematic approach is valuable not only in reducing current feelings of distress and hopelessness but also in preparing the patient to deal better with future problems. Counselling can be given by all doctors or by paramedical staff; it lasts usually for six sessions or less.

(b) **Cognitive-behaviour therapy** deals with ways of thinking or behaving that exacerbate or prolong a disorder. The behavioural procedures are simpler to carry out, for example, assisting patients to return repeatedly to situations that provoke anxiety and which they have been avoiding. The cognitive methods include ways of changing irrational fears and beliefs. For example, if the patient is convinced that physical sensations are evidence of serious physical illness, the therapist examines the evidence on which the patient supports his beliefs, helps the patient to see that the ideas are irrational and that there is a more rational way of thinking. Cognitive-behavioural treatment is carried out by psychiatrists, clinical psychologists, and psychiatric nurse specialists.

(c) **Dynamic psychotherapy** helps patients understand the origins in earlier life of their present problems, and the unconscious elements of these problems. This aim is achieved by encouraging patients to talk about their problems, and encouraging them to identify occasions in the past when they experienced similar feelings. Hypotheses are made about the ways in which past experiences (e.g. rejection by a parent) explain present problems (e.g. difficulty in establishing close relationships); hypotheses of this kind are called interpretations.

Dynamic psychotherapy is carried out mainly by psychiatrists and clinical psychologists. For most patients, treatment is weekly for 6–9 months (so called brief dynamic psychotherapy). A few patients need more intensive and prolonged treatment lasting for 18 months or more. When dynamic psychotherapy is intensive and lengthy and closely modelled on the methods developed by Freud, it is called psychoanalysis.

Social treatment
The term social treatment is used in two ways. First, it refers to methods in which the influences of a social group are used to bring about beneficial changes in patients. The second is to describe attempts to arrange a suitable environment for the patient, for example by finding suitable work and living conditions. Social treatment in either of these senses is to be distinguished from social work, which is the name for the various activities carried out by social workers. The latter are concerned with people with social difficulties (especially children and old people); they organize and supervise community resources such as hostels and old people's homes; they arrange the provision of services such as meals-on-wheels for the old; and they provide counselling for people who need this.

A special form of social treatment is called a therapeutic community. This term is used to describe a group of patients (usually about 20) who share a common problem, such as difficulty in relationships or drug dependence. These people live together, take part in communal activities, and engage in group discussions. The focus of the discussions is the patients' problems in their relationships with one another, for example inappropriate aggression or unwillingness to take responsibility. Because the patients are resident, it is possible to arouse strong emotional responses in group therapy that might be hazardous in people returning home from out-patient treatment. It is the hope that changes brought about in these problems within the therapeutic community will generalize to everyday life when the patient is discharged.

Psychiatric services
In every branch of medicine, the provision of services depends on social conditions as well as clinical considerations. This is particularly true of psychiatry, because the scale and type of provision required for mentally ill people are determined in part by the willingness of a society to tolerate unusual behaviour and to care for its handicapped members. The number of hospital places needed for people with chronic mental disorder depends crucially on these social factors.

The organization of services
Patients with chronic psychiatric disorder treated outside hospital require accommodation, occupation, supervision, and treatment. Accommodation may be with the family, or in a hostel or shared house (a 'group home'). Occupation may be in ordinary employment but often sheltered work is needed; patients who cannot undertake even sheltered work require occupational therapy. These activities may be provided in a centre in the community

or at a hospital. Supervision and treatment are provided by general practitioners and psychiatrists, community nurses and social workers, working in clinics in the community, or in day hospitals. Clinical psychologists and occupational therapists are other members of the 'community team', which aims to provide in the community most of the treatments available in hospital, and to support and counsel the families of patients living at home. When these provisions work well, treatment in hospital is needed for only the most ill patients who require intensive nursing or a degree of security for their own safety or that of other people.

Psychiatric research
In the UK there are academic departments of psychiatry in every medical school. In this short article, it is possible only to consider the subject very briefly from three viewpoints: subject matter, advances in knowledge, and educational activities.

Psychiatric research is concerned with the description, causes, and treatment of psychiatric disorders, and with their distribution in the community. Effective enquiries into these issues involve the use of the research methods of *genetics, experimental psychology, neurophysiology, *pharmacology, *biochemistry, and *sociology. Psychiatric research contributes to the solution of some of the problems in these other fields of knowledge, for example, to questions about the ways that drugs act on the healthy brain, and psychiatric research groups often include members of one of these other disciplines.

*Epidemiology is the study of the distribution of disease in the population. Differences in this distribution can point to the causes of psychiatric disorder; for example, attempted suicide is more frequent among people living in areas with overcrowding and poor social amenities, suggesting that social factors may play a causal role.

Genetic studies begin with enquiries into the frequency of a disease in people with different degrees of kinship to patients with the disease in question. For example, the finding that schizophrenia is more common among identical twins of schizophrenics than among non-identical twins of schizophrenics, suggests a hereditary cause, because identical twins have identical genes but non-identical twins do not. Genetic influences act through biochemical mechanisms, and in mental disorders the relevant mechanisms are likely to be in the brain. It is considerably more difficult to investigate the chemical processes in the living human brain than it is to study the similar processes in other organs, because the skull makes the brain inaccessible. For this reason, two indirect methods of investigation are often used. One method is to study a brain function that is known, from studies of animals, to depend on a particular biochemical process. One such mechanism is that which controls the release of *hormones into the bloodstream. Measuring levels of hormones in the blood provides an indirect measure of the controlling brain mechanisms. The second approach is to use one of the new methods of brain imaging, which can assess the metabolic activity of various parts of the brain and identify some of the chemical processes within it.

Another approach is to study the structure and the chemistry of the brains of people who have died in the course of mental illness. These methods have limitations because death in mental illness usually occurs after many years of treatment (so that any changes could be due to treatment rather than to illness), and because some, but not all, of the chemical processes in the brain change after death. Despite these limitations, such methods have yielded valuable information about dementia, and are beginning to yield important facts about schizophrenia.

A third approach to understanding changes in the brain in mental illness is to study the effects of drugs that control the symptoms of illness. Since drugs may suppress symptoms rather than correct the primary cause, such studies do not necessarily reveal the basic abnormality, but they can reveal how primary cause is translated into the symptoms and signs that cause so much suffering to patients.

As well as these genetic and biochemical studies (often called 'biological' studies) social and psychological investigations are needed to explain how mental disorders develop. For example, schizophrenia is provoked by stressful circumstances of life, and the course of the illness depends partly on the patient's personality and on the psychological reactions of people with whom the patient is in close contact. Psychological and social investigations are even more relevant to the study of neuroses and personality disorders, in which ways of thinking and behaving in stressful circumstances are of central importance.

Some recent advances in knowledge

Because psychiatric research is advancing rapidly, it is impossible to review here even a small proportion of the recent advances in knowledge. Instead, four brief representative examples will be given, two concerned with treatment, two with causes.

Striking progress has been made in developing and evaluating new treatments for serious mental disorders. Drugs are now available to reverse the symptoms of depressive disorders, reduce acute symptoms of schizophrenia, and control mania. It is also possible to prevent many recurrences in schizophrenia, mania, and depressive disorders. These beneficial effects have been demonstrated in controlled clinical trials. At the same time, substantial progress has been made in finding out how these drugs work.

Psychological treatments have also advanced. Cognitive-behaviour therapies have been developed using knowledge and techniques derived from experimental psychology. Most anxiety and obsessional neuroses can now be treated in this way without the use of drugs, and effective treatments have been developed for some sexual problems, some kinds of eating disorder, and many other abnormal behaviours. Like the new drug treatments, these cognitive-behavioural methods have been tested in controlled clinical trials.

New knowledge has also been gained about the causes of mental illness. For example, schizophrenia has been shown to have multiple causes. Genetic factors are of major importance, and structural changes have been found in the temporal lobes of the brain, which could be the basis of a vulnerability to schizophrenia. It has also been demonstrated that stressful life events play an important (and measurable) part in precipitating the illness in predisposed people, and provoking relapses.

Important progress has been made in unravelling the complicated causes of mental illness in the elderly. It used to be supposed that all serious mental diseases in old people were caused by degenerative changes in the brain. Now it is known that schizophrenia, depressive disorders, and mania occur in late life and generally respond to the same treatments used in younger people. At the same time, the disorders caused by brain degeneration have become better understood through the application of methods of cell biology and molecular genetics.

Conclusion

It is important to end by emphasizing the close links that exist between psychiatry and the rest of medicine. These are most apparent—and most important—in the area of professional standards, education, and training. They are also evident in the use of common methods of research (e.g. biochemical methods). Finally, methods of treatment are moving closer as psychiatrists develop new and effective drugs, and physicians pay increasing attention to psychological and social aspects of care, which are a central concern of psychiatrists.

M. G. GELDER

Further reading

Andreasen, N. C. (1985). *The broken brain: the biological revolution in psychiatry*. Harper and Row, New York.

Bloch, S. (1982). *What is psychotherapy?* Oxford University Press, Oxford.

Clare, A. (1980). *Psychiatry in dissent*, (2nd edn). Tavistock, London.

Gelder, M. G. (1986). Psychiatry. In *The Oxford companion to medicine* (ed. J. Walton, P. B. Beeson and R Bodley Scott). Oxford University Press, Oxford.

Gelder, M. G., Gath, D. H., and Mayou, R. (1994). *The concise Oxford textbook of psychiatry*. Oxford University Press, Oxford.

PSYCHIATRY: A SHORT HISTORY OF ITS DEVELOPMENT

The ancient world

The treatment of mental illness has not always been the province of doctors. For long periods of recorded history, mental disorders have been thought of, not as illness, but as the result of divine or demonic possession. It is true that Graeco-Roman medical writings contain some references to mental illnesses and that these illnesses were generally regarded by the writers as having bodily causes and requiring medical treatment. However, in the ancient world generally and throughout the Middle Ages, mental illness was more often ascribed to possession by supernatural forces. As such it was not generally thought to be the concern of doctors. Instead, many mentally ill people were either given religious help or persecuted as witches.

New beginnings

In the 16th and 17th centuries a more scientific approach to mental disorders began to develop. Several doctors wrote about the less severe mental disorders that physicians encountered among their patients. For example, Timothy Bright published a *Treatise on melancholy* in 1586, Thomas *Willis referred to *melancholia and hysteria in his lectures in 1663, and Thomas *Sydenham wrote about hysteria and *hypochondriasis. However, most doctors had little to do with the care of patients with severe mental illness, and there were hardly any hospital provisions for such treatment. Indeed, until the beginning of the 18th century the only hospital in England devoted solely to the care of the insane was the *Bethlem Hospital. At this time, most psychotic patients were not treated in hospital, but lived as best they could in the community, often as beggars or vagabonds. Others were in prison.

In the first half of the 18th century, small signs of progress began to appear. In England three other hospitals began to provide for the mentally ill. These were Bethel Hospital (1724) in Norwich, and *Guy's Hospital (1728) and the French Protestant Hospital (1737) in London. In Ireland, a mental hospital was founded in Dublin with money left for this purpose in the will of Jonathan Swift, who died in 1745.

In 1751 St Luke's Hospital was opened in London. The physician to this new hospital was William Battie, a distinguished medical man who served as president of the Royal College of Physicians from 1764 to 1765. He instituted courses of clinical instruction in psychiatry at St Luke's and later published them. His book was the first significant English medical text devoted solely to psychiatric disorders. In the introduction, Battie explained that one purpose of the founders of St Luke's was to 'introduce more gentlemen of the faculty to the study and practice of one of the most important of branches of physick'. In his writings, Battie warned against the excessive use of many of the treatments of the day, such as *emetics, *purges, and *blood-letting. He stressed that even severe mental illness often recovers spontaneously if the patient received good nursing.

Battie's book was followed by others which reflected a growing interest among doctors in the problems of mental illness. Meanwhile the interest of the general public

in psychiatry was increased by the news of the illnesses of George III, whose first mental illness occurred in 1788–9. At the same time, a few psychiatric hospitals were founded by public subscription. Many of these were associated with a general hospital—foreshadowing arrangements that are thought desirable today. In addition, small private *asylums for the mentally ill (called 'mad-houses') flourished in many parts of the country. Some of these were supervised by doctors, others by laymen. Although a number were the subject of scandals, many provided efficient and humane care.

Hospital reform

It was not only in the UK that many mentally ill people were treated in poor conditions. In France conditions in the mental hospitals of Paris were equally unsatisfactory. In 1793 Philippe *Pinel set out to reform the Bicêtre, a hospital in which many patients were restrained in chains. Pinel released them from their chains and instituted a more liberal form of care. He made the important observation that the abnormal behaviour of mentally ill patients can be caused as much by unsuitable treatment as by illness.

In the UK, the pioneer of similar reforms was a layman Quaker philanthropist, William *Tuke. In 1796 he established a new kind of institution in York, calling it The Retreat. Here, restraint was seldom used, neither were any of the harsh physical treatments of the day. Instead, patients were nursed in quiet, friendly surroundings in which they stayed until their illness abated. This 'moral' (i.e. psychological) treatment was intended to foster self-control, so reducing the need for external restraint.

Despite this example, conditions in many hospitals continued to be very unsatisfactory. Those in the Bethlem Hospital eventually provoked a public inquiry in 1807. The subsequent report was followed in 1808 by legislation for England and Wales. This allowed each country to provide, at public expense, an asylum for the mentally ill.

Although the County Asylum Act of 1808 encouraged the building of asylums, progress was slow. For this reason, a further Act was passed in 1845, requiring counties to take action. In the new county asylums that resulted, patients were at first managed with 'moral' treatment. As time passed, more and more were admitted because the public was becoming less willing to tolerate the mentally ill in the community, or to pay for their maintenance in *poor-law institutions. The resulting overcrowding led to less satisfactory care and to an increasing use of restraint in inadequately staffed wards. It therefore became necessary to restate the liberal ideas of the earlier pioneers. Between 1835 and 1837 Charlesworth and Hill, working at Lincoln asylum showed, once again, that mental hospitals could be conducted without the use of restraint. Similar principles were subsequently expounded by John *Conolly in an important book *The treatment of the insane without mechanical restraints*, published in 1856.

The birth of academic psychiatry

In the early 19th century the academic study of psychiatric disorders developed most strongly in France and Germany. In France, Pinel published his *Traité de la manie* in 1801. This influential text was followed in 1838 by another important book written by Pinel's pupil *Esquirol. Pinel's book was notable for the quality of the descriptions of disease and for the use of simple statistics of the frequency of various forms of mental illness. However, it was in Germany that psychiatry first became firmly established as a subject for university study. In 1811, J. C. A. Heinroth was appointed to the first chair of 'mental therapy' in Leipzig, a post renamed the chair of psychiatry in 1828. In 1865 William *Griesinger was appointed first professor of psychiatry and neurology in Berlin and developed a university department for the study of mental disorders. Other chairs were established in Göttingen (1866), Heidelberg (1871), Leipzig (1882), and Bonn (also 1882); and in Zurich (1869) and Vienna (1877).

With these academic developments, the study of psychiatric disorder began to flourish in German-speaking countries. Several themes were important. First, study of the natural course of psychiatric disorder, notably by Kahlbaum and *Kraepelin. It was mainly on the basis of these outcome studies that Kraepelin developed a comprehensive classification of mental illness which is the basis of schemes now in use throughout the world.

The second theme was concerned with the relationship of psychiatric disorder to brain pathology. Enquiries of this kind were encouraged by the progress then being made in identifying pathological lesions in *neurological disorders. Among similar studies applied to mental disorders, the work of *Meynert and *Wernicke was particularly influential. The discovery of *general paralysis of the insane (GPI) encouraged this line of research. However, the scientific methods of the day were not adequate, and further progress was limited.

The third theme was also concerned with the causes of mental disorder. It developed from the work of a Frenchman, Morel, who in 1809 proposed ideas which came to be known as the 'theory of degeneration'. This postulated first that mental illness is inherited, and secondly that it tends to appear in an increasingly severe form as it is transmitted to successive generations. These ideas flourished for a time. They had the unfortunate effect of encouraging a pessimistic approach to treatment, and supported those who wished to remove the mentally ill from society. Partly as a reaction, the last part of the 19th century saw an increasing interest in the psychological causes of mental disorder.

The rise of psychoanalysis

The most important step in developing ideas about psychological factors in mental illness was taken by a neurologist. Sigmund *Freud began his professional career as a research worker, changing to the clinical practice of neurology in his late twenties. In his new work, he often saw patients whose symptoms could not be explained by organic disease. Some had hysteria, and were particularly difficult to treat. Freud therefore visited the clinic of the distinguished French neurologist *Charcot to learn about his use of *hypnotism in hysteria. When he returned to practise in Vienna, Freud began to use hypnosis with similar patients. However, he was not a natural hypnotist and experimented with an alternative technique of his own. In this, no attempt was made to induce a hypnotic trance; instead, patients simply spoke aloud the thoughts that came into their minds (free association). From this simple beginning, Freud gradually developed the elaborate techniques of *psychoanalysis.

Freud was not content simply to treat patients but also tried to discover the psychological causes of their symptoms. Finding little to help in the textbooks of the time, he developed his own psychological theory. Freud's ideas were complex and ingenious. They were particularly controversial because he referred repeatedly to sexual motives. He also stressed the role of the unconscious and irrational parts of the mind, and the effects of childhood experience on the behaviour of adults. None of these ideas was wholly original, but Freud welded them together in a novel and imaginative way.

These broad aspects of Freud's theories have had a great influence on the arts and literature, as well as on the ways in which ordinary people think about the mind. In psychiatry they were important in directing attention to the role of psychological factors in mental disorder. In addition, his practical discoveries about the technique of psychoanalysis laid the foundation of modern psychotherapy. These were important contributions. However, the details of Freud's theory were less satisfactory. Despite frequent revisions, the theory has not provided a satisfactory explanation for most mental disorders. Furthermore, it was not constructed as a set of scientific hypotheses which could be tested, so that it has not fitted easily with the scientific ideas on which medicine is generally based.

Freud's own contributions were outstanding in their breadth and ingenuity, but several of his colleagues and successors also did important work. Among these, *Jung made the most significant independent contribution. Jung had read some of Freud's papers and decided to apply the ideas to the study of schizophrenia. Before long the two men were collaborating closely, but in 1914 Jung left the psychoanalytical movement as he disagreed strongly with some of Freud's most important ideas, notably his emphasis on sexual motivation. Jung's 'analytic psychology' has not equalled psychoanalysis in its influence on psychiatry and psychology, partly because his writings were often less clear and compelling than those of Freud. Another distinguished Swiss psychiatrist, Eugen *Bleuler resigned from the International

Psychoanalytic Association in 1930. He made important contributions to the understanding of the symptomatology of schizophrenic patients. His departure from psychoanalytical circles removed from Freud an important early opportunity to establish psychoanalysis in the universities. It was not until the 1930s, and in America rather than Europe, that this came about.

Not all those who were interested in the psychological cause of mental illness worked with Freud. The most important of the others was the French psychiatrist Pierre *Janet. His theories were less elaborate, in that he recognized an unconscious part of the mind, and his theory was also concerned with mental forces. He differed from Freud in seeking the causes of neurosis mainly in contemporary events rather than in the experiences of childhood.

Psychiatry between the wars

Inevitably the First World War interrupted the development of psychiatry. The return of peace marked the beginning of a period of increasing interest in prevention and treatment of mental disorders. In the UK a most important event was the opening of the *Maudsley Hospital. Henry Maudsley had worked as a psychiatrist at the Manchester Lunatic Asylum (Cheadle Royal) before becoming professor of medical jurisprudence at University College, London. He wrote three important textbooks and was a most influential teacher in his day, but his lasting achievement was an imaginative plan for a new kind of psychiatric hospital concerned with early treatment, teaching, and research. Maudsley gave a substantial endowment which helped establish the hospital and the associated academic developments.

In the post-war years, gradual progress was made in opening out-patient clinics for treatment with psychotherapy of the less severe mental disorders. Some such—child guidance clinics—were devoted to the care of children. As well as seeking to relieve their immediate problems, it was hoped that treatment in childhood would prevent mental illness in adult life. Unfortunately, these hopes proved overoptimistic.

By the 1930s further developments were taking place, notably the introduction of new forms of physical treatment for serious mental disorders. In 1933 Sakel described insulin coma treatment for schizophrenia. Injections of *insulin were used to cause a temporary fall in *blood sugar. Repeated treatments benefited some schizophrenic patients. Subsequently the beneficial effects were shown to be non-specific, probably resulting from increased nursing attention. For this and other reasons, insulin treatment is no longer used.

Another treatment introduced in the 1930s is still in use. Convulsive treatment for severe states of depression was described in 1938 by Cerletti and Bini. At first a drug, cardiazol, was used to produce the convulsions, but this was soon replaced by electrical stimulation, so that the method became known as *electroconvulsive treatment (ECT). The

new treatment produced dramatic improvement in severe depressive disorders—conditions which, up to that time, often lasted for months or even years and had a significant death rate from suicide or self-starvation.

*Leucotomy was the third treatment to be introduced in the 1930s; the first operation was performed in 1935 by *Egas Moniz. It is a form of brain surgery which has the immediate effect of reducing aggressive behaviour, anxiety, severe depression, and obsessional symptoms. Although often effective, the original operation was often followed by undesirable changes in personality. Although modified operations have largely eliminated these personality changes, they are seldom used today because equal benefit can usually be obtained from drug treatment.

In the 1930s, psychoanalysis was developing in important ways. This development owed much to the migration to the USA of a number of influential German analysts, including Franz Alexander, Erich Fromm, and Karen Horney. These people did two things of note: first, they modified Freud's theories by placing less emphasis on sexual instincts and on the events of early childhood, and more on contemporary social forces; secondly, they began to establish psychoanalysis as an important ingredient of American psychiatry.

The UK also received many psychoanalysts fleeing from Nazi persecution and they, too, found opportunities to re-establish their work. Nevertheless, psychoanalysis never assumed the dominant place in British psychiatry that it attained in North America. That a more eclectic view prevailed in the UK was, no doubt, partly a reflection of national temperament, but it also reflected the influence of two outstanding teachers. These were D. K. (later Sir David) Henderson of Edinburgh and A. J. (later Sir Aubrey) *Lewis of the Maudsley Hospital in London. Both had trained in America with Adolph *Meyer, a Swiss psychiatrist who was professor of psychiatry at *Johns Hopkins Medical School. Meyer was an influential teacher who championed an approach to psychiatry which stressed the interplay of psychological, social, and physical causes of mental disorder and discouraged an excessive preoccupation with any one set of theories. These ideas, known as psychobiology, became the mainstay of British psychiatry through the teaching of Henderson and Lewis.

Psychiatry after the Second World War

The post-war period was marked by two important therapeutic advances. The first, which originated in experiences gained from the practice of psychiatry in the armed forces, was the use of social rehabilitation using small and large groups. These methods were increasingly used to treat the schizophrenic patients resident in overcrowded mental hospitals. Reforms were introduced which in many ways repeated those of the early 19th century. Locked doors were opened, restrictions removed, and patients encouraged to take more personal responsibility. These liberalizing steps were aided in 1952 by the second therapeutic advance: the discovery in France of the beneficial effects of *chlorpromazine. This drug suppresses many of the most troublesome symptoms of schizophrenia, including the overactive and aggressive behaviour which had been the main reason for restrictions imposed on schizophrenic patients in earlier years. As a result of these two advances, the number of in-patients in psychiatric hospitals in England and Wales, which had been rising progressively, began to fall. Similar changes took place in other countries as these new methods were introduced.

The discovery of chlorpromazine was soon followed by the development of other valuable drugs. In the early 1950s, *isoniazid was being used to treat *tuberculosis. Related compounds were tested and one of these—iproniazid—was found to produce euphoria in some patients, although it was less effective as an antitubercular agent (see CHEST MEDICINE). Subsequently iproniazid and similar compounds were used to treat depression. In 1957 Kuhn found that another drug, imipramine, also had antidepressant properties. Since that time, imipramine and related drugs have transformed the treatment of depressive illness, which can now often be treated in its early stages by family doctors. Soon after this, Cade discovered that *lithium carbonate can prevent relapses of manic-depressive disorders. This was another important milestone.

Another feature of the post-war period was the development of community services designed to enable mentally ill patients to live outside hospital. Such people need help with work and accommodation as well as continuing psychiatric treatment. To provide this help, rehabilitation units, hostels, and sheltered workshops were developed (see PSYCHIATRY).

In the UK, a most important feature of post-war medicine was the development of a comprehensive system of good general practice. This was becoming well-established by the time that safer and more effective drugs enabled general practitioners to undertake the treatment of many people with less serious mental disorders, including many who in other countries would be treated by specialists. At the same time, the new policies of treating patients in the community involved family doctors increasingly in the care of people with chronic mental illness and with the mentally handicapped. Indeed, a survey showed that general practitioners refer to specialists only about 1 in 20 of the patients who consult them with problems which have an important psychiatric component.

At the same time that patients with minor disorders were being treated more by family doctors, the care of patients with major mental illness was increasingly undertaken in small psychiatric units attached to general hospitals rather than in large mental hospitals. However, recurrent financial shortages held back ambitious plans for replacing all the old psychiatric hospitals in this way.

While in the UK in the post-war years, psychiatrists were particularly concerned with improving the care of patients with severe mental disorders, psychiatrists in the USA were developing psychoanalytical ideas. In the post-war period, psychoanalysis became strongly represented in the American medical schools and training in psychoanalysis became a general requirement for a successful career in psychiatry. These developments led to good provisions for psychotherapy and fostered an interest in less severe psychological problems, including those of physically ill people. These were some of the benefits of these developments. However, the extreme reliance on psychoanalysis in the USA had disadvantages. One problem was that psychoanalysts began to claim too much. The assertions that they could explain a wide range of human behaviour, from physical illnesses such as *asthma to social phenomena such as the behaviour of crowds, led to increasing scepticism on the part of other doctors and informed laymen. Because some laymen wrongly equated psychoanalysis with psychiatry, they became sceptical of the subject as a whole. By the 1970s the influence of psychoanalysis in American psychiatry began to wane and it is now one force among many, as it has always been in the UK.

The mentally handicapped

Until the second half of the 19th century few provisions were made for mentally handicapped people. By the end of the century many of these people were confined in large hospitals in which they were segregated from society, partly with the intention of preventing them from having children. Many such hospitals were understaffed, and provided insufficient variety and stimulation for their patients. While hospital provisions were often inadequate, arrangements for care in the community were generally lacking and many of the mentally handicapped remained in hospital for much of their lives.

These conditions persisted until well after the Second World War when, as many of the mentally ill were being discharged from hospital, more attention was given to the possibility of discharging mentally handicapped people as well. Gradually, hostels, special schools, and sheltered work were provided. Progress was slow and many hospitals continued to be overcrowded and understaffed. Even today, in many hospitals for the mentally handicapped, hard-pressed staff are attempting to cope with impossible demands.

Developments in psychiatry and the law

The law is concerned with mentally ill and mentally handicapped people in two ways. First, there are provisions concerned with mentally ill offenders whose illness appears to have reduced their responsibility for illegal actions. Those which most often come to public notice are concerned with the killing of another person by someone who is, or is claimed to be, mentally disordered. Secondly, the law defines circumstances in which mentally disordered or mentally handicapped people can be admitted to hospital and kept there, against their own wish. In general, this is permissible by law when a person is suicidal or dangerous to others as a result of mental illness (or, in certain circumstances, severe personality disorder or mental handicap). This legislation has two aims: it prevents the improper admission to a psychiatric hospital of a person who does not need to go there; and it ensures that people who do not realize that they are ill receive the treatment they require. It has always been difficult to balance these considerations. In the 19th century public concern was aroused by reports of cases in which people had been admitted to mental hospitals against their will and without adequate reason. This led to the requirement that all admissions to a mental hospital must be 'certified' by a magistrate. This requirement continued until 1930 by which time it had become clear that it was preventing the admission to hospital of other people whose illness was in an early stage and who were likely to benefit if they could enter hospital in a more informal way. The *Mental Treatment Act of 1930 allowed the admission of voluntary patients, though retaining the requirement that a magistrate should be involved in the admission to a psychiatric hospital of those unwilling to enter.

In 1959 a new *Mental Health Act was introduced in England and Wales. A magistrate was no longer involved in compulsory admission; instead, the procedure was usually completed by the nearest relative (or a social worker) and two doctors. By this time, more effective methods of early treatment had reduced substantially the need for compulsory admission. Thus in the 1980s, only a few patients are admitted in this way to a psychiatric ward, most being voluntary admissions carried out with no more formality than entry to a medical or surgical ward. In 1983 a further Mental Health Act came into force requiring, for example, a statutory second opinion prior to the administration of certain forms of treatment in patients incapable of giving informed consent.

M. G. GELDER

Further reading
Ackernecht, E. H. (1968). *A short history of psychiatry*, trans. S. Wolf. Hefner, New York.
Hunter, R. and MacAlpine, I. (1963). *Three hundred years of psychiatry*. Oxford University Press, London.

PSYCHIC SURGERY, not to be confused with *psychosurgery, is the alleged performance of surgical procedures (e.g. removal of supposed *tumours) by paranormal methods which do not involve physical intervention. It has been reported particularly from the Philippines.

PSYCHOANALYSIS is a system of psychiatric theory and practice based on the ideas of Sigmund *Freud. Its basic tool is the technique of free association, in which the patient is encouraged to express his thoughts,

ideas, emotions, and memories with the minimum of intervention by the psychoanalyst, who listens, records, and eventually interprets. The final interpretation, when communicated to the patient, is intended to provide him with the insight into his motivation and behaviour necessary for him to solve his life problems.

PSYCHOANALYST. A psychiatrist trained in *psychoanalysis. See PSYCHIATRY.

PSYCHOGALVANOMETER. A version of the *polygraph, for recording physiological changes associated with mental and emotional reactions.

PSYCHOLINGUISTICS is the branch of *linguistics dealing with the interrelation between the acquisition, use, and comprehension of language, and the processes of the mind. See LANGUAGE, COGNITION, AND HIGHER CEREBRAL FUNCTION.

PSYCHOLOGY IN RELATION TO MEDICINE
Introduction
In what still remains the finest textbook of psychology yet written, William James (1890) writes, 'Psychology is the Science of Mental Life, both of its phenomena and of their conditions.' 'The phenomena', he continues, 'are such things as we call feelings, desires, cognitions, reasonings, decisions, and the like; and, superficially considered, their variety and complexity is such as to leave a chaotic impression on the observer.' In his endeavour to bring some order to this chaos, James distinguished between two broad traditions that were often seen as in competition with each other: faculty psychology and associationist psychology.

The former tradition (which derives from Aristotle and the early Church fathers) seeks to decompose the mind into discrete faculties of perception, imagination, reasoning, memory, and will, etc., each generic power obeying its own laws. The latter tradition (which derives from Hartley, Hume, and Herbart) seeks to reconstruct the richness of mental life from 'atomic' sensations (and 'ideas'), according to associative laws of spatial contiguity and temporal succession which range indiscriminately over all external objects and events. Although much of the sound and fury has evaporated from the debate, the contrast between the two approaches can still be seen in the tension between modern information-processing psychology (Neisser 1966) and the 'new' connectionism (Quinlan 1991).

As in faculty psychology, the primary thrust of information-processing psychology resides in the attempt to isolate a particular mental function, such as short-term memory (STM), and then further to fractionate that function into its component parts; those parts may include a capacity-limited visuospatial scratchpad, a temporally limited phonological or articulatory loop, and a central executive that controls the switching of attention between two or more concurrent tasks. By contrast, the distinguishing feature of current connectionism in this domain resides in the attempt to model (with matrix algebra) the competitive interactions between elements stored in a (limited-capacity) STM; as in earlier days, the system as a whole is conceived as an 'associative network' with the elements and connections thereof having different 'strengths'. Whether or not these two approaches are complementary or contradictory remains in doubt. In some areas, connectionist models are simply implementations of classical information-processing theories. In other cognitive domains there seems little chance that rule-governed behaviour will reduce to associative connections; the systematic, combinational, and, above all, productive character of language and logical reasoning appear to demand formal syntactic and semantic representations that cannot be simulated by any kind of purely associative learning.

Proponents of modern connectionism often claim a 'biological reality' for their theories on the basis that (computational) 'associative nets' look like (real) nerve-nets. But this is merely a category-mistake. As William James, once again, reflected, 'if we make a symbolic diagram on the blackboard of the laws of association between ideas, we are inevitably led to draw circles, or closed figures of some kind, and to connect them by lines. When we hear that the nerve centres contain *cells which send off *fibres, we say that Nature has realized our diagram for us, and that the mechanical substratum of thought is plain. In some way, it is true our diagram must be realized in the brain, but surely in no such visible and palpable way as we at first suppose' (James 1890). No traditional faculty theorist was ever in any doubt that the material substrate of cognition was the brain. It is, as Reid (1787) wrote, 'a law of our nature, that we perceive not external objects, unless certain impressions be made by the object upon the organ, and by means of the organ upon the nerves and brain'. The problem lies not in admitting this dependence but rather in formulating the correct fractionation (functional architecture) of human cognition, discovering the principles that govern each cognitive domain, and then showing how particular neuronal architectures (anatomical, physiological, and pharmacological) realize those principles (Shallice 1988).

Cognition and the brain

The Hippocratic treatise *On the sacred disease* (*epilepsy) was clear that, in health, 'Men ought to know that from nothing else but the brain come joy, despondency and lamentation . . . and by this [organ], in an especial manner we acquire wisdom and knowledge, and see and hear . . .'. And likewise in disease, 'By the same organ we become mad and delirious and fears and terrors assail us, some by night and some by day; and dreams and untimely wanderings, and cares

that are not suitable, and ignorance of present circumstances, desuetude, and unskillfulness. All these things we endure from the brain when it is not healthy.'

The history of early Graeco-Roman medicine records many examples of specific cognitive disorder consequent upon disease or *trauma. Thucydides (471–404 BC) reports cases of severe memory loss following famine and *typhus in the Doric Wars; two millennia later *Korsakoff provided a more detailed account of how nutritional deficits can cause *amnesia. The elder Pliny (AD 23–79) reports how a man who fell from a high roof could no longer recognize his mother, his friends, and close relatives; two millennia later, Bodamer coined the expression 'prosopagnosia' for such a deficit in the recognition of familiar faces. Seneca (AD 1–65) observed a woman with acquired blindness who appeared unaware, and indeed firmly denied, that she was blind; two millennia later, Anton likewise described cortical blindness with denial thereof. Maximus (*c.* AD 30) described an Athenian scholar who, after closed head injury, lost the ability to read words or letters while apparently retaining intact the rest of his knowledge and skills; two millennia later, Dejerine began to report similar cases of isolated acquired reading disorder after *stroke and brain *tumour.

Prior even to the Hippocratic corpus, Egyptian surgeons, some three and a half millennia ago, recorded on papyrus their observation that loss of language could result from injury to the head. They interpreted the correlation as showing that 'the breath of an outside god or death' had entered the brains of their patients who henceforth became 'silent in sadness'. This spiritual interpretation of the phenomenon did not prevent *surgeons from adopting a physical approach to the amelioration of the patient's symptoms; the practice of trepanning (removal of a bone flap from the skull) was instituted in Egypt and in many other areas of the Old and New Worlds.

Much later, the Hippocratic corpus contained numerous references to the fact that injury to one side of the head frequently results in spasm or *paralysis of the opposite side of the body; it was also observed that loss of speech was often associated with paralysis of the *right* arm and leg. The conjunction of these two observations carries, for us, the implication that the *left* hemisphere of the brain must be more intimately bound up with the exercise of basic language skills than is the right hemisphere. That is to say, the brain as a whole is not the material substrate for language, but rather a particular subpart of the brain subserves this function. The notion that the grey and white matter of the human brain are characterized by localization of function is, of course, now a commonplace concept of neuroscience, but the Greeks did not succeed in obtaining this insight.

With respect to higher mental capacities, we distinguish between focal localization of function within the cerebral hemispheres (the frontal lobes have different functions from the occipital lobes) and lateralization of function between the hemispheres (the left temporal lobe subserves different functions from the right temporal lobe). Yet the first of these concepts played little role in neuroscience until the work of Franz-Joseph *Gall, and the second played no role until the work of Paul *Broca and John Hughlings *Jackson. The central dogma of modern neuropsychology, the complementary specialization of the left and right hemispheres for core linguistic and visuospatial skills, respectively, was established by the latter two physicians in the second half of the 19th century. Graeco-Roman neuropsychology fell into the trap of associating cognitive functions with the flow of 'vital fluids' through the cerebral ventricles; later generations of physicians could not resist analogizing the *anatomy of the cerebral hemispheres to that of other paired organs (eyes, ears, lungs, kidneys) in which similarity of form is indeed associated with identity of function.

Once we move beyond the very crudest of anatomo-clinical correlations (e.g. the association of aphasic language disorder with lesions of the left perisylvian region), the importance of establishing a valid basis for describing the patterns of impaired and preserved cognitive skills seen after neurological (and psychiatric) pathology becomes manifest. As Vygotsky (1934–1965) so presciently wrote, the 'lack of an adequate system of psychological analysis of the functions localized in the brain is now one of the most significant obstacles in the development of the theory of functional localization which made a marked progress due to the progress of modern *histology, *cytoarchitectonics, and clinical *neurology.' More recent studies with *in vivo* imaging of the normal brain (*positron-emission *tomography and functional *magnetic resonance) have only served to highlight how technological sophistication at the physiological level can so easily mask inadequate specifications of functions at the psychological level. Similarly, the emphasis on localization of *pathology in the diseased brain can, all too easily, obscure the fact that much of the patient's overt symptomatology must arise from the interaction between normal and impaired tissue; in the extreme case (when cells in particular regions are dead rather than malfunctioning), there is the danger, as Smith (1979) writes, of 'focussing on the hole rather than the doughnut' in our interpretation of signs and symptoms. Studies of cognitive *rehabilitation have accordingly placed justified stress on elucidating whether, for a particular patient, therapy should concentrate on the direct remediation of deficit or on the acquisition of compensatory strategies to bypass the primary impairment (Riddoch and Humphreys 1994).

Clinical cognitive neuropsychology

Current investigations of cognitive impairments have close methodological and theoretical affinities with late 19th century work in behavioural neurology. As in classical work by the German, French, and English diagram makers, the main thrust of modern research (Heilman and Valenstein 1993) has concentrated on the description and interpretation of: acquired disorders of language (*aphasia), reading and writing (dyslexia and dysgraphia), mathematics (dyscalculia), object recognition (*agnosia), familiar face recognition (prosopagnosia), space perception (neglect and simultanagnosia), long-term and autobiographical memory (amnesia), skilled voluntary action (*apraxia), and problem-solving and planning (frontal lobe pathologies). In all of these areas, much more precise, well-controlled experimental data are now available than could be found even 20 years ago; the traditional symptom-complexes of behavioural neurology have been shown to fractionate into a wide variety of clinically distinct (and theoretically meaningful) forms. The overall aim has been to effect an integration of clinical neuropsychology (the principled description of disorders consequent upon brain pathology) and normal cognitive psychology (the construction and empirical validation of general models of complex mental functions). The distinctive character of cognitive neuropsychology lies in the explicit endeavour to interpret disorders of cognition in relation to formal information-processing models of normal (brain/mind) systems.

Seen in this light, the study of pathologies of cognition serves a threefold purpose:

1. Neuropathological fractionations of cognition impose strong constraints upon theories of the normal system. The striking dissociations of impaired and preserved performance seen after brain damage indicate which overt behavioural abilities must *not* be analysed together as manifestations of a single underlying function.
2. The interpretation of pathological performance by reference to normal theory allows the investigator to move beyond the mere description of overt symptomatology to accounts of the underlying processes that are impaired.
3. In any complex system, identical *overt* failures and errors can arise from malfunction of different underlying components. Such ambiguities must be resolved by linking the patterns of impaired and preserved performance to specified (and justified) information-processing components.

Studies of language disorders (investigated within the above framework) are reported in Blanken *et al*. (1993). Vallar and Shallice (1990) outlined current thinking on the relationship of short-term memory disorders to impairments of language processing. Acquired disorders of reading, writing, and spelling are described in Coltheart *et al*. (1987) and Patterson *et al*. (1985). Dehaene (1993) included much relevant work on disorders of numerical cognition. Farah (1990) provided an up-to-date account of disorders of visual object-recognition, while Bruce *et al*. (1992) outlined the more restricted syndromes of face-recognition impairments. Disorders of spatial cognition are covered by

Grüsser and Landis (1991) and Robertson and Marshall (1993). Parkin and Leng (1993) summarized the range of memory disorders in a wide variety of organic pathologies. Roy (1985) described praxic impairments, and Passingham (1993) discussed many of the planning and control problems that can follow frontal lobe lesions.

Much of this work has involved patients with relatively well-localized lesions (due to cerebrovascular accident, space-occupying lesions, penetrating or closed head injury). More recently, the behavioural consequences of progressive degenerative diseases of the central nervous system (including *Alzheimer's disease, *Huntington's disease, *Parkinson's disease, and *Pick's disease) have also been investigated in detailed cross-sectional and longitudinal studies. As in cases with more focal lesions, these investigations of diffuse pathology or systemic disease have shown that it is, as Martin (1988) wrote, mistaken to assume that 'homogeneity with respect to one category [medical/biological] will ensure homogeneity with regard to another category [cognitive/behavioral]'. Studies of Alzheimer's disease, in particular, have revealed a large range of behavioural subtypes and clinical courses; the debilitating consequences of some of these deficits of memory, language, visuospatial perception, and planning can be significantly ameliorated by therapies targeted on remaining areas of cognitive strength.

More recently still, the discipline of neuropsychiatry has been invigorated by the application of methods of cognitive testing derived from experimental psychology and neuropsychology. Studies of frankly psychiatric conditions, e.g. the *schizophrenias (David and Cutting 1994) and of many pathologies that lie in the hazy borderzone between neurology and psychiatry have been fractionated into discrete impairments of cognitive processes that are firmly established in normal psychology. Advances have been made in the understanding of auditory, tactile, and visual *hallucinations after brain damage. The causes of reduplicative delusions, including such rare conditions as the *Capgras syndrome and various confabulation syndromes, for example. Some recent studies of psychiatric phenomena are consistent with the conjecture that *delusions can arise from the patient's effort to interpret his or her organically provoked abnormal experiences by reasoning processes that are themselves normal (Young *et al.* 1993). In other conditions and cases, specific deficits of reasoning (including probabilistic inference) have been found to contribute to pathological belief formation and maintenance (Garety *et al.* 1991).

The attempt to understand pathology is not confined to the examining physician: the patient is also concerned to form 'a bridge of meaning between illness and dysfunction' (Fulford 1989). It would not, therefore, be surprising if future studies began to dissolve the purported incompatibility between 'psychodynamic' and 'physicalist' approaches to neuropsychology and psychiatry. Although brain disease can itself alter personality, the venerable notion that premorbid personality is one determinant of florid psychopathology is surely correct. Considerable progress has been made in understanding the organic bases of the emotions (Watts 1993), an area in which the combination of evidence from neuropsychology, *neurophysiology, and psychopharmacology is mandatory for further advances. Studies of the interaction between cognitive and affective disorder seem set to play a major role in future neuropsychiatric enquiry.

The new organology

The constraint that disorders of higher cognitive functioning cannot be reduced to more elementary impairments of sensory and motor processes is explicit in classic definitions of neuropsychological syndromes. But it was the much-maligned 'phrenologist', Franz-Joseph *Gall, who first conjectured that the human brain might contain organs specialized to deal with all cognitive aspects of particular content-domains, from perceptual processing to response organization. Gall's insight was that such traditional faculties as perception, memory, attention, etc. were philosophical abstractions devoid of any biological reality; rather, Gall argued, the higher organization of the mind/brain was into special-purpose organs devoted to such domains as language, topography, music, and mathematics, and that perceptual, memorial, and praxic systems would fractionate according to the content that they encoded. Gall accordingly hypothesized that distinct cortical organs devoted to the analysis of size, shape, and colour would be discovered in the human brain.

On the whole, subsequent developments in psychology and neuropsychology have supported (and further refined) Gall's conjectures. For example, perceptual processing mechanisms that deal with language in any modality, spoken or signed, are tailored to the structural principles (phonological and syntactic) that govern the linguistic system. Neuropsychological fractionations that confirm a basically Gallist position are numerous. Consider the case of aphasia without amusia in a musician blind from the age of two, reported by Signoret, Van Eeckhout, Poncet, and Castaigne (1987). This man, who suffered a large *infarct in the territory of the left middle cerebral artery, had been accustomed to read both French and music in braille. Subsequent to his stroke, he lost the former ability but not the latter; this dissociation held even for the identical dot patterns that could represent either a letter (f) or a note (mi).

Studies of long-term memory and impairments thereof have provided compelling evidence for a distinction between knowledge systems (semantic memory) and event memory (the recall of past episodes). Within the latter system (episodic memory), there may be distinct encoding and retrieval mechanisms for autobiographical events and public events. Within semantic memory, numerous category-specific disorders have now been reported; these include impairments of expression or comprehension specific to such domains as the common names of living things, artefacts, actions, colours, and body parts, and to the proper names of people or places (McCarthy and Warrington 1990). Even auditory short-term (or working) memory may contain special-purpose routines committed to the initial parsing and semantic analysis of spoken language (Vallar and Shallice 1990).

In the realm of skilled praxis, high-level motor disorders can likewise show domain specificity. Basso and Capitani (1985) have reported the case of a well-known Venetian conductor who suffered an extensive left hemisphere corticosubcortical infarct. He displayed global aphasia and gross ideomotor apraxia of the left arm and hand; simple movements (and sequences thereof) could not be imitated correctly and there was a striking deficit in the execution of such overlearned gestures as demonstrating the use of a toothbrush. He was none the less able to conduct a performance of Verdi's *Nabucco* that the Italian opera critics (not known for their generosity of soul) praised as an outstanding interpretation.

The perception of conspecific faces provides one of the best examples of a Gallist 'mental organ'. The ontogenetic development of face recognition is triggered by simple well-defined stimulus configurations, and thereafter follows a relatively invariant course to the mature state in which thousands of faces can be effortlessly distinguished. After brain damage, prosopagnosia without visual object agnosia has been frequently reported. Many neuropsychologists have argued that this dissociation merely reflects the fact that faces are the most extreme example of stimuli where small physical differences make a large psychological difference. They therefore interpret the dissociation as an index of overall perceptual difficulty: very slight differences between faces are crucial to the identity of the individual, while by contrast, the recognition of a chair as a chair does not depend upon precise discrimination of the relative sizes and positions of component parts.

This line of argument would appear to be false. There are severely prosopagnosic patients who can discriminate adequately between very similar coins, purses, and even animals within a flock or herd. Completing the *double* dissociation, there are patients with gross visual object agnosia (who cannot, for example, distinguish between a dart and a feather duster) who none the less have intact recognition of familiar conspecific faces. These dissociated patterns of performance constitute strong evidence for a dedicated face-recognition module with a discrete neuronal locus. Within the face-module, there is further evidence for dissociable perceptual mechanisms devoted to facial identity and facial expression.

At lower levels of perceptual analysis, recent research showing an ever-increasing proliferation of distinct visual (and auditory) areas in the primate brain would have come as no surprise to Gall; the principal problem now

is to show how these prestriate areas, which are differentially sensitive to form, colour, position, orientation, depth, movement, and so forth, intercommunicate and give rise to the experience of an orderly world of objects in space.

Consciousness

Current emphasis upon the neurological patient as a conscious agent derives in part from studies of subjects with complete transections of the *corpus callosum (for the relief of otherwise intractable epilepsy). Although the brain is a modular system of domain-specific processors, 'human beings enjoy what appears to be a unified and unitary experience of conscious awareness' (Gazzaniga 1989). Gazzaniga continues, 'Patients who have undergone brain bisection have the same basic awareness of unity even though it is demonstrably the case that each disconnected half-brain can have separate and isolated experiences.' How then is 'their sense of conscious unity developed and maintained' (Gazzaniga 1989)? One possibility is that the linguistically sophisticated left hemisphere contains an 'interpreter' that attempts to make sense of the full range of the patient's behaviour, including those more 'automatic', 'unconscious' actions that derive from right-hemisphere mechanisms (Gazzaniga 1989).

There is now unequivocal evidence that many neurological pathologies can leave quite complex cognitive functions relatively intact while resulting in a dramatic lack of 'conscious access' to the information computed. The most famous example of lack of awareness of the grounds on which behaviour is based, comes from an anecdotal report by Claparède in 1911 (see Parkin and Leng 1993). The physician shook hands with a patient with *Korsakoff's disease (and a consequent dense amnesia) while concealing a pin in his hand. The consequent pain was such that when Claparède returned some moments later the patient refused to shake his hand and thereafter attempted to avoid him; yet the patient had no conscious recall of the specific event that had caused her to behave in this way. Subsequent experimental studies have amply documented how many amnesic patients can show good perceptual and perceptuomotor learning in the absence of episodic memories of the events upon which the learning was based (Parkin and Leng 1993).

In the perceptual domain, similarly counterintuitive phenomena have been reported. Thus some patients with partial loss of striate (occipital visual) cortex (and hence dense visual field deficits on conventional testing) show 'blindsight'. When stimuli are presented in the blind part of the field, patients (very reasonably) say that they do not see anything. Yet, if instructed to 'guess', these patients can reliably point to objects in the blind field and even discriminate between the orientation (horizontal or vertical) of a small object in that field. The patients are as surprised as their examiners at their above-chance performance, and they continue to insist that the tasks they have been set are ridiculous; phenomenologically, the patients claim that they are merely 'guessing' the answers to questions that a (partially) blind person could not possibly answer correctly.

Such 'seeing without believing' can also be found in some patients with severe prosopagnosia. Patients with prosopagnosia cannot recognize the faces of people who were well known to them before their accident, and seem to experience no feeling of appropriate familiarity. None the less, some of these patients can, for instance, learn correct pairings of (unrecognized) famous faces and (recognized) names far faster than they learn sequences of incorrect pairings (e.g. the face of Prince Charles with the name Nigel Mansell). They may also show significant priming effects in which a consciously unrecognized face speeds reaction-time to a conceptually related name.

Similar covert or tacit perception has been reported in some cases of left visuospatial neglect after right parietal infarcts. Patients with neglect seem unable to detect or respond to stimuli in spatial locations contralateral to the damaged cerebral hemisphere. One such case when presented simultaneously with a drawing of a normal house and a drawing of the same house with bright red flames emerging from the left-hand side thereof, insisted that the two drawings were identical. On subsequent trials, she was requested to indicate which house she would prefer to live in. In response, she forthrightly stated that this was a very stupid question because no rational person could possibly have a preference for one of two identical houses. None the less, when asked to 'guess', she reliably picked the non-burning house, insisting all the time that she was choosing at random. Similar 'covert' recognition of 'neglected' stimuli has now been reported in priming studies; a stimulus that is not 'consciously' seen in the left 'neglected' field can speed the recognition of semantically related stimuli presented in the normal right visual field (see Robertson and Marshall 1993, for references). The therapeutic implications of high-level, but preconscious, processing remain to be determined.

After many decades in which the mere mention of the topic was taboo in psychology, there is now hope that some aspects of consciousness may eventually yield to scientific inquiry. The twin problems of unawareness of deficits and unawareness of competences (Prigatano and Schachter 1991) in neuropsychological syndromes are far from solved, but they can at least be posed with greater clarity than in the days when psychology was a purely introspective endeavour.

The training of clinical psychologists

*Clinical psychologists in the UK have an undergraduate degree in general psychology (and often the higher research degree of Ph.D). Their subsequent training is regulated by the British Psychological Society; it includes completion of a master's degree in clinical psychology and in-service training (within the *National Health Service) under the guidance of more senior practitioners. Comparable criteria must be met in the USA (under the governance of the American Psychological Association), and usually include a Ph.D in some branch of clinical psychology. In some centres, specific instruction in neuropsychology is provided to the master's or doctoral level. Training, practice, and research will often be team-based with major input from both behavioural neurologists and experimental psychologists. In neuropsychology, most clinical psychologists work in specialist neurological or psychiatric units where, with the responsible physicians, they contribute to diagnostic assessment, remedial retraining, and longer-term follow-up assessments.

J. C. MARSHALL
JENNIFER M. GURD

References

Basso, A. and Capitani, E. (1985). Spared musical abilities in a conductor with global aphasia and ideomotor apraxia. *Journal of Neurology, Neurosurgery and Psychiatry*, **48**, 407–12.

Blanken, G., Dittmann, J., Grimm, H., Marshall, J. C., and Wallesch, C.-W. (ed.) (1993). *Linguistic disorders and pathologies: an international handbook*. de Furceyter, Berlin.

Bruce, V., Cowey, A., Ellis, A. W., and Perrett, D. I. (ed.) (1992). *Processing the facial image*. Clarendon Press, Oxford.

Coltheart, M., Patterson, K., and Marshall, J. C. (ed.) (1987). *Deep dyslexia*, (2nd edn). Routledge and Kegan Paul, London.

David, A. S. and Cutting, J. (ed.) (1994). *The neuropsychology of schizophrenia*. Erlbaum, Hove.

Dehaene, S. (ed.) (1993). *Numerical cognition*. Blackwell, Oxford.

Farah, M. J. (1990). *Visual agnosia*. MIT Press, Cambridge, Mass.

Fulford, K. W. M. (1989). *Moral theory and medical practice*. Cambridge University Press.

Garety, P. A., Hemsley, D. R., and Wessely, S. (1991). Reasoning in deluded schizophrenic and paranoid patients: Biases in performance on a probabilistic inference task. *Journal of Nervous and Mental Disease*, **179**, 194–201.

Gazzaniga, M. S. (1989). Organization of the human brain. *Science*, **245**, 947–52.

Grüsser, O.-J. and Landis, T. (1991). *Visual agnosias and other disturbances of visual perception and cognition*. Macmillan, London.

Heilman, K. M. and Valenstein, E. (ed.) (1993). *Clinical neuropsychology*, (3rd edn). Oxford University Press, Oxford.

James, W. (1890). *Principles of psychology*. Holt, New York.

McCarthy, R. A. and Warrington, E. K. (1990). *Cognitive neuropsychology: a clinical introduction*. Academic Press, New York.

Martin, A. (1988). The search for the neuropsychological profile of a disease state: a mistaken enterprise? *Journal of Clinical and Experimental Neuropsychology*, **10**, 22–3.

Neisser, U. (1966). *Cognitive psychology*. Appleton-Century-Crofts, New York.

Parkin, A. J. and Leng, N. R. C. (1983). *Neuropsychology of the amnesic syndrome*. Erlbaum, Hove.

Passingham, R. (1993). *The frontal lobes and voluntary action*. Oxford University Press, Oxford.

Patterson, K., Marshall, J. C., and Coltheart, M. (ed.) (1985). *Surface dyslexia*. Erlbaum, Hove.

Prigatano, G. P. and Schachter, D. L. (ed.) (1991). *Awareness of deficit after brain injury*. Oxford University Press, Oxford.

Quinlan, P. (1991). *Connectionism and psychology*. University of Chicago Press.

Reid, T. (1785). *Essays on the intellectual power of man*. MIT Press (1969), Cambridge, Massachussetts.

Riddoch, M. J. and Humphreys, G. W. (ed.) (1994). *Cognitive neuropsychology and cognitive rehabilitation*. Erlbaum, Hove.

Robertson, I. H. and Marshall, J. C. (ed.) (1993). *Unilateral neglect: clinicial and experimental studies*. Erlbaum, Hove.

Roy, E. A. (ed.) (1985). *Neuropsychological studies of apraxia and related disorders*. North Holland, Amsterdam.

Shallice, T. (1988). *From Neuropsychology to mental structure*. Cambridge University Press, Cambridge.

Signoret, J. L., Van Eeckhout, P. H., Poncet, M., and Castaigne, P. (1987). Aphasie sans amusie chez un organiste aveugle. *Revue Neurologique*, **143**, 172–81.

Smith, A. (1979). Practices and principles of clinical neuropsychology. *International Journal of Neuroscience*, **9**, 233–8.

Vallar, G. and Shallice, T. (ed.) (1990). *Neuropsychological impairments of short-term memory*. Cambridge University Press, Cambridge.

Vygotsky, L. S. (1934–1965). Psychology and localization of functions. *Neuropsychologia*, **3**, 381–6.

Watts, F. N. (ed.) (1993). *Neuropsychological perspectives on emotion*. Erlbaum, Hove.

Young, A. W., Reid, I., Wright, S., and Hellawell, D. J. (1993). Face-processing impairments and the Capgras delusion. *British Journal of Psychiatry*, **162**, 695–8.

PSYCHOMOTOR. Descriptive of the motor expression of mental activity.

PSYCHONEUROSIS is a synonym of *neurosis.

PSYCHOPATHOLOGY is the study of the nature and causes of mental disorder.

PSYCHOPATHY is a personality disorder independent of *intelligence, characterized by impulsive, egocentric, irresponsible, and antisocial behaviour; there is difficulty in forming normal relationships, and a manner which is either aggressive or charming or which alternates between the two.

PSYCHOPHARMACOLOGY is the branch of pharmacology concerned with the effects of drugs on mental processes and behaviour. See PHARMACOLOGY.

PSYCHOSEXUAL means pertaining to the mental and emotional aspects of sexual behaviour.

PSYCHOSIS is a term for any of the more serious mental disorders recognized by the lay public as constituting insanity, the defining features of which are loss of contact with reality and derangement of the personality. They include some attributable to organic disorders, although these are a small minority. Thought disorganization, profound *mood alterations, *hallucinations, and *delusions are characteristic manifestations. *Schizophrenia and *manic-depressive psychosis are examples. See PSYCHIATRY.

PSYCHOSOMATIC DISEASE. Disease in which both mind (*psyche*) and body (*soma*) are involved. The term usually refers to disorders which, although of an unquestioned organic physical nature, are also strongly influenced by emotional and psychosocial factors. Examples include bronchial *asthma, *peptic ulcer, *migraine, *hypertension, *colitis, menstrual disorders, sexual dysfunction, skin diseases such as *eczema and *psoriasis, and many more.

PSYCHOSURGERY. Brain surgery, of which *leucotomy is an example, undertaken with the object of altering behaviour in patients with severe chronic mental disorders refractory to other forms of treatment. See NEUROSURGERY; PSYCHIATRY.

PSYCHOTHERAPY is the treatment of psychiatric disorders by psychological methods, without the use of drugs or other physical interventions. It consists essentially in listening and talking to the patient. *Psychoanalysis is an example, but most psychotherapy consists of much simpler techniques, such as encouragement or reassurance. See PSYCHIATRY.

PSYCHOTROPIC DRUGS. Drugs that have an effect on the mind, altering the mental or emotional state, for example *tranquillizers, *antidepressants, *hypnotics, etc.

PTOMAINE is a general term formerly applied to nitrogenous products of putrefied flesh (*ptoma* = corpse) considered to be poisonous.

PTOSIS is the drooping of one or both upper eyelids; it is sometimes also applied to downwards displacement of other organs or parts.

PUBERTY is the onset of the reproductive period of life, marked in girls by the *menarche and in both sexes by the development of the *secondary sexual characteristics.

PUBLIC HEALTH ACT 1848. A major piece of British public health legislation, sometimes referred to as 'the Chadwick Act' after Sir Edwin *Chadwick, the civil servant who was largely responsible for framing its provisions. These provisions invested local authorities with important responsibilities, including the paving of streets, the construction of drains and sewers, the collection of refuse, and the procurement of water supply both for domestic use and for other purposes such as street cleaning and fire-fighting. The Act also instituted the *General Board of Health.

PUBLIC HEALTH ACTS 1875, 1936, 1961. Three major and comprehensive enactments concerning public health in England and Wales (the first is known as 'The Great Public Health Act'). They encompassed a huge variety of provisions. Among them were: sewerage and sewage disposal, including private sewers and cesspits; the sanitation of buildings; refuse; scavenging; the keeping of animals; public conveniences; verminous premises and persons; nuisances and offensive trades; water supply; preventing and notification of disease; registration and inspection of nursing homes; notification of births; maternity and child welfare; child life protection; baths, wash-houses and bathing places; common lodging houses; canal boats; water courses, ditches, and ponds; tents, vans, and sheds; hop-pickers; trade effluents; cleaning and paving of highways; inspection of markets and slaughterhouses; and other matters, including the administration of all the foregoing.

PUBLIC HEALTH IN THE USA. In the mid-19th century there were a few individuals in the USA who were groping to establish a public health movement, but they concerned themselves primarily with defensive measures instituted locally to ward off epidemics or to correct environmental conditions that had become intolerable. Responsibility for action was a matter that had barely begun to be discussed. The times were ripe for the new concepts and policies that came in rapid succession—with consequences that inspired the president of an American university to reflect, in the mid-20th century, on the importance of public health:

. . . A historian a thousand years hence examining the records of our culture will conclude perhaps that the goal of physical well-being was one of the unifying forces of the twentieth century . . . A widespread concern with alleviating or eliminating suffering and a firm belief that suffering can be reduced by human efforts are certainly characteristic of America today.

. . . it is clear that if we are to attain the social objectives of making the new knowledge equally effective in the lives of all the people of a nation—let alone of the entire world— improving our methods of curing disease is not enough. The problem today is keeping people well . . .

. . . as the profession of public health advances . . . the entire people of a free and prosperous society will enjoy a state of health undreamed of even by the kings and nobles and the privileged classes of a few centuries ago.

Today one can easily see that public health has its foundations not only in the biological and natural sciences, but also in the realm of social and political affairs. This article begins with a very brief indication of the kinds of scientific advances that gave rise to the first great successes of public health in the USA.

Origins of basic concepts
Successful preventive measures most often depend on accurate information about the cause and factors influencing the course of a disease. This precept is vividly illustrated by the consequences of applying new information about communicable diseases: the proof that *micro-organisms and *parasites can cause disease in man and animals; the recognition of the role of *carriers in certain diseases; the discovery of the many animal reservoirs of human diseases; the proof that certain *arthropods can transmit disease agents and sometimes serve as intermediate *hosts; and the demonstration that control measures appropriately designed and adapted to the habits and life cycle of an arthropod *vector can sharply reduce the *incidence of the disease in question.

Prodigious results accompanied the application of advances in the science of *immunology. A glance at the list of vaccines currently recommended for public use indicates the firm place attained by active *immunization. American scientists had central roles in the development of several vaccines on the list, notably those against *yellow fever, *poliomyelitis, *louse-borne *typhus fever, *influenza, *measles, and *rubella. In addition to the basic knowledge permitting the development of vaccines, immunological research provided many diagnostic procedures now indispensable in public health as well as clinical medicine.

By the mid-point of the 20th century the application of the findings of *microbiology and immunology enabled public health to lift a great burden of communicable diseases from large segments of society. Meanwhile, ideas and recommendations put forward in 1850 by Lemuel Shattuck, in his monumental report, gradually won acceptance in the USA. Scores of individuals, both doctors and laymen, participated in the process of working out an acceptable and effective *modus operandi* for the practice of public health. The basic principles in the USA today are that:

1. The health of people generally can best be protected and improved by *organized community actions*.
2. Such actions must draw not only upon doctors, dentists, and nurses, but also upon experts from such diverse fields as chemistry, education and communications, engineering, entomology, laboratory sciences, law, *nutrition, *pharmacy, public affairs, *social work, *veterinary medicine, and, more recently, management sciences; in brief, *public health consists of a mosaic of professions*.
3. The most effective way to deal with complex health problems whether local, state, or national is to *mobilize the relevant experts for collaboration with community leaders* in analysing the particular problems and developing appropriate measures.

These principles have been put to use in hundreds of ways in the USA, ways that include programmes of governmental agencies, voluntary organizations, industries, even international groups. An excellent illustration is the *American Public Health Association* (APHA), formed in 1872, growing in size and influence to become, in 1992, a voluntary association of thousands of members from the mosaic of more than a score of the disciplines comprising public health. Particularly in recent decades, the APHA has spoken to the policy makers of cities, states, and the federal government, sometimes with a single voice, but at other times there have seemed to be divergent views among its leaders. The record of its accomplishments, however, is impressive— it has influenced government policies, set standards for professional education, devised ways to evaluate the performance of local and state health agencies, and, even more importantly, recommended actions well before the medical profession or the general public recognized the importance of new issues. The *American Journal of Public Health* (often referred to as the *Journal of the APHA*) from time to time publishes a 'Public policy forum'; the most recent one (July 1992, vol. 82) presents Sir Richard Doll's statement, 'Health and the Environment in the 1990s' containing wise and forthright advice for the policy makers in the USA as well as in the UK and Europe.

One might infer that public health now has all the administrative inventions it needs to deal with any problems that arise. Such may not be the case, however, because there are several very complex issues demanding the attention of society in general, not just the health professions.

Comprehensive health care

Comprehensive health care and how it is to be provided are the first such issues. While the principal causes of death and disability in the USA were shifting from communicable diseases to chronic degenerative and neoplastic disorders, the nature of medical practice also changed. Doctors spent more time attempting to arrest the progression of chronic disease. Then came new methods of paying for medical care, methods that have had great impact on people's behaviour. Soon patients began to expect personal health care to include both preventive and curative services; further, they wanted them to be provided in a single setting. Many doctors and patients alike now think that prevention should pervade all of the medical specialties.

The goal of comprehensive health care is utopian. A principal obstacle to its attainment is the fact that medical students and their teachers are traditionally attracted much more strongly by the tangible satisfactions of direct patient care than they are by the abstract satisfaction of knowing that one's efforts have helped to keep large numbers of people from getting sick, a situation lacking personal patient contact. One cannot realistically expect a sudden change in attitude of doctors such that they will devote adequate attention to preventive measures in all facets of medical practice. Thus, the health care of tomorrow will still be of better quality in its therapy than in its prevention.

Consequently there will still be a need for those who do derive satisfaction from keeping people well, and who make it their careers, whether as teachers, researchers, or practitioners.

Health a universal human right

This is the second new issue confronting society, and especially its political elements. The idea took form slowly, through times of prosperity and depression, wars and their consequences, struggles over civil rights, and women's liberation. It gained support from campaigns to reduce infant mortality, to educate the public in matters of personal hygiene, to establish nursing services for the poor, to provide care for the elderly, the handicapped, and the unemployed. By 1946 it had such a degree of public approval that it appeared as the basic tenet in the Preamble to the Constitution of the newly created *World Health Organization (WHO). The USA formally endorsed the concept along with most of the nations of the world. The language in the preamble is simple, direct, and clear, yet revolutionary to a degree not appreciated by all the governments when they signed the document, nor even now, decades later:

The States Parties to this Constitution declare, in conformity with the Charter of the United Nations, that the following principles are basic to the happiness, harmonious relations and security of all peoples:
   Health is a state of complete physical, mental and social well-being and not merely the absence of disease or infirmity. The enjoyment of the highest attainable standard of health is one of the fundamental rights of every human being without distinction of race, religion, political belief, economic or social condition . . .
   Governments have a responsibility for the health of their peoples which can be fulfilled only by the provision of adequate health and social measures.

What was the effect in the USA of endorsement of this WHO charter concept? To what extent have federal, state, and local governments provided people of all economic levels, religions, and races with access to health services? One must say, not enough, and point to the perplexing paradoxes of the health-care situation in the nation. See also GOVERNMENT AND MEDICINE IN THE USA.

Rapid population growth

This issue rivals nuclear warfare in its implications for the world. It affects public health directly and indirectly, in the USA as well as in every other nation, now and far into the future. It affects environmental resources, agricultural practices, nutrition, hunger, the quality of life, and even the stability of governments. Gradually over the past few decades the health professions have become involved in several aspects of the control of human fertility. (See below on 'Contributions to public health activities world-wide'.)

*AIDS

The acquired immune deficiency syndrome has become a pandemic that poses enormous problems, for its victims and their families, for health providers, for scientists who are vigorously seeking the basic facts needed to devise both effective therapy and immunological means of prevention, for hospitals, for industries, for government officials, both local and national, and for taxpayers (see AIDS). The vice-chairman of the USA's National Commission on AIDS has summarized the remarkable scientific progress that has been made since 1981 in research; he states vividly and concisely what has not yet been accomplished by government and voluntary agencies, and what actions the Commission recommends as the first priority (Rogers 1992). At the international conference on AIDS in Amsterdam, July 1992, the cost of caring for the numbers of patients expected in the USA in 1995 was anticipated to be close to US$15 billion (£10 billion); furthermore, the total number of persons newly infected with the HIV virus in that year was predicted to be about 50 000—approximately the same as the number of deaths from AIDS expected to occur in the same twelve-month period. The bad news arising from the AIDS *pandemic must include the rapid increase in *tuberculosis that is resistant to the whole range of currently available chemotherapeutic combinations, a most unwelcome development facing the health professions.

*Substance abuse

This term subsumes drug addiction, intravenous injection by individuals of cocaine, its derivatives, or other substances, alcoholism, and inhalation of various mind-altering chemicals, etc. In the USA authorities have declared war on drug smugglers and dealers in the attempt to curb the rising toll taken by drugs on health and many other aspects of human affairs. Nearly 30 per cent of new infections by the AIDS virus each year, for example, are directly related to needle-sharing among intravenous drug users. Likewise, transmission of *hepatitis B has been caused by this practice. Despite widespread efforts and expenditure of large sums of money, the problems related to drugs and 'substance abuse' continue to constitute a vexing issue for the health professions and society in general.

Contributions to public health activities world-wide

The USA first became directly involved in international health activities as a consequence of its success in the control of *yellow fever in Havana and in Panama during the construction of the canal. That involvement led in 1902 to participation in forming the International Sanitary Bureau (later the Pan-American Health Organization). The USA also supported the Office International d'Hygiène Publique from its origin in 1907 until it was absorbed into the WHO. Several Americans worked vigorously to assure the establishment of the WHO as an effective instrument for achieving common objectives for human health. Thomas Parran, when surgeon-general of the United States Public Health Service, was particularly effective in negotiations that preceded adoption of the charter of WHO.

The extent of commitment of the USA to the success of the WHO can be measured in part by the fact that in its first three decades approximately 30 per cent of WHO's regular annual budget came from the USA, a larger proportion than the total provided by the four next largest contributions, the Soviet Union, West Germany, the UK, and France.

Over and above its annual contributions to WHO, the United States government has expended several billion dollars to support programmes in other countries for health and nutrition through the State Department; the Department of Health and Human Services (chiefly by the Public Health Service's Center for Disease Control); and nearly a score of other federal agencies. Private organizations also spent substantial sums in this same period to promote the health and nutrition of other nations. One example follows.

Malaria

In the 1930s the Rockefeller Foundation became involved in work that proved to be a landmark for international health. The *malaria-transmitting mosquito, *Anopheles gambiae*, while indigenous to Africa, had not been observed in the western hemisphere until it appeared in Brazil in 1930. Within a few years this species established itself in north-east Brazil, where it caused a disastrous outbreak of malaria in 1938. A veteran malariologist described the situation in these terms:

> There is no doubt that this invasion of *gambiae* threatens the Americas with a catastrophe in comparison with which ordinary pestilence, conflagration, or even war are but small and temporary calamities. *Gambiae* literally enters into the very veins of a country and may remain to plague it for centuries.

The International Health Division of the Rockefeller Foundation launched a campaign against *A. gambiae* in Brazil in 1939 under the direction of Fred L. Soper. Before the end of 1940, *A. gambiae* had been eliminated. This had repercussions extending far beyond Brazil: the results showed that a task presumed to be hopeless could be done, given skilful leadership with adequate financial support. Advocates of global campaigns to eradicate malaria and smallpox cited this success as a forceful argument in favour of their proposals. The argument was further strengthened when another incursion by *A. gambiae*, this time into Egypt from Sudan, was repulsed in the early 1940s, again under Soper's direction.

In 1946 the Rockefeller Foundation and the government of Italy began an intensive campaign against malaria on the island of Sardinia, using residual spraying of the walls of all human dwellings. The insecticide was *dichlorodiphenyltrichloroethane (DDT). Before 1946 Sardinia was rated as one of the three most malarious areas in the world; the termination of malaria transmission on the island in 1949 was therefore a spectacular accomplishment.

Although the extensive use of DDT in the early 1950s reduced the incidence of malaria in many regions, the disease continued to be a serious problem. In 1955 the World Health Assembly decided to implement a programme having world-wide eradication as its goal. By 1968 data collected by WHO indicated that of 1700 million people living in malarious areas 1350 million had been protected by the campaign and were living in improved economic conditions as a consequence. The appearance of DDT-resistant anopheline mosquitoes and the emergence of strains of malaria resistant to various forms of chemotherapy were setbacks to the campaign, as were the administrative and financial problems encountered in individual countries. Unfortunately, global eradication is still a distant goal.

*Smallpox

The USA contributed both funds and experts to the world-wide campaign against smallpox. This disease had been eliminated from several countries in the 1950s, but national smallpox efforts had varied so greatly in effectiveness that eradication seemed only a dream. Nevertheless, WHO launched its campaign in 1958 and intensified the work a few years later by establishing regional reference centres, including the Center for Disease Control (CDC) in Atlanta. Several members of the CDC staff were soon involved in eradication activities in West and Central Africa. By May 1970, after 3.5 years of intensive field work in 20 African countries, they showed that smallpox was no longer occurring in this formerly endemic region, equal in size to the continental USA. Furthermore, they found that epidemiologically directed surveillance and containment activities were more effective than mass vaccination, an observation of great value to eradication programmes in other regions. The goal of zero cases was reached in 1979—a triumph of international co-operation in which the USA played a very significant part.

Malaria and smallpox are by no means the only examples of far-reaching contributions to international health by the USA, its official and voluntary organizations, its scientists and administrators. Accomplishments in prevention of yellow fever, poliomyelitis, epidemic typhus, or measles could readily be cited to illustrate the point. Similarly, the many advances in nutrition and reduction of deficiency diseases are worthy of close attention.

World-wide population increase

The USA has participated in efforts to reduce the burdens of rapid population growth that press upon most of the developing nations of the world. The magnitude of

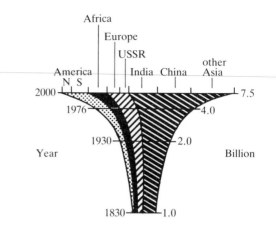

Fig. 1 Actual and predicted population growth, showing regional differences, 1830–2000. (Adapted from the *New York Times*, 20 April 1970 and from Rudel, W., Kinel, F. A., and Henzl, M. R. (1973). *Birth control: contraception and abortion.* New York.)

the problem is awesome as to both sheer numbers and complexity. According to present and projected growth rates, the world's population is expected to reach 10 billion by 2030 and approach 30 billion by the end of the 21st century. Figure 1 shows the changes in the size and distribution of the world's population since 1830 and a projection to the year 2000.

The official representatives of 135 nations meeting at the World Population Conference in Bucharest in 1974 endorsed without opposition the principle that all people have the basic human right to decide freely and responsibly the number and spacing of their children and to have the information, education, and means to do so. Acceptance of this principle means that members of the health professions, as public servants, must assist in providing the necessary information and services for fertility control. A start has been made in this direction and it is a significant one. American scientists have been intimately involved in the development of the contraceptives and *intrauterine devices that so many millions of healthy women are using in the USA and in scores of other countries. In 1980, the United States Government donated approximately 187 million dollars for support of population and family planning assistance in other countries; contributions by two major foundations in the USA raised the figure to 200 million dollars, about half the total funds donated by the industrialized nations for population assistance. Much is still to be done: at least 50 million women not using oral contraceptives in less-developed countries would do so if they were readily obtainable; equally large numbers of people would accept sterilization, terminate their pregnancies, or use one of the other effective methods of birth control if generally and appropriately available.

Some observers believe that voluntary programmes

of family planning will not succeed in bringing population growth to a halt. Garrett Hardin concluded that mankind must adopt 'mutual coercion, mutually agreed upon' as the solution. Mark Twain lamented the advent of improvements in medical practice because, he said, doctors had done so much in former times to keep population growth in check. Both Hardin and Mark Twain, however, would surely agree that the health professions in concert with national leaders should strive to stabilize the total world population at a level low enough to permit people everywhere to enjoy a life of peace, civility, dignity, and meaning.

Status of public health in the USA

Widely voiced concern about rising costs of medical care might lead one to infer that the health of people in the USA is worsening. Some statistics that are often used to assess health status show striking differences between 1870, for example, and the present. The nation grew in total population more than sixfold. Live births per 1000 women aged 25–44 dropped to less than half the figure for 1870, as did the crude death rate. The greatest change occurred in the number of infant deaths—in 1990 the figure was one-fifteenth of that a century ago. As an accompaniment to these developments, life expectancy at birth nearly doubled, the proportions of the population across the age range became more evenly distributed, and the median age increased by 10 years.

Comparing the principal causes of death, now and a century ago, reveals that the five communicable diseases accounting for such a large proportion of deaths in 1870 (pulmonary tuberculosis, typhoid fever, *diphtheria, *measles, and smallpox) do not appear among the chief causes of death now—these being heart disease, *cancer, accidents, *cerebrovascular disease, and chronic pulmonary obstructive diseases.

Changes in causes of mortality of this magnitude, affecting millions of people in such a short time, were unknown in previous eras. It is probable, moreover, that changes also occurred in the duration of disability from preventable disorders, especially in childhood and early adulthood.

Statistics such as these tempt one to think that the present status of human happiness and the quality of life now are better than they were 100 years ago. It would be unwise, however, to make assertions because there are as yet no generally accepted definitions or quantitative criteria for measurement. Indeed, questions raised by the Secretary of Health, Education, and Welfare in 1972 concerning the impact of federal programmes resulted in an 18-page paper by his staff. Their report stressed the imperfections of current data, outlined disagreements over criteria for evaluation of the quality of life, and predicted the futility of any federal attempt in the near future to establish indices for measuring the impact of governmental programmes on health and welfare.

The lack of criteria has not deterred discussion of the issues. Health is widely assumed to consist of far more than the absence of disease or physical disability. Just as the physical health of people is clearly affected by housing conditions, environmental defects, automobiles, and conditions of employment, so too are mental health and well-being affected by the social changes accompanying rapid urbanization and technological developments (see SOCIOLOGY). The special issue of *Daedalus* in 1977 presented 18 essays on various aspects of health in the USA, ranging from the perceptions and expectations of people regarding health and medical care to the impact of technological advances on the economics and growth of the health care industry (Knowles *et al.* 1977).

That health care *has* become an industry is now beyond question: its more than 5 million employees make health the largest industry in the USA in terms of workers and the third largest in terms of income produced. Total expenditures for health care in 1990 amounted to more than 12 per cent of the gross domestic product of the USA. But the benefits of the industry are not equally distributed among the population. By what means can access be provided to all the people regardless of their status? What methods of financing should be used? The furore over ways to resolve these problems in the USA can be appreciated by a glance at the indices published in the *New England Journal of Medicine* for the twelve month period from 1 July 1991 to 30 June 1992. The reader will find editorials, reviews of recently published books on several aspects of the subject, cost-benefit analyses, advantages (or disadvantages) of health care under various systems of delivery, statements bearing on public policies, etc., in all a total of more than 50 articles for just a single year in only one of the numerous journals that have the topic under surveillance.

William B. Schwartz, physician and expert analyst of medical care in the USA, illustrated concisely these issues in a contribution to a forum in the *New York Sunday Times*, 19 July 1992, Section 3, p. 11:

The choice is clear: we either must pay the staggering bill imposed by new medical technology or we must ration expensive services. The prime target should be tests or treatments for which costs are high and prospective benefits small. For example, under tight budget constraints, admission to the intensive care unit might be denied to the patient who has only a small prospect of survival. To contain costs effectively, managed care will force wrenching decisions on who gets what kind of care.

No matter how painful the effort, the process of ordering national priorities for the expenditure of public funds for health must soon begin. To succeed in this process, ways must be found to escape from the political tyranny of single-issue minorities with their militant intolerance and their unwillingness even to let other viewpoints be heard.

Furthermore, there must be innovations in the art and science of educating the public in matters of health. The accomplishments of the health sciences have but slight effect until incorporated into the practices of considerable segments of the population. The key elements in changing the perception of people and their behaviour are accurate information, skilful communication thereof, and, finally, motivation of those leaders in a community who will use the information to influence the behaviour of those around them.

Success in these undertakings will go far toward improving the health of the public at large. It will also reduce the enormous expense of operating the health-care system itself, a matter that will surely continue to be of concern to the taxpayers everywhere.

The Clinton administration's health-care policy

On 22 September 1993, the Clintons presented to Congress their extensive plans for major changes in the nation's health-care system. The *New York Times* devoted three pages the following day to summaries of various aspects of the proposed new structure, citing the opinions *pro* and *con*, voiced by powerful segments of the public at large during the preceding 6 months. A few features of these summaries indicate the broad scope of the plan and the concessions made to obtain wide support of the undertaking:

Health insurance for all citizens of the USA is to be achieved over the next few years, under the aegis of a seven-member, presidentially appointed 'National Health Board'. This group will monitor compliance by the States and the functioning of the States' new regional health alliances; it will interpret to the public the standard health insurance packages that are to be offered by the health alliances and recommend new benefits reflecting changes in technology and in needs of the public. In order to promote informed choices by citizens, the National Board will develop and publicize indicators of quality of services and care, as these are offered by the many differing health plans of the competing health maintenance organizations in each regional alliance. Costs of prescription drugs will be under continuous scrutiny so that the Board can inform the pharmaceutical companies of its evaluation of both cost and usefulness of those drugs deemed unreasonably expensive.

A 'Health Security Card' is to be issued to every American, but not to illegal immigrants. The card will guarantee benefits in the 13 categories that are listed; it will also specify those services that are excluded from coverage. Individual choice of personal physicians will be retained except for those who are unable to pay the individual's share of the insurance, perhaps 20 per cent of the total. Government subsidy will cover the insurance costs of those who are unable to pay. Employers will be required to provide 80 per cent and employees 20 per cent (tax deductible) of the costs of employees' insurance to be purchased from the competing physicians' health maintenance organizations approved by their regional health alliances. Insurance coverage will continue when people change jobs or

become unemployed. Medical schools will be under pressure to send a larger proportion of their graduates into primary care rather than the specialties.

The expense of this restructuring is to be met in part by taxes on tobacco (and perhaps also alcohol), in part by greatly simplifying the management of records and payments, and in part by ceilings on allowable fees for various procedures in different regions; the ceilings will not apply to private physicians who opt not to join the practice groups authorized by the regional health alliances.

Lobbyists for powerful special interest groups have already besieged members of Congress, both by personal conferences and through widely circulated accounts in the news media and on television broadcasts—each group stressing the potentially damaging consequences they anticipate for their interests if this or that part of the whole plan is passed by Congress. Many individuals, including some legislators, publicly elected officials, and economists, regard the costs as prohibitively expensive. There is only a slight chance that all the details in their present form as requested by the Clintons will be voted into law by Congress. Possibly, however, compromises will be reached that preserve some of the important features of the new policy.

J. C. SNYDER

References

Many of the statements and quotes above were obtained from the references cited by the five articles that follow:

Doll, Sir Richard, (1992). Health and the environment in the 1990s. *American Journal of Public Health*, **82**, 933–41.

Knowles, J. (guest ed.) (1977). Doing better and feeling worse. *Daedalus: Journal of the American Academy of Arts and Sciences*, **106**, (1), 1–278.

Rogers, D. E. (1992). Report card on our national response to the AIDS epidemic. *American Journal of Public Health*, **82**, 522–4.

Snyder, J. C. (1976). Public health and preventive medicine. In *Advances in American medicine: essays at the bicentennial*, (ed. J. Z. Bowers and E. F. Purcell), Vol. 1, pp. 384–457. Josiah Macy Jr. Foundation, New York.

Snyder, J. C. (1986). *Public health in the USA*. In *The Oxford companion to medicine*, (ed. J. N. Walton, P. B. Beeson, and R. B. Scott), Vol. 2, pp. 1171–9. Oxford University Press.

PUBLIC HEALTH LABORATORY SERVICE (PHLS)

A government-funded statutory body responsible in England and Wales for the surveillance of communicable diseases and for the provision of a microbiological laboratory service for the diagnosis, control, and prevention of such diseases. In addition to the Central Public Health Laboratory, which provides specialized microbiological reference services and to the Communicable Disease Surveillance Centre, both of which are based at Colindale, north-west London, the PHLS operates 52 regional and area laboratories, a number of which also offer specialized reference services. The information collected by the CDSC is disseminated in the weekly publication *Communicable Disease Report*. The monthly publication *Communicable Disease Review* contains articles on communicable disease epidemiology, and the *PHLS Microbiology Digest* is published quarterly.

PUBLIC HEALTH MEDICINE IN THE UK. One of the difficulties in discussing public health medicine is in defining the term, as it seems to have changed continuously. The 1988 government Committee of Inquiry into the future development of the public health function defined public health as 'the science and art of prolonging life and promoting health through the organised efforts of society'. The Faculty of Public Health Medicine of the *Royal College of Physicians of the UK has defined it most recently (1991) as:

the science and art of preventing disease, prolonging life and promoting health through organised efforts of society. Its chief responsibilities are the surveillance of the health of a population, the identification of its health needs, the fostering of policies which promote health, and the evaluation of health services.

The central tasks of public health physicians are:

1. To provide epidemiological advice on the setting of priorities, planning of services, and evaluation of outcomes.
2. To develop and evaluate policy on prevention, health promotion, and *health education involving all those working in this field, and to undertake surveillance of non-communicable disease.
3. To co-ordinate the control of communicable disease.
4. To act as chief medical adviser to an authority.
5. To publish an annual report on the health of the population.
6. To act as spokesperson for the health authority on appropriate public health matters.
7. To provide public health and medical advice to, and link with, the local authorities.

To understand the present state of public health medicine it is necessary to review the history and development of the specialty. Primitive man believed that disease was sent by the gods as punishment, with the consequence that there was little search for either cure or prevention. *Hippocrates took the first steps towards a modern view of medicine by separating it from religion and philosophy. The ancient Greeks linked disease to an imbalance between man and his *environment, placed importance on education and developed an excellent system of personal *hygiene. The Romans advanced civic planning and engineering, and provided both water supply and sewage disposal.

During the Middle Ages public health measures such as isolation, *quarantine, and the cleaning of streets were introduced. During the Renaissance, interest in science revived, ecclesiastical registration of births and deaths began in Britain, and Bills of Mortality, consisting of lists of trials, marriages, and baptisms, were compiled weekly by parish clerks. In 1532 the London City Council ordered that a record of deaths from *plague should be kept.

Health statistics in the modern sense began with John Graunt, a London haberdasher and politician, who was the first to study the Bills of Mortality, classify deaths and death rates by causes, and note the seasonal and annual variations in the death rate. His study showed that the rate of *mortality was higher in towns and was rising.

As plague repeatedly appeared in the 17th century, quarantine became a common method of preventing the spread of disease, although in 1665 the village of Eyam in Derbyshire isolated itself and almost all the inhabitants died in an attempt to prevent plague from ravaging the district. In 1720 the government sought the advice of Richard Mead, who recommended the appointment of a Council of Health with extensive powers to enforce a system of quarantine, which was not realized until the 19th century.

In the 18th century new methods of prevention were developed, the first of which was environmental control. John *Pringle in the army, James *Lind in the navy, and John *Howard in the prisons, showed how improvements in environmental conditions could reduce the toll of disease, which in the forces caused a greater loss of life than warfare, and in the prisons caused more deaths than public executions. But the most important advance came with the discovery of *vaccination by Edward *Jenner. This not only provided a safe and effective means of preventing *smallpox, but it also laid the foundations for *immunology. Progress in the 18th century was remarkable, but the impact was limited because the civic apparatus necessary to exploit the advances was still lacking.

The Industrial Revolution led to the appearance of densely populated industrial communities, which were characterized by destitution and squalor, conditions ideal for the outbreak of *epidemics of *typhus and other fevers. The high mortality levels in towns previously identified by Graunt intensified, contrasting with the improvement in the health of the country as a whole. Concerted action to protect the weaker members of the community was contrary to the *laissez-faire* economic theories of the day, but eventually, after almost a century of efforts at reform, an effective framework of public health control was implemented. The social reforms, however, were introduced not out of compassion but to ensure a healthy workforce.

After 1830 two events stimulated further progress. In 1832 a Royal Commission was appointed, with Edwin *Chadwick as secretary, to examine and reform the Elizabethan Poor Law system. Chadwick argued that relief given to the poor must be lower than the wages of a paid labourer. The new law was harsh but, from the public health point of view, it was important because it created the post of medical officer to the Poor Law union and established central medical inspectors. All this had a profound effect on the future organization of health care. The second event was the passing of the 1836 Act making civil registration of births, deaths, and marriages obligatory in England and Wales. Public health advanced further with Edwin Chadwick's *Report on the labouring population of Great Britain* (1842), which called for sanitary reform, an idea supported by a Royal Commission appointed in 1843 to inquire 'into the state of the large towns'. Edwin Chadwick's report was significant because it was the first ever English social survey.

In 1848 the Public Health Act established the *General Board of Health with the power to create local boards. Medical officers of health (MOHs), the earliest career specialists in public health medicine, were appointed under private acts, notably to Liverpool (William Duncan, 1847) and the City of London (John *Simon, 1848). The Public Health Act 1848 authorized their appointment to all local boards, although the appointments were not obligatory.

In 1855 the 38 newly formed London vestries were required to appoint medical officers, and Leeds appointed an MOH in 1866, Manchester in 1868, Birmingham in 1872, and Newcastle in 1873. At first no special qualifications were required, but Trinity College, Dublin, provided a diploma in public health in 1870 and Cambridge University in 1875, and other universities followed suit. The Local Government Act of 1888 required every MOH of a county or district with a population of 50 000 or more to be a qualified practitioner, with a diploma in public health, and conforming to rules prescribed by the *General Medical Council.

The threat of *cholera was another spur to action as it led to John *Snow's classic epidemiological studies, which demonstrated the transmission of cholera infection by contaminated water supplies. Snow successfully used epidemiological analysis to show the relationship between the source of water supplies from the Thames (either above or below the heavily contaminated section of the river) and cholera. He demonstrated a much higher rate of mortality and morbidity from cholera in the households supplied from the more heavily contaminated water.

The appointment of John Simon as Medical Officer to the new General Board of Health and subsequently to the Privy Council was another significant event. He set in motion a series of inquiries into disease which were notable forerunners of contemporary epidemiological studies. Simon investigated a wide range of health problems and transformed the practice of public health into a scientific discipline.

In 1869 a Royal Commission made recommendations which this time led to the establishment of a firm and permanent foundation of public health. Sanitary law was consolidated in the Public Health Act of 1875, and the country was divided into urban and rural sanitary district authorities, which were required to appoint an MOH.

By the turn of the century it was becoming clear that environmental sanitation was not enough to secure an adequate standard of health for the great mass of the people, but that services directed specifically towards the needs of vulnerable groups were needed.

Public concern over the fitness of the nation led to the establishment by Balfour's Conservative government of the Committee on Physical Deterioration. The immediate outcome of this Report was the provision of school meals in 1906 and the founding of the school medical service in 1907. A school medical department was established at the Board of Education and the MOH became the principal school medical officer for his district. From 1912 the Board of Education made grants to local authorities for the establishment of minor ailment clinics. These provided treatment for conditions of the skin, ears, nose, mouth and throat, and also provided dental treatment and spectacles.

Lloyd George established the National Health Insurance Scheme to tackle poverty and sickness. It was a compulsory contributory scheme paid for by a weekly deduction from the worker's pay, supplemented by a contribution from the employer and the Treasury. It provided the wage-earner with medical care from a *general practitioner without payment, and provided a cash benefit to help to compensate for loss of earnings during sickness. The two deficiencies were that it did not provide either hospital treatment for workers or any assistance for their dependants. The National Insurance Act of 1911, which embodied the National Health Insurance Scheme, was, however, the first step towards the provision of medical care for all.

By 1918 the Chief Medical Officer to the Local Government Board, Sir George Newman, was arguing that preventive medicine must be given a greater role in the education of every medical student, and urged for greater co-operation between those concerned with curative medicine and preventive medicine. Public health doctors welcomed this wider recognition, but it became increasingly difficult to distinguish between this public philosophy and the practice and work of other medical practitioners. Public health doctors and general practitioners were particularly in conflict, since the former ran public health clinics and the latter accused them of encroaching on to their private practices. Further problems arose because the hospitals provided through local government were under the control of the public health departments.

In 1929 the Local Government Act was passed, which abolished the Boards of Guardians and transferred their powers and duties to the local authorities, which were required to set up committees to administer 'public assistance', as poor relief was now called. The Act of 1929 transferred all the institutions of the Poor Law to the local authorities, including the infirmaries. In time, these were to become municipal hospitals under the executive control of the MOH, who was also responsible for curative and preventive medicine. This was the position the MOH was to hold until the coming of the *National Health Service (NHS) in 1948. But public health failed to establish its own identity within the medical profession, with the consequence that in the post-war reorganization of the health service the government decided against using the public health service as a model for the new NHS. In addition, the public health preoccupation with the hygiene of the individual and the administration of a growing number of services resulted in a neglect of the traditional task of the MOH, i.e. that of community watchdog over people's health.

In 1939 the MOH was instrumental in the evacuation of children and in coping with the effects of bombing. Fears of large-scale epidemics were met by the expansion of the *immunization programme and of radiology. A network of laboratories, covering the whole country, was also established to provide diagnostic and other services to local public health departments, which in due course became a permanent part of the public health establishment (Public Health Laboratory Service).

With the establishment of the NHS in 1948 the MOHs lost their responsibility for hospitals. This transfer of control to the regional hospital boards, boards of governors, and hospital management committees created new opportunities, new challenges, and saw the development of what came to be called 'modern public health'. The opportunities were the ability to provide caring and supportive services to meet the needs of an ageing population and for the physically and mentally handicapped. The challenges were the changing pattern of disease, as the *infectious diseases of the past gave way to what may be called the 'behaviourally based' conditions of the present, such as lung *cancer, *coronary heart disease, and death and disablement on the roads. All this demanded new approaches, methods of detection, and prevention, while removing from the MOH responsibility for the management of the institutional 'disease' service. It also saw a new importance attached to health education as a potentially valuable instrument of prevention and health promotion.

There were also environmental improvements. The 'smog' episode in London in December 1952, as a result of which 4000 people died, led to the passing of the Clean Air Act in 1956. In 1960 the Noise Abatement Act was passed, which made excessive noise a statutory nuisance that could be dealt with under public health law. However, on the negative side, in 1970 social work was hived off to the new Social Services Departments and the MOH lost half his staff and budget. Increasingly, the MOHs found themselves squeezed by pressures from within, in the form of the local government hierarchy and the desire of *sanitary inspectors, *health visitors, and *social workers for greater professional freedom,

and external pressures, such as the role of general practice and hospitals.

The Report of the Royal Commission on Medical Education (Todd Report) in 1968 made the first reference to the community physician as the practitioner of community medicine. The job specification was spelt out in detail in 1970 by the Hunter Committee (*Report of the Working Party on Medical Administrators* 1972), by which time a training course for the new specialist had been started at the London School of Hygiene and Tropical Medicine under Professor J. N. Morris. In 1972, the Royal Colleges of Physicians of the UK collaborated in founding the Faculty of Community Medicine, thus signifying the formal recognition of the new specialty.

The *community physician formally came into being with the reorganization of the NHS on 1 April 1974, as the public health departments of the local authorities were closed. Community physicians were appointed to key positions at every level of the service, including the district. Their functions were: first, to provide information to clinicians and to advise them on possible approaches to care; secondly, to be concerned with the planning of services, with the supply and interpretation of information, with the maintenance and evaluation of services and programmes, and with the development of measures for the prevention of disease and the promotion of health; thirdly, as an adviser to local authorities. Community physicians were considered specialist advisers, but with specific skills in *epidemiology and management responsibilities. The community physician was required to have a basic understanding of *clinical practice, and a thorough knowledge of epidemiological principles and methods, and of the epidemiology of communicable and non-communicable disease. A familiarity with statistical methods, aspects of the social sciences and the principles of administration and management, and the ability to apply this knowledge to the management of health services and the study of disease, were also required.

However, the community physicians did not achieve the success expected of them. There are many possible reasons for this, one of which was undoubtedly the name. Practitioners, other than community physicians, thought the term meant medicine within the community and thus misunderstood the role of its practitioners, while community physicians themselves did not feel that they were the only advocates of medicine within the community. The most important reason, however, was that they were not necessarily trained for some of the tasks that they were expected to perform. Many of them considered that power lay in management, for which they were not trained, and thus neglected those areas where they could have exercised most influence. In many authorities the staff that they had formerly worked with and managed were taken from them, so that they were unable to achieve some of their objectives. Finally, many of the best pre-war practitioners who had flourished in the past were disenchanted with not being 'in control' and took the opportunity of early retirement.

Between 1974 and 1988 there was a significant loss of morale. This was partly due to the problems of the reorganization and restructuring that occurred in the health service between 1974 and 1989 and the fact that community physicians were the only medical practitioners who always had to re-apply for their posts after any reorganization. Although recruitment to the specialty began to improve, many of the entrants came for negative reasons, and some of those who were keen to join associated the subject with change in the structure of society and the delivery of health services.

The important policy documents of the 1980s showed little awareness or appreciation of the community physician's role. The 1979 government document, which signalled the 1982 reorganization of the NHS, and the Griffiths Report (NHS Management Inquiry) of 1983 clearly emphasized the need for a better management of hospitals and made virtually no mention of community medicine.

Public health medicine had to adapt to two developments. The first one was the Acheson Inquiry into public health in England, which was established by the Secretary of State in 1986, following two major outbreaks of communicable disease—*Salmonella food poisoning at the Stanley Royd Hospital in Wakefield, and *Legionnaire's disease at Stafford in 1985. Two public inquiries had indicated a decline in medical expertise in environmental health and in the investigation and control of communicable disease. The second development was the reorganization of the health service in 1991 and the separation of the provision from the purchasing of health services. Separating these functions enabled public health to establish its identity more clearly.

There have been a number of successes in public health medicine over recent years, which are too easily forgotten. One is the promotion of health services evaluation, which owes much to community medicine specialists, most notably *Cochrane. Public health medicine has also led to environmental improvements, such as clean air, and consequently to improvements in mortality and morbidity from respiratory disease. It has also led the fight against cigarette-smoking, not only through such pioneering work as that of Hill and Doll, but also through the commitment of public health physicians to changing behaviour and attitudes towards smoking.

There have also been some notable successes in health service organization. The recommendations of the Resource Allocation Working Party were criticized, but the suggested approaches, which were based on epidemiological principles, were a significant advance in tackling the problems inherent in the equitable distribution of health services. Public health medicine has also been active in developing health promotional activities, as well as in creating a more suitable balance of care between the institution and the community, and

in prevention, care, and cure. Other areas where it has achieved success include the evaluation of nutritional policies, which has led to improvements in nutritional intervention. It is now rare to see children who are underfed; indeed, if anything children are increasingly obese. We now know a great deal about the aetiology of a variety of diseases, although it is true that there has been only limited success in changing the incidence of common diseases or significantly improving the treatment of these conditions.

Despite these successes, public health medicine has failed to achieve several of its objectives. This is because, first, too much time has been spent by the specialty in developing committee and management structures, rather than on developing its own skills. Much effort has been expended on creating niches in the belief that it would attain power through management positions. As a result, it has failed until recently to develop a clear identity and to demonstrate that its prime interest is in the health of groups. It has also aroused fear and suspicion amongst many medical colleagues. In particular, its concern with effectiveness has not made it many friends, since few people like having to justify their actions. It is also confused about when it should be acting as an executive and when its role should be purely advisory.

The development of appropriate methods of training, based on gaining experience of practical applications and then incorporating this into theory, has proved much more difficult to design than originally envisaged, but is now in place. It is difficult to show how the basic skills of epidemiology and medical *statistics, for example, can be applied to the service situation. Trainees in public health medicine, after their general professional training, have about 1 year's theoretical training, followed by 3 years' experience under supervision, including the submission of a dissertation which has to include two examples of how the theoretical aspects of the subject have been applied in practice. This training is considered by trainees to be of a high standard, and the specialty has been successful in attracting recruits of high calibre.

The attraction of power and politics has also hindered the advance of public health medicine. It has often failed to identify who holds power and what the real political issues are. It has also often been unsuccessful in identifying the groups that could assist in promoting the specialty's goals. A final problem has been internal division. On one side are the academics and on the other the practitioners, and co-operation between them is often difficult, partly because, in contrast to the clinical disciplines, separation in universities and service authorities has been greater than between clinical academic and service practitioners. It also has long-term possible dangers for public health medicine unless firm links are maintained with other clinical colleagues. The separation of provider and purchaser in the 1991 reorganization has helped to create a clear identity, with the creation of a role that has been recognized and appreciated both by other medical colleagues and by lay authorities.

To overcome these past difficulties, the future aims of public health medicine are to establish a clearer identity and develop greater expertise. Public health physicians will gain the respect and recognition of their colleagues only by demonstrating that they are as expert in their own specialty as are their colleagues in theirs. It is also important to appreciate the extent to which the success of the work of public health physicians is dependent on the co-operation and involvement of clinicians and other professional groups. While they do not need to develop expertise in, for example, *sociology, *economics, or medical *statistics, they must be willing to work with multidisciplinary groups, including experts in all these subjects.

A major problem is to decide upon the balance between general public health and specialist public health. As a result of the reforms of the health service, public health medicine plays an important role in the purchasing of health care, in defining health-care needs, and in evaluating the effectiveness of health-care services, as well as in the orthodox old style public health activities of control, prevention, and the surveillance of disease. But this means that much greater expertise is required both in these specific tasks, as well as in individual specialties, such as *paediatrics and *mental illness. Furthermore, advances in the physical, biological, and molecular sciences which will impact on both clinical and public health activities will require both continual up-dating as well as specialization as it is unlikely that any generic practitioner will be able to cope with all such aspects.

The challenge is to be able to monitor and influence the health service of a local population, and to be able to demonstrate perceptible health gains. To achieve this, practitioners will need detailed health information for a population, to ensure co-ordination between the different sectors of the health system and to assess and improve the efficiency and effectiveness of health care.

Many different approaches will clearly be needed, but a start can be made by the preparation of a report on the health of the population which indicates where there is unmet need, inefficient provision, and opportunities for more effective resource use. This work must be capable of having a direct influence upon the health system. The preparation of annual public health reports can be a powerful tool and public health practitioners are beginning to exploit this.

There have obviously been significant changes in public health medicine in recent years. This has been assisted by the publication of *The health of the nation* (Secretary of State for Health 1992) which has done an enormous amount to focus peoples' ideas on prevention and health promotion, rather than simply on disease treatment. It has, furthermore, led to the appreciation of the need for interspecialty working and thus for the development of co-ordination between a very large variety of different disciplines. Thus the future is bright.

W. W. HOLLAND
S. HILDREY

Further reading
Faculty of Public Health Medicine (1991). *Standing orders*. Royal College of Physicians, Faculty of PHM, London.
NHS Management Inquiry (1983). *Recommendations for action*. DHSS, London.
Report of the Working Party on Medical Administrators (1972). HMSO, London.
Secretary of State for Health (1992). *The health of the nation: a strategy for health in England*. Command Paper cmnd 1986. HMSO, London.
The Committee of Inquiry into the Future Development of the Public Health Function (1988). *Public health in England*. Command Paper cmnd 289. HMSO, London.
The Report of the Royal Commission on Medical Education, 1965–68 (1968). Command Paper cmnd 3569. HMSO, London.

PUBLIC VACCINATOR. The office of public vaccinator was created in 1871, when England and Wales were divided into districts each under the charge of a public vaccinator, a general practitioner under contract to vaccinate without a fee.

PUDENDA. The external *genitalia, particularly of females.

PUERPERAL FEVER is fever after childbirth, due to *streptococcal infection of the birth canal and surrounding tissues, leading to *septicaemia—the once deadly 'childbed fever'. The incidence and the danger of this complication have been drastically reduced by *aseptic methods and *antibiotics, respectively, although in the UK puerperal fever is still a *notifiable disease. See also OBSTETRICS AND GYNAECOLOGY.

PUERPERIUM. The period following *childbirth, which lasts until the maternal pelvic organs and tissues have returned to their normal condition.

PULEX IRRITANS, the human *flea, is parasitic on the skin of man. Individual sensitivity varies, but pulicine bites can be very irritant, causing flea-bite *dermatitis. Unlike some other species, notably the rat flea *Xenopsylla* which transmits *plague, *Pulex irritans* is not normally a vector of infectious disease.

PULHEEMS is the acronymic classification of medical fitness used by the British army, the letters representing: physical capacity (P); upper limbs (U); lower limbs (L); hearing (H); visual acuity (EE); mental capacity (M); and emotional stability (S). A numerical grade is assigned to each letter.

PULMONARY ARTERY. The blood vessel which conducts deoxygenated blood from the right *ventricle of the *heart to the lungs. It consists of a main trunk and right and left pulmonary arteries going to the right and left lungs, respectively.

PULMONARY DISEASE. See CHEST MEDICINE.

PULMONARY OSTEOARTHROPATHY is *clubbing of the fingers, painful swelling of the distal joints of the extremities with associated soft tissue swelling, and radiological evidence of subperiosteal new bone formation in the shafts of the long bones: it is also known as hypertrophic pulmonary osteoarthropathy. It almost invariably signifies serious disease of the lungs or heart, particularly *bronchial carcinoma, of which it may be the first manifestation, or chronic lung sepsis (*abscess, *empyema, *bronchiectasis). Finger clubbing alone, without new bone formation, occurs in *infective endocarditis, cyanotic *congenital heart disease, pulmonary arteriovenous malformations, and some diseases of the intestine and liver (e.g. *Crohn's disease, *ulcerative colitis, and some types of liver *cirrhosis). It may also be congenital and of no pathological significance.

PULSE. A pressure wave in a blood vessel, corresponding to the heart beat; it can be seen or felt, or both. The arterial pulse is easily felt at several sites and its rate is commonly used as an index of heart rate; careful and skilled examination can provide other valuable information about the state of the heart, circulation, and arteries. The central venous pulse can usually be seen (but not felt) just above the inner third of the clavicle, and similarly repays detailed study.

PULSUS ALTERNANS is an arterial *pulse in which the beats are of alternating strength, owing to a corresponding alternation in left ventricular (and thus arterial) systolic pressure. The phenomenon may be detected on routine palpation of the radial pulse, or may be first noticed when taking the blood pressure: as the *sphygmomanometer cuff is deflated, the arterial sounds abruptly double in rate as the systolic pressure achieved by the weaker beats is reached. Pulsus alternans occurs in left ventricular failure, and although the precise mechanism is not understood, it is recognized to be of poor prognostic significance.

PULSUS PARADOXUS. A marked decrease in amplitude of the arterial pulse during inspiration. This physical sign, particularly characteristic of *pericardial effusion and constrictive *pericarditis, is badly named, as it represents an exaggeration of a normal phenomenon. Normally, the inspiratory fall in intrathoracic pressure sucks in a greater volume of blood to the right side of the heart, augmenting its output and partially compensating for the simultaneous increase in pulmonary vascular capacity; the output from the left heart either falls a little, or not at all. Pulsus

paradoxus indicates that the right heart is unable to achieve this compensatory output increase usually because its expansion is limited by a tense or rigid pericardium but sometimes because the myocardium itself is rigid ('constrictive' *cardiomyopathy, or extreme right ventricular dilatation). The sign may also occur when the respiratory swing in intrathoracic pressure is exaggerated, as in obstructed or stertorous breathing.

PUNCH-DRUNK SYNDROME. The syndrome exhibited by certain professional boxers resulting from repeated *trauma to the head. The manifestations are those of chronic *encephalopathy, with muscular incoordination, hesitancy of speech, slowness of thought, and memory loss.

PUNCTURE BIOPSY involves the removal of a sample of tissue from a patient for histological examination by needle puncture and aspiration (also known as needle or aspiration *biopsy).

PUPIL. The circular opening enclosed by the *iris that admits light into the eye.

PURGATION is the administration of a purgative or *laxative to induce defaecation.

PURGATIVE is a synonym for *laxative.

PURINES are substituted derivatives of purine, a bicyclic organic base with the formula $C_5H_4N_4$ related to uric acid. Their biological importance is due to their presence in *adenosine triphosphate (ATP) and *nucleic acids. Adenine and guanine, two of the nucleotide bases of *deoxyribonucleic acid (DNA) and *ribonucleic acid (RNA) are examples of purines.

PURKINJE (PURKYNE), JAN EVANGELISTA (1787–1869). Czech physiologist. A histologist of distinction, he was the first to use a *microtome and *Canada balsam. He described the cells in the *cerebellum (1837) and the fibres in the *myocardium (1839), both of which bear his name. He noted *ciliary action in 1835. His physiological research was centred on sensory phenomena, especially vision, and the maintenance of equilibrium and posture. He invented the term *protoplasm' (1846). In 1823 he analysed and classified fingerprints.

PURKINJE CELL, FIBRES, VESICLE, ETC. Among the structures and physiological phenomena to which the name of *Purkinje is attached, the most important are: Purkinje cells (also Purkinje corpuscles, Purkinje layer), large branching neurones in the cortex of the *cerebellum; Purkinje fibres (also Purkinje network), specialized subendocardial myocardial fibres responsible for conducting the exciting impulse to the ventricular muscle of the *heart; and Purkinje vesicle, which is the nucleus of an *oocyte.

PUROMYCIN is an *antibiotic produced by the fungus *Streptomyces alboniger* with antineoplastic and antiprotozoal activity. It has been used to treat *tumours, *trypanosomiasis, and *amoebiasis. See also ANTIINFECTIVE DRUGS.

PURPURA is a condition marked by multiple spontaneous capillary haemorrhages, chiefly in skin and mucous membranes. It is distinguished morphologically from the smaller pin-point or punctate haemorrhages known as *petechiae and from the larger black-and-blue haemorrhages of bruising known as *ecchymoses. There are many causes usually classified into two main groups, namely, those associated with a low circulating level of *platelets, the thrombocytopenic purpuras, and those not so associated, the vascular purpuras.

PURULENT means associated with the presence or the formation of *pus.

PUS is a yellowish fluid of varying consistency formed as a product of *inflammation, notably with particular species of bacteria known on that account as pyogenic. Its main constituents are white blood cells, bacteria, necrotic tissue, the debris of all these, and tissue fluid.

PUSTULE. A pimple containing visible *pus.

PUTREFACTION is enzymatic and bacterial decomposition of organic material.

PYAEMIA (PYEMIA) is the presence of pus-forming (pyogenic) micro-organisms in the blood circulation; it may be associated with the formation of *abscesses remote from the site of original infection: a form of *septicaemia.

PYELITIS is inflammation of the renal pelvis, a frequent result of bacterial infection. Since the kidney substance is inevitably also involved to some extent, the term pyelonephritis is virtually synonymous. See NEPHROLOGY.

PYELOGRAPHY is *radiographic visualization of the pelvis of the kidney after it has been filled with a radiopaque dye. There are two main methods. The first is known as intravenous pyelography (or excretory urography). An iodinated contrast medium which is both excreted and concentrated by the kidney is injected intravenously, and X-ray films are then taken at appropriate intervals; initially, the kidneys are seen in outline and then the dye concentrates in the renal pelves and *ureter, revealing any anatomical abnormality. Impaired renal function may be suggested by delayed or deficient excretion by one or both kidneys. The other method, known as retrograde pyelography, is independent of the state of renal function. A *cystoscopy is performed and a catheter inserted under direct vision into one or other ureteric orifice, allowing contrast medium to be injected directly into it; the medium spreads in a retrograde fashion to fill the rest of the collecting system of the kidney.

PYELONEPHRITIS. See PYELITIS.

PYKNIC. One of the constitutional types described by Kretschmer, the pyknic habitus is a short, stocky build associated with a cheerful extraverted social temperament and swings of mood. When those of pyknic constitution suffer a mental breakdown, the illness is likely to be of the *manic-depressive variety. Kretschmer's 'pyknic' is roughly equivalent to Sheldon's '*endomorph'.

PYKNOLEPSY is a name sometimes given to *petit mal epilepsy when attacks are very frequent, of the order of 100 or more a day.

PYKNOSIS is cell degeneration in which the cell nucleus contracts into a dense, featureless mass.

PYLORIC STENOSIS is an outflow obstruction from the *stomach due to contraction of the pyloric orifice. In adults this may result from scarring due to *peptic ulceration or from a *tumour in the pyloric region. Congenital pyloric stenosis of genetic origin occurs in newborn infants.

PYLOROPLASTY is the surgical re-formation of the pylorus, the narrow muscular tube connecting the *stomach to the *duodenum.

PYLOROSPASM is spasm of the pyloric muscle.

PYODERMA is any skin disease associated with *pus formation.

PYOGENIC. *Pus-forming.

PYOMYOSITIS is *myositis with *pus and *abscess formation, usually due to *staphylococci and occurring more commonly in the tropics.

PYONEPHROSIS is suppurative infection of the kidney, in which the renal parenchyma is partly or completely destroyed by a collection of *pus.

PYOPNEUMOTHORAX is the simultaneous presence of air and *pus in the *pleural cavity.

PYORRHOEA (PYORRHEA) is any flow of *pus; when otherwise unqualified, it usually means pyorrhoea alveolaris, purulent *periodontitis.

PYRAZINAMIDE is an antibacterial drug used in the treatment of *tuberculosis, normally in combination with other drugs. Its value is limited by the development of drug resistance and by its side-effects, notably liver damage.

PYREXIA is a synonym for *fever.

PYRIMIDINES are substituted derivatives of pyrimidine, an organic base with a heterocyclic six membered ring structure (formula $C_4H_4N_2$). Cytosine, thymidine, and uracil, nucleotide bases found in *nucleic acids, are pyrimidines.

PYROGEN. An agent which produces *fever.

PYROSIS is a synonym for *heartburn.

PYURIA is the presence of *pus in the *urine.

Q FEVER is a severe but self-limiting influenza-like illness due to the micro-organism *Coxiella burnetii. C. burnetii* is a species of **Rickettsia*, but Q fever differs in two respects from other rickettsial infections such as *typhus: first in being transmitted to man by inhalation, and secondly in not being marked by a rash. The organism, moreover, is remarkably resistant to drying and to exposure in soil and dust. A reservoir exists in wild animals, maintained through transmission by *arthropod vectors; man becomes liable to infection when this spreads to domestic animals, particularly cattle, sheep, and goats. Clinically, the illness gives high fever, malaise, muscle pains, and headache; a mild pneumonia is not uncommon. The overall mortality rate is less than 1 per cent, and the response to antibiotics is favourable. The only serious complication is *endocarditis, and this is rare. Q stands for query.

QUACKS. Medical impostors or charlatans. See MEDICAL CULTS AND QUACKERY.

QUADRIPLEGIA is paralysis of all four limbs.

QUADRUPLETS. Four offspring from a single gestation. See MULTIPLE BIRTH.

QUAIN, SIR RICHARD, Bt (1816–98). Anglo-Irish physician. He was president of the *General Medical Council from 1891 to 1896.

QUARANTINE is a period, originally (for a ship) of 40 days (derived from the French *quarante*), of compulsory isolation or detection in order to prevent contagion or infection. The term is now used extensively in other contexts, as for example in relation to the period of 6 months for which an imported dog must be kept 'in quarantine' in the UK in order to prevent the importation of *rabies.

QUARANTINE LAWS. Improvements in knowledge, sanitation, therapy, and prophylactic *immunization during the 20th century have led to increasing relaxation of various quarantine regulations for infectious diseases. To replace these, and in the light of increasing international air travel, the *World Health Organization

(WHO) in 1969 issued International Sanitary Regulations to set standards for reporting of diseases and quarantine measures, including maximum quarantine requirements that could be imposed on international traffic. These regulations were concerned with six designated 'quarantinable diseases', namely *cholera, *plague, *yellow fever, *smallpox, louse-borne *relapsing fever, and louse-borne *typhus. Subsequently, WHO International Health Regulations revised the standards applicable to the first four of these diseases, and downgraded the two last to 'diseases under surveillance' (along with *malaria, *influenza, and *poliomyelitis). A quarantine law which remains strictly in force is that governing the importation of live animals into the UK, which has been free of endemic *rabies for over 70 years. Under the Rabies (Importation of Dogs, Cats and Other Animals) Order 1974 it is an offence to import into the UK most mammals except with an advance licence, which requires the animal to be retained in approved quarantine premises for 6 months. This applies to any animal that has been in a foreign port, regardless of whether or not it actually landed and whether or not it has been vaccinated against rabies. Contravention can result in a prison sentence and destruction of the animal.

QUARANTINE PERIOD. A period of isolation or detention imposed on those who have or may have been in contact with an infectious disease, in order to prevent further transmission; the period being normally equal to the maximum *incubation period of the particular infection. With the common infections, quarantine periods are now rarely strictly observed, ordinary medical surveillance of contacts being regarded as adequate; however, it may be advisable in some instances to keep contacts away from, for example, schools and places of public entertainment.

QUARTAN FEVER is a fever recurring at 72-hour (not 96-hour) intervals, as in the type of *malaria due to *Plasmodium malariae*, a parasite which has an asexual life cycle of 72 hours.

QUECKENSTEDT, HANS HEINRICH GEORG (1876–1918) German physician. In 1916 he devised a test to show whether the *spinal canal is blocked (see QUECKENSTEDT'S TEST). He was killed by an army wagon on the last day of the First World War.

QUECKENSTEDT'S TEST. A hollow needle with a pressure-measuring device is introduced into the *cerebrospinal fluid by *lumbar puncture. The jugular veins in the neck are then compressed. This dams back blood in the cranial cavity. Cerebrospinal fluid is therefore compressed and the rise in pressure is transmitted to the spinal canal. If there is a block, the pressure does not rise. If there is a partial block, the pressure rises and falls back more slowly than normal.

QUERVAIN, FRITZ DE (1868–1940). Swiss surgeon. He described a non-suppurative form of thyroiditis (1904) and chronic stenosing vaginitis of the thumb (1895).

DE QUERVAIN'S DISEASE is painful *stenosing vaginitis of the thumb.

DE QUERVAIN'S THYROIDITIS is an inflammatory condition of the *thyroid gland, also known as subacute granulomatous thyroiditis: it usually follows a viral infection and is characterized by painful swelling of the gland. Disturbance of thyroid function, if it occurs, is transient and the disease is self-limited.

QUETELET, LAMBERT ADOLPHE JACQUES (1796–1874). Belgian statistician and astronomer. The founder of *vital statistics and the first to conceive of the 'average man', he devised a technique for the application of statistics to the data of biology and the social sciences.

QUICKENING. The first perception by the mother of fetal movement, usually early in the fifth month of pregnancy.

QUINCKE, HEINRICH IRENAEUS (1842–1922). German physician. He described the capillary *pulse (1868) and *angioneurotic oedema (Quincke's disease, 1822). He was the first to use *lumbar puncture for therapy and diagnosis (1895).

QUINIDINE is a *cinchona alkaloid, used mainly for its antiarrhythmic and myocardial depressant effects.

QUININE was the first, and is still one of the medicinally important quinoline *alkaloids of cinchona bark, obtained from South American trees of the genus *Cinchona*. Although for most antimalarial purposes quinine has been superseded by synthetic compounds, it remains valuable in the treatment of malignant tertian (falciparum) *malaria resistant to *chloroquine. Its wide variety of pharmacological actions finds other therapeutic applications, for example in controlling night *cramps.

QUINSY is an *abscess in the peritonsillar region and is an occasional complication of pharyngeal infections.

QUINTUPLETS. Five offspring from a single gestation. See MULTIPLE BIRTH.

RABELAIS, FRANCOIS (?1494–?1553). French physician and writer. In 1532 he was appointed physician to the Hôtel-Dieu in Lyon, where he lectured on anatomy. Here he wrote the works which have made his memory imperishable, *Pantagruel* (1533) and *Gargantua* (1535).

RABIES is an almost uniformly fatal viral infection transmitted to man by the bite of an infected animal, usually a dog. In many countries, the virus (a large, bullet-shaped ribonucleic acid (RNA) virus belonging to the *rhabdovirus group) is enzootic in wild warm-blooded animals; the chief danger to man occurs in communities where rabies in domestic animals is inadequately controlled. Some countries (e.g. the UK and Japan), which have been able to eliminate the disease, maintain this situation by stringent control of the importation and *quarantine of animals. Once signs of infection appear (the incubation period varies from 1–2 weeks to several years), treatment has little or no influence on the ultimate outcome. It is, however, possible to reduce the likelihood of infection after the bite of a rabid animal by a combination of active and passive *immunization.

RACE, ROBERT RUSSELL (1907–83). British haematologist. Race made a memorable contribution, with *Fisher, to the genetics of blood group inheritance, particularly of the *rhesus factors. He introduced the CDE/cde system, which has helped illuminate many aspects of *haematology.

RACHISCHISIS is the absence of the vertebral arches of the spine in the lumbar region, a severe form of *spina bifida.

RACIAL FACTORS IN DISEASE. Like other genetically determined characteristics, such as skin colour, facial appearance, height, etc., disease of genetic origin, or having a contributory genetic component, may vary in incidence between different racial groups. For instance, *sickle-cell anaemia does not occur among Caucasians and *cystic fibrosis is rare in those of Negro origin; *gout is common among Maoris; *phenylketonuria is rare in Jews but *Tay–Sachs disease is fairly common:

*thalassaemia occurs chiefly in people from South-East Asia and the Mediterranean littoral; and there are many other examples. See also GENETICS.

RAD. A unit of absorbed dose of ionizing *radiation. One rad is equal to an energy absorption of 0.01 joule per kilogram of irradiated material. In current clinical practice it has been replaced by the SI unit gray (Gy) equal to 1.0 joule per kilogram. Thus 1 Gy = 100 rad.

RADCLIFFE, JOHN (1650–1714). British physician. Radcliffe was the original owner of the gold-headed cane and left a large fortune to Oxford University, from which were built the Radcliffe Camera, the *Radcliffe Infirmary, and the Radcliffe Observatory.

RADCLIFFE INFIRMARY, Oxford, England, is named after the physician John *Radcliffe who graduated from Oxford and practised in London. The infirmary was opened in 1770 and named after him. Clinical instruction for undergraduates occurred sporadically there, occasionally disappearing. Henry Acland in the 19th century seemed to feel that a medical education should consist of basic sciences in the university, followed by clinical education elsewhere, a pattern which was adopted against some opposition. William *Osler came from the USA as regius professor of medicine and an illustrious period began at the Radcliffe and in Oxford leading ultimately to the opening of an Oxford clinical school. Lord Nuffield (see MORRIS) made major benefactions in the 1930s and clinical chairs in surgery, medicine, obstetrics, and anaesthesia were founded and filled by the distinguished Hugh *Cairns, L. J. Witts, Chassar Moir, and R. R. Macintosh. Further renowned names associated with the infirmary were J. Trueta in traumatic surgery (from experience in the Spanish Civil War), John *Ryle, who held the first chair of social medicine in the UK, and Sir George *Pickering. A clinical medical school is now firmly established in Oxford using the new John Radcliffe Hospital and the Radcliffe Infirmary, amongst others, for teaching.

RADIATION is the emission of any rays, wave motion, or particles (e.g. *alpha particles, *beta particles, *neutrons) from a source.

RADIATION, IONIZING: ITS BIOLOGICAL EFFECTS

Introduction

The biological effects of ionizing radiation are better known than those of any other physical or chemical agent. Knowledge of such effects—and, in turn, the development of principles and procedures for protecting against radiation injury—have helped us to cope with the health hazards of other environmental agents.

Historical background

Within months after its discovery by *Roentgen, in 1895, the *X-ray was introduced widely into the diagnosis and treatment of disease. As a result of ignorance of the dangers of overexposure, ulceration of the skin and other harmful effects of radiation were encountered almost immediately in early workers and patients.

In 1902, skin *cancer was recognized as a potential late-occurring complication of radiation injury, ultimately afflicting scores of pioneer radiation workers. Because such cancers were characteristically preceded by long-standing and progressive radiation damage of the underlying skin, it was generally assumed that they would not be produced in the absence of gross injury. By the middle of the century, however, the frequency of *leukaemia in A-bomb survivors, *radiologists, and certain groups of medically irradiated patients was thought to increase in proportion to the dose, without a threshold dosage being defined. The implication that any dose of radiation, however small, might increase the risk of cancer aroused concerns which still persist.

The nature of ionizing radiation

Ionizing radiation consists of electromagnetic radiations (e.g. X-rays and gamma rays) and particulate radiations (e.g. electrons, protons, neutrons, alpha particles, and other atomic particles) of varying mass and charge. These radiations, in contrast to other forms of radiation, impart enough localized energy to materials in which they are absorbed to cause ionization, as well as excitation, of atoms and *molecules.

Sources and levels of radiation in the environment

Ionizing radiation is ubiquitous, coming from three main natural sources:

(1) cosmic rays, originating in outer space;
(2) terrestrial radiations, emitted by *radium, thorium, *uranium, and other radioactive elements in the Earth's crust; and
(3) internal radiations, emanating from *potassium-40, *carbon-14, and other radionuclides present in living cells themselves.

The average dose received annually from all three sources by a person at sea-level is slightly less than 1.0 mSv (the sievert (Sv) as a unit of radiation has replaced the curie) (Fig. 1). It is noteworthy, however, that the

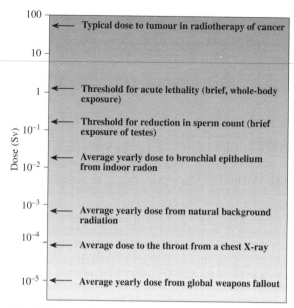

Fig. 1 Levels of exposure to ionizing radiation from different sources, in relation to the thresholds for various forms of acute radiation injury.

dose to the respiratory tract from inhaled *radon is several orders of magnitude larger, especially in smokers, who receive additional radiation from polonium-210, which is present naturally in tobacco smoke.

In addition to natural background irradiation, people are exposed to radiation from artificial sources, the largest of which is the dose from different types of medical and dental examinations. The annual dose to the population from such examinations in developed countries approaches that received from natural sources. Lesser sources of man-made radiation include radioactive minerals in crushed rock, building materials, and phosphate fertilizers; radiation-emitting components of TV sets, smoke detectors, and other consumer products; radioactive fall-out from atomic weapons; and nuclear power.

Interaction of radiation with matter

As radiation penetrates matter, it gives up its energy through random collisions with atoms and molecules in its path, causing the formation of ions and reactive radicals which, in turn, break chemical bonds and cause other molecular changes, resulting in biological injury. The spatial distribution of the ionization events along the path of an impinging radiation varies, depending on the energy, mass, and charge of the radiation, as well as the density of the absorbing tissue. In general, X-rays and *gamma rays produce ions sparsely along their tracks and tend to penetrate deeply, whereas charged particles produce ions densely and penetrate poorly. Alpha particles, for example, generally cannot even penetrate the skin. Since the production of injury is correlated with the density of energy deposition in the affected cells, protons and alpha particles are generally higher in relative biological effectiveness (RBE) than X-rays and gamma rays.

The anatomical distribution of the dose delivered by an internally deposited radionuclide depends on its uptake, tissue distribution, retention, and metabolism, which tend to be relatively radionuclide-specific. In the case of radioiodine, for example, the pattern of uptake and retention by the *thyroid gland is so predictable that this radionuclide is used clinically for assaying thyroid function.

Effects of radiation on cells
At the cellular level, radiation injury can take various forms, including inhibition of *cell division, damage to *chromosomes, *gene *mutation, neoplastic transformation, and various other changes. Any living cell can be killed by radiation if exposed to a large-enough dose.

Although radiation can alter essentially any molecule within the cell, *deoxyribonucleic acid (DNA) is the most critical target, since damage to a single gene can profoundly affect the cell. Many of the changes in DNA are reparable, but the type of lesion caused by a densely ionizing radiation is likely to be less reparable than that resulting from a sparsely ionizing radiation.

Damage to chromosomes
Radiation can cause the breakage and rearrangement of chromosomes and can interfere with the normal segregation of chromosomes to daughter cells at the time of cell division, thereby giving rise to changes in chromosome number and structure. The frequency of such chromosome aberrations increases as a linear non-threshold function of the radiation dose in the low-to-intermediate dose range, approximating 0.1 cell Sv in human blood lymphocytes irradiated in culture. Only a small percentage of all chromosome aberrations is attributable to natural background radiation, however; other causes include certain *viruses, chemicals, and drugs.

Damage to genes
Since Muller's pioneer studies with the fruit fly, in 1927, *mutagenic effects of radiation have been investigated extensively in many types of organism. In mouse spermatogonia and *oocytes, for example, the frequency of mutations per genetic locus is increased by about 100 per cent per Sv, depending on the conditions of irradiation. Heritable effects of radiation on human germ cells remain to be demonstrated as yet, but the fact that no increase in genetic abnormalities has been detected in the children of atomic bomb survivors is not unexpected, given their relatively small number (78 000) and the small size of the average dose (0.5

Sv) to their parents. On the basis of the available data, it has been estimated that the dose required to double the frequency of mutations in the human species probably exceeds 1.0 Sv, from which it is inferred that only a small percentage (0.1–2.0 per cent) of all genetically related diseases in the general population is attributable to natural background irradiation.

Effects on cell survival
The susceptibility of cells to irradiation increases with their rate of proliferation, a relationship which accounts for the radiosensitivity of cancer cells as a class. In most tissues, 1–2 Sv suffices to reduce the number of dividing cells by 50 per cent. In tissues characterized by relatively rapid cell proliferation (e.g. the *bone marrow, *gonads, lymphoid system, skin, lining of the gastrointestinal tract, and lens of the eye), inhibition of cell division may be detected immediately after intensive irradiation, to be followed months or years later by *fibrosis and other degenerative changes. Because cells depleted by irradiation may be replaced in time by the compensatory proliferation of uninjured cells, a given dose generally causes less damage to tissue if it is accumulated over a period of days or weeks than if it is received in a single brief exposure. By the same token, a given dose generally causes greater injury if delivered to a whole organ or to the whole body than if delivered to only a small part of an organ or of the body.

Radiation sickness
Intensive irradiation of a major part of the blood-forming organs (i.e. the haemopoietic system) or of the gastrointestinal tract may kill sufficient numbers of cells in these tissues to cause radiation sickness (the 'acute radiation syndrome'). In both the haemopoietic and intestinal forms of the syndrome, loss of appetite, nausea, and vomiting typically occur within a few hours after intensive irradiation, to be followed by a symptom-free interval until the main phase of the illness.

In the intestinal form of the syndrome, which may result from a dose in excess of 10 Sv, the main phase of the illness typically begins 2–3 days after irradiation, with severe diarrhoea, followed rapidly by prostration and death. In the haemopoietic form of the syndrome, which may result if the dose exceeds 1–2 Sv, the main phase typically begins 2–3 weeks after irradiation, with reduction in the white blood cell count and other complications of radiation-induced damage to the bone marrow; if the injury is sufficiently severe, death is likely to ensue 4–6 weeks after irradiation, from *infection or *haemorrhage. A third form of the acute radiation syndrome, the cerebral form, results from rapid exposure of the brain to a dose in excess of 50 Sv. In this syndrome, *anorexia, nausea, and vomiting occur almost immediately after irradiation, followed within hours by drowsiness, loss of equilibrium, confusion, *convulsions, loss of consciousness, and death.

Effects on growth and development of the embryo

Embryonal, fetal, and juvenile tissues are highly radio-sensitive. Rapid exposure to 0.25 Sv during a critical stage in embryonic development has been observed to cause birth defects in laboratory animals, and such effects have been encountered at higher doses in pre-natally irradiated children. For example, atomic-bomb survivors who were irradiated during the second tri-mester of prenatal development have shown a dose-dependent increase in the incidence of severe mental handicap.

Effects on cancer incidence

In atomic-bomb survivors, patients exposed to radia-tion for medical purposes, and various occupationally exposed groups, certain types of cancer have been observed to increase in frequency with increasing dose. Such cancers typically have not appeared, however, until years or decades after irradiation, and they have possessed no distinguishing features which identify them individually as having resulted from radiation, as opposed to some other cause. The increase in cancer rates has been observed predominantly at relatively high doses (0.5–2.0 Sv), moreover, and in no instance over a wide-enough range of doses and dose rates to define precisely the shape of the dose–incidence curve. Thus, the *carcinogenic risks of low-level irradiation can be estimated only by extrapolation from observations at relatively high doses and high dose rates, on the basis of assumptions about the dose–incidence relationship.

Although the data do not exclude the possibility that there may be no carcinogenic risks at the low dose rates characteristic of natural background irradiation, the risks are generally assumed for *public health pur-poses to increase in proportion with the dose, even at the lowest levels of exposure. On this basis, up to 3 per cent of all cancers in the general population are estimated to be attributable to natural background radiation, a somewhat larger percentage of lung cancers being attributed to inhalation of radon. The hypothesis that the risks extend to the lowest doses has prompted growing efforts to minimize all unnecessary exposures to ionizing radiation.

A. C. UPTON

Further reading

Hall, E. J. (1984). *Radiation and life*, (2nd edn). Pergamon Press, Elmsford, New York.

National Academy of Sciences Advisory Committee on the Biological Effects of Ionizing Radiation (BEIR) (1990). *The effects on populations of exposure to low levels of ionizing radiation*. Washington, DC.

United Nations Scientific Committee on the Effects of Atomic Radiation (1988). *Sources, effects and risks of ionizing radia-tion*. Report to the General Assembly, with annexes, New York.

Upton, A. C., Shore, R. E., and Harley, N. H. (1992). The health effects of low-level ionizing radiation. *Annual Review of Public Health*, **13**, 127–50.

RADICAL. A group of atoms, usually incapable of independent existence, forming part of a molecule and maintaining its identity during chemical changes affec-ting the rest of the molecule (e.g. NH_4^+, the ammonium radical).

RADICLE, meaning a small root, is a term applied anatomically to the smallest subdivisions of a branching structure.

RADICULITIS is inflammation of a spinal nerve root.

RADIOACTIVE SUBSTANCES ACT 1960. This UK Act regulated the keeping and use of radioactive sub-stances and radiation equipment and the accumulation and disposal of radioactive waste.

RADIOACTIVITY is the property of spontaneous dis-integration possessed by certain unstable atomic nuclei, this being accompanied by the emission of either *alpha or *beta particles and/or *gamma rays.

RADIOBIOLOGY is the branch of biology concerned with the effects of *radiation on living organisms and the behaviour of radioactive substances in biological systems.

RADIOCOBALT UNIT. Megavoltage apparatus for the *radiotherapy of cancer which uses as the radiation source an *isotope of cobalt, ^{60}Co; this isotope, easy to produce in a reactor, emits *gamma rays with a penetration equivalent to *X-rays from a 3 million volt X-ray machine, but can be contained in a much more compact unit (also known as a cobalt teletherapy or cobalt bomb unit). ^{60}Co decays at a rate of about 1 per cent a month (half-life 5.3 years); the source must therefore be replaced after 5–10 years. The radiocobalt unit was developed in Canada in 1951 and is now one of the two major types of megavoltage equipment in general use (the other being the *linear accelerator).

RADIOGRAPHY is the formation of images on photo-graphic material or fluorescent screens by short wave-length radiation such as *X-rays or *gamma rays. See RADIOLOGY.

RADIOIMMUNOASSAY is a technique for measuring minute quantities of any substance to which an *anti-body can be produced. A preparation of the antibody is first saturated with a known quantity of the substance which has been tagged with *radioactivity. The extent of displacement of the radioactive label by the test material when this is added is a measure of how much of the non-radioactive substance it contains.

RADIOISOTOPE. An *isotope possessing *radioactiv-ity, which can be used in physiological and diagnostic studies or for therapeutic radiation of tissues in which it is concentrated.

RADIOLOGICAL PROTECTION ACT 1970. This Act created a National Radiological Protection Board for the UK, with the functions of undertaking research and providing advice and services in connection with protection from *radiation hazards. It provided that the new Board would take over the Radiological Protection Service, formerly administered by the *Medical Research Council, and the Radiological Protection Division of the UK Atomic Energy Authority's Health and Safety Branch; the Board also took over the functions of the Radioactive Substances Advisory Committee appointed under the Radioactive Substances Act 1948, which was thereby repealed. The Board is subject to the directions of the Health Ministers of England, Scotland, Wales, and Northern Ireland.

RADIOLOGIST. A specialist in the use of electromagnetic radiation for diagnostic imaging. See RADIOLOGY.

RADIOLOGY
Window on the world of disease
Radiology is the field of medicine in which electromagnetic waves are used to produce images of normal and abnormal organs in order to permit the accurate diagnosis of disease. In *roentgenography*, X-rays generated in an X-ray tube penetrate a selected region of the body, are absorbed to different degrees by different tissues (depending on their specific density), and, finally, as remnant unabsorbed radiation, blacken a film to produce an image. The chest X-ray is a familiar example. *Fluoroscopy* (or radioscopy) utilizes a tube and a fluorescent screen (as a substitute for film) so that moving organs can be viewed in real time. *Diagnostic *ultrasound* directs a sonic beam at organs and produces an image of reflected waves that depends on structural characteristics and tissue interfaces to define 'density' differences. *Computed *tomography* (CT) (sometimes called computerized axial tomography or CAT scanning in the UK) uses an external beam to produce transmitted and attenuated X-rays that register on multiple detectors, are digitized by a *computer, and are finally reconstructed to give a cross-sectional view. *Magnetic resonance imaging* (MRI) depends on electromagnetic pulses to perturb a magnetic field, with measurement of 'relaxation' times and spin density to depict proton distribution and concentration in tissues. An image is then reconstructed in cross-section, sagittal section, coronal section, or other planes with relative ease. In *nuclear radiology* (*nuclear medicine), an internal source of radiation—a radioactive *isotope—is injected into the body and then registers on external detectors (such as a gamma camera), producing an image that depicts the distribution of the isotope in tissue.

There are many other specialized branches of radiology, including *arteriography*, *cardioangiography* (or angiocardiography), *venography*, *mammography*, and *interventional radiology*, all of major clinical importance.

How and where did it all begin?

The past
On 8 November 1895, Wilhelm Conrad *Roentgen, during an experiment with the Hittorf–Crookes tube, observed a bright fluorescence of barium platinocyanide crystals. He assumed initially that the fluorescence might be caused by cathode (beta) rays. Using a fluorescent screen, he removed it beyond the range of cathode rays; when the fluorescence persisted, he realized that the effect was produced by a new kind of ray. Not long afterwards, he replaced the screen by a recording photographic plate and soon obtained an image of his wife's hand. On 28 December 1895, Roentgen delivered the manuscript reporting his discovery of X-rays to the Physical Medical Society of Würzburg.

By early January 1896, word of Roentgen's discovery and its importance had spread around the world. Almost immediately the possibilities of applying the new 'photography' to traumatic lesions of bone fired the imagination and, within a month, X-rays of *fractures had been obtained and published. Early in the year, Edison and many others began intensive work on the fluoroscope. In 1896, Walter B. *Cannon, then a medical student, later to become a great Harvard physiologist, undertook a study of the movement of bismuth subnitrate through the feline gastrointestinal tract. He subsequently described in detail the nature and site of peristaltic activity as visualized on the fluoroscopic screen. The usefulness of contrast agents was already becoming apparent. Before the year ended, the first textbook on the subject of X-rays appeared.

By 1900 a volume by Borden entitled *The use of the roentgen ray by the medical department of the U.S. army in the war with Spain* had been published. Gunshot fragments in the soft tissues and traumatic lesions of bone were illustrated in large plates in this volume.

Important technical improvements early in the 20th century made radiography safer and more effective, and new areas became more accessible. In 1918, Dandy of Johns Hopkins performed the first air *ventriculogram, demonstrating enlarged ventricles in children with *hydrocephalus. The discovery that intravenous sodium iodide was not only excreted by the kidneys but opacified the urine, led to the description of clinical *urography in 1923. At about the same time, arteries and veins were visualized following contrast injection.

Bronchography (visualization of the bronchi) in 1922, gall-bladder visualization in 1924, carotid arteriography (demonstration of the blood vessels to the brain) in 1928, and angiocardiography (contrast visualization of the cardiac chambers and great vessels) in 1931 were all important milestones in the development of the field. Image-amplified fluoroscopy constituted the major technical advance of the 1940s and the 1950s.

The present

Radiology today, besides shedding important light on disordered *physiology, represents the most important approach to delineating gross pathological anatomy in living man. It is literally the foundation of every creative new surgical therapeutic approach of the 20th century. Without sophisticated radiology, there could be no advanced surgery of the central nervous system, the lungs, the stomach, duodenum, and large bowel, the kidneys, and certainly not of the heart or vascular bed.

The radiologist as a consultant and a teacher may work with medical students and residents, but his or her teaching is also levelled at the *internist specialist (physician in internal medicine), the *paediatrician, the surgeon, and, indeed, all of the specialists in medicine, though perhaps less useful to the psychiatrist.

The field goes well beyond the application of external radiation to the diagnosis and characterization of human disease. *Nuclear medicine, with its internal sources of radiant energy, has become an important method because of its imaging yield and also because of its capacity for dynamic retrieval of physiological data.

Another important growth sector within the discipline is diagnostic ultrasound, which has become the centre of an explosion in technology. The logarithmic growth rate in application of this technique to *obstetrics is based not only on its ability to locate the *placenta and characterize fetal growth and development, but also on the fact that it does not expose patients to ionizing radiation.

Radiological methods have become so integral an element in our approach to visceral disease in man that it seems highly likely that many of the conventional radiological examinations now in use will continue to be applied for a long period. The special procedures are equally important in their yield of diagnostic and physiological information.

During the past 15 years, the field of 'interventional' radiology has become an important component of patient care. The intravascular *catheter is used today not only to inject contrast agents so as to define the site of gastrointestinal or intracranial bleeding, but also, in some circumstances, to infuse pharmacological agents that constrict the vascular bed and stop the bleeding. A whole new field of pharmacoangiography has thus developed. Similarly, the radiologist has become concerned with the technology of balloon catheters, as a means of obstructing flow in circulatory beds in which uncontrolled haemorrhage is a threat to life. Such catheters are also used to overcome narrowing or *stenosis in important arteries such as the coronaries. There has also been increased interest in the character of intravascular embolic materials, and the delivery of these materials to control local bleeding without rendering other segments ischaemic has become both an art and a science.

Using ultrasound or CAT scanning, the radiologist

has become involved in biopsy of the *liver, *pancreas, *lymph nodes, retroperitoneum, and *kidney. He or she can drain abdominal and pelvic *abscesses non-operatively, and leave catheters *in situ* for longer-term evacuation of pus, remove gallstones, actively intervene in treating *intussusception and *volvulus of the *colon, and infuse chemotherapeutic agents and/or embolic materials into neoplastic beds. Percutaneous lung biopsy performed with the image-amplified fluoroscope is now a standardized procedure. In the patient threatened with pulmonary embolism from peripheral venous thrombosis, the radiologist may now place a filter in the inferior vena cava to stop the progress of a clot towards the lung. When the intestine is deprived of adequate blood supply because of vasoconstriction of its vascular bed, it may be necessary for the radiologist to infuse vasodilator drugs.

An important area of research in radiology focuses on decreasing the *radiation dose and increasing the information yield. Concern for the impact of radiological examinations on clinical management and health outcome has brought the radiologist directly into the field of utilization and cost-effectiveness studies.

The future

The past two decades have seen the most important developments in the imaging field since image-intensified fluoroscopy became a reality. The initial application of CT scanning was to the brain because the scanning time was relatively long and the skull could be immobilized for long periods. Once cranial CT had proved useful, it was only a matter of time before the method was applied to body scanning. CT has proved to be highly accurate in diseases of the lungs, mediastinum, liver, pancreas, *adrenal gland, *bladder, *uterus, *ovary, the retroperitoneum, the *spleen, and the kidneys.

Meanwhile, MRI has undergone a period of rapid technological development, still unfolding, in which it has shown its capacity not only in detection and assessment of diseases of the brain and spinal cord, but also of the musculoskeletal system, bones and joints, heart, and vascular bed. Magnetic resonance *spectroscopy remains in an investigative stage, but is sure to provide important information in the future. Similarly, emission tomography using radioisotopes has steadily improved and is being widely applied to investigation and to some clinical problems.

Thus, the field of radiology employs multiple modalities in order to define both the character and extent of disease and to participate in its management. In less than a century it has become a critically important tool in the exploration and treatment of illness and *trauma in living man.

H. L. ABRAMS

RADIOPAQUE SUBSTANCES are impervious to *X-rays and are therefore employed as contrast media to outline hollow structures in various radiographic techniques. See RADIOLOGY.

RADIOSCOPY is examination of structures and their movement by *X-ray images projected on to a fluorescent screen (also called fluoroscopy).

RADIOTHERAPIST. A specialist in the application of ionizing radiation to the treatment of disease. See RADIOTHERAPY.

RADIOTHERAPY, the branch of clinical medicine concerned with the application of ionizing radiations in the treatment of disease, is now devoted almost entirely to the treatment of *cancer, and this is indicated by its more modern designation of *radiation *oncology, which forms an integral part of *clinical oncology*. The success of irradiation in the cure of a malignant *tumour depends on a greater ability of normal tissues to recover under suitable conditions from a given radiation dose, compared with that of the tumour. Either electromagnetic radiations (photons), such as *X-rays or gamma rays, or corpuscular radiations (particles), such as electrons, neutrons, protons, or pions, may be employed, all with sufficient energy to produce ionization in living matter, and the biological effects depend on the intensity and distribution of this ionization. The method of radiotherapy used depends on the type of tumour, on its size and position, and on the extent of spread. External beams of high-energy radiation may be directed at a defined volume of the body; or radioactive sources inserted in or around the tumour; or, less commonly, radioactive *isotopes may be administered. Treatment may be prescribed with a view to possible cure of the tumour, or as a palliative measure to control local tumour deposits and relieve symptoms when, because of spread, cure is not feasible. Radiotherapy is used in over half of the 200 000 patients who develop cancer in the UK each year, and has a curative role in at least half the cases.

When a beam of X-rays impinges on tissue, the penetration depends on the energy, and the megavoltage beams needed for treating deeply placed tumours have energies of over 1 million electron volts (1 MeV). Linear accelerators for clinical use (Fig. 1) produce X-rays of 4–35 MeV, compared with the 1.25 MeV of the gamma radiation from a radiocobalt unit. The ionization effect being fundamental, this is used in the measurement of the quantity of radiation: the modern (SI) unit of absorbed dose is the gray, one centigray (cGy) being equivalent to an energy absorption of 100 ergs/g (and corresponding to the previous dosage unit of the rad). In cancer therapy the summated dose to the tumour is commonly in the range of 3500–6500 cGy (with treatment being given daily, or three times per week, for 3–6 weeks).

The biological effects of radiations are complex because many parts of the intricate cellular mechanism

are affected. While the visible changes depend on the tissue and organ irradiated, their severity is determined by the total radiation dose, its distribution in time and space, and the size of the volume irradiated. *Chromosome aberrations lead to cell death after an attempt at mitotic division, so that both normal tissues and tumours show radiation response at a pace proportional to their rate of reparative or proliferative cellular turnover.

The effects of irradiation on normal tissues have been studied in great detail both clinically and experimentally, for in essence they are the limiting factor in the local cure of cancer by this means. Rapidly replicating tissues show their responses early: local skin reaction, shown by redness, may appear after 8–14 days, then gradually subside with scaling and perhaps residual pigmentation; when the mouth or upper airways are irradiated a similar surface (but mucosal) reaction occurs; and during abdominal or pelvic irradiation diarrhoea may occur from the effect on intestinal mucosa. When large volumes of tissue are irradiated, blood-forming marrow depression is often the limiting factor, the circulating *lymphocytes being rapidly affected, then the *platelets, and a little later the granular cells. A large body of information has been acquired over the years on the radiation tolerance of normal tissues under various conditions, enabling a dose schedule to be chosen which allows them to recover. The ultimate dose-limiting effects are those on small blood vessels and

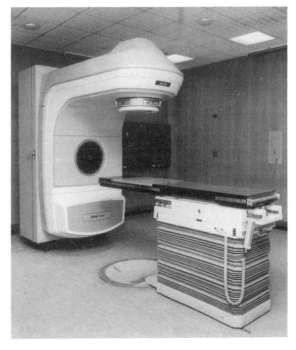

Fig. 1 A modern linear accelerator producing beams of X-rays at 6 MeV energy for megavoltage radiotherapy.

connective tissue, with the consequent impairment of blood supply aggravating a direct effect on *connective tissue cells to produce *fibrosis and *atrophy after latent periods of from a few months to several years. Certain 'critical organs' are particularly vulnerable to radiation, importantly the eyes, the lungs, the spinal cord, and the kidneys, and appropriate measures have to be taken to shield them during routine radiotherapy. *Testes and *ovaries are also highly radiosensitive, and for both somatic and genetic reasons particular care is taken to avoid their being inadvertently irradiated.

Tumours, which are characterized by their histo-genesis and morphology, vary greatly in their clinical response to irradiation, and in general the more cellular the tumour and the more primitive the cell type, the greater the likelihood of radiosensitivity. Their growth is the result of a complex balance between cell production and cell loss. The average time for a human tumour to double in size varies widely: often about 3 months, it may be as short as 1 week in embryonal tumours or as long as several years for *adenocarcinoma. The effect of radiotherapy depends on the relative kinetics and sensitivities of tumour and normal tissues within the beam: after a radiation dose capable of sterilizing a high proportion of malignant cells, an embryonal tumour (with high growth-fraction and cell-loss factor) may regress within days, while a well-differentiated adenocarcinoma with low growth parameters may take months to regress. Large tumours are more difficult to control locally than are small ones, partly because of the number of cells to be sterilized, but also because (from outstripping the blood supply, and spontaneous cell-death) they have regions which are practically anoxic (lacking oxygen) and in which the cells can survive the largest dose of radiation tolerable by normal tissues.

In practice three grades of responsiveness have been recognized. The most sensitive, mainly tumours of embryonal or lymphoid origin, respond to dosage which may be tolerated by a large volume of tissue, and can be treated even when extensive; examples are the primitive tumours of childhood and the *lymphomas (including *Hodgkin's disease). Tumours of moderate radiosensitivity arise mainly in surface epithelium or glands, e.g. *carcinomas of skin, upper respiratory tract, breast, and uterus, and they can be sterilized by high radiation dosage if confined to a reasonable volume. Those of low radiosensitivity are a heterogeneous group including bone *sarcoma, malignant *melanoma, and gastrointestinal cancer, but, by applying recent research, radiotherapy can have an adjunctive role in controlling such tumours after surgery.

The question is often asked as to why courses of radiotherapy have to be so prolonged. Clinical experi-ence over the past 70 years has shown that *fractionation*, the spreading of dose over a period, is more effective than is a single dose in eradicating tumours for a mini-mum of normal tissue damage. Radiobiological studies have revealed the mechanisms by which giving multiple

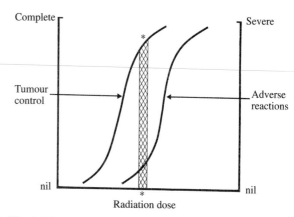

Fig. 2 The degree of tumour control and the adverse responses of normal tissues appear as S-shaped curves when plotted against radiation dose. The skill of the radiation oncologist is to choose a dose regimen (such as *) giving the best differentiation between good and adverse responses.

smaller doses amplifies this therapeutic differential: by repair of cellular injury, repopulation of surviving viable cells, cell-cycle redistribution, and re-oxygenation of the tumour.

The relationship between radiation dose and the probability of curing the tumour is indicated in Fig. 2. There is a threshold dose below which no tumours are controlled but above which control increases steeply. A similar curve applies to normal tissue damage, but dose fractionation and other biological and physical strata-gems displace it to the right. The greater the separation between these curves, the greater the 'therapeutic ratio'. The skill of the radiation oncologist is to select, in the circumstances of the individual patient, an effective dose and technique (such as in Fig. 2) giving optimal differentiation between good and adverse responses.

Present scope and application of radiotherapy

The strategy of treatment of a neoplastic disorder depends essentially on the type of tumour, its patho-logical degree of malignancy, and the extent of spread, while the role of radiotherapy depends additionally on the radiosensitivity of the tumour type relative to that of adjacent tissues. Preliminary clinical and special investi-gations to determine as accurately as possible the extent of spread are thus essential, and at the same time the patient's general condition is assessed.

In certain instances, radiotherapy alone may be the treatment of choice (as in early laryngeal cancer), but it is now frequently administered in association with sur-gery, or with the phased use of *cytotoxic drugs. When combined with surgery it may be given preoperatively to reduce the tumour mass, or postoperatively to sterilize any residual tumour seedlings. *Chemotherapy before irradiation may be used, not only against the whole disease process, but specifically to reduce the mass of tumour (and hence of normal tissue) to be irradiated. However, if such agents are used simultaneously with irradiation, there is considerable risk of enhanced toxicity. With quite a different aim, cytotoxic drugs or hormones may be combined with surgery or radiotherapy to control 'silent' remote deposits (micrometastases) before they become apparent. Multimodal treatment is exemplified in the modern management of breast carcinoma, which involves both the treatment of the tumour to prevent local recurrence and the control of possible blood-borne micrometastases. By depending on the efficacy of megavoltage X-ray therapy and brachytherapy, the initial excisional surgery can be much less extensive, and it is often possible to conserve the breast; in cases deemed from the pathological data to be at risk of metastases, 'adjuvant' chemotherapy may then be administered using a combination of cytotoxics or a hormonal agent such as *Tamoxifen.

Once the full clinical and pathological data are available, the treatment strategy can be defined for the individual patient. The nature of the disorder, what radiotherapy may involve, and the likely reactions are explained at the outset. Unfortunately, the diagnosis and treatment of cancer involve, for both patient and relatives, varying degrees of anxiety and stress which the medical, nursing, and radiographic staff do all in their power to allay. The patient is encouraged to discuss such problems with the consultant and his or her associates, both initially and throughout the course of treatment. In the UK, BACUP (British Association of Cancer United Patients) is a registered charity providing advice and information on all aspects of cancer, as well as emotional support for patients and their families. Their admirable booklet *Understanding radiotherapy* (BACUP 1992) gives informed guidance, with details of the Cancer Information Service and a list of facilities offered by similar organizations, and can be valuable in supplementing advice given verbally.

While superficial skin carcinoma is very successfully treated by medium-voltage X-irradiation, the treatment of deep tumours calls for the use of highly penetrating X-ray beams. Whichever method of radiotherapy may be used to achieve adequate and uniform tumour irradiation while sparing normal tissues, the treatment plan is the end-result of a detailed process taking into account the biological nature of the tumour and its spatial distribution within the body as seen in various cross-sections. This 'treatment planning' is carried out by the radiation oncologist in collaboration with a physicist or radiation dosimetrist (see also PHYSICS, MEDICAL). A 'treatment simulator', a special diagnostic X-ray machine, enables tumour-imaging data (often obtained from *CT and *MR studies) to be related to exact landmarks, and for checks to be made on the final accuracy. When the tumour-bearing area has been delineated, together with the position of 'critical organs', such as the spinal cord or

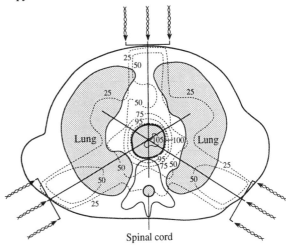

Fig. 3 Composite isodose plan of 8 MeV X-ray therapy for cancer of the oesophagus. Three incident radiation beams summating at the tumour are so arranged as to maximize dose to the 'target volume' and to minimize dose to the vulnerable lungs and spinal cord.

kidneys, which need to be avoided, from data supplied by the planning computer an appropriate technique is selected (Fig. 3).

For small, accessible tumours the most suitable treatment may be *brachytherapy*, the application of radioactive sources within or close to the tumour. The interstitial implantation of tumours such as those of the mouth or breast has been practised successfully for many years, *radium needles now having been superseded by iridium-192 wires or caesium-137 needles for greater geometric accuracy and for ease of personnel protection. In intracavitary therapy for gynaecological tumours such as carcinoma of the *uterus, radioactive sources are placed within the natural body cavities. Also originally carried out with radium, this treatment is now delivered by radiocaesium, or by the Cathetron technique, which uses high-activity cobalt-60 sources.

In contradistinction, the whole body may be irradiated by high-energy X-rays in a single or a few fractions in conjunction with alkylating agents (commonly *cyclophosphamide), in preparation for *bone marrow *transplantation in patients with *leukaemia or lymphoma. The aim is both to produce immunosuppression, to allow allogeneic marrow engraftment, and to eliminate any residual tumour cells, and such treatment can be curative.

The outcome for a given type and site of cancer is mainly related to its stage, and for localized cancer the results of radiotherapy can be highly satisfactory. In early carcinoma of the larynx 80 per cent of irradiated patients are cured and retain a normal voice; a similar proportion of early cases of uterine cervix carcinoma are curable with radiocaesium; and carcinomas of the skin and lip, and those of the anus, are particularly radiocurable. Technical innovation has brought increased cure rates in more advanced tumours, ranging from those of the head and neck to those of the uterus or prostate. While some deeply placed tumours, such as those of the *bladder, frequently respond well, others, for example of the *oesophagus, are difficult to control. Again, in others, such as lung cancer, a satisfactory local response is often vitiated by the appearance of remote *metastases. For such highly responsive conditions as Hodgkin's disease and *seminoma, cure rates of over 90 per cent are regularly reported for early stage disease; both are also highly responsive to cytotoxic drugs, which are employed in more advanced disease, and the role of each modality in the management of an individual patient (following the preliminary staging investigations) has now become well-defined. Irradiation also plays an important part (often in association with chemotherapy) in the cure of childhood cancer, including *medulloblastoma of the brain, *rhabdomyosarcoma of the head and neck or pelvis, *Wilms tumour, *neuroblastoma, and acute leukaemia. With less responsive or more advanced disease, or that with high metastatic potential, irradiation has a prominent role in multimodality curative treatment, e.g. for breast carcinoma, rectal carcinoma, and soft-tissue sarcoma.

When actual cure has not been attained, there may still be valuable long-term relief of symptoms, and especially in head and neck tumours the best palliation may come from a frustrated attempt at cure. Unfortunately about half of the patients presenting at radiotherapy departments have no prospect of cure because of the advanced stage at the outset. Beneficial palliation of symptoms may nevertheless be achieved in a wide variety of situations, ranging from the healing of *ulceration, the rapid relief of pain from bone metastases, to the control of *dysphagia, and the avoidance of *paralysis from spinal deposits.

Prospects

The remarkable development of radiotherapy in recent decades has come not only from clinical studies and the application of physical technology, but also from qualitative and quantitative understanding of the underlying biological processes. Current research builds on the progress achieved by the general application of megavoltage methods, the increased knowledge of tissue tolerances, and the manipulation of dose fractionation. While megavoltage beams can now provide adequate depth doses at any part of the body, one factor limiting the prescribed dose is the volume of normal tissue within a rectangular target volume. If this volume were reduced (without excluding tumour cells) it could reduce the risk of normal tissue damage or permit an increase in radiation dose. This is being investigated with precise three-dimensional imaging and

by using linear accelerators with multi-leaf collimators to obtain 'conformation therapy' with the summated shaped beams. Similar principles are particularly developed in the external stereotactic radiotherapy of small brain tumours (including *angiomas), whereby a high dose of radiation is applied in a small and carefully defined volume.

The overall protraction of treatment and the number, size, and distribution of the individual doses are of critical importance in protecting the host's vasculo-connective tissue and in preventing late radiation damage such as tissue *necrosis. Preferential sparing of such late-responding *normal tissues* is afforded by reducing the radiation dose per fraction: however, some *tumours* may require a larger dose of radiation each day to prevent tumour-cell repopulation during the course of treatment, but such an escalation would increase the risk of tissue damage. A solution is to give several small doses of radiation per day, a promising method known as 'accelerated fractionation', now under trial for the treatment of head and neck tumours.

The prediction of tumour control from a given treatment regimen is based on clinical and pathological features of the tumour (such as site of origin, type and grade, size, morphology, pattern of invasion, and stage), parameters obtained from retrospective studies of groups of cases. It would be helpful to have separate predictive information on the tumour in an individual patient, in the form of intrinsic tumour cell radiosensitivity, metabolic and microenvironmental data, and tumour cell proliferation kinetics and ploidy (see CELL AND CELL BIOLOGY). Flow cytometric methods quantitating responses of human tumour cells to irradiation employ single-cell techniques applicable to biopsy specimens. Important questions are whether *in vitro* tumour measurements can predict local recurrence, e.g. in carcinoma of the cervix, and whether such assay data could form secondary prognostic factors of use in multivariate analysis. The other side of the therapeutic equation concerns the response of the host tissues, which may vary significantly from person to person. *In vitro* cellular sensitivity of fibroblasts has been correlated with such normal tissue responses, and an improved assay could ultimately lead to improved results through a more individual prescription of radiation dose.

Fully oxygenated tumour cells can be sterilized experimentally by about one-third of the dose necessary for anoxic cells, but despite a vast amount of effort it has proved difficult to exploit the 'oxygen effect' clinically. While benefit has been recorded from irradiation of head and neck tumours in *hyperbaric oxygen, the method is difficult to apply generally. Heavy particles, such as neutrons, producing very densely ionizing tracks in tissue, are less dependent on the oxygen effect and can result in increased control of certain tumours (e.g. of *salivary glands and advanced head and neck cancer), but an effect on the 'therapeutic ratio' is still undecided. On the other hand, protons, also produced by the *cyclotron, have achieved an established place in the treatment of melanoma of the eye. Extensive and continuing studies of chemical radiosensitizers of anoxic cells have not yet resulted in determination of a consistent role, their activity being limited by side-effects.

The question of combining radiotherapy with chemotherapy is complicated by the wide variety of drugs and radiotherapeutic schedules that can be associated, always remembering the risk of enhanced toxicity when used in temporal proximity. A number of collaborative clinical trials are in progress in, for instance, carcinoma of the head and neck, cervix and lung, and carcinoma of the rectum.

The complicated interplay with the drug treatment of cancer requires the closest collaboration between the respective specialties, to formulate strategies, investigate interactions, and evaluate results, and this has resulted in much greater understanding of the problems. The major advances in chemotherapy in dealing with diffuse and often widespread disease have nevertheless highlighted the importance of a residually active primary tumour. In contrast to its success in lymphoma and in germ-cell tumours, in few adult solid cancers can the use of cytotoxic drugs alone ablate the primary tumour, without which cure can never be achieved. This has two important implications: with expansion in the use of cytotoxic drugs there will be *pari passu* an increased need for measures dealing with the primary tumour; and accordingly there is every reason for seeking to improve the efficacy of local radiotherapy.

Whatever the form of impending improvements in radiotherapy, it is certain that future advances in the care of patients with cancer will come from multimodal therapy in which the individual agents of surgery, radiation, and cytotoxic drugs will be used to their best advantage in planned schedule—selected not only from knowledge of their effects on groups, but also with reference to the clinical and biological features of the tumour in the individual patient.

ARTHUR JONES

Further reading
BACUP (1992). *Understanding radiotherapy*. BACUP, 3 Bath Place, Rivington Street, London EC2A 3JR, UK.
Moss, W. T. and Cox, J. D. (1989). *Radiation oncology*. Mosby, St Louis.
Perez, C. A. and Brady, L. W. (1992). *Principles and practice of radiation oncology*, (2nd edn). Lippincott, Philadelphia.
Sikora, K. and Halnan, K. E. (ed.) (1990). *Treatment of cancer*, (2nd edn). Chapman and Hall, London.

RADIUM is a naturally occurring radioactive element (symbol Ra; atomic number 88, and, for the most stable isotope, with a half-life of 1620 years, relative atomic mass 226). It is a rare metal, chemically resembling barium. For decades it was used as a source of *beta particles and *gamma rays in *radiotherapy.

RADON is a short-lived radioactive gaseous element (symbol Rn; atomic number 86, and, for the most stable isotope, with a half-life of 3.825 days, relative atomic mass 222). The immediate decay product of *radium, it belongs chemically to the inert (noble) gases.

RAGWORT is the name for various flowering plants of the genus *Senecio* (family Compositae), the commonest species being *S. vulgaris*. Ragwort (or ragweed) pollen is highly allergenic and a common cause of allergic rhinitis (see ALLERGY). The common ragwort has yellow daisy-like flowers and is widely distributed in dry grassland.

RALES are moist bubbling sounds heard on *auscultation of the lungs, coarser than *crepitations, indicating fluid in the air-passages.

RAMAZZINI, BERNARDINO (1633–1714). Italian physician. He was the first physician to be interested in *occupational disease. In *De morbis artificum diatriba* (1700), he described some 40 industrial diseases. He was also a pioneer of *epidemiology.

RAMON Y CAJAL, SANTIAGO (1852–1934). Spanish neuroanatomist. He improved *Golgi's staining methods and studied systematically the microscopic structure of the central nervous system, confirming the *neurone doctrine. His researches were published in Spanish and were not generally available, but they were embodied in his work *Textura del sistema nervioso del hombre y de los vertebrados* (1904). He received the *Nobel prize with *Golgi in 1906.

RAMUS is the anatomical term for a branch.

RANITIDINE is, like *cimetidine, an *H_2 receptor antagonist used to treat *peptic ulcer and other conditions where reduction of gastric acidity is likely to be of benefit, such as *reflux oesophagitis and the *Zollinger–Ellison syndrome. It is more potent than cimetidine, and has fewer side-effects; it does not cause anti-androgen effects such as *gynaecomastia and *impotence.

RANSON, STEPHEN WALTER (1880–1942). American neuroanatomist. He and colleagues demonstrated neural connections between the *hypothalamus and the *pituitary gland.

RANVIER, LOUIS ANTOINE (1835–1922). French anatomist. He wrote a successful textbook of pathology (1869–76), described the constrictions on medullated *nerve fibres (nodes of Ranvier, 1878), and suggested the concept of the *reticuloendothelial system (1900), and the name 'clasmatocyte' for what is now called the *macrophage.

RAPE is sexual intercourse, usually with a woman, but occasionally with a man or child, without consent. See SEXUAL OFFENCES ACTS.

RASH. Any temporary skin eruption.

RAT-BITE FEVER is an uncommon condition occurring under poor sanitary conditions where *rats flourish, due to either of two distinct micro-organisms, *Streptobacillus moniliformis* and *Spirillum minus*. The mortality is low, and the infection responds well to antibiotic treatment.

RATHKE, MARTIN HEINRICH (1763–1860). German embryologist. He is known for Rathke's pouch, a depression in the roof of the embryonic mouth, from the walls of which the anterior hypophysis (*pituitary) is developed.

RATIONALISTS are those who regard reason as the chief source and test of knowledge.

RATIONALIZATION is the mental defence mechanism whereby actions or attitudes are justified after the event by finding reasons for them.

RATS are small rodents of the genus *Rattus*, of which the best known are the black rat (*Rattus rattus*) and the brown rat (*Rattus norvegicus*). They live in close relationship to man and are the vectors of a number of communicable diseases, including *leptospirosis, *plague, *typhus, *relapsing fever, *rat-bite fever, and several forms of *helminthiasis, as well as *food poisoning. Various inbred strains are used as laboratory animals.

RAVITCH, MARK M. (1912–89). An early and prominent American paediatric surgeon. Apart from his surgical prowess, his literary labours were prodigious, including the two-volume history of the American Surgical Association and the editing of the collected papers of Alfred *Blalock.

RAY. The rectilinear path along which directional energy (e.g. electromagnetic, particulate) travels from its source.

RAYNAUD, MAURICE (1834–81). French physician. He described intermittent cyanosis and/or pallor of the extremities very occasionally progressing to gangrene (*Raynaud's disease or phenomenon, 1862).

RAYNAUD'S DISEASE OR PHENOMENON. Raynaud's phenomenon is characterized by intermittent restriction of blood supply to the fingers and toes (and sometimes the ears and nose), most often in response to cold. There is numbness, tingling, pain, and obvious pallor of the affected extremities, occasionally with blueness. Warmth relieves the symptoms after some minutes or hours as the blood vessels dilate again, and this phase may itself be painful. The phenomenon is a nuisance, but rarely harmful; occasionally it is progressive, causing atrophic changes or rarely even *gangrene in the terminal extremities. It may be a symptom of more serious underlying vascular, neurological, or collagen disorder; it may be occupational, classically in those who operate pneumatic drills; or it may be due to the action of certain drugs or chemicals. More often, it is 'idiopathic', i.e. no cause is found, when it is termed 'Raynaud's disease'.

REACTION, in *psychology, is any mental, emotional, or *psychomotor response to the stimulus of an event or situation; in chemistry, it is any process involving chemical change.

REAUMUR, RENE-ANTOINE FERCHAULT DE (1683–1757). French scientist, naturalist, entomologist, and physician. He is mainly remembered for his thermometric scale, now obsolete, which took the freezing point of water as zero but the boiling point as 80°. The *Celsius scale takes the boiling point as 100°.

RECEPTORS. The term 'receptor' is used in two different senses in medicine: first, to describe a specialized nerve ending which detects and responds to a particular stimulus such as touch, light, heat, pain, etc.; secondly, to describe a chemical component of a molecule or cell which has an affinity for a particular substance (e.g. hormone, toxin, antigen, neurotransmitter, etc.) and therefore binds with it, with consequent chemical, immunological, or cellular effects.

RECERTIFICATION. Periodic relicensing of medical practitioners, as required by some states in the USA.

RECESSIVE describes a genetically determined characteristic manifest only in *homozygotes, i.e. individuals who inherit the responsible *gene from both parents. It is not detectable, except sometimes by special tests or in X-linked disorders, in *heterozygotes, who possess only one such gene. See GENETICS.

RECIDIVIST. A habitual criminal, who persistently relapses into crime despite punishment or attempts at reform.

RECKLINGHAUSEN, FRIEDRICH DANIEL VON (1833–1910). German pathologist. Much of his research was on diseases of bone and tumours. He described multiple *neurofibromatosis (1882), adenomyosis of the uterus (1896), and *osteitis fibrosa cystica (1891).

VON RECKLINGHAUSEN'S DISEASE, when otherwise unqualified, is synonymous with multiple *neurofibromatosis; 'von Recklinghausen's disease of bone' is another name for osteitis fibrosa cystica, the bone condition which results from *hyperparathyroidism.

RECOMBINANT DNA TECHNOLOGY. See GENETIC ENGINEERING; GENETICS.

RECORD LINKAGE is the process of combining terms of information or sets of data relating to the same subject but obtained from different sources. The essential requirement of record linkage, which has been developed as a technique of medical epidemiology, is that the individual subject or patient must be uniquely identifiable either by name and other personal data or by a code of some sort. Medical record linkage has been defined as 'the process of bringing together selected data of biological interest for a population commencing with the conception and ending in death, into a series of personal cumulative files, the files being so organized that they can also be assembled in family groups' (Acheson, E. D. (1967), *Medical record linkage*, London.)

RECTUM. The terminal portion of the large intestine, joining the pelvic *colon to the *anus.

RECURRENT LARYNGEAL NERVE. This nerve is an important branch of the *vagus (tenth cranial) nerve; it supplies motor fibres to the intrinsic muscles of the *larynx (except the cricothyroid). Lesions of the nerve cause *dysphonia, and are not uncommon; because of its anatomical course (it leaves the vagus in the thorax and runs upwards into the neck, behind the *thyroid gland), it is vulnerable to damage by neck tumours, bronchial carcinoma, and operations on the thyroid. The nerve on the left side may be damaged by an *aneurysm of the *aortic arch.

RED BLOOD CELL. See ERYTHROCYTE.

RED CRESCENT. In Muslim countries, a red crescent replaces a red cross as the symbol of the International *Red Cross.

RED CROSS, INTERNATIONAL, AND THE BRITISH RED CROSS SOCIETY
The International Red Cross
In July 1859 at Solferino, Italy, a bloody battle raged between Piedmontese, French, and Austrian troops. In one day 40 000 men were killed or seriously injured, and witness to it all was a young Swiss, Henry Dunant. Appalled by the scenes of the helpless injured, Dunant aided the wounded of both sides and persuaded others to help him.

Afterwards Dunant wrote a book, *A memory of Solferino*, pleading for neutral status for the wounded, their carers, and the premises used to house them. He also suggested that countries train volunteers in peacetime to supplement the army in wartime. The book was a great success and in October 1863, the first National Society meeting was held in Geneva. In August 1864 the first Geneva Convention was signed. It was at this meeting that the Red Cross symbol was adopted. In 1919 the International Red Cross extended its activities to help the victims of natural disasters. By 1983, the International Red Cross's 120th anniversary, the movement had over 200 million members and practically every independent state in the world was a signatory to the Geneva Convention.

Although National Red Cross Societies are autonomous, they are bound by the principles and statutes of the Red Cross. National societies are involved in peacetime programmes appropriate to that country's need. Primary health care is an important aspect in most societies, while other main services range from blood donation to welfare services.

The British Red Cross
The British Red Cross, founded in 1870, was first known as the National Society for Aid to the Sick and Wounded in War. Its first task was to give help in the Franco-Prussian war. In 1880 the first group of eight nurses went to the military hospital in Netley, to be trained for wartime nursing duty. In 1882, the Foreign Office made its first request for Red Cross nurses to go to Egypt.

The society became the British Red Cross in 1905, at which time the relationship it had with the military medical services was informal. Official status was conferred when the Territorial and Reserve Forces Act defined its role as that of 'providing supplementary aid to the Territorial Medical Services to meet the needs of war'.

During the First World War, Voluntary Aid Detachments (VADs) of both men and women served on the battlefield, helping the injured, and in convalescent homes, helping the wounded recover. The role played during the Second World War was different: Red Cross personnel concentrated on welfare operations for prisoners of war. The all-Swiss International Committee of the Red Cross was able to visit camps and ensure that the parcels and messages sent to all prisoners of war (POWs) were being received.

Since the end of the 1939–45 war the British Red Cross has been able to focus more on domestic projects and international aid and welfare programmes. Domestically, the British Red Cross is now involved in much more than traditional first aid. There are now five key areas of work on which the society centres its efforts in the UK.

(1) The community programme provides: first-aid cover at events, large or small; an escort service to enable housebound people to make journeys which would otherwise be impossible; medical equipment such as wheelchairs and bedrests on short-term loan to people in urgent need; boost to the morale of sick and elderly people in hospitals, homes, and day-care support. Many other services are organized according to local need.

(2) The British Red Cross provides training courses in first aid for members and the public. Courses

in nursing, welfare, and other care skills are also available.
(3) Each branch has a team of highly trained members ready to respond to unexpected local or national emergencies. Members have provided first aid, transport, escort, or comfort for the survivors, bereaved relatives, and rescuers in almost all the technological accidents, floods, and storms which have occurred in Britain in recent years.
(4) The development of knowledge and skills for youth members which can be applied to service in the community.
(5) International tracing services work to reunite close relatives who have been separated through war or natural disaster.

Internationally, the British Red Cross is involved in aid and welfare programmes. The provision of emergency assistance to the victims of war, conflict, and natural disasters remains a priority. Where possible, schemes are now being initiated to prevent the worst excesses of foreseeable events, such as crop failure or monsoon.

The society operates through local branches in England, Scotland, Wales, Northern Ireland, the Channel Islands, the Isle of Man, and the UK's remaining colonies and dependencies. The society's governing body is the council, which is responsible for its policies, for the formation of branches, and for presenting the conditions of membership. The trustees who manage the society's affairs, at national and local level, discharge all the responsibilities laid down by law on charity trustees (see CHARITIES ACT, 1992). It relies on donations from the public to pay for training its members, and maintaining its services.

JAMES M. MURRAY

REDI, FRANCESCO (1626–97/8). Italian physician and a pioneer parasitologist. In 1668 he disproved the widely held belief in the spontaneous generation of insects, showing that maggots developed from eggs laid by flies. He made valuable studies of *toxicology and *snake venoms.

RED TIDE is a red discoloration of sea water due to the presence of enormous numbers of dinoflagellates, *protozoal organisms of the order Dinoflagellata, class Phytomastigophora. Red tides may be very destructive of fish and invertebrate life; species of the genus *Gonyaulax* are neurotoxic, and their ingestion by bivalve molluscs leads to 'paralytic shellfish poisoning' in man, a severe form of food poisoning which may be fatal following, for example, the investigation of mussels. The neurotoxic alkaloid involved is saxitoxin.

REED, WALTER (1851–1902). American military medical officer. In 1898 he was appointed head of a medical commission to Cuba, charged with study of the cause and mode of transmission of *yellow fever, which was causing serious morbidity and mortality among American troops. By 1900, using human volunteers (members of the commission and soldiers), Reed's group established that the disease is contracted by the bite of an infected mosquito. This led directly to control of the disease in Cuba, and, shortly thereafter, in Panama, by eliminating mosquito breeding places. It is believed that the Panama Canal could not have been built without control of yellow fever. (See also TROPICAL MEDICINE.)

REFLEX. Any involuntary or automatic response to a stimulus. The nervous pathway mediating a reflex is termed a reflex arc and represents a circuit by which the *receptor, which has been stimulated, is connected to the effector organ, which responds.

REFLEX ARC. See REFLEX.

REFLUX. Retrograde flow.

REFLUX OESOPHAGITIS (ESOPHAGITIS) is inflammation of the lower part of the *oesophagus caused by regurgitation of gastric contents containing acid and *pepsin. See also HEARTBURN, HIATUS HERNIA.

REFRACTION is the deflection of light waves as they pass from one medium to another of different optical density, the deflection occurring at the boundary between the two.

REFRACTIVE ERROR is any impairment of the lens function of the eyes, such as *myopia, *hypermetropia, *presbyopia, etc. See OPHTHALMOLOGY.

REFSUM, SIGVALD (1907–91). Norwegian neurologist. He succeeded *Monrad-Krohn in the chair of neurology at Oslo in 1954. In 1946 he described in his MD thesis a disease which he called heredopathia atactica polyneuritiformis, now called *Refsum's disease. He was President of the World Federation of Neurology from 1973 to 1981.

REFSUM'S DISEASE is a rare *recessive disorder associated with an inability to metabolize a particular *fatty acid (phytanic acid). The chief manifestations are motor and sensory *neuropathy, *deafness, *ataxia, *retinal degeneration, *cardiomyopathy, and *ichthyosis. A diet free of derivatives of *chlorophyll is of value in treatment.

REGENERATION is the replacement or regrowth of a substance or structure in its original form and by natural processes.

REGIMEN. A course of diet, exercise, or mode of living prescribed for health reasons.

REGIMEN SANITATIS SALERNITANUM. The *Salernitan guide to health* is a famous and popular work of the

12th century *Salerno school of medicine, probably by several authors. Written in verse, the *Guide* appeared in many versions, editions, and translations, one of which includes the well-known couplet:

> Use three physicians still, first Doctor Quiet,
> Next Doctor Merryman and Doctor Diet.

The *Guide* was essentially a home medical handbook. It is said to have been written for the crusader, Robert, Duke of Normandy, when he visited Salerno.

REGIONAL ANAESTHESIA. See LOCAL ANAES-THESIA.

REGIONAL ILEITIS. See CROHN'S DISEASE.

REGISTRAR. One whose responsibility it is to maintain records. In many organizations in the UK, such as universities and the *General Medical Council, for example, the registrar is the chief administrative officer. In the context of hospital medicine in the UK, a registrar is a doctor undergoing further training with a view eventually to attaining consultant status, that is to becoming a recognized specialist in one of the branches of medicine. 'Registrar', when otherwise unqualified, denotes a person usually in the third or fourth year following graduation in medicine (second or third year following full registration), whereas a 'senior registrar' is already likely to have served as a registrar for 2 years and to be undertaking a final period of training and preparation while awaiting a *consultant post. The former grade of 'junior registrar' has been replaced by 'senior house officer'. The fact that many present-day registrars complete and ensure the accuracy of case-records recalls the origin of the term. See MEDICAL EDUCATION, POST-GRADUATE AND CONTINUING.

REGISTRAR GENERAL. An officer who superintends registration of all births, deaths, and marriages in England and Wales. He is appointed by the Queen under the Registration Service Act 1953, which obliges him to supply registrars of births and deaths with durable register books, strong fire-resisting storage boxes, and forms for certified copies. The Registrar General is also responsible for making arrangements for a population census when an Order in Council made by the Queen so directs. See also OFFICE OF POPULATION, CENSUSES, AND SURVEYS.

REGISTRARS OF BIRTHS AND DEATHS. Under the UK Registration Service Act 1953, each county, or other local council is obliged to make a scheme, known as 'the local scheme', for the organization of the registration service in its area and to have the scheme approved. The area of each council is divided into districts and subdistricts. For each district, a superintendent registrar of births, deaths, and marriages is appointed, and for each subdistrict a registrar of births and deaths, who may also have conferred on him by the local scheme the function of a registrar of marriages for the purposes of the Marriage Act 1949. A registrar of births and deaths in England and Wales must register the birth of every child within his subdistrict within 6 weeks of its occurrence. Deaths must also be registered within a similar period.

REGISTRATION in UK medicine is a responsibility of the *General Medical Council (GMC), the statutory professional body which governs the professional standards and conduct of doctors. Registration involves keeping the *Medical Register* which is the official reference of enquiry as to whether a person is qualified in medicine or not. Unless a doctor's name is on the *Register*, he is precluded from filling a public office, from using dangerous drugs, from signing death certificates, and from performing certain other duties such as the issue of statutory certificates. Registration requires satisfactory completion of a course of study approved by the GMC. After the final graduating examination, provisional registration is granted. Before the student proceeds to full registration, he or she must work as a house officer for 1 year in a recognized hospital, 6 months in surgery and 6 months in medicine (with certain alternatives). Registration of Commonwealth and foreign medical graduates wishing to work in the UK is also the responsibility of the GMC. An indicative (i.e. non-compulsory) register of completion of specialist training has been introduced recently.

In other countries, registration of medical graduates is sometimes carried out by a similar national body, sometimes by ministries or departments of health, sometimes by registration authorities of individual states (as in the USA, Canada, and Australia), and sometimes by local medical associations.

REGISTRATION ACT 1836. The Births and Deaths Registration Act 1836 was an enactment which provided for the registration of births, deaths, and marriages in England. It has been superseded by subsequent Acts, the latest being the Births and Deaths Registration Act 1953.

REGURGITATION is retrograde flow, particularly referring to the return of swallowed food and drink into the mouth or to the backwards leakage of blood across an incompetent cardiac valve (e.g. mitral regurgitation, aortic regurgitation).

REHABILITATION. The word 'rehabilitation' has many uses. It can be applied to things as diverse as crumbling buildings, convicted prisoners, frail old ladies, disgraced politicians, and soldiers injured in battle. The word conjures up a picture of restoring, renovating, and reclothing an object of misfortune so that it regains its previous function and identity. In *medical practice, the word is both more technical and broader in its meaning. The sense of optimism is retained, but medical rehabilitation concerns not only people who are getting better from an illness or an injury, but people whose disability can be prevented from getting worse, or whose rate of deterioration can be slowed by a programme of treatment and training. Medical rehabilitation does its best not to stigmatize disabled people as objects as misfortune, and seeks to help them establish or re-establish full independence.

Rehabilitation has been defined by the *World Health Organization (WHO) as the application of all measures aimed at reducing the impact of disabling and handicapping conditions and enabling disabled and handicapped people to achieve social integration. This definition draws attention to the importance of changing the environment and behaviour of non-disabled people in achieving such integration. The term is also used in a different and more personal sense to denote a process of active change by which a person who has become disabled acquires the knowledge and skills needed for optimal physical, psychological, and social function. That definition implies that some development of personal capacities has taken place.

Traditionally, medicine has adopted a 'bio-medical model' of disability, in which the aim of rehabilitation is to restore a person's physical or psychological functions to as near the 'normal' or non-disabled condition as possible. However, such an aim is not necessarily espoused by the disabled person, who may feel devalued by being categorized as a rehabilitation failure and would prefer to be valued as a human being who happens to have a physical or cognitive impairment that he or she might or might not wish to change. The contrasting 'social model' of disability defines the social and day-to-day difficulties experienced by disabled people more neutrally as a mis-match between their abilities and their environment. An environment that is hostile to disabled people, such as one which has many steps, nowhere to sit down, and poor signposts, is there by virtue of connivance by non-disabled people. By creating such an environment they have excluded those with disabilities from participation. That such environments are not inevitable is demonstrated by the large stores that have become fashionable in developed countries in recent years which have ready access for children in pushchairs and frail elderly people, with gentle slopes and electrically operated doors to encourage mothers with pushchairs to use them. Why are these features not standard for all social venues, so that wheelchair-dependent people could have open access to them? Since many disabilities cannot be reversed, the 'bio-medical' model of disability is criticized for implying that it is the duty of the disabled person to change, thus reinforcing prejudice in society at large.

Medical rehabilitation

Those involved in medical rehabilitation recognize the importance of these arguments but see their contribution as helping to optimize the disabled person's ability to function autonomously, by integrating medical and surgical treatments with therapy, training, and the use of specialized or adapted equipment.

Theoretically, rehabilitation is part-and-parcel of the process of convalescence from all medical and surgical treatment. For example, the Act of Parliament establishing the UK *National Health Service specified prevention, treatment, and rehabilitation as its three principal elements. In the event, perhaps because of the dominant influence of the medical profession, treatments using drugs or surgery have been more successful in attracting resources than treatments that relieve suffering or disability by other means. Research, training, and the allocation of resources for the non-medical therapies have tended to lag behind, and have been weakly linked to the basic sciences needed to underpin and develop them. In most developed countries, rehabilitation medicine has therefore emerged as a medical specialty for the treatment of people with established disabilities that are particularly complex, or whose management requires a high degree of technical skill and integrated work by a number of professions, including medicine.

Attitudes to disability and patterns of disablement in different countries

Since the aim of rehabilitation is to help the disabled person assume or re-assume his or her role in society, the objectives that are actually selected are crucially dependent upon the nature of the society in which the person lives. In some cultures, disability brings shame on the family and is something to be hidden away. Treatment may contain elements of punishment and exclusion for the patient. The way the disability is managed may also reflect the social status of the patient. Thus, a man whose judgements, memory, and ability to make consistent decisions have been impaired by traumatic brain injury would be treated as an outcast in many developing countries of Africa. However, in an Arabic state, where the head of the household is afforded special status and privileges, his position in the household would be upheld and it would be the duty of his family to accommodate his eccentricities with the minimum of protest. Most developed Western countries would adopt an approach somewhere between these extremes, and would aim to guide the patient to a greater insight into his behaviour. Concurrently, the other members of the family would be encouraged to reflect the realities of the situation to the patient and to negotiate appropriate changes in his behaviour.

Another contrast, this time between two highly developed countries, Japan and the USA, demonstrates the range of different attitudes to frailty and disability in elderly people. In the USA, as in western Europe, many elderly people live alone (or at least apart from their children) and are fiercely independent. They see it as one of their rights to be helped to maintain this independence. In Japan, by contrast, many couples on retirement expect to move in with the family of their eldest son. Their daughter-in-law both expects and is expected to care for them if they become ill or frail. Frailty and illness are both managed traditionally by retiring to bed. Thus approximately 10 per cent of the Japanese population over the age of 70 years in 1992 were 'bed-bound'. It is self-evident that the objectives and expectation of rehabilitation for an elderly disabled person are very different in the two countries, despite the availability of similar professional expertise in both.

Further intriguing contrasts emerge when the physical measures needed to enable a wheelchair-dependent person to remain independent in the same two countries are considered. Japanese houses tend to be smaller than North American ones and have traditional layouts and floor coverings that have considerable social and cultural significance, embracing concepts of etiquette and hygiene. It is impossible to travel in the same wheelchair from the front door, through the living area and into the toilet of a traditional Japanese house without transgressing important rules. Either a much more complicated mode of progression has to be introduced, or 'Western style' furnishings adopted, which may impose an additional social disability on the whole family.

Causes of disability

Quite apart from such important cultural factors, both the causes of disability and the resources available to overcome it are fundamentally different in developing and developed countries. *Infection and *trauma are major causes of disability in developing countries. It has been estimated that appropriate *public health measures and effective treatment of infections would prevent two-thirds of all cases of disability world-wide.

In developed countries, chronic disorders contribute to a much larger proportion of cases, and the percentage of people with a disease who are disabled by it is greatest for neurological diseases. Thus, in the population of the UK approximately 80 per cent of those with *stroke, *parkinsonism, or *multiple sclerosis are disabled, compared with 14 per cent of those with *arthritis. However, four times more people in the UK are disabled by arthritis, because arthritis is 20 times more prevalent than the three neurological disorders combined.

For all age-groups in all countries, combinations of physical and mental impairment cause a far greater degree of dependency than either physical or mental impairment alone. A large survey of the UK population conducted between 1986 and 1988 showed that 14 per cent of the population have a disability of some kind. Most of these disabilities were relatively mild, but severe disability was shown to become increasingly common with advancing age. This is because of the combined effects of frailty and the various degenerative diseases which commonly occur at that time of life. Thus, in developed countries, where the population has a long life expectancy, two-thirds of all disabled people are over the age of retirement, and many of the services geared to rehabilitation and support of disabled people have been designed primarily for those beyond retirement age.

However, younger disabled people have very different social aspirations and thus different objectives for their rehabilitation. The most successful model of medical rehabilitation of younger people was the service developed for spinal injury by Ludwig Guttman at Stoke Mandeville Hospital in England in the 1950s. By meticulous attention to detail, refinement in treatment, and comprehensive training in self-care and personal independence, the life expectancy of people recovering from spinal injury was transformed from 18 months in 1950 to 30 years or more by 1980.

However, not all young disabled people have seen such improvements in the services available. Many problems are still encountered by those suffering lasting cognitive impairment as a result of head injury. Special difficulties are also encountered by those with congenital disability, because their education is often interrupted by the time spent in coping with the disability, and they are unable ever to establish their potential in society or to amass the personal wealth that is available to adults who become disabled only after years of paid employment.

Basic objectives for rehabilitation

Therapy is directed towards restoring independence in daily life at home, then in moving outside the home and participating in social activities, and then (usually) in employment and recreation. The precise objectives, and the therapy and training needed to meet them, will depend upon the patient's pattern of impairment and aspirations.

Objectives are most often formulated in relation to independent mobility, independence in personal care (washing, dressing, and continence), *communication with others, the management or avoidance of *pain, and the development of physical and mental stamina. When disturbances of cognitive function or behaviour are present, they often confer a much greater handicap than coexisting physical disabilities. It is essential that these 'invisible' impairments receive appropriate attention.

Another set of objectives relates to the selection and use of special equipment. Some of this equipment may be applied to the patient, for example, to replace a missing part (a prosthesis) or to stabilize or guide the movement of the limbs or trunk (an orthosis). A much more extensive range of equipment is available to help the disabled person to react more effectively with the environment. Ideally, all such equipment should be specifically tailored to the patient's needs, and training in its use is usually essential.

Principles of rehabilitation practice

Some principles involved in medical rehabilitation are summarized below, taking as an example a disability that has been acquired suddenly in adult life.

1. The *prognosis (probable outcome) of the condition must be accurately defined, together with an estimate of the effects that therapy will have in improving function and in preventing deterioration or other complications. This assessment will inevitably need to take account of the person's attributes and expectations.

2. This information must be communicated effectively to the patient and, normally, to the family. Any disputed aspects of interpretation or prediction need to be resolved. Comprehensive information must be provided. Reaching a consensus may take time and often has to proceed concurrently with the early stages of treatment.

3. A set of long-term aims and short-term objectives is then agreed with the patient (and, as appropriate, with the family), through discussion and negotiation.

4. A programme of therapy and training is then given according to an agreed timetable.

5. If the disability or the treatment needed is particularly complex, these aims and objectives must be espoused by the whole of the rehabilitation team. The therapy needs to be reinforced. Thus the ability to dress one's own top half independently, for example, or to communicate effectively, should be encouraged and not restricted to periods during which 'formal therapy' is being given.

6. Delays in moving on to the next objective or stage of treatment must be minimized. This is often a difficulty when the person has to transfer from one environment to another, for example, from a hospital rehabilitation ward back to their home, or from a hospital-based out-patient therapy department to an employment retraining centre.

7. It is essential to establish a relationship of personal trust between the patient and those who are trying to help. Skilled listening and recognition of the validity of the patient's feelings are essential. This too may take a long time. If the patient shows obvious denial or underlying fear or anger, support must continue to be given in the hope that these feelings will eventually be recognized and worked through.

Medical rehabilitation teams and teamwork
A wide range of skills has developed in several professions which make an essential contribution to rehabilitation. They include, in alphabetical order: clinical *psychology, education and employment training, medicine, nursing, occupational therapy, orthotics and prosthetics, physiotherapy, psychotherapies (including a very wide range of practice from counselling to analytical psychotherapy and the arts-based therapies), rehabilitation engineering, *social work, and speech and language therapy.

Each of these professions has a potential part to play in assessing the disabled person's condition and estimating the probable response to treatment, preventing unwanted consequences of the disability, and providing treatment or training to help overcome it. A brief guide to the work of some of these professions is given in Table 1.

It is clear that rehabilitation is quite different from other branches of medicine in that treatment is effective only in so far as the disabled person is willing to accept it and able to co-operate. A medical condition such as raised *blood pressure can be readily controlled with the simple expedient of taking tablets regularly. The changes are then brought about by a drug without further effort on behalf of the patient. Rehabilitation, by contrast, often means the patient adopting time-consuming procedures each day and practising skills that require the sort of concentration and commitment usually associated with learning to play a musical instrument. Just as a musical instrument has to be practised regularly to maintain the player's skill, so a disabled person may need to continue to adopt regular 'maintenance training' in order to maintain the gains that have been achieved through therapy.

In many cases, a person's disability is circumscribed. Hence, contact with only one profession may be needed and the necessity of teamwork between the professions does not arise. However, for more complex cases, medical treatment needs to be integrated with the acquisition of specific skills and the provision of detailed information; specialized equipment and training are used, and adjustments are made in the life of the family and the home environment of the patient. The plethora of assistance available as listed in Table 1 can help the disabled person achieve excellent rehabilitation—but if badly organized, will leave him and his family confused, demoralized, and angry. The pitfalls of such large teams are that if team management and teamwork skills are poor, its various members will work to different objectives, competing with each other and giving conflicting advice. There will be a tendency for physical elements of a person's disability to be concentrated upon to the exclusion of the psychological or social ones, which are actually more disabling. Patients may find their personal wishes brushed aside in the pursuit of biological excellence. If no one member of the team takes responsibility for the package of help that is provided, the patient is likely to feel increasingly disempowered.

Effective teamwork requires clear guidelines, agreed working practices, supervision and support for its members, clear allocation of responsibilities, and leadership. A pattern of work in which each member acts as an independent contractor must be avoided.

Various patterns of teamworking are currently being evaluated. 'Multidisciplinary' working implies that each profession performs within its traditional boundaries, collaborating at the boundary with the others. 'Interdisciplinary' implies sharing work and responsibilities across professional boundaries, with responsibility for segments of the treatment being retained by individual

Table 1 Illustration of some of the areas of assessment, prevention, and treatment in which individual members of rehabilitation teams have particular skills and experience

Profession	Aspects of patient that are assessed	Complications of disability that are to be prevented	Treatment or service given
Arts-based therapies (art, music, and drama therapy)	Capacity for expression of feelings and non-verbal communication; need for such forms of communication and for emotional and creative expression	Withdrawal, isolation, depression, apathy	Encouragement to enjoy creative communication in a supportive environment; facilitation of the expression of feeling, hopes, fears, anger, and loneliness
Clinical psychology	Cognitive strengths and weaknesses; appropriateness of behaviour	Deterioration of behaviour and other functions due to lack of understanding or cognitive impairment; social isolation; stress in relatives	Educating and informing patients of cognitive strengths and weaknesses; negotiating objectives and appropriate strategies for improving performance and circumventing cognitive deficits; modifying behaviour
Medicine	Overall prognosis; interaction between any diseases present and disabilities; interaction between the various treatments being employed; overview of patients' overall expectations, objectives and need for information	Medical complications of underlying disease or of continuing disability; side-effects of medication; contradictory advice from team	Explanation of prognosis with and without treatment; advice on avoidance of complications; giving and monitoring of medical treatment; negotiation of disagreements between team members if necessary; clinical responsibility for the service provided by the team as a whole
Occupational therapy	Dependency and prospects for independence in essential activities of daily living; the disabled person's environment; selection of appropriate equipment and adaptations of environment	Dependency and loss of autonomy; unnecessary restriction of activities; loss of fitness and function, especially of upper limbs; misuse of equipment; avoidable accidental injury; social isolation	Training in the performance of daily living activities using different techniques or specialized equipment; supervision of environmental adaptations and provision of equipment; training in basic activities needed for recreation, social interaction, and employment; training in practical tasks affected by cognitive impairment using appropriate cognitive strategies

Table 1 (*cont.*)

Profession	Aspects of patient that are assessed	Complications of disability that are to be prevented	Treatment or service given
Physiotherapy	Impairment of mobility; certain forms of musculoskeletal pain; posture; physical fitness	Deformities associated with immobility, muscle spasm, or paralysis; loss of muscle strength and physical fitness due to immobility or disuse; pain resulting from inappropriate physical activity and poor posture; avoidable accidental injury; dependency	Mobilization of joints; stretching of muscles; acquisition of motor skills, especially in relation to mobility and muscular strength; building up stamina; advice on mobility aids
Rehabilitation engineering	Possibility of engineering solutions to current or anticipated problems; review of current equipment, especially in relation to mobility and interaction with environment	Use of inappropriate or potentially dangerous equipment; unnecessary expenditure of time and resources on problems to which there is a ready engineering solution	Provision of appropriate equipment or specific adaptations to current equipment or to environment, and guidance on training requirements
Speech and language therapy	Disorders of swallowing, voice production, speech, communication, and the use of language; assessment of suitability for communication aids and specialized communication equipment	Aspiration into the lungs due to impairment of swallowing; isolation, dependency, and frustration	Helping the patient understand the nature of the defects; providing practice in overcoming or avoiding them; exercises to improve articulation and clarity of speech; practice in communication, both verbal and non-verbal; selection of appropriate equipment and training in use of specialized communication equipment; education of family and others wishing to communicate with the patient

members. 'Transdisciplinary' implies shared responsibility and application of therapies without being restricted by professional boundaries, undertaken to an agreed programme by any member of the team, while formally recognizing that the special skills and experience of each discipline are resources for the other members.

Impairment, disability, handicap, and need

The World Health Organization's definition of impairment, disability, and handicap provides a useful conceptual framework for rehabilitation. Impairment is the loss of a part of a function. Disability is the inability to perform a function in the manner or to the level considered normal for a human being. Handicap is the restriction of the social role that would otherwise be considered normal for the disabled person, allowing for cultural factors.

Handicap is a broad and complex concept, since, as we have seen, major restrictions of social role often result more from the environment or from the prejudice of non-disabled people than from impairment or disability *per se*.

'Need' is even harder to define. There is a difference between wanting something and needing it, but the border between these two concepts is often hotly disputed. Need has to be assessed from at least three perspectives—that of the disabled person, the main family or carer, and of the rehabilitation professional. Because of the potential for interaction among different disabilities and the unique situation of each individual, impairments, disabilities, handicaps, and needs cannot accurately be predicted from each other. For example, impairment of control of the detrusor muscle of the bladder does not *necessarily* lead to the disability of incontinence. Mild incontinence does not *necessarily* lead to handicap. The only way of establishing the *needs* of a person with detrusor instability is purposefully to make a specific assessment of what they are, based on an analysis of the particular case.

Environments for rehabilitation

It is rarely possible to pursue rehabilitation effectively in an environment that is geared primarily to acute medical or surgical treatment. The surroundings need to encourage social interaction, flexibility of therapy programmes, and the exercise of autonomy in day-to-day life. Ideally, rehabilitation should be conducted in the environment in which the disabled person is hoping to live or work. This ideal should not be lost sight of, but in practice a compromise has to be reached with the cost and logistics of deploying the expertise and other resources that are required. In addition, recently disabled patients may need time to become accustomed to their new situation before facing up to an environment that may be rather ill-prepared for them.

Community-based rehabilitation

Because of scarcity of resources, developing countries are establishing a pattern of practice that can achieve real gains at relatively low cost. Recognizing that there are simply not enough professional staff to provide the therapy that is needed, selected members of the local population are trained in very basic principles of assessment and management of the commonest forms of disability, without attempting to incorporate advanced technology or complex medical or surgical procedures. Health promotion and secondary prevention are important parts of this work. A trained member of staff responsible for a region visits towns and villages on a regular basis, providing basic training, advice, and monitoring for lay volunteers. These volunteers can monitor events and consult regularly with professional staff as they visit. Local technology can be adopted to solve certain problems—for example, a basic artificial leg made from local materials is far better than no prosthesis at all. This dissemination of appropriate attitudes and basic skills could perhaps bring about gradual changes in general attitudes to disability and disabled people that might, in the long term, release their potential even more effectively than the individual treatment given.

Conclusion

Medical rehabilitation had its origins in the retraining given to injured servicemen during the First World War which, to everyone's surprise, enabled infantrymen to recover from their injuries faster than the officers who were receiving gentler treatment. Since that time, considerable improvements have occurred in medical treatment, therapies, and equipment, and the specialty of rehabilitation medicine has grown up to assist the rehabilitation of people with particularly complex disabilities. In the past 15 years there has been a fundamental shift in general attitudes towards disability, especially in developed countries, with the beginnings of a general recognition of the need to make society fully accessible to people whose impairments cannot be reversed. New research methodologies have been developed, mainly by cognitive and behavioural psychology, which have opened the way to definitive scientific research into the mechanisms and effectiveness of the various treatments employed in rehabilitation. In some countries, undergraduate training of all the various caring professions now takes place in universities where it is more effectively integrated with the work of the scientific and academic community. This has allowed rehabilitation to become a respectable academic discipline. However, until these changes are accompanied by corresponding improvements in the attitude of non-disabled people towards those who are disabled, neither disabled people's potential contribution to society nor their potential for personal fulfilment will be fully realized.

D. L. McLELLAN

Further reading

Gianutsos, R. and Gianutsos, J. (1987). Single-case experimental approaches to the assessment of interventions in rehabilitation psychology. In *Rehabilitation psychology*, (ed. B. Caplan). Aspen Corporation, Rockville, MD.

Kottke, F. J. and Lehmann, F. F. (ed.) (1990). *Krusen's handbook of physical medicine and rehabilitation*, (4th edn). W. B. Saunders, Philadelphia.

Martin, J., Mettzer, H., and Elliot, D. (1988). *The prevalence of disability among adults*. OPCS Surveys of Disability in Great Britain, Report 1. HMSO, London.

The national concept of rehabilitation medicine. Proceedings of a conference of the Disablement Services Authority and the Royal College of Physicians of London (1991). Royal College of Physicians, London.

REICHERT, KARL BOGISLAUS (1811–83). German anatomist. He introduced the cell theory into *embryology and made valuable studies of the germ layers.

REIL, JOHANN CHRISTIAN (1759–1813). German physician. He described the *insula (island of Reil) in the brain, and was a leading medical educator, but later immersed himself in nature-philosophy and metaphysical speculation. He died of *typhus acquired while in charge of a military *lazarette.

REINFORCEMENT. The strengthening of a response to a stimulus by some means.

REINNERVATION. The attachment or growth of a living nerve into a denervated and paralysed muscle with the object of restoring its function.

REITER, HANS (1881–1969). German physician. Reiter described the *sexually transmitted disease now named after him (see REITER'S SYNDROME).

REITER'S SYNDROME is the association of *non-specific urethritis, *conjunctivitis, and *polyarthritis, occurring most commonly in young men and usually of venereal origin with a similar aetiological pattern to that of non-specific urethritis itself. The causal agent is unknown.

REJECTION is the process by which the body destroys tissue which has been transplanted into it, unless the donated tissue is genetically identical (syngeneic) with that of the host, or unless the host's *immune system is depressed. Rejection serves as a defence against invasion by pathogenic micro-organisms but is a major obstacle to successful organ *transplantation. Except for incompatible *blood transfusion, where immediate rejection results due to pre-existing host *antibody to *antigens on the transfused cells (ABO antigens), rejection is caused by host reaction to the major histocompatibility (MHC) antigens on the surface of the transplanted cells (see HLA). The host lymphocytes (T and/or B cells, with their non-specific adjuncts such as complement and macrophages) attack the graft; antibody generated by B cells destroys free cells and

vascular endothelium, initiating inflammation; while T cells attack solid tissue directly or via macrophages. The experience gained with kidney grafting has shown that rejection can be classified as: immediate, due to ABO incompatibility or MHC presensitization; acute (weeks or months), due to B-cell (antibody) or T-cell response to MHC antigens; or chronic (months to years), usually due to immune complex deposition. Immunosuppressive drugs nevertheless now enable the successful survival of many transplants other than those from identical twins. Tissues such as cornea and cartilage, which do not naturally contain blood vessels, are not normally rejected after transplantation. See GENETICS; IMMUNOLOGY; TRANSPLANTATION.

REJUVENATION is the restoration of youthfulness, or of some of the mental or physical characteristics of youth: the aim and claim of innumerable popular remedies.

RELAPSE. The recurrence of illness after partial or complete remission.

RELAPSING FEVER is an infection marked by recurrent fever, in which haemorrhage and jaundice are common, due to *spirochaetal organisms of the genus *Borrelia*. There are two forms, with different *arthropod vectors; epidemic or louse-borne relapsing fever, due to *B. recurrentis* and transmitted from person to person (there is no animal reservoir) by the *body louse *Pediculus humanus humanus*; and endemic or tick-borne relapsing fever due to various *Borrelia* species, notably *B. duttoni*, which is primarily a *zoonosis and is transmitted to man by various *tick species of the genus *Ornithodorus*. The former infection is world-wide, whereas the distribution of the latter is determined by that of the tick vectors and is restricted to certain endemic regions, mostly tropical and subtropical. Louse-borne relapsing fever is internationally *notifiable to the *World Health Organization.

RELAXATION is a lessening of muscular tension or tone, which occurs when muscular contraction has ceased. Total relaxation can be achieved by preventing excitatory nervous stimuli from reaching the muscles. Drugs such as *curare have this effect, and are often used with general anaesthesia to facilitate surgical operations; since spontaneous breathing is then no longer possible, pulmonary ventilation must be artificial. The severe and life-threatening muscular contractions of *tetanus can be similarly controlled. The word 'relaxation' is also used to mean lessening of mental and emotional 'tension'. Here the group of drugs known as '*tranquillizers' may be of value.

RELIGIO MEDICI was the first published work (1642) of Sir Thomas *Browne, believed to have been written during the 4 years he was engaged in medical practice in Oxford (1634–37) before he settled at Norwich in 1637. *Religio medici* is essentially an examination and an affirmation of Browne's religious faith, a private document written, it is said, without any thought of publication, this being forced by the appearance of a pirated version.

REM (roentgen equivalent man) is the unit dose of ionizing radiation that gives the same biological effect as that due to 1 roentgen of *X-rays. In the case of beta particles, and gamma and X-radiations, the rem is equivalent to the rad, which is equivalent to an energy absorption by irradiated tissue of 0.01 joule per kilogram. The rad has now been supplanted by the gray (Gy): 1 Gy=100 rad. See RADIATION, IONIZING; RADIOTHERAPY.

REMEDIAL GYMNASTS. A small group of UK professionals who use graduated gymnastic methods to treat musculoskeletal disorders; they merged with the physiotherapists in 1986.

REMEDY. Any means of counteracting a disease process.

REMISSION. Temporary abatement of the manifestations of a disease.

REM (RAPID EYE MOVEMENTS) SLEEP is a phase of normal sleep, also known as 'paradoxical sleep'. During this period, rapid eye movements, *hypotonia, muscle twitching, and dreaming occur; it is an essential component of human sleep. REM sleep is cyclical and refreshing and normally accounts for about 25 per cent of the normal night, although this proportion may be varied by the administration of hypnotic and stimulant drugs. It is the phase during which a subject is most difficult to arouse. See SLEEP.

RENAL COLIC is severe *colic, due usually to impaction of a *stone in the urinary tract.

RENAL DISEASE. Disease of the kidney. See NEPHROLOGY.

RENAL FAILURE describes the situation in which the *kidneys, because of disease or destruction, are no longer able to maintain physiological *homeostasis for their several functions, in particular the excretion of nitrogenous and other waste products and the regulation of water, electrolyte, and acid–base equilibrium. The terms *azotaemia and uraemia (or uraemic syndrome) are virtually synonymous with renal failure. See NEPHROLOGY; RENAL FUNCTION TESTS.

RENAL FUNCTION TESTS. Many tests can help to evaluate kidney function and the presence, extent, and type of renal functional impairment. They include: examination of the urine (particularly for *albumin and blood cells); assessment of concentrating and diluting capacity in response to varying water loads; measurement of urinary *electrolyte concentrations; assessment of acidifying capacity in response to administered ammonium chloride; blood biochemistry (particularly *acid–base balance, electrolyte concentrations, and concentrations of urea, creatinine, and serum proteins); *clearance tests; radiographic visualization of the urinary tract; other imaging techniques; and histological study of renal tissue removed by percutaneous needle *biopsy.

RENAL TUBULE. The basic functional unit of the kidney, also known as the nephron, of which there are about a million in each kidney. Each tubule, consisting of a *basement membrane lined with *epithelium, begins in the cortex (outer layer) as an expansion (*Bowman's capsule) surrounding a *glomerulus, and ends in a collecting tubule in the medulla (inner layer), merging with others to drain into one of the calyces of the renal pelvis. In between, the tubule is divided into sections from above downwards: proximal convoluted tubule, Henle's loop with descending and ascending limbs, distal convoluted tubule, arched collecting tubule, and straight collecting tubule. See also NEPHROLOGY.

RENIN is an *enzyme secreted by the juxtaglomerular cells of the kidney in response to lowering of renal arterial *blood pressure. It catalyses the formation of *angiotensin-1 from a fraction of *plasma *globulin.

REOVIRUS. A group of *ribonucleic acid (RNA) *viruses causing enteric and respiratory infections, including the common *cold.

REPRESSION is a common concept in psychiatry, denoting an unconscious mechanism whereby thoughts, ideas, memories, and impulses unacceptable to the conscious mind are banished from it and prevented from re-entering. Repression is the means by which the true nature of an emotional conflict may be concealed from the individual.

RESEARCH. Investigation towards the acquisition of new medical knowledge is broadly divided into basic or fundamental research, which may involve almost any branch of science, its application being unlikely to be planned or even foreseen; and applied research, itself divided into clinical research and research into methods and systems of health care (operational research). Financial support comes from many public and private sources, the main agencies through which government funds are provided being the *National Institutes of Health in the USA and the *Medical Research Council in the UK. See EXPERIMENTAL METHOD; FOUNDATIONS, ETC. IN THE UK; RESEARCH INSTITUTES.

RESEARCH INSTITUTES, MEDICAL. Independent medical research institutes emerged in a number of countries in the late 19th and early 20th centuries. The first such body, founded in 1888, was the Pasteur Institute in Paris, which became the model and inspiration for similar ventures across Europe, North America, and, very soon, the world (Table 1). The impetus behind these early institutes was to develop bacteriological research and to spread its practical benefits. Thus, the Pasteur Institute sought to institutionalize the achievements of Louis *Pasteur and initially acted as an antirabies serum dispensary as well as a research institute. The Koch Institute for Infectious Diseases in Berlin was created to extend the bacteriological ideas and techniques of Robert *Koch and opened with a flourish announcing a purported remedy for *tuberculosis—*tuberculin. Both institutes were created outside existing universities and medical schools, and attempted to associate medical innovation with national, if not imperial, social and economic progress. The Pasteur Institute was the product of a populist newspaper campaign and voluntary fund-raising, whereas the Koch Institute was supported by the state. All of the institutes founded at this time followed one or other of these patterns, although it soon became common for private institutes to rely upon a single large donation from wealthy benefactors, as was the case with the Lister and Rockefeller Institutes.

The thinking behind this burst of institution building was that if such recent achievements in medical science as germ theories of disease, *antisera, and *vaccines had been achieved by the *ad hoc* activities of isolated individuals, what more might be expected from organized, well-supported and perhaps mission-oriented teamwork. A second assumption was that the future understanding and control of disease would emerge from the work of laboratory-based, biomedical scientists rather than from clinicians or *public health doctors. In other words, one could invest in and expect results from research, and that the place to invest in was the laboratory; thus, in these developments the modern meaning of medical research was created.

The *Rockefeller Institute was the first to adopt the term 'medical research' in its title. The idea for such an agency came from a board of scientific directors, which had been called together by John D. Rockefeller to advise on the creation of a permanent arrangement for his philanthropy in medicine. Rockefeller was one of a number of wealthy business magnates in the USA who, for various motives, chose to distribute some of their accumulated wealth to what they saw as worthwhile causes and activities. At the turn of the century the endowment of the sciences, especially the applied sciences, was a particularly favoured subject. The other great philanthropist of the time, Andrew *Carnegie, invested heavily in the physical sciences, leaving medicine to Rockefeller. For a short time grants were distributed to individuals, before policy shifted to

Table 1 Selected research institutes founded before 1910

Institution	Year of foundation	Location
Pasteur Institute	1888	Paris
Koch Institute for Infectious Diseases	1890	Berlin
Russian Institute for Experimental Medicine	1890	St Petersburg
British Institute of Preventive Medicine (Lister Institute)	1893	London
Institute for Medical Research	1900	Kuala Lumpur
Rockefeller Institute for Medical Research	1901	New York
Oswaldo Cruz Institute	1907	Rio de Janeiro

the establishment of a separate institute. The Rockefeller Institute opened its laboratories in 1904, moved to permanent quarters in 1906, and produced its first notable innovation—spinal injection of cerebrospinal meningitis serum—in 1907. A permanent endowment followed, some of which was used to found a hospital for clinical research.

The Rockefeller Institute, like the Carnegie, was deliberately established without a link to a university or medical school. The aim was to avoid the competing pressures of teaching and administration, and to free medically qualified researchers from private clinical practice. The provision of full-time posts in medical schools had been an issue in the USA for some time, as medical schools broke with the tradition of employing local practitioners on a part-time basis to teach preclinical subjects. Without the state support, long histories of endowment, or affiliation with universities enjoyed by their European counterparts, American schools were vulnerable financially and professionally. Most were private colleges that relied on student fees for income, and in the late 19th century they were finding it increasingly difficult to keep up with the expertise and expense demanded by the new laboratory medicine. The first full-time post was held by Henry P. Bowditch at *Harvard, but the major breakthrough came in 1893 when *Johns Hopkins created the first full-time department to teach the preclinical sciences. Other colleges and universities soon followed. This created a new group of medical scientists with both time and the facilities to become researchers in subjects such as *physiology, experimental *pathology, *bacteriology, and *immunology.

As a dedicated research agency, the Rockefeller Institute differed from medical institutes in Europe as well as from earlier public health laboratories in the USA. Other institutes had been involved in servicing public health measures (for example, the production of antisera, vaccines, and regulatory functions) and research had evolved from, and to support, these activities. Thus, the Pasteur Institute quickly produced a spectacular innovation in *diphtheria antitoxin, becoming involved in its production and standardization. The Koch Institute also worked on an antitoxin for diphtheria as well as that for *tetanus. Paul *Ehrlich, whose work was integral to these successes and who subsequently went on to pioneer modern *chemotherapy, left the Koch Institute to establish rival institutes with similar missions, first to head the State Institute for the Investigation and Control of Sera, and then to the Institute for Experimental Therapy at Frankfurt in 1899. In its early years the Lister Institute could not claim obvious successes from its research programmes, although its teaching of preventive medicine and production of vaccines and sera were valued. In 1904, a second medical research institute was founded in London when the *Imperial Cancer Research Fund charity opened laboratories with the specific aim of identifying the cause of *cancer and hence a solution to this growing problem.

In the USA the Rockefeller endowments stimulated similar ventures, most notably the McCormick Memorial Institute for Infectious Diseases at Chicago in 1902, and the Henry Phipps Institute for the Study, Treatment and Prevention of Tuberculosis at Philadelphia in 1903. However, the latter was not supported at the level promised and in 1910 it became a unit of the University of Pennsylvania. This was part of a new pattern of associating endowments with universities or medical schools rather than creating independent establishments. Henry Phipps subsequently made further donations for a tuberculosis clinic and a psychiatric clinic at Johns Hopkins University. The Henry Kirke Cushing Laboratory of Experimental Medicine (1906) was attached to Western Reserve University, and the Russel Sage Institute of Pathology (1907) went to New York Hospital.

In the late 1900s the fate of medical research institutes was caught up in the wider reform of medical education as, with the 'carrot' of Rockefeller money and the 'stick' of the criticisms of reformers like Abraham *Flexner, attempts were made to establish the training of doctors on a more rigorous scientific basis. The strategy, as part of the wider philanthropic gospel of applied science, was to create high-powered institutions that would train doctors and give them the necessary weapons to become effective agents in the fight to improve the health, and hence the wealth, of nations. However, it was acknowledged that a medical school could not simply relay knowledge; it also had to be engaged in its development. Hence, medical education and research became increasingly tied to universities, a trend exemplified by such new foundations as the Otho S. A. Sprague Memorial Institute, which went

to the University of Chicago (1911), and the George Williams Hooper Foundation for Medical Research at the University of California, San Fransisco (1913).

A novel source of funding for research emerged in the USA—that of clinicians themselves establishing institutes to investigate a particular treatment or disease. For example, Edward L. *Trudeau successfully appealed for funds to establish the Saranac Laboratory for the Study of Tuberculosis based at the Adirondack Cottage Sanitorium. A more entrepreneurial and significant venture was the *Mayo Clinic, founded in Rochester, Minnesota by William J. and Charles H. Mayo. With finance accumulated from their highly successful and lucrative practice, the brothers created the Mayo Foundation for Medical Education and Research at the University of Minnesota in 1915. The Rockefeller endowment of research was widely emulated, but their particular organizational model was not; the founders of other institutes felt it essential to link applied research to a university, medical training, a hospital, or all three.

In Europe in the early part of this century, there was far less private and philanthropic support for medical research. Universities and medical schools were less entrepreneurial and government played a far greater role in medical training and research. In Britain state support and policies were developed through the *Medical Research Council (MRC), or Committee as it was between its inception in 1913 and 1919. With responsibility for medical research in the country as a whole, the MRC had to wrestle with issues that would loom ever larger in years to come:

(1) the balance between supporting research work at a central research establishment (intramural) as against work at institutions across the country (extramural); or

(2) whether to fund the long-term work of individuals and groups (grants-in-aid) or to support only projects with specific outcomes (applied research contracts).

In 1914 the MRC decided to create a central institute independent of both medical schools and universities. The First World War delayed matters and it was not until 1920 that the *National Institute for Medical Research (NIMR) opened in its own buildings. Initially, there were departments of bacteriology, applied physiology, biochemistry and pharmacology, and medical *statistics, all of which pursued lines of research largely chosen by their staff. In its extramural support the Council, influenced by the ideas of its secretary, William Morley Fletcher, came to see its role primarily as the support of fundamental research. The Council, and Fletcher in particular, tried to direct the whole of medical research in Britain in this direction, and to this end worked closely with philanthropists and the international wing of the Rockefeller Foundation. However, there was friction with other bodies, for example, the *Royal Colleges of Physicians and Surgeons, interest groups such as the cancer charities, and even the *Ministry of Health, all of which had other ideas about the aims and organization of medical research.

Another important development in the 1920s was the growth of industrial research laboratories devoted to medical research, especially in the pharmaceutical industry. The most notable in Britain was the Burroughs Wellcome and Co. Research Laboratory whose first head, Henry *Dale, following his work on insulin, became head of the NIMR in 1928. Also between the wars, important work was performed in Britain by the May and Baker Company, which, with Lionel Whitby, based at an MRC unit at the Middlesex Hospital, developed the new *sulphonamide—sulphapyridine or M&B 693. Similar developments occurred elsewhere, especially in Germany and the USA. The Bayer Company had supported a research group, headed by Gerhard *Domagk, in experimental pathology, which from the 1920s explored antibacterial drugs. After many false dawns they identified a substance that killed streptococci in mice, which was then developed in Germany, France, and Britain as the sulpha drugs. In the USA the involvement of Eli Lilly and Company in *insulin production transformed not only that company, but the whole attitude of the pharmaceutical industry to in-house research and to collaborative projects with universities, medical schools, and institutes. An early success for such links came from Merck's support of *Waksman's research on *antibiotics that produced *streptomycin.

The Koch Institute remained at the centre of German medical research in the early decades of this century, a role that continued during the Nazi period and the racialization of medicine. The only counterweight of note was the Kaiser Wilhelm Society for the Promotion of Sciences, intended as a German version of the Rockefeller Foundation, and established with donations from industrialists. However, this concentrated on promoting the 'pure' sciences and sought to preserve the unity of the sciences by avoiding the support of specialized institutes. Its role in the development of medical research institutes was small until after the Second World War. The Society was then renamed in honour of Max Planck, and eventually established no fewer than 22 autonomous Max Planck institutes concerned with research in the medical and biological sciences. In France the Pasteur Institute system also continued to hold centre stage. However, the central Paris laboratory lost its dynamism in the 1910s and 1920s, and took many years to re-establish itself as a world centre of medical research, which it became once again after 1945.

An enduring problem for medical research institutes was the linking of laboratory work and its results to clinical practice. The Pasteur Institute opened a hospital for clinical investigation in 1900 and the Rockefeller a similar facility in 1910. In 1914 it was anticipated that the NIMR would have a hospital for clinical research. However, for reasons of cost, likely public resistance,

and fears of a divorce from higher teaching, the plan was dropped. Instead, a Department of Clinical Research and Experimental Medicine was supported at University College Hospital, London, and the MRC promoted the establishment of academic units in teaching hospitals nationwide, to provide both research and higher postgraduate teaching. However, in the 1930s this policy was challenged by leading clinicians, notably Thomas *Lewis and Lord *Moynihan, who called for the creation and long-term support of clinical researchers. Several important issues concerning medical research were at stake. First, the differing weights to be placed upon the basic sciences ancillary to medicine, as against studies with patients in clinical settings. Secondly, the extent to which it was appropriate to associate research and education. Thirdly, who was qualified to undertake medical, and especially clinical, research, and whether careers and full-time posts in clinical research should be fostered. Ultimately, these issues were settled, if not resolved, by the massive expansion of support for medical research after 1945, when it became possible to support many of the diverse interests that had previously competed for scarce resources. In the 1960s the MRC established a Clinical Research Centre (CRC) in association with a district general hospital at Northwick Park in Harrow. Despite several successes, it probably suffered from lack of association with a university, and in the 1990s its units were dispersed around various hospitals and universities, and it closed.

Central government also moved into medical research in the USA in the 1930s, when the Roosevelt administration transformed the Hygiene Laboratory of the Public Health Service into the *National Institute of Health (NIH). By 1940, following the addition of the National Cancer Institute, the NIH budget stood at US$700 000, (£467 000) still barely a seventh of the US$4.7 million (£3.13 million) spent by foundations. But this was soon to change. The success of the investment in science and technology during the Second World War ushered in what has been called the era of 'Big Science'; that is, large-scale state support of research and development across the scientific spectrum, summed up in Vandevaar Bush's phrase—'Science: the endless frontier'. In the USA most of the new federal money went to the physical sciences and was linked with defence. However, medicine benefited too, able to boast its own research successes of the war—the production of *penicillin and antimalarial drugs for example, and found its own influential champions in Congress. (Although penicillin was a British discovery—see FLEMING; FLOREY; and CHAIN—and was first produced in Oxford, UK, commercial production was initiated in the USA.) By 1946 the NIH budget had increased to US$3 million (£2 million) and in 1948 it was US$26 million (£17 million). A National Heart Institute was added in 1948 and the overall title of NIH was changed to the plural—National Institutes of Health. Its home, Bethesda in Maryland, became, if not quite a 'science city', then certainly a large medical research suburb. In the late 1960s NIH central laboratories employed 13 000 full-time researchers and took about 20 per cent of the total NIH budget, which had by then climbed to over US$1 billion.

In the post-war period the NIH, through the award of extramural grants and contracts, took on a major role in the development of the biomedical sciences and the support of medical schools. By the end of the 1960s a third of all medical school income came from external research grants, and much of this was from the NIH. The growth of state funding was matched by that from philanthropy and industry, so that in the late 1980s the now huge NIH budget (over US$6 billion, £4 billion) accounted for only a third of all health research and development spending, then standing at around US$15 billion (£10 billion). The 1940s and 1950s had seen a continuing proliferation of privately endowed, medical research institutes. Unlike the earlier institutes with a dedicated endowment, the new wave depended upon mixed sources of funding—endowments, federal grants, research contracts for private, industrial, voluntary, and public bodies. The role of in-house research by pharmaceutical and other industrial corporations also grew in importance, as too has their support of research in institutes and universities.

The rapid expansion of medical research has been questioned on a number of occasions. In the mid-1960s there was a reaction to what was seen to be research for its own sake, and the NIH was given responsibility, in the context of Medicare and Medicaid, for the regional medical programmes, that aimed at spreading the results of medical progress to people at all levels of American society. In the early 1970s there were claims that years of investment had brought no major changes to the prospects of cancer patients, and it was argued that a new mission-oriented programme, similar to that which had put humans on the moon, was needed. The passing of the National Cancer Act, 1972 was intended to galvanize and support research scientists to these ends, although this raised the question of the extent to which medical research could be directed, and signalled the growing and overt politicization of medical research, only too evident in the 1980s in AIDS research.

One of the most famous new medical institutes in the post-war period has been the Salk Institute for Biological Studies in California, which opened in 1960. Like many of the earlier institutes, this was based on the work and innovation of a distinguished researcher—Jonas Salk of the polio vaccine—and once again sought to provide the opportunity for the pursuit of fundamental research without the distractions of routine university or clinical work. However, it was a new-wave body in the sense of being a diverse, multidepartment institute, without a single goal or particular disease problem in view. But while this reassertion of independence was happening on the west coast, on the east coast the Rockefeller Institute was moving the other way to integrate its research into postgraduate training, a position formalized in 1977 when it became the Rockefeller University.

The aims of the Salk Institute can be seen as a reaction to the new pattern of post-war funding of medical research, which had seen a loss of the relative autonomy that had previously allowed medical research staff to decide research goals. There was never a golden age of complete independence; institutes always had their own internal policies and financial controls, but, often and within the limits of their overall mission, staff had been able to set their own agenda and to follow this with some flexibility. However, the quantum rise in the scale of funding after 1945 brought greater calls for greater accountability. Several aspects of this new situation caused and continue to cause, concern:

1. The possible neglect of long-range and long-term research.
2. The effects of the growing bureaucratization of research. Medical scientists spend ever more of their time writing research-grant applications, refereeing the applications of others, and serving on research policy and grant committees.
3. Whether the link between 'laboratory' and 'clinic' has grown too wide. The typical medical researcher in the late 20th century holds a Ph.D., not an MD. However, while the original aim of medical research institutes had been to free medical researchers from the pressures of teaching and clinical practice, neither of these aims proved wholly possible or desirable, and it subsequently became the norm to associate research with postgraduate training and clinical research in what were seen to be more productive ways.

The post-war growth in medical research coincided with a switch in research goals from attempts to understand and combat infectious diseases to the different problems of chronic, degenerative diseases. For many years after 1945 it was successfully maintained that the first item on this new agenda had to be understanding of the biological processes of chronic diseases, and that the work of biomedical scientists in institutes and laboratories would provide the keys to unlock these secrets. While political, public, and medical faith in this model of medical research is still strong, it no longer has the tacit and perhaps unquestioning public support it once enjoyed. The unease, first evident from the cost–benefit concerns of mid-1960s, has become more challenging in the 1970s, 1980s, and 1990s. First, more and more people have asked whether reductionist laboratory research is the best means of improving the quality of life and longevity. From both within medicine and outside, the claims of the benefits of life-style changes, especially diet and exercise, have pointed to the importance of non-medical factors in the prevention of disease. Many now say that more community health centres would make a greater contribution to health than more medical research institutes. Secondly, ethical issues have come to the fore at every level, from *vivisection and animal rights through to asking about the personal and public costs of the search for perfect physical health and the postponement of death. Thirdly, the medicine of advanced, industrialized countries offers little that is applicable or transferable to third world countries, where health problems are very serious. Finally, and as a consequence of one of the recent and more promising aspects of biomedical research—*genetic engineering—people are questioning the ecological and moral dangers of altering genetic material. Some have gone so far as to ask what right biomedical scientists now have to 'play God'. Clearly, the work of medical research institutes in the late 20th century suffers from problems related to their very success, as their work is much more public than it was when they were founded a century ago. But the underlying issues are little changed: basic versus mission-oriented research; freedom and accountability; competing pressures of teaching, clinical practice, and administration; links between laboratory innovation and clinical medicine; ambivalent public perceptions; and increasingly the relative value of different means of improving health.

MICHAEL WORBOYS

Further reading
Austoker, J. and Bryder, L. (ed.) (1989). *Historical perspectives on the role of the MRC.* Oxford University Press, Oxford.
Blake, J. B. (1957). Scientific institutions since the Renaissance: their role in medical research, *Proceedings of the American Philosophical Society*, **101**, 31–62.
Delaunay, A. (1962). *L'Institut Pasteur, des origines à aujourd' hui.* France-Empire, Paris.
Harden, V. A. (1986). *Inventing the N.I.H.: Federal biomedical research policy, 1887–1937.* Johns Hopkins University Press, Baltimore.
Strickland, S. P. (1974). *Politics, science and dread disease. A short history of United States medical research policy.* Harvard University Press, Cambridge, MA.

RESECTOSCOPE. A surgical instrument designed for transurethral resection of the *prostate gland, employing an electrically powered wire loop for cutting tissue. See UROLOGICAL SURGERY.

RESERVOIR. A store, or place used for storage. In *infectious diseases, reservoir denotes the place or manner in which the causative agent is perpetuated between outbreaks of clinical infection. Such a reservoir of infection may be provided by symptomless human carriers of the disease, as with *typhoid fever, or by animals acting as alternate or intermediate hosts to the particular micro-organism, as with *rabies and many other infectious and parasitic diseases.

RESIDENT is a US term for a medical graduate who has completed an *internship and who is undertaking specialized hospital training under supervision.

RESIDENT HOSPITAL APPOINTMENTS are training posts for medical graduates that require full- or part-time residence in hospital.

RESIDENT HOUSE OFFICERS are junior doctors undergoing further training and normally responsible for the day-to-day care of patients. In both the UK and the USA, a period spent as a resident house officer is essential for admission to independent medical practice, that is in the UK for admission to the full, rather than provisional Medical Register (see GENERAL MEDICAL COUNCIL REGISTRATION). House officers are usually resident in their first year after graduation, but many are also resident (i.e. living in hospital) for up to 2 more years.

RESISTANCE, ANTIBIOTIC. *Antibiotic resistance refers to the property possessed by some bacteria which enables them to combat the effect of a drug which kills or prevents the growth of most other members of that species. Thus some *staphylococci produce an enzyme, penicillinase, which destroys benzoylpenicillin. Since resistance is genetically determined, resistant strains may emerge through *natural selection during treatment of an infection with an antibiotic. Resistance may also be transferred from one organism to another by the independent units of genetic material known as *plasmids or resistance transfer factors (RTF).

RESOLUTION is discrimination between objects or values that are close together, usually applied to optical systems. Resolving power, that is the ability to distinguish between two points or objects, is limited by the wavelength of the light employed; however great the magnification of the system, objects which are closer together than about half the wavelength of the light cannot be distinguished. Hence the magnification of *microscopes employing ordinary light cannot usefully be greater than about 1500 times. Finer detail can be resolved only by decreasing the wavelength of the illumination. Electrons have a very short wavelength, explaining the high resolution which can be achieved by electron microscopes.

The word 'resolution' is also used in medicine in respect of pathological states, for example *pneumonia, to mean subsidence, clearing, or disappearance of the abnormal features.

RESONANCE is the slightly ringing, hollow sound elicited by *percussion when no solid or dense structure or substance (such as the liver or fluid in the pleural cavity) underlies the body surface area on which the *pleximeter finger is placed; resonance is increased over an air-containing viscus or cavity. Vocal resonance refers to the quality of the voice sounds heard on *auscultation.

RESPIRATION is the exchange of gases which results from oxidative metabolism, by which *oxygen is taken up and *carbon dioxide released. This gas exchange occurs between the atmosphere and the blood circulation in the lungs through pulmonary ventilation (sometimes called external respiration), and similarly between blood and tissue in the peripheral circulation (tissue or internal respiration).

RESPIRATOR is a term sometimes used, though less so than formerly, to describe apparatus for artificially ventilating the lungs (see INTENSIVE CARE). It also meant a device for filtering or otherwise modifying the composition of the air breathed; during the Second World War 'respirator' was the official term for gas-mask.

RESPIRATORY DISTRESS SYNDROME is an alternative term for *hyaline membrane disease; a similar syndrome associated with *atelectasis but without hyaline membrane formation is called idiopathic respiratory distress of the newborn. Severe rapidly progressive respiratory failure in the adult is sometimes termed adult respiratory distress syndrome.

RESPIRATORY EXCHANGE RATIO. See RESPIRATORY QUOTIENT.

RESPIRATORY FAILURE occurs when the respiratory system is unable to maintain normal body *homeostasis, notably for arterial gas tensions of oxygen and carbon dioxide, indicating extensive impairment of lung function.

RESPIRATORY INFECTION is a term embracing all conditions resulting from invasion by micro-organisms of part of the respiratory tract, from nasal air passages to lung parenchyma. It includes many trivial and self-limiting conditions, and many that are life-threatening. See CHEST MEDICINE.

RESPIRATORY QUOTIENT is the volume of *carbon dioxide excreted by the lungs divided by the volume of *oxygen taken up, usually abbreviated to RQ. The RQ is alternatively termed the respiratory exchange ratio (RER).

REST. Physical rest has long been an established principle of therapy, and remains so. There are many instances, of which cardiac decompensation can be a striking example, where rest alone can visibly reverse the course of an illness. In others, the nature of the condition itself, whether influenza, a sprained ankle, or a slipped disc, dictates that rest be part of the treatment. However, appropriate and graduated activity is an important stimulus to repair and growth after injury; and the deleterious physical and mental consequences of prolonged immobility are well-known. Complete rest should therefore be ordered only when judged strictly necessary, and should not last too long. Modern surgical and obstetric practice accords with these principles.

Similar considerations apply to mental and emotional rest, as when induced by tranquillizing agents.

RESURRECTIONISTS were professional criminals, also known as 'resurrection men' or 'body-snatchers', whose trade was the clandestine exhumation of recently buried corpses and their profitable sale to teachers of anatomy before the *Anatomy Act 1832 provided medical schools with a legitimate source of bodies for dissection. See ANATOMY; BODY-SNATCHERS.

RESUSCITATION is the restoration by artificial means of pulmonary ventilation and effective circulation when these vital functions have ceased (cardiopulmonary arrest). The immediate first aid steps are: establishment of an airway; artificial ventilation with the operator's expired air (mouth-to-mouth or mouth-to-nose); and maintenance of circulation with external cardiac compression. Where necessary, more sophisticated life-support techniques can then take over.

RETARDATION, when otherwise unqualified, usually means 'mental retardation', a term equivalent to *mental subnormality or handicap. 'Psychomotor retardation' means the abnormal slowness of thought and movement seen in patients with depressive disorders (see DEPRESSION).

RETE. Anatomically, a network or *plexus.

RETENTION OF URINE is accumulation of urine within the *bladder as a result of failure to urinate. The bladder becomes distended, and can be detected above the pubis by palpation and percussion through the abdominal wall. The cause may be mechanical obstruction, for example urethral compression by an enlarged *prostate gland, or it may be neurogenic bladder dysfunction. In the latter case, retention may be accompanied by *incontinence ('retention with overflow').

RETICULOCYTE. An immature *erythrocyte, distinguished by a fine network (reticulum) on basophilic staining. Large numbers in the circulation (reticulocytosis) indicate active *erythropoiesis, such as that which follows blood loss from *haemorrhage or *haemolysis.

RETICULOENDOTHELIAL SYSTEM (RES) is the body-wide system of *phagocytic cells, of which the *macrophage is the essential unit, together with other cells of similar type and function derived from the *bone marrow via the blood *monocyte (*histiocytes, *Kupffer cells, microglial cells, and others). Reticular cells (the supporting cells of lymphoid organs) and endothelial cells (lining blood vessels), although not so derived, are also phagocytic and are part of the RES. The main function of the RES is scavenging of foreign particulate matter, bacterial debris, degenerate cells, etc.

RETICULOENDOTHELIOSES are proliferative disorders of the *reticuloendothelial system.

RETICULOSIS is any proliferative disorder of the *reticuloendothelial system (a system of cells and tissues with marked *phagocytic properties which forms part of the immune defence mechanism).

RETINA. The retina is the light-sensitive structure of the eye, a membrane lining its interior; it has an outer pigmented layer and an inner transparent nervous layer next to the vitreous body. The nervous layer contains two kinds of sensitive nerve-endings, the rods and the cones. The latter, themselves of three types, are sensitive to colour and function only in strong light; the rods function in poor light, and are sensitive only to blue and green. The nerve cells are continuous with the *optic nerve, which carries impulses back to the visual cortex of the brain. The retina is embryologically part of the brain. It develops as a hollow outpouch of the brain wall, the end of which is invaginated to form a two-layered cup which becomes the two layers of the retina, its stalk forming the optic nerve. See OPHTHALMOLOGY.

RETINACULUM is an anatomical term for a band or sheet of *connective tissue which holds a structure in place.

RETINITIS PIGMENTOSA is a genetically transmitted degeneration of the *retina characterized by *atrophy, attenuation of blood vessels, clumping of pigment, and contraction of vision. The pattern of *genetic transmission varies.

RETINOL. See VITAMIN A.

RETINOPATHY is any pathological condition of the *retina.

RETINOSCOPY is measurement of the refractive power of the eye by observation of the movement of a beam of light reflected from the retinal surface.

RETRACTOR. A surgical instrument, of which there are many designs, for restraining and separating the edges of an incised wound and the structures underlying it.

RETROCOLLIS is a form of *torticollis or wryneck in which muscular spasm displaces the head and neck backwards.

RETROLENTAL FIBROPLASIA is due to the administration of excessive concentrations of *oxygen to newborn infants, in whom intense spasm of retinal vessels leads to necrosis and fibrosis of the retinal tissue; a fibrous mass develops at the back of the eye. Since the aetiology of retrolental fibroplasia was elucidated in the 1940s, oxygen has been administered to premature infants with great caution, intermittently, and in dilute concentrations.

RETROPULSION is a physical sign sometimes demonstrated by patients with *parkinsonism: if the standing patient is suddenly pulled backwards, he cannot prevent himself taking a few more backward steps.

RETROVERSION is backwards displacement or rotation of an organ, and is usually used with reference to the upper part of the *uterus.

RETROVIRUS. A member of a group of RNA viruses, the RNA of which is copied during viral replication into DNA by a reverse transcriptase (see MOLECULAR BIOLOGY). The viral DNA is then integrated into the host chromosomal DNA. Retroviruses are thus potentially *oncogenic. The *acquired immune deficiency syndrome (AIDS) is due to the human immunodeficiency (HIV) retrovirus.

RETZIUS, ANDERS ADOLF (1796–1860). Swedish anatomist. He described the space in front of the *urinary bladder which allows it to expand and contract freely, a space now known as the cave of Retzius. He made many new observations in animals; certain *gyri in the brain were named after him, as was a *ligament of the ankle joint; he discovered the canals in the *cornea which were later named after Schlemm. He was an anthropologist who measured physical features of the body and introduced craniometry, the measurement of skulls, on which skull indices could be based and which distinguishes brachycephalic, mesocephalic, and dolichocephalic human types.

REVERSION is used in respect of the *tuberculin test to denote a return to a negative reaction in an individual who was previously positive ('Mantoux reversion', the opposite of 'conversion').

REYE'S SYNDROME. An acute toxic *encephalopathy of children, causing nausea, vomiting, lethargy, or delirium, and sometimes seizures. It is fatal in 10–40 per cent of cases and patchy degeneration of the liver may be found at post-mortem. It may follow influenza and may be precipitated by *aspirin or other salicylates.

RHABDOMYOMA. A non-malignant *tumour of skeletal muscle.

RHABDOMYOSARCOMA. A rare, highly malignant tumour derived from primitive striated muscle cells.

RHABDOVIRUS. A group of rod- or bullet-shaped ribonucleic acid (RNA) *viruses, including the causative agent of *rabies.

RHAZES (ABU BAKR MUHAMMAD IBN ZAKA-RIYYA) (*c.* 864–925/35). Persian physician. He distinguished *smallpox from *measles, giving excellent accounts of each. He described the *guinea worm (*Dracunculus medinensis*), the *recurrent laryngeal nerve, and *spina ventosa. He is best known for his Graeco-Arabic encyclopaedia of medicine, *Kitab al-hawi*, translated into Latin as *Liber continens* in 1279. It was antireligious and critical of *Galen. The ninth book was the main source of therapeutic knowledge for three centuries.

RHEOLOGY is the science of the deformation and flow of matter; it is used in medicine to describe the study of blood flow in the *circulatory system.

RHESUS FACTOR is a complex of blood group *antigens of particular importance because of the association of one of them (possessed by 85 per cent of the population, termed 'rhesus-positive', the remainder being 'rhesus-negative') with *haemolytic disease of the newborn. A rhesus-positive baby may be born with the condition if its mother is rhesus-negative and has developed antibodies as a result of a previous rhesus-incompatible pregnancy or blood transfusion. See also GENETICS; HAEMATOLOGY.

RHEUMATIC FEVER is an acute febrile illness with a marked tendency to recur, associated with haemolytic (group A) *streptococcal infection and occurring predominantly in childhood and early adult life. The chief manifestations are in the joints (migratory *polyarthritis), the skin and subcutaneous tissues (*erythema and palpable *nodules), the heart (*endocarditis), and the central nervous system (*chorea). Its importance lies in its frequent legacy of permanent damage to heart valves; it was formerly the major cause of acquired *valvular heart disease. The risk was greater the younger the age at the first attack, and when attacks were recurrent; antibacterial prophylaxis against further streptococcal infections in susceptible patients was an essential part of management. The likelihood of adult heart disease is little correlated with the severity of the acute rheumatic episodes, which may pass unnoticed altogether or be dismissed as 'growing pains'. The condition, once common in Europe and the USA, is now rare, but still occurs in the disadvantaged and particularly in the Third World. See also RHEUMATOLOGY.

RHEUMATISM is a generic term for a number of disparate conditions, whose common denominator is pain, with or without signs of inflammation in joints, muscles, tendons, and connective tissues. It embraces, for example, *rheumatic fever, *rheumatoid arthritis, other forms of *arthritis, and conditions with such imprecise labels as *fibrositis. See RHEUMATOLOGY.

RHEUMATOID ARTHRITIS is a chronic and often progressive *polyarthropathy of unknown aetiology, affecting primarily joint *synovial membranes, although other tissues and organs may also be involved. There may be extensive deformities and corresponding disability in advanced cases. There is evidence that a disordered *immune system plays a part in pathogenesis. See RHEUMATOLOGY.

RHEUMATOLOGIST. A specialist in the rheumatic disorders. See RHEUMATOLOGY.

RHEUMATOLOGY
Introduction and historical perspective
The term 'rheumatology' designates both the science (the knowledge of the diseases of the musculoskeletal system and rheumatic diseases) and the art (the practising specialty as a guild). It is impossible to separate these two aspects because developments in the art and organization depend on social need and also, to a considerable extent, on the science and its technical advances. The field of rheumatology has moved from its origins in 19th century *hydrotherapy with the internal and external application of spa water, through a phase of developing recognition of rheumatic diseases such as *gout and *rheumatic fever, to its present explosion into a scientific field that is globally recognized. Today rheumatology has developed into an important topic that is at the brink of defining the important interactions between our genetic predispositions and environmental factors such as drugs and infectious agents.

The expansion in knowledge in rheumatology has paralleled that in medicine. The fields of *immunology and *molecular biology, most particularly, have led to a rapid increase in the understanding of rheumatological disorders, especially the *connective tissue disorders such as *rheumatoid arthritis (RA) and *systemic lupus erythematosus (SLE), and the seronegative spondyloarthropathies such as *ankylosing spondylitis. The field of rheumatology has progressed from a initial phase of description to one of the definition of the basic *pathophysiology of many of the disorders within its purview. For years, *infection has been a common aetiological theme with regard to the causation of joint disorders. Not only has that concept persisted, but we now feel that infectious agents stimulate inflammatory and immunological processes in genetically predisposed hosts. While we have failed to define the causal infectious agent(s) in diseases such as RA and SLE, a systemic disorder such as Lyme disease is now known to be caused by a syphilis-like *spirochaete called *Borrelia burgdorferi*, which is injected into the patient via the bite of an *Ixodes* *tick. Almost all Lyme patients treated early, and most patients treated late in the course of the illness, are cured of their disease with the use of penicillin, penicillin-like, or tetracycline-type *antibiotics. Chronic inflammatory disorders such as RA and SLE do not appear to be responsive to antibiotics, and thus an initial infectious process may very well have set into motion a self-perpetuating, immunological disease process. Thus, the initiating agent may no longer need to be present for the disease process to persist or worsen. In those disorders, some 'immunological switch' may need to be 'turned off' for the systemic process to be curtailed. Since both antibodies and immunologically active cells appear to play a role in inflammatory joint disorders, modern therapeutic approaches include the inhibition of action of those immunological factors. Future avenues for defining the pathogenesis of, and immunotherapy for, joint and connective tissue disorders will involve advances in immunology, *virology, *genetics, and molecular biology.

The rheumatologist deals primarily with the treatment of musculoskeletal disorders, most commonly involving joints. There are more than 100 joints in the body, and these joints can be affected by a myriad of disorders. While some of the disorders are localized to a few joints, others affect many joints and internal organs and are associated with constitutional symptoms such as fatigue, fever, and weight loss. It is the pattern of such involvement that enables the rheumatologist to diagnose a disorder and treat it appropriately (Table 1).

Rheumatological disorders and their treatments
Osteoarthritis (OA)
(a) Cause and clinical presentation. This is the most common rheumatological disorder, and by 55–64 years of age, 85 per cent of people have radiographical changes of OA in one or more joints. After age 55, OA is more common in women than in men. It is important to note that there is a very poor correlation between the presence or extent of OA X-ray abnormalities, and joint complaints or limitation in function. The causes of OA probably include both mechanical (e.g. trauma, obesity, developmental abnormalities, joint laxity) and biological factors (ageing, metabolic, immunology, and genetic). The characteristic joint abnormalities include changes in components of the joint (including *cartilage and bone) and remodelling of bone to form bony spurs. OA is generally progressive, although its clinical course is variable and unpredictable. The primary complaint is joint pain, but patients can also develop bony deformities (obvious in the first joints at the tip of the fingers or the base of the thumb), or limitation in range of motion or function (primarily if the knee or hip is involved). OA is not associated with systemic symptoms such as fatigue, fever, or weight loss. The outcome and effect of OA are quite dependent upon the site and extent of joint involvement. If the primary problems involve the fingers, the effect upon function is clearly less than if there is involvement of a weight-bearing joint such as the knee or hip. Other common areas of involvement include the low back and the neck. Low back and neck strain can lead to persistent pain, and can also be associated with pinched nerve symptoms in the arm or leg.

Table 1 Treatment of rheumatic diseases

Rheumatic disorders	Disease-modifying drug?
Osteoarthritis	No (negative effect?)
Rheumatoid arthritis	Maybe (methotrexate, gold, Cytoxan®)
Gout	Yes (allopurinol)
Seronegative spondylo-arthropathies	Maybe (methotrexate, Azulfidine®)
Systemic lupus erythematosus	At times (steroids, Cytoxan®, antimalarial drugs)
Vasculitides	Yes (steroids, Cytoxan®)
Lyme disease	Yes, in most cases, (amoxycillin, doxycycline, ceftriaxone)

(b) Treatment of osteoarthritis. Avoiding joint abuse, weight reduction, counselling on occupation and sports-related activities, as well as an appropriate exercise programme are necessary to preserve joint function. Physical therapy, directed at improving motion, increasing strength, and reducing pain are fundamental components of any treatment plan. While there is no medication that can change the course of OA, medications can help to control pain, improve function, and allow for optimal physical therapy. If pain is mild, acetaminophen can be used. If pain or disability persists, non-steroidal anti-inflammatory drugs (called NSAIDs) such as *aspirin and aspirin-like drugs (e.g. naproxen, ibuprofen) may be used, beginning with the lowest dose possible. Older patients should be aware that they are at increased risk for NSAID-induced stomach irritation (called gastritis) or even stomach ulcers. Other uncommon, but potential, side-effects include kidney and liver inflammation. Patients should consult their physician before starting such medications. Local injections of *corticosteroids into involved joints, such as the knee and the bottom joint of the thumb, are helpful in controlling flares of local pain and inflammation that are unresponsive to the above measures. Such injections should not be given more frequently than three times a year.

Rheumatoid arthritis (RA)
(a) Cause and clinical presentation. RA, as opposed to osteoarthritis, is a systemic, inflammatory disorder. While the symmetrical (both sides of the body) inflammation of the small and large joints of the arms and legs is the predominant manifestation, RA patients also may develop fatigue, *anaemia, and weight loss. Throughout the world, RA occurs in 2 per cent of people, primarily in women. The present concept of the cause of this disorder involves an initial infectious (?viral) trigger in a genetically predisposed person that leads to a self-perpetuating illness. Immunologically

active cells, such as *lymphocytes and *macrophages, and antibodies appear to play an important role in the persistence of joint and organ inflammation. The development of joint damage (called erosions) is caused by *enzymes that arise from the inflammatory process. The typical presentation is in a woman between 20 and 50 years of age who complains of morning stiffness, and swelling, warmth, or redness of the small joints of the hands, wrists, ankles, and feet on both sides of the body. Twenty per cent of patients develop nodular swellings on the forearms, called rheumatoid nodules. Less commonly, RA can also be associated with internal organ inflammation, presenting with chest pain on breathing due to inflammation of the lining of the lung, or nerve involvement with pins and needles in the feet. The diagnosis is usually defined by this characteristic presentation, but 80 per cent of RA patients also have, in their blood, protein antibodies called rheumatoid factors. It is not uncommon for patients to have an anaemia (low red blood cell count) due to inflammation, and an elevated sedimentation rate (a blood test that demonstrates the level of inflammation). Regarding the course and prognosis of RA, 50–70 per cent of patients will continue to have some level of joint inflammation and change in joint structure over time. Ten per cent of patients may have an acute onset, with a gradual clearing of the inflammation. A small group of patients will develop more severe disease, at times necessitating surgical intervention in order to correct joint deformities and dysfunction.

(b) Treatment of rheumatoid arthritis. The management of RA involves the following goals:

(1) education regarding the disorder, its manifestations, and the therapies used to treat it;
(2) suppression of the joint and systemic inflammation and immunological process that leads to damage;
(3) maintenance of joint function and prevention of deformities; and
(4) repair of joint damage if it will relieve pain, improve the range of motion, or facilitate function.

The patient should become familiar with all of the possible treatments, along with the likelihood of response and potential side-effects. The patient must balance between the quality of their life, and the potential side-effects of the therapy. All patients should receive an evaluation and guidance by a physical and *occupational therapist for a regular exercise programme, with goals being the maintenance of the maximal range of motion, preservation of joint function, and education in the principles of joint protection. All patients will be placed, initially, on one type of non-steroidal anti-inflammatory drug, such as aspirin or aspirin-like drugs (e.g. Naprosyn®, salsalate, or ibuprofen), in order to control inflammation and pain. NSAIDs do not have the capacity to alter the natural history of RA, but are an important component in the control of joint inflammation. Over the past 10 years, there has been a significant change in the rheumatologist's approach to RA, a potentially aggressive disorder in which irreversible joint erosions can occur within the first 2 years. It is now commonplace to introduce early what are called disease-modifying anti-rheumatic drugs (DMARDs). Unlike NSAIDs, these drugs *have* the capacity to alter the natural progression of RA (i.e. stop the development or progression of joint erosions, or lead to their healing). While there is some debate about the extent of the ability of DMARDs to effect such a positive outcome, RA patients should be given one or more of these drugs once the definitive diagnosis is established. Rheumatologists differ on the choice or order of use of DMARDs, but such drugs are usually added to an already prescribed NSAID. DMARDs include sulphasalazine (Azulfidine®), an antimalarial drug called hydroxychloroquine (Plaquenil®), gold salts, including an oral form (Ridaura®, auranofin) and one given by intramuscular injection (Solganal, Myocrisin®), and two immunosuppressive (chemotherapy) drugs, methotrexate (Rheumatrex®) and azathioprine (Imuran®). Because all of these medications have significant potential side-effects, patients must make a therapeutic decision based upon a balance between the quality of their lives and the potential side-effects of the medication.

Corticosteroid-type medications are quite effective in controlling inflammation, but their long-term side-effects (e.g. thinning of the bones (*osteoporosis), stomach irritation or *ulcer, *diabetes, increased risk of infection) demand either short courses of medication to control disease flares, or the lowest dose possible. Steroids can also be injected into a joint in order to control local inflammation, and avoid systemic side-effects.

Occasionally surgery may be needed to improve the functional capacity of a person with RA; total knee and hip replacements are remarkably successful in improving functional limitations.

Newer approaches to the treatment of RA include the use of agents that suppress or control specific lymphocytes involved in the immunological process leading to RA.

*Connective tissue diseases
This term describes a group of systemic disorders in which tissue injury and inflammation are caused by immunological mechanisms. The initial disease trigger, as in RA, is thought to be a viral infection in a genetically predisposed host. Diseases in this category include *systemic lupus erythematosus (SLE) (presenting with joint inflammation, rash, fever, blood count abnormalities, kidney and nervous system dysfunction), scleroderma or *systemic sclerosis (presenting with skin tightening, lung inflammation and scarring), a swallowing disorder, and colour change in the fingers on cold exposure (called *Raynaud's phenomenon), *dermatomyositis/polymyositis (with muscle weakness and rash), and

types of *vasculitis (manifested by organ damage due to inflammation of the blood vessels). All of these disorders are multisystem diseases, a term that reflects the wide range of tissues and organs affected by the underlying immunological process. The goal in all of them is to control the inflammatory state, and thus prevent organ damage. In SLE and scleroderma, joint inflammation is treated with non-steroidal anti-inflammatory drugs. Antimalarial drugs such as hydroxychloroquine (Plaquenil®) may be highly effective in SLE for the control of joint inflammation, fatigue, and in preventing disease flares. In more severe cases of SLE (e.g. with kidney disease), dermatomyositis, and types of vasculitis such as *polyarteritis nodosa, corticosteroids are used in an attempt to control the inflammatory process. In certain cases, unresponsive to steroids, immunosuppressive drugs such as *methotrexate, *azathioprine, or *cyclophosphamide are used to further suppress the damaging immunological reaction. As noted above, all of these drugs have significant potential side-effects that must be appreciated by the patient and the physician.

*Gout and pseudogout
In some genetically predisposed patients, chemicals in the body may form into crystals, and these crystals can trigger severe episodes of joint inflammation. In gout, the crystal involved is composed of *uric acid; in pseudogout, it is calcium pyrophosphate. Both disorders lead to the rapid onset of redness, warmth, and swelling of one joint in the body. While in gout this is usually localized to the great toe, in pseudogout it most commonly involves the knee. Less commonly, more than one joint may be involved. Patients with gout commonly have an elevated uric acid level in their blood, and also a family history of gout or uric acid kidney stone. Some patients with pseudogout have a metabolic abnormality that leads to an elevated level of calcium or iron. The definitive diagnosis of both disorders is made when the characteristic crystals are found within the joint fluid. Treatment of these disorders involves control of the acute inflammatory state with non-steroidal anti-inflammatory drugs. In gout, *colchicine may be used to prevent recurrent attacks of joint inflammation. In difficult cases of gout with large tissue collections of uric acid (called tophi) or in the setting of uric acid kidney stones, uric acid-lowering medications such as *allopurinol (Zyloprim® or Zyloric®) may be used.

Arthritis caused by infections
While RA is thought to be triggered by an as yet undefined infectious agent, such a concept remains only theoretical. However, some patients do develop well-defined infections that lead to joint inflammation.

(a) **Rheumatic fever.** In this systemic disorder, a streptococcal throat infection sets up a systemic, inflammatory reaction that can lead to joint inflammation. This problem is called a 'reactive arthritis' because the actual bacteria cannot be found within the joint itself and the disease process is thought to represent an immunological 'reaction' to the 'strep' organism in the throat.

(b) **True infectious (septic) arthritis** involves the actual direct infection of a joint, usually due to the migration of a bacterium into the joint. The most common bacteria include gonococci (in the setting of gonorrhoea), staphylococci, and streptococci. Whereas rheumatic fever commonly presents with inflammation migrating from joint to joint, septic arthritis most commonly involves one joint, and is associated with fever and chills. The joint is markedly inflamed, with severe limitation in range of motion. The most commonly involved joint is a hip or a knee. The diagnosis is usually defined by the clinical presentation, the type of joint involvement, and synovial fluid analysis and cultures. Such joint infection necessitates the rapid institution of intravenous *antibiotics. With such medication in association with drainage of fluid from the joint, an optimal outcome of normal function and range of motion is expected.

(c) **Lyme disease** is another type of infectious arthritis, in this case caused by the injection of a *spirochaetae infectious agent, called *Borrelia*, into the person via the bite of a deer tick. The most common early manifestation is an expanding red rash with a central clearing called *erythema chronicum migrans (ECM); while this is characteristic of early Lyme disease, a history of a tick bite or the ECM rash may be found only in 60 per cent of patients. Often patients will also have flu-like symptoms and fatigue, low-grade fever, aches, and pains. Many months after the initial infection, patients may develop abnormalities of the electrical system of the heart, neurological disorders such as *Bell's palsy of the face, or arthritis. The most common type of late-onset arthritis involves a waxing and waning inflammation of a knee. Despite the fact that this is a true infectious arthritis and often involves a single joint such as the knee, it differs from infectious arthritis in that it is not associated with a septic presentation (i.e. fever, chills), and is more like the chronic type of inflammation found in RA. The diagnosis is usually based upon the history (of a tick bite, the ECM rash, or living or visiting an area known to be infested with Lyme-infected ticks) and the clinical presentation. While blood tests are used to detect a prior infection with the Lyme *Borrelia* organism, the test may turn positive weeks or months after the infection, and, rarely, may remain negative. Thus, the diagnosis is a clinical one, supported by the blood test. While most patients with Lyme disease do respond to treatment with tetracycline, penicillin, or penicillin-like antibiotics, some patients may have persistent joint inflammation necessitating arthroscopic removal of the synovial membrane.

(d) **Viral infections** can also lead to joint inflammation. *Hepatitis B infection can lead to a self-limited, RA-like inflammatory joint disorder with an associated rash in the early stages of the illness. Joint inflammation can occur in the setting of *rubella infection or immunization. Some children, and their parents, can develop a short-lived, RA-like illness in the setting of a viral infection due to parvovirus (called fifth disease, erythema infectiosum, or slapped-cheek disease).

Overuse syndromes

The soft tissues surrounding the joint include tendons (connecting muscles to bones), bursae (sacs of fluid cushioning the space between skin and bone), and muscles. All of these tissues can become inflamed if overused. Such overuse can occur in the late setting of one's occupation, sports activities, or with wear and tear over time. The most common areas of tendinitis and bursitis include the shoulder, the elbow, and the outer aspect of the thigh. Patients most commonly present with pain on activity, or, in the setting of shoulder and thigh inflammation, at night. Most commonly, *radiography of the involved areas will be either normal or will demonstrate small flecks of calcium in the site of inflammation. Treatment of these disorders often involves the use of non-steroidal anti-inflammatory drugs to control the inflammatory process, decrease in local trauma or overuse, and physical therapy to improve the range of motion.

Thus, while musculoskeletal problems may present in a similar fashion, with joint pain, there are many different underlying causes and treatments. The diagnosis is usually based upon an assessment of the patient's overall medical status, the clinical presentation and pattern of joint involvement, with the aid of radiography of blood and/or synovial fluid testing.

STEPHEN A. PAGET

Further reading
McCarty, D. J. and Koopman, W. J. (ed.) (1993). *Arthritis and allied conditions. A textbook of rheumatology.* Lea and Febiger, Philadelphia.
Paget, S. A. and Fields, T. R. (ed.) (1992). *Summaries in clinical practice. Rheumatic disorders.* Andover, Boston.

RHINITIS is inflammation of the nasal mucous membrane, as in the common *cold.

RHINOLOGY is the specialty concerned with disorders of the nose. See OTORHINOLARYNGOLOGY.

RHINOPHYMA is a disfiguring irregular enlargement of the nose due to sebaceous hyperplasia, occurring in *rosacea.

RHINOPLASTY is any *plastic surgical procedure on the nose.

RHINORRHOEA (RHINORRHEA) is any discharge from or through the nose.

RHINOSCLEROMA is a chronic granulomatous condition of the mucous membrane of the nose and upper respiratory tract occurring in south-east Europe and South America, due to a bacterium, *Klebsiella rhinoscleromatis*.

RHINOVIRUS. A large and widely distributed group of small ribonucleic acid (RNA) *viruses causing respiratory infections in man, including about half of all common *colds.

RHODES SCHOLARS are recipients of scholarships awarded annually since 1902 (the year of Cecil Rhodes's death) to students from the USA, the British Commonwealth, South Africa, and Germany for study at the University of Oxford.

RHODOPSIN is a visual pigment of the *retina, also called visual purple, occurring in the cellular elements responsible for dim-light vision (rods). It consists of a *protein (opsin) combined with a prosthetic group synthesized from *vitamin A.

RHONCHUS. An extra sound heard accompanying the breath sounds on *auscultation of the chest in patients with partial obstruction of the air-passages by bronchoconstriction or relatively dry exudate; rhonchi are of variable pitch and have a whistling or wheezing quality.

RHYTHM is the pattern displayed by recurrent events, for example that of the *pulse beats felt at the wrist, the heart sounds heard over the precordium, the galvanometric deflections seen in the *electroencephalogram, etc. A regular rhythm is one in which the same event or sequence of events is repeated at uniform intervals, for example the arterial pulse. A biological rhythm is one arising from any recurrent biological phenomenon. *Circadian rhythm implies a frequency of about 24 hours. Other adjectives may be descriptive (gallop rhythm, triple rhythm), may indicate the origin of the events (cardiac rhythm, sinus rhythm, ventricular rhythm), may simply be an arbitrary classification (alpha, beta, gamma rhythm), or may give an indication of the cycle length (circadian, ultradian, infradian). See also ARRHYTHMIA.

RIBES, CAMILLE LOUIS ANTOINE CHAMPETIER DE (1848–1935). French obstetrician. He is remembered for devising a balloon which, in its collapsed state was introduced through the uterine *cervix, and then inflated by injecting fluid along its attached tube. The idea was to help the lower uterine segment to distend; after the bag was expelled the birth canal would be open enough to allow the presenting part of the fetus to follow. With a small weight or gentle traction on its protruding tube it could be made to bring pressure on to a bleeding *placenta praevia and so reduce bleeding. The method is no longer used, but was valuable in its time when operative intervention in pregnancy and labour was so dangerous to mother and child (see OBSTETRICS).

RIBOFLAVIN. See VITAMIN B.

RIBONUCLEIC ACID (RNA), a vital component of all living *cells, consists of a large number of nucleotides attached together in single file to form a long strand. Each nucleotide contains the sugar ribose and one of four different bases, namely adenine, guanine, cytosine, and uracil (the same as in *deoxyribonucleic acid (DNA) except that uracil replaces thymine). RNA translates the structure of inherited DNA into that of protein molecules. In some viruses RNA is the inherited material itself but undergoes translation into DNA before replication in the host cell.

RIBOSOMES are granules of *protein and *ribonucleic acid (RNA) present in the cytoplasm of all living organisms, often attached to *endoplasmic reticulum. They are the site of protein synthesis. See CELL AND CELL BIOLOGY.

RICH, ARNOLD RICE (1893–1968). American pathologist. His principal interest was in the inflammatory reaction, especially as it pertained to the advantage or disadvantage to the host of *hypersensitivity to agents such as the tubercle bacillus. He also showed that lesions morphologically identical with those of *polyarteritis nodosa could be induced in experimental animals with drugs or foreign proteins.

RICHARDS, ALFRED NEWTON (1876–1966). American pharmacologist. His best-remembered scientific contribution was in the study of renal function, where he and colleagues developed the technique of micropuncture of *renal tubules.

RICHARDS, DICKINSON WOODRUFF (1895–1973). American physician. With Cournand he developed the technique of right heart catheterization, which made possible precise measurements of *cardiac output in various disease states. For this work Richards, Cournand, and *Forssman (of Germany, who had first succeeded in inserting a *catheter into his own right heart, via peripheral veins) were awarded the *Nobel prize in 1956.

RICHET, CHARLES ROBERT (1850–1935). French physiologist. His earlier researches were on gastric secretion (1878), muscular contraction (1884–89), and the nervous control of the body temperature. His late interests were in *blood transfusion after immunization of the donor against the recipient's infection (1888) and in sensitization against foreign proteins (1895). He invented the term '*anaphylaxis'. For this work he was awarded the *Nobel prize in 1913.

RICKETS is the defective development and growth of bones due to inadequate absorption and utilization of *calcium. The usual cause is *vitamin D deficiency in childhood. Vitamin D promotes calcium absorption from the intestine and its incorporation into bone structure; many diets contain only a small amount, but it is also formed by the action of ultraviolet light on 7-dehydrocholesterol in the basal layers of the skin. Rickets may therefore result from the combination of inadequate light exposure and insufficient vitamin D intake; it is now rare in Western urban communities except in certain special groups such as coloured immigrant children. It may also be caused by certain *inborn (inherited) errors of metabolism. Its clinical features are soft and fragile bones, inadequate growth, deformities of the limbs, thoracic cage, pelvis, and skull, and characteristic radiographical changes. *Hypocalcaemia and *tetany may occur.

RICKETTS, HOWARD TAYLOR (1871–1910). American microbiologist and epidemiologist. He carried out important field studies of *Rocky Mountain spotted fever, succeeding in transmitting the disease from man to laboratory animals, and demonstrating the causative organism, which was subsequently named for him: *Rickettsia*. He showed that this organism is carried by *ticks and transmitted to man by their bites. In Mexico in 1910, while studying *typhus fever, another rickettsial infection, he succumbed to it himself.

RICKETTSIA. A genus of very small intracellular *bacteria (at one time considered intermediate between bacteria and *viruses) transmitted by *arthropod vectors and responsible for *typhus fever and related diseases.

RICORD, PHILLIPE (1799–1889). French venereologist. He was the leading venereologist of the century. He finally proved, by innumerable inoculation experiments, that syphilis and *gonorrhoea were different diseases. He described the three stages of syphilis and published a standard book on venereal diseases (1838).

RIEDEL, BERNHARD MORITZ KARL LUDWIG (1846–1916). German surgeon. He described ligneous or woody thyroiditis (*Riedel's thyroiditis, 1896) and *Riedel's lobe of the liver.

RIEDEL'S LOBE is an anatomically anomalous tongue of tissue protruding from the lower edge of the right lobe of the liver. It may be palpable on examining the abdomen and, if not recognized as a normal variant, may cause diagnostic confusion.

RIEDEL'S THYROIDITIS is a rare condition of unknown aetiology in which the *thyroid gland and surrounding structures are invaded by hard sclerotic tissue, producing a strikingly firm neck enlargement (and sometimes tracheal obstruction) which may be mistaken for thyroid *carcinoma.

RIFAMPICIN is a powerful antibiotic, effective against many bacteria including *mycobacteria. Its use is largely confined to treating *tuberculosis and *leprosy. See ANTI-INFECTIVE AGENTS.

RIFAMYCIN is a generic name for a group of *antibiotics, including *rifampicin, originally obtained from the mould *Streptomyces mediterranei.*

RIFT VALLEY FEVER is an *influenza-like illness of farm animals and man endemic in certain areas of Africa, originally described from the Rift Valley of Kenya. It is due to an *arbovirus.

RIGIDITY is inflexibility of the body or limbs due to increased muscular tone. It is typical of extrapyramidal disorders such as *parkinsonism.

RIGOR is the sensation of shivering experienced when the body temperature rises sharply.

RIGOR MORTIS is the increasing stiffness of muscles which develops after death.

RINDERPEST. Cattle plague; it caused a disastrous epidemic in the UK in 1865–66. See VETERINARY MEDICINE.

RINGER, SYDNEY (1835–1910). British physician and physiologist. He showed that isolated organs survived longer when calcium and potassium were added to the saline perfusate (Ringer's solution).

RINGER'S SOLUTION is a physiological *saline solution with potassium and calcium chlorides added.

RINGWORM is a common term for various *tinea infections in which centrifugal spread of the fungus in the skin accompanied by central healing of the lesion leads to a circular rash (tinea circinata).

RINNE'S TEST was first described by the German otologist Heinrich Adolf Rinne (1819–63). It determines whether *deafness is due to disease of the middle ear (conductive deafness). A tuning fork is set into vibration and alternately held half an inch from the external auditory meatus to assess air conduction and then placed on the mastoid process behind the ear to assess bone conduction. Normally (and in sensorineural deafness such as that due to a lesion of the auditory nerve) the sound is heard louder and longer through the air. Should the reverse be the case, conductive deafness is indicated.

RIO-HORTEGA, PIO DEL (1882–1945). Spanish neurohistologist. In 1918 Rio-Hortega developed a silver impregnation stain which identified two new glial elements: the microglia and the oligodendroglia (see NEUROGLIA). Working at the National Institute for Cancer in Madrid he reclassified the *gliomata (1919).

RIOLAN, JEAN (1580–1637). French physician. His slavish veneration for *Galen led him to oppose any new current in medical thought. He recorded his disapproval of *Harvey's views in *Encheiridium* (1648) to which Harvey replied in 1649.

RIPPLE BED. A bed with a mattress containing several compartments which can be separately inflated and deflated, so varying the points at which pressure bears on the patient's body.

RIVA-ROCCI, SCIPIONE (1863–1937). Italian physician. In 1896 he devised the type of mercury *sphygmomanometer still in general use today.

RIVERS, THOMAS MILTON (1888–1962). American microbiologist. In 1922 he joined the staff of the Rockefeller Institute, and began a lifelong investigation of viral diseases of man. He thus played an important part in establishing virology as a discipline separate from bacteriology. He studied *measles, *varicella, lymphocytic choriomeningitis, *psittacosis, and *smallpox. His books on animal viruses were standard references for many years.

RNA. See RIBONUCLEIC ACID.

ROAD ACCIDENTS. See SURGERY OF TRAUMA.

ROBINSON, ROBERT A. (1914–90). American orthopaedic surgeon. He and Michael Watson were the first to demonstrate the structure of the apatite crystal and the collagen-crystal relationship in bone. He investigated the microstructure of cartilage and bone matrix, the ultrastructure of bone cells, the morphology of the osteon, and the water content of bone. He developed a method of anterolateral fusion of the cervical spine which played a major role in the evolution of spine surgery.

ROCKEFELLER, JOHN DAVISON (1839–1937). American industrialist and philanthropist. Towards the end of the 19th century he turned his attention to philanthropy, and began to give large sums of money to religious and educational institutions. On the advice of his friend and clergyman, Frederick T. Gates, he founded the Rockefeller Institute for Medical Research in New York City in 1904. Later he established the General Education Board and the *Rockefeller Foundation, agencies which contributed to biomedical research, medical education, and control of world health problems, such as *malaria, *yellow fever, and *malnutrition.

ROCKEFELLER FOUNDATION. The Rockefeller Foundation was endowed by John D. *Rockefeller in 1913 'to promote the well-being of mankind throughout the world'. In its early years its main thrust was in public health and medical education. Now its work has expanded to include agriculture, natural and social sciences, and the arts and humanities. It has a board of trustees and officers concerned with the main activities, with headquarters in New York. Its work is carried out by making grants, supporting fellowships, and field operations in which expert teams help developing countries until they are capable of managing their problems out of their own resources. In medicine it has concern with reproductive biology, contraceptive technology, and social factors of significance in population control. It also supports research into neglected diseases afflicting mainly the developing world, into epidemiology and other quantitative approaches to disease control and their incorporation into medical education, and into the efficient use of biomedical information.

ROCKEFELLER INSTITUTE AND UNIVERSITY. See FOUNDATIONS IN THE USA; RESEARCH INSTITUTES.

ROCKY MOUNTAIN SPOTTED FEVER. Tick-borne *typhus, due to *Rickettsia rickettsii*.

RODDICK, SIR THOMAS GEORGE (1846–1923). Canadian surgeon. His greatest work was in forming the Medical Council of Canada, after 18 years of frustrating work through professional organizations (he was president of the Canadian and British Medical Associations in turn). As a result, a medical graduate is able to take examinations which permit him to practise anywhere in Canada.

RODENT ULCER. Basal cell *carcinoma of the skin, almost always situated on sun-exposed parts of the face. It begins as a small nodule, which then breaks down in the centre to form an ulcer with firm raised edges. Although locally malignant, it rarely metastasizes, and is eminently curable.

RODS are the specialized *retinal structures containing the visual pigment *rhodopsin which are the receptors for vision at low levels of light intensity, sensitive to blue and green light only.

ROENTGEN. The amount of *gamma or *X-radiation that will produce *ions carrying 2.58×10^{-4} coulomb of electric charge per kg of dry air.

ROENTGEN, WILHELM CONRAD (1845–1923). German physicist. On 8 November 1895, while experimenting with a highly evacuated vacuum tube on the conduction of electricity through gases, he noted fluorescence of a barium platinocyanide screen lying nearby.

Further investigation of this radiation showed that it could pass through some substances impervious to light. In view of its unusual features he suggested the name X-rays. For this discovery he was awarded the *Nobel prize for physics in 1901.

ROGER OF PALERMO (Ruggiero Frugardi) (*fl*. 12th century). Roger was the most distinguished surgeon of the school of *Salerno. He published *Practica chirurgiae* (*c*. 1170) which became the standard textbook at Salerno. He used seaweed or burned sponge for treating *goitre and believed *suppuration was essential for wound healing.

ROGERS, SIR LEONARD (1868–1962). British physician and pathologist. A pioneer of *tropical medicine, he identified *Entamoeba histolytica* as the cause of *amoebiasis and introduced *emetine in its treatment; he was the first to use *antimony in treating *kala-azar and hypertonic intravenous saline in *cholera.

ROGET, PETER MARK (1779–1869). Anglo-Swiss physician and savant. Roget was one of the founders of London University and secretary of the Royal Society from 1827 to 1848. He made many contributions to the *Encyclopaedia Britannica*, but his main claim to fame is his *Thesaurus of English words and phrases* (1852), of which there had been 76 impressions by 1983.

ROKITANSKY, KARL FREIHERR VON (1804–74). Austrian pathologist. His *Handbuch der pathologischen Anatomie* (1842–46), enjoyed a large circulation, although neglecting morbid histology. The doctrine of 'crases' and 'stases' it contained was demolished by *Virchow. When he retired he had carried out more than 30 000 autopsies. He was the first to describe *acute yellow atrophy of the liver (1843) and acute dilatation of the stomach (1842).

ROLANDO, LUIGI (1773–1831). Italian physician and anatomist. He described the *fissure of Rolando (the Rolandic fissure). After excising the *cerebrum and *cerebellum in animals he concluded that the first presided over voluntary and the second over involuntary movements.

ROLLESTON, SIR HUMPHRY DAVY, BT (1862–1944). British physician. Rolleston was a scholarly and widely read physician and medical historian and co-editor with Sir Clifford *Allbutt of *A system of medicine* (1905–11, 9 vols).

ROMANOWSKY, DIMITRI LEONIDOVITCH (1861–1921). Russian physician, remembered chiefly for the eosin–methylene blue stain he developed (Romanowsky's stain), the forerunner of other similar stains used for blood smears and malarial parasites (e.g. *Leishman's stain).

ROMANOWSKY'S STAIN. See ROMANOWSKY.

ROMBERG, MORITZ HEINRICH (1795–1873). German physician and neurologist. He published the first formal textbook of neurology, *Lehrbuch der Nervenkrankheiten* (1840–46). He was first to describe *achondroplasia (1817). He is now chiefly remembered for *Romberg's sign.

ROMBERG'S SIGN. Swaying or falling on closing the eyes while in a standing position with the feet together. It indicates sensory *ataxia, that is ataxia due to impaired *proprioception (lack of position and joint sense) in the legs which is compensated by vision; ataxia is therefore aggravated by closing the eyes.

ROONHUYZE, HENDRICK VAN (b. ?–1625). Dutch surgeon. He was noted for his operations on *hare-lip, for his obstetric skills, and for championing *caesarean section. His son, Rogier, also an obstetrician, is said to have bought the secret of the *obstetrical forceps from Hugh *Chamberlen the elder.

RORSCHACH TEST. This psychodiagnostic method, also known as the 'inkblot test', was devised by the Swiss psychiatrist Hermann Rorschach (1884–1922). The subject is shown a series of 10 cards (each of which bears a bilaterally symmetrical inkblot, five of which are in black and white, three in black and red, and two multicoloured) and is invited to interpret what he or she sees on each card. Scoring and analysis are complicated, but the test is said to be helpful in assessing personality, intellect, and emotion, and in the differential diagnosis of psychiatric disorders. Objective validation of these claims has been disappointing.

ROSACEA is a chronic disorder of the skin of the nose, cheeks, and forehead—the 'blush area'—marked by persistent capillary dilatation, papule and pustule formation, and, in some longstanding cases, *rhinophyma. See DERMATOLOGY.

ROSEOLA is an infection of infancy (also called exanthema subitum or roseola infantum) presumed to be due to an as yet unidentified *virus. It is marked by fever for 3–4 days followed by a rose-coloured macular rash. Recovery is uneventful.

ROSS, SIR RONALD (1857–1932). British malariologist. He undertook research into *malaria with Sir Patrick *Manson, observing the parasite in the stomach of the anopheline *mosquito in 1897. He was awarded the *Nobel prize in 1902 for his work on malaria.

ROTAVIRUS. A group of double-stranded *ribonucleic acid (RNA) *viruses associated with acute non-bacterial *gastroenteritis.

ROUNDWORM. Any *nematode worm parasitic in man or animals. Roundworms, when long and slender, such as *Oxyuris*, may also be referred to as *threadworms.

ROUS, FRANCIS PEYTON (1879–1970). American experimental pathologist. In 1911 he demonstrated that a *sarcoma of chickens could be transmitted by an agent in cell-free sterile filtrates of the tumours, that is, a *virus. For this work he received the *Nobel prize 55 years later. In addition, he made significant discoveries with respect to other animal tumours caused by viruses, as well as those induced by irritation, for example tar cancers of the skin. During the First World War he conducted studies on the preservation of blood, and showed that by bleeding into a solution of citrate and sugar, blood could be maintained in fluid state, with cells fairly undamaged, for weeks. The reagent he helped to devise was called the Rous–Turner solution. This finding enabled the later practical development of *blood banks.

ROUS SARCOMA is a type of virus-induced *sarcoma occurring in fowls, described in 1911 by Francis Peyton *Rous.

ROUX, PIERRE PAUL EMILE (1853–1933). French bacteriologist. With von *Behring he demonstrated the value of treatment with *diphtheria antitoxin and of immunization with toxin.

ROYAL APOTHECARIES. There are, by tradition, five general medical attendants in the *Royal Medical Household in the UK. They are: the apothecary to the Queen and to her Household; the apothecary to Household at Windsor; the apothecary to Household at Sandringham; the apothecary to Household at Balmoral; and the apothecary to Household at the Palace of Holyrood.

ROYAL BROMPTON NATIONAL HEART AND LUNG HOSPITAL, THE. This new hospital, opened in London in 1991, brought together on one site two postgraduate specialist hospitals, the Brompton Hospital for Diseases of the Chest and the National Heart Hospital, both of which had been founded in the mid-19th century. They are closely associated with the National Heart and Lung Research Institute which occupies an adjacent site.

ROYAL COLLEGE OF ANAESTHETISTS. See MEDICAL COLLEGES, ETC. OF THE UK.

ROYAL COLLEGE OF GENERAL PRACTITIONERS. See MEDICAL COLLEGES, ETC. OF THE UK.

ROYAL COLLEGE OF NURSING. See MEDICAL COLLEGES, ETC. OF THE UK; NURSING IN THE UK.

ROYAL COLLEGE OF PATHOLOGISTS. See MEDI-CAL COLLEGES, ETC. OF THE UK.

ROYAL COLLEGE OF PHYSICIANS AND SUR-GEONS OF CANADA began in 1929 after the usual negotiations, arguments, and counter-arguments inseparable from the founding of such professional corporations. The general model adopted was that of the Royal Colleges of the UK (see MEDICAL COLLEGES, ETC. OF THE UK). The Act which went through Parliament made it clear that the College was intended to stimulate postgraduate education and 'to act as an incentive to medical men, both physicians and surgeons, to aspire to higher qualifications and therefore higher standards of service to the public'. It does this still, as similar predominantly educational bodies do, by setting standards of experience required for admission to the stiff examinations for the fellowship. These are conducted in both English and French for many specialties. There are now many committees for the specialties and regional committees across the country, all accountable to the Council which is the governing body. Naturally there are relationships established with many other bodies concerned with medicine nationally and internationally.

ROYAL COLLEGE OF PHYSICIANS AND SUR-GEONS OF GLASGOW. See MEDICAL COLLEGES, ETC. OF THE UK.

ROYAL COLLEGE OF PSYCHIATRISTS. See MEDI-CAL COLLEGES, ETC. OF THE UK.

ROYAL COLLEGE OF RADIOLOGISTS. See MEDI-CAL COLLEGES, ETC. OF THE UK.

ROYAL COLLEGES OF PHYSICIANS. See MEDI-CAL COLLEGES, ETC. OF THE UK.

ROYAL COLLEGES OF SURGEONS. See MEDICAL COLLEGES, ETC. OF THE UK.

ROYAL FREE HOSPITAL. The Royal Free Hospital, London, will be remembered for its prime place in the history of medical education for women. Before the middle of the 19th century there was no medical education available to women in the UK, but in the first *Medical Register*, published as a result of the *Medical Act of 1858, there was the name of one woman, Elizabeth *Blackwell, who had obtained a medical degree in the USA. Mrs Elizabeth Garrett *Anderson in 1865 had complied with all the requirements for qualification of the Society of Apothecaries. Almost immediately, the Society changed its rules to exclude women. Sophia *Jex-Blake and others had persuaded Edinburgh University to educate them medically, but by technicalities they too were excluded from practice. This aroused concern in London, where a medical school for women was

set up in 1874, and among the governors were the Earl of Shaftesbury, Charles *Darwin, and Thomas Henry *Huxley. However, there was still no clinical instruction. Then in 1877 the Royal Free Hospital agreed to admit students of the school to its wards. Under an Act of 1876, Examining Boards were empowered to open their examinations to women. The Royal College of Physicians of Ireland did this in 1887, and in the same year the University of London admitted women to its degrees. In 1900 the University recognized the Royal Free Hospital School of Medicine as one of its schools. By the later 1940s men were first admitted to the school, just as women had to be admitted to the previously all-male schools in London.

The hospital moved in 1982 from its more central site to one in Hampstead, a northern suburb of London. This brought together the whole school in its preclinical and clinical parts.

ROYAL HOSPITAL, CHELSEA, by the Thames in London, is not a medical hospital but a home for old soldiers. It was founded in 1682 by King Charles II, and the original building, still standing, was designed by Sir Christopher Wren. The foundation was modelled on the Hôtel des Invalides in Paris, started by Louis XIV in 1670 for similar purposes. The Royal Hospital is run by a Board of Commissioners appointed by the Crown and supported by parliamentary grant since 1847. There are about 450 pensioners, almost all over the age of 65. They are familiar about London in their long scarlet coats with small black military caps. On ceremonial occasions the headgear is a tricorn. There is an infirmary of about 80 beds for the weak and ill.

ROYAL MARSDEN HOSPITAL, THE, founded by Dr William Marsden in 1851, was the first hospital in the world to be devoted exclusively to the diagnosis and treatment of cancer. It operates from two sites, one on Fulham Road, London, the other at Sutton in Surrey, and is closely associated with the Chester Beatty Institute for Cancer Research.

ROYAL MEDICAL HOUSEHOLD. The doctors serving the Queen in the UK are appointed by the Lord Chamberlain, who has overall responsibility for the Royal Medical Household.

ROYAL NATIONAL INSTITUTE FOR THE BLIND (RNIB) began in 1868 when Thomas Rhodes Armitage of London lost his sight and then determined to help the blind to read. The British and Foreign Society for Improving the Embossed Literature of the Blind was formed. In 1914 it became the National Institute for the Blind and took over the Moon works, which produced a form of embossed type that can be printed individually but not written by hand. It is easier to read than braille, but the latter system has prevailed, with help from the

RNIB, as it can be printed and written–a great advantage for communication. In 1915 the Institute founded St Dunstan's Hostel for Blinded Soldiers and Sailors and this became independent in 1922. In the following few years the RNIB took over education in massage for the blind and this has developed into a School of Physiotherapy; it started after-care and home industries; published a journal; started the Sunshine Homes for Blind Babies; and opened the Chorleywood College for Girls. The Talking Book Service came in 1935, mainly for the elderly blind (a large group) who find learning braille particularly difficult. Now there are homes of recovery for those recently blinded, training centres for telephonists, typists, braille shorthand writers, and computer operators, homes for those with multiple handicaps, and a British Foundation for Research into Prevention of Blindness. Braille books are produced for undergraduates, the first braille book was translated by computer in 1968, and the advanced autobraille printing press has been in use since 1982. Books, tapes, and other facilities are available to the blind at subsidized prices. Its financial support comes mainly from donations and legacies. See also OPHTHALMOLOGY.

ROYAL NATIONAL ORTHOPAEDIC HOSPITAL,

London, was formed in 1905 out of the amalgamation of three small metropolitan hospitals, under some pressure from the King Edward VII Hospital Fund, which contributed money to all of them. The Fund wished for a new hospital to be built in central London, and another one in the country, in that order. After the First World War traumatic surgery gave a fillip to this development. The town branch was established in Great Portland Street, and a convalescent home at Stanmore, in the northern suburbs, was acquired for the country branch, and opened in 1922. A chair of orthopaedics was founded, with a benefaction from the National Fund for Research into Poliomyelitis and other Crippling Diseases, in the University of London, during 1965. Before this the university had started an Institute of Orthopaedics at the hospital in 1948. Because the lease of the Great Portland Street branch terminated during 1984, it was decided not to continue with it, but to transfer some clinical facilities and the work of the Institute to the nearby Middlesex Hospital, with which there have long been close associations. The branch at Stanmore continues and a Spinal Injuries Unit is available there.

ROYAL PHARMACEUTICAL SOCIETY OF GREAT BRITAIN.

The professional body for the pharmaceutical profession in the UK. The Council of the Society is responsible for publishing the *British Pharmaceutical Codex* (now the *Pharmaceutical Codex*). See PHARMACY ACTS 1852, 1868, 1954; PHARMACY AND PHARMACISTS.

ROYAL POSTGRADUATE MEDICAL SCHOOL.

The Royal Postgraduate Medical School is associated with the Hammersmith Hospital in west London. The establishment of such a school was recommended by a committee under the chairmanship of the Earl of Athlone. In 1930 another committee recommended the siting of the school at Hammersmith, where it was opened in 1935, and it was granted a Royal Charter in 1966. At first it was part of the London University's British Postgraduate Medical Federation but seceded from it in 1974 to become a School of the University of London. The hospital is almost entirely staffed by academics, except for juniors, who are provided by the *National Health Service. The school conducts advanced research in all major specialties of medicine and has extensive teaching commitments to postgraduate students from all over the world. The hospital provides a major service to the population in its immediate vicinity, as do other hospitals in the *National Health Service, and because of the advanced nature of its work, it provides a consultative service for anyone referred to it.

ROYAL SOCIETY. The national academy of science for the UK and one of the oldest scientific societies of Europe. Its origins date back to the middle of the 17th century when a group of scholars began a series of meetings in London from about 1645. The Civil War and the Protectorate divided the group, some going to Oxford, where meetings continued in Wadham College, others remaining in London. After the Restoration, the group came together again in London and resumed their meetings. The foundation of the Society is regarded as having occurred in November 1660, at a meeting at which '. . . Something was offered about a designe of founding a Colledge for the Promoting of Physico-Mathematicall, Experimentall Learning'; this was the first meeting to be recorded in the Society's journal book. The Society's first Charter was granted by Charles II on 15 July 1662, and a second Charter granted less than a year later extended the Society's privileges; in the latter the Society is referred to by its full title as 'The Royal Society of London for Improving Natural Knowledge'. Medical men were among the founding fellows, and have continued to play an important role in the Society's affairs. The Society, which engages in a wide range of national and international scientific activities, is partly financed by an annual parliamentary grant-in-aid, administered as part of the UK government budget for civil science.

ROYAL SOCIETY OF MEDICINE grew out of the Medico-Chirurgical Society founded in 1805 which received a Royal Charter in 1834. In 1907 it combined with 14 other medical societies in London to form the present Royal Society of Medicine. Its purpose was and is 'for the promotion of physic and surgery and of the branches of science connected with them'. It has an international membership and includes scientists and interested lay people. It carries out its work through many sections and forums, each devoted to a wide aspect of medical and surgical practice. Each holds regular meetings on topics within its interest. Its headquarters in London incorporates a club with some bedrooms and restaurants and maintains one of the best and most comprehensive medical libraries in the UK. Its purposes are essentially educational in the organization of meetings and symposia, in publishing a journal of proceedings and much other material, and in the production of audio-visual materials for teaching and learning. It is non-political, and continues to flourish as an independent educational body.

ROYAL TOUCH. See KING'S EVIL.

ROYAL VICTORIA HOSPITAL, Belfast, Northern Ireland, arose out of the Fever Hospital started in 1797. It became the Belfast General Hospital in 1848. A first charter changed the name to Belfast Royal Hospital in 1875 and a further charter in 1899 brought the present title. Because of the workload a new hospital was built in Grosvenor Road and was opened in 1903 by King Edward VII. Its in-patient work has increased 14-fold since that time. It is now a major regional centre for the whole of Northern Ireland for patients with complicated disorders, and for such specialties as radiotherapy, neurosurgery, and cardiology. It includes all the specialties of medicine and is the teaching hospital of the Queen's University of Belfast. The civil strife in Northern Ireland, especially since 1970 and often in Belfast, has given the hospital staff unrivalled experience in *surgery of trauma caused by many forms of weaponry and fire.

ROYAL VICTORIA HOSPITAL, Montreal, Canada, was founded in 1887, Queen Victoria's jubilee, by Sir George Stephen and Sir Donald Smith, who gave a million dollars for a hospital for the sick poor, without distinction of race or creed. There were also to be facilities for medical and nursing education. By 1894 seven beds were in use and soon the full complement of 260 beds was open. In 1926 a maternity hospital began and is now known as the Women's Pavilion. Later came the Psychiatric (Allan Memorial) Institute in 1944, a large surgical wing in 1956, and a medical one in 1959. All specialties are represented, with special interests in high-risk obstetrics, reconstructive surgery, emergency medicine, endocrinology, and geriatrics. Much research is carried out in all departments. It is a major centre (along with Montreal General Hospital) for the teaching of medical students of *McGill University, which has an innovative educational programme that has attracted interest world-wide. There is teaching for all other health care professions.

ROYAL VICTORIA INFIRMARY (RVI), Newcastle upon Tyne, England, began in 1751 because of the concern of local dignitaries and doctors for the sick poor. The new hospital was opened to patients in 1753 on a site close to the river, near a poor part of the city. A College of Medicine made a stuttering start in 1832 but became established in 1834, and the clinical facilities of the RVI were used for teaching students. The Medical School was at first part of the University of Durham, but from 1962 of the University of Newcastle upon Tyne. In 1896 Queen Victoria's diamond jubilee was approaching and a public appeal was launched. The foundation stone of the new hospital, on its present site (Leazes), was laid in 1900 by the Prince of Wales, Albert Edward, and the Royal Victoria Infirmary was named, being opened in 1906. From the 1940s onwards there was rising specialization and chairs in various clinical subjects were founded. Now it is but one part of a wide teaching hospital complex serving the medical school. In the hospital George Murray first treated *myxoedema with thyroid extract and famous surgeons of the first half of the 20th century included James Rutherford Morison and George Grey Turner.

RUBBER GLOVES. Latex rubber gloves are worn to prevent transmission of micro-organisms from and to the wearer's hands. The introduction of rubber gloves as part of *aseptic technique in surgical practice is credited to the surgeons of *Johns Hopkins Hospital, Baltimore, USA.

RUBEFACIENT is descriptive of agents causing *erythema.

RUBELLA is a common and mild virus infection, also known as German measles, affecting principally children and young adults. One attack usually confers lifelong immunity. The main features are slight fever, inflammation of *lymph nodes particularly behind the ears and below the occiput, and a transient pink *macular rash on face, trunk, and hands and feet in that order. Rapid recovery without complications is the rule. The incubation period varies between 14 and 21 days. The fleeting nature of the rash (which may not be overt) and the mildness of the illness mean that the clinical diagnosis is rarely certain without recourse to laboratory investigations. Its major importance lies in the tragic consequences it produces in the fetus when a mother is infected during the first 3 or 4 months of pregnancy. Transplacental infection occurs, and the infant has a high probability (more than 50 per cent if infection is within four weeks of conception) of being born with *congenital heart disease, *mental handicap, eye *cataracts, *deafness, or a combination of these. Active *immunization with live attenuated virus is effective. Girls who have not acquired natural immunity (ascertainable by serology) should be immunized before the reproductive period. Rubella during the first 4 months of pregnancy is an indication for therapeutic *abortion.

RUBNER, MAX (1854–1932). German physiologist. He first described the specific dynamic action of foodstuffs.

RUELLE, JEAN DE LA (du Ruel; Ruellius) (1474–1537). French physician. He translated *Dioscorides in 1516 and in *De natura stirpium* (1536) gave a full description of many plants, including many new species.

RUFFER, SIR MARC ARMAND (1859–1917). Anglo-French palaeopathologist. Going to Cairo to convalesce, Ruffer was appointed professor of bacteriology in the medical school and became the pioneer *palaeopathologist. He described *tuberculosis of the spine, *arteriosclerosis, *gallstones, and *schistosomiasis in mummies of 3000 BC.

RUPTURE is the usual lay term for *hernia.

RUSH, BENJAMIN (1746–1813). American physician and political figure. He took an active interest in matters of public policy, including abolition of slavery and the temperance movement. He was a member of the Continental Congress, and a signatory of the Declaration of Independence. After the War of Independence he became a professor of medicine at the University of Pennsylvania. During the terrible *yellow fever epidemic of 1793 in Philadelphia he bravely remained in the city, caring for hundreds of victims. He became convinced of the value of drastic purgation, and engaged in a violent controversy with medical colleagues about the benefit of this treatment in patients with yellow fever.

RUTHERFORD, WILLIAM (1839–99). British physiologist. He was known for his theory of hearing, as well as other physiological researches. The resonance theory of *Helmholtz noted the varying fibre lengths of the cochlear membrane, so that notes of varying pitch were assumed to cause vibration of only selected fibres. This accounted for only some of the observed phenomena. Rutherford proposed a telephone theory, in which the whole membrane was thought to vibrate in response to sound, as in the diaphragm of a telephone microphone, which then generates electrical impulses in bursts.

RUXTON, BUCK (*fl.* 1935). British medical practitioner and murderer. Ruxton killed his wife and nursemaid, then dismembered their bodies in a bath, extracted some of their teeth, cut off ears and parts of the face, as well as finger tips, all to make recognition difficult. The parts of the two bodies were distributed widely on moors near Edinburgh. More than 70 pieces were ultimately discovered. The forensic investigation was brilliant in reconstructing the two bodies as the parts turned up. The mode of dismemberment showed that the person responsible must have had medical and anatomical knowledge since joints were neatly disarticulated and features were removed to make identification difficult. After the remains were found on 29 September 1935 and the forensic work was done, it was discovered that two women had disappeared from Ruxton's household on 15 September of the same year. Search of the house revealed hair and bloodstains in the bathroom and on various parts of the stairs, and human remains in the drainage system. Ruxton was found guilty of murder and was hanged.

RUYSCH, FREDERIK (1638–1731). Dutch anatomist. He was the first to demonstrate the valves in the *lymphatics (1665) and developed a method of displaying blood vessels by injecting them post-mortem with a material which solidified. He suggested that the *thyroid secreted some substance into the bloodstream.

RYLE, JOHN ALFRED (1889–1950). British physician. He renounced one of the largest consulting practices in London to become a pioneer of social and *preventive medicine.

S

SABIN, FLORENCE RENA (1871–1953). American biologist. She helped to elucidate the path of lymph flow through lymph nodes, and developed techniques for staining and observing living blood cells.

SABOURAUD, RAYMOND JACQUES ADRIEN (1864–1938). French dermatologist. His studies of mycotic infections were of great value and he devised a culture medium for pathogenic fungi (Sabouraud's medium).

SACCHARIN is a non-nutritive sweetening agent manufactured from toluene. Pure saccharin has about 550 times the sweetening power of sugar.

SACHER-MASOCH. LEOPOLD VON (1836–95). Austrian novelist. Sacher-Masoch described the sexual pleasure derived from being treated cruelly, now known as masochism. This is to be contrasted with sadism—sexual pleasure from causing pain in others.

SACRED DISEASE was a name for *epilepsy, although to *Hippocrates it was 'nowise more divine nor more sacred than other diseases'.

SACROILIAC JOINTS. The two fairly rigid articulations between the sacrum (the bone formed by the five fused sacral vertebrae of the *spine) and the right and left iliac bones, through which the weight of the body is transmitted to the legs. Little movement occurs at the sacroiliac joints, which are supported almost entirely by ligaments, but some relaxation, allowing expansion of the pelvis, takes place during later pregnancy; aching of the lower back at this time may be due to tension of the ligaments supporting the joints. Inflammation of the sacroiliac joints produces important early radiological changes in *ankylosing spondylitis.

SADE, COUNT DONATIEN ALPHONSE FRANCOIS (1740–1814). French writer commonly known as le Marquis de Sade. The term 'sadism', a sexual perversion marked by love of cruelty, is derived from his name.

SADISM is the derivation of sexual pleasure from the infliction of pain or humiliation on another.

SAFE PERIOD. The 'safe period' is that period of the menstrual cycle during which conception is least likely to occur, usually taken as the 10 days preceding *menstruation and the 7 days following. In other words, sexual intercourse is avoided during the periovulatory period of the cycle. As menstruation may not itself be strictly regular, the safe period is best related to the actual time of *ovulation; women who are not aware of its occurrence, for example by experiencing *mittelschmerz may detect the accompanying slight pyrexia by taking daily measurements of body temperature. Restricting intercourse to the safe period is the so-called 'rhythm method' of contraception. It is unreliable, and can result in up to 20 pregnancies per 100 woman-years.

SAFETY OF DRUGS. See MEDICINES ACT 1968; MEDICINES COMMISSION; FOOD AND DRUG ADMINISTRATION; PHARMACEUTICAL INDUSTRY; PHARMACOLOGY.

ST ANTHONY'S FIRE is *erysipelas, to the nursing of which disease an entire monastic order (the Antonines, or Hospital Brothers of St Anthony) was exclusively devoted. The order was founded in 1095 by a Gaston de Dauphine, who believed he owed his recovery from erysipelas to the intervention of the saint, and over the next few centuries erysipelas hospitals were built by the order throughout Europe. They disappeared from England and France when religious orders were suppressed in those countries. St Anthony's fire has also been taken to refer to *ergotism.

ST BARTHOLOMEW'S HOSPITAL, London, was founded with the Priory of the same name in 1123, by Rahere, an Augustinian canon. It remains on its original site, from where it has ministered to the sick of the City of London for 860 years. The first carers were monks and nuns. Some of their patients came from the nearby notorious Newgate Prison. In 1539 the Priory was closed at the Dissolution of the Monasteries by Henry VIII. He confiscated the property of the hospital, but allowed it to remain open. Under pressure from the City and his own surgeon Thomas *Vicary, Henry re-established the Royal Hospitals of St Bartholomew's, *St Thomas's, *Bethlem, and Bridewell. Nothing remains of the medieval hospital. James Gibbs designed a new hospital in the 18th century. There is a magnificent Great Hall in the North Wing. The staircase leading to it is decorated with murals by William Hogarth, who was a governor. In 1609 William *Harvey was appointed to the staff. Percivall *Pott was on the staff in the 18th century. John *Abernethy founded the Medical College in 1822, and James *Paget was the first warden. In 1877 a school of nursing was started. The Medical College is now part of the University of London.

ST COSMAS AND ST DAMIEN were twin brothers, early Christian martyrs of Cyrrhus in Syria, who practised medicine without fees and came to be regarded as patron saints of doctors. There are several versions their lives, and even the fact of martyrdom is uncertain; but their cult adapted the ancient Greek practice of incubation (see TEMPLE MEDICINE) to the Christian faith, their patients sleeping overnight in their churches in order to dream of a cure.

ST FIACRE is the patron saint of *haemorrhoids. He was the son of an Irish king; he emigrated to France and lived there as a hermit for many years.

ST GEORGE'S HOSPITAL was founded in 1733 at Hyde Park Corner in the West End of London, on which site its buildings were a London landmark for more than two and a half centuries. Edward *Jenner was trained there, and among the many illustrious members of staff were John *Hunter, Matthew *Baillie, Thomas *Young, Benjamin *Brodie, and Stewart *Duke-Elder. St George's Hospital and its associated medical school have been relocated in new buildings in Tooting, a southern suburb of London, a move which took place in phases during the 1960s and 1970s. The facilities at Hyde Park Corner were finally closed in 1980.

ST JOHN, ORDER OF; KNIGHTS HOSPITALLER; ST JOHN AMBULANCE
Historical background: the Knights Hospitaller
When the first Crusaders captured Jerusalem in 1099, they found a *hospice which cared for sick and weary pilgrims to the Holy Land, run by a group of monastic brothers. The Crusaders gave this hospice money and estates in the Holy Land and Europe. In 1113 the Hospitallers became an independent religious order, recognized by the Pope: the Order of the Hospital of St John of Jerusalem. Its precincts and hospital were near the Church of the Holy Sepulchre. The brothers followed a monastic rule and made a vow to honour Our Lords the Sick. Hospitaller nuns did not usually undertake nursing duties.

Late 12th century rules of the Order show that they employed four wise doctors, qualified to examine urine and diagnose different diseases, and able to administer appropriate medicines. They also employed surgeons. The Knights laid great stress on the importance of *hygiene, good *nursing, *diet, and a knowledge of herbs and drugs.

By the mid-12th century, the Hospitallers had developed a military role, protecting travellers and pilgrims, and defending the states set up by the Crusaders from the attacks of the Saracens. The Knights garrisoned huge crusader castles, like Krak des Chevaliers and Margat (in Syria) and employed mercenaries.

Jerusalem fell in 1187 and the Order moved its headquarters to Acre. The Knights later captured the island of Rhodes, which became a busy trading harbour and a noted port-of-call for travellers and pilgrims *en route* to the Holy Land. Its *hospital was renowned for the quality of its care. The 15th century building, now the National Museum in Rhodes, had wards for *infectious diseases, an *obstetric ward, and cots for children born to pilgrims, as there had been in Jerusalem. Every Knight, including the Master of the Order, worked in the wards, although orderlies were employed, as well as specialist *physicians, *surgeons, and *pharmacists. During the Rhodian period, the Organization of the Order became more structured, as its international affairs became more complex. Rhodes fell to the Turks after a prolonged siege in 1522, following which the Knights were forced to leave.

For some years they were without a base, until Malta was given to them by Charles V, King of Spain and Holy Roman Emperor. In 1565, under their Grand Master, Jean de la Valette, they withstood a massive Turkish siege. Soon afterwards, a new capital city was built—Valletta—with strong fortifications, a conventual church, *auberges* or inns to house the Knights, a Grand Master's Palace, and a major hospital, the Holy Infirmary. Wounded and sick Knights, Maltese, slaves, and travellers were all cared for in the Order's several hospitals on Malta. In 1676 a school of *anatomy and *surgery was founded by the Grand Master, which produced a number of qualified Maltese practitioners, including such pioneers as Michel' Angelo Grima, who became apprenticed when he was 12. There was no shortage of corpses for *dissection, as it was directed that the bodies of Knights and patients from the Holy Infirmary should automatically be sent to be dissected by the physicians and surgeons. In the 18th century Grand Master Vilhena introduced a quarantine hospital to counteract the spread of *plague and other infectious diseases.

The Order owned a great deal of property throughout Europe. This was organized into priories, each with a prior at its head. Estates administered by the priories were subdivided into commanderies or preceptories. Few ran hospitals but all had the monastic duty of hospitality. In England the Order established its headquarters at Clerkenwell, just outside the city walls of London; the 12th century English Knights of St John were few in number and frequently holders of high office under the Crown. St John's Gate, the entrance to the Priory of Clerkenwell, still stands, as does the 12th century crypt and part of the church. It now houses the headquarters of the Most Venerable Order of St John and its library and museum. The Order in England was dissolved by Henry VIII in 1540, as part of his dissolution of the religious orders. Mary Tudor restored the Order briefly in the last year of her reign, but it fell into abeyance again under Elizabeth I. The French Revolution undermined the Order's failing finances internationally and in 1798 Malta fell to Napoleon's troops. The Order entered a period of decline and disarray until, eventually, a new headquarters was established in Rome.

The Sovereign Military Order of St John of Jerusalem, called of Rhodes, called of Malta

Today, the members of the Sovereign Military Order of Malta, as it is commonly known, still have their headquarters in the Via Condotti in Rome. Its Grand Master is the head of a Sovereign Order that sends ambassadors to many countries and whose members are of aristocratic origin. Its role is entirely humanitarian: the care of pilgrims to Lourdes and to Rome, aid to refugees, and the care of leprosy patients are examples of the Order's world-wide charitable concerns. It has National Associations in most countries, including the UK.

The Johanniterorden

The knightly order of St John of Jerusalem (Bailiwick of Brandenburg) is based on a former province of the Hospitallers which adopted the reformed faith and continued in being. It was constituted as a separate order by King William IV of Prussia in 1852. It has commanderies in France, Switzerland, Finland, and Hungary, and runs hospitals, a first-aid service (Johanniter-Unfall-Hilfe), and a nursing service.

The Order of St John in Sweden

Formerly part of the Johanniterorden, declared a separate order in 1920 under the Crown of Sweden. It runs charitable projects.

The Order of St John in the Netherlands

Formerly part of the Johanniterorden, declared a separate Order in 1945, under the Dutch monarchy. It undertakes hospitaller and welfare work.

The Most Venerable Order of the Hospital of St John of Jerusalem

In the early 19th century a move to restore the Priory of England resulted in an 1888 Charter by Queen Victoria in recognition of the valuable work done by the British Order of St John. Since then a member of the Royal family has held the position of Grand Prior, at present HRH the Duke of Gloucester. The British Order of St John has priories and commanderies in many, mainly Commonwealth, countries such as Australia, Canada, and New Zealand.

The St John Ambulance Association

Founded in 1887, had the aim of training the public in 'aid to the injured', later called first aid. Association centres were set up all over the country, particularly along the industrial backbone of England, in the Midlands, Yorkshire, and Lancashire, in the collieries, the main railway centres, and the manufacturing centres.

Today the St John Ambulance Association still has the major responsibility for training industry, the police, the fire brigade, and the public in first aid. The training is intended to save life, to the point where superior medical knowledge and training may take over. A major responsibility is the provision of textbooks which are compiled jointly with the British *Red Cross and the St Andrew's Ambulance Association (which provides similar services to Scotland). Training is provided by qualified medical staff, who give their services voluntarily. Each registered first aider must know the basic methods for saving and prolonging life and the procedures to be followed at an accident.

St John Ambulance Brigade

Founded in 1887 as a uniformed body of trained volunteers proficient in first aid, present at public events to provide instant cover for accident and injury. They also provide a valuable supporting service to the statutory *ambulance services in times of emergency, for example, a major industrial accident. The Brigade is organized on a country structure with local ambulance, nursing, cadet, and combined divisions and centres. Its headquarters are in Grosvenor Crescent, London, alongside those of the Joint Committee of St John and the Red Cross.

In 1899 the Brigade was required to support the army medical services, by providing hospital orderlies for the Boer War. During the First World War a Joint Committee of St John and the Red Cross was formed, which provided the Voluntary Aid Detachments (VADs), who acted in support of the Royal Army Medical Corps, the Military Home Hospitals Reserve, and the Royal Naval Sick Berth Reserve. The Brigade also ran its own hospital in the First World War, at Etaples. The St John roles in civil defence and the armed services medical reserves were clearly established and work continued throughout the Second World War. The Joint Committee still exists, providing hospital welfare services and care of war disabled.

The St John Cadets, founded in 1922 as a youth movement to train and interest young people in the medical, nursing, and ancillary professions, also participate in welfare work. The St John Ambulance Overseas Relations Department co-ordinates and channels information to and from the many countries world-wide in which St John Ambulance operates.

The St John Ambulance Association and Brigade were amalgamated in 1968 to form St John Ambulance.

St John Ophthalmic Hospital

In 1882 the British Order of St John founded an eye hospital in Jerusalem. The hospital, now in the Sheik Jarrah district of Jerusalem, continues its work of aiding those with eye disease, regardless of race, colour, or creed. Its work is supported by the other Orders of St John, especially the American Society of the Most Venerable Order. Poor Arabs make up the majority of the patients, and the hospital provides training facilities for Arab nurses and orderlies. Doctors and surgeons are usually British or American, on short-term contracts. The hospital is run by the warden and matron under the direction of the hospitaller. It also has an 'outreach' programme to tackle eye problems in outlying areas.

The long tradition of caring for the sick established by the Knights Hospitaller continues today in the work of the Orders of St John.

PAMELA WILLIS

Further reading
Sainty, G. S. (1991). *The Orders of Saint John*. American Society of the Order of the Hospital of Saint John, New York.

ST MARY'S HOSPITAL, London, is in the Paddington district. After being mooted from 1841, the building began in 1846, and 5 years later the hospital was opened for 50 in-patients. Two years later the medical school was established, as part of the University of London. Now in the hospital group under the NHS are Paddington Green Children's Hospital, Princess Louise Hospital for Children, St Luke's Hospital, Bayswater (terminal care), The Samaritan Hospital for Women (gynaecology), and the Western Ophthalmic Hospital. It was in the microbiological laboratory that Alexander *Fleming discovered *penicillin in 1928. The tradition of investigation of infections had long been established, mainly by Almroth *Wright, who was appointed in 1902, and who introduced *vaccine therapy for many diseases. A. D. *Waller of the physiology department played a major part in the development of *electrocardiography. Lord Moran (see WILSON, CHARLES McMORAN), Winston Churchill's physician, was at one time dean of the medical school.

ST THOMAS'S HOSPITAL, London, has one of the longest records of service to the sick of any institution in the world. Its origin has been placed in the Priory of St Mary the Virgin in about AD 1106. This was on the south bank of the Thames near the only bridge over the river from the City. Richard (Dick) Whittington, Mayor of London, established a ward for unmarried mothers there (provided they would mend their ways!). Miles Coverdale printed the first full English translation of the Bible in the hospital precincts. At the Dissolution of the Monasteries by Henry VIII it was virtually closed, but was restored by Edward VI in 1553. Since then its doors have never been closed.

Richard *Mead was appointed physician in 1703 and was contemporary with William *Cheselden, the surgeon. Thomas *Guy, the bookseller, was a governor and he built a hospital in the grounds of St Thomas's to take incurable and mental cases in 1721. Teaching of students took place from very early in the foundation, and John *Keats, the poet, is variously claimed as having studied first at St Thomas's and then *Guy's. Sir Astley *Cooper had established a fine anatomy school early in the 19th century and students of both St Thomas's and Guy's hospitals were taught there. But tensions were rising between them, and when Guy's students were prevented from witnessing operations at St Thomas's unless they produced tickets, there was a riot which produced a total rift between the two hospitals. In 1847 the site of St Thomas's was compulsorily bought for £296 000 (US$444 000) by the Charing Cross Railway, and a new position had to be found. The present prime position opposite the Houses of Parliament, was obtained for £100 000 (US$150 000) through the good offices of Sidney *Herbert, a member of the government, under pressure from Florence *Nightingale, who wanted a place for her proposed school of nursing, which she thought was essential after her experiences in the Crimean War. The school was founded, revolutionizing concepts of nursing, ultimately throughout the world.

During the Second World War the hospital suffered severe damage from enemy bombing, and a few members of staff but no patients were killed. For much of the war many in-patient wards were evacuated to the country, although out-patient work continued in London, and there were emergency operations for casualties. By the 1970s several local hospitals had been incorporated into St Thomas's and it was partly rebuilt on its site near Westminster Bridge. The medical schools of Guy's and St Thomas's have combined once more to face the 1980s and beyond.

ST VITUS'S DANCE is Sydenham's *chorea (rheumatic encephalopathy), from the reputed power of St Vitus over nervous and hysterical afflictions.

SALBUTAMOL, known in the USA as albuterol, is a selective beta$_2$–adrenergic stimulant used as a *bronchodilator in bronchial *asthma and states of reversible airways obstruction. It is best administered by inhalation (of an *aerosol solution or in powder) but is also effective by oral and parenteral routes.

SALERNO, on the west coast of Italy, just south of Naples, is famous in medical history for housing the first medical school of real pretensions in Europe, flourishing in the 11th and 12th centuries. Southern Italy, and especially Sicily, were much influenced both by Greek and Islamic cultures, as they moved along the Mediterranean. Several medical books were published from Salerno, and there were both male and female physicians and students. The practice of medicine came under the jurisdiction of the Emperor Frederick II, who in 1221 decreed that doctors would have to pass examinations set by the masters in Salerno. Moreover, no one was allowed to start an education in medicine until the age of 21, the prior 3 years being spent in the study of logic; the medical course lasted 5 years.

There is a famous poem, *Regimen Sanitatis Salernitanum*, with editions varying from several hundred to a few thousand verses. It is literally a regimen of health and has references to healthy living, diet, liquor, sleep, and remedies of many kinds, including surgical. *Castiglioni (a medical historian) thought it 'the backbone of all practical medical literature up to the time of the Renaissance'.

SALICETTI, GUILIELMO (Guilelimus di saliceto) (c. 1210–77). Italian surgeon. He reintroduced the knife in place of the *cautery favoured by the Arabs and regarded suppuration, inevitable after use of the cautery, as undesirable. He recorded *crepitus as a sign of fracture, distinguished between arterial and venous bleeding, noted contralateral paralysis in skull wounds, and appreciated the venereal origin of *chancres and *bubos.

SALICYLATE. Any salt of salicylic acid: preparations of aspirin (*acetylsalicylic acid) are examples.

SALINE. A solution of salt (sodium chloride: $NaCl$). Saline containing 0.9 g $NaCl$ per 100 ml has the same *electrolyte strength as blood and is referred to as normal, physiological, or isotonic saline.

SALIVA is the fluid secreted by the parotid, submaxillary, and sublingual salivary glands. As well as assisting mastication by moistening the mouth, saliva contains an *enzyme, salivary amylase which initiates *digestion by hydrolysing starch to maltose.

SALIVARY GLANDS. The three main pairs of glands which, together with small accessory glands, secrete *saliva; they are the *parotid, sublingual, and submandibular glands.

SALK VACCINE is inactivated *poliomyelitis vaccine, administered by injection.

SALMON, DANIEL ELMER (1850–1914). American veterinary pathologist. He is chiefly remembered because of the bacteria (*Salmonella*) which bear his name, but among his other scientific contributions was the discovery (in 1886 with Theobald *Smith) that bacteria could produce protective *immunity despite having been killed by heat.

SALMONELLA is a genus of *bacteria comprising many different species responsible for several diseases in man and animals, including *typhoid and *paratyphoid fever and some types of food poisoning.

Salmonella (named after Daniel Elmer *Salmon) are rod-shaped, Gram-negative bacilli, which are distinguished from other enteric bacilli by their inability to ferment lactose.

SALPETRIERE (Hospice de la Vieillesse (femmes)) was founded in Paris by royal decree in 1656. The king gave the grounds and some buildings where there had been a small arsenal, and where saltpetre had been made. The intention was to lodge women and children in need, and at first there were 628 women and 192 children aged from 2 to 5 years supervised by 27 male and female officers. By 1684 a special quarter for debauched women, female criminals, and prostitutes was established. In 1780 letters patent were issued which forbade the inmates of Salpêtrière being taken, when ill, into the Hôtel-Dieu, so an infirmary was built in the grounds.

Matters improved when the Salpêtrière came under the control of a council for the hospitals of Paris; 4000 of the prostitutes, criminals, and children were discharged elsewhere, and the mortality dropped to one-quarter of its previous figure. The treatment of the mentally ill became renowned throughout Europe and attracted many students. Jean-Martin *Charcot was physician there from 1862. The original humanitarian purpose of caring for ageing indigent women also continued. Today the Salpêtrière functions as a major teaching hospital in which all major specialties are represented and many new buildings function alongside the old.

SALPINGITIS is inflammation of the *Fallopian (uterine) tube.

SALT is a compound formed when the hydrogen of an acid is replaced by a metal. A salt is produced by the reaction of an acid with a base, water being formed at the same time. In common use the word salt refers to sodium chloride ($NaCl$).

SALT DEPRIVATION. A condition of salt deprivation arises when too much salt (sodium chloride) is lost from the body, as in heavy sweating and in some pathological conditions. Salt deprivation is common after exertion in a hot environment, causing weariness, prostration, and painful muscular cramps ('stoker's cramp'). It may be prevented by salt tablets.

SALVARSAN is an *arsenic-containing organic compound, also known as arsphenamine, formerly used in the treatment of *syphilis.

SAL VOLATILE is ammonium carbonate or smelling salts, a traditional remedy for faintness.

SANATORIUM. An establishment for the reception and treatment of invalids, particularly those with *tuberculosis. Since the advent of antituberculous chemotherapy obviated the need for special tuberculosis hospitals the word has largely fallen into disuse. It is still occasionally used for convalescent homes and private hospitals for the treatment of, for example, *alcoholism.

SANDFLY is the name commonly applied to various species of the genus *Phlebotomus*, small, biting dipterous flies common in tropical and subtropical countries. Female sandflies transmit *kala-azar and other forms of *leishmaniasis, a South American bacterial infection called *Oroya fever (bartonellosis), and sandfly fever. Sandfly (or pappataci) fever is an acute self-limiting febrile illness without any obvious diagnostic features, and is difficult initially to distinguish from other causes of fever such as influenza, malaria, etc. It lasts, however, only 3–4 days, and requires symptomatic treatment only. It is caused by a group of viruses transmitted by *Phlebotomus papatasii*. The sandfly is infected by biting a patient with the acute illness, and remains infective for the rest of its life. There is no animal reservoir and maintenance of the virus is thought to be due to transovarial transmission within the sandfly population.

SANDFLY FEVER. See SANDFLY.

SANGER, MARGARET (1883–1966). American feminist leader, and world figure in *birth control. As a nurse in a poor district of New York City she became concerned about problems of uncontrolled fertility in conditions of poverty. She established birth control clinics in the New York area; she was prosecuted for violations of the law and spent one 30-day term in gaol. Nevertheless she founded the American Birth Control League in 1921; this later became part of a larger organization, the Planned Parenthood Federation of America.

SANITARY INSPECTOR. A professional officer concerned with environmental sanitation and responsible for sanitary inspection. The designation of this officer varies widely from country to country, for example health inspector, public health officer, environmental health officer, etc. The term 'sanitarian' is sometimes used to cover all types of sanitary inspection personnel.

SANITATION. The establishment and maintenance of conditions favourable to health, particularly toilet facilities, drainage, and sewage disposal.

SANTORINI, GIOVANNI DOMENICO (1681–1737). Italian anatomist and physician. One of the outstanding anatomists of his time, his name is attached to some ten anatomical structures. He published *Observationes anatomicae* (1724).

SANTORIO, SANTORIO (Sanctorius) (1561–1636). Italian physician and physiologist. He was one of the architects of the iatrophysical school of medicine. His main interest was in *mensuration and he tried to make it a support for humoral pathology. He devised an 'air thermometer', a hygroscope, and a device which he called the 'pulsilogium' for indicating the pulse rate. He invented instruments for extracting bladder *stones and a *trocar and *cannula. However, he is best known for his observations, published in *De medica statica* (1614), on his own changes in weight due to 'insensible perspiration' resulting from such physiological activities as eating, sleeping, and digestion.

SAPPHISM. See LESBIANISM.

SARCOIDOSIS is a chronic disease of unknown cause marked by the development of granulomatous tissue in various parts of the *reticuloendothelial system. Pulmonary infiltration, enlargement of mediastinal *lymph nodes, and involvement of the skin, eye, and nervous system are the commonest presenting manifestations.

SARCOMA. A malignant *tumour arising from bone, connective tissue, muscle (*sarco* denotes 'flesh'), and other tissues, the embryonic origin of which is the *mesoderm. Sarcomas are much less common than *carcinomas (which arise from epithelial tissue) but are often highly malignant. An appropriate prefix is attached to indicate the tissue of origin when known, for example osteosarcoma (bone), chondrosarcoma (cartilage), lymphosarcoma, fibrosarcoma, etc.

SARCOPLASM is the substance in which the fibrils making up a muscle fibre are embedded.

SATURNISM. *Lead poisoning.

SATYRIASIS is pathologically increased sexual activity in men, the equivalent of *nymphomania in women.

SAUCEROTTE, NICOLAS (1741–1814). French army surgeon. He was a skilled neurosurgeon and experimentally confirmed contralateral innervation (e.g. the left side of the brain controls the right side of the body). He described *acromegaly in 1772.

SAUERBRUCH, ERNST FERDINAND (1875–1951). The leading German surgeon of his time, he was a pioneer of thoracic surgery (see CARDIOTHORACIC SURGERY) and devised a positive-pressure cabinet in which he operated. He much improved the technique of *thoracoplasty. Interested and concerned with the broader issues of medicine, he constantly warned surgeons against becoming mere technicians.

SAVE THE CHILDREN FUND, THE, started in 1919 in the UK, and has a headquarters in London. Its aims are to secure the welfare of children, wherever threatened by natural disasters, hunger, poverty, and disease. It is entirely non-political, and charity is its only source of finance. Funds are raised by branches and volunteers throughout the country. Now there are similar funds in many developed countries, including the USA, Canada, Australia, Denmark, and Norway, and others exist in some parts of the developing world, all with similar aims. Expert teams of agronomists, engineers, educationists, doctors, nurses, and others work in the field in many places. Their tasks are to help, but more especially to educate local people to help themselves, with the hope that various enterprises can later be handed over to local initiative. There are campaigns for maternal and child welfare, nutrition, education, and against infectious diseases, particularly gastroenteritis. There are teams for emergency relief and for refugees. In the UK there are special centres for help with children and their problems in inner city areas.

SAXITOXIN is the neurotoxic *alkaloid secreted by dinoflagellates of the genus *Gonyaulax* and responsible for paralytic shellfish or gonyaulax poisoning. See RED TIDE.

SCABIES is skin infestation with the itch mite *Acarus scabiei*, also *Sarcoptes scabiei*. The condition causes intense itching and is contagious.

SCAN. The record produced by a *scanner, or the procedure of scanning.

SCANNERS are instruments which make pictorial records of particular events (such as radioactivity, X-rays, ultrasound, etc.) by measuring different areas in turn and producing an integrated picture of variations over a body part or an organ, such as the liver or the thyroid gland. In common parlance, 'scanner' when unqualified is usually taken to mean 'CT or MRI scanner', i.e. a machine for *computerized tomography or *magnetic resonance imaging. Thus 'head scanner' and 'body scanner'. See also NUCLEAR MEDICINE; RADIOLOGY.

SCAR. The new fibrous tissue that remains after an injury has healed.

SCARLATINA is a synonym for *scarlet fever.

SCARLET FEVER is a streptococcal infection, usually of the throat, with certain strains of group A haemolytic *streptococci which elaborate 'erythrogenic' toxins, so that the usual manifestations of acute *pharyngitis are accompanied by a generalized *rash. This is a diffuse *erythema with punctate darker papules, the skin around the mouth typically being spared (circumoral pallor). Also typical is peeling or desquamation which follows fading of the rash.

SCARPA, ANTONIO (?1714–1832). Italian surgeon and anatomist. Although best remembered for his description of the *femoral (Scarpa's) triangle, his work on the ear, the olfactory apparatus, and the cardiac nerves was more important. He was a brilliant anatomical draughtsman as shown by his *Tabulae neurologicae* (1794).

SCHÄFER, SIR EDWARD ALBERT SHARPEY. See SHARPEY-SCHÄFER.

SCHAUDINN, FRITZ RICHARD (1871–1906). German protozoologist. In 1902 he claimed to have seen a *malarial sporozoite entering a red blood cell. The following year he distinguished the pathogenic *Entamoeba histolytica* from the (often) harmless *Escherichia coli*, and in May 1905, together with Hoffmann, he discovered *Spirochaeta pallida*, now known as *Treponema pallidum*, the causative organism of *syphilis.

SCHIFF, MORITZ (1823–96). German physician and physiologist. His main investigations were into the nervous system and dealt with the pathways for sensations of pain and touch in the *spinal cord. In 1856 he showed that *thyroidectomy in dogs and guinea-pigs was followed by death. He made unsuccessful attempts to graft *thyroid tissue.

SCHISMATIC MEDICAL COLLEGES. See NESTORIAN MEDICINE.

SCHISTOSOMIASIS is *bilharziasis.

SCHIZOID is a term describing a personality which is withdrawn and introspective, with marked dissociation between the emotions and the intellect; the personality resembles that of *schizophrenia, but is within the bounds of normality.

SCHIZOPHRENIA is the commonest psychotic illness, accounting for some 80 per cent of patients under the age of 65 who have been in hospital for 2 years or more. The term 'schizophrenia' was introduced by *Bleuler in 1911, replacing the older name 'dementia praecox', in order to describe the apparent splitting of the mind which is typical of the condition, part remaining in touch with reality and part not. The manifestations are protean, the commonest being withdrawal, regression, infantilism, asocial or antisocial behaviour, aberrant ideas, delusions, and hallucinations. Several clinical types are recognized: simple, paranoid, catatonic, hebephrenic, and mixed. The onset is usually in adolescence or early adult life and the course is chronic, sometimes with remissions. Despite intensive research its aetiology and pathogenesis are still not understood. It is clear, however, that there is a strong genetic factor.

SCHLEIDEN, JACOB MATTHIAS (1804–86). German physician and botanist. He was a popularizer of science, and his textbook *Grundzüge der wissenschaftlichen Botanik* (1842) had great influence. He showed that plant tissues were made of groups of cells and he realized the importance of the nucleus, although he thought that it gave rise to young cells. Discussions with Schleiden inspired his friend, Theodor *Schwann, to formulate the 'cell theory'.

SCHMIEDEBERG, OSWALD (1838–1921). German pharmacologist. He had many distinguished pupils including J. J. *Abel and A. R. *Cushny. He showed the *vagus to contain accelerator fibres (1871); extracted *muscarine from *Amanita muscaria* (1869); carried out important studies on *digitalis (1883); and deduced the formula of *nucleic acid (1896).

SCHÖNLEIN, JOHANN LUCAS (1793–1864). German physician. He was the founder of the school that believed that medicine could be studied like botany or zoology and that diseases could be classified like plants and animals. He was an outstanding clinician, one of the first to make *auscultation and *percussion a routine, and to exploit clinical pathology. He described *peliosis rheumatica (Schönlein's disease) in 1837 and discovered the causative organism of trichophytosis (*Achorion schönleinii*) in 1839.

SCHOOL DENTAL SERVICE. Part I, Section 5, of the *National Health Services Act 1977 lays upon the Secretary of State for Social Services the responsibility in England and Wales for providing for the dental inspection and treatment of pupils in attendance at schools maintained by local education authorities. Before the 1974 reorganization of the NHS, the school dental service (which had existed in some form since 1907) was the responsibility of local education authorities, a principal school dental officer with a staff of school dental officers being responsible to the *Medical Officer of Health. These staff were transferred to health authorities under the *National Health Service (Reorganization) Act 1973.

SCHOOL MEDICAL SERVICE. Like the *school dental service, a school medical service existed in the UK from 1907. It is now the responsibility of the Secretary of State, under the *National Health Service Act 1977, and delegated by him to local health authorities, who provide regular medical inspection and treatment of pupils in schools maintained by local education authorities. Before the 1974 NHS reorganization, this responsibility rested with local education authorities.

SCHWANN, THEODOR AMBROSE HUBERT (1810–82). German physiologist. His early researches were into muscular activity and metabolism. He described *pepsin and the *neurilemma and hinted at the germ theory of disease. In 1837 he published his classic declaration of the *cell theory in a book of microscopical investigations into the similarities of the structure and growth of animals and plants.

SCHWANN CELLS are large nucleated cells responsible for the production of *myelin in peripheral nerve fibres.

SCHWEITZER, ALBERT (1875–1965). German-French philosopher, theologian, and physician. After appointment as principal of the theological faculty in Strasbourg, he decided that his duty lay in the medical care of the sick poor in Africa and trained in medicine. He settled in Lambaréné, Gabon, French Equatorial Africa, in 1913, built a hospital with his own hands, and maintained it. He was interned briefly in 1914 as a German subject but he returned to Africa to work in his hospital in 1925. In 1952 he was awarded the *Nobel peace prize.

SCIATICA is pain in the distribution of the *sciatic nerve, that is, radiating from the buttock down the back and outside of the thigh and lower leg. See PROLAPSED INTERVERTEBRAL DISC.

SCIATIC NERVE. The largest nerve in the body, derived via the sacral plexus from the 4th and 5th lumbar and the 1st, 2nd, and 3rd sacral segments of the *spinal cord. Through its two main divisions, the tibial and the common peroneal nerves, it supplies motor fibres to the posterior (flexor) thigh muscles and to all muscles below the knee; and sensory fibres to the posterolateral aspects of the leg and all the foot except the medial border.

SCINTILLATION COUNTER. A device for measuring *ionizing radiation. The radiation energy is absorbed by a phosphor, a substance which is luminescent, that is after a brief storage period it releases the absorbed energy as light; the flashes of light are then converted into electrical pulses by a photomultiplier, counted, and recorded.

SCLERA. The thick white outer coat which covers most of the eyeball, merging into the *cornea in front and the sheath of the *optic nerve behind.

SCLERITIS is inflammation of the *sclera.

SCLERODERMA. See SYSTEMIC SCLEROSIS, PROGRESSIVE.

SCLEROSIS. Literally hardening; it is applied to any pathological process of which hardening is a feature, for example *fibrosis. See also MULTIPLE SCLEROSIS; SYSTEMIC SCLEROSIS, PROGRESSIVE.

SCOLIOSIS is spinal deformity due to curvature in a lateral direction.

SCOPOLAMINE is the alternative name for *hyoscine.

SCORPIONS are venomous arachnids found in many tropical and subtropical parts of the world, envenomation by which can sometimes cause serious reactions and even occasionally death.

SCOTOMA is a blind spot in the visual field (see OPHTHALMOLOGY).

SCRAPIE is an *encephalopathy occurring in sheep and goats, one of the prototypes of 'slow' infection of the nervous system (the incubation or latent period is up to 4 years). It can be shown to be due to a transmissible agent, now believed to be a *prion.

SCREEN. The device employed for visualizing *X-ray images in *radioscopy.

SCREENING

General principles

Screening means testing people for early signs of an illness for which they have not yet sought medical help. Sometimes the purpose of screening may be to protect other people, for example in testing the contacts of patients with *infectious disease such as *tuberculosis, *typhoid, or *AIDS, so that, if infected, steps can be taken to prevent them spreading the infection to others. But more usually, in developed societies, screening is performed for the purpose of finding and treating a disease in its very early stages and thereby preventing the individuals concerned from developing its full-blown consequences. This article is concerned solely with this latter purpose.

In screening, unlike normal clinical practice, it is not the patient who goes to the doctor for help, but rather the doctor who goes to the public, recommending that they be tested for their own good. This pro-active role, which is like that of a missionary or a salesman, puts a particular ethical responsibility on the doctor or public health authority to be sure that the prospect of a person benefiting from screening greatly exceeds the prospect of him or her being harmed.

The main benefit of screening is an improved prognosis for those found to have early signs of a potentially serious, even life-threatening, disease which can be cured by early treatment. The disadvantages of screening accrue mainly to the screened people who do *not* have the disease in question, who usually outnumber the diseased people by thousands to one. Some may suffer from hazards of the test itself, e.g. accidental *miscarriage following *amniocentesis, and some may suffer anxiety caused by a false positive result and morbidity from its further investigation, e.g. an unnecessary *biopsy operation. These side-effects of screening are usually minor, but because they may affect so many people the total sum of *morbidity must be weighed against the major benefit to a few. Moreover, screening is usually a very expensive form of medical care because so many people have to be tested for every one helped.

Therefore before introducing screening as a service it should be fully evaluated by research to measure how many people will benefit, to quantify that benefit, in terms of years of life gained or quality of life improved, and to measure how many people will suffer the harmful side-effects of screening, and to assess its costs.

An important factor influencing both benefit and cost is the validity of the screening test. In diagnosing a patient with an overt complaint the doctor uses information derived from several sources, including the patient's history, physical signs, and specialized investigations which he may order and which he may repeat. But in screening he has only the result of a single test at one point in time, and on the basis of this has to sort out those who probably have the disease, 'positives', from those who probably do not, 'negatives'. People with positive results need a full diagnostic work-up to clarify whether they really do have the disease or whether they are false positives. A test which gives many false positives is said to have a low *specificity*. Conversely, a test may fail to detect some people with the disease, thereby giving false negative results. A test which gives many false negatives is said to have a low *sensitivity*. Many screening tests are based on measuring a continuously distributed variable, such as *blood pressure or serum phenylalanine, and so the cut-off point to distinguish positives from negatives can be varied. If it is made less stringent, sensitivity will improve but specificity will decrease, giving more false positives; if it is made more stringent, specificity will improve but sensitivity will be lower, giving more false negatives.

In seeking the very earliest indicators of disease it is often found that even a full diagnostic work-up cannot tell which individuals with positive results will go on to develop overt disease, and which will not—there is a borderline group whose future is uncertain, and the size of this group is usually much larger than the group with obvious early disease. The management of people in this borderline group poses problems because it is impossible to distinguish those with progressive disease requiring treatment from those with non-progressive disease. Hence all must be treated even though some will not benefit from it, and may even be harmed by being incorrectly labelled as having the disease in question.

Antenatal screening

The long-revered system of repeated antenatal visits is itself a form of screening, although it was introduced long before the need for evaluation was recognized. Its precise role in bringing down maternal, fetal, and infant *mortality cannot be ascertained since so many other factors, such as improved *nutrition and better housing, have been happening at the same time. Comparison of mortality among mothers who used antenatal care with others who did not is beset by a behavioural selection bias inherent in all screening programmes, namely that screening is used most by those least at risk.

In recent years a number of screening tests for specific fetal abnormalities have been developed and evaluated. This is a field which is rapidly expanding as a result of developments in imaging and in *molecular genetics, enabling identification of fetuses with severe inherited diseases and other *congenital abnormalities. Some of the tests, e.g. *ultrasound detection of intestinal atresia, enable treatment *in utero* or in the immediate neonatal period. But most are directed against conditions for which there is no effective treatment and in which the prognosis for the *fetus is so poor that termination of pregnancy is offered to the prospective parents. The benefits of this policy are avoidance of a lifetime of handicap in the child, and greatly improved quality of life for the parents. This form of screening raises ethical issues for some, but is relatively easy to evaluate in terms of the number of handicapped children avoided; it has been shown, for *neural tube defects and for *Down's syndrome, that it is cost-effective for society, the saving in costs of care for affected children being greater than the costs of screening. Its unwanted side-effects are serious, but fortunately very rare, being the loss of a normal fetus either because of a false positive result or as a result of physical *trauma from the screening and follow-up procedures.

Screening in infancy and childhood
*Phenylketonuria and congenital *hypothyroidism, two important causes of severe *mental handicap, can be prevented by screening blood samples taken from infants at 6–10 days of age. The screening tests are measurement of serum phenylalanine, and *thyroid-stimulating *hormone, respectively. Infants with confirmed positive results can be successfully treated for phenylketonuria by a low phenylalanine diet, and for hypothyroidism by thyroid hormone. The screening programme reaches 99 per cent of new born infants, and most patients with each of these conditions are now of normal intelligence. The only drawback to these highly cost-effective screening programmes is overdiagnosis (and consequent overtreatment) of some children who would have developed normally. This is evidenced by the fact that the incidence of known cases of both these abnormalities has nearly doubled since the introduction of screening.

Infants are also routinely screened at 6 weeks of age for congenital *dislocation of the hip, although the effectiveness of treatment (by immobilization or traction) in preventing later hip disease has never been tested. Screening tests for hearing impairment and for *squint are routinely applied later in infancy, and early correction of these conditions is accepted as being beneficial, even though they too have not been formally researched. Other tests, for example for motor development, *congenital heart disease, and undescended testicle, are also widely used. In older children the emphasis of screening shifts away from congenital and inherited diseases to acquired conditions, such as dental

*caries and chronic ear infections. Screening schoolchildren for spinal *scoliosis by visual examination is advocated by some, but there is considerable doubt about the efficacy of treatment and probably most cases are non-progressive. It is unfortunate that, given the uncertainty about much screening in children, randomized controlled trials of effectiveness have never been done.

Screening adults
Screening for the chronic diseases of middle-age such as vascular disease and *cancer has been more extensively researched, with somewhat disappointing results in terms of its value. Nevertheless, it is widely practised within primary care on the assumption that regular surveillance of a person's risk factors for disease must be beneficial. The lack of precision about the ultimate aims of health surveillance make it intuitively difficult to monitor and evaluate. For example, when a *general practitioner enquires about a patient's smoking habit, should this be rigorously evaluated as a screening test, with reduction in *heart disease and lung cancer as the end-point, or is it sufficient to regard it as a common-sense measure leading to individually targeted health education which may be of benefit and probably does no harm? Within primary care, 'case-finding', i.e. screening a patient who is consulting the doctor for some other complaint, is generally preferred to organized systematic screening, because it is cheap, easy, and establishes a relationship between doctor and patient that facilitates long-term advice about changes in lifestyle. But it is extremely difficult to monitor even its short-term aims, such as adequate coverage of the target population, much less its outcome. Moreover, in cancer screening it has been shown that, to achieve maximum effect, screening has to be systematically organized with quality control of every step, from the method of inviting people to be screened, to the sensitivity and specificity of the test, to the adequacy of investigation of positives, and the treatment of those found to have early disease. Disorganized screening programmes without quality control wastefully dissipate resources and the screening programme fails to achieve its potential. There is, for instance, no continuing evidence to indicate that the vogue, especially prevalent in the United States, for regular estimation of prostate antigen or for biannual sigmoidoscopy is successful in identifying early prostatic or colonic cancer.

There are only two cancers for which screening has been shown to be effective, namely cancers of the uterine *cervix and the *breast. The 'Pap' smear for cervical cancer, repeated at intervals of 3–5 years, has the theoretical capacity to detect about 90 per cent of cancers when they are in the pre-invasive intraepithelial phase, and thus to make a very large impact on morbidity and mortality from this cancer, which is increasing in frequency. The main constraint to its effectiveness is that the women who are most at risk are also the least likely to be screened. Its principal disadvantage is overdiagnosis and overtreatment of women with minor degrees of intraepithial *neoplasia, most of which would never progress to invasive cancer. This problem is exacerbated by overfrequent screening and it has been shown that annual as opposed to three yearly screening adds hardly any benefit in terms of preventing invasive cancer.

Screening for breast cancer, using *mammography at intervals of 2–3 years among women aged 50–74, has been shown in several research trials to reduce subsequent breast cancer mortality by up to 40 per cent. It appears to be ineffective under the age of 50 mainly because mammography is less sensitive in premenopausal women who have a greater density of breast tissue.

Trials of screening for lung cancer, using chest X-rays and sputum *cytology, repeated as frequently as six-monthly, have shown that even this intensive screening cannot influence the prognosis of this aggressive form of cancer. Screening programmes for other cancers, including colorectal, ovary, prostate, skin *melanoma, and cancers of the mouth, are still being evaluated.

The purpose of screening for vascular disease is to reduce the incidence of coronary heart disease and of *stroke. Unfortunately, direct tests (electrocardiogram and carotid bruit) to detect early coronary or cerebral arterial disease lack both sensitivity and specificity. One therefore has to fall back on screening for earlier risk factors such as *hypertension, hypercholesterolaemia, obesity, and smoking habit. While blood pressure and serum *cholesterol are known to be valid tests for their respective risk factors, judged by their ability to predict future coronary and cerebrovascular events they, too, lack sensitivity and specificity. Nevertheless, it has been shown that screening for mild to moderate hypertension does result in a modest reduction in the incidence of stroke, but not heart disease, and, similarly, among people with very high cholesterol levels, early treatment has been shown to reduce heart attacks. The main drawback to these two screening tests is that most people with positive results are not going to suffer heart attacks or strokes, but nevertheless have to undergo long-term drug treatment and endure the anxiety and side-effects accompanying it, a similar problem to that of screening for cervical cancer. Most authorities now recommend screening for hypertension in middle-age, at intervals of 3–5 years, but there is more controversy about hypercholesterolaemia as a 'stand alone' screening test. A cautious approach is to include serum cholesterol in a package of risk-factor tests, but only to regard as positive those subjects who have at least one other risk factor.

Conclusions

Most of the disorders for which screening can clearly be recommended are identified very early in life. The benefits can be quickly realized, they result in cost savings which offset the costs of screening, compliance (of parents) is good, and often a single screen is all that is needed. By contrast, in screening adults the benefits tend to be limited and do not appear for many years, compliance is lower, the test needs to be repeated at intervals and hence is much more costly, and over-treatment of people, who in the absence of screening would not develop overt disease, is a common problem. As a strategy for controlling chronic disease, screening has a limited role and comes a poor third, after primary prevention and effective therapy.

JOCELYN CHAMBERLAIN

SCROFULA is *tuberculosis of the cervical *lymph nodes or skin (scrofuloderma).

SCROTUM. The pouch of skin, fascia, and smooth muscle containing the *testes and their accessory structures, enabling them to be maintained at a slightly lower temperature than the core of the body.

SCURVY is the condition which results from a deficiency of vitamin C (*ascorbic acid) in the diet. It is now rare except in groups at special risk, such as the isolated elderly and the mentally handicapped. Its clinical manifestations (as opposed to the non-specific symptoms ascribed to putative 'subclinical' states) include follicular *hyperkeratosis of the skin, perifollicular *petechial haemorrhages, ecchymoses (bruising), swollen gums which bleed easily, *subperiosteal haemorrhages (in children), *hypotension, and *anaemia. Ascorbic acid is widely available in most fruits and vegetables.

SCUTARI (now Uskiidar) was the suburb of Constantinople (Istanbul) in which were the military hospitals serving the Crimean battlefields, the scene of Florence *Nightingale's first and greatest achievement. The accommodation, for more than 1000 men, had not been secured until many months after the war began and was in a parlous condition when Miss Nightingale, with 38 nurses, arrived on 4 November 1854. Of the main hospital, Lytton Strachey later wrote:

In these surroundings, those who had long been inured to scenes of human suffering—surgeons with a world-wide knowledge of agonies, soldiers familiar with scenes of carnage, missionaries with remembrances of famine and of plague—yet found a depth of horror which they had never known before. There were moments, there were places, in the Barrack Hospital at Scutari, where the strongest hand was struck with trembling, and the boldest eye would turn away its gaze. (*Eminent Victorians*, London, 1918.)

The transformation brought about by Miss Nightingale during the following 6 months represents a landmark in British history, military, medical, social, and administrative.

SEAT-BELTS are restraining belts which buckle across the chest and/or waist of passengers in aircraft, motor vehicles, etc. and which are designed to prevent the body being propelled forward in the event of an impact. The wearing of seat-belts by those in motor cars is required by law in the UK and many other countries.

SEBACEOUS CYST. A swelling of the skin, often on the scalp, neck, or forehead, due to blockage of the *duct of a sebaceous gland and distension with sebaceous secretion. These cysts, commonly called wens, are often unsightly, but are readily removed by minor surgery.

SEBACEOUS GLAND. Any of the small glands found in the dermis or true *skin in relation to hair follicles; they secrete *sebum, which lubricates the skin and keeps it supple.

SEBORRHOEA (SEBORRHEA) is excessive production of *sebum by the sebaceous glands of the dermis. See SKIN.

SEBORRHOEIC DERMATITIS is a skin disorder affecting particularly the scalp and skin flexures in individuals with *seborrhoea. The lesions are red and irritable, and shed loose, greasy scales.

SEBUM is the yellow, greasy, semi-solid secretion of the *sebaceous glands.

SECONDARY HEALTH CARE is health care normally provided by consultants and their departments of a general hospital, to which patients are referred when necessary by those providing *primary health care, i.e. general practitioners.

SECONDARY SEXUAL CHARACTERISTICS are the physical manifestations of sexual maturity which begin to appear at *puberty. In girls the most obvious include: rounding of body contours; development of the breasts; and growth of axillary and pubic hair. In boys the most obvious signs are: deepening of the voice (due to laryngeal enlargement); growth of pubic and facial hair; enlargement of the external genitalia; and body growth spurt.

SECRETIN is a hormone secreted by glands in the wall of the *duodenum in response to an acid stimulus; secretin in turn stimulates the *pancreas to produce pancreatic juice which is high in volume and bicarbonate concentration.

SECTION means cutting, or cut segment; sometimes it is an abbreviation for *caesarean section. Occasionally it is used in the UK as a slang abbreviation for the process of compulsory admission to hospital of a patient under a specific section of the *Mental Health Act.

SEDATIVE. Any agent which slows down mental and physical activity and has a calming, relaxing effect; not significantly different from the later designation *tranquillizer.

SEDGWICK, WILLIAM THOMPSON (1855–1921). American public health authority. He was one of the early advocates of pasteurization of milk, and of the addition of chlorine to drinking water. See also PUBLIC HEALTH MEDICINE IN THE USA.

SEIZURE. A seizure is any sudden attack of illness, such as a *fit or *stroke.

SELF-EXPERIMENTATION has a long history among doctors and medical scientists. At one level, it is a variety of the more general phenomenon of human experimentation, but with its own special characteristics. Using oneself as the experimental subject can be a public demonstration of the importance and/or safety of the experiment; it allows the experimenter direct access to the subjective results of the experiment; it neutralizes some of the ethical ambiguity surrounding the use of a new technique, drug, or procedure; it ensures the reliability of the subject; and it can seem 'natural' even if it is uncomfortable, painful, or even dangerous. Animal experiments may establish the relative safety, effectiveness, or importance of new discovery, but if the results are to be applied to a human situation, someone must go first. Ethical protocols governing human experimentation are recent and revolve, *inter alia*, around the issue of informed consent. No one is better able freely to give informed consent than the actual investigator, although recently special protocols have been devised even here.

Although certain branches of medicine, e.g. surgery, do not readily lend themselves to self-experimentation, most areas of medical knowledge and practice have been influenced by a few classic, and hundreds of routine, examples. Many of these relate to what Claude *Bernard (1813–78) described as the three pillars of medical science: *physiology, *pharmacology, and *pathology.

Physiology

One of the most disciplined of all self-experimenters was *Sanctorius (Santorio Santorio, 1561–1636). His quantifying impulse led him to devise an elaborate balance chair where, for 30 years, he took frequent careful measurements of his body weight, and the weight of his food, drink, and excreta. From this he calculated the amount of fluid lost in insensible perspiration. He also routinely recorded his pulse and temperature. Sanctorius' balance chair was the forerunner of the advanced metabolic chambers which Theodore *Bischoff, Carl *Voit, and others constructed in 19th century Germany, using themselves in relating controlled diets and exercise to measure oxygen consumption and the elimination of *carbon dioxide, *urea, and other waste products through the lungs, kidneys, and bowels.

Many of the basic principles of respiratory physiology and adaptation to high altitude were established from the 1870s by Paul *Bert, both in a pressure chamber and in the Peruvian Andes. Bert's self-experiments on respiration were continued by J. S. *Haldane, who habitually used himself as his principal subject, and made important contributions to the identification of the occupational hazards of miners and sewage workers, invented the haemoglobinometer, and developed the decompression chamber to treat *caisson disease in divers.

Cardiac catheterization has become a routine diagnostic procedure and has led to a variety of minimally invasive therapeutic innovations. The German surgeon, Werner *Forssman, who first developed the technique, was discouraged by his superiors from that line of inquiry. Instead, following animal experiments, he used himself as his first human subject, in 1929. His work led to much condemnation and little immediate interest and he abandoned it, although he later shared the *Nobel prize with two other investigators who carried on his work in the early 1940s.

A classic investigation of the physiology of pain was carried out by Sir Henry *Head and Wilfred *Trotter, who had nerves in their arms severed so that they could observe the gradual return of sensation. Trotter's colleague at University College Hospital, Sir Thomas *Lewis, established the sequence of events occurring after local skin irritation (the 'triple response') and, with J. H. Kellgren, conducted an elaborate series of self-experiments, aimed at providing a classification of the varieties of pain and the patterns of referred pain.

Long before William *Beaumont's creative use of the gastric fistula in his patient Alexis St Martin in the 1830s, Lazzaro *Spallanzani (1729–99) had investigated his own digestion, training himself to swallow bags of food tied to a string and to regurgitate food at will. A modern parallel was W. B. *Castle's search for the cause of pernicious anaemia. He showed through regurgitating minced beef that his own normal stomach secreted a substance ('intrinsic factor') missing in patients suffering from *pernicious anaemia. *Vitamin and nutrition research have also lent themselves to self-feeding (and deprivation) experiments. Modern pioneers in this approach include Robert McCance and Elsie Widdowson, Victor Herbert and John H. Crandon. Joseph Goldberger tried to convince dubious colleagues that *pellagra is a nutritional, rather than an infectious, disorder, by injecting himself with blood and swallowing capsules containing urine, faeces, and skin from patients suffering from the condition.

Pathology

Goldberger's experiments demonstrate how close physiological and pathological methods can be, and are one series in many aimed at elucidating the causes, mechanisms, and/or prevention of disease. A classic instance is John *Hunter's report of a man (probably himself) whom he inoculated with some pus taken from a patient suffering from *gonorrhoea. When the subject

subsequently developed signs of both gonorrhoea and *syphilis, Hunter concluded that these two are simply stages of a single venereal disease.

*Koch's postulates specified an animal model in establishing the bacteriological causes of disease, but diseases spread through insect vectors have produced some of the most dramatic self-experiments. Several early advocates of the mosquito hypothesis of *malaria transmission allowed themselves to be bitten by mosquitoes which had fed off malarious patients, or injected malarious blood into themselves. *Yellow fever was without known treatment, but the same mosquito procedure was used by an American team in Havana, with the accidental death of Jesse Lazear and the permanent incapacitation and premature death of James Carroll, two of the team. More recently, Ralph Lainson's work on *leishmaniasis and Claude Barlow's investigations of *schistosomiasis involved deliberately contracting the disease.

*Vaccine development has been another common source of autoexperimentation, to test whether the vaccine is safe and actually protects. Louis *Pasteur volunteered to test *rabies vaccine on himself. In the end, he did not, although Jacques Graucher, who accidentally stuck himself with a syringe containing rabies virus, and two other of Pasteur's assistants, did. Waldemar Haffkine tested his *cholera and *plague vaccines on himself; Almroth *Wright tried out his *brucellosis and *typhoid vaccines; and a number of workers first tested the variety of *polio vaccines which were produced from the 1930s.

Pharmacology

Observing and measuring the effects on oneself of ingested or injected drugs have long been mainstays of experimental pharmacology. During the 19th century, many *anaesthetic agents were first used on the experimenter: the subjective effects of *nitrous oxide were described long before the substance was actually employed during surgery, and Crawford Long had experienced *ether socially before he used it professionally. In the 1860s, Benjamin Ward Richardson used himself in investigating a series of compounds of known chemical composition. Amyl nitrite was one of them, later taken up for the treatment of angina pectoris because Richardson reported intense flushing and other signs of vasodilatation.

Other 19th century self-experimentalists include Enoch Hale Jr, who injected himself with castor oil; J. E. Purkinje, who described digitalis toxicity; and P. J. Touéry, who showed that charcoal was a useful antidote against arsenic and strychnine poisoning. In the present century, A. Hoffmann reported the hallucinogenic effects of LSD; H. Osmond worked with amphetamine, mescaline, and other hallucinogens; and S. M. Smith and F. Prescott allowed themselves to be completely paralysed with curare, under monitored conditions.

These examples represent merely the tip of a large iceberg. The circumstances are usually routine, but occasionally extreme. The results, too, are generally simply part of normal science. Nevertheless, self-experimentation is embedded within the fabric of research and, governed by the ethics of human experimentation, is certain to retain its importance.

W. F. BYNUM

SELF-HELP ORGANIZATIONS (IN THE UK)
Introduction
In an age when, in the UK, the general perception of medicine and health is that 'The State should take care of it', it is perhaps surprising that voluntary self-help organizations should not only be thriving, but should be increasing more rapidly than at any other time. And yet, paradoxically, the State has given rise to their proliferation. As more conditions and diseases are defined and diagnosed, so the desire increases among those whose families are affected to learn more and to meet others with the same problems. Such organizations with many varied objectives have long existed in North America and in other parts of the world.

The earliest British self-help organizations in the medical field were, in the main, those dedicated to research. Parents and families who could do little to help their affected children or adults banded together to form groups or associations whose principal aim was the funding of research to eradicate the conditions. Today, many of these have expanded their role to include care, and many new bodies have been founded exclusively to care for those directly involved. Thus, in the 1990s, the self-help organizations fall into three main groups: those whose sole or primary interest is in medical research; those whose primary interest is in care; those whose interest is in both. Recently, there has also been a trend towards some self-help organizations becoming pressure groups.

Research
The largest self-help organizations in medical research in the UK are the Imperial Cancer Research Fund and the Cancer Research Campaign, which raised respectively £44 (US$66) million and £40 (US$60) million from their members and supporters in 1991. The next largest is the British Heart Foundation, raising £24 (US$36) million.

While most of the organizations funding medical research go to the general public for donations, it is usually their voluntary branches which provide the stimulus. In the rarer conditions, it is often those who are affected and their families who found the organizations and run them.

The most difficult areas for self-help groups are in mental health and *AIDS. The large cancer and heart organizations have a vast natural constituency, in that most people believe themselves to be at risk of contracting some form of cancer or heart disease. In the case of mental health and AIDS the constituencies are far smaller, since most people convince themselves, or at least pretend to themselves, that they are not at risk.

Care
There are three principal types of caring groups: the institutional, the community care, and the support groups. There is a feeling that care should now be given in the community wherever possible and that institutional care should be a last resort. Thus the Leonard Cheshire Foundation now attempts to provide care in the home wherever it can: similarly, MacIntyre, founded by parents of children with a mental disability, now works to provide homes in the local community for those for whom they care, although they also provide institutional facilities for those who still need them. The Spinal Injuries Association is a good example of a self-help group. Its officers, staff, and members are themselves people who have sustained a spinal injury and who help others in the same situation to learn about and come to terms with their condition.

Most of the support groups for individual medical conditions also try to help in the same way. The Jennifer Trust for Spinal Muscular Atrophy started when Ken and Anita Macaulay lost their infant daughter. They found themselves isolated and frightened. When their own grief began to abate, they realized that other parents must be going through the same fears: they founded their support group, first as a telephone 'listening' service, just to provide an ear into which others could pour out their own pent-up grief, and later as a meeting-ground for parents, children, and adults with spinal muscular atrophy.

In fact, most support groups for individuals and families with specific diseases have started in the same way. They provide a much-needed source of information, advice, and comfort at a time when the extended family has effectively ceased to be the type of unit which can cope alone. Macmillan nurses, who keep patients with a terminal illness at home for as long as possible, and the *hospice movement, which has done so much to assist these same people when home care ceases to be possible, are other examples.

There are support groups for almost every known disease. Contact-a-Family, an umbrella organization, often helps to found these groups and keeps a register of all those that are active. They publish a *Directory of specific conditions and rare syndromes in children* which has information on almost 200 conditions such as Wolf–Hirschhorn syndrome and dystrophia epidermolysis bullosa.

Research and care
Most charities in the field of health and medicine are active both in research and care. The Muscular Dystrophy Group, the Multiple Sclerosis Society, the British Diabetic Association, and the Chest, Heart, and Stroke Association all fund research and all provide information and support, as do a hundred or more disease-specific organizations. As new conditions develop, or come to the public attention, so new self-help groups are formed: for example, the Foundation for the Study

of Infant Deaths and the Psoriasis Association, both of which fund research and offer support.

Pressure groups
Finally, within the various types of organization described, there are pressure groups such as DIG (the Disabled Income Group) and GIG (the Genetic Interest Group). The former is permanently campaigning, the latter campaigns only when there is a specific issue that affects it. GIG was especially active at the time of the embryo research debate in Parliament in 1989–90 because, had research on the pre-embryo been banned, there would have been no opportunity to learn how parents whose children would be at risk from such diseases as *tuberous sclerosis, Duchenne *muscular dystrophy, and *cystic fibrosis could be given the opportunity, through IVF (*in vitro fertilization) to produce children who could be guaranteed not to inherit the condition.

PAUL F. WALKER

Details of the organizations mentioned and of many more can be obtained from:
The Association of Medical Research Charities, Tavistock House South, Entrance D, Tavistock Square, London WC1H 9LE, UK.
Contact-a-Family, 16 Strutton Ground, London SW1P 2HP, UK.
The Charities Aid Foundation, 48 Pembury Road, Tonbridge, Kent TN9 2JD, UK.

SEMANTICS is the science of the relationship between language and meaning.

SEMEN is seed-fluid, the white viscous secretion of the male genital organs; it is composed chiefly of *spermatozoa produced by the *testes, with contributions from the accessory reproductive glands (prostate, seminal vesicles, etc.).

SEMICIRCULAR CANALS. The three looped bony canals of the *labyrinth of the ear which lie in different planes at right angles to each other. Acceleration of the head in any direction causes movement of the fluid in one or more of them; this can be detected by the fine sensory receptors they also contain. Together with the otolith organ, they comprise the vestibular apparatus, subserving the functions of posture and balance via the vestibular division of the eighth cranial (auditory) nerve. See also OTORHINOLARYNGOLOGY.

SEMICOMA is *stupor, distinguished from *coma by the fact that the patient will respond to sufficiently vigorous stimuli.

SEMINAL VESICLE. The organ which stores sperm in the male. It is attached to the back of the *bladder and its duct joins the *vas deferens to form the ejaculatory duct.

SEMINOMA. A malignant *neoplasm of the *testis.

SEMIOLOGY is the study of symptoms and signs.

SEMMELWEISS, IGNAZ PHILIPP (1818–65). Hungarian obstetrician. In 1846 when working at the *Allgemeines Krankenhaus in Vienna, he noted that the maternal mortality in the ward attended by students was far higher than in that staffed by nurses. He suspected that this was due to students coming directly from the dissection room and infecting the parturient women they examined. When he enforced their thorough washing, the maternal mortality fell from 9.9 per cent to 1.3 per cent. His views were not acceptable to his superiors and he left Vienna for Budapest, where he became professor of obstetrics in 1855. In 1861 he set out his findings in *Die Aetiologie der Begriff, und die Prophylaxis des Kindbettfiebers*. It was badly received and in 1865 he suffered a mental breakdown and died, ironically from *septicaemia from a wound infection.

SEMON, SIR FELIX (1849–1921). Anglo-German laryngologist. Semon was a highly skilled operator and worked with *Horsley on the thyroid. He enunciated Semon's law: 'a destructive lesion of the motor nerve to the intrinsic laryngeal muscles causes abductor weakness before adductor weakness'. See also OTORHINOLARYNGOLOGY.

SENILE DEMENTIA is an insidious and progressive *dementia occurring in old age and affecting some 10 per cent of persons over 80; the onset is usually some time in the early 70s. The first and almost invariable manifestation is loss of memory, particularly for recent events, names, and places. A decline in all mental faculties follows, with disintegration of personality and deterioration of habits. Paranoid and persecutory ideas are common, together with disorientation and confusion. Urinary and faecal *incontinence usually develop. Senile dementia is associated with demonstrable *cerebral atrophy and neuronal loss. The pathological process is not reversible; it is usually that of *Alzheimer's disease.

SENILITY. See AGEING; GERIATRIC MEDICINE; SENILE DEMENTIA.

SENIOR HOUSE OFFICER is the grade of UK hospital appointment normally filled when the first (preregistration) year after medical qualification has been completed; it was formerly known as 'junior registrar'.

SENIOR REGISTRAR. See REGISTRAR.

SENIUM. The period of old age, marked by deteriorating mental and physical powers.

SENSATION is awareness of a physical experience, dependent upon stimulation of sense receptors and transmission of impulses to the sensorium of the brain. This definition excludes 'sensations' experienced in dreams and *hallucinatory states, which represent cerebral activity occurring in the absence of the appropriate afferent impulses.

SENSE. Any of the faculties, or any combination of the faculties, by which perception takes place.

SENSITIVITY is the level of responsiveness to sensory or other stimuli.

SENSORIUM. The whole nervous system apparatus involved in sensation considered collectively; or that part of the brain concerned with sensation; or the brain itself.

SENSORY DEPRIVATION is the removal of the external stimuli to which a person is normally subjected.

SENSORY SYSTEM. That part of the *nervous system, peripheral and central, concerned with the reception and appreciation of sensory stimuli.

SEPSIS is the infection of blood or other tissues by pathogenic bacteria.

SEPTICAEMIA (SEPTICEMIA) is the presence and multiplication of pathogenic micro-organisms in the bloodstream.

SEPTUM. An anatomical structure which serves as a dividing wall or partition.

SEPULCHRE (SEPULCHER). A tomb or burial place.

SERJEANT-SURGEON. The chief surgeon of the UK *Royal Medical Household.

SEROLOGY is the laboratory analysis and study of *antibodies in the blood circulation, for which blood *serum is conveniently used as the sample.

SEROTONIN is a vasoactive amine and local *hormone also known as 5-hydroxytryptamine; widely distributed in the body, it is found in high concentrations in the intestinal mucosa, the *pineal gland, and central nervous system. It has several physiological roles: these include *haemostasis (it is released by platelets and acts as a powerful vasoconstrictor); inhibition of gastric secretion; and neurotransmission in the brain (either excitatory or inhibitory according to site). It is derived from the *amino acid tryptophan.

SERPENT. The use of a serpent as a medical emblem derives from *Aesculapius, who was classically depicted, cloaked but bare-breasted, holding a staff with a serpent coiled round it. This emblem is not to be confused with the two entwined serpents of the *caduceus, which have

no particular medical relevance. The Aesculapian snake is a species of rat-snake, *Elaphe longissima*, native to south-east Europe and Asia Minor. The present isolated populations which exist in Germany and Switzerland are the descendants of specimens brought to health resorts in those countries by the Romans. In ancient Greece, the Aesculapian snake was venerated as a symbol of renewal and treated as sacred; specimens kept in temples were encouraged to lick the wounds of the injured and sick as a means of promoting healing.

SERTÜRNER, FRIEDRICH WILHELM ADAM (1783–1841). German pharmacologist. He isolated *morphine from opium in 1806 and published this in the *Journal der pharmacie* of Leipzig. The work was overlooked for a time but in 1817 the chemist Gay-Lussac drew attention to it.

SERUM, when otherwise unqualified, means blood serum, which is the clear, slightly yellow fluid which separates from blood when it clots. In composition it resembles blood *plasma, but with fibrinogen removed. Sera containing *antibodies and antitoxins against infections and toxins of various kinds (antisera) have been used extensively in prevention or treatment of various diseases (such as *tetanus and *diphtheria).

SERUM SICKNESS is an immune reaction to injected foreign serum or serum protein characterized by fever, *urticaria, joint pains, oedema, and lymph node enlargement. See ALLERGY; ANAPHYLAXIS.

SERVETUS, MICHAEL (Miguel Serveto) (?1511–53). Spanish physician and theologian. He studied medicine in Paris and, although he is known to have practised in Charlieu and Avignon, it is not certain that he graduated. He wrote many contentious theological works in which he opposed the doctrine of the Trinity. In one of them, *Restitutio christianismi* (1553), in order to explain the introduction of the divine spirit into the body, he suggested that blood passed through the lungs to the left ventricle and was then distributed to the arteries. He was denounced by Calvin to the authorities in Geneva and burned at the stake.

SESAMOID BONE. A bone embedded in a tendon or joint capsule; the *patella is an example.

SETON. A thread of silk or other material laid in a wound so as to initiate a passage for drainage.

SEVENTH DAY ADVENTISTS are the adherents of the largest of the Adventist churches, who keep the seventh day of the week (Saturday) as the sabbath rather than the first. Like other adventists, they are messianists, that is they believe in a Second Coming and the fulfilment thereupon of millennial expectations derived from their interpretation of the Bible. Seventh Day Adventists eschew meat, alcohol, tobacco, and the non-medical use of drugs. The sect operates over 325 medical units throughout the world.

SEX CHANGE is a phrase used to denote the simulation, usually by a combination of surgical and pharmacological methods, of the secondary and external sexual characteristics of the opposite sex in patients suffering from persistent paradoxical gender identification.

SEX LINKAGE. A characteristic is said to be sex-linked when the gene that produces it is carried on one of the two sex chromosomes. See GENETICS.

SEXOLOGIST. A specialist in the management of sexual disorders.

SEXUAL INTERCOURSE. Sexual union, involving penetration of the vagina by the penis and usually, but not necessarily, seminal emission.

SEXUALITY AND MEDICINE. Medical disorders and their treatments often interfere with sexuality and may cause persistent sexual problems. Such problems may arise because of the direct effects of illness or treatment on the anatomical or neurophysiological components of sexual function. In some cases sexual difficulties develop because of emotional responses to illness or treatment. Commonly both types of association are relevant. Thus, a patient who suffers from a disorder which partially interferes with sexual function may react to this with anxiety or embarrassment such that the sexual problem is amplified. Illnesses sometimes precipitate sexual problems because of poor previous sexual adjustment. Thus how a couple adjusts sexually to a physical disorder in one partner will depend partly on the quality of their sexual relationship prior to the illness.

A further important influence on sexual adjustment to illness is the way this topic is addressed by doctors and their colleagues. For example, lack of discussion or advice about sexuality following a heart attack may result in a couple abandoning their sexual relationship because they fear, albeit usually erroneously, that sexual activity is likely to be dangerous because it might precipitate another heart attack.

Types of sexual problems

Sexual difficulties can affect any of three aspects of sexual function: sexual desire, sexual arousal, and orgasm. The most important sexual problems (or 'dysfunctions' as they are known technically) are shown in Table 1.

Nearly all illnesses are likely to be associated with reduced interest in sex, but this usually returns. However, certain conditions, especially those that are debilitating, are likely to be associated with persistent low sexual desire, perhaps reflecting depression or generally reduced energy levels. Many cases of erectile dysfunction, especially in older men, are due to organic factors. A history of a gradual onset to the problem, with a persistent pattern of erectile difficulties and absence of full erections in masturbation is strongly suggestive of an organic cause. Female impaired sexual arousal can reflect hormonal disturbance. This may be associated with the *menopause, especially following removal of the ovaries, or recent childbirth, particularly in breast-feeding mothers. Retarded or absent ejaculation and orgasmic dysfunction can be caused by certain types of medication (see Table 3).

Dyspareunia means that sexual intercourse is painful. While this can be due to anxiety and reduced arousal, it can be symptom of a physical disorder such as *endometriosis. *Vaginismus is usually a psychologically determined problem, the woman being unable to have sexual intercourse because of a phobia about vaginal penetration. However, it can also result from pain caused by, for example, an unsatisfactory *episiotomy scar.

The dysfunctions most commonly caused by illnesses or their treatments are low sexual desire, erectile dysfunction and impaired sexual arousal, retarded (or absent) ejaculation, orgasmic dysfunction, and dyspareunia.

Medical causes

Medical disorders that commonly cause sexual difficulties are listed in Table 2. Erectile dysfunction is particularly common in men with *diabetes mellitus, 30–50 per cent of such men eventually experiencing erectile difficulties. This occurs because diabetes can cause both

Table 1 Types of sexual dysfunction

Aspect of sexuality affected	Men	Women
Sexual desire	Low sexual desire	Low sexual desire
Sexual arousal	Erectile dysfunction	Impaired sexual arousal
Orgasm	Premature ejaculation Retarded/absent ejaculation	Orgasmic dysfunction
Other		Vaginismus Dyspareunia

Table 2 Examples of medical disorders that often cause sexual dysfunction

System	Examples	Possible sexual dysfunctions
Endocrine	Diabetes mellitus	Erectile dysfunction Impaired sexual arousal
	Hypogonadism	Low sexual desire Retarded/absent ejaculation Erectile dysfunction
Cardiovascular	Arteriosclerosis Myocardial infarction	Erectile dysfunction Low sexual desire
Neurological	Spinal cord damage	Erectile and orgasmic dysfunction
	Multiple sclerosis	Absent ejaculation

circulatory problems and *neuropathy (impaired nerve conduction). *Hypogonadism in men can be caused by any condition that damages the testes or affects production of the hormones produced by the pituitary gland, which stimulate the testes. Its effects are due to reduced production of the male sex *hormone, *testosterone. This hormone is also important in female sexuality (being produced by both the ovary and the adrenal cortex in women) since it influences levels of sexual desire.

*Arteriosclerosis is a common cause of sexual difficulties in older men, narrowing of the pelvic blood vessels reducing the blood supply to the penis and hence the ability to obtain and sustain an erection. Total section of the *spinal cord will cause erectile and orgasmic dysfunction. Partial damage to the spinal cord, through injury or a disease such as *multiple sclerosis, may result in difficulty, but not inability, to obtain erections and reach orgasm.

Surgical causes

Surgery may affect sexuality because of direct interference with sexual anatomy. Examples include surgery to the rectum or bladder, which may disrupt nervous pathways to the genitals, major surgery involving the genitalia, and surgical procedures involving the spinal cord. Surgery may also affect sexuality because of the disfiguring effects of certain operations. Examples include *mastectomy, *amputation, and creation of an 'ostomy' (e.g. *colostomy) because of bowel disease.

Effects of medication

Many drugs used to treat physical or psychiatric conditions can affect sexuality. The more important drugs in this regard are listed in Table 3. Antihypertensives, *diuretics, tricyclic *antidepressants, and major *tranquillizers often cause erectile dysfunction. Monoamine-oxidase inhibitors and antidepressants which act on the *serotonin system may cause delayed or absent ejaculation or orgasm. Long-term use of steroids and *anticonvulsants can cause diminished sexual interest, the latter because of induction of sex hormone-binding globulin, which binds with testosterone in the bloodstream and thereby inactivates it.

Other physical causes of sexual dysfunction

Excessive *alcohol consumption is an important cause of sexual problems. In addition to its potential disruptive effects on relationships, it may cause peripheral neuropathy, hypogonadism, and liver damage (which may interfere with the metabolism of sex hormones). Sexual problems are common in drug *addiction, probably because of the effects of consequent general debility on sexual desire. Sexual difficulties, particularly erectile dysfunction, may also be linked to *smoking because of the increased risk of arteriosclerosis.

Psychological cause

Sexual problems often occur because of the adverse psychological effects of physical illness or treatment on sexual adjustment. An individual may develop anxieties about sexual activity because of fears that it might cause a relapse of a physical condition, or because of concerns about the perceived effects of illness or

Table 3 Medication that may cause sexual dysfunctions

Antihypertensives (e.g. propranolol)
Diuretics (e.g. bendrofluazide)
Antidepressants, including tricyclics (e.g. imipramine), monoamine oxidase inhibitors (e.g. phenelzine), and serotonergic antidepressants (e.g. fluoxetine)
Major tranquillizers (e.g. chlorpromazine)
Hormones (e.g. steroids)
Anticonvulsants (e.g. phenytoin)

Table 4 Help for people with sexual problems caused by medical disorders or their treatments

Psychological	Sexual aids
Advice	Vacuum constriction device
Sex therapy	
Surgical	**Medication**
Penile prosthesis	Intracavernosal injections
Vascular surgery	of vasoactive drugs
	(e.g. papaverine)
	Sex hormones
	Yohimbine

surgery on sexual attractiveness. The partner may have similar concerns. Changes in roles because of illness in either partner may affect a couple's relationship. Depression following a severe illness is a common cause of reduced sexual desire. Lastly, the ways in which the implications of physical illness are managed by clinicians may be very important in determining subsequent sexual adjustment.

Treatment

Management of sexual problems must be based on very careful assessment. It is usually appropriate and necessary to involve both partners in this. The clinician should endeavour to establish the extent to which physical and psychological factors have contributed to the problem. When treatment is provided for a member of a couple, both partners should be seen whenever possible.

Specific treatments that may help people with sexual problems caused by physical disorders or their treatments are listed in Table 4. For many people with medically related sexual problems, careful explanation and advice may be of considerable assistance. Explaining that a sexual problem is a recognized effect of a disorder (e.g. diabetes) can reassure the patient. Advice may then be given about the benefits of spending more time on foreplay, and a couple may perhaps be encouraged to modify their sexual relationship if sexual intercourse is unlikely to be possible.

Sex therapy was developed at the beginning of the 1970s following the work of Masters and Johnson in the USA. In this approach, specific instructions are given to the couple about gradually rebuilding their sexual relationship, beginning with simple caressing. The aim is partly to remove the pressure the couple might be experiencing because of their not being able to have a full and satisfying sexual relationship, and also to help them to begin to enjoy their physical relationship in a non-demanding fashion. Improved *communication is a major goal in this treatment. The therapist has to use skilful psychological intervention to help the couple when they encounter difficulties with the home-work programme. Education about sexuality is another

important element of treatment. Sex therapy can be particularly helpful for couples whose sexual difficulties are the result of a psychological response to an illness or surgery, or where psychological factors are amplifying the sexual consequences of a medical disorder.

Surgical procedures are reserved for people with special indications, such as young men with diabetic erectile dysfunction, or men with vascular abnormalities affecting the blood supply to the genitals. The vacuum constriction device is a relatively new and safe sexual aide for men with erectile dysfunction. Intracavernosal injections are used widely for men with organic erectile dysfunction but do have the risk of priapism (excessively prolonged erections) which can be harmful. Sex hormones are usually reserved for men with hypogonadism. Oestrogen can be helpful for women with vaginal dryness associated with either a natural or a surgical menopause. The drug yohimbine may help some men with erectile dysfunction.

Where medication has caused a sexual problem, other types of medication might be tried. It is important that the minimal effective dose of medication is used. Doses of a drug might be timed so that it causes as little interference as possible with sexual activity.

Sources of help

Treatment for sexual problems may be obtained from several sources. Some general practitioners take a particular interest in providing such help. Some specialists in a variety of clinical disciplines, including *psychiatry, clinical *psychology, gynaecology, *family planning, and *urology, will have special expertise in this type of work. In the UK the Relate organization has many trained sex therapists. There are also private therapists, although people seeking help should ensure that they only consult properly trained therapists providing bona fide treatments.

KEITH HAWTON

Further reading
Bancroft, J. (1989). *Human sexuality and its problems*, (2nd edn). Churchill Livingstone, Edinburgh.
Hawton, K. (1985). *Sex therapy: a practical guide*. Oxford University Press, Oxford.
Rosen, R. C. and Leiblum, S. R. (1992). *Erectile disorders: assessment and treatment*. Guilford Press, New York.
Schover, L. R. and Jensen, S. B. (1988). *Sexuality and chronic illness: a comprehensive approach*. Guilford Press, New York.

SEXUALLY TRANSMITTED DISEASE. In recent years it may have seemed to the casual observer that *AIDS has somewhat eclipsed other sexually transmitted diseases. However, the UK Department of Health publication *The health of the nation* has highlighted sexually transmitted diseases, not only in their role in the causation of ill-health but in relation to their possible long-term consequences, including *infertility, *ectopic pregnancy, and genital *cancers. It is now well known that the concurrent presence of some sexually transmitted diseases (STDs) may facilitate the transmission of human immunodeficiency virus (HIV). HIV/*AIDs, STDs, drug misuse, and sexual health, including family planning and contraception, have been identified as key areas in *The health of the nation*.

STDs used to be called venereology, but venereal diseases often have legal classifications, usually established in developed countries at the turn of the 20th century. Venereal diseases are generally considered to include *syphilis, *gonorrhoea, *chancroid, and, in some countries, *granuloma inguinale and *lympho-granuloma venereum (LGV). In the past 40 years a wide range of infections have been seen to be sexually transmissible, so over 20 years ago the term genito-urinary medicine was adopted to describe the study and management of sexually transmitted diseases, or venereology, in the UK, which still remains the principal country to have full-time specialists in this group of disorders.

The situation, however, is very different in other countries. In Europe, Latin America, and many countries in Asia, venereology is a subspecialty of dermatology, dermato-venereology. In some other countries the treatment of sexually transmitted diseases is even more fragmented. Urologists treat men who have a urethral discharge. Gynaecologists treat the female patient. Elsewhere, notably in parts of the USA, venereology is considered to fall within the scope of *infectious disease. This last trend has occurred elsewhere in recent years because of the need to care for patients with HIV/AIDS.

Origins and development

There are records of STDs, most notably gonorrhoea, from the earliest times. Only with the development of the city and the concept of travel, be it in the context of war, commerce, or expedition, can it be said that there has been some practice of venereology. Gonorrhoea was mentioned by the ancient Egyptians, being described in the papyrus discovered by Ebers. It was mentioned in the Old Testament in Leviticus 15: 2–33: 'the man who has a running of the reins is unclean, even though his defilement, at certain times, dries up and causes a stoppage' (Knox translation). The Greek and Roman writers, notably Herodotus, *Celsus, and *Galen, described gonorrhoea and its sequelae. In the Middle Ages *Avicenna of Baghdad wrote at length on urethral discharge, recommending irrigations. Moses *Maimonides of Cordoba aptly described gonorrhoea as fluid escaping without erection or feeling of pleasure, doughy, and the result of disease including amorousness and excesses. By that time complications of gonorrhoea such as epididymo-orchitis were recognized. The infectiousness of gonorrhoea was realized and records note measures taken by civic authorities to control it, both in cities abroad such as Avignon (1347) and in London from the 12th century onwards. *Scabies

and louse infestation were also recognized at an early date, although the concept of different causes for skin disease has developed only in the past 300 years. Genital warts, condylomata acuminata, venereally acquired, have been recognized for 2000 years. Anal warts as a result of sodomy were exemplified by Juvenal in his satires. Much later they were described by the Restoration surgeon Richard Wiseman (1676) and the French physician John Astruc (1736).

Syphilis is among the most interesting of diseases from a historical standpoint, not only because of arguments about its origin, but because of its influence on morality and measures towards public health and hygiene. There are conflicting views as to its origin in Europe. The pre-Columbian (Europeanist) theory is that syphilis was somehow endemic in Europe throughout the Middle Ages, becoming pandemic at the end of the 15th century and venereally acquired. The Columbian (Americanist) theory is that in 1493 after the return of Christopher Columbus from the New World to Spain, his sailors brought back with them this new disease. Another idea is the Unitarian theory of Hudson (1946). *Yaws, a treponemal infection, is widespread in equatorial regions. It has many similarities in its manifestations to syphilis. Hudson emphasized the evolutionary relationship of yaws, *pinta, endemic syphilis, and sporadic syphilis, regarding them all as varieties of one disease caused by one parasite, *Treponema pallidum*. This concept considers sub-Saharan Africa to be the area where treponematosis originated. Whatever the origin of syphilis, its passage was well described after the siege of Naples (1495) and the disbandment of mercenaries throughout Europe. Public health edicts against the disease stemmed from that time. One such was at Nuremberg (1496) which inspired the celebrated drawing attributed to Durer of a syphilitic man (Fig. 1).

Physicians very soon described the signs and symptoms of early syphilis as well as accepting the concept of congenital syphilis. From its first epidemic ravages, treatment for syphilis had been by inunction with *mercury ointment (unguentum Saracenicum) (Fig. 2). Preparations of mercury had long been in favour for the treatment of skin diseases. They had been used for this purpose by the Arabian physicians. Mercury was also given in pill form, by inhalation and fumigation (Fig. 3), and, much later in the 19th century, by hypodermic injection. Among the many references to syphilis in Shakespeare is one to fumigation which was carried out in the sweating tub, the patients often being confined for this purpose to the 'spital', the equivalent of the subsequent lock-hospital, and successor to the old lazar house. In *Henry V*, II. i Pistol tells us that Doll Tearsheet is in the 'powd 'ring tub of infamy', and that '. . . my Nell is dead, the spital of malady of France' (*Henry V*, v. i). Guaiacum, an organic substance derived from a South American tree, was later introduced as an alternative treatment. It was imported into Europe by the mercantile house of Fugger of Augsburg. Its most

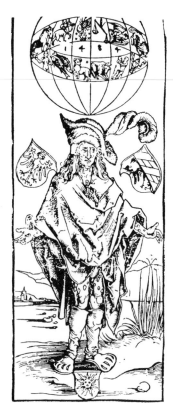

Fig. 1 A syphilitic man (Dürer).

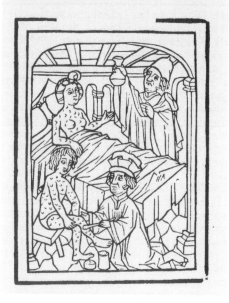

Fig. 2 From Parent-Duchatelet (1837), *De la prostitution dans la ville de Paris*, Paris—an early epidemiological work on prostitution and STDs.

celebrated advocates were *Fallopius (1564) and Fernel (1579). The dread of mercury was such that guaiacum was kept in the pharmacopoeia for 400 years, together with two other drugs used in treatment, sarsaparilla and sassafras.

Early descriptions called syphilis the Great Pox or Morbus Gallicus, the French disease (Fig. 2), or, in France, The Neapolitan disease or Spanish disease. Jacques de Bethencourt of Rouen was the first to use the term venereal disease (lues venerea) in 1527. In 1530 Girolamo *Fracastoro of Verona wrote the celebrated poem *Syphilus sive morbus gallicus*. Syphilus, a swineherd, was smitten when he refused to make sacrifices to Apollo. Syphilis must be the only disease to be named after an imaginary person in a poem. The term was not used in English literature until 1686 when the poet laureate Nahum Tate translated the work of Fracastoro. The first mention in English medical writing was the work of the surgeon-dermatologist Daniel Turner *On syphilis* (1717).

Although in modern times gonorrhoea and syphilis have been regarded as different diseases, this has not always been so. The confusion between syphilis and gonorrhoea seems to have been compounded during the first part of the 16th century. For the next 300

years, until the final proof of their difference by the French physician Phillipe *Ricord (1838), the medical world was split into two on the pathology of venereal diseases. There were monists, such as the celebrated 17th century English physician Thomas Sydenham, who believed that syphilis and gonorrhoea were one and the same disease, and dualists who stuck out for their being two distinct conditions. The frequent association of gonorrhoea with syphilis, as well as the discharge due to a urethral chancre, doubtless explains the tendency of the old writers to regard 'clap' as the early stage and syphilis the late stage of 'the pox', a view idealized by Pope, 'Time that at last matures a clap to pox'.

To understand the development of STDs an appreciation of important discoveries and progress in the field in the past 400 years is required. After the early events there was a long period in the history of syphilis in the 17th century during which nothing of special merit occurred. A posthumous publication of work by Lancisi (1728) correlated dilatation of the heart with syphilis—'aneurysma gallicum'. In the same year the great innovative physician *Boerhaave of Leiden implicated syphilis as a cause of cardiovascular disease. In 1736

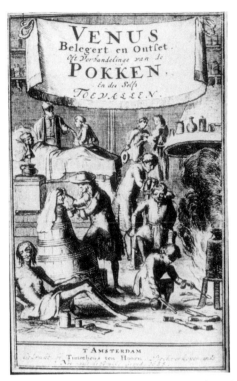

Fig. 3 Frontispiece of Stephen Blankaart's (1684) *Venus Belegert en Ontset*, Amsterdam.

Jean Astruc, physician to Louis XV, summarized the whole corpus of knowledge on venereal disease to that time, in the most comprehensive and scholarly work on the subject yet written. He argued strongly for the American origin of the disease, but at the same time shared the then current belief that gonorrhoea and syphilis were two stages of the same venereal disease. Among his descriptions of other STDs is an accurate one of genital *herpes. Van Swieten, a pupil of Boerhaave, reinvigorated the teaching and practice of medicine in Vienna after 1749 and popularized more liberal treatment of syphilitics, as well as the introduction of graduated dosage with mercury in its treatment, thus preventing troublesome side-effects such as over-salivation (ptyalism), the shakes (tremor), and renal disease.

John *Hunter's book of 1786 *A treatise on the venereal disease*, although notable for scientific objectivity, is not one of his greatest works, but such was his eminence that perhaps more importance has been attached to it than would have been the case with a publication by a lesser man. Hunter's most important error was, however, adhesion to the monist doctrine. Until recently it was thought that in the celebrated experiment of 1767, Hunter, to prove the view of the single identity of gonorrhoea and syphilis, inoculated himself with

matter of gonorrhoea on to his prepuce and glans. Unfortunately, he chose the inoculum from a patient suffering from both syphilis and gonorrhoea, after which he further strengthened his single-identity view. Two modern commentators, Qvist and Dempster, state that the experiment is described in the third person and they argue that there are reasons for believing that the experiment was done on a patient. Hunter thought that the only difference between the two diseases depended on the nature of the surface to which the inoculum was applied, that it caused ulceration when it acted on a cutaneous surface, but only a purulent discharge without breach of surface, when applied to a mucous membrane. In Edinburgh, Benjamin Bell (1793) carried out inoculation experiments on medical students, showing that gonorrhoea and syphilis were different diseases, but, at last, Philippe Ricord in Paris in 1838 showed conclusively, by experiments on 667 patients in a mental hospital, that gonorrhoea and syphilis were different diseases. Ricord also classified syphilis into three stages: primary, secondary, and tertiary. He was the founder of a remarkable school of venereology in France in the 19th century.

Much progress in sexually transmitted diseases was made in the 19th century, often secondary to advances in scientific medicine using laboratory techniques such as microscopy and the disciplines of *microbiology, *serology, *immunology, and inorganic chemistry. Between 1857 and 1863 Jonathan *Hutchinson of the London Hospital described the entities now known as Hutchinson's triad (interstitial keratitis in the cornea, eighth cranial nerve deafness, and Hutchinson's teeth (notching of the incisor both in the juvenile and adult dentitions)), important signs of established congenital syphilis. It was left to Alfred *Fournier in Paris in 1875 to propose that syphilis was a cause of the symptoms of paralysis, motor incoordination, and progressive locomotor ataxia. Fournier formed the concept of parasyphilis—those diseases of which syphilis was essentially the cause, but which were not directly the result of the syphilitic organism, namely *general paralysis, *tabes dorsalis, *taboparesis, and primary *optic atrophy.

Albert *Neisser in 1879 at Breslau, using Koch's staining methods, conclusively described the causal agent of gonorrhoea. Advances in the field of diagnosis and treatment of gonorrhoea progressed quickly after Neisser's discovery. In 1881 Credé of Leipzig introduced instillation of silver nitrate drops into the eyes of the newborn to prevent gonococcal *ophthalmia neonatorum, in those days a common cause of blindness in infants. *Gram's stain (1884) provided a reliable staining technique for the microscopic diagnosis of gonorrhoea. For about 100 years several commentators had noticed *urethritis which did not seem like gonorrhoea in its true sense. In 1907 Halberstaedter and Prowazek found inclusions in the eyes of infants with neonatal conjunctivitis, and then found genital discharge in their mothers. Lindner (1909) in Vienna advanced knowledge into the aetiology of non-gonococcal urethritis when he demonstrated elementary bodies, morphologically indistinguishable from those seen in inclusion conjunctivitis, in urethral discharge. Thus by the beginning of the 20th century the realization of the aetiology of gonorrhoea and non-gonococcal urethritis was well under way.

In 1903 *Metchnikoff and Roux showed that syphilis could be consistently transmitted to chimpanzees (Fig. 4). Fritz *Schaudinn, a protozoologist, collaborated with Erich Hoffmann, a dermatologist, in examining specimens of preparations of primary and secondary syphilis stained with aniline dye. On 3 March 1905, in the Charité in Berlin, Schaudinn was able to demonstrate *spirochaetes in one of Hoffman's slides. Using dark-field microscopy, Landsteiner and Mucha recognized, in 1906, the spirochaete responsible for syphilis, *Treponema pallidum*.

Their method is still in use today. In 1913 Noguchi and Moore, using a silver staining method, were able to demonstrate *Treponema pallidum* in the brains of 12 patients with general paralysis of the insane, thus proving its causation by syphilis.

Immunology came into its own in the latter years of the 19th century. In 1901 Bordet and Gengou described the *complement fixation test, by means of which an infection could be diagnosed by finding its antibody in the serum. *Wassermann (1906) in Berlin was able to show the value of the complement fixation test in the diagnosis of syphilis. Over the next 40 years many different serological tests for syphilis were devised. However,

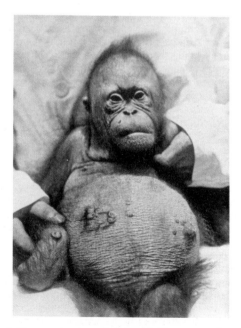

Fig. 4 Orang-utan inoculated with *Treponema* by Albert *Neisser *et al.*, Java, 1906.

it was not until the early 1940s that it was fully realized that many diseases could be responsible for a positive Wassermann reaction. The introduction of the test for specific antibody, the *treponemal immobilization test by Nelson and Mayer in 1949, inaugurated an era of more accurate serological diagnosis.

In 1909 Paul *Ehrlich in Frankfurt found salvarsan (arsphenamine), his 'magic bullet' to be effective as a cure for syphilis. This was superseded in 1943 when Mahoney and co-workers from the USA demonstrated that penicillin was effective and without serious side-effects in the treatment of syphilis.

A new era was ushered in; despite antibiotic resistance the pharmaceutical industry has managed to maintain effective therapies for those sexually transmitted diseases caused by bacteria, namely syphilis, gonorrhoea, chancroid, granuloma inguinale, lymphogranuloma venereum, and non-gonococcal urethritis.

The more common sexually transmitted diseases
Gonorrhoea

(a) Cause. *Neisseria gonorrhoeae.* This may cause uncomplicated urogenital infection in both sexes. In addition, especially after homosexual activity or oropharyngeal contact, there may be rectal and pharyngeal infections, respectively. If left untreated in the male, epididymo-orchitis and prostatitis may result, and in the female, pelvic inflammatory disease may occur, with resultant sterility. Disseminated infection may occur infrequently with variable skin, joint, and blood-spread manifestations. Adult *conjunctivitis is rare in developed countries, where spread may be via fomites. An untreated mother may give rise to a baby born with neonatal conjunctivitis. In recent years various strains of *N. gonorrhoeae* have developed which are completely resistant to penicillin and to some other antibiotics; they are found throughout the world.

(b) Treatment. Uncomplicated infections:

1. Penicillin-sensitive strains: penicillin and its analogues and probenecid in high doses by mouth or intramuscular injection; alternatively other antibiotics may be used with care.
2. Penicillin-resistant strains: spectinomycin or some *cephalosporins by injection. Rectal, pharyngeal, and systemic infections usually require more prolonged courses of treatment with appropriate antibiotics.

Non-specific genital infection
This is the name often used synonymously with non-gonococcal urethritis and non-specific urethritis.

(a) Cause. In 30–60 per cent of cases, the causative organism is *Chlamydia trachomatis; Ureaplasma urealyticum* and *Mycoplasma hominis* are also implicated. These organisms may cause non-gonococcal urethritis, post-gonococcal urethritis, *epididymitis, *proctitis, cervicitis, infection of Bartholin's ducts, *salpingitis, and perihepatitis.

Infrequently in males, mostly after a urethritis, *Reiter's syndrome may occur with associated *arthritis, conjunctivitis, and other variable manifestations.

(b) Treatment. Tetracycline or doxycycline by mouth for at least 7 days. If tetracyclines are contraindicated, *erythromycin or azithromycin is given for several days.

Syphilis
(a) Cause. *Treponema pallidum.*

1. Early infections: the primary stage gives rise to sore, or chancre, with regional lymphadenopathy at the site of inoculation, i.e. the genitals, ano-rectum, mouth, or pharynx; the secondary stage gives rise to systemic manifestations, especially rashes.
2. Early latent: latent syphilis of not more than 2 years' duration.
3. Latent: no manifestations but specific serological tests for syphilis are positive.
4. Late syphilis (tertiary or late syphilis): may lead on to cardiovascular, neurological, and systemic complications.
5. Congenital syphilis: acquired infection of the newborn from an untreated mother.

(b) Treatment, according to stage, but generally with benzathine penicillin or procaine penicillin by injection of varying dosages. If the patient is allergic to penicillin, tetracycline, doxycycline, or erythromycin can be given by mouth in prolonged courses of treatment. Follow-up after treatment is necessary. HIV infection with immunodeficiency may complicate the treatment.

Genital *herpes simplex virus infections
(a) Cause. Herpes simplex virus (types 2 and 1). Genital herpes infection is a viral disease that may be chronic and recurring. Symptoms are variable, starting with a small blister (vesicle) leading on to recurrent, small, genital sores. There may be systemic complications. There is a potential danger to the child born to a pregnant woman who has had herpes genitalis. Her clinical attendants should be informed of her history.

(b) Treatment. As yet there is no totally effective therapy. *Acyclovir may help in a particular event, but does not cure for ever.

Venereal warts (condylomata acuminata)
(a) Cause. Genital wart virus. Soft infectious warts may occur in the anogenital region after sexual contact with a person also infected with genital warts. Atypical warts should be biopsied. Cervical cytology should be performed in women with genital warts, which may be a factor in various genital cancers.

(b) Treatment. Tincture of podophyllotoxin should be applied to the warts. Other alternatives are cryotherapy, electrosurgery, or surgical removal.

Molluscum contagiosum
(a) Cause. A pox virus. This is not infrequently found in the genital region. Small, horny papules which may be mistaken for warts, are found in groups. It may occur on the face in AIDS.

(b) Treatment. By simple removal using various techniques.

Trichomoniasis
(a) Cause. *Trichomonas vaginalis*, a protozoon. This causes an unpleasant vaginal discharge. Men are symptomless carriers.

(b) Treatment. With *metronidazole for the patient and her sexual partners.

Non-specific vaginitis: Gardnerella vaginalis
(a) Cause. *Gardnerella*, *Haemophilus vaginalis*, and various anerobic organisms. This may cause a variable vaginal discharge.

(b) Treatment. The patient should be treated with metronidazole.

Genital candidiasis (thrush)
(a) Cause. This is a common disorder caused by a yeast, *Candida albicans*, which is often found on the skin and in the intestines, and symptomless carriage is reported in the vagina. It may be associated with other systemic disease, especially in recurrent cases. It may occur after antibiotic treatment for other conditions. It is not a venereal disease, but as it may present with genital symptoms is included in this list for completeness. It commonly occurs:

(1) in women, when it may present with a vaginitis;
(2) in men, when it may present with a balanoposthitis, i.e. inflammation of the glans and prepuce.

Oral thrush may occur in AIDS.

(b) Treatment. With intravaginal pessaries or creams. Effective therapy can be achieved with antibiotic—nystatin or newer synthetic imidazole derivatives such as clotrimazole or miconazole. Genital candidiasis can be treated with oral azoles.

Skin parasite infections, sexually transmissible
(a) Scabies. Caused by a mite *Sarcoptes scabiei*. This causes an itchy rash. It is passed on by close body contact, which may include coitus. It can be treated with benzyl benzoate or 1 per cent gamma benzene hexachloride lotions to the body. Close contacts should be treated.

(b) Pediculosis pubis (vulgarly 'crabs'). Caused by a louse, *Pediculosis pubis*, which makes the patient itch. It may be found in the anogenital area and also in pubic, abdominal, and axillary hair. The treatment for this is similar to that for scabies.

Tropical sexually transmitted disease
The following diseases are more commonly found in the tropics (see TROPICAL MEDICINE). Travellers may occasionally bring them back to more temperate latitudes.

Lymphogranuloma venereum
(a) Cause. Lymphogranuloma venereum (LGV) serotype of *Chlamydia trachomatis*. After an initial transient genital lesion, inguinal adenitis occurs, followed by various constitutional symptoms. There may be late complications resulting from fibrotic changes to the lymph vessels draining from the genitals.

(b) Treatment is by prolonged courses of tetracycline or sulphonamides. In addition, surgical intervention may be needed for late cases.

Chancroid
(a) Cause. Ducrey's bacillus (*Haemophilus ducreyi*). This may cause painful genital sores which lead on to inguinal buboes (swellings with abscess formation in the groins). It must be differentiated from syphilis, genital herpes, and granuloma inguinale (see below).

(b) Treatment. Administration of co-trimoxazole, tetracyclines, or erythromycin by mouth. According to the geographical area of infection, other antibiotics may also be used.

Donovanosis (Granuloma inguinale)
(a) Cause. *Calymmatobacterium granulomatis* (Donovan body)—a bacterium. This disease was first described by tropical medicine specialists in the Indian Medical Service at the turn of the 20th century. Ulcerating, enlarging, granulating sores leading to inguinal pseudobuboes occur.

(b) Treatment is by administration of tetracycline or co-trimoxazole by mouth.

Some other viral diseases in which a sexually transmissible organism (and route) has been implicated
*Epstein–Barr virus
The cause of a glandular fever-like illness in young adults. It may be passed on by oral transmission at the time of coitus.

*Cytomegalovirus
It causes mild glandular fever-like symptoms in young adults. It is a serious cause of neonatal congenital infection, and causes serious eye disease and blindness in patients with AIDS.

*Hepatitis A
The cause of faecally transmitted jaundice, especially in homosexuals.

*Hepatitis B
The cause of jaundice and chronic ill-health, especially in homosexuals. There may be asymptomatic carriers. It can be prevented by an effective vaccine. Other rarer forms of hepatitis may be transmitted sexually.

Present situation in the United Kingdom
In 1917 the recommendations of the Royal Commission on Venereal Disease came into force. Its guiding principles were that free and confidential treatment under the supervision of qualified medical practitioners should be available to all who required treatment for what are now regarded as STDs.

This service is an essential part of the *National Health Service and it is more than ever required, not only for the treatment of these conditions but also to aid in the prevention of STDs and HIV/AIDS and their effects on morbidity and mortality.

Apart from the treatment of bacterial infections, the control of STDs in women and of sexually transmitted viral disease, such as genital herpes and genital warts, takes up more and more time. Partner notification and skilled contact tracing of these conditions are essential, coupled with informing the public about these conditions. Since 1982 most STD specialists in the UK have also taken on a major role in the care of patients with HIV/AIDS and play a major part in sexual health programmes.

Postgraduate training is rigorous and follows that of any other medical specialty, with the added input of gynaecological training. Clinics in genitourinary medicine are found throughout the UK, and the specialty has grown, with increasing numbers of consultants in the past 10 years, due to the problems of HIV/AIDS and rising expectations of good sexual health in the population. Research has flourished. Professorial chairs have been instituted. There is a postgraduate medical society in the UK, the Medical Society for the Study of Venereal Diseases, with similar societies throughout the world. There are two thriving UK journals: *Genitourinary Medicine* and *The International Journal for STDs and AIDS*. As long as humans continue to behave as they do, it looks as though there will be STDs and a need for specialist medical care for those affected.

M. A. WAUGH

SEXUAL OFFENCES ACTS 1956, 1967, 1976. The UK Sexual Offences Act 1956 was amended by the Sexual Offences Act (Amendment) 1976. Among the provisions of the statutes, the following may be noted. In rape or unlawful carnal knowledge, the offence is committed by penetration only without emission, even when penetration is slight; consent is no defence when intercourse is unlawful. Rape is defined as intercourse with a woman who does not at the time consent to it, by a man who knows she does not or who is reckless as to whether she does; a husband separated from his wife under a separation order or agreement may be guilty of rape if he has intercourse with her without her consent. More recent legal judgements suggest that rape within marriage may also, under certain circumstances, be an offence. In rape, the anonymity of the complainant is preserved and other restrictions are placed on evidence. Other sexual offences include: intercourse after facilitation by the administration of drugs; intercourse with a girl under 13, or between 13 and 16; intercourse with an idiot, imbecile, or defective (these terms are now defunct and would be covered by 'severe subnormality'); incest; and the general offence of indecent assault.

The Sexual Offences Act 1967 concerned *homosexual practices, removing the prohibition on these provided they take place in private and between consenting adults. In 1994 the UK Parliament reduced the legal age for consent to homosexual acts from 21 years to 18.

Before these several enactments, to which should be added the Indecency with Children Act 1960, the misdemeanours they concern were offences under the Common Law and under the Offences Against the Person Act of 1861. It should be noted that an assault with intent to commit rape is still often prosecuted under the 1861 Act.

SHAMAN. A primitive healer, tribal physician, or witch doctor.

SHARPEY-SCHÄFER, SIR EDWARD ALBERT (1850–1935). British physiologist. He was a man of powerful personality who carried out important work on *cerebral localization and devised a method of *artifical respiration (Schafer's prone pressure method).

SHATTUCK, LEMUEL (1793–1859). See PUBLIC HEALTH MEDICINE IN THE USA.

SHEATH is an anatomical term denoting an enveloping tubular structure; it is also commonly used as a synonym for *condom, to mean an occlusive latex rubber cover for the penis worn during sexual intercourse to prevent conception and/or to provide protection against sexually transmitted diseases. High reliability and ready availability are its chief merits as a *contraceptive.

SHELLFISH POISONING. Shellfish are particularly liable to be agents of bacterial *food poisoning (e.g. *Salmonella, Shigella*), since their breeding grounds may be contaminated by sewage and they filter large quantities of water. Another type of shellfish poisoning, in which muscular paralysis may follow ingestion of neurotoxic material, is due to dinoflagellates (see RED TIDE). In certain individuals shellfish can cause a severe *allergic reaction.

SHELL-SHOCK was a term used during the First World War to describe psychiatric disturbances developed by some soldiers in reaction to battle conditions, a form of war *neurosis, or battle exhaustion.

SHERRINGTON, SIR CHARLES SCOTT (1857–1952). British neurophysiologist. In 1932, jointly with Lord *Adrian, he was awarded the *Nobel prize in physiology for his work on the nervous system. After a few years as a pathologist, Sherrington turned to physiology, particularly of the nervous system. His researches over a period of 50 years explained *reflex action and laid the foundation of our present knowledge of *neurophysiology. They were embodied in his book *The integrative action of the nervous system* (1906).

SHIFTING DULLNESS. Impaired resonance on *percussion of the abdominal flanks, the line of demarcation of which shifts when the patient is rolled to one side. This physical sign indicates the presence of fluid in the peritoneal cavity (*ascites).

SHIGA, KIYOSHI (1870–1957). Japanese microbiologist. He carried out valuable work on *plague and *tetanus but his name was made by isolating the *dysentery bacillus now known as *Shigella*.

SHIGELLA is a genus of Gram-negative *bacilli responsible for bacillary *dysentery.

SHINGLES. See HERPES ZOSTER.

SHIVERING is a physiological method of heat production by involuntary muscle contractions. See also RIGOR.

SHOCK. Medically, 'shock' is acute circulatory failure from whatever cause (e.g. blood loss, fluid loss, trauma, sepsis, myocardial infarction, cardiac arrhythmias, pulmonary embolism, pericardial effusion, burns, anaphylaxis, etc.). The common denominator is a fall in arterial blood pressure to 90 mmHg or less. The rest of the clinical picture varies with the cause, but typically includes signs of generalized peripheral vasoconstriction, with cold clammy skin, pallor, peripheral cyanosis, rapid thready pulse, oliguria, hyperventilation, and confusion. This meaning must be distinguished from the loose use of the term to mean any sudden mental or emotional disturbance.

SHOPE, RICHARD EDWIN (1901–66). American virologist. His chief study was viral diseases of animals. He showed that swine influenza is a complex infection caused by a filterable *virus and the bacterium *Haemophilus influenzae*. That virus was later shown to be related to some strains of human influenza virus, and there was serological evidence that it was related to the virus responsible for the world pandemic of influenza in 1918–19. In the early 1930s he found that certain natural *tumours of wild rabbits, a fibroma and a papilloma, were caused by filterable viruses; these were later shown to be related to *myxomatosis. This work was later pursued by Peyton *Rous, who used it to add substance to the growing body of evidence that some animal and human tumours result from viral infections. During the Second World War Shope headed a team which developed an effective *vaccine against a highly contagious disease of cattle: *rinderpest.

SHORT-SIGHTEDNESS. See MYOPIA; OPHTHAL-MOLOGY.

SHUNT. A short-circuit or bypass, usually between blood vessels, whereby blood flows from that with the higher intravascular pressure to that with the lower. A shunt may be physiological or pathological (congenital, acquired, or created surgically).

SIALOGRAM. An X-ray picture of the *salivary ducts produced by injecting radiopaque material into them.

SIAMESE TWINS are a developmental anomaly of monozygotic *twins in which there is a varying degree of fusion of the two bodies; they are also known as conjoined twins.

SIBBALD, SIR ROBERT (1641–1722). British physician and antiquary. He practised in Edinburgh, founding the Botanical Gardens at Holyrood in 1667. In 1680 he obtained a Royal Charter to found the Royal College of Physicians of Edinburgh, of which he was president in 1684. He was the first professor of medicine in Edinburgh (1665).

SIBILUS. A *rhonchus of whistling character.

SIBLING (or sib). Brother, sister, or litter-mate.

SICK-ABSENCE is absence from employment due to illness. In the UK, sickness benefit can be claimed for medically certificated sick-absence under the state national insurance scheme by Class 1 (employed) and Class 2 (self-employed) contributors. Sickness benefit is paid for up to 28 weeks only, then being replaced by invalidity benefit.

SICKLE-CELL DISEASE is a lifelong disorder due to an inherited abnormality of the *haemoglobin molecule, characterized by chronic *haemolytic anaemia, a sickle-shaped deformity of red blood cells, and intermittent 'vaso-occlusive crises' due to aggregations of sickled *erythrocytes blocking vessels and causing *infarction

in various tissues and organs of the body. The disease is fully expressed only in the *homozygous state, that is when the abnormal gene has been inherited from both parents. The very high gene frequency in certain parts of the world, notably across the middle third of Africa and in populations elsewhere deriving from that area, is explained by the fact that the *heterozygous state (one abnormal gene only) confers some protection against the effects of falciparum *malaria in early life. The term 'sickle-cell trait' is used to distinguish the relatively asymptomatic heterozygous state from homozygous sickle-cell disease.

SICKNESS. Illness.

SIDE-EFFECTS are the unwanted pharmacological consequences of drug administration; they may be minor (e.g. dryness of the mouth, slight constipation) and considered acceptable in view of the therapeutic value of the drug, or may, because of discomfort or danger, require it to be withdrawn.

SIDS. See SUDDEN INFANT DEATH SYNDROME.

SIGMOIDOSCOPY is inspection of the interior of the pelvic *colon with an *endoscope.

SIGN. A manifestation of disease perceptible to an observer, as opposed to a symptom, which is a manifestation of disease perceived by the patient.

SILICOSIS is a serious form of *pneumoconiosis due to inhalation of particles of silica (crystalline silicon dioxide), characterized by extensive damage to lung tissue.

SIMON, SIR JOHN (1816–1904). British pathologist and sanitary reformer (his name is pronounced Simone). In 1848 he was appointed the first *Medical Officer of Health to the City of London, and was successively, Medical Officer to the *General Board of Health (1855), to the *Privy Council (1858), and finally the first Chief Medical Officer to the *Local Government Board (1871). His reports on the state of sanitation, the water supply, *vaccination, and *cholera had an immense influence on the public health of the nation.

SIMON, THEODORE (1873–1961). French psychologist. With Alfred *Binet he introduced graded tests for patients with mental retardation, relating mental age to growth and chronological age. See PSYCHOLOGY.

SIMPSON, SIR JAMES YOUNG, BT (1811–70). British obstetrician. He introduced *chloroform as an anaesthetic in 1847, inhaling it experimentally with his assistants Matthews *Duncan and George Keith. He was the leading obstetrician of his day and one of the founders of *gynaecology. He invented the *uterine sound.

SIMS, JAMES MARION (1813–83). American gynaecologist. He practised medicine in Alabama, gaining attention by surgical skill in treatment of *vesicovaginal fistula. He devised the duckbill vaginal *speculum, and introduced the 'Sims position' for vaginal examinations: patient on left side, with right thigh drawn up.

SINGER'S NODES are small white nodules which develop on the *vocal cords of those who are required to use their voices excessively.

SINISTRAL means left-handed, or on the left side of the body.

SINOATRIAL NODE. The normal cardiac *pacemaker, also called the sinus node. It is a collection of specialized myocardial cells situated high up in the wall of the right atrium, near the opening of the superior vena cava. It has a higher inherent rhythmicity than any other part of the myocardium and initiates the wave of excitation which produces each contraction of the heart.

SINUS, in the anatomical sense, is applied to a variety of channels or cavities (e.g. the *paranasal sinuses); in the pathological sense, sinus denotes a blind channel opening (and usually discharging pus) on to the surface of the body.

SINUS ARRHYTHMIA is a physiological waxing and waning of heart rate due to respiratory variation in vagal (parasympathetic) tone: the pulse quickens with inspiration and slows with expiration. This influence of breathing on heart rate is quite normal, but tends to be more marked at the extremes of age.

SINUSITIS is inflammation of one or more of the *paranasal sinuses.

SINUS NODE. See SINOATRIAL NODE.

SINUS THROMBOSIS is *thrombosis of a venous sinus, particularly of one of the large intracranial sinuses of the *dura mater. Any of the latter may be involved, but most notable are cavernous, lateral, and superior sagittal sinus thromboses. Before *antibiotics, septic *thrombophlebitis was a relatively common cause but is now less so than aseptic *phlebothrombosis associated with various states that cause hypercoagulability.

SISTERS OF CHARITY OF ST VINCENT DE PAUL. Pre-eminent among the religious orders founded after the Renaissance with the aim of tending the sick and needy (hence anticipating the modern nursing profession), St Vincent de Paul's order, the Sisters of Charity, was established in Paris in 1634.

SITUS INVERSUS is *dextrocardia combined with transposition of the abdominal viscera.

SI UNITS. The Système International d'Unités was adopted in 1960 as the internationally agreed coherent system of measurement for all scientific purposes. It replaces previous systems, such as the centimetre–gram–second (cgs) system and the foot–pound–second (fps) system.

There are seven basic units as follows: metre (m), length; kilogram (kg), mass; second (s), time; ampere (A), electric current; kelvin (K), temperature (absolute); mole (mol), amount of substance; and candela (cd), luminous intensity. In addition, there are two supplementary units: radian (rad), plane angle; and steradian (sr), solid angle. There are also a number of derived units, that is which can be stated in terms of basic units. These include: newton (N), force; pascal (Pa), pressure; coulomb (C), electric charge; farad (F), capacitance; ohm (Ω), electric resistance; siemens (S), electric conductance; weber (Wb), magnetic flux; tesla (T), magnetic flux density; henry (H), inductance; hertz (Hz), frequency; degree Celsius (°C), temperature; lumen (lm), luminous flux; lux (lx), illuminance; becquerel (Bq), radioactivity; and gray (Gy), absorbed dose (of radioactivity).

Decimal multiples are given by metric prefixes, and where possible a prefix representing 10 raised to a power that is a multiple of three should be used, for example kilo- (10^3), mega- (10^6), giga- (10^9), etc. and milli- (10^{-3}), micro- (10^{-6}), nano- (10^{-9}), etc.

SJÖGREN'S SYNDROME is a condition, almost certainly *autoimmune, in which there is progressive destruction of *salivary and *lacrimal gland tissue. The major features are dryness of the mouth (xerostomia) and eyes (keratoconjunctivitis sicca), often with enlargement of the *parotid glands. There is an association with *rheumatoid arthritis and *systemic lupus erythematosus, and the condition is much more common in women.

SKELETON. The bony framework of the body; all the bones collectively.

SKIN, the external covering or integument of the body, consists of two distinct layers: the outer epidermis (derived from ectoderm) and the inner dermis or corium (derived from mesoderm). The epidermis, which is avascular, has a basal layer of growing cells which migrate outwards, becoming flattened and losing their nuclei to become the outermost horny layer or stratum corneum in about 2 weeks from their formation; after about another 2 weeks they are shed completely, so that the total turnover time of epidermal cells is approximately 1 month. During migration and differentiation the cells form a fibrous protein called *keratin, which is an integral component of the protective epidermal layer. The cells are therefore called keratinocytes. Mingled with them are some melanocytes, which produce pigmentation. Beneath the epidermis, resting on a cushion of fat tissue, is the main mass of skin, the dermis (sometimes called the 'true skin', or corium). It largely consists of vascular connective tissue, containing, along with blood vessels, fibrous protein, mucopolysaccharide, elastic fibres, and collagen, all the other structures found in skin: lymph channels, nerves, sweat and sebaceous glands, hair follicles, and a few cells, largely fibroblasts, mast cells, and histiocytes. See also DERMATOLOGY.

SKIN TESTS determine an individual's immunological reactivity to a substance by bringing it into contact with the skin by local application or by intra- or subcutaneous injection. See, for example, TUBERCULIN TEST.

SKODA, JOSEPH (1805–81). Austrian physician. His chief contribution was to correlate physical signs with pathological lesions. His *Abhandlung über Perkussion und Auskultation* (1839) is a medical classic and one of the foundations of physical diagnosis. A popular teacher and a therapeutic nihilist, he was the first in Austria to teach in German. He described the hyperresonant *percussion note above a *pleural effusion (Skodaic resonance).

SKODAIC RESONANCE is increased resonance on *percussion of the chest wall above the level of a *pleural effusion.

SKULL. The bony casing enclosing the *brain, also known as the cranium. The skull consists of a number of individual bones rigidly articulated to each other, with mobile articulations with the vertebral spine and the lower jaw.

SLEEP
Introduction
We evolved upon a rotating Earth in which light and dark, warmth and cold, came and went about every 24 hours. In common with other animals we have within our genetic design an inherent rhythmicity that combines in a sensible manner with the alternation of light and dark. Some creatures have specialized and are nocturnal in habit, but man is among the majority; during the light he is active and during the dark he rests. His nervous system imposes rest, sleep being a positive state of inertia and unresponsiveness to the environment.

Biological rhythms of about a 24-hour periodicity (circadian rhythms) can be found in isolated tissues but are normally co-ordinated in the whole body by the brain. If we fly to the other side of the northern hemisphere, our biological rhythm continues to make us sleepy and inefficient at times when those around us are alert, and it makes us wakeful while they rest.

The mental life of sleep has always held a special fascination and in most cultures the soul has been thought to leave the body during sleep, to mingle with supernatural beings, so to receive guidance for the future. The interpretation of dreams for prophetic purposes is familiar, in the story of the boy Joseph, who grew to interpret Pharoah's dream, and in the dream-books of 19th century Europe. Sigmund *Freud considered his greatest work to be his book *The interpretation of dreams* (1899) in which he saw the dream as a guardian against disturbance of sleep, and as revealing not the future, but the hidden personality traits of the individual.

Until the 1950s sleep was often seen as a negative state, of mere absence of arousal. It was a decade in which the regulatory role of the *brainstem reticular formation came to be understood. Formerly, *Pavlov, the Russian physiologist, for example, had supposed that wakefulness was determined by the intensity of sensory information reaching the cerebral cortex. It emerged that this was not the case, and that there is a key part of the brain, situated in the central core of the brainstem, excitement of which would lead to ascending and descending impulses that would activate the forebrain and the *spinal cord, raising their responsiveness to wakeful levels.

Characteristics of sleep
The most important determinant of falling asleep is to have arrived at that phase of the circadian cycle during which we have learned to fall asleep. Falling asleep is, however, also promoted by sheer lack of sleep, by immobility, monotony, warmth, or lack of immediate purpose. The heart slows, the blood pressure falls, the muscles relax, the electrical resistance of the skin rises as insensible sweating diminishes, the pupils become small, and the electrical brain waves (*electro-encephalogram or EEG) change in appearance. We first flit to and fro between wakefulness and drowsiness, while imperceptibly the control of our thoughts escapes us. Environmental cues become missed and reactions delayed whenever, for a second or more, the EEG displays slower waves. The tired car driver may at such a point leave the road without any reason other than his inattention.

As sleep deepens, the EEG displays the characteristic sleep spindles or groups of waves at 12–14 cycles per second (Hz), while slower waves of 1–3 Hz become more and more prominent. The body's *oxygen consumption falls and reaches its lowest while the EEG's slowest waves prevail. During this same slow-wave sleep of the early night the brain's blood flow and *glucose consumption fall and *growth hormone is secreted in greatest amounts. Circulating *cortisol and *adrenaline have by this time fallen to their lowest levels of the 24 hours. Soon afterwards body temperature falls to its lowest and near the end of the sleep period, cortisol begins to rise again in pursuit of its after-breakfast peak.

Within sleep there can readily also be seen an ultradian rhythm of about 100 minutes, periodicity with recurring periods of paradoxical (rapid eye movement, *REM) sleep. In this form of sleep there are EEG waves in appearance near to those of drowsiness, jerky eyeball movements, extreme muscular relaxation, penile erection, enhanced brain blood flow, and irregularity of heart, blood pressure, and respiration. Although, in statistical terms, mental life most often deserves to be described as dreaming just after the very moment of one of the rapid eye movements during paradoxical sleep, mental life at any other time of sleep can be indistinguishable.

The function of sleep

There is a widespread intuitive belief that sleep renews and restores. The apparent renewal is most evident for the brain. If total wakefulness is deliberately imposed on volunteers for several days and nights, they become unable to sustain attention or coherent thought because of brief 'microsleeps' that would lead them directly into full sleep were it not for relays of vigilant watchers. Judgment becomes impaired, visual and other misperceptions intrude, irritability and *paranoid ideas erupt, volition diminishes, energy is conserved, body temperature and muscular strength fall, while *nitrogen excretion rises and the *immune system that fights infection functions less effectively. A couple of subsequent nights of unbroken sleep, during which long periods of slow-wave sleep have priority, restore normal function. We need to sleep.

Tissues such as skin or the epithelium of the *gut are constantly worn away and renew themselves by cell division, whereas the brain renews its structural components, not by making new cells but by replacement of *protein molecules ('turnover'). Most research into these renewal processes has been conducted in rodents, in which, in all tissues, there has been found to be a higher rate of renewal by cell division or by protein synthesis during that time of the 24 hours when rodents sleep, and this is true of brain protein synthesis.

Poor sleep

The complaint of poor sleep is one of the commonest any doctor encounters. Dissatisfaction with sleep is more frequent among women, among persons of anxious temperament, and among older age-groups.

A reduction of sleep duration below normal, with greater brokenness of sleep, is commonly a consequence of enhanced *anxiety arising out of problems in daytime life. As worries recede, sleep improves again. Sometimes sleep is reduced for weeks or months as a result of mental illness, severely so in *mania, characterized as it is by excess energy and confidence. The obverse disorder, *depressive illness, is more common

and, especially in middle or later life, unaccustomed and persisting *insomnia accompanied by a black cloud of gloomy worries unjustified by the circumstances of daily life should provide a proper reason for seeking medical advice.

Drugs

Drugs taken to promote sleep were formerly provided by *alcohol, the *poppy, and extracts from plants containing *hyoscine and related compounds, the *mandrake root being the most famous. Conversely, *caffeine and other xanthines in *coffee and *tea have been natural substances capable of delaying and disturbing sleep, especially for the middle-aged or older.

Chemical compounds of non-plant origin have come into use in the past two centuries as promoters of sleep: *paraldehyde, *chloral, *bromides, *barbiturates, and, most often used nowadays, *benzodiazepine derivatives. They relieve anxiety and promote sleep.

The regular intake of any sleep-promoting, anxiety-relieving compound leads to compensatory adjustments in the brain. If intake of the drug ceases suddenly, then, as a consequence of the prior use of the drug, there is unnatural insomnia, with restlessness, anxiety, and an enhanced liability to fits. If large daily doses have been taken, the withdrawal picture may even be that of *delirium tremens, although the less extreme syndrome is much commoner after benzodiazepines. Several weeks are then needed before the *withdrawal phenomena fade and for return to a natural level of anxiety and a natural duration of sleep.

Sleep disorders

Although complaints of insomnia are commoner among older adults, some 5 per cent of adolescents regard themselves as sleeping badly, with associated feelings of unhappiness and low self-esteem. In even younger children, no fewer than 40 per cent of parents of children under 4 years of age regard their child as having a sleep problem, with rapid improvement after that age.

Nightmares are common at any age and the true nightmare is a phenomenon of paradoxical sleep, made up of a relatively prolonged and fearful sequence within a dream, coupled with inability to move, and generally arising in the later night. Neither nightmares nor *night terrors denote mental disorder, although they are commoner when daytime life is anxious, and nightmares are frequent after recent withdrawal of sleep-promoting drugs. Night terrors are features of the early night: they arise during EEG slow-wave sleep and are coupled with unelaborated mental life, such as a brief experience of being entrapped, and may be accompanied by shrieking and lashing out. Night terrors run strongly in families, together with a liability to sleep-walking and nocturnal shouting. They often begin around *puberty and occasionally persist into adult life. The affected child remembers almost nothing of the nocturnal experience. The most important need is for reassurance of the family, together with simple precautions against injury while sleep-walking. It must be noted that any drug that acts upon the brain may provoke night terrors and sleep-walking in occasional individuals.

Daytime sleepiness
While many people complain of lack of sleep, there are a few who complain of falling asleep too readily. In some cases this must be attributed to a constitutional need for more than the average hours of sleep, or to getting up early for work and then trying to remain awake in the evening in company with other family members. Sometimes, however, the liability to fall asleep must be regarded as a disorder, usually of unknown origin. Often it is manageable only by attempts at losing weight, and by the judicious use of deliberate naps and of caffeine or *amphetamine derivatives. Two syndromes that the average doctor may expect to encounter can, however, be defined.

One is known as idiopathic *narcolepsy with *cataplexy. It can begin at any age and is usually first manifested by spells of irresistible sleep, each lasting for about 10 minutes, a couple of times a day. The same person may during the day suddenly find himself or herself partly or totally paralysed for a brief moment in response to an emotion characteristic for him or her, be it laughter, triumph, or anger. These brief paralyses are known as cataplectic attacks. About one person in a thousand suffers from idiopathic narcolepsy and the disorder should be more widely recognized as one that causes embarrassment and a liability to road accidents. Another reason for excessive sleepiness, particularly among males, is obstructed breathing that develops only during sleep. Children with large and infected *tonsils and *adenoids may be affected and also some obese adults. The obstruction means that every 20 seconds or so the sleeper almost awakens while engaging in violent snorting efforts to breathe, thereby greatly disturbing sleep.

Hypnosis
The Greek god of sleep was Hypnos and because many people during hypnotic trances look like sleep-walkers, the term '*hypnosis' came into use. However, despite the conventional instructions, 'You are falling asleep, you are falling asleep', the trance that is induced by the *suggestions of the hypnotist is not a state of sleep, but one of wakefulness and enhanced suggestibility.

Hints for good sleep
It is advisable to keep regular hours for getting up and going to bed. We should minimize alcohol intake and smoking, avoid evening caffeine, take plenty of regular exercise, and avoid being underweight or severely overweight. We should take evening meals at regular times and let them be of easily digestible food. Above all, we should seek to be satisfied with ourselves as we are, accepting our failures and disabilities, and being forgiving of others. We should not worry about how many hours of sleep we get; the brain will look after its needs.

I. OSWALD

Further reading
Empson, J. (1989). *Sleep and dreaming*. Faber, London.

SLEEP APNOEA (APNEA). Cessation of breathing during sleep due either to insensitivity of the respiratory centre or to inspiratory obstruction by the relaxed walls of the oropharynx (obstructive sleep apnoea). Also see CHEST MEDICINE; SLEEP.

SLEEPING DRAUGHT. A dose of medicine taken in order to promote sleep. See SLEEP.

SLEEPING SICKNESS. See TRYPANOSOMIASIS.

SLEEP PARALYSIS is temporary loss of muscle power on arousal from *REM sleep.

SLEEP WALKING. See SLEEP.

SLIT LAMP. An instrument which enables minute inspection of the structures of the eye by projecting into it a flat light-beam of high intensity.

SLOANE, SIR HANS, Bt (1660–1753). British physician. In 1687 he was appointed physician to the Duke of Albemarle, Governor of the West Indies, where he made a large collection of plants and natural curiosities. He attended Queen Anne and became physician-general to the army in 1722 and physician to George II in 1727. He was secretary to the Royal Society from 1693 to 1712 and president from 1727 to 1741; from 1719 to 1735 he also occupied the position of president of the Royal College of Physicians of London. In 1712 he bought the manor of Chelsea where several streets still bear his name. He published in two volumes an account of his voyage to the West Indies and of the natural history of Jamaica (1707, 1725). After his death his collection was bought by the nation for £20 000 (US$30 000) and went to form the basis of the British Museum.

SLOW VIRUS INFECTIONS are infections, now known to be due to *prions, rather than viruses, which have a very long incubation period, possibly lasting many years. *Kuru, *scrapie and *Creutzfeldt–Jakob disease are examples.

SMALLPOX (or variola), a devastating and pestilential scourge all over the world and at all known periods of history until the present, was finally eradicated as a human disease by the time the *World Health Organization made its historic declaration in May of 1980. Since there is no animal reservoir of infection, the virus, one of the group of orthopoxviruses which includes *vaccinia and a number of related animal poxviruses, can be assumed to exist no longer except where it is maintained in laboratories under the strictest security precautions.

SMEGMA is a soapy, cheesy secretion derived mainly from *sebaceous glands, particularly that which occurs under the *prepuce.

SMELL is the faculty of detecting odours. Loss of this sense is termed anosmia. It is sometimes due to local disease of the nose and is a not uncommon sequel of head injury. There are some rare causes, for example *cerebral tumour, and occasionally the sense is congenitally absent.

SMELLIE, WILLIAM (1697–1763). British obstetrician. He was a pioneer '*man-midwife'; he described a manoeuvre for delivering the after-coming head (Mauriceau–Smellie–Veit method) and devised special craniotomy scissors. See OBSTERICS AND GYNAECOLOGY.

SMELLING SALTS. See SAL VOLATILE.

SMITH, SIR GRAFTON ELLIOT (1871–1937). Anglo-Australian anatomist and anthropologist. Elliot Smith was an anatomist of distinction who was fired with an interest in anthropology by working in Egypt, during which time he supervised the anthropological survey of Nubia.

SMITH, NATHAN (1762–1829). American physician. He is best remembered for a classic clinical description of *typhoid fever (then called typhus fever).

SMITH, THEOBALD (1859–1934). American bacteriologist and immunologist. His discoveries in veterinary medicine were of seminal importance to the study and understanding of human diseases. A list of his accomplishments includes: demonstration that an infectious anaemia of cattle (Texas cattle fever) is conveyed by an insect *vector, introduction of the fermentation tube in bacteriology, differentiation between the typhoid bacillus and coliforms on the basis of gas formation, use of lactose and sucrose fermentation to differentiate Gram-negative bacteria, cultivation of *anaerobes, determination of thermal lability of tubercle bacilli, differentiation between human and bovine strains of tubercle bacilli, induction of immunity in pigs by injection of heat-killed bacilli, discovery of *Vibrio fetus* in contagious abortion of cattle, recognition of bacterial dissociation resulting from serial *passage *in vitro*, differentiation of the flagellar and somatic antigens, standardization of *toxin and *antitoxin of *diphtheria and *tetanus, and demonstration of presence of *antibody in *colostrum. See also MICROBIOLOGY.

SMITHWICK, REGINALD H. (1899–1987). American surgeon. He developed lumbodorsal sympathectomy and splanchnicectomy (the Smithwick operation) for the treatment of essential hypertension. He devised the combined operation of vagotomy and antral resection for peptic ulcer disease.

SMOG is a combination of smoke and fog, a form of air pollution which occurs in industrial areas where motor vehicles are in heavy use (such as Los Angeles), particularly when temperature inversions are frequent. A layer of warm air is trapped close to the ground, so preventing the escape or dilution of chemical pollutants.

SMOKING AND HEALTH. Tobacco was introduced to Europe from the New World at the end of the 15th century. In 1604 King James I of England, in *A counterblaste to tobacco*, said that smoking is 'A custome lothsome to the eye, hatefull to the Nose, harmefull to the braine, daungerous to the Lungs, and in the blacke and stinking fume thereof, neerest resembling the horrible Stigian smoke of the pit that is bottomelesse'. In 1605 the members of the Royal College of Physicians—pipes in hands—dismissed the king's views and smoking spread rapidly and was long regarded as having medicinal value. Smoking became a mass habit as mechanization of the manufacture of cigarettes made them cheaper. The first half of the 20th century saw a steep rise in smoking—particularly in men during the First World War and women during the Second (Fig. 1)

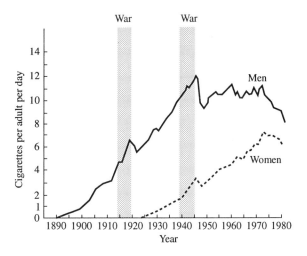

Fig. 1 Tobacco consumption in the UK 1890–1981, given as the average number of cigarettes per adult per day for men and women separately (the average number is calculated on the basis of the number of adults in the population, not on the number of adult smokers.)

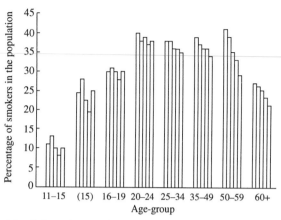

Fig. 2 Prevalence of smoking by age-group 1982–90. Successive bars show the results of biennial surveys in 1982, 1984, 1986, 1988, and 1990.

Two large-scale studies published in 1954 confirmed the hypothesis that smoking is a major cause of lung *cancer. However, it was the 1962 Royal College of Physicians (RCP) report, *Smoking and health*, that brought home the risks of smoking to the layman. For the first time in a decade, cigarette sales fell. The RCP report recommended the restriction of tobacco advertising, increased taxation on cigarettes, more restrictions on the sales of cigarettes to children and smoking in public places, and more information on the tar/nicotine content of cigarettes. Two years later Doll and Hill's nationwide prospective survey on 'Mortality in relation to smoking: 10 years' observation in British doctors' reported that about half the UK's doctors who smoked had given up and had been rewarded by a dramatic fall in lung cancer incidence.

In January 1971 the RCP, frustrated by government inaction on smoking, set up Action on Smoking and Health (ASH) to make non-smoking the norm in society and to inform and educate the public about the death and disease caused by smoking. This followed the publication of its second report, *Smoking and health now*, which received widespread publicity and caused a permanent drop of 5 per cent in cigarette consumption. In April 1971 the Department of Health unveiled the first in a series of voluntary agreements on tobacco advertising between it and the tobacco industry.

The debate on smoking and its health effects focused mainly on the harm done to smokers until March 1988 when the fourth report of the Independent Scientific Committee on Smoking and Health was published. It concluded that, in the UK, several hundred non-smokers die each year of lung cancer caused by passive smoking. Thereafter, the issue of the non-smoker's right to breathe smoke-free air became central to the campaign against tobacco use.

According to the latest figures about 13½ million adults in the UK smoke cigarettes—29 per cent of men and 28 per cent of women. The decline in smoking in recent years has been heavily concentrated in older age-groups, i.e. young people continue to take up smoking—23 per cent of 15-year-old boys and girls smoke cigarettes regularly (Fig. 2). Men and women in the unskilled manual socio-economic group are nearly three times more likely to smoke than people in the professional group. Approximately 11 million adults, or 25 per cent of the population, are ex-smokers.

Tobacco is the only legally available consumer product which kills people when it is used entirely as intended. It kills over 111 000 smokers each year in the UK. One in four smokers will die prematurely as a result of their smoking. Deaths from smoking dwarf all other forms of premature death—killing five times more people in the UK than road and other accidents, murder, suicide, illegal drug use, and AIDS all put together (Fig. 3)

Smoking causes 30 per cent of all cancer deaths, including 90 per cent of all deaths from lung cancer. Cancers other than lung cancer which are linked to smoking include cervical cancer; cancers of the mouth, lip, and throat; cancer of the *pancreas; *bladder cancer; cancer of the *kidney; and *stomach cancer. In addition, 90 per cent of all deaths from chronic *bronchitis and *emphysema, and 20–25 per cent of all deaths from heart disease are due to smoking. Cigarette-smoking increases the risk of having a heart attack by two or three times, compared with the risk to non-smokers. Nine out of 10 cases of peripheral vascular disease, leading to amputation of one or both legs, are caused by smoking—about 2000 amputations a year.

Women who smoke and take the contraceptive pill have 10 times the risk of a heart attack, *stroke, or other cardiovascular disease compared with those who take

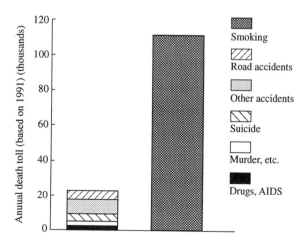

Fig. 3 Smoking's death toll—five times all other avoidable deaths.

the pill but are non-smokers. In pregnant women, smoking leads to an increased risk of spontaneous *abortion, *premature birth, and *sudden infant death syndrome (cot death).

The risks of smoking pipes and cigars compared with cigarettes depend on whether the smoker inhales the smoke or not. Smokers who inhale pipe and cigar smoke are just as much at risk of developing lung cancer as cigarette smokers. All cigar- and pipe-smokers have a higher risk than non-smokers of developing cancers of the lip, mouth, and throat. Giving up smoking can reduce the risk of developing many of these problems. Within 10–15 years of giving up smoking, an ex-smoker's risk of developing lung cancer is only slightly greater than that of a non-smoker.

Smoking costs the *National Health Service £437 million ($656 million) a year for hospital admissions alone. The state also pays for out-patient costs, costs of care in the community, social security payments, etc. At least 50 million working days are lost to British industry every year from smoking-related sick leave, at an estimated yearly cost of between £2.2 and £3.2 billion ($3.3 and $4.8 billion).

MARK FLANNAGAN

SMOLLETT, TOBIAS GEORGE (1721–71). British physician and novelist. His rough contentious manner proved unacceptable to many patients, but his lively and original novels have enjoyed lasting popularity. His best known works are *Roderick Random* (1748), *The adventures of Peregrine Pickle* (1751), and *The expedition of Humphrey Clinker* (1771).

SNAILS AS VECTORS OF DISEASE. Certain freshwater snails are of considerable medical and public health importance as vectors of *helminthic diseases, most notably of schistosomiasis (*bilharziasis) but also of other trematode infestations such as *paragonimiasis, for which the snails are intermediate hosts. The most important genera are *Bulinus*, *Planorbarius*, *Biomphalaria*, *Australorbis*, and *Tropicorbis*.

SNAKE BITE. More than 2500 species of snakes have been described, but less than one-quarter are venomous and have in their upper jaw enlarged teeth (the fangs) which are either grooved or contain a venom channel to introduce the *venom into their prey during a bite. Most snakes of medical importance belong to two families. The Elapidae include cobras, kraits, mambas, coral snakes, and Australasian snakes such as tiger snakes, taipans, and death adders. The Viperidae comprise the Old World vipers and adders (subfamily Viperinae), and the pit vipers of Asia and the lance-headed vipers, moccasins, and rattlesnakes of the New World (subfamily Crotalinae) which possess a heat-sensitive pit organ, situated between the eye and the nostril, for detecting their warm-blooded prey. Other families of venomous snakes are Hydrophiidae (sea snakes), Atractaspididae

(burrowing asps or stiletto snakes), and Colubridae. Venomous snakes occur in most parts of the world except in icy regions, altitudes above 4000 m, and on some islands. Sea snakes frequent the Indian and Pacific Oceans between latitudes 30°N and 30°S.

Most snake venoms would be harmful if injected into humans, but bites by fewer than 200 species have proved either life-threatening or likely to cause permanent disability. Snake bite is an uncommon accident in industrialized countries. The number of bites and deaths each year is a few thousand and less than 100, respectively, in Europe; 7000 and 12–15 in the USA, and 1000–3000 and 2 in Australia. However, snake bites are common in tropical countries which are densely inhabited both by 'irritable' species of snakes (those which readily strike when disturbed) and humans. Snake bite is a major medical problem in parts of West Africa, the Indian subcontinent, South-East Asia (especially Burma, where snake bite has been the fifth most common single cause of death), and Latin America. In some localities, such as north-eastern Nigeria, the incidence of bites and deaths may be as high as 500 and 50 per 100 000 population per year, respectively. The global annual total of snake bite deaths is probably around 100 000, but the incidence of chronic morbidity from loss or dysfunction of digits or limbs is unknown. Seasonal increases, often dramatic, in the incidence of snake bite are related to rains, flooding, or agricultural activity.

Venomous snakes are not aggressive

They bite humans only when inadvertently trodden upon, picked up or cornered, or when intentionally handled. World-wide, the most frequent victims of snake bite are agricultural workers, herdsmen, hunter-gatherers, and children. These inhabitants of the rural tropics are usually bitten on the feet or ankles when they tread on a snake in the dark or in undergrowth. The snake's venom apparatus may be mechanically inefficient when it strikes reflexly at the intrusive human limb; this may explain why only about half the cases of bites by venomous snakes result in significant envenoming.

Snake venoms

Snake venoms are rich sources of enzymes and fascinating pharmacologically active *peptides. They are 90–95 per cent protein and consist of many components: polypeptide *toxins (e.g. postsynaptic and other neurotoxins, endothelin-like sarafotoxins, membrane-damaging 'cardiotoxins'); enzymes (e.g. neurotoxic, muscle- and membrane-damaging phospholipases A_2, procoagulant enzymes, vascular endothelium-damaging haemorrhagins); non-toxic proteins (e.g. nerve growth factor), *carbohydrates, metals, lipids, free *amino acids, nucleotides, and biogenic amines.

Clinical effects of snake venoms

Clinical effects of snake venoms in humans represent an aberration of the biological function for which they have

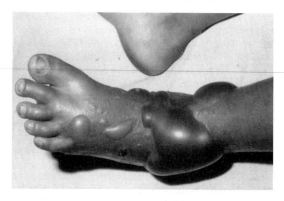

Fig. 1 Local swelling and blistering developing 24 hours after a bite on the dorsum of the foot by a Brazilian lance-headed viper, the jararaca (*Bothrops jararaca*).

evolved, i.e. to immobilize and predigest their natural prey. When a snake bites a human the dose of venom injected in relation to body weight, and the specific binding of toxins to their tissue target *receptors, are different from when it bites its prey.

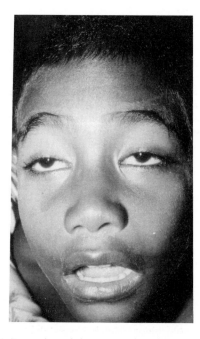

Fig. 2 Drooping of the eyelids (ptosis), paralysis of eye movements (external ophthalmoplegia), and inability to open the mouth wide and protrude the tongue in a boy bitten by a taipan (*Oxyuranus scutellatus canni*) in Papua New Guinea.

Local tissue damage (caused by many Viperidae; some Elapidae, such as African spitting cobras and Asian cobras; Atractaspis)

Cytolytic and *necrosis-inducing factors damage tissues, *membranes, and muscle, and cause leakage of *blood and *plasma into the tissues, swelling, blistering, local bruising and lymphangitis of the bitten limb (Fig. 1), and painful enlargement of draining *lymph nodes. *Gangrene and secondary bacterial *infections may lead to life-threatening *septicaemia, necessitating *amputation or result in crippling deformity and development of a chronic *ulcer which may become cancerous.

Neurotoxic (paralytic) effects (caused by many Elapidae and Hydrophiidae; some Viperidae)

There is progressive paralysis of muscles innervated by the cranial nerves (Fig. 2): first drooping of the eyelids (ptosis) and paralysis of eye movements (external *ophthalmoplegia), followed by inability to open the mouth, protrude the tongue and speak, paralysis of the muscles of swallowing and breathing, and finally generalized *paralysis. In human victims, snake venom neurotoxins affect the peripheral *nerves only, not the *brain and *spinal cord.

Generalized breakdown of skeletal muscle (rhabdomyolysis) (caused by most Hydrophiidae, some Elapidae such as the Australian tiger snake, some Viperidae)

Muscle pigment (myoglobin), muscle enzymes, and potassium leak from the damaged muscles into the circulation. Patients pass brown urine (myoglobinuria). Muscles are painful and tender and the jaws are clenched shut (trismus).

Kidney damage (caused by some Viperidae, especially Russell's viper and sea snakes)

Venoms can damage the kidney in many ways, e.g. by blocking the small blood vessels with fibrin, through the effect of products of damaged muscles and red blood corpuscles, and through direct effects on the renal tubules.

Bleeding and blood clotting abnormalities (caused by many Viperidae, Australian Elapidae, some Colubridae)

Some snake venoms contain *enzymes which activate specific steps of the blood clotting cascade (e.g. activators of clotting factors I (fibrinogen), II, V, X, XIII, etc.) (see HAEMATOLOGY), resulting eventually in such depletion of these factors that the blood will not clot (consumption coagulopathy, disseminated intravascular coagulation, or defibrination syndrome). Other venom components affect *platelet function, and 'haemorrhagins' damage vascular *endothelium, resulting in bleeding from the gums (Fig. 3) and into the gut, brain, lungs, kidneys, or heart.

Cardiovascular effects (caused by many Viperidae and Atractaspididae, some Elapidae)

*Blood pressure may fall and *shock develops from loss of circulating blood volume by leakage into the tissues. Some venoms have direct actions on the heart itself, or on the calibre of blood vessels and on endogenous systems controlling the blood pressure (such as brady-kinin and *angiotensin), which usually result in a fall in blood pressure. The sarafotoxins from *Atractaspis* venoms are potent vasoconstrictors (like endothelin, which they closely resemble in structure) and may cause constriction of the coronary arteries and *heart block.

Traditional first-aid methods for snake bite

Traditional first-aid methods for snake bite, such as the use of tight bands or *tourniquets, cuts at the site of the bite, and attempts to suck out the venom, have been largely abandoned as dangerous and ineffective. Patients should be reassured and transported to hospital as quickly as possible, with the bitten limb immobilized with a *splint or sling. 'Pressure immobilization' of the bitten limb with a crepe bandage and splint may delay the spread of venom from the site of the bite. Anti-venoms, which were introduced at the beginning of this century, are the only specific *antidotes for treating snake bite. They consist of *serum from horses or sheep which have been immunized with increasing doses of specific venoms to stimulate production of neutralizing *antibodies. Antivenoms are effective only against the specific venom or venoms used in their production, or against a limited range of venoms from related species. They have been effective in reducing mortality from up to 50 per cent to less than 5 per cent in the case of patients envenomed by the most deadly species. Anti-venoms may produce serious reactions and so should

be used only by medically qualified people. Ancillary treatments for snake bite include mechanical *ventila-tion (for patients with respiratory paralysis), surgical excision of dead tissue, and treatment of kidney failure, shock, and other complications in *intensive care units.

DAVID A. WARRELL

Further reading
Harvey, A. L. (ed.) (1991). Snake toxins. In *International encyclopedia of pharmacology and therapeutics*, Section 134. Pergamon Press, New York.
Lee, C.-Y. (ed.) (1979). Snake venoms. In *Handbook of experimental pharmacology*, Vol. 52. Springer-Verlag, Berlin.
Sutherland, S. K. (1983). *Australian animal toxins. The crea-tures, their toxins and care of the poisoned patient*. Oxford University Press, Melbourne.
Warrell, D. A. (1987). Venoms and toxins of animals and plants. In *Oxford textbook of medicine*, (2nd edn (ed. D. Weatherall, J. Ledingham, D. A. Warrell)). Oxford University Press, Oxford.

SNEEZING is the abrupt audible expulsion of air from the nose, reflexly induced by irritation of the nasal mucosa.

SNELLEN, HERMAN (1834–1903). Dutch ophthal-mologist. Snellen is known today for his printed *test types for testing visual acuity, which are still in use.

SNOW, JOHN (1813–58). British anaesthetist and hygienist. Snow introduced *ether to the UK and administered *chloroform to Queen Victoria for the births of Prince Leopold and Princess Beatrice in 1853 and 1857. From his observations of the *cholera epidemic in 1848 he deduced that the infection was spread by the water supply and recommended the removal of the handle of the Broad Street pump to control it, although the epidemic was subsiding before this was done. He published his views in *On the mode of communication of cholera* (1849).

SNUFF is ground *tobacco leaf or stalk, perfumed with a variety of essential oils, taken by insertion into the nostrils; *nicotine absorption occurs through the nasal mucous membrane.

SOCIAL MEDICINE. See PUBLIC HEALTH MEDI-CINE; SOCIOLOGY IN RELATION TO MEDICINE; SOCIAL WORK AND MEDICINE.

SOCIAL SECURITY ACTS 1973, 1975. The 1973 Act repealed nearly all existing English national insurance (other than industrial injuries) legislation and substi-tuted a new system embodying the essential purpose of the original but with certain changes and improvements. Among these were: wholly earnings-related contribu-tions for employed earners instead of the previous hybrid structure of flat-rate and graduated contribu-tions; earnings-related contributions for self-employed

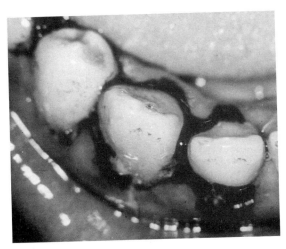

Fig. 3 Bleeding from the tooth sockets in the lower jaw in a boy bitten by a saw-scaled viper (*Echis ocellatus*) in Nigeria.

earners with earnings above a certain level, in addition to weekly flat-rate contributions; voluntary contributions for people who would otherwise be unable to qualify for basic pension and some other benefits; winding up of the previous state graduated pension scheme; recognition of occupational pension schemes for purpose of exemption from the reserve pension scheme; preservation of occupational pension rights on change of employment; an independent Occupational Pensions Board to administer the new arrangements affecting occupational pension schemes; a reserve pension scheme managed by an independent board to provide earning-related pensions for employees not covered by recognized occupational schemes.

The 1975 Act consolidated for England, Wales, and Scotland as much of the 1973 Act as established a basic scheme of contributions and benefits, together with the National Insurance (Industrial Injuries) Acts 1965 to 1974 and other enactments relating to social security.

SOCIAL WORK AND MEDICINE
Introduction
Social work became an established profession in the 20th century in many countries, but this article refers mainly to the UK. Most social workers are employed in agencies which may be statutory (e.g. Local Authority Social Services Departments (SSDs) or the Probation Services in England and Wales, in Scotland the Social Work Departments, and in Northern Ireland the Social Services and Probation Board) or voluntary (e.g. national or local charities). In every situation, their objectives are to help alleviate problems of psychosocial adjustment and to enhance the social functioning of individuals, groups, families, and communities. Often they will do this within a framework explicitly set by the law; frequently, the agency will have its own objectives, policies, and preferred ways of working; always, the actions of the social workers will be shaped by their professional education and training, the broad outlines of which are determined by the Central Council for Education and Training in Social Work (CCETSW). This central government body confers its own Diploma in Social Work in addition to the Master's or Bachelor's degree in social work or equivalent qualification which successful students may obtain from the university or comparable higher education institution in which they study.

The education of social workers and probation officers invariably includes a combination of theory and supervised practical experience. The theoretical background will include a knowledge of relevant aspects of *psychology, *sociology, social policy, the law, social work theory, and professional values. At the professional qualifying level, practical experience will be with a variety of client groups, but social work is increasingly developing training of a more specialized nature at postqualifying level.

Social work comes into relationship with medicine in many different ways. We may distinguish between social work in primary health care (more or less the equivalent of community care) and that in secondary (i.e. hospital) settings, social work with patients with predominantly somatic disorders and those with predominantly psychological disorders, and social work with patients with acute problems and those with chronically disabling conditions or handicap.

Social work in primary health care
Virtually everyone will consult a *general practitioner at some time in their life—some people, particularly at some stages, will consult frequently. But only a proportion of the population will ever be clients of a social worker. Among these, however, many have significant medical problems. Research over the past 25 years has demonstrated from various viewpoints the tendency for those with psychosocial problems also to have a concentration of medical problems: population surveys in the community have found this to be true; studies of social workers' case-loads suggest that typically something of the order of 40 per cent of unselected cases in local authority SSDs, and perhaps 25 per cent of probation cases, will have significant medical problems; studies of social work referrals generally show that more cases arrive in social work agencies by referral from health services personnel, and are referred by social workers to health services, than cross any similar inter-agency boundary. Thus, members of the primary care health team and social workers starting from different standpoints will frequently find themselves contributing simultaneously to the care of the same client—and where such clients have multiple problems, not infrequently they will be felt by all the professionals involved to be among the more demanding of their cases.

Such overlapping responsibilities suggest a need for collaboration. The extent of such collaboration informally in contemporary practice is unknown; it is desirable that it should occur often, although from both the health and the social work sides individual practitioners occasionally complain that it is insufficient. Among the problems that may arise are: (1) the sense of trust among professionals of different disciplines; (2) the issue of the identity of the team leader; and (3) questions of confidentiality. Increasingly in the past decade such difficulties have been tackled by instituting formal *case conference* procedures. In some situations (e.g. proceedings in England and Wales under the Children Act 1989) these have become mandatory. In the 1970s there was a vogue for specific schemes to attach social workers to general practices, and a number of demonstration projects showed that this was an excellent way for social work to pick up relevant referrals and for doctors to become more sensitive to their patients' psychosocial needs; nevertheless, this organizational solution has not become widespread and most co-working remains informal.

At an abstract level, social work usually involves a

combination of interventions into the clients' social and psychological worlds; that is, problems of psychosocial adjustment can be tackled from either side. More concretely this requires, on the one hand, social care planning and either obtaining or providing social resources—money, accommodation, substitute family care, day care, and the like—and, on the other hand, some form of advice-giving, counselling, behaviour modification, or *psychotherapy. Any of this repertoire may contribute in appropriate fashion to any of the four main approaches taken by social work: *casework* (where the individual or family is dealt with 'case by case'), social *group work*, *residential* or *day-care*, or *community work* (where the target of intervention may be a local neighbourhood or larger social unit, or a particular client group such as alcohol or drug abusers, or sufferers from *HIV or *AIDS).

Medical social work

Although the term is not currently used, this type of work persists, chiefly in hospitals for predominantly somatic disorders. In 1896 the first hospital '*almoner'. was appointed at the *Royal Free Hospital, London, to assess patients' abilities to pay for their medical treatment. In the course of this work she, and the colleagues who began shortly thereafter to be employed in other hospitals, came into possession of a good deal of information concerning patients' psychosocial circumstances, and where problems emerged they attempted to respond to them. A Hospital Almoners Association, formed in 1905, began in 1907 to grant a diploma on the basis of 1 year's course at the London School of Social Science, plus 1 year of practical experience. This body became the Institute of Almoners in 1917, changed its title to the Institute of Medical Social Workers (IMSW) in 1963, and in 1970 was absorbed into the newly formed British Association of Social Workers (BASW). By the 1950s the Institute had become the largest professional training body for social work in Britain, and its Membership qualification (MIMSW) continued to be awarded until CCETSW came into being in 1971. Historically, therefore, medical social work played a major part in the formation of the larger social work profession and in establishing its educational basis.

Up to 1974, social workers in hospitals were employed by the *National Health Service; thereafter their employer became the local authority SSDs. Controversy surrounded this change, but in the event social workers in increasing numbers continued to function in hospitals, and most clinical teams in acute and long-stay wards will now have access to social work services. One study of medical social work characterized its tasks as shown in Table 1. Changes in the management and funding arrangements taking place in both the NHS and local government social services during the final decade of the 20th century will mean that the precise form of the relationship between the two will continue to call for debate and experimentation.

Table 1 The tasks of medical social work (after E. H. Law (1982), *Light on hospital social work: A major study in Manchester* Social Work Services, DHSS).

	Cases (%)
Financial advice	15
Relationship problems	19
Diagnostic reports	21
Adaptation to illness	23
General advice	25
Emotional and therapeutic support	42

Mental-health social work

Psychiatric social work began in Britain in the early 1920s, predominantly in the context of the child guidance movement (later to evolve into child and adolescent *psychiatry). The Association of Psychiatric Social Workers, formed in 1930, although never as large as the IMSW, also developed a parallel professional training and qualification (an associateship—the AAPSW). This organization was similarly absorbed into BASW and its qualification into that awarded by CCETSW.

From the beginning, psychiatric social workers strongly identified themselves with the notion of the multi-disciplinary clinical team. In child psychiatry the minimum team would be a psychiatrist, a psychiatric social worker and an educational psychologist: to characterize their respective tasks as lying with the children individually, their families, and their schools would be no more than partly true, since teamwork always involves some, often substantial, overlap of functions. Frequently, child psychiatry teams nowadays will include a wider variety of professionals—*speech therapists and remedial teachers among others. Administratively, child and adolescent psychiatry are provided through the NHS, while child guidance clinics, mainly administered through local education authorities, are diminishing in numbers. However, contributions from *psychiatry and psychology (and also from general practice and *paediatrics) are increasingly made to the work of children and families teams in local authority SSDs, where social workers have statutory responsibility for child protection in, for example, cases of child abuse.

Teamwork is also a typical feature of mental health practice of adults, both those with acute problems and the chronically mentally disabled, including the growing number of elderly and very elderly persons. Most NHS psychiatric teams will include at least a part-time social worker, and here the predominating ethos will be medical. But local authority SSDs also have mental health social workers and teams where the starting point for the assessment and management of mental health problems is their social aspects. Specific duties arise under the Mental Health Act 1983 (and corresponding legislation for Scotland and Northern Ireland) for specially trained approved social workers, who may, and generally do, make the application, where this is required, for the compulsory admission to hospital of a person suffering from mental disorder. Such an application has normally to be supported by two medical recommendations (in urgent circumstances, by one) and the conditions under which compulsory admission and continuing detention occur are strictly controlled by law.

Probation officers operating in the community or in hostels or prisons collaborate with forensic psychiatry services in work with mentally disordered offenders. This may involve the early detection of such persons and their diversion from the criminal justice system, reference to mental health issues in pre-sentence reports, or the supervision of offenders on probation orders. The possibility was introduced in 1948 of adding to such orders a concomitant condition of psychiatric treatment, naturally requiring the consent of both the offender and the psychiatrist, and this is retained in the Criminal Justice Act, 1991. Probation officers also supervise offenders on release from custodial sentences, including life sentences, which can involve ongoing support of psychiatric management in the community. The supervision of patients released under the Mental Health Acts from forensic psychiatric institutions, the special hospitals, and regional secure units, is a task also invariably demanding multidisciplinary teamwork.

The National Health Service and Community Care Act, 1990 codified a policy which had been developing over 2 decades; broadly, that the NHS should be chiefly responsible for the diagnosis and management of acute psychiatric disorders, but that community care for those with long-term disabilities arising from both mental illness and mental handicap should be increasingly the responsibility of social services departments. (The same is true of persons with physical disability.) Social workers would have a major role as care managers whose function is to assess need and to act as purchasers of the requisite services on behalf of their clients. Providers of such services might include the SSDs themselves, other statutory agencies such as the NHS, and organizations in the voluntary and private sectors; social workers in all these settings are responsible for the range of functions noted above.

Conclusion
The social dimension of all types of medical problems has been increasingly emphasized in recent decades. While social workers have no monopoly of the knowledge of, or control over, such factors, they certainly have a key part to play alongside colleagues in the health professions in making available a social or psychosocial contribution to diagnosis and management wherever this may be appropriate in the health field.

D. W. MILLARD
COLIN ROBERTS

Further reading
Barclay Report (1982). *Social workers; their roles and tasks.* National Institute of Social Work, London.
Butrym, Z. and Horder, J. (1983). *Health, doctors and social workers.* Routledge and Kegan Paul, London.
Harris, R. (1992). *Crime, criminal justice and the probation service.* Tavistock/Routledge, London.
Younghusband, E. (1978). *Social work in Britain: 1950–1975.* George Allen & Unwin, London.

SOCIETY OF APOTHECARIES. See APOTHECARIES; MEDICAL COLLEGES, ETC. OF THE UK; PHARMACY AND PHARMACISTS.

SOCIOLOGY IN RELATION TO MEDICINE
Introduction
Sociology is only one of several social sciences, most of which have been in existence a good deal longer than has sociology. Sociology seriously emerged as a distinct discipline only towards the end of the 19th century and at the beginning of the 20th, as a result mainly of the work of Saint-Simon, Comte, Marx, Durkheim, Spencer, and Weber. *Psychology, political science, and social *anthropology had all begun to develop their own elaborate methodological and theoretical traditions before sociology emerged, and modern sociological theory and methods retain clear and close links with these other social science disciplines. Despite the differences between these social sciences, all are concerned with one common subject matter, that of the explanation and understanding of human social behaviour. There are, to this day, no hard-and-fast lines between the social sciences. Sociology is distinctive as a discipline in that it gives particular emphasis and focus to human behaviour as conditioned by membership of social groups, cultures, and societies. But the different divisions of the social sciences are only relative, and research within any one may be vital to another: thus sociologists draw upon research in social psychology, political science, social anthropology, and even *economics to inform their understanding of their own areas of study; likewise other social sciences draw on sociological theory and research. Sociology itself has been subject to the same process of specialization as the other social sciences, with the development of specialist 'domains', of which medical sociology has been of particular importance in Britain. Other major domains are: sociology of education, urban sociology, social stratification, sociology of the family, sociology of crime and deviance, ethnic and race relations, and political sociology.

Sociology of medicine
The sociology of medicine is concerned with the application of sociological research methods and theories to both medicine as a social institution and to the nature, explanation, and significance of health, illness, and disease for individuals, groups, and societies. This means that the sociology of medicine includes the study of

beliefs and norms about health and illness, social factors which assist in or limit the attainment of health, or result in the diagnosis of illness and disease. Studies of the differential distribution of *mortality and *morbidity rates in relation to social conditions, health-care facilities, and resources are also part of the discipline (see ENVIRONMENT AND MEDICINE II). It also includes the study of the organizational, social policy, and professional context in which medicine and health services function, and the relationship between health occupations and the wider society. Four areas of study in the sociology of medicine are of particular note: social conditions and disease, health and illness beliefs and behaviour, relationships and interactions between patients and medical staff, and medical professions and the organization of health care.

Social conditions and disease
Some of the earliest studies of disease and the environment, carried out in the 19th century (e.g. *Chadwick, and Farr), identified the association between poor social conditions and disease. Such studies continue to be of particular importance in the sociology of medicine and provide important links with other studies of the causes of disease (see EPIDEMIOLOGY). They also provide evidence of the interrelationship between social conditions and other key factors which affect health and disease (see DEMOGRAPHY). Contemporary sociological studies of social conditions emphasize the importance of differential vulnerability, how different patterns of social factors affect different diseases, and how some societal structures adversely affect life-chances (see Townsend and Davidson 1988). Identification of the range of social factors in a person's past and present which render them vulnerable to, or protect them from, potentially adverse factors in their current environment and which are causally linked to disease and ill-health, is of particular importance. The extent to which different diseases (such as *rheumatoid arthritis and *depression) can be identified as responding directly to the same social factors or conditions is also important. There is evidence that *diabetes, *peptic ulcer, and myocardial infarction (*coronary thrombosis), for example, are over-represented among those having stressful and highly responsible occupations. Such sociological studies are becoming increasingly significant as part of the scientific endeavour to track down the multivariate causes of a wide range of diseases.

Health and illness, beliefs and behaviour
Sociological studies have demonstrated that certain aspects of the attitudes and behaviour of individuals and groups cannot be properly understood without reference to the culturally determined beliefs, values, and norms pertaining to conditions and behaviours. Hence the states and conditions which are 'normal' or 'pathological', or 'healthy' or 'ill', are partly culturally determined. The growing evidence of the importance of psychosocial factors in the disease process has added significance to the study of the sociological determinants of health and illness. Sociologists have emphasized the importance of distinguishing between disease, as a biomedical condition, and illness as the everyday perception and expression of a culturally recognized condition. From this perspective a wide range of sociological studies have been undertaken which have examined gender and ethnic differences, occupational, social class and social mobility variations, and, particularly, cross-cultural or societal differences in both the perception and the response to health and illness.

Relationships and interactions between patients and medical staff
Some sociologists have studied the interaction of individuals with other individuals and groups, from both the perspective of the roles and role expectations, and also from the structural and situational constraints on interaction. Both of these perspectives have been important in the study of the interactions and relationships between patients and medical staff (doctors, nurses, paramedics, ancillaries, etc.) for example, in tracing the process of becoming a patient. Other studies focus on the interactions and relationships between and within medical-staff groups. Many studies of this type have identified the degree of role conflict experienced by medical staff, in both their interactions with patients and with other staff. They have also frequently emphasized the difficulties experienced in differentiating between professional roles and values, and personal ones, and the tendency towards individualism and particularism as a means of resolving dilemmas and ethical issues.

Medical professions and the organization of health care
The sociological study of professions and organizations has been particularly important in respect of medicine and health care. Studies have concentrated on the characteristics of the medical profession in relation to other professions, and in particular to paramedical professions (especially nurses). Studies have examined both the essential elements of professions in terms of skills, knowledge, training, codes of conduct, etc., but also the elements concerning autonomy, control over work, and self-regulation. The organizational scale and complexity of hospitals and other health-care facilities have led to a wide range of studies of the organizational context within which medicine and health care operate. Studies have shown how behaviour in organizations depends on both an analysis of the formal structure of the organization (the way tasks are specified, the organizational rewards available, the way authority is structured, etc.) and of the way individuals or groups within it perform their organizational tasks, define such tasks, and behave in relation to other groups and the wider society. Studies of health-care systems, and particularly the current re-organization within the *National Health Service in the

UK, have identified how reorganization which reflects a managerial, cost-effective, and mechanistic orientation is likely to induce non-participative attitudes and behaviours in staff at the lower levels and service-delivery points of the organization.

Sociology and medical education

It is now some years since the bodies responsible for medical education in the UK recommended that the sociology of medicine should be included in the medical curriculum (*General Medical Council 1967: Royal Commission on Medical Education (the *Todd report) 1968). It became commonplace by the late 1970s for all medical students to undertake a course in the sociology of medicine as an integral part of their medical course. The importance of this component in medical education, although frequently questioned, was further endorsed in 1980 by the General Medical Council's Education Committee, which re-emphasized the importance of sociological teaching and recommended that the students should 'learn to assess and consider together the biological and sociological bases of human behaviour'. The education of nurses, particularly in degree courses, now also includes teaching of the sociology of medicine.

Sociological associations and journals

The British Sociological Association established a Medical Sociology Group in 1969, and since then medical sociology has grown in importance and continues to provide a significant contribution to the annual British Sociological Association Conferences. The *British Journal of Sociology* and the journal *Sociology*, contain regular articles on medical and health topics. There is a 'specialist' British journal on the sociology of medicine entitled *Sociology of Health and Illness–A Journal of Medical Sociology*. Both the *British Medical Journal* and the *British Journal of Psychiatry* frequently contain sociological articles. In 1982 a register of research and teaching entitled *Medical Sociology in Britain* was first published, and this is regularly up-dated and published by the British Sociological Association.

COLIN ROBERTS
D. W. MILLARD

Further reading

Armstrong, D. (1989). *Outline of sociology: as applied to medicine*. Wright, London.
Field, D. and Woodman, D. (1991). *Medical sociology in Britain*. British Sociological Association, Medical Sociology Group, London.
Freidson, E. (1988). *Profession of medicine: a study of the sociology of applied knowledge*. University of Chicago Press, Chicago.
Illich, I. (1990). *Limits to medicine: medical nemesis, the expropriation of health*. Penguin Books, London.
Patrick, D. and Scambler, G. (ed.) (1991). *Sociology as applied to medicine*. Baillière, London.
Townsend, P. and Davidson, N. (1988). *Inequalities in health: the Black report*. Penguin, Harmondsworth.
Tuckett, D. (ed.) (1976). *An introduction to medical sociology*. Tavistock Publications, London.

SODIUM (symbol Na, atomic number 11, relative atomic mass 22.990), is a soft, silvery, white, very reactive, metallic element which reacts violently with water forming *hydrogen gas and sodium hydroxide. Its compounds are widely distributed in nature, the commonest being common salt or sodium chloride (NaCl). Sodium has a fundamental role in physiology as the main extracellular *cation (cf. *potassium); *depolarization of excitable tissue is accompanied by an influx of Na$^+$ ions across the cell membranes.

SODIUM, SERUM. Normal range: 136–146 mmol/l of the blood serum. See also HYPERNATRAEMIA; HYPONATRAEMIA.

SODOMY is anal intercourse, particularly between males.

SOEMMERRING, SAMUEL THOMAS (1755–1830). German neuroanatomist. He described the crossing of the fibres of the *optic nerves in 1786 and published a classification of the *cranial nerves. He was one of the inventors of the electric telegraph.

SOFTENING is degeneration, particularly of brain tissue (encephalomalacia).

SOFT SORE is a synonym for *chancroid.

SOLIDISM was an early doctrine which referred all diseases to the state of, or to morbid changes in, the solid parts of the body.

SOMATOSTATIN is a polypeptide hormone (with 14 amino acids), secreted by the delta cells of the *islets of Langerhans and by cells in the *hypothalamus; it has an inhibitory effect on the release of several other hormones. These include *growth hormone (GH), *adrenocorticotrophic hormone (ACTH), and *thyroid stimulating hormone (TSH) from the anterior *pituitary; *gastrin; *secretin; *glucagon; *insulin; and *renin.

SORE. Any circumscribed area of skin or mucous membrane which is tender, injured, ulcerated, or in some other way diseased.

SOUND is a physiological sensation received by the ear, generated by a vibrating source with a frequency in the range 20–20 000 Hz (cycles per second) and transmitted as a longitudinal pressure wave motion through a material medium (e.g. air).

SOUTHWOOD SMITH, THOMAS (1788–1861). English Unitarian minister. He came under the influence of Jeremy Bentham, and became an ardent health reformer, working with Edwin *Chadwick. He made a report to the *Poor Law Commissioners in 1838 on the physical causes of sickness and mortality among the poor. These he had observed during epidemic fevers in Nottingham during 1837–38. He was a founder of the Epidemiological Society in 1850, previously having written a treatise called *Philosophy of health* in 1835. He was a member of the original *General Board of Health which evolved over the course of time into the *Ministry of Health in 1917.

SPA. A mineral-water resort or mineral spring (after Spa in Belgium). See MINERAL SPRINGS.

SPALLANZANI, LAZZARO (1729–99). Italian physiologist. His wide-ranging achievements have been underrated. He studied respiration and the circulation, distinguished between putrefaction and fermentation, disproved spontaneous generation, and established the digestive power of saliva and gastric juice. He undertook artificial insemination in dogs and proved that spermatozoa were essential for fertilization of the ovum.

SPANISH FLY. See CANTHARIDES.

SPASM. Sustained involuntary contraction of a muscle or group of muscles, or sustained constriction of a small vessel or other channel.

SPASTIC DIPLEGIA, or Little's disease, is the condition afflicting many patients loosely known as 'spastics' or as suffering from *cerebral palsy. It is impairment or paralysis of voluntary movement affecting both legs. The muscles involved exhibit increased resistance to passive movement (spasticity); this heightening of muscle tone tends to keep the legs extended and the feet in plantar flexion (pointing downwards). The legs tend to cross when the body is supported, and during walking (the 'scissors' gait). There are no sensory changes, the arms are relatively unaffected, and mental handicap is less common than in other forms of cerebral palsy. The condition is present from birth, or from soon afterwards, although the diagnosis may not become apparent for some time. There is a strong association with prematurity, and it is thought that perinatal *hypoxia plays an aetiological role. Spastic diplegia is becoming less common as a result of improvements in the management of premature babies.

SPASTICITY. Increased tone of skeletal muscle, with exaggeration of the *tendon jerks or reflexes.

SPECIALIST. See MEDICAL EDUCATION, POST-GRADUATE AND CONTINUING; MEDICAL PRACTICE.

SPECIALIST PRACTICE. See MEDICAL PRACTICE.

SPECTROPHOTOMETER. A *photometer for comparing at various wavelengths the light emission from two sources (or the light absorption of two substances).

SPECTROSCOPY is the observation and analysis of spectra.

SPECULUM. An instrument designed to assist the examination of body cavities and passages. Some specula include reflecting mirrors.

SPEECH is the utterance of vocal sounds codified into meaningful language.

SPEECH DISORDERS may be due to disturbances of articulation (anarthria, *dysarthria); of phonation (aphonia, *dysphonia); of language function (*aphasia, dysphasia); or to psychiatric illness. See LANGUAGE, COGNITION, AND HIGHER CEREBRAL FUNCTION.

SPEECH THERAPISTS are staff professionally trained in the application and use of special techniques aimed at improving language and speech function. See LANGUAGE, COGNITION, AND HIGHER CEREBRAL FUNCTION; PROFESSIONS ALLIED TO MEDICINE (IN THE UK).

SPENCE, SIR JAMES CALVERT (1892–1954). British paediatrician and pioneer of social paediatrics. In 1942 he became the first Nuffield professor of child health in the University of Durham (the second chair in this subject in the UK). His interests, which had earlier related to the scientific aspects of his discipline, such as *clinical trials (e.g. his report in 1933 to the *Medical Research Council on the effect of calciferol in *rickets), later turned towards the larger issues of child development, growth, nutrition, and health (the classic 1000-family survey began in 1947, following his 1939 analysis of the causes of infant mortality, and a smaller but important investigation of the health and nutrition of children between the ages of 1 and 5 years). Among his many other contributions was his widely emulated innovation of admitting mothers along with their sick children into single hospital rooms, eliminating the then considerable hazard of cross-infection and providing a kinder and more efficient, as well as a safer, environment for hospital care.

SPERM. *Semen: or *spermatozoon.

SPERMATOZOON. A male gamete or germ cell, the essential generative component of *semen.

SPHINCTER. A circular muscle guarding the orifice of an organ and controlling passage through it, e.g. the anal sphincter.

SPHINGOMYELIN is one of a group of phospholipids (see LIPIDS) found in membranes and in brain and nervous tissue.

SPHYGMOGRAPH. Any instrument for recording the arterial *pulse.

SPHYGMOGRAPHY is the recording of arterial *pulse waves.

SPHYGMOMANOMETRY is the measurement of arterial *blood pressure. See KOROTKOFF SOUNDS.

SPICA. A spiral, figure-of-eight bandage, so called because of its resemblance to an ear of barley, often applied to anatomical features of differing dimensions, such as the thumb and the hand. A hip spica is a complicated *plaster-of-paris cast used in immobilization of fractures near, or dislocation of, the *hip joint.

SPIDERS are arthropods of the class Arachnida, order Araneida, suborders Labidognatha (true spiders) and Orthognatha (tarantulas or bird spiders). Almost all spiders envenomate their prey, but very few are of medical importance in the sense of biting and envenomating man. Of these, the best known are members of the genus *Latrodectus* (including the *black widow spider) and the genus *Loxosceles* (brown spiders).

SPILSBURY, SIR BERNARD (HENRY) (1887–1947). British forensic pathologist. He showed in the notable *Crippen trial that the murder was due to hyoscine hydrobromide, and thereafter was continually in the public eye. Regarded by many as the doyen of his subject in the UK, he was a man of infinite patience in his search for evidence, which he sifted with an uncanny flair for 'the upper limits of reasonable inference'.

SPINA BIFIDA is a condition which results from defective development of the posterior wall of the spinal canal, that is the neural arches (see SPINE), and thus one or more vertebrae remain incomplete. The defect may be minor and symptomless, discovered only on X-ray (spina bifida occulta). In more serious cases there is herniation of the meninges through the opening (meningocele); the spinal cord itself may be involved (meningomyelocele), with varying degrees of neurological disorder, including total paralysis of the lower part of the body and incontinence. Sometimes an associated anomaly prevents normal circulation of *cerebrospinal fluid, causing *hydrocephalus, which may add mental handicap to the already formidable medical and social problems facing these babies if they survive. Spina bifida is a relatively common congenital abnormality (approximately 1 in 300 live births). There has been much controversy about its causation, particularly with regard to the relative importance of genetic and environmental factors but recent evidence strongly suggests that multivitamin supplementation of the diet during pregnancy may be important in prevention. Prenatal detection is possible in some cases by examination of the amniotic fluid (see ALPHAFETOPROTEIN; AMNIOCENTESIS; ANENCEPHALY).

SPINAL ANAESTHESIA is a variety of regional *anaesthesia in which a *local anaesthetic agent is injected into the *subarachnoid space round the *spinal cord.

SPINAL CARIES is tuberculous *osteitis of the vertebrae and intervertebral cartilages.

SPINAL CORD. That part of the *central nervous system contained within the spinal canal of the vertebral column (see SPINE). It is continuous above with the medulla oblongata of the brain, beginning at the level of the foramen magnum of the skull and extending down the canal as far as the first lumbar vertebra. It comprises a central core of grey matter (nerve cells) surrounded by an outer layer of white matter (myelinated nerve fibres). In this grey matter incoming sensory fibres (neurones) form connections (synapses) with the cell bodies of other neurones, some of which give rise to fibres which synapse in turn with anterior cells in the anterior horn of grey matter, from which motor fibres (lower motor neurones) arise and pass into the anterior roots. Other fibres carry sensation upwards in the columns of white matter to the brain. The posterior columns are concerned with fibres carrying fine touch, tactile discrimination, and position and joint sense, while the spinothalamic tracts of the lateral columns contain ascending fibres which have crossed the midline of the cord close to the central canal (which is continuous above with the fourth ventricle of the brain) and which carry the sensations of pain and temperature. There are also several descending pathways in the lateral columns, such as the corticospinal (pyramidal) tract, which carries messages from the brain to the anterior horn cells in order to initiate movement. Thirty-one pairs of spinal nerves arise from the cord (8 cervical, 12 thoracic, 5 lumbar, 5 sacral, and 1 coccygeal). These spinal nerves are formed by the union of posterior roots, which carry incoming sensory impulses from peripheral nerves into the spinal cord (via cell stations attached to these roots in each intervertebral foramen, called the posterior root ganglia), and anterior roots, which carry outwards from the cord impulses that pass down the motor nerves to supply the voluntary muscles (see NEUROMUSCULAR DISEASE). The cord is surrounded by three protective membranes or *meninges, the innermost pia mater, the arachnoid, and the outermost dura mater.

SPINAL DYSRAPHISM is a *neural-tube defect related to spina bifida.

SPINAL FUSION is surgical *ankylosis of one or more vertebral joints of the *spine.

SPINAL TUMOUR. A variety of neoplasms may arise either within the spinal cord itself (the commonest being *astrocytoma and *ependymoma) or outside the cord but within the spinal canal (most commonly *neurofibroma and *meningioma). Tumours arising outside the canal, for example in the vertebral bodies, may invade or compress the cord and its roots; these are usually metastatic (from the breast, lung, prostate, kidney, etc.).

SPINA VENTOSA is *tuberculous dactylitis (inflammation of the digits) occurring in infants and young children and affecting one or more fingers and toes. It causes a hard, red, spindle-shaped swelling of the digit, usually with *abscess formation. Permanent deformity may result.

SPINE. The spinal or vertebral column, or backbone, is the distinguishing characteristic of vertebrates. It may be described as a jointed hollow rod enclosing the *spinal cord. In man, the spine consists of 33 vertebrae (7 cervical, 12 thoracic, 5 lumbar, 5 sacral, and 4 coccygeal), the upper 24 of which form separate bones with flexible joints occupied by the intervertebral *discs. Each *vertebra consists of a main weight-bearing rounded body, from the back of which projects a neural arch forming part of the spinal canal containing the *spinal cord. The neural arch has three projections, right and left transverse processes and a posterior spinous process, which serve as points of attachment for muscles.

SPIRITS, in the medical context, usually implies a solution in *ethanol (ethyl alcohol): alternatively, it means any liquid obtained by distillation.

SPIROCHAETES (SPIROCHETES) are spiral *bacteria. Spirochaetales is one of the 10 orders of the class Schizomycetes (bacteria); it has two families (Spirochaetaceae and Treponemataceae), each subdivided into three genera and many species. The term 'spirochaete' therefore applies to many different bacteria and most are of no medical importance. Those that are include the agents of *syphilis, *yaws, *bejel (non-venereal childhood syphilis), *pinta (a skin disease of tropical South America), *relapsing fever, *rat-bite fever, and the various forms of *leptospirosis.

SPIROMETER. An instrument for measuring the volume of air taken in and out by the lungs during breathing.

SPLEEN. A large unpaired organ situated in the left upper part of the abdominal cavity between the stomach and the left kidney, behind the left lower ribs and underneath the left hemidiaphragm. It is purple and pliable, oblong and about 125 mm along its long axis. It is rarely palpable in health, but readily becomes so in several pathological conditions leading to an increase in size (splenomegaly) and a firmer consistency. It has a fibrous structure occupied by blood and lymphoid tissue. The spleen has several functions: in fetal life and in the newborn it is a site of red blood cell formation, a function to which it can revert in later life under certain conditions; it acts as a reservoir of blood; it sequesters and destroys ageing or imperfect red blood cells; it is part of the immunological system, producing *antibodies, *plasma cells, and *lymphocytes; it is also part of the *reticulo-endothelial system. None of these functions, however, is vital or unique, and surgical removal of the spleen (occasionally necessary, e.g. after abdominal trauma) does not usually produce obvious ill-effects in adults. Removal is also needed in some blood diseases (see HAEMATOLOGY).

SPLENOMEGALY is enlargement of the *spleen.

SPLINT. Any device for immobilizing part of the body.

SPONDYLITIS is inflammation of the vertebrae. See also ANKYLOSING SPONDYLITIS.

SPONDYLOSIS is any non-inflammatory (e.g. degenerative) disorder of the spine.

SPONGIFORM ENCEPHALOPATHY is a term descriptive of the pathological appearance of the brain in certain putative *slow virus or, more correctly, *prion infection of the central nervous system, such as *kuru, *scrapie, and *Creutzfeldt–Jakob disease.

SPORE. A resting or dormant form assumed by certain bacteria (e.g. species of *Clostridium) in which they are able to survive a wide variety of environmental changes.

SPOROTRICHOSIS. A mycosis due to the fungus *Sporothrix schenckii*, commonly found as a mould on vegetation and wood. The infection is a chronic *granulomatous process usually limited to the skin and regional *lymphatics, but like other mycoses it may become disseminated under certain conditions, notably during *immunosuppression from any cause. A rare pulmonary form may follow inhalation of spores. Sporotrichosis occurs most frequently in Central and South America.

SPORT. An unusual variant appearing as a result of *genetic mutation.

SPORT AND MEDICINE. Sport, being essentially both physical and competitive, makes physical and mental demands on the participant which he or she may or may not be able to sustain. Medical interest in sport derives from the consequences of such, and the practice of sports medicine has become one of the growth areas in medicine in the latter part of the 20th century. Sport now plays an essential part in the lives of many individuals, to say nothing of the community in general and the country as a whole. The interest aroused by, for example, the Olympic Games and each country's tally of medals is well known.

Sports medicine

Over the years the notion of sports medicine as a specific specialty within medicine has gained a measure of support, but it must be regarded as suspect. Sports medicine is better considered as the application of the various specialties of medicine and their basic sciences to the preparation for, and consequences of, participation in sport. Thus sports *cardiology of necessity demands a thorough grounding in cardiology as a whole before the practitioner can practise it in the sporting context. The term 'sports physician' as an indication of some sort of *specialist is, therefore, probably misleading, while the term 'consultant in sports medicine' is even more so, in so far as it is humanly impossible to achieve a consultant level of expertise throughout the whole of medicine as would be needed before such a designation could be justified.

Sports medicine is, therefore, best regarded as a *specialism* and as such exhibits a number of specific components. These have been simply described as: (1) man (or woman) as an athlete; (2) the athlete as a man (or woman); (3) the athlete as a patient; and (4) the patient as an athlete.

Man (or woman) as an athlete

Man (or woman) as an athlete relates essentially to the human biology of sport, embracing at the same time a number of important scientific disciplines. The ability of an individual to cope with a physically very demanding programme of training and competition depends on many factors. Although attempts have been made to formulate the work demands of certain types of activity, such formulae remain essentially paradigms rather than directly applicable instructions. The basic characteristics that determine physical performance, particularly those that can be modified, are, however, relatively easy to define. The scientific fields covering them, include applied *physiology, *psychology, *anatomy, biomechanics (mechanics of movement in living creatures), kinesiology (the scientific study of human movement relating mechanics to an athlete), and biochemistry.

Essential components of physical fitness can be considered in two groups, one general and the other specific. General components are common to all activities and involve physiological (for example, cardiovascular fitness) and psychological health. Specific components are those of speed, strength, local endurance, skill, and flexibility, all of which relate in a very particular way to the specific activity in question (while yet relating in a general way to activity as a whole). Physical capacity, and indeed mental capacity, may be improved by the process of training. This is the deliberate manipulation of human biology to modify the resting state to that which permits the highest level of activity with a minimum of physical and psychological disturbance. In general, the body's response to activity is two-stage.

Immediate, or primary, physiological changes are directed towards returning the body to the status quo before exercise and these responses are fast, an example being the increase in pulse rate that follows exercise, which then returns to the resting rate when the activity is over and recovery complete.

Secondary changes resulting from training involve a process of adaptation which alters the pre-exercise resting state so as to diminish the need for so great a primary response. Continuing the cardiovascular example, this is represented by the physiological dilatation of the heart, which increases the stroke volume to enable a lower pulse rate to be required for a given cardiac output. This consequently admits a higher minute volume at maximum pulse rate.

This first major area of sports medicine studies the physical and psychological components of training that allow the human sports person to engage in feats of skill, strength, and endurance way beyond those of which the ordinary untrained human is capable.

The athlete as a man (or woman)

Sport is typically an activity of the second and third decades, and it is within these decades that most problems arise. Nevertheless participants' ages vary widely. Children are now being taught to swim before they can run and the foundations of competitive careers in sport may be laid among 6- to 8-year-olds. This gives rise to problems, particularly in relation to overuse and stress effects which do not form part of normal *paediatric practice. By the same token, continued participation in sport by veterans is becoming more popular, and indeed many individuals take up physical activity of a sporting type such as jogging and long distance running for the first time in the latter part of their lives. The ambivalent relationship of physical activity to maturity is manifested on the one hand by the apparent benefits of long-term exercise in prevention of cardiac disease, and on the other by the effects of degenerative change on the locomotor system, while the unwillingness of some sportsmen and to women to accept the consequences of advancing age is well known.

Differences in gender introduce important problems. Fundamental differences between men and women are hardly to be denied, but peculiarly the definition of femininity does not rest absolutely on any single biological parameter. From a sporting point of view this produces difficulties in gender determination in areas where biologically there is an established difference between male and female performance.

In recent years the role of women in sport has undergone dramatic change, in part as a result of sympathetic understanding in re-evaluation of women's physical capacity, but there still remain, and will remain in many sports, significantly higher levels of performance to be achieved by men than by women, simply because the sports in question have been designed to emphasize and reward specifically masculine characteristics. It is true that there are many sports in which men and women can complete on equal terms, and in fact do so today, but there are others in which they cannot, and feminists do themselves no justice by arguing that they can. The day when the lady's champion at Wimbledon is able to challenge the men's is so far away as to be virtually unimaginable.

Female athletes face additional problems in the biological consequences to their sports capacity of their primary and secondary sexual characteristics. The phenomena of menstruation themselves have a significant effect on the performance capacity of the female athlete, and problems may occur. The increased femoral obliquity in women is a factor in the development of chondromalacia patellae (anterior knee pain syndromes). Although women with markedly oblique femora do not normally achieve the highest levels in competitive sport, they are found among the fun runners and joggers in mass marathons, and can be a rich source of 'clinical material'.

Apart from such obvious influences on athletic activity as age and gender, the specific environment in which the athlete competes is also highly significant. Modification of physiological response due to variation in climate is well recognized and factors such as temperature, humidity, and altitude are all important. These environmental factors may influence athletic activity either advantageously or disadvantageously, and a proper understanding of these factors and the methods by which the disadvantages can be offset, is an essential component of the scientific preparation of sportsmen. Other environmental factors of significance include sportswear, clothing, and sports footwear, much of which may be unsuitable for the activity in question. The scientific design and selection of suitable equipment as implements for sports (for example tennis, squash, and badminton) is also an area of significance. Sportsmen may be hampered in their performance and, perhaps more importantly, put at risk by the use of unsuitable sportswear or equipment.

Much interest is shown in diet for sport, although in recent years considerable confusion has arisen. As an example, the method of 'glycogen loading' by the so-called Åstrand diet has been due to a misunderstanding of the nature of the original experiment—in fact glycogen loading does not require starvation. The scientific and accurate application of principles of *dietetics to sport keeps the sports person healthy and able to achieve.

In addition to the use of normal food substances, much attention continues to be paid to the artificial modification of performance by alien materials, or natural materials in alien doses. The practice of doping still plagues sport, particularly at the highest levels, and some sports are indeed notorious in this respect. Doping control seeks, on the one hand, to define what is and is not permissible in terms of the use of medication, and, on the other, to monitor participants in sport to make certain that dangerous and forbidden substances are not used. The object of sport is in effect to establish a controlled clinical trial. The object of dope control is to keep the effects of drugs in the controlled element of the experiment and not to admit them as variables. So much is this the case that dope control has become a growth industry in support of sport from the Olympic Games downwards, and many sophisticated tests have evolved to trap the athlete who resorts to the use of drugs in attempts to improve performance artificially.

The athlete as a patient

The third element of sports medicine covers the athlete as a patient and embraces three major fields: sports traumatology, internal medicine, and sports psychiatry.

Sports traumatology

Inevitably, perhaps, when people think of sports medicine they think of injuries, largely because many are dramatic, frequently affecting well-known and important sports personalities. By providing an immediate interruption of sporting activity, with inevitable subsequent disability, injuries create a demand for instant action. Many that occur in sport are no different from those that occur in other activities. When the mechanism of injury is the same, the type of tissue damage that follows is also the same. The severity may be different since the effects of injury on exercising tissue (with a high blood perfusion rate) will be more dramatic, with, for example, much more extensive *haematoma formation than would occur in the sedentary individual.

Most injuries in sport are instantaneous, that is to say they occur as a result of a sudden immediate stress to the body. These are most common in body-contact sports or vehicular sports, where the forces are applied from outside the body and are relatively large. Some of these injuries are direct, due to the application of violence to the immediately damaged area, (for example, a fractured tibia as a result of a kick from a horse), while others are indirect, occurring at a site other than that at which the external force is applied. An example of the latter is O'Donaghue's triad in the knee in a patient whose injury is due to trapping of the foot. It is useful to classify injury by *aetiology since this gives a guideline to the mechanism of tissue damage, and hence is of assistance in considering management.

It is the *mechanism* that matters rather than the activity in which the mechanism is found, so to talk of 'football injuries' or 'athletic injuries' is not teleologically sound. Sport is peculiar in the extent to which self-inflicted or intrinsic injuries occur. These do not involve external forces or outside agents but occur as a result of excessive force generation within the body. They are often due to incoordination and are an exhibition of inadequate skill.

By contrast, other intrinsic injuries common in sport (sometimes referred to as 'technopathies' or 'athlopathies') are the overuse injuries, due to the repeated application of stresses to a part of the body, not allowing time for recovery from the effects of each episode of stress or exercise. Injuries in this group are essentially *inflammatory in soft tissue, with oedematous reactions in the acute phase and chronic *fibrosis and scarring in the chronic. The overactivity may occur either at a time when the individual is taking up exercise *ab initio* or as a result of a drastic change in the training programme which, while not overloading the body as a whole, has the effect of overloading one particular part or system.

Patterns of injury in sport are readily established and make it possible to identify significant problems which can be tackled by appropriate preventive means. The management of injury in sport, as elsewhere, involves both prevention and treatment, the former demanding an understanding of the relationship of the injury to the mechanism of activity involved in training and competition. Unfortunately, one difficulty with preventive measures is that they may, of themselves, denature the sport—a classic example is *boxing.

Many sports carry risks that, in some sections of the population, are regarded as unacceptable. This presents a real moral problem and some may see abolition as the solution. In most instances, however, a high measure of safety may be achieved by proper drafting and administration of the rules of the game or sport. The concept of prevention by regulation of the manner in which a sport is conducted is readily accepted, and the laws of most sports, particularly the most vigorous, contain specific regulations to control violence. It is a sad fact that in some areas these rules are flouted, and even governing bodies themselves seem unwilling collectively to take concrete appropriate steps (e.g. extended disqualification), particularly in those sports which depend for their existence on input from paying spectators.

In fact, most sports are safe and injury does not occur if the rules are followed, if the participant is properly fit for the activity (including having a sufficiently well-developed level of skill), is properly clothed and shod, uses the right type of equipment, and, finally, uses a little common sense.

The treatment of injury in sport logically follows accurate diagnosis along clearly defined and well-tried lines. Sportsmen and -women as a whole, however, tend to differ from the population at large in that many are impatient of delay and require to return to sporting activity as soon as possible. Management of injury, therefore, involves selection of those methods that offer the most rapid recovery, not those that require the least effort on the part of the sportsman's medical advisers. Unqualified advice to rest, for example, is often given in cases of the average sports injury and is too often an indication of the physician's ignorance or lack of interest. Even when the injury manifestly precludes further immediate training, much can be done to preserve morale and general fitness by the development of an appropriate programme of activity involving other parts of the body.

As a result of pressures for early return to sport, plus the effects of excessive training in the form of overuse injuries, new methods of treatment of sports injuries have evolved of necessity, based on concepts of *pathology which appear valid, and these have been dramatically successful in returning patients safely and effectively to activity at an early stage. A useful spin-off is that these methods can also be applied in a work situation, to enable workers to get back to their own jobs more quickly.

The majority of injuries in sport are relatively minor, but 10 per cent are sufficiently severe to cause time off work, while a few cause very severe disabilities. There is no justification for treating sports injuries lightly, any more than any other sort of injury. Early and effective treatment, even at the simplest levels, will dramatically reduce morbidity and the associated economic costs. Many injuries, particularly the more severe ones, may be treated along generally accepted and proven lines, provided that medical attendants recognize that return to normal function at the earliest possible moment is the object, particularly in patients who are professional sportsmen or women.

Finally it must be accepted at all levels that there is a small but well-defined group of patients where problems are associated with sport and sport alone, and require a specific expertise and knowledge for their proper management. Unless and until the teaching of such management (in for example, overuse injury) becomes a regular part of *orthopaedic training (to say nothing of other medical and paramedical training), athletes will suffer unnecessarily and at the same time fringe 'specialists' will flourish. There can be no substitute whatsoever for appropriate specialist knowledge and experience in the treatment of injured or diseased sportsmen and women.

Internal medicine

General medical problems in sport are not uncommon, and previously held views that many diseases were incompatible with sporting activity have had to be revised. Physical activity is possible even at a very high level, provided that the nature of the disease is clearly understood and its effects are properly offset. Patients particularly at risk should be identified and channelled into appropriate and less dangerous areas of activity.

Sports psychiatry

Psychological disorders occur in athletes and sportsmen and women as much as in the population as a whole. It is true that supreme athletic prowess is unlikely to be found except in a psychologically well-balanced individual, but in sport in general a wide variety of personality types is to be found and personality disorder may manifest itself in problems relating to sporting activity. Some athletes may present bizarre motor disorders which are finally revealed to be hysterical or to relate consciously or subconsciously to attempts at secondary gain, while *psychopaths may find their release in sporting activity, often to the disadvantage of other players. Sporting activity, particularly at a high level, induces intense stresses, which often bring to the surface latent psychological as well as physical disorders. The young athlete is particularly vulnerable to severe pressure from parents and coach.

The patient as an athlete

The final area in which medicine and sport impinge, embraces two fields, the use of sport as therapy and sport for the disabled.

Sport may be extremely valuable as therapy, since it may be programmed to provide controlled exercise in what should be a pleasant and mentally stimulating context. As a rule it should be prescribed only for individuals who are normally genuinely physically active and who are interested in physical recreation. The evolution of sports therapy was extended by the encouragement of sport for the disabled in its own right by Sir Ludwig *Guttmann, who devised the programme of sports for paraplegics which led to the Stoke Mandeville Games and later to the Paralympics.

The general principle underlying sport for the disabled is straightforward. It involves a selection of recreational physical activities within the capacity of the disabled individual, the practice of which will not further prejudice or put at risk the health of the participant. The ideal object is the integration of the disabled individual with the able-bodied in the same sporting environment. Quite apart from the immediate pleasure and satisfaction gained, this leads to reintegration of the participant into society as a whole. Unfortunately, disabled people frequently find themselves isolated from the mainstream of society, and sports for the disabled, where disabled persons are segregated, have a similar negative effect.

Sport is now playing an established and increasing part in the social and economic life of every community. Whatever personal attitudes to sport may be, it is here to stay and has an significant influence in human life. It throws up its own problems, which present a variety of interfaces with medicine. Hitherto these interfaces have often been neglected. Happily they are now attracting an informed and responsible attention within the general umbrella of sports medicine.

This is a specialism involving the application of skills, knowledge, and experience in different fields of clinical medicine and related applied sciences to the problems engendered by sporting activity. It is full of challenge and interest, and offers opportunity to push back the frontiers of knowledge in the study of high-performance human beings.

J. G. P. WILLIAMS

Further reading
Bloomfield, J., Fricker, P. A., and Fitch, K. D. (1992). *Textbook of science and medicine in sport*. Blackwell Scientific Publications, Oxford.
Ryan, A.J. and Allman, F. L. (1989). *Sports medicine* (2nd edn). Academic Press, San Diego.
Williams, J. G. P. (1990). *A colour atlas of injury in sport* (2nd edn). Wolfe Medical, London.
Williams, J. G. P. and Sperryn, P. N. (1976). *Sports medicine*, (2nd edn). Edward Arnold, London.

Journals of interest
American Journal of Sports Medicine. (105 Physicians Building, Columbus, Georgia 31901, USA.)
British Journal of Sports Medicine. (Butterworth-Heinemann Ltd, 59/60 Grosvenor Street, London WIX 9DA, UK).
Journal of Sports Medicine and Physical Fitness. (Corso Bramante 83–5, 10126 Torino, Italy).
Medicine and Science in Sports. (1440 Monroe Street, Madison, Wisconsin 53706, USA.)
Sports Medicine. (Suite B-30, Oxford Court Business Centre, 582 Middletown Boulevard, Langhorne, PA 19047, USA.)
The Physician and Sportsmedicine. (4530 West 77th Street, Minneapolis 55435, USA.)

SPOT. See MACULA; TACHE.

SPRAIN. A joint injury which results in partial rupture of one or more supporting *ligaments.

SPRUE is adult *coeliac disease, or *gluten-sensitive enteropathy. A condition with similar features of intestinal malabsorption called tropical sprue occurs in some tropical regions; its cause is uncertain but it is not due to gluten sensitivity and it responds to treatment with vitamin supplements and antibiotics.

SPUTUM is matter ejected from the respiratory tract, the product of coughing or hawking. Expectoration of sputum indicates inflammation of the lungs, bronchi, or trachea. The material varies in colour, consistency, and volume according to the nature of the underlying infection, but is basically a mixture of *pus and *mucus. Microbiological and cytological studies can help in diagnosis.

SQUINT. Faulty alignment of the visual axis of one eye, also known as strabismus. Squint is described as convergent, divergent, or vertical, according to whether the squinting eye is deviated inwards, outwards, or either upwards or downwards. Most squints are congenital, and due to faulty insertion of the eye muscles; the visual axes then move together and the squint is therefore called 'concomitant'; the degree of squint remains constant whatever the direction of gaze. But where squinting is due to damage to one of the nerves supplying the eye muscles, the squint varies with the position of the eyes and is termed 'nonconcomitant' or paralytic; this variety is usually accompanied by double vision (diplopia). See also OPHTHALMOLOGY.

STACPOOLE, HENRY DE VERE (1863–1951). Irish physician and novelist. Stacpoole trained in London, but practised only briefly before devoting himself to authorship. He wrote many novels, of which the best-known is *The blue lagoon* (1908), which was reprinted 23 times in 12 years.

STAGING OF DISEASE refers to the classification of *malignant disease according to the anatomical extent of the primary *neoplasm, of involved regional *lymph nodes, and of *metastases. Accurate staging before the initiation of treatment is important for several reasons: it allows prognosis to be estimated; it determines the programme of treatment most likely to be effective; it provides a reference point by which the efficacy of treatment can subsequently be measured; and it allows comparison of different treatment regimens and of the same regimen at different times and in different medical centres. Staging usually requires not only careful clinical examination but a range of ancillary investigations which may include *laparotomy or *laparoscopy. It is of obvious advantage if staging criteria can be internationally agreed; for *Hodgkin's disease, for example, this was achieved at the Ann Arbor Conference of 1971.

STAHL, GEORGE ERNST (1660–1743). German physician. He denied that the body was governed by physicochemical laws, holding that the soul or 'anima' presided over all bodily activities and that when it departed death and putrefaction resulted. Interested in chemistry, he believed that something he called '*phlogiston' was given up when combustion took place. This hypothesis was widely accepted and delayed the advance of chemistry for half a century.

STAINS AND STAINING METHODS. See MICROBIOLOGY; PATHOLOGY.

STALLARD, HYLA BRISTOW (1901–73). English eye surgeon. He had a distinguished career as practitioner, writer, editor, and athlete. He represented England in athletics (1921–27), Great Britain in the Olympic Games of 1924, and the British Empire against the USA in 1924.

STAMMERING, in English usage, is synonymous with stuttering, a common speech disorder occurring in about 1 per cent of children of school age, much more often in males. It may be a temporary condition associated with anxiety during early childhood but sometimes persists in a chronic form into adult life. It consists of either an explosive repetition of the initial letter of a word before the word is finally achieved or of a total blocking of speech followed by a rush of words; the two may occur together, and are often combined with a compulsion to finish a word once embarked upon. There is no clear agreement about causation; probably psychological and physical factors are both involved, but in any event psychological problems for the sufferer from established stammering can be severe.

STANDARDIZATION is the formulation and observance of standards in respect of quality, potency, ingredients, method of preparation, etc. of biological and pharmaceutical substances.

STANDARDIZED MORTALITY RATIO. The ratio of observed to expected deaths in a subpopulation (e.g. cigarette smokers) multiplied by 100, the expected deaths being calculated as the sum of the expected deaths in each age-group on the basis of the overall population mortality for that age-group. Sometimes abbreviated to SMR. See also EPIDEMIOLOGY.

STAPEDECTOMY is surgical excision of the *stapes, a method of treating deafness due to *otosclerosis. The stapes is replaced with a small plastic rod, restoring mobility to the system.

STAPES. The innermost of the chain of three tiny bones (auditory ossicles) which transmit sound vibrations from the *tympanic membrane across the *middle ear cavity to the inner ear.

***STAPHYLOCOCCUS*.** Spherical, Gram-positive bacteria with a tendency to grow in clusters resembling bunches of grapes. They are widely distributed in the environment and are often present on the skin and in the nasal cavity of healthy subjects. They vary in their capacity to produce infection; most that do so belong to a species called *Staphylococcus aureus* (or *S. pyogenes*). Staphylococci are responsible for many types of superficial infection, particularly those in which *pus formation is a feature (*boils, *carbuncles, *impetigo, etc.). They also cause many more serious deep infections, including *septicaemia, *osteomyelitis, *enteritis, *pneumonia, and *abcesses in almost any part of the body. Certain strains elaborate an *enterotoxin which produces *food poisoning. Many staphylococci have acquired resistance to particular antibiotics and are therefore especially dangerous; this is often the case in nosocomial (hospital-acquired) infections.

STAPHYLOCOCCUS AUREUS is an important *pathogen responsible for many *pyogenic infections. See *STAPHYLOCOCCUS*.

STARCH is the principal storage form of *carbohydrate in plants (cf. *glycogen in animals). Starch is an insoluble mixture of two *polysaccharides, amylose and amylopectin.

STARLING, ERNEST HENRY (1866–1927). British physiologist. He worked in close association with Sir William *Bayliss on the discovery of *secretin (1902). He enunciated his 'law of the heart' which stated that the energy of contraction is a function of the length of the muscle fibres. He was the author of the standard textbook *The principles of human physiology* (1912).

STARVATION. In total starvation, the energy expenditure necessary for existence leads to progressive consumption of the body's energy reserves: when *carbohydrate and *fat are exhausted, then *protein must be consumed. The duration of survival in total food deprivation is variable, but averages between 4 and 6 weeks, at which time body weight has been about halved. See FAT; ENERGY REQUIREMENTS; HUNGER STRIKE; KWASHIORKOR; MARASMUS; NUTRITION.

STATISTICS
The role of statistics in medical research
In everyday use the term 'statistics' is often used as a synonym for numerical information of any sort, and the common misuse of such information has given statistics a bad name. The term is most usefully applied to numerical summaries of information (called data) from groups of individuals—medical examples are the infant *mortality rate, the prevalence of high blood pressure (*hypertension) in an age-group, or the average serum *cholesterol level among adult males in the UK. In medical research statistics is also the name given to the methodology used to decide how best to collect data (called research 'design') and the techniques that are applied to analyse and interpret research data. Statistical methods also underlie other areas of medicine to varying degrees, including *diagnosis and decision-making in general (for example, genetic counselling), interpretation of laboratory results, quality control, and *audit. In essence, statistical methods are relevant to any medical activity that involves numerical information, from fetal ultrasound scans to forensic studies. Statistics are particularly important in the study of causes of disease (*epidemiology), the evaluation of new treatments or technologies, studies of diagnostic ability, and studies to evaluate individual patient prognosis. Medical statistics as now practised is a recent discipline, and is still evolving. The modern era can probably be dated from the publication in the *Lancet* of a series of expository articles by Austin Bradford-Hill in 1937, still in print in book form (Hill and Hill 1991).

If one key idea underlies all medical research, it is that we make observations on a sample of individuals and use them to make inferences about the population of interest. The term 'population' here does not mean the general population but a specific group of people. In medical research the population is often patients with a particular disease, such as *epilepsy or *diabetes. The validity of any inferences based on a sample of patients with a disease relies upon the sample being representative of all patients with the disease. Systematic lack of representativeness is one form of *bias*, which is the main impediment to valid research. For example, a study of diabetic patients attending a hospital diabetes clinic may not be relevant to all patients with the same disease because they are a highly selected subgroup. Bias can also arise from a representative sample if observations are not obtained from some individuals: patients who do not agree to participate in a study or who do not complete their treatment often have characteristics different from those who do comply. In a study comparing two or more groups it is desirable also to try to avoid systematic differences between the characteristics of the patients in the different groups, as these might bias the comparison.

Design of research
Medical research may be passive, in which patients are simply observed, or active, in which therapies or other interventions are evaluated. The choice of research design depends upon circumstances and sometimes also on ethical considerations. The relative strengths of different types of study design can be assessed largely in relation to the potential for avoiding bias. The most reliable research results come from controlled trials, often called *clinical trials.

Controlled trials are comparative studies of different ways of treating patients with some condition or disease. It is important that the groups of patients receiving each treatment differ only in the nature of their treatment; otherwise the comparison would not be a fair one. The key feature of the controlled trial is that each patient's treatment should be chosen at random, eliminating bias. ('Random' is a technical term meaning that all patients have the same chance of getting each of the treatments—it is equivalent to tossing a coin, although more sophisticated procedures are used.) The ethical basis for this approach is that the trial is being carried out because doctors do not know which treatment is better.

Many controlled trials compare a new treatment with the current best treatment; for convenience these are called the treatment group and control group, although often all patients are in fact treated. When there is no standard treatment for a condition it is usual to give an inert treatment, or placebo, to the control group, although this is not always possible. Ideally, neither the doctor nor the patient should know which treatment is being given, so that neither is biased by this knowledge—this is then a 'double blind' trial. *Placebos and double blindness are usually feasible in drug trials, but their use may not be possible for other treatments, notably in surgery. Controlled trials are also used to assess measures for preventing disease, such as *health education or screening of apparently healthy people for early signs of life-threatening disease, some cancers for example.

Despite the clear superiority of randomized trials as the appropriate way to evaluate treatments, many studies are carried out with controls selected in a non-random way or without any controls. The results of such studies are much less reliable. It is essential that treatment and control groups are studied at the same time to isolate the effect of treatment from various other possible influences, and random allocation ensures that the treatment groups are not systematically different.

Whereas controlled trials are used to assess treatments, observational studies are needed to study the causes of disease. Such 'epidemiological' studies can be either retrospective, in which existing data are used, or prospective, when data are usually collected specifically for the study. Observational studies often involve relating different pieces of information obtained from a single group of individuals or comparing information from two pre-existing groups. These studies are prey to a wide number of potential problems that can lead to systematic differences between the groups and so to misleading findings.

The three main types of epidemiological study can be illustrated in the context of a hypothetical study to see if there is an association between eating carrots and good eyesight. In a *cross-sectional* study, people would be interviewed or complete a questionnaire to ascertain consumption of carrots and probably other foods, as well as demographic and clinical information. Eyesight could be assessed by asking them, or preferably by testing their eyes. It is then simple to see if there is a relationship between the quantity of carrots consumed and visual acuity. However, such a study could not establish cause-and-effect even if an association was found. In particular, it is possible that carrot consumption and eyesight are both affected by something else. In a (retrospective) *case–control* study, groups of individuals with poor eyesight (cases) and good eyesight (controls) would be identified and asked about their history of consumption of carrots. In a (prospective) *cohort* study, subjects with good eyesight would be classified according to their consumption of carrots and then followed up, perhaps for many years, to see which of them develop poor eyesight. All of these designs have potential problems. The cohort design is the most reliable, but such studies take much longer to carry out.

The crucial distinction between randomized controlled trials and these other research designs is that only with the former is it valid to infer a causal link from an observed association. If a clinical trial shows a clear difference in outcome between treatment groups, we can reasonably conclude that the difference was the result of the treatments given. Findings from other types of study are open to many potential biases, and so their findings must be treated much more cautiously. Some of the potential problems can be anticipated and thus avoided by careful study design.

Sometimes observed associations can be useful even when we cannot infer causality. For example, in many diseases much research effort goes into identifying *prognostic* or *risk* factors, variables which predict outcome to some degree. While some of these associations will probably be causal (such as *smoking in many cases) others, such as age or social class, may act more as markers for unknown risk factors. Nevertheless, they can still be useful in the context of predicting a patient's prognosis.

Basic principles of statistical analysis

The preceding section referred in vague terms to drawing conclusions from data. This topic is now considered more thoroughly, through discussion of the two basic approaches to statistical analysis.

The more obvious of the two principal ways of analysing data is known as *estimation*. Here we measure the aspect of interest in the sample and infer that the same applies in the population of similar subjects. For example, we may observe the average (mean) reduction in blood pressure in a sample of patients treated with a particular drug, or the difference between such means for groups of patients treated with different drugs. A further, crucial aspect is that each estimate, such as a mean or a proportion, is accompanied by a measure of its uncertainty. Thus a range of values is obtained extending either side of the observed value, which is highly likely (usually 95 per cent) to include the true population value. This range of values is known as a *confidence interval*. Put simply, the estimation approach is one of measurement plus explicit assessment of uncertainty.

The alternative approach of *hypothesis testing* is rather less intuitive. First, a 'null hypothesis' is set up, which is usually the opposite of the research hypothesis. Thus, the null hypothesis might be that two drugs are equally effective, or that smoking does not increase the risk of developing *cancer of the colon. The second step is to calculate the probability of getting the observed data if the null hypothesis was in fact true. If this probability, P, is very small the null hypothesis is rejected in favour of the alternative—for example, that the two drugs do differ or that smoking is associated with an increased risk of colon cancer. By convention, a P value of 0.05 (i.e. 5 per cent, or 1 in 20) is taken as the cut off point for such an interpretation, so that if the P value is less than this level ($P<0.05$) the difference or association is termed 'statistically significant'. The value of 0.05 is, however, quite arbitrary and has no clinical relevance.

The hypothesis testing approach dominated medical research for many years. Recently estimation has become more popular, although most papers still contain P values. The two approaches are in fact closely related mathematically, but their interpretations are rather different. There are several difficulties associated with hypothesis testing (often called significance testing). First, the precise meaning of P is not well understood (a common error is to interpret P as the probability that the observed difference is due to chance).

Secondly, the *P* value measures the strength of the evidence against the null hypothesis, it does not give any information about the strength of the effect (such as the magnitude of the difference between the observed effects of two treatments). Thirdly, there is, by definition, a 5 per cent chance of getting $P<0.05$ when the null hypothesis is true, i.e. a false positive finding. Likewise a non-significant result ($P>0.05$) should not be interpreted as evidence of no effect, but rather that there is no convincing evidence that there is an effect.

The inflexible use of the *P* value to determine whether an observed effect is significant or not significant can lead to major differences in interpretation when the data change slightly. If we study two groups of patients and observe 27 out of 49 (55 per cent) with a certain attribute in one group and 14 out of 41 (34 per cent) in the other group, the appropriate calculation gives $P = 0.047$. If there were one further patient in the first group so that the proportion was 27/50 (54 per cent) we get $P = 0.058$. By strict use of the 5 per cent convention the first comparison is significant and the second is not, but it is ridiculous to draw opposite conclusions from virtually identical data. By contrast, the difference between the proportions is 21 per cent in the first case and 20 per cent in the second, and the 95 per cent confidence intervals for the difference are 1–41 per cent and 0–40 per cent. In other words, the estimation approach gives virtually the same results whether or not the extra patient is included, which accords with common sense. These and other arguments make the use of estimates and confidence intervals preferable to *P* values, so the recent changes in presentation are most welcome. In general, however, for the foreseeable future the most common presentation is likely to be a mixture of both forms of analysis.

The preceding example also illustrates that estimates based on small samples have considerable uncertainty, as shown by the wide confidence intervals. Sample sizes are frequently too small to allow a clear interpretation of research results. This is one of the motivations behind the recent development of methods to carry out a systematic overview of all the available research evidence on a topic, as discussed below.

Statistical methods of analysis
In statistics textbooks (Altman 1991; Hill and Hill 1991) a considerable amount of space is devoted to describing the various techniques that have been developed for analysing different types of data. It is not appropriate to consider those specific methods here. However, it may be helpful to explain briefly what types of analysis can be performed.

Many of the simpler forms of analysis involve comparing two or more groups of patients. The data could be measurements, such as serum cholesterol or birth weight (known as continuous variables); they could be attributes, such as blood group, presence of a certain disease or symptom, or whether or not the individual was a smoker (known as categorical variables); or they might be the time elapsed since some event, such as diagnosis of a disease; and there are also some other types of data. Different methods of analysis are used according to the type of data, but all fall within the estimation and hypothesis-testing framework outlined above.

The usual case is to have one observation of each variable per person. However, often more than one measurement is taken from each person. For example, patients may be assessed before and after treatment. Here the change is of primary interest. With several measurements per person, usually taken over an extended period of time, it may be advisable to try to summarize each individual's data before applying a simpler analysis to these summaries. For example, we might use the average of all the observations, or the largest, depending on the context.

A large body of research takes a rather different line, looking at the relationship between the values of different variables measured in the same individuals. In its simplest form *correlation* is used to assess how strong is the association between two variables, for example between serum cholesterol and blood pressure. A more useful (although closely related) approach is to use *regression* to try to predict one variable from another. Thus, for example, it is possible to obtain an equation to predict someone's blood pressure from their age. This type of analysis underlies the use of ultrasound measurements of a fetus to estimate the elapsed duration of the pregnancy and thus the expected date of delivery.

Regression is also used to make predictions based on values of several variables. An important aspect of this type of analysis is to know how well the regression 'model' predicts the outcome of interest for individuals. Unfortunately, in many circumstances it is not possible to make accurate predictions even when several individual prognostic variables have been identified. There remains major uncertainty in predicting birth weight, for example, even though it is well known that birth weight is affected by the length of the pregnancy, the number of previous children, the sex of the baby, whether the mother smokes, and some other factors. When the outcome is not a measurement but an event which may or may not occur, the uncertainty is usually considerable. It is common to relate the risk of the event for an individual with a risk factor to the risk for someone without the factor. Thus we can say that a heavy smoker has a relative risk of about 10 for developing lung cancer. In other words, they are 10 times as likely to get lung cancer as a non-smoker. Even though one cannot make precise predictions for an individual, it may still be valuable to make predictions based on data from large groups. A 'prognostic index' can be derived from the regression model, giving an index of relative risk of some event. One such is the Dundee coronary risk score, used to estimate the risk of *coronary heart disease within 5 years in relation to age, blood pressure, serum cholesterol, and smoking behaviour (Tunstall-Pedoe 1991).

Diagnosis

Considerable research effort is devoted to the development of improved ways of diagnosing a disease (Sackett *et al.* 1991). The ideal *diagnostic test* is one which always gives a positive result for subjects who do have the disease in question, and always gives a negative result among those who do not. Such tests are exceptionally rare. The usual case is that the test will miss some patients with the disease (called false negatives) and wrongly identify some patients who do not have the disease (called false positives). The question then arises as to whether the test is reliable enough to be used in clinical practice. Various clinical considerations come into play here, as does the true prevalence of the condition among patients with the symptom in whom the test will be used. An example of a diagnostic test is the use of acute abdominal pain as a means of diagnosing *appendicitis. Because such pain is not specific to appendicitis, some patients will have healthy appendices removed.

Some tests yield a continuous measurement, such as the level of some substance in the blood. The problem is then to define the best value for distinguishing those who do or do not have the disease. This choice must consider the relative costs (in the widest sense) of false positive and false negative findings.

Similar considerations apply when *screening apparently healthy people for possible disease, such as cancer of the large bowel or heart disease. However, because disease is rare in the general population even a small false positive rate can lead to the vast majority of patients with positive tests being free of disease. For example, suppose that 1 per cent of the population has the disease of interest, that a test correctly identifies 95 per cent of those with the disease, and that only 2 per cent of healthy people are wrongly diagnosed. This seems like a good test, but in fact only about 1 in 20 patients identified will have the disease, with serious implications of unnecessary worry and financial cost.

Uncertainties of medical research

Research rarely provides clear answers to scientific problems. The usual pattern is a slow evolution of understanding until the truth emerges. Even the association between smoking and lung cancer, which is easily the strongest known effect of a common environmental influence, was not suspected before 1948, and was not widely accepted until 20 years or more after the first report suggesting the link. Most associations are much weaker, and so advances in the understanding of disease and the development of improved treatments are inevitably slow. Also, it is unavoidable that various false trails will be followed until the truth emerges. The history of therapeutic medicine is full of abandoned 'wonder' treatments. Often the first reports arise from small uncontrolled series of patients, only for subsequent controlled studies to show that the new treatment is ineffective, or at least no advance on existing treatments. An example was the use of gastric freezing as a treatment for ulcers, which was introduced, widely adopted, and then abandoned within 8 years. Many treatments in current use have never been properly evaluated in controlled trials, such as epidural *anaesthesia in childbirth.

Also, because medical research studies tend to be much too small, the inevitable consequence is that there will be much confusion, misunderstanding, and controversy. Some apparent controversies are simply due to the expected variation among several small studies, especially if using different methodologies. Others are, at least in part, due to inadequate statistical design or analysis. Medical journals make increasing use of statisticians to assess the statistical acceptability of papers submitted to them. Nevertheless, it is an unfortunate fact that the general standard of statistics in medical papers is poor, largely because there are too few statisticians in research institutes.

Individual studies rarely provide a definitive answer to a research question. It is common for several similar studies to be carried out over several years, probably in several countries. It makes sense to try to combine the information from them all, and in recent years there has been a growth of this type of analysis. A systematic and objective overview (sometimes called a meta-analysis) uses all the available reliable data to assess the evidence. Usually such studies relate to controlled trials of a particular treatment, but the same principles are becoming more widely adopted for combining the results of other types of study.

DOUGLAS G. ALTMAN

References

Altman, D. G. (1991). *Practical statistics for medical research*. Chapman and Hall, London.

Hill, A. B. and Hill, I. D. (1991). *Bradford Hill's principles of medical statistics*. Edward Arnold, London.

Sackett, D. L., Haynes, R. B., Guyatt, G. H., and Tugwell, P. (1991). *Clinical epidemiology: a basic science for clinical medicine*, (2nd edn). Little, Brown, Boston.

Tunstall-Pedoe, H. (1991). The Dundee coronary risk-disk for management of change in risk factors. *British Medical Journal*, **303**, 744–7.

STATUS EPILEPTICUS is a series of successive epileptic fits lasting for hours or even days, without return of consciousness between attacks.

STEATORRHOEA (STEATORRHEA) is the occurrence of pale bulky frothy *stools, indicating the presence of excessive fat in the faeces, typical of intestinal malabsorption syndromes (e.g. *coeliac disease and *sprue).

STENOSING TENOVAGINITIS. A painful localized form of *tenosynovitis involving the common sheath of the tendons of two thumb muscles (abductor pollicis longus and extensor pollicis brevis).

STENOSIS is abnormal narrowing of a passage or orifice.

STENSEN, NIELS (Nicolaus Steno) (1638–86). Danish anatomist. He described the *parotid duct (Stensen's duct, 1661) in sheep and gave an account of his researches in *De musculis et glandulis* (1664). He was also a notable geologist. In 1667 he joined the Catholic church, was ordained in 1675, and renounced medicine to become Bishop of Titiopolis.

STEREOTAXIS is precise positioning in space; in stereotactic, or stereotaxic, surgery, a lesion is produced deep in the brain in a group of cells which has been localized in three dimensions.

STERILITY, in the microbiological context, is the state of being free from living micro-organisms. Otherwise, sterility means inability either of male or female to produce offspring.

STERILIZATION, in the microbiological context, means the total elimination of all living micro-organisms by physical or chemical methods. Otherwise it means the act of rendering an individual incapable of reproduction, usually by obliteration of the *vasa deferentia in men or of the uterine (Fallopian) tubes in women.

STERNBERG, GEORGE MILLER (1838–1915). American military surgeon and bacteriologist. His main scientific interest was in bacteriology, and he was one of several workers who independently discovered the *pneumococcus. He developed the technique of *photomicrography, and published a manual which became the authoritative American work on the subject. As surgeon-general he organized and supported Walter *Reed's *yellow fever commission in Cuba, which established the role of the mosquito in transmitting the causative agent.

STERNBERG, KARL (1872–1935). Austrian pathologist. He described the characteristic giant cells of *Hodgkin's disease (Sternberg cells, 1898) and published an account of the disorder (sometimes called Paltauf–Sternberg disease), and of '*lymphosarcoma cell' leukaemia (Sternberg's leukosarcoma).

STERNUM. The breast bone, the central structure of the front of the bony thoracic cage, to which the cartilages of the upper ribs are attached.

STEROIDS are a group of chemically similar but biologically diverse derived *lipids, being saturated hydrocarbons with 17 carbon atoms arranged in four linked rings (three six-membered and one five-membered, with six atoms shared between rings). Steroids include sex hormones, adrenal hormones, bile acids, cardiac glycosides, sterols such as cholesterol, and other substances of biological importance. See also CORTICO-STEROIDS.

STETHOSCOPE. An instrument for coupling the examiner's ear to the patient's body surface for purposes of *auscultation. The stethoscope, invented in 1816 by *Laënnec, enabled direct auscultation to be replaced by the more elegant, hygienic, and efficient technique of 'mediate' or indirect auscultation. Laënnec employed a single rigid wooden tube, and a not dissimilar monaural instrument is still employed in obstetrics for listening to fetal heart sounds. The familiar modern stethoscope, however, is binaural and has two flexible tubes connecting the earpieces to a chestpiece which is either an open bell or a closed diaphragm or (best) a combination of the two. The bell, especially when loosely applied, is sensitive mainly to lower sound frequencies, the diaphragm to high frequencies. The overall efficiency of a stethoscope relates directly to the area in contact with the body surface (i.e. the area of the diaphragm, or of the opening of the bell) and inversely to the total volume of the system, which should therefore be kept to a minimum (e.g. by using tubing of small internal calibre and keeping it as short as possible).

STIGMA. Any identifying mark or 'fingerprint' characteristic of a particular condition. The plural form 'stigmata' when otherwise unqualified refers to marks, usually haemorrhagic or purpuric, located in the sites of the wounds of the crucified Christ; such marks are recorded as having appeared on the bodies of numerous saints, mystics, and others over the past 2000 years, as for instance those impressed on St Francis of Assisi on 15 September 1224 by a seraph with six wings. The full set of stigmata includes marks corresponding to the crown of thorns and to the spear wound as well as to those on the hands and feet.

STILBOESTROL (STILBESTROL) is a synthetic *oestrogen, now used mainly in the treatment of neoplastic conditions such as postmenopausal breast cancer (although here it has been replaced by the oestrogen antagonist *tamoxifen) and cancer of the prostate. Toxic side-effects are common, including nausea, fluid retention, and arterial and venous thrombosis; in the male, it causes impotence and *gynaecomastia. The use of stilboestrol should be avoided in pregnancy, as high doses are associated with the development of vaginal carcinoma in female offspring.

STILL, SIR GEORGE FREDERIC (1868–1941). British paediatrician. Still was the outstanding British paediatrician of his day; he described juvenile *rheumatoid arthritis ('Still's disease') in his MD thesis.

STILLBIRTH. Birth of a dead child. In the UK, the arbitrary division between spontaneous abortion and premature stillbirth is drawn at 28 weeks' *gestation.

STIMULANT. An agent which increases the activity of an organ, tissue, system, or function. The term when otherwise unqualified usually means '*central nervous system (CNS) stimulant'. That most widely used is *caffeine, present in tea, coffee, and cola beverages. Others include *pemoline, *fencamfamin, and *meclofenoxate. *Cocaine and the *amphetamine drugs are more powerful stimulants of the CNS but are, on that account, dangerously *addictive; they have no place in the management of *depression.

STING, INSECT. The reaction which follows envenomation by stinging insects, notably species of Hymenoptera (e.g. bees, wasps, hornets); although unpleasant and often very painful, it is normally localized to the region of the sting. Systemic manifestations usually indicate *anaphylaxis but may also arise as a result of the direct action of the venom toxins in cases where multiple stings have been inflicted. Severe stings may also be due to non-insect arthropods such as *scorpions. See also ALLERGY.

STITCH. A sharp, pricking, painful sensation in the side of the lower chest due to *cramp of the intercostal muscles.

STOKE MANDEVILLE HOSPITAL. A general hospital has existed at Stoke Mandeville near Aylesbury in Buckinghamshire, UK, since the Second World War, but the name 'Stoke Mandeville' is generally associated with the world-famous spinal injuries centre established by Sir Ludwig *Guttmann in 1944. See also REHABILITATION; SPORT AND MEDICINE.

STOKES, WILLIAM (1804–78). Irish physician. With *Graves he reformed clinical teaching in Dublin. He described *Cheyne–Stokes respiration (1846) and *Stokes–Adams syndrome (1846).

STOKES–ADAMS SYNDROME is characterized by attacks of unconsciousness due to cerebral *anoxia as a result of (usually) temporary cessation of cardiac ventricular contraction (*asystole) in patients with atrioventricular *heart block. The patient suddenly blanches and falls to the ground. After a few seconds, acute cerebral anoxia often causes convulsive movements. If asystole persists, life ceases. More often, probably as a result of anoxic stimulation of the myocardium, ventricular contraction resumes spontaneously. Return of circulation is accompanied by characteristic flushing. Artificial 'pacing' of the heart (see PACEMAKER) in patients with atrioventricular heart block removes the risk of this serious complication.

STOMACH. An important organ of *digestion, an expansion of the upper gastrointestinal tract situated in the upper abdomen below the *diaphragm, connecting the lower end of the *oesophagus with the *duodenum, the beginning of the small intestine. It has a muscular wall which churns the mixture of food and digestive enzymes, and conveys it onwards into the duodenum. The lining, or mucous layer, contains glands responsible for the secretion of *mucus itself, *hydrochloric acid, the digestive enzyme *pepsin, and a protein promoting *vitamin B$_{12}$ absorption, called '*intrinsic factor', together with various other substances. Nervous control is mediated by the *autonomic nervous system. Hormonal influences are also important. See GASTROENTEROLOGY.

STOMACH PUMP. A device for washing out the *stomach contents.

STOMATITIS is inflammation of the *mucous membrane of the mouth.

STOMATOLOGY is the study of the mouth and its diseases.

STONE. A stone, or calculus, is an abnormal concretion or hard mass developing in a duct or hollow organ. The commonest stones are those which occur within the renal and the biliary tracts, where they predispose to infection and may cause obstruction. Stones may also develop within the ducts of *exocrine glands, such as the pancreas, salivary glands, and breast. They vary in composition according to site and the factors which led to their formation, but usually involve the precipitation of *calcium salts.

STOPES, MARIE CHARLOTTE CARMICHAEL (1880–1958). British pioneer of contraception. She was trained as a botanist and in 1911 she was married for the first time. The marriage was annulled in 1916 for non-consummation and in 1918 she married Humphrey Verdon-Roe, who was also interested in *birth control. She founded the first contraceptive clinic in the UK in 1921. She wrote many books on sex and contraception; the first, *Married love* (1918), was translated into 13 languages.

STORAGE DISORDER denotes any disease in which a metabolic defect results in the abnormal accumulation within the body of a substance or class of substance, for example the *lipidoses. Many such disorders are known, involving *fat, *carbohydrate, *protein, or other substances, such as *iron in *haemochromatosis. Storage disorders are usually associated with absent or defective *enzymes and are genetically determined. See also INBORN ERRORS OF METABOLISM.

STRABISMUS. See SQUINT.

STRAIN. A group of organisms within a species sharing some defining characteristic. An alternative usage is synonymous with *sprain.

STRANGULATION is killing by compression of the throat, interrupting arterial circulation to the head and/or ventilation of the lungs. It is also applied to circulatory obstruction of an organ or part due to compression of the blood vessels supplying it, as in 'strangulated *hernia'.

STRANGURY is slow, difficult, and painful discharge of urine.

STRAWBERRY MARK. A vascular *naevus, bright red in colour, which eventually shrinks and disappears spontaneously.

STREPTOCOCCUS is one of a large and heterogeneous group of Gram-positive spherical bacteria named for their common tendency to grow in chains. They can be classified in several ways, one of which is their capacity to cause *haemolysis when grown on an appropriate blood *medium. Alpha-haemolytic streptococci, which cause partial haemolysis, are particularly associated with *infective endocarditis and *dental caries. Beta-haemolytic streptococci cause complete haemolysis and are further subdivided on the basis of a polysaccharide antigen into 18 groups, labelled A to T; of these, group A organisms (also known as *Streptococcus pyogenes*) cause over 90 per cent of human infections, particularly of the upper respiratory tract (e.g. *tonsillitis, *scarlet fever, *otitis media), skin and subcutaneous tissues (e.g. *cellulitis, *erysipelas, *wound infections), and blood (*septicaemia), and are also responsible in an indirect way for *rheumatic fever and *glomerulonephritis. Gamma-streptococci cause no haemolysis; they include most of those found in the gastrointestinal tract, and are sometimes involved in urinary tract infections.

STREPTOKINASE. An enzyme derived from streptococci which can break down blood clots by converting plasminogen to plasmin. It and its derivatives have been shown to be of value in the treatment of *coronary thrombosis (see CARDIOLOGY).

STREPTOMYCES is a genus of micro-organisms, many free-living or saprophytic in soil, some of which have proved valuable as sources of *antibiotics such as *streptomycin and the *tetracyclines.

STREPTOMYCIN is an *antibiotic produced by the soil micro-organism *Streptomyces griseus*, discovered by *Waksman in the USA in 1943 and obtained in pure crystalline form in 1944. It is active against a range of bacteria, including Gram-negative and acid-fast organisms, such as that of *tuberculosis. Streptomycin is pH-sensitive and is little absorbed from the alimentary tract, so that for systemic infections it must be administered by parenteral injection. Its major side-effect is damage to the auditory nerve, which may be permanent. It should be given with caution, particularly in elderly patients and those with impaired renal function. See also ANTI-INFECTIVE AGENTS.

STREPTOTHRIX was formerly the name of a genus of micro-organisms, the species of which have now been reclassified under different genera such as *Streptomyces*, *Nocardia*, *Actinomyces*, etc.

STRESS is the totality of the physiological reaction to an adverse or threatening stimulus, or the stimulus itself. Such stimuli include all forms of physical, mental, and emotional trauma, in fact any event which threatens to disturb the body's *homeostasis. The hormones of the *adrenal cortex play a particularly important role in adaptation to stress. It has been suggested that failure of the system to cope with stress may lead to so-called 'stress diseases'.

STRIA. A linear streak on the surface of the body due to weakening of elastic tissue and suggesting past or present stretching of the skin and subcutaneous layers. Abdominal striae are common in women who have been pregnant (striae gravidarum) and can follow abdominal distension from any cause. Characteristically purplish striae occur in the flanks and on the thighs of patients suffering from *hyperadrenalism or who have been given *corticosteroids.

STRIATED MUSCLE. See MUSCLE.

STRICTURE. An abnormal constriction of a duct or other passage.

STROKE. A sudden impairment of brain function due to haemorrhage from or obstruction of one or more cerebral blood vessels. Also called apoplexy.

STROKE VOLUME is the volume of blood ejected by the heart at each beat, which may be calculated by dividing the *cardiac output (minute volume) by the *pulse rate.

STROMEYER, GEORG FRIEDRICK LOUIS (1804–76). German surgeon. He was one of the early *orthopaedic surgeons and popularized the subcutaneous *tenotomy devised by *Delpech.

STRONGYLOIDES is a genus of *nematode worms, species of which are intestinal parasites of man and animals; the species infecting humans is *Strongyloides stercoralis*, occurring mostly in tropical and subtropical regions. Mild infestation, which because of autoinfection may persist over many years, may be asymptomatic; heavier infection causes abdominal symptoms and *malabsorption. A dangerous hyperinfection syndrome can occur in patients whose immune defences become depressed, as in *AIDS.

STRÜMPELL, ERNST ADOLF GUSTAV GOTTFRIED VON (1853–1925). German neurologist. Although first interested in biochemistry, he turned to neurology and published many clinical papers. He described spondylitis deformans (Strümpell–Marie's disease, 1884), acute polioencephalitis (Strümpell–Leichtenstern disease, 1891), and 'pseudo-sclerosis' (Westphal–Strümpell disease, 1897).

STRYCHNINE is a highly poisonous *alkaloid obtained from the seeds of a tropical tree *Strychnos nux-vomica*, small doses of which have traditionally been used as an ingredient of 'tonic' medicines. In larger amounts, it produces a condition resembling *tetanus, with violent muscle contractions, *convulsions, and *opisthotonos leading to death from *asphyxia.

STUPOR is a state of depressed consciousness in which only vigorous stimuli will elicit an observable response. Cf. COMA.

STURGE–WEBER SYNDROME is the combination of a congenital port-wine stain (capillary *haemangioma) on the face in the distribution of the *trigeminal nerve and a similar vascular malformation in a part of the *meninges and *cerebral cortex. The latter leads to *calcification (seen on X-ray), *epilepsy, and *cerebral atrophy on the affected side. Other congenital anomalies, including buphthalmos or 'ox-eye', may be associated.

STUTTER. Stammer. See STAMMERING.

STYE. A purulent *staphylococcal infection of the *sebaceous glands of the eyelids.

SUBACUTE BACTERIAL ENDOCARDITIS. See INFECTIVE ENDOCARDITIS.

SUBACUTE COMBINED DEGENERATION. See PERNICIOUS ANAEMIA.

SUBACUTE MYELO-OPTIC NEUROPATHY (SMON) is a disorder characterized by numbness and weakness of the legs, with difficulty in walking and impairment of vision. The condition is progressive over a few weeks. The pathological changes seem mainly to be in the dorsal and lateral columns of the spinal cord, the peripheral nerves, and the optic nerves. Many cases were reported from Japan, with sporadic cases elsewhere. It is now evident that the cause was the chemical antibacterial agent *clioquinol (iodochlorhydroxyquinoline), known under the proprietary name Enterovioform®, used as an antidiarrhoeal agent. The marked decrease in the incidence of SMON is presumed to be due to withdrawal of this compound for other than topical use.

SUBACUTE SCLEROSING PANENCEPHALITIS is a rare, progressive encephalitis affecting children and young adults, in which mental and neurological deterioration leads to death within months or a year or two. A viral aetiology is now established, usually involving an altered form of the *measles virus.

SUBARACHNOID HAEMORRHAGE (HEMORRHAGE). Haemorrhage into the *subarachnoid space is usually due to rupture of a small ('berry') aneurysm on one of the arteries on the surface of the brain, or to bleeding from a congenital arteriovenous malformation. It is an important cause of sudden death or unconsciousness; but when consciousness is retained, the characteristic manifestations are severe headache combined with those due to meningeal and spinal root irritation. *Lumbar puncture reveals bloodstained *cerebrospinal fluid.

SUBARACHNOID SPACE. The space between the *arachnoid mater and the *pia mater, which is crisscrossed by a cobweb-like network of fine threads through which the *cerebrospinal fluid circulates. See also MENINGES.

SUBDURAL HAEMORRHAGE (HEMORRHAGE). Bleeding into the subdural space (i.e. between the *arachnoid and *dura mater) is usually a complication of *head injury. A chronic subdural *haematoma may follow relatively minor injury, especially in older patients; cerebral dysfunction due to compression of the brain develops gradually, often over several weeks, by which time the original injury has often been forgotten. This type of subdural haemorrhage notoriously presents diagnostic difficulty.

SUBLIMATION, in psychoanalytic *psychology, is the process of modifying instinctual impulses into socially acceptable activity. Thus, for example, aggression is sublimated by playing rugby football.

SUBPERIOSTEAL HAEMORRHAGE (HEMORRHAGE) is the extravasation of blood beneath the periosteum, the connective tissue sheath which envelops bone; subperiosteal haemorrhage is a common and painful consequence of *trauma.

SUBSTANCE ABUSE
General consideration
Substance abuse is one of many terms used to designate a particular type of problematical behaviour that is characterized by an unusually intense relationship to an object. The classes of objects that may become the focus of such a relationship include substances (such as alcohol or other drugs), activities (such as work, gambling, and exercise), ideas or clusters of ideas (such as nationalism, racism, and patriotism), and, some would

say, other individuals. The intensity of the relationship is sufficiently extreme that it may persist despite undeniable evidence that it is harming the individual and those who are close to him or her. Terms such as *abuse*, *dependence*, *habituation*, *addiction*, and *obsession* are used to characterize the quality of such relationships. While these terms have somewhat different meanings, they all attest to the tendency of the relationship to the chosen object to grow increasingly dominant in the life of the individual over time. Partly for this reason such behaviours are sometimes viewed as beyond the control of the individual who manifests them, though this is a matter of active dispute.

Although increased attention has been given to these behaviours in the modern era, they have been noted throughout history. Some see in the episode of the lotus-eaters in the *Odyssey* an early reference to *opium. The Judeo-Christian Bible records examples and warnings against the excessive use of alcohol, and the Koran absolutely prohibits it. Shakespeare spoke of Marc Antony as being 'addicted to revels', and in *Hamlet* remarks upon individuals who 'by some habit that too much o'erleavens the form of plausive manners' are censured by others. Thomas de Quincey's *Confessions of an English opium eater* is a classic work from the early 19th century. A contemporary (1992) American dictionary speaks of addiction to 'hot cars' and to rock music. The behaviour is quintessentially human, although animals that are subjected to various kinds of training regimens or to selective breeding can be induced to display behaviour that closely resembles similar behaviour in humans; this is useful in understanding certain aspects of such behaviour.

Despite long acquaintance with this behaviour, many aspects of it are not well understood even at present. This lack of knowledge is no doubt what keeps so many different terms alive. (Multiple terms are not an exclusively contemporary phenomenon in this area; Benjamin *Franklin, for example, published in 1737 a list of 228 terms that were in current use for being drunk.) An important, and as yet unresolved, issue has to do with whether so broad a spectrum of behaviours is best understood by considering them all together, or by considering them individually.

On the one hand, the manner in which some people relate to such activities as work or gambling, or to other people, bears a close resemblance to how others relate to alcohol or to drugs. This raises the very interesting question as to whether the cause of the problem resides in the individual or in the properties of the object he or she chooses for this sort of intense relatedness. If it is legitimate to classify activities together with substances, ideas, and other people, it becomes more difficult to argue that the cause resides primarily in the object, since the classes of objects are so different. Rather, the cause would seem to lie primarily in the propensity of some individuals to form this sort of intense relationship. In addition more than one of these behaviours tend to occur in the same individual, a good example being the very high correlation between the excessive consumption of alcohol and the excessive *smoking of cigarettes.

On the other hand, there are also important differences between individual behaviours and the manner in which they are customarily dealt with; for example, in most Western societies the use of alcohol is legal while the use of opiates is not. Work is socially productive (some writers have referred to it and to other socially productive but excessive behaviours, such as exercise, as 'positive addictions') but gambling is not. Some recent writers have gone so far as to say that the structure of society itself can be addicting, and in that sense virtually everyone is engaged in this sort of behaviour. Such broad definitions, while provocative, tend to deprive specific behaviours of any particular meaning.

In reality it is not necessary to choose between these points of view. Each behaviour is like the others in some respects and is unique in other respects. Both the differences and the similarities can be illuminating. In practice, however, many people feel more comfortable in limiting their perspective, and use terms and concepts that accomplish this goal.

'Substance abuse' is among these terms. It links the excessive use of alcohol and the excessive use of drugs, and opts for these two problems as the principal focus of study and action. But the term excludes other similar behaviours. Tobacco is technically a substance, for example, but is excluded from 'substance abuse' in common usage. Perhaps this is because tobacco smoke is too insubstantial. In any case, the meanings of terms in practice are often not governed by logical principles; as Lewis Carroll's Humpty Dumpty remarked, 'When I use a word it means just what I choose it to mean—neither more nor less'. Food and water are also indisputably substances and may be abused even in the narrow sense under consideration here, but are not a part of the usual understanding of the term substance abuse. The term is in disfavour in certain governmental agencies in the USA because it is thought to give insufficient weight to alcohol problems, and the phrase 'alcohol and other drugs' is at present the preferred designation. This is in part a reaction to the 'war on drugs' that is periodically waged by rival governmental agencies in the USA, which characteristically excludes any consideration of alcohol.

Finally, its focus upon 'abuse' differentiates substance abuse from some alternative terms. Abuse covers the mid-portion of a spectrum of consumption that extends from use at one pole to the most extreme indulgence at the other pole, variously termed dependence, addiction, or (to give an example involving a single substance) alcoholism at the other pole. Terms other than abuse are used in differing classification systems. For example, the official diagnostic language of American *psychiatry speaks of these behaviours as psychoactive substance use disorders, while the more extreme pole in the instance of alcohol is referred to by the *World Health Organization (WHO) as alcohol dependence. However, in general usage it is reasonably clear that the term substance abuse excludes use but includes everything else, including the more severe end of the spectrum.

Particular substances
Alcohol

It is a tribute to its importance that we know ethyl alcohol or ethanol by the name that designates a whole class of substances: alcohol. Among the many other alcohols is, for example, wood alcohol (methanol or methyl alcohol), a by-product of the breakdown of wood. Ethanol is produced by the fermentation of fruit, grain, or some other compound containing *carbohydrates (e.g. honey, sugar-cane) by yeasts. The yeasts that are capable of producing this change occur naturally; and, correspondingly, there is evidence that alcohol (as we shall refer to it) has been known since prehistory. In the commercial manufacture of alcoholic beverages, highly developed and pure yeast cultures are used for the most part, although certain beverages, such as the lambic beers of Belgium, still make use of wild yeasts. Fermentation alone produces beverages with an average alcohol content of approximately 5 per cent (in the case of most beers, fermented from grains) to 12–15 per cent (in the case of most wines, fermented from grapes or other fruits). The alcohol content of a fermented liquid can be greatly increased by the process of distillation, which uses heat to drive off other constituents and has been employed since approximately AD 800. Distillation is used to produce such beverages as whisky, gin, rum, vodka, and others, and for this reason these products are commonly referred to as distilled spirits. The concentration of alcohol in distilled spirits is commonly around 40 per cent.

'Alcohol', a perceptive proverb instructs us, 'is both man's oldest friend and his oldest enemy; if there is truth in wine, there is also destruction.' In more recent times there has been an increasing and almost exclusive emphasis on the adverse effects of alcohol use, but up until approximately the 18th century the opposite was the case, even though the adverse effects were well known. Cotton Mather (1663–1728), a clergyman in colonial America, referred to alcohol as 'the good creature of God'. Although the hazard to public health produced by excessive alcohol consumption is very real and very large, the fact that most individuals are able to limit their consumption to reasonable quantities and derive nothing but pleasure and benefit from alcohol is frequently overlooked. The manufacture of the many varieties of alcoholic beverages has a long and honourable history, and alcohol plays a positive and traditional part in many social settings. Its production provides a substantial level of employment and yields enormous tax revenues to most modern states. The hospitality, restaurant, and tourism industries would not exist without alcohol. If it were an unmitigated evil, dealing with

alcohol would be a relatively simple matter. But because it is both so beneficial and so harmful it has proved difficult for most societies to evolve a reasonable and balanced alcohol policy.

The generally positive picture of alcohol that had prevailed until the 18th century was probably altered by the development of international commerce on a broad scale. For the first time, distilled spirits became widely available at a low price. In England, for example, the widespread consumption of inexpensive gin imported from The Netherlands became a sufficiently serious problem—'drunk for a penny, dead drunk for tuppence'—that the trade had to be suppressed. In the USA, the document that formed the basis for the temperance crusade in the 19th century, which lead to the 'great experiment' with national prohibition in the 20th century, was published first in 1785. Its author was Benjamin *Rush, the only physician signer of the Declaration of Independence and the former surgeon-general of the victorious Continental Army.

Governments have frequently attempted to control the manufacture, distribution, and sale of alcoholic beverages, using a variety of methods, including taxation and state-owned and -operated wholesale and retail sales monopolies. Absolute prohibition of alcoholic beverages has also been attempted from time to time, most notably in the period immediately following the First World War in the USA. Swept in on a tide of patriotism, prohibition was stoutly resisted by widespread bootlegging and illicit distilling. The jury is still out on whether it resulted in social and health benefits to the population, a difficult question to resolve because of the incomplete collection of relevant measures at that time. As increasingly harsh enforcement measures were instituted, the cure soon became more of a problem than the disease. Ultimately, prohibition seemed too much an intrusion of government into private behaviour, particularly with respect to a practice so deeply ingrained in the social fabric. While in most jurisdictions some kinds of restrictions on alcohol consumption continue (for example, the prohibition of sale to minors), the 'great experiment' was a political failure. But it taught a valuable lesson. We learned that we could not live without alcohol, and that we would have to learn to live with it. Prohibition on a large scale is no longer a viable option in Western society even though it survives and is fully implemented in some fundamentalist Muslim communities.

A fairly elaborate apparatus for helping those having serious difficulties with alcohol had developed in most countries prior to prohibition. When prohibition was repealed—in the USA, as late as 1933—a treatment apparatus had to be re-established all over again. Considerable progress has been made in this direction. But the scope and coherence of the treatment effort even now are unable to cope with the dimensions of the problem. Most of those with serious alcohol problems receive no treatment of any kind. It is true that, as with many other health problems, a considerable proportion do not view themselves as needing treatment. But many such persons could be persuaded to be helped if treatment were widely available.

One particular form of assistance with severe alcohol problems is nevertheless ubiquitous, at least in the Western world. Alcoholics Anonymous, founded shortly after prohibition was repealed (in 1935) is a lay fellowship that has developed and elaborated a stepwise approach with a spiritual reawakening at its core. Although AA (as it is familiarly called) does not wish to be viewed as competitive with professional assistance, and insists that it is not a form of treatment, it would nevertheless meet most definitions of that term. The scope of AA is impressive (for example, more than half a million members in North America, and a presence in 90 countries), and there is little doubt that it has assisted more people to deal with their difficulties than any other form of help. It has also proved to be an important model, and there are now 12-step programmes for almost all of the problems that the widest definition of this area of behaviour could encompass (e.g. Narcotics Anonymous, Gamblers Anonymous, Overeaters Anonymous, Shoppers Anonymous, and many others). Nevertheless, Alcoholics Anonymous is not a programme that appeals to all. Many prefer to be treated on an individual rather than a group basis, and many find the spiritual dimensions of AA unacceptable. Most individuals who enter AA drop out after a small number of sessions. No one doubts that AA is effective for some people with alcohol problems, but it clearly is not effective for most. However, the same could be said for any known form of treatment for these problems.

It is fortunate, then, that many different kinds of treatment for alcohol problems have been developed. Some are pharmacological methods, which employ drugs such as disulfiram (*Antabuse®). Some take place in a hospital or residential setting, while others are offered on an out-patient basis. Some assume that serious alcohol problems, termed by them alcoholism, constitute a disease, while others view them as learned responses to life situations. None of these treatments is universally successful, but all are successful with some individuals. Therefore the broadest possible variety of treatments is necessary to achieve good results, and future progress in treatment will involve the careful matching of each individual with the treatment that is most appropriate for his or her problems. Although the development of prevention activities, aimed both at assuring that those who do not have problems in relation to alcohol will remain problem free (primary prevention) and at the prompt detection and effective response to problems when they first develop (secondary prevention), lags behind the development of treatment, there is reason for optimism in this area as well. Effective prevention is of the greatest importance; although much can be accomplished through treatment, reduction in the burden sustained by society from alcohol problems can be accomplished only through prevention.

Opiates

Raw opium, collected from the scored seed pod of the opium poppy, is a mixture of many different active ingredients, termed opiates. These drugs constitute an important segment of substance abuse. The most important is *morphine, isolated from opium at the beginning of the 19th century. Further advances in chemistry made it possible to produce wholly artificial drugs whose effects were very similar to those of the naturally occurring opiates. Examples include meperidine (Demerol®, pethidine) and methadone (Dolophine®). It also became possible to alter naturally occurring compounds artificially; at the close of the 19th century, two extra molecular groups were added to naturally occurring morphine to produce diacetyl morphine, given the trade name Heroin® in appreciation of its powerful effects. The term 'opioids' has been suggested as a designation for the group of drugs, both natural and artificial, that have effects similar to those of opium.

The effects of opiates were long known, and formed the basis of medical therapeutics for many centuries. A classic description of serious involvement with them, *Confessions of an English opium eater*, by Thomas de Quincey (1785–1859), first appeared in magazine form in 1821. But it was not until the introduction of the hypodermic syringe in approximately 1858 that serious involvement of a widespread nature began to be appreciated. During the Civil War in the USA (1861–65) an unusually high proportion of painful and debilitating wounds was produced by regular confrontations between outmoded military tactics and modern firepower. Morphine by syringe was very widely used, and its protracted self-administration became known as 'the soldier's disease'. Ironically, it had been felt that the syringe, by avoiding the stomach, 'the organ of appetite and habituation', would prevent problems of this kind. But by 1870 physicians such as Sir Clifford *Allbutt in England observed that 'injections of morphia, though free from the ordinary evils of opium eating, might, nevertheless, create the same artificial want'.

Concerns of this sort surfaced on a world-wide basis and eventually led to strict control of opiates in virtually every country. The controls imposed were generally effective until the emergence of widespread recreational drug use in the 1960s. Since that time problems associated with these drugs have been a matter of major concern. Indeed, although problems related to alcohol are at least 10 times more frequent, problems related to opiates and opiate-like drugs have been far more widely advertised and are feared to a much greater extent. The emergence of the acquired immune deficiency syndrome (*AIDS) in the 1980s greatly enhanced these concerns, because of the well-documented propensity of the virus to spread through the shared use of non-sterilized injection equipment that is traditional in this group.

A number of treatments are available for those with serious opiate problems, although considerably less is known about treatment here than is known about the treatment of alcohol problems. Long-term, intense, residential treatment programmes called 'therapeutic communities', historically descended from Alcoholics Anonymous but profoundly modified from that approach, have been a significant treatment innovation. The synthetic opiate, *methadone, has also become prominent as an element of effective treatment. Its introduction in the 1960s meant that withdrawal from drugs prior to treatment was no longer a necessary condition for obtaining help. Individuals were given a sufficient dose of this long-acting and orally effective artificial opiate to prevent the effects of the usually less potent drugs, illegally obtained, to allow them to resume productive employment, and to preclude the necessity of criminal activity in order to sustain an adequate level of use. While questions remain about the effectiveness of both of these major treatment approaches, their introduction and development have enhanced the probability of successful outcomes. As with alcohol, the prevention of problems with opiates and opiate-like drugs is a necessity for the eventual resolution of the problem. Regrettably, most of the work on prevention in this area lies before us.

Other drugs

Additional families of drugs are subsumed by the term substance abuse, but can only be granted minimal space in a brief general review. Drugs derived from the plant *Cannabis sativa*, including marihuana and hashish, had an enormous vogue in the late 1960s and early 1970s as a symbol of differences in outlook between the older and younger generations, although they had been well known throughout the world for many centuries. Stimulants of various kinds, including both the natural (e.g. *cocaine) and the artificial (e.g. *amphetamines), have also gone through cycles of use at different times in history. Recently a new and highly potent crystalline preparation of cocaine, called 'crack' because of the sound made when it is melted, is in widespread use in major metropolitan centres in the West, while the use of other forms of cocaine is declining. Hallucinogens, like the artificial *lysergic acid diethylamide (LSD) and the natural *mescaline and *psilocybin (derived from particular kinds of cactus and mushrooms respectively), have had their vogue, largely in the 20th century. Barbiturates, a class of drugs once much used as sleeping 'pills', had effects similar to alcohol; these drugs are not now commonly prescribed. Little is known about the treatment of these kinds of drug problems.

Finally, mention should be made of problems that are not considered to be included under the term substance abuse, but which bear a close resemblance to those that are. By far the most important are problems that arise from the use of tobacco products, particularly cigarettes. Only tobacco products can successfully compete with alcoholic beverages as a threat to the public health. The awesome strength of the bond between the smoker (or chewer) and his or her tobacco is something to which most individuals can testify on the basis of personal experience in themselves or in others. Recent advances have been made in assisting chronic smokers to stop through the application of techniques derived from behavioural *psychology, and through newly developed pharmacological agents, such as nicotine-containing chewing gum and nicotine skin patches. In some countries (e.g. the USA) where a vigorous anti-smoking campaign has been actively pursued over a prolonged period of time, with visible leadership from the federal health establishment, significant overall reductions in cigarette-smoking have been achieved. Nevertheless, the use of tobacco continues and is increasing in certain groups, such as younger women. On a global basis, and particularly in developing countries, the picture is far less favourable.

In the past 25 years, increasing attention has been paid to the deliberate inhalation of a diverse group of organic compounds, including gasoline, solvents (particularly toluene) contained in glues and paint thinners, and fluorinated hydrocarbons used as propellants in aerosols. These compounds can produce changes in consciousness ranging from mild intoxication to sleep, often accompanied by vivid hallucinations. They are widely available, relatively inexpensive, and, unlike alcohol, often have no age or other restrictions attached to their sale. Unfortunately they are, for the most part, highly toxic. Serious damage can be done to the central nervous system and other organ systems by their prolonged use and, especially in the case of the fluorinated hydrocarbons, acute death from severe irregularities of the heartbeat has been reported frequently. Little is known about the effective treatment of these problems or their relationship to other similar problems, such as the use of alcohol, opiates, or tobacco.

As noted above, neither cigarette-smoking nor the inhalation of organic compounds is generally understood as being included under the term substance abuse, perhaps because of their use in the form of a vapour or gas rather than as a solid. Yet history records episodes of problems with many similar drugs including *ether, *chloroform, *nitrous oxide, most other general anaesthetics, and *amyl nitrate, the vapours of which were once used as a treatment for acute asthmatic attacks. In time the nature of problems that have to do with the intense relationships that may be formed between individuals and a wide class of objects, including but not limited to alcohol, drugs, activities, ideas, and still other objects, will become better understood. New and more encompassing terms may be used to designate this kind of human behaviour, and many of the terms that are currently used may well become obsolete. In future, alcohol and tobacco, although they will continue to be available legally, will be recognized as the principal problem areas for public health that require to be understood and dealt with. When this occurs a term that does not encompass both of these problems, such as substance abuse, may be viewed as unacceptably narrow.

FREDERICK B. GLASER

SUBSULTUS TENDINUM is a convulsive twitching movement of the muscles and tendons seen in some severe fevers.

SUCCUSSION SPLASH is a splashing sound produced when a patient is shaken or moves suddenly, indicative of fluid and air in a body cavity. The splash heard when gas and fluid (usually pus) are present in the pleural cavity is traditionally termed 'Hippocratic succussion'.

SUDDEN INFANT DEATH SYNDROME (SIDS or cot death). Babies not more than a few months old, and apparently healthy, may be found dead in their cots. The cause seems to be respiratory failure of acute onset, although why this should happen is still not known. Suggested possible causes have included acute virus infection, allergy to milk, an incorrect sleeping position, or some failure of response of the respiratory centre in the brain to fluctuations in the gases normally being carried in the blood (oxygen and carbon dioxide). No fully satisfactory explanation has been found to cover all cases. There are usually no clues to be found at *autopsy. Parents are shattered when this tragedy befalls them. They feel guilt and remorse particularly painfully, yet in reality they should neither be blamed nor blame themselves, although this last is a natural and usual reaction. Their grief is great and often hidden. Subsequent babies are a source of continuous anxiety until the child is well into its second year. The major mortality is at 3–4 months of age and diminishes up to 1 year. It is particularly unfortunate that at one time cot deaths were often assumed to be caused by parents smothering their children. This notion still lingers in some members of the public and sometimes in the police, who may be called in cases of sudden death. They, and others, can make the parents unnecessarily and miserably unhappy, when their need is for comfort and understanding. An association of parents who have suffered such a loss has been formed in the UK in order to promote research and greater public understanding.

SUFFOCATION is the interruption of breathing by deprivation of air.

SUGAR is, in general, any sweet soluble monosaccharide or disaccharide. In particular, the word is applied to *sucrose, the sugar of cane-sugar, beet sugar, maple sugar, etc., a white sweet crystalline disaccharide of melting point 160–186 °C and formula $C_{12}H_{22}O_{11}$; sucrose, also known as saccharose, is found in many plants but not in animals (except in the alimentary tract after ingestion).

SUGGESTION is the process of influencing an individual so that he or she shows uncritical acceptance of an idea or belief. Suggestion plays a large part in *hypnosis and *faith healing.

SUICIDE is a major social, psychological, and medical problem, and in most developed nations it is among the first 10 causes of death. Each year about 25 000 people in the USA and about 5000 people in England, Wales, and Scotland kill themselves. The suicide rate in men goes up with age, and in women the rate reaches a peak in their fifties and then gradually declines.

The history of suicidal behaviour

During the early history of Greece, suicide was in disfavour except under a few specific circumstances, such as incurable illness, old age, grief, or some other calamity. In the Roman Republic, with its emphasis on civic duty, moral virtue, and individual sacrifice, recorded suicide was predominantly of the heroic type; however, it was also permissible as an alternative to shame or *chronic incurable disease. Early Christians, such as St Augustine, considered that suicide was a mortal sin and a crime because it precluded the possibility of repentance and because it violated the Sixth Commandment against killing. Social condemnation of suicidal behaviour became embodied in legal and religious prohibitions.

Not until the social upheavals accompanying the Renaissance and the Reformation was there some softening of the harsh medieval attitude towards suicide. Early studies linked *insanity, *alcoholism, physical illness, family troubles, and love problems with suicide. As medical studies enhanced understanding of the deep-seated psychological reactions that precede suicidal acts, cultural attitudes began to change. Gradually the laws against suicide behaviour have been repealed, until at present few nations or states retain such legal restrictions.

The modern era of the study of suicide began at about the turn of the 20th century, with two main types of investigation, psychological and sociological, associated with the names of Sigmund *Freud and Emile Durkheim, respectively.

In his classic sociological study, Durkheim (1952) used statistical comparative studies of suicide rates among different groups to support his argument that suicide is the result of a society's strength or weakness of control over the individual. He postulated three basic types of suicide, each associated with an individual's relationship to his society. One type, the 'altruistic' or institutionalized suicide, is required by the customs of the society. In India, since time immemorial, *suttee has been practised, influenced by the religious belief that death was followed by living again with the lost one. The suttee practice of burning with the dead on the funeral pyre was committed most often by wives, but sometimes by mothers, to avoid separation from the lost loved one. Although the altruistic type of suicide is rare today, it was more common in the past.

Most suicides in Western countries are 'egoistic'—Durkheim's second category. Egoistic suicide is brought about by the individual's weak ties to, or integration with, the social group. The high rate among unmarried older men is accounted for in Durkheim's theory by their lack of ties to social groups.

The last category, 'anomic' suicides, occur when there is a traumatic disruption of the accustomed relationship between an individual and society. This results in weak social control and the resultant emergence of unrestrained self-destructive forces in the individual (e.g. the divorced or those with loss of money or status).

Investigations in the USA and Europe show that suicide, as well as some other forms of social deviance, tends to occur more frequently in the central business districts and contiguous areas of large cities. Suicidal behaviour tends to be associated with urban districts that have high levels of social disorganization and social isolation.

Psychiatric and psychoanalytical contributions

Freud (1917) emphasized the importance of unconscious hostility and unresolved grief over lost loved ones (bereavement) as causes of suicidal reactions. The loss, or threatened loss, of a loved person often causes the individual unconsciously to turn his aggression back upon the self in self-destructive ways.

The many psychiatric studies of *depression and suicidal behaviour have contributed to our understanding, but have not produced a theory which has broad acceptance as an explanation of the complexities of suicidal behaviour. The conscious and unconscious meanings of suicide vary with individuals, both in the same society and between different cultures. Some of the more important, predominantly unconscious, suicidal motivations include the following:

(1) a desire for escape, sleep, surcease, or death;
(2) a guilt wish for punishment, atonement, or sacrifice;
(3) a hostile wish for revenge, power, and control, or to punish and to commit murder;
(4) an erotic wish for masochistic surrender or for reunion with a dead loved one; and
(5) a hope for rescue, rebirth, *rehabilitation, or a new life.

Systematic psychiatric studies in Great Britain and the USA demonstrate that at least 94 per cent of those who commit suicide have some kind of serious psychiatric illness. About half have a serious depressive illness, approximately one-quarter suffer from chronic alcoholism, and a smaller but significant number suffer from *schizophrenia or drug *addiction.

Attempted and completed suicide compared

About 10 times as many people make unsuccessful suicide attempts as commit suicide. More men than women commit suicide (about 3 to 1) and more women than men attempt suicide (again about 3 to 1). The average age of completed suicides (about 50) is considerably older than the mean age (roughly about 34) of those who attempt suicide (often called parasuicide). In general, completed suicides tend to use more lethal methods, such as firearms and hanging, than do the attempters, who often employ drugs.

A basic difference between the attempted and completed suicide populations is the degree of suicidal intent. Persons in the attempted suicide category show a continuum of suicidal intent ranging from a suicide gesture group who show little or no suicidal intention, through a large group of ambivalent attempters, and finally a serious suicide-attempt group who, like the completed suicides, have a high degree of intent to kill themselves. Many serious suicide attempters would die were it not for intensive medical efforts to save their lives.

Facts and fables about suicide

Shneidman (1976) wrote about popular misconceptions of suicide and these are listed below, together with the authenticated facts demonstrated by those who have done research on suicide in the past 60 years.

1. *People who talk about suicide do not commit suicide.* Fact: 8 out of 10 individuals communicate their intention to kill themselves before they commit suicide. Usually, they express their intention explicity, although sometimes they may make indirect and non-verbal communications about their suicide wishes.
2. *Suicide occurs precipitously and without warning.* Fact: studies reveal that nearly all suicidal persons give many clues, warnings, and threats concerning suicidal intentions.
3. *Suicidal individuals are fully committed to dying.* Fact: most suicidal persons are ambivalent and undecided about living or dying, and they 'gamble with death', leaving it to others to rescue them.
4. *Suicide is a problem of lifelong duration.* Fact: individuals who wish to kill themselves most often are suicidal only for a limited period of time.
5. *Improvement after a suicidal crisis means that the suicidal risk is over.* Fact: remobilization of suicidal morbidity can ensue after apparent improvement. The individual should be considered vulnerable for several months following a suicidal crisis.
6. *The poor or the rich are most likely to kill themselves.* Fact: all socio-economic strata are proportionately represented.
7. *The propensity to commit suicide is inherited.* Fact: there is no scientific evidence that a self-destructive potential is inherited.

8. *All suicidal persons are insane.* Fact: studies demonstrate that a minority of individuals who commit suicide are *psychotic at the time of their death. Most suicidal persons are extremely unhappy and depressed.

Treatment and prevention

Individuals posing a serious suicide risk are often referred to a psychiatrist and hospitalized in psychiatric hospitals. The specific treatment measures used depend on the patient's needs and the clinical diagnosis. Individual, group, and family *psychotherapy, *electroconvulsive therapy, and the use of *antidepressant drugs are the main therapeutic approaches to the treatment of the suicidal.

The pioneer suicide prevention service, the Samaritans, was founded in 1953 in London, and has more than 150 centres in the UK. In the USA, the crisis intervention work and the suicide prevention services of the Los Angeles Suicide Prevention Service, established in 1955, have been widely emulated. Today there are more than 320 suicide prevention centres in the USA. Typically they are 24-hour telephone answering centres that use both professional and lay volunteer staff to provide short-term crisis intervention services.

The study of suicide as an interdisciplinary subspecialty has developed since 1950. Most of those involved are also mental health professionals, that is *psychiatrists, *psychoanalysts, *psychologists, or *social workers. Some are anthropologists, sociologists, clergy, or other professionals, and they, together with mental health professionals, are involved in suicide research, education, prevention, and intervention.

T. L. DORPAT

References
Durkheim, E. (1952). *Suicide: a study in sociology*. Routledge and Kegan Paul, London.
Freud, S. (1917). Mourning and melancholia. In *Standard edition of the complete psychological works of Sigmund Freud*, Vol. 14. Hogarth Press, London.
Shneidman, E. (ed.) (1976). *Suicidology: contemporary developments*. Grune and Stratton, New York.

SULPHONAMIDES (SULFONAMIDES) introduced into medicine by *Domagk in 1935, ushered in the modern era of *chemotherapy. They have been used since then against a wide variety of bacterial and protozoal infections and are still important, although less so than formerly, since they have been largely superseded by *antibiotics. Sulphonamides, which are derivatives of the original sulphanilimide and contain the sulphonamide group $-SO_2NH_2$, exert their antibacterial action by preventing bacterial uptake of para-aminobenzoic acid which is required for the synthesis of folic acid and essential for bacterial metabolism. They are effective by mouth. Sulphonamides are toxic and side-effects are, unfortunately, common, occasionally serious.

SULPHUR (SULFUR) is a non-metallic element (relative atomic mass 32.064, atomic number 16, symbol S) occurring in nature in several allotropic forms. It is present in the *amino acids cysteine and methionine and hence in many *proteins. Sulphur atoms form cross-links between amino acids containing them, either in the same chain (as in *oxytocin and *vasopressin) or between two chains (as in *antibodies and *insulin). The amino acid resulting from a sulphur bond between two molecules of cysteine is called cystine. Inorganic sulphur preparations have been used in medicine, particularly in skin diseases; as have some sulphur-containing compounds (e.g. the *sulphonamides).

SUMMERSKILL, EDITH CLARE (Baroness Summerskill of Kenwood, life peeress) (1901–80). British physician and politician. From 1938 to 1955 she sat as a Labour Member of Parliament, first for Fulham and later for Warrington. She was parliamentary secretary to the Ministry of Food from 1945 to 1950 and Minister of National Insurance in 1950 and 1951. In 1954 she was chairman of the Labour Party. Throughout her life she was a vigorous champion of feminist causes.

SUN YAT-SEN (1866–1925). Chinese statesman and physician. In 1894 he left China during the Sino-Japanese war but returned in 1895 to lead an unsuccessful armed rising. When this failed he fled to Japan, then the USA and Europe, living for part of the time in England (1896–97) before returning to Japan in 1897. Shortly after his arrival in London he was kidnapped by members of the Chinese Legation, being released only after he had smuggled a message to his former medical school principal in Hong Kong, Dr James Cantlie. Later he was involved in organizing many Chinese uprisings, of which that of October 1911 was successful. The Manchu dynasty was deposed and Sun became the first president of the Chinese Republic, resigning in 1912. He then founded the Nationalist party (the Kuomintang) and spent the remainder of his life trying to bring unity to China.

SUNBURN is the familiar syndrome provoked by excessive exposure to sunlight, of which the ultraviolet component is chiefly responsible. It is characterized by erythema, tenderness, and discomfort and in severe cases vesiculation, followed by desquamation and variable pigmentation. Individual susceptibility varies, and may be enhanced by drugs (e.g. *sulphonamides) and by disease (e.g. *lupus erythematosus, *porphyria). Repeated exposure to sun over long periods accelerates ageing in skin, and confers an increased liability to skin cancer. Sunburn is sometimes termed actinic dermatitis.

SUNSTROKE. See HEAT AS A CAUSE OF DISEASE.

SUPEREGO is a psychoanalytical term designating a hypothetical structure built up in the unconscious by early experience, mainly parental, which acts rather in the manner of a conscience, causing guilt and anxiety when primitive impulses are gratified.

SUPERIOR SAGITTAL SINUS. One of the major venous sinuses of the *dura mater, an unpaired channel which runs anteroposteriorly in the midline. See also SINUS THROMBOSIS.

SUPPORTIVE CARE is the provision of assistance and facilities to the elderly and infirm in respect of everyday living requirements.

SUPPOSITORY. A medicated plug of material, solid at room temperature but designed to melt at body temperature, for insertion into the rectum, vagina, or urethra; the purpose is either to introduce a drug into the systemic circulation by absorption from the mucous membrane or to exert a local action on the mucous membrane itself. The base of the suppository is cocoa butter, gelatin, or some other substance with suitable physical characteristics.

SUPPRESSION has various senses: in *immunology, it is the inhibition by suppressor T-cells of B- and T-cell responses, or the depression of immune responses generally by drugs or other immunosuppressive agents such as irradiation; in *genetics, it is the restoration of a character lost by *mutation by the occurrence of a secondary mutation; in *psychoanalysis, it is the deliberate dismissal from consciousness of unpleasant thoughts, memories, and ideas, as opposed to the unconscious mechanism of *repression.

SUPPURATION is the process of *pus formation. See also INFLAMMATION.

SUPRARENAL GLAND is synonymous with *adrenal gland.

SURFACTANT. A surface-active agent, which when introduced into a liquid affects those properties which depend on surface tension, i.e. spreading, wetting, etc. Detergents are surfactants. Pulmonary surfactant refers to the phospholipid secretion of alveolar cells which reduces the surface tension of fluid within the lungs.

SURGEON. Literally, one who treats disease with his hands. See SURGERY, GENERAL.

SURGERY, GENERAL
Origins and traditions in prehistory
The origins of surgery in prehistory cannot be separated from speculation and fantasy. Trepanning or *trephining is one of the early operations of which we have definite proof. There seems no reason to doubt the popular notion that it was to release some demon entrapped in the skull. Examples have been found dating back to

10 000 BC in which the growth of new bone around the site of trepanning suggests that some subjects lived following the operation. The practice had evidently spread widely and trepanned skulls have been found not only in Europe but also in Mexico and Peru. However, none has been found in India, China, or Egypt.

The instruments used would clearly have been the implements available at the time and not specifically designed. Initially, flints are likely to have been employed but eventually metal instruments would have become available. Flints would also have been suitable for the practice of scarification. *Cautery at the site of an *abscess or as a counter irritant over a *dermatome related to a deeper internal pain (which is still common in the Middle East and the African continent) may also have been undertaken, but no proof remains.

The primitive and ancient world
Speculation gives way to pictorial and written record about 2000 BC in Babylon, with the seal of the surgeon Urlugaledin and the stele of the great law-giver Hammurabi defining a code of medical practice with some quite specific instructions, which serve to illustrate the development of the art of surgery by that time, as the example below shows.

If a physician operates on a man for a severe wound (or makes a severe wound upon a man) with a bronze lancet and save a man's life, or if he opens an abscess (in the eye) of a man with a bronze lancet and saves that man's eye, he shall receive 10 shekels of silver (as his fee).

It was from this time that the rod and serpent Sachan, the signs of the god Ninazu and his son, Ningischzida, were used as symbols of healing. The existence of surgical implements from Nineveh fashioned in bronze with both smooth and serrated edges confirm the transition of medicine from something magical to a developing art determined by the experience of those engaged in its practice.

Accounts of Egyptian surgery are to be found in various papyri dating from about 2000 to 1500 BC. The *Edwin Smith papyrus, somewhat speculatively attributed to *Imhotep, physician to King Zoser, gives a good but limited account of the practice of medicine in the 2nd millennium, and also suggests a link with Babylonian and Assyrian medicine. It is interesting in that it demonstrates that the art of examination and observation at this time was already regarded as important in the clinical assessment which, in the developing science of surgery, had to precede treatment. In the papyrus there are records of detailed examinations of 48 patients and from these we know that the *pulse was thought to be important in assessing patients with head injuries, and the probing of wounds in establishing their depth before treatment was undertaken. Following such an examination it became possible for the surgeon to give some prediction of the probability of cure. Methods of wound closure and *splinting are also given in some detail.

The *Ebers papyrus is a collection of medical texts. Some of the material belongs to an earlier period but the rest records the extensive practice at the time. It is of surgical interest because there is an account of *circumcision which was apparently carried out at the age of 14 and was practised amongst Egyptians, Ethiopians, and Copts. Whether the reason was for *hygiene or supposed increased *fertility is obscure.

The Kahun medical papyrus from the Faiyum, which is entirely devoted to *gynaecology, may mean that there was some specialization and instruction organized in schools or through apprentices, as was known to be the custom in surgical training in the Middle Ages. From the 3rd millennium BC, knives were probably used for evisceration before burial, as well as circumcision and other simple operations. Formal anatomical records were not made until the Alexandrian School in the 3rd century BC.

Between the third and first millennium BC there were significant migrations into the Mediterranean Basin, bringing primitive civilization and culture which then spread to India. There was, therefore, a certain uniformity of medical practice spreading centrifugally from the eastern Mediterranean.

The development of Indian surgery, however, seems to have been in advance of that of classical Greece in many respects. An operation for *fistula in ano and some plastic operations on ears, nose, and cheeks are described in sacred Indian texts such as the *Susruta*. These included the most suitable incisions in different regions, indicating some knowledge of lines of stress and tension, which anticipate the formal description of Langer's lines. The use of metals in India and China preceded that in Europe and the Mediterranean Basin, and the availability of instruments must, to some extent, have dictated the development of surgery.

There is a tradition that *acupuncture with metal needles was started in China by the Emperor Shen Nung in the 3rd millennium BC, as recorded in the *Nei Ching*, but a more widely held view is that this practice dates from the 3rd century BC. *Castration was certainly practised at this time and was accomplished by a combination of *ligation and *amputation.

Classical times

The speculation about medical practice in the 3rd millennium BC gives way to more detailed documentation in the Greek world, about 500 BC. Initially, we learn from the Homeric writings such as the *Iliad* that, by this time, wounds were accurately described and that there was considerable knowledge about extracting foreign bodies and stopping *haemorrhage. Achilles binding Patroclus' wound is illustrated on the bowl of Sosia (5th century BC) and is, incidentally, an early example of the application of a *spica (figure-of-eight) bandage.

However, the cult of *Aesculapius, which came to dominate medical thinking in Greece and Asia Minor, being introduced in Athens in 429 BC, was to a large extent mystic, with little relevance to the development of surgery. Such medicine as was practised was once more in the hands of the priests rather than the laity, as had been the case in the Homeric period.

From the many cult centres in the Aegean a form of cleansing and treatment developed, which was to herald the start of medicine and surgery as both an art and a science. Traditionally, the school at Cos with *Hippocrates was the most important, although others, such as that of *Alcmaeon of Croton, who practised anatomical dissection, must surely have contributed to the growing knowledge.

The Hippocratic writings describe a number of surgical instruments—sounds, knives, curettes, trephines, forceps, and specula—which indicate an increasing range of surgical skills. Some of the procedures, such as the reduction of *dislocated joints, operations for fistula in ano, *haemorrhoids, and *cataracts, are also described in some detail. It was known that pure, boiled water or wine benefited the healing of wounds, although there was no knowledge of *asepsis.

The empirical school at Alexandria, and particularly *Herophilus of Chalcedon, who, around 300 BC, practised both animal and human dissections, advanced anatomical knowledge. The period of greatest development in this school came when *Heracleides of Tarentum in the 2nd century BC undertook operations for *hernia, vesical *calculi (bladder stones), and cataracts. With the development of the Roman Empire it was inevitable that medicine should reach a certain preeminence and the documentation of this we owe largely to Aulus Cornelius *Celsus, who died about AD 50. In the sixth and seventh book of *De artibus* we find particularly detailed accounts of surgical procedures. The techniques he records, and of which there was no good evidence previously, are the resection of protruding fragments of bone in open *fractures and of the *omentum following penetrating injury of the abdomen. Operations for *phimosis, abdominal *paracentesis, gut *anastomosis, and certain plastic operations, including one for *exophthalmos, are also described. In discussing breast *cancer, although he recommends excision for an early lesion, he records that surgery aggravates the problem when the *tumour is advanced. A Greek physician who came to Rome was Galen (AD 138–201). He had been born in *Pergamum, an ancient shrine of Aesculapius, and was destined to dominate medical thought for some centuries to come. Of surgical interest, he records that an escape of air from the *thorax indicates that a penetrating injury has perforated the lung, and the new technique of resection of the ribs and sternum for *empyema and *tracheotomy is described. Undoubtedly, procedures of this complexity were being attempted in various centres within the Roman Empire and perhaps even in the Orient. The lack of development of *analgesia and *anaesthesia were among the factors that clearly were to limit the possibility of undertaking more major operations. It is likely that

*Hua T'o (AD 115–205), accepted as the father of Chinese surgery, had a greater knowledge and access to *opiates, allowing him to perform relatively major procedures under the influence of *narcotics. He is known to have had a powder which effervesced in wine and produced a certain degree of anaesthesia. *Antyllus, also from Pergamum, gave a good account of arterial *aneurysms and details of exposure and ligation above and below. He discussed indications for *plastic surgery of the eyelid, nose, and cheek.

Actinus of Amida, a Byzantine writer of the 6th century, who studied medicine in Alexandria, described *tonsillectomy and ligation above an aneurysm of the brachial artery. The importance of Alexandria as a centre of medical learning continued into the 7th century. The last great Byzantine physician, *Paul of Aegina, who studied there in the mid 7th century, discussed in his *Eptome* cancer of the *uterus and breast, for which he recommended surgery. He gives detailed accounts of *lithotomy with the patient positioned in what was to become the classical lithotomy position, and also repair of *inguinal hernia by reducing the intestines with a sound and uniting the bulges on either side with *sutures.

Surgical writings of importance gradually dwindled. Medicine, which had thrown off empirical priestly and mystic associations, to flower in the period of Hellenic philosophy and science and to be consolidated during the great period of the Roman Empire, declined. Many of the ideas and traditions of Greek medicine, however, were to be kept alive in the Arab world.

Arab legacy
The schismatic dispute in AD 431 involving *Nestorius, the Patriarch of Constantinople, caused him to flee with followers to Mesopotamia, and a medical school was eventually established there. This had far-reaching implications for surgery in that the Greek writings and thought were preserved. Even when the *Nestorians were subsequently expelled from Edessa, they took their libraries with them to Jundishapur, which was to become the important nucleus of the Muhammadan tradition of surgery. Some of the Greek documents were translated by Hunain ibn Ishaq, and when he was eventually appointed court physician to Al-Mamun, Caliph of Baghdad, the centre of learning was transferred there, and it became an important centre with a large hospital. It was here that Ar-Razi (*Rhazes) came from Teheran to study in the late 9th century, and it was from Baghdad that he published his encyclopaedic medical work, *Hawi*, or *Continens*. This records bleeding by *cupping and the application of *leeches. It also suggests the use of animal gut for suturing abdominal wounds, which is therefore traditionally attributed to Rhazes.

Amongst the writings at this time is the *Canon* of *Avicenna. His *Canon* contains the suggestion that pig bristles should be used for sutures, and also the first main reference to *obstetric forceps for extracting a dead fetus. Despite the advances for which he was responsible, his acceptance that surgery was a separate branch of medicine to be practised by those in an inferior position, took centuries to eradicate and undoubtedly hindered surgical progress.

The Arab world embraced the Mediterranean Basin not only in the east but also in the west, with an important presence in Spain. Albucasis, born in Cordoba in AD 936, kept alive the ideas of Paul of Aegina, and they were disseminated in his *Altasrif* within the western Arab world. It became a valuable surgical source book with good accounts of the techniques of cautery, lithotomy, and amputation.

Medieval renaissance
The reawakening of surgical interest and practice which took place in Europe was, on the whole, in a climate of thought created by religious dogma that was certainly restrictive, if not openly hostile. Although St Benedict of Nusia had, in AD 529, founded a monastery at Monte Cassino whose work was, to a large extent, directed towards healing, the belief in the evils and uncleanliness of the body was firmly held. It was considered wrong even to cut for stone—especially as the site of the operation required the exposure of parts of the body not fit to be observed. A further blow was dealt in 1215 by Pope Innocent III, who formulated the views of the Church in *Ecclesia abhorret a sanguine*. The shedding of blood was thought to be so abhorrent that occupations which entailed bloodshed were relegated to the lowly strata of society. It was with this background of opinion that surgical activities, even of monks committed to surgical work, had been restricted by the Council of Tours in 1163. However, the Church was unable to stop the Arab influence coming back into European culture. Constantine the Moor, born in Carthage in AD 1010, eventually arrived in Monte Cassino in AD 1072 and translated the *Pantegni* of Heli ibn al Abbas, an Arabic version of an original Greek text, into Latin. The section which is devoted to surgery discusses suturing methods, the ligating of blood vessels, fractures, and inflammation. None of this was new, but when reintroduced to Europe after a dormant period it was natural that it would be looked at objectively. One of the centres where this happened was *Salerno. Constantine himself had been there before going to Monte Cassino and the city was already a centre of healing and destined to have one of the first universities. *Regimen sanitatis Salernitanum*, by tradition compiled and edited by John of Milan, was published from Salerno. This and *Practica chirurgiae*, compiled in 1170 by Guido Aretino (a pupil of Roger Frugardi who was one of the most distinguished surgeons of this period in Salerno), bear witness to the pre-eminence of this university in the field of medicine and surgery. This remained so for some 150 years, with the *Practica*, or *Rogerina*, being developed through several editions (e.g. *Glossulae quatuor magistorum super*

chirurgium Rogerii et Rolandi) as the most important working surgical treatise of the time, with sections on wounds of the head, fractures of the skull, and diseases of the neck and limbs.

In addition to the preoccupation of surgeons with wounds received in battle, they were now beginning to think about such matters as the merits of *incision as opposed to cautery in healing (Guglielmo *Salicetti in *Cyrurgia*, 1210) and the differential diagnosis of benign breast lumps and cancer (Lanfranck *Chirurgia magna*).

European enlightenment

The French school was pre-eminent and started with Lanfranck. In addition to his technical achievements he clearly understood that a knowledge of medicine was also essential for the surgeon. The belief that he should not merely be a technician but a physician who practises surgery—and able to appreciate and be able to meet the whole needs of the patient and his family—was suggested by Lanfranck's contemporary Henri de *Mondeville. He wrote about the qualites of the ideal surgeon, including the need to counsel both the patient and relatives about prognosis.

Some small technical advances were made at this time. Lanfranck's pupil Jehan Yperman was appointed surgeon in Ypres in 1308 and described a metal shield for allowing cautery at relatively small and precise points. The great Guy de *Chauliac, surgeon to three popes, wrote a comprehensive textbook of surgery (1363) in which he described radical cure of hernia, but he is perhaps popularly remembered now for the chain hoist still seen hanging over many surgical beds. His textbook of surgery was translated into English (the *Questyonary of surgeons*), French, Provençal, Dutch, and Hebrew. It maintained its importance until the writings of Ambroise *Paré 200 years later.

In England, the Guilds of Barbers and Surgeons (officially recognized in 1368) increased in importance and began to exercise jurisdiction over the practice and standards of the profession. A system of apprenticeship was established by the early guilds, but it was not until 1629 that this was eventually supplemented by a series of lectures.

Barber-surgeons performed *venesections and many operations in France, Ambroise Paré was at first refused admission to the College of St Come because he could not write Latin and was, therefore, considered unworthy of the honour. The court, Church, and universities had a somewhat greater influence on the structure of the developing profession in the rest of Europe than the guilds and colleges in England.

Some important English surgeons emerged at this time. John of *Gaddesden, physician to Edward II and probably the model of Chaucer's doctor of physic, and John of Mirfield (d. 1407) spanned the 14th century. From their writings, *Rosa anglica* and *Breviarium Bartholomei*, respectively, we get a good idea of clinical practice at this time. They described injuries, hygiene, diet, and dressings. The development of surgical techniques clearly changed little during this time but John of Mirfield is credited with observing that an injury on the right side of the head may lead to *paralysis on the left side of the body.

The greatest English contribution during the 14th century was that of John of *Arderne. His experience was obtained largely on the battlefield, but the writings for which he is justly remembered were on fistula in ano. Until his detailed account of treating it with a grooved probe, ligature, and scalpel, his contemporaries considered it as largely incurable. His manuscript *De arte phisicale et de chirurgia* (1412) remains as a good record of his practices.

Despite the importance of surgeons to the armies of Europe, over many generations they remained socially and academically inferior to physicians. The development of specialized surgical techniques did nothing to remove this trend.

It was not unnatural that surgeons and barbers, being denied university education, should protect their interests by the formation of guilds. In France during the 13th century the College of St Come was founded (or refounded, for Malgaigne states that it was originally established in 1033) and to some extent protected the interests of surgeons. In England a Company of Barbers and the Guild of Surgeons fulfilled a similar function between 1300 and 1540, when the two merged and were incorporated in the city of London as the Company of *Barber-Surgeons with Thomas *Vicary as first Master. It was not until 1745 that the definitive Company of Surgeons was founded, and 1840 before it was dignified by having a royal charter. Progress towards academic and social acceptance had been somewhat faster on the continent, and, as early as 1672, Louis XIV of France had ordained that public demonstrations of surgery be given annually in the royal garden.

By the mid-16th century, the barber-surgeons, *phlebotomists, and the travelling *lithotomists were fused into a recognizable profession in Europe, with leaders emerging in each country. One of the greatest of these was Ambroise Paré.

He started life as a military surgeon and arrived in Paris in 1532, ignorant of Latin and Greek but with an intelligence and originality which were to dignify surgery and leave us with the important and immortal concept that, although the surgeon dressed wounds, God healed them. Compared with his personality and independent mind, and the fact that he helped release surgery from dogma, his reintroduction of ligatures in amputation and belief that treating gunshot wounds with boiling oil was harmful to the tissues were comparatively modest advances. His contemporaries in England were William Clowes (b. 1540), who described ligating an omental mass and leaving long tails on the ligatures so that they could be extruded, and William *Chamberlen, a Huguenot, who designed *midwifery forceps. An ingenious technique was introduced about this time by Jean Tagout of Belgium who, in 1543, described the injection of alum and silver into a *sinus tract to find where a bullet had lodged. These were, however, minor advances and somewhat pedestrian when compared with the art of lithotomy or cutting for stones so skilfully practised by Jermain Colot, Pierre Franco, and Frère Jacques, who developed an approach lateral to the midline to avoid damaging central structures.

Anatomical awareness

The rising status of surgeons and commitment to their profession inevitably led to an interest in *anatomy. Andreas *Vesalius and his contemporaries in the Italian school founded the modern science of anatomy in the 16th century. This had been stifled by religious scruples between the 2nd and 16th centuries, except for the remarkable textbook of anatomy written in 1316 by Mondino de Luzzi (*Mundinus) of Bologna. Vesalius performed dissections in Bologna, Pisa, Basle, and Padua, which formed the basis of his book *De humani corporis fabrica* published in Basle in 1543. Gabriel *Fallopio, a pupil of Vesalius, succeeded him as professor in Padua in 1551. He is chiefly remembered for his description of the human oviducts.

Although a human body had been dissected publicly in Venice in 1308, resistance remained, largely from the Church, and in England it was not until 1540 that the barber-surgeons were given permission to have four bodies each year to dissect, although it was known that clandestine dissection had been carried out frequently in the past. The first proposal that the Company of Surgeons in England should build an anatomical theatre, was by Michael Andrews in 1636; it was opened 2 years later.

Surgeons were understandably preoccupied with the organization of their profession, for raising standards of surgical practice and improving the education of barber-surgeons' apprentices. Society was still served by quacks and pseudo-surgeons, including cutlers, cooks, tooth-drawers, sow gelders, and witches, who had little honesty and skill in surgery. However, out of the disorder significant figures emerged, whose surgical stature was to serve as a foundation for the great developments that were to come. John *Woodall is remembered surgically for abandoning the method of amputating *gangrenous limbs by cutting through the dead tissue below the line of demarcation of viability; he recommended cutting through the healthy tissue above. His *The surgeon's mate* (1617) was a comprehensive surgical handbook for ships' surgeons, their mates, and probably ships' captains who found themselves without a surgeon on board and might need information about instruments and their use in accident surgery, bowel obstruction, and other medical topics. The range of operations was very limited and the art of surgery still comparatively primitive as a result of *sepsis and the lack of *anaesthesia.

Many leading surgeons, despite the knowledge in basic sciences developing in parallel, were both critical and scornful of attempts to investigate the causes of disease rather than concentrating on surgical technique. Operations without anaesthesia on a delicate organ such as the eye demanded great manual dexterity. It was understandable, therefore, that many should feel that surgery was not capable of further refinement or advance. In 1745 Percivall *Pott, assistant surgeon to St Bartholomew's Hospital, took a contrary view:

Many and great are the improvements which the chirurgical art has received in the last 50 years, and many thanks are due to those who contributed to them; but when we reflect how much still remains to be done it should rather excite our industry than inflame our vanity.

This reference to vanity reflected the mental attitude of many of his contemporaries, who were not only individualists but had fixed ideas which prevented their accepting or seeking any innovations apart from minor modifications in technique.

Surgery at this time largely entailed removal of any affected part. The lack of knowledge about the cause and treatment of infection prevented surgery from being used for anything but relatively minor conditions such as hernias. Operations on the body cavities were extremely dangerous. However, developments took place during the 18th century which mark a significant advance in the surgical approach to various serious clinical problems.

The true founder of scientific surgery in the 18th century, was undoubtedly John *Hunter. The method of his scientific argument, with a clarity of inductive and deductive reasoning, allowed him to approach and solve problems far ahead of others of his generation. This was seen not only in his ability to advance surgical technique, but also in his enunciation of the general principles of inflammation and their application to various diseases. He always tried to link structure and function and to know not only the diseases but their causes. He was the founder of the science of experimental and surgical pathology, and was able to convince his generation, and subsequent generations, that there were processes of disease which could be studied scientifically.

The scientific approach to pathology and the understanding of function is most strikingly displayed in John Hunter's (*Hunterian) Museum at the College of Surgeons in London. It has rightly been described as a treasury of experience and a storehouse of facts in a visible and palpable form, to which the young medical student may resort to increase, and the old one to refresh, his knowledge.

Hunter's legacy was left at a time when there was still religious prejudice which prevented official legislation from allowing the lawful supply of bodies for dissection in England and Europe. Thomas *Burke was hanged in 1828 for assisting the death of aged inmates of a hostel in Edinburgh in order to supply bodies for dissection. It took nearly three centuries in England, from 1540, when the barber-surgeons were allowed four corpses of criminals each year for public dissection, until the Anatomy Act of 1832, for the legal supply of bodies for medical students to be assured.

World growth

Within Europe there had been a tradition of travel between centres such as Salerno, Padua, Montpellier, Basle, and London. The time had now arrived for the European tradition to be carried to the New World. Philip Syng *Physick was an American pupil of John Hunter who, having qualified in Edinburgh, returned to Philadelphia in 1792. His inventive and unrestricted American mind brought many modifications in techniques and instrumentation. He became, with Alexander *Monro of Edinburgh, the first to wash out the stomach, and was known to have undertaken *caesarean section in 1824. He designed a wire snare for removing tonsils, and a flexible pewter cannula for insertion into the *ventricle of the brain through a trephine hole. He was the first full professor of surgery at the University of Pennsylvania—a position that he held for 13 years. It is interesting to speculate on the restrictive practices within the profession in England which delayed the establishment of the first chair of surgery within the University of London until 1919, when George Gask was appointed as professor at St Bartholomew's Hospital.

A great American tradition developed. Henry Jacob *Bigelow of Boston was an inventive genitourinary surgeon who favoured the crushing of bladder stones and bladder irrigation, designing his own instruments. A similarly ingenious surgeon, John B. *Murphy, developed a 'button' for end-to-end anastomosis of the intestine. Charles *McBurney is remembered in the annals of clinical surgery for his grid-iron abdominal incision for appendicectomy. The international pre-eminence of W. S. *Halsted and of Harvey *Cushing, the leading neurological surgeon, both of *Johns Hopkins Hospital, consolidated the position of American surgery. Halsted introduced his radical *mastectomy in 1882 and Cushing's classic monograph on *pituitary diseases and surgery was published in 1912.

International standardization of practice

In 1881, a year after von *Mikulicz had operated on a patient with a perforated *peptic ulcer, Theodore *Billroth performed the successful resection of a *carcinoma of the pylorus (distal aperture of the *stomach). This was a momentous step in surgery, acclaimed the world over. It was, however, the third hazardous operation he had introduced, for in 1872 he resected the *oesophagus and in 1873 performed a laryngectomy. It was not until 1897 that total *gastrectomy was undertaken by Schlatter. Such developments attracted many visitors from around the world. Travel was not easy, but these visitors were then able to reproduce the sophisticated operations in their own countries.

Pain and *anaesthesia

Many potions and concoctions have been used through the ages to relieve the pain and suffering of injury and surgery. *Opium prepared from poppy seeds and Indian hemp (*Cannabis indica) were known to the ancients, as well as *mandrake (*Atropa mandragora*) and *henbane (*Hyoscyamus*). In more recent times *alcohol was employed for its analgesic and paralytic qualities. Joseph *Priestley discovered *nitrous oxide in 1772, and Humphry *Davy experienced its ethereal qualities in 1799 and suggested that the gas might be used for the relief of pain. The discovery of *morphine and its soporific effects by Friedrich Wilhelm *Sertürner in 1806 was an important milestone.

In January 1842 Wiliam Clarke, a medical student, used *ether while a tooth was extracted from a friend, and *Long, of Athens, Georgia, gave ether later in 1842. William *Morton used it in a public demonstration in Boston in 1846. Chloroform was popularized by James *Simpson of Edinburgh when, on 15 November 1847, he anaesthetized a 4-year-old patient. The benefits that followed the introduction of general and local anaesthesia were quite inestimable. They were to release the patient from fear and pain, and surgeons from the need to exercise excessive speed. Anatomical dissections were to become possible and injury to tissue less. The surgeon was allowed to seek a better anatomical and physiological solution to operative problems. Anaesthesia was to prove the catalyst of surgical development between 1850 and 1950, when John Gillies introduced *hypotensive anaesthesia to reduce the loss of blood during surgery. Since then the supportive role of anaesthetics has diversified even further, with *resuscitation and *intensive care.

Infection

The tide of history has often been ruled by disease and plague. In surgery, infection remained, after anaesthesia, as the factor preventing its advance. The key to a greater understanding of surgical infection had existed since Alexander Gordon of Aberdeen claimed in 1795 that infection and fever was carried from woman to woman by the *midwife. However, it was not until Ignaz Philipp *Semmelweiss in 1846 had formulated his doctrine of *puerperal fever that the message was clearly received.

Joseph *Lister started his medical studies at *University College Hospital the year after Semmelweiss published his views on puerperal fever. As a child he had developed an interest in *microscopy from his father who had been made a fellow of the Royal Society for work on microscopical lenses. By 1860 Joseph Lister was appointed regius professor of surgery at Glasgow. His contributions to general surgery were significant by any standards, devising an amputation of the thigh through the *condyles (1860), a new operation for excision of the wrist joint (1865), radical mastectomy planned on anatomical principles (1867), and various operations and instruments for *urethral surgery. However, as we read in the *Lancet* in 1855, the excision of the wrist joint led to six cases of gangrene and one of *pyaemia.

Fortunately, Lister was acquainted with the growing influence of the ideas of *Pasteur. This led him to speculate about how micro-organisms could be destroyed by some chemical agent. Lister himself had seen *carbolic acid used to disinfect sewage at Carlisle, and as a result of this he tried carbolic acid in a case of compound fracture in 1865. Initially it was applied undiluted with lint. This damaged the tissue, so in 1866 he mixed the carbolic acid with linseed oil and common whitening. The cases of compound fracture on which he used this less-damaging mixture were recorded in the *Lancet* in 1867. Nine of the 11 patients were alive with intact limbs at 6 months after surgery. With the confidence of this success he recommended that even silk ligatures should be carbolized to prevent secondary sepsis and haemorrhage at the site of ligated vessels.

Lister, in an attempt to kill the micro-organisms in the air which might settle on wounds and lead to infection, attempted to create a bactericidal microcosm by operating within a sterile environment created and maintained by a small hand-spray filled with dilute carbolic acid. Even though this was developed into a more powerful steam-projected spray, Lister abandoned it in 1887. However, his recommended simple gauze dressings impregnated with carbolic acid were used widely until 1889, and thereafter were replaced by gauze impregnated with mercuric cyanide and zinc. His thinking was generally accepted and immediately led to developments such as that by Karl *Thiersch of Munich who, in 1874, introduced a method of skin *grafting which would otherwise have been impossible.

Although this method did much to reduce sepsis, the latter still occurred, and Lister's shrewd surgical judgement led him to advocate the adoption of India-rubber drains, first used by Chassaignac in 1859, to allow any pus that might form to drain away freely. Lister's great contribution to surgery resulted from his ability to relate advances in other fields to those of his own, and to solve problems that had eluded surgeons for generations. Perhaps this can be described as genius, or perhaps explained in the words of Pasteur, to whom he owed so much; 'In the field of experimentation, chance favours only the prepared mind.' Lister's mind was certainly prepared and, happily, it was not as inward-looking as those of his surgical contemporaries, and therein lay his greatness.

Modern times

The surgery of trauma and war has always been a sad and urgent necessity and has, through the ages, led to advances. One notable development, which became an important and life-saving advance, resulting from the impetus of war, was the science of *blood transfusion. This had been anticipated in the 16th century when Hieronymus Cardanus and Magnus Pegeius suggested cross-transfusion. Between 1814 and 1836 James *Blundell at *Guy's Hospital in London demonstrated the value of cross-transfusion in resuscitating exsanguinated dogs. George *Crile of Cleveland in 1907 successfully performed transfusions in seven patients. Thereafter, work on *blood groups, *anticoagulation, and the preservation of blood enabled transfusion to become a realistic possibility, and the collection and preservation of blood was an important by-product of the First World War.

*Plastic surgery was stimulated by the work of plastic surgeons, such as Harold *Gillies at this time and subsequently Archibald *McIndoe in rehabilitating badly burned air-crew during the Second World War in England.

The miracle of *penicillin, discovered by Alexander *Fleming and later developed during the Second World War with dedication and single-mindedness by Howard *Florey and E. B. *Chain, would not have been possible in a time of peace and security. Apart from the impetus of two world wars, steady progress in elective surgery was being made. Ingenious surgeons began to take liberties and make advances which established them as pioneers of the new science. This was justified once the pain, *mortality, and *morbidity of infection, as well as *shock, had been reduced to an acceptable level. Almost all organs now became amenable to elective surgery.

In 1885 Sir Victor *Horsley carried out physiological experiments on the function of various parts of the brain. He developed an antiseptic modelling wax from beeswax and almond oil to reduce the bleeding from the edges of the cranial bones. Although he did not fully appreciate the mechanism, he found that the application of living *muscle tissue to the bleeding surface of the brain reduced haemorrhage. In 1887 he successfully removed a tumour of the *spinal cord—the first operation of its kind.

Chest disease in the form of *tuberculosis was a widespread scourge. Various methods of draining tuberculous abscesses were devised, in conjunction with artificial *pneumothorax which temporarily rested the lungs. Occasionally chest disease appeared to demand pulmonary resection. This reached a sufficiently advanced stage in 1931 for Rudolf Nissen to achieve complete resection of one lung.

Following the initial success with intestinal surgery in the second half of the 19th century, Vincenz Czerny resected the upper oesophagus in 1877 for cancer, and Franz Torek resected the thoracic oesophagus in 1913. Resection of the small and large bowel for tumours, *diverticular disease, vascular lesions, and regional *enteritis became common practice. Success was dependent on great skill and also on a ritual of technique learned from those who were thought of as the old masters, but who were, in effect, merely the great men of the previous generation; the field was moving fast.

Paediatric surgery did not lag behind, despite the rather specialized anaesthetic techniques required. Conrad Ramstedt in 1912 described two cases of pyloromyotomy for congenital hypertrophic *pyloric stenosis. The abundance of vascular injuries over the centuries produced an early interest in vascular surgery. Von Eck undertook the first portacaval anastomosis in 1877, and Berkeley *Moynihan, in 1895, excised an aneurysm of the subclavian artery. It was not, however, until 1944 that John Alexander and F. X. Byron successfully resected a *coarctation of the aorta. The modern age of vascular surgery was ushered in when, in 1964, DeBakey used synthetic Dacron vascular grafts.

Elective, or so-called 'cold' surgery (as distinct from emergency surgery), had, understandably, been preoccupied in the early days with solving mechanical problems. Stones had been removed from the bladder from early times, and by 1905 Howard Lilienthal had reported 31 suprapubic transvesical *prostatectomies without death. This had been refined by Terence Millin, who in 1945 described retropubic prostatectomy. Intestinal obstruction from a variety of causes and perforated peptic ulcers posed little problem now for surgeons, and the mortality of caesarean section, even for *placenta praevia, first undertaken by A. C. Bernays in 1893, was now acceptably low. Delicacy of technique and perfection of sutures allowed the restoration of continuity of even small structures such as the *bile duct, which was accomplished by W. J. Mayo in 1905.

Classically, operations had primarily been directed towards solving mechanical problems, and clinical benefit resulted with restoration of function. Many interesting physiological observations were ultimately made on the alteration of function of organs before and after such surgery. *Renal failure and *diuresis, for example, were studied in patients after surgery for urinary obstruction. Astley *Cooper undertook experimental thyroidectomies in animals to elucidate the changes that were seen after the technical problems of thyroidectomy (for *goitre causing laryngeal obstruction) had been mastered by pioneers such as Theodor Kocher, who published a series of 13 thyroidectomies in 1872 with only two deaths. In studies of function following surgery, physiologists and physicians worked closely with surgeons. It soon became evident that surgery was a tool by which normal function could be altered, and also through which physiological normality could be restored, after removal of an abnormally functioning organ.

An early example of normal function being altered by surgery was *castration, which had been practised from the earliest times—initially on those in charge of harems and subsequently to prevent the breaking of voices of ecclesiastical choristers. In 1881, tubal ligation for *sterilization was introduced by W. P. Langren and, in recent times, both *oophorectomy and *adrenalectomy have been used to alter the *hormone environment of certain tumours, such as breast cancer, in an attempt to reduce their dissemination.

Following a greater understanding of *thyroid function and its control of the *basal metabolic rate, Sir Patrick Watson in 1872 undertook a partial thyroidectomy for exophthalmic goitre. The first subtotal thyroidectomy for this condition was undertaken by Ludwig Rehn in 1884. The possibility of ablative endocrine surgery having far-reaching metabolic consequences led to a close association between physicians and surgeons, which was to herald a new co-operation between specialists who had differing, but essentially complementary, expertise.

A similar co-operation was to exist in the field of heart surgery. The optimal timing of surgery was clearly within the discretion of the physician as well as that of the surgeon. Such a co-operation enabled Henry Souttar in 1925 to attempt digital fracture (i.e. breaking open with a finger) of a mitral valve stenosis (see CARDIOTHORACIC SURGERY) via the auricular appendage of the atrium. Subsequently, success with instrumental dilatation of the mitral valve was achieved by Dwight Harken of Boston in 1948. Two other successes in cardiac surgery took place, first when Robert Gross in 1939 successfully ligated a patent *ductus arteriosus in children, and later when Alfred *Blalock in 1949 anastomosed the left subclavian and left pulmonary artery to reduce the effect of the congenital abnormality of *Fallot's tetralogy.

After the development and insertion of artificial, mechanical, and denatured animal valves into failing hearts, which had considerable clinical success, the ultimate goal in cardiovascular surgery appeared to be the *transplantation of a healthy heart from a donor who had suffered irreversible brain damage (see CARDIOTHORACIC SURGERY). Such a dramatic achievement was accomplished in man by Christiaan Barnard in 1967. This followed considerable pioneering work in many laboratories throughout the world, which was possible only as a result of enormous advances in our understanding of *immunology. However, many scientific and ethical problems were posed by the achievement; techniques had, to some extent, advanced too rapidly.

The concept of organ transplantation had been a dream for generations and had become a reality in the mid-1950s when Hume performed nine kidney homotransplants in patients and Goodrich undertook the first successful liver transplant in man. However, despite the initial enthusiasm for spare-part transplantation surgery, the problems of immunological *rejection, availability of organs, finance, and ethics all dictated that what originally appeared to be the ultimate goal might not be so. In 1982 the first artificial hydraulic heart was inserted into a patient.

The field of *orthopaedics illustrates what has, in many respects, been a happier revolution, raising less controversial ethical and financial problems. In addition, the surgical techniques have developed in parallel with related disciplines, such as those of immunology. After the days of external fixation of fractures, the inevitable progress to internal fixation took place with plates and intramedullary nails. By the mid-1960s, the development of biologically inert implantable material was such that very satisfactory artificial hip joints of varying design were being widely inserted, following pioneering work in many centres. These demanded a high technical ability and a close liaison with mechanical engineers and chemists, who developed biological cements.

Clearly, such a stage of sophistication and technical expertise has been reached in various branches of surgery that the classic concept of general surgery is somewhat outmoded. It will, however, always remain the training ground of all superspecialists, and within it there will always be areas of special expertise, demanding skills and experience equal to those of what are now regarded as the specialized branches of surgery. These have previously been organ-specific, such as *ophthalmology, or system-specific, such as *gynaecology and *gastroenterology, but may now also need to be disease-related.

Although all general surgeons treat cancer, for example, the multidisciplinary approach required now dictates that, at least in some specialized centres, there should be surgeons who have a greater commitment and knowledge in this field. At one time cancer surgery meant merely more radical surgery, as when *Wertheim in 1900 developed his radical *hysterectomy or when Ernest Miles of the Royal Marsden Hospital, London, undertook the first synchronous combined abdomino-perineal excision of the *rectum. Now, however, cancer surgery is undertaken in close association with physicians who supervise *chemotherapy and *radiotherapy. A new area of specialization within general surgery has been born and is now called surgical *oncology.

Technical developments in *fibre-optics, microvascular anastomosis (*microsurgery), and *lasers are being introduced into general surgery, allowing 'minimally invasive' surgery on such organs as the gall bladder and appendix. The contention of Percivall Pott that 'much still remains to be done' and that this should 'excite our industry' is as true today as it was in 1745. See also ARTERIES AND VIEWS, THEIR DISEASES AND VASCULAR SURGERY; CARDIOTHORACIC SURGERY; KEY-HOLE SURGERY; NEUROSURGERY; ORTHOPAEDICS; PLASTIC AND MAXILLOFACIAL SURGERY; UROLOGY.

HARVEY WHITE

Further reading

Bennion, E. (1979). *Antique medical instruments*. Sotheby Parke Benet, London.

Bishop, W. J. (1960). *The early history of surgery*. R. Hale, London.

Cartwright, F. F. (1967). *The development of modern surgery*. Barker, London.

Casrtiglioni, A. (1936). *Storia della medicina* Milan. (Translation: Krumbhaar, E. B. (1941). *A history of medicine*. Ryerson Press, New York.)

Cope, Z. (1959). *The Royal College of Surgeons of England: a history*. Blond, London.

Dennis, F. S. (1905). *The history and development of surgery during the past century*. (Reprinted from *American Medicine*, **9**, Nos 4–7.)

Graham, H. (1939). *Surgeons all*. Rich and Cowan, London.

Hurwitz, A. and Dagensheim, G. A. (1958). *Milestones in modern surgery*. Harper, London.

Meade, R. H. (1968). *Introduction to the history of general surgery*. Saunders, Philadelphia.

Power, D. A. (1933). *Short history of surgery*, John Bale & Sons and Danielsson Ltd, London.

Richardson, R. G. (1968), *Surgery, old and new frontiers*. Scribner, New York.

Zimmerman, L. M. and Veith, J. (1961). *Great ideas in the history of surgery*. Williams & Wilkins, Baltimore.

SURGERY OF TRAUMA, see TRAUMA AND ITS MANAGEMENT.

SURGERY, OPEN HEART. Operative surgery on the dry, non-beating heart, cardiopulmonary function being temporarily taken over by a *heart–lung machine (extracorporeal oxygenator). See CARDIOTHORACIC SURGERY.

SUTHERLAND, EARL WILBUR (1915–74) American biochemist. His first investigations were on carbohydrate metabolism in muscle and liver tissue. In the course of this he discovered the presence, in almost all cells, of adenosine-3′,5′-phosphoric acid (cyclic adenosine monophosphate (*cyclic AMP)). Much subsequent work by Sutherland and colleagues showed that cyclic AMP mediates the action of many extrinsic *hormones on the intrinsic processes of cells—the so-called 'second messenger' concept. For this work he was awarded a *Nobel prize in 1971.

SUTTEE is the Indian custom of widow-suicide by self-immolation on the husband's funeral pyre (see SUICIDE).

SUTURE is the surgical insertion of a stitch or stitches, the stitch itself, or the material employed for stitching; the inflexible fibrous articulations between the skull bones are also called sutures.

SWAB. A wad of cotton wool or other absorbent material for mopping up blood or other fluids, cleaning a patient's mouth, applying antiseptics to the skin, taking bacteriological specimens, etc.

SWAMMERDAM, JAN (1637–80). Dutch biologist. Swammerdam never practised medicine, spending his brief life in physiological and biological research. He devised a muscle–nerve preparation and showed that there was no increase in muscle bulk with contraction. He made many observations on insects and their development and described the red blood cells in a frog's web (1658). His great work *Bijbel der Natuure* was published nearly 80 years after his death by *Boerhaave (1757–58).

SWEATING is the secretion of a weak saline solution by the sweat glands of the skin, the evaporation of which plays an important part in thermoregulation. In extreme climatic circumstances, such fluid loss may be as much as 10 litres a day.

SWIETEN, GERARD VAN (1700–72). Dutch physician. Van Swieten practised in Leiden, but, as a Catholic, was debarred from a university appointment in The Netherlands. He moved to Vienna and completely reorganized the medical faculty, establishing the great Vienna School. He was much influenced by *Sydenham and *Boerhaave, publishing a commentary in five volumes on the aphorisms of the latter (1754–55).

SWIMMING. Surface swimming (i.e. excluding deep diving) in pools, rivers, and the sea is a valuable form of symmetrical whole-body exercise which presents few medical hazards. In Europe, fear of infection, probably well-justified at that time, led to a decline in popularity of bathing during the Middle Ages, which recovered only in the 19th century; now, only bathing in highly polluted rivers is likely to result in enteric or other infections. The sea, given calm water and an absence of dangerous currents, presents chiefly the possibility of occasional envenomation by certain marine animals, notably coelenterates, molluscs, echinoderms, and venomous fishes; their stings can be unpleasant but, in temperate waters at least, only rarely dangerous. 'Swimmer's itch' is a skin reaction to invasion by cercariae of *Schistosoma* spp. (see BILHARZIASIS), non-human as well as human, which can result from bathing in infested lakes in certain parts of the world, including North America. Conjunctival irritation is a well-known consequence of using highly chlorinated swimming-pools. Chlamydial *conjunctivitis can also occur rarely, the organisms being transferred from the genital tract of the swimmer or his or her companions ('swimming-pool conjunctivitis'). Lastly, severe spinal injury, including *haematomyelia, can result from diving into unexpectedly shallow water.

SYCOSIS is suppurative infection of the hair follicles, particularly in the beard area of the face (sycosis barbae).

SYDENHAM, THOMAS (1624–89). British physician. Sydenham has often been called 'the English Hippocrates'. He established the value of clinical observation in the practice of medicine and based his treatment on practical experience rather than upon the theories of *Galen. He was a sufferer from *gout, of which he left a classic description (1649). He published *Methodus curandi febris* (1666) and *Observationes medicae* (1676).

SYLVIUS, FRANCISCUS (Franz de la Boë) (1614–72). Dutch physician. A renowned anatomist, he described the Sylvian *aqueduct and the *middle cerebral (Sylvian) artery. A leader of the *iatrochemical school, he studied salts and ascribed all vital activity to a balance between acid and alkali. He was the first to institute laboratory teaching.

SYMBIOSIS is the living together of two dissimilar organisms in close association, the relationship being mutually beneficial. Examples are the association between cellulose-digesting bacteria and the herbivorous animals in whose alimentary tract they reside, and that between nitrogen-fixing bacteria and leguminous plants.

SYMBOLISM, in psychiatry, is the unconscious mental mechanism whereby an object, person, or idea is substituted for another that is causing an emotional or mental problem. Symbolism is an important component of dreams. It is also a characteristic of *schizophrenic thought disorder.

SYME, JAMES (1799–1870). British surgeon. Syme was, in his time, the acknowledged leader of surgery in Europe; he devised an operation for *amputation through the ankle joint (Syme's amputation). He was Lord *Lister's father-in-law.

SYMONDS, SIR CHARLES PUTNAM (1890–1978). British neurologist. He was the first to describe clearly the clinical picture of spontaneous *subarachnoid haemorrhage and was a brilliant clinical teacher.

SYMPATHECTOMY is the surgical interruption of part of the *sympathetic nervous system, cutting off sympathetic impulses to a part, organ, or region.

SYMPATHETIC NERVOUS SYSTEM. Part of the *autonomic nervous system, which regulates the involuntary automatic functions of the body. The sympathetic nerves are derived from the thoracolumbar regions of the spinal cord (cf. the *parasympathetic system, which comes from the craniosacral portions of the neuraxis) and run in the first instance to a series of cell junctions or ganglia situated in longitudinal chains on either side of the spine; from here the sympathetic nerves, running mostly in conjunction with arteries, spread out to supply the whole body. In general, sympathetic stimuli produce effects directly opposed to those of parasympathetic stimulation. They include: dilatation of the pupils; stimulation of sweat glands; dilatation of muscle arteries but constriction of those supplying the skin and digestive organs; stimulation of the heart; increased ventilation of the lungs; and inhibition of digestive function. Similar effects (hence 'sympathomimetic') are produced by the circulating *catecholamines, adrenaline and noradrenaline, liberated by the *adrenal medulla.

SYMPATHOMIMETIC. See SYMPATHETIC NERV-OUS SYSTEM.

SYMPTOM. A disease manifestation of which the patient complains, as opposed to one observed by others (cf. *sign).

SYMPTOMATOLOGY is most often used in respect of the totality of symptoms, either of a particular disorder or manifested by a particular patient; it is also the study of symptoms generally. Unfortunately the term is being used increasingly as a pompous alternative to symptoms.

SYNAPSE. The site of impulse transmission between one nerve cell (*neurone) and another, where a nerve fibre (axon) of the first neurone terminates in close apposition to the cell body or a branch (dendrite) of the second. When excited, the first, or presynaptic, neurone releases a chemical *neurotransmitter substance which diffuses across the synaptic cleft to bind with receptors on the postsynaptic cell membrane, initiating *excitation (depolarization) in the postsynaptic cell.

SYNCOPE is a sudden temporary loss of consciousness due to transient cerebral *anoxia; it is synonymous with faint.

SYNDROME. A collection of symptoms and signs which tend to occur together and form a characteristic pattern, but which may not necessarily always be due to the same pathological cause.

SYNERGISM is the combination of two agents to pro-duce an effect greater than the sum of their separate individual actions.

SYNGRAFT. A transplant of organ or tissue between genetically identical individuals, which in man means between monozygotic (uniovular or identical) *twins (cf. *allograft, *autograft, and *xenograft).

SYNOVIAL MEMBRANE is the lining membrane of joints, bursae, and tendon sheaths; it secretes the alka-line viscid synovial fluid, which acts as a lubricant.

SYNOVITIS is inflammation of a *synovial membrane.

SYPHILIS. Until *HIV infection emerged, this was the most serious and the most feared of the sexually transmitted diseases. It is due to infection with the spiral bacterium (*spirochaete) *Treponema pallidum*. Apart from *congenital syphilis, it is only acquired by close contact, almost always venereal. The primary manifes-tations of the disease (see CHANCRE) are minor and usu-ally pass off without incident even when untreated; they are sometimes unnoticed altogether. The second stage, weeks or months later, takes the form of a mild general illness with lymph node enlargement and various types of rash, often mucocutaneous (see CONDYLOMA). Dur-ing these first two stages, the patient remains infectious and able to pass the disease on to others. There follows a latent period, which may last for years, or even a lifetime. Late, or tertiary, syphilis then supervenes, bringing with it the tragic and destructive lesions for which the disease has justly acquired its evil reputation. Late syphilis can affect almost any system of the body (see GUMMA), but those of most importance involve the central nervous system (see GENERAL PARALYSIS OF THE INSANE; NEUROSYPHILIS; TABES DORSALIS) and the heart and great vessels (particularly aortitis, aortic aneurysm, and aortic valve incompetence). The advent of *penicillin, to which *T. pallidum* has remained sensitive, has revolutionized the former unsatisfactory treatment of syphilis with various metal preparations, which began in the 16th century with mercury and further developed (1910) with *Ehrlich's 'magic bullet' arsphenamine (*salvarsan). In theory, since no animal reservoir for the organism is known to exist outside man and one or two higher primates, syphilis should be completely eradicable. Although reduced in incidence, however, it remains a major public health problem. See also BEJEL; PINTA; SEXUALLY TRANSMITTED DISEASE; YAWS.

SYRINGE. An instrument for injecting or withdrawing liquids or gases, usually with manually applied pressure. The common form is a cylinder, in which the internal pressure is varied with a piston; the outlet of the cylinder is connected to a tube or hollow needle.

SYRINGOMYELIA is a neurological condition, often progressive, in which an abnormal cavity (or syrinx) develops in the centre of the *spinal cord, usually most marked in the cervical region. The resultant interfer-ence with motor and sensory tracts causes muscular weakness and wasting, with loss of *tendon jerks or reflexes in the arms and a characteristic type of sen-sory impairment known as dissociated anaesthesia, in which pain and temperature appreciation are lost while touch and tactile discrimination are preserved. When the signs suggest that the defect extends upwards into the medulla oblongata, the term syringobulbia is used. See also HAEMATOMYELIA; NEUROSURGERY.

SYRINX. A tube or channel, particularly a *fistula.

SYSTEM. Any one of the major physiological subdivi-sions of the whole organism, each comprising a set of cells, tissues, and organs subserving a broad general function (e.g. cardiovascular system, nervous system, endocrine system, immune system, reproductive system, etc.).

SYSTEME INTERNATIONAL. See SI UNITS.

SYSTEMIC LUPUS ERYTHEMATOSUS is a chronic generalized inflammatory disorder, which may or may not be associated with a rash resembling that of local *lupus erythematosus. It is usually classified with the collagen or connective tissue disorders (e.g. *rheumatoid arthritis, *dermatomyositis, *polyarteritis nodosa, *systemic sclerosis, etc.); and *autoimmunity is clearly involved in its pathogenesis. The clinical manifestations are varied and may affect, apart from the skin, the joints, other serous membranes, the kidneys, the central nervous system, and other organs and systems of the body. See RHEUMATOLOGY.

SYSTEMIC SCLEROSIS, PROGRESSIVE is a chronic and serious disease of unknown aetiology, also and less accurately known as scleroderma, which appears to be primarily a disorder of *collagen. There is gradual and progressive thickening, hardening, and contraction of skin, particularly of the hands and face (acrosclerosis); at the same time, a similar process invades other organs and structures and may cause important damage to the digestive tract, the kidneys, the lungs, and the heart. *Morphoea, or true scleroderma, is a localized form in which the pathological process is limited to the skin.

SYSTOLE is the contraction period of the heart, corresponding to the time interval between the beginning of the first heart sound to the end of the second. During this period, the atrioventricular valves are closed and blood is ejected from the right and left ventricles through the open pulmonary and aortic valves into the pulmonary artery and the aorta respectively (cf. *diastole).

T

TABES DORSALIS is one of the classic expressions of *neurosyphilis, now uncommon, of which the major manifestations are due to degeneration of the posterior columns and nerve roots of the *spinal cord. It is a late complication, which may not develop until 20 or more years after the primary infection. Symptoms and signs include: 'lightning' pains; tabetic 'crises' with severe abdominal pain and vomiting which may be mistaken for a surgical emergency; sensory *ataxia causing unsteadiness in the dark and a positive *Romberg's sign; loss of pain sensation and joint position sense; painless enlargement and disorganization of joints (*Charcot's joints); absent tendon reflexes; muscular hypotonia; and small irregular unequal pupils which react to accommodation but poorly or not at all to light (*Argyll Robertson pupils). Unless *general paralysis of the insane coexists (taboparesis), the plantar responses are flexor and the mental state is unaffected.

TABLET. The usual form in which a drug or drug combination is presented for oral administration, an accurately measured dose being combined with a suitable *excipient and compressed into a convenient and preferably identifiable shape. It may be designed either for chewing or swallowing.

TABOO is a word of Polynesian origin denoting something prohibited, or restricted to a particular class of person, or sacred.

TABOPARESIS is *neurosyphilis with features of both *tabes dorsalis and *general paralysis of the insane.

TAB VACCINE is a killed *vaccine for active immunization against the *Salmonella organisms responsible for *typhoid fever and *paratyphoid fevers A and B.

TACHE. A stain, spot, or *macula.

TACHYCARDIA is a rapid heart rate, whether a physiological or pathophysiological reaction (e.g. to emotion, exercise, fever) or due to an inherent cardiac *arrhythmia.

TACHYPHYLAXIS is the phenomenon whereby repeated doses of a drug result in progressively smaller effects, or progressive increases in dosage are required to produce the same effect.

TADDEO, ALDEROTTI (also known as Taddes of Florence or Thaddeus Florentinus) (1223–1303). He was an early medical teacher at *Bologna, and Dante may have been among his students. He introduced the system of analysing case histories to include all the features of disease in particular patients as a teaching method.

TAENIA is a genus of large *tapeworms (or cestodes) parasitic in mammals including man. There are many species, the two of most medical importance being *Taenia saginata* (the beef tapeworm) and *T. solium* (the pork tapeworm); for both, man is the only natural definitive host. Intestinal infection occurs from eating raw or insufficiently cooked beef or pork contaminated with the intermediate or larval stage of the parasite; since completion of the life cycle depends on intimate contact between cattle or pigs and human faeces, indigenous infection is uncommon in the USA and western Europe. Despite the sometimes massive size of the worms (up to 10 m for *T. saginata* and up to 4 m for *T. solium*), intestinal infections cause little disturbance except revulsion, and are recognized by the discovery of the gravid mobile segments in the faeces. In the case of *T. solium*, however, man may also become the intermediate host with more serious consequences. This can sometimes result from autoinfection from faecal contamination. The larvae migrate to all parts of the body, die, and calcify, causing symptoms perhaps many years after infection. These depend on the site; if in the brain, for example, epilepsy may result. This condition is called cysticercosis.

TAGLIACOZZI, GASPARE (1546–99). Italian surgeon. Tagliacozzi is accounted the 'father of *plastic surgery' and was famed for *rhinoplasty, an operation condemned by the church. He also recorded plastic repairs of the lips, ear, and tongue using the predecessor of the pedicle graft.

TAIT, ROBERT LAWSON (1845–99). British gynaecologist. He was a pioneer of operative *gynaecology and one of the first to operate for tubo-ovarian abscess (1872), *hysterectomy for *fibroids (1873), and *ectopic pregnancy (1883).

TAKAYASU'S DISEASE is a condition, also known as 'pulseless disease' and 'aortic arch syndrome', in which there is progressive obliteration of the major arteries arising from the *aortic arch. It is fairly common in Japan, and affects women more often than men.

TALIPES is any congenital foot deformity (club-foot).

TALIPES EQUINOVARUS is a common variety of *talipes in which the foot is plantar-flexed and adducted, with the medial border raised.

TALISMAN. An *amulet or charm.

TALKING BOOKS are voice recordings of written material, made for the blind. See OPHTHALMOLOGY.

TAMOXIFEN is an *oestrogen antagonist which blocks receptor sites in target organs. It has become the drug of choice in the palliative or adjuvant treatment of postmenopausal breast cancer. See PHARMACOLOGY.

TAMPON. A plug of cotton wool or other absorbent material for insertion into body orifices in order to control *haemorrhage or a flow of secretions.

TAMPONADE is compression of the heart by an accumulation of fluid in the *pericardial cavity sufficient to embarrass cardiac function; this is particularly likely to be the case when the fluid accumulates rapidly, as with bleeding into the pericardium (haemopericardium).

TAPEWORM. Any cestode worm, i.e. a member of the subclass Cestoda of the class Cestoidea. True tapeworms have a head (or scolex) and many segments (or proglottides). Adult worms are parasitic in the alimentary tract of vertebrates; the larval stages occur in the organs and tissues of animals acting as intermediate hosts. The subclass has 11 orders, of which two, the Cyclophyllidea and the Pseudophyllidea, contain species of medical importance. The species are *Diphyllobothrium latum* (fish tapeworm), *Taenia saginata* (beef tapeworm), *Taenia solium* (pork tapeworm), *Hymenolepis nana* (dwarf tapeworm), and *Echinococcus granulosus* (the agent of *hydatid disease). Infestation of man by other species is rare.

TARANTISM was an epidemic form of dancing mania prevalent in parts of Italy from the 15th to the 17th century. It was popularly supposed either to be caused by or to cure the effects of a bite of a spider.

TARANTULA. See SPIDERS.

TARSORRHAPHY is the surgical suturing together of the upper and lower eyelids along all (total tarsorrhaphy) or part (partial tarsorrhaphy) of their length.

TASTE is the sensation produced by particular substances coming into contact with specialized *receptors (taste-buds) on the mucous membrane of the tongue and palate. Impulses from the taste-buds are carried to the brain by fibres running in the *facial and *glossopharyngeal nerves.

TATTOOING produces an indelible mark or design on the skin by introducing permanent dyes with a needle through the *epidermis into the *dermis. Transmission of *hepatitis B is an obvious hazard when instruments are inadequately sterilized. The word 'tattoo' is derived from the Tahitian *tatu*, which means a puncturing. In the UK, except for Northern Ireland, tattooing persons under the age of 18 years is forbidden by law under the *Tattooing of Minors Act 1969.

TATTOOING OF MINORS ACT 1969. This UK Act prohibited the tattooing of persons under 18 years of age, except in Northern Ireland, and except when undertaken for medical reasons by a qualified medical practitioner. Tattooing was defined as the insertion into the skin of any colouring material designed to leave a permanent mark.

TATUM, EDWARD LAWRIE (1909–75). American geneticist. He was awarded the *Nobel prize (with G. W. Beadle and J. Lederberg) for work leading to the 'one gene–one enzyme' concept, that is, that biochemical processes are regulated by genes.

TAUSSIG, HELEN BROOKE (1898–1986). American paediatric cardiologist. Head of the first paediatric cardiac clinic at the Johns Hopkins Hospital. With Alfred *Blalock she helped to develop the Blalock–Taussig operation for tetralogy of Fallot. She probably did more towards the development of paediatric cardiology than any other person.

TAXIS is the locomotor movement of an organism or cell in response to a directional stimulus (as in phototaxis, chemotaxis, etc.); also, the reduction by manipulation of a fracture, dislocation, or displacement of a part or organ.

TAXONOMY is the science of classification of organisms according to their resemblances and differences.

TAY, WARREN (1843–1927). British ophthalmologist. Tay described cherry-red spots seen by ophthalmoscopy at the back of the eyes, now known as part of

*Tay–Sachs disease. He was one of the last men in London to combine the practice of general surgery with that of ophthalmology. He was also an authority on diseases of the skin and of childhood.

TAYLOR, JOHN 'CHEVALIER' (1703–72). English surgeon and oculist. Taylor was a bombast, who advertised his skills with little propriety and prefaced his operations with prolonged harangues about his prowess, which was in fact operatively good. He was well known in his time and was referred to by Dr Johnson as 'an instance of how far impudence will carry ignorance'. He was the author of several treatises on the eye.

TAY–SACHS DISEASE is an inherited metabolic disorder (once called amaurotic family idiocy), the infantile form of cerebral sphingolipidosis (abnormal *storage of sphingolipids). It causes progressive *dementia, paralysis, blindness, and death, the usual age of onset being 4–6 months. A cherry-red spot on each retina is characteristic. It is an autosomal *recessive trait, and occurs mainly among the *Ashkenazi (i.e. Jews of middle and northern Europe). Detection of *heterozygote carriers is possible by serum enzyme studies in high-risk populations, and the *homozygous state can be detected prenatally in the fetus by *amniocentesis.

T CELL. T *lymphocyte.

TEA is an infusion made from the dried and prepared leaves of a small evergreen tree of the genus *Camellia* (particularly *C. sinensis*), widely used as a beverage. Tea, which was known in China at least as far back as 2373 BC, contains tannic acid and the pharmacologically active substances *caffeine and *theophylline. Other herbal infusions, for example 'bush tea', may contain plant derivatives which are toxic (see POISONOUS PLANTS).

TEARS are the aqueous saline secretion of the *lacrimal glands.

TECHNICIANS are those whose profession concerns the technical aspects of medical and scientific work, such as the operation and maintenance of equipment, the laboratory procedures involved in biochemical analyses, histological preparations, etc. Special technical qualifications are normally required, although an increasing number of technicians also possess university degrees in science and occasionally doctorates. North American usage equates 'technologist' with 'technician'. In UK hospitals staff formerly called technicians are now called medical laboratory scientific officers (MLSOs). See PROFESSIONS ALLIED TO MEDICINE (IN THE UK; IN THE USA).

TEETH. The main constituent of teeth is *dentine, which is identical to ivory. A layer of hard inorganic material, enamel, covers the dentine of the exposed portion, or crown, of each tooth; a layer of softer cement covers the concealed, or root, portion. Dentine resembles bone but contains no cells and no blood vessels. The cavity of the tooth is filled with the pulp, soft connective tissue containing blood vessels and nerves. In man, the deciduous, or milk, teeth begin to erupt at about 6 months of life; there are 20 teeth in all, five in each quadrant of the mouth (two incisors, one canine, and two molars). They have all usually appeared by the age of 2 years. From the sixth year onwards, they begin to be replaced by the permanent teeth, the full set of which numbers 32, eight in each quadrant (two incisors, one canine, two premolars, and three molars). The first to appear are the first molars, and the last milk teeth (the canines) have normally been replaced by the twelfth year. The third molars, or wisdom teeth, do not appear for a few more years and may not erupt at all.

TELANGIECTASIA. Dilatation of small blood vessels.

TELEOLOGY is the doctrine of causes, or interpretation in terms of purpose.

TELEPATHY. Extrasensory thought transference. See EXTRASENSORY PERCEPTION; PARAPSYCHOLOGY.

TEMPERAMENT is a combination of the characteristic qualities of an individual's emotional nature, his or her constitutional tendency to react to the environment in a certain way, and the quality and lability of mood. *Galen recognized four types of temperament reflecting a preponderance of one or other of the supposed four body *humours', namely sanguine, choleric, melancholic, and phlegmatic. There have been other more recent attempts to categorize temperamental differences. One such proposes a dimension based on proneness to a particular type of mental disorder: at one extreme is the 'cyclothymic personality', often jovial, friendly, and outgoing but with swings of mood, and prone in the event of breakdown to develop *manic-depressive psychosis; the associated bodily habitus is 'pyknic', that is short, thick, and stocky. At the other end of this spectrum is the 'schizothyme', who is introverted, withdrawn, and shy, and liable to develop *schizophrenia; here the habitus is tall, thin, and 'leptosomatic'.

TEMPERATURE is the measure of hotness, which can be defined as a property determining the rate at which heat will be transferred to or from a body. Temperature is thus a measure of the kinetic energy of the molecules, atoms, or ions of which matter is composed. The basic physical quantity, the thermodynamic temperature, is expressed in kelvins. Other scales of temperature are the *Celsius (centigrade), *Fahrenheit, and *Réaumur scales. The normal body temperature when measured orally averages 37 °C (98.6 °F). It fluctuates slightly, being lowest in the early morning and highest in the evening. It also varies with the menstrual cycle, being lowest during menstruation and highest at ovulation.

TEMPLE MEDICINE. The temple medicine of ancient Greece probably began in the 8th century BC, when temples were first erected to *Aesculapius, the god of medicine; they were called *asclepieia* (singular *asclepieon*). The medicine practised was known as 'incubation'. The patient, after sacrifice and purification, lay down to sleep near the altar of the god, whereupon the remedy for the illness was revealed, either in a dream or by a priest dressed to represent Aesculapius. On recovery, thank-offerings were presented to the temple, including models of the affected part in gold, silver, and wax, and a tablet was erected describing the illness and treatment. Other persons than the patient could incubate on his or her behalf, and in some temples there were professional dreamers who could be hired. More than 300 such temples were mentioned by classical writers, the most famous being at *Epidaurus, Cnidus, *Cos, and *Pergamum. *Hippocrates is said to have been indebted to the clinical material accumulated on the tablets at Cos, but the Hippocratic school, though partly contemporaneous with the temple movement, was independent of it.

TEMPLE OF HEALTH. The principal temple of *Aesculapius, the god of medicine, in *Epidaurus.

TEMPORAL BONE. The paired skull bone which forms the flat part of the side of the head (temple) above the check-bone or zygoma; it houses the structures of the *middle and *inner ear and the *Eustachian tube.

TENDON. A fibrous cord, largely composed of *collagen, attaching muscles to bone; also called a sinew.

TENDON JERK (or reflex) is a spinal reflex elicited by tapping a *tendon to stimulate its stretch receptors; this evokes an involuntary contraction of the associated muscle or muscle group.

TENNIS ELBOW is characterized by pain over the outer aspect of the elbow, localized to the attachment of the common extensor tendon to the lateral humeral epicondyle but sometimes also present over the neck of the radius. It is associated with repetitive pronation and supination of the forearm, and with sports and occupations that require this movement (cf. 'golfer's elbow', which is medial humeral epicondylitis).

TENON, JACQUES RENE (1727–1816). French surgeon and ophthalmologist. He joined the army as a surgeon in 1744 and later acquired renown as an anatomist and ophthalmologist, describing several structures in the eye, including the fascial sheath of the eyeball (Tenon's capsule). In 1788 he published memoirs on Paris hospitals exposing their overcrowding, squalor, and the total disregard for sanitation. These led the authorities to introduce great improvements.

TENOSYNOVITIS is inflammation of a *tendon sheath.

TENOTOMY is the surgical incision or division of a *tendon.

TENOVAGINITIS is synonymous with *tenosynovitis.

TENSION has various senses: stretching, the degree of stretching, or the state of being stretched; the partial pressure of a gas in a liquid (e.g. the oxygen tension of blood); a mental state of suppressed emotion, or conflicting ideas.

TERATOGENIC. Producing abnormal embryos. See TERATOLOGY.

TERATOLOGY is the branch of science which deals with the production, development, and classification of abnormal *embryos and/or *fetuses. The word 'teratology' is derived from the Greek word 'teras', meaning monster, so that the subject matter of teratology is literally the 'study of monsters'.

TERATOMA. A *tumour arising from several different types of tissue, or from persistent embryonic remnants.

TERMINOLOGY. See CLASSIFICATION; INTERNATIONAL CLASSIFICATION OF DISEASE.

TERRY, LUTHER LEONIDAS (1911–85). American physician. Surgeon-General of the USA, 1961–65. Chairman, Study Group on Smoking and Health, 1964; he was among those who identified cigarette-smoking as a cause of lung cancer and as a risk factor for coronary heart disease.

TERTIAN FEVER recurs at intervals of 48 (not 72) hours, particularly the type of malaria due to *Plasmodium vivax* (benign tertian *malaria).

TERTIARY HEALTH CARE. The third order of medical care, namely that provided by 'super'-specialist physicians and surgeons (e.g. neurosurgeons, paediatric cardiologists) and by departments, not found in all general hospitals, into which expensive resources and skilled staff are concentrated (e.g. oncology, renal dialysis, cardiac surgery); patient reference to this level of health care is from both the *primary and *secondary tiers, but chiefly the latter.

TEST. Any examination, trial, or biochemical analysis.

TESTAMENTARY CAPACITY is the capacity of an individual to make a will. It depends on an individual's ability to be aware of his estate and to express his or her wishes concerning its disposal to family, friends, charities, etc. Mental illness does not necessarily impair testamentary capacity, which may need to be judged by expert psychiatric and legal opinion.

TESTICLE. Synonymous with *testis.

TESTIS. The male reproductive organ or gonad, which produces *spermatozoa and (in vertebrates) sex hormones.

TEST MEAL. A meal given to facilitate subsequent biochemical analysis of *stomach contents as an aid to diagnosis. As a diagnostic method, the procedure has been largely superseded.

TESTOSTERONE is the main male sex hormone (*androgen), secreted by the Leydig (or interstitial) cells which constitute the endocrine tissue of the *testis. It promotes the formation of *semen, development of the accessory sexual organs (*epididymis, *vas deferens, *seminal vesicle, and *prostate), and of male *secondary sexual characteristics. Testosterone is secreted in response to stimulation by the *luteinizing hormone (LH) of the anterior *pituitary gland, and in turn exerts a negative feedback action on LH secretion.

TESTS OF PATERNITY. Blood group analysis was once widely used in order to disprove putative paternity (it would not prove paternity), but it has now been superseded by *DNA fingerprinting.

TEST-TUBE BABY. See FERTILIZATION *IN VITRO*.

TEST TYPES are letters of varying sizes printed on a card, used in the measurement of visual acuity. See also SNELLEN.

TETANUS, or 'lockjaw' is due to the anaerobic spore-bearing bacillus *Clostridium tetani*, which, when allowed to multiply under conditions where little or no oxygen is available, produces a powerful and dangerous *neurotoxin. The vegetative organism lives freely (and harmlessly) in the intestine of animals and man, accounting for the wide distribution, particularly in well-manured soil, of tetanus spores; the spores, resistant to destruction by heat and other agents, remain viable for many years. Conditions favourable to their germination occur in necrotic tissue and in deep puncture wounds; when this happens, although the bacteria remain at the local site, the neurotoxin that they elaborate spreads along the peripheral nerves to reach the central nervous system. Here its effect is to cause uncontrolled bombardment by nervous impulses of the muscles, resulting in sustained and spasmodic contractions. The result is similar to that of *strychnine poisoning. Without treatment, death may occur from respiratory difficulty or from metabolic exhaustion. Active *immunization with

a preparation of modified toxin is an effective method of prevention; and *antitoxin is an important component of treatment which now also requires assisted ventilation, muscle relaxant drugs, and nursing in an *intensive care unit.

TETANY is characterized by abnormal neuromuscular irritability leading to cramps and muscular spasm. In latent cases, the patient may complain of numbness and tingling in the extremities, especially around the lips; and heightened neuromuscular excitability can be demonstrated by tapping over the *facial nerve to induce contraction of facial muscles (Chvostek's sign) or compressing the upper arm to occlude the blood supply, when the hand assumes the *main d' accoucheur* position (flexion of the wrist and metacarpophalangeal joints with extension of the fingers and adduction of the thumb: Trousseau's sign). When tetany is fully developed, the hands go into this position spontaneously, and there is plantar flexion of the feet (carpopedal spasm), contraction of the facial muscles (causing the 'risus sardonicus'), contraction of the laryngeal muscles with hoarseness and stridor ('laryngismus stridulus'), and sometimes generalized convulsions. The condition is almost always caused by a decrease in the circulating concentration of ionized *calcium. Possible causes include: low calcium intake, as in *vitamin D deficiency and *malabsorption syndromes; *hypoparathyroidism, either idiopathic or *iatrogenic following *thyroidectomy; respiratory *alkalosis due to overbreathing; metabolic alkalosis due to prolonged vomiting or excessive intake of alkali; impairment of renal function in certain cases; and several other rarer conditions such as hypomagnesaemia (reduced *magnesium in the blood).

TETRACYCLINES are a group of broad-spectrum natural (from *Streptomyces aureofaciens*) and semi-synthetic antibiotics; they were formerly effective against many organisms, but increasing bacterial resistance has lessened their usefulness. They remain the first line of treatment for infections due to *Brucella*, *Rickettsia*, *Mycoplasma*, and *Chlamydia*, and are also useful in chronic bronchitis because of their activity against *Haemophilus influenzae*. They are deposited in growing bones and teeth (causing staining), and should not be given to children under 12 years or to pregnant women. They are also contraindicated in patients with kidney disease. See also ANTI-INFECTIVE AGENTS.

TETRAHYDROCANNABINOL. See CANNABIS.

TETRALOGY OF FALLOT. See FALLOT'S TETRALOGY.

TETRAPLEGIA. See QUADRIPLEGIA.

THACKRAH, CHARLES TURNER (1795–1833). British physician. He was a founder of the Leeds

Medical School and author of the first book in England on *occupational diseases (1831).

THALAMUS. A region of the *brain, situated between the cerebral hemispheres at the upper end of the brainstem, which acts both as a sensory relay station and as a centre for *pain perception.

THALASSAEMIA (THALASSEMIA) is the name for a group of inherited *anaemias in which the basic abnormality is defective synthesis of one or other of the globin chains of *haemoglobin. The name derives from its first recognition in people of Mediterranean origin (*thalassa* is Greek for 'sea'), but forms have since been described in several other racial groups. The two main types are labelled according to which of the two adult chains is affected, that is alpha- and beta-thalassaemia. The *heterozygous, partially expressed, or carrier state is sometimes referred to as thalassaemia minor (or thalassaemia trait), the fully expressed *homozygous disease as thalassaemia major. The molecular genetics of thalassaemia is a rapidly advancing topic.

THALIDOMIDE ($C_{13}H_{10}O_4$) is a drug which gained favour as a sedative and hypnotic following its introduction in Germany in 1958, but was withdrawn from use 3 years later when it became apparent that it caused serious congenital abnormalities in children born of women who had taken it during pregnancy. Prominent among these abnormalities was the otherwise rare condition of *phocomelia, in which the arms and legs fail to develop. It also caused a severe sensory *neuropathy. The use of thalidomide is now restricted to one particular condition, a complication of *leprosy known as erythema nodosum leprosum, in which it is very effective. It was never licensed for use in the USA.

THAYER, WILLIAM SYDNEY (1864–1932). American physician. He described the third heart sound, and wrote about various cardiac *murmurs.

THECA. An enclosing sheath, particularly the *dura mater of the spinal cord. See MENINGES.

THEILER, MAX (1899–1972). South African/ American virologist. His greatest achievement was in attenuating a strain of *yellow fever virus, so that a live virus vaccine, suitable for large-scale immunization of human beings, could be developed. For this work he was given the *Nobel prize in 1951.

THEOPHAGY is the sacramental and symbolic eating of a god as part of a religious ritual, such as that which takes place during the mass or communion service in the Christian church.

THEOPHYLLINE is a xanthine *bronchodilator drug, now mainly used in oral sustained-release preparations for bronchial *asthma.

THEORY. A hypothesis; or the principles of a science as opposed to the practice.

THERAPEUTIC NIHILISM is an attitude of extreme scepticism on the part of a doctor as to the value of treatment, particularly with drugs. It may sometimes conceal a lack of familiarity with modern *pharmacology.

THERAPEUTICS. The science of the treatment of diseases. See PHARMACOLOGY.

THERAPIA STERILISANS MAGNA is the theory of treating disease with an agent which destroys infecting organisms without harming the host, proposed by *Ehrlich.

THERAPY is the treatment of disease.

THERIAC is a supposed *antidote to venomous bites.

THERMODYNAMICS is the study of the laws governing heat changes and the conservation of energy.

THERMOGRAPHY is the pictorial representation of an area in terms of its temperature and temperature differences. The most commonly used method detects and records infra-red radiation from the body surface, but other techniques are possible. It can be used to study superficial vascularity and to detect underlying pathological processes such as some breast tumours.

THERMOMETER. An instrument to measure *temperature. Any physical property of a substance that varies with temperature can be used, such as volume, pressure, electrical resistance, electromotive force, and so on, instruments being designed with regard to the desired temperature range, accuracy, and convenience. The clinical thermometer of today was introduced by Sir Clifford *Allbutt in 1867.

THIAMINE is vitamin B_1, an essential dietary component also known as aneurin, deficiency of which results in *beriberi. It is required for the synthesis of the *coenzyme thiamine pyrophosphate, necessary for one step in energy metabolism, and the body's requirement is approximately related to energy (i.e. *carbohydrate) intake. It is widely distributed in the diet, and deficiency in the West is virtually confined to chronic *alcoholics (who have a large energy intake in the form of alcohol but little or no normal food).

THIERSCH, KARL (1822–95). German surgeon. He was a strong supporter of Listerian doctrine and reawakened interest in the subject by his method of skin grafting (*Thiersch graft) introduced in 1874. He wrote on cancer (1865) and also described phosphorus necrosis of the jaw ('phossy jaw') in 1867.

THIERSCH GRAFT. A very thin skin (split-skin) graft, which, unlike the thicker *flap, does not need to retain its own blood supply during the period following transfer to the new site. See PLASTIC AND MAXILLO-FACIAL SURGERY.

THIOURACIL is a drug which inhibits the synthesis of thyroid hormone by the *thyroid gland and is thus of value in treating *thyrotoxicosis.

THIRD ORDER OF ST FRANCIS. This entirely lay Order, also known as the Franciscan Tertiaries, numbered many famous men and women among its members, including the physicians and polymaths Luigi *Galvani and Roger *Bacon.

THIRST is the sensation of wanting to drink, mediated through osmotic and volume receptors and a thirst centre situated in the anterior *hypothalamus. The stimulus is plasma hyperosmolality; a 2 per cent rise is sufficient to cause thirst.

THOMAS, HUGH OWEN (1834–91). British orthopaedic surgeon. He devised the universally known Thomas's *splint, advocated passive congestion before *Bier, and used silver wire for internal fixation of fractures (1873). His work was largely unrecognized until revealed by his pupil and nephew Sir Robert *Jones.

THORACIC DUCT. The major vessel of the *lymphatic system, which empties into the venous system at the junction of the left internal jugular and left subclavian veins.

THORACIC SURGERY. See CARDIOTHORACIC SURGERY.

THORACOPLASTY is a surgical operation in which several ribs are removed, allowing the underlying lung to collapse, once widely used in the treatment of pulmonary *tuberculosis.

THORACOSCOPY is inspection of the pleural cavity with an *endoscope.

THORAX. The region of the body enclosed by the rib cage, extending from the first rib at the root of the neck to the *diaphragm.

THREADWORM. Any slender thread-like *nematode (roundworm), but the term usually refers to the small parasite *Enterobius* (or *Oxyuris*) *vermicularis*, also called the pinworm, which commonly infests the lower intestine, particularly in children. Infestation is usually asymptomatic, apart from *pruritus ani due to nocturnal laying of eggs by the female in the perianal area. Transfer of the eggs to the fingers on scratching and subsequent ingestion is the mode both of person-to-person transmission and auto-reinfection. Diagnosis and treatment are straightforward.

THRILL. Vibrations at the body surface which can be felt on palpation. The hand is relatively poor at appreciating high-frequency vibrations, of which most thrills consist, and ability to detect them varies between observers. Over the precordium, thrills are cardiac *murmurs, which can be felt as well as heard, with this additional significance: while a systolic murmur may or may not be due to heart disease, a systolic thrill is always pathological. At the apex of the heart, it indicates mitral incompetence; localized to the lower sternal area, either tricuspid incompetence or ventricular septal defect; at the base, either aortic or pulmonary stenosis. See VALVULAR HEART DISEASE.

THROMBIN is an enzyme, formed from the precursor substance *prothrombin, which catalyses the conversion of the soluble fibrinogen into *fibrin. See HAEMATOLOGY AND BLOOD TRANSFUSION.

THROMBOANGIITIS is *inflammation with *thrombosis of blood vessels. Thromboangiitis obliterans is an obliterative vascular condition chiefly of the lower extremities, also known as Buerger's disease; it occurs more often in younger men and is aggravated by smoking. Indeed, it is said not to occur in non-smokers but is particularly common in Ashkenazi Jews.

THROMBOEMBOLISM is *embolism due to a detached *thrombus.

THROMBOPHLEBITIS. See PHLEBITIS.

THROMBOSIS is intravascular blood coagulation during life. The resultant clot, called a thrombus, consists of *fibrin and *platelets, along with other blood cells; it may completely occlude the vessel within which it forms, causing obstruction to blood flow. Thrombosis occurs when flow is sluggish or stagnant, when the integrity of the vascular endothelium has been damaged by trauma, inflammation, or another pathological process, or when blood coagulability is abnormally increased; sometimes these factors operate in combination.

THROMBOXANE is an endogenously produced substance related to the *prostaglandins, derived from arachidonic acid in the *platelets. In its active form, known as thromboxane A_2, it is a potent stimulator of *platelet aggregation and constrictor of arteries, including the cerebral and coronary arteries. It rapidly hydrolyses to an inactive form, thromboxane B_2. *Acetylsalicylic acid (aspirin) exerts its anti-platelet-aggregating effect by blocking the production of thromboxane A_2.

THROMBUS. The intravascular clot of blood formed during the process of *thrombosis.

THROW-AWAY JOURNALS are journals distributed free of charge to the medical profession, or selected members of it, that depend for their income on revenue from advertising, chiefly of 'ethical' products of the *pharmaceutical industry. The opprobrious designation is sometimes, but not always, justified. See also MEDICAL JOURNALS.

THRUSH is oral *candidiasis, characterized by creamy white patches accompanied by *erythema on the oropharyngeal mucosa.

THYMECTOMY. Surgical removal of the *thymus.

THYMUS. A lymphoid organ of vertebrates, usually situated in the pharyngeal or neck region. In man, as in other mammals, it lies in the upper anterior *mediastinum, behind the *sternum. From birth to puberty it doubles in size to reach a maximum, and thereafter gradually undergoes involution. Since *Galen declared the thymus to be the site of the soul, its function has been the subject of much speculation. Although still not fully elucidated, it is now known to play an important part in the body's cell-mediated immunological processes. *Myasthenia gravis, an autoimmune disorder, is sometimes cured by thymectomy. See IMMUNOLOGY.

THYROID. The important endocrine gland situated in the front of the neck which controls the overall rate of the body's metabolism. It has two lobes lying on either side of the *trachea, joined by a small isthmus crossing the midline; it is normally neither visible nor palpable except occasionally through physiological enlargement (e.g. during adolescence or pregnancy). Stimulated by the *thyroid-stimulating hormone (TSH) of the anterior *pituitary gland, the thyroid secretes the iodine-containing hormones *thyroxine and *tri-iodothyronine. It also secretes *calcitonin. See ENDOCRINOLOGY.

THYROIDECTOMY is surgical removal of all or part of the *thyroid gland.

THYROIDITIS is inflammation of the *thyroid.

THYROID-STIMULATING HORMONE (TSH) is the *hormone of the anterior *pituitary gland which controls the function of the *thyroid gland. TSH is also known as thyrotrophin.

THYROTOXICOSIS is overactivity of the *thyroid gland, also known as hyperthyroidism. The abnormally raised *metabolic rate causes weight loss (despite an often large appetite), heat intolerance and sweating,

emotional lability and nervousness, tremor, and tachycardia. In most cases the aetiology is unknown, although both *autoimmunity and genetic factors play a part; this group of patients often suffer from ophthalmopathy, chiefly *exophthalmos, as well as thyroid overactivity, a syndrome known as *Graves' disease. In the remainder, thyrotoxicosis is the result of *thyroiditis or of various types of thyroid or pituitary tumour.

THYROXINE is one of the two main *thyroid hormones, also called tetra-iodothyronine (T4), the other being *tri-iodothyronine (T3). T4 is at least partly converted into T3 by deiodinating enzymes in the tissues, and T3, which is about four times more active than T4, probably accounts for most of the metabolic effects of *thyroid secretion.

TIC. A tic, sometimes also known as a habit spasm, is a repetitive spasmodic movement involving a particular group of muscles, particularly of the face, neck, and shoulders. It is compulsive and unintentional, but not strictly involuntary as it can often be suppressed for a time by an effort of will. It may be aggravated by adverse psychological factors such as anxiety, and diminished by *tranquillizing drugs. It is to this category that the habitual winking, grimacing, and shrugging sometimes observed in otherwise normal individuals belongs. Vocal tics also occur. Although similar repetitive movements may sometimes occur in *encephalitis, or in the rare *Gilles de la Tourette syndrome, tics are usually held to be nervous mannerisms which have become persistent. Childhood tics often disappear with maturity.

TIC DOULOUREUX, also known as trigeminal neuralgia, is a syndrome affecting mainly older adults, characterized by intense one-sided facial pain in the distribution of one or more divisions of the *trigeminal nerve. The pain is spasmodic, dagger-like, and very severe; it is often precipitated by local stimuli such as eating, speaking, touching of certain areas on the face known as 'trigger points', and cold draughts. Attacks occur at varying intervals, and tend to become more frequent with increasing age. The causation is often obscure; in many patients there is a mechanical lesion of the trigeminal nerve or its ganglion (pressure from an aberrant artery) and *multiple sclerosis is an infrequent association, which should nevertheless be suspected in younger age-groups. Spontaneous remissions are usually only temporary, and medical or surgical treatment is required for its amelioration.

TICKS. An order of *arachnids closely related to, but larger than, mites; they are blood-sucking and can act as vectors of several diseases of both animals and man. These include forms of *typhus, *relapsing fever, *Lyme disease and virus *encephalitis. Tick paralysis is a type of ascending motor paralysis reported from certain parts of the world and thought to be due to a toxin secreted by the tick (*Dermacentor andersoni*) itself.

TIMOTHY GRASS is a group of six grasses with sausage-shaped flower-spikes similar to the foxtails, the two commonest being *Phleum pratense* and *Phleum bertolinii*. Their pollen is a cause of *hay fever.

TINCTURE. An alcoholic solution.

TINEA is any fungal infection of the skin. The site (or other characteristic) is usually designated, as for example in tinea barbae (beard), tinea capitis (scalp), tinea pedis ('athlete's foot'), tinea cruris (crotch), tinea circinata ('ringworm'), etc.

TINNITUS is a sensation of ringing, buzzing, or hissing in the ears. It can occur in many conditions, particularly those involving the *cochlea and the *auditory nerve, and as a side-effect of certain drugs (e.g. *quinine, *salicylates), but is often unexplained, especially in the elderly. As an isolated symptom it can be intractable and distressing.

TISSOT, SIMON ANDRE (1728–97). Swiss physician. He wrote on *epilepsy and nervous disease but was chiefly renowned for his popular works on personal hygiene, *balneotherapy, and *masturbation.

TISSUE. A collection of cells of similar type fulfilling a similar function, together with organizing and supportive elements such as connective tissue cells, blood vessels, etc.

TISSUE BANK. A stored supply of human tissues for future use, for example for grafting, tissue culture, etc.

TISSUE CULTURE is the maintenance of living tissue under artificial conditions separately from the organism from which it was derived.

TOBACCO is prepared in various ways, from the leaves and stalks of the tobacco plant, a solanaceous shrub *Nicotiana tabacum*. Tobacco is consumed chiefly by *smoking, in which form it is a potent cause of disease because of tar and carbon monoxide formation. These products are lacking when tobacco is used in ways not involving combustion (e.g. *snuff, *tobacco chewing), which nevertheless allow absorption of the addictive alkaloid *nicotine; undesirable effects may then be only those related to local irritation, as it has not been shown that nicotine itself plays a major part in the pathogenesis of the important smoking diseases.

TOBACCO AMBLYOPIA is a particular type of visual defect associated with heavy use of certain tobaccos. The mechanism is uncertain, but cyanide in smoke is probably a factor and alcohol may also play a part (tobacco–alcohol amblyopia).

TOBACCO CHEWING is one form of tobacco use, less common now than formerly, in which the material is chewed and retained in the mouth for a time before being expectorated; *nicotine absorption occurs from the oral mucosa. The chewing of tobacco mixtures in certain parts of the world is associated with oral *cancers, although it is not established that tobacco itself is the cause.

TOCOPHEROL is a fat-soluble *vitamin (vitamin E), essential for the correct synthesis of *porphyrins and *haemoglobin. Deficiency in human diets is unusual.

TODD REPORT. The report of a UK Royal Commission on medical education set up in 1956 under the chairmanship of Lord Todd, published in 1968. It contained a number of major recommendations concerning undergraduate and postgraduate medical education generally, and the reorganization of the London medical school system in particular. See MEDICAL EDUCATION, UNDERGRADUATE.

TOGAVIRUSES form a subgroup of the *arboviruses; they are ribonucleic acid (RNA) viruses named because of their host-derived envelope.

TOLERANCE, in pharmacology, is the ability to withstand without ill-effect relatively large doses of a drug. It may be acquired as a result of previous administration of the drug (see TACHYPHYLAXIS) or of a substance related to it (illustrated by the resistance of chronic alcoholics to certain anaesthetic agents). Immunological tolerance refers to lack of reactivity on the part of the lymphoid *immune system to a specific *antigen (as distinct from general *immunosuppression).

TOMOGRAPHY is a *radiographic technique which, by altering the geometrical relationship between the X-ray tube and the film during exposure, allows visualization of structures in a single plane (or 'cut') and blurs images in other planes.

TONE usually refers to muscular tone (or tonus), the slight degree of tension normally present in healthy muscles when stretched, which can readily be assessed by passively moving the limbs.

TONICS. A term used to describe various medicinal preparations formerly prescribed with the intention of restoring tone and vigour to the system of those supposedly suffering from a deficiency of these qualities. Such *nostra often contained substances of therapeutic value when used under appropriate circumstances in correct dosage, such as *vitamins and *iron salts, along with colouring, flavouring, *ethanol, and a variety of other ingredients (for example, harmless quantities of *strychnine or *arsenic salts). It is debatable whether the use of such *placebos is ever justified.

TONOMETRY. The measurement of tension, particularly the indirect measurement of intra-ocular tension.

TONSILLECTOMY is surgical removal of the *tonsils.

TONSILLITIS is inflammation of the *tonsils; a common accompaniment of viral and bacterial infections of the upper respiratory tract.

TONSILS. Two small almond-shaped masses of lymphoid tissue situated on either side of the throat, between the pillars of the *fauces.

TONUS. See TONE.

TOPHUS. Tophi are localized deposits of crystalline monosodium urate monohydrate, typical of *gout; they occur in relation to cartilages, bones, tendons, and joints, and may be visible in subcutaneous tissues, particularly over the external ear.

TORSION. Twisting about a long axis.

TORTI, FRANCESCO (1658–1741). Italian physician. He established the value of *cinchona bark (quinine) in his widely read book on intermittent fevers (1712). He introduced the term '*malaria'.

TORTICOLLIS is abnormal persistent or intermittent contraction of neck muscles causing the head to be held in an unnatural and twisted position. Torticollis is also known as wryneck.

TORULA is an earlier name for *Cryptococcus neoformans*. See CRYPTOCOCCOSIS.

TOTAL ALLERGY SYNDROME is a condition in which there is supposed allergy to innumerable substances normally present in the environment, from which sufferers must therefore be protected by controlled, filtered ventilation, specially prepared food, etc. In fact, the condition is 'neither allergic nor total' (see ALLERGY) and other explanations should be sought for the patient's symptoms.

TOTAL PARENTERAL NUTRITION (TPN) is the administration through a catheter placed in a central vein of a patient's whole nutritional requirements, in conditions in which feeding via the alimentary canal is not possible.

TOURNIQUET. A constricting band encircling a limb, usually in order temporarily to interrupt the arterial blood supply and to prevent *haemorrhage from a site distal to the point of compression.

TOXAEMIA (TOXEMIA) is the liberation of toxic bacterial products into the bloodstream. The word assumes a rather different meaning in the term 'toxaemia of pregnancy' (now called pre-eclampsia), as bacteria are not involved in the causation of this syndrome (*oedema, *proteinuria, and *hypertension sometimes progressing to *encephalopathy and occurring during pregnancy or the puerperium: see OBSTETRICS AND GYNAECOLOGY).

TOXICOLOGY is the study of poisons and their effects. See POISONING.

TOXIN is any poison, but particularly a protein poison of animal or bacterial origin.

TOXOCARA CANIS is a common intestinal *nematode parasite of dogs, which can occasionally infect man with serious consequences. See DOGS AS CARRIERS OF DISEASE.

TOXOID. A bacterial *toxin which has been modified for purposes of *immunization.

TOXOPLASMOSIS is infection with the *protozoan parasite *Toxoplasma gondii*, common in birds and mammals; the domestic cat is particularly important in transmission. Human infection is widespread in most communities in dry and temperate zones, although often producing only mild and transient disturbances. In two groups, however, infection is serious: fetuses, transplacentally infected; and patients with generalized depression of the *immune system. The eye (retinochoroiditis) and brain are among the many organs and tissues which may be damaged by congenital toxoplasmosis.

TRACE ELEMENTS. Elements (metals and nonmetals), found in only minute amounts in the tissues of the healthy body, which are nevertheless essential components of the human diet (for example, copper, manganese, fluorine, chromium, selenium, molybdenum) or which may be harmful if taken in excess.

TRACHEA. The windpipe, the tube connecting the *larynx to the right and left main *bronchi and forming part of the *airway by which atmospheric air reaches the lungs. Its wall is membranous and elastic, and lined with mucous membrane; it is kept patent by a series of incomplete rings of *cartilage.

TRACHEITIS is inflammation of the *trachea, common in upper respiratory infections.

TRACHEOSTOMY is the surgical creation of an opening into the *trachea from the front of the neck, an operation described by *Galen in the 2nd century AD and said to have been performed by Alexander the Great with the point of his sword. Present-day indications include: upper respiratory obstruction and failure of laryngeal function; provision of an airway for *artificial respiration; and provision of access to the bronchial tree.

TRACHOMA is a chronic infectious eye disease due to a *chlamydia (*Chlamydia trachomatis*), a common cause of blindness in hot, arid regions of the world. The organism is carried in the genital tract, and infection may occur at birth, in childhood, or in adult life.

TRACT. A collection of nerve *fibres travelling in the same direction and serving a similar function.

TRACTION is the exertion of a pulling force on a part, for example, to maintain bone position during the healing of a fracture.

TRACTOTOMY is surgical division of a nerve *tract, an operation sometimes undertaken in order to interrupt the pathways responsible for severe and intractable pain.

TRAINEE ASSISTANTS. See GENERAL MEDICAL PRACTICE.

TRAIT is a term used to denote any inherited characteristic, such as the relatively asymptomatic *heterozygous state in *sickle-cell disease.

TRANQUILLIZERS. A term used to describe a group of drugs used to calm the emotions but with lesser sedative and hypnotic actions than the *bromides and *barbiturates formerly employed for this purpose. The tranquillizers are sometimes subdivided into major and minor, but the so-called 'major tranquillizers' (exemplified by the *phenothiazine derivatives, the butyrophenones, the thioxanthenes, and pimozide) are better termed 'antipsychotic drugs' (or 'neuroleptics'); they are used primarily for the treatment of *psychoses. The alternative and perhaps better term for minor tranquillizers is 'anxiolytics', since their primary use is in the treatment of *anxiety states. They are almost all derivatives of *benzodiazepine (e.g. chlordiazepoxide or Librium®, diazepam or Valium®; oxazepam or Serenid-D®; lorazepam or Ativan®; clorazepate or Tranxene®; and many others, all with essentially the same action and differing only in speed and duration of action). Tolerance, dependence, and addiction all occur with these drugs. Other anxiolytics include benzoctamine, meprobamate, and beta-blocking agents such as *propranolol.

TRANSAMINASE is the name for any of the *enzymes that catalyse the transfer of an amino group between an *amino acid and a keto acid (transamination).

TRANSDUCTION is a technique of *genetic engineering whereby *deoxyribonucleic acid (DNA) is exchanged between bacteria.

TRANSFER FACTOR. An extract of *leucocytes originally thought to transfer specific immunocompetence to T *lymphocytes; the specificity, however, is now doubted.

TRANSFORMATION is a term used to denote the change undergone by a *cell when it becomes *malignant.

TRANSFUSION is the *infusion of whole blood or blood components. See HAEMATOLOGY AND BLOOD TRANSFUSION.

TRANSILLUMINATION is the examination of a part by placing a light source behind it and observing it from the front.

TRANSLOCATION is the exchange of genetic material between different *chromosomes. See GENETICS.

TRANSMISSION has various biomedical senses; it refers particularly to the passage of nervous impulses from one nerve cell to another or to a receptor organ (see NEUROTRANSMITTERS); to the transfer of *communicable diseases between individuals; or to the transfer of genetically determined characteristics to and through offspring.

TRANSPLANT. An organ or piece of tissue removed from its native site and re-established elsewhere, either in the same individual or in another individual of the same or another species: synonymous with *graft. For terminology, see ALLOGRAFT; see also TRANSPLANTATION OF HUMAN ORGANS.

TRANSPLANTATION OF HUMAN ORGANS
History
In 1800 the Italian surgeon Baronio reported the first clearly defined scientific experiment on tissue grafting. He showed that free '*autografts' of skin taken from the animal to be grafted took permanently if the surgery was skilful, but skin '*allografts' taken from another individual were destroyed after a few days (Fig. 1).

More than a century later, in the classic experiments of Gibson and Medawar (1943), this process was shown to be an immune reaction. These researchers found that after skin grafts taken from a donor rabbit were rejected by the recipient, 'second-set' grafts from the same donor were destroyed more rapidly. As a result of exposure to the donor's skin, the recipient becomes specifically sensitized in a manner analogous to the immunity to *measles that follows infection with the measles *virus.

Billingham *et al.* (1956) showed that the destructive immune response could be prevented if the donor *antigens were presented to the recipient *in utero* or during the neonatal period before the *reticuloendo-thelial cells, the *lymphocytes, and *macrophages of the immune system had developed. The recipient animals were unable to recognize these grafts as foreign and accepted subsequent grafts from the same donor origin. They had developed specific 'immunological tolerance'.

Technical developments
No progress was possible until a reliable method of joining blood vessels together was devised by Alexis *Carrel at the turn of the century, which permitted surgeons to investigate grafted organs. In a series of experimental kidney grafts, Carrel concluded that if the surgery was correctly performed, renal autografts were accepted permanently whereas allografts were destroyed after a period of function of a few days. Thus, he duplicated Baronio's experiments but with a vascularized kidney instead of skin. Further studies of kidney grafting in the dog along similar lines led Dr Murray and his colleagues to perform the first clinical renal transplant at the Peter Bent Brigham Hospital in Boston.

Confidence in the surgical technique of kidney grafting had become established. Some of the early patients still have functioning transplants after more than 30 years, demonstrating that when rejection is avoided, the kidney graft can remain in excellent condition. These two unrelated early experiments were a signal to many surgeons that organ grafting might one day become a more general form of surgical therapy, but tentative trials of allografts from both unrelated and familial donors were extremely disappointing. Initially, large doses of total body X-irradiation were given to the recipient, which damaged the immune system but was extremely toxic and usually did not prevent rejection. However, there were two important exceptions; both of these grafts were between non-identical twins, one was performed in Paris, the other at the Brigham. The advantage of familial donors has been established subsequently and the main transplantation tissue groups, the major *histocompatibility complex (MHC), have been unravelled to a large extent.

Graft rejection
It became clear that without immunosuppressive treatment, rejection was to be expected of all grafts except those between identical twins, and that total body X-irradiation could not prevent rejection except in recipients of particularly well-matched familial donors. Rejection in the kidney is manifested by two destructive processes. Lymphocytes from the blood penetrate the capillary walls of the graft and divide rapidly in the substance of the kidney, causing swelling of the organ and impaired function. This cellular infiltration can often be dispersed with high doses of *corticosteroid drugs, leaving little damage behind. The second immune response is due to circulating *antibodies secreted by *plasma cells (secretory B lymphocytes) in the *lymph nodes and *spleen. The antibodies are specifically active

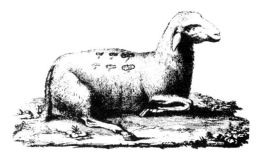

Fig. 1 Baronio's skin-grafting experiemnt. Autografts, below, took satisfactorily; allografts, above, were rejected.

against the graft blood vessels, causing destruction of their lining and eventually blocking their lumina. This humoral response is not easily controlled and much of the damage is irreversible.

Schwartz and Dameshek (1959) reported experiments on rabbits challenged with bovine gamma-globulin (BGG) and given the antileukaemia drug 6-mercaptopurine for the first 2 weeks after the protein injection. Antibody production was inhibited, and subsequent injections of BGG after the 6-mercaptopurine treatment had been stopped still failed to produce an immune response. However, a different protein, human serum albumin, elicited normal antibody production. A 'drug-induced immunological tolerance' had been produced. The rejection of renal allografts in dogs was also impaired by 6-mercaptopurine (Calne 1960) but did not produce a tolerant state.

Elion *et al.* (1951) at Burroughs Wellcome Laboratories, New York, had synthesized a number of anti-metabolite analogues of purine bases; one of them, *azathioprine, a derivative of 6-mercaptopurine, was more effective than 6-mercaptopurine and this, combined with corticosteroids, became the sheet anchor of clinical immunosuppressive treatment for recipients of organ grafts.

Transplantable organs
The kidney was the first organ to be transplanted successfully because the surgery is straightforward. In addition, patients dying from kidney disease (see NEPHROLOGY) can be restored from a moribund state to reasonable health by recurrent *haemodialysis, which can also be used to maintain the patient if the graft is slow to function or suffers from an rejection crisis. With the same immunosuppression, grafts of heart and liver were performed, the results initially being poor as there were no adequate substitutes for function corresponding to dialysis for kidney failure. With the *liver, rejection is less severe than with other organs, an intriguing observation that in some species can be remarkable. In man, immunosuppressive drugs are needed but the

main danger is the operation itself, which is a major trauma in an already sick patient.

With the exception of renal transplantation, organ grafting did not really enter into general therapy until a new immunosuppressive agent, *cyclosporin, was introduced. This agent was discovered in 1976 by Borel at Sandoz Laboratories, Basle, to have powerful immunosuppressive properties. Experiments in animals with organ grafts confirmed the efficacy of cyclosporin, and when it was first used in human renal transplantation in Cambridge, the functional graft survival at a year increased from around 60 to 80 per cent. Unfortunately, cyclosporin was found to be toxic to the kidney and therefore, the dose has to be watched very carefully. In order to reduce toxicity of all the agents used to prevent rejection, a strategy of multiple therapy has been adopted by most centres, giving small non-toxic doses of azathioprine, corticosteroids, and cyclosporin together, so that the agents' immunosuppressive effects are additive but side-effects are minimized.

Organ preservation

This is an important requirement if the benefits of tissue typing are to be applied. Throughout the world there is a shortage of *donor organs, and in many countries superstitious taboos preclude cadaveric transplantation. The ideal donor is a person, otherwise healthy, who has died as a result of head injury, intracranial *haemorrhage, or primary *cerebral tumour, who does not harbour sepsis or an extracranial neoplasm. Such cases managed on a ventilator can be maintained so that the organs to be grafted are in perfect condition until they are removed and cooled. They may then be stored in ice for several hours. The cooling of the organs is accomplished by immersion in cold fluid and perfusion through the blood vessels of special cooling solutions which slow down the inevitable damage which occurs with time. Using modern perfusion fluids, the kidney can be kept in good condition for 36–48 hours, the liver and *pancreas for 12–24, and the heart and lungs for 4–6 hours. These time intervals are important in order to make use of the advantages of getting good tissue matches and also to move the organs to the appropriate recipients.

The world-wide shortage of donor organs means that many potential recipients do not get a chance of a graft.

The present state of organ transplantation

Current control of rejection is by treatment with cyclosporin and triple therapy, together with the use of biological antilymphocyte preparations produced by injecting human lymphocytes into animals. The animal serum is given to prevent or treat rejection. New monoclonal antibodies produced by biological culture techniques may become more effective than standard *antilymphocyte sera, since they are more selective in their targets. Clinicians now have effective control of rejection, so that liver and heart grafting have become routine and lungs can be transplanted with or without the heart.

The pancreas is usually grafted together with the kidney in patients with diabetic renal failure, and results are good. The functional survival of most organ transplants is around 70–80 per cent at 1 year, although with well-matched kidneys, more than 90 per cent functional survival is expected at 5 years. Really long-term survival has now been achieved in recipients of allografts as opposed to identical twin transplants. Throughout the world there are a number of patients with renal transplants still living between 20 and 25 years after transplantation from cadaver donors. The longest surviving recipient of a liver transplant is 23 years and of a heart 20 years; pancreas, 10 years; heart and lungs, 8 years. Thus prolonged survival is possible and *rehabilitation can be excellent. Recipients of all organ grafts can lead normal lives and have children.

Future developments

Despite the rapid advances recently in effective immunosuppression, rejection and infection are still the main causes of failure of all types of organ grafts. Infection is a side-effect of immunosuppressive drugs used to try to prevent rejection. There are now several new agents being studied in man and animals. The drug FK506, related to the *antibiotic *erythromycin, was found to be immunosuppressive by the Fujisawa company in Japan, and has been used extensively in organ allograft recipients in Pittsburgh. The agent is effective in remarkably low doses and has a very similar effect and side-effects to cyclosporin. FK506 is being evaluated in comparison with cyclosporin to determine whether it has advantages.

Interest is now returning to the possibility of achieving tolerance in man. As mentioned above, the Medawar type of immunological tolerance required injection into the *fetus or immediately after birth; however, now there are laboratory models of tolerance produced in adult animals achieved by the use of donor cells together with short courses of powerful immunosuppression. It is expected that there will be advances in the next few years so that application of tolerance to man may be achieved in patients. We would then avoid the necessity of taking long-term potentially dangerous immunosuppressive drugs. Other organs will be grafted, and already the results of intestinal transplants are beginning to look encouraging from London, Ontario, and Pittsburgh.

As the results of organ transplantation improve, so the demand for this form of treatment becomes more and more insistent; already there are many ethical worries concerning the payment of living donors who are not related to the patients, inducing them to give organs or parts of organs; the question of coercion, the use of organs from executed criminals, and how to decide on priorities in organ allocation are all difficult problems.

As immunosuppression improves, so there will be an inevitable extension of the organ graft repertoire to transplantation of other tissues, possibly limbs and gonads. Transplantation of testes and ovaries would certainly cause many new ethical and moral concerns.

The world-wide donor organ shortage inevitably led to attempts to use alternative sources, namely, organ *xenografts from animals. In the 1960s a number of kidneys were transplanted from chimpanzees to man, and one of the chimp kidneys functioned in a human patient for more than 9 months. More recently, a liver has been transplanted from baboon to man; this functioned for 70 days, when the patient died from infection. Transplantation from non-human primates to man is between two relatively closely related species, and overcoming rejection would seem to be a goal that might be achieved in the near future, the so-called 'concordant' xenograft. Grafts from widely disparate species, for example pig to man, are destroyed almost instantaneously, and understanding and overcoming this 'discordant' reaction is currently the subject of intense research. However, the barriers to be overcome are probably great, and even if they were achieved, it is possible that the physiology and metabolism of the organs from a foreign species would not be suitable for man. For example, proteins produced from a baboon's liver would be different and might not be able to sustain the health and well-being of the human.

Research will be focused on these questions in the next decade, and no doubt unforeseen advances, which have always occurred in the progress of science, will continue to surprise us.

ROY CALNE

References
Billingham, M. E., Brent, L., and Medawar, P. B. (1956). The antigenic stimulus in transplantation immunity. *Nature (London)*, **178**, 514.

Calne, R. Y. (1960). The rejection of renal homografts. Inhibition in dogs by 6-mercaptopurine. *Lancet*, **i**, 417.

Elion, G. B., Hitchings, G. H., and van der Werff, H. (1951). Antagonists of nucleic acid derivatives. IV. Purines. *Journal of Biological Chemistry*, **192**, 505.

Gibson, T. and Medawar, P. B. (1943). The state of skin homografts in man. *Journal of Anatomy*, **77**, 299.

Schwartz, R. and Dameshek, W. (1959). Drug induced immunologic tolerance. *Nature (London)*, **183**, 1682.

TRANSPOSITION usually refers to an abnormal anatomical relationship of the great vessels, a developmental anomaly of the heart in which the *aorta arises from the right (instead of the left) ventricle and conversely the *pulmonary artery is on the left (instead of the right) side. The result is severe functional impairment of the circulation. Surgical amelioration is possible.

TRANSSEXUAL. An individual suffering from persistent paradoxical gender identification, or such a person who has undergone *sex change procedures.

TRANSUDATE is the fluid extruded from a tissue or through a membrane.

TRANSVESTISM is a morbid compulsion, also known as 'cross-dressing', to wear the clothing of the opposite sex. Transvestites are usually males who wear female underclothing in order to induce sexual excitement. There is a strong, though not exclusive, association with repressed *homosexuality. They may come to notice because of their tendency to steal ladies' underwear. The condition may be regarded as a form of *fetishism.

TRANYLCYPROMINE is an *antidepressant drug of the *monoamine-oxidase inhibitor (MAOI) group. Like other MAOIs, tranylcypromine has a number of side-effects and can have potentially dangerous interactions with other drugs and with certain foodstuffs (see TYRAMINE).

TRAUBE, LUDWIG (1818–76). German physician. He was the founder of experimental pathology in Germany, publishing his *Gesammelte Beiträge zur experimentelle Pathologie* (1871–78). He studied the pulmonary effects of vagal section (1846), suffocation (1847), and rhythmic variations in vasomotor tone (Traube–Hering waves, 1865). He popularized new methods of physical examination, introduced the *thermometer into clinical medicine (1850), described *pulsus alternans (1872), and the area of resonance to *percussion over the gastric air bubble (Traube's space).

TRAUMA AND ITS MANAGEMENT. Trauma is an injury to the body, especially one resulting from external force.

History
The history of trauma management is mainly the history of military *surgery. Written evidence is scanty before the end of the 18th century, but Ambroise *Paré wrote in 1545 of the benefit of wound exploration and debridement. However, his advice was largely ignored for almost 400 years, because of the surgical obsession with closing wounds.

*Larrey created the first army medical team in 1792, by providing ambulances with trained attendants and equipment to collect the wounded on the battlefield. However, the mortality from wounds in battle was horrendous. An open *fracture was regarded as a sentence of death, with the only question being would death occur before or after an *amputation? The *mortality rate for all kinds of open fractures in the Franco-Prussian war (1870–71) was 41 per cent. Of 13 173 amputations performed on the French side, 10 006 patients died.

Up until 1915 it was policy in all armies that penetrating abdominal wounds should be treated non-operatively. In the American Civil War, there was an 82 per cent mortality rate following penetrating abdominal wounds treated in this way. The concept of exploration for penetrating abdominal wounds was developed by the Russian army in the Russo-Japanese war (1903–5), but it was not until 1915 that operative care of abdominal wounds became the rule. However, there was no concept of the cause of *shock and the reported mortality rate, even with surgical exploration, remained between 50 and 60 per cent. As the First World War evolved, the role of wound excision became regulated and wounds were excised and left open. In 1917, the Allies issued an edict that all war wounds should be left open.

However, at this time the *physiology of shock was not appreciated and the importance of blood volume replacement was not recognized until the late 1930s. During the Spanish Civil War and Second World War, the concept of early blood volume replacement became established and was a major factor in reducing the mortality after penetrating wounds. The American army also paid particular attention to reducing the time between injury and treatment and the mortality rate after penetrating abdominal wounds fell to 24 per cent.

In the Korean War, the American army introduced the widespread use of the helicopter, together with mobile army surgical hospitals to further reduce the therapy-free interval. The mortality rate following abdominal wounds fell to under 12 per cent. During the Vietnam War, advances in understanding of the pathophysiology of shock and pulmonary failure led to vastly improved systemic care of the patient, with data showing that the mortality rate after abdominal wounds in the American army was under 9 per cent.

Knowledge and interest in the management of the injured were much slower to develop in civilian practice. Gissane established the Birmingham Accident Hospital in 1941; this was an experiment designed to improve the care of the injured by providing continuous cover by trained consultant surgeons and *anaesthetists, supported by appropriate technical and transfusion services. In the USA, the stimulus to improve trauma care came with the end of the Vietnam War and the return into civilian practice of experienced surgeons, anaesthetists, and paramedics, who translated their military experience into the care of the civilian injured.

In 1976 the Committee on Trauma of the American College of Surgeons called upon hospitals to commit themselves to provide facilities and personnel to deal with the seriously injured. This group has set standards for staffing and equipment for hospitals dealing with injuries in North America, and has also been a major force in pioneering the concept of trauma centres, where the management of severely injured patients is concentrated in suitably staffed and equipped units.

The Federal Republic of Germany also set up an integrated trauma care system in the early 1970s. This was based on 35 designated trauma centres, each supported by a sophisticated air/ground ambulance system. Skilled medical care was deployed to the scene of accidents, and patients were rapidly transported back to the designated trauma centres.

However, the lessons learnt from North America and central Europe have not been widely accepted within the UK, which continues to lag behind other Western nations in provision of care for the injured.

Modern concepts in trauma care

The aim of a comprehensive trauma care programme is to provide optimum care of the injured from the moment of injury until full physical and mental health is regained. The objective must be to reduce preventable mortality and *morbidity to the lowest possible level.

Death from trauma has a tri-modal distribution. The first peak of death is within minutes of injury. The second death peak occurs within the first 2–3 hours after injury; this time window of opportunity has been referred to as the 'golden hour'. Appropriate intervention during this time can save the lives of the seriously injured. The third peak of death occurs days or weeks after injury and is most often due to pulmonary failure or multiple organ system failure. It is well recognized that failure of initial *resuscitation is a major factor in the development of these two conditions, and therefore early and aggressive resuscitation during the 'golden hour' can improve the survival prospects of those who reach *intensive care alive.

Within the UK, nearly 15 000 people die every year following trauma, of whom 5000 die as a result of road-traffic accidents. Trauma is the most common cause of deaths in adults under the age of 35 years—the most economically active segment of the population. The cost of the 5000 road-traffic accident deaths alone has been estimated at £2.5 billion (US$3.75 billion) annually, giving an estimated cost for the 15 000 deaths annually from all trauma of £7.5 billion (US$11.25 billion). When the cost to the nation of the morbidity following injury is assessed, the total cost to the UK of all accidents annually is equivalent to 1 per cent of the gross national product.

Pre-hospital care

There are two main requirements for the care of the seriously injured—the first is to get the seriously injured person to hospital alive, and the second is to provide that patient with expert surgical and anaesthetic care immediately on arrival. Pre-hospital care within the UK is mainly the responsibility of the various ambulance services, although in some parts of the country local *general practitioners are active in locally organized immediate care schemes. Within the USA, Australia, and South Africa, pre-hospital care is increasingly provided by specially trained *paramedics, who have skills in airway management and fluid resuscitation. In European countries such as France, Belgium, and Germany, doctors are usually involved in the provision of field care.

Within the UK, paramedic training schemes first became established in the mid 1970s and have gradually spread across the country. The *National Health Service Training Directorate has been involved in producing a standardized training manual for paramedic training and this is now used by all ambulance services throughout the country. The *Department of Health has set a target of every emergency vehicle having one trained paramedic aboard by the end of 1995, and currently ambulance services around the country are working hard to achieve this target. However, there is still concern about the intervention of paramedics within the field. Some groups have expressed concern that delay while carrying out certain tasks in the field may delay the patient's transfer to hospital and some authorities have advocated a return to the 'scoop and run' policy.

The Pre-Hospital Trauma Life Support (PHTLS) programme, which was developed in the USA by the National Association of Emergency Medical Technicians, concentrates on training paramedics to recognize rapidly those patients with severe injuries who need rapid extrication from the scene of the accident and rapid transfer to an appropriate receiving hospital. It also teaches a logical resuscitation system which integrates with the Advanced Trauma Life Support (ATLS) programme, currently in widespread use as a resuscitation protocol in hospitals.

The military experience has clearly shown the value of rapid transfer from scene of injury to definitive care, and within the military environment transport by helicopter is almost universal. Within parts of North America and Europe sophisticated air transport is also widely used. There are a number of pilot schemes now being evaluated within the UK, and it is likely that the role of helicopter transfer of the injured to definitive care centres will increase within the UK.

Hospital care

The improvement in training and resources available for pre-hospital care should ensure that all those who survive beyond the first few minutes of their accident will be able to reach hospital alive. However, there is evidence from a number of studies within the UK that there are serious deficiencies in the provision of care for those who reach hospital alive after serious injury. The *Royal College of Surgeons of England produced data in 1988 that showed that up to 30 per cent of those who died of injury following admission to hospital, died from potentially treatable causes. Further studies have confirmed these findings, and preventable death rates of between 20 and 40 per cent have been reported from various centres within the UK.

The system also needs to ensure that a rare commodity—the seriously injured patient—is brought into rapid association with a rarer resource—experienced surgeons and anaesthetists, capable of undertaking life-saving intervention. In its report of 1988, the *Royal College of Surgeons reported on a prospective study carried out in four hospitals in the UK. Of 150 consecutive trauma patients admitted to hospital, 71 per cent of the initial consultations were at *senior house officer level, and in only 11 per cent were such patients seen by a *senior registrar or *consultant. Of the 71 patients

requiring surgery for their injuries, a consultant surgeon was present in only four cases. Out of the 150 patients, 21 per cent died and analysis showed that one-third of these deaths were potentially preventable.

Traditionally, within the UK the supervision of care in accident and emergency departments was formerly the responsibility of *orthopaedic surgeons. However, in 1970 the accident Services Review Committee indicated that from the staffing point of view, the orthopaedic solution had failed. It revealed that consultant cover in the accident and emergency department was often nominal.

As a result, in 1971 the Joint Consultants Committee recommended that accident and emergency departments be placed under the control of a new type of specialist—namely a consultant in accident and emergency medicine. Three years later, positive benefit had been reported from all the appointments initiated under the pilot scheme. A further report from the Joint Consultants Committee in 1978 stated that the new system was developing well and this report confirmed that all accident and emergency departments should be placed under the direction of consultants in accident and emergency. Since then, the specialty has grown rapidly and now the vast majority of accident and emergency departments in the UK are supervised by consultants in accident and emergency medicine. However, most of these departments have only one such consultant and this is clearly inadequate for a service required for 24 hours a day, 7 days a week. New training programmes at senior registrar and registrar level have helped to improve the provision of middle-grade cover, where such units are approved for training. Nevertheless, it remains the case that in most accident and emergency departments in the UK, the initial medical contact would inevitably be with an inexperienced senior house officer.

The Department of Health has approved plans for expanding the specialty of accident and emergency medicine, with a view to seeing that all accident and emergency departments are supervised by trained consultants. In some areas of the UK, health authorities are trying to move further. In its framework for hospital medical services in the year 2000, the Oxford Regional Health Authority has recently recommended that all hospitals providing accident and emergency cover should ensure that the departments are supervised by a trained consultant in accident and emergency for 24 hours a day, 7 days a week. Clearly, the application of such recommendations across the country will require significant resources. However, if care can be supervised by trained consultants, then the standard of resuscitation and treatment should be improved.

Until such a radical change occurs, the current thrust is to ensure that training of junior medical staff is such that they are able to assess and initiate resuscitation of the severely injured. The ATLS programme was introduced to the UK in 1988. This programme, developed by the American College of Surgeons in the late 1970s, is designed to teach an individual doctor the skills of assessment and treatment necessary to manage safely a severely injured patient during the 'golden hour'. The scheme within the UK is administered by the *Royal College of Surgeons of England and has proved extremely successful. In the first 5 years of the programme, over 2500 doctors have successfully completed ATLS provider courses and a further 250 have gone on to train as ATLS instructors, to develop the programme further. Both the Royal College of Surgeons of England and the *Royal College of Anaesthetists are seriously considering making possession of an ATLS certificate a requirement for higher specialty training. The current emphasis of the programme is now to train junior doctors (at senior house officer and registrar level) in the principles of assessment and resuscitation of the seriously injured.

It has become increasingly clear over the past 15 years that to manage the seriously injured, multidisciplinary teams are required. The complexity of modern trauma care is such that no one individual surgeon or anaesthetist can hope to retain all the knowledge or skills necessary for optimum care.

The current concept, used in many hospitals internationally, is that of the 'trauma response team'. Individual hospitals are responsible for defining the composition of their team, together with the criteria for call-out. Typically, a trauma response team will consist of junior doctors from accident and emergency, anaesthesia, general surgery, and *orthopaedic surgery departments, led by a more senior doctor from one of these specialties as the trauma team-leader. Recent work by Driscoll and Vincent has clearly shown the benefit to patients derived from the development of trained trauma response teams under effective leadership.

The importance of the definitive care specialties being involved in the initial assessment is, first, to bring their requisite skills to the patient and to ensure that there is no delay in the provision of any necessary anaesthetic and surgical skills for resuscitation. Secondly, the involvement of the definitive care specialty at an early stage ensures that correct decisions about definitive care are taken and patients can proceed rapidly to the operating theatre or intensive care unit if required.

To develop the concept of trauma care further in the UK, it will obviously be necessary for some consultants in the definitive care specialties (anaesthesia, general surgery, trauma and orthopaedic surgery, *neurosurgery, and *plastic surgery) to make the care of the injured their main professional area of expertise. Between 60 and 80 per cent of patients admitted to UK hospitals with multiple trauma will have musculoskeletal injuries, and some trauma and orthopaedic surgeons have given up elective orthopaedic work to concentrate solely on the management of the injured. It is likely that over the next 5–10 years this trend will also become apparent in other definitive care specialties and the

number of trained consultants with a special interest and expertise in injury management will steadily increase.

Such developments obviously require assessment; the Department of Health has made it a priority in the UK for hospitals who receive the injured to *audit their performance. It is currently trying to encourage all such hospitals to participate in the national Major Trauma Outcome Study (MTOS). This is an audit programme, run by the North-Western Injury Research Centre in Manchester. Participating hospitals enter data relating to injury pattern, physiological disturbance on arrival in hospital, and age; these data are compared with both the national database and the North American database. On a regular basis, the participating units receive data analysis, which allows them to evaluate their own performance against national and international standards. The system also allows such hospitals to identify unexpected survivors and unexpected deaths from major injury for further evaluation of their individual performance. The involvement of the Department of Health in this programme is encouraging, and it is likely that it will be a requirement that all hospitals receiving the injured participate in this programme. It is to be hoped that routine participation in such an audit programme will lead to development of further audit and evaluation packages so that changes in provision of care can be evaluated.

Another major deficiency in the provision of trauma care within the UK is the relative lack of dedicated *rehabilitation facilities. It has been said that the three 'Rs' of trauma management are resuscitation, reconstruction, and rehabilitation. The first two proceed simultaneously from the time of injury, but the third is all too often neglected following initial surgical reconstruction. In contrast, sophisticated trauma systems in North America and Europe have integrated rehabilitation units in their programmes. These ensure that following surgical management, intensive physical and *occupational therapy are provided for the patient to restore optimum function. In the past few years, it has become appreciated that the psychological impact of trauma is often the major determinant regarding how patients will function after major injury. There are units in North America and Europe (and now at least one in the UK) that are actively looking at psychological intervention during the hospital stay and subsequently are trying to minimize the psychological/psychiatric effects of major injury. Such developments are long overdue, bearing in mind that the overall objective of the trauma care system must be to provide the necessary resources to ensure that all patients are restored to full physical and mental health as quickly as possible.

Conclusion

In the developed world, trauma continues to be a major cause of preventable mortality and morbidity, especially amongst the economically active segment of the population. Unfortunately, despite the major financial cost to society, there has been a lack of will to focus on the problem in most developed countries. With the exception of the former West Germany, which has a highly integrated system, the response in most Western countries to the injured is piecemeal.

Over the past 10 years there have been major strides forward in the provision of trauma care, particularly in North America and western Europe. Unfortunately, the UK has lagged behind in the developments that have occurred. The task for the next decade must be to improve the standards and quality of care offered to the injured throughout the UK, in an attempt to reduce dramatically the massive financial and human cost to the nation.

PETER WORLOCK

Further reading
American College of Surgeons (1989). *Advanced trauma life support provider manual*. American College of Surgeons, Chicago.
Border, J. R., Allgower, M., Hansen, S. T., and Ruedi, T. P. (ed.) (1990). *Blunt multiple trauma–comprehensive pathophysiology and care*. Marcel Dekker, New York.
British Orthopaedic Association (1992). *The management of skeletal trauma in the United Kingdom*. British Orthopaedic Association, London.
McMurtry, R. Y. and McLellan, B. A. (ed.) (1990). *Management of blunt trauma*. Williams and Wilkins, Baltimore.
Royal College of Surgeons of England (1988). *Report of the Working Party on the management of patients with multiple injuries*. Commission on the Provision of Surgical Services, Royal College of Surgeons of England, London.

TREATMENT. The application of remedies to disease; the general management of illness. This is the central purpose and *raison d'être* of the profession of medicine; its objectives were set down by the anonymous author of the 15th century folk-saying: *guérir quelquefois, soulager souvent, consoler toujours* (to cure sometimes, to relieve often, to comfort always).

TREMATODE. See FLUKES.

TREMOR is a form of involuntary movement in which there is a constant high-frequency rhythmic oscillation of a body part or parts. The commonest type is postural tremor, most easily observed (and palpated) in the fingers with the arms outstretched and the fingers separated. A very slight tremor can usually be detected in normal subjects; it is part of the physiological mechanism for maintaining posture. More obvious tremor can have several causes: it occurs in *anxiety states, *thyrotoxicosis, chronic *alcoholism (an important sign), as a result of certain *sympathomimetic and *antidepressive drugs, and in heavy metal poisoning; it may also result from structural brain disease (e.g. *neurosyphilis, *cerebellar disease, *Wilson's disease); one form, termed 'benign essential', is inherited and a similar tremor is characteristic of senility. Other types are rest or static tremor, which occurs in *Parkinson's

disease and other extrapyramidal disorders, and intention tremor, which is greatly intensified towards the end of a purposive movement; the latter indicates cerebellar or brainstem disease, due for example to *multiple sclerosis.

TRENCH FEVER is an infectious disease due to a *rickettsia-like organism (*Rochalimaea quintana*) transmitted by the human *body louse (*Pediculus humanus humanus*). As the name implies, trench fever flourished in Europe during the First World War; it remains endemic in parts of Europe, Africa, Asia, and America. It has features resembling *typhus but is rarely fatal; the course is characteristically recurrent, with eventual complete recovery. Like other diseases in the typhus groups, it has many synonyms, for example five-day fever, quintan fever, Meuse fever, shin bone fever, Volhynia fever, and His–Werner disease.

TRENCH FOOT. See IMMERSION FOOT.

TRENDELENBURG, FRIEDRICH (1844–1924). German surgeon. He was the first to administer endotracheal *anaesthesia through a *tracheostomy (1869), to undertake gastrostomy (1877), and to operate for pulmonary *embolism (1908). His position of the supine patient with the pelvis elevated, his test for competence of the long saphenous vein, and his sign for dislocation of the hip are all familiar.

TRENDELENBURG'S POSITION. Lying on the back on a table which is angulated at the knees so that the thighs, trunk, neck, and head are sloping backwards and downwards at an angle of about 40° and the lower legs forwards and downwards by about the same amount.

TREPAN. An obsolete cylindrical saw for removing a circle of bone from the skull.

TREPHINE is the modern version of the *trepan: a crown saw with a central guiding pin, designed to remove a circular disc of bone, usually from the skull.

***TREPONEMA* IMMOBILIZATION TEST.** A specific serological test for *syphilis, in which a positive result is the immobilization of a live motile culture of *Treponema pallidum* in the presence of *complement by *antibody in the patient's serum. Though highly accurate when properly performed, the test is expensive and laborious, and one of the many other tests available for detecting treponemal antibody is usually preferred.

TREPONEMA PALLIDUM is the spiral bacterium (spirochaete) which causes *syphilis.

TREVES, SIR FREDERICK Bt (1853–1923). British surgeon. Treves operated on King Edward VII for acute *appendicitis on 24 June 1902, which led to the coronation being postponed. He was the author of several textbooks as well as books of travel and *belles-lettres*. He was also the holder of a 'master mariner's ticket'. Also see ELEPHANTIASIS

TRIAGE is the assortment of casualties according to severity, urgency, nature of treatment required, and proposed disposal. See TRAUMA AND ITS MANAGEMENT.

TRIAMCINOLONE is a potent synthetic *glucorticoid available in preparations for oral, intramuscular, intraarticular, and topical use.

TRIBADISM is mutual genital friction, or more elaborate simulation of heterosexual intercourse employing a prosthetic penile device, between female homosexuals (lesbians).

TRICHINELLA SPIRALIS. See TRICHINIASIS.

TRICHINIASIS, also known as trichinosis and trichinellosis, is due to infestation with the small parasitic *nematode worm *Trichinella spiralis*. Infection, which is common and often passes unnoticed, is acquired by eating inadequately cooked infected meat, usually pork. Ingested larvae develop in the intestine into adult forms (sometimes causing gastrointestinal symptoms) and produce a second generation of larvae; these then disseminate widely throughout the body via the blood and lymphatic circulation causing systemic symptoms, usually between 7 and 14 days after the initial infection. Among the various manifestations, fever, malaise, periorbital oedema, petechial haemorrhages, and muscle pain and tenderness are prominent. Complications are rare but can be serious; they include *pneumonia, *myocarditis, and *meningoencephalitis. In their absence, the condition resolves in a few weeks. Larvae persist mostly in skeletal muscle, where they become encysted and eventually calcified. The prevalence of trichiniasis in pigs can be greatly reduced by not feeding them raw garbage.

TRICHOLOGY is the study of hair.

TRICHOMONIASIS is infection with one of the mobile flagellated protozoal organisms belonging to the genus *Trichomonas*. The important species in man is *T. vaginalis*, which causes irritation and discharge in the urogenital tract, mainly the vagina and male urethra. Trichomoniasis is often transmitted by sexual intercourse. As it may be asymptomatic, it is important to investigate, and if necessary to treat, both members of a sexual partnership.

Other trichomonad species are found in man (*T. hominis, T. tinax*) but are not pathogenic. Some cause disease of animals and are of importance in veterinary medicine, for example, those causing mortality among young turkeys (*T. gallinarum*) and abortion in cattle (*T. fetus*).

TRICHOPHYTON is a genus of fungi, some species of which cause superficial infections of the skin, nails, and hair, including some cases of *ringworm.

TRICHROMAT. An individual with normal *colour vision.

TRICUSPID VALVE. The right atrioventricular valve. See VALVES, CARDIAC.

TRIGEMINAL NERVE. The fifth cranial nerve, which through its three divisions (ophthalmic, maxillary, and mandibular) carries nerve fibres responsible for sensation over the face, within the mouth and nasal cavity, and from the teeth; the mandibular division also carries motor fibres to the muscles of the jaw. See also TIC DOULOUREUX.

TRIGEMINAL NEURALGIA. See TIC DOULOUREUX.

TRI-IODOTHYRONINE is one of the two main *thyroid hormones, the other being *thyroxine. Tri-iodothyronine (T_3) is four times more active than thyroxine and accounts for most of the metabolic effects of thyroid secretion.

TRI-ORTHO-CRESYL PHOSPHATE is a toxic organophosphorus compound which has caused outbreaks of polyneuropathy by contamination of bootleg liquor or illicit cooking oil. See POISONING.

TRISMUS is spasm of the jaw muscles, which may be due to a local inflammatory lesion or to the muscular rigidity of *tetanus; it may cause inability to open the mouth (lockjaw).

TRISOMY is a chromosomal abnormality in which an extra (third) *chromosome is present with one of the normal 23 pairs, so that the total chromosome complement is 47 instead of 46. Trisomy 21 results in *Down's syndrome or mongolism; other developmental anomalies are produced by trisomy at other locations. See also GENETICS.

TROCAR. A stout surgical needle employed in conjunction with a *cannula to puncture body cavities, the trocar being subsequently withdrawn to allow the drainage of fluid.

TROCHANTERS. Two large protuberances below the neck of the femur (known as the greater and lesser trochanters) to which muscles are attached.

TROILISM is the involvement of three individuals simultaneously in sexual activity.

TROPHOBLAST. The outer epithelial layer which encloses all embryonic structures in the placental mammal, from which the *chorion, the *amnion, and the embryonic side of the *placenta, are derived.

TROPHOBLAST BIOPSY (CHORIONIC CELL BIOPSY) is removal of a fragment of *trophoblastic tissue at an early stage of pregnancy (before *amniocentesis is possible) so that cells of embryonic origin can be subjected to genetic analysis.

TROPICAL MEDICINE AND PARASITOLOGY
Introduction
Tropical medicine is remarkable among the specialties of medicine in being defined neither by the organ of the body affected, nor the age of the patient, nor the agent of disease, but by the part of the world where the illness was acquired. It has been affected far more than most specialties, in its history and definition, by political realities and social values, and can best be understood in a historical perspective. A clear perception of the origins of the concepts may explain the confusion and clarify the future of the subject. The ties of tropical medicine to *public health of developing countries (traditionally called tropical hygiene) are so close that they have to be considered together, and both are related to the natural history of the agents and vectors of warm climate diseases: the science known as parasitology. For the first half of the 20th century tropical medicine and parasitology were closely intertwined and almost synonymous.

History
Although medical practice in the tropics originally comprised the traditional medical systems of indigenous peoples, except for the use of *quinine as an antimalarial originally among the Incas, indigenous medical systems had little impact on 'tropical medicine', as usually defined, until recently. Rather, the subject arose from the problems encountered by explorers and the military, and developed as a necessary aspect of the colonial system.

Mortality amongst Europeans visiting the tropics, from the time of the earliest Portuguese and Spanish explorers, was very high. In addition to the nutritional problems of long sea voyages, visits to tropical ports were accompanied, or shortly followed, by fevers with or without *jaundice, diarrhoeal diseases, and many other illnesses. In both West Africa and the Caribbean the most lethal were what we would now call *malaria and *yellow fever, with men of the garrisons in Jamaica dying at the rate of 13 per cent per year in the early 19th century. Even in South and South-East Asia, where yellow fever was absent, 45 per cent of a military expedition to Burma in 1824 died of disease. With so high a mortality, there was a clear need for understanding and control of the diseases of these tropical areas, and the military medical services had a large role in this.

The initial discovery that linked medicine in the tropics to specific biological processes was, however, made by a civilian British physician working in Amoy (Xiamen) in China, on the spread of *elephantiasis (swelling of the limbs) which had been shown by Lewis and by Bancroft to be caused by a filarial *worm. Patrick Manson (1878) demonstrated that the embryos of the worm were found in the peripheral blood only at night and that they underwent development in a night-biting mosquito which was responsible for transmission of the infection. This was the first demonstration of an insect vector of human disease, adding two further connotations to the idea of tropical disease: first, that many are transmitted by insect vectors, and, secondly, that the life cycle of many agents of tropical disease involves development outside the human body, and that this stage is temperature-dependent. Where the extrinsic part of the cycle (outside the human body) is in an insect or other organism living at environmental temperature, the association of the disease with a warm climate is explained.

In the decades that followed, corresponding to the golden age of *bacteriology, mosquitoes were shown to be responsible for the transmission of malaria and yellow fever, and many other diseases peculiar to the tropics were shown to be insect-borne, while the role of ticks and snails in the transmission of infections was discovered, together with the role of mammalian reservoirs of viral, bacterial, and parasitic diseases. The strong zoological and natural history component of tropical medicine was thus established.

Parasitology
Although the Greek origin of the word 'parasite' simply applies association, parasitism is used by scientists to imply that one organism lives in or on another and is usually nutritionally dependent on it. To the concept of dependence is often added that of doing harm, or pathogenicity, especially when considering the organisms parasitic on man. Those that simply share man's food, such as the intestinal microbes, are usually called commensals, and where the relationship is one of mutual dependence (as with the alga and fungus that together comprise a lichen), it is known as *symbiosis. Now, although plants, animals, *fungi, and other organisms down to the viruses may be parasitic, the science of 'parasitology' has come to mean the study of a much reduced subset of these, the parasites belonging to the animal kingdom. Most of these are either protozoa, acellular small animals, or helminths, the parasitic worms. In addition, parasitic arthropods (insects, ticks, and mites) which live on the outside of the body (ectoparasites) are included. Beyond that, the definition of parasitology seems to be culture-dependent. Blood-sucking insects and other arthropods that bite man are often included in the USA, even though they usually do not stay on people after feeding. However, many act as vectors of protozoa and helminths. In France, it is

customary to deal with the fungi that infect man as part of human parasitology, whereas they are part of *micro-biology in anglophone countries. Because the animal parasites of man almost all have an extrinsic cycle which is temperature-dependent, the classic tropical diseases are predominantly parasitic, often vector-borne, diseases and it is easy to see how tropical medicine and parasitology became so intertwined.

Epidemic disease control

The 19th century scientific advances in understanding parasitic disease transmission were accompanied by, and sometimes due to, concern for practical problems of *epidemic disease control in the tropics. Interest in tropical countries moved from exploration to colonization, and the period 1890–1910 was marked by disease outbreaks on a scale that could not be ignored by governments. In particular, *sleeping sickness was responsible for the death of perhaps one-third of the population of southern Uganda. India was affected by epidemics of *plague and of *kala-azar, while the great Punjab malaria epidemic of 1908 led to an intensified interest in malariology. In the New World the building of the Panama canal depended on adequate measures for control of yellow fever and malaria. The complex life cycles of the major parasitic and other vector-borne diseases were elucidated, usually by the military or by expeditions from industrial countries, but the life cycle of *schistosomiasis was first determined by Japanese workers in their own country.

To control epidemics in the absence of adequate *chemotherapy, emphasis had to be placed on the environmental control of vectors. It had been found that malaria was transmitted only by anopheline mosquitos, and that in a given area only a few species are important vectors, with specific breeding habitats: some species lived in swamps, others in small sunlit pools, and yet others in shaded streams. Environmental modifications directed to removing the specific habitats of the major vectors often achieved good results at moderate cost, an approach known as species sanitation. Sleeping sickness was similarly controlled by selective removal of vegetation to make the area unattractive to tsetse flies.

Tropical health-care systems

As colonial governments became involved with the welfare of indigenous populations as well as colonists, there was a gradual expansion of health-care systems to the major towns, while the concept of a medical officer with responsibility for the defined population of a district developed. The doctors were expatriates, of military or civilian origin, depending on the country. Thus in the French African territories a military system operated and has continued; in India the Indian Medical Service was primarily military, but doctors could be seconded to the civil service; and in British parts of Africa a civil Colonial Service provided medical care.

To train European doctors in the diseases peculiar to the tropics, schools of tropical medicine were set up at the beginning of the 20th century, gradually taking over the lead in this area from the military. They reflected the shift from military to trading ventures and colonization, and were usually sited at major ports. They gradually became more associated with imperial power (e.g. the Royal Tropical Institute in Amsterdam), and the corresponding national colonial territories. France and the UK, with a widespread distribution of their colonies around the globe, tended to have a world-wide interest.

Research laboratories were often established in the tropics in response to a particular problem, but some had a broader function, such as the Institute for Medical Research in Kuala Lumpur, founded at the beginning of the century. The *Rockefeller Foundation founded laboratories specifically to study yellow fever in Belem, Trinidad, Poona, and several places in Africa. Other research institutes were of indigenous origin, such as the Oswaldo Cruz Institute in Brazil. In the UK, the early part of the 20th century saw the emergence of the London and Liverpool Schools with a focus on East and West Africa, respectively, as the intellectual centres. The Indian Medical Services provided bases for research on malaria under such workers as Christophers, Sinton, and Shortt, who extended the pioneer work of *Ross; on cholera by *Rogers; on kala-azar by Shortt; and on dysentery by *Boyd. They were gradually replaced in the field by a distinguished group of Indian national research workers.

The American tradition in tropical hygiene has a strong military component, exemplified by the outstanding work of Walter *Reed on the transmission of yellow fever and of *Gorgas on its control, together with malaria, in Cuba and Panama. Civilian parasitological work, involving biologists rather than doctors, focused particularly on helminthology in the USA, and then in China and the Philippines. The Second World War was a notable stimulus to tropical medicine. It speeded up the introduction of residual insecticides, synthetic antimalarials, and antibacterial chemotherapy. Whereas before the Second World War the British focus in tropical medicine was in India, the post-war focus was on Africa, for the obvious reason of Indian political independence. The focus also shifted from sleeping sickness, epidemics of which had wrought such havoc in Uganda and the West African Sahel but were now under control, to the other parasitic diseases. Malaria and filariasis were studied, and especially the extreme degree of malarial endemicity seen only in sub-Saharan Africa and New Guinea.

The recent past
Malaria

Malaria dominated much of the world scene in tropical medicine until the 1960s and is returning to this position at present. Indeed, the largest international meetings in this subject area were known as the 'International Congresses of Tropical Medicine and Malaria' and the picture of malaria as constituting half the subject was realistic. During the post-war decade, *DDT became widely available and its use in the Mediterranean islands controlled malaria to a dramatic extent because its persistent insecticidal properties reduced mosquito numbers but also reduced the long-term mosquito survival which is needed for malaria transmission. It was found that when spraying was discontinued after several years, in some instances malaria did not recur, as the reservoir of infection in man had died out. This was developed into deliberate national campaigns aimed at malaria eradication within specific time limits, rather than control. These were capital projects of immense cost in relation to national health resources, and organized separately from the general health services of developing countries. They required international financing and specialized expertise, often provided through the *World Health Organization (WHO), which achieved international importance through malaria eradication which dominated its activities in the 1960s. The programme was highly successful in Europe and North America and on many islands. An initially successful campaign in Asia was followed by a resurgence of infection in the 1970s, while in the highly *endemic areas of stable malaria in sub-Saharan Africa little impact was made on the disease. The problems of malaria control increased with the emergence of insecticide resistance among vectors and drug resistance among the parasites, twin problems of so many control campaigns.

Medicine in the tropics

As this intensive public health endeavour developed, medicine in Africa and the Caribbean moved in other directions. Medical colleges were founded in the post-war period, often in partnership with UK expatriate staff from the UK medical academic scene, with a few from the field research workers of the Colonial Medical Service. There was strong emphasis on comparability of graduates with those from UK medical schools, and the research interests of the teaching staff initially derived from UK medicine. Heart disease and *cancer in Africa were investigated and many important and fascinating new diseases and syndromes were studied, such as Burkitt's *lymphoma. There grew an interest in what has been called 'medicine in the tropics' to distinguish it from those parasitic infections which were the traditional content of 'tropical medicine'. The two approaches remained relatively separate in Africa, with the consequence that medical students were educated in the first tradition, and for too long the focus of the first generation of indigenous physicians educated in modern medicine was not primarily upon the tropical parasitic diseases. Nutritional research, after the early description of tropical vitamin deficiency syndromes, was given new impetus by the description of *kwashiorkor by Cicely Williams in Ghana.

The late stages of WHO's efforts at malaria eradication prepared the way for changes in the perception of tropical medicine. By 1970 it was clear that a prerequisite for the consolidation phase of eradication was effective health service coverage. This required better management and organization. The focus of attention moved away from building up excellence in medical schools and towards the periphery, with emphasis on health centres rather than large hospitals. Medical schools acquired teaching health centres and their adjacent small communities as pilot or demonstration areas, and during the 1960s can be thought of as discovering the 'population denominator' with all its implications: effective coverage, or access by people to the health services; recognition that disease control and health promotion may be the only feasible routes to follow; attention directed towards childhood where mortality is greatest; and an implied use of lower-cost approaches if coverage was to be achieved.

The medicine of poverty

These issues were first crystallized in such books as *Medical care in developing countries* by Maurice King (1966). It emphasized coverage, and achieving it by health care largely delivered by paramedical workers. The reflection of the community diagnosis concept, recently introduced, meant that the key causes of death and disability emerged as cosmopolitan infections such as *tuberculosis and acute gastrointestinal and respiratory infections, the ages most at risk were the very young and mothers during delivery, and the importance of *malnutrition was apparent. These were not intrinsically tropical problems—similar diseases predominated in the poverty-sticken parts of temperate countries, most dramatically during the industrial revolution—but they were the principal health problems of the tropics. Thus a third view of tropical medicine emerged, as the 'diseases of poverty', and this predominated during the 1970s. It clearly united health with development, although in the converse of the earlier way. Instead of health being viewed as a prerequisite for economic productivity, disease in the tropics was thought of as primarily being a consequence of poverty, with socio-economic development representing the road to health. Thus, malnutrition might be reduced more effectively by land reform than by specifically nutritional supplementation. This change of viewpoint had three major implications for tropical health. If disease was due to poverty, the reduction of disease was, in the long run, not primarily a matter of medical professional intervention. Either the doctor accepted that his role was peripheral or else he became involved in developmental issues requiring more than clinical skills. To achieve the necessary population coverage the doctor could no longer practise on a traditional doctor–patient basis; his role became that of a teacher and manager of paramedical workers. Thirdly, if tropical medicine comprises the diseases of poverty, it follows that the resources available to provide medical care will be extremely limited, and only low-cost interventions will be feasible: the 'medicine of poverty' for the diseases of poverty. These problems attract a different sort of person from the clinically oriented physician. There is a strong component of humanitarian administration and a tendency to minimize professional skills of *diagnosis and one-to-one patient care, while the elements of social engineering are often uncongenial to the independently minded physician. This approach grew out of the charities such as Oxfam, and such non-governmental organizations played an increasing role along with charismatic individuals, outside the government health services and in remote places. Religious groups often led the way. Meanwhile, the WHO had progressed from the faltering attempts at malaria eradication to an emphasis on building up basic health services, then on self-help and 'community participation', leading to locally recruited and trained paramedical staff providing preventative as well as curative 'primary health care'. This global programme, launched at a meeting at Alma Ata in 1978, marked the extreme of de-professionalizing tropical medicine in an effort to improve access to health care for the entire populations of tropical and other developing countries. This needed cheap, simple, and effective interventions.

Treatment and control interventions

A prototype of what is involved in a 'medicine of poverty' is oral rehydration therapy for the acute watery *diarrhoeas. This was developed from work on the physiological mechanisms whereby a mixture of saline and glucose allowed fluid absorption. A series of investigations has determined how far other sugars or starches could be substituted for glucose; the possible replacement of bicarbonate by citrate for easier storage; whether packets of salts will be made up correctly in villages, and how far domestic ingredients can substitute; as well as how best to make the therapy both available and widely used in villages of the tropics. Such studies have something in common with the research needed for successful environmental control of malaria vectors: a detailed understanding of the ecological and cultural milieu, precise definition of a relatively simple and low-cost intervention, and through field study of its operational deployment. Other agents for the treatment and prevention of tropical infections have involved more complex laboratory work.

Towards modern parasitology

During the first half of the 20th century the study of animal parasites reached maturity. Although helminth infections were recorded in ancient Egypt and parasitic protozoa in man from the first microscopes in the 17th century, the elucidation of their life histories was closely related to the foundation of tropical medicine. The complexity of the life cycles was often great, involving up to four hosts in sequence (for example, man, a snail, and freshwater crabs for the lung fluke *Paragonimus westermani*), and only gradually did attention shift from these, and the problems of parasite survival in nature, to the regulation of parasite numbers in the host, as *immunology developed. The host in which the sexual stages of the parasite take place is called the definitive host (man for schistosomiasis; the anopheline mosquito for malaria). Where another vertebrate host as well as man is involved in the life cycle, either in series or as an alternative to man, the infection is known as a zoonosis.

Protozoa differ markedly from helminths. The parasitic protozoa resemble bacteria and other microparasites in their small size and high rate of multiplication within the host, so that in a non-immune host a small inoculum of the parasite can lead to a heavy infection in a few days. Helminths have a longer generation time and usually do not multiply in the human host, so that re-exposure is needed if worm numbers are to build up. Helminth infections must be considered quantitatively, and illness usually results from heavy infections. Many parasites have evolved along with their hosts and are now very host-specific. For example, the malaria parasites of man will not infect other primates (other than splenectomized apes). Acquired resistance by the individual host to repeated parasitic infections usually develops slowly and may never be complete. Sometimes there is a balance between protective and blocking responses. Many protozoan parasites are widespread in human populations but usually cause little disease. They are becoming apparent as a result of *immunosuppression, either in transplant recipients or now as a result of *AIDS. *Pneumocystis* is an example.

The animal parasitic infections, both with protozoa and with helminths, have posed particularly difficult chemotherapeutic and immunological problems. They are eukaryotic organisms and hence resemble their hosts in their metabolic pathways more closely than do most bacteria and rickettsiae, so that safe chemotherapy of tropical parasites has been an elusive goal. The size and complexity of parasites are associated with multiple *antigens, so that although the infected host produces multiple *antibodies, to determine which are protective and then to purify the corresponding antigens for use as vaccines has been very difficult until recently, when there has been, in the past decade, a resurgence of interest by basic scientists in the problems of parasitic disease. The recent advances in molecular *genetics have come in time to contribute substantially to progress in this field, with the use of monoclonal antibodies in the identification of pathogens, and the production of biosynthetic antigens for diagnosis, as well as the promise of vaccines. The USA, with its relative lack of post-colonial responsibilities and field experience of the tropics, has been particularly active in these new areas.

Tropical disease *chemotherapy goes back (apart from quinine) to the antitrypanosomal arsenic compounds studied by *Ehrlich. Synthetic antimalarials date from the 1930s but in general the chemotherapy of parasitic infections has moved slowly; thus, there are still no good drugs available for killing the South American trypanosomes causing *Chagas' disease, and malaria parasites are becoming resistant even to the newest antimalarials. During the 1970s anthelminthic agents against intestinal worms and schistosomes greatly improved.

There is as yet no operationally available vaccine against any human parasitic disease, but recent intensive efforts, most successfully against malaria, and the possibility of bioengineering methods for synthesizing large quantities of protective antigens, make this an area of rapid progress. Vaccines against other tropically important infections, such as neonatal *tetanus (prevented by maternal immunization) and *poliomyelitis, are an important component of primary health-care strategy, and the development of a relatively heat-stable *measles vaccine has made this an important way to reduce child mortality in the tropics.

The deployment of child immunization has been encouraged by the WHO, and grew out of its dramatically successful *smallpox eradication campaign. WHO's recent programme in tropical parasitic disease research has developed the interest of biomedical research workers in the problems of drug and vaccine development against malaria and other parasites; the diarrhoeal diseases programme has focused attention on oral rehydration and other aspects of the control of these major killing diseases; and a respiratory disease programme is beginning, directed at the largest single cause of tropical mortality. There has also been a revived interest in environmental health, with renewed concern for the improvement of water supplies and sanitation, and for habitat control of disease vectors, all of which were neglected in the post-war enthusiasm for insecticides and chemotherapy. The regulation of human population growth has repeatedly been raised, too, in discussion of the health of tropical populations. The infectious diseases scene is rapidly becoming dominated by HIV–AIDS, first in Africa and now in Asia. In these areas heterosexual transmission predominates, and urban infection rates in people of reproductive age may reach 25 per cent. The disease appears more virulent than in industrial countries, with 23 per cent mortality in 2 years, and tuberculosis as the main cause of death. This is associated with rising overall tuberculosis rates in Africa.

The present day

The field once known as tropical medicine is now full of activity. The different aspects and perceptions of the subject—as parasitic disease, as diseases of poverty, as tropical variants of disease, and as the medicine of poverty—are all jostling for position in a rapidly evolving scene. The traditional subject is breaking up. It has been the last 'vertical' specialty of medicine, where it was possible for one person to have expert knowledge and do research while working at the cellular level, the level of the sick patient, and the level of the community. The rate of progress in all these fields is now such that this is no longer possible.

After a difficult transition, especially in career structures in the post-colonial era, the subject is settling into three main parts: molecular parasitology has become an accepted aspect of basic scientific research; international health has developed greatly, with links to development studies—the continuum of problems from the least developed countries through to affluent ones is now more apparent than the previous dichotomous approach; and clinical tropical medicine is becoming closely aligned with the specialty of *infectious diseases.

Internationally, the dominance of WHO in the field of health is being challenged by the activist approach of UNICEF, with its tendency towards vertical programmes and emphasis on child mortality, and by the World Bank in policy analysis. The Bank reflects the economic approach to health interventions. The role of non-governmental organizations is now accepted. Tropical health continues to be a rapidly moving topic conceptually, while what is happening on the ground moves slowly. The public in richer countries are better informed. Many tropical health issues are easy to explain visually, and television has increased their visibility. The health consequences of famine, environmental change, refugee situations, and poverty are now well known. The challenge of the next decade is not only to develop new and cost-effective interventions to control the major diseases of developing countries, but also to make them effectively available to the people of the tropics.

D. J. BRADLEY

Further reading

The original reports of many tropical medicine discoveries are in journals that are difficult to access. However, the majority of them have been reprinted in:

Kean, B. H., Mott, K. E., and Russell, A. J. (1978). *Tropical medicine and parasitology: classic investigations*, 2 vols. Cornell University Press, Ithaca, New York.

There is no wholly satisfactory history of tropical medicine, the fullest now available in English is:

Scott, H. H. (1939). *A history of tropical medicine*. London.
There are several large textbooks of tropical medicine for those wishing to go into greater detail on the subject matter. The three listed here are the longest-standing British and American texts, respectively, and the most recently written ones:
Manson-Bahr, P. E. C. and Bell, D. R. (1987). *Manson's tropical diseases*, (19th edn). Ballière Tindall, London.
Strickland, G. T. (ed.) (1984). *Hunter's tropical medicine*, (7th edn). Saunders, Philadelphia.
Warren, K. S. and Mahmoud, A. A. F. (ed.) (1990). *Tropical and geographical medicine* (2nd edn). McGraw-Hill, New York.

On the community aspects of tropical health:

King, M. H. (1966). *Medical care in developing countries*. Oxford University Press, Nairobi.

Lucas, A. O. and Gilles, H. H. (1984). *A short textbook of preventative medicine for the tropics*, (2nd edn). London.

Macdonald, G. (1965). On the scientific basis of tropical hygiene. *Transactions of the Royal Society of Tropical Medicine and Hygiene*, **59**, 611–20.

TROPISM is a growth response to a stimulus, the direction of growth being either towards the stimulus (positive tropism) or away from it (negative tropism).

TROTTER, WILFRED BATTEN LEWIS (1872–1939). British surgeon and philosopher. In addition to his superlative technical skill as a surgeon, his diagnostic acumen and his ability as a teacher, Trotter possessed intellectual qualities of a high order. His essays *The instincts of the herd in peace and war* (1916) had a great influence on sociological thought.

TROTULA (11th century). Italian physician. The existence of Trotula is uncertain. Some authorities held that she was a teacher at *Salerno and wife of Johannes Platerius, others that 'Trotula' was a nickname for all Saliternan midwives. Extensive writings, especially on gynaecology and *midwifery, are attributed to her.

TROUSSEAU, ARMAND (1801–67). French physician. He was the first to undertake *tracheostomy in Paris (1831), published an important monograph on laryngeal *tuberculosis (1837), and popularized pleural *paracentesis (1843) and *intubation (1851). He suggested the eponymic titles of *Graves' disease (1860) and *Addison's disease (1856), and described the spasm produced by compression of the nerves in latent *tetany (Trousseau's sign, 1864). His publication *Clinique médicale de l'Hôtel-Dieu de Paris* (1861) enjoyed immense success.

TRUDEAU, EDWARD LIVINGSTON (1848–1915). American physician. He began practice in New York City, but soon developed symptoms of pulmonary *tuberculosis. He went to the Adirondack Mountains to rest, expecting to die of the disease, but his health gradually improved and he attributed that to rest and mountain air. He remained there, founding and directing the Saranac Lake Sanatorium. He carried out some laboratory and animal experiments on tuberculosis, following discovery of the organism by *Koch. He became a leading US authority on the disease.

TRUNK. The main undivided part of an anatomical structure, for example the trunk of the body, to which the neck, the four limbs, and the genital appendages are attached.

TRUSS. A device for maintaining pressure over a weak area of the abdominal wall in order to prevent a *hernia from protruding.

TRYPANOSOME. Any protozoal organism belonging to the genus *Trypanosoma* (see TRYPANOSOMIASIS). Those important to man include *T. gambiense* and *T. rhodesiense* (agents of African sleeping sickness); *T. cruzi* (Chagas' disease); and *T. vivax*, *T. congolense*, and *T. brucei* (trypanosomiasis of cattle and other domestic animals).

TRYPANOSOMIASIS is the name of a group of parasitic diseases of man and animals caused by various species of protozoa of the genus *Trypanosoma*. Transmission occurs through certain tropical insects in which the trypanosomes spend part of their life cycle and which inoculate the vertebrate hosts by biting or faecal contamination. In man, the principal types of trypanosomiasis are: African sleeping sickness, which has two distinct clinical forms due to *T. gambiense* and *T. rhodesiense*, and which is transmitted by *tsetse flies; and American trypanosomiasis or *Chagas' disease, due to *T. cruzi* and transmitted in the faeces of insects belonging to the family Reduviidae (variously known as cone-nose, kissing, or assassin bugs). Animal trypanosomiasis is also important to man, as in certain regions it severely impairs the farming of cattle and other domestic animals; the organisms chiefly concerned are *T. vivax*, *T. congolense*, and *T. brucei*.

TRYPARSAMIDE. An arsenical preparation used in the treatment of trypanosomiasis.

TRYPTAMINE. See SEROTONIN.

TRYPTOPHAN is one of the eight 'essential' *amino acids; i.e. it cannot be synthesized by the body and is therefore a necessary component of the human diet. It is a metabolic precursor of nicotinic acid (tryptophan deficiency is thus of equal importance to that of *niacin in the causation of *pellagra), and of *serotonin; and it is required for normal growth and nitrogen metabolism.

TSETSE FLY. A genus (*Glossina*) of biting flies native to tropical Africa, some species of which (most notably *G. palpalis* and *G. morsitans*) transmit *trypanosomiasis to man and animals.

TSH. See THYROID-STIMULATING HORMONE.

TUBAL TIE. Tubal ligation: sterilization of the female by *ligation of the *Fallopian tubes.

TUBE. Any hollow cylindrical structure, particularly the Fallopian (or uterine) tube, the long slender tube which extends from the upper lateral angle of the *uterus to the region of the *ovary on each side and which provides a passage for shed ova into the uterine cavity.

TUBERCULIN is an extract prepared from tubercle bacilli used in diagnostic tests for *tuberculosis. See TUBERCULIN TEST.

TUBERCULIN TEST. A test to determine whether *tuberculous infection has occurred in a subject. It involves the intracutaneous or subcutaneous injection of an extract of tubercle bacilli (tuberculin), then studying any local and systemic reaction. The standard test, also known as the Mantoux test, requires the intracutaneous injection of 0.1 ml of the purified protein derivative (PPD) of tuberculin, containing 5 tuberculin units, the reaction being read 48–72 hours later; induration of more than 10 mm in diameter is interpreted as a positive reaction, indicating prior infection with *Mycobacterium tuberculosis*. A negative test may be repeated with a larger dose. False negatives are not uncommon, probably as a result of non-specific immune depression. False positives, when they occur, are usually the result of infection with other *mycobacterial species.

TUBERCULOMA. A tuberculous *granuloma.

TUBERCULOSIS is infection with one of the two variants of the tubercle bacillus which commonly parasitize man (*Mycobacterium tuberculosis hominis* and *bovis*). It can involve almost any organ or tissue of the body, and remains a common and serious disease, but both its terrors and its prevalence have been vastly reduced by the discovery and application of tuberculostatic chemotherapy. See also CHEST MEDICINE.

TUBERCULOSIS OFFICER. An appointment created by the UK Public Health Act 1913. The Act, aimed chiefly at tuberculosis, required county councils to prepare schemes for prevention and treatment that included, as well as the provision of dispensaries and sanatoria, nurses for home visiting, and other facilities, the appointment of a tuberculosis officer.

TUBEROSITY. A bony protuberance.

TUBEROUS SCLEROSIS is one of the *phacomatoses, also known as epiloia and Bourneville's disease. It is inherited as an autosomal *dominant characteristic, although with incomplete penetrance. The main features are fibrotic and depigmented skin lesions (adenoma sebaceum), mental deficiency, and *epilepsy, often with associated defects of brain, kidney, heart, lungs, and other organs.

TUBOCURARINE is a neuromuscular blocking agent, the active alkaloid of *curare.

TUBULE. Any small *tube.

TUFFIER, MARIN THEODORE (1857–1929). French surgeon. He was noted for his work in urology and the operative treatment of fractures and was a pioneer of thoracic surgery. He popularized *spinal anaesthesia in France.

TUKE, WILLIAM (1732–1822). British philanthropist. Tuke was inspired to found The Retreat for the insane at York after a friend had died in the County Asylum, possibly from maltreatment. He 'struck the chains from lunatics'. See PSYCHIATRY.

TULARAEMIA (TULAREMIA) is a rare infectious disease known to occur in the USA, Japan, and Russia and having some resemblance to *plague, except that the animal reservoir is mainly in rabbits. When infection is due to the bite of an infected tick or deerfly, there is a local lesion at the site associated with regional *lymphadenopathy. A pneumonic form also occurs. In many cases, the disease is mild and self-limiting; and the response to antibiotics is good. The causative organism is a small Gram-negative bacillus, *Francisella tularensis*.

TULP, NICOLAAS (1593–1674). Dutch physician and anatomist. Born Pieterz, he assumed the name of Tulp (= tulip) from sculptures on his house. He practised in Amsterdam, where he also held civic office and acquired immortality in Rembrandt's painting, *The Anatomy Lesson of Dr Tulp* (1632). He gave an early account of *beriberi (1652) and instituted the first Dutch *pharmacopoeia.

TUMOUR. Strictly, any swelling; but it normally signifies a new growth (neoplasm), either benign or malignant. See ONCOLOGY.

TUPPER, SIR CHARLES (1821–1915). Canadian physician and politician. From 1884 to 1886 he was High Commissioner for Canada in London, returning to Canada as Minister of Finance to be responsible for floating the large loan through which the Canadian Pacific Railway was completed to the west coast of Canada. He returned to London to represent Canada, but was subsequently brought back to Ottawa as Prime Minister of Canada. It was Tupper's courage and determination which brought his native province of Nova Scotia into the Canadian confederation. *Osler wrote in his obituary notice: 'His life is an illustration of the brilliant success of the doctor in politics.'

TÜRK, WILHELM (1871–1916). Austrian physician. He published a large number of observations in clinical *haematology and described a circulating *plasma cell (Türk cell).

TURNER'S SYNDROME results from failure of the *gonads (ovaries) to develop as a result of deletion (or other anomaly) of the second X chromosome; in classic Turner's syndrome, the chromosome complement is therefore 45,XO and the patient is chromatin-negative on *nuclear sexing although phenotypically female. The cardinal features become obvious at *puberty: they include primary *amenorrhoea; *dwarfism; sexual *infantilism; webbing of the neck, low-set ears, and a wide carrying angle at the elbow; and associated anomalies, of which an important one may be *coarctation of the aorta. See also GENETICS.

TWILIGHT SLEEP is a popular term for a state of semi-narcosis induced by *morphine and *scopolamine during labour; this drug combination produces both *analgesia and *amnesia, and was once widely employed in obstetric practice.

TWINS are two offspring produced in the same pregnancy. Dizygotic (fraternal or non-identical) twins result from the fertilization and implantation of two ova at the same time. A tendency to produce more than one ovum at *ovulation can be inherited, so that fraternal twins can run in families; multiple ovulation can also be stimulated by drugs and hormones administered to counteract infertility and may thus result in multiple pregnancy (see FERTILITY DRUG). Monozygotic or identical twins, however, develop from the two halves of a single fertilized ovum formed after its first division. Hence monozygotic twins have identical *karyotypes and are genetically identical, whereas the genetic relationship of dizygotic twins is no closer than that of ordinary siblings and they are often of opposite sex.

TYMPANIC MEMBRANE. The eardrum, the membrane separating the external from the *middle ear; it transmits sound vibrations from the air to the chain of auditory *ossicles in the middle ear.

TYPHOID FEVER is a serious febrile infectious disease caused by one of the *Salmonella organisms, *S. typhi*. Infection is from person to person, being transmitted by the urine or faeces of patients or symptomless carriers. The typhoid bacilli first multiply in the lymphoid tissue of the small intestine (typhoid is also called enteric fever), whence they invade the bloodstream, causing high fever and severe general illness, often marked by delirium or stupor. Abdominal pain, splenic enlargement, and a rose-coloured macular rash are common, but almost any organ can be involved and serious complications may ensue; the commonest are intestinal haemorrhage and perforation of the small intestine. In favourable cases, improvement begins at about the fourth week. The untreated mortality rate is up to 25 per cent; modern antibiotic therapy reduces this to less than 5 per cent. Some recovered patients become chronic typhoid *carriers, and unless the persistent infection is eliminated (by intensive *antibiotic therapy and sometimes removal of the *gall bladder), constitute a public health problem.

TYPHUS, or typhus fever, also known as epidemic, louse-borne, or classic typhus, and as gaol fever, is caused by a species of *Rickettsia* (*R. prowazekii*), a group of small intracellular organisms intermediate between bacteria and viruses. The only known reservoir of *R. prowazekii* is man, transmission being by the human *body louse (*Pediculus humanus humanus*). Epidemics of typhus occur in dirty, overcrowded conditions, favouring lice and their transfer between people. The disease is characterized by sudden onset, headache, prostration, high fever, a generalized macular rash, and signs of central nervous system involvement. In patients who recover, the condition resolves in about 16 days; the mortality, however, can be high, particularly in patients over 40 when *antibiotic treatment is not available. Several allied infections are due to other species of *Rickettsia*, with other arthropod vectors, such as scrub or mite-borne typhus (*R. tsutsugamushi*), murine or flea-borne typhus (*R. typhi*), and Rocky Mountain spotted fever or tick-borne typhus (*R. rickettsii*). Unlike epidemic typhus, these are all zoonoses having animal reservoirs of infection. Interepidemic survival of *R. prowazekii* is due to persistence in the tissues of recovered patients, in whom subsequent recrudescence (known as Brill–Zinsser disease) sometimes occurs.

TYRAMINE is a substance derived from the *amino acid *tyrosine, closely related to *adrenaline and *noradrenaline; it is found in some articles of diet, notably ripe cheese, yoghurt, bananas, wine, and decaying meat. Its importance lies in its interaction with *antidepressant drugs of the *monoamide-oxidase inhibitor (MOAI) group, producing abrupt *sympathomimetic effects and paroxysmal *hypertension. Patients taking MAOIs should be instructed as to which foods they must avoid.

TYROSINE is a white crystalline *amino acid present in most proteins and important in body metabolism as a precursor of various physiological substances (e.g. *thyroxine, *catecholamines').

U

ULCER. A breach or discontinuity in skin or mucous membrane, usually one that is persistent.

ULCERATION is the formation of an *ulcer, or the ulcer itself.

ULCERATIVE COLITIS is a chronic relapsing inflammatory condition of the large bowel, usually including the rectum, involving the mucosal and submucosal layers and characterized by ulceration. The cardinal symptoms are rectal bleeding, diarrhoea, abdominal pain, weight loss, and fever. Patients are usually young or in early middle age, with a slight preponderance of women; remission and relapses are common. The disease is a serious one, with a significant mortality rate. The cause is unknown, and has been the subject of much speculation. It is now generally thought that a disturbance of immunological mechanisms is involved. In most cases the condition can be controlled by the use of *corticosteroids and the drug sulphasalazine has proved useful. If medical treatment fails, surgical exteriorization of the terminal ileum to the abdominal surface (ileostomy), with or without colectomy, has been performed, but such heroic procedures are less often required than in the past.

ULTRACENTRIFUGE. A precision *centrifuge capable of very high speeds (up to 75 000 r.p.m.) at controlled temperatures. Preparative ultracentrifuges are used for the separation of large molecules or small particles from liquids, as in the isolation of viruses, the preparation of cell fractions, or the separation of protein mixtures. Analytical ultracentrifuges allow the determination of relative molecular masses (molecular weights).

ULTRAMICROSCOPY. An ultramicroscope demonstrates the presence of particles too small to be seen with the conventional microscope. A powerful beam of light is brought to a focus in the liquid being examined in such a way that suspended particles scatter the light and appear as bright specks (the Tyndall effect). The term is sometimes also used, less accurately, for electron microscopy.

ULTRASONICS. See ULTRASOUND.

ULTRASOUND IN MEDICINE
History of ultrasound
The early research on the *physics of ultrasound was undertaken in the first two decades of the 20th century, but its possible role in medicine was not considered until the 1940s and the first clinically useful images were produced in the early 1950s (Howry and Bliss 1952). By the early 1960s (Donald and Brown 1961) the quality of the images produced was sufficiently good for ultrasound to begin to find a role in *diagnosis. The early scanners were cumbersome and the image was produced by the operator moving the probe by hand over the surface of the patient. During the past 20 years many automated mechanical and electronic devices have been invented which perform the scanning very quickly, producing 15–25 images per second. These are displayed in real time, to give the effect of a live moving image.

Nature of ultrasound
All sound is mechanical vibration; audible sound has frequencies in the range of 20–20 000 cycles (20 hertz (Hz) to 20 kilohertz (kHz)). All sound with a frequency above 20 kHz is ultrasound but medical applications make use of very high frequencies in the range of 3.5–20 megahertz (1 MHz is 1 million oscillations/sec). Sound of this frequency can be focused into a fine beam, which is directed through the patient by the scanner. As the sound strikes discontinuities in the tissue, small portions of it are reflected to give echoes. Some of these echoes return to the surface and are received by the scanning probe. Sound travels at an almost constant speed within the patient, and therefore, if both the direction in which the beam was transmitted and the time taken for the echo to return are known, it is possible for the scanner electronics to calculate where, from within the patient, the echo originated. Ultrasound images are composed of thousands of echoes collected in the space of about 1/25 sec.

Diagnostic ultrasound
Ultrasound imaging is now applied to almost every area of the body. In addition, the echoes returning from moving structures can now be detected using the Doppler principle, and thus blood flow can be monitored at many

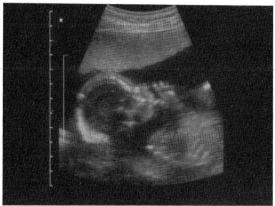

Fig. 1 Ultrasound scan of a normal fetus at 16 weeks of pregnancy.

sites in the body. The prime applications of diagnostic ultrasound are summarized below.

Gynaecology

This was the first specialty to make use of ultrasound (Donald and Brown 1961) and remains one of the main users. Ultrasound is used for the diagnosis of ovarian cysts and tumours, uterine *fibroids, and pelvic infections. It is also now used widely in the management of *infertility, especially using small probes which can be passed into the vagina so that they are only 1 to 2 cm from the ovaries. Such probes use high frequencies and give pictures with superb resolution. Special adaptations now make it possible to use the probe to guide a needle into an ovary to suck out the eggs necessary for *in vitro* fertilization.

*Obstetrics

Virtually every pregnancy in the developed world is now scanned to establish the duration of gestation, to confirm the presence of a live baby (Fig. 1), and to exclude twins. Many patients now receive special detailed scans to check for abnormalities of the baby, and scans may be performed late in the pregnancy to confirm continuing normal growth. The Doppler technique is also now used to confirm a normal blood supply to the *placenta from both the maternal and fetal circulations.

Abdominal organs

Ultrasound imaging is essentially a technique for producing pictures of *anatomy. It is therefore mainly used to assess the size and shape of organs and to look for cysts and tumours (Fig. 2). The *liver, *gall bladder, *spleen, *kidneys, and urinary *bladder are well seen with ultrasound, and this has now substantially replaced previous *X-ray methods for imaging these organs. In addition, the *pancreas, *aorta, *adrenal glands, and several other structures can often be seen well.

The presence of gas within the intestinal tract prevents adequate imaging of the stomach and bowel.

Small parts

This term is used to describe a range of structures such as the breasts, eyes, *thyroid gland, and *testes, which are now all investigated by suitable high-frequency ultrasound scanners.

The heart

Cardiac ultrasound is a specialty area of its own and generally requires special dedicated scanners (see CARDIOLOGY). It has replaced many of the previous highly invasive techniques for investigating the heart, and is used for studying both its anatomy and function. The Doppler technique is used to give additional information about the speed with which blood is moving in the heart and to help find and grade the severity of abnormal holes and leaky valves.

Doppler ultrasound

When the sound pulses bounce off moving structures such as red *blood cells their frequency is slightly altered, in proportion to the speed of the movement. This Doppler shift frequency is used to permit the moving blood to be detected, and a graph of the frequency changes with time can be printed out to show the changes in flow over the cardiac cycle. These graphs are very useful for detecting disease in vessels and in the organs supplied by the vessels.

A recent development is colour Doppler imaging in which the frequency-shifted information is used to produce a colour overlay on the conventional image, to give a colour 'road map' of the vessels. The colour is used to code both the speed and direction of the blood flow.

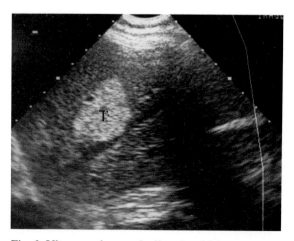

Fig. 2 Ultrasound scan of a liver in which a tumour (T) is present.

Therapeutic ultrasound
Ultrasound with a power of 0.1 to 10 watts is used by physiotherapists to assist the healing of a range of soft-tissue problems, including the effects of mild trauma. All professional football teams now have an ultrasound therapy machine to help players return to activity as soon as possible. Therapy ultrasound may also help in a range of other conditions such as *fibrositis (fibromyalgia) and the healing of burns. The mechanism by which ultrasound exerts these beneficial effects is uncertain, but it appears to be associated with an increase in the local blood flow.

Biological effects of ultrasound
The fact that ultrasound can be used to help soft-tissue healing proves that it can have an effect on tissues. Fortunately this is usually beneficial, but if very delicate tissues, such as those of the *fetus, were exposed to the high-power levels used in therapy it is quite likely that they would be damaged. The large majority of diagnostic scanners produce power levels very much lower than those used in therapy and are very safe in normal clinical use.

However, higher power levels are used for Doppler scans and for higher probe frequencies. For extracorporeal scanning this is almost certainly of no significance, but for transvaginal scanning in early pregnancy it is possible that the ultrasound dose reaching the fetus could be sufficient to cause adverse effects. For this reason such scans should only be undertaken when there is a strong clinical indication for the scan, and the operator should take steps to ensure that the power is as low as possible and that the duration of the scan is as short as possible.

Advantages of ultrasound
The main advantage is complete freedom from the ionizing radiations used in X-ray diagnosis. In addition, the vast majority of scans do not rely on organ function for the production of images, and can thus be used to examine organs such as the kidneys even if they are not working. Similarly, it is virtually never necessary to inject anything into the patient to help with ultrasound scanning.

Disadvantages of ultrasound
The main disadvantage derives from the fact that ultrasound is totally reflected by gas and almost totally by bone; therefore the sound does not reach the tissues beyond, no echoes are derived from these tissues, and thus they are not seen in the images. This prevents ultrasound from being of any value for imaging the lungs or for seeing through bones or bowel gas. It can, however, be used with some limitations, in brain imaging, but has been largely supplanted by *CT and *MRI imaging.

Its freedom from reliance on organ function is generally an advantage, but conversely the scans seldom give any clues as to the state of organ function.

Finally, the technique is highly dependent on the skill of the operator. Even the most sophisticated scanner is useless unless the operator is skilled in its use.

HYLTON MEIRE

Further reading
Those readers who wish to learn more about the subject may wish to read a recently published small, simple, and inexpensive book which covers the basic aspects of ultrasound physics and clinical applications in more detail (Meire and Farrant 1994).

References
Donald, I. and Brown, T. (1961). Demonstration of tissue interfaces within the body by ultrasonic echo sounding. *British Journal of Radiology*, **34**, 539.
Howry, D. H. and Bliss, W. R. (1952). Ultrasonic visualisation of soft tissue structures of the body. *Journal of Laboratory and Clinical Medicine*, **40**, 579.
Meire, H. B. and Farrant, P. (1994). *Basic ultrasound*. Wiley and Sons, Chichester.

ULTRAVIOLET LIGHT is electromagnetic *radiation of shorter wavelength than the shortest perceptible by the human eye (violet) but longer than that of *X-rays, the range being 5–400 nanometres. Sunlight is rich in ultraviolet radiation, but most is absorbed by the *ozone layer of the upper atmosphere. Acting on the skin, UV rays produce *sunburn and stimulate the formation of *vitamin D_2 from ergosterol (see RICKETS). UV radiation can be generated artificially by the mercury vapour lamp.

UMBILICAL CORD. The structure, containing the two umbilical arteries and the umbilical vein, together with supporting tissues, which connects the fetal circulation with the maternal *placenta.

UMBILICUS. The scarred pit in the centre of the abdomen, also called the navel, marking the point of former attachment of the *umbilical cord.

UNCINATE ATTACKS are an uncommon variety of epileptic attacks associated with neuronal discharge arising in the uncal gyrus of the temporal lobe. The typical manifestations are unpleasant olfactory hallucinations, thought to be related to the physiological function of the *uncus.

UNCONSCIOUSNESS is a state of insensibility and unawareness. See COMA.

UNCUS. An anatomical region of the *cerebral cortex, part of one of the convolutions on the inferior surface of the temporal lobe.

UNITED STATES NAVY MEDICAL CORPS. See ARMED FORCES OF THE USA.

UNITS. A unit may be defined as the quantity by reference to which other quantities are measured, the unit being taken as one. See, for example, SI UNITS.

UNIVERSITIES FUNDING COUNCIL. See UNIVERSITY GRANTS COMMITTEE.

UNIVERSITY COLLEGE HOSPITAL (UCH), London, arose partly out of reform of university education in general. Until 1826 this had been open in England only to members of the Anglican Church. The Council of the University of London was formed in that year and admission of students to the university was not based on religious discrimination. University College was opened in 1828 with a medical school to which Charles *Bell, of the *Middlesex Hospital, had been invited as professor of physiology and surgery. There were then no clinical facilities for medical students; it was soon realized that a new hospital had to be built. The foundation stone was laid in 1833 and patients were admitted to the new hospital in 1834, opposite the College.

At the start the staff included David Daniel Davis in midwifery, Robert *Liston (invited from Edinburgh) in clinical surgery, and Richard *Quain in anatomy. Joseph *Lister was a student when Liston performed the first surgical operation in England under anaesthesia. A strong investigative and scientific tradition has continued at UCH. Of recent years famous physicians have included Sir Thomas *Lewis and Lord Rosenheim.

UNIVERSITY GRANTS COMMITTEE (UGC). This UK body was formerly responsible for allocating government funds to universities. The Committee received a block grant from the government and formerly allocated it between individual universities on a quinquennial basis, after discussing their financial requirements with them during five-yearly 'grand visitations'. In the 1980s, owing to a change in government policy and cuts in spending, allocations were made annually. The size of the overall government grant was determined after consideration of a submission by the UGC to the Secretary of State for Education and Science. In 1988 it was superseded by the Universities Funding Council, whose responsibilities were taken over in turn by Higher and Further Education Funding Councils in 1992 when the former UK polytechnics became universities.

UNIVERSITY HEALTH (OR MEDICAL) CENTRES provide *primary health care for university students, sometimes with specialized services as well (e.g. psychiatry, family planning, etc.).

UNNA, PAUL GERSON (1850–1929). German dermatologist. After early pathological research he turned to the biochemistry of skin disease. He described *seborrhoeic eczema (1887–93) and introduced icthyol, resorcin, and zinc oxide paste (Unna's paste) into treatment (1886).

URAEMIA (UREMIA) is synonymous with *azotaemia.

URANIUM is a hard, white, naturally occurring, radioactive, metallic element (relative atomic mass 238.03, atomic number 92, symbol U). The natural element consists of a mixture of 99.3 per cent of the isotope uranium-238 (half-life 4.5 thousand million years) with 0.7 per cent of the isotope uranium-235 (half-life 710 million years); the latter is of greater importance in nuclear reactors and nuclear weapons. The principal ore is pitchblende.

UREA (NH_2CONH_2), also known as carbamide, is the end-product of protein *metabolism and the principal form in which nitrogen is excreted by the body. On an average daily dietary intake of about 100 g of protein (about 16 g of nitrogen), about 30 g of urea (14 g of nitrogen) are excreted in the urine, urea being formed in the liver from the breakdown of *amino acids. Urea was the first organic compound to be created artificially in the laboratory (by Wohler in 1828).

URETER. The tube, with muscle as well as fibrous tissue in its wall, leading from each kidney to the *urinary bladder. In the adult, it is 40–45 cm long.

URETHRA. The membranous tube connecting the *urinary bladder to the exterior, through which the urine is voided. The female urethra is short (3.7 cm), passing below the pubis to open in front of the *vagina. In males it is much longer (about 20 cm), running downwards through the *prostate gland before turning forwards to traverse the length of the *penis. The male urinary tract is accordingly better protected from retrograde infection.

URETHRITIS is inflammation of the urethra. In many cases, though by no means all, it is a manifestation of *sexually transmitted disease. See also GONORRHOEA; NON-SPECIFIC URETHRITIS.

URETHROSCOPE. An *endoscope for inspecting the interior of the *urethra.

URIC ACID is the end-product of *nucleic acid metabolism, up to 1 g being normally excreted in the urine each day. Having a very low solubility, it is often implicated in the formation of urinary *calculi; it is also involved in the pathogenesis of *gout.

URINARY BLADDER. The distensible and contractile

muscular bag lying in the anterior part of the pelvic cavity which acts as a storage receptacle for the *urine before its intermittent discharge; it receives a continuous inflow from the kidneys via the two *ureters, the openings of which are guarded by valves; it empties through a *sphincter of the *urethra.

URINATION is the act of voiding *urine.

URINE is the excretory product of the *kidneys, of which about 96 per cent is water (daily volume under normal conditions varying between about 1 and 2 litres). Volume and solute content reflect the critical role of the kidney in regulating the water, *electrolyte, and *acid–base composition of the body and body fluids (see NEPHROLOGY). The urine also contains many waste products, notably those resulting from protein, muscle, and nucleic acid metabolism and products of hormonal degradation. Examination of the urine is an essential part of physical examination, as abnormal constituents may give important diagnostic leads. Among those detected by simple inspection and routine testing by the examiner are: blood; haemoglobin; pus; bile; protein; sugar; ketone bodies; crystals of certain recognizable types; tubular *casts; epithelial cells; and some parasites.

UROGRAPHY is *radiography of part of the urinary tract using a contrast medium, for example *nephrography, *pyelography, etc.

UROLITHIASIS is the occurrence of *calculi in the urinary tract.

UROLOGY or urological surgery encompasses the care of the urinary tract and the male genitourinary system, including *infertility and *impotence. It overlaps *nephrology in the care of *renal disease; *endocrinology in male infertility, *adrenal diseases, and metabolic stone disease; and *gynaecology in the care of female incontinence.

The symptoms of urological disease are most commonly disturbances in the voiding pattern. Frequent voidings (frequency), pain or burning with voiding (dysuria), and the urgent need to void (urgency) are the most common, usually indicating inflammation or irritation of the lower urinary tract. A slow stream or the need to strain to urinate is indicative of lower tract obstruction, while back or flank pain, nausea, and vomiting may accompany upper tract obstruction. Chills and fever are usually indicative of *kidney or *prostate infections. Foul-smelling blood in the urine may be a sign of early *cancer. All of them should be investigated.

The development of urology was inseparable from the technological explosion of the late 19th and 20th centuries. Its practitioners were the intellectual descendants of the lithotomists (stone-cutters), the venereologists, and the surgeons. They became expert in the diagnosis of urinary tract disease through their mastery of urethral instrumentation, which included the use of the *cystoscope. This gave them the opportunity to compete with general surgeons in certain cases, and eventually urology became a subspecialty of *surgery.

Stone disease
Some of the most colourful urological history concerns the treatment of urinary calculus, or stone disease. Cutting for stone (which until 100 years ago included only bladder calculi) was separated from the main body of medicine and surgery long ago by *Hippocrates, who stated in his oath 'I will not cut persons labouring under the stone but will leave this to be done by practitioners in this work'. Hippocrates regarded wounds of the bladder as fatal ('Death commonly follows wounds of the brain, spinal cord, liver, diaphragm, bladder, and the great vessels'), and apparently preferred that his disciples should not be involved.

The earliest descriptions of the operations for stone were those in the Susruta Samhita from India and of *Celsus, both written before AD 600, describing essentially the same operation, with a perineal exposure, going up through the bladder floor. The operation had changed little by the time of Frère Jacques (1651–1714). He was an itinerant French lithotomist, setting up operating clinics in villages. Here he would line up his patients and prepare them for several days with *clysters, *bloodletting, and *purges. On the day of surgery, he and four assistants operated on all his patients, and then moved on before the results of the surgery became known. After a long struggle with the medical establishment, he was finally granted hospital privileges, where his errors caught up with him. Operating before crowds of up to 200 people, he 'cut' 60 patients in a four-month period. Twenty-five died soon after surgery and 13 were cured. The remaining 22 were 'beyond cure'. On one day seven patients died. He then went back to his itinerant practice, learned some more anatomy, modified his operation, and is said to have operated on 5000 people by the end of his career.

For a while the leadership in lithotomy went to England where *Cheselden, a trained anatomist who was also a lithotomist, tried the suprapubic approach (through the lower abdomen), only to abandon it because of problems with patients straining. Straining was a help in the perineal approach since it helped to push the stone out of the incision, but with a suprapubic approach straining tended to push bowel into the incision and made it difficult to avoid opening the *peritoneum. With adequate relaxation the suprapubic approach is by far the safest and easiest, but it did not come into popular use until *anaesthesia was available, and at that point the treatment of stones came into the mainstream of surgery.

A completely non-invasive treatment of renal calculi,

the electro-hydraulic *lithotriptor, was developed in the late 1970s. In this technique the patient is placed in a tub of water and an underwater spark-gap is used to produce a shock wave, which is then focused by an ellipsoidal reflector on the stone. The stone is strong to compression, but as the shock wave passes through, a negative pressure pulls off small fragments which are then carried away by the urine.

Understanding of the metabolic causes of stone disease has progressed along with surgical treatment. In the 1950s, apart from the stones which developed as a result of infection, the mechanism of their formation was understood in only a small proportion of cases. Now in only about 5 per cent of cases is the mechanism of formation obscure. The commonest cause of stone formation is an excess of *calcium in the urine (hypercalciuria), which may be classified into absorptive (too much calcium from the gut), resorptive (excess mobilization of calcium from the bone), or renal (tubular wasting and loss of calcium from the kidney). Increased oxalate (hyperoxaluria) or *uric acid (hyperuricosuria) occurs less frequently but can easily be determined by testing a 24-hour urine specimen. Improved capacity to prevent stone means that surgical treatment is less often necessary.

Instruments

The age-old problem of an obstructed, over-filled bladder has been relieved by *catheters made of reeds, straws, palm leaves, or the leaves of the onion family. The double-lumened retention catheter, with a balloon on the end to keep it in place, was invented in the 1820s by Reybard in France, although Foley designed the modern version in 1933.

Although the first *cystoscope was invented by Bozzini in 1804 and Nitze developed the first adequate lens system in 1879, the first really useful cystoscope had to await invention of the Edison electric-light bulb in 1880. In 1887 Harwig of Berlin and Leiter of Vienna both placed Edison's light in Nitze's scope and the interior of the bladder could be routinely and safely visualized. Modification of these instruments by Brown of Baltimore allowed insertion of catheters into the ureters, and when *X-rays were available contrast medium could be injected into the ureter to obtain an image of it for the first time. In the 1960s the Hopkins solid-rod lens system increased clarity considerably. *Fibre-optic light bundles increased the amount of light available and were much more reliable. The use of coherent fibre-optics allowed the image-carrying portion of the 'scope' to be flexible and led to the development of nephroscopes and ureteroscopes, permitting direct visualization of the entire urinary tract.

Percutaneous surgery of the kidney, especially for larger stones, is now done with an instrument introduced through the flank directly into the kidney, and laparoscopic surgery of the peritoneum and pelvis is replacing some of the open surgical procedures.

Tumours

The era of modern open urological surgery, as with all surgery, began with the development of anaesthesia and asepsis. Simon carried out the first planned *nephrectomy in 1869 and the development of X-ray techniques made possible the preoperative diagnosis of most larger lesions. Smaller tumours may now be demonstrated much earlier with the use of computerized tomography (*CT) scans, magnetic resonance imaging (MRI), and ultrasonography (see ULTRASOUND). Since the incidence of metastatic spread is proportional to the size of the primary renal tumour, this early diagnosis should carry with it a better prognosis.

In childhood renal tumours (Wilms' tumour, or nephroblastoma), even though the diagnosis is still made relatively late after the discovery of an abdominal mass, the prognosis has changed from less than 40 per cent survival to better than 90 per cent, largely due to a combination of surgery, antineoplastic *chemotherapy, and *radiation.

Bladder

The first recognized cause of bladder tumour was the so-called aniline dye workers' tumour described by Rehn in a German chemical plant in 1895. Actually, the tumour was probably produced by exposure to beta-naphthylamine, a by-product in the manufacture of alpha-naphthylamine, but that was not shown until the 1930s when Heuper produced tumours in dogs by feeding beta-naphthylamine. Rats and mice metabolize naphthylamines by a different pathway than humans and dogs, and the same carcinogenic effects cannot be demonstrated in rodent experiments. Since then many chemicals, and even bracken fern, have been reported to be *carcinogenic to the bladder. However, the most important clinical factor is cigarette *smoking, which increases the incidence of bladder cancers fourfold.

Such tumours can now be produced reliably in animal models by several agents. The carcinogen is thought to be conjugated and detoxified in the liver, and excreted in an inactive form in the urine, where the conjugate is broken up by urinary *enzymes to release the active carcinogen.

This hypothesis fits with clinical experience in two important respects: first, bladder tumours are 10 times as common as tumours of the renal pelvis where the urine rests for only a short time, and the carcinogen has not been released from its conjugated form; secondly, the clinical behaviour of the tumour, with multiple recurrences over time in different parts of the bladder, and even in the lining of the kidney and ureter, can best be explained by exposure of the lining of the urinary tract to the same carcinogenic stimulus. Because of their tendency to recur, bladder tumours require close follow-up with cystoscopy. This is often supplemented by urine *cytology, which can detect malignant cells in the urine, much as is done with early detection of cervical carcinoma.

Tumours limited to the mucosal lining of the bladder may be treated locally with cautery or intravesical agents, but invasive tumours require radiation or surgical removal of the bladder. Removal of the bladder creates the problem of how to manage (divert) the urine. One solution was to bring the ureters to the skin as performed by LeDentu in 1889; but this frequently resulted in stenosis or infection. Over the next 100 years almost all segments of the intestinal tract, from the stomach to the rectum, were used; it is now possible to build a continent pouch which is emptied by catheterization, avoiding the need for a collection bag.

Prostate gland
The prostate gland is that part of the sexual apparatus which is responsible for *ejaculatory contractions. It might be considered as the weak link of the male urinary tract as it suffers from three common diseases: benign prostatic *hyperplasia, which affects one-third of men over 60 years of age; *carcinoma of the prostate, which is the second commonest male cancer and is present at least in some form in 80 per cent of men over 80 years of age; and prostatitis, which is one of the more common male complaints between the ages of 25 and 50 years.

The first reported *prostatectomy as such was performed by Amussat, who in 1827 incidentally removed an obstructing intravesical prostate while removing a bladder calculus. The patient recovered completely. Eugene Fuller of New York, in 1894, was the first to describe a technique for the complete suprapubic removal of a prostatic *adenoma. Fryer popularized the operation in the UK. In 1904 Young described his perineal approach to prostatectomy, and then Terence Millen in 1947 described the retropubic approach, coming down in front of the bladder directly on to the anterior prostatic capsule. However, the most common type of prostatectomy in the USA at present is the transurethral resection. The first resectoscope was developed by Maximilian Stern in 1926, using a square-wave (spark gap) current for cutting and a sine-wave current for coagulation. Some operators were able to remove several hundred grams of prostatic tissue at a single procedure, but usually the large glands were dealt with by open surgery. The advantage of the transurethral approach is that there is little discomfort and the patient may be out of the hospital in a few days. Many new methods of control of prostatic enlargement have been proposed, ranging from medical treatments to *laser surgery. None has been tested over a prolonged period of time.

Cancer of the prostate is now a leading cause of cancer deaths in men, second only to that of the lung. Until the 1940s very little could be done for these patients, except for the fortunate few (usually less than 5 per cent of patients) in whom the disease was diagnosed while still localized. The treatment for localized cancer was then surgical removal by a radical prostatectomy. This differs from simple prostatectomy in that the entire gland is removed and the bladder is then re-attached to the urethra; while in a simple prostatectomy only the central obstructing portion is removed, leaving the outer capsule intact.

In 1941 Huggins (an American urologist) published his work describing the hormonal control of the prostate in dogs and the use of *stilboestrol or *orchidectomy as a clinical treatment for widespread carcinoma of the prostrate. The results of orchidectomy were immediate, with dramatic relief of severe bone pain within a few hours. Huggins later received a *Nobel prize for his work, the first surgeon to do so since Alexis *Carrel. Bagshaw reported on the use of megavoltage treatment in localized prostatic cancer. It seemed to be as good as radical surgery for up to 10 years, but was followed by an increased number of recurrences after this period. Another approach has been implantation of *radioactive material into the prostate, but the long-term results are still not available.

Significant side-effects occur after all forms of treatment for carcinoma of the prostate. *Impotence is expected after hormonal therapy or surgery, and occurs in up to 60 per cent of patients after external beam therapy. Recent anatomical studies and investigations by Walsh in Baltimore suggest that careful preservation of the nerves on either side of the prostate may make it possible to maintain potency after a radical prostatectomy. Incontinence can follow radical surgery in 1–5 per cent of cases. Rectal and bladder irritability may occur following radiation therapy.

Recently, screening for prostate cancer with prostate-specific antigen (PSA) in the blood and digital rectal examination, supplemented by ultrasonically guided needle biopsies, has multiplied the percentage of operable lesions found by a factor of at least four. The use of complete androgen ablation by luteinizing hormone-releasing hormone (LHRH) antagonists and anti-androgens offers to those men reluctant to undergo an orchidectomy, an alternative therapy, albeit an expensive one.

Paediatric urology
Studies have shown that about 40 per cent of the more serious congenital malformations occur in the genito-urinary tract, and most of the urological surgery in the young is concerned with their correction. In the past the management of these problems was in the hands of general surgeons and until Meredith Campbell published his textbook on paediatric urology in 1937 there was little concerted effort to pay special attention to paediatric urology. David Innes Williams held a similar position in the UK, as did Gregoire in France.

Obstruction, with dilated urinary tracts above the obstruction, is the most common problem. These obstructions are being recognized earlier, partly because of the availability of ultrasound scans, which are non-invasive. It is now not unusual to diagnose obstruction *in utero* and efforts are being made to drain some of these obstructions *in utero* so that upper tract damage is less severe at the time of birth.

Neurogenic bladder and urodynamics

It is important that urine is delivered to the outside at a low pressure and without infection. The recognition that urine flow is not simply a matter of static pressure but of dynamic flow has led to the development of a field of urology called urodynamics.

In spite of the incompleteness of our theoretical knowledge, much has been done in the practical treatment of *incontinence. Female stress incontinence due to perineal relaxation has been a longstanding problem, often related to after-effects of childbearing. For years it was treated with *pessaries inserted into the vagina to hold the bladder in place. Then anterior vaginal repairs advocated by Kelly gave considerable relief. In the 1950s the Marshall–Marchetti–Krantz procedure was devised. This involved suturing the periurethral and bladder neck tissue to the underside of the pubis to give a solid support to the bladder neck. Later, Perrera developed a simpler technique, inserting a long needle down either side of the bladder neck and placing a stitch to lift the bladder neck up towards the abdominal wall. This procedure has gained wide popularity because of reliability and lack of morbidity.

In some cases an artificial *sphincter may be used. This consists of an inflatable silastic cuff which is placed around the urethra, a reservoir, and a pump or control valve which controls the flow between the reservoir and the cuff. Fluid is pumped into the inflatable cuff to hold the urine and is released into the reservoir to empty the bladder.

The importance of these problems and the results of increased understanding are most obvious in the improved prognosis, both early and late, in patients with *spinal cord injury. Before the 1960s if the patient survived the acute injury or the first few years of life, the major cause of death was renal failure, usually from a combination of obstruction, infection, and stone. Expectant treatment is now begun immediately and the disastrously damaged urinary tracts that were so common in *paraplegics 15–20 years ago are now seen infrequently.

In patients with acute spinal cord injury, a programme of intermittent catheterization is begun almost immediately. Without the initial insult of an over-distended, often infected bladder, they are managed with either an intermittent catheterization programme, a sphincterotomy (cutting the sphincter to allow continual flow of urine), or a timed voiding programme.

The situation is much the same in patients with *spina bifida and *meningomyelocoele. Previously, almost 100 per cent of the latter patients had some urinary tract abnormality noted by the age of 4 years. Now many patients can be kept free of difficulty, either with medication or with intermittent catheterization.

W. H. CHAPMAN

URTICARIA is a rash due to *allergy, also known as nettle rash or hives. Itchy blotches appear on the skin, with raised *erythematous patches of cutaneous *oedema (weals).

US PHARMACOPOEIA. Like its British equivalent, the *US Pharmacopoeia* (abbreviated to *USP*) is an official compilation of approved names and standards for substances and preparations used in medicine and pharmacy. It is published by the United States Pharmacopoeial Convention.

UTERINE SOUND. A slender surgical *probe or *bougie designed to be introduced into the *cervix uteri for exploration and dilatation.

UTERUS. The womb. In the non-pregnant woman the uterus is an elongated muscular organ about 8 cm long lying more or less vertically in the *pelvis behind the *urinary bladder. Above, its cavity communicates with the right and left *Fallopian tubes; below, the narrow lower section (the *cervix) protrudes into and communicates with the *vagina. Physiological changes during pregnancy are associated with an increase of 30-fold or more in the weight of the uterine muscle (myometrium). See also ENDOMETRIUM; MENSTRUATION.

UVEA. The vascular middle coat of the eye, comprising the *iris, the ciliary body, and the *choroid. See OPHTHALMOLOGY.

UVEITIS is inflammation of one or more of the structures comprising the *uvea; it has many causes. See OPHTHALMOLOGY.

UVEOPAROTITIS is one clinical presentation of *sarcoidosis, in which the inflammatory process involves the *parotid gland and structures of the *uvea; it is also called uveoparotid fever.

UVULA. The small downwards midline projection of the soft *palate.

VACCINATION is immunization against any infectious disease by exposure to an appropriate *vaccine. The term was originally applied to immunization against *smallpox with *vaccinia virus, but *Pasteur extended the meaning to include all forms of active immunization with micro-organisms or their products.

VACCINE is any preparation of micro-organisms, killed or living but modified so as to reduce pathogenicity, administered to stimulate the production of *antibodies and hence to prevent or ameliorate the effects of infection with the natural or 'wild' organisms. Some vaccines, such as the Sabin vaccine against *poliomyelitis, are effective by mouth, but most have to be given parenterally.

VACCINIA is the localized papulovesicular eruption which occurs at the site of inoculation with vaccinia virus (see COW-POX); it was widely employed in immunization against *smallpox but now that the disease has been eradicated it is indicated only in a few special groups, such as laboratory workers who handle *poxviruses. Rarely, the eruption became generalized due to blood-borne spread of the virus ('generalized vaccinia') but without serious effects. 'Progressive vaccinia' or 'vaccinia gangrenosa' was a much rarer and often fatal complication which followed vaccination of those whose *immune system had been depressed by disease or drugs.

VACUOLE. A small space within the cytoplasm of a *cell, initially formed by invagination of the cell membrane; material on the cell surface is thus engulfed—the process of *phagocytosis.

VAGINA. The sheath-like passage between the *vulva and the *cervix uteri which receives the *penis during sexual intercourse. Its mucous lining is under hormonal (*oestrogen) control.

VAGINISMUS is painful spasm of the muscles around the *vagina, making sexual intercourse difficult or impossible.

VAGINITIS is inflammation of the *vagina. *Candidiasis and *trichomoniasis are common causes. Atrophic (or senile) vaginitis can occur in postmenopausal women due to *oestrogen deficiency.

VAGOTOMY is the surgical division of one or both *vagus nerves.

VAGUS. The tenth cranial nerve, a major component of the *parasympathetic nervous system. The vagus is also a mixed nerve, so that, as well as supplying parasympathetic fibres to and visceral afferents from the thoracic and abdominal organs, it carries sensory fibres from the ear, tongue, *pharynx, and *larynx and motor fibres to the pharynx, larynx, and *oesophagus.

VALERIAN is the dried rhizome and roots of the plant *Valeriana officinalis*, formerly used as an extract, infusion, or tincture (often with *bromides, *chloral hydrate, *phenobarbitone, or other sedatives) to treat nervous conditions.

VALSALVA, ANTONIO MARIA (1666–1723). Italian physician and anatomist. His *De aura humana tractatus* (1704) contained an excellent account of the anatomy of the ear in which he named the *Eustachian tubes. He first described the aortic sinuses (sinuses of Valsalva). *Valsalva's manoeuvre provides a simple test of circulatory function.

VALSALVA MANOEUVRE. Forced expiration against a closed *glottis, a simple bedside test of circulatory function. In the normal subject, the increase in intrathoracic pressure hinders venous return to the heart, causing a fall in *cardiac output and hence in arterial *blood pressure; the resultant reflex *tachycardia can be detected in the *pulse at the wrist. When the manoeuvre is terminated (after about 10 seconds), the accumulated venous blood is pumped by the heart into a constricted vascular bed, causing an 'overshoot' of arterial pressure above the normal level and consequent reflex *bradycardia. An alternative method of inducing a forced expiratory effort is to ask the subject to blow into the tube of a *sphygmomanometer against the mercury column, maintaining it at a level of about 40 mmHg for 10 seconds.

VALVE. In general, any fold or flap, or a system of these, in the lumen of a vessel, channel, or orifice which permits flow in only one direction. Many such valvular structures exist in the body: of particular note are those scattered throughout the veins (see VARICOSE VEINS) and those controlling the flow of blood between the chambers of the heart (see VALVES, CARDIAC).

VALVES, CARDIAC. A pair of *valves on each side control blood flow into and out of the right and left *ventricles of the *heart. They are the right and left atrioventricular valves (known as tricuspid and mitral valves, respectively), which open during *diastole to allow blood to flow into the ventricles from the atria and close during *systole to prevent retrograde flow; and the valves guarding the outflow tracts of each ventricle (aortic and pulmonary valves), which open during systole to allow blood to flow into the pulmonary artery and aorta and close during diastole to prevent backwards leakage. Each valve has three segments (cusps or leaflets) except the mitral, which usually has only two.

VALVULAR HEART DISEASE. Disease affecting the heart *valves, sometimes abbreviated to VHD. Defective valve function is of two types: stenosis, in which narrowing of the orifice restricts flow in the normal (forward) direction; and incompetence (or regurgitation), in which the defective valve fails to prevent retrograde flow. Its major causes are *congenital heart disease, *rheumatic fever, and *infective endocarditis.

VAN SLYKE, DONALD DEXTER (1883–1971). American biochemist. He developed many gasometric methods for *biochemical analyses. His two-volume work, (with J. P. Peters) *Quantitative clinical chemistry* was a standard reference for many years. Van Slyke was especially interested in acid–base balance, and the equilibria between gases and electrolytes. He and associates made noteworthy contributions to measurement of urea clearance by the kidney, and in the identification of glutamine as the source of urinary ammonia. See CHEMISTRY, CLINICAL.

VAPOUR BATHS. Steam baths.

VARICELLA. See CHICKENPOX.

VARICOCELE. Varicosity (see VARICOSE VEINS) of the veins draining the *testis, usually the left. When symptomatic, the condition is easily dealt with surgically.

VARICOSE ULCER. A skin ulcer on the lower leg above the ankle associated with *varicose veins, due to impaired blood flow and hence impaired nutrition of the skin and subcutaneous tissues.

VARICOSE VEINS are abnormally dilated and tortuous veins associated with conditions or circumstances causing persistently high venous pressure when defective venous *valves allow retrograde flow. Varicose veins are commonly manifest in the subcutaneous tissue of the legs, but may occur in other situations due to prolonged venous obstruction. There is usually held to be a genetic component in aetiology, and predisposing conditions include obesity, pregnancy, ascites, and occupations which involve prolonged standing. Apart from cosmetic disfigurement, varicose veins can cause aching of the legs and swelling of the ankles. Venous *thrombosis and *ulceration of the skin over the lower parts of the legs (varicose ulcer) are troublesome complications.

VARIOLA. See SMALLPOX.

VARIX (pl. varices). A *varicose vein.

VAROLIO, CONSTANZO (1543–75). Italian anatomist. He described the ileocaecal valve (between the *ileum and *caecum) and, in *De nervis opticis* (1573), the pons Varolii.

VASCULITIS is inflammation of blood vessels; it is equivalent to *angiitis.

VASCULOTOXIC. Having a damaging effect on blood or lymph vessels.

VAS DEFERENS. The duct carrying *spermatozoa from the testis; after uniting with the duct from the *seminal vesicle, it joins the *urethra.

VASECTOMY is interruption of the *vasa deferentia by ligation or removal of a portion, often performed as a method of male sterilization; the operation is simple, because for part of its course the duct lies subcutaneously.

VASOCONSTRICTION is contraction of blood vessels with narrowing of their calibre, particularly of the *arterioles, which are the main determinant of peripheral vascular resistance and the means by which adjustments in regional *perfusion occur.

VASODILATATION is relaxation of blood vessels with widening of their calibre, particularly of the *arterioles (cf. VASOCONSTRICTION).

VASOMOTOR. Affecting the calibre of blood vessels, particularly of *arterioles.

VASOPRESSIN is an alternative name for *antidiuretic hormone (ADH). See PITUITARY GLAND.

VAULT. Any structure with an arched roof, for example the vault of the *skull.

VECTOR is used in two medical senses: the usual scientific meaning of any quantity that requires a direction to be stated in order to define it completely; and alternatively to denote an animal carrier of the agent of a communicable disease (e. g. the anopheline *mosquito in the case of *malaria).

VECTORCARDIOGRAPHY is recording and analysis of the *electrocardiogram in terms of a series of instantaneous mean *vectors, that is in terms of the moment-to-moment average magnitude and direction of the electrical forces generated during cardiac contraction.

VEGAN. A strict *vegetarian, i.e. one who abstains from eating flesh and also from all other foods of animal origin, including milk, milk products, eggs, and honey.

VEGETARIANISM, strictly speaking, is abstention from all foods of animal origin, including dairy products, eggs, milk, and honey as well as meat and fish. In practice, most vegetarians abstain only from meat and fish; such a diet, provided it is adequately varied, is compatible with normal health. The term 'vegan' is used to denote one who is strictly vegetarian; instances of *vitamin B_{12} deficiency have been reported in such individuals.

VEGETATION. One of the warty aggregations of *platelets, *fibrin, *erythrocytes, and sometimes *bacteria which form on the *endocardium of the heart *valves in rheumatic, bacterial, and other forms of *endocarditis.

VEHICLE. A non-active substance in which a drug or other medicinal agent is incorporated to ease administration; an *excipient.

VEIN. Any of the blood vessels in which blood returns from the tissues (and lungs) to the heart. Veins are distinguished from *arteries in having walls which are much thinner (the intravascular pressure being correspondingly lower) and collapsible, in carrying (except in the case of the pulmonary veins) deoxygenated blood, and in having many *valves along their course.

VENAE CAVAE. The two main venous channels which return blood to the right *atrium of the heart, known as the superior vena cava and the inferior vena cava. The former drains venous blood from the head, neck, arms, and chest; the latter from the legs, pelvis, and abdomen. The two vessels enter the right atrium separately.

VENEPUNCTURE. See VENESECTION.

VENEREAL. Transmitted by sexual intercourse. See SEXUALLY TRANSMITTED DISEASE.

VENEREAL DISEASE ACT 1917. This UK Act was passed to prevent the treatment of venereal disease (defined as *syphilis, *gonorrhoea, and soft chancre or *chancroid) otherwise than by duly qualified medical practitioners, to prohibit advertisements for the treatment of venereal disease, and to control the supply of venereal disease remedies.

VENESECTION is the cutting of a vein to draw off blood or to insert, for example, a *cannula. The term is synonymous with 'phlebotomy'. It is sometimes used interchangeably with the more precise 'venepuncture', the puncturing of a vein with a needle to obtain a specimen of venous blood or to deliver an injection.

VENOGRAM. A *radiograph obtained by *phlebography.

VENOM is the poisonous material secreted and injected by certain stinging or biting *arthropods, reptiles, and fish.

VENO-OCCLUSIVE DISEASE OF THE LIVER is a syndrome produced by certain toxic substances; it has been reported from Jamaica after ingestion of plant alkaloids in so-called 'bush teas', and following *antineoplastic chemotherapy, for example with *cytarabine. The smaller branches of the hepatic veins are occluded by thrombosis, causing centrilobular *necrosis of the liver, fibrosis, and *portal hypertension.

VENTILATION is the movement of air in and out of the lungs during breathing.

VENTILATOR. Any device for artificially ventilating the lungs. See also RESPIRATOR.

VENTOUSE. A cupping glass. See CUPPING.

VENTRICLE. A small cavity. The term ventricle usually means one of the several cavities of the *brain; or one of the two lower chambers of the *heart, from which blood is expelled at each heart beat by the forcible muscular contraction of the ventricular walls.

VENTRICULAR FIBRILLATION is the most serious of all the cardiac *arrhythmias, in which normal coordinated contraction of the ventricular *myocardium ceases and is replaced by chaotic uncoordinated electromechanical activity at many independent foci. There is no effective *cardiac output, and it is therefore incompatible with life for more than a minute or two unless the circulation is artificially restored and maintained. It is the usual mode of sudden death following *coronary thrombosis. It can be reversed by *defibrillation, provided the circulation can be adequately supported until the appropriate apparatus is available.

VENTRICULAR SEPTAL DEFECT is a developmental anomaly in which there is an abnormal opening in the interventricular septum of the heart, allowing blood to shunt from the chamber of higher pressure (normally the left ventricle) across to the other side. Ventricular septal defect (VSD), either alone or in combination with other cardiac malformations, is a common form of *congenital heart disease and is what is usually meant by 'hole in the heart'.

VENTRICULOGRAM. See VENTRICULOGRAPHY.

VENTRICULOGRAPHY is the *radiographic visualization of the *cerebral ventricles by replacing the *cerebrospinal fluid with a contrast medium such as air. This technique, unlike *pneumoencephalography (air encephalography) in which the air is injected into the lumbar canal after lumbar puncture, involves direct injection into a lateral ventricle via a needle inserted through a burr-hole in the skull. Since the advent of *computerized tomography (CT) scanning, it is rarely needed.

VENULES are the smallest vessels of the venous system, connecting the *capillaries to the *veins.

VERATRINE is a derivative of the hellebore plants (*Veratrum viride* and *V. album*), formerly used in the treatment of arterial *hypertension.

VERMIS. The central portion of the *cerebellum.

VERNEUIL, ARISTIDE AUGUSTE STANISLAS (1823–95). French surgeon. A distinguished anatomist, his contribution to surgery was in the treatment of *cold abscesses by instilling *iodoform. He was the founder in 1881 of the influential *Revue de chirurgerie*.

VERRUCA. A wart, a small benign epidermal tumour caused by a *papovavirus.

VERSION is conversion, usually by manipulation, of an abnormal fetal position into a normal one.

VERTEBRA. See SPINE.

VERTIGO is a sensation of dizziness in which it seems to the sufferer that the immediate environment is rotating; the cause usually lies in the structures of the inner ear or their central connections.

VERVET MONKEY DISEASE. A synonym for *Marburg disease.

VESALIUS, ANDREAS (1514–64). Flemish anatomist. Vesalius studied in Louvain and Paris, before enrolling at *Padua, where on graduation he was appointed demonstrator of anatomy. He established a great reputation as a teacher with unorthodox views. In 1543 he published his *De humani corporis fabrica*, probably the most influential of all medical works. He supervised its production himself, selecting the paper, the draughtsman, the block-cutters, and the printer. The anatomical descriptions, founded on his own observations and frequently differing from those of *Galen, aroused bitter antagonism, not least from his old teacher Johannes *Sylvius. Possibly on this account he left Padua in 1543 to serve the Emperor Charles V and, after his abdication in 1555, his son Philip II. He also achieved renown in practice. He introduced surgical drainage of pleural *empyema (1547). In 1564 he was taken ill and shipwrecked on a voyage home from Palestine and died on the island of Zante.

VESICLE. A small blister, a localized epidermal swelling containing clear fluid. Cf. BULLA.

VESICOVAGINAL FISTULA. A *fistula connecting the *urinary bladder with the *vagina.

VESSEL. An *artery, *vein, or *lymphatic channel.

VESTIBULE. An anatomical space at the entrance to a canal.

VETERANS' ADMINISTRATION, US, AND ITS MEDICAL PROGRAMME. The Veterans' Administration (VA) makes a significant contribution to medical care in the USA. It operates about 170 hospitals, and more than 230 clinics throughout the country. Some 16 million clinic visits are made each year, and 1.3 million patients are treated in VA hospitals each year, amounting to about 7 per cent of all hospital admissions. US programmes for the care and pensioning of veterans of military service (i.e. all former members of the armed forces) began after the American Revolutionary War. By the early part of the 19th century there were 'homes' for elderly and disabled veterans in many parts of the nation, in which medical care often had to be provided. Following the American Civil War several veterans' hospitals were created, and maintained by the government, and by the early part of the 20th century these had increased to some 50. More hospitals were created after the two world wars. At present, more than 30 per cent of US men over the age of 17 may be eligible for VA medical care. A system of priorities has been established. The highest priority is for illness or disability incurred in military service. The second category is the veteran who has been disabled to some extent in military service, but who needs care for some other form of disability. In the third category is the veteran with non-service connected disability who claims to be unable to pay for medical care in other institutions. The question of inability to pay is answered largely by a statement made by the veteran. At the end of the Second World War, arrangements were made for affiliation between VA hospitals and various medical schools. Now about three-quarters of all VA hospital staff members have medical school faculty appointments. This has been advantageous to both parties, and has undoubtedly accounted for a general upgrading of the quality of medical care provided in veterans' hospitals.

The VA Department of Medicine and Surgery also sponsors biomedical research; this source of research funding is important in the overall research activity in the USA today. Two VA scientists, R. S. Yalow and A. V. Schally, received *Nobel prizes in recognition of their work. The system of VA hospitals has provided an excellent base for multicentre programmes to evaluate forms of therapy, for example the *chemotherapy of *tuberculosis, and *coronary bypass surgery. Several agencies of government were responsible for funding veterans' benefits, pensions, and care in the early history of the USA, but these were all combined in 1930 with the formation of the Veterans' Administration. It was made an independent agency responsible directly to the President of the USA; it is exceeded only by the Defense Department and the Postal Service in its number of federal employees. The motto of the Veterans' Administration is a phrase from the second inaugural address of Abraham Lincoln: 'To care for him who shall have borne the battle and for his widow, and his orphan'.

VETERINARY MEDICINE IN RELATION TO HUMAN MEDICINE. The special relationship between animal and man is one of antiquity, and with the evolution of relatively static man–animal cultures from about 9000 BC onwards there was increasing evidence that animals were given special acknowledgement of their role in society. In Egypt they were deified, being mummified and given ceremonial burial, as exemplified by the Apis bull cult of Memphis. The Serapeum, the large special burial site for Apis bulls begun by the Pharaoh Amasis in 574 BC, is an example of the importance of the cult. The supreme goddess, Hathor, the cow, the earth mother of upper and lower Egypt, was the deity from which the Pharaohs claimed their legitimacy to the throne.

In these early cultures the art and science of healing animals and man coincided, and priests became healers of both the animal and human gods; in early civilizations the treatment of animals was well ahead of that of humans. Specialism was recognized throughout the ancient cultures and, indeed, separate identities were given to the practice of healing various species, and veterinary hospitals were established, for example the pasuciktsa by the Buddhist emperor Asuka, well before the creation of human hospitals.

These examples of comparative medicine were also fostered by Greek mythology, in which Chiron, the

Chief Centaur, played an important role, as did *Aesculapius the god of medicine, son of Apollo, and entrusted to Chiron for his upbringing. But the advent of the Christian era brought a substantial change in outlook, animals being relegated to an inferior position, and the Cartesian doctrine of *Descartes epitomized the concept that animals were automata, like clocks, capable of complex behaviour but devoid of speech, constructive reasoning, and, especially, of feeling pain. During this nadir of relationships with animals, those who dealt with them were held in similar low status, for example veterinarians were 'cow leeches', but with the establishment of veterinary schools, first in Lyon in France (1762) then in London (1791), followed by many in several European countries, the science of the 'art and science' increasingly predominated, but not without set-backs along the way. The name 'veterinary surgeons' derived in 1796 from the need by the British Army's Board of General Officers to distinguish them from human surgeons. Previously they had been called farriers.

Laboratory animal medicine
Veterinarians are increasingly involved in providing advice and undertaking duties concerning the health, care, and welfare of laboratory animals, and serving in an official capacity as Named Veterinary Surgeon in the UK under the *Animals (Scientific Procedures) Act 1986. The Named Veterinary Surgeon, who may be a full-time staff member of an institution or part-time from private general practice, is increasingly recognized as an important participant in providing the best possible health care to experimental animals, thereby ensuring the maximum opportunity for effective research. Apart from the skills applicable to disease prevention and control, breeding, and feeding, he also frequently collaborates with research workers by providing surgical and other manipulative expertise. While the *Cruelty to Animals Act of 1876 served a most useful purpose for over 100 years, the need for change was increasingly demanded. In the 1970s and 1980s, the veterinary profession played an important role in introducing change by the provision of advice to legislators and joining with animal welfare societies for the effective coming together of minds on the many issues concerning experimental animals.

Indeed, the profession played a substantial role in the events leading to the promulgation of the 1876 Act. For example, in 1863 it became known that students in the veterinary schools in Alfort and Lyon in France were required to perform dissections to gain surgical dexterity on live horses without anaesthesia. A petition signed by 500 British veterinary surgeons was delivered to Alfort by a Mr James Cowie and the practice was eventually stopped. Much of the effort to bring legislative control to animal experimentation (vivisection) was provided by the Royal Society for the Prevention of Cruelty to Animals, an organization founded in 1824. The importance placed on animal welfare in Britain may be gauged by the fact that the National Society for the Prevention of Cruelty to Children was not established until some 60 years later.

Food hygiene

The traditional role of the veterinarian in this field has been, and still is, the inspection of slaughtered animals and condemnation of those unfit for human consumption. While the UK has trained overseas personnel for this discipline and established effective systems in other countries through aid programmes, it is an anomaly that until recently in England and Wales meat inspection was largely in the hands of local authority environmental health officers, and veterinary responsibility occurred only when meat was intended for export. This anomaly has been removed with the Single European Act, but the role of the veterinarian in ensuring a healthy and wholesome meat product, produced under conditions of good welfare, has greatly expanded, and the veterinarian is now responsible for ante-mortem inspection of animals, the hygiene of the slaughter house, and the immediate healthiness of the carcase. Indeed, the increasing role of the veterinarian in the food chain may involve him 'from conception to consumption', in view of his increasing inputs to breeding, selection of genetic material, rearing, and feeding of animals. The veterinary surgeon has yet to have a major input to the wholesale marketing and customer interface, but it is perceived that in order to provide a sound and whole-some end-product, a food chain should have substantial veterinary input. Fundamental changes in the production of human foods of animal origin have occurred over the past few decades, many resulting from intensive methods of husbandry. This has greatly increased the incidence of certain infections, e.g. *Salmonella, and feed additives for growth promotion, pesticide residues, antibiotic residues, heavy metals, and fungal toxins also pose problems in the safety of food.

New challenges in this field will be the health and wholesomeness of animal products from hitherto unusual farmed species, including fish, shellfish, duck, camelids, and the like.

Companion animals

Increasing numbers of companion animals are kept by an increasing number of households in the Western world. In the UK every second household owns a pet (or preferably a companion animal), amounting to 7.5 million dogs, some 7 million cats, and a range of other species, including fish, amphibians, and reptiles. The human–companion animal bond is increasingly recognized as an important component in the normal everyday life of people, and an indispensable part of life for many elderly persons or the handicapped or disabled. Maintaining the health of this population of animals devolves on the private veterinary practitioners, 60 per cent of whom are largely or wholly occupied by this work. While pet health insurance schemes exist and are increasing in number, as is the number of animals covered, the majority are still not so insured. It is noteworthy that the veterinary profession provides a national animal health service at little or no cost to government in this respect.

Apart from companionship and emotional rewards, pets can exert a distinct and positive influence on the health of humans. Such medical benefits include increased survival rates in pet-owning heart attack patients, and significantly lower *cholesterol and triglyceride levels and lower systolic *blood pressure than in equivalent individuals who do not own dogs or cats. More recently, it has been shown that individuals suffer significantly fewer minor medical complaints if a companion animal is in the household. The UK pet owner is typically young to middle aged with children, not the affection-deprived elderly social group often associated with pet-keeping. The phenomenon is not new, for it is recorded that William of Wykeham, the founder of Winchester College in 1387, sternly admonished the Abbess of Romsey to discourage her nuns from keeping 'birds, rabbits, hounds and such frivolous creatures to which they have given more heed than to the offices of the church, and frequent hindrance . . . to the grievous peril of their souls'.

Zoonoses

These are diseases naturally transmitted between vertebrate animals and man, and where contact is close, as in the human–companion animal relationship, it is to be expected that disease agent transmission is facilitated. Examples of this are visceral larva migrans of children, caused by the migratory larval stages of the *nematode *Toxocara canis and congenital *toxoplasmosis of children derived from *Toxoplasma gondii*, an intestinal parasite of the cat. In the first example, regular antiworm treatment of puppies and of pregnant bitches in the later stages of gestation can greatly reduce environmental contamination of gardens and public parks, playgrounds, etc. Recent research has identified the nursing bitch as an important source of parasite eggs which, when embryonated and then ingested accidentally by children, cause either the visceral or ocular form of larva migrans.

The treatment of cats infected with *Toxoplasma* is less satisfactory, and although immunity to the infection in cats develops quickly, several million oocysts may be shed in the faeces before a cat becomes refractory to infection. Humans may become infected by accidental ingestion of sporulated (infective) oocysts through contaminated vegetables, cleaning of litter trays, etc., but an additional source is the ingestion of infected meat containing other infective developmental stages. Should this occur in a pregnant woman, previously unexposed to *Toxoplasma*, congenital toxoplasmosis may result in the child. Vaccines against toxoplasmosis have been developed for sheep, in which abortion occurs, and recent research has focused on the development of a vaccine for cats using recombinant *DNA technology.

The outstanding zoonosis of dog origin is *rabies. In the UK since 1922 there has been no case of rabies in animals not undergoing quarantine. The situation is quite different on the continent of Europe. In the first quarter of 1993, 2119 cases were reported, but countries such as Portugal, Spain, Greece, Denmark, The Netherlands, Finland, and Ireland remained free of rabies. Of the 2119 cases, 1627 occurred in wild animals (76.8 per cent) and 490 in domestic animals, such as dogs, cats, cattle, small ruminants, horses, etc. Two human cases occurred in the European part of the Russian Federation, compared with 16 and 3 cases in that area in the previous 2 years, respectively.

*Vaccination of dogs (and other domestic animals) has greatly reduced the incidence of rabies in these animals and in man in many countries. When coupled with vaccination of humans at possible risk, rabies in man is rare. However, the large number of infected wild animals, especially foxes, poses a potential problem of 'spill-over' into domestic carnivores with a result-ant threat to man. This possibility is much reduced by the oral vaccination of foxes using a recombinant *vaccinia–rabies vaccine offered in a bait which can be distributed by small aeroplanes at low altitudes or by ground personnel. Such vaccination, using a re-combinant vaccinia–rabies virus or an SAD (Street–Alabama–Dufferin) double mutant vaccine, is a power-ful tool, and for the first time rabies has been eradicated from large areas of Europe. Some 9 million baits have been deposited over an area of more than 300 000 km^2. In France oral vaccination was used in 1992 to protect young foxes over the entire area of rabies infection (111 600 km^2).

Some zoonoses, for example bovine *tuberculosis, *brucellosis, and salmonellosis, are of great economic importance in animal production, as well as being a threat to human health. Control programmes have resulted in the near eradication of the first two, but in the case of salmonellosis intensive livestock systems and the use of antimicrobial feed additives present difficulties in achieving the desired control.

Control of animal diseases

The veterinary profession has an excellent record in the control and eradication of animal diseases. Major plagues affecting domestic animals, such as rinder-pest, contagious bovine pleuropneumonia, glanders of horses, and more recently, foot-and-mouth dis-ease and warble fly infestation of cattle, have been eradicated from the UK. They present object lessons in surveillance, diagnosis, and control, and although not zoonoses (with the exception of glanders), they are important indirectly to the economic health and well-being of the nation: this was possibly summed up by the then Archbishop of Canterbury who, during 1865, when cattle plague (rinderpest) entered the country and

killed half a million cattle, sought the ear of the Lord in a prayer 'Stay we pray Thee, this plague . . . shield our homes from its ravages'.

It is worth mentioning that the control of cattle plague was beset with contention between medical and veterin-ary authorities, by attempts to treat affected animals, by prejudice, and by taking political capital from the situation. Nevertheless, with the acceptance of a slaugh-ter policy for affected animals, the disease was rapidly brought under control.

Elsewhere in the world *pandemics of disease, destructive to organized livestock farming and con-ducive to human distress, poverty, and famine, have been brought under control by veterinary research and the application of control, vaccination, or eradication policies. Particularly severely affected is the peasant farmer of developing countries, who so frequently is totally reliant on oxen, buffalo, or other draught animals for his livelihood. Should illness befall these animals then disaster may be the result. Examples of the *successful control of animal diseases are the eradication of Texas fever (babesiosis) from cattle in the USA, through a determined arsenical dipping programme against the transmitting tick *Boophilus annulatus* over the first quar-ter of this century; and the control of tick-transmitted diseases in tropical countries in Africa and elsewhere by regular routine dipping.

Major progress has been made over the past few decades in the production of vaccines for the control of animal diseases which threaten the national economy of many countries. Examples of such vaccines include an in-feed Newcastle disease vaccine for poultry for use by small farmers in South-East Asia, prepared from a heat-resistant strain of the virus; an attenuated, and more recently a recombinant, vaccine for babesiosis of cattle in Australia; a tick vaccine based on immunization of cattle with 'concealed antigens', namely tick-gut cell antigens; a cell culture rinderpest vaccine for cattle; an *anthrax vaccine; one for hog *cholera or swine fever; vaccines from the several strains of foot-and-mouth disease; and so on. Indeed, there is now scarcely an infectious disease of animals for which there is not an effective vaccine. Parasitic helminths are an exception to this, other than the vaccine against bovine lungworm.

Comparative medicine

This is the advancement of the understanding of human diseases by studies of analogous conditions in animals. Many animal models of human disease exist naturally and they assist greatly in the understanding of human disorder. They provide opportunities for study of the environmental, genetic, and nutritional factors, for example, leading to expression of disease, and allow experimental manipulation not applicable to the human form of the condition. It is likely that most human disorders have an animal counterpart, although the animal kingdom has not yet been fully explored in this respect. Alternatively, animal models may be created experimentally. In some cases, the induced animal disease behaves similarly in man, and hence is a valuable research entity, but it may not always do so; nevertheless, the reasons for this difference may be important in understanding the disease.

Examples of naturally occurring animal models assisting the understanding of human disease include the infection of cats by the feline immunodeficiency virus, which closely resembles *HIV in structure, its genome, and its tropism for T lymphocytes. The infection in cats mirrors *AIDS in a number of respects, as the animals suffer a variety of immunodeficiency syndromes. However, sexual transmission is not thought to be of major importance. There are also several genetically determined disorders in animals which have a counterpart in man, such as, for example, *X-linked dystrophin deficiency in mice and dogs, comparable with the X-linked *muscular dystrophies in man.

Scrapie, a degenerative neurological disorder of sheep, has many similarities to 'slow virus disorders' of man, such as *Creutzfeldt–Jakob syndrome, Gerstmann–Straussler syndrome, and *kuru. However, the identity of the infectious agent is unknown. Various propositions have been advanced for the nature of the infectious particle, from an infectious protein, or '*prion', to a nucleic acid or 'virino'. Research on scrapie has identified a susceptibility gene in mice and sheep, and has also provided essential information on the pathogenesis of these neurological disorders. In the case of kuru, cannibalism of human brains was responsible for transmission, and it was of particular interest that *bovine spongiform encephalopathy (BSE or 'mad cow disease') can be traced to the feeding of animal-derived protein, mainly from sheep heads and offal. The prohibition of feeding animal-derived protein to cattle will eventually lead to the eradication of the disorder, although this is likely to take several years, due to the prolonged incubation period of BSE.

Many *cancers of animals resemble those of humans in location and character (e.g. mammary tumours of dogs). They offer a unique opportunity to investigate the breed or genetic susceptibility of dogs, for example, to mammary tumours, and new approaches to treatments such as radiotherapy.

Whereas hitherto artificially created animal models of human disease have been achieved by deliberate infection with micro-organisms or surgical or other manipulations of the animals, in the future, animal models may be created by genetic modifications, so as to create a specific target for pharmaceutical investigations, thereby lending a degree of accuracy to investigations previously unavailable with conventional animals.

An area of veterinary research that has direct benefit to human medicine is veterinary parasitology. Almost all antiparasitic compounds in use today were developed initially for veterinary use and were evaluated in parasite-infected animals. This is because the antiparasitic compound market is both lucrative and essential for the control of parasitic diseases of livestock, while the countries that need antiparasitic compounds for human patients are the least able to afford them, or their development costs.

One medicine

In past centuries the medical and veterinary professions have evolved separately, and their respective skills of healing and the empirical use of remedies for different types of patients have maintained this distinction. However, the two professions now share and contribute to the same body of scientific knowledge, and each is as much at home as the other in biomedical research laboratories. Animal health and welfare contribute very importantly to their human counterparts, and can be best expressed as 'one medicine' for the benefit of all.

SOULSBY

Further reading

Beveridge, W. I. B. (1978). The need for closer collaboration between medical and veterinary professions. *Bulletin of the World Health Organization*, **56**, 849–58.
Edny, A. (1992). Companion animals and human health. *Veterinary Record*, **130**, 285–87.
Pattison, I. (1984). *The British Veterinary Profession. 1791–1948*. J. A. Allen, London.

VIBRIO is a genus of motile curved and rod-shaped Gram-negative *bacteria which includes the causative agent of *cholera, *Vibrio cholerae*.

VIBROMASSAGE is a method of *massage employing an electrically powered vibrating pad.

VICARY, THOMAS (d. 1561). British surgeon. He features in Holbein's painting, receiving from Henry VIII in 1541 the Act of Incorporation of the Company of *Barber-Surgeons, in the formation of which he was instrumental.

VICQ D'AZYR, FELIX (1748–94). French physician and anatomist. A distinguished anatomist, his name is attached to the mammillothalamic fasciculus which joins the *mammillary bodies to the *thalamus (Bundle of Vicq d'Azyr).

VIDIUS, VIDUS (1508–69). See GUIDI, GUIDO.

VIERORDT, KARL VON (1818–84). German physiologist. He was the first to devise a method of enumerating the red blood cells (1851) and worked on cardiovascular and respiratory physiology. He made the first *sphygmograph (1855).

VIEUSSENS, RAYMOND (*c.* 1635–1715). French physician and anatomist. He was first to describe *aortic incompetence and its characteristic pulse wave (1695) and *mitral stenosis (1705).

VILLEMIN, JEAN ANTOINE (1827–92). French physician. In 1868 he firmly established the infectivity of *tuberculosis by transferring it from man to rabbit. This was before *Koch had isolated the mycobacterium and Villemin's work was discounted.

VILLUS. A projection from a *membrane, usually with a rich blood supply.

VINBLASTINE is one of several *alkaloids extracted from the plant *Vinca rosea*, collectively known as the vinca alkaloids. They are cytotoxic, causing *metaphase arrest by interfering with *microtubule assembly, and are used as *antineoplastic agents. Vinblastine is used particularly against *lymphomas and malignant *teratomas. It may cause toxic depression of *bone marrow.

VINCI, LEONARDO DA. See LEONARDO DA VINCI.

VINCRISTINE is a vinca alkaloid (see VINBLASTINE), used in the treatment of *leukaemias and *lymphomas and of some solid tumours. It may cause neurotoxic side-effects.

VINYL CHLORIDE (C_2H_3Cl), or chloroethylene, is also known as VCM (vinyl chloride monomer). The toxic effects of vinyl chloride, which is extensively used in the manufacture of PVC (polyvinylchloride, to which it polymerizes) and other vinyl polymers and was also employed as a propellant in aerosol sprays and cosmetics, were recognized in man only after it had been shown to induce *tumours in animals. It is now known that exposure to this chemical causes angiosarcoma of the liver, an otherwise unusual malignant tumour, as well as an unrelated condition called acro-osteolysis, a form of finger *clubbing associated with *scleroderma and *Raynaud's phenomenon. Occupational exposure in industry to vinyl chloride is now limited to a concentration of 10 parts per million, and its use as an aerosol propellant and in cosmetics is prohibited (1976 Directive of the Council of the European Communities). See also OCCUPATIONAL MEDICINE.

VIRCHOW, RUDOLF KARL (1821–1902). German pathologist. An outstanding figure in 19th century medicine, he has been accounted the greatest pathologist of all time. Although not of great originality, he avoided metaphysical speculation and his opinions were founded on his own observations and experience. His most famous work *Die Cellularpathologie* (1858) applied the *cell theory to *pathology and allowed him to proclaim his doctrine of 'omnis cellula e cellula'. He regarded all disease as disease of cells. He described *leukaemia (1845), invented the term *amyloid', studied *thrombosis and introduced the idea of *embolism (1846–56), and observed and defined *leucocytosis. He first described the *neuroglia (1846) and the cerebral perivascular spaces (Virchow–Robin spaces, 1851). In his later years he became interested in anthropology and wrote widely on the subject. In 1847 he founded the still extant *Archiv für pathologische Anatomie* (*Virchows Archiv*). Virchow was a man of powerful personality, unbounded energy, and strongly held opinions. At the end of his life he not only enjoyed unparalleled renown in the international world of medicine, but was one of the great folk heroes of Germany. See also PATHOLOGY.

VIRILISM is synonymous with *masculinization.

VIROLOGY is the branch of *microbiology concerned with *viruses. See MICROBIOLOGY.

VIRULENCE is the ability of a particular micro-organism (bacterium, virus, protozoan, etc.) to cause infection or death. Epidemiologically, virulence is judged by severity of clinical disease or by case fatality rate. In the laboratory, virulence is quantified by measuring the dose of micro-organisms required to kill one-half of a population of experimental animals (the median lethal dose or LD_{50}) or to produce some observable effect other than death (the median effective dose or ED_{50}).

VIRUS. An infectious micro-organism smaller than a *bacterium, usually beyond the resolution of the light *microscope, and consisting simply of a nucleic acid (*deoxyribonucleic acid (DNA) or *ribonucleic acid (RNA), but never both) genome in a protein envelope. Unlike bacteria, viruses can only reproduce inside host cells. See MICROBIOLOGY, MEDICAL.

VISCOSITY is the property of a fluid whereby it tends to resist relative motion within itself. A viscous liquid (i.e. one of high viscosity) drags in a treacle-like manner. Viscosity is measured in newton seconds per square metre (SI units).

VISCUS. Any of the large organs of the body (plural: viscera).

VISION is the faculty of sight, or the act of seeing. Visual acuity, or sharpness of sight, depends on the ability of the eye to adjust its total refractive power so that both near and distant objects can be brought into focus on the retina (see LENS; OPHTHALMOLOGY). Too strong a refractive power relative to the anteroposterior length of the eye causes short-sight (myopia), too weak long-sight (hypermetropia).

VISNA is a slow virus infection of the central nervous system in sheep, characterized by progressive paralysis and pathological changes of inflammation and demyelination; it is due to a ribonucleic acid (RNA) *retrovirus (cf. SCRAPIE).

VISUAL ACUITY is sharpness (i.e. power of *resolution) of vision, usually measured by means of standard *test types.

VISUAL FIELD. The area, assessed for each eye separately with the visual axis aimed straight forward, within which visual stimuli can be perceived; it can be roughly but usefully assessed at the bedside by 'confrontation' testing, that is by comparison with the examiner's (contralateral) visual field.

VISUAL PURPLE. See RHODOPSIN.

VITAL CAPACITY is the maximum volume of gas which can be expelled from the lungs after maximal inspiration.

VITALISM is the doctrine that the origin and manifestations of life are produced by a vital force or principle distinct from chemical and physical forces.

VITAL STATISTICS is that branch of statistics, sometimes known as biostatistics, which deals with demographic data (birth rate, death rate, morbidity, etc.). See EPIDEMIOLOGY.

VITAMIN A, also known as retinol, is a fat-soluble vitamin, which, together with its precursor substance (or pro-vitamin) carotene, is widely distributed in foodstuffs, particularly dairy products, fish liver oils, and vegetables. It is essential for the normal functioning of skin and mucous membranes and for adequate night vision (see CAROTENE; XEROPHTHALMIA; NIGHT BLINDNESS; RHODOPSIN). Very large doses of vitamin A are toxic.

VITAMIN B covers a number of essential water-soluble dietary components, collectively known as the vitamin B complex. They include thiamin, also known as aneurin or vitamin B_1 (see BERIBERI; THIAMIN); riboflavin or vitamin B_2, which functions as a *coenzyme in the processes of oxidative metabolism and which is plentiful in the normal Western diet; niacin or vitamin B_3, sometimes also called vitamin PP for 'pellagra-preventing', which is a mixture of nicotinic acid and nicotinamide (see NIACIN; PELLAGRA); pantothenic acid or vitamin B_5, essential as part of the coenzyme A molecule for normal metabolism, but so available in the human diet that spontaneous deficiency does not occur; pyridoxine and related substances, collectively known as vitamin B_6, which are concerned particularly with amino acid metabolism and lack of which may be a cause of anaemia; and cyanocobalamin or vitamin B_{12} (see CYANOCOBALAMIN; PERNICIOUS ANAEMIA). Other substances usually classified with the vitamin B complex are *biotin (or vitamin H), *choline, and *folic acid, although spontaneous deficiency of the first two probably does not occur in man and choline is not strictly a vitamin (see MEGALOBLASTIC ANAEMIA).

VITAMIN C. See ASCORBIC ACID; SCURVY.

VITAMIN D. See CALCIFEROL; OSTEOMALACIA; RICKETS.

VITAMIN E. See TOCOPHEROL.

VITAMIN K. A group of fat-soluble vitamins which promotes the synthesis in the liver of *prothrombin and several other blood coagulation factors (see HAEMATOLOGY). Although the dietary content of vitamin K is normally adequate (and is supplemented by bacterial synthesis in the gastrointestinal tract), a deficiency may develop in conditions associated with *malabsorption of fat. Newborn infants may also suffer from a haemorrhagic state due to deficiency of vitamin K, while oral anticoagulant drugs such as the *coumarin group achieve their effect by inhibiting the K- dependent hepatic synthesis of clotting factors.

VITAMINS, or accessory food factors, comprise a group of unrelated organic compounds which have in common the twin attributes of being necessary in trace amounts to the normal metabolic functioning of an organism and yet cannot be synthesized by it; to remain healthy, the organism must therefore obtain them from the environment, in man normally from the diet. Vitamins are peculiar to species; what is a vitamin for one organism may be synthesized by another and is not therefore a vitamin for that species. For example, vitamin C (*ascorbic acid) is an essential part of man's diet but of few other animals. The defining qualifications 'organic' and 'in trace amounts' should be noted. Essential *amino acids and essential *trace elements are not vitamins.

Adequate amounts of the various vitamins are necessary to the human diet to prevent corresponding deficiency disorders. For recommended daily dietary allowances, see NUTRITION. There is no good evidence that excessive amounts are ever beneficial, and, as in the case of vitamins A and D, they may be harmful. Sir Frederick Gowland *Hopkins first proposed the existence of accessory food factors in 1906, although deficiency diseases such as *scurvy, *beriberi, and *rickets had been treated empirically with appropriate foodstuffs for many years before that.

VITILIGO is a skin disorder in which there is progressive destruction of epidermal melanocytes (*melanin-producing cells), probably as a result of an *autoimmune process, causing patches of depigmentation. The white areas are usually symmetrical, sharply defined, and with a scalloped and hyperpigmented border. Other autoimmune disorders may be associated.

VITREOUS. The transparent gel-like substance that occupies the posterior cavity of the eye, between the *lens and the *retina. See OPHTHALMOLOGY.

VIVISECTION is the performance of experiments on living animals involving surgical procedures. See

LICENCES FOR ANIMAL EXPERIMENTATION; VETERI-NARY MEDICINE.

VOCAL CORDS. The two mucous membrane-covered ridges which form the V-shaped opening within the *larynx known as the *glottis, through which the breath passes; their length and tension determine the pitch of the voice; they are drawn together as the glottis closes during swallowing.

VOIT, KARL VON (1831–1908). German physiologist. Much of his working life was devoted to metabolic research and especially to the chemistry of *nutrition. He worked with *Pettenkofer in devising a method of studying simultaneously the utilization of food, heat production, and respiratory exchange in large animals. Together they proved the conservation of energy in living animals.

VOLKMANN, RICHARD VON (1830–89). German surgeon. A supporter of *Lister's views, he was the first to excise the rectum for cancer (1878). He described the fibrosis of muscle resulting from *ischaemia (Volkmann's ischaemic contracture, 1881), and recommended cod liver oil in surgical tuberculosis. He was also a poet of distinction (under the name Richard Leander).

VOLVULUS. Twisting of a loop of *intestine and its mesenteric attachment, causing intestinal *ischaemia and obstruction.

VOMITING is the forcible regurgitation and ejection through the mouth of the contents of the stomach. It is a reflex action of obvious protective value when due, for example, to ingestion of an irritant substance, and is preceded or accompanied by retching, nausea, sweating, and pallor. It involves reverse peristaltic contractions of the stomach and spasmodic contractions of respiratory and abdominal muscles. It is controlled by vomiting centres in the *medulla oblongata of the brain, and can be precipitated by various stimuli.

VORONOFF, SERGE (1866–1951). French physiologist and surgeon. Born in Russia, he became a naturalized French citizen in 1897. He worked on the grafting of organs, with special reference to rejuvenation and the prevention of ageing through grafting testicular tissue.

VOYEURISM is a sexual deviation (or variation as some have it) in which vicarious pleasure is obtained from observation of the sexual activity of others, even sometimes of animals. It includes *troilism and the peeping-tom syndrome.

VULVA. The female external genitalia, bounded by the mons veneris (mons pubis) and the two folds of skin and subcutaneous fat known as the *labia majora or greater pudendal lips and enclosing the labia minora or lesser pudendal lips, the *vaginal and *urethral orifices, and the clitoris.

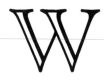

WAGNER-JAUREGG, JULIUS (1857–1941). Austrian psychiatrist. He was interested in the beneficial effect of *fever in psychotics, especially in those with dementia paralytica (*general paralysis of the insane). In 1917 he inoculated such a patient with benign tertian *malaria and noted striking improvement. He continued to develop the method for the next 20 years. In 1927 he was awarded the *Nobel prize for his work.

WAKLEY, THOMAS (1795–1862). British physician, reformer, and editor. Wakley was a friend of William Cobbett and well aware of the jobbery and nepotism in the medical profession. He founded the *Lancet* in 1823, publishing reports of hospital lectures and operations and attacking hospital administration and the Royal College of Surgeons. Involved in many law suits, he was coroner for West Middlesex from 1839 until his death and sat as Member of Parliament for Finsbury from 1835 until 1852. He obtained a pardon for the Tolpuddle Martyrs. Clauses from his Private Member's Bill were adopted in the *Medical Act 1858. He reduced adulteration by publishing analyses of foods in the *Lancet* (1851). His life was an unremitting battle against injustice, favouritism, and charlatanism. See also MEDICAL JOURNALS.

WAKSMAN, SELMAN ABRAHAM (1888–1973). American microbiologist. His field of study was the microbiology of soil. From various soil organisms he isolated *antibiotics, including *streptomycin, *neomycin, and *actinomycin. For his work on streptomycin, the first effective treatment for *tuberculosis, he received many honours, including the *Nobel prize in 1952.

WALDEYER-HARTZ, HEINRICH WILHELM GOTTFRIED VON (1836–1921).German anatomist. He studied the spread of *tumours and the mechanism of *metastasis (1867–72), discovered the germinal epithelium (1870), and described the pharyngeal lymphoid tissue (Waldeyer's ring). He suggested the terms '*chromosome' and '*neurone', showing that the second was the basic unit of the nervous system.

WALE, JOHANNES DE (WALAEUS) (1604–49). Dutch physician. Wale was a strong supporter of *Harvey's views on the circulation. He confirmed these by showing that blood spurted from a ligated artery if an incision were made proximal to the ligature, but only oozed through one which was distal (1640).

WALLER, AUGUSTUS DESIRE (1856–1922). English physiologist. He investigated many topics with scrupulous accuracy. Most concerned the electrical response of tissues to stimulation. He used the capillary electrometer and the string galvanometer, but his favourite instrument was the reflecting galvanometer. Among important advances in cardiac electrophysiology, he was the first to suggest the electric dipole model of the heart (1898), showing how the varying cardiac potentials could be measured at the body surface and how the human *electrocardiogram could be obtained. He also studied nerve excitation and the effect of narcotic and other drugs; and was led on from this to a consideration of the problems of general anaesthesia. Publishing much, his books included *Introduction to physiology* in 1891 which was highly praised, and another book on *Animal electricity*.

WALLER, AUGUSTUS VOLNEY (1816–70). British physiologist. He demonstrated the vasoconstrictor action of *sympathetic nerves and the function of the *posterior root ganglia. He described the *diapedesis of *leucocytes (1846) and the degeneration of the *myelin sheath of a *nerve after its section ('Wallerian degeneration', 1851).

WALSHE, SIR FRANCIS MARTIN ROUSE (1885–1973). British neurologist. His interests lay in the correlation of clinical and experimental findings, but in later years, he gained an international reputation as an acutely critical writer on *neurology.

WARBURG, OTTO HEINRICH (1883–1970). German biochemist. His researches covered a wide field: he made many contributions to biochemical methods; he identified cytochrome oxidase (1934) and *nicotinamide (1938); and he studied *photosynthesis, tissue *respiration, and the metabolism of *cancer cells. He was awarded the *Nobel prize in 1931.

WARD, JOSHUA (1685–1761). British quack doctor. Although Ward was returned as Member of Parliament for Marlborough in 1716, he never took his seat and had to flee to France because of electoral irregularities. While abroad he devised his celebrated 'drop and pill' and returned to England with a pardon from the king, whose dislocated thumb he had reduced. Ward, known as 'Spot' because of a facial birthmark, converted three houses in Pimlico into a hospital for the poor. He was exempted by name from the Apothecaries Act (1748), which disallowed unregistered prescription. His pill, which contained *antimony, is said to have killed as many as it cured.

WARDROP, JAMES (1782–1869). British surgeon. He was renowned for the operation of resection of the lower jaw and for distal ligature for *aneurysm.

WARFARIN is one of the *coumarin group of oral *anticoagulants used in the prophylaxis and treatment of venous thrombosis and its complications, and in other situations where it is desired to inhibit blood coagulation. It is also used as rat poison.

WARREN, JOHN (1753–1815). American surgeon. Born in Roxbury, Massachusetts, USA, he took an active part in the Boston Tea Party of 1773. He was prominent in helping to control *smallpox and *yellow fever epidemics. He gave anatomical lectures at the military hospital in Boston, helped found the Boston Medical Society, and established the first school of medicine associated with *Harvard in 1782, becoming the first professor of anatomy and surgery there.

WARREN, JOHN COLLINS (1778–1856). American surgeon. Warren performed the first operation for *strangulated hernia in the USA, and in 1846 invited the dentist *Morton to administer ether *anaesthesia to a patient, from whom he removed a tumour of the neck. The Warren Museum of Harvard Medical School was founded on the geological, palaeontological, and other specimens he left. He was also a founder of the *New England Journal of Medicine and Surgery*.

WARREN, W. DEAN (1924–89). American surgeon. He made major contributions to the pathophysiology of portal hypertension. He was appointed Chairman of the Department of Surgery at the University of Miami, and served as President of the Society of Surgery of the Alimentary Tract, the Allen O. Whipple Society, the American Surgery Association, and the American College of Surgeons.

WART. See VERRUCA.

WASSERMANN, AUGUST-PAUL VON (1860–1925). German bacteriologist. He studied *complement fixation and described his test for syphilis in 1906 (Wassermann reaction). In later years he turned his attention to the *chemotherapy of cancer.

WASSERMANN REACTION. One of several serological tests for *syphilis which depend upon the fact that syphilitic patients (and occasionally those with other diseases) develop *antibodies to a normal component of many tissues called cardiolipin. See KAHN TEST.

WATER (H_2O) is the normal oxide of *hydrogen. Pure water (natural water is never quite pure) is a colourless, odourless liquid of melting point 0 °C and boiling point 100 °C, with a maximum density of 1.000 gram per cubic centimetre at 4 °C. The human body (70 kg) contains about 40 litres of water.

WATER BED. A water-filled rubber mattress, the object of which is to ensure that the patient's weight is distributed evenly.

WATERBRASH is *regurgitation into the throat and mouth of acid sour-tasting fluid from the stomach, often accompanied by *heartburn.

WATER CLOSET. A device for flushing excreta into a drain by discharging the contents of a water cistern. Water closets first came into limited use in the latter half of the 18th century, when they constituted a potent source of infection because of the dry brick-built drains into which they emptied.

WATER-HAMMER PULSE is the term (named after a Victorian toy) given to a type of arterial *pulse wave in which there is an unusually sharp upstroke followed by a similarly abrupt *diastolic collapse, so that the percussion wave gives a palpable shock to the examining fingers. The sign, also known as a collapsing pulse or Corrigan's pulse (see *CORRIGAN), is most marked in *aortic incompetence.

WATERHOUSE, BENJAMIN (1754–1846). American physician. Waterhouse studied medicine at Edinburgh, Leiden, and *Harvard. He practised in Boston, and became professor of the theory and practice of physic at Harvard. From about 1800 he began using *Jenner's method of cow-pox *vaccination, to protect against *smallpox. This caused much controversy. He was supported in the matter by President Thomas Jefferson, and lived to see himself vindicated.

WATER SUPPLY. The object is to supply the community with an adequate quantity of clean, pure, odourless, and palatable water. The two most important medical aspects of water supply are chemical and microbiological. *Dental caries is markedly influenced by the *fluoride content of water; areas in which the supply contains one part per million or more have a very low prevalence of caries compared with those in which the content is much less. Hardness or softness, governed by the content of calcium and magnesium salts, may also be important; a positive correlation between soft water and the incidence of sudden death from *coronary heart disease has been suggested. Iodine deficiency in water is a possible cause of *goitre.

Numerous viral, bacterial, and parasitic diseases may be transmitted by contaminated water. They include viral hepatitis, poliomyelitis, gastroenteritis, enteric fever, bacillary dysentery, leptospirosis, cholera, amoebiasis, hookworm, bilharziasis, filariasis, and many others.

WAVE. A periodic disturbance in a medium or in space that involves the elastic displacement of material particles or a periodic change in some physical quantity (e.g. temperature, pressure, electric potential, etc.).

WAX BATHS. A technique of *physiotherapy for applying heat to a part of the body by immersing it in heated liquid wax.

WEAKNESS. Lack of strength, feebleness, ill health.

WEAL (alternative spelling, wheal). A raised streak or patch of cutaneous *oedema accompanied by *erythema, due to *trauma or *urticaria.

WEATHER AND DISEASE. See ECOLOGY; ENVIRONMENT AND MEDICINE I; FAMINE; FROSTBITE; HEAT AS CAUSE OF DISEASE; TROPICAL MEDICINE AND PARASITOLOGY.

WEBER, ERNST HEINRICH (1795–1878). German anatomist and physiologist. Weber was appointed professor of anatomy at Leipzig (1821) and was one of three brothers holding chairs there. With one of them, Eduard Friedrich Weber (1806–71), he applied the study of hydrodynamics to the circulation and measured the velocity of the *pulse wave (1825). They were the first to demonstrate the inhibitory effect of *vagal stimulation (1845). His later researches were into sensory functions, especially those of touch and temperature.

WEBER, FRIEDRICH EUGEN (1832–91). German otologist. In Weber's test for *deafness a vibrating tuning fork is applied to the vertex of the skull. If the air passages are blocked on one side the sound is best heard there. If the internal ear is affected by disease the sound is best heard on the unaffected side.

WEBER, FREDERICK PARKES (1863–1962). English physician. He was a supreme collector and describer of medical rarities, and his name is linked with familial *telangiectasia, cerebral *angioma, and relapsing

*panniculitis (*Weber–Christian disease). In his life of close on 100 years, he saw much and forgot little; his millenary of papers seem little more than the gleanings of his vast store of knowledge. He attended medical meetings well into his 80s, and published papers and annotations into his 90s.

WEBER, SIR HERMANN (1823–1918). London physician. Weber described the syndrome of *hemiplegia together with *paralysis of the *oculomotor nerve on the opposite side due to a lesion of the cerebral peduncle.

WEBER–CHRISTIAN DISEASE is a rare condition characterized by recurrent patches of inflammation in the subcutaneous fat (panniculus adiposus), resolution of which leaves puckered dimples on the skin. The chief features are summarized in the alternative name: relapsing febrile nodular non-suppurative panniculitis. The aetiology is unknown but the prognosis is generally good.

WEEPING describes a wound or surface which is discharging clear, serous fluid.

WEIGERT, KARL (1845–1904). German pathologist. He devised special stains for *myelin sheaths (1884), *fibrin (1887), and *elastic fibres (1898), and made valuable contributions on miliary tuberculosis, smallpox, and nephritis.

WEIGHT is defined as the force of attraction of the Earth on a given mass. It is therefore properly expressed in units of force, such as the newton (N), and not in units of mass (g or kg), though the latter are in general use.

WEIL'S DISEASE. See LEPTOSPIROSIS.

WELCH, WILLIAM HENRY (1850–1934). American pathologist and microbiologist. He moved to *Johns Hopkins Hospital and Medical School when that institution opened in 1889, as the first professor of pathology. He exerted a powerful influence upon the incorporation of the scientific method and thought into the teaching and practice of medicine in the USA. His special interest was in *infectious diseases. He demonstrated that *Staphylococcus epidermidis could cause wound infections, and was the first to describe an anaerobic organism—*Clostridium welchii—isolated from patients with *gas gangrene.

WELLCOME, SIR HENRY SOLOMON (1853–1936). Anglo-American patron of science and medicine. With his compatriot, E. M. Burroughs he founded the pharmaceutical firm of Burroughs Wellcome in 1880. In 1924 he endowed the Wellcome Trust.

WELLCOME FOUNDATION. This foundation ultimately arose from the partnership of two American pharmacists, Silas M. Burroughs and Henry S.

*Wellcome in the firm of Burroughs Wellcome & Co. in London in 1880. This inaugurated a new era in pharmacy as American methods were introduced into the UK. Both partners became British subjects, and Wellcome was later knighted. Burroughs died in 1895, and in 1924 Wellcome brought together all his now extensive business interests into the Wellcome Foundation Ltd. On his death in 1936 the profits of the company were transferred under his will to the Wellcome Trust, which is the largest endowed charitable trust supporting research in medicine in the UK. The business interests are of large scale and world-wide. They conform with the ideas of the founders in 'the discovery, development, manufacture, and sale of products to promote the health and hygiene of man and animals'. The headquarters remains in Euston Road in London, with research and production facilities round the UK and abroad in many countries, including the USA in North Carolina. In the London building is housed the *Wellcome Institute for the History of Medicine.

WELLCOME INSTITUTE FOR THE HISTORY OF MEDICINE arose from the Wellcome Historical Medical Museum and Library set up by Sir Henry *Wellcome in the 40 years before he died in 1936. His will founded the Wellcome Trust, a charity devoted to supporting medical, scientific, and medical historical research. Its funds come from the trading profits of the international pharmaceutical company, the *Wellcome Foundation, whose sole shareholders are the trustees. Wellcome had made a collection of books and artefacts with a major theme of medical history, and this forms the basis of the present library and museum, both of which have been added to in subsequent years. There is also a Wellcome Research Institution, and the present Institute includes this and the Library. Because of several factors, especially shortage of space at the building in Euston Road, London, the Museum has been loaned permanently to the Science Museum in South Kensington, where parts of it are on display. The Library remains at Euston Road and is probably the best library in Europe on medical history, with many rare documents and volumes among its 400 000 printed works. Research in medical history has been enhanced by links with the Unit of the History of Medicine of University College, London, where a chair in the subject, created in 1992, is held jointly.

WELLCOME TRUST. See WELLCOME FOUNDATION.

WELLS, HORACE (1815–48). American dentist. Wells practised in Hartford, Connecticut, USA. Gardner Colton, a chemist, visited the town in 1844, and demonstrated laughing gas—now known as *nitrous oxide. Wells saw a person in the audience who hurt his leg while under its influence and yet felt no pain. The next day he induced Colton to administer the gas to him while Riggs, a fellow dentist, extracted a molar tooth. Wells felt no pain and used the gas in his practice. He gave a public demonstration of it, which unfortunately failed lamentably. This discredited the gas and also Wells himself. He left the practice of dentistry as a result and later commited suicide in despair about the episode. See ANAESTHESIA.

WELLS, SIR THOMAS SPENCER, Bt (1818–97). British surgeon. He was one of the earliest of the great abdominal surgeons, particularly skilled in *ovariotomy, which he had carried out over 1000 times by 1880. He devised the well-known Spencer Wells artery *forceps.

WEN. A *sebaceous cyst of the skin.

WENCKEBACH, KAREL FREDERIK (1864–1940). Dutch physician. He described a collection of fibres running from the superior *vena cava to the right atrium (Wenckebach's bundle), but his reputation was founded on his studies of the cardiac *arrhythmias (1903, 1914). He described a form of atrioventricular block with progressive lengthening of the PR interval (see ELECTROCARDIOGRAPHY) until conduction fails (Wenckebach periods, 1899). See also CARDIOLOGY.

WERLHOF, PAUL GOTTLIEB (1699–1767). German physician. He described *purpura haemorrhagica or Werlhof's disease, in which there are spontaneous *haemorrhages into the skin and mucous membranes and many other tissues and organs. This is now known to be caused by a diminution of *platelets (thrombocytes) in the blood. Its modern name is idiopathic thrombocytopenic purpura.

WERNICKE, KARL (1848–1905). German neuropsychiatrist. He described sensory *aphasia (Wernicke's aphasia), the encephalopathy known by his name (*Wernicke's encephalopathy), and the hemianopic pupil reaction.

WERNICKE'S ENCEPHALOPATHY, sometimes known as cerebral *beriberi, is a syndrome caused by brain damage due to deficiency of *thiamin (vitamin B_1) and commonly, though not invariably, associated with chronic *alcoholism. The main features are *ophthalmoplegia, *nystagmus, and cerebellar *ataxia, together with the *amnesia and *confabulation characteristic of *Korsakoff's syndrome. Pathological examination of the brain shows widespread symmetrical areas of *necrosis, *demyelination, *capillary proliferation, and *haemorrhage, especially in the *brainstem and *mammillary bodies. The condition is dangerous, and requires urgent administration of thiamin.

WERTHEIM, ERNST (1864–1920). Austrian gynaecologist. He devised his radical pan-*hysterectomy for *cervical carcinoma (Wertheim's operation) in 1898.

WESBROOK, FRANK FAIRCHILD (1868–1918). Canadian physician and educator. In 1913 he became founding president of the University of British Columbia in Vancouver. He died in the influenza epidemic of 1918 aged 50. In five hectic years he changed life on the west coast of Canada as much as any other Canadian in history.

WEST, CHARLES (1816–98). British physician. In 1852 he founded the Hospital for Sick Children in Richard *Mead's house in *Great Ormond Street and was physician there for 23 years. Those who helped the foundation included Lord Shaftesbury and Charles Dickens.

WESTMINSTER HOSPITAL was founded in London in 1716 by public subscription, in response to the needs of the sick poor of the time. At first it was opposite Westminster Abbey, but moved about half a mile away in 1939 before moving again to the Westminster and Chelsea Hospital in 1993. When the *National Health Service started it incorporated the Westminster Children's Hospital (1948).

WET NURSE. A woman who suckles another's child.

WHIPPLE, GEORGE HOYT (1878–1976). American pathologist. In his early work at Johns Hopkins he described a chronic inflammatory disease of the bowel, still called Whipple's disease. His later research concerned liver injury, protein regeneration, and iron metabolism. His finding that dogs with *anaemia due to exsanguination recovered rapidly when fed liver led to the use of liver in treating patients with *pernicious anaemia by *Minot and Murphy. The *Nobel prize in 1934 was given to these three, for this discovery.

WHITE, PAUL DUDLEY (1886–1973). American physician. He limited his practice to the field of diseases of the heart, and over his long career he trained scores of young physicians in that specialty. His textbook *Heart disease* was a standard reference work for many years.

WHITE BLOOD CELLS. See LEUCOCYTES.

WHITLOW. A purulent infection of the terminal phalanx of a finger, around or underneath the nail; *paronychia.

WHOOPING COUGH. See PERTUSSIS.

WHYTT, ROBERT (1714–66). British physician. He attracted attention by attempting to dissolve stones in the bladder with lime water. He was strongly opposed to the doctrines of *Stahl, who attributed vital activities to an all-pervading 'anima' or soul. Whytt held that involuntary movements in animals were due to a 'stimulus acting on an unconscious sentient principle'.

WIDAL, GEORGES FERNAND ISIDORE (1862–1929). French microbiologist and serologist. He made many studies of infections and described acquired *haemolytic anaemia (Hayem–Widal haemolytic jaundice, 1907). He is best known, however, for his work on *typhoid fever. With Chantemesse he pointed out the significance of coliform bacilli which did not ferment lactose (1887), devised the diagnostic *agglutination test (Widal's reaction, 1896), and initiated preventive *vaccination (1888).

WILDE, SIR WILLIAM ROBERT WILLS (1815–76). Irish surgeon and antiquary. He practised in Dublin as an ophthalmologist and otolaryngologist. He was the father of Oscar Wilde.

WILLAN, ROBERT (1757–1812). British dermatologist. He was the first to devise a systematic description of skin diseases. It was set out in his classic work *The description and treatment of cutaneous diseases* (1798–1814). See DERMATOLOGY.

WILLIS, THOMAS (1621–75). British physician. He was one of the founders and an original fellow of the Royal Society. He was the first to note the sweet taste of the urine in *diabetes mellitus. Richard *Lower assisted him in the preparation of *Cerebri anatome nervorumque descriptio et usus* (1664), in which he described the arterial system at the base of the brain (the *circle of Willis).

WILMS' TUMOUR. A malignant tumour of the kidney, typically occurring in childhood; also called nephroblastoma.

WILSON, CHARLES McMORAN (1st Baron Moran of Manton, created 1943) (1882–1977). English physician. He served with distinction in the First World War, and in 1945 he published *The anatomy of courage*. He became president of the Royal College of Physicians in 1941, and retained this office until 1950, covering the period of medico-political struggle which attended the formation of the *National Health Service. He also had the distinction of being physician to Winston Churchill during and after the Second World War; and this part of his experience he narrated, not without raising some ethical misgivings, in *Winston Churchill, the struggle for survival* (1966).

WILSON, EDWARD ADRIAN (1872–1912). British physician, explorer, and ornithologist. Wilson accompanied Captain R. F. Scott on Antarctic expeditions, first in 1901–2, when he became an expert on Antarctic bird life, and secondly in 1911, dying with him on about 29 March 1912.

WILSON, SAMUEL ALEXANDER KINNIER (1874–1937). British neurologist. In 1912, he described the syndrome of familial hepatolenticular degeneration which bears his name (*Wilson's disease). He founded the *Journal of Neurology and Psychopathology* in 1920. His writings were marked by unusual clarity, and he was a gifted lecturer.

WILSON, SIR WILLIAM JAMES ERASMUS (1809–84). British surgeon and dermatologist. He paid for the transport of Cleopatra's needle (a carved granite obelisk, *c*. 1475 BC) from Egypt to London.

WILSON'S DISEASE is a rare disorder of copper metabolism. The disease, also known as hepatolenticular degeneration, is inherited as an autosomal *recessive trait and is marked by copper deposits in various tissues and organs, notably the liver, brain (especially the basal ganglia), kidney, and cornea. The major clinical manifestations are hepatic *cirrhosis, widespread neurological disturbances (in which slurred speech, tremor, muscular rigidity, and mental deterioration usually predominate), and pigmented rings at the corneal rims (Kayser–Fleischer rings). Treatment with a *chelating agent is of benefit if started early; *penicillamine is the drug of choice.

WIND is air or gas (flatus) in the gastrointestinal tract. It may cause discomfort because of distension and is relieved by expulsion through the anus or oropharynx.

WINDPIPE. See TRACHEA.

WINE is the fermented juice of the grape used as a beverage. The therapeutic value of wine, although often extolled ('Drink no longer water, but use a little wine for thy stomach's sake and thine other infirmities,' I Timothy 5:23) is in most applications less certain than is the damaging effect of the abuse of *ethanol in any form. However, epidemiological evidence now suggests that modest regular consumption, particularly of red wine, reduces the incidence of coronary artery disease.

WINTROBE, MAXWELL MEYER (1901–86). American physician and haematologist. Developer of many techniques for use in clinical haematology. Author of *Clinical hematology*, long the standard textbook in the field. he made fundamental contributions to the study of anaemia, nutritional and vitamin deficiencies, Wilson's disease, and neutrophil kinetics.

WISDOM TEETH. The third molar teeth, the last of the permanent dentition to erupt; they often do not appear until early adult life, and may not do so at all. See TEETH.

WISEMAN, RICHARD (?1622–76). British surgeon. He was the first of the great surgeons and did much to raise the craft of surgery to the status of a profession.

WISH FULFILMENT. In Freudian psychology, the attainment of an objective, the desire for which is not acknowledged by the conscious mind.

WISTAR INSTITUTE, THE, in Philadelphia was founded in 1892 as a result of a benefaction of the Wistar family and the initiative of the University of Pennsylvania. At first it was dependent on the income from the endowment but now receives a major contribution from the US *National Institutes of Health. It has no clinical facilities but co-operates with many hospitals. Its work is essentially devoted to the study of biological phenomena at cellular and subcellular levels. In these it has a world-wide reputation, and it has produced *vaccines against *rubella and *rabies which are now used universally, through sales by pharmaceutical companies. Current concerns are with ageing, nutrition, the cause of tumours, and the actions of viruses on cells.

WITCHCRAFT. Magic or sorcery; the supposed exercise of supernatural powers by witches and *witchdoctors.

WITCH DOCTOR. One who professes to cure disease by *magic arts. Alternatively, among some African tribes, one who professes to detect witches and to counteract the effects of their magic.

WITHDRAWAL SYMPTOMS are those experienced by drug and alcohol addicts during the early stages of abstinence from the addictive substance. See SUBSTANCE ABUSE.

WITHERING, WILLIAM (1741–99). British physician and botanist. A distinguished botanist, he was the first to use *digitalis, learning that foxglove was 'good for the dropsy' from an old country woman. He published *An account of the fox-glove* (1776) and *The botanical arrangement of all the vegetables naturally growing in Great Britain* (1776).

WOLFF–PARKINSON–WHITE SYNDROME is the combination of paroxysmal *tachycardia with characteristic *electrocardiographic (ECG) abnormalities consisting of a short PR interval and a wide QRS complex. It is due to the presence of an accessory bundle of conducting tissue, which short-circuits the normal atrioventricular conducting system and causes premature excitation of the right ventricle; thus the ventricles contract asynchronously and the ventricular complex is splayed out. A re-entry mechanism using the accessory bundle accounts for the paroxysmal tachycardia.

WOLFSON FOUNDATION, THE, was started in 1955 out of the munificence of the businessman, Sir Isaac (later Lord) Wolfson. It has a distinguished board of trustees and makes grants to education, technology, health, and social welfare, the arts, and historic buildings. In 25 years from its founding, over £10 million

($15 million) was granted to health and social welfare projects, about half being for education and research; £17 million (US$25.5 million) went to universities and £10 million (US$15 million) to technology.

WOLLASTON, WILLIAM HYDE (1766–1828).

British physician and chemist. His many discoveries included the metals palladium (1803) and rhodium (1804); how to render platinum malleable; that *gouty joints contained urates; and that some *calculi were composed of cystine. From his own visual disorders he suggested the semi-decussation of the *optic nerves (1824).

WOMB. See UTERUS.

WOMEN IN MEDICINE (WOMEN DOCTORS)
Introduction
Women have always practised the art of healing and have also always been responsible for the care of children, the sick, and the dying. In primitive societies illness and the supernatural were often linked. Women often took a leading part in both magical rituals and medical treatments. Herbs and plants such as sacred mistletoe were used to try to dispel illness or exorcise devils. Women also carried out massage and manipulation as part of early medical treatment. There was no medical profession in the formal sense, as we have it today. Simple medical care was carried out by women as part of their role as wife and mother, using basic and practical skills. Remedies were passed down from one woman to another in a family and mostly consisted of home and herbal remedies. Many women must have endeavoured to alleviate pain and suffering with little or no formal knowledge.

Medicine was also practised by women in religious orders. Deaconesses in the early Christian Church were women whose task was to visit the sick in their homes and care for the sick in hospital. Caring for the sick and needy was a well-recognized role of women, with some believed to have a special gift for healing. Some of those in religious orders came from influential and wealthy families, being well-educated, intelligent nuns who had pledged their lives to God and the care of the sick and needy.

The early history of women doctors
Following the Norman Conquest of England, a traditional pattern of care for the sick developed, including both castle and cottage. There was a role for the lady of the manor, who dispensed remedies, as well as a loose network of local women, helping each other in times of crisis and sickness. A number of the most influential women came from aristocratic families. Some women were practitioners of domestic medicine, some could reduce *fractures, probe and dress wounds or burns, and prepare herbal remedies. This traditional pattern

was similar in Europe from the 5th to 15th century. Women physicians were trained by apprenticeship, by reading medical texts, and by practice. Surgeons were more likely to be men, who would be employed to assist in the treatment of those fighting battles, and in dealing with wounds. There were no reports of famous women physicians during this period in Britain, unlike the women professors reported to be working in Salerno. At the time of the Crusades a plan was suggested to Edward I of England that a band of women doctors should be sent with the Crusaders to the Holy Land in order to win the confidence of the local inhabitants. Although this suggestion was not carried out, it suggests that there were women practitioners at that time, who would presumably have been a mixture of nun, *apothecary, *general practitioner, and *nurse.

Among the very poor there were always local women who lacked basic medical and nursing skills apart from what they had acquired from experience and observation in their own parish or locality. They attended at births and were present at deaths. Such women have been well recognized over the centuries as contributors to the care of the sick.

Development of an organized medical profession
Medicine changed as the scientific approach developed and became more dominant. Women were not excluded from the sciences, and many became interested in such areas as the study of botany, flora and fauna, and astronomy. Women with a basic knowledge of science were found among those intelligent women who had received some education and had the time, capability, opportunity, and money to pursue this special interest. Two factors hindered the possibility of women making a major impact in scientific medicine. The first was the lack of any formal structure for the education of women, apart from a few privileged by birth. The second factor was that several countries had restricted medical practice by introducing some form of regulation and control. For example, distinctions between *surgeons and apothecaries became apparent in Europe from 1311, when the University of Paris decreed 'No surgeon or apothecary, man or woman, shall undertake work for which he or she has not been licensed or approved'. Approval was given by examination. In England the Surgeons' Guild (1368) restricted the practice of barbers and surgeons. In 1390 the Mayor of London appointed four surgeons to scrutinize both men and women surgeons, presumably to see whether they were competent for the job at that time.

With the advent of medical professionalism, and greater emphasis on university training, women began to be excluded and no longer could become members of guilds such as the *barber-surgeons. In the 15th century the Surgeons' Guild in England became more powerful and began to press for the exclusion of women. In 1421 that guild petitioned parliament to legislate that no man should practise without having graduated from a school of physic within a university, and that no woman should practise at all, and the penalty for doing so would be imprisonment. After repeated petitions by the guild, an Act of Henry V finally repealed the Law of Edgar, which had given medical women legal status in Britain from the 10th century. For centuries there had been some women doctors, but with new rules and regulations they slowly lost their equal role in medicine. This was followed by a period where women could continue in their role as apothecaries but they were forced to withdraw from full medical practice.

Changes in health in the population

The Industrial Revolution had long-lasting effects, as many people moved from closely knit rural communities into large industrial cities and towns. Many small, local village groups and families were broken up, with many younger members seeking their fortune in cities or other countries. This huge population shift to urban life led to changes in the types of jobs carried out by men and women. This was accompanied by poor housing, poor sanitation, poverty, and overcrowding. Women continued to have to work exceedingly hard despite still having large families. *Birth control was virtually non-existent so the burden of motherhood associated with poverty, disease, and overwork left many women poorly nourished and exhausted, and many remained chronically ill. The very high maternal and infant death rates confirmed the grimness of pregnancy and childbirth for many poor women. The chances of surviving early childhood were small, and many children succumbed to infections. Poverty, lack of knowledge about hygiene, health, and prevention of pregnancy, and poor social circumstances were overwhelming. All these contributed to the short life expectancy as there were few effective medicines or treatments. Death rates were high for men, too, particularly from infections and accidents, but the risks associated with pregnancy and childbirth made them higher for women.

The development of the scientific approach in medicine, and the introduction of rules and regulations controlling licences to practise in some countries, limited the role of women. Medicine no longer relied solely on household remedies, magic, or superstition. Women were gradually excluded from *medical practice. Women were necessary for nursing care but the advent of more male doctors, particularly in *midwifery, changed what was originally an exclusive role for women into a secondary one. In particular, many of the special practical and managing skills provided by women were eventually to be viewed as non-scientific.

The plight of the poor

Educated women were aware of the very poor care (or, in many cases, no care at all) received by large numbers of poor women. They also realized that some of these conditions could be helped or alleviated if the women themselves were better educated. They considered that

such women might sometimes wish to get advice from a person of their own sex who could understand and who had had some experience of their problems, for example, when they had *obstetrical and *gynaecological problems. There remained a need for women physicians. One of the groups to draw attention to some of the burdens that women suffered, often in silence, were the early suffragettes. Contemporary literature gives many graphic accounts of the illnesses of women, often following childbirth, or their death from *consumption (tuberculosis). Society, too, could be cruel to unmarried pregnant women. Florence *Nightingale in England (although not a doctor) was a nurse, a powerful administrator, and statistician. She showed that intelligent women could make major changes in the care of the sick. She came from a wealthy family, was well educated, and, over half a century, brought about changes by writing clear and succinct reports, and providing statistics which could not be faulted. She had considerable organizational skills and knew how to influence those who were making decisions, and she persisted until she got her way. Those who campaigned for women to practise medicine were essentially asking for their reinstatement into medicine. Their arguments often focused on the plight of women and their poor health. There was a long struggle, but ultimately reason prevailed. Women proved that they could be capable doctors and this became more apparent during the two world wars (1914–18 and 1939–45).

The effects of war

Many countries had to rely on women medical auxiliaries and nurses during wartime. Some of these women were given greater responsibilities and were determined that the positions held during wartime should not be eroded. During the Crimean War (1854–56) they proved their medical skills and ability to work in difficult conditions and to care for the sick and wounded. The advent of asepsis, and better organization, recruitment, and training by the followers of Florence Nightingale led to better hygiene, with more effective surgical treatment. After the Crimean War the Russians became aware that they required women doctors for the medical care of Muslim Cossacks and their families. They decided specifically to train women doctors in Russia. This training started with some acrimony in St Petersburg. Subsequently France, Germany, and Switzerland followed and introduced the training of women doctors.

Formal registration of medical practitioners

In 1858 the Medical Act was passed in Britain and Ireland and formal registration was instituted. A minimum standard of training was needed before registration. This register of practitioners was held by the *General Medical Council. It did not exclude women doctors initially, but they could not gain admission into universities or medical schools, or take qualifying examinations. This registration was essentially for the protection of the public. Only 'registered medical practitioners' could sign a death certificate or claim legal protection in their work. The Medical Act did not stop anyone from practising medicine, but he or she could not be employed by the state or recover legal fees and were not allowed to call themselves 'doctor'. Women doctors who had qualified outside Britain were able to practise but were not able to register. This was a barrier to full equality. Elizabeth *Blackwell was the first woman to be admitted to the GMC register (in 1859); she came to England from the USA (see below).

The development of medical education for women

The 19th century saw the beginning of changes in the education of women. These initially affected those women whose families were relatively wealthy and whose fathers held more liberal views on the role of education for women. Women themselves were beginning to see the benefits that a higher education could provide. In addition, major social changes were opening up new horizons. With better and increased travel they were discovering for themselves that there were many places to visit in Europe and elsewhere around the world. They were no longer confined to a small circle of family and friends and the place where they lived. They discovered that they could, with effort, make changes in their own lives. Sometimes this was so despite strong opposition. For some, the suffragette movement provided a platform for change in their lives. The particular difficulties women had to undergo to obtain the vote are well documented.

These opportunities were open to upper middle-class women who did not wish to stay at home, nor get married, nor become a governess. They did not affect most women, who remained poor, who continued to have large families and live in poverty. At the end of the 19th century there were some feelings of discontentment and resentment held by a few women and enlightened men. They did not consider that women were given fair and equal opportunities to do some of the things that they were capable of doing. The earliest women doctors had shown that it was possible to practise medicine and provide a satisfactory service, particularly for women and children. This was done in the USA by Elizabeth Blackwell and, in a different way, by Miranda (James) Barry in the British Empire (Table 1). In the early 1870s on the strength of a foreign degree, Louisa Atkins, Edith Pechey, and Eliza Walker were able to practise, but were not allowed to have their names on the GMC register. They did not have recognized qualifications for entry to the register because they were prevented from obtaining them. The difficulty in being registered was a formal barrier preventing the acceptance of women as equals in the profession.

Although women could theoretically become licensed to practise, for a long time it was very difficult for them to receive a proper medical training as medical students. There was overt discrimination against them to prevent

them from entering the profession. Many methods of obstruction were used, including changing rules and denying scholarships. A medical school, the London School of Medicine for Women, was set up in 1874, but at that time no examining body or general hospital would accept women students. In 1876 the Enabling Bill was passed and this removed any statutory ban on accepting women students. A year later the school faced closure but the Kings and Queens College of Physicians of Dublin (subsequently the *Royal College of Physicians of Dublin, later of Ireland) accepted foreign students and recognized the course at the London School of Medicine for Women. In 1877 clinical teaching was arranged at the *Royal Free Hospital, London. Later, a second school for women was founded in Edinburgh by Sophia *Jex-Blake, who was originally involved with Elizabeth Garrett *Anderson in the founding of the medical school for women in London. The first established medical school to accept female medical students was Queen's University, Belfast. In 1878 the University of London accepted women, and Edinburgh did so in 1894. By 1947 all medical schools in the UK accepted and had some women students. The number of women students steadily rose, and today roughly 50 per cent of new students are women.

Some notable early women practitioners

James (Miranda Stewart) Barrie (Barry) (1797–1865)

The first woman doctor in the UK entered medical school dressed as a man. She practised as such and rose to high rank in the army. This was not discovered until she died in 1865, having been qualified as a doctor for 53 years. Dr Barrie graduated from Edinburgh in 1812 and 1 year later joined the British Army. She was assigned to hospital work and was promoted to the rank of assistant surgeon at the Battle of Waterloo in 1815. Later she was promoted again and became the Inspector General of Hospitals in 1858. She served in many countries, including the Crimea. She was noted for her concern for soldiers and their families. Dr Barrie was small and looked rather feminine but was well known for her temper and skilled marksmanship with a pistol.

Elizabeth Blackwell (1821–1910)

Elizabeth Blackwell was born in Bristol into a family of non-conformists and political reformers, prominent in the anti-slavery movement. When she was 11 years old her family moved to the United States. She was determined to practise medicine, and in 1847 enrolled as a medical student at Geneva College in New York, qualifying there 2 years later. In 1850 she visited England and was generally well received by the medical profession. She then went to Paris to study obstetrics and while there she lost an eye in an accident. She then returned to the USA and practised in New York City, opening a clinic for immigrant women and their children. She never married but in 1852 adopted a daughter Katherine (Kitty) Barry. In 1859, after practising for 8 years, she visited England again and became the first woman on the General Medical Council *Medical Register. She also visited Florence Nightingale, who impressed on her the importance of hygiene and preventive medicine. She lectured about her work and articles appeared about her in the *English Women's Journal*. She became a role model for English women who had aspirations to become doctors. She settled in London and practised there. In 1874 she was appointed to the chair of *gynaecology in the London School of Medicine for Women.

Elizabeth Garrett Anderson (1836–1917)

Elizabeth Garrett Anderson was born in Whitechapel, London. Her father was a self-made businessman who became wealthy. The family moved to Suffolk, whence they had originally come. The family was large and Elizabeth the second child. Elizabeth was sent to the academy for the daughters of gentlemen in Blackheath and was considered a bright pupil. When staying with her schoolfriend, Jane Crew, she met Emily Davies, who later founded Girton College, Cambridge. In 1859 they became involved with the Society for Promoting the Employment of Women and also with the *English Women's Journal*, which was then active and influential in the cause for women.

Elizabeth Garrett was introduced to, and was much influenced by, Elizabeth Blackwell and decided to become a doctor. In 1860 she became a student nurse and an unofficial student at the Middlesex Hospital but was asked to leave. She then pursued her medical studies privately, both in Scotland, at St Andrews and Edinburgh, and in London. In 1865 she became a licentiate of the Society of Apothecaries. This was not achieved without a struggle and came about only when her father threatened to sue the Apothecaries if they refused. Her name was added to the Medical Register in 1866. (This was the first time that a woman had qualified legally as a doctor in England.)

She opened and practised at a dispensary for women and children at St Mary's Marylebone. For a short time she was involved in the women's suffrage movement, but later withdrew. Later she studied for and obtained an MD from Paris in 1870 and in the same year was appointed to the East London Hospital for Children. In 1871 she married Mr J. G. S. Anderson, who was in shipping in the City. She had two children, Louisa in 1873 and Margaret in 1874. She resigned her hospital appointment but continued to be active in promoting the cause of women in education and medicine. A new hospital for women was started in 1872 above the Marylebone dispensary and Elizabeth Garrett Anderson, as she now was, operated there. Later it moved to larger premises and she was asked to join the Council of the London School of Medicine for Women. She became Dean in

Table 1 Some notable dates and early women practitioners

Year		
1812	UK, Edinburgh	James Miranda Barry (a woman posing as a man) qualified; she became a senior army medical officer
1848	USA	Elizabeth Blackwell qualified. First woman in the USA acknowledged as a doctor. Specialty: women and children
1859	UK	Elizabeth Blackwell became the first woman on the UK Medical Register
1865	UK	Elizabeth Garrett (Anderson) requalified. Specialty: women and children
1865	Switzerland	The Faculty of Medicine in Zurich accepted women with foreign medical qualifications to sit examinations. Basel and Geneva followed
1869		Universities in Germany and Paris permitted women to take examinations
1870	Sweden	Women medical students accepted
1871	The Netherlands	Women medical students accepted
1872	St Petersburg	College for women medical students was set up
1874	London	Sophia Jex-Blake founded the London School of Medicine for Women
1877	Copenhagen/Denmark	
1877	Paris	
1879	University of London	
1884	Norway	Women medical students accepted
1889	Spain/Portugal/Austria	
1894	Edinburgh	
1908	Germany	
1947	All UK medical schools	

1883 when she was 47 years old and stayed in this post for 20 years.

Cicely Wiliams (1893–1992)

Cicley Williams was primarily responsible for identifying, in the 1920s, kwashiorkor, a nutritional deficiency disease which had ravaged children in drought and war-torn areas of maize-eating Third World countries. As a paediatrician and nutritionist, she was a pioneer of women's progress in the medical profession. She was the first adviser in maternal and child health to the *World Health Organization, from 1948 to 1951. She was a forceful protagonist of breast feeding and, in a blistering speech in 1939 entitled 'Milk and murder' accused proprietary-brand baby-food manufacturers of causing infant deaths.

Recent developments

In developed countries over the past two centuries greatly improved standards of care, associated with improvements in literacy and sanitation, have led to improved health, with a marked reduction in infant *mortality rates and increased longevity. The surgeon's previous nightmare of sepsis has been controlled with good *hygiene and *aseptic and *antiseptic techniques. *Antibiotics have been discovered which can further control infections. *Blood transfusion has enabled sick patients to have safer surgery, reduced fatal haemorrhages at childbirth, and is life-saving in major accidents. Technological changes have assisted women in the control of their own fertility. The 'pill' has enabled many women to lead very different lives from those of previous generations; better education, equal job opportunities, and social mobility have influenced these changes. The reduction in family size has been another factor leading to improvement in the health of women in general. These changes will continue to influence the type and quality of medicine, and numbers and type of medical personnel, that will be needed in the future.

In the 20th century women doctors have regained their proper place in the medical profession and are now to be found in all branches of it. In 1979 the British Medical Association elected its first woman president, Dame Josephine Barnes, and in 1989 the Royal College of Physicians of London elected Professor (later Dame) Margaret Turner-Warwick as its president. Nevertheless, there are still too few women doctors serving in the super-specialties and in the highest echelons of the profession in the UK and in North America, although the situation is improving steadily.

BEULAH R. BEWLEY

Further reading
Blake, C. (1990). *The charge of the parasols, Women's entry to the medical profession*. The Women's Press, London.
Bowden, R. (1986). *Women in medicine*. In *The Oxford companion to medicine* (ed. J. Walton, P. B. Beeson, and R. Bodley Scott) Oxford University Press, Oxford.
Lorber, J. (1984). *Women physicians. Careers, status and power*. Tavistock, London.
Lyons, A. S. and Petrucelli, R. J. (1978), *Women in medicine an illustrated history*. H. N. Abrams, New York.
Manton, J. (1965). *Elizabeth Garrett Anderson*. Methuen, London.

WOOD, PAUL HAMILTON (1907–62). Anglo-Australian physician. He established a world-wide reputation as a cardiologist with an original and acute mind. He published a classic textbook *Diseases of the heart and circulation* (1950).

WOODALL, JOHN (?1556–1643). British surgeon. He published *The surgeon's mate* (1617), in which he recommended lemon juice for the treatment of *scurvy, and *Viaticum, being the pathway to the surgeon's chest* (1628).

WORLD HEALTH ORGANIZATION (WHO) was established in 1948 by the United Nations. It took over the functions of the Health Organization of the League of Nations and the International Office of Public Health in Paris. These had been concerned with control of epidemics, quarantine measures, and drug standardization. Now the WHO has a remit which covers all aspects of health of all peoples, and in many ways assists countries to improve the health of their own populations. The head office is in Geneva, Switzerland, and there are regional offices in Egypt, the Congo, Denmark, India, the Philippines, and the USA. There is a staff of over 3500 in these offices and in the field, supported by contributions made by member states of the World Health Assembly, which determines broad policy annually. Its tools for assistance to countries include information and education on all aspects of health; sponsoring measures for the control of epidemics and other disorders by mass programmes, particularly of vaccination, immunization, antibiotics, and chemotherapy, and the setting up of laboratory and clinical facilities for early diagnosis and prevention of disease, improving water supplies and health education; and helping to strengthen *public health administration locally in countries where this is needed. The work of WHO was largely responsible for the eradication of *smallpox from the world. It also sponsors doctors and health-care professionals of all kinds to go to countries to help with their problems and to teach. Its resources are miniscule by comparison with the tasks that lie ahead of it in the drive for international good health, but its help is often visible in areas where it is most needed. In 1981, at Alma Ata, the World Health Assembly adopted a policy of health for all by the year 2000. This requires the recognition of health as a fundamental right; the elimination of inequalities in health care; community involvement in health care and attention to the socio-economic factors on which it depends; political commitment by states to health care; national self-reliance in health care; integration of health care with all other factors, such as agriculture, culture, animal husbandry, food, education, housing, public works, and communications; and better use of the world's resources.

WORLD MEDICAL ASSOCIATION, THE, with headquarters in Ferney-Voltaire, France, was founded in 1947. It represented the coming together of representatives from National Medical Associations, which have to be free associations for doctors and bona fide medical students only, and not subject to or controlled by any organ of government. 'The purpose of the Association shall be to serve humanity by endeavouring to achieve the highest international standards in medical education, medical science, medical art, and medical ethics, and health care for all people of the world.' It has few direct powers, and is unable to enforce its decisions on its member associations without their agreement. Nevertheless, the WMA has attained considerable prestige and influence by many of its pronouncements. These have been issued from time to time from various places where the WMA Assembly has met, for there are regional organizations covering Europe, Asia, the Pacific region, Latin America, Africa, and North America.
Among the successful publications have been:

Regulations in time of armed conflict (Havana, 1956; Istanbul, 1957).
Declaration of Tokyo (1975). 'Guidelines for medical doctors concerning torture and other cruel, inhuman or degrading treatment or punishment in relation to detention and imprisonment.'
Declaration of Helsinki (1964): revised Tokyo (1975). 'Recommendations guiding medical doctors in biomedical research involving human subjects.'
Declaration of Sydney (1968). Statement on death especially with regard to the use of organs for transplantation.
International code of medical ethics (London, 1949; Sydney, 1968) which includes (a) *Duties of doctors in general*, (b) *Duties of doctors to the sick*, (c) *Duties of doctors to each other*.
Declaration of Geneva (1948; Sydney 1968). This is a form of updating of the ancient *Hippocratic Oath to meet modern conditions.

WORMS parasitic in man (helminths) fall into one of three broad groups: roundworms or nematodes; flukes or trematodes; and tapeworms or cestodes. (The latter two groups both belong to the phylum of flatworms or platyhelminths.) Also see FLUKES; NEMATODES; and TAPEWORMS; and the names of individual worms and their diseases.

WOUND INFECTION. Postoperative wound infections vary in incidence and type with the nature of the surgical procedure, the degree of surgical skill, and the adequacy of aseptic technique before, during, and after the operation. Staphylococci and coliform bacilli are the commonest organisms responsible but others, including haemolytic streptococci, may be identified: all are potentially dangerous.

WOUNDS. Lesions produced by external mechanical force involving damage to the normal continuity of tissues, such as bruises (contusions), cuts (incisions), tears (lacerations), stabs (punctures), breaks (fractures), etc.

WRIGHT, SIR ALMROTH EDWARD (1861–1947). British bacteriologist. He introduced routine antityphoid vaccination into the army. He developed and exploited therapeutic immunization by vaccines at his Institute at *St Mary's Hospital and his work inspired Bernard Shaw's *The Doctor's Dilemma*.

WRITER'S CRAMP. See OCCUPATIONAL CRAMP.

WRY-NECK. See TORTICOLLIS.

WUNDERLICH, KARL REINHOLD AUGUST (1815–77). German physician. He made the thermometer an indispensable clinical tool, describing his findings in *Das Verhaltern der Eigenwärme in Krankheiten* (1868).

WYNDHAM, SIR CHARLES (1841–1919). British physician and actor. He was manager of the Criterion Theatre in London from 1876 until 1899, when he opened Wyndham's Theatre.

X

XANTHINE is a nitrogenous base from which a number of pharmacologically active compounds are derived; they include *caffeine, *theophylline, theobromine, and aminophylline. Xanthine derivatives have *bronchodilator, myocardial stimulant, respiratory stimulant, and *diuretic properties.

XANTHOCHROMIA is a yellowish discoloration, particularly with reference to the normally colourless *cerebrospinal fluid.

XANTHOMA. A yellow plaque or nodule in the skin, due to the deposition of *lipids.

XENOGRAFT. A *transplant of organ or tissue between individuals of different species. Cf. ALLOGRAFT; AUTOGRAFT; SYNGRAFT.

XENOPHOBIA is a pathological fear of strangers or a dislike of foreigners.

XENOPSYLLA is a genus of rat *fleas, many species of which are vectors of human disease, particularly *plague (notably the Asiatic rat flea, *Xenopsylla cheopis*).

XENOPUS PREGNANCY TEST. An outdated *urinary test for *pregnancy, based on the rate of egg deposition by the female African toad (*Xenopus laevis*) following the injection of 2 ml of the woman's urine specimen into the dorsal lymph sac.

XERODERMA is any condition in which the skin is abnormally dry, for example *ichthyosis.

XERODERMA PIGMENTOSUM is a recessively inherited defect of the *enzyme system for *deoxyribonucleic acid (DNA) repair, resulting in a syndrome of sun-sensitivity with freckling, dryness, and atrophy of the skin, *telangiectasia, and the development of cutaneous malignant tumours. The condition becomes apparent in early childhood and death from *metastases or intercurrent infection is usual by the third decade.

XEROGRAPHY is a dry process for producing *radiographs.

XEROPHTHALMIA is dryness of the conjunctiva and cornea due to *vitamin A deficiency. See also NIGHT BLINDNESS.

X-LINKED DISEASE. *Sex linkage in which the abnormal gene responsible for the disease is carried on the X chromosome. In the case of a dominant gene, an affected father will transmit the condition to all his daughters but none of his sons, an affected *heterozygous mother to half her children of whatever sex. Recessive X-linked conditions are much more common; they occur only in males, who are hemizygous, and are transmitted only through heterozygous females (the classic example being *haemophilia); females are affected only in the very rare case of a homozygote, resulting from the union of a male sufferer with a female carrier. See also GENETICS.

X-RAY MICROANALYSIS is the analysis of minute quantities of material by *X-ray spectra.

X-RAYS are electromagnetic *radiation (i.e. radiation of the same non-particulate type as light, *gamma rays, and radio waves) whose wavelength is shorter than that of *ultraviolet light but longer than that of gamma rays, ranging from 5 nanometres to 6 picometres. See also RADIATION, IONIZING; RADIOLOGY; RADIOTHERAPY.

XXX SYNDROME. Females with the triple X syndrome, that is with 47 chromosomes due to the addition of an extra X or female chromosome, are not uncommon, since the XXX *genotype is found in about 1 in 2000 of all live births. Many are clinically normal, and may be fertile, but this genotype is significantly associated with low intelligence.

XYY SYNDROME is a common genetic abnormality (one in 700 live male births) in which the patient's cells have 47 chromosomes, the extra one being an additional male or Y chromosome. Many normal individuals possess this *genotype, but there is an established association with tallness; and studies of populations of men with aggressive, psychopathic, and criminal tendencies have shown an increased incidence of XYY constitution.

YANG AND YIN are the two opposing principles or essences of Chinese philosophy and medicine, influencing destiny and health. Yin is negative, feminine, and dark, dominating earth, moon, winter, and water; Yang is positive, masculine, and light, dominating heaven, sun, summer, and fire. For good health, the two must be perfectly balanced; imbalance leads to disease. An elaborate system of interrelationships between tissues and organs is constructed from this simplistic concept, and deductions about them are made by studying the character of the arterial pulse.

YAWN. A semi-voluntary wide opening of the mouth, which may be associated with deep inspiration and sometimes with stretching of the limbs; a manifestation of fatigue, boredom, or anxiety.

YAWS is a chronic non-venereal spirochaetal infection of the tropics, usually acquired in childhood, which has many features resembling *syphilis. The causative organism is *Treponema pertenue*, very similar to *Treponema pallidum*.

YEAST is a general term for single-celled fungi belonging to the class Ascomycetes. Yeasts typically multiply by budding.

YEAST EXTRACT is a preparation derived from a culture of *yeast, a by-product of the brewing and baking industries. It is a source of *protein and *vitamins of the B complex.

YELLOW FEVER is an acute viral infection of tropical Africa and America transmitted by biting mosquitoes of the *Aedes* and *Haemagogus* genera; the causative agent is an enveloped ribonucleic acid (RNA) *virus of the flavivirus group. Yellow fever varies in severity from a mild influenza-like episode to a dangerous and sometimes fatal illness marked by jaundice due to liver *necrosis, haemorrhagic manifestations, and renal failure. Immunization with live attenuated vaccine provides safe, effective, and long-lived (at least 10 years) protection, and is essential for travellers to endemic areas. Yellow fever is one of the six diseases internationally notifiable to the *World Health Organization.

YERSIN, ALEXANDRE (1863–1943). Swiss bacteriologist. He found the cause of *plague (*Pasteurella pestis*, now known as *Yersinia pestis*) independently of *Kitasato (1894) and made an effective serum (1896). He did much to control epidemics in Indo-China and became director of the Pasteur Institute in Annam.

YOGA is a system of mental concentration, abstract meditation, asceticism, and physical discipline derived from Hindu philosophy and practised with the object of emancipating the soul and achieving union with a supreme spirit.

YOUNG, FRANCIS BRETT (1884–1954). British physician and novelist. He practised little, but wrote many novels, the best known of which were *Portrait of Clare* (1927), *My brother Jonathan* (1928), and *They seek a country* (1937).

YOUNG, HENRY ESSON (1867–1939). Public health pioneer and educator. He was 'the father of the University of British Columbia', and a pioneer in mental health; he established the provincial library, archives, and museum, and a civil service based on merit. With advice from Osler and *Sherrington he selected *Wesbrook to be first (outstandingly successful) president of the university.

YOUNG, HUGH HAMPTON (1870–1945). American urological surgeon. Young wrote scores of articles on urological diseases, and on surgical treatment, and edited the *Journal of Urology* for many years.

YOUNG, THOMAS (1773–1829). British physician and polymath. He was the founder of physiological optics (Young's theory of *colour vision); he supervised the *Nautical Almanac*; he propounded the first theory of capillary action; and deciphered part of the demotic text of the Rosetta stone. As a mathematician he devised Young's modulus.

YULE, GEORGE UDNY (1871–1951). British statistician. He wrote the standard textbook, *Introduction to the theory of statistics* (1911), and made many contributions of lasting value to the subject, and to Mendelian *inheritance and *epidemiology. Because of authorship controversies he proposed the statistical study of works of doubtful authorship and published *The statistical study of literary vocabulary* (1944).

Z

ZEISS, CARL (1816–88). German optician. In 1846 he opened his optical glass works in Jena, in the east of Germany, and produced the finest of optical instruments, including *microscopes. Abbe, a physicist, joined him, and so did Schott, a glass chemist who developed over 100 types of optical and heat-resistant glass. After the death of Zeiss, Abbe gave the firm, in which he was then a partner, to start the Carl Zeiss Foundation. Schott added his share later to the same cause. Zeiss instruments are still among the best in the world for scientific purposes, and are widely used in medicine.

ZENKER, FRIEDRICH ALBERT (1825–98). German pathologist. He is best known for his description of waxy degeneration in muscle (Zenker's degeneration). He gave an excellent description of *trichiniasis in 1860.

ZIDOVUDINE. An antiviral drug which inhibits retroviral reverse transcriptase. It is of limited value in treating *AIDS.

ZIEGLER, ERNST (1849–1905). Swiss pathologist. One of the leading morbid anatomists of his time, his textbook of pathological anatomy (1881) circulated widely. He founded the influential journal *Beiträge zur pathologischen Anatomie* (1886).

ZINC is a hard, bluish-white, metallic element (relative atomic mass 65.37, atomic number 30, symbol Zn). It is a constituent of a several important body *enzymes and an essential dietary *trace element; deficiency is associated with dwarfism, *hypogonadism, *anaemia, and impaired wound healing. A congenital defect of zinc absorption accounts for the severe and ultimately fatal disease of infancy, acrodermatitis enteropathica. Zinc salts are mildly astringent and antiseptic and are used in various lotions, ointments, and dusting powders (*calamine is zinc oxide).

ZINSSER, HANS (1878–1940). American bacteriologist and immunologist. Much of his research was directed toward elucidating the role of immunological mechanisms in *infectious diseases. During the First World War he served in Europe on the Typhus Commission; thereafter he maintained an intense interest in *rickettsial diseases. By using epidemiological information he produced persuasive evidence that *Brill's disease is a recrudescence, in older adults, of *typhus fever contracted in early life. His popular book, *Rats, lice and history* was enjoyed by both medical and lay readers.

ZOLLINGER–ELLISON SYNDROME is due to a *gastrin-secreting tumour, situated usually in the *pancreas, which causes marked gastric hypersecretion and in most cases, a *peptic ulcer in the *duodenum or stomach. Other endocrine abnormalities are often also present.

ZONDEK, BERNHARD (1891–1966). German gynaecologist. He worked with *Aschheim on the first reliable *pregnancy test. He left Germany as a result of Nazi persecution and in 1934 was made professor of obstetrics and gynaecology at the Hebrew University-Hadassah Medical School in Jerusalem.

ZOOLOGY IN RELATION TO MEDICINE. Ever since *Galen dissected apes and pigs, the advance of medicine has depended crucially on the scientific study of animals. This debt is not confined to human anatomy, embryology, and physiology, although zoology remains an important premedical subject in the education of most doctors. Pharmacology, nutrition, microbiology, genetics, experimental pathology, operative surgery, psychology, parasitology, and the human zoonoses are but a few of the branches of medicine where animal studies have always been of paramount importance. See also VETERINARY MEDICINE.

ZOONOSIS. Any disease of animals which may be transmitted to man, for example, *rabies, *plague, *brucellosis, *ornithosis, and many others.

ZOSTER. See HERPES ZOSTER.

ZUCKERKANDL, EMIL (1849–1901). Viennese anatomist. He described paraganglia (now known as *chromaffin tissue) in the vicinity of the abdominal *aorta, the subcallosal sulcus of the brain, and a vein running between the nasal cavities and the brain.

ZYGOTE. The cell produced by fusion of male and female *gametes (spermatozoon and ovum respectively), i.e. the fertilized ovum.

APPENDIX I

MAJOR MEDICAL AND RELATED QUALIFICATIONS

AAPSW	Associate of the Association of Psychiatric Social Workers
AB	Bachelor of Arts
ABPsS	Associate of the British Psychological Society
AFOM	Associate of the Faculty of Occupational Medicine
AIMBI	Associate of the Institute of Medical and Biological Illustration
AIMI	Associate of the Institute of Medical Illustration
AIMLS	Associate of the Institute of Medical Laboratory Science
AIMSW	Associate of the Institute of Medical Social Workers
AM	Master of Arts
ARPS	Associate of the Royal Photographic Society
BA	Bachelor of Arts
BAO	Bachelor of the Art of Obstetrics
BC	Bachelor of Surgery
BCh	Bachelor of Surgery
BChD	Bachelor of Dental Surgery
BCL	Bachelor of Common Law
BChir	Bachelor of Surgery
BDS	Bachelor of Dental Surgery
BDSc	Bachelor of Dental Science
BHyg	Bachelor of Hygiene
BM	Bachelor of Medicine
BMedSc	Bachelor of Medical Science
BPharm	Bachelor of Pharmacy
BPhil	Bachelor of Philosophy
BS	Bachelor of Surgery; Bachelor of Science
BSc	Bachelor of Science
BVMS	Bachelor of Veterinary Medicine and Surgery
CChem	Chartered Chemist
ChB	Bachelor of Surgery
ChM	Master of Surgery
CM	Master of Surgery
CPH	Certificate in Public Health
CRCP(C)	Certificant, Royal College of Physicians of Canada
CQSW	Certificate of Qualification in Social Work

DA	Diploma in Anaesthesia
DABR	Diplomate of the American Board of Radiology
DASS	Diploma in Applied Social Studies
DBA	Doctor of Business Administration
DC	Doctor of Chiropractic
DCCH	Diploma in Child and Community Health
DCD	Diploma in Chest Diseases
DCH	Diploma in Child Health
DCh	Doctor of Surgery
DCL	Doctor of Common Law
DCMHE	Diploma of Contents and Methods of Health Education
DCMT	Diploma in Clinical Medicine of the Tropics
DCP	Diploma in Clinical Pathology
DCR(R)	Diploma of the College of Radiographers (Diagnostic Radiology)
DCR(T)	Diploma of the College of Radiographers (Radiotherapy)
DD	Doctor of Divinity
DDM	Diploma in Dermatological Medicine
DDO	Diploma in Dental Orthopaedics
DDPH	Diploma in Dental Public Health
DDR	Diploma in Diagnostic Radiology
DDS	Doctor of Dental Surgery
DDSc	Doctor of Dental Science
D en M	Docteur en Médecine
DGO	Diploma in Obstetrics and Gynaecology
DHMSA	Diploma in the History of Medicine (Society of Apothecaries)
DHyg	Doctor of Hygiene
DIH	Diploma in Industrial Health
DipBMS	Diploma in Basic Medical Science
DipSW	Diploma in Social Work
DipVen	Diploma in Venereology
DLO	Diploma in Laryngology and Otology
DM	Doctor of Medicine
DMD	Diploma in Medical Dentistry
DMHS	Diploma in Medical and Health Services

DMJ	Diploma in Medical Jurisprudence	FAAFP	Fellow of the American Academy of Family Physicians
DMJ(Path.)	Diploma in Medical Jurisprudence (Pathology)	FAAN	Fellow of the American Academy of Nursing
DMR	Diploma in Radiology	FAAP	Fellow of the American Academy of Pediatrics
DMRD	Diploma in Medical Radiological Diagnosis	FACC	Fellow of the American College of Cardiology
DMRE	Diploma in Medical Radiology and Electronics	FACCP	Fellow of the American College of Chest Physicians
DMRT	Diploma in Medical Radiotherapy	FACD	Fellow of the American College of Dentistry
DMSA	Diploma in Medical Service Administration	FACDS	Fellow of the Australian College of Dental Surgeons
DMV	Doctor of Veterinary Medicine	FACFP	Fellow of the American College of Family Practice
DNS	Doctor of Nursing Science		
DNSc	Doctor of Nursing Science	FACG	Fellow of the American College of Gastroenterology
DO	Diploma in Ophthalmology; Doctor of Osteopathy	FACN	Fellow of the American College of Nutrition
D Obst RCOG (or DCROG)	Diploma in Obstetrics, Royal College of Obstetricians and Gynaecologists	FACO	Fellow of the American College of Otolaryngology
DOMS	Diploma in Ophthalmic Medicine and Surgery	FACOEM	Fellow of the American College of Occupational and Environmental Medicine
DOrth	Diploma in Orthodontics	FACOG	Fellow of the American College of Obstetricians and Gynecologists
DPD	Diploma in Public Dentistry		
DPH	Diploma in Public Health		
DPhil	Doctor of Philosophy	FACP	Fellow of the American College of Physicians
DPM	Diploma in Psychological Medicine	FACPM	Fellow of the American College of Preventive Medicine
DR	Diploma in Radiology		
DRD	Diploma in Restorative Dentistry	FACR	Fellow of the American College of Radiologists
Dr PH	Doctor of Public Health	FACS	Fellow of the American College of Surgeons
Dr Phil	Doctor of Philosophy		
DS	Doctor of Science	FACTM	Fellow of the American College of Tropical Medicine
DSc	Doctor of Science		
DSM	Diploma of Social Medicine	FAGO	Fellowship in Australia in Gynaecology and Obstetrics
DSN	Doctor of the Science of Nursing	FAMA	Fellow of the American Medical Association
DTCD	Diploma in Tubercular and Chest Diseases		
DTCH	Diploma in Tropical Child Health	FAMS	Fellow of the Academy of Medical Sciences
DTD	Diploma in Tubercular Diseases	FAPA	Fellow of the American Psychiatric Association
DTH	Diploma in Tropical Hygiene		
DTM	Diploma in Tropical Medicine	FAPHA	Fellow of the American Public Health Association
DTM&H	Diploma in Tropical Medicine and Hygiene	FBPsS	Fellow of the British Psychological Society
DTPH	Diploma in Tropical Public Health	FCAP	Fellow of the College of American Pathologists
DV&D	Diploma in Venereology and Dermatology		
DVM	Doctor of Veterinary Medicine	FChS	Fellow of the Society of Chiropodists
DVMS	Doctor of Veterinary Medicine and Surgery	FCMA	Fellow of the Chartered Institute of Management Accountants
DVS	Doctor of Veterinary Surgery		
DVSc	Doctor of Veterinary Science		
		FCMS	Fellow of the College of Medicine and Surgery
EdD	Doctor of Education		
EOPH	Examined Officer in Public Health		

FCOG(SA)	Fellow of the South African College of Obstetricians and Gynaecologists	FLS	Fellow of the Linnean Society
		FPS	Fellow of the Pharmaceutical Society
FCOphth	Fellow of the College of Ophthalmologists	FRACDS	Fellow of the Royal Australian College of Dental Surgeons
FCP(SoAf)	Fellow of the College of Physicians, South Africa	FRACGP	Fellow of the Royal Australian College of General Practitioners
FCSP	Fellow of the Chartered Society of Physiotherapists	FRACMA	Fellow of the Royal Australian College of Medical Administrators
FCSSA	Fellow of the College of Surgeons, South Africa	FRACO	Fellow of the Royal Australian College of Ophthalmologists
FCST	Fellow of the College of Speech Therapists	FRACOG	Fellow of the Royal Australasian College of Obstetricians and Gynaecologists
FDS	Fellow in Dental Surgery		
FDSRCPS(Glasg.)	Fellow in Dental Surgery, Royal College of Physicians and Surgeons of Glasgow	FRACP	Fellow of the Royal Australasian College of Physicians
FDSRCS	Fellow in Dental Surgery, Royal College of Surgeons of England	FRACR	Fellow of the Royal Australasian College of Radiologists
FDSRCS(Ed.)	Fellow in Dental Surgery, Royal College of Surgeons of Edinburgh	FRACS	Fellow of the Royal Australasian College of Surgeons
FFARACS	Fellow of the Faculty of Anaesthetists, Royal Australasian College of Surgeons	FRANZCP	Fellow of the Royal Australian and New Zealand College of Psychiatrists
FFARCS	Fellow of the Faculty of Anaesthetists, Royal College of Surgeons of England	FRCA	Fellow of the Royal College of Anaesthetists
FFARCS(Irel.)	Fellow of the Faculty of Anaesthetists, Royal College of Surgeons in Ireland	FRCGP	Fellow of the Royal College of General Practitioners
		FRCN	Fellow of the Royal College of Nursing
FFCM	Fellow of the Faculty of Community Medicine	FRCOG	Fellow of the Royal College of Obstetricians and Gynaecologists
FFDRSC(Irel.)	Fellow of the Faculty of Dentistry, Royal College of Surgeons in Ireland	FRCOphth	Fellow of the Royal College of Ophthalmology
FFHom	Fellow of the Faculty of Homoeopathy	FRCP	Fellow of the Royal College of Physicians of London
FFOM	Fellow of the Faculty of Occupational Medicine	FRCPA	Fellow of the Royal College of Pathologists of Australia
FFPHM	Fellow of the Faculty of Public Health Medicine	FRCPath	Fellow of the Royal College of Pathologists
FHA	Fellow of the Institute of Health Service Administrators	FRCP(C)	Fellow of the Royal College of Physicians of Canada
FIBiol	Fellow of the Institute of Biology	FRCP(Ed.*or* Edin.)	Fellow of the Royal College of Physicians, Edinburgh
FICS	Fellow of the International College of Surgeons	FRCP(Glasg.)	Fellow of the Royal College of Physicians and Surgeons of Glasgow
FIHE	Fellow of the Institute of Health Education	FRCPI	Fellow of the Royal College of Physicians of Ireland
FIHospE	Fellow of the Institute of Hospital Engineers	FRCP&S(Canada)	Fellow of the Royal College of Physicians and Surgeons of Canada
FIMLS	Fellow of the Institute of Medical Laboratory Sciences	FRCPsych	Fellow of the Royal College of Psychiatrists
FInstP	Fellow of the Institute of Physics	FRCR	Fellow of the Royal College of Radiologists
FIPHE	Fellow of the Institute of Public Health Engineers	FRCS	Fellow of the Royal College of Surgeons of England
FLA	Fellow of the Library Association		

FRCS(C)	Fellow of the Royal College of Surgeons of Canada	LRCPI	Licentiate of the Royal College of Physicians of Ireland
FRCS(Ed.*or* Edin.)	Fellow of the Royal College of Surgeons of Edinburgh	LRCPS(Glasg.)	Licentiate of the Royal College of Physicians and Surgeons of Glasgow
FRCS(Glasg.)	Fellow of the Royal College of Physicians and Surgeons of Glasgow	LRCS	Licentiate of the Royal College of Surgeons of England
FRCS(Irel.)	Fellow of the Royal College of Surgeons in Ireland	LRCS(Ed. *or* Edin.)	Licentiate of the Royal College of Surgeons of Edinburgh
FRCVS	Fellow of the Royal College of Veterinary Science	LRCS(Irel.)	Licentiate of the Royal College of Surgeons in Ireland
FRIPHH	Fellow of the Royal Institute of Public Health and Hygiene	LSA	Licentiate of the Society of Apothecaries
FRPhamS	Fellow of the Royal Pharmaceutical Society	MA	Master of Arts
		MACP	Master of the American College of Physicians
FRPS	Fellow of the Royal Photographic Society	MAO	Master of the Art of Obstetrics
FRS	Fellow of the Royal Society	MAOT	Member of the Association of Occupational Therapists
FRSC	Fellow of the Royal Society of Canada	MB	Bachelor of Medicine
FRSE	Fellow of the Royal Society of Edinburgh	MB BS	Bachelor of Medicine and
		(or MBCLB)	Bachelor of Surgery
FRSH	Fellow of the Royal Society for the Promotion of Health	MC	Master of Surgery
		MCh	Master of Surgery
FRSTM&H	Fellow of the Royal Society of Tropical Medicine and Hygiene	MChD	Master of Dental Surgery
		MChir	Master of Surgery
FSA	Fellow of the Society of Antiquaries	MChOrth	Master of Orthopaedic Surgery
		MChOtol	Master of Otology
		MChS	Member of the Society of Chiropodists
HDD	Higher Dental Diploma		
KLJ	Knight of St Lazarus of Jerusalem	MClSc	Master of Clinical Science
		MCommH	Master of Community Health
KSTJ	Knight of the Order of the St John	MCR(R)	Member of the College of Radiographers (Diagnostic Radiography)
LAH	Licentiate of the Apothecaries' Hall, Dublin	MCR(T)	Member of the College of Radiographers (Radiotherapy)
LCh	Licentiate in Surgery	MCSP	Member of the Chartered Society of Physiotherapists
LCST	Licentiate of the College of Speech Therapists	MD	Doctor of Medicine
LDS	Licentiate in Dental Surgery	MDentSc	Master of Dental Science
LHD	*Literarum Humaniorum Doctor*, Doctor of Literature	MDS	Master of Dental Surgery
		MFCM	Member of the Faculty of Community Medicine
LicMed	Licentiate in Medicine		
LLB	Bachelor of Law	MFHom	Member of the Faculty of Homoeopathy
LLD	Doctor of Law		
LM	Licentiate in Midwifery	MFOM	Member of the Faculty of Occupational Medicine
LMCC	Licentiate of the Medical Council of Canada		
		MFPHM	Member of the Faculty of Public Health Medicine
LMed	Licentiate in Medicine		
LMSSA	Licentiate in Medicine and Surgery of the Society of Apothecaries	MHyg	Master of Hygiene
		MIH	Master of Industrial Health
		MIPR	Member of the Institute of Public Relations
LRCP	Licentiate of the Royal College of Physicians of London		
		ML	Licentiate in Medicine
LRCP(Ed.*or* Edin.)	Licentiate of the Royal College of Physicians, Edinburgh	MMed	Master of Medicine
		MMedSc	Master of Medical Science

MMSA	Master of Midwifery (Society of Apothecaries)	MSA	Member of the Society of Apothecaries
MNAS	Member of the National Academy of Sciences	MSc	Master of Science
		MScD	Master of Dental Science
MO&G	Master of Obstetrics and Gynaecology	MSUP	Master of Science in Urban Planning
MPH	Master of Public Health	MTD	Midwife Teacher's Diploma
MPhil	Master of Philosophy		
MPS	Member of the Pharmaceutical Society	ND	Doctor of Nursing
		NP	Nurse-practitioner
MPSI	Member of the Pharmaceutical Society of Ireland	OHNC	Occupational Health Nursing Certificate
MPSNI	Member of the Pharmaceutical Society of Northern Ireland	OSTJ	Officer of the Order of St John
MPsyMed	Master of Psychological Medicine		
MRACP	Member of the Royal Australasian College of Physicians	PD	Doctor of Pharmacy
		PhB	Bachelor of Philosophy
		PhD	Doctor of Philosophy
MRACS	Member of the Royal Australasian College of Surgeons	PhM	Master of Philosophy
		PRCOG	President of the Royal College of Obstetricians and Gynaecologists
MRad	Master of Radiology		
MRCGP	Member of the Royal College of General Practitioners	PRCP	President of the Royal College of Physicians of London
MRCOG	Member of the Royal College of Obstetricians and Gynaecologists	PRCP(Ed.*or* Edin.)	President of the Royal College of Physicians, Edinburgh
MRCP	Member of the Royal College of Physicians of London	PRCS	President of the Royal College of Surgeons of England
MRCPA	Member of the Royal College of Pathologists of Australia	PRCS(Ed.*or* Edin.)	President of the Royal College of Surgeons of Edinburgh
MRCPath	Member of the Royal College of Pathologists	PRS	President of the Royal Society
		PRSE	President of the Royal Society of Edinburgh
MRCP(Ed.*or* Edin.)	Member of the Royal College of Physicians, Edinburgh		
MRCP(Glasg.)	Member of the Royal College of Physicians and Surgeons of Glasgow	RCNT	Registered Clinical Nurse Teacher
		RFN	Registered Fever Nurse
		RGN	Registered General Nurse
		RHV	Registered Health Visitor
MRCPI	Member of the Royal College of Physicians of Ireland	RM	Registered Midwife
MRCPsych	Member of the Royal College of Psychiatrists	RMN	Registered Mental Nurse
		RN	Registered Nurse
MRCP(UK)	Member of the Royal Colleges of Physicians of the UK	RNMD	Registered Nurse for Mental Defectives
MRCR	Member of the Royal College of Radiologists	RNMH	Registered Nurse for the Mentally Handicapped
MRCS	Member of the Royal College of Surgeons of England	RNMS	Registered Nurse for the Mentally Subnormal
MRCS(Ed.*or* Edin.)	Member of the Royal College of Surgeons of Edinburgh	RNT	Registered Nurse Tutor
		RSCN	Registered Sick Children's Nurse
MRCS(Irel.)	Member of the Royal College of Surgeons of Ireland		
		SB	Bachelor of Science
MRCVS	Member of the Royal College of Veterinary Science	ScD	Doctor of Science
		SCM	State Certified Midwife
MRPharmS	Member of the Royal Pharmaceutical Society	SEN	State Enrolled Nurse
		SM	Master of Science
MRSH	Member of the Royal Society for the Promotion of Health	SRN	State Registered Nurse
		SRP	State Registered Physiotherapist
MS	Master of Surgery; Master of Science		

Selected honours in the UK and Commonwealth conferred by the Crown (including awards for gallantry in military service).

AFC	Air Force Cross
Bart	Baronet
BEM	British Empire Medal
Bt	Baronet
CB	Companion of the Order of the Bath
CBE	Commander of the Order of the British Empire
CH	Companion of Honour
CMG	Companion of the Order of St Michael and St George
CVO	Companion of the Royal Victorian Order
DBE	Dame Commander of the Order of the British Empire
DCB	Dame Commander of the Order of the Bath
DCM	Distinguished Conduct Medal
DCMG	Dame Commander of the Order of St Michael and St George
DCVO	Dame Commander of the Royal Victorian Order
DFC	Distinguished Flying Cross
DL	Deputy Lieutenant
DSM	Distinguished Service Medal
DSO	Companion of the Distinguished Service Order
ERD	Emergency Reserve Decoration (Army)
GBE	Knight or Dame Grand Cross of the Order of the British Empire
GC	George Cross
GCB	Knight Grand Cross of the Order of the Bath
GCMG	Knight or Dame Grand Cross of the Order of St Michael and St George
GCVO	Knight or Dame Grand Cross of the Royal Victorian Order
GM	George Medal
KBE	Knight Commander of the Order of the British Empire
KCB	Knight Commander of the Order of the Bath
KCMG	Knight Commander of the Order of St Michael and St George
KCVO	Knight Commander of the Royal Victorian Order
KG	Knight of the Order of the Garter
KT	Knight of the Order of the Thistle
Kt	Knight
MBE	Member of the Order of the British Empire
MC	Military Cross
MVO	Member of the Royal Victorian Order
OBE	Officer of the Order of the British Empire
OM	Order of Merit
TD	Territorial Efficiency Decoration
VC	Victoria Cross
VD	Royal Naval Volunteer Reserve Officers' Decoration (now VRD)

MEDICAL ABBREVIATIONS

A	argon	AEA	Atomic Energy Authority
A$_2$	second heart sound, aortic area	AEG	air encephalogram
AA	(i) Alcoholics Anonymous	AERE	Atomic Energy Research
	(ii) achievement age		Establishment
AAA	aneurysm of the abdominal aorta	aet.	*aetas* (age)
AAAS	American Association for the	AF	atrial fibrillation
	Advancement of Science	AFB	(i) American Foundation for the
AADR	American Association for Dental		Blind
	Research		(ii) acid-fast bacillus
AAMC	Association of American Medical	AFIP	Armed Forces Institute of Pathology
	Colleges	AFP	alphafetoprotein
AAP	Association of American Physicians	AFRC	Agriculture and Food Research
AAV	adenovirus-associated virus		Council
Ab	antibody	Ag	(i) silver
ABG	arterial blood gases		(ii) antigen
ABN	Association of British Neurologists	A/G ratio	albumin/globulin ratio
ABP	arterial blood pressure	AGL	acute granulocytic leukaemia
ABPI	Association of the British	AGN	acute glomerulonephritis
	Pharmaceutical Industry	AHA	(i) Area Health Authority
ABRC	Advisory Board for the Research		(ii) American Heart Association
	Councils	AHG	antihaemophilic globulin
Ac	actinium	AI	(i) aortic incompetence
a.c.	*ante cibum* (before meals)		(ii) artificial insemination
ACCME	Accreditation Council for	AID	artificial insemination from donor
	Continuing Medical Education	AIDS	acquired immunodeficiency syndrome
ACD	acid–citrate–dextrose	AIH	artifical insemination from husband
ACE	angiotensin-converting enzyme	AIIMS	All India Institute of Medical
ACG	apex cardiogram		Sciences
ACGIH	American Conference of	AJ	ankle jerk
	Governmental Industrial Hygienists	AK	above knee
ACGME	Accreditation Council for Graduate	Al	aluminium
	Medical Education	Ala	alanine
ACh	acetylcholine	ALAC	Artificial Limb and Appliance
ACOST	Advisory Council for Science and		Centre
	Technology	ALG	antilymphocytic globulin
ACP	American College of Physicians	ALL	acute lymphoblastic leukaemia
ACS	(i) American Cancer Society	ALS	(i) antilymphocytic serum
	(ii) American College of Surgeons		(ii) amyotrophic lateral sclerosis
ACTH	adrenocorticotrophic hormone	ALT	alanine aminotransferase
ACTH-RH	ACTH-releasing hormone	alt. dieb.	*alternis diebus* (every other day)
ADA	American Dental Association	AM	actomyosin
ADH	antidiuretic hormone	AMA	American Medical Association
ADI	acceptable daily intake	AMI	acute myocardial infarction
ADMS	Assistant Director of Medical	AML	acute myelogenous leukaemia
	Services	AMP	adenosine monophosphatae
ADP	(i) adenosine disphosphate	AMS	Army Medical Service
	(ii) automatic data processing	a.m.u.	atomic mass unit
ADTA	American Dental Trade Association	ANF	(i) antinuclear factor
A & E	accident and emergency		(ii) American Nurses' Foundation

ANP	arterial natriuretic peptide	BAL	(i) British Anti-Lewisite
AP	(i) anteroposterior		(ii) blood alcohol level
	(ii) artificial pneumothorax	BaM	barium meal
APA	American Psychiatric Association	BBA	born before arrival
APC	aspirin, phenacetin, and caffeine	BBB	(i) bundle branch block
APE	anterior pituitary extract	BBB	(ii) blood–brain barrier
APGAR	(see text entry)	BBSRC	Biotechnology and Biological
APH	antepartum haemorrhage		Sciences Research Council
APKD	adult polycystic kidney disease	BC/BS	Blue Cross/Blue Shield
APT	alum-precipitated toxoid	BCG	(i) bacille Calmette–Guérin
APTT	activated partial thromboplastin		(ii) ballistocardiogram
	time	BCS	British Cardiac Society
APUD	(see text entry)	b.d.	*bis die*(twice a day)
AQ	achievement quotient	BDA	British Dental Association
AR	(i) Analytical Reagent	BDL	below detectable limits
	(ii) artificial respiration	Be	beryllium
	(iii) aortic regurgitation	BERBOH	British Examining and Registration
ara-A	adenine arabinoside		Board in Occupational Hygiene
ara-C	cytosine arabinoside	BGG	bovine gamma globulin
ARC	Arthritis and Rheumatism Council	BHL	biological half-life
ARD	acute respiratory disease	Bi	bismuth
ARDS	adult respiratory distress syndrome	BIBRA	British Industrial Biological
Arg	arginine		Research Association
ARI	acute respiratory infection	BID	brought in dead
ARIA	automated radioimmunoassay	b.i.d.	*bis in die* (twice daily)
ARM	artificial rupture of the membranes	BIPP	bismuth, iodoform, and paraffin
ARV	AIDS-associated retrovirus		paste (Morison's paste)
AS	(i) aortic stenosis	BLAR	British League Against Rheumatism
	(ii) ankylosing spondylitis	BMA	British Medical Association
As	arsenic	BMI	body mass index
ASA	(i) American Surgical Association	BMR	basal metabolic rate
	(ii) acetylsalicylic acid	BMSA	British Medical Students'
ASB	anencephaly and spina bifida		Association
ASD	atrial septal defect	BNA	*Basel Nomina Anatomica*
ASH	Action on Smoking and Health	BNF	*British National Formulary*
ASME	Association for the Study of Medical	BNO	bowels not opened
	Education	BO	(i) bowels opened
Asn	asparagine		(ii) body odour
ASO	antistreptolysin-O	BOD	biological oxygen demand
Asp	aspartic acid	BP	(i) *British Pharmacopoeia*
ASS	anterior superior spine		(ii) blood pressure
AST	aspartate transaminase	b.p.	boiling point
ATA	antithyroglobulin antibody	BPA	British Paediatric Association
ATP	adenosine triphosphate	BPC	*British Pharmaceutical Codex*
ATPase	adenosine triphosphatase	BPH	benign prostatic hypertrophy
Au	gold	BPMF	British Postgraduate Medical
AV	(i) atrioventricular		Federation
	(ii) arteriovenous	BR	*Birmingham Revision*
AVB	atrioventricular block	Br	bromine
AVP	arginine vasopressin	BS	(i) breath sounds
A & W	alive and well		(ii) blood sugar
AZT	Aschheim–Zondek test	BSA	body surface area
		BSI	British Standards Institution
B	boron	BSP	bromsulphthalein
Ba	barium	BSR	(i) blood sedimentation rate
BAAS	British Association for the		(ii) British Society of Rheumatology
	Advancement of Science	BSS	buffered saline solution
BaE	barium enema	BT	bleeding time

BTG	Biotechnology Group	CDH	congenital disease of the heart
BUN	blood urea nitrogen	CDSC	Communicable Disease Surveillance
BUPA	British United Provident		Centre
	Association	CEA	(i) cost-effectiveness analysis
BV	(i) blood vessel		(ii) carcinoembryonic antigen
	(ii) blood volume	CEC	Central Ethical Committee (BMA)
BW	(i) body water	CERD	chronic end-stage renal disease
	(ii) body weight	CF	(i) cystic fibrosis
			(ii) complement fixation
C	carbon	CFA	(i) complement-fixing antibody
C_1, C_2, etc.	cervical vertebrae		(ii) complete Freund's adjuvant
C_5	pentamethonium	CFT	complement fixation test
C_6	hexamethonium	CFU	colony-forming unit
C_{10}	decamethonium	CGH	chorionic gonadotrophic hormone
CA	(i) chronological age	CGL	chronic granulocytic leukaemia
	(ii) cardiac arrest	CGN	chronic glomerulonephritis
Ca	(i) calcium	c.g.s.	centimetre–gram–second system
	(ii) carcinoma	CHA	chronic haemolytic anaemia
CABG	coronary artery bypass graft	CHAMPUS	Civilian Health and Medical
CACMS	Committee on Accreditation of		Program of the Uniformed Services
	Canadian Medical Schools	CHB	complete heart block
CAH	(i) chronic active hepatitis	CHC	Community Health Council
	(ii) congenital adrenal hyperplasia	CHD	coronary heart disease
CALLA	common acute lymphoblastic	ChE	cholinesterase
	leukaemia antigen	CHF	congestive heart failure
CAM	chorio-allantoic membrane	CHO	carbohydrate
cAMP	cyclic adenosine monophosphate	CI	(i) cardiac index
CAMR	Centre for Applied Microbiology		(ii) colour index
	and Research	CID	cytomegalic inclusion disease
CAPD	continuous ambulatory peritoneal	C_{in}	inulin clearance
	dialysis	CIOMS	Council for International
CASPE	Clinical Accountability, Service		Organizations of Medical Sciences
	Planning, and Evaluation	CJD	Creutzfeldt–Jakob disease
CAT	computerized (computed) axial	CK	creatine kinase
	tomography	Cl	chlorine
CBA	cost–benefit analysis	CLL	chronic lymphocytic leukaemia
CBC	complete blood count	CLT	clot lysis time
CBD	common bile duct	CMA	Canadian Medical Association
CBF	cerebral blood flow	CMB	Central Midwives' Board
CBG	corticosteroid-binding globulin	CMC	carpometacarpal
CBR	complete bed rest	CMI	cell-mediated immunity
CBW	chemical and biological warfare	CML	chronic myeloid (myelogenous)
CCCM	Central Committee for Community		leukaemia
	Medicine (BMA)	CMN	cystic medial necrosis
CCCR	closed chest cardiac resuscitation	CMO	Chief Medical Officer
CCF	congestive cardiac failure	CMR	cerebral metabolic rate
CCHMS	Central Committee for Hospital	$CMRO_2$	cerebral metabolic rate for oxygen
	Medical Services	CMV	cytomegalovirus
CCK	cholecystokinin	CNA	Canadian Nurses Association
CCL	carcinoma cell line	CNAA	Council for National Academic
C_{cr}	creatinine clearance		Awards
CCS	casualty clearing station	CNS	central nervous system
CCSC	Central Consultants and Specialists	CO	(i) cardiac output
	Committee (BMA)		(ii) carbon monoxide
CCU	coronary care unit	CO_2	carbon dioxide
CD	controlled drug	Co	(i) cobalt
Cd	cadmium		(ii) coenzyme
CDC	Center for Disease Control		(iii) *compositus* (compound)

C/O	complains of	CS	caesarean section
CoA	coenzyme A	Cs	caesium
COAD	chronic obstructive airways disease	CSF	cerebrospinal fluid
COBT	chronic obstruction of the biliary tract	CSM	(i) Committee on Safety of Medicines
COD	(i) cause of death		(ii) cerebrospinal meningitis
	(ii) chemical oxygen demand	CSOM	chronic suppurative otitis media
COHb	carboxyhaemoglobin	CSP	Chartered Society of Physiotherapy
COLD	chronic obstructive lung disease	CSSD	Central Sterile Supply Department
COMA	Committee on Medical Aspects of Food Policy	CST	(i) cavernous sinus thrombosis
			(ii) convulsive shock therapy
COMT	catechol-O-methyltransferase		(iii) Council for Science and Technology
CON	cyclopropane, oxygen, and nitrogen		
COOH	carboxyl group	CSU	catheter specimen of urine
COP	colloid osmotic pressure	CT	(i) computerized (computed) tomography
COPD	chronic obstructive pulmonary disease		(ii) coronary thrombosis
			(iii) cerebral thrombosis
COphth.	College of Ophthalmologists		(iv) cerebral tumour
CoR	Congo red	CTC	Clinical Trial Certificate
CP	(i) chemically pure	CTR	cardiothoracic ratio
	(ii) cor pulmonale	CTS	carpal tunnel syndrome
C/P	cholesterol/phospholipid ratio	Cu	copper
C & P	cystoscopy and pyelography	CV	(i) cardiovascular
C_{pah}	*para*-aminohippurate clearance		(ii) cerebrovascular
CPAP	continuous positive airway pressure	CVA	cerebrovascular accident
CPB	cardiopulmonary bypass	CVD	cerebrovascular disease
CPC	clinicopathological conference	CVP	central venous pressure
CPD	(i) cephalopelvic disproportion	CVR	cerebrovascular resistance
	(ii) citrate–phosphate–dextrose	CVS	cardiovascular system
CPE	chronic pulmonary emphysema	CWI	cardiac work index
CPK	creatine phosphokinase	CX	cervix
CPKD	childhood polycystic kidney disease	CXR	chest X-ray
CPM	counts per minute	CyA	cyclosporin A
CPME	Council for Postgraduate Medical Education	Cys	cysteine
		Cys–Cys	cystine
CPP	cerebral perfusion pressure		
CPPB	constant positive pressure breathing	D	deuterium
CPPV	continuous positive pressure ventilation	DA	(i) developmental age
			(ii) dopamine
CPR	cardiopulmonary resuscitation	DADMS	Deputy Assistant Director of Medical Services
c.p.s.	cycles per second		
CPU	central processing unit	DAH	disordered action of the heart
CR	(i) conditioned reflex	DAO	Duly Authorized Officer
	(ii) crown–rump	DBP	diastolic blood pressure
Cr	chromium	DBW	desirable body weight
C & R	convalescence and rehabilitation	D & C	dilatation and curettage
CRAO	central retinal artery occlusion	DCS	dorsal column stimulation
CRC	(i) Cancer Research Campaign	DD	(i) dangerous drug
	(ii) Clinical Research Centre		(ii) differential diagnosis
CRE	cumulative radiation effect	DDMS	Deputy Director of Medical Services
CRF	corticotrophin-releasing factor	DDRB	Doctors' and Dentists' Review Body
CRH	corticotrophin-releasing hormone	DDS	dapsone (diamino-diphenyl-sulphone)
CRL	crown–rump length		
CRM	cross-reacting material	DDSO	diamino-diphenyl-sulphoxide
CRP	C-reactive protein	DDST	Denver Developmental Screening Test
CrP	creatine phosphate		
CRS	congenital rubella syndrome		
CRT	cathode ray tube	DDT	dichloro-diphenyl-trichloroethane

DEA	dehydroepiandrosterone	DS	(i) disseminated (multiple) sclerosis
DEC	diethylcarbamazine		(ii) Down's syndrome
decd.	deceased		(iii) dead space
decub.	*decubitus* (lying down)	D/S	dextrose saline
DES	(i) diethylstilboestrol	DSA	digital subtraction angiography
	(ii) Department of Education and Science	DSS	(i) dioctyl sodium sulphosuccinate
			(ii) Department of Social Security
DF	degrees of freedom	DST	dexamethasone suppression
DFE	Department for Education		test
DFO	District Finance Officer	DT	delirium tremens
DFR	(dihydro) folate reductase	DTP	(i) distal tingling on percussion
DGAMS	Director General, Army Medical Services		(ii) diphtheria, tetanus, pertussis
		DTR	deep tendon reflex
DGMS	Director General, Medical Services	DU	duodenal ulcer
DH	Department of Health	D & V	diarrhoea and vomiting
DHA	District Health Authority	DVT	deep vein thrombosis
1,25-DHCC	1,25-dihydroxycholecalciferol	D/W	dextrose in water
DHE	dihydroergotamine	Dx	diagnosis
DHEW	Department of Health, Education and Welfare	DXR	deep X-ray
		DXRT	deep X-ray therapy
DHHS	Department of Health and Human Services	DZ	dizygotic
DHR	delayed hypersensitivity reaction	EACA	epsilon-aminocaproic acid
DHSS	Department of Health and Social Security	EAE	experimental allergic encephalomyelitis
DI	diabetes insipidus	EAHF	eczema, asthma, hay fever
DIC	disseminated intravascular coagulopathy	EAM	external auditory meatus
		EB	epidermolysis bullosa
DIP	distal interphalangeal joint	EBF	erythroblastosis fetalis
DLE	(i) discoid lupus erythematosus	EBI	emetine bismuth iodide
	(ii) disseminated lupus erythematosus	EBS	Emergency Bed Service
		EBV	Epstein–Barr virus
DLF	Disabled Living Foundation	EC	(i) electron capture
DM	(i) diabetes mellitus		(ii) European Community
	(ii) diastolic murmur	ECAT	emission computerized (computed)
DMF	decayed, missing, and filled (teeth)		axial tomography
DMO	District Medical Officer	ECBO	(i) enteric cytopathic bovine orphan
DMP	dimethylphthalate		(virus)
DMS	Director of Medical Services		(ii) European Cell Biology
DMSO	dimethyl sulphoxide		Organization
DNA	(i) deoxyribonucleic acid	ECF	extracellular fluid
	(ii) did not attend	ECFMG	Educational Commission for
DNMS	Director of Naval Medical Services		Foreign Medical Graduates
DNO	District Nursing Officer	ECG	electrocardiogram
DNOC	dinitro-*ortho*-cresol	ECHO	(i) Equipment to Charity Hospitals
DNR	do not resuscitate		Overseas
D_2O	deuterium oxide (heavy water)		(ii) enteric cytopathic human orphan
DOA	dead on arrival		(virus)
DOB	date of birth	ECoG	electrocorticogram
DOC	11-deoxycorticosterone	ECT	electroconvulsive therapy
DOCA	deoxycorticosterone acetate	ECV	extracellular volume
DOE	(i) dyspnoea on effort	ED	erythema dose
	(ii) Department of the Environment	ED_{50}	median effective dose
dopa	dihydroxyphenylalanine	EDD	expected date of delivery
Dp	data processing	EDM	early diastolic murmur
DPAG	Dangerous Pathogens Advisory Group	EDP	(i) end-diastolic pressure
			(ii) electron dense particles
DRG	diagnostic-related group	EDS	Ehlers–Danlos syndrome

EDTA	(i) ethylenediamine tetraacetic acid (edetic acid)	ERV	expiratory reserve volume
	(ii) European Dialysis and Transplant Association	ESF	European Science Foundation
		ESN	educationally subnormal
EDV	end-diastolic volume	ESP	(i) extrasensory perception
EEC	European Economic Community		(ii) end-systolic pressure
EEE	eastern equine encephalitis	ESR	(i) electron spin resonance
EEG	electroencephalogram		(ii) erythrocyte sedimentation rate
EFA	essential fatty acids	ESRC	(i) Economic and Social Science Research Council
EFE	endocardial fibroelastosis		(ii) European Science Research Councils
EGDF	embryonic growth and development factor	ESRD	end-stage renal disease
EGF	epidermal growth factor	ESV	end-systolic volume
EHC	enterohepatic circulation	ETC	estimated time of conception
EHL	effective half-life	ETEC	enterotoxigenic *Escherichia coli*
EHV	equine herpes virus	ETO	estimated time of ovulation
EIA	enzyme immunoassay	ETR	effective thyroxine ratio
EIS	Epidemic Intelligence Service	ETT	exercise tolerance test
EJ	elbow jerk	EU	European Union
EKG	see ECG	EUA	examination under anaesthesia
ELISA	enzyme-linked immunosorbent assay	EULAR	European League Against Rheumatism
ELSS	Emergency Life Support system	EWL	evaporative water loss
EM	electron microscopy		
E–M	Embden–Meyerhof pathway	F	fluorine
EMAS	Employment Medical Advisory Service	FA	fluorescent antibody
		Fab	fragment, antigen-binding (of IgG molecule)
EMBL	European Molecular Biology Laboratory	FAD	familial autonomic dysfunction
EMBO	European Molecular Biology Organization	FAH	Federation of American Hospitals
		FANY	First Aid Nursing Yeomanry Service
EMF	(i) electromotive force	FAO	Food and Agricultural Organization (United Nations)
	(ii) endomyocardial fibrosis	FAS	fetal alcohol syndrome
EMG	electromyogram	FB	foreign body
EMRC	European Medical Research Councils	FBC	full blood count
		Fc	fragment, crystallizable (of IgG molecule)
EMS	Emergency Medical Service	FCA	Freund's complete adjuvant
EN	erythema nodosum	FCM	Faculty of Community Medicine
ENL	erythema nodosum leprosum	FCO	Foreign and Commonwealth Office
ENT	ear, nose, and throat	FDA	Food and Drug Administration
EOA	examination, opinion, and advice	FDIU	fetal death *in utero*
EOG	electro-oculogram	FDP	fibrin degradation products
EOL	end of life	Fe	iron
EORTC	European Organization for Research into the Treatment of Cancer	FEUO	for external use only
		FEV	forced expiratory volume
EP	*Extra Pharmacopoeia*	FEV_1	forced expiratory volume in one second
EPA	Environmental Protection Agency		
EPP	end-plate potential	FF	filtration fraction
ERA	oestrogen (estrogen) receptor assay	FFA	free fatty acids
ERBF	effective renal blood flow	FFD	focus–film distance
ERCP	endoscopic retrograde cholangiopancreatography	FFI	fit and free from infection
		FFP	fresh frozen plasma
ERPC	evacuation of retained products of conception	FFT	flicker fusion threshold
		FH	(i) family history
ERPF	effective renal plasma flow		(ii) familial hypercholesterolaemia
ERT	oestrogen (estrogen) replacement therapy		(iii) fetal heart

FHH	fetal heart heard	GCMS	gas chromatography with mass spectrometry
FHNH	fetal heart not heard	GCS	Glasgow Coma Score
FHR	fetal heart rate	GCSE	General Certificate of Secondary Education
FIF	fibroblast interferon		
FIGLU	formiminoglutamic acid	GD	gonadal dysgenesis
FIP	Fédération Internationale Pharmaceutique	GDB	Guide Dogs for the Blind
FIUO	for internal use only	GDC	General Dental Council
FMDV	foot-and-mouth disease virus	GDH	glutamate dehydrogenase
FMS	fat-mobilizing substance	GDMO	General Duties Medical Officer
F–N	finger–nose	GE	gastroenterology
FOB	faecal occult blood	GET	gastric emptying time
FOM	Faculty of Occupational Medicine	GF	(i) growth factor
f.p.	freezing point		(ii) glomerular filtrate
FPA	Family Planning Association	GFR	glomerular filtration rate
FPB	femoropopliteal bypass	GGT	gamma-glutamyl transpeptidase
FPC	(i) Family Practitioner Committee	GH	growth hormone
	(ii) family planning clinic	GHRF	GH releasing factor
FPHM	Faculty of Public Health Medicine	GI	gastrointestinal
f.p.s.	foot–pound–second system	GIG	Genetic Interest Group
FRC	functional residual capacity	GIK	glucose, insulin, and potassium
FRF	see FSH-RF	GIP	gastric inhibitory peptide
FRJM	full range of joint movement	GIS	gastrointestinal series
FSD	focus–skin distance	GITT	glucose insulin tolerance test
f.s.d.	full-scale deflection	GLC	gas–liquid chromatography
FSH	follicle-stimulating hormone	Gln	glutamine
FSH-RF	FSH releasing factor	Glu	glutamic acid
FSH-RH	FSH releasing hormone	Gly	glycine
FT	(i) full term	GM	Geiger–Müller
	(ii) formol toxoid	GMAG	Genetic Manipulation Advisory Group
FT_4	free thyroxine		
FTA	fluorescent treponemal antibody test	GMC	General Medical Council
FTBD	full term, born dead	GMSC	General Medical Services Committee
FT_4I	free thyroxine index		
FTE	full-time equivalent	GN	glomerulonephritis
FTM	fractional test meal	GNC	General Nursing Council
FTND	full term, normal delivery	GNP	gross national product
FTT	failure to thrive	GOS	Great Ormond Street
FU	follow up	GOT	glutamic-oxaloacetic transaminase
FUO	fever of uncertain origin	GP	general practitioner
FVC	forced vital capacity	G-6-P	glucose 6-phosphate
Fx	fracture	GPB	glossopharyngeal breathing
		G-6-PD	glucose 6-phosphate dehydrogenase
GA	(i) general anaesthesia	GPI	general paralysis (paresis) of the insane
	(ii) gestational age		
GABA	gamma-aminobutyric acid	GPT	glutamic-pyruvic transaminase
GADS	gonococcal arthritis/dermatitis syndrome	GRAS	generally recognized as safe (food additives)
Gal	galactose	GRID	gay-related immunodeficiency
GALT	gut-associated lymphoid tissue	GSD	glycogen storage disease
GB	gall-bladder	GSE	gluten-sensitive enteropathy
GBM	glomerular basement membrane	GSW	gunshot wound
GBS	Guillain–Barré syndrome	GTH	gonadotrophic hormone
GC	(i) gas chromatography	GTP	glutamyl transpeptidase
	(ii) gonococcal	GTT	glucose tolerance test
GCE	General Certificate of Education	GU	(i) gastric ulcer
GCFT	gonococcal complement fixation test		(ii) genitourinary
		GVH	graft-versus-host(reaction, disease)

GY	gray (see RADIATION, text entry)
H	hydrogen
HA	haemagglutination
HAA	(i) Hospital Activity Analysis
	(ii) hepatitis-associated antigen
HAI	haemagglutination inhibition
HAV	hepatitis A virus
Hb	haemoglobin
HbA	adult haemoglobin
HBAB	hepatitis B antibody
HBAg	hepatitis B antigen
HB$_c$Ag	hepatitis B core antigen
HBD	has been drinking
HBF	hepatic blood flow
HbF	fetal haemoglobin
HbH	haemoglobin H
HbO$_2$	oxyhaemoglobin
HbS	sickle-cell haemoglobin
HB$_s$Ag	hepatitis B surface antigen
HBV	hepatitis B virus
HC	hereditary coproporphyria
HCC	hepatocellular carcinoma
HCD	heavy chain disease
HCG	human chorionic gonadotrophin
HCL	hairy-cell leukaemia
HCVD	hypertensive cardiovascular disease
HD	Hodgkin's disease
HDA	Hospital Doctors' Association
HDL	high-density lipoprotein
HDLC	high-density lipoprotein cholesterol
HDN	haemolytic disease of the newborn
HDU	haemodialysis unit
He	helium
H & E	(i) haematoxylin and eosin
	(ii) haemorrhages and exudates
HEA	Health Education Authority
HEC	Health Education Council
HeLa	Helen Lake (tumour cell line)
HEFC	Higher Education Funding council
HFIF	human fibroblast interferon
HFPPV	high-frequency positive-pressure ventilation
Hg	mercury
HGG	human gamma-globulin
HGH	human growth hormone
HHT	hereditary haemorrhagic telangiectasia
5-HIAA	5-hydroxyindole acetic acid
His	histidine
HJR	hepatojugular reflex
HJSC	Hospital Junior Staff Council (BMA)
HLA	(see text entry)
HLH	human luteinizing hormone
HMD	hyaline membrane disease
HMMA	4-hydroxy-3-methoxymandelic acid
HMO	Health Maintenance Organization
HMP	hexose monophosphate
HNA	higher nervous activity
HNP	herniated nucleus pulposus
HOCM	hypertrophic obstructive cardiomyopathy
HP	house physician
Hp	haptoglobin
HPA	hypothalamus–pituitary–adrenal
HPG	human pituitary gonadotrophin
HPI	history of present illness
HPL	human placental lactogen
HPLC	high-pressure liquid chromatography
HPNS	high-pressure nervous syndrome
HPOA	hypertrophic pulmonary osteoarthropathy
hPRL	prolactin
HR	heart rate
HRH	hypothalamic releasing hormone
HRT	hormone replacement therapy
HS	house surgeon
HSA	human serum albumin
HSC	Health and Safety Commission
HSE	(i) Health and Safety Executive
	(ii) herpes simplex encephalitis
HSR	health services research
HSRB	Health Services Research Board
HSV	herpes simplex virus
5-HT	5-hydroxytryptamine
HTLV	human T-cell lymphoma (leukaemia) virus
HUS	haemolytic-uraemic syndrome
HV	*Herpesvirus*
HVA	homovanillic acid
HVG	host-versus-graft
HVH	*Herpesvirus hominis*
I	iodine
IA	intra-arterial
IADR	International Association for Dental Research
IAEA	International Atomic Energy Agency
IAM	Institute of Aviation Medicine
IAPB	International Agency for the Prevention of Blindness
IARC	International Agency for Research on Cancer
IASP	International Association for the Study of Pain
IBRO	International Brain Research Organization
IBS	irritable bowel syndrome
IBW	ideal body weight
IC	internal conversion
ICD	(i) International Classification of Disease

ICF	(ii) immune complex disease intracellular fluid	IPPR	intermittent positive pressure respiration
ICLA	International Committee of Laboratory Animals	IPPV	intermittent positive pressure ventilation
ICP	intracranial pressure	IQ	intelligence quotient
ICRF	Imperial Cancer Research Fund	IR	infra-red
ICRP	International Commission on Radiological Protection	Ir	iridium
		IRDS	idiopathic respiratory distress syndrome
ICSH	interstitial cell-stimulating hormone	IRMA	International Rehabilitation Medicine Association
ICSU	International Council of Scientific Unions		
ICU	intensive care unit	IRV	inspiratory reserve volume
I & D	incision and drainage	ISD	interventricular septal defect (also IVSD)
IDD	insulin-dependent diabetes		
IDK	internal derangement of knee	ISE	ion-sensitive electrode
IDL	intermediate density lipoprotein	ISF	interstitial fluid
IDU	idoxuridine	ISO	International Standards Organization
IDV	intermittent demand ventilation		
IEM	inborn error of metabolism	ISQ	*in statu quo* (unchanged)
IEP	immunoelectrophoresis	IST	insulin shock therapy
IF	intrinsic factor	IT	isomeric transition
IFA	immunofluorescence assay	ITP	idiopathic thrombocytopenic purpura
Ig	immunoglobulin		
IgA	immunoglobulin A	ITT	insulin tolerance test
IgD	immunoglobulin D	IU	international unit
IgE	immunoglobulin E	IUD	(i) intrauterine device
IgG	immunoglobulin G		(ii) intrauterine death
IgM	immunoglobulin M	IUGR	intrauterine growth retardation
IHD	ischaemic heart disease	IUP	intrauterine pressure
ILAE	International League Against Epilepsy	IUT	intrauterine transfusion
		IV	intravenous
Ile	isoleucine	i.v.	iodine value
ILO	International Labour Organization	IVC	inferior vena cava
IM	(i) intramuscular	IVCD	intraventricular conduction defect
	(ii) infectious mononucleosis	IVD	intervertebral disc
IME	Institute of Medical Ethics	IVF	*in vitro* fertilization
IMLS	Institute of Medical Laboratory Science	IVGTT	intravenous glucose tolerance test
		IVH	intraventricular haemorrhage
IMS	Indian Medical Service	IVP	intravenous pyelogram
In	indium	IVS	interventricular septum
INH	isoniazid (isonicotinic acid hydrazide)	IVSD	interventricular septal defect
		IVT	intravenous transfusion
INI	intranuclear inclusion	IZS	insulin zinc suspension
INM	Institute of Naval Medicine		
I & O	intake and output	JACNE	Joint Advisory Committee on Nutrition Education
IOD	injured on duty		
IOFB	intraocular foreign body	JCC	Joint Consultants' Committee
IOM	Institute of Medicine	JCHMT	Joint Committee on Higher Medical Training
IOP	intraocular pressure		
IP	(i) *International Pharmacopoeia*	JCHST	Joint Committee on Higher Surgical Training
	(ii) interphalangeal		
IPD	intermittent peritoneal dialysis	JDM	juvenile diabetes mellitus
IPPA	inspection, palpation, percussion, ausculation	JEE	Japanese equine encephalitis
		JG	juxtaglomerular
IPPF	International Planned Parenthood Federation	JGA	juxtaglomerular apparatus
		JHDA	Junior Hospital Doctors' Association
IPPNW	International Physicians for the Prevention of Nuclear War		
		JHMO	Junior Hospital Medical Officer

JHU	Johns Hopkins University
JJ	jaw jerk
JNA	*Jena Nomina Anatomica*
JND	just noticeable difference
JOD	juvenile onset diabetes
JV	jugular vein
JVP	jugular venous pressure (or pulse)
K	potassium
17-K	17-ketosteroids
KA	King–Armstrong (units of alkaline phosphatase)
KB	ketone bodies
kb	kilobase
kcal	kilocalorie (1000 calories or 1 Calorie)
K_e	exchangeable body potassium
K-F rings	Kayser–Fleisher rings
17-KGS	17-ketogenic steroids
KJ	knee jerk
KLS	kidney, liver, spleen
KO	knock-out
KP	keratin precipitates (in keratitis punctata)
Kr	krypton
KS	Kaposi's sarcoma
17-KS	17-ketosteroids
KUB	kidney, ureter, bladder
K-WS	Kimmelstiel–Wilson syndrome
L1, L2 etc.	lumbar vertebrae
LA	(i) left atrial
	(ii) latex agglutination
L & A	light and accommodation
LAA	leucocyte ascorbic acid
LAD	(i) left axis deviation
	(ii) lactic acid dehydrogenase
LAF	laminar air flow
LAH	left anterior hemiblock
	(ii) left atrial hypertrophy
LAIT	latex agglutination inhibition test
LAP	(i) leucine aminopeptidase
	(ii) leucocyte alkaline phosphatase
L-ASP	L-asparaginase
LAT	latex agglutination test
LATS	long-acting thyroid stimulator
LATS-P	LATS-protector substance
LBB	left bundle branch
LBBB	left bundle branch block
LBF	liver blood flow
LBH	length, breadth, height
LBL	lymphoblastic lymphoma
LBM	lean body mass
LBP	low back pain
LBW	low birth weight
LCD	liquid crystal display
LCFA	long-chain fatty acid

LCM	lymphocytic choriomeningitis
LCME	Liaison Committee on Medical Education
LCMV	LCM virus
LD	legionnaires' disease
LD_{50}	median lethal dose
LDH	lactate dehydrogenase
LDL	low-density lipoprotein
LDLC	low-density lipoprotein cholesterol
LE	lupus erythematosus
LED	light-emitting diode
LES	lower oesophageal (esophageal) sphincter
LET	linear energy transfer
Leu	leucine
LFD	least fatal dose
LFT	(i) liver function tests
	(ii) latex fixation test
LFV	Lassa fever virus
LGH	lactogenic hormone
LGV	lymphogranuloma venereum
LH	luteinizing hormone
LHC	Local Health Council
LHRF	luteinizing hormone releasing factor
LHRH	luteinizing hormone releasing hormone
LHS	left heart strain
Li	lithium
LIG	left iliac fossa
LIH	left inguinal hernia
LKS	liver, kidney, spleen
LLO	*Legionella*-like organisms
LLQ	left lower quadrant
LMC	Local Medical Committee
LMN	lower motor neurone
LMP	last menstrual period
LOC	length of stay
LOM	limitation of movement
LOPS	length of patient stay
LP	lumbar puncture
LPF	low-power field
LPH	left posterior hemiblock
LPL	lipoprotein lipase
LRF	see LHRF
LRH	see LHRH
LRT	lower respiratory tract
LRTI	LRT infection
LSCS	lower segment caesarean section
LSD	lysergic acid diethylamide (lysergide)
LSF	lymphocyte-stimulating factor
LSK	liver, spleen, kidney
LSMW	London School of Medicine for Women
LTC	long-term care
LTF	lymphocyte-transforming factor
LUQ	left upper quadrant
LV	left ventricle

LVEDP	left ventricular end-diastolic pressure	MEC	minimum effective concentration
LVEDV	left ventricular end-diastolic volume	MED	(i) minimum effective dose
LVF	left ventricular failure		(ii) minimum erythema dose
LVH	left ventricular hypertrophy	MEDLARS	Medical Literature Analysis and Retrieval System
LVN	low viscosity nitrocellulose	MEDLINE	MEDLARS on-line
LVS	left ventricular strain	MEF	mean expiratory flow rate
L & W	living and well	MELAS	mitochondrial encephalomyopathy, lactic acidosis, and stroke
Lys	lysine		
LZM	lysozyme	MEN	multiple endocrine neoplasia
		MEP	motor end-plate
M_1	first heart sound, mitral area	MEPP	miniature end-plate potential
M_2	second heart sound, mitral area	MERRF	Mitochondrial encephalomyopathy with ragged-red fibres
MA	mental age		
MABP	mean arterial blood pressure	Met	methionine
MAC	maximum allowable concentration	metHb	methaemoglobin
MAF	macrophage activating factor	MF	myelofibrosis
MAHA	microangiopathic haemolytic anaemia	M/F	male/female
		MFD	minimum fatal dose
MAKA	major karyotypic abnormality	MG	macroglobulinaemia
MAL	mid-axillary line	Mg	magnesium
mal	malate	MGH	Massachusetts General Hospital
MAO	monoamine oxidase	MHC	major histocompatibility complex
MAOI	monoamine oxidase inhibitor	MHD	minimum haemolytic dose
MAP	(i) mean arterial pressure	MHI	malignant histiocytosis of the intestine
	(ii) muscle action potential		
MAS	Medical Advisory Service	MI	(i) myocardial infarction
MASC	Medical Academic Staff Council (BMA)		(ii) mitral incompetence
			(iii) medical inspection
MASH	Mobile Army Surgical Hospital	MIC	minimum inhibitory concentration
MBC	maximum breathing capacity	MICU	mobile intensive care unit
MBD	minimal brain dysfunction	MID	minimum infective dose
MBL	(i) Marine Biological Laboratory	MIF	migration-inhibition factor
MBL	(ii) menstrual blood loss	MIFR	maximum inspiratory flow rate
MBP	mean blood pressure	MIKA	minor karyotypic abnormalities
MCAT	Medical College Admission Test	MIMS	Monthly Index of Medical Specialities
McB	McBurney's point		
MCCU	mobile coronary care unit	MIO	minimum identifiable odour
MCD	mean corpuscular diameter	MIT	mono-iodotyrosine
MCH	mean corpuscular haemoglobin	MK	monkey kidney
MCHC	mean corpuscular haemoglobin concentration	m.k.s.	metre–kilogram–second system
		MLC	mixed lymphocyte culture
MCKD	multicystic kidney disease	MLD	minimum lethal dose
MCL	midclavicular line	MLSO	medical laboratory scientific officer
MCP	metacarpophalangeal	MLV	murine leukaemia virus
MCQ	multiple-choice question	MM	(i) multiple myeloma
MCT	mean circulation time		(ii) mucous membrane
MCTD	mixed connective tissue disease	mmHg	millimetres of mercury
MCV	mean corpuscular volume	MMPI	Minnesota Multiphasic Personality Inventory
MD	(i) mentally deficient		
	(ii) muscular dystrophy	MMR	mass miniature radiography
MDM	mid-diastolic murmur	Mn	manganese
MDH	malic dehydrogenase	MND	motor neurone disease
M-dopa	methyl-dopa	MO	medical officer
MDQ	minimum detectable quantity	Mo	molybdenum
MDR	minimum daily requirement	MOC	maximum oxygen consumption
MDU	Medical Defence Union	MOD	(i) maturity onset diabetes
MEA	multiple endocrine adenomatosis		(ii) Ministry of Defence

MOH	Medical Officer of Health	NAS-NRC	NAS-National Research Council
MOUS	multiple occurrence of unexplained symptoms	NAWCH	National Association for the Welfare of Children in Hospital
m.p.	melting point	NBI	no bone injury
6-MP	6-mercaptopurine	NBM	nil by mouth
MPB	male pattern baldness	NBME	National Board of Medical Examiners
MPC	maximum permissible concentration		
MPD	maximum permissible dose	NBTS	National Blood Transfusion Service
MPE	maximum possible error	NCD	normal childhood disorders
MPGN	membranoproliferative glomerulonephritis	NCI	National Cancer Institute
		NCIB	National Collection of Industrial Bacteria
MPI	maximum permissible intake		
MPL	maximum permissible level	NCTC	National Collection of Type Cultures
MPU	Medical Practitioners Union		
MPV	mean platelet volume	ND	Nomenclature of Disease
MR	mitral regurgitation	NDA	no detectable activity
MRC	Medical Research Council	NDE	near death experience
MRD	minimal residual disease	NDI	nephrogenic diabetes insipidus
mRNA	messenger RNA	NDV	Newcastle disease virus
MRV	minute respiratory volume	NE	niacin equivalent
MS	(i) multiple sclerosis	Ne	neon
	(ii) mitral stenosis	NEC	necrotizing enterocolitis
MSG	monosodium glutamate	NED	no evidence of disease
MSH	melanocyte-stimulating hormone	NEFA	non-esterified fatty acids
MST	mean survival time	NERC	National Environment Research Council
MSU	mid-stream specimen of urine		
MSUD	maple syrup urine disease	NET	nasoendotracheal tube
MSV	murine sarcoma virus	NF	*National Formulary*
MTC	medullary thyroid carcinoma	NFTD	normal full-term delivery
MTP	metatarsophalangeal	NGF	nerve growth factor
MTT	mean transit time	NGU	non-gonococcal urethritis
MTU	methylthiouracil	NHI	National Health Insurance
MTX	methotrexate	NHL	non-Hodgkin lymphoma
MV	mitral valve	NHLBI	National Heart, Lung and Blood Institute
MVP	mitral valve prolapse		
MVR	mitral valve replacement	NHS	National Health Service
MW	molecular weight	Ni	nickel
MWF	Medical Women's Federation	NIA	National Institute of Aging
MZ	monozygotic	NIADDK	National Institute of Arthritis, Diabetes, and Digestive and Kidney Diseases
N	nitrogen		
NA	(i) *Nomina Anatomica*	NIAID	National Institute of Allergy and Infectious Diseases
	(ii) numerical aperture		
Na	sodium	NIAMD	National Institute of Arthritis and Metabolic Diseases
NAA	no apparent abnormalities		
NAD	(i) nicotinamide adenine dinucleotide	NIB	National Institute for the Blind
		NIBSC	National Institute for Biological Standards and Control
	(ii) nil abnormal discovered		
NADP	nicotinamide adenine dinucleotide phosphate	NICHHD	National Institute of Child Health and Human Development
Na$_e$	exchangeable body sodium	NICM	Nuffield Institute of Comparative Medicine
NAHAT	National Association of Health Authorities and Trusts		
		NICU	neonatal intensive care unit
NAI	non-accidental injury	NIDD	non-insulin-dependent diabetes
NALP	neuroadenolysis of the pituitary	NIDR	National Institute for Dental Research
NANBH	non-A, non-B hepatitis		
NAR	nasal airway resistance	NIH	National Institutes of Health
NAS	National Academy of Sciences	NIHL	noise-induced hearing loss

NIMH	National Institute of Mental Health	O & G	obstetrics and gynaecology
NIMR	National Institute for Medical Research	OGTT	oral glucose tolerance test
		25-OHCC	25-hydroxycholecalciferol
NINDB	National Institute of Neurological Diseases and Blindness	17-OHCS	17-hydroxycorticosteroids
		17-OHP	17-hydroxyprogesterone
NINDS	National Institute of Neurological Diseases and Stroke	OHS	obesity hypoventilation syndrome
		OI	opsonic index
NIOSH	National Institute for Occupational Safety and Health	OIHP	Office International d'Hygiene Publique
NLM	National Library of Medicine	OND	other neurological disorders
NLN	no longer needed	ONTR	orders not to resuscitate
NMR	nuclear magnetic resonance	OP	(i) out-patient
NND	neonatal death		(ii) over proof
NNR	New and Non-official Remedies	OPCA	olivopontocerebellar atrophy
NOPWC	National Old People's Welfare Council	OPCS	Office of Population, Censuses and Surveys
NP	nurse practitioner	OPD	out-patient department
n.p.	*nomen proprium* (label with its own name)	OPV	oral poliomyelitis vaccine
		OR	operating room
NPHT	Nuffield Provincial Hospitals Trust	O–R	oxidation–reduction
		ORIF	open reduction with internal fixation
NPL	National Physical Laboratory	Orn	ornithine
NPN	non-protein nitrogen	ORT	oral rehydration therapy
NRPB	National Radiological Protection Board	OS	opening snap
		OSHA	Occupational Safety and Health Administration
NRS	normal rabbit serum		
NS	normal saline	OSRD	Office of Scientific Research and Development
NSAID	non-steroidal anti-inflammatory drug	OST	Office of Science and Technology
NSD	(i) normal spontaneous delivery	OT	(i) occupational therapist
	(ii) nominal standard dose		(ii) old tuberculin
NSR	normal sinus rhythm	OVX	ovariectomized
NSU	non-specific urethritis	o/w	oil in water
NTD	neural tube defect		
NTG	nitroglycerine	P	phosphorus
NTP	normal temperature and pressure	*P*	probability
N & V	nausea and vomiting	P_1	pulmonary first sound
NVM	non-volatile matter	P_2	pulmonary second sound
NWB	non-weight-bearing	PA	(i) pernicious anaemia
NYD	not yet diagnosed		(ii) pulmonary artery
NZB	New Zealand Black (mice)	PABA	*para*-aminobenzoic acid
		P_aCO^2	arterial partial pressure of carbon dioxide
O	oxygen		
OA	osteoarthropathy (osteoarthritis, osteoarthrosis)	PAF	platelet activating factor
		PAG	(i) polyacrylamide gel electrophoresis
OAD	obstructive airways disease		(ii) periaqueductal grey matter
OB	(i) obstetrics	PAH	*para*-aminohippuric acid
	(ii) occult blood	PAHO	Pan-American Health Organization
OBD	organic brain disease	PAL	posterior axillary line
OC	oral contraceptive	PAM	penicillin aluminium monostearate
O & C	onset and course	PAMA	post-amputation mobility aid
OD	overdose	PANLAR	Pan-American League Against Rheumatism
ODA	(i) Overseas Development Administration (FCO)		
	(ii) Overseas Doctors' Association	P_aO^2	arterial partial pressure of oxygen
OECD	Organization for Economic Cooperation and Development	PAP	peak airway pressure
		Pap	Papanicolaou (smear, etc.)
OER	oxygen enhancement ratio	PAPP	pregnancy-associated plasma protein

PARU	post-anaesthetic recovery unit
PAS	(i) *para*-aminosalicylic acid
	(ii) periodic acid–Schiff
PASB	Pan-American Sanitary Bureau
PAT	paroxysmal atrial tachycardia
PAWP	pulmonary artery wedge pressure
Pb	lead
PBC	primary biliary cirrhosis
PBG	porphobilinogen
PBI	protein-bound iodine
PBP	progressive bulbar palsy
PBV	pulmonary blood volume
PBZ	phenylbutazone
p.c.	*post cibum* (after food)
PCA	passive cutaneous anaphylaxis
PCB	(i) post-coital bleeding
	(ii) polychlorinated biphenyls
PCC	(i) phaeochromocytoma
	(ii) Professional Conduct
	Committee (GMC)
PCD	polycystic disease
PCE	pseudocholinesterase
PCG	phonocardiogram
PCH	paroxysmal cold haemoglobinuria
PCKD	polycystic kidney disease
PCL	persistent corpus luteum
PCM	protein–calorie malnutrition
pCO_2	partial pressure of carbon dioxide
PCP	phencyclidine
PCS	post-cardiotomy syndrome
PCT	(i) prothrombin consumption test
	(ii) porphyria cutanea tarda
PCV	packed cell volume
PD	(i) potential difference
	(ii) pupillary difference
PDA	patent ductus arteriosus
PECT	positron emission computerized
	(computed) tomography
PEEP	positive end-expiratory pressure
PEF	peak expiratory flow rate
PEG	pneumoencephalogram
PEM	protein–energy malnutrition
PERLA	pupils equal, react to light and
	accommodation
PES	pre-excitation syndrome
PET	(i) positron emission tomography
	(ii) pre-eclamptic toxaemia
PETN	pentaerythritol tetranitrate
PEV	peak expiratory volume
PFK	phosphofructokinase
PFO	patent foramen ovale
PFP	platelet-free plasma
PFR	peak flow rate
PFT	pulmonary function tests
PG	prostaglandin (also PGA, PGB,
	etc.)
PGC	primordial germ cell
PGH	pituitary growth hormone

PGM	phosphoglucomutase
PGN	proliferative glomerulonephritis
PH	previous history
pH	(see text entry)
PHA	phytohaemagglutinin
Phe	phenylalanine
PHI	permanent health insurance
PHK	post-modern human kidney
PHLS	Public Health Laboratory Service
PHR	peak heart rate
PHS	Public Health Service
PI	pulmonary incompetence
PICU	paediatric intensive care unit
PID	(i) prolapsed intervertebral disc
	(ii) pelvic inflammatory disease
PIE	pulmonary infiltration with
	eosinophilia
PIF	prolactin-inhibiting factor
PIFR	peak inspiratory flow rate
PIP	proximal interphalangeal (joint)
PISCES	percutaneously implanted spinal
	cord epidural stimulation
PIV	parainfluenza virus
PK	(i) pyruvate kinase
	(ii) Prausnitz–Kustner (reaction)
pK	dissociation constant
PKD	polycystic kidney disease
PKU	phenylketonuria
PLAB	Professional and Linguistic
	Assessment Board
PLG	plasminogen
PLM	polarized light microscopy
PM	(i) photomultiplier
	(ii) post-mortem
PMA	progressive muscular atrophy
PMB	post-menopausal bleeding
PMC	pseudomembranous colitis
PMF	progressive massive fibrosis
PMI	point of maximum impulse
PML	progressive multifocal
	leucoencephalopathy
PMO	Principal Medical Officer
PMR	polymyalgia rheumatica
PMRAFNS	Princess Mary's Royal Air Force
	Nursing Service
PMT	premenstrual tension
PN	percussion note
Pn	plutonium
PNA	*Paris Nomina Anatomica*
PND	paroxysmal nocturnal dyspnoea
PNH	paroxysmal nocturnal
	haemoglobinuria
PNO	Principal Nursing Officer
pO_2	partial pressure of oxygen
POA	primary optic atrophy
PoE	portal of entry
PoM	prescription-only medicine
POMR	problem-orientated medical record

POP	plaster of Paris	PVP	polyvinylpyrrolidone (providone)
POSM	patient-operated selector mechanism	PVR	(i) peripheral vascular resistance (ii) pulmonary vascular resistance
POSSUM	patient-operated selector mechanism	PVT	paroxysmal ventricular tachycardia
		PWM	pokeweed mitogen
PP	placenta praevia	PWP	pulmonary wedge pressure
PPC	Preliminary Proceedings Committee (GMC)	PZ	pancreozymin
		PZI	protamine zinc insulin
PPD	purified protein derivative (tuberculin)	QALYs	quality-adjusted life years
PPF	pellagra-preventing factor	QARANC	Queen Alexandra's Royal Army Nursing Corps
PPH	post-partum haemorrhage		
PPLO	pleuropneumonia-like organisms	QARNNS	Queen Alexandra's Royal Naval Nursing Service
p.p.m.	parts per million		
PR	(i) *per rectum* (ii) pulse rate (iii) pre registration (year)	q.i.d.	*quater in die* (four times a day)
		QNS	quantity not sufficient
		q.s.	sufficient quantity
PRA	(i) progesterone receptor assay (ii) plasma renin activity	QT	Quick's test
PRF	prolactin-releasing factor	RA	(i) right atrium (ii) rheumatoid arthritis
p.r.n.	*pro re nata* (as and when required)		
Pro	proline	Ra	radium
PROM	premature rupture of membranes	RACGP	Royal Australian College of General Practitioners
PRP	platelet-rich plasma		
PRU	peripheral resistance unit	RACP	Royal Australasian College of Physicians
PRV	polycythaemia rubra vera		
PS	pulmonary stenosis	RACS	Royal Australasian College of Surgeons
P/S	polyunsaturated/saturated ratio		
PSGN	post-streptococcal glomerulonephritis	RAD	right axis deviation
		rad	(see text entry)
PSS	progressive systemic sclerosis	RADAR	Royal Association for Disability and rehabilitation
PSVT	paroxysmal supraventricular tachycardia		
		RAIU	radioactive iodine uptake
PSW	psychiatric social worker	RAM	relative atomic mass
Pt	platinum	RAMC	Royal Army Medical Corps
PTA	prior to admission	RANZPsych	Royal Australian and New Zealand College of Psychiatrists
PTC	(i) phenylthiocarbamide (ii) plasma thromboplastin component (factor IX)		
		RAP	right atrial pressure
		Rb	rubidium
PTD	permanent total disability	RBB	right bundle branch
PTF	plasma thromboplastin factor (factor X)	RBBB	right bundle branch block
		RBC	red blood cell(s)
PTH	parathyroid hormone	RBE	relative biological effectiveness
PTT	partial thromboplastin time	RBF	renal blood flow
PTU	propylthiouracil	RNN	retrobulbar neuritis
PTx	parathyroidectomy	RBP	retinol binding protein
PU	(i) passed urine (ii) peptic ulcer	RCAMC	Royal Canadian Army Medical Corps
PUFA	polyunsaturated fatty acids	RCF	relative centrifugal force
PUO	pyrexia of uncertain (or unknown or undetermined) origin	RCGP	Royal College of General Practitioners
PUVA	psoralens and ultraviolet A	RCM	red cell mass
PV	(i) *per vaginam* (ii) polyoma virus	RCN	Royal College of Nursing
		RCOG	Royal College of Obstetricians and Gynaecologists
PVB	premature ventricular beat		
PVC	polyvinyl chloride	RCOphth	Royal College of Ophthalmology
PVD	peripheral vascular disease	RCP	Royal College of Physicians of London
PVG	periventricular grey matter		

RCPath	Royal College of Pathologists	RPMS	Royal Postgraduate Medical School
RCP(Ed. *or* Edin.)	Royal College of Physicians, Edinburgh	RPP	retropubic prostatectomy
RCPI	Royal College of Physicians of Ireland	RPS	renal pressor substance
		RQ	respiratory quotient
RCPS(C)	Royal College of Physicians and Surgeons of Canada	RRA	radioreceptor assay
		rRNA	ribosomal RNA
RCPS(Glasg.)	Royal College of Physicians and Surgeons of Glasgow	RRP	relative refractory period
		RS	Royal Society
RCPsych	Royal College of Psychiatrists	RSF	rheumatoid serum factor
RCR	Royal College of Radiologists	RSM	Royal Society of Medicine
RCS	Royal College of Surgeons of England	RSO	resident surgical officer
		RSR	regular sinus rhythm
RCS(Ed. *or* Edin.)	Royal College of Surgeons of Edinburgh	RSV	respiratory syncytial virus
		RT	reaction time
RCS(Irel.)	Royal College of Surgeons in Ireland	RTA	renal tubular acidosis
		RTF	resistance transfer factor
RCT	randomized clinical trial	RTI	respiratory tract infection
RD	(i) relative density	RV	(i) right ventricle
	(ii) reaction of degeneration		(ii) residual volume
R & D	research and development	RVH	right ventricular hypertrophy
RDA	recommended daily allowance	RW	Rideal–Walker (coefficient)
RDE	receptor-destroying enzyme		
rDNA	recombinant DNA	S	sulphur
RDS	respiratory distress syndrome	SACE	serum angiotensin-converting enzyme
redox	reduction–oxidation		
REF	renal erythropoietic factor	SAH	subarachnoid haemorrhage
REM	rapid eye movements	SAN	sinoatrial node
rem	roentgen equivalent man	SAS	sterile aqueous suspension
RER	respiratory exchange ratio	SB	stillbirth
RES	reticuloendothelial system	Sb	antimony
R factor	resistance factor	SBA	sick-bay attendant
RH	relative humidity	SBE	subacute bacterial endocarditis
Rh	rhesus	SBP	systolic blood pressure
RHA	Regional Health Authority	SBR	strict bed rest
RHB	Regional Hospital Board	SC	subcutaneous
RHD	(i) rheumatic heart disease	SCA	sickle-cell anaemia
	(ii) rhesus haemolytic disease	SCAN	suspected child abuse and neglect
RHF	right heart failure	SCAT	sheep cell agglutination test
RI	refractive index	SCBU	special care baby unit
RIA	radioimmunoassay	SCD	subacute combined degeneration
RIF	right iliac fossa	SCE	sister chromatid exchange
RIH	right inguinal hernia	SCI	spinal cord injury
RLC	residual lung capacity	SCG	sodium cromoglycate
RLF	retrolental fibroplasia	SCM	State Certified Midwife
RMM	relative molecular mass	SCU	Special Care Unit
RMO	(i) resident medical officer	SCUBA	self-contained underwater breathing apparatus
	(ii) Regional Medical officer		
RMS	root mean square	SD	standard deviation
RMV	respiratory minute volume	SDA	specific dynamic action
Rn	radon	SDHD	sudden death heart disease
RNA	ribonucleic acid	SE	standard error
RNase	ribonuclease	Se	selenium
RNIB	Royal National Institute for the Blind	SED	skin erythema dose
ROM	rupture of membranes	SEM	scanning electron microscope
RPF	renal plasma flow	SEN	State Enrolled Nurse
RPGN	rapidly progressive glomerulonephritis	SEP	systolic ejection period
		Ser	serine

SES	socio-economic status	STD	(i) sexually transmitted disease
SFD	small for dates		(ii) skin test dose
SG	specific gravity	STEM	scanning transmission electron
SGOT	serum glutamic-oxaloacetic		microscopy
	transaminase	STH	somatotrophic hormone
SGPT	serum glutamic-pyruvic	STI	serum trypsin inhibitor
	transaminase	STOP	suction termination of pregnancy
SH	(i) serum hepatitis	s.t.p.	standard temperature and pressure
	(ii) social history	SV	stroke volume
SHHD	Scottish Home and Health	SVC	superior vena cava
	Department	SVR	systemic vascular resistance
SHMO	Senior Hospital Medical Officer	SVT	supraventricular tachycardia
SHO	Senior House Officer	SWD	short-wave diathermy
SI units	(see text entry)		
Si	silicon	T1, T2, etc.	thoracic vertebrae
SIADH	syndrome of inappropriate ADH	$T_{1/2}$	half-life
	secretion	T_3	triiodothyronine
SIDS	sudden infant death syndrome	T_4	thyroxine
sig.	*signetur* (let it be labelled)	T & A	tonsils and adenoids
SIW	self-inflicted wound	TAB	typhoid, paratyphoid A and B
SK	streptokinase	TAF	toxin–antitoxin floccules
SLE	systemic lupus erythematosus	TAH	total abdominal hysterectomy
SLR	straight leg raising	TAPV	totally anomalous pulmonary
SM	systolic murmur		veins
SMAC	Standing Medical Advisory	TAT	Thematic Apperception Test
	Committee	TB	tuberculosis
SMD	senile macular degeneration	TBE	tick-borne encephalitis
SMO	Senior Medical Officer	TBG	thyroxine-binding globulin
SMON	subacute myelo-optic neuropathy	TBI	total body irradiation
SMR	standardized mortality rate	TBM	tuberculous meningitis
SMX	sulphamethoxazole	TBP	thyroxine-binding pre-albumin
Sn	tin	TBW	total body water
S/N	signal to noise ratio	Tc	technetium
SOB	shortness of breath	TCA	(i) tricyclic antidepressant
SOL	space-occupying lesion		(ii) trichloroacetic acid
SOP	standard operating procedure	TCB	tumour cell burden
sp.	species (singular)	TCI	to come in
SPA	stimulus-produced analgesia	T-CLL	T-cell chronic lymphatic leukaemia
SPECT	single photon emission	TCO	carbon monoxide transfer factor
	computerized (computed)	TCT	thyrocalcitonin
	tomography	TDD	thoracic duct drainage
SPF	specific pathogen-free	TDE	total digestible energy
SPP	suprapubic prostatectomy	t.d.s	*ter die sumendum* (to be taken three
spp.	species (plural)		times a day)
SPV	Shope papilloma virus	TE	alpha-tocopherol equivalent
SR	(i) Senior Registrar	Te	tellurium
	(ii) sinus rhythm	TEAB	tetraethylammonium bromide
Sr	strontium	TEAC	tetraethylammonium chloride
SRN	State Registered Nurse	TED	threshold erythema dose
SRNS	steroid-responsive nephrotic	TEE	total energy expenditure
	syndrome	TEM	transmission electron microscopy
SRR	Society for Research in	TES	transcutaneous electrical stimulation
	Rehabilitation	TEV	talipes equinovarus
SRS-A	slow reacting substance of	TF	transfer factor
	anaphylaxis	TFA	total fatty acids
SSPE	subacute sclerosing panencephalitis	TFS	testicular feminization syndrome
SSS	sick sinus syndrome	TG	(i) triglycerides
stat.	*statim* (at once)		(ii) thyroglobulin

TGA	transposition of the great arteries
TGE	transmissible gastroenteritis
TGT	thromboplastin generation time
TGV	transposition of the great vessels
THC	tetrahydrocannabinol
Thr	thrionine
THRF	thyrotrophic hormone releasing factor
TI	tricuspid incompetence
Ti	titanium
TIA	transient ischaemic attack
TIBC	total iron-binding capacity
t.i.d.	*ter in die* (thrice a day)
TJ	triceps jerk
TK	thymidine kinase
Tl	thallium
TLC	(i) thin-layer chromatography
	(ii) total lung capacity
TLD	thoracic lymph duct
TLE	thin-layer electrophoresis
TLV	(i) total lung volume
	(ii) threshold limit value
T_M	maximum tubular reabsorption
TMA	thyroid microsomal antibody
TME	total metabolizable energy
TMJ	temporomandibular joint
TMP/SMX	trimethoprim/sulphamethoxazole
TMV	tobacco mosaic virus
TNF	tumour necrosis factor
TNS	transcutaneous nerve stimulation
TNT	trinitrotoluene
TNTC	too numerous to count
TOF	tetralogy of Fallot
TOP	termination of pregnancy
TPI	*Treponema pallidum* immobilization test
TPN	total parenteral nutrition
TPR	total peripheral resistance
TR	tricuspid regurgitation
TRCH	tanned red cell haemagglutination test
TRH	thyrotrophin-releasing hormone
TRIAC	triiodothyroacetic acid
TRIC	trachoma-inclusion conjunctivitis
tRNA	transfer RNA
TRP	(i) tubular reabsorption of phosphate
	(ii) total refractory period
Trp	tryptophan
T_3RU	triiodothyronine resin uptake test
TS	tricuspid stenosis
TSA	tumour-specific antigen
TSH	thyroid-stimulating hormone
TSH-RF	thyroid-stimulating hormone-releasing factor
TSI	thyroid-stimulating immunoglobulin
TSP	total serum protein
TSS	toxic shock syndrome

TT	(i) tetanus toxoid
	(ii) tuberculin tested
TURP	transurethral resection of prostate
TVF	tactile vocal fremitus
TVP	tricuspid valve prolapse
TVU	total volume of urine (24 hours)
TX	thromboxane
Tyr	tyrosine
U	uranium
UCD	usual childhood diseases
UCG	urinary chorionic gonadotrophin
UCH	University College Hospital
UCR	usual, customary, and reasonable
UFAW	University Federation for Animal Welfare
UFC	Universities Funding Council
UGC	University Grants Committee
UICC	Union Internationale Contre le Cancer (International Union Against Cancer)
UKCC	United Kingdom Central Council (for Nursing, Midwifery, and Health Visiting)
UMN	upper motor neurone
UMT	unit of medical time
UNEP	United Nations Environment Programme
UNESCO	United Nations Educational, Scientific and Cultural Organization
UNICEF	United Nations Children's Fund (originally United Nations International Children's Emergency fund)
UNRRA	United Nations Relief and Rehabilitation Administration
UO	urinary output
UP	under proof
URF	uterine relaxing factor
URI	upper respiratory infection
URT	upper respiratory tract
USAN	United States Adopted Name
USNF	*United States National Formulary*
USP	*United States Pharmacopoeia*
USRDA	United States Recommended Dietary Allowance
USS	ultrasound scanning
UTI	urinary tract infection
u.v.	ultraviolet
UVA	ultraviolet light, long wave
V	vanadium
VA	Veterans' Administration
V_a	alveolar ventilation (1/min)
VAD	Voluntary Aid Detachment
Val	valine
VAT	ventricular activation time
VBL	vinblastine

VC	vital capacity	WD	Wallerian degeneration
VCC	vasoconstrictor centre	WDLL	well-differentiated lymphatic
VCG	vectorcardiogram		lymphoma
VCO$_2$	carbon dioxide production (1/min)	WEE	Western equine encephalitis
VCR	vincristine (Oncovin®)	WFME	World Federation of Medical
VD	venereal disease		Education
VDC	vasodilator centre	WFN	World Federation of Neurology
VDH	valvular disease of the heart	WFNS	World Federation of Neurosurgical
VDRL	Venereal Disease Reference		Societies
	Laboratory Test	WHML	Wellcome Historical Medical
VE	vaginal examination		Library
VEB	ventricular ectopic beats	WHO	World Health Organization
VEE	Venezuelan equine encephalitis	WISC	Wechsler Intelligence Scale for
VER	visual evoked response		Children
VF	ventricular fibrillation	WL	waiting list
VGH	very good health	WMA	World Medical Association
VI	virgo intacta	WNL	within normal limits
VIC	vasoinhibitory centre	WO	wash out
VIP	vasoactive intestinal peptide	w/o	(i) water in oil
VLDL	very low-density lipoprotein		(ii) without
VLP	virus-like particle	WPW	Wolff–Parkinson–White (syndrome)
VMA	vannillylmandelic acid	WR	Wassermann reaction
VMC	vasomotor centre	WS	water soluble
VNA	Visiting Nurse Association	wt.	weight
VO$_2$	oxygen consumption (1/min)		
VOD	veno-occlusive disease	Xan	xanthine
VON	Victorian Order of Nurses	XDH	xanthine dehydrogenase
VOR	vestibulo-ocular reflex	XDP	xeroderma pigmentosum
VP	variegate porphyria	Xe	xenon
VPB	ventricular premature beat	XLP	X-linked lymphoproliferative
VR	vocal resonance		syndrome
VRI	viral respiratory infection	XO	xanthine oxidase
VS	vesicular sounds	XR	X-ray
VSD	ventricular septal defect	XRT	X-ray therapy
VSS	vital signs stable	XS	cross-section
VT	ventricular tachycardia	XX	sex chromosomes (normal female)
V_t	tidal volume	XY	sex chromosomes (normal male)
VU	varicose ulcer	Xyl	xylose
VUR	vesicoureteric reflex		
VWD	von Willebrand's disease	Y	yttrium
VWF	von Willebrand factor	yr	year
Vx	vertex	YS	yellow spot (macula retinae)
V-Z	varicella-zoster	ZES	Zollinger–Ellison syndrome
V-ZV	varicella-zoster virus		
		ZF	zona fasciculata
WAIS	Wechsler Adult Intelligence Scale	ZG	zona glomerulosa
WBA	whole body activity	ZN	Ziehl–Neelsen
WBC	white blood cell(s)	Zn	zinc
WBR	whole body radiation	ZR	zona reticularis
WBS	whole body scan	Zr	zirconium
WBT	wet bulb temperature		